Lewin, Weinstein, and Riddell's

Gastrointestinal Pathology and Its Clinical Implications

SECOND EDITION

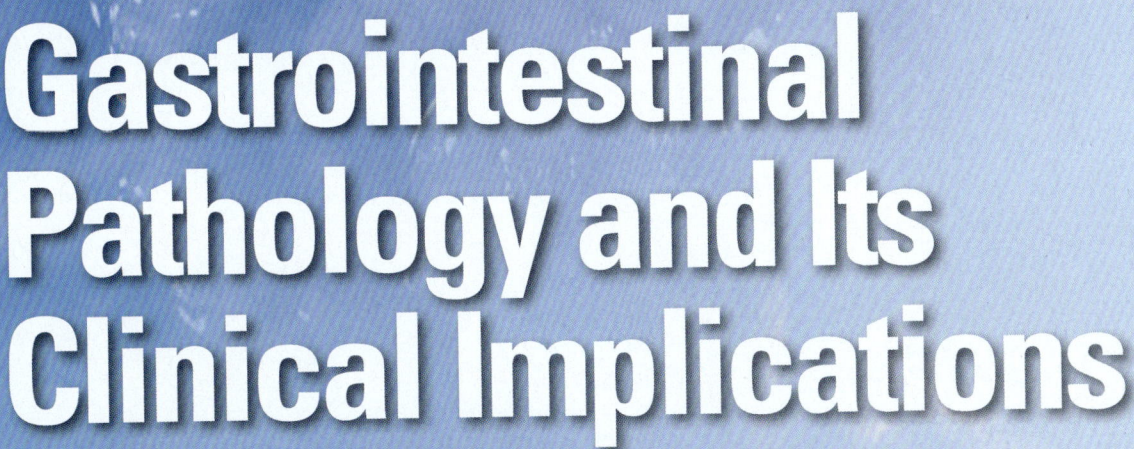

VOLUME I

Lewin, Weinstein, and Riddell's

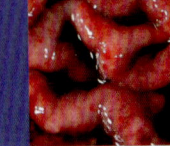

Gastrointestinal Pathology and Its Clinical Implications

SECOND EDITION

VOLUME I

Robert Riddell, MD, FRCPath, FRCPC
Professor of Laboratory Medicine and Pathobiology
University of Toronto
Mount Sinai Hospital
Toronto, Ontario, Canada

Dhanpat Jain, MD
Professor of Pathology
Director, Program in Gastrointestinal and Liver Pathology
Department of Pathology
Yale University School of Medicine
New Haven, Connecticut, USA

Clinical Editors
Charles N. Bernstein, MD
Professor of Medicine
University of Manitoba
Head, Section of Gastroenterology
Director, University of Manitoba of IBD Clinical and Research Centre
Bingham Chair in Gastroenterology
Winnipeg, Manitoba, Canada

Sushovan Guha, MD, PhD
Associate Professor and Director of Research
Division of Gastroenterology, Hepatology, and Nutrition
Department of Internal Medicine
The University of Texas Medical School and Health Science Center at Houston
Houston, Texas, USA

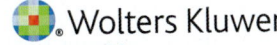

Health
Philadelphia · Baltimore · New York · London
Buenos Aires · Hong Kong · Sydney · Tokyo

Acquisitions Editor: Ryan Shaw
Product Manager: Kate Marshall
Production Project Manager: Marian Bellus
Senior Manufacturing Coordinator: Beth Welsh
Marketing Manager: Dan Dressler
Designer: Stephen Druding
Production Service: SPi Global

© 2014 by LIPPINCOTT WILLIAMS & WILKINS, a WOLTERS KLUWER business

Two Commerce Square
2001 Market Street
Philadelphia, PA 19103 USA
LWW.com

First Edition © 1992 by Igaku-Shoin Medical Publishers, Inc.
All rights reserved. This book is protected by copyright. No part of this book may be reproduced in any form by any means, including photocopying, or utilized by any information storage and retrieval system without written permission from the copyright owner, except for brief quotations embodied in critical articles and reviews. Materials appearing in this book prepared by individuals as part of their official duties as U.S. government employees are not covered by the above-mentioned copyright.

Printed in China

Library of Congress Cataloging-in-Publication Data
Lewin, Weinstein, and Riddell's gastrointestinal pathology and its clinical implications / [edited by] Robert Riddell, Dhanpat Jain. — 2nd ed.
   p. ; cm.
   Gastrointestinal pathology and its clinical implications
   Rev. ed. of: Gastrointestinal pathology and its clinical implications / Klaus J. Lewin, Robert H. Riddell, Wilfred M. Weinstein. c1992.
   Includes bibliographical references and index.
   ISBN 978-0-7817-2216-2
   1. Gastrointestinal system—Diseases. I. Riddell, Robert H., 1943- II. Jain, Dhanpat. III. Lewin, Klaus J. IV. Lewin, Klaus J. Gastrointestinal pathology and its clinical implications. V. Title: Gastrointestinal pathology and its clinical implications.
   [DNLM: 1. Gastrointestinal Diseases—pathology. WI 100]
   RC802.9.L48 2011
   616.3'3—dc22

2011011658

Care has been taken to confirm the accuracy of the information presented and to describe generally accepted practices. However, the authors, editors, and publisher are not responsible for errors or omissions or for any consequences from application of the information in this book and make no warranty, expressed or implied, with respect to the currency, completeness, or accuracy of the contents of the publication. Application of the information in a particular situation remains the professional responsibility of the practitioner.

The authors, editors, and publisher have exerted every effort to ensure that drug selection and dosage set forth in this text are in accordance with current recommendations and practice at the time of publication. However, in view of ongoing research, changes in government regulations, and the constant flow of information relating to drug therapy and drug reactions, the reader is urged to check the package insert for each drug for any change in indications and dosage and for added warnings and precautions. This is particularly important when the recommended agent is a new or infrequently employed drug.

Some drugs and medical devices presented in the publication have Food and Drug Administration (FDA) clearance for limited use in restricted research settings. It is the responsibility of the health care provider to ascertain the FDA status of each drug or device planned for use in their clinical practice.

To purchase additional copies of this book, call our customer service department at (800) 638-3030 or fax orders to (301) 223-2320. International customers should call (301) 223-2300.

Visit Lippincott Williams & Wilkins on the Internet: at LWW.com. Lippincott Williams & Wilkins customer service representatives are available from 8:30 am to 6 pm, EST.

10 9 8 7 6 5 4 3 2 1

Dedication

Robert Riddell
To my immortal parents Harry and Joyce.
To my wife Hala, who wrote the gastritis chapter, contributed to numerous others and whose constant love, support, and encouragement is greatly appreciated.
To Mark, Juliet, and Mike, and grandchildren Alannah, Natalie, Paisley, and Eli, all of whom we are so proud of and who give us more pleasure than they will ever know.

Dhanpat Jain
To my teachers who always showed me the right path.
To my parents Milap Chand and Biraj who always led me to the right path.
To my wife Shilpa without whom nothing would have been possible.
To my daughters Nimisha and Anisha for whom it was all worthwhile.

Charles N. Bernstein
I dedicate any accolades I receive for the hard work put into this book to Evelyn, Matthew, and Lexie Bernstein. They provide me with the constant entertainment, support, and love that reminds me constantly of what is really important in life.

Sushovan Guha
I would like to dedicate this to my wife Sarmistha, to our children Siddarth and Shivani, to my father Sukumar, and to my mother Dolly for their collective wisdom, unflinching support, utmost dedication, and unbridled joy. Also I would like to offer my deepest gratitude to Fred, Klaus, and all the great teachers that I had at UCLA. Finally I would offer my thanks to all the patients that motivated me to be a good doctor.

Contributors

Henry D. Appelman, MD
M.R. Abell Professor of Surgical Pathology
Department of Pathology
University of Michigan
Ann Arbor, Michigan, USA

Charles N. Bernstein, MD
Professor of Medicine
University of Manitoba
Head, Section of Gastroenterology
Director, University of Manitoba of IBD Clinical
 and Research Centre
Bingham Chair in Gastroenterology
Winnipeg, Manitoba, Canada

Hala El-Zimaity, MD, MS (Epidemiology)
Professor
Department of Laboratory Medicine
 and Pathobiology
University of Toronto
Gastrointestinal Pathology Consultant
University Health Network
Toronto, Ontario, Canada

Karel Geboes, MD, PhD, AGAF
Professor Emeritus
Emeritus Clinical Chief
Department of Pathology
KU Leuven University
University Hospitals Gasthuisberg
Leuven, Belgium

Joel Kasle Greenson, MD
Professor of Pathology
Department of Pathology
University of Michigan Medical School
Director of Gastrointestinal Pathology
Department of Pathology
University of Michigan Health System
Ann Arbor, Michigan

Sushovan Guha, MD, PhD
Associate Professor and Director of Research
Division of Gastroenterology, Hepatology,
 and Nutrition
Department of Internal Medicine
The University of Texas Medical School
 and Health Science Center at Houston
Houston, Texas, USA

Dhanpat Jain, MD
Professor of Pathology
Director, Program in Gastrointestinal
 and Liver Pathology
Department of Pathology
Yale University School of Medicine
New Haven, Connecticut, USA

Richard Kirsch, MBChB, PhD, FRCPath(SA), FRCPC
Associate Professor
Department of Laboratory Medicine
 and Pathobiology
Mount Sinai Hospital
Toronto, Ontario, Canada

Hiroyoshi Ota, MD, PhD
Professor
Department of Biomedical and Laboratory Sciences
Shinshu University
Staff Pathologist
Department of Laboratory Medicine
Shinshu University Hospital
Matsumoto, Nagano, Japan

Robert Riddell, MD, FRCPath, FRCPC
Professor of Laboratory Medicine and Pathobiology
University of Toronto
Mount Sinai Hospital
Toronto, Ontario, Canada

Masanori Tanaka, MD
Director
Department of Pathology and Laboratory Medicine
Hirosaki City Hospital
Hirosaki, Japan

Michael Vieth, Dr. med habil. Dr. med
Professor of Pathology
Institute of Pathology
University of Magdeburg
Magdeburg, Germany
Director
Institute of Pathology
Klinikum Bayreuth
Bayreuth, Germany

Preface to the First Edition

The decision to write a textbook of pathology coupled with clinical implications came primarily because of the increasing interdependence of the pathologist and clinician in the investigation and management of gastrointestinal disorders where modern gastrointestinal pathology plays a dynamic role. In many instances, it is no longer sufficient for the pathologist to simply make a morphological diagnosis. Conversely, we hope that clinicians with gastroenterology interests will view this book as a requisite companion for a general textbook of gastroenterology.

Pathologists can achieve their full potential by understanding the clinical scenarios in which they are playing a part and by appreciating the effect of their decisions in clinical management. We hope that the clinicians who read this book will more readily maximize the information they obtain from gastrointestinal biopsies through an understanding of the indications, by appreciating the need for providing relevant clinical information, which specific questions to ask the pathologist, and also to understand when biopsies are likely to be of limited value.

We have done our best not to perpetuate some of the myths of pathologist uncritically. In areas where issues are controversial, we have tried to state this; we have also frequently offered our own "solutions" to these problems in situations that lack data on which they can satisfactorily be based.

We hope that the greatest criticism that can be leveled against this book is that it assumes that each gastroenterologist, whether medical or surgical, adult or pediatric, has an interested pathologist with whom to work and vice versa. We know that this is frequently not the case. However, by appreciating the necessity of such a working relationship for the best in patient care, we hope that pathologists and clinicians will see the overwhelming benefits of this relationship and will try to foster it.

Klaus J. Lewin
Robert H. Riddell
Wilfred M. Weinstein

Preface

The first edition of this book was published over 20 years ago in 1993. The driving force behind that book came from Klaus Lewin, and was that, to do pathology well, pathologists have to understand the clinical implications of their diagnoses, which explains the title of the book. At the same time clinicians need to understand when to biopsy, where to biopsy, which questions to ask, as well as which cannot be answered by pathology, and what to expect from the pathologist. The book was thus written as a guide for pathologists and clinicians for circumstances that they have to deal with on a day-to-day basis, and also as a resource for any unusual lesion, for difficult diagnoses, and for those issues where good guidelines are lacking. It also explained the unconventional authorship of the book, especially having Wilfred (Fred) Weinstein as both an author and clinical contributor. The book tried to provide answers for such situations and gave rationale for what we did and why, sometimes finding that we did them differently ourselves. Teaching new gastroenterologists where to sample and why and also to teach them how to interpret the pathologist's reports, which are highly variable themselves, is a challenging task. Pathologists can be just as guilty of providing defensive and unhelpful descriptions that are not easily understood and leave the clinician trying to guess how to interpret the findings of the report, especially when told that "clinical correlation is required"—in practice the statement that tends to be a hedge for "I have no idea why you took these biopsies or what I should be looking for."

Most will not be aware that a second edition of this book was well underway in 2000 when it gradually became clear that Klaus was unable to continue. He died a few years later in 2005, and we miss him and his sense of both the important and his sense of the ridiculous, tremendously. However there was always encouragement from friends, colleagues, and strangers alike to bring forth a new edition. With much encouragement, it began to take shape when Dr. Dhanpat Jain from Yale accepted the Co-Editorship. Fred Weinstein, the third member of the team, decided that the book would not really be the same without Klaus; he did suggest that two of "his boys" Charles N. Bernstein (now in Winnipeg) and Sushovan Guha (at MD Anderson at that time) could fill in his shoes. They agreed to become the "clinical editors" and it has been an absolute pleasure to work with them.

Our goal for the second edition was to keep the philosophy similar to the first edition, the challenge being to incorporate the explosion of knowledge in molecular pathology, cancer biology, and genomics that continues to change our field on a daily basis, and to keep this all relevant for the practicing pathologists and clinician. Since the last edition, images have changed from B&W and "Kodachromes" to digital, so the challenge was to replace these figures and endoscopic photomicrographs. The number of tables and management algorithms has also increased substantially. While adding new material, we were also conscious not to omit important historical details, the challenge being to keep the book to a reasonable size. We have also tried to keep the book relevant on a global level, and international experts helped to write some of the chapters; indeed, it could not have happened without them. We hope that we have been able to fulfill the purpose of the book as a resource not only for practicing and academic pathologists, but also for those in training in pathology and gastroenterology, and our clinical colleagues of all stripes—endoscopists and imagers, gastroenterologists, and surgeons.

Robert Riddell
Dhanpat Jain

Acknowledgments

So many people have been involved in ensuring that this book becomes a reality that it is difficult to know where to begin. Family and spouses inevitably are first on the list for their huge support and for bearing with our relative absence during this time for the cause.

We thank our clinical editors Drs. Charles N. Bernstein and Sushovan Guha who went through each chapter and were wonderfully responsive in carrying out their roles in a very efficient manner, provided illustrations where needed, and made our lives much easier. They have, in turn, expressed their thanks for the opportunity.

We thank all our authors, who not only contributed their respective chapters but allowed us to "bend" their chapters out of recognition to avoid the stylistic issues that can arise with multiple authors.

We are grateful to our colleagues and friends at each institution for their encouragement, for lending their material to be used, moral support, and valuable advice. We are deeply indebted to our numerous trainees and pathology assistants who took excellent gross photographs, which are an invaluable resource for teaching and worth their weight in gold. We owe a lot of gratitude to our support staff at Photographics division, Yale University, Department of Pathology for their services.

Lastly, we thank the numerous people with Lippincott Williams & Wilkins, but especially Kate Marshall whose unmerciful cajoling helped to get this done as quickly as was possible, and also the expertise of Satheesh Velayutham and his team for their help with the page proofs.

Contents

Contributors *vii*
Preface to the First Edition *ix*
Preface *xi*
Acknowledgments *xiii*

Volume I

1 Dialogue, Biopsies–Taking and Handling; Resected Specimens; Protocols — 1
ROBERT RIDDELL, CHARLES N. BERNSTEIN, SUSHOVAN GUHA, AND DHANPAT JAIN

2 Vascular Disorders and Related Diseases — 28
KAREL GEBOES AND DHANPAT JAIN

3 Immunodeficiency Disorders — 88
JOEL KASLE GREENSON AND DHANPAT JAIN

4 Lymphoproliferative Disorders of the Gastrointestinal Tract — 123
DHANPAT JAIN

5 Disorders of Endocrine Cells — 190
HENRY D. APPELMAN

6 Motility Disorders — 226
ROBERT RIDDELL, HALA EL-ZIMAITY AND DHANPAT JAIN

7 Mesenchymal Tumors — 290
RICHARD KIRSCH

8 Gastrointestinal Manifestations of Extraintestinal Disorders and Systemic Disease — 378
RICHARD KIRSCH

9 Esophagus: Normal Structures, Developmental Abnormalities, and Miscellaneous Disorders — 422
MICHAEL VIETH AND DHANPAT JAIN

10 Inflammatory Disorders of the Esophagus: Reflux and Nonreflux Types — 450
MICHAEL VIETH AND ROBERT RIDDELL

11 Polyps and Tumors of the Esophagus — 505
MASANORI TANAKA AND ROBERT RIDDELL

12 Stomach: Normal Structures and Developmental Abnormalities — 552
HALA EL-ZIMAITY

13 Stomach and Proximal Duodenum: Inflammatory and Miscellaneous Disorders — 570
HALA EL-ZIMAITY AND ROBERT RIDDELL

14 Gastric Epithelial Polyps and Tumors — 705
HIROYOSHI OTA AND ROBERT RIDDELL

Volume II

15 Appendix — 795
ROBERT RIDDELL

16 Small and Large Bowel Structure: Developmental and Mechanical Disorders — 875
DHANPAT JAIN

17 Small Bowel Mucosal Disease — 929
JOEL KASLE GREENSON AND DHANPAT JAIN

18 Inflammatory Bowel Diseases — 983
KAREL GEBOES, ROBERT RIDDELL AND DHANPAT JAIN

19 Enteric Infections and Associated Diseases — 1209
DHANPAT JAIN

20 Small and Large Bowel Polyps and Tumors — 1327
DHANPAT JAIN AND ROBERT RIDDELL

21 The Anal Canal — 1547
HENRY D. APPELMAN

Index *I-1*

Lewin, Weinstein, and Riddell's

Gastrointestinal Pathology and Its Clinical Implications

SECOND EDITION

VOLUME I

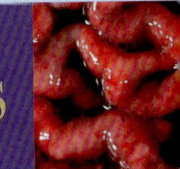

Dialogue, Biopsies—Taking and Handling; Resected Specimens; Protocols

Chapter Outline

- **MUCOSAL BIOPSY**
- **USUAL ENDOSCOPIC PINCH BIOPSIES**
  - Hot Biopsy Forceps
  - Cold Biopsies
- **ELECTROCAUTERY SNARE BIOPSY**
  - Snare Polypectomy
  - Snare Polypectomy after Submucosal Injection ("Lift-and-Cut" Technique)
  - Shave Biopsy
  - Endoscopic Mucosal Resection and Endoscopic Submucosal Dissection
    - Endoscopic mucosal resection
    - Endoscopic submucosal dissection
    - Submucosal lesions
- **ANCILLARY TECHNIQUES USED AT ENDOSCOPY**
  - Diagnosis of Infections—Smears, Brushings, Aspiration, and Culture
  - Cytology
    - Direct-vision brush cytology
    - Balloon mesh cytology
    - Fine-needle aspirates
  - Chromoendoscopy
    - Barrett's esophagus
    - Inflammatory bowel disease
    - Screening and surveillance colonoscopy for adenomas in otherwise healthy individuals
  - Virtual Histology
    - Biopsy specimen handling and processing
- **HANDLING OF THE BIOPSY SPECIMEN PRIOR TO IMMERSION IN FIXATIVES**
  - Handling Polyps
- **ROUTINE FIXATION**
- **TISSUE PROCESSING, EMBEDDING, AND CUTTING**
- **DESCRIPTION OF ENDOSCOPIC FINDINGS**
- **BIOPSY SPECIMEN LOCATION**
- **NUMBER AND SIZE OF BIOPSY SPECIMENS**
- **THE HISTORY AND THE QUESTION FOR THE PATHOLOGIST**
- **APPROACH TO THE MICROSCOPIC EXAMINATION**
- **A SYSTEMATIC APPROACH TO BIOPSY SPECIMEN INTERPRETATION**
- **TECHNICAL PROBLEMS IN INTERPRETATION**
  - Mucosal Hemorrhage and Edema
  - Pseudoerosions
  - Other Artifacts
- **THE PATHOLOGIST'S INTERPRETATION**
  - Mild Nonspecific Chronic Inflammation
- **SPECIAL FIXATIVES, STAINS, OR STORAGE CONDITIONS**
  - Immunohistochemical Applications in Gastrointestinal Disorders
  - Interpretation of Immunohistochemical Stains
  - Infections
  - Tuberculosis and Mycobacterium avium-intracellulare
- **SURGICALLY RESECTED SPECIMENS**
  - Examination of the Specimen
- **FROZEN SECTIONS**
- **PHOTOGRAPHY**
- **OPENING THE SPECIMEN**
- **FIXATION**
  - Insufflation with Fixative
    - Injection studies for vascular diseases
    - Examination and dissection of the fixed specimen
- **REEXAMINATION OF THE FIXED SPECIMEN**
- **DISSECTION**
  - Dissections of Tumors
  - Lymph Node Dissections
  - Depth of Tumor Penetration
  - Venous Invasion by Tumor
  - Sections of Resected Margins
  - Incidental Findings

MUCOSAL BIOPSY

Most tissue specimens from the gastrointestinal tract are in the form of mucosal biopsy specimens obtained at endoscopy. The pathologist can provide a diagnosis for many polyps and tumors. However, for inflammatory lesions he or she can provide a description, but cannot provide a meaningful interpretation of the biopsy specimen without the relevant clinical information, endoscopic findings, and a precise description of the biopsy sites. The endoscopist must also be specific concerning the information requested from the biopsy review. He or she must also be aware of the criteria the pathologist uses to make specific diagnoses and provide those biopsies. This is rarely taught in standard endoscopy training unless there are regular meetings at which such requirements can be discussed. This chapter stresses the coordination and dialogue, which must exist between the clinician who obtains the biopsy specimens and the pathologist who interprets them. Table 1-1 summarizes a method that can be used to obtain high-quality biopsy specimens and to maximize their clinical value.

Table 1-1 Recipe to Improve Biopsy Quality and Interpretation Dramatically

I. ENDOSCOPIST–PATHOLOGIST DIALOGUE
  1. *Endoscopist*
     A. Describe the bowel preparation used.
     B. Provide brief but relevant clinical information.
     C. Use simple, noninterpretive terms to describe appearance of biopsy specimen (*see Table 1-2*).
     D. Use standardized biopsy site descriptions.
     E. Ask specific questions on the pathology requisition.
     F. Include endoscopic photos.
     G. Give the pathologist important relevant papers from the gastroenterology literature.
  2. *Pathologist*
     A. Explain the terms you use (e.g., *acute, chronic, dysplasia, atypia*).
     B. Do not sign out normal biopsy specimens as "mild nonspecific chronic inflammation."
     C. Provide feedback regarding the quality of specimen.
     D. In the report, answer the specific questions asked by the endoscopist.
     E. Give the endoscopist important relevant papers from the pathology literature.

II. HANDLING TISSUE
  1. *In the endoscopy unit*
     A. Make the endoscopy assistant responsible for monitoring uniformity of the terminology used in reports.
     B. The endoscopy assistant is responsible for ensuring the labeling on specimen jars is accurate.
     C. Endoscopy assistant keeps up-to-date on ancillary techniques (e.g., culture transport conditions).
  2. *In the pathology laboratory*
     A. Designate one or two small-piece technologists.
     B. Technologist embeds oriented biopsy specimens on edge but polyps en face.
     C. Technologist recognizes when the central core is reached during sectioning.

Surgical or autopsy pathology often deals with advanced inflammatory or neoplastic processes. Mucosal biopsies are often used in a more dynamic dimension, namely, to assess the patient's response to therapy or to alter the direction of an investigation. An example of the latter is the workup of a patient with diarrhea. The clinician may decide to begin the investigation with endoscopy and biopsy of the large bowel. However, if the biopsy specimen is normal, he or she may then direct their attention to the small bowel as a possible source of symptoms.

USUAL ENDOSCOPIC PINCH BIOPSIES

Endoscopic pinch biopsy forceps are by far the most commonly used instruments to obtain gastrointestinal mucosal biopsy specimens to the point that the word "pinch" is invariably omitted. Most specimens taken with these instruments yield the full thickness of the mucosa down to the muscularis mucosae. They may contain a small amount of submucosa or none at all. In the esophagus, the basal layer of the squamous epithelium is usually included and sometimes the lamina propria, but rarely the muscularis mucosae.

The forceps have two cup-shaped jaws and most contain a central pin (Fig. 1-1). The opened cups are thrust against the mucosa and closed, and then the forceps is rapidly withdrawn, avulsing the enclosed mucosa. Forceps with smaller cups are used in "skinny" (pediatric) endoscopes with narrow biopsy channels, yielding inferior biopsy specimens that are often small and shallow. They may be the only option for endoscopic biopsy in very young or they may be used in unsedated upper endoscopies (easier to swallow). Large biopsy forceps (also referred to as "jumbo") require a larger endoscope with a larger (3.5 mm) endoscopic biopsy channel (Fig. 1-1). It yields biopsy specimens approximately twice as long (5–8 mm) as those obtained with conventional forceps, but they are not much deeper. A variety of developments include large-capacity biopsy forceps that can pass through a regular (2.8 mm) biopsy channel but can yield a biopsy specimen close to the size obtained from jumbo biopsy forceps. (They can also be hinged jaws allowing excellent positioning of these forceps on the target [Fig. 1-1B].). It is often helpful to gently suction the tissue that needs to be biopsied into the cusps of the biopsy forceps prior to removal. This technique provides a cleaner bite and reduces crush artifact. We recommend the largest forceps possible as they provide better biopsies, but especially when "tissue is the issue" at endoscopy.

In certain parts of the gastrointestinal tract, it may be more difficult to obtain sufficiently deep mucosal

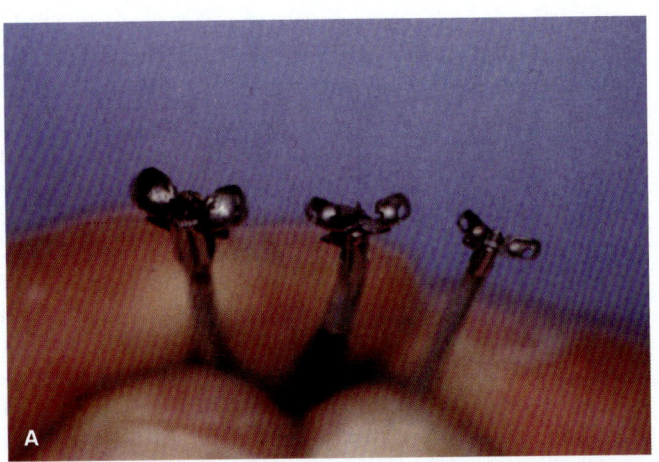 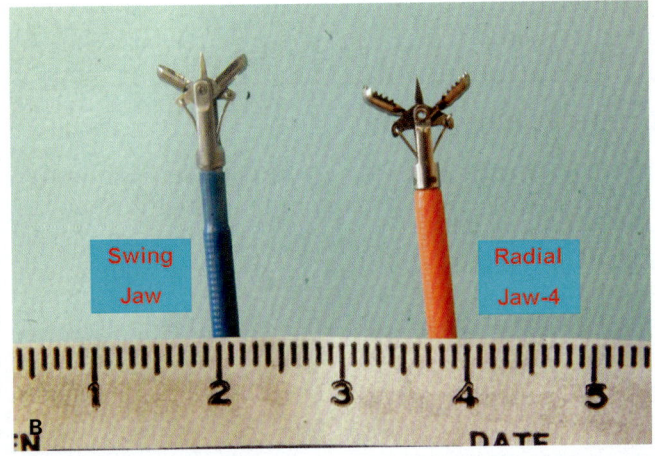

Figure 1-1. **A:** Endoscopic pinch biopsy forceps. These are passed through a side channel in the endoscope. The forceps on the right is small and fits into a 1.8-mm pediatric-sized scope but commonly yields suboptimal biopsy specimens. The middle forceps is often the standard size fitting into a 2.8-mm endoscopy channel. The forceps on the left has an 8-mm open span and is the best; it requires a larger biopsy channel and hence a slightly larger-diameter endoscope. Most of these forceps have a central spike to help impale the mucosa. **B:** Biopsy forceps that produce larger biopsies. The swing jaw mechanism enables easier cup positioning for biopsy sites approached tangentially such as in the esophagus. That on the right produces jumbo biopsy-sized pieces of tissue but fits down a scope's standard 2.8-mm biopsy channel.

biopsy specimens. These are areas, which normally lack folds or valves, especially the esophagus, gastric antrum, and duodenal bulb. In these areas, the endoscopist should partially collapse the lumen by suctioning out insufflated air just prior to biopsy. In the esophagus, the tip of the endoscope may be deflected 90 degrees against the wall, thus allowing the forceps to be advanced *en face* from close up ("turn-and-suction" biopsy technique). The esophageal mucosa is still the most difficult area in the gastrointestinal tract from which to obtain sufficiently deep, high-quality biopsy specimens.

Hot Biopsy Forceps

Some endoscopists use the *hot biopsy* technique, whereby coagulation current is passed through the jaws of an insulated pinch biopsy forceps. This is most commonly used for removal and simultaneous obliteration of diminutive colonic polyps, that is, those <6 mm in diameter. The forceps is used to grasp and tent the mucosal lesion upward and then to heat the localized area for several seconds with electrocoagulation current before pulling off the specimen contained in the cups of the forceps. This seemingly innocuous technique is not without potential complications, and some investigators have suggested more limited use.[1] An issue with only using forceps without coagulation to remove polyps is the potential for local recurrence.

When the hot biopsy forceps is used to fulgurate adenomas, the assumption is made that any residual adenoma has been destroyed. With the hot biopsy technique, the pathologist may expect to see some coagulation necrosis artifact with streaming of nuclei at the edges of the sections. Some endoscopists use conventional biopsy forceps to remove diminutive polyps and then use the argon plasma coagulation technique to ablate the remaining area instead of using hot biopsy forceps. However, one or more large forceps biopsy specimens can be taken with a conventional forceps to remove these diminutive polyps or to use a mini snare to guillotine these lesions (without cautery). The hot biopsy forceps is most useful when it is used simply to obliterate multiple tiny polyps after a few of them have been taken for histological interpretation.

Cold Biopsies

Diminutive polyps (5 mm or less in diameter) can be removed using hot biopsies as in the previous section or without the use of cautery—cold biopsies. Morphology is better preserved as there is no cautery artifact, although the lack of cautery also results in a slightly higher recurrence rate (29% vs. 21% in one study).[2] Larger polyps can also be removed with cold snare, in which the snare is placed over the polyp, which is mechanically strangulated and removed. The risk of perforation is reduced, but the risk of bleeding increased, so that cold biopsy is relatively contraindicated in patients with bleeding abnormalities.

ELECTROCAUTERY SNARE BIOPSY

Snare Polypectomy

The electrocautery snare wire is used for endoscopic polypectomy. Its main application is for pedunculated colonic polyps. The electrocautery snare can also be used to remove the much less commonly encountered pedunculated polyps of the upper gastrointestinal tract. The wire is looped over the polyp to encircle the stalk (Fig. 1-2A) and is progressively tightened until it firmly grasps the stalk of the polyp. At that point, electrical current is applied to resect the stalk. It is important to recognize that the full length of the polyp stalk is underrepresented in the specimen because the endoscopist intentionally keeps the snare away from the bowel wall in order to prevent intramural or transmural burns (Fig. 1-2B). Thus, a small amount of cauterized polyp stalk often remains after snare polypectomy removal. To avoid postpolypectomy bleeding specially after resection of large polyps (>2 cm) or in the right colon, endoscopists often inject submucosally 1:10,000 epinephrine/saline to achieve immediate hemostasis followed by placement of endoscopic hemoclips when necessary. Other methods of hemostasis can also be successful including bipolar cautery and band ligation. This technique can also be used for large sessile polyps.

The technique recommended to identify the stalk zone of endoscopically removed polyps is referred to later in this chapter. Small polyps can be sucked into the biopsy/suction channel and retrieved by having a special trap placed where the wall suction attaches to the endoscope. An alternative for larger polyps is to grasp them with a device passed through the biopsy channel of the endoscope and to remove the endoscope. This device can be either a tri-pronged device or a mesh basket (Roth Retrieval Net). Sometimes these resected polyps are lost. A variety of creative stool-straining techniques have been used to retrieve them, often after the patient takes (reluctantly) additional lavage solution. These delayed-delivery polyps often retain surprisingly good morphology.

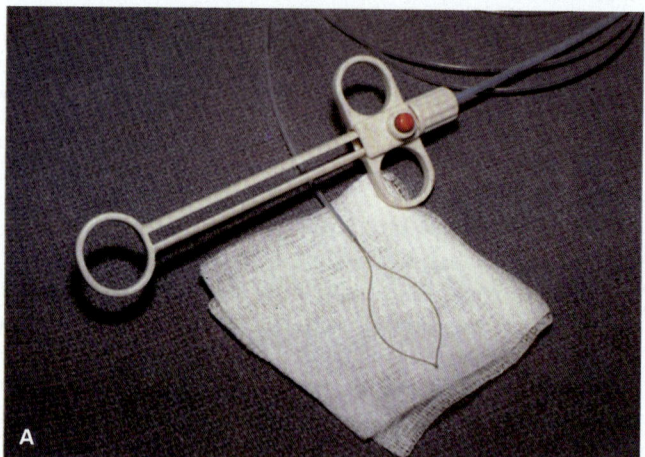

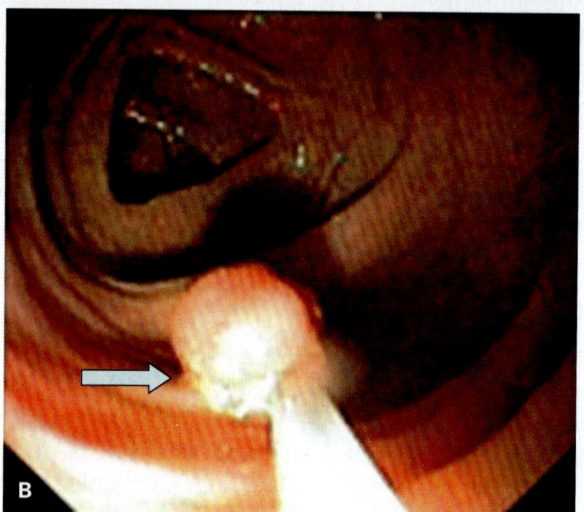

Figure 1-2. Electrocautery snare used for polypectomy. **A:** The device is attached to an electrocautery unit. The handle is used to extend and retract the snare. **B:** Snare tightened around the stalk of a polyp in transverse colon. Some stalks can be intentionally left behind (*arrow*) to avoid cauterizing too close to the wall (possibly making a mockery of proximity to the cauterized margin as an indication of nodal metastases if this can be deliberately varied).

Snare Polypectomy after Submucosal Injection ("Lift-and-Cut" Technique)

Flat or depressed polyps are increasingly identified during colonoscopies using either improved imaging techniques (chromoendoscopy) or after excellent bowel preparation. These polyps can be resected using snare polypectomy technique described above or after submucosal injection. The fluid lifts the polyp and increases the distance between the base of the polyp and the muscularis propria and serosa. This submucosal "cushion" of fluid (bleb formation) has been shown to prevent deeper thermal injury during polypectomy. The most commonly used fluid is saline (normal or hypertonic), with or without 1:10,000 epinephrine. With time, this fluid will be reabsorbed; thus, other fluids have been used in an attempt to prolong the effect, including 10% glycerol/5% fructose, 50% dextrose, sodium hyaluronate, and hydroxypropyl methylcellulose. It is preferable to inject the proximal (far) aspect of the polyp first.

If the distal aspect (closest to the endoscope, and the most tempting) is injected first, the polyp can be tilted away from the colonoscope, making subsequent resection more difficult. If a bleb does not immediately form, the needle can be slowly withdrawn and lifted slightly while injecting until bleb formation is observed. It is often helpful to inject at the lateral margin of the cushion produced by the previous injection (which has already separated the mucosal layer from the muscularis propria). However, if a bleb does not form, the needle may have penetrated the colon wall and so the fluid is being injected into the peritoneum. Alternatively, the failure to lift may indicate the presence of invasive cancer that is tethering the polyp to the underlying muscularis propria. This is called the "nonlifting sign."[3]

Shave Biopsy

A shave biopsy technique is occasionally used to remove large, sessile, adenomatous polyps from the colon. This is reserved mainly for high-risk surgical patients. The technique involves serial loopings and excisions of parts of the sessile lesion until it is completely removed. The main concern is always whether there is residual submucosal or deeper involvement by the adenomatous process.

Endoscopic Mucosal Resection and Endoscopic Submucosal Dissection

These are techniques developed in Japan that are used for removing large lesions endoscopically. These can be large adenomas or areas of glandular or squamous dysplasia, mucosal or early submucosal carcinomas, or primary submucosal tumors. The area to be resected may be tattooed if not obvious (e.g., an area of dysplasia). These techniques are extraordinarily safe, with virtually no mortality and minimal morbidity, which often contrasts with its surgical counterparts to the point that it is the preferred mode of therapy for many lesions that would otherwise require surgical resection.[4-6]

Endoscopic mucosal resection. *Endoscopic mucosal resection* (EMR) is a technique in which the submucosa is raised by injection with fluid (see above), and, using one of a variety of techniques the entire lesion is removed in one or more pieces that include part of the submucosa. Currently, the most popular technique uses a specially designed cap that is placed over the lesion to facilitate resection. A disadvantage is that lesions are commonly removed piecemeal, so that while the submucosal margin can be identified in the retrieved fragments, it can be very difficult to piece the fragments back to be certain that the entire lesion has been removed. In North America and Europe, endoscopic resections of dysplastic lesions in Barrett's esophagus are the most common use of this technique.[7]

Endoscopic submucosal dissection. *Endoscopic submucosal dissection* (ESD) is a technique in which the lesion is removed using an endoscopic knife, again at the level of the submucosa. The advantage of this technique is that the entire lesion can be removed in one piece, pinned out, and sent to pathology, so that even circumferential esophageal lesions can be removed using this technique. The disadvantage is that it takes far longer, which can be one or more hours, so it is difficult to accommodate into the schedule of a busy endoscopy unit. It also needs considerable more training than EMR (which itself is quite considerable).

Submucosal lesions. Some discourage the biopsy of large submucosal lesions of the esophagus. The reason is that if the lesion is a smooth muscle tumor, fascial planes will be disturbed, making it difficult to shell out at surgery. In other sites, it is often desirable to biopsy endoscopically benign-appearing submucosal lesions. One reason is to prove that the lesion is submucosal by documenting the presence of a normal overlying mucosa. A second reason is to determine the type of lesion (e.g., in the stomach, to differentiate between stromal tumor, pancreatic rest, cacinoid, and a submucosal metastasis). Some biopsy specimens taken with the jumbo pinch biopsy forceps reach the upper submucosa and thus reveal the nature of the tumor if it involves that zone. Another technique that some endoscopists use is to take multiple biopsy specimens from the same site directed progressively deeper.[8] The optimal practice, where available, is to have the lesion assessed by endoscopic ultrasound (EUS). Then, using a special cap placed over the tip of the endoscope and a snare technique, termed *endoscopic mucosal resection* (EMR), these lesions can be shelled out and removed in total endoscopically, if <1.8 cm, and piecemeal, if larger. In ESD, mucosal lesions are removed by the dissection of submucosa under the lesion using endoscopic knives, such as the insulated-tip diathermy knife and hook knife. Large specimens can be removed in toto (Fig. 1-3), and pinned out for pathology (Fig. 1-4). These techniques have been used throughout the gastrointestinal tract, but ESD is mostly practiced by Japanese endoscopists and is less used in the West. In practice, virtually identical specimens are obtained when rectal tumor are removed by transanal excision.

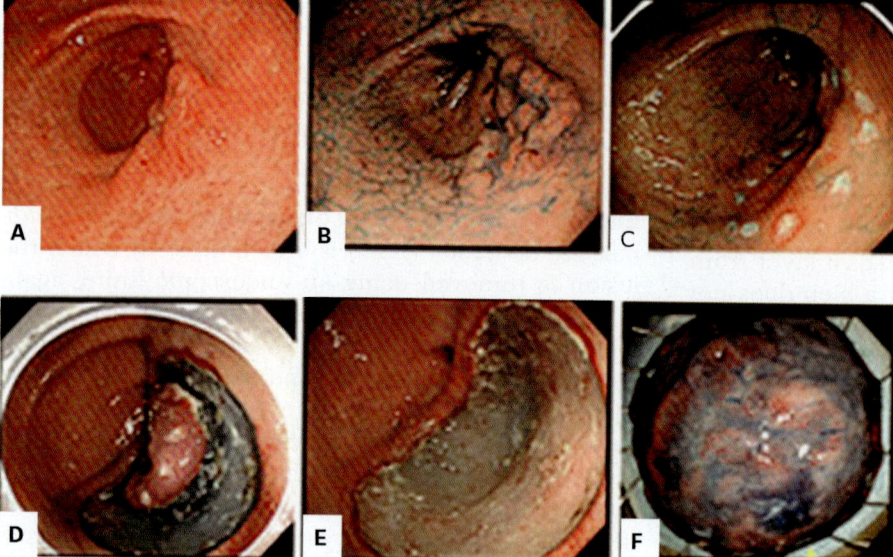

Figure 1-3. Endoscopic submucosal dissection. **A:** Large bowel lesion to be resected. **B:** The lesion is highlighted using chromoscopy. **C:** The limitation of the dissection is outlined by tattooing. **D:** The lesion has almost been removed. **E:** Removal is complete leaving a smooth base (**F**) pathology specimen. (Courtesy: Dr. C. Streutker.)

ANCILLARY TECHNIQUES USED AT ENDOSCOPY

Diagnosis of Infections—Smears, Brushings, Aspiration, and Culture

The diagnostic specificity of endoscopic biopsy may be enhanced markedly by other techniques used at the same endoscopy session. In the case of gastrointestinal infections, ancillary techniques such as cultures and smears of exudates and of biopsy tissue are often superior to biopsy.

In order to obtain samples from ulcerative or exudative lesions from the gastrointestinal tract, brushes (Fig. 1-5) may be passed through the same channel of the endoscope that is used to pass biopsy instruments. The material on the brush can be smeared on slides for direct examination for fungi or parasites (especially amebae) and for preparation of cytology smears when herpes infection or malignancy is a concern. Similarly, brushes with their adherent material can be swirled in transport media for appropriate cultures. In this regard, the most common purposes are to exclude herpes simplex infection of the esophagus and rectum and *Chlamydia* infection of the distal rectum.

When upper endoscopy is done in patients who have a suspected parasitic infestation (e.g., *Giardia* or *Cryptosporidium*), aspirated duodenal fluid can be obtained by attaching a suction trap between

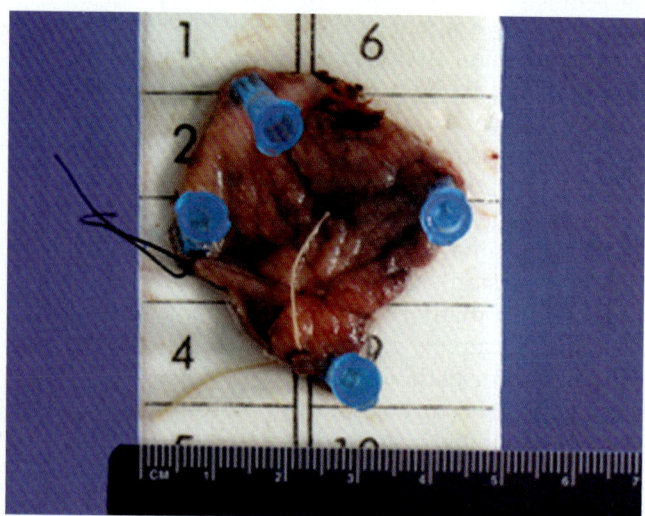

Figure 1-4. Pinned out specimen from rectum obtained by transanal excision.

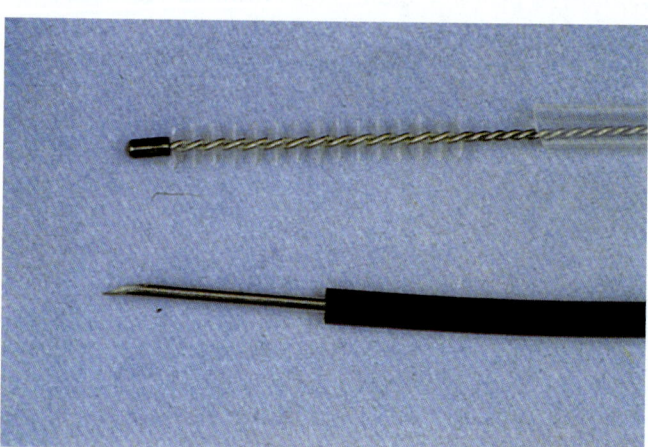

Figure 1-5. Accessories used to complement endoscopic biopsy. **Top:** Cytology brush. This is passed through the biopsy channel enclosed in a plastic sheath and is then advanced, using a handle at the head end. **Bottom:** A 21-gauge needle or thinner is used for fine-needle aspiration, usually under ultrasound guidance for submucosal or deeper lesions.

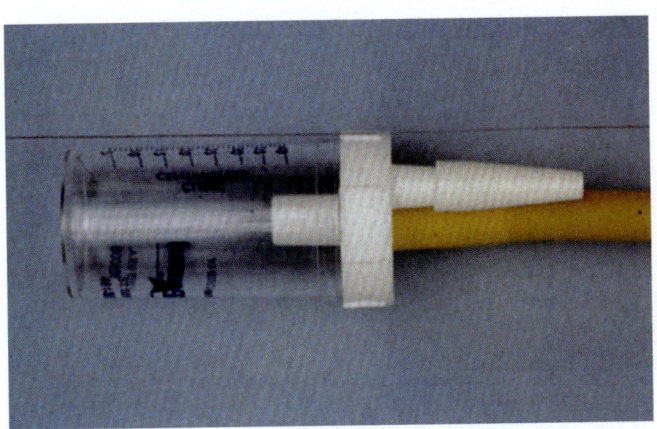

Figure 1-6. A suction trap is attached to the suction line of the endoscope to obtain luminal fluids, especially from the duodenum.

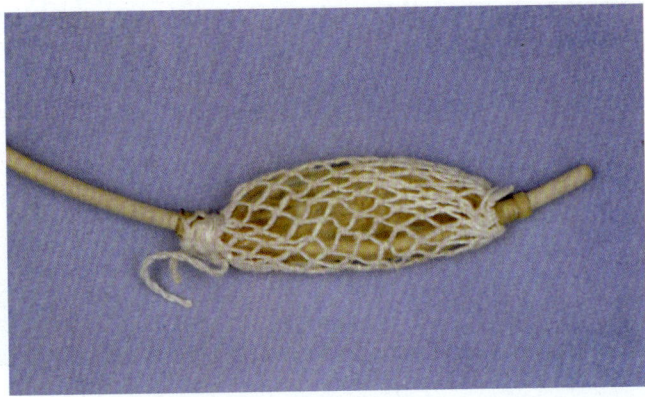

Figure 1-7. Balloon surrounded by mesh for esophageal cytology. This is used to screen for esophageal cancer, especially in certain high-prevalence provinces in China. The device is passed perorally into the stomach; the balloon is inflated and then removed while inflated. Thus, the surface cells are trapped in the mesh.

the endoscope and the suction line (Fig. 1-6). If the duodenum is "dry," a segment of mucosa can be rubbed with the cytology brush and smears prepared for parasite examination. It can be useful to obtain aspirated material or brush smears from the duodenum whenever small-bowel biopsies are being done in the evaluation of patients with diarrhea.

Cytology

The utility of cytology is almost totally dependent upon the cytologist's interest integrating the clinical and histological information. Without this interest, cytology usually adds very little information or may even be misleading because of false-positive diagnoses or the frequent diagnosis of "suspicious for malignancy." Cytology has gained increasing importance with the advent of EUS and passage of needles via EUS into mass lesions and lymph nodes. In fact, in many EUS centers, a designated cytology assistant is present in the endoscopy suite to perform the smears and confirm that analyzable cells are present. By far its most frequent use is in lesions of the pancreatico-biliary tree.

Direct-vision brush cytology. *Direct-vision brush cytology* can enhance diagnostic accuracy in malignancy when it is used as an adjunct to biopsy.[9] Sometimes brush cytology is the only technique available to establish a diagnosis of malignancy, especially when there are very tight strictures of the esophagus, stomach, or colon.

Balloon mesh cytology. *Balloon mesh cytology* (Fig. 1-7) is used to screen for squamous carcinoma in high-risk groups.[10]

Fine-needle aspirates. Fine-needle aspirates can be obtained from thickened folds or submucosal lesions. This is done by passing a needle attached to hollow plastic tubing through the biopsy channel of the endoscope (Fig. 1-5). The needle is pushed into the wall, suction is applied with a syringe attached to the proximal end of the plastic sheath, and the needle is jiggled back and forth two or three times. The needle is then retracted into the sheath and removed from the endoscope, and the contents are blown onto a slide. A second slide is apposed, and a smear is prepared just as for a blood smear. It is useful to repeat this procedure one or two more times so that four to six slides are available for cytology review. Experience with this technique has grown with the advent of EUS for the evaluation of submucosal lesions, for infiltrative disorders (e.g., lymphoma) associated with a normal overlying mucosa, and for assessing nodes adjacent to tissues accessible at EUS (i.e., mediastinum, paragastric, paraduodenal, celiac axis, paracolic, and pararectal).

Chromoendoscopy

Chromoendoscopy (the use of dye stains or an image system that changes the color visualized at endoscopy to enhance visualization of potential neoplastic lesions) either with a magnifying endoscope or without has been increasingly explored as an approach in both Barrett's esophagus and inflammatory bowel disease (IBD) colitis dysplasia screening (Fig. 1-8). Methylene blue as chromogen is taken up by actively absorbing intestinal-type epithelial cells and dysplastic cells but not by squamous or gastric mucosa. A lighter intensity of staining would highlight an area of dysplasia. So while methylene blue was introduced as an agent to distinguish inflammation from normal colonic mucosa in the mid-1980s,[11,12] it has been studied as an adjunctive technique for identifying neoplastic from nonneoplastic mucosa in the esophagus

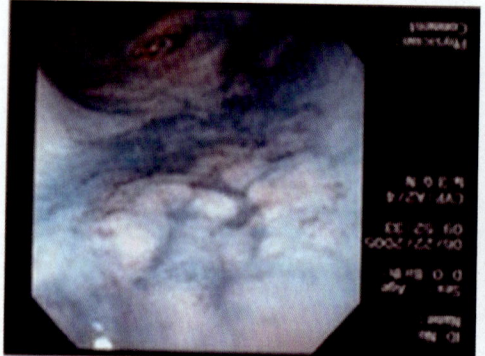 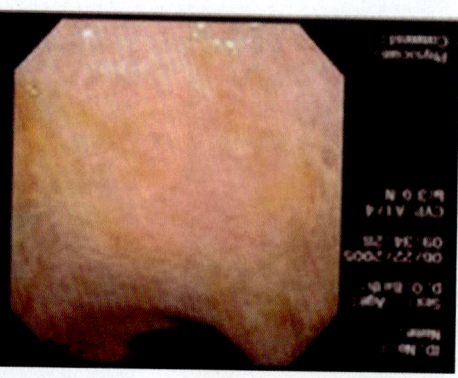

Figure 1-8. Chromoscopy in UC. The lesion on the **left** has been highlighted using methylene blue. In the prechromoscopy image (**right**), it is barely visible.

and the colon. Missing some foci of inflammation in an otherwise obviously inflamed organ has much less clinical implication than missing neoplastic foci in either an inflamed or a noninflamed organ. Indigo carmine as chromogen enhances the mucosal surface by pooling in the grooves between the mucosal villi enabling the visualization of the pattern formed by the mucosal folds and pits. Acetic acid achieves the same goal by means of reversible desaturation of superficial mucosal proteins. The bottom line is that these dyes or acetic acid can accentuate mucosal pit patterns so that neoplastic ones become more evident.

Because the spraying of solutions can be time consuming and messy, the advent of narrow band imaging (NBI) had the potential to be a major advance. NBI involves light of a short wavelength (blue light in the visible spectrum) penetrating superficially into the mucosa allowing for improved surface detail. As blue light is highly absorbed by hemoglobin, the vascular pattern is especially accentuated. The major advantages of NBI are that it involves merely the switch of a button on the head of the endoscope and hence requires little time and also lacks mess. Further it is uniformly applied, whereas dye spraying can be nonuniform.

Autofluorescence imaging (AFI) uses blue light for excitation of endogenous tissue fluorophores which emit fluorescent green light of longer wavelength. It can also highlight neoplastic tissue without the need for exogenous fluorophores. These latter two modalities have the potential advantage of not just identifying neoplasia when present that might be missed by white light endoscopy, but also by highlighting the superficial pit patterns of the lesion in question. This could help the endoscopist identify if a lesion is in fact neoplastic or is merely hyperplastic.

Endoscopes are currently available that are trimodal. These scopes have the usual high-definition white light endoscopy with buttons that allow conversion to either NBI or AFI.[13] These imaging systems are already widely available, whereas more sophisticated modalities such as confocal microscopy remain mostly available in research centers.

Confocal endomicroscopy allows visualization of individual cells and their nuclei, so that the enlarged stratified nuclei of dysplasia may be directly identified. While chromoendoscopy with dye spraying or other novel imaging systems exist, do they actually improve the detection of neoplasia in any of Barrett's esophagus, chronic colitis, or simply for routine screening or surveillance colonoscopy in the search for adenomas or dysplasia? This is discussed subsequently.

Regardless of how they are identified, whenever a neoplastic or presumed neoplastic lesion is removed and when there is a question of having to return sooner rather than later for repeat endoscopic assessment, it is prudent for the endoscopist to inject India ink (Spot) at the site of lesion removal. This helps for subsequent targeted biopsies either during surveillance or to provide a map for the surgeons who will resect that area. Endoscopists must notify pathologists that biopsies were performed from previously tattooed areas.

Barrett's esophagus. Methylene blue staining was reported to be highly accurate in identifying dysplasia in Barrett's esophagus.[14] In one report, methylene blue enhanced the detection of the extent of the Barrett's but not necessarily of finding dysplastic lesions, most of which were visible endoscopically.[15,27] In another Barrett's esophagus study, methylene blue staining was only 37% sensitive in picking up dysplastic lesions compared with routine histological assessment of four-quadrant biopsies. Although the specificity was good in this latter study (97%), to obviate the need for multiple biopsies, sensitivity would have to be excellent.[16] Therefore high rates of predictive value of methylene blue for identifying dysplasia are either operator dependent or may require specialized magnifying endoscopes. In one randomized crossover study of methylene blue versus random four-quadrant biopsy in patients with dysplasia in Barrett's found methylene blue directed biopsies to be significantly less sensitive in detecting dysplasia than routine biopsies in Barrett's esophagus.[17] Methylene blue identified dysplasia in 9 of 18 subjects while random biopsy with white light endoscopy found dysplasia in 17 of 18 leading these authors to suggest that methylene blue dye spray with targeted biopsies was inferior to random nontargeted biopsies. Further, a higher percentage of biopsies in the random biopsy group were dysplastic (36%) compared to that of the methylene blue targeted group (26%, $p = 0.05$).[17] A meta-analysis of nine studies comparing methylene blue chromoendoscopy with routine white light endoscopy plus biopsy revealed no incremental benefit of methylene blue chromoendoscopy over white light endoscopy.[18]

A series of studies have explored the role of NBI for detecting dysplasia in Barrett's esophagus. One of the first observational studies showed a benefit of using NBI in defining nondysplastic and high-grade dysplastic Barrett's epithelium.[19] In a prospective tandem study of 65 patients with Barrett's esophagus, NBI identified more subjects with higher grades of dysplasia than white light endoscopy (18% vs. 0), while standard endoscopy was associated with more biopsies (8.5 vs. 4.7, $p < 0.001$).[20] While NBI is easy to use, a study of 8 endoscopists scoring 1,600 NBI images of Barrett's esophagus found moderate interobserver agreement at best, including for high high-grade dysplasia. This suggests that NBI could not replace histological evaluation for neoplasia in Barrett's.[21] Perhaps the most sobering of studies for enhanced imaging in Barrett's esophagus was a study comparing white light endoscopy with the enhancement of any of indigo carmine chromoendoscopy, acetic acid chromoendoscopy, and NBI. Twelve endoscopists examined 22 areas, all assessed with the four techniques. The chromoendoscopy techniques added nothing to the interobserver agreement achieved on white light endoscopy. So while endoscopists appreciated the enhancement techniques as revealing more appealing images, the images did not enhance clinical outcomes over and above white light endoscopy.[22]

Inflammatory bowel disease. The first randomized controlled trial of dysplasia surveillance in IBD was performed in Germany, where approximately half the subjects underwent routine dysplasia surveillance and half underwent dysplasia surveillance with chromoendoscopy.[23] Chromoendoscopy was performed by spraying methylene blue 0.1% on the colonic mucosa in 30-cm segments and observing the mucosa with a special magnifying endoscope. Biopsies were directed to the paler, less blue, or white areas since neoplastic epithelium is less likely to take up the dye. During the course of the chromoendoscopy, the mucosa was scored for inflammation. The investigators found that chromoendoscopy better delineated the extent of inflammation by an average of 14 cm. More importantly, chromoendoscopy identified significantly more neoplastic lesions (35 in 13 cases, of which 32 were dysplastic and 3 were cancers, vs. routine endoscopy plus biopsy where neoplasia was detected 11 times in 6 cases, of which 10 were dysplastic and 1 was cancer). However, chromoendoscopy did not identify significantly more *patients* with dysplasia than routine endoscopy. Chromoendoscopy did lead to some false positives and even a few false negatives.

Overall the Kiesslich study has been considered a success of chromoendoscopy in ulcerative colitis (UC) which may relate simply to the use of methylene blue, which could be widely adopted by endoscopists with little extra cost. However, based on the experience with Barrett's esophagus, it may have reflected the use of the specialized magnifying endoscopes in combination with the dye. The availability of this technique may be dependent on the availability of these specialized endoscopes, and their widespread purchase will likely depend on further validation of this method. Elsewhere, the application of indigo carmine dye immediately after a standard surveillance endoscopy in 100 patients enhanced the yield of finding dysplasia in 2 patients to 7 in UC.[24]

The dye spraying technique may help target biopsies, so considerably fewer biopsies will be necessary. This technique may also help solve the problem of identifying at endoscopy those lumps that are neoplastic and not simply inflammatory; this would be a major advance. However, in colons widely studded with inflammatory (pseudo)polyps, the effects of the dye may be obscured.[23] False positives are also evident with chromoendoscopy as both highly inflamed areas and neoplastic areas do not take up the methylene blue dye.[23] Thus, chromoendoscopy will likely not aid in the dilemma of distinguishing dysplasia histologically in the setting of severe inflammation.

Some studies evaluating dye spraying did not employ a magnifying endoscope or mucolytics. The potential of chromoendoscopy without magnification endoscopy was evaluated in 102 chronic colitis patients undergoing surveillance. Each patient underwent two passes of the colonoscope; the first pass involved random biopsies with targeted biopsies of raised lesions. The second pass was after spraying of methylene blue dye and targeted biopsies of only raised or suspicious lesions. The dye spray method yielded 17 patients with dysplasia versus 9 with the targeted nondye technique and only 3 with the random biopsy technique. This group advocated consideration of abandoning random biopsies in favor of targeted biopsying only as directed by dye spraying.[25] In practice, chromoendoscopy, as described without a magnifying endoscope, can identify raised lesions that may only be inflammatory and not neoplastic (Fig. 1-8) but may also accentuate raised lesions that are neoplastic facilitating more focused biopsies (Fig. 1-9). Chromoendoscopy is typically not helpful with widespread inflammatory (pseudo) polyps (Fig. 1-10).

NBI identifies vascular changes and is very good at identifying the extent of inflammation (areas that

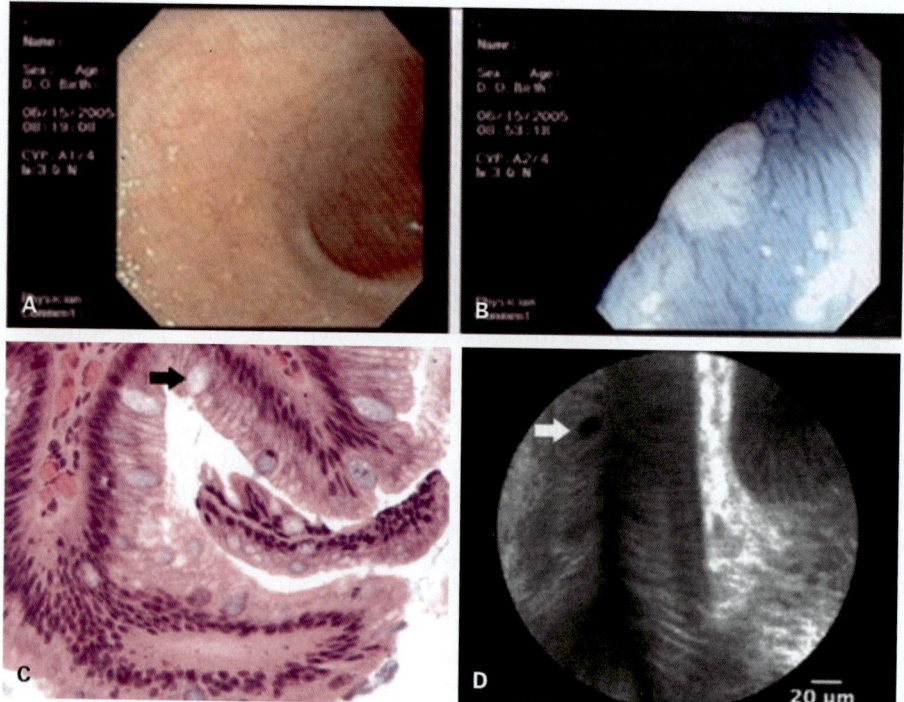

Figure 1-9. Chromoscopy in UC demonstrating how neoplastic lesions may be virtually invisible using white light (**A**) but highlighted using methylene blue (**B**). **C:** Histopathologic image demonstrating Barrett esophagus with no dysplasia. The surface, columnar epithelial cells are aligned in a neat row with small, basally oriented nuclei. The *black arrow* points out a goblet cell—the rounded bluish cell—that is the diagnostic feature of intestinal metaplasia of Barrett esophagus. **D:** Confocal laser endomicroscopy image of the corresponding tissue in vivo. The *whiter areas* are the lamina propria where fluorescein is in the highest concentration. Orderly, columnar epithelial cells line in the lamina propria as seen in the histopathologic image. The *white arrow* indicates a goblet cell.

are endoscopically normal may actually have subtle vascular changes and NBI may identify this). It may not be as effective at identifying mass lesions as dye-based chromoendoscopy, although this requires further study. In one study, 50 patients with UC were endoscopically inspected with a scope that had the capacity for usual white light endoscopy, NBI, as well as autofluorescence—AFI (trimodal endoscopy).[26] NBI can help determine the extent of inflammation and hence target where increased biopsy sampling should be undertaken. It is not clear that NBI is as good as dye spraying for colitis-associated neoplasia.

Screening and surveillance colonoscopy for adenomas in otherwise healthy individuals. Methylene blue staining with and without magnifying endoscopy has been used to identify flat and raised adenomas in noninflamed colons in persons who would be undergoing usual screening colonoscopy.[27,28,33,34] More recent studies have focused on the role of NBI in routine colon cancer (and adenoma) screening. In endoscopy units trying to push through a large volume of screening colonoscopies, it is easy to see how dye spraying and the extra time required to undertake this would be unpopular. In one study, 100 patients at high risk for having adenomas underwent trimodal endoscopy (see previous paragraph). AFI did not reduce the adenoma miss rate compared to white light endoscopy. Further, both NBI and AFI were somewhat disappointing in terms of diagnostic accuracy.[26] In a study of 276 patients who underwent tandem colonoscopy either with a second white light endoscopy or NBI after white light endoscopy, NBI did not enhance the pickup rate, which was approximately 12% for the second endoscopy.[29] In a 6-center study of 1,256 patients randomized subjects to either NBI or white light endoscopy, there was no difference on adenoma detection between these two modalities (?33%). There was a significantly longer withdrawal time in NBI.[30] These studies suggest that high-resolution white light endoscopy with careful

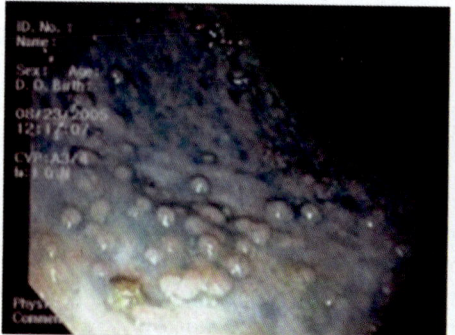
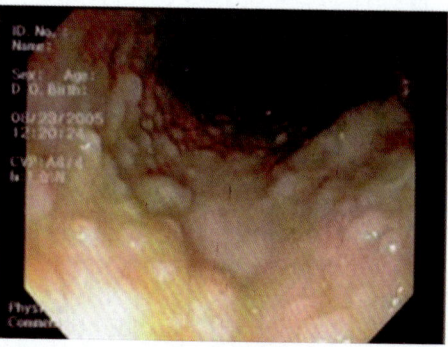

Figure 1-10. Inflammatory (pseudo) polyps can be highlighted using methylene blue but are of no clinical significance.

endoscopic examination is so good that it is hard to improve upon it with the various novel methods for polyp detection currently available.

Could NBI facilitate real-time assessment of which polyps are likely adenomas (and hence require resection) versus hyperplastic and hence can be left in situ reducing endoscopy time and costs of histopathology examination? One hundred subjects underwent screening colonoscopy with high-definition white light endoscopy followed by NBI. NBI had a high degree of accuracy at determining that polyps were adenomatous versus hyperplastic.[31] These findings were corroborated in a single investigator study by Rex.[32]

Virtual Histology

Despite the possibilities of chromoendoscopy, a dream of the endoscopist is to obtain virtual histology, which means "real-time" in vivo histology. The endoscopist can decide what the area of interest is and, if necessary, can remove the lesion in a targeted fashion. Many new optical developments may further advance early diagnosis of gastrointestinal cancer. Raman spectroscopy, optical coherence tomography, light scattering spectroscopy, confocal laser fluorescence endoscopy, and immunofluorescence endoscopy are some of the newer methods with different advantages and disadvantages which have been under development for considerable time.[33,34] However, these techniques potentially allow the pathologists and endoscopists to work closely together for the proper diagnosis of the targeted biopsies. The best studied to date of these techniques is confocal laser endomicroscopy. It enables in vivo microscopy of the mucosal layer of the gastrointestinal tract with subcellular resolution during ongoing endoscopy. Different types of diseases can be diagnosed with optical surface and subsurface analysis. This can be used for targeting biopsies to relevant areas, and subsurface imaging can unmask microscopic diseases or bacterial infection.[35,36] In a randomized study compared to conventional endoscopy in UC patients, the presence of neoplastic changes could be predicted by endomicroscopy with high accuracy (sensitivity, 94.7%; specificity, 98.3%; accuracy, 97.8%). Endomicroscopy was associated with a 4.75-fold increase in neoplasias detected ($p = 0.005$) than with conventional colonoscopy, although with 50% fewer biopsy specimens ($p = 0.008$). Hence endomicroscopy could increase the diagnostic yield and reduce the need for biopsy examinations.[37] This technique has been explored in a variety of neoplastic conditions of the gastrointestinal tract.[38]

Biopsy specimen handling and processing. Despite the major advances in endoscopy and diagnostic pathology, it is disheartening to observe that the general quality of gastrointestinal tract biopsy specimens continues to be poor. In fact, their quality seems to have remained relatively unchanged over the past three decades. The lack of interest by endoscopists and pathologists in improving this situation is difficult to understand because it often influences diagnosis and therapy. Those who choose to improve the quality of biopsy specimens for interpretation find that it requires some motivation, very little extra effort, and an ongoing dialogue between endoscopists, endoscopy nurses, pathologists, and technologists. It is surely time to "legislate" that when a specific clinical question is being asked, a minimum biopsy set is required for the pathologist to have the best chance of answering the question. While these are discussed in more detail in the specific chapters, a summary is provided in Table 1-2, which (one could argue) should be on the wall of every endoscopy suite.

HANDLING OF THE BIOPSY SPECIMEN PRIOR TO IMMERSION IN FIXATIVES

Biopsy specimens from different levels or sites of the large bowel should be placed in different fixative bottles (see Table 1-2). One creative approach for reducing the number of blocks is to use standardized marking ink colors for specimens from different parts of the gut (e.g., brown for rectum, red for cecum). The different colors of the inks are recognizable around each specimen on microscopic examination.

Even when multiple specimens are taken from the same site, we avoid placing more than three or four of them in any bottle, although in many labs more than this are placed in >1 block anyway. Whenever there is more than this number in the block, sectioning through the full face of all specimens becomes increasingly difficult because the specimens vary in size and are not fully represented in the final histological slide. Each bottle is labeled with a separate letter followed by a bracketed number indicating the number of specimens in that bottle. The pathology requisition is labeled in a similar fashion. The pathologist should expect that in 99% of endoscopy units, biopsy forceps are merely swirled in formalin to shake off the specimen without any mounting.

Handling Polyps

Polyps removed with the electrocautery snare with a good stalk can just be immersed in formalin. Because stalks are usually short and retract quickly, most of the time the pathologist/technologist does their best to find the cauterized margin and bisect the polyp in

Table 1-2 Guide to Sites for Taking Biopsies

Esophageal biopsies for gerd
a) Immediately above Z-line (neutrophils, eosinophils)
b) Edge of any erosions ulcers
c) Number of cm above Z-line (reactive changes)
d) Mid esophagus (in case numerous eosinophils are present in the distal biopsy to include/exclude eosinophilic esophagitis (in the setting of undiagnosed dysphagia or when endoscopic findings are suggestive of eosinophilic esophagitis, then biopsies should always be taken from the distal and mid esophagus and at least five biopsies in total should be taken)

Barrett's esophagus—Any tongues, SSBE, or LSBE—at first endoscopy to confirm the diagnosis and exclude dysplasia/carcinoma. Subsequent endoscopies for dysplasia/carcinoma only
   Intestinalization (if required) is best closest to the squamo-Barrett junction
     For dysplasia—any endoscopic irregularity/lesion, then four-quadrant biopsies every 2 cm

Gastric biopsies for Helicobacter[a]
Two biopsies of the antrum and two of oxyntic mucosa—organisms migrate proximally under numerous circumstances (see Chapter 13). It is usually OK to put these in one container, although wisdom/experience suggest the 2 antral in one and the 2 body in a second
Any areas of redness, erosions, or ulcers

Gastric polyps
Remove/sample polyp and take biopsies from background mucosa as for *Helicobacter* (overt gastric fundic gland polyps may be excluded from this, unless the question of *Helicobacter* is also an issue), but it frequently saves an additional endoscopy if the "soil" is included automatically

Duodenum for celiac disease
Four biopsies of second part and two or more of the bulb (5%–10% of adults/children have changes limited to the bulb and need to be taken into account (see Chapter XX)

Terminal ileal biopsies for Crohn's disease
Edge of any erosions/ulcers, plus two close by for focal disease
Biopsies of cecum/ascending colon (backwash ileitis must have similar disease in continuity and so demonstrate its presence or absence)

Colitis—Query nature of underlying colitis (including microscopic colitis). Demonstrate distribution and focality of disease throughout the colon—Minimum are biopsies from terminal ileum (microscopic disease), right colon, transverse colon, descending colon, sigmoid colon, and rectum. Put EACH site in separate containers or distribution changes are lost. Also inflammation is greatest in right colon and to a lesser extent the rectum (see Chapters 16 and 18)

Surveillance in IBD
Any suspicious lesions (targeted biopsies)
If polypectomy is carried out take biopsies around its base to demonstrate the adequacy (or not) of polypectomy and whether any dysplasia exists in the flat mucosa adjacent to the polyp which would be an indication for colectomy as opposed to ongoing surveillance
Four biopsies every 10 cm from cecum to rectum. The distance may be decreased in the rectosigmoid as this is the prime site for dysplasia and carcinoma. Ideally each site into separate containers (see Chapter 18)

[a]Whenever the stomach or proximal duodenum is biopsied, the issue of whether any changes found are *Helicobacter*-related arises, so anticipate it and take biopsies accordingly.

---

this plane. In some units, a dye is used to identify this (bright colors work best), and this greatly facilitates cutting the polyp in the correct plane so that, should invasive carcinoma be present, its proximity to the cauterized margin can be assessed.

ROUTINE FIXATION

Formalin is now used almost exclusively. Nonformalin fixatives such as Bouin's solution or Hollande's modification of Bouin's solution for gastrointestinal biopsy specimens cause leaching out the granules of eosinophils and other cells such as Paneth and mast cells and cause major problems with immunohistochemistry, and are not recommended. Fixation for 6 hours usually suffices, although this is basically alcohol fixation and overnight fixation is preferred, especially for polyps.

TISSUE PROCESSING, EMBEDDING, AND CUTTING

All too often, biopsy specimen interpretation is severely compromised or impossible because of technical flaws that are readily preventable. These include misorientation during embedding, sections that are too thick, and shattering by dull microtome knives or by overcooling of blocks prior to cutting (Fig. 1-11). In any pathology laboratory, it is invaluable to have one or two technologists assigned primarily to biopsies. All technologists should be aware that biopsies need to be embedded on edge and not en face, to be able to cut into its core. Polyps are embedded en face by sectioning them in the plane of the stalk (Fig. 1-12).

During the embedding process, the technologist can check to ensure that the number of biopsy specimens designated for a given cassette is correct. When several specimens are embedded in the same tissue block, they should be closely aligned in a straight row to make viewing of the stained sections easier (Fig. 1-13). They must be embedded quickly so that they are placed at approximately the same level in the paraffin block.

The paraffin block should be trimmed with straight parallel edges. Trimming should be done fairly close to the tissue so that only a small rim of paraffin surrounds the specimens. This allows multiple sections

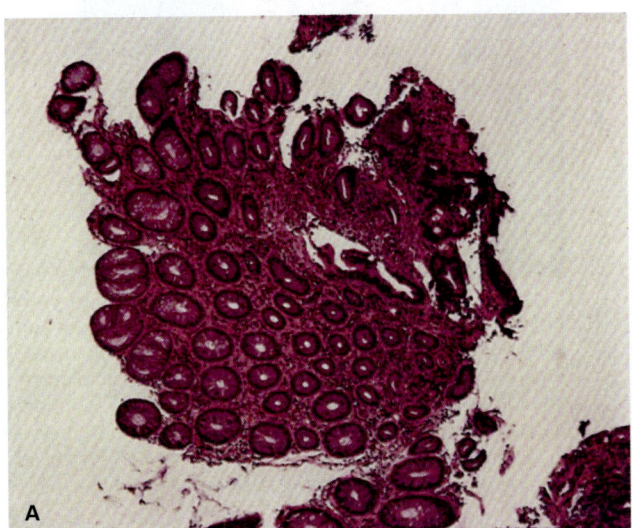
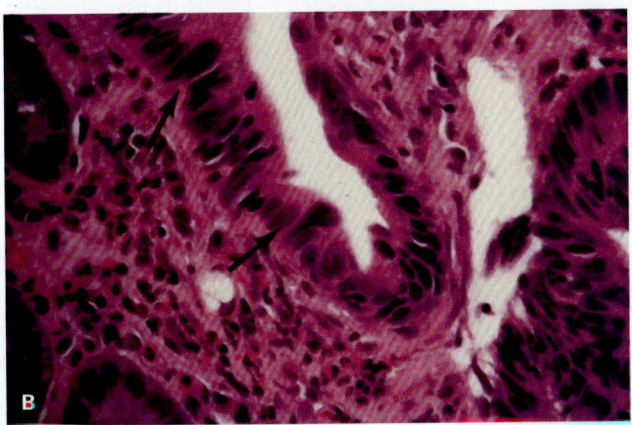
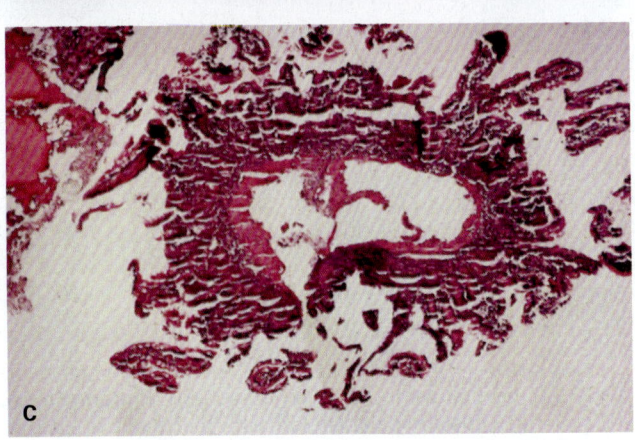
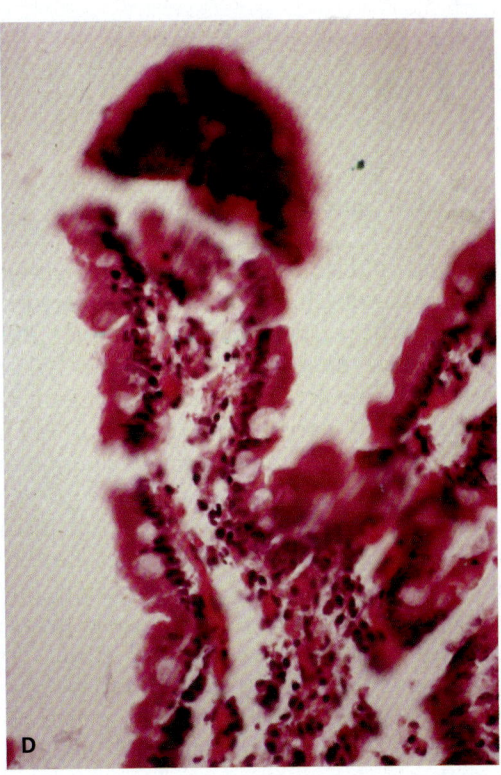

Figure 1-11. Examples of poor processing and cutting techniques. **A:** This slide was submitted for a second opinion concerning dysplasia in UC. Any possibility of assessing architectural change was precluded by the fact that the biopsy specimen was sectioned completely tangentially. **B:** Detail of Figure 1-11A. The section is also overstained and too thick, so that there is a lack of nuclear detail (*arrows*) in the area that was suspicious for dysplasia. **C:** Biopsy section of duodenal mucosa from a patient with chronic diarrhea. Severe chatter and poor orientation are obvious at this low power. **D:** The chatter and wrinkles are even more obvious at this power. Villi with these sorts of artifacts make it virtually impossible to diagnose abnormalities such as untreated celiac sprue, while abnormalities such as intraepithelial lymphocytosis that might provide a clue to the cause of the chronic diarrhea similarly cannot be assessed.

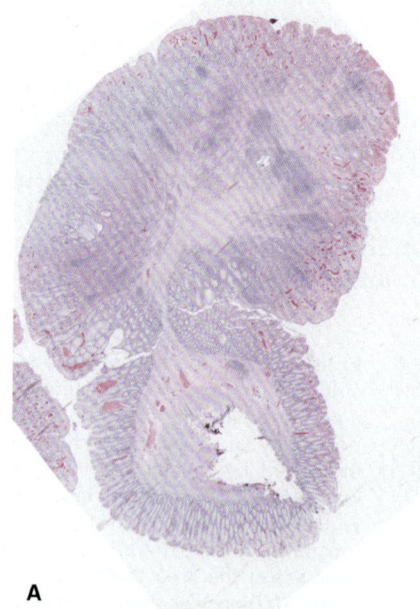
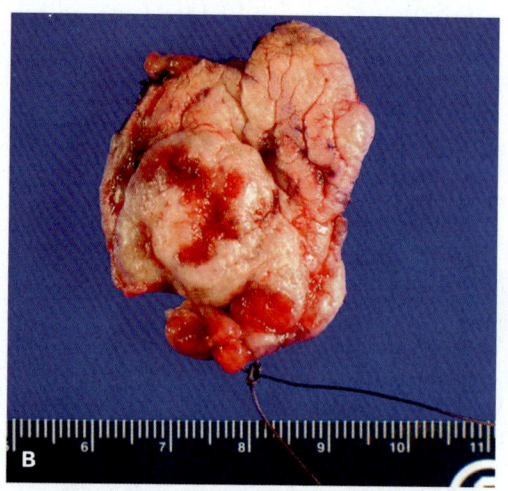
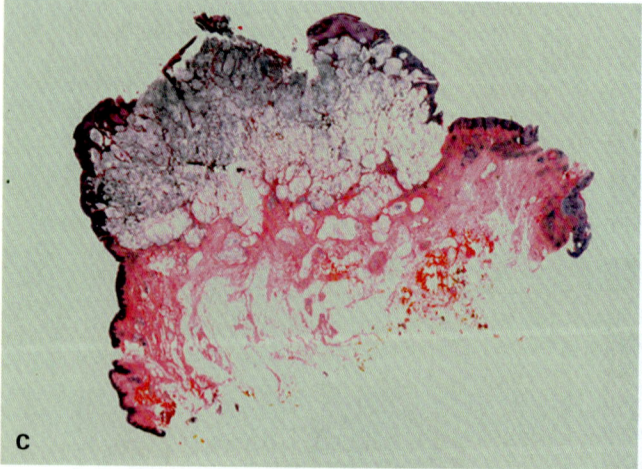

Figure 1-12. Handling endoscopically removed polyps. **A:** A stalk as long as the one shown here is very uncommon for the reason outlined in Figure 1-2B. **B:** Macroscopic picture of polyps showing the stalk at its base suture. **C:** Polyp sectioned through its stalk so that the resected margin is visible in the section.

from each ribbon, and sometimes more than one row on a slide.

Sections should be 3 to 5 μm thick. High-quality sections cannot be obtained without very sharp knives. Technologists who section gastrointestinal mucosal biopsy specimens must learn to recognize what the central oriented core looks like in each region of the gut. Although rarely carried out, this involves checking *each group of wet, untrained sections under a microscope* to ensure that core sections are represented; the ghost-like patterns of normal mucosal histology in each part of the gastrointestinal tract can be recognized (Fig. 1-14). The major landmarks are the dermal papillae in the esophagus, the gastric pits, small intestinal villi and their crypts, and rectal crypts. The technologist must recognize that cross-sectioned "doughnuts" are seen at the edges of biopsy specimens (necessitating further cutting into the block) or in specimens that have been improperly oriented, either

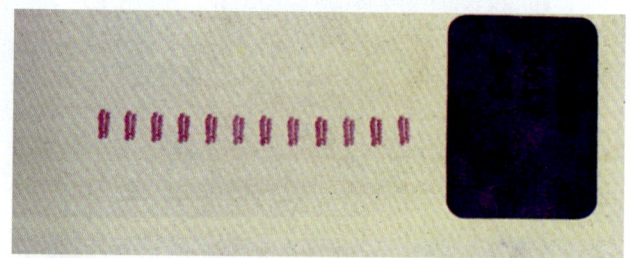
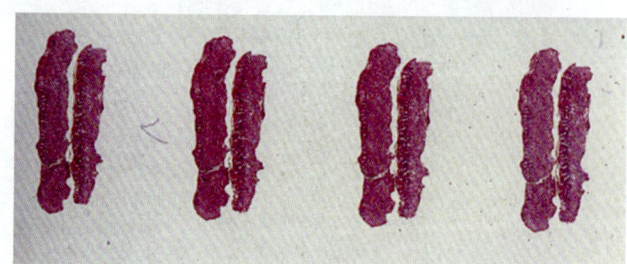

Figure 1-13. Two tissue specimens in a single block. **Top:** A representative ribbon of serial sections. **Bottom:** Embedding the biopsy specimens close to each other helps to ensure they will both be represented with the best orientation.

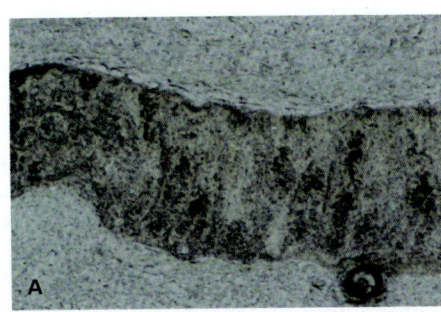 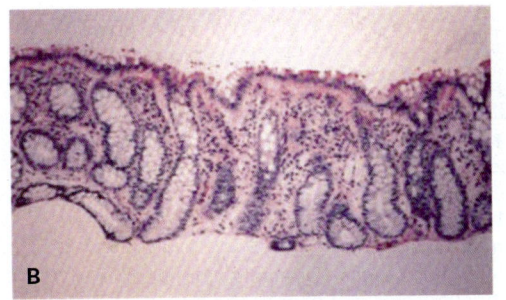

Figure 1-14. **A:** Appearance of a rectal biopsy section in the unstained "wet" state. The technologist must look for the landmark (oriented crypts) that indicates that the section is in the oriented core of the specimen. **B:** The stained section.

in the endoscopy unit or in the pathology laboratory (Fig. 1-15).

Up to 30 (two ribbons, each containing 15 sections) serial sections can be obtained from the best-oriented core of each mucosal biopsy specimen (Fig. 1-13). If serial sections are not prepared, a plan for the minimum number of random (serial-step) sections through the central core of each specimen must be established. One approach is to cut groups of sections from at least three different levels of the central core of the biopsy specimen. While we routinely perform only hematoxylin and eosin stains, if the biopsy concerns require special stains (e.g., *Helicobacter*), a strip of sections from the central core is set aside in advance. Unless carried out routinely, this requires the technologist to survey all the pathology requisitions before beginning to section.

If multiple serial sections are not routinely prepared, the pathologist must be prepared to provide levels/deepers as required. This also presupposes that the clinician has alerted the pathologist to specific questions, such as concern about the presence of granulomas or parasites, both of which may be sparsely distributed.

In the final analysis, it is clearly better to have several well-cut, well-oriented sections from the thickest part of the biopsy specimen than strips of multiple misoriented sections laden with scratch marks and folds.

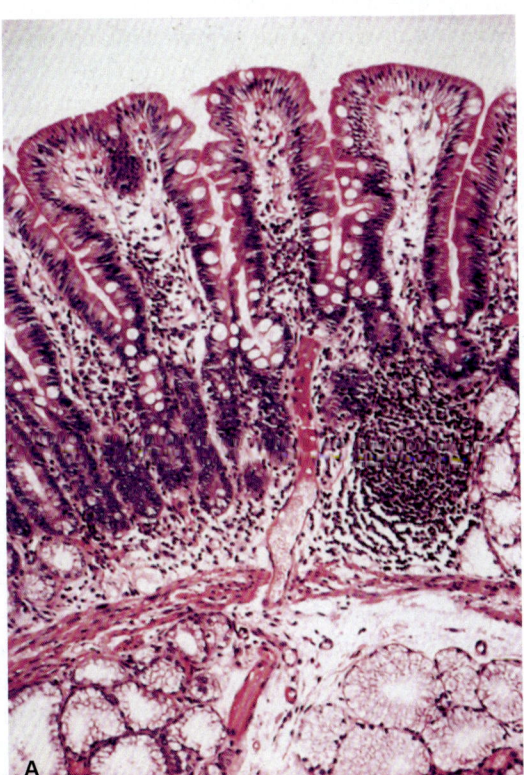 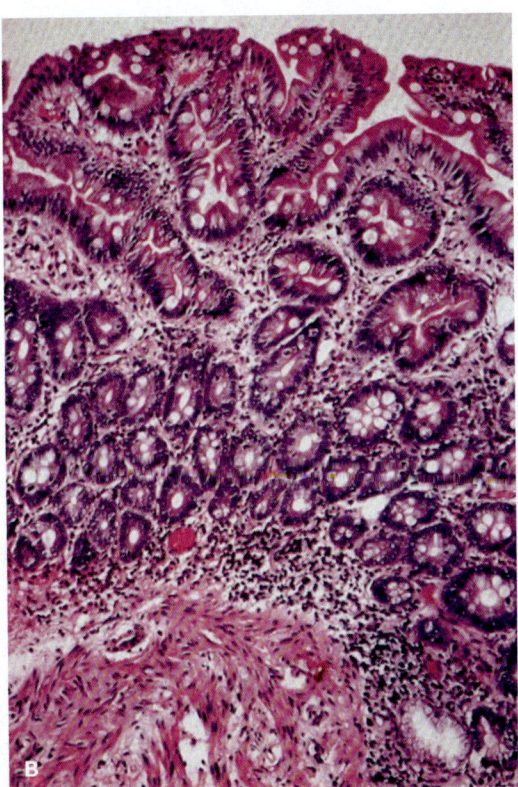

Figure 1-15. Duodenal biopsy specimen illustrating orientation artifacts. **A:** Normal duodenal bulb specimen. **B:** The edge of the same specimen away from the central core gives the false impression of villous blunting because of tangential artifact. Here the clue to tangential sectioning is the presence of numerous multilayered, cross-sectioned crypts in the bottom half of the section. A similar appearance is produced when the specimen is improperly oriented during embedding. There is also no reason for a flat mucosa as the inflammatory cell component is normal, there is no intraepithelial lymphocytosis and no surface damage.

Table 1-3	Suggested Descriptive Terms for Benign-Appearing Lesions at Endoscopy

To replace "-it is"
  Absent vascular pattern—especially in the colon
  Erythema—streaks, patches
  Friability—blood ooze or petechiae?
    —after wiping mucosa?
  Subepithelial hemorrhages—punctate, confluent
  Exudates—qualify color and degree of adherence
  Erosions—depressed or nondepressed
    —white based; black based

To replace "edema"
  Swelling—localized, diffuse
  Cobblestone appearance
  Prominent folds

To replace "scar"
  Depressed or nondepressed, white, stellate, or linear streak

To replace "atrophy"
  Thin folds (e.g., in body of stomach)
  Pallor
  Prominent vessels

To replace "ectasia" or "angiodysplasia"
  Describe the actual lesion (e.g., "3-mm smooth, nonraised cherry-red spot")

Note: For each lesion, a description of the size, extent, or both should be given.
Source: Weinstein WM, Hill TA. Gastrointestinal mucosal biopsy. In: Berk J, ed. *Bockus Textbook of Gastroenterology*. Philadelphia, PA: W.B. Saunders; 1985:626–644.

DESCRIPTION OF ENDOSCOPIC FINDINGS

The endoscopist and pathologist must establish an understanding for the description of mucosal appearances. For the endoscopist, this is essential so that all persons concerned can develop a mental picture of what was seen. For the pathologist, this is important in order to integrate the gross pathology (endoscopic appearance) with the microscopic findings. Table 1-3 lists terms that have a simple descriptive connotation, rather than some of the commonly used editorial jargon, which is subject to a variety of interpretations or misinterpretations. Simply describing the appearance of a mucosal biopsy specimen as gastritis or duodenitis can embrace a perception of factors ranging from color changes to distinct erosions. Concerning the latter, the pathologist must be aware of the fact that the endoscopic distinction between ulcers and large erosions may be purely arbitrary. Endoscopists can still interpret their descriptive findings provisionally at the end of the endoscopy report and in the clinical history section of a pathology requisition.

Some centers have specially designed gastrointestinal pathology requisitions that include diagrams of endoscopy sites, findings, or both. This or any other mechanism is acceptable, assuming that it permits the interpretation of what was actually seen and provides a precise description of biopsy specimen locations. In this era of video endoscopy, it may be easy to include pictures in the endoscopy report that can go with the pathology requisition. Every requisition should include the question/issues being addressed. The photos may be present in electronic records, but it takes far more time to look up, the pictures may not be available, and there may be sufficient delay that it may not be available when the pathologist is signing out the case. Most pathologists will not bother to pull up the endoscopic report, so if it accompanies the pathology requisition that is a great advantage for the pathologist. As discussed subsequently, it is also useful for pathologists to see how biopsy specimens are taken and how polyps are snared in order to understand the source of some of the histological artifacts they encounter.

BIOPSY SPECIMEN LOCATION

The histological appearance of the mucosa in a given organ may vary according to the location of the biopsy specimen within that organ. This is especially true in the upper gastrointestinal tract. The best way to ensure that different endoscopists in a given endoscopy unit provide uniform information is to make the endoscopy assistant aware of the prerequisites for location description. Precise, uniform descriptions of lesion and biopsy specimen locations also permit other clinicians to interpret the findings. The dilemma for many pathologists is that they are simply given the organ source, with no specific description of sites within that organ. Table 1-4 outlines the minimum requirements for describing lesion and biopsy sites.

NUMBER AND SIZE OF BIOPSY SPECIMENS

For many disorders, the number of biopsy specimens provided influences the ease or precision of interpretation (see Table 1-2). The endoscopy assistant should be trained to recognize what constitutes an acceptably sized biopsy specimen and to provide ongoing feedback during the procedure. For example, it is useful if a biopsy specimen is reported as tiny or shallow when it is only 2 or 3 mm in diameter or when it is transparent when placed on the finger. The latter indicates marked shallowness, except for squamous esophageal biopsy specimens, which are commonly transparent.

Table 1-4 Recommended Approach to Describe the Locations of Endoscopic Lesions and Biopsy Sites

Esophagus—Give all as number of centimeters from the incisor region
    Location of the region of the squamocolumnar junction (Z-line)
    Location of the lesion or biopsy site

Stomach
    Fundus
    Body—For each, proximal, mid, or distal
    Antrum—For each, give curvature or wall

Duodenum
    Bulb
    Descending portion—proximal, mid, or distal
    Third and fourth portions—need x-ray confirmation for precise localization

Colon
    Cecum
    Ascending colon
    Hepatic flexure
    Transverse colon—proximal, mid, or distal
    Descending colon
    Sigmoid colon
    Rectum—number of centimeters from anal verge

Note: These are minimum prerequisites; in many circumstances, additional descriptions are required to depict the location accurately.
Source: Weinstein WM, Hill TA. Gastrointestinal mucosal biopsy. In: Berk J, ed. *Bockus Textbook of Gastroenterology*. Philadelphia, PA: W.B. Saunders; 1985:626–644.

When the endoscopy assistant reports that only a tiny fragment has been obtained, the endoscopist should rebiopsy the same site. Even the most skilled endoscopists using large biopsy forceps have to go back to a given site periodically to get a better-quality specimen. Increasingly large forceps can be passed through standard 2.8-mm channels (see Fig. 1-1B).

THE HISTORY AND THE QUESTION FOR THE PATHOLOGIST

In biopsy specimens taken for malignancy, the question is self-evident. However, in benign diseases, especially suspected infections and inflammatory bowel diseases, enough clinical details should be provided so that the pathologist can give an informed diagnosis or differential diagnosis. In addition, the specific question should be clearly outlined for the pathologist to help guide the direction and intensity of the pathologist's review.

For all biopsy specimens taken from the colon, it is helpful if the type of purgative preparation used is stated and also whether the patient is taking anti-inflammatory drugs is recorded on the pathology requisition. The reason for the former is that certain irritant laxatives used for flexible sigmoidoscopy may create epithelial and inflammatory changes.[39] The large-volume purging solutions used prior to colonoscopy do not appear to create any morphologic havoc. Oral sodium phosphate preparations may also create "skid marks" in the colon. In relation to corticosteroids, especially in enema form, the histology for a disorder such as UC might be different in the treated compared to the untreated state.

Sometimes clinicians are disappointed because they fail to obtain histological confirmation of their endoscopic interpretations. The pathologist must communicate the limitations of the ability to make a histological diagnosis in certain disorders. One example is in the case of red streaks or even frank tiny erosions in the stomach, where the histology may be very nonspecific or even normal (see Chapter 13). It is not uncommon for endoscopists to use the term gastritis and colitis when in fact there might simply be some redness that others might view as within normal limits. This is especially a problem in the stomach, and gastritis is one of the most overused endoscopic diagnoses. The pathologist should not feel bullied into overinterpreting normal gastric biopsies because of an endoscopic diagnosis of gastritis. A second example concerns appearances believed to represent small vascular ectasia. The clinician may not realize that the histological verification of such vascular lesions may be possible in only 50%[40] or less of these cases. The factors responsible for this low yield include tissue shrinkage and vessel collapse in the fixative, failure to represent the lesion in the sections that were stained, or the location of the vascular abnormality in the submucosa (see Chapter 2). When polyps have been biopsied, it may be necessary either to cut through the entire block or re-embed it. When the latter was actually carried out in large-bowel polyps showing normal mucosa, 10% were found to have lesions.[41]

APPROACH TO THE MICROSCOPIC EXAMINATION

It is possible to adopt very different approaches to the initial microscopic examination. Both approaches will be described, and the reader can decide which is preferred.

One view holds that the histology is examined first, without prior review of the clinical information. A systematic initial examination "without expectation bias" is believed to be more accurate. After this initial review, the clinical information is incorporated into a final interpretation. If a firm diagnosis is made, the issue is whether the clinician got it right. One gets very good at identifying the precise sites, but sometimes the diagnosis cannot be made without knowledge of the precise site (intestinal metaplasia in the stomach vs. gastric metaplasia in the proximal duodenum vs. Barrett's esophagus).

A second view is that a more relevant clinical diagnosis can be obtained more quickly and with equal detachment by analyzing the histology with prior knowledge of the clinical findings. Here the analogy is that of a physical examination, targeted to some extent after one takes a history. The disadvantage is that if the requisition states, for example, "? UC," the pathologist is already trying to find evidence for that diagnoses, and the likelihood of other (correct) diagnoses overlooked, or just about anything in the biopsy/biopsies stated to be "consistent with" whatever is on the requisition form. The issue is whether complete detachment really can be obtained from the information on the requisition form before looking at the slide.

A SYSTEMATIC APPROACH TO BIOPSY SPECIMEN INTERPRETATION

Interpretation of biopsy specimens from different areas of the gastrointestinal tract is dealt with in the individual chapters. The theme, however, is the same for each area: try to maintain a uniform and systematic approach. Much of the examination is done at low power to get an impression of the overall architecture and lymphoid aggregates and to determine whether there are striking inflammatory or neoplastic changes.ABnormal-appearing areas are focused on selectively. One purpose of serial sections is to follow suspicious lesions such as granulomas and early crypt abscesses. With experience, such lesions can also be scanned for at low power; higher magnification is used only to confirm their presence.

Table 1-5 outlines a systematic approach to mucosal biopsy examination, beginning with the examination of luminal contents (i.e., cell fragments, exudate, and organisms adherent to or near the surface epithelium). Within exudate, there may be superficial fragments of a carcinoma or evidence of infection. The organisms found in luminal contents or attached to the surface epithelium are listed in Table 1-6. Some other infections are recognized in an intracellular location in surface epithelium (e.g., *Isospora belli*) or as transformed cells in deeper zones of granulation tissue (e.g., cytomegalovirus).

TECHNICAL PROBLEMS IN INTERPRETATION

Mucosal Hemorrhage and Edema

Biopsy specimens for benign disorders are usually taken after a complete examination of the region in question. In a sense, the mucosa is "massaged," sometimes vigorously, by repeated passage back and forth in order to examine all areas. Biopsy specimens are then usually taken at the end of the procedure. Thus, theoretically, a certain amount of mucosal edema and congestion can be induced by the endoscopy procedure itself. Also, most pinch biopsy forceps do not have sharp cup edges; the mucosa is pinched off and avulsed rather than cut. Trauma can be induced by this procedure. Additional congestion and hemorrhage may be induced by a maneuver called *tenting*, in which the mucosa is pinched and then slowly retracted to produce a mucosal "tent" in order to obtain some reassurance that the tissue sample

Table 1-5 Example of a Systematic Approach to the Examination of Gastrointestinal Biopsy Specimens

Low power
  Identify/confirm biopsy site
  Uniformity or lack of it between biopsy specimens or within a specimen (i.e., tumor, focal inflammation)
  Architecture
  Lymphoid aggregates (focal, diffuse)

High power
  Lumen: organisms
  Surface epithelium
    Organisms
    Type—any dysplasia
    Cells within epithelium?—neutrophils, intraepithelial
    Lymphocytes
    Subepithelial collagen
  Crypt/pit epithelium
    Height
    Mitoses, any dysplasia
    Paneth/endocrine cells
  Lamina propria
    Predominant cells
    Abnormal cells (histiocytes, pigment cells, carcinoma)
    Eosinophils
    Fibrosis
  Submucosa if present
    Inflammation
    Ganglion cells
    Vessels (amyloid, ectasia)

Table 1-6 Some Infections That May Be Found in Exudate or as Attachments to the Surface Epithelium

SITE OF BIOPSY	ORGANISMS
Esophagus	*Candida*, herpes simplex
Stomach	*Helicobacter pylori, Candida*
Small intestine	*Giardia, Cryptosporidium*
Large bowel	*Amoeba, Cryptosporidium*, spirochetes

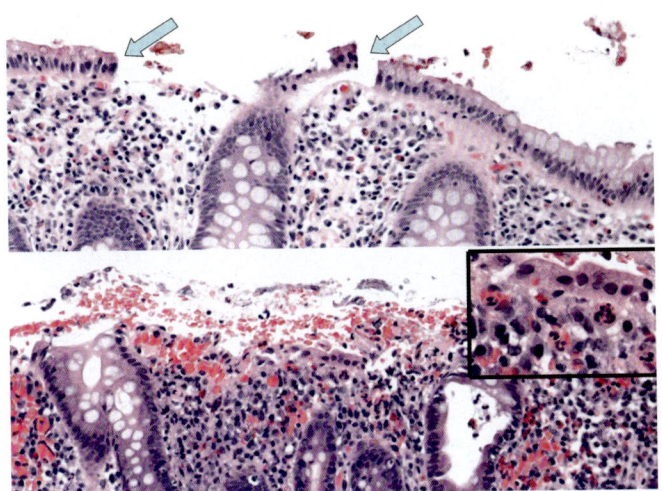

Figure 1-16. Artifact. Pseudoerosions versus early erosions. **Top:** Large-bowel biopsy in which the surface mucosa has been artifactually stripped. The clue is the abrupt cessation of epithelium (*blue arrows*) without acute inflammation, fibrin, hemorrhage, restitution, or reactive changes in the underlying crypts. **Bottom:** Early erosion. Surface epithelium is markedly attenuated, with hemorrhage, reactive changes in the adjacent crypts and usually (not always) neutrophils (**inset**).

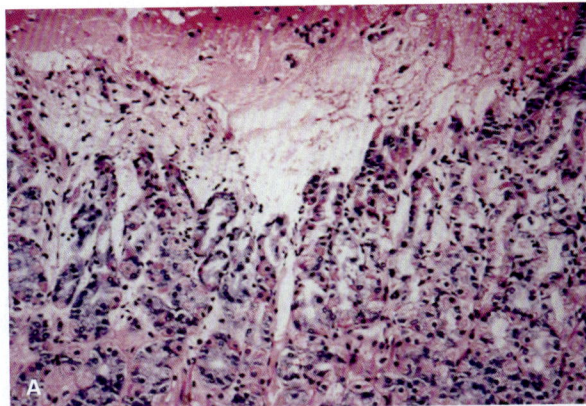
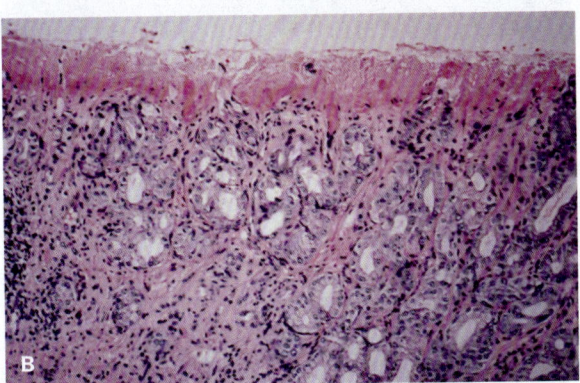

Figure 1-17. Gastric biopsy specimen with NSAID erosion and denudation of surface epithelium. However there are marked reactive changes with mucin depletion suggesting that this is not artifact. The lack of lamina propria inflammation is a feature of many NSAID/ASA erosions as seen in (**B**). **A:** There is superficial loss of epithelium with a loose pseudomembrane superficially. **B:** True erosion of gastric mucosa. Surface epithelium is absent, and there is only a superficial fibrin exudate only, without inflammatory cells or granulation tissue.

is not too deep. The ideal way to take the biopsy specimen is to retract the forceps back quickly after it is closed on a given area of mucosa.

Given these technical considerations, we tend to ignore focal congestion, hemorrhage, and edema in mucosal biopsy interpretation because we cannot exclude the possibility that they were induced by trauma. For example, in the stomach, up to one-quarter of the horizontal span of a biopsy specimen may contain lamina propria hemorrhage and edema that are presumed to be due to some or all of the above factors.[42] When there is extensive hemorrhage or edema in a biopsy specimen, especially if it is present in a focal lesion seen at endoscopy and not in adjacent grossly uninvolved mucosa, we mention it in the biopsy report.

Pseudoerosions

In a similar vein, there is a problem in relation to apparent microscopic erosions. Portions of the surface epithelium of mucosal biopsy specimens are commonly detached (Fig. 1-16). Erosions should not be diagnosed histologically unless there are other accompanying features—specifically, thin restituting epithelium that may cease abruptly, evidence of necrosis, fibrin over the erosion, neutrophils, or granulation tissue beneath the area of denuded epithelium (Fig. 1-17). Traumatic artifact with surface epithelial denudation and crush is especially common at the edges of biopsy specimens. This is because of compression of the tissue at the point of closure of the biopsy forceps. This compression may cause inflammatory cells to appear dense and may concentrate connective tissue, simulating fibrosis (Fig. 1-18). Some conditions (e.g., collagenous colitis) are frequently stripped of epithelium but lack fibrin or neutrophils or any reaction.

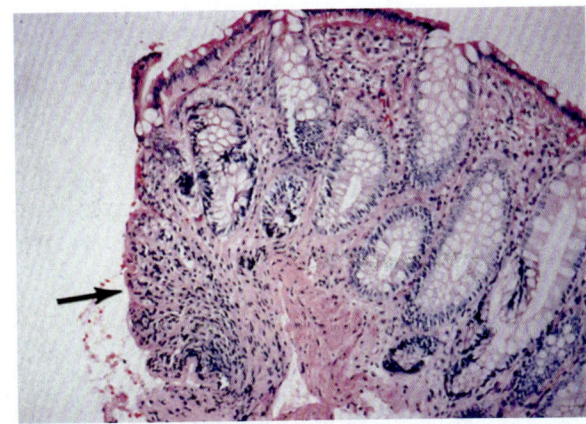

Figure 1-18. Artifact. Compression artifact at the edge of a rectal biopsy specimen (*arrow*). This is almost the rule in all pinch biopsy specimens obtained at endoscopy. The crush can simulate lymphoid aggregates and fibrosis.

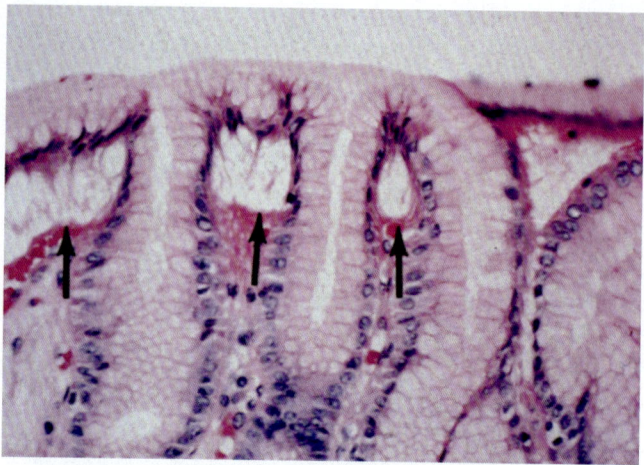

Figure 1-19. Artifact. Intraepithelial tears (*arrows*).

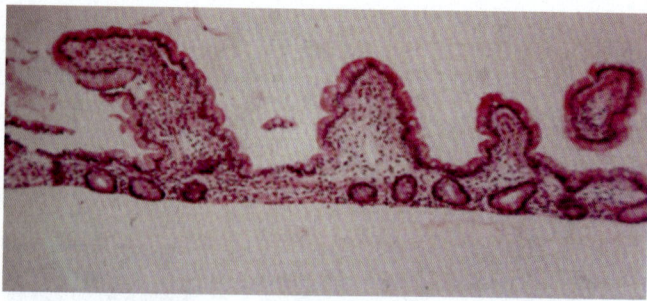

Figure 1-21. Artifact. Shallow small-bowel biopsy specimen creates an illusion of villous blunting. (Courtesy of Cyrus E. Rubin.)

Other Artifacts

In the surface epithelium, there may be dramatic intraepithelial spaces (Fig. 1-19), which could theoretically be labeled as intracellular edema but probably represent a technical artifact's. Another artifact is air-lined spaces[43] in the mucosa and submucosa (Fig. 1-20). This appearance is common enough that it is usually recognized, but it can be mistakenly attributed to fat or to dilated lymphatics. During endoscopy, air is routinely insufflated to permit visualization; presumably it penetrates the mucosa.

Biopsy specimens that are shallow may create an illusion of villous blunting in the small intestine (Fig. 1-21) or of sparse crypts in the large intestine.

THE PATHOLOGIST'S INTERPRETATION

All too often, the pathologist is given biopsy specimens that are overly traumatized or too small for interpretation. The final pathology report should indicate

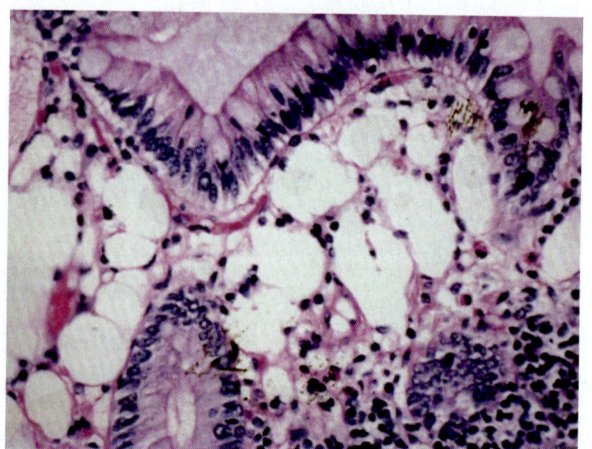

Figure 1-20. Artifact. Air-filled spaces in duodenal mucosa.

clearly that this was the case and should only indicate which features or diagnoses, if any, can be excluded on the basis of the available suboptimal material.

Well-intentioned pathologists are sometimes overly helpful in relation to their friends, the endoscopists. One example is when an endoscopist submits a biopsy specimen of a "polyp" that proves histologically to be normal mucosa. The pathologist should resist the urge to assuage the endoscopist and not sign out such a case as a "mucosal tag," a "redundant fold," or, even worse, a "polypoid fold." In such a situation, the truth cannot be ascertained. The possibilities include endoscope suction artifact, a submucosal lesion, a true mucosal polyp that the endoscopist did not target accurately and that did not appear in the sections examined, or a "wrinkle" equivalent.

The pathologist's final interpretation should address the specific questions raised by the clinician either positively or negatively. A provisional differential diagnosis can be added, based on the history, endoscopic findings, and microscopic findings. Terms such as *nondiagnostic* should be avoided. In the investigation of benign disease of the gastrointestinal tract, the issue is often not whether a given lesion is nondiagnostic, since many are, but whether there is any mucosal abnormality at all. When a biopsy specimen, is normal, we encourage the use of the word *normal* in the final diagnosis.

Mild Nonspecific Chronic Inflammation

One of the greatest challenges for even the most experienced morphologist is to differentiate between a normal appearance and one that is very mildly abnormal. "Mild chronic inflammation" is an excessively used final diagnosis for many biopsy specimens that are actually normal. The term "nonspecific" as a descriptor of inflammation is a waste of words, as all inflammation is nonspecific. Granulomas have numerous causes, and even Warthin–Finkeldy giant cells are not specific for measles. One of the most common complaints that endoscopists have in relation to interpretation of their specimens is that the pathologists in their institution never call anything normal and sign out virtually all cases as "mild nonspecific chronic inflammation." At one end of the spectrum, the clinicians, in turn, may ignore this diagnosis, perhaps doing the patient a disservice. At the other, in the presence of a normal colonoscopy, this may be interpreted as evidence of microscopic colitis, and the whole therapeutic armamentarium for this swung into place. One general rule is that mild inflammation is rarely an isolated finding in a biopsy specimen, and virtually never is the cause of symptoms unless part of more general disease (e.g., Crohn's disease). Bona fide microscopic inflammation in the colon can contribute to diarrhea but in the absence of other findings is not cause of abdominal pain or gastrointestinal bleeding. There are also usually other accompaniments, such as epithelial changes. For certain disorders, namely, gastritis and duodenitis, "mild chronic inflammation" has undefined clinical implications. On the other hand, in the small bowel and colon, this finding may point the clinician to the source of the symptoms or may dictate the need for an additional search for the cause of this change (e.g., parasitic infestation or Crohn's disease).

Overdiagnosis of normal biopsy specimens is avoided when the pathologist gains experience with the normal histological spectrum and the technical artifacts. In badly oriented and traumatized material, it is virtually impossible to make a diagnosis of mild abnormalities with certainty. A study of biopsies in the cecum and rectum in healthy individuals has shown that there is increased inflammation in health in the right colon.[44] Hence pathologists need to be careful in assessing what they consider to be increased inflammation when the biopsies are from the right colon.

The pathologist must communicate with the clinicians he or she works with concerning the meaning of certain terms that are used in biopsy reports. Otherwise, the findings may be misinterpreted in their clinical context. For example, the terms *acute* and *chronic inflammation*, as used by the pathologist, usually refer to the nature of the inflammatory cell infiltrate. The clinician should not interpret these terms as necessarily having a temporal connotation.

Effective communication is also important in conditions such as Barrett's esophagus and UC when surveillance biopsy specimens are taken. The clinician must understand that the term *dysplasia* refers to a neoplastic change in the epithelium and that high-grade dysplasia in the gastrointestinal tract may be equated with carcinoma in situ. Another term, which requires clarification to avoid misunderstanding and needless worry, is *atypia*. We prefer to use it in the context of nonneoplastic change, and that in pathology reports it be prefaced with a reassuring term such as *reactive* or *inflammatory*.

SPECIAL FIXATIVES, STAINS, OR STORAGE CONDITIONS

Table 1-7 outlines conditions that may require special fixatives, stains, or storage conditions. For some disorders, such as lymphomas and endocrine cell tumors, the diagnosis is not apparent until the first set of biopsy specimens is obtained. Rebiopsy may then be done to obtain additional tissue specimens, as outlined in Table 1-2. For gastrointestinal infections, nonbiopsy techniques (e.g., examination of smears or cultures) are often more definitive for diagnosis than the examination of biopsy sections.

Immunohistochemical Applications in Gastrointestinal Disorders

Immunohistochemical methods are used in the everyday practice of diagnostic pathology. The application of this technology has been facilitated by the development of highly sensitive immunohistochemical methods and the production of antibodies to new markers that can be identified in paraffin-embedded tissue. The main value of immunohistochemistry in the gastrointestinal tract is in the diagnosis of tumors and hyperplasias and, to a lesser extent, infections and motility disorders.

Immunohistochemistry or in situ hybridization is often of great help in determining the cell of origin of poorly differentiated tumors such as gastric carcinomas, lymphomas, carcinoids, and gastrointestinal mesenchymal tumors including stromal tumors. The primary objective of this section is to outline certain principles that have special relevance to gastrointestinal tract pathology.

Interpretation of Immunohistochemical Stains

Immunohistochemistry can be carried out with antibodies requiring dilution and optimal titration, prediluted, and in kit form. Kits contain all the necessary reagents to be applied to the tissues and are generally as reliable as methods using individually purchased reagents. However, whichever is used, one must still be constantly aware of potential artifacts, that is, false positives and false negatives. With an ever-increasing number of antibodies available for diagnosis, it is useful to check with an expert in the field concerning sensitivity and specificity before using a newly touted reagent, and ensuring that appropriate controls and dilutions are used.

Table 1-7 Disorders That May Require Special Fixatives, Stains, or Storage Conditions

DISORDERS	TECHNIQUE[a]
I. NEOPLASMS	
1. Lymphoma and other immunoproliferative disorders	Some tissue for (a) ideally frozen for RNA/DNA/gene rearrangement, translocation studies, (b) for flow cytometry, possibly microbiology
2. Endocrine cell tumors	Diagnosis usually established histologically. Confirmed with immunohistochemistry (chromogranin A, synaptophysin—silver stains can be used but are largely obsolete). Cell type(s) determined with immunohistochemistry for specific peptides. Electron microscopy may be of primary value in undifferentiated endocrine tumors.
3. Undifferentiated tumors and to help distinguish from (1) and (2) above	As for disorders (1) and (2) above. Electron microscopy is also sometimes used. Increasingly most studies are carried out from paraffin if required.
4. GISTS	Molecular sequencing (mutations in CD117, PDGFRα genes)
II. INFECTIONS	
1. Fungi	Methenamine silver stain or periodic acid-Schiff (PAS)
2. Parasites	
A. *Giardia lamblia*	In addition to conventional histology for all parasites, prepare Giemsa or other stain of mucus removed from the duodenal biopsy specimen or duodenal aspirate.
B. *Isospora belli* (Coccidiosis)	Giemsa stain of tissue sections
C. *Cryptosporidium*	Biopsy cases can be diagnosed in conventional sections. Electron microscopy rarely used in doubtful cases.
D. Amebiasis	PAS and iron hematoxylin stains make organisms stand out.
3. Tuberculosis, *Mycobacterium avium-intracellulare*	Stain for acid-fast bacilli. Sometimes PCR
4. Spirochetes	Silver impregnation test for syphilis; fluorescent antibody techniques[b]
5. Whipple's disease	PAS and acid-fast stain for confirmation; electron microscopy may be done but is not essential for diagnosis. PCR for *T. whippelii*
6. Bacterial	Modified Giemsa, Warthin–Starry, or other stains for *Helicobacter pylori*; Gram's stain in rare circumstances (e.g., phlegmonous gastritis, necrotizing enterocolitis). Immunohistochemistry
7. Viruses: cytomegalovirus, Herpes	Immunohistochemistry in situ hybridization
III. HYPOGAMMAGLOBULINEMIA (COMMON VARIABLE IMMUNODEFICIENCY)	Immunohistochemistry to confirm reduction or absence of plasma cells and to demonstrate the marked reduction of IGA-containing cells.
IV. INFILTRATIVE AND METABOLIC DISORDERS	
1. Amyloidosis	Congo Red stain with polarized light; crystal violet stain. Immunohistochemistry
2. Eosinophilic gastroenteritis and Mastocytosis	Immunohistochemistry. Formalin-fixed biopsies are fine.
3. Lipid storage diseases	Electron microscopy may be used to confirm the presence of deposits in foamy-appearing ganglion cells initially seen with routine fixatives and stains. Specific enzyme studies
4. Abetalipoproteinemia, hypobetalipoproteinemia, chylomicron retention disease	Diagnosis made in conventional sections; fat stain of fresh-frozen tissue can be done.
V. HIRSCHSPRUNG'S DISEASE	Frozen tissue as some laboratories use acetylcholinesterase histochemistry as an adjunct for mucosal biopsies

[a] Unless otherwise indicated, formalin is adequate.
[b] Pathologist should make clinician aware of other possible preferred fixatives and transport conditions.

Infections

Table 1-6 lists conditions in which special techniques may be employed to aid in the diagnosis of certain infections of the gastrointestinal tract, and histopathological examination may play a secondary role in diagnosis. In some gastrointestinal infections, the pathology does not provide a primary diagnosis. This is especially true for the nonparasitic infectious causes of colitis. In other infections, the examination of luminal fluid smears (e.g., from duodenal aspirate or surface exudate) is an easier way to make a diagnosis than the examination of multiple tissue sections. Also, these materials, plus biopsy tissues, may be submitted for culture to provide a definitive diagnosis. Under appropriate circumstances, smears of exudate or a brushing of mucosa can be prepared for slide smears. One smear is air dried and stained using the modified Ziehl–Neelsen technique,[45] primarily for *Cryptosporidium* and *Isospora belli*. A second smear is placed immediately in Schaudinn's fluid, and a trichrome or Giemsa stain is performed to screen for the other commonly occurring intestinal parasites.

Tuberculosis and *Mycobacterium avium-intracellulare*

Tuberculosis and *Mycobacterium avium-intracellulare* may be proven with culture of biopsy material but are readily suspected on the basis of the biopsy or surgical specimen morphology. This is especially true of *Mycobacterium avium-intracellulare*, which has a pathognomonic appearance in sections stained with acid-fast techniques. PCR for *Mycobacterium tuberculosis* is increasingly available, although, as elsewhere, a negative is no guarantee that the infection is not present. Wet mount examination of stool or small intestinal fluid for helminths or eggs is the best diagnostic method.

SURGICALLY RESECTED SPECIMENS

Examination of surgically resected specimens is essentially a two-stage procedure: (a) that carried before fixation and (b) that related to fixation and the taking of sections. There are four basic laws that all pathology trainees should be taught:

- Law 1. Examine the specimen as soon as possible after it has been obtained.
- Law 2. Photograph it (it is rarely possible to know which specimens will come up for rounds, which will be rare diseases, or which will be required for lectures or for publication).
- Law 3. Anticipate any special studies (electron microscopy, frozen tissue for special studies, flow cytometry for lymphoma, culture for microbiology, etc.).
- Law 4. If possible, treat it as a museum specimen when dissecting. That is, try to preserve the structures and relationships; avoid hacking it to bits.

Examination of the Specimen

Ideally, all specimens should be examined directly after resection because unexpected findings may immediately alter the intraoperative management of the patient. For example, gross examination may reveal unexpected tumors (or second tumors) requiring radical lymphadenectomy in that segment. The proximity of a tumor to a resected margin may require extension of the resection when possible.

FROZEN SECTIONS

Frozen sections are not part of the routine examination of the resected specimen. They are indicated in the following circumstances:

1. At the proximal resected margin of all gastric or esophageal resections for carcinoma to ensure that an anastomosis is not being carried out through residual tumor, usually in submucosal lymphatics.
2. For any tumor when the diagnosis is in doubt. Unexpected findings of a lymphoma necessitate more extensive sampling of lymph nodes for immunological markers or gene rearrangement studies. However, samples taken to assess for lymphoma at endoscopy are rarely frozen and usually placed in saline for handling as soon as possible.
3. When special studies are anticipated, both frozen and fresh tissue can be taken for a variety of procedures, such as flow cytometry, mutational analysis, translocations where fresh tissue is preferable to paraffin-embedded tissue, and microbiology culture.

PHOTOGRAPHY

In our opinion, at least one photograph should be taken of most major resections (e.g., for tumors, IBD, and ischemia). Most often the area of interest is in the internal (opened) surface of the specimen, but occasionally (e.g., Crohn's disease) the outside is also worth a photograph. Photographs provide a permanent record, which is especially valuable if the diagnosis proves to be unusual or controversial. In that event, the photographs can be sent along with the histology slides for additional opinions.

OPENING THE SPECIMEN

Most specimens should be opened in the fresh state. Sometimes it is desirable to fix the specimen by inflation or, more rarely, to inject in order to demonstrate vascular abnormalities. Clearly, the least desirable method is to place the unopened specimen in a container of fixative.

If the resection is for a tumor, care should be taken not to cut through the tumor unless it is circumferential. Even if it is circumferential, digital palpation will often suggest which wall is least involved; the incision should be through the least involved side so that the region of deepest tumor penetration remains intact. This can be facilitated, as discussed subsequently.

Esophageal tumors can easily be palpated through the esophageal wall prior to opening unless there is a coexisting benign stricture, as in Barrett's esophagus. Failing this, the proximal esophagus can sometimes be everted to reveal the proximal extent of gross tumor; again, the least affected wall should be utilized. If the tumor is polypoid, the esophagus should be opened directly opposite the epicenter. If there are no distinguishing features but the proximal stomach is included, the greater curve should be utilized.

Stomachs are opened along the greater curve to produce the usual butterfly shape; this also preserves the lesser gastric vessels, where most lymph nodes are encountered. However, circumscribed tumors on the greater curve should be avoided by taking the incision either anteriorly or posteriorly. For example, if the epicenter of the tumor appears to be on the posterior wall, the anterior wall is opened, and vice versa. Incisions for diffusely infiltrating carcinoma or linitis plastica are usually best carried out along the greater curve.

If the duodenum is resected for an ampullary or periampullary lesion, it should be opened anteriorly from the vicinity of the antroduodenal junction, proceeding distally and perhaps deviating a little to the medial wall to allow easy photography of the tumor. If the tumor is intraampullary or periampullary, probes should be introduced down both the bile and pancreatic ducts. Cuts should be made over the probes to reveal the duct systems, and then a cut should be made through the tumor, using a large knife, and beginning at the ampulla.

Small and large intestinal and anal tumors are also best displayed by cutting through the noninvolved or least involved wall.

Resection specimens from patients with Crohn's disease often prove more difficult because tight strictures preclude opening the bowel to visualize easily the entire circumference of the mucosa, particularly in the ileum. Sometimes this is facilitated either by using two incisions in a V shape with a wide base or by bisecting the bowel in the plane of the mesentery.

In resections for UC, the specimen is opened either on the mesenteric or on the anterior border. The latter is sometimes easier if a reasonable amount of mesentery is included. If the patient with UC is in the high-risk clinical group for carcinoma, the mucosa should be examined carefully for plaques or irregular mucosal lumps or bumps that may harbor an underlying carcinoma. We prefer to incise these lesions with a scalpel, looking for pools of mucin or indentations of white or yellow tissue into the submucosa or beyond that might be the site of a carcinoma. Frozen section examination of suspicious lesions may allow lymphadenectomy to be carried out where the large bowel was taken close to the bowel wall.

For total mesorectal excisions, a careful examination for tears into the mesorectum from outside, especially those that penetrate into the muscularis propria or tumor, need to be searched for and recorded. It is wise to ink the external surface of all nonperitonealized margins.

The appendix is usually sectioned by taking a longitudinal section through the tip (to detect unsuspected carcinoids macroscopically), along with two transverse sections, one of them at the proximal margin that needs to be marked (inked, separate cassette, one side of the section cut through). The appendix is usually bisected in the plane of the mesoappendix over its distal half and then sectioned (ideally at 1–2 mm to find diverticula) transversely. Inclusion of the proximal resected margin is a useful routine practice (ink for identification) as most tumors are incidental findings; if one is going to take cross sections, they might as well be of value. For the same reasons, inclusion of the mesoappendix precludes the embarrassing situation of not knowing whether unexpected tumors reach the surgical margin. If tumor is seen or strongly suspected, numerous transverse sections should include the greatest depth of penetration of the tumor. This is particularly important with tumors that have infiltrated through the muscularis propria, because this is where tumor may have escaped into the peritoneal cavity. The presence of mucin on the external surface or a dilated appendix containing mucin ("mucocele") should immediately draw attention to the possibility of a mucinous neoplasm within and careful examination for any rupture.

FIXATION

We believe that ideal morphology for most surgical resection specimens is achieved by pinning out the opened specimen, washing it in saline, and fixing it overnight. Some prefer to carry out lymph node dissections before fixation on the grounds that they are easier to palpate; some also take the sections for fixation directly in order to save a day.

It should be noted that specimens removed at night, and even on weekends, survive surprisingly well if refrigerated immediately. If a specimen needs to be transferred between hospitals and it is clear that some fixation will be required, the specimen should be opened, washed, and immersed in fixative.

Insufflation with Fixative

This procedure is used especially in some centers for colorectal carcinomas, for diverticular disease, and for some cases of strictured bowel in Crohn's disease. The specimen is flushed through with buffered saline to remove fecal matter, the distal end is clamped, and the specimen is slowly inflated with fixative. When the specimen is reasonably distended, the proximal end is tied off or clamped, and the entire specimen is immersed in fixative for overnight fixation (sometimes for several days for carcinomas). Transverse sections are often best to demonstrate diverticula, and either transverse or longitudinal sections are optimal to demonstrate strictures in Crohn's disease. For carcinomas, whole-mount sections provide spectacular overviews, and sections that show the extent of infiltration as well as node deposits, and proximity to margins, but require separate storage for the slides and blocks.

Although insufflation may produce spectacular morphology, it has some notable disadvantages. If an unexpected carcinoma is present, the option of intraoperative lymphadenectomy is lost. If there is a tight stricture, it may be difficult to get enough buffered saline through to clean the specimen adequately; consequently, fixation will be poor.

Injection studies for vascular diseases. These studies are not commonly performed; they are described elsewhere (see Chapter 2).

Examination and dissection of the fixed specimen. This is usually carried out following overnight fixation.

REEXAMINATION OF THE FIXED SPECIMEN

This should always be the first step, because ill-defined mucosal abnormalities are often easier to see following overnight fixation. It is frequently helpful to rephotograph such lesions or to photograph the specimen after fixation if this is the usual practice of the institution. Areas of superficial ulceration or erosion, foci of mucosal carcinoma, and diminutive polyps may be more easily seen.

DISSECTION

Sections are taken to confirm the nature of the underlying disease and any associated lesions. They are also taken, if appropriate, to determine the extent, staging, and adequacy of local excision and resections.

Dissections of Tumors

Accurate staging of the disease is required to determine the prognosis and devise a management plan. When resection of gastric or esophageal adenocarcinoma is being contemplated, some surgeons begin by taking a biopsy specimen from the celiac axis nodes for frozen section analysis. If it is positive for tumor, only a palliative resection may be undertaken.

Lymph Node Dissections

These are best carried out first, when the anatomy and vessels are intact. If a certain therapeutic protocol is being used, the sections may need to be tailored to ensure that the entire protocol is covered; this is facilitated by a well-labeled diagram of the tumor showing where both tumor and node sections were located. While each physician develops his own method of finding nodes by palpation, the best general method is to make multiple sections through the mesentery as close together as possible. The most common errors are to leave large pieces of mesentery unsampled, to slice them at inordinately large intervals such as 1 cm or more rather than a few millimeters, and to fail to continue the dissection into the tumor. The last is especially important, because the greatest number of involved nodes may be found adjacent to the tumor. Whole-mount sections of tumor that are close together are one method of minimizing this.

Evidence of a good nodal dissection is the finding of nodules of lymphoid tissue in the 1- to 3-mm range, with a sprinkling of pieces of fibrofatty tissue and small vessels in cross section. Conversely, inadequate sampling is characterized by the finding of only a few nodes measuring 5 mm or more.

A variety of techniques can be used to enhance visibility of nodes including clearing the fat and injection of the artery with methylene blue, which works surprisingly well, but it is unclear if makes a clinical difference to staging.

Depth of Tumor Penetration

This is assessed by sectioning the area where tumor appears grossly to extend farthest through the wall, as revealed by inspection, particularly of the external surface, or by palpation. A series of parallel cuts are then made through the tumor as close together as possible, taking full-thickness sections through the area(s) of maximum penetration. If some of the cuts are left intentionally incomplete, the specimen is less likely to fall apart. This allows preservation of the original anatomy. In addition, especially if a diagram is used, it allows a return to interesting areas with some precision, so that further sections can be taken if necessary.

Venous Invasion by Tumor

It is useful to obtain a section routinely, looking for involvement of extramural veins by tumor. It is also useful to ensure that one tumor section is taken directly across the venous return on the deep aspect of the tumor. A particularly helpful feature microscopically is to look for the *orphan arteriole* in microscopic sections. Normally, arterioles are accompanied by at least one and often two venules. The lack of any veins and the presence of adjacent well-circumscribed nodules of tumor imply that the accompanying venules have been infiltrated and largely destroyed (orphan arteriole sign) or tongues of tumor, especially those pushing through the muscularis propria into the subserosa (protruding tongue sign). The elastic stain may demonstrate remnants of their walls. Although it is logical to use endothelial or lymphatic markers (CD31, D2-40) to identify this, in practice markers for muscle (actins, desmin) identify preserved walls of vessels when the endothelium has been lost.

Sections of Resected Margins

These are extremely important in most esophageal, gastric, and duodenal resections. In the large bowel, the proximal and distal margins are usually much further removed from the tumor or other pathology than in the upper gastrointestinal tract. However, examination of remote resection margins of colon may reveal other incidental disease.

Incidental Findings

Other macroscopic lesions or areas of mucosal irregularity should be sought and sectioned. It is amazing how synchronous lesions, such as polyps and even small carcinomas, may escape detection because of preoccupation with the largest lesion. Depending on the underlying condition, some sections of apparently uninvolved mucosa should be sampled. A convenient but uncommonly employed way to sample large areas is the *Swiss roll* technique, whereby two parallel cuts are made in the mucosa about 3 mm apart, and the ensuing strip of mucosa, which can be 10 cm or more in length, is dissected from the submucosa and rolled up concentrically and placed in a single block. This is particularly useful for identifying very small adenomas in familial adenomatous polyposis and the metaplastic mucosa in gastrectomy or esophageal specimens. Should anything resembling a neoplasm be found, the procedure is terminated for that segments and full-thickness sections taken.

In resections for IBD, apart from any obvious lesion, it is worthwhile to take about one section for every 5 to 10 cm of resected bowel, beginning at the proximal resected margin, to document the distribution and morphology of the disease together with a sampling of the lymph nodes. Such sampling may prove invaluable, particularly when the primary diagnosis is questionable and occasionally when there are areas of dysplasia and even occult carcinoma. If focal disease is present, sections should be taken specifically to demonstrate it. Tables 1-1 and 1-2 give the recipe for success.

References

1. Wadas DD, Sanowski RA. Complications of the hot biopsy forceps technique. *Gastrointest Endosc.* [Comparative Study]. 1988;34(1):32–37.
2. Woods A, Sanowski RA, Wadas DD, et al. Eradication of diminutive polyps: a prospective evaluation of bipolar coagulation versus conventional biopsy removal. *Gastrointest Endosc.* 1989;35(6):536–540.
3. Ishiguro A, Uno Y, Ishiguro Y, et al. Correlation of lifting versus non-lifting and microscopic depth of invasion in early colorectal cancer. *Gastrointest Endosc.* 1999;50(3):329–333.
4. Cao Y, Liao C, Tan A, et al. Meta-analysis of endoscopic submucosal dissection versus endoscopic mucosal resection for tumors of the gastrointestinal tract. *Endoscopy.* 2009;41(9):751–757.
5. Bourke. Current status of colonic endoscopic mucosal resection in the west and the interface with endoscopic submucosal dissection. <http://www.ncbi.nlm.nih.gov/pubmed/19691728?itool=EntrezSystem2.PEntrez.Pubmed.Pubmed_ResultsPanel.Pubmed_RVDocSum&ordinalpos=61>. *Digest Endosc.* 2009;21(1 suppl):S22–S27.
6. Inoue H, Minami H, Kaga M, et al. Endoscopic mucosal resection and endoscopic submucosal dissection for esophageal dysplasia and carcinoma. *Gastrointest Endosc Clin N Am.* 2010;20(1):25–34.
7. Lauwers GY, Forcione DG, Nishioka NS, et al. Novel endoscopic therapeutic modalities for superficial neoplasms arising in Barrett's esophagus: a primer for surgical pathologists. *Mod Pathol.* 2009;22(4):489–498.
8. Altman AR, Finkel S, Waye JD. Multiple "spot" biopsy technique for infiltrative gastric carcinoma [Case Reports]. *Mt Sinai J Med.* 1977;44(4):570–573.
9. Vidyavathi K, Harendrakumar ML, Lakshmana Kumar YC. Correlation of endoscopic brush cytology with biopsy in diagnosis of upper gastrointestinal neoplasms. *Indian J Pathol Microbiol.* 2008;51(4):489–492.
10. Tsang TK, Hidvegi D, Horth K, Ostrow JD. Reliability of balloon-mesh cytology in detecting esophageal carcinoma in a population of US veterans. *Cancer.* [Research Support, Non-U.S. Gov't]. 1987;59(3):556–559.
11. Tada M, Katoh S, Kohli Y, Kawai K. On the dye spraying method in colonofiberscopy. *Endoscopy.* 1977;8(2):70–74.
12. Baldi F, di Febo G, Biasco G, et al. Methylene blue dye spraying method in patients with ulcerative proctitis: a comparative study with morphological findings and functional capacity of the rectal epithelium [Comparative Study]. *Endoscopy.* 1979;11(3):179–184.
13. van den Broek FJ, Fockens P, van Eeden S, et al. Endoscopic tri-modal imaging for surveillance in ulcerative colitis: randomised comparison of high-resolution endoscopy and autofluorescence imaging for neoplasia detection; and evaluation of narrow-band imaging for classification of lesions. *Gut.* 2008;57(8):1083–1089.
14. Canto MI, Setrakian S, Willis JE, et al. Methylene blue staining of dysplastic and nondysplastic Barrett's esophagus: an in vivo and ex vivo study [Clinical Trial Research Support, Non-U.S. Gov't]. *Endoscopy.* 2001;33(5):391–400.

15. Kiesslich R, Hahn M, Herrmann G, Jung M. Screening for specialized columnar epithelium with methylene blue: chromoendoscopy in patients with Barrett's esophagus and a normal control group. [see comment] [Clinical Trial]. *Gastrointest Endosc.* 2001;53(1):47–52.
16. Egger K, Werner M, Meining A, et al. Biopsy surveillance is still necessary in patients with Barrett's oesophagus despite new endoscopic imaging techniques.[see comment][comment] [Comment Comparative Study]. *Gut.* 2003;52(1):18–23.
17. Lim CH, Rotimi O, Dexter SP, et al. Randomized crossover study that used methylene blue or random 4-quadrant biopsy for the diagnosis of dysplasia in Barrett's esophagus.[see comment] [Comparative Study Randomized Controlled Trial]. *Gastrointest Endosc.* 2006;64(2):195–199.
18. Ngamruengphong S, Sharma VK, Das A, et al. Diagnostic yield of methylene blue chromoendoscopy for detecting specialized intestinal metaplasia and dysplasia in Barrett's esophagus: a meta-analysis [Meta analysis]. *Gastrointest Endosc.* 2009;69(6):1021–1028.
19. Kara MA, Ennahachi M, Fockens P, et al. Detection and classification of the mucosal and vascular patterns (mucosal morphology) in Barrett's esophagus by using narrow band imaging. *Gastrointest Endosc.* 2006;64(2):155–166.
20. Wolfsen HC, Crook JE, Krishna M, et al. Prospective, controlled tandem endoscopy study of narrow band imaging for dysplasia detection in Barrett's Esophagus. [see comment] [Randomized Controlled Trial]. *Gastroenterology.* 2008;135(1):24–31.
21. Herrero LA, Curvers WL, Bansal A, et al. Zooming in on Barrett oesophagus using narrow-band imaging: an international observer agreement study. *Eur J Gastroenterol Hepatol.* 2009;21(9):1068–1075.
22. Curvers W, Baak L, Kiesslich R, et al. Chromoendoscopy and narrow-band imaging compared with high-resolution magnification endoscopy in Barrett's esophagus. *Gastroenterology.* 2008;134(3):670–679.
23. Kiesslich R, Fritsch J, Holtmann M, et al. Methylene blue-aided chromoendoscopy for the detection of intraepithelial neoplasia and colon cancer in ulcerative colitis. *Gastroenterology.* 2003;124(4):880–888.
24. Rutter MD, Saunders BP, Schofield G, et al. Pancolonic indigo carmine dye spraying for the detection of dysplasia in ulcerative colitis [see comment]. *Gut.* 2004;53(2):256–260.
25. Marion JF, Waye JD, Present DH, et al. Chromoendoscopy-targeted biopsies are superior to standard colonoscopic surveillance for detecting dysplasia in inflammatory bowel disease patients: a prospective endoscopic trial. *Am J Gastroenterol.* 2008;103(9):2342–2349.
26. van den Broek FJ, Fockens P, Van Eeden S, et al. Clinical evaluation of endoscopic trimodal imaging for the detection and differentiation of colonic polyps. *Clin Gastroenterol Hepatol.* 2009;7(3):288–295.
27. Masaki T, Sheffield JP, Talbot IC, et al. Non-polypoid adenoma of the large intestine. *Int J Colorectal Dis.* 1994;9(4):180–183.
28. Kudo S, Tamura S, Nakajima T, et al. Diagnosis of colorectal tumorous lesions by magnifying endoscopy. *Gastrointest Endosc.* 1996;44(1):8–14.
29. Kaltenbach T, Friedland S, Soetikno R. A randomised tandem colonoscopy trial of narrow band imaging versus white light examination to compare neoplasia miss rates. *Gut.* 2008;57(10):1406–1412.
30. Adler A, Aschenbeck J, Yenerim T, et al. Narrow-band versus white-light high definition television endoscopic imaging for screening colonoscopy: a prospective randomized trial. *Gastroenterology.* 2009;136(2):410–416 e1; quiz 715.
31. Rastogi A, Keighley J, Singh V, et al. High accuracy of narrow band imaging without magnification for the real-time characterization of polyp histology and its comparison with high-definition white light colonoscopy: a prospective study. *Am J Gastroenterol.* 2009;104(10):2422–2430.
32. Rex DK. Narrow-band imaging without optical magnification for histological analysis of colorectal polyps. *Gastroenterology.* 2009;136(4):1174–1181.
33. Dacosta RS, Wilson BC, Marcon NE. New optical technologies for earlier endoscopic diagnosis of premalignant gastrointestinal lesions. *J Gastroenterol Hepatol.* 2002;17(suppl):S85–S104.
34. Kiesslich R, Neurath MF. Endoscopic detection of early lower gastrointestinal cancer. *Best Pract Res Clin Gastroenterol.* 2005;19(6):941–961.
35. Borschitz T, Kiesslich R. Confocal chromolaser endomicroscopy: a supplemental diagnostic tool prior to transanal endoscopic microsurgery of rectal tumors? *Int J Colorectal Dis.* 2010;25(1):71–77.
36. Kiesslich R, Goetz M, Neurath MF. Confocal laser endomicroscopy for gastrointestinal diseases. *Gastrointest Endosc Clin N Am.* 2008;18(3):451–466, viii.
37. Kiesslich R, Goetz M, Lammersdorf K, et al. Chromoscopy-guided endomicroscopy increases the diagnostic yield of intraepithelial neoplasia in ulcerative colitis. *Gastroenterology.* 2007;132(3):874–882.
38. Goetz M, Kiesslich R. Confocal endomicroscopy: in vivo diagnosis of neoplastic lesions of the gastrointestinal tract. *Anticancer Res.* 2008;28(1B):353–360.
39. Meisel JL, Bergman D, Graney D, et al. Human rectal mucosa: proctoscopic and morphological changes caused by laxatives. *Gastroenterology.* 1977;72(6):1274–1279.
40. Stamm B, Heer M, Buhler H, Ammann R. Mucosal biopsy of vascular ectasia (angiodysplasia) of the large bowel detected during routine colonoscopic examination. *Histopathology.* 1985;9(6):639–646.
41. Calhoun BC, Gomes F, Robert ME, Jain D. Sampling error in the standard evaluation of endoscopic colonic biopsies. *Am J Surg Pathol.* 2003;27(2):254–257.
42. Laine L, Weinstein WM. Histology of alcoholic hemorrhagic "gastritis": a prospective evaluation [Research Support, U.S. Gov't, P.H.S.] *Gastroenterology.* 1988;94(6):1254–1262.
43. Snover DC, Sandstad J, Hutton S. Mucosal pseudolipomatosis of the colon. *Am J Clin Pathol.* 1985;84(5):575–580.
44. Paski SC, Wightman R, Robert ME, Bernstein CN. The importance of recognizing increased cecal inflammation in health and avoiding the misdiagnosis of nonspecific colitis. *Am J Gastroenterol.* 2007;102(10):2294–2299.
45. Garcia LS, Bruckner DA, Brewer TC, Shimizu RY. Techniques for the recovery and identification of Cryptosporidium oocysts from stool specimens. *J Clin Microbiol.* 1983;18(1):185–190.

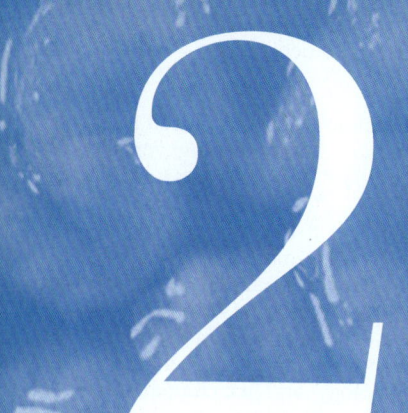

Vascular Disorders and Related Diseases

Chapter Outline

VASCULARIZATION OF THE DIGESTIVE TRACT—OVERVIEW
VASCULARIZATION OF THE SPECIFIC SEGMENT OF THE DIGESTIVE TRACT
Esophagus
Stomach, Small Intestine, and Large Intestine
  Intramural circulation
  Extramural (Splanchnic) circulation
  Venous drainage
  Collateral blood supply
ISCHEMIA OF THE GASTROINTESTINAL TRACT
Pathophysiology
Etiology and Clinical Manifestations
  Esophageal ischemia
  Gastric ischemia
  Acute mesenteric ischemia
  Chronic mesenteric ischemia
Pathology
  Gross features
  Microscopy
  Ischemic colitis
  Ischemic proctitis
INFLAMMATORY VASCULAR DISORDERS OF THE GASTROINTESTINAL TRACT (VASCULITIDES)
Introduction
Classification

Clinical Presentation
Different Types of Vasculitides
  Large vessel vasculitides
  Infectious vasculitides
  Medium vessel vasculitides
  Medium and small vessel vasculitis (ANCA-associated vasculitides)
  Small vessel vasculitis
  Miscellaneous conditions
  Malignant-atrophic papulosis (Kohlmeier–Degos Syndrome)
Biopsy Diagnosis of Ischemic Colitis and Differential Diagnosis
Stercoral ulcers
MECHANICAL OBSTRUCTION AND ISCHEMIA OF THE DIGESTIVE TRACT
Pathogenesis and Clinical Features
Adhesions
Hernias
  Hernia of the anterior abdominal wall
  Inguinal and femoral hernia.
  Umbilical hernia
  Internal hernias
Volvulus
Intussusception
IATROGENIC DISORDERS OF THE VASCULAR SYSTEM
Iatrogenic Intestinal Ischemia
  Arterial obstruction or constriction

  Drug-induced vascular lesions
  Neutropenic colitis
Iatrogenic Gastrointestinal Bleeding
Radiation Injury
  Pathophysiology
  Acute radiation injury
  Chronic (late) radiation injury
VASCULAR ABNORMALITIES OF THE GASTROINTESTINAL TRACT
Vascular Ectasia (Angiodysplasia)
Gastric Antral Vascular Ectasia
Dieulafoy Malformation (Caliber-Persistent Arteriole)
Telangiectasias
  Hereditary hemorrhagic telangiectasia (Rendu–Osler–Weber Syndrome)
Arteriovenous Malformation
Phlebectasia
Diseases Affecting Blood Vessels
Disorders of Connective Tissue Affecting Blood Vessels
  Pseudoxanthoma elasticum
  Ehlers–Danlos syndrome
HANDLING OF SPECIMENS
Endoscopic Biopsies
Surgical Specimens
  Ischemic disease
  Vascular malformations

VASCULARIZATION OF THE DIGESTIVE TRACT—OVERVIEW

The splanchnic circulation is well developed and composed of major intramural and extramural pathways. Under resting conditions, the splanchnic circulation receives 30% of the total blood flow. During the process of digestion, the superior mesenteric artery blood flow increases by more than 100%.[1] Conversely, exercise reduces both resting and postprandial blood flow. The blood flow through these pathways is subject to a complex interplay of extrinsic and intrinsic controlling mechanisms including hemodynamic factors (cardiac output, systemic arterial pressure), the autonomic nervous system, hormones (vasopressin, vasoactive intestinal polypeptide, somatostatin), and locally produced metabolites. Alterations of the various control mechanisms can lead to occlusive or non-occlusive disease and limited or extensive ischemic damage.

VASCULARIZATION OF THE SPECIFIC SEGMENT OF THE DIGESTIVE TRACT

Esophagus

The extramural arterial supply of the human esophagus is divided into three major segments, the cervical, thoracic, and abdominal esophagus, with numerous anastomoses. The pharyngoesophageal transition and cervical esophagus are supplied by the lower thyroid artery, a branch of the thyrocervical trunk. An additional, individually variable supply is provided by small branches of the subclavian, common carotid, vertebral, and superior thyroid arteries and the costocervical trunk. The thoracic esophagus receives blood from branches of the aorta, the bronchial arteries, and the right intercostal arteries. At the level of the bifurcation of the trachea, the main supply comes from branches of the bronchial arteries, which descend on the ventral side of the esophagus. Below the bifurcation of the trachea, the blood supply originates from two esophageal branches that arise directly from the ventral side of the aorta. Both branches run to the dorsal side of the esophagus where they anastomose with the descending branches of the lower thyroid and ascending branches of the left gastric and left lower phrenic arteries. The abdominal esophagus is supplied by esophageal branches of the left gastric and left lower phrenic arteries. An additional blood supply may be provided by branches of the aorta, the splenic artery, the celiac trunk, and an aberrant left hepatic artery.[2,3]

The intramural arterial pattern is characterized by a well-developed subepithelial capillary network in the stromal papillae of the mucosa (intraepithelial channels), supplied by a prominent submucosal arterial plexus, composed of longitudinally oriented arteries with lateral anastomoses. Submucosal arteries are formed by penetrating branches arising from a minor extrinsic plexus in the adventitia. These branches pass through the muscle layer and give off branches to the muscle tissue and the myenteric plexus.[4,5]

Esophageal veins are classified into three groups: (a) intrinsic veins including subepithelial and submucosal veins, which join the gastric veins below, and perforating veins, which pierce the muscular wall to join the extrinsic veins; (b) extrinsic veins formed by the union of groups of perforating veins, which join the left gastric vein below and the systemic veins above; and (c) venae concomitantes, which run longitudinally in the adventitia.[6,7]

The subepithelial or superficial venous plexus drains the stromal papillae; lies in the lamina propria, close to the epithelium; and extends over the whole length of the esophagus.[6] At the esophagogastric junction, the veins lie predominantly superficially in the lamina propria.[7-9] Numerous small veins perforate the muscularis mucosae to join larger veins of the submucosal plexus (deep intrinsic veins) and constitute the palisades vessels seen endoscopically. The submucosal plexus consists of 10 to 15 longitudinal veins, evenly distributed around the circumference of the esophagus and connected by numerous anastomoses. In its proximal part, this plexus drains the longitudinally oriented veins from the ventral and dorsal pharyngoesophageal subepithelial plexus. At the distal end of the esophagus, the longitudinal submucosal veins increase in number but decrease in diameter. At the cardia, they become tortuous and aggregate in the longitudinal folds of the mucosa before joining the submucosal veins of the stomach. Perforating veins arise from the longitudinal submucosal plexus and pass through the muscle layer, which they drain also, at regular intervals.

The greater extrinsic periesophageal veins include two larger and several smaller veins. The larger veins run longitudinally on the outer surface in close proximity to the vagus nerves and connect the left gastric vein to the azygos or hemiazygos veins. Other veins are the cervical periesophageal veins draining into the inferior thyroid, vertebral, and deep cervical veins; small esophageal veins at the cardia joining the superior and inferior phrenic veins; and small abdominal esophageal veins draining into the left gastric vein as well as the vena phrenica inferior, gastroepiploica, and splenica.[6]

Stomach, Small Intestine, and Large Intestine

Intramural circulation. The gastric blood supply is derived from the common hepatic, left gastric, and splenic arteries arising from the celiac trunk (Fig. 2-1). The fundus and left margin of the greater curve are supplied by short gastric arteries derived from the splenic artery. The right gastric artery and the right gastroepiploic artery supply the lesser and distal greater curve, respectively. The proximal greater curve is supplied by the left gastroepiploic artery and arteries from the splenic artery. These vessels form two extrinsic arcading anastomotic loops. The loops give off a series of short branches to the anterior and posterior walls. They form a subserosal plexus.[10-12] Perforating branches originating from this plexus pass through the external muscle layers to reach a richly anastomotic submucosal arterial plexus. Small side branches are given off to the external muscle layers and to Auerbach's plexus en route, but the majority of arterioles to the external muscle come from the submucosal plexus. The mucosa is supplied by small branches from the submucosal plexus, which pass perpendicularly through the muscularis mucosae. In the lamina propria, the arterioles branch into capillaries, which run toward the lumenal surface between the gastric glands. There are frequent cross anastomoses between adjacent capillaries. Just underneath the surface epithelium, the capillaries form a polygonal network around the necks of the gastric pits.[13-17] Mucosal venules drain into the submucosal venous plexus, which is continuous with a similar plexus in the esophagus and duodenum. In the gastric cardia the submucosal venous plexus is composed of a series of parallel veins oriented toward the esophagogastric junction. Drainage of the muscle layers occurs to the submucosal venous plexus and partly to perforating veins, which pass to subserosal veins. The latter drain toward the portal system.

The duodenum is supplied chiefly by the pancreaticoduodenal artery. The jejunum and the ileum are supplied by a dozen branches of the superior mesenteric artery. These branches divide and anastomose several times in the mesentery forming arcades. The last of these forms a marginal artery along the small intestine. The marginal artery is defined as the artery closest to and parallel with the wall of the intestine. From the marginal artery, blood reaches the intestine by way of short, straight branches or "vasa recta." They penetrate the external muscle layers to reach a profusely anastomotic submucosal arterial plexus from which arterioles originate for the mucosa, submucosa, and muscular layers. The submucosal plexus gives off two types of mucosal branches: long or villous arterioles and short or cryptal ones. Arterioles to the villi pass without branching in the lamina propria. At the tip of the villus, the arteriole splays into a network of capillaries that subsequently course down along the sides of the villus in a fountain-like pattern. The crypts receive their arterial supply adjacent to the muscularis mucosae. The lymphoid tissue is supplied by the submucosal plexus through interfollicular arteries between the lymphoid follicles and through follicular arterioles originating from the interfollicular arteries. Venous drainage of each of the small intestinal capillary beds passes to the submucosal venous plexus, which anastomoses both longitudinally and

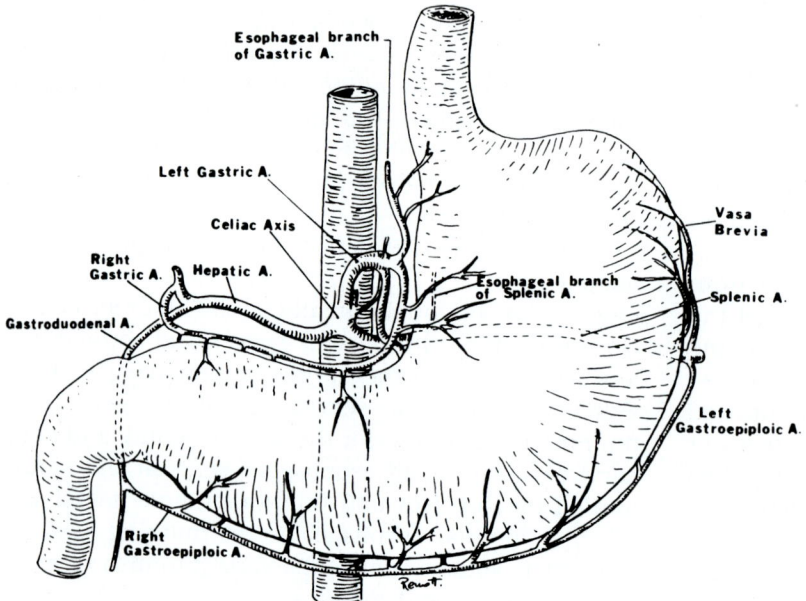

Figure 2-1. Arterial blood supply of the stomach.

circumferentially in the bowel wall. This plexus is drained by short veins, which penetrate the external muscle layers, chiefly along the mesenteric margin and then pass to branches of the superior mesenteric vein in the mesentery. The superior mesenteric vein receives venous drainage of the distal duodenum, the jejunum, the ileum, the appendix and cecum, the ascending and transverse colons and a right gastroepiploic vein draining the stomach, before joining the splenic vein to form the hepatic portal vein.[13,15,18]

The ascending and transverse colons are supplied by three branches of the superior mesenteric artery (ileocolic and right and middle colic arteries), whereas the splenic flexure, descending colon, and sigmoid are nourished by branches of the inferior mesenteric artery (left colic and sigmoid arteries). These vessels form arcades that are less numerous and complex than those in the small intestine. Within 2 cm of the colon wall, a single large anastomotic marginal artery is formed. This marginal artery runs retroperitoneally, extending from the ileocecal junction down to and into the sigmoid mesocolon close to its attachment to the colon wall, thus forming an anastomotic channel between ileocolic; right, middle, and left colic; and sigmoid arteries. The rectum has a richly anastomosing arterial system derived from the inferior mesenteric and internal iliac arteries. Through the superior rectal artery, it forms an anastomosis with the marginal artery of the colon. Short vasa recta pass from the marginal artery to the colon wall, with few or no anastomoses en route. Upon reaching the wall, they divide to form subserosal branches, which pass circumferentially around the bowel wall, and other branches, which form a subserosal anastomosing plexus. The subserosal plexus gives off branches that traverse the external muscle coat to reach the submucosal arterial plexus. There is extensive anastomosis in the submucosa both longitudinally and circumferentially. Arteriolar branches from the submucosal plexus penetrate the muscularis mucosae and then break up in a leash of capillaries. These capillaries ascend along the glands and reach the surface of the mucosa where they form a honeycomb pattern around the openings of the glands, just beneath the surface epithelium. The muscularis contains capillaries derived from both the subserosal and submucosal plexuses and is perforated by larger arteries coming from the serosa and subserosa. The venous drainage largely parallels the arterial supply.[13,19]

Extramural (Splanchnic) circulation. *The celiac trunk* is a short (2 cm) but larger caliber (5–8 mm) artery, which arises from the front of the aorta. It divides almost immediately into three branches: the common hepatic, splenic, and left gastric arteries. There are however many variations of the typical origin. The most striking of these is a common origin of the celiac trunk and the superior mesenteric artery in a celiacomesenteric trunk (in ~2% of cases). In this situation, a single artery is the sole source of vascularization of the supramesocolic organs. Collateral flow is possible only from the inferior mesenteric, phrenic, esophageal, and retroperitoneal arteries.[10]

The common hepatic artery arises on the right side of the celiac trunk, giving off branches to the stomach, duodenum, and pancreas. The right gastric artery arises from hepatic artery and less frequently from the gastroduodenal artery (8%). It descends to the pylorus along the lesser curvature of the stomach where it usually anastomoses with the left gastric artery. The right gastric artery frequently gives rise to the supraduodenal artery (of Wilkie).

The gastroduodenal artery usually arises from the common hepatic artery (75%) but may arise from the left or right hepatic artery or superior mesenteric artery. It divides into the right gastroepiploic and the anterior superior pancreaticoduodenal arteries. This artery anastomoses with the posterior inferior pancreaticoduodenal artery to form the pancreaticoduodenal arcade supplying the posterior surface of the entire duodenum and the head of the pancreas. The anterior pancreaticoduodenal arcade is formed by the anterior superior pancreaticoduodenal artery and the anterior inferior pancreaticoduodenal artery, which arises from the superior mesenteric artery. The right gastroepiploic artery is the final continuation of the gastroduodenal artery. After supplying one or more branches to the pylorus, it passes to the left along the greater curvature of the stomach. Ascending branches supply the greater curvature of the stomach and anastomose with descending branches of the right and left gastric arteries.

The left gastric artery courses toward the gastric cardia. It supplies part of the stomach and the inferior esophagus. The anastomosis with the right gastric artery may be absent.

The splenic artery from the celiac artery gives off branches to the pancreas and stomach. Often, a branch of the dorsal pancreatic artery descends below the inferior border of the pancreas to communicate with the superior mesenteric artery. Occasionally, this branch gives rise to the middle colic artery (artery of Riolan). The left gastroepiploic artery arises from the splenic artery prior to its terminal divisions or from a terminal division itself. It gives off the left epiploic artery, which anastomoses with the right epiploic artery, a branch of the right gastroepiploic artery, to form the arcus epiploicus magnus of Barkow, in the great omentum below the colon. Short gastric arteries originate from the distal splenic artery and supply the fundus and cardia of the stomach.

The superior mesenteric artery originates from the aorta at the level of the first lumbar vertebra, behind the body of the pancreas (Fig. 2-2). It emerges from under the lower border of the pancreas, passes forward anteriorly over the upper border of the third portion of the duodenum, and descends anteriorly into the mesentery. Usually, the middle colic artery arises from the superior mesenteric artery just before it enters the mesentery. The middle colic artery can arise as a separate branch or be derived from a common right colic–middle colic trunk (53% of the cases). Occasionally, it arises directly from the celiac artery. When the middle colic artery has a large branch running parallel and posterior to it in the transverse mesocolon, this branch is often described as the arc of Riolan. The right colic artery can arise directly (38%) from the superior mesenteric artery. The middle and right colic arteries supply the right half of the transverse colon and the ascending colon. Within the mesentery, the superior mesenteric artery courses to the right iliac fossa, curving to the left to end in the ileocolic artery by forming an anastomosis. Major side branches of the superior mesenteric artery originating usually on the right side are the inferior pancreaticoduodenal arteries supplying the lower part of the duodenum. These arteries connect with the superior pancreaticoduodenal arteries. The inferior pancreaticoduodenal artery can also arise from or can be in common with the first jejunal artery. To the left, four to six jejunal arteries and nine to thirteen intestinal branches that supply the ileum can be identified. These are often called "intestinal arteries."

They divide into two branches, forming a first-order arcading anastomosis with the neighboring branches. Subsequent anastomes form second- to fourth-order arcades. Branches of these arcades finally form the marginal artery. The marginal artery may thus be composed of arteries that range from third- or fourth-order arcades to the parent colic artery itself. The middle colic artery is often the marginal artery for the major portion of its distribution. Fine branches originating from the marginal artery reach the bowel wall as "vasa recta." The vasa recta of the small intestine are shorter, closer together, and less straight in appearance than the large bowel vasa recta. The terminal branch of the superior mesenteric artery is the ileocolic artery. It distributes branches to the terminal ileum, the cecum, and the lower third or half of the ascending colon. In its distal distribution the ileal and colic branches of the ileocolic artery often form an "ileocolic loop." The anterior and posterior cecal arteries and the appendicular artery arise separately from this loop.

The inferior mesenteric artery arises from the aorta anteriorly at the level of the third lumbar vertebra (Fig. 2-3). Major side branches are the left colic artery and the sigmoid arteries. The descending branch of the inferior mesenteric artery becomes the superior rectal artery. The left colic artery is usually an ascending branch from the inferior mesenteric artery. This branch bifurcates at the splenic flexure, its right branch joining the middle colic artery from the superior mesenteric artery and its left branch joining the marginal artery. Sigmoid arteries can originate from the ascending branch in common with the left colic or arise from a descending branch of the inferior mesenteric artery. A few sigmoid arteries may arise from a middle branch. The number of sigmoid arteries varies from one to five. The superior rectal artery divides

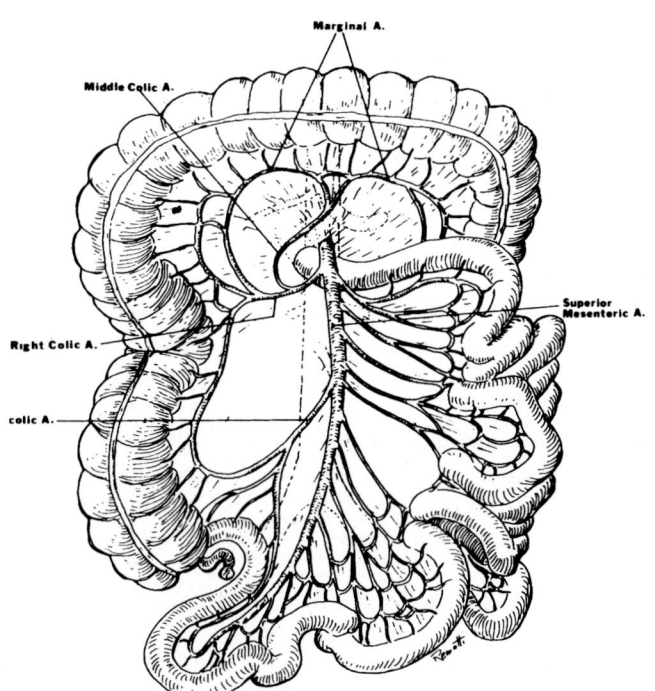

Figure 2-2. Distribution of the superior mesenteric artery.

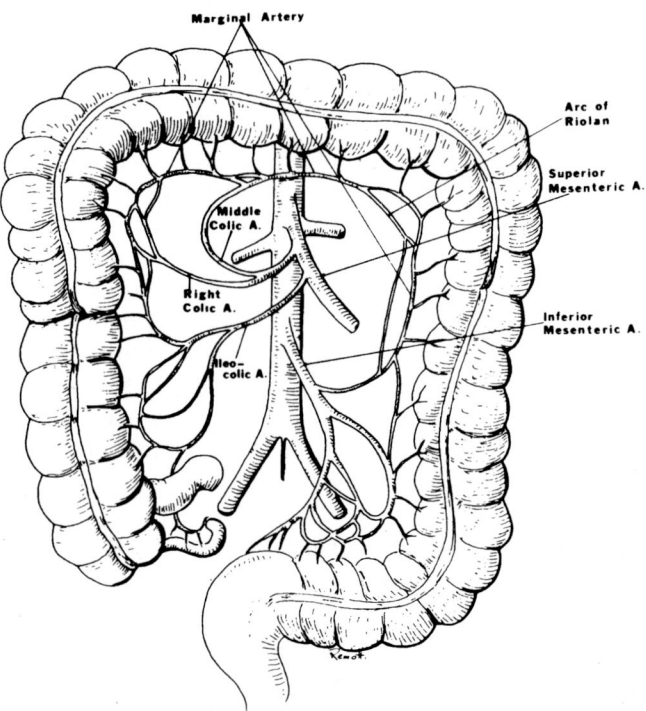

Figure 2-3. Arterial blood supply of the colon.

into two branches of unequal size at the level of the second or third sacral vertebra, commonly at the bottom of the pouch of Douglas. The larger right branch divides into several branches, which descend on the posterior and lateral surfaces of the rectal ampulla. The smaller left branch deviates to the left and supplies the lateral and anterior surfaces. In contrast to the small and large intestinal arteries, the branches of the rectal arteries do not form arcades but enter the gut wall directly and independently.

The branches of the superior rectal artery further anastomose with the middle and inferior rectal arteries originating respectively from the internal iliac and pudendal arteries.[10-12]

Venous drainage. The venous blood from the gastrointestinal (GI) organs and spleen is drained by the hepatic portal circulation through the liver before it returns to the heart. The hepatic portal vein is formed by the union of the superior mesenteric and splenic veins. The superior mesenteric vein drains blood from the pancreas, the stomach, the small intestine, and portions of the large intestine through the pancreaticoduodenal, right gastroepiploic, jejunal, ileal, ileocolic, right colic, and middle colic veins. The splenic vein drains blood from the stomach, the pancreas, and portions of the large intestine through the short gastric, left gastroepiploic, pancreatic, and inferior mesenteric veins. The inferior mesenteric vein, which passes into the splenic vein, drains portions of the large intestine through the superior rectal, sigmoid, and left colic veins. The right and left gastric veins, which open directly into the hepatic portal vein, drain large portions of the stomach. The cystic vein, which drains the gallbladder, also opens into the hepatic portal vein.

Collateral blood supply. The various pathways can be subdivided into six categories: channels between the celiac trunk and the superior mesenteric artery; channels between the celiac trunk and the aorta; channels between the different celiac branches; channels between superior mesenteric branches; connections between the superior and inferior mesenteric artery; and routes between the inferior mesenteric artery and parietal branches of the aorta. There are thus many anastomoses between the different arterial networks, but there are several weak points or "watershed" zones prone to vascular compromise in the setting of hypoperfusion. The collateral circulation between the hypogastric arteries and the inferior and superior mesenteric arteries is for instance most tenuous at the splenic colonic flexure (Griffith's point) and in the ileocecal region (Sudeck's point). These relatively underperfused sites are therefore preferentially involved in ischemic insults. Any vascular compromise from hypovolemia or splanchnic shunting during exercise can affect these zones.

ISCHEMIA OF THE GASTROINTESTINAL TRACT

Pathophysiology

There are many causes of GI tract ischemia (Table 2-1) that result in varied clinical manifestations. However, many, if not most, of these conditions result from a combination of arterial damage, usually atherosclerosis, and hypotension/hypovolemia/shock (nonocclusive mesenteric ischemia—NOMI). The other major

Table 2-1 Causes of Acute and Chronic Mesenteric Ischemia

ACUTE

Nonocclusive
  Cardiac failure with low output (arrhythmias, myocarditis, congestive heart failure)
  Hypotension (shock, dehydration, hemorrhage)
  Sepsis
  Drugs
    Thrombotic: oral contraceptives, NSAIDs
    Vasoconstrictive: ergotamine, cocaine, methysergide
    Hypotensive/hypovolemic: digitalis, diuretics, catecholamines, antihypertensives
  Vasculitic
    Hypersensitivity: antibiotics, diazepam, griseofulvin
    Toxic: gold, amphetamines
    Others: kayexalate, meloxicam, alosetron

Occlusive
  Arterial thrombosis
  Arterial embolism
  Iatrogenic (ligation, embolization, postaortic bypass graft)
  Arterial dissection
  Venous thrombosis
  Trauma
  Hypercoagulable states (disseminated intravascular coagulation)
  Cholesterol emboli
  Large and small vessel vasculitis
  Degenerative disorders of the vessel wall (atherosclerosis, diabetes mellitus)
  Amyloid
  Fibromuscular hyperplasia—dysplasia
  Radiation
  Neuroendocrine tumors
  Extrinsic compression (tumor, dissecting aneurysm)
  Intestinal obstruction/pseudo-obstruction
  Strangulation and torsion (adhesions, hernia, volvulus)
  Internal or external hernia
  Trauma
  Pressure necrosis (increased intraluminal pressure leading to decrease intramural flow)
  Carcinoma
  Diverticular disease
  Intussusception
  Fecal impaction

causes include adhesions or internal and external hernias causing strangulation and intussusception.

When a major vessel is severely narrowed, the fall in arterial pressure distally opens up collaterals in the vascular arcades, which remain open until the blood flow normalizes. Bowel ischemia develops following further narrowing or thrombotic occlusion of the major vessels, to the point where the collaterals cannot supply the additional blood flow needed or, more commonly, if additional strain is placed on the marginal blood supply—for example, following a fall in blood pressure, due to congestive heart failure, shock, or a myocardial infarct.[20]

Ischemia may also result following sudden occlusion of the mesenteric arteries by a thrombus or embolus, because collateral circulation cannot be established in time. The terminal branches from the marginal arteries and the intramural arteries have only a marginally adequate collateral circulation. Thus, occlusion of these vessels, as may occur in vasculitis or embolism following trauma, strangulation, or irradiation, is more likely to result in focal ischemic injury. Similar mechanisms occur also at the venous side of the circulation, where problems such as venous stagnation and thrombosis are ultimately transmitted to the arterial end.[21]

Generally, the mucosa of the GI tract receives half of the intestinal blood flow, while the muscularis propria, although accounting for half of the mass of the wall, receives only 30%. The mucosa is therefore more vulnerable. Local regulation of the mucosal vasculature plays an important role in the prevention of ischemic damage. The GI mucosa has a higher capillary density and more collateral vessels than any other organ, and the venous pressure is higher in the portal than the peripheral circulation. Oxygen extraction can also increase if blood flow is compromised. For the mucosa, the flow is governed by prearteriolar sphincters in the submucosal plexus. The responsiveness of these sphincters to local pO_2, pCO_2, and metabolites dictates perfusion of mucosal capillaries. It has been estimated that only one-fifth of the mucosal capillaries are open at any one time. Therefore, it is possible for an agent to constrict prearteriolar sphincters and arterioles without reducing the oxygen diffusion into cells, as long as the total blood flow does not fall more than 75%. Significant ischemia is seen when mesenteric pressure falls below 30 mm Hg. The splanchnic sympathetic nervous system is the main mediator of the autoregulation. However, oxygen diffusion within the villus is not determined by blood flow rates and the patency of capillaries alone. The close proximity of villus arteries and veins and the permeability of their walls suggest a possible countercurrent exchange in the villi, which allows direct transfer of oxygen between artery and vein at the base of the villus. This would establish an oxygen gradient up the villus and explain the increased susceptibility to hypoxic injury of cells at the surface.

Prolonged ischemia results in a variety of cellular metabolic and ultrastructural changes causing ultimately degeneration of enterocytes (Table 2-2). Hypoxia causes membrane degeneration leading to altered permeability and diminished activity of ATPase-dependent ionic pumps. This induces disturbed osmoregulation and an influx of fluid into epithelial cells with subsequent hydropic degeneration. Lysosomal rupture increases the damage. Within 30 minutes of total ischemia the intestinal villi are damaged, and after 8 to 16 hours irreversible transmural injury occurs.

The ischemic injury has a hypoxic and reperfusion component. In many cases, occlusion is not complete and even in occlusive disease much of the mucosal injury develops when normal perfusion and oxygenation have been more or less restored. This is called "reperfusion injury." Reperfusion damage is mediated by "free radical formation," inflammation, and exhaustion of antioxidant defense mechanisms. Oxygen-derived free radicals are oxygen molecules that have an unpaired electron in excess. The most important sources of O_2-radicals in the intestinal mucosa are xanthine oxidase, mitochondrial electron transport chain, prostaglandin synthetase, and activated neutrophils. Increasing hypoxia and diminished energy levels in the cell results in the utilization of adenosine triphosphate (ATP) and accumulation of adenosine 5' monophosphate (AMP). AMP is catabolized into adenosine, which diffuses out of the cell where it is broken down into inosine and hypoxanthine. Normally, hypoxanthine is oxidized by xanthine dehydrogenase to xanthine. Xanthine dehydrogenase is present in high concentration in the intestine with an increasing gradient of activity from villus base to tip. Under hypoxic conditions, xanthine dehydrogenase is converted into xanthine oxidase by proteolysis, which is an irreversible process. In experimental conditions in rats, it is almost complete within a minute of ischemia. Unlike xanthine dehydrogenase, which uses nicotinamide adenine dinucleotide as its substrate, xanthine oxidase

Table 2-2 Cellular Effects of Ischemia

Altered membrane potential
Altered ion distribution (increase of intracellular Ca^{2+}/Na^{2+})
Cellular swelling
Cytoskeletal disorganization
Increased hypoxanthine
Decreased ATP
Decreased phosphocreatine
Decreased glutathione
Cellular acidosis
Apoptosis

uses oxygen and therefore, during ischemia, is unable to catalyze the conversion of hypoxanthine to xanthine, resulting in a buildup of excess tissue levels of hypoxanthine. When oxygen is reintroduced during reperfusion, conversion of the excess hypoxanthine by xanthine oxidase results in the formation of toxic reactive oxygen species (ROS). These are potent oxidizing and reducing agents that directly damage cellular membranes by lipid peroxidation. In addition, ROS stimulate leukocyte activation and chemotaxis by activating plasma membrane phospholipase A_2 to form arachidonic acid. They also stimulate leukocyte adhesion molecule and cytokine gene expression via activation of transcription factors such as nuclear factor-κb. In addition to causing direct cell injury, ROS thus increase leukocyte activation, chemotaxis, and leukocyte–endothelial adherence. Ischemia reperfusion also results in complement activation and the formation of several proinflammatory mediators.

Etiology and Clinical Manifestations

Esophageal ischemia. Esophageal infarction with or without perforation is extremely rare. It has been reported to occur secondary to traumatic aortic transection, as a complication of spontaneous rupture of the thoracic aorta and in the anticardiolipin antibody syndrome (Fig. 2-4).[22–24]

Gastric ischemia. This is also very rare, largely because of the protective collateral circulation. The rare cases of gastric infarction reported in the literature have usually followed severe occlusive three-vessel disease (celiac artery and superior and inferior mesenteric arteries), volvulus, and therapeutic selective transcatheter embolization of the right gastric artery for gastric bleeding (Fig. 2-5A–E). Patients usually present with severe gastric bleeding.[25–27] Rarely chemoembolization beads that are injected into the hepatic artery for the treatment of hepatocellular carcinoma may accidentally enter gastric artery leading to gastric ischemia and ulceration.

Erosive gastritis due to chronic mesenteric ischemia has been documented in a number of case reports. The lesions occur primarily in the antrum. Biopsies will show epithelial desquamation, but otherwise the lesions are not very characteristic (see Fig. 2-5C,D).[28–32]

Ischemia can also occur in a less severe way resulting in lamina propria fibrosis, while the crypt epithelium is shed into the lumen of the pits. If the cells produce mucus, then this can resemble signet ring carcinoma, especially in antral mucosa, akin to the changes seen in pseudomembranous colitis. In the oxyntic mucosa the parietal cells collapse into the lumen, and the resulting disorganization can be mistaken for a parietal cell carcinoma (see Fig. 2-5A–E). The gastric changes are further discussed in Chapter 14. Rarely the stomach can be involved in severe NOMI. When very severe, it is found to affect the entire GI tract from the gastroesophageal junction to the rectum.

Acute mesenteric ischemia. Acute mesenteric ischemia is an abrupt decrease of mesenteric blood flow that may result in intestinal infarction. It can be caused by arterial (acute mesenteric embolism and thrombosis) or venous occlusion (Table 2-3). Venous ischemia results in vascular engorgement and hemorrhagic infarction. NOMI can be observed with systemic hypoperfusion, hemoconcentration including severe sepsis, and low flow states or as a result of vasoactive drugs. More exceptionally mesenteric ischemia is caused by vasculitis affecting the main mesenteric arteries. Venous mesenteric thrombosis can occur in patients with thrombophilia due to genetic or acquired coagulation disorders.[33] All types of genetic coagulation disorders, including factor V Leiden, prothrombin mutation, proteins C and S deficiencies, and antithrombin-III deficiency, carry the risk of venous occlusion. In the western populations, factor-V Leiden is most prevalent.[33,34] Acquired coagulation disorders associated with mesenteric venous thrombosis include autoimmune disease with lupus anticoagulants, heparin-induced thrombocytopenia, polycythemia vera, and hemoconcentration. In general, in 50% of patients with genetic coagulation disorders, the venous thrombosis is triggered by an external cause (intercurrent disease, estrogen intake, pregnancy). Abdominal trauma is an established but rare cause of intestinal ischemia. Postoperative mesenteric ischemia is most typically associated with open aortoiliac aneurysm surgery and cardiac surgery.[35,36]

Some 10% to 50% of all small intestinal ischemias are thought to be "nonocclusive," indicating that upon diagnostic workup no critical stenosis can be found. The damage to the ischemic intestinal segments evolves rapidly and becomes irreversible within a few hours, which necessitates immediate diagnostic evaluation

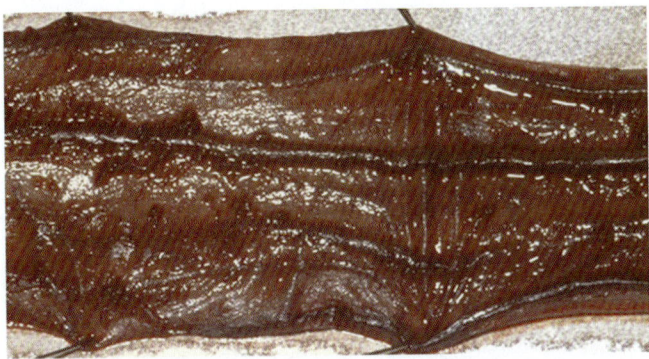

Figure 2-4. Acute esophageal infarction. Gross appearance of the opened esophagus showing a diffusely dark and necrotic mucosa.

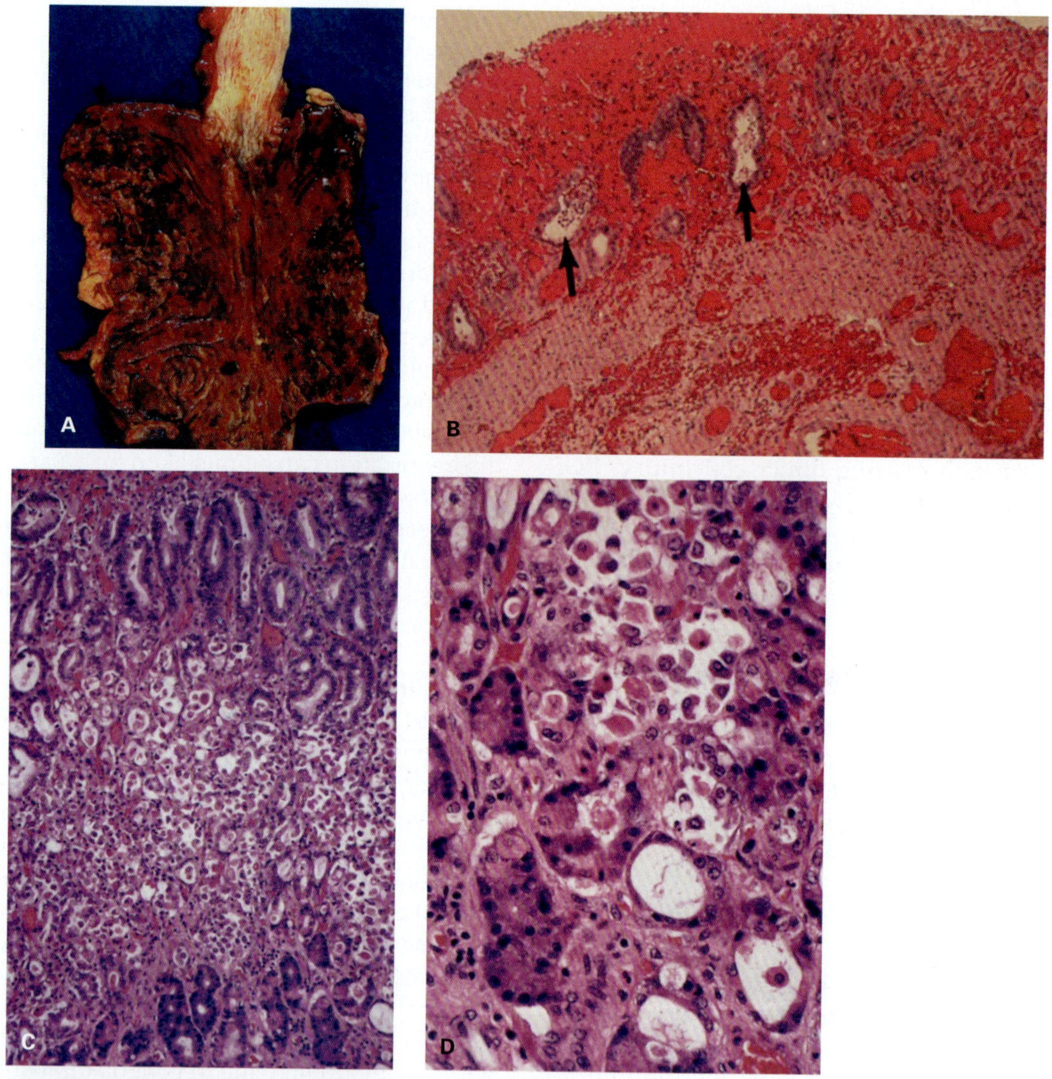

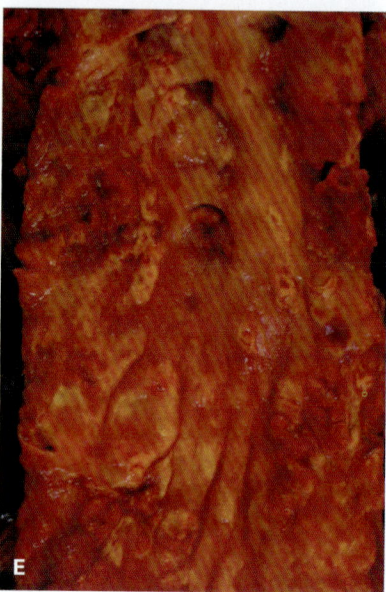

Figure 2-5. Acute gastric infarction. **A:** Gross appearance of the opened stomach and lower third of the esophagus. The mucosa is swollen, hemorrhagic, and partially covered by pseudomembranes. **B:** Section of mucosa and superficial submucosa showing intense congestion and hemorrhage. The outline of many atrophic gastric glands is still visible (*arrows*). **C:** Another area of gastric fundic mucosa showing desquamation of glandular epithelium. **D:** Higher-power magnification of part **(C)** showing desquamated parietal and chief cells lying within the space formerly occupied by the gland. Sometimes the desquamated epithelial cells may resemble malignant cells of early gastric cancers. **E:** Abdominal aorta from the same patient with gastric infarction showing virtual occlusion of the origin of the celiac axis and the superior mesenteric artery.

Table 2-3	Major Causes of Acute Mesenteric Ischemia
Nonocclusive mesenteric ischemia	50%
Superior mesenteric artery embolism	25%–30%
Superior mesenteric artery thrombosis	15%
Mesenteric vein thrombosis	5%–10%
Other	<5%

and prompt therapeutic decisions. Intestinal ischemia accounts for an estimated 0.2% of all hospital admissions and 1% of all laparotomies. The true incidence of mesenteric ischemia is probably higher.[37] The recent increase in acute mesenteric ischemia is most likely explained by improved abdominal imaging and by the aging population. Ischemia due to venous occlusion occurs in lower age groups. The symptoms and signs of acute mesenteric ischemia vary depending on the multitude of underlying vascular events. Arterial thromboembolism results in the most dramatic presentation, while the symptoms of NOMI and venous thrombosis tend to develop gradually over hours to days.[38] The clinical picture of typical acute mesenteric ischemia can be subdivided into four stages.[39] The hyperreactive state is characterized by severe abdominal pain in the absence of major abdominal findings at physical examination. In this stage there is hyperperistalsis and sudden vomiting or passage of loose stools. In the paralytic stage, the pain spreads over the abdomen and becomes continuous. The abdomen distends and loses its bowel sounds. The last two stages are nonspecific and are related to generalized peritonitis. In the third stage massive fluid and electrolyte losses occur due to capillary leak and a disturbed intestinal barrier. In the final stage shock rapidly evolves and the patient's general state deteriorates rapidly. NOMI and venous thrombosis present more nonspecifically, and of all the early clinical signs only abdominal pain is seen in the majority of the patients. Recognition of vascular abdominal rest pain, defined as severe and persisting for more than 2 hours without recent caloric intake in the absence of peritoneal signs, is the key to early diagnosis.

Laboratory analysis can be helpful in the diagnosis. Leukocytosis and metabolic acidosis with elevated lactate levels are common. Elevated serum enzymes include lactate dehydrogenase, creatine kinase, and amylase. However, no single enzyme is specific and they all carry low negative predictive value. Although abdominal imaging can help and is usually routine practice it should never delay medical and surgical treatment. Abdominal Doppler ultrasound is noninvasive and can be diagnostic for occlusive mesenteric ischemia. Emergency digital substraction angiography (DSA) is at present the gold standard for the detection of mesenteric occlusive disease. In selected cases, immediate endovascular revascularization can be performed. However, DSA cannot exclude transmural ischemia, and careful and repeated clinical examination of the abdomen is the key to performing a laparotomy or a laparoscopy. The other main value of DSA in assessing acute mesenteric ischemia is found in the handling of nonocclusive disease. In a patient with high suspicion of intestinal ischemia and with radiological signs of NOMI, the arterial catheter can be left in situ for vasodilator therapy. Computerized tomography (CT) scan carries a relatively short examination time and again in experienced hands has a sensitivity of 85% for proximal occlusion of the superior mesenteric artery and for mesenteric vein thrombosis. It is currently proposed as a standard test for the evaluation of acute abdominal pain. Magnetic resonance imaging (MRI) provides better anatomical resolution but is, due to longer examination times, in general not indicated in the acute management. Angiographic signs of nonocclusive disease include narrowing of the orifices of arterial branches, alternate narrowing and dilatation of intestinal branches (string of sausage), spasms of arteries in the arcade of Riolan, and impaired filling of intramural vessels.

When intestinal ischemia is being considered in an emergency setting, early fluid resuscitation is critical. When signs of generalized peritonitis are present, intravenous antibiotics should be started.[40] Surgery with revascularization of the ischemic segment (embolectomy, thrombectomy, arterial reconstruction) should be performed as soon as possible and preferably within 12 hours. The surgeon will have to decide if the affected intestinal segment is viable or should be resected immediately.[41]

Intraoperative assessment of intestinal viability remains a problem. The usual criteria employed after vascular repair are the return of bowel coloration and the peristalsis and pulsation of the mesenteric vessels. In cases of questionable viability, second-look operations within 24 to 48 hours have been advocated in order to prevent complications.

When there is evidence of nonocclusive ischemia without signs of peritonitis, in a stabilized patient intra-arterial papaverine in the superior mesenteric artery should be administered during the angiography. The management of venous thrombosis is more controversial, although intravenous heparin has also been indicated. Surgery with venous thrombectomy has been attempted but experience is limited.

Acute mesenteric ischemia portends a poor prognosis. Although decrease in mortality from 80% to 50% has been reported with early diagnosis and emergency surgery, the mortality rates still remain very high. Mortality with venous thrombosis is estimated to vary between 20% and 40%. Part of the poor prognosis is associated with the advanced age of most patients and associated comorbidities. Interestingly, most of this relates to superior mesenteric artery territory, and involvement of inferior mesenteric territory is less dramatic, possibly due to collateral circulation. For the clinician, a key to early diagnosis of mesenteric ischemia or mesenteric venous thrombosis is to keep a low threshold to consider it in the differential diagnosis since symptoms or signs may be nonspecific. If clinicians wait for dramatic signs of mesenteric ischemia like lactic acidosis, it may be too late.

Chronic mesenteric ischemia. Chronic mesenteric ischemia (also known as intestinal angina) is relatively uncommon. It is caused by atherosclerotic occlusion of the large mesenteric arteries. Due to the elaborate collateral circulation, usually two or three of the major mesenteric arteries have to be severely affected before patients become symptomatic. Even if abdominal imaging demonstrates severe stenoses in the large arteries, it can be hard to correlate these changes with symptoms. Patients with a suspected diagnosis of chronic mesenteric ischemia and generalized atherosclerosis are at increased risk for acute mesenteric ischemia with lethal prognosis. The true prevalence can probably be inferred only from angiographic studies of an atherosclerotic population.[42-44] It is estimated that in such a population between 8% and 15% may meet the radiological criteria. Fibrodysplasia and large vessel vasculitis are rare causes. The existence of the celiac axis compression syndrome as a possible cause of chronic mesenteric ischemia remains controversial.

Clinically, it appears that 75% of the patients presenting with chronic mesenteric ischemia are women, generally heavy smokers and middle-aged. Postprandial abdominal pain and weight loss dominate the clinical presentation. The increased mucosal blood flow in the postprandial phase with a steal effect toward nonatherosclerotic vessels probably explains the postprandial ischemic pain. The pain can start as early as 15 minutes after the start of a meal and usually subsides within 1 to 2 hours. Weight loss may be a result of intestinal malabsorption due to villous atrophy, altered motility, or food avoidance due to pain triggered by meals. The classical triad, postprandial abdominal pain, epigastric bruit, and weight loss, is present in a minority of the patients. In more than 75% of patients, the celiac artery has an orificial stenosis, and ischemic gastritis with ulcerations can occur.

Although the final proof of chronic mesenteric ischemia lies in the response of the symptoms to successful surgical revascularization, abdominal imaging is helpful in evaluating patients with clinical suspicion of chronic splanchnic ischemia.[45] Aortography and selective injection of all mesenteric arteries will allow to detect high-grade stenosis or occlusion.[46]

Superior Mesenteric Artery Syndrome This syndrome is thought to arise when rapid weight loss occurs. The fat surrounding the mesentery diminishes and the angle at which the superior mesenteric artery comes off the aorta becomes more acute. A loop of duodenum can become trapped in the angle and create an acute obstruction. Patients may report worsening of symptoms when lying supine and a relief when sitting upright and leaning forward (and hence bringing the superior mesenteric artery forward off the trapped bowel).

Pathology

Gross features. Ischemic lesions in the small intestine may be single, multifocal, or diffuse, depending on the cause of the vascular impairment and the state of the collateral circulation. Either occlusive or nonocclusive mesenteric ischemia can produce widespread infarction. In general, superior mesenteric vascular insufficiency involves the small and large bowels to the level of the transverse colon; inferior mesenteric insufficiency involves the splenic flexure and distal colon. Thrombi may extend into the mesenteric veins and extrude from the veins when transected. Ischemic lesions are, however, often patchy and irregular and do not necessarily conform to the area supplied by the major vessel. Extrinsic causes of intestinal ischemia may sometimes be apparent, for example, adhesion bands. In ischemia due to blunt trauma, there is often a hematoma in the mesentery and sometimes the bowel separates from the mesentery.

In early ischemia (including hemorrhagic enterocolitis), all that may be seen is purple discoloration of the bowel wall, the serosa retaining its normal glistening appearance. Later the viscus becomes dilated, thinned, and dark red or purple in color, and the serosa rapidly becomes dull and granular (Fig. 2-6). In more advanced ischemic injury, the bowel wall becomes thickened, rigid, and intensely hemorrhagic. Full-thickness infarction ensues leading to perforation and peritonitis. Most surgically resected specimens consist of bowel with only a thin rim of mesentery with vessels that are usually patent. Consequently, the patency of the larger, more proximal mesenteric vessels, which are more likely to be involved, cannot be examined, and the cause of the infarction (i.e., whether due to occlusive or nonocclusive vascular insufficiency) remains unclear on gross examination. However, sometimes atheromatous emboli can be identified in smaller arterioles, although by themselves they rarely give rise to anything other than minor transient lesions.

The appearances of the bowel following mesenteric vein thrombosis are similar to those of arterial insufficiency, except that there is more intense congestion and hemorrhage, and the thrombosed mesenteric veins are thickened and prominent. Lesions following mesenteric vein thrombosis tend to have indistinct borders compared to those due to arterial insufficiency.

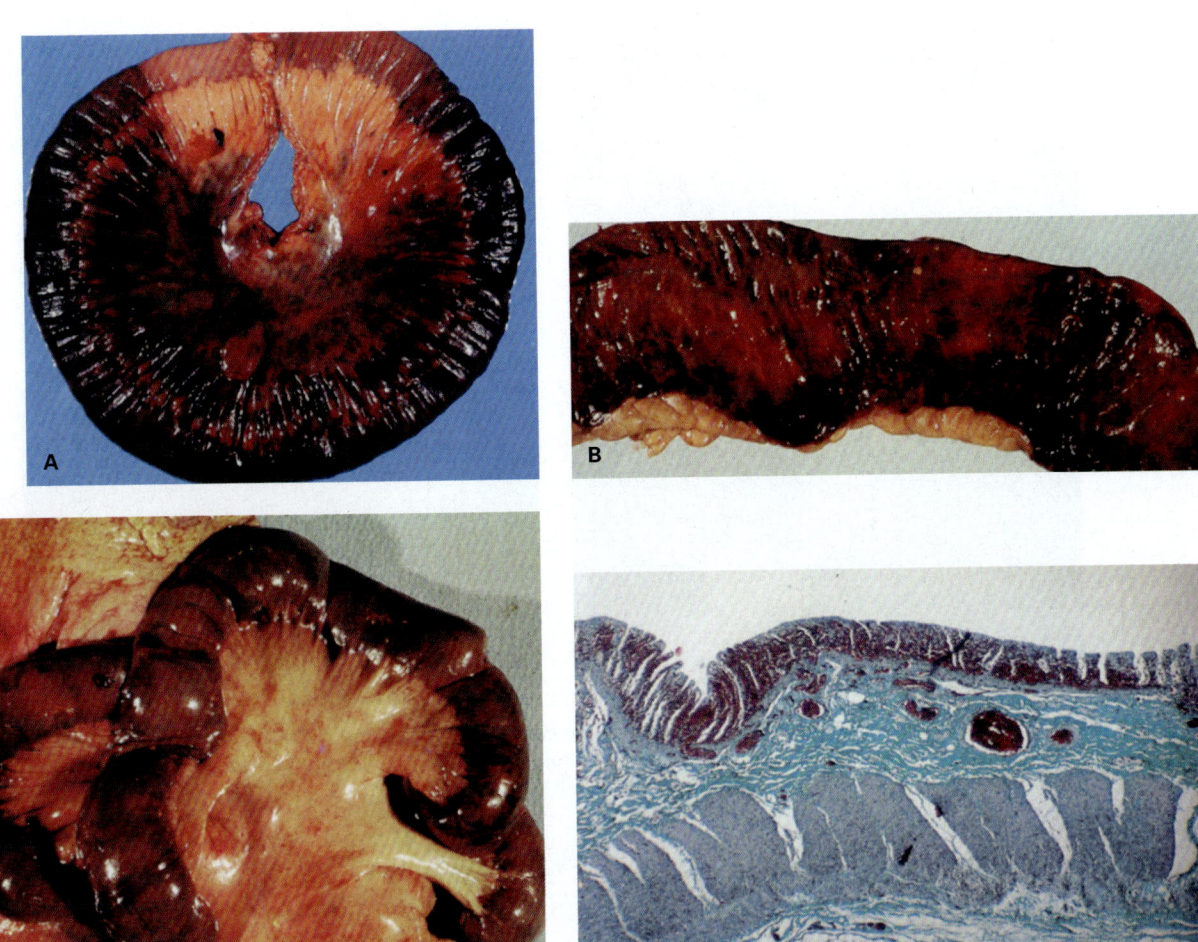

Figure 2-6. Focal segmental infarction of ileum. **A:** Intense congestion and hemorrhage of the loop of bowel and the attached mesentery. Note that the serosal surface has retained its shiny quality. **B:** Opened ileum showing the intense purple discoloration of the mucosa. Hemorrhagic enterocolitis. **C:** Autopsy specimen of small bowel showing diffuse purple discoloration. The serosa is uninvolved and maintains its sheen. **D:** Full-thickness section of intestine showing mucosal hemorrhage and submucosal congestion of vessels.

The appearance of the mucosa also depends on the severity and extent of the ischemic injury. At one end of the spectrum (acute hemorrhagic enterocolitis), the injury remains confined to the mucosa and submucosa, with intense congestion and hemorrhage and scattered superficial mucosal erosions. There is also extensive hemorrhage into the lumen.[47] The more common pattern of ischemic injury consists of severe mucosal congestion, hemorrhage, and edema, often with deep linear ulcerations (Fig. 2-7). This results in boggy, coarse cobblestoning of the mucosa, which has a rather characteristic x-ray appearance, namely, blunt semiopaque projections into the intestinal lumen with a margin of half-shadowing, so-called thumbprinting (Fig. 2-8). The more severe forms of ischemia result in extensive mucosal necrosis, often with pseudomembrane formation. The necrotic mucosa is dark green or black in color due to bile staining or adherent altered blood. There is also thickening of the bowel wall due to marked interstitial hemorrhage. In full-thickness infarction, the bowel wall becomes gangrenous and friable and may perforate.

If the bowel is only partially infarcted, the ulcerated mucosa is replaced first by granulation tissue and later by an atrophic mucosa, which may contain superficial serpiginous ulcers. The submucosa and

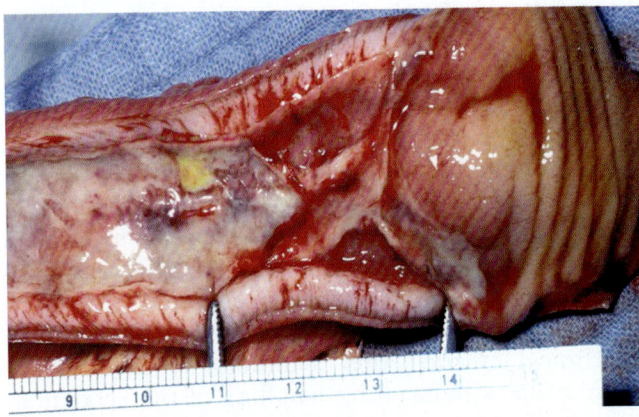

Figure 2-7. Segmental infarction of the terminal ileum showing a large mucosal ulceration. The demarcation between normal and involved segment is fairly sharp in arterial lesions as seen here.

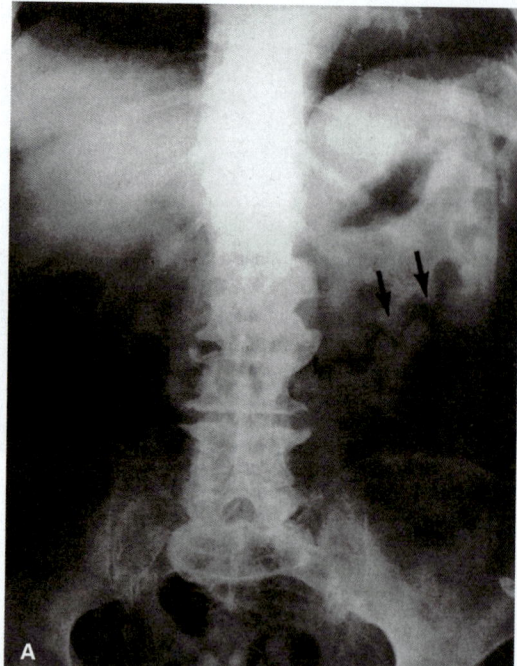
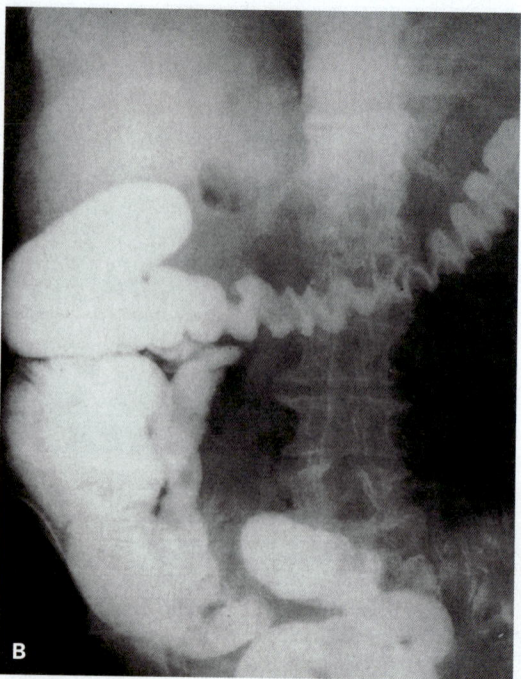

Figure 2-8. x-Ray appearances of ischemic colitis corresponding to the colon illustrated in Figure 2-9. **A:** Preliminary film showing the thickened mucosal folds, described as thumbprinting (*arrows*). **B:** Barium examination showing thickened mucosal folds. (Courtesy M. Weiner, M.D.)

muscle coats are replaced by fibrous tissue, resulting in strictures, which may be concentric or eccentric, depending on the extent of the ischemic necrosis.

Microscopy. There are two principal histologic patterns of intestinal ischemia: congestion, hemorrhage, and necrosis confined mainly to the (a) mucosa or (b) extending beyond mucosa and sometimes the full thickness of the bowel wall. Vascular injury affects the mucosa first. Marked mucosal and submucosal congestion, hemorrhage, and edema are the initial features. This may be all that is seen in some patients, and if the patient does not die from massive intestinal hemorrhage, the intestine is capable of complete resolution without scar formation when necrosis is limited to the mucosa.[20]

The microscopic mucosal lesions of acute ischemia have been studied in animal models mainly for the small intestine and were later confirmed in samples from patients.[48] Fluid accumulation between the surface epithelial cells and the basement membrane may be found as early as 60 minutes after ischemic injury, but is best seen ultrastructurally.[49] The earliest microscopic lesion is the formation of a subepithelial space underneath the epithelial cells lining the top of the villi, the Gruenhagen–Mingazzini space (Fig. 2-9). In clinical practice, this is difficult to differentiate from artifacts induced by handling of the specimen. The space progressively increases with lifting of the epithelial layer and separating it from the underlying lamina propria, followed by desquamation of the surface epithelium, with sparing of the deeper portion of the crypts. In the human small intestine, detachment and disruption of the lining epithelium at the villus tip are observed after 4 hours of absolute ischemia.[50] Subsequently the basement membrane becomes damaged and ruptures with disintegration of the lamina propria, vascular congestion, and hemorrhage. The villi become shorter and progressively disappear (Fig. 2-10). When hypoxia/reperfusion is mild small intestinal villi may not disappear but just become shorter, in a diffuse way. The epithelial cells lining the

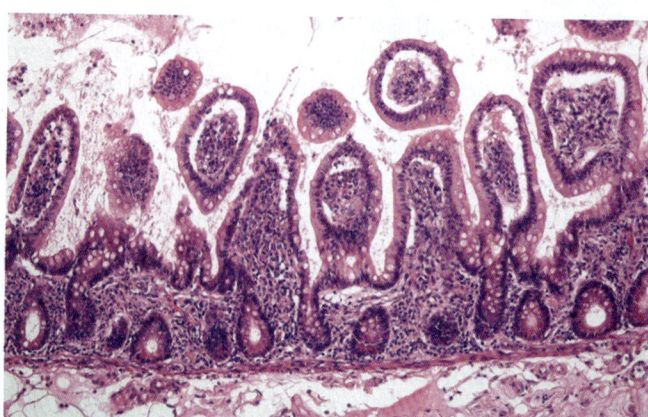

Figure 2-9. Early phase of small intestinal ischemia characterized by extensive lifting of the villous surface epithelial cells. This change cannot be reliably differentiated from artifacts that commonly occur in surgical or autopsy specimens.

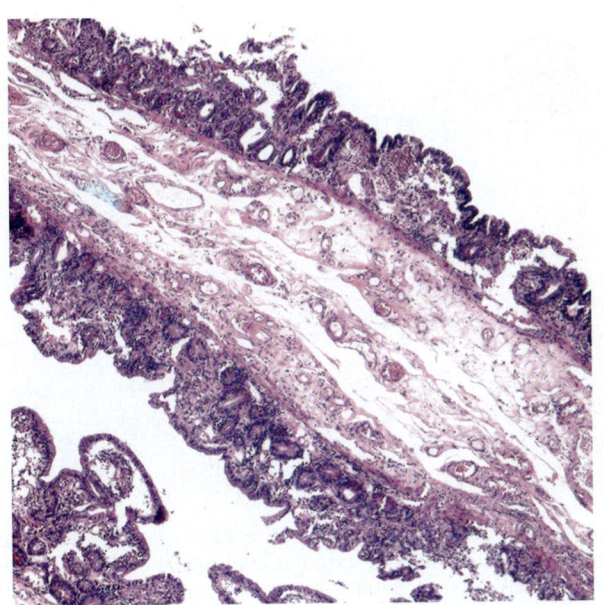

Figure 2-10. Diffuse flattening of the mucosa with loss of villi in the early recovery phase of small intestinal ischemic necrosis.

villi appear low cuboidal or flat with a basophilic cytoplasm. The crypts become mucin depleted, undergo coagulative necrosis, and eventually become detached from the basement membrane and extruded. Complete necrosis of the small intestinal mucosa in man is observed after about 44 hours of ischemia (Fig. 2-11).[50]

More extensive ischemic damage varies from superficial erosions to large ulcers to complete denudation of the mucosa. In severe cases, the sloughed mucosa is covered by a pseudomembrane composed of pus intermixed with mucus, blood, fibrin, and necrotic tissue, and frequently the devitalized tissue contains large numbers of mucosal bacterial colonies, both superficial and deep. Residual viable crypts often have extensive apoptosis, and epithelial cells slough into the lumen, sometimes producing a signet-ring

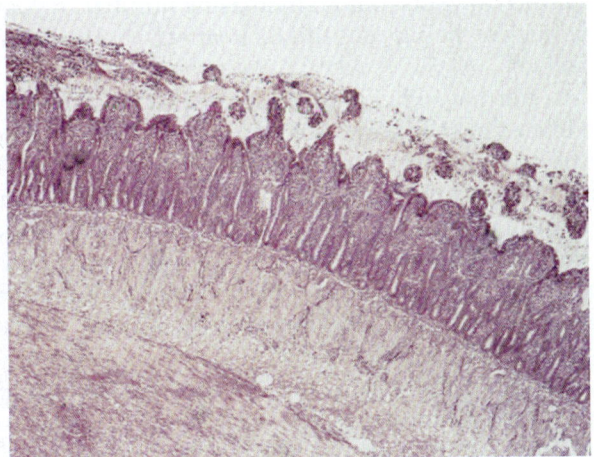

Figure 2-11. Extensive small intestinal ischemic necrosis in an experimental animal model.

appearance similar to that seen in the large bowel and stomach. Extensive hemorrhage is common, especially in the submucosa, and there may be platelet thrombi in capillaries. Occasionally, only vague outlines of the mucosa and the other layers of the bowel wall can be identified. In the early stages, there is only moderate leukocytic infiltration. Later, a secondary acute inflammatory infiltrate develops. The ischemic changes in the muscle coats are similar to those seen in myocardial infarcts. The earliest changes consist of poor staining of the muscle fibers, loss of nuclei, and thinning and separation of muscle fibers. The smooth muscle cells may show contraction bands, wavy fibers, thick waves, and coagulation necrosis.[51,52] "Contraction bands" are characterized by (hyper-)contraction of the smooth muscle cell with irregular eosinophilic bands and are a marker of cell death. With immunostaining, contraction bands are not reactive with antibodies against vimentin, desmin, actin, or myosin, indicating myofibrillar degeneration.[53] Typical coagulative necrosis, often accompanied by a dense neutrophilic infiltration, is a late event.

The histologic changes in mesenteric venous thrombosis are similar, except that sometimes there is more intense transmural congestion and hemorrhage (Fig. 2-12A,B), and while the veins are thrombosed, the arteries are patent.[54] However, even when thrombosed veins are found, it is not always certain that they represent the primary event. Presence of organization of the blood clot indicates a thrombus of some duration, which favors mesenteric venous thrombosis rather than an artifact or postmortem clot (Fig. 2-12C).

In the cases of resolution, fibrosis may result in stricture formation. Ischemic strictures are usually concentric. They can be short or long and single or multiple. They are relatively common in the left colon. They may be characterized by patchy mucosal ulceration. Histology shows irregularity of crypts without much inflammation. This may be confused with inactive or quiescent inflammatory bowel disease (IBDs). However, the degree of mucosal inflammation is still generally milder compared to IBD. Often one has to resort to clinicopathologic correlation with history suggesting predisposition to ischemia, endoscopic findings, presenting signs and symptoms, IBD serologies, and follow-up to rule out IBD. The submucosa is widened in the earlier phases but gradually becomes thinner and fibrotic. The fibrosis is hypocellular and extends downward between the smooth muscle cells of the circular muscle. Macrophages containing hemosiderin pigment are sometimes a prominent feature, but are not pathognomonic for ischemia and can also be seen in hemorrhagic IBD.[55] Transmural lymphoid aggregated, fissuring, and fibromuscular obliteration of the submucosa are conspicuously absent, which help to differentiate it from Crohn's disease.

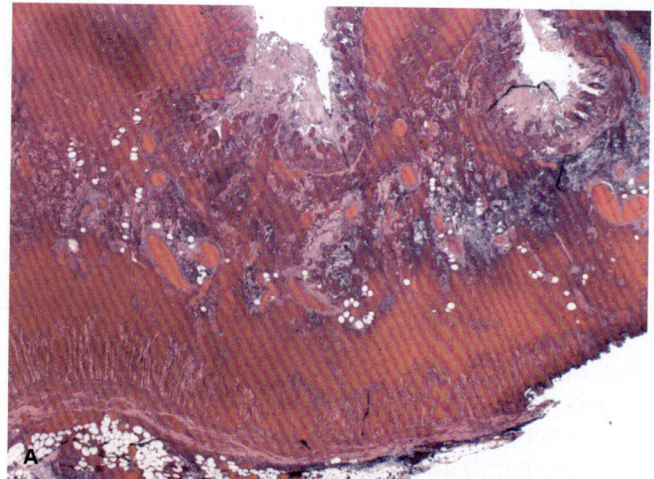
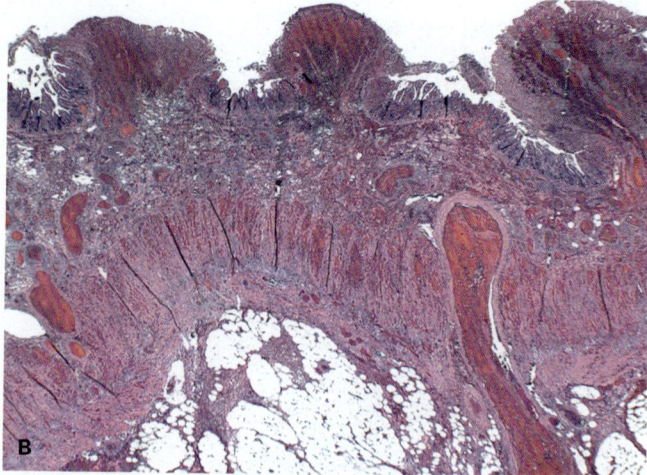
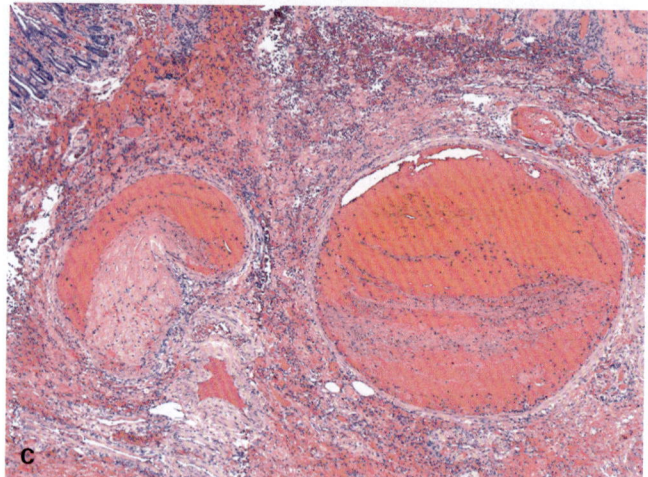

Figure 2-12. Low magnification in a case of mesenteric vein thrombosis (**A**) with marked vascular congestion and hemorrhage obscuring architectural details, which is more typical of venous obstruction compared with arterial obstruction. **B:** Another case of mesenteric venous thrombsis showing similar features. However, the hemorrhage is less intense and the thrombosis in veins is evident even at this magnification. **C:** Higher magnification showing varying degrees of organization of the thrombi in veins, differentiating this from a postmortem/postsurgical clot or an artifact.

Finally, it should be realized that sometimes transient ischemic episodes may occur in which no morphologic changes are found, although changes at the ultrastructural and biochemical levels could conceivably produce GI symptoms.

Ischemic colitis

Clinical Features The large bowel accounts for roughly half of all episodes of GI ischemia. Three major manifestations of colonic ischemia can be distinguished. Ischemic colitis (nongangrenous colitis) accounts for the large majority of the cases. Massive bowel infarction (gangrenous colitis) is noted in 15% to 20% of the cases and hemorrhagic enterocolitis is rare. Massive bowel infarction results from occlusive or nonocclusive vascular insufficiency, usually in association with small bowel infarction. Hemorrhagic enterocolitis is a variant of NOMI, with lesions confined to the mucosa and submucosa, occurring usually in the severely debilitated elderly individuals. Ischemic colitis is usually due to subacute colonic ischemia and can be reversible or irreversible. It can be mucosal (ulceroinflammatory pattern) or transmural (cobblestoning and stricture forming). It represents about 50% to 60% of all vascular disorders in the GI tract and 3% to 10% of lower GI tract bleeding.[56] The incidence is underestimated because many patients have mild or transient disease.[57] It occurs most frequently in the elderly and represents almost half of the colitides in patients aged over 50 years, but an increasing number of young patients are being identified. It affects both genders equally.[58]

In normal individuals, the rate of GI blood flow is the lowest in the colon. Colonic ischemia occurs when the blood flow is temporarily diminished in patients who already have a preexisting impaired blood flow because of arterial or venous thrombi, low flow states, diseases of the small vessels, or an elevated intraluminal pressure caused by colonic obstruction. Older patients with cardiovascular disorders; patients on various medications such as antihypertensives, oral contraceptives, or nonsteroidal antiinflammatory drugs (NSAIDs); people taking recreational drugs, for example, cocaine; patients with obstructing lesions of the colon such as carcinomas or diverticulitis; and patients with systemic conditions including vasculitis, infections (cytomegalovirus [CMV],

Escherichia coli [*E. Coli*] O157:H7), or coagulopathies are at risk. Intestinal vasculitis rarely occurs in the absence of systemic manifestations of vasculitis.

The etiology of ischemia in young people (< 45 years) differs from that in the elderly (Table 2-4). In young patients, drugs, hypercoagulable states, infections, and hypovolemia/hypoperfusion constitute the major etiologies.[59] Ischemic colitis has been reported following strenuous exercise such as running a marathon.[60-62] About one-fourth of males and females show occult blood in stool after a marathon run and occasionally will present with overt ischemic colitis. The mechanism is likely diversion of blood away from the bowel. However, other factors are likely involved as young trauma victims with extensive splanchnic vasoconstriction rarely develop ischemic colitis. Infections like *E. coli* (O15:H7), *C.difficle*, and CMV that cause endothelial damage also cause ischemia in young. A variety of drugs that include nasal decongestants (pseudoephedrine), cocaine, ergot alkaloids, sumatriptan, oral contraceptives, kayexalate, and Alosetron have been associated with ischemic colitis.[63-70] Young patients should also be screened for protein C and S deficiencies, antithrombin-III deficiency, or activated protein C resistance, and possibilities of vasculitis should be considered in the differential.[71-73] Colonic ischemia can also occur in young people following anorexic behavior.[74] Other rare causes of ischemia include carbon monoxide poisoning, sickle cell disease, scuba diving, and even colonoscopy itself.[75-78]

The most common presentation of ischemic colitis is where no clearly precipitating cause is identified other than older age. Colonic ischemia is frequently observed after aortic or cardiac bypass surgery.[57,79] The intestinal permeability is affected by the ischemia, which causes failure of the immunologic barrier and bacterial translocation.[79]

Any patient who has one or more of the above conditions and develops mild-to-moderate abdominal pain, diarrhea, or lower intestinal bleeding with minimal to moderate abdominal tenderness should be investigated for colonic ischemia. In cases of gangrenous ischemic colitis, the physical findings are more severe with acute abdominal pain, peritonitis, and hypovolemic shock. The clinical presentation, however, does not always correlate with the degree of ischemia. Colonic ischemia comprises a spectrum of disorders: (a) reversible colopathy (submucosal or intramural hemorrhage), (b) transient colitis, (c) chronic colitis, (d) stricture, (e) gangrene, and (f) fulminant colitis.[57]

Laboratory findings are nonspecific. Barium enema had been the primary diagnostic tool to diagnose colonic ischemia for a long time. Demonstration of "thumbprinting" (indentation of the barium due to submucosal swelling), transverse ridging (narrow contractions caused by spasm of the muscles in the colonic wall), loss of the colonic haustration pattern, ulcerations and spicula, intramural barium, strictures, sacculations, or pseudotumors reflect different stages of the disease. Serial studies are required to confirm the diagnosis.[57,79] Currently, this diagnosis is most often considered at colonoscopy first and confirmed by the clinical evaluation of disease and by typical biopsy findings. Sometimes CT scan is the initial investigation revealing evidence of colitis and followed by colonoscopy. The changes are not specific and may be similar to those seen in acute infectious colitis or acute presentations of IBD.[58] Colonoscopy should always be carried out with caution as insufflation of air causes an elevation of intracolonic pressure with further impairment of blood flow.[57,79,80] Occasionally ischemic lesions may masquerade as carcinoma. Biopsy-negative tumors require reendoscopy; ischemic lesions will change dramatically within a week or two.[81]

Treatment varies with the severity of the disease. Most cases of ischemic colitis resolve spontaneously. Such patients have what is called "transient or evanescent ischemic colitis." In patients with more severe symptoms, general supportive measures, fluid replacement, bowel rest, and correction of possible precipitating conditions are recommended.[82] There is no clinical evidence of beneficial effects of antibiotics, although they protect against bacterial translocation, which has been shown to occur with the loss of mucosal integrity. The progression of ischemic damage to gangrene is unpredictable and is another reason for the use of antibiotics at presentation.[57]

Pathology

Gross features. Ischemic colitis can affect all parts of the colon. In a study of 313 cases of biopsy-proven ischemia, the distribution of involvement was right colon in 25.2%, transverse colon in 10.2%, left colon in 32.6%, rectosigmoid in 24.6%, and pancolonic in 7.3%.[83] Splenic flexure area appears to be the most common single site of involvement in the colon. The involved segments may be small or large, single or multifocal, or rarely pancolonic. The pathologic changes range from mild, reversible mucosal injury to severe, irreparable damage with fibrous scarring and stricture

Table 2-4	Etiology of Ischemic Colitis in Young Adults (*n* = 42)
Drugs	31%
Low-flow state (hypovolemia, dehydration)	9.5%
Vascular thrombosis	9.5%
Collagen vascular disease	5%
Unidentified	45%

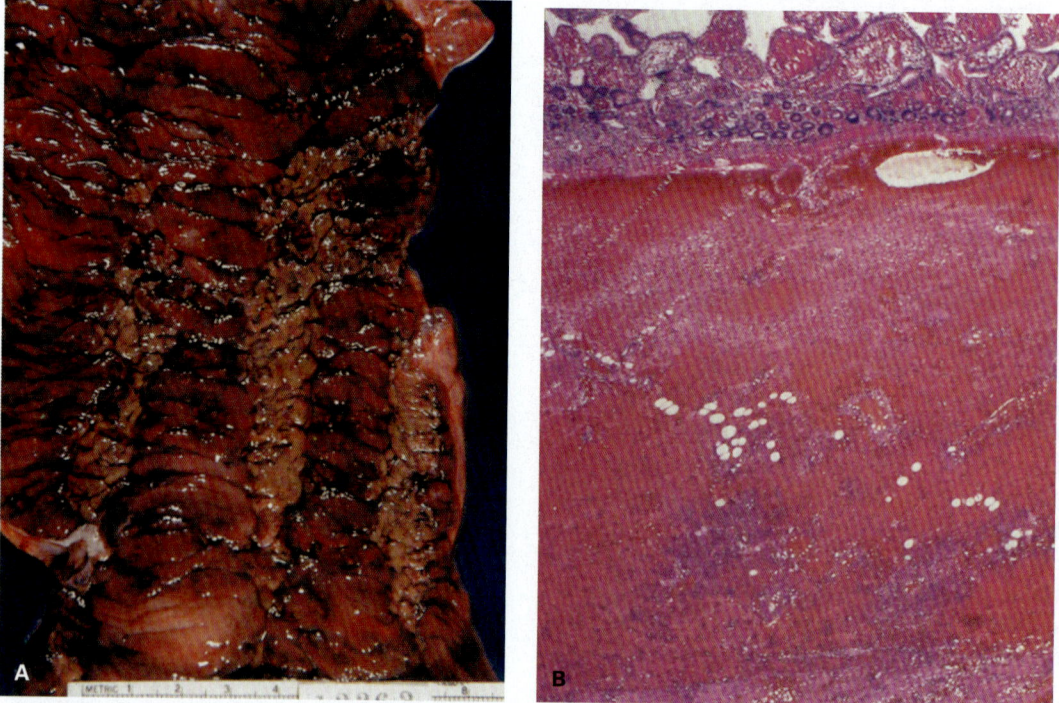

Figure 2-13. Acute ischemic colitis. **A:** Opened colon showing dilatation of the bowel wall and focal mucosal necrosis. Note the marked purple discoloration of the mucosa due to congestion and hemorrhage and the areas of greenish-brown discoloration. The latter result from bile staining of the necrotic mucosa. **B:** Full-thickness section of bowel showing transmural hemorrhage.

or, rarely, gangrene and perforation (Figs. 2-13 and 2-14). In some cases, ischemia produces pseudomembranes (Fig. 2-15) characterized by yellowish mucosal plaques. However, most of these cases occur in patients on antibiotic therapy and are thought to be caused by *C. difficile* colitis, but can be seen in other severe infections especially verotoxin-producing organisms.

The initial changes consist of pinpoint petechiae and patchy areas of hyperemia alternating with pale areas. Later the mucosa becomes swollen, edematous, and purplish blue in color, and there may be contact bleeding. Multiple small superficial ulcers (<1 cm) follow; these may become large and serpiginous and resemble those of Crohn's disease (see Fig. 2-13).

In *resection specimens* in the acute stage the colon is thickened and rigid. There is surface hemorrhage and a coarse cobblestoning of the mucosa due to linear ulceration and submucosal edema (Fig. 2-15A). In more advanced cases the necrotic mucosa shows a greenish discoloration, and the serosal surface varies in color from plum to black. In healed or chronic lesions, tubular or fusiform strictures with fibrous thickening of the submucosa, often with shallow ulcers, are seen.[84,85]

Microscopy. The histologic changes range from mild mucosal and submucosal edema and hemorrhage to transmural destruction. The outcome of ischemia is also variable. About 50% of patients develop some degree of necrosis, followed by granulation tissue, scarring, and fibrous stricturing. The *earliest mucosal changes* appear to be mucosal congestion and hemorrhage, followed shortly afterward by lifting of the surface epithelial cells and coagulative necrosis of the surface and crypt epithelium. At this point, one may still see the ghost outline of the crypts or surviving crypt bases in the shape of tear drops, but shortly afterward the entire epithelium is sloughed, and one may then see crypt spaces devoid of epithelium (Fig. 2-16A,B). Similar changes may occur in an autolyzed bowel, though without the hemorrhage. This change may result in pseudomembranes composed of necrotic mucosa, fibrin, and blood. Histologically, there are subtle differences between genuine *C. difficile*–associated pseudomembranous colitis and ischemic necrosis. Hyalinization of the lamina propria such that the normal loose connective tissue punctuated with plasma cells, lymphocytes, and eosinophils is replaced with dense eosinophilic hyalinized matrix is characteristic of genuine ischemia (Figs. 2-17 and 2-18). Usually the residual glands become more closely spaced (lamina propria "collapse"). Atrophic-appearing microcrypts, lamina propria hemorrhage, full-thickness mucosal necrosis, and a diffuse microscopic distribution of pseudomembranes are more common in ischemia (Fig. 2-19). In genuine *C. difficile*–associated pseudomembranous colitis, neutrophils are more common, the upper parts of the

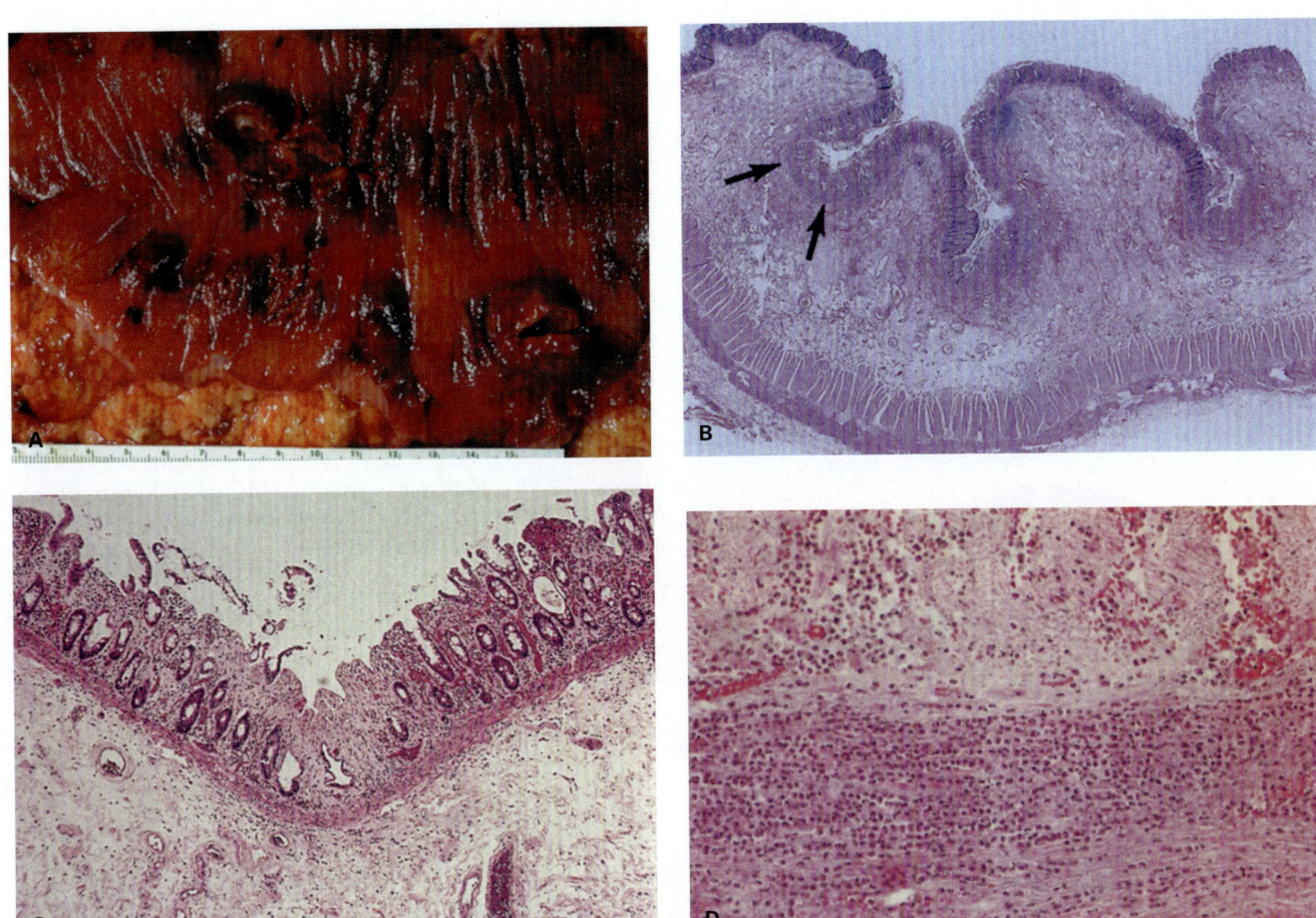

Figure 2-14. Acute ischemic colitis. **A:** Mucosal surface showing hemorrhage and swelling producing multiple polypoid nodules. **B:** Full-thickness longitudinal section of colon showing marked thickening of the bowel wall due to submucosal edema. The mucosa is focally ulcerated (*arrows*) and shows focal loss of glandular epithelium. **C:** Higher-power magnification of the mucosa in (**B**) showing focal loss of surface and glandular epithelium. **D:** Higher-power magnification of the muscularis propria in (**B**) showing the neutrophilic infiltration of the ischemic muscle coat.

crypts are dilated, and necrosis is mainly present in the upper half of the mucosa.[86]

It is also important to be aware that crypt epithelial cells can collapse into the lumen where they can become rounded up and resemble signet ring cells.[87,88] This trap is seen primarily in pseudomembranous colitis, but the resemblance to signet ring carcinoma can be striking; with only the realization that the signet ring cells are still confined to lumen of the crypts, an overall misdiagnosis can be prevented.

In the *healing phase* granulation tissue becomes prominent. The mucosa regenerates but is often atrophic, with shortened and branched crypts, and is subject to recurrent ulceration. The changes are usually patchy. At this stage, it may resemble chronic treated or quiescent IBD. However, despite the similarities in practice this is seldom a problem. Any mucosal destruction resolves with distorted crypts, but the chronic inflammation of IBD is not present. The submucosa and muscularis propria are markedly widened initially by the granulation tissue and later replaced by fibrosis. This results in stricture formation, often with thinning of the viscus (Fig. 2-20). Sometimes the submucosal fibrosis may extend into the mucosa, frequently in a diffuse manner. Hemosiderin-laden macrophages may be found in the scarred tissue and have been described as a hallmark of ischemia (Fig. 2-21).[89] However, in our experience, these are few and far between; they are also of little value in the distinction from other IBDs. Occasionally cholesterol emboli can be seen that may have traveled from proximally located ulcerated atherosclerotic plaques (Fig. 2-22). The overlying mucosa sometimes appears normal, and the patient can be asymptomatic, although GI symptoms occur in about one-third of cases. Limited ischemic bowel necrosis, occasionally with subsequent stricture formation, can however occur.[90]

Ischemic proctitis. It was thought that the rectum is spared from ischemic injury because of its ample collateral circulation. However, rectal ischemia does occur either in conjunction with colonic ischemia or

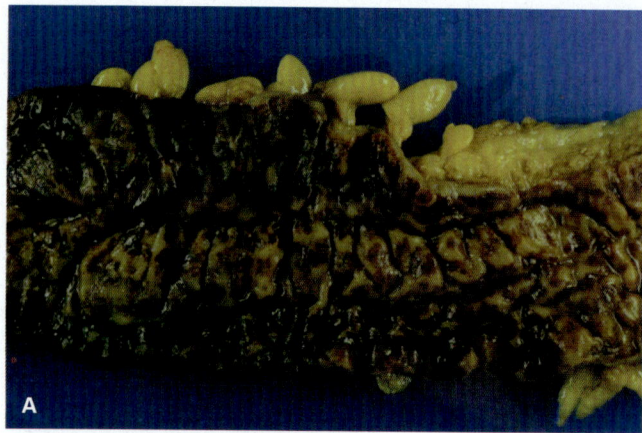
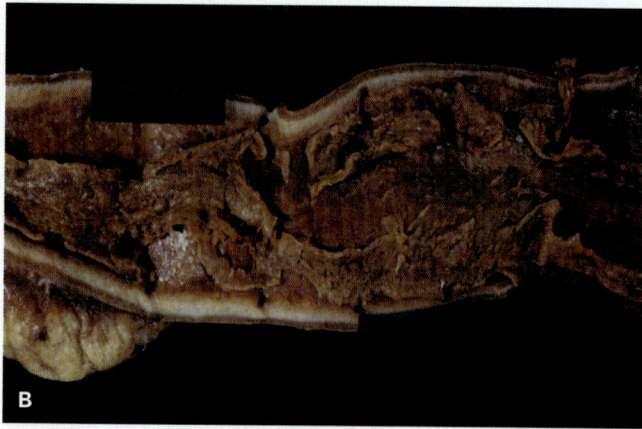
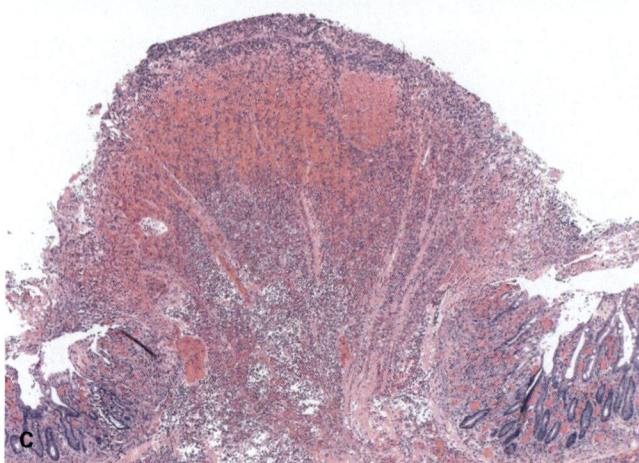

Figure 2-15. Ischemic colitis with pseudomembranes. **A:** Opened bowel showing green discoloration of the mucosa and adherent yellowish pseudomembranes. **B:** Opened colon from another patient showing loosely adherent greenish pseudomembranes. The underlying tissues are markedly inflamed. (Courtesy of Maureen Duffield, Johannesburg) **C:** Histologic section of mucosa and pseudomembrane. The mucosa is necrotic, and most of the glandular epithelium is gone. The pseudomembrane, which is in the center of the section, is composed of a fibrinous exudate mixed with necrotic tissue and inflammatory cells.

by itself and represents about 10% of all cases of large bowel ischemia. Rectal ischemia occurs in patients with occlusive internal iliac artery disease. Acute presentation may follow the ligation of the inferior mesenteric artery (operations of the lower aorta) or other iatrogenic interventions including sclerotherapy for hemorrhoids.[91] The endoscopic features and pathology of ischemic proctitis are the same as those of ischemic colitis.[92,93] It must be differentiated from other causes of rectal inflammation such as the solitary rectal ulcer syndrome or rectal lesions due to abuse of suppositories.

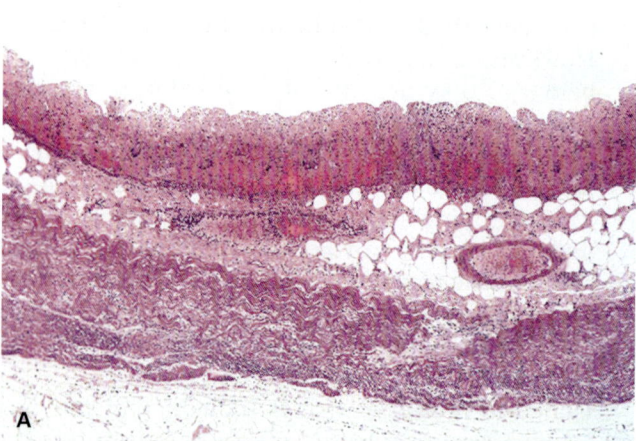
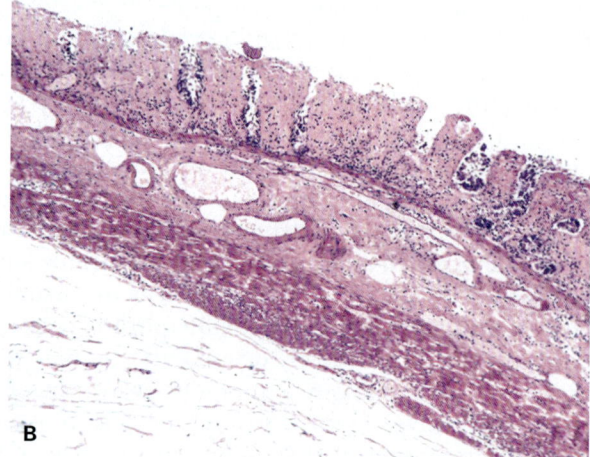

Figure 2-16. A: Extensive large bowel infarction with diffuse transmural necrosis and complete loss of glands. **B:** Epithelial cells can persist in some crypts.

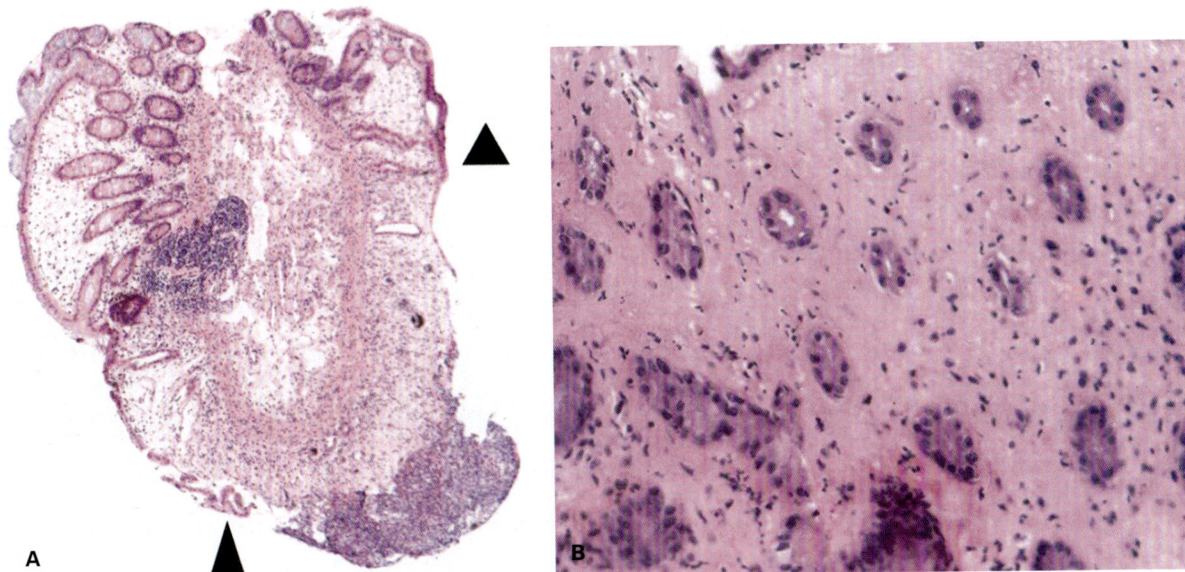

Figure 2-17. **A:** Endoscopic biopsy from ischemic colitis showing the well demarcated lesion with mucosal necrosis (*arrowheads*). **B:** Hyalinization of the lamina propria characterized by dense eosinophilic and paucicellular matrix and microcrypts are specific markers for a diagnosis of ischemic colitis.

INFLAMMATORY VASCULAR DISORDERS OF THE GASTROINTESTINAL TRACT (VASCULITIDES)

Introduction

Genuine "vasculitis" is characterized by fibrinoid degeneration (eosinophilic degeneration) of the vessel wall and infiltration of the vessel wall by leukocytes, with neutrophils, nuclear dust, and extravasated red cells in the vessel wall and the adjacent stromal tissue.[94,95]

The term "vasculits" is applied to "noninfectious inflammatory" disorders of blood vessels. Vasculitis has many causes, which result in only a few limited histologic patterns (Table 2-5). Vasculitis can affect any caliber blood vessel in the GI tract (Table 2-6), and the frequency of GI tract involvement varies among different types of vasculitides (Table 2-7). It is characterized by general symptoms such as fatigue, fever, weight loss, and arthralgias and abdominal symptoms such as pain, nausea, vomiting, diarrhea, intestinal bleeding, and perforation. If GI manifestations occur in a patient with established vasculitis, endoscopy, angiography, and histology are generally sufficient to demonstrate the involvement of the GI tract. Endoscopy may reveal minimal abnormalities or ulceration and strictures. Angiography shows stenoses, aneurysms, and infarctions. Histology may show inflammation and necrosis of blood vessels and perivascular inflammation. In a patient, not previously diagnosed as suffering from vasculitis, diagnosis is more difficult. The physician should be alerted especially if general symptoms point toward systemic disease. In addition, other organ systems may show signs of inflammation such as the skin, eyes, lungs, nervous system, and kidneys.

Complete biologic screening involves testing for evidence of inflammation and immunologic deficiencies; screening for immune complexes and complement, autoantibodies, infections, and factors that promote clotting; and testing for the evidence of vascular endothelial damage (Table 2-8). Involvement of large- and medium-sized vessels by vasculitis can be demonstrated by means of arteriography and other imaging techniques. Skin, muscle, nose, and kidney biopsies can reveal signs of vasculitis.[96] Endoscopic

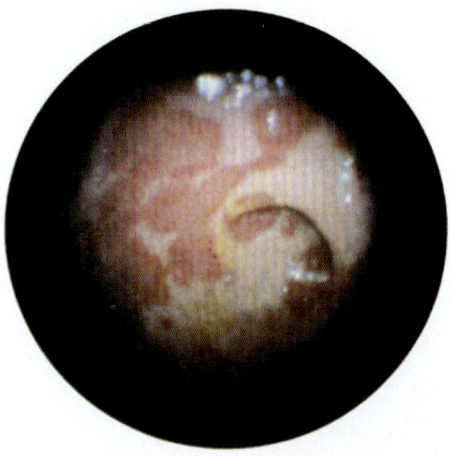

Figure 2-18. Ischemic colitis following aortofemoral bypass surgery. Endoscopic appearance showing a serpentine, white-based exudate in the rectum.

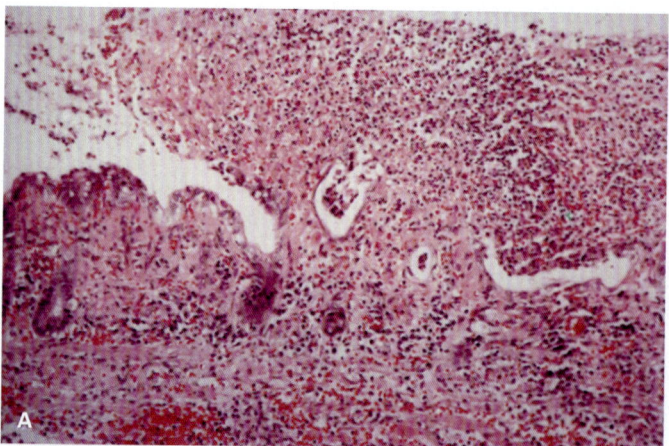 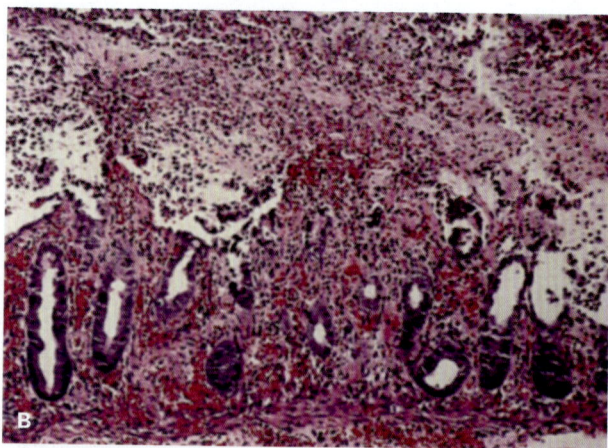

Figure 2-19. Comparison of ischemic colitis with pseudomembranes and pseudomembranous colitis due to *Clostridium difficile* toxin. **A:** Ischemic colitis with pseudomembranes shows full-thickness necrosis of the mucosa below the adherent pseudomembrane. **B:** Pseudomembranous colitis showing the characteristic explosive necrosis of the upper half of the mucosa with preservation of the lower half of the gland crypts.

biopsies of the GI tract are more likely to be negative as very little submucosa is included, and they merely show features of mucosal ischemia. Rectal biopsies were indeed negative in many patients with established systemic vasculitis.[97] The establishment of the involvement of larger vessels requires surgical samples. The presence of isolated GI vasculitis is extremely uncommon in the absence of other systemic features of vasculitis.[98]

The minimum criteria for a microscopic diagnosis of vasculitis remain controversial, but it is generally accepted that there must be two components: (a) an inflammatory cell infiltrate and (b) vascular injury. The absence of inflammation thus precludes the diagnosis of vasculitis, although in a late, healing state, inflammatory infiltration may be minimal. Like many other inflammatory conditions, vascular injury is a continuum. The spectrum ranges from endothelial cell swelling and leakiness to frank fibrinoid necrosis and fibrin deposition. Pathologists require a certain degree of histologic evidence of injury manifested by deposition of fibrinoid material, necrosis

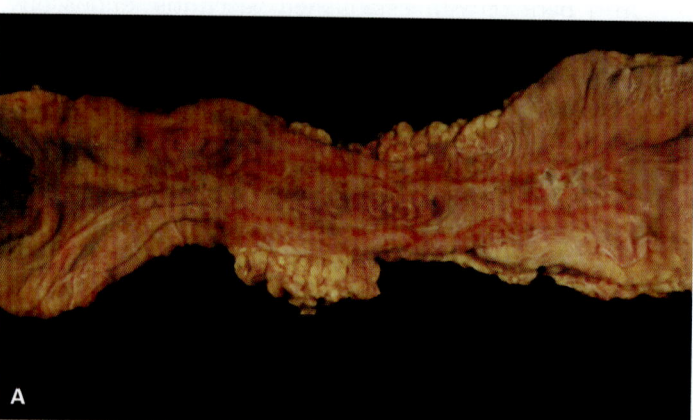

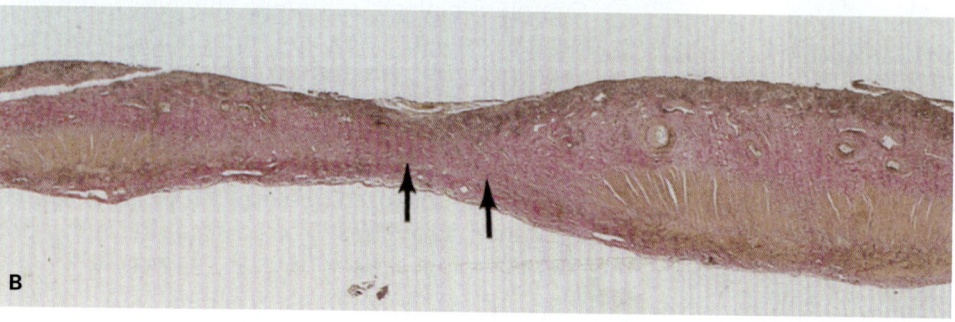

Figure 2-20. Ischemic stricture of the colon. **A:** Opened segment of the colon, showing stricturing and narrowing of the lumen. The central portion of mucosa is atrophic and surrounded by an irregular hyperemic margin. **B:** Full-thickness section of the colon showing marked thinning of the bowel wall and replacement of the muscularis propria by fibrous tissue (*arrows*).

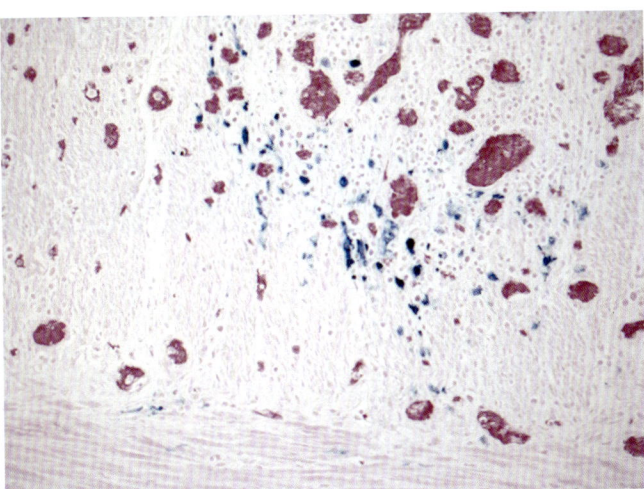

Figure 2-21. Recovery following ischemic damage can be characterized by abnormal crypt architecture and the presence of iron-laden, Perls-positive macrophages which are stained blue.

of the vessel wall, or both. However, certain changes such as extravasation of erythrocytes and edema due to leakiness, thrombosis, and infiltration of the vessel wall can occur without fibrinoid necrosis of the vessel wall.

The term "vasculopathy" has been used to describe vascular alterations without clear inflammation. Another problem is the difference between primary and secondary vascular injury. Secondary vascular injury should be distinguished from secondary vasculitis, a term which is used by clinicians for vasculitis associated with rheumatic or other connective tissue disorders, malignant diseases, infections or exposure to toxic substances.[99] Secondary vascular injury can occur in different inflammatory conditions, such as a peptic ulcer of the stomach and cholecystitis, when local blood vessels are affected

Table 2-5	Classification of Vasculitis According to Histologic Pattern
I: Vascular damage—vasculopathy: scant inflammatory cells	
II: Vasculitis: Lymphocytes predominant	
"Lymphocytic vasculitis"	
Lupus erythematosus	
Angiocentric lymphomas	
Cytomegalovirus inclusion disease	
Behçet's syndrome	
III: Vasculitis: Neutrophils predominant	
Small vessel leukocytoclastic vasculitis	
Polyarteritis nodosa	
Behçet's syndrome	
III: Vasculitis: Mixed cell types: granulomas	
Churg–Strauss syndrome	
Wegener's granulomatosis	
Giant cell arteritis	
Secondary vasculitis	

by the inflammatory process. The occurrence of vascular lesions in otherwise severely inflamed tissue should therefore not be confused with a genuine vasculitis. Thus, it is always helpful to look in areas away from severe inflammation and necrosis to identify genuine vasculitis.

There is also considerable overlap in the histologic appearances of different genuine forms of vasculitis. A reliable histologic classification is thus difficult because of lack of histologic specificity and the variability of histologic changes depending on the stage of the disease, its activity, and any prior treatment. In some cases a differential diagnostic scheme based on the histology can be helpful, but in general this type of classification is not very useful clinically (see Table 2-5).

Classification

Large vessel vasculitis was also the first type to be described.[100] For years, vasculitis was known as "periarteritis nodosa," a term initially used to characterize a nodular inflammatory lesion in medium- and small-sized arteries throughout the body. The name was later changed to "polyarteritis nodosa (PAN)." By the 1950s, it was realized that a variety of clinically distinct forms of vasculitis existed and that small vessels could also be involved. Small vessel vasculitis was referred to as either "hypersensitivity vasculitis" or "microscopic periarteritis."[101] The latter is now commonly known as microscopic polyangiitis (MPA). Since then the classification of vasculits has evolved and become more complex.

Despite many causes, vasculitis has limited histologic patterns.[102] The histologic lesions vary with time,

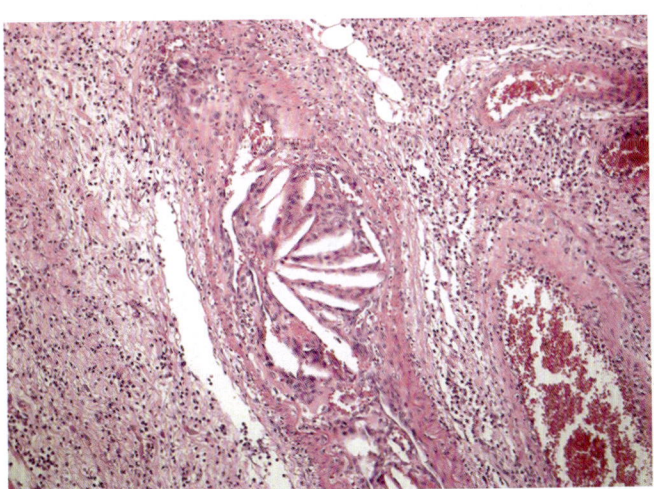

Figure 2-22. Cholesterol emboli that result from the release of material from atherosclerotic plaques in a submucosal artery.

Table 2-6 Classification of Vasculitides by Caliber of the Vessel

Vasculitides involving large- and medium-sized vessels
 Temporal arteritis (Giant cell arteritis)
 Takayasu arteritis
 Buerger's disease
 Infectious vasculitis

Vasculitides involving medium- and small-sized vessels
 Polyarteritis nodosa
 Kawasaki's disease
 ANCA-associated vasculitis
 – Churg–Strauss syndrome
 – Wegener's granulomatosis
 – Microscopic polyangiitis
 Vasculitis associated with rheumatic diseases
 – Rheumatoid arthritis
 – Systemic lupus erythematosus
 – Systemic sclerosis
 – Dermatomyositis
 – Sjögren's syndrome
 – Sarcoidosis
 – Autoimmune hepatitis
 – Primary biliary cirrhosis
 – Crohn's disease
 – Behçet disease
 – Mixed essential cryoglobulinemia
 Vasculitis associated with infectious disorders
 – Bacteria (*Staphylococcus*, streptococci, *Treponema*, *Borellia*, *Mycoplasma*, etc.)
 – Viruses (Hepatitis B and C, HIV, coxsackie, etc.)
 – Fungi (*Zygomycosis*, *Aspergillus*)
 – Parasites
 Vasculitis associated with drugs
 – Antirheumatic drugs (gold, chloroquine, D-penicillamine)
 – Carbimazole
 – Dextran
 – Angiotensin-converting enzyme inhibitors
 – Cytotoxic drugs
 Paraneoplastic

Small vessel vasculitis
 Henoch–Schönlein purpura

Table 2-7 Frequency of Intestinal Involvement in Different Vasculitides

TYPE OF VASCULITIS	FREQUENCY OF INTESTINAL INVOLVEMENT (%)
Polyarteritis nodosa	40–60
Churg–Strauss syndrome	20–50
Takayasu's arteritis	up to 15
Wegener's granulomatosis	5–11
Giant cell arteritis	1
Thromboangiitis obliterans	1
Henoch–Schönlein purpura	50–90
Systemic lupus erythematosus	up to 50
Rheumatoid arthritis	up to 10

an international conference, and attempts have been made to combine the classification according to the vessel size and etiology (see Table 2-6).[103] This was followed by a proposal for uniform terminology and definitions.[104] It is clinically important to identify the type and size of inflamed vessels and to determine

Table 2-8 Laboratory Parameters Important for Patients Clinically Suspected of Vasculitis

Nonspecific evidence for inflammation
 – Erythrocyte sedimentation rate
 – C-reactive protein
 – Leukocyte and eosinophils count
 – α-2 globulins
 – Haptoglobin

Organ-specific
 – Creatinine
 – Urinalysis
 – Transaminases
 – Creatine phosphokinase

Immunologic data
 – Electrophoresis
 – Quantification of immunoglobulins

Other
 – Antineutrophil cytoplasmic antibodies
 – Antiendothelial cell antibodies
 – Antinuclear antibodies
 – Antiphospholipid antibodies
 – Rheumatoid factor
 – Cryoglobulins
 – Antiphospholipids
 – Complement (CH50, C3, C4)
 – Hepatitis B and C antigen and antibodies
 – Other infections: parvovirus, HIV, *Rickettsia*, streptococci, etc.
 – Blood cultures

and the clinical presentation depends upon the size of the vessels involved as well as distribution of the disease. The protean clinical manifestations, combined with the etiologic nonspecificity of the histologic lesions, complicate the diagnosis of specific forms of vasculitis. This is problematic because different vasculitides with indistinguishable clinical presentation (e.g., Henoch–Schönlein and MPA) may have different prognosis and treatment. A general classification covering all these aspects and easily applicable in clinical practice is at present not available. One approach is to categorize the noninfectious vasculitides on the basis of the predominant type of vessel affected. Such a classification has been proposed by whether the inflammation is focal or extensive.[102,104] These variables have an influence upon the clinical presentation and the diagnostic techniques used.[94,95] Involvement of larger vessels is frequently associated with more severe clinical syndromes; for example, involvement of larger "mesenteric vessels" results in complications such as bowel necrosis, infarction, and perforation.

Etiologic classification of vasculitis also remains problematic. Some of the "noninfectious inflammatory" disorders of blood vessels are the result of inflammation secondary to an immunologic reaction at the endothelial surface of the affected vessel. This can be induced by an infection, but in many cases the underlying pathogenesis is poorly understood. Based on the pathogenesis, "vasculitis" can be subdivided into secondary vasculitis, immune-mediated vasculitis, and vasculitis of uncertain origin. Abnormal immunoglobulin deposition is detected in some distinct forms of vasculitis such as "Henoch–Schönlein purpura." Viral antigens such as hepatitis B antigen (or bacterial and fungal antigens) can be found in immune complexes or in association with vasculitis in PAN. In vitro studies have shown the occurrence of a separate class of antibodies against endothelial cell antigens in lupus and Wegener's granulomatosis.

In recent years the identification of the antineutrophil cytoplasmic antibodies (ANCAs) has greatly aided the subclassification of vasculitis. ANCAs are common in Wegener's granulomatosis, in Churg–Strauss vasculitis (CSV) (70%), and in MPA (80%). They are rare in Kawasaki's disease and occasionally found in lupus and Takayasu's disease. ANCAs are specific for antigens in neutrophil granules and monocyte lysosomes. They can be detected with indirect immunofluorescence microscopy by using alcohol-fixed neutrophils as substrate. This produces two major staining patterns: cytoplasmic ANCA (c-ANCA) and perinuclear ANCA (p-ANCA). Specific immunochemical methods demonstrate two major antigen specificities in patients with vasculitis: antimyeloperoxidase (MPO-ANCA) and antiproteinase-3 (PR3-ANCA). The majority of c-ANCAs (90%) react with proteinases, and most p-ANCAs (90%) are specific for myeloperoxidases (MPO-ANCA). Wegener's granulomatosis is usually associated with c-ANCA (PR3-ANCA) and only rarely with p-ANCA, whereas MPA (see PAN) and Churg–Strauss show the opposite pattern (more likely p-ANCA positive). The p-ANCA of ulcerative colitis is distinct from the p-ANCA of vasculitis in that the ulcerative colitis p-ANCA is DNAse sensitive, meaning that in the presence of DNAse the immunofluorescence pattern disappears. The p-ANCA of ulcerative colitis is thought to be responding to either a histone or a bacterial antigen.

Clinical Presentation

Vascular injury can result in lesions of variable severity, depending on the number, size, and type of vessels involved (arterial vs. venous); the extent of vascular damage; the intensity of the inflammation; the type of inflammatory infiltrate (neutrophils vs. lymphocytes); and other parameters. The GI involvement in different vasculitides varies, and the incidence of GI involvement in some of the common forms of vasculitis is shown in Table 2-7.[105] In the GI tract, severe occlusive vascular damage leads to necrosis, ulceration, or both. Nonocclusive vascular disease may be associated with damage to the structural integrity of the vessel wall and may lead to leakage of blood, resulting in edema and hemorrhage (clinically seen as purpura or petechiae or as GI bleeding). There may be a combination of both types of lesions. The clinical presentation of GI vasculitis is equally variable.[95,97] Most often patients do have involvement of other organ systems, and isolated GI involvement is uncommon. Eighteen patients (27%) out of a series of sixty-five patients with systemic vasculitis had major GI complaints. These included 13/25 patients with PAN (8 classic PAN, 17 microscopic PAN), 4/36 with Wegener's granulomatosis, and 1/4 with Churg–Strauss disease. In a subsequent study of 62 patients with systemic necrotizing vasculitis, GI involvement was seen in 50 (81%) patients. The study included patients with PAN ($n = 38$), microscopic PAN ($n = 4$), Wegener's granulomatosis ($n = 6$), Churg–Strauss syndrome (CSS) ($n = 11$), and rheumatoid arthritis (RA)-associated vasculitis ($n = 3$). The difference in the two studies in the percentage of GI manifestation may be due to different proportion of various vasculitides in the study groups. Abdominal pain is the most common symptom present in almost all patients.[105] Overt lower or upper GI bleeding, ulcers in any segment of the GI tract, appendicitis, cholecystitis, acute pancreatitis, chronic occult blood loss, diarrhea, and intestinal obstruction are other major GI manifestations. Some patients may present with acute surgical abdomen. The diagnosis is primarily made on the basis of renal or skin biopsies.[106] The mortality of patients with GI involvement used to be very high; however, it has decreased over the years. Adverse outcomes are more common in those presenting with an acute abdomen requiring immediate surgery (surgical abdomen).[105]

Different Types of Vasculitides

Large vessel vasculitides. *Giant cell arteritis (synonyms: cranial arteritis, temporal arteritis)* occurs predominantly in elderly people. The estimated incidence is 18.8 per 100,000 people aged over 50 years.

T lymphocytes play a crucial role in the pathogenesis.[107] Major diagnostic criteria proposed by the American Rheumatological Association include age >50 years, recent localized headache, temporal artery tenderness, a positive biopsy, and erythrocyte sedimentation rate >50 mm/h. When three of these criteria are met, a positive diagnosis is likely. For the GI tract, a positive histology can only be obtained in surgical specimens, given the size of the vessel involved. This vasculitis may be associated with polymyalgia rheumatica, a condition primarily manifested as muscle weakness and also associated with elevated serum transaminases.

Histologically, the involved arteries show an inflammation that may extend throughout the entire arterial wall. It is composed mainly of lymphocytes, macrophages, and sometimes multinucleated giant cells. Neutrophils may be present. The infiltrate is unevenly distributed. There is fragmentation of the elastic lamina and elastophagocytosis by the giant cells. In later stages there may be only thickening of the intima. GI involvement is rare, and manifestations include chronic mesenteric ischemia and intestinal perforation. In a series of 248 patients with giant cell arteritis, 15% had involvement of the aorta including the superior mesenteric artery.[106,108]

Takayasu arteritis (Takayasu's disease) occurs especially in young females (before the age of 40) and mostly affects the aortic arch and its major branches. The estimated incidence in Japan is 2 to 3 per million per year. In the Western world, it is probably less frequent. In 10% to 15% of the patients, the celiac trunk and its major branches are involved; however, GI symptoms are infrequent consisting of abdominal pain, diarrhea, or rarely perforation and may mimic IBD. Splanchnic involvement may occur.[105] The pathologic features consist of a chronic inflammatory process extending from the outer aspect of the artery (lymphocytes and macrophages, some giant cells, and plasma cells), with most changes seen in the adventitia and media. Thrombosis is uncommon. The elastic structure of the media is destroyed. The intima is thickened by edematous connective tissue with little cellular infiltration. In the later stage, there is fibrosis.[106]

Thromboangiitis obliterans (Buerger's disease) is a nonatherosclerotic segmental occlusive disease of the small- and medium-sized vessels of unknown etiology.[109] It affects both arteries and veins. The disease is more common in male smokers in their third and fourth decades. Pathologically, there is occlusion of the vessels by distinctive inflammatory thrombi with microabscesses and giant cells. Familial cases occur, and cell-mediated sensitivity to type I and III collagen may be found. Limb ischemia is common but the GI tract is only rarely affected. There are a few well-documented cases of mesenteric involvement leading to small bowel and colonic disease (segmental) with inflammation, ulceration of transverse and sigmoid colons, and even perforation and peritonitis.[109-112] Pathologic findings are often nonspecific except in the acute stage, when tissues are usually not available for diagnosis.

Infectious vasculitides. A variety of infections have been associated with vasculitis (see Table 2-6). The vasculitis can be caused by direct invasion of the endothelial cells by the pathogen, immune complex deposition, and B- or T-cell–mediated vascular injury or both, secondary to molecular mimicry or superantigens.[113,114] For example, *Rickettsia* and *Staphylococcus aureus* can directly infect the endothelium of small arteries and veins resulting in vasculitis.[115,116] *Treponema pallidum* causing syphilis leads to vascular injury largely due to endarteritis obliterans of the vasa vasorum of the large arteries, particularly aorta.[117] Hepatitis C virus (HCV) leads to immune complex deposition and vasculitis in about 5% to 10% of the cases. HCV, in addition, also stimulates the B cells directly that contributes to vascular damage.[114,118] Hepatitis B virus (HBV) also causes vasculitis in about 10% of the infected patients. The mechanism is largely immune complex–mediated and resembles PAN.[119] HCV infection has also been rarely associated with PAN, although the association is less convincing than HBV. Parvovirus B19 has been associated with Henoch–Schönlein pupura, PAN, Wegner's granulomatosis, giant cell arteritis, and Behçet's disease.[120,121] The mechanism is immune complex–mediated and possibly also direct injury to the vessel wall due to infection. The vascular endothelium expresses erythrocyte P antigen, which is the receptor for this virus. CMV is well known to infect the vascular endothelium directly, resulting in intestinal ulcers and perforation.[122] Other microorganisms that have been associated with vascular injury include *Salmonella* species, mycobacteria, zygomyces, and *Aspergillus fumigatus*.

In many of these conditions, the diagnosis of the infection is obvious on the clinical and pathologic grounds, while in some recognition of the vasculitis (e.g., PAN) may initiate the search for the infection (HBV or HCV). The diagnosis of infectious vasculitis is based on clinical findings, positive blood cultures, serologies, and identification of the pathogen on tissue examination.

Medium vessel vasculitides

Kawasaki's Disease Kawasaki's disease (mucocutaneous lymph node syndrome) is an Oriental disease. Caucasian and African American children are rarely affected. The annual incidence in Japan is 700 to 800 per million, which rises to 4,000 to 5,000 in epidemics; however, no known infectious agent has been identified. Most of the children are below the age of 5. In addition to the principal symptoms of high fever, variable exanthema, oral and skin lesions, cervical lymphadenopathy, and bilateral conjunctival congestion can be seen. GI complications can cause deterioration of the general condition can be seen. In the acute phase, abdominal pain, vomiting, and diarrhea are seen. The angiitis inherent with these complications can be separated into four stages: intensive perivasculitis, focal panvasculitis, ongoing inflammation, and finally stenosis and formation of aneurysms.[123]

Polyarteritis Nodosa The first description of PAN dates back from 1866 when a case of a 27-year-old man with fever, abdominal pain, muscle disease, peripheral neuropathy, and renal disease was reported.[100] The authors termed the fatal illness "periarteritis nodosa" because of the cellular infiltrate at the periphery of the vessel wall and referring to nodular protuberances along the course of medium-sized muscular arteries. In 1903 the term "polyarteritis" instead of periarteritis was proposed because inflammation was present at all levels of the affected vessel. Classic PAN is a systemic, necrotizing vasculitis, primary affecting muscular arteries and resulting in lesions of various ages, often with focal aneurysms. Over the years, different forms have been distinguished. These include the "classic" and the "microscopic" forms. The microscopic form now has been recognized as a separate entity unrelated to classic PAN.

Classic PAN characteristically involves medium- and small-sized arteries. Small segments of the muscular arteries are involved, and the lesions at a given time appear in different stages of development. Early lesions are characterized by degeneration of the arterial wall—partial to complete destruction of the external and internal elastic laminae; deposition of fibrinoid material; and infiltrate in and around the vessel composed largely of neutrophils (showing evidence of leukocytoclasis or white blood cell necrosis), often with some eosinophils (Fig. 2-23A,B). In the later stage, there is intimal proliferation, thrombosis leading to ischemia with ulceration, and an infiltrate composed of lymphocytes, histiocytes, and plasma cells. GI complaints are noted in about 25% to 80% of the patients. They include abdominal pain, nausea, vomiting, anorexia, and diarrhea. Vascular occlusion can lead to ischemia with ulceration, bowel infarction, and hemorrhage. In a series of 30 cases 17% had melena and 10% hematemesis.[124] GI bleeding was also noted in another series in 50% of the patients.[125] Serious complications such as "intestinal infarction" occur in about 6% to 15% of all patients.[106] "Related lesions" have been described such as "cryptogenic multifocal stenosing ulcerations of the small intestine."[126]

Medium and small vessel vasculitis (ANCA-associated vasculitides). Wegener's granulomatosis, CSS, and MPA belong to the so-called ANCA-associated vasculitides. There are however ANCA negative cases. The three types are histologically very similar. Wegener's granulomatosis is differentiated from the other two by the presence of necrotizing granulomatous inflammation in the absence of asthma; CSS is differentiated by the presence of asthma, eosinophilia, and necrotizing granulomatous inflammation, and MPA is differentiated by the absence of granulomatous inflammation and asthma.

Wegener's Granulomatosis It is defined by a triad of features: systemic necrotizing "angiitis," necrotizing inflammation of the respiratory tract, and necrotizing glomerulonephritis (limited forms without glomerulonephritis may occur).[102,127] GI involvement is uncommon.[128,129] GI manifestations were present in 4 of 36 patients, but only one had bleeding. In an autopsy review of 59 fatal cases of patients with Wegener's granulomatosis, histologic evidence of GI involvement was found in 23, but symptoms (nausea, abdominal pain, blood loss) were infrequent.[92]

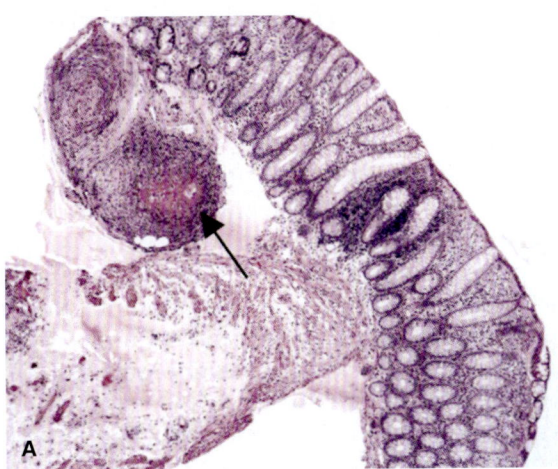
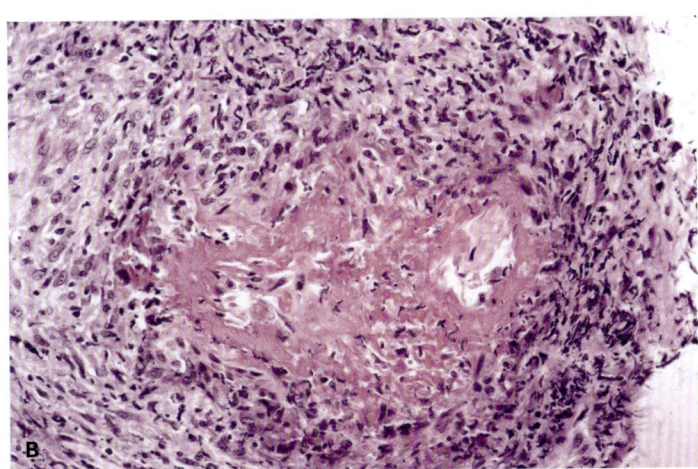

Figure 2-23. Rectal biopsy showing necrotizing vasculitis **(A)** low magnification and **(B)** higher magnification of a submucosal arteriole (*arrow*) in a patient with PAN.

Churg–Strauss Vasculitis (Synonyms: Churg–Strauss Syndrome, Allergic Granulomatous Angiitis, Allergic Granulomatosis, and Angiitis) This is a nonhereditary disease with unclear underlying pathogenic mechanisms. Immunologic defects have been reported, but because of the rarity of the disease there are no data in large studies. Immunologic alterations reported include derangement of CD95 system (resistance to apoptosis) and an increase in CD4– and CD8– T cells.[130] The definition of the disease is unclear because of an overlap with other systemic vasculitides such as PAN and Wegener's granulomatosis and with other inflammatory conditions exhibiting increased eosinophils. Clinically CSS is often defined by the presence of asthma, hypereosinophilia (>10% eosinophils in the blood or 1.5 × 10⁹ eosinophils per liter), and systemic vasculitis involving two or more extrapulmonary organs.[131,132] Approximately 70% of patients with CSS have ANCA (MPO-ANCA in the majority of cases). The incidence of CSS is largely similar in males and females with mild predilection for males. CSS usually presents in the third or fourth decade of life, although it can also occur in children. It presents in several phases (asthma or allergic rhinitis: prodromal phase; hypereosinophilia with eosinophilic pneumonitis or gastroenteritis: second phase; systemic vasculitis: third phase). The three phases not necessarily occur sequentially. GI involvement has been reported in two larger series, one including 154 patients with CSS and one with 146 cases.[133,134] In a Japanese series 21 cases had multiple ulcers (stomach $n = 11$; small intestine $n = 16$; colon $n = 7$) sometimes presenting with perforation (12/21 cases).[134] The small intestine was the most common site of involvement (Figs. 2-24 and 2-25). Endoscopically, colonic ulcers were shallow and irregular in size. Other clinical manifestations are cholecystitis, gastric ulcer, pseudopolyps in the colon similar to ulcerative colitis, and allergic granulomas in the stomach, liver, and omentum.[106] The intestinal lesions may show features similar to eosinophilic gastroenteritis (see Fig. 2-25). Histologically necrotizing vasculitis (infiltration of the wall by eosinophils and granulomatous lesions in the wall of the vessels) and granulomas in the extravascular tissue are present (see Fig. 2-24A–C). The granulomas are composed of histiocytes, and frequently multinucleated giant cells centered around degenerating collagen fibers. In the central portion, there may also be disintegrated cells, particularly eosinophils. Extravascular granulomas in the Japanese series were reported in 48% of cases. The granulomas are not a prerequisite for the diagnosis.[95] The colitis of CSS can mimic ulcerative colitis because the repeated ulcerations can cause diffuse architectural distortion. However, the chronic inflammatory infiltrate is less, and the erosions may be pseudomembrane-like. The vascular lesions are very difficult to detect on endoscopic mucosal biopsies, and just show ischemia with lamina propria fibrosis (see Fig. 2-25). Some patients who present with GI and possibly respiratory symptoms with eosinophilia meet the criteria for CSS and may be labeled as having hypereosinophilic syndrome. GI biopsies may show significant eosinophilic infiltrates in the absence of a definite vasculitis. These patients respond rapidly to corticosteroids.

Related lesions have been reported as "necrotizing granulomatous vasculitis—isolated or limited form of CSS in the GI tract."[133] In this case, involvement of small arteries and veins was noted, and the lesions were limited to the digestive tract. Whether this can be regarded as genuine CSS is unclear.

Microscopic Polyarteritis Nodosa This was formerly called microscopic PAN; however, it differs from classic PAN by the presence of extensive glomerular involvement and involvement of smaller caliber vessels. It is defined as necrotizing vasculitis with few or no immune complexes affecting small vessels including capillaries, venules, or arterioles. Involvement of medium-sized arteries may also be present. Serologic tests for p-ANCA are often positive. GI involvement is common and seen in 30% to 55% of patients.[135,136] Abdominal pain, nausea and vomiting, diarrhea, and blood loss are common manifestations, and some patients may even present with surgical abdomen.

Connective tissue diseases (CTDs) such as *rheumatoid arthritis (RA)* and *systemic lupus erythematosus (SLE)* may have vascular involvement as a major clinical manifestation. Vasculitis rarely precedes other manifestations of the CTD. Most patients with CTD-associated vasculitis have small-vessel involvement affecting the skin, kidneys, or both. In some cases, mesenteric vasculitis similar to that in PAN is found. In RA, GI involvement is observed in approximately 10% of patients[137,138] (Fig. 2-26). The usual presentation is acute abdominal pain due to intestinal ulceration and sometimes perforation and peritonitis. Symptoms can also be the result of amyloid depositions. Rectal or other GI biopsies may help to identify the lesions. Staining with Congo red, Sirius red, or thioflavin T can identify amyloid deposits if sufficient vessels are present in the biopsies.[139,140] In SLE, intestinal manifestations are recognized in more than 50% of the patients. In contrast, systemic vasculitis is uncommon in patients with localized cutaneous chronic discoid lupus erythematosus. In SLE, anorexia and weight loss may occur in more than 50% of patients with active disease. Lupus can affect the entire GI tract, although the small and large intestines are more commonly involved. GI vasculitis occurs in approximately 2% of patients with SLE (Fig. 2-27). Adhesions, ulcers, ileus, protein-losing

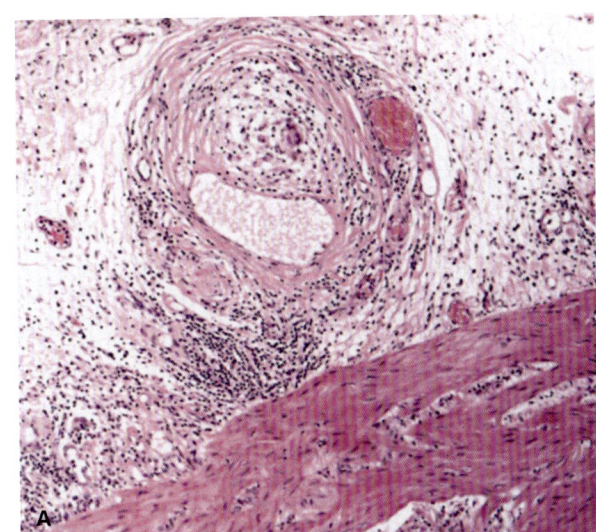
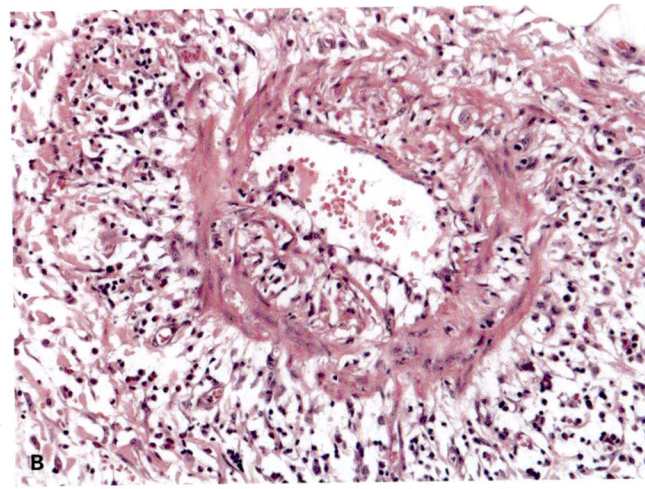

Figure 2-24. A: Granulomatous vasculitis in a subserosal artery of the colon in a patient with (less active) of CSS. CSS is characterized by **(B)** necrotizing vasculitis, and can be associated with impressive transmural inflammation **(C)**.

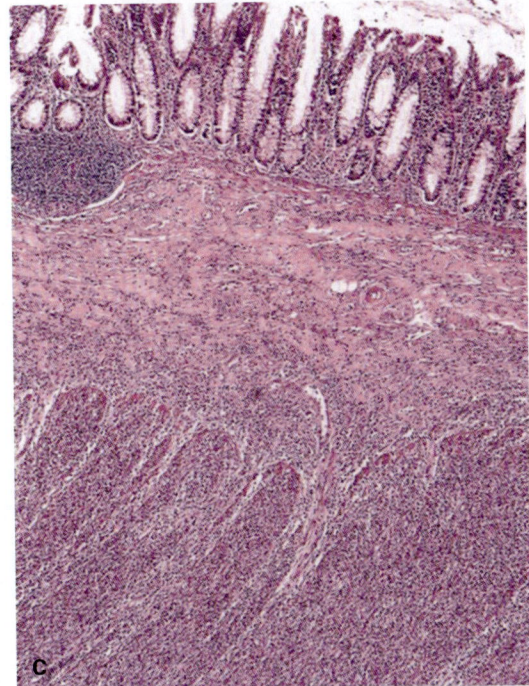

enteropathy, malabsorption, and variable degrees of small and large bowel ischemia are known to occur.[141] Acute abdominal pain may be a result of serositis, pancreatitis, and intraabdominal abscess. Furthermore, patients may have intestinal infarction due to the so-called antiphospholipid syndrome, a disease characterized by arterial and venous thrombosis, thrombocytopenia, recurrent pregnancy loss, and the presence of antiphospholipid antibodies.[142,143] The syndrome can, however, also occur in other CTDs and vasculitides or in the absence of any CTD or vasculitis (primary antiphospholipid syndrome).[144]

Small vessel vasculitis

Henoch–Schönlein Purpura (Anaphylactoid Purpura)
It is the most common form of vasculitis of childhood, presenting usually between 3 and 10 years of age. It usually affects only the smallest blood vessels. Organs commonly involved are the GI tract, skin, joints, and kidneys. The disease affects patients of any age but is most often found in young children (mean age: 4 years). The estimated annual incidence varies between 6.2 and 24 per million children in different parts of the world and also varies depending on the race.[127] The diagnostic criteria include (a) abdominal pain, (b) leukocytoclastic vasculitis with predominant IgA deposition or proliferative glomerulonephritis with predominant IgA deposition, (c) arthritis or arthralgia, and (d) renal involvement with proteinuria or hematuria or the presence of red cell casts. The diagnosis is based on clinical findings. Tissue diagnosis is required only in atypical cases and rests on demonstration of

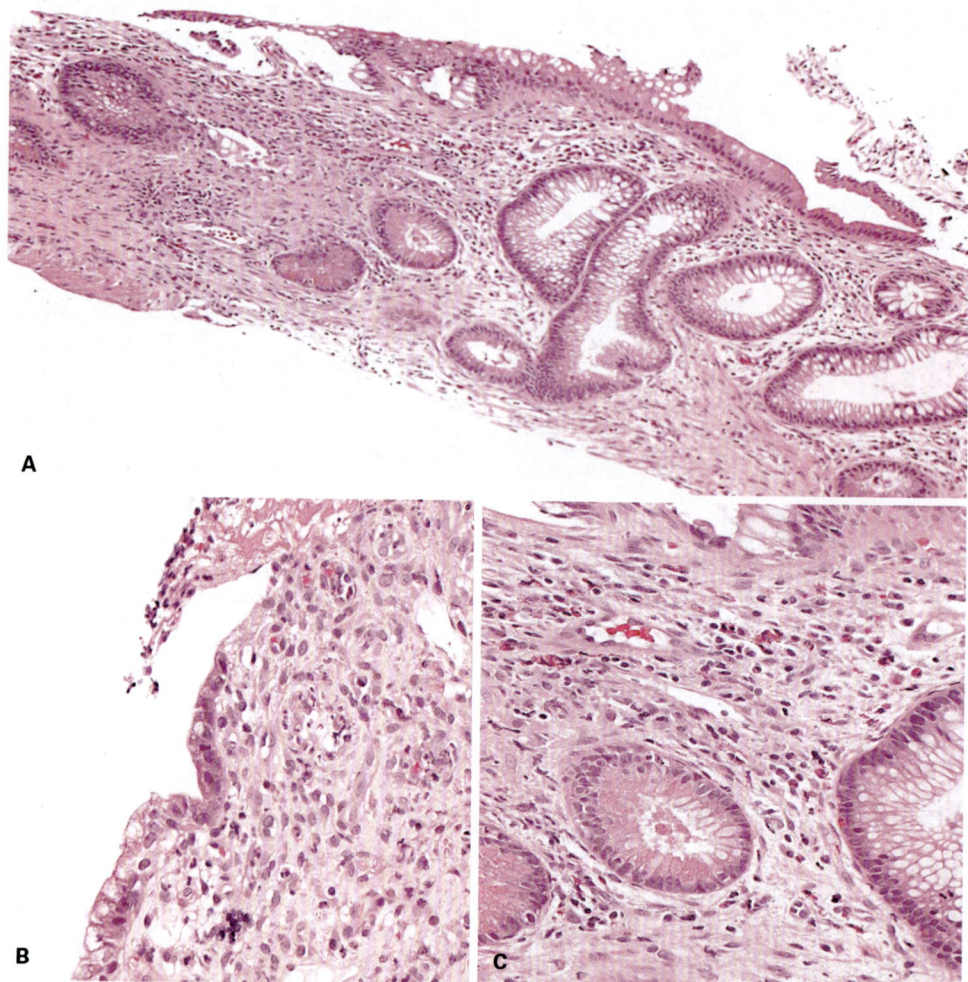

Figure 2-25. A: Biopsy in a 9-year-old child with peripheral eosinophilia and CSS showing colonic ulceration, inflammation, crypt loss and distortion **B,C:** The lamina propria shows increased neutrophils and eosinophils and inflammation around small vessels. Often a specific diagnosis of vasculitis is difficult to make on such mucosal biopsies and correlation with the clinical findings is essential.

IgA deposits in either skin or kidney biopsies.[127] Occasionally, the leukocytoclastic vasculits and IgA deposition may be seen in intestinal biopsies. About 50% to 75% of the patients have GI symptoms such as colicky abdominal pain, nausea, vomiting, melena, or hematemesis. Histologically, the venules are primarily involved, showing a mixed infiltrate composed of neutrophils and mononuclear cells. Nuclear debris is often present within the vessel wall, giving rise to the term "leukocytoclastic vasculitis." Less frequent manifestations include intussusception and bowel infarction, resulting in perforation.[145] Henoch–Schönlein purpura is related to hypersensitivity vasculitis, a heterogeneous group of conditions, associated with immune complexes. Leukocytoclastic vasculitis, not associated with classical Henoch–Schönlein purpura, can also affect the GI tract (Fig. 2-28).[146,147]

Miscellaneous conditions

Paraneoplastic Vasculitis Neoplasias are rarely associated with vasculitis syndromes. Overall, cancer is found in approximately 5% of patients with vasculitis. Only a few reports of vasculitis associated with adenocarcinoma have been published. These include cases of adenocarcinoma of the colon with cutaneous vasculitis in two patients and mesenteric vasculitis (necrotizing) in two other patients. The pathogenesis of vasculitis in cases with malignancy is unknown. It has been suggested that tumor antigens may provoke host reactions and give rise to antigen–antibody complexes that produce inflammation. Another possible mechanism is a direct destructive effect of cancer cells on the vascular wall.[148] Lymphoproliferative and myeloproliferative disorders can also induce vasculitis.

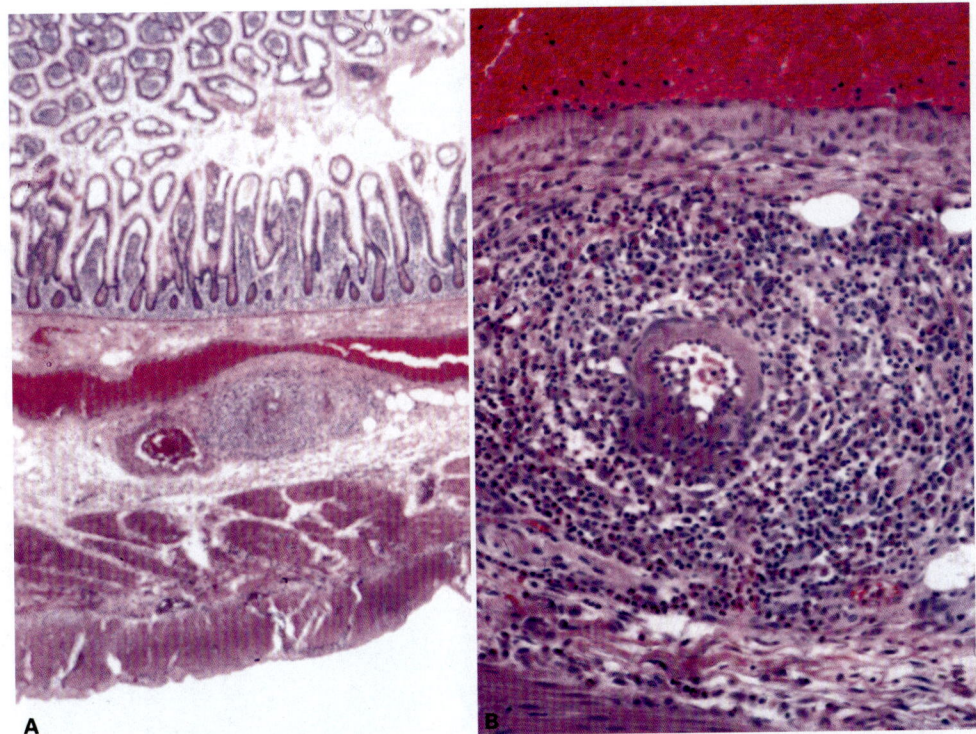

Figure 2-26. **A:** Low magnification showing a section of the small bowel resected for ischemia in a patient with RA. A submucosal artery is seen surrounded by inflammatory cells at this magnification. **B:** Higher magnifications of the same artery showing perivascular mixed inflammatory infiltrate and fibrinoid necrosis of the wall.

Enterocolic Lymphocytic Phlebitis

LYMPHOCYTIC PHLEBITIS (MESENTERIC INFLAMMATORY VENOOCCLUSIVE DISEASE, MYOINTIMAL HYPERPLASIA OF MESENTERIC VEINS). This condition is characterized by a diffuse lymphocytic inflammation involving the veins of the small and large bowels (Fig. 2-29A–C), fibrinoid necrosis, and secondary thrombosis, with lack of systemic involvement.[149] The lymphocytic infiltrate is composed of a mixture of T and B lymphocytes. This condition is probably related to two other conditions reported as "mesenteric inflammatory venoocclusive disease" and "myointimal hyperplasia of mesenteric veins." Mesenteric inflammatory venoocclusive disease is characterized by polymorphonuclear inflammation and subsequent thrombosis involving arteries as well as veins.[150] Idiopathic myointimal hyperplasia of mesenteric veins is a descriptive term for a microscopic lesion consisting of proliferation of smooth muscle cells in a proteoglycan matrix (Fig. 2-29 D,E). It was first described in four previously healthy patients with a short history of abdominal pain, diarrhea, and often blood in stools. Colonoscopy showed changes consistent with colitis. Mucosal biopsies usually do not confirm or refute a clinical suspicion of IBD, but may show dilated, thick-walled blood vessels or ulceration. No vasculitis is seen. A relation with heterozygous factor V Leiden has been suggested.[151] It may be speculated that there also exists minor forms such as the entity called "lymphocytic vasculitis."[152] Rare cases have been described that show necrotizing granulomatous inflammation of veins (Necrotizing granulomatous phlebitis) that may be limited to mesenteric vessels.

Behçet's Disease Behçet's disease (Behçet's syndrome) is a multisystemic disorder of unclear etiology that can also involve the GI tract in two main forms. (a) In Europe and North America, the GI involvement is indistinguishable from large bowel Crohn's disease pathologically, and usually no vasculitis is identified. (b) However, in Japan, in particular, there are large, often solitary, ulceroinflammatory lesions primarily involving the terminal ileum and cecum (see Chapter 18). The problem is that NSAIDs were clearly not excluded as a possible etiology for the ileocecal ulcers in the Japanese patients, especially in the setting of an arthritis for which NSAIDs may well have been taken. It is therefore difficult to know whether these ulcers are the results of Behçet's-associated vasculitis or NSAIDs, unless a resection is carried out and vasculitis found to support the diagnosis of Behçet's disease. Even when vasculitis is seen, it is unclear if this is primarily a vasculitic disease. The vasculitis can involve any sized blood vessel and typically represents a lymphocytic vasculitis, although in cases neutrophils may be prominent (Fig 2-29 F,G).[153]

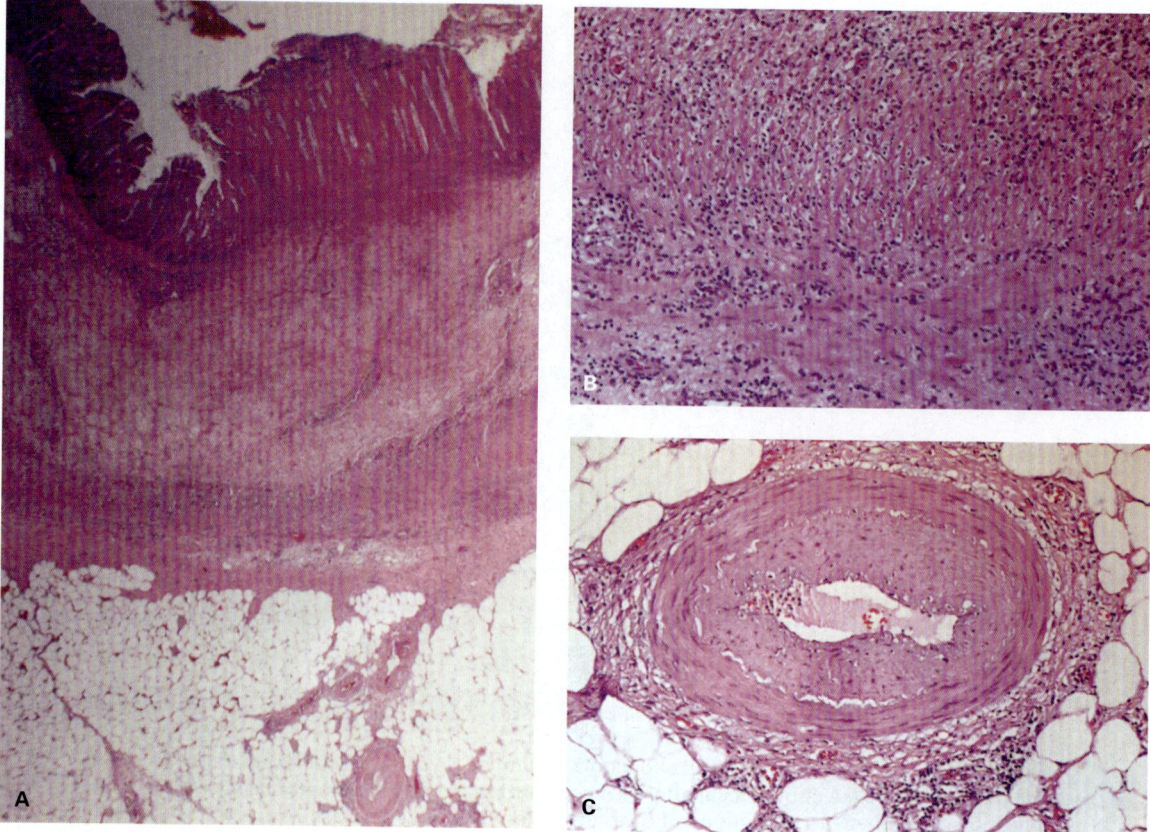

Figure 2-27. Focal ischemic necrosis due to SLE. **A:** Low-power view of full thickness of colon showing ischemic necrosis of the mucosa and part of muscularis propria. **B:** High-power view of muscularis propria showing necrosis of inner circular muscle coat and neutrophilic infiltrate. **C:** High-power view of small serosal artery showing severe endarteritis obliteration and periadventitial inflammation.

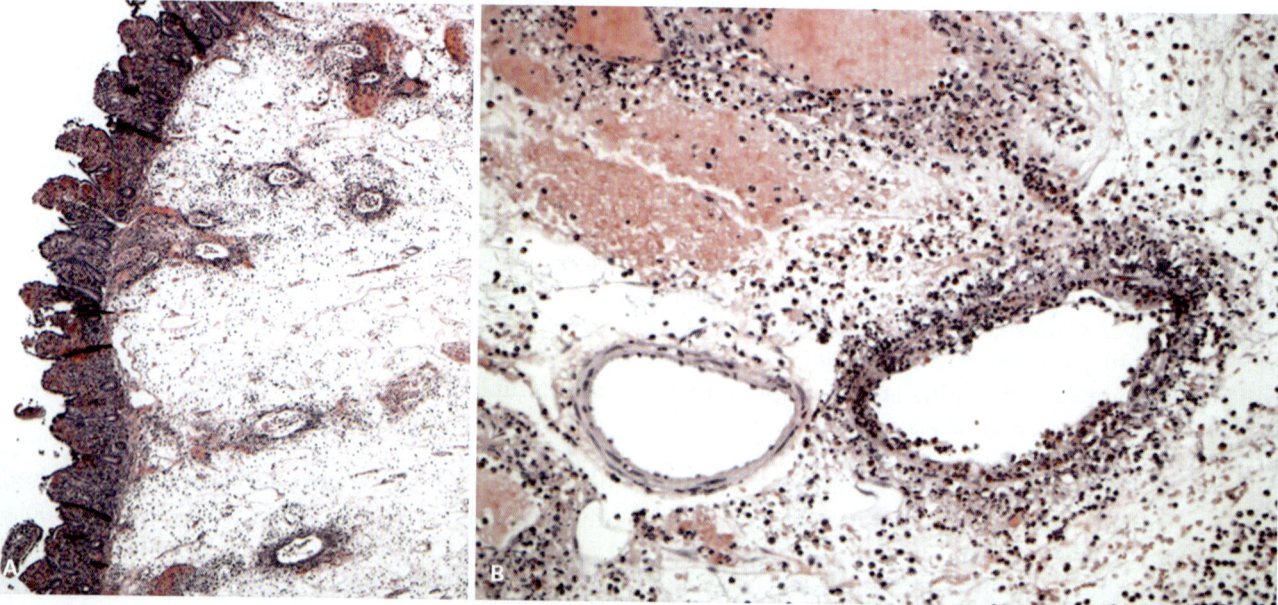

Figure 2-28. **A:** Low magnification of the small bowel showing ischemic changes in the mucosa, edema and perivascular inflammatory infiltrates around the submucosal vessels. **B:** Higher magnification showing the neutrophils and lymphocytes, and prominent nuclear fragmentation typical of leukocytoclastic vasculitis. This patient did not have Henoch–Schönlein purpura, although the histologic changes would be identical.

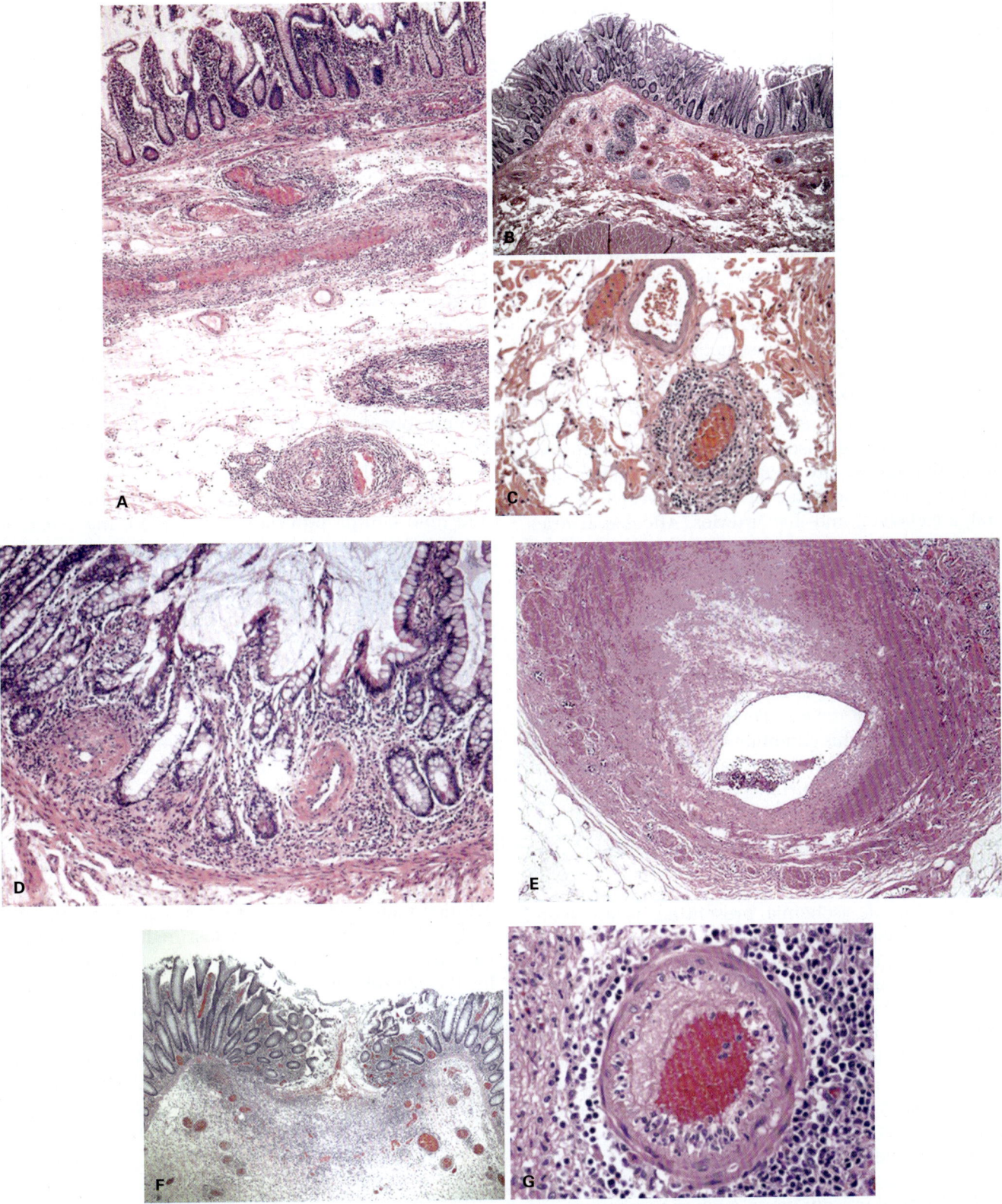

Figure 2-29. **A:** Lymphocytic phlebitis involving small intestine showing diffuse perivascular inflammation and secondary thrombosis. **B:** Lymphocytic phlebitis involving colon showing diffuse perivascular inflammation at low magnification, and **(C)** higher magnification showing lymphocytic infiltrate in the vein wall. Note that an adjacent artery appears completely uninvolved. Lymphocytic phlebitis is probably related with "myointimal hyperplasia of mesenteric veins," a condition characterized by a thickening of the tunica intima in mesenteric veins but sometimes also in mucosal blood vessels **(D)** or mesenteric vessels **(E)**. Behçet's disease showing colonic ulcer with overhanging edges **(F)**. Close up the submucosa showing lymphocytic vasculitis in the same case **(G)**.

Usually, the submucosal veins and sometimes the arteries are involved. ANCA is generally negative, and granulomas are not seen.

Malignant-atrophic papulosis (Kohlmeier–Degos Syndrome). This is a rare cutaneovisceral disease of young adults, commonly involving the GI tract, conjunctiva, and choroid plexus.[154,155] It is characterized by progressive, occlusive vascular disease of small- and medium-sized vessels showing endothelial cell swelling, intimal proliferation, thrombosis, and sometimes fibrinoid necrosis. The diagnosis is usually established in conjunction with the clinical setting. GI manifestations include patchy necrosis, infarction, peritonitis, and intestinal obstruction.[156,157]

Fibromuscular Arterial Dysplasia This is an uncommon though well-recognized nonatherosclerotic cause of stenosing vasculopathy and hypertension, which frequently involves the renal arteries and less frequently the internal carotid, vertebral, visceral, subclavian, and iliac arteries. Affected arteries tend to be occlusive primarily, and secondary events include aneurysm, dissection, and arteriovenous fistula. Excess of smooth muscle or fibrous tissue with thickening of the wall causes stenosis. Alternatively deficiencies of elastic or fibromuscular tissue can cause aneurysm and dissections. Several pathogenic mechanisms have been proposed, including hormonal effects on smooth muscle, genetic factors, and mural ischemia. Rarely, this condition can involve GI vessels such as the superior mesenteric artery, in children and adults.[158] A familial occurrence has been noted.[159–161]

Biopsy Diagnosis of Ischemic Colitis and Differential Diagnosis

Cases of colonic ischemia presenting as an acute emergency, with abdominal pain and rectal bleeding, usually pose no diagnostic problem. Histologic examination of endoscopic biopsies or a surgical specimen will confirm the diagnosis. The majority of problematic cases, however, are due to less severe forms of ischemia. The presence of specific lesions such as hyalinization of the lamina propria and atrophic-appearing crypts is however highly diagnostic. If these lesions are observed in biopsies in a clinical setting of an elderly patient, with sharply demarcated lesions on endoscopy, the diagnosis is obvious. With atypical clinical presentations, such as those in young patients, or when the clinical information is not available, we usually sign out these biopsies as "ischemic-type" colitis. In such a situation other conditions such as drug-induced lesions, adhesions, the presence of peritoneal metastases, and other less common causes of ischemic colitis including vasculitis and amyloidosis, should be considered. Various drugs can, for example, cause ischemic lesions either through vasculitis or through an impairment of the blood flow (see also iatrogenic lesions). In several cases, the presentation and histology of ischemic colitis may be less typical. The acute clinical presentation may mimic acute infectious colitis, pseudomembranous colitis, and even ulcerative colitis. Later in the course of the illness it may clinically resemble Crohn's disease or a carcinoma. In some of these cases, the biopsy will still show the typical features of ischemia. Histology may also show simple necrosis or ulceration with mild inflammation in the adjacent mucosa or mucosal fibrosis in association with hemosiderin-laden macrophages, which are not diagnostic. Occasionally, the biopsy may show changes suggestive of IBD such as diffuse glandular distortion and atrophy (which is probably due to earlier injury with necrosis and loss of crypts followed by repair) and inflammation with neutrophils in the lamina propria and cryptitis. Superficial cryptitis, a normal mucosal architecture and mild lamina propria inflammation, may suggest acute infectious colitis. Rarely, granuloma formation can be observed.[162] The inflammatory reaction may be explained by a disturbed mucosal permeability and bacterial translocation. This inflammatory pattern can be observed in samples from patients with vasculitis and in the so-called obstructive colitis.

"Obstructive colitis" occurs usually in the elderly in a background of generalized atherosclerosis. The obstruction is most frequently secondary to a tumor or in the setting of diverticular disease, but any disturbance of motility can be responsible. The histology is essentially the same as that for the earlier stages of ischemic colitis, but in addition, inflammation is more prominent. The histologic changes such as a mixed inflammatory infiltrate, crypt abscesses, and mucosal ulceration and fibrosis are not diagnostic, and the diagnosis is often "colitis unclassified."[85] In less typical cases, a diagnosis of ischemia may be suggested by the age of the patient, associated cardiovascular disease, and x-ray appearances such as thumbprinting. In many patients, a diagnosis of ischemia may have to await the outcome of the disease. For example, resolution of the symptoms within several weeks is suggestive of a reversible ischemic episode. The development of strictures within 1 to 3 months of the onset of symptoms also suggests ischemia, providing, of course, that the clinical setting is right.

Stercoral ulcers

Impacted hard feces can result in ischemia of the underlying mucosa leading to ulceration referred to as stercoral ulcers. They are associated with constipation and most commonly occur in the rectosigmoid.[163] Clinically, stercoral ulcers are usually asymptomatic

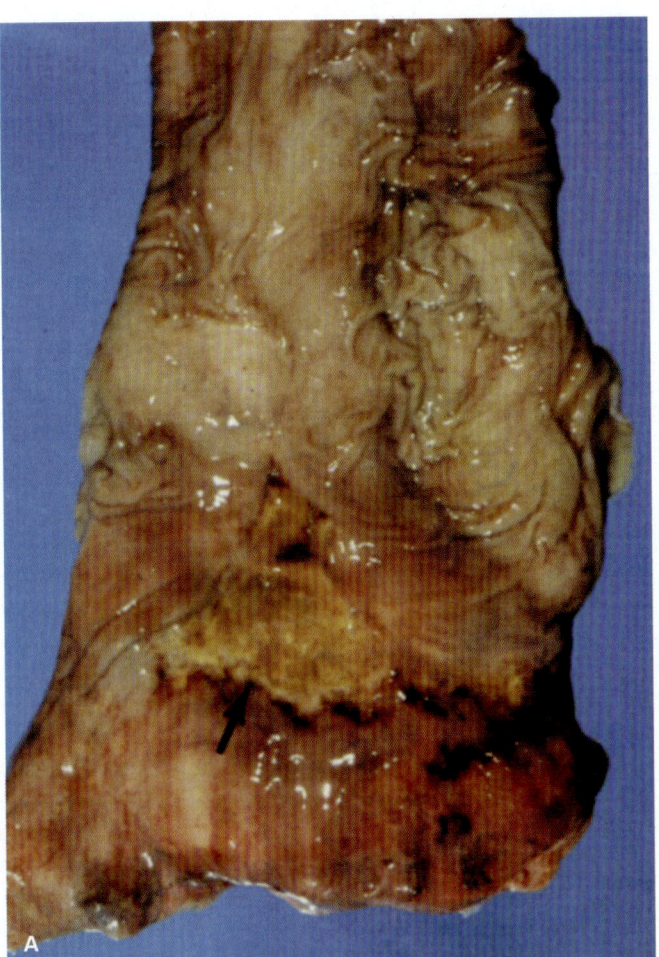
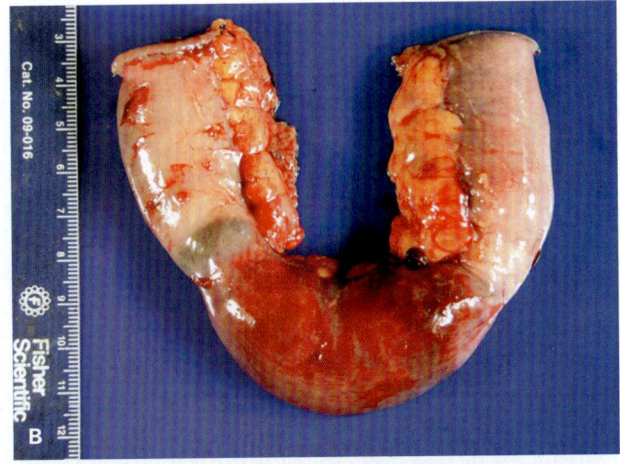
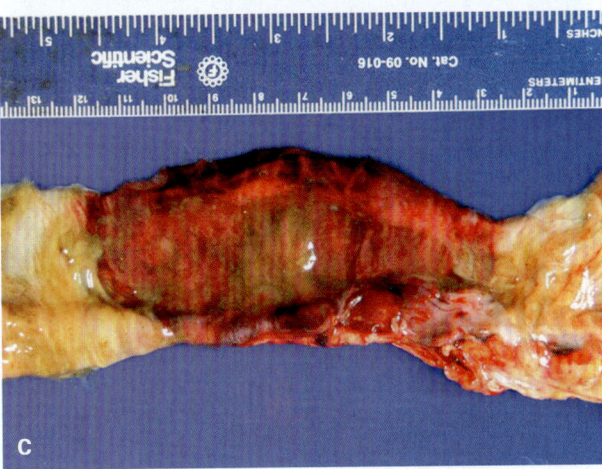

Figure 2-30. **A:** Stercoral ulceration of the lower rectum. The ulcer bed is slightly depressed and greenish brown in appearance, with an irregular margin (*arrow*). Intestinal ischemia due to mechanical obstructions. **B:** Segmental ischemia of small intestine due to strangulation in a hernia sac. Note the intense red-purple discoloration due to hemorrhage and the dulling of the serosal surface of the infarcted bowel. **C:** Same specimen when opened up also shows similar sharply demarcated areas of mucosa necrosis.

for long periods, unless complications ensue, which include occult bleeding, occasionally massive hemorrhage, or rarely perforation and peritonitis. Rarely the perforation and peritonitis can be fatal.[163,164] It is a relatively common condition in the elderly, with a reported incidence of about 5% in one study of 175 consecutive adult autopsies.[165] Some of the patients with constipation and underlying renal disease with hyperkalemia tend to develop stercoral ulcers, due to ingestion of nonabsorbable antacids (especially magnesium and aluminum hydroxide) and cation-exchange resins.[166] Usually, the ulcers are single, but they can be multiple, and often the impacted stool is still attached at the ulcer site in the resected specimens (Fig. 2-30A). The ulcer has an irregular margin, and its base is depressed and has a yellow-gray to greenish discoloration. The histology of the ulcer is entirely nonspecific, and the inflammation may extend into the underlying muscularis propria or deeper. The bowel wall beneath the ulcer may be thinned and stretched and is susceptible to perforation. Vascular changes are not striking, although fibrin thrombi may be seen. Treatment of uncomplicated stercoral ulceration consists of careful removal of the impacted fecal mass, care being taken to avoid perforation of the thinned bowel. Treatment of perforation is surgical and is accompanied by a high mortality rate.

MECHANICAL OBSTRUCTION AND ISCHEMIA OF THE DIGESTIVE TRACT

Pathogenesis and Clinical Features

Mechanical obstructions due to adhesions, carcinoma, hernias, volvulus, and intussusception are important causes of acute intestinal obstruction and vascular compromise. Adhesions are by far the most common cause, accounting for approximately 75% of these cases, followed by malignancy (10%), hernia (10%), and others (5%).[167] The introduction of laparoscopic surgery reduces, the incidence of adhesions and incisional hernias.[168-171] All the types of mechanical obstruction listed above initially cause compression of veins, producing vascular congestion and edema. With progression, further compromise of the vascular supply occurs, ultimately occluding the arterial blood supply, often with accompanying thrombosis of veins and arteries. This results in intestinal infarction and, depending on the site of obstruction, may lead to perforation and peritonitis. Nonoperative treatment may be used for 24 to 48 hours provided that no signs of strangulations develop.[172] Preoperative detection of intestinal ischemia due to adhesions or hernia and intraoperative assessment of the viability of the intestinal segment are difficult. A systemic inflammatory response may suggest advanced ischemia. CT examination is a sensitive but not completely specific preoperative indicator of intestinal ischemia.[173]

Adhesions

Adhesions are an important postoperative complication.[174] The incidence of adhesion formation after a single abdominal operation is high, with an incidence over a lifetime of 47% after appendectomy and up to 91% after pelvic surgery.[175] The incidence is however reduced with laparoscopic surgery.[168] Adhesion formation is a form of peritoneal wound healing. The injury of the peritoneum may be inflammatory or surgical and may include exposure to infection or to intestinal contents. Ischemia or irritation from foreign materials such as sutures, gauze particles, or glove dusting powder; abrasion; desiccation; and overheating by lamps or irrigation fluid may also lead to adhesions. Rarely, congenital fibrous bands occur in the absence of inflammation. Adhesions often create fibrous bridges through which loops of bowel may slide and become trapped, thus predisposing them to the same complications as a hernia sac. Volvulus is another complication.

Hernias

Hernias consist of intestinal protrusions through weaknesses or defects in the wall of the peritoneal cavity. They can be either external or internal. External hernias are far more common and are due to defects in the anterior abdominal wall. Internal hernias occur either within the abdominal cavity or into the retroperitoneum through defects in the posterior wall of the abdominal cavity. Segments of viscera, usually small intestine, often become trapped in these sacs. The narrowed necks of the hernia sacs frequently obstruct venous return, producing congestion and edema. This increases the bulk of the tissues, which then become trapped in the hernia sac, a so-called irreducible or incarcerated hernia. Continued vascular impairment results in infarction (Fig. 2-30B,C). A *Richter's* hernia occurs when only part of the circumference of the bowel becomes incarcerated in the hernia sac.

Clinically, patients with incarcerated hernias have the signs and symptoms of acute or subacute intestinal obstruction, which if unrelieved may progress to intestinal strangulation, infarction, and gangrene.[176,177] Some hernias, especially the internal ones, may be difficult to diagnose even at operation, because the trapped loops of bowel may have been reduced spontaneously by the time of investigation or operation.

Hernia of the anterior abdominal wall. These consist of the *inguinal* and *femoral hernias*, the *incisional* or *ventral hernias* occurring at sites of previous operation, the rare *epigastric hernias* through the linea alba, and the *umbilical hernias*. Almost all are associated with increased intra-abdominal pressure.

Inguinal and femoral hernia. These hernias are by far the most common, accounting for about 80% of all hernias. They may be congenital or acquired and may result from any condition that chronically increases intra-abdominal pressure, such as marked obesity, abdominal strain from heavy exercise or lifting, or a chronic cough. Complications are more frequent with femoral hernias because of their narrow, unyielding necks.

Umbilical hernia. These hernias can be acquired or congenital. Most umbilical hernias in adults are in fact paraumbilical protrusions through the linea alba and occur in females who have had multiple pregnancies with prolonged labor. True acquired umbilical hernias are rare and occur most frequently in cirrhotic patients with ascites.[178,179]

Internal hernias. Internal abdominal hernias account for 0.2% to 0.9% of all cases of intestinal obstruction.[180,181] They develop when one or more viscera extrude through an intraperitoneal orifice but remain within the peritoneal cavity. The orifice may be normal (Winslow foramen, the opening between the lesser and greater omenta) or paranormal (peritoneal fossae: paraduodenal, ileocecal, inter- and mesosigmoid, paracolic, supravesical, of the large ligament of the uterus). All these hernias possess a sac and are true hernias. The orifice may be abnormal or pathologic in origin if formed in a mesentery or an omentum (transmesenteric, transmesocolic, transomental, by colo-omental disinsertion) or in the form of an anomalous orifice if it occurs in a congenital anomaly of a ligament (falciform ligament of liver) or a mesentery (mesentery of Meckel's diverticulum). All these hernias lack a sac and are "internal prolapses or procidentia."[181]

Internal herniations include (a) herniations into anomalous defects through the mesenteries, especially the mesocolon and omentum; (b) herniations into the foramen of Winslow, the opening between the greater and lesser omenta; and (c) retroperitoneal hernias (see Chapter 16).

Volvulus

Volvulus occurs when a portion of intestine twists on itself, causing marked distention and obstruction of the rotated segment and compromising blood flow through the mesentery. Volvulus of the colon occurs most commonly in the sigmoid colon, followed by the cecum and proximal colon.[182] Sigmoid volvulus is infrequent in children and more common in the elderly. The incidence is higher in male patients. Two clinical presentations have been reported: an acute fulminant presentation with the sudden onset of severe cramping abdominal pain, distension, nausea, and vomiting, and another type characterized by recurrent abdominal pain. Volvulus of the sigmoid colon is usually associated with an excessively mobile long mesentery with a narrow attachment zone. Such a dolichomesocolon (wider than long) is more common in men.[183,184] Aggravating factors include adhesions and overloading of the luminal contents of the sigmoid. The number of ganglion cells in the Meissner's and Auerbach's plexuses in specimens from patients operated for volvulus is not different from those found in control samples.[185] Cecal volvulus is an axial twist of the cecum, ascending colon, and terminal ileum around a mesenteric pedicle. Its original description was by Rokitansky in 1837 as a cause of intestinal strangulation. Cecal volvulus is relatively uncommon with an incidence of 2.8 to 7.1 per million people per year.[186] It results from defects in peritoneal fixation, leading to laxity and mobility of the cecum and the right side of the colon. Volvulus can also involve the stomach, small intestine, and Meckel's diverticulum. Volvulus of the stomach is most often seen in patients with large diaphragmatic hernias; rotation occurs around the axis of the pylorus and cardia, the two fixed points of the stomach. Midgut volvulus occurs primarily in the neonate because of malrotation and fixation defects of the small intestine. Intestinal volvulus can also occur as a result of adhesion formation following intestinal inflammation.[187]

Intussusception

Intussusception develops when a portion of the bowel (intussusceptum) telescopes or invaginates into a distal portion (the intussuscipiens) resulting in venous congestion leading to intestinal obstruction (Fig. 2-31). As the intussusceptum pulls its mesentery along with it, it causes compression of the vessels and vascular compromise. Intussusception is the most common cause of intestinal obstruction in children younger than 2 years. The incidence varies. In Denmark, a decrease from 16 cases per 10,000 person-years in 1980 to 8.5 cases in year 2000 was noted. The clinical presentation is usually acute, with the sudden onset of intermittent colicky pain. Predisposing conditions are inverted Meckel's diverticula and appendicitis. Viral infections such as those caused by adenovirus, rotavirus, and human herpes virus 6, and oral vaccines against rotavirus have been reported to be associated with intussusception. Lymphoid hyperplasia around the ileocecal region has been suggested as often the "lead point" in the pathogenesis. In older children and adults a demonstrable lesion at

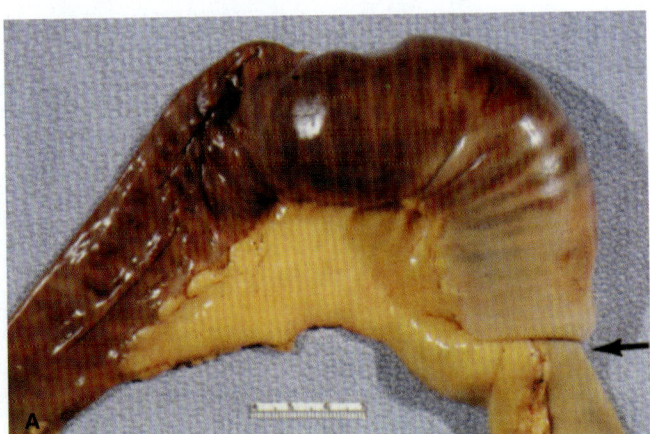 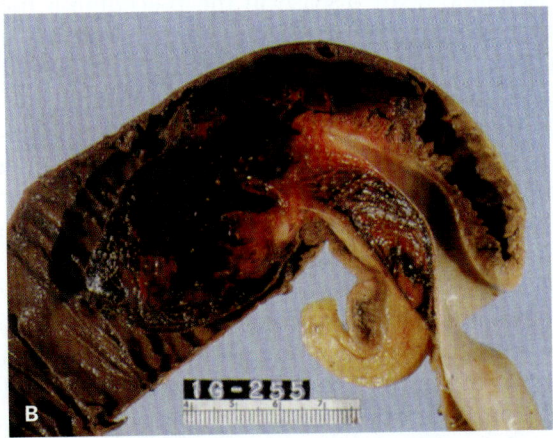

Figure 2-31. Intussusception of the small bowel. **A:** External appearance showing swelling and hemorrhage due to vascular compromise of the intussuscepted bowel. The point of intussusception can be seen at the right margin of the specimen (*arrow*). **B:** Same specimen as part (**A**) opened longitudinally to show the infarcted and intussuscepted portion of small bowel.

the lead point is present in over 90% of cases, with neoplasms accounting for 65% of them in adults. The likelihood of a malignancy is greater in the colon. Less common etiologies include postoperative factors (adhesion, suture line, tubes) and miscellaneous causes (Meckel's diverticulum, sprue, human immunodeficiency virus, duplications, intramural hematoma). Adult patients present more commonly with recurrent bowel obstruction and pass blood per rectum. Fewer than 20% present acutely with complete bowel obstruction.[188] In adults, it can be difficult to localize the site of intussusception at the time of presentation with imaging (such as by CT scan, by transcutaneous ultrasound, or with barium imaging). It is recommended that when the diagnosis is suspected, an ultrasound be obtained as soon as possible. This is a simple, cheap, noninvasive method for diagnosing the problem. An alternative is to get a plain abdominal x-ray at the time of the acute pain at least to document that some type of obstruction is occurring.

IATROGENIC DISORDERS OF THE VASCULAR SYSTEM

Causes of iatrogenic disorders of the vascular system of the GI tract include drugs, trauma and irradiation, and chemotherapy-induced injury. They can be responsible for either ischemia or GI bleeding, but may also cause obstruction and strictures.

Iatrogenic Intestinal Ischemia

Iatrogenic intestinal ischemia involves mostly the colon, although all segments of the GI tract can be affected. Clinically evident colonic ischemia arises preferentially in people with prior abdominal complaints, a history of ischemic heart disease in the preceding 6 months, abdominal surgery in the past month, and the use of drugs with a side effect of constipation (e.g., anticholinergics, opioids, etc.). Many of the patients already have intrinsic vascular disease.[189] In young adults, drugs may be more important (see Table 2-4).[59] Iatrogenic intestinal ischemia falls into two categories: (a) secondary to arterial obstruction or constriction or both and (b) due to reduction in blood pressure and blood volume.

Arterial obstruction or constriction. Arterial obstruction can be due to ligation or trauma of vessels during surgery, other therapeutic or diagnostic procedures, and drugs. Intestinal infarction may sometimes result from the unintentional embolization of adjacent vessels during embolization for treating GI bleeding (Figs. 2-32 and 2-33). For example, embolization of the left gastric artery can result in extensive gastric infarction.

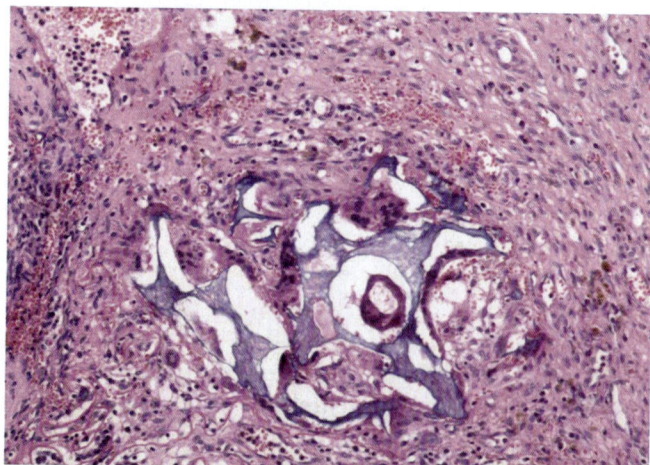

Figure 2-32. A case of ischemic gastric ulceration showing foreign body embolus (gelfoam) in a medium-sized artery following therapeutic embolization for severe GI bleeding in a patient with Henoch–Schönlein pupura.

Angiography may induce arterial obstruction, through contrast medium injected into the wall of a major vessel or when atheromatous plaques or thrombi are dislodged. This usually affects the aorta or superior mesenteric artery.

Drug-induced vascular lesions. Drug-induced vascular lesions can be due to coagulation, vasoconstriction, low blood flow, or vasculitis. Drug-induced obstruction or vasoconstriction can be due to oral contraceptive pills, nonselective NSAIDs and selective cyclooxygenase (COX)-2 inhibitors (rofecoxib, meloxicam), ergot alkaloids, cocaine, vasopressin and other vasoconstrictors, neuroleptics, sumatriptan succinate (a serotonin-1/5-hydroxytryptamine-1 receptor agonist), Alosetron hydrochloride

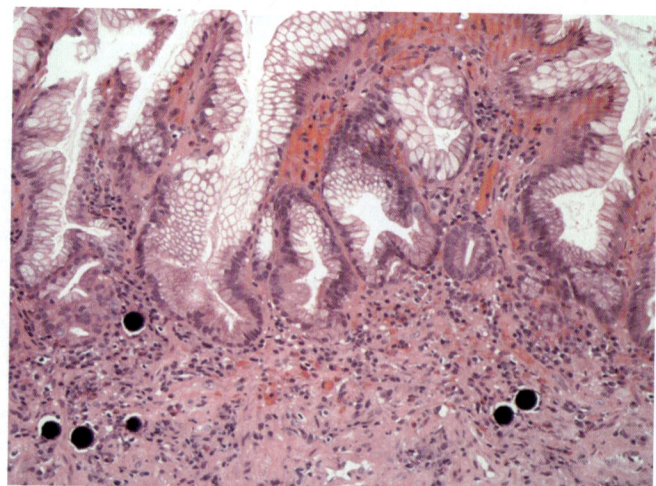

Figure 2-33. Endoscopic biopsy from a stomach with ischemic erosions in a patient who underwent chemoembolization of a hepatocellular carcinoma chemotherapeutic beads accidentally entered the left gastric artery. The round beads are easily identified within the vessels.

(a selective 5-hydroxytryptamine-3 receptor antagonist) used for the treatment of diarrhea-predominant irritable bowel syndrome, and some hormonal drugs such as flutamide (antiandrogenic).[65,190–195] While irritable bowel syndrome is said to be associated with increased rates of ischemic colitis, the use of alosteron further increases the risk. The absolute risk is less at approximately 1 case per 1,000 patient-years.[69] Estrogen and oral contraceptives are causes of iatrogenic hypercoagulation disorders, and these may be potentiated by anticoagulants.[196–198] Hypercoagulation can involve all vessels, including those of the gut, especially the superior mesenteric artery. There is evidence that the risk is related to the dosage of estrogen, especially dosages >0.5 mg daily. Recent formulations of oral contraceptives seem much safer. Smoking and hypertension are additional risk factors.[198] On histologic examination, in addition to finding recent thrombotic occlusion, there is frequent evidence of previous thrombosis characterized by focal marked intimal proliferation and an intact internal elastic lamina indicating the absence of an underlying vasculitis. For nonselective NSAIDs, an effect upon the isozymes COX-1 and COX-2 has been proposed. These isozymes catalyze the conversion of arachidonic acid to eicosanoids, which play a role in the platelet–vessel wall interaction. Thromboxane, the major COX-1 product of arachidonic acid metabolism in platelets, causes platelet aggregation and vasoconstriction.

Ergot compounds are generally safe, but in some instances colitis with rare perforations and strictures have been recorded as a result of vasoconstriction. Sumatriptan may induce vasopressor responses that are distinct from the cranial circulation. The relationship between the drug and ischemia is, however, not always clear. Marketing of Alosetron, a drug developed for irritable bowel syndrome, was suspended after reports of colonic ischemia. Subsequent studies showed that rates of colonic ischemia among patients with a diagnosis of irritable bowel syndrome are higher than those in the general population. Colonic ischemia may therefore constitute a distinct part of the irritable bowel natural history or alternatively be a consequence of therapy.[195]

Reduction in blood pressure or volume can be due to a variety of drugs (antihypertensive drugs, diuretics, digoxin) (see Table 2-1). Local reduction of blood flow may play a role in Kayexalate–sorbitol (sodium polystyrene sulfonate)–induced necrosis. Kayexalate is given as an enema or orally for the treatment of hyperkalemia. It has been reported to induce intestinal necrosis in uremic patients. Necrosis is the common lesion observed in endoscopic and surgical specimens of the stomach, small intestine, and colon. The mechanism of the mucosal damage is unclear. Experimental evidence suggests that the sorbitol component of the drug, rather than Kayexalate itself, is involved in the pathogenesis of the necrosis. Sorbitol is metabolized by colonic bacteria to short-chain fatty acids. If the concentration of these acids exceeds the patient's absorption capacity, osmotic entrance of fluid into the GI lumen occurs with subsequent necrosis. It has indeed been shown that rats receiving enemas of Kayexalate in water developed no lesions while 6 in 10 rats receiving sorbitol enemas showed transmural colonic necrosis. Nevertheless, the lesions induced by Kayexalate can be recognized due to the presence of characteristic Kayexalate crystals (Fig. 2-34).[199,200] The crystals on hematoxylin and eosin stains are polygonal, opaque, slightly basophilic to amphophilic and are not birefringent. It must be remembered that other resins besides Kayexalate are also used clinically. For instance, Questran (cholestyramine) is an orally administered resin that binds to bile acids. The histologic changes induced

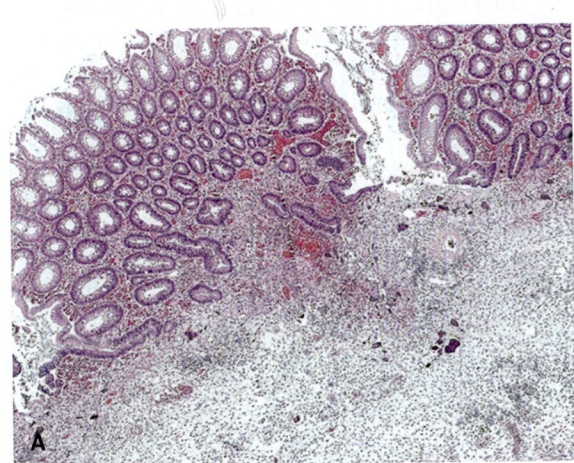
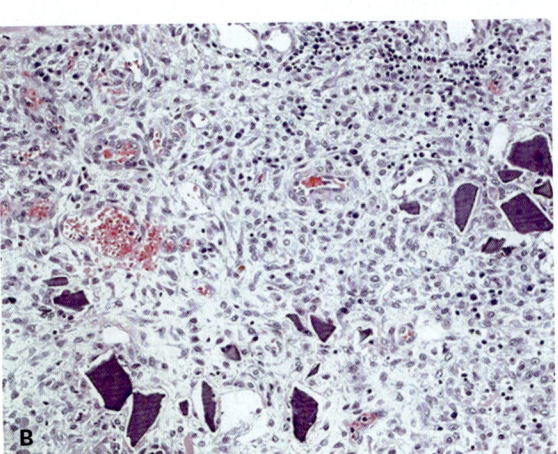

Figure 2-34. Biopsies in a patient with ischemic colitis secondary to Kayexalate use. **A:** Low magnification showing mucosal ulceration and presence of multiple kayexalate crystals in embedded in the submucosa. **B:** Higher magnification to show the typical morphology of the crystals.

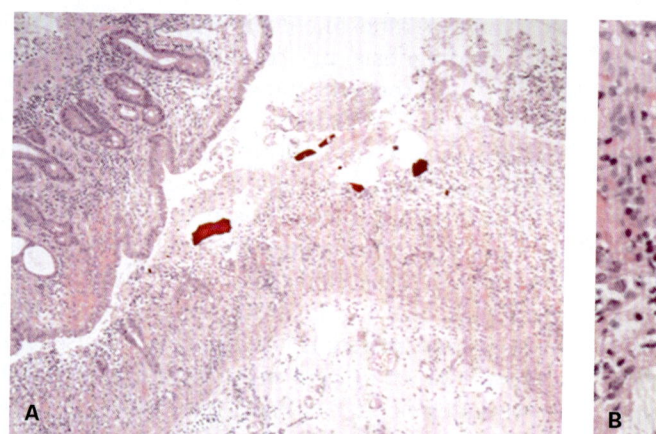 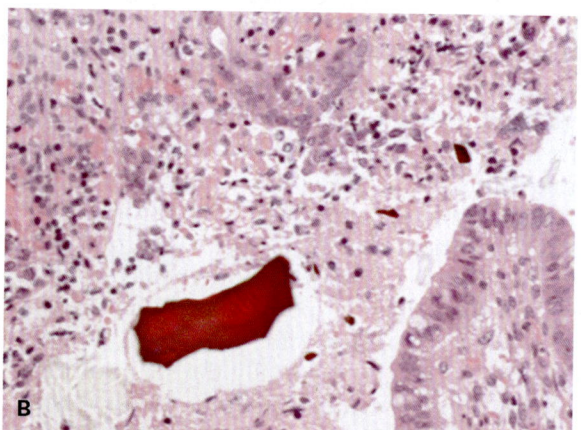

Figure 2-35. Biposies in a patient with ischemic colitis secondary to Questran use. **A:** Low magnification showing mucosal ulceration and presence of multiple Questran crystals embedded in surface exudate. **B:** Higher magnification to show the typical morphology of the crystals.

by Questran are very similar to those induced by Kayexalate, except that Questran tends to be more opaque and more pinkish (Fig. 2-35). With acid-fast stains, Kayexalate crystals are more maroon while Questran is more pink.[201]. Biopsies from cases with drug-induced ischemic colitis are indistinguishable from those with other ischemic conditions.

Drug-induced vasculitis consists of two types: hypersensitivity and toxic. Hypersensitivity vasculitis may develop after the patient has been on drugs for months or years or after a short interval following cessation of medication, for reasons that are unclear. A growing list of drugs has been implicated including numerous antibiotics such as penicillins, tetracyclines, chloramphenicol and sulfonamides, griseofulvin, isoniazid, but also other products such as diazepam and spironolactone. Histologically, the lesions involve primarily arterioles, capillaries, and venules, with sparing of the larger vessels. They are characterized by a severe mononuclear infiltrate of the vessel wall and surrounding perivascular tissues, without fibrinoid necrosis.[202]

Toxic vasculitis involves primarily small- and medium-sized arteries. Morphologically, it is similar to PAN and results in similar complications. The major causes of toxic vasculitis are injection of heterologous serum (serum sickness) and nonprotein drugs such as penicillins and sulfonamides. Toxic vasculitis has also been seen in intravenous drug users, such as those injecting amphetamines.

Neutropenic colitis. Neutropenic colitis or enterocolitis (synonyms: ileocecal syndrome and typhlitis) is a special type of therapy-related necrotizing colitis (see also Chapter 19). It occurs in patients who have been rendered neutropenic by drugs (particularly cancer chemotherapy) or other marrow suppressants. It is characterized by bowel-wall necrosis, occurring during the treatment of hematologic malignancies (lymphoma, leukemia) but also during aplastic anemia and cyclic neutropenia. Histologically, one may see only numerous luminal bacteria, extensive edema, reactive crypt changes, and a lack of neutrophilic response. Degree of necrosis is variable. A CT scan is a favored method of investigation to clinch the diagnosis as colonoscopy carries increased risk for perforation in these patients, and often colonic resection is undertaken.[203] It has also been reported in transplant patients and in patients with AIDS, usually secondary to an infection occurring in a patient with neutropenia.[204,205]

Iatrogenic Gastrointestinal Bleeding

GI hemorrhage may take several forms. The most frequent one is associated with ingestion of NSAIDs and is due to gastric erosions and ulcers. Another important cause is intramural hematoma, which may rupture through the mucosa, producing GI hemorrhage; this can be seen in patients taking anticoagulants such as warfarin. Patients taking ASA also have an intrinsic tendency, which can potentiate any other source of bleeding. Retroperitoneal hemorrhage is uncommon and may extend into the mesentery. Common causes of hemorrhage other than the NSAIDs are therapeutic endoscopic procedures such as polypectomy and mucosectomy, abdominal trauma, and spontaneous hemorrhages occurring in patients on medications such as anticoagulants, thrombolytic agents, and antineoplastic agents, which produce thrombocytopenia.[206–210] In the majority of cases, the bleeding is relatively harmless, but in a few patients severe abdominal pain with ileus or intestinal obstruction ensues.[211,212] The site of hemorrhage varies. About one-half originate in the upper GI tract, one-third from the lower bowel, and the remainder from undetermined sites. When apparent, the hemorrhagic lesions, unassociated with peptic ulceration, are usually well localized to a small segment of intestine and may occupy part or the full circumference of the bowel. In the latter case, obstruction ensues rarely.[213] Histologically, the hemorrhage occurs mainly into the submucosa and the muscularis propria, with sparing of the mucosa. This sparing of the mucosa, which grossly looks pink, is often helpful to the surgeon in distinguishing intramural hemorrhage from infarction. Another unusual cause of GI bleeding associated with colonic injury is from shock wave lithotripsy where the right colon in the case reported was obviously injured by being in the field of the shock waves. The lesion resolved on its own over time.[214]

Another important cause of intramural hematoma is blunt trauma from causes including motor vehicle accidents and seat belt injuries. It occurs principally in the duodenum and proximal jejunum because the bowel is fixed in the latter location.[215,216] The combination of trauma and hemorrhage may sometimes result in separation of the viscus from the mesentery.

Radiation Injury

Many forms of cancers are treated with radiotherapy, chemotherapy, or both. However, these also have significant dose-limiting toxicities. Radiation damage of the GI tract can be the result of a remote (abscopal) effect of the treatment of malignancies located in other organ systems (e.g., lung, gynecologic malignancies, prostate, etc.) or a direct complication of the treatment of primary GI malignancies. Intestinal complications of pelvic and abdominal radiation are function of the volume of the treatment field, total radiation dose, fraction size, overall treatment time, radiation energy used, and treatment technique. In general, higher doses over short intervals given to a larger volume with large fraction size contribute to an increased incidence of complications. The incidence of severe rectosigmoid sequelae was 4% or less with doses below 8,000 cGy to the rectum, 7% to 8% with doses of 8,000 to 9,500 cGy, and 13% with doses above that level.[217] It is generally accepted that a total dose of 4,500 to 5,000 cGy in 180 to 200 cGy daily fractions can be delivered safely to a standard pelvic field.[218] During a 6-week course of radical radiotherapy for pelvic cancer, approximately 80% of patients will develop GI symptoms. These acute symptoms are supposed to settle within 3 months. Symptoms persisting at that time or arising subsequently are considered to be late toxic effects. Approximately 20% of the patients will be referred to a gastroenterologist for late symptoms.[219] Previous surgery increases the risk by 2.5- to 3-fold because adhesions cause the same segments of bowel to be irradiated each time. Concomitant chemotherapy may increase the damage. Conditions that cause impaired blood supply to the intestines such as hypertension, arteriosclerosis, diabetes mellitus, and cardiovascular disease are also associated with a higher risk of developing complications. Patients with IBD may also have an increased risk for acute radiotherapy-related complications.[220]

Pathophysiology. Radiation-induced damage can be acute or chronic. Some also include a subacute phase between about 6 months and 1 year after start of therapy, and the chronic phase being 1 to 5 years later. The morphologic alterations can also be subdivided into acute and chronic, or rather delayed injury. The effect of ionizing radiation in the GI tract is also twofold. There is a direct toxic effect, responsible for the acute injury, and then an indirect effect, which is mainly due to progressive obliterative vascular damage and submucosal fibrosis, responsible for the late effects.[220]

The sequence of events has been studied in animal models. Intestinal mucositis appears to pass through a number of developmental stages. There is a short initial inflammatory phase during which cellular infiltration occurs, but epithelial cell numbers are unaltered. Then, a period of apoptosis and restitution follows. Subsequently, there may be a stage in which there is almost complete ablation of the absorptive epithelium. Finally, there is a period of reepithelialization, re-formation of gut structure, and restoration of functionality.

During the initial period, radiation causes DNA damage. The rapidly dividing progenitor cell populations in the crypts are particularly affected by this effect. Concomitant chemotherapy, blocking for instance DNA synthesis, may aggravate the process. Cell division stops within a few hours of commencement of therapy and is followed by an increase in apoptosis around 24 hours. The rate of apoptosis relates to radiation-induced increase in the expression of the p53 tumor suppressor gene. Migration of epithelial cells out of the crypts may not be inhibited.[221] Free radical damage, mediated by radiation, will affect additional epithelial and also subepithelial cell populations. These processes lead to mitotic inhibition, disruption of cell–cell and cell–matrix interactions, epithelial denudation, and impaired epithelial integrity. There is a collapse of crypts and loss of villus or absorptive surface over 2 to 4 days. The process is associated with a loss of goblet cells and a marked reduction of intestinal trefoil factor m-RNA.[222] In the small intestine, pancreatic secretions with proteolytic enzymes may aggravate the mucosal injury. The loss of epithelial integrity appears to trigger a rapid influx of immune and inflammatory cells into the lamina propria. The loss of epithelial cells from the crypts and absorptive surface triggers "restitution." Restitution is a rapid process capable of restoring the continuity of the epithelial surface. Cells next to the damaged area reorganize their cytoskeletons, create specialized structures known as pseudopodia, and loosen their linkage to the underlying matrix. This enables them to migrate and spread over the damaged area. Shrinking of the underlying layers facilitates closure of the damaged site. Goblet cell numbers increase transiently between 24 and 48 hours after irradiation. Goblet cells appear to be preferentially spared during chemotherapy compared to radiation.

If aggressive therapies are used, the cell loss may be extensive leading to an almost complete loss of barrier integrity, absorptive epithelial structure, or both. This can lead to bacterial invasion and colonization and inflammation. Significant cellular proliferation restarts at around 3 to 4 days after the onset of therapy. This leads to the restoration of functional crypts and increased crypt numbers. The structure of the villi and absorptive surfaces of the gut can return to normal after around 1 week. Goblet cell numbers may return to normal at around 4 to 7 days posttherapy. Paneth cells may be spared during therapy.

Factors predisposing to intestinal mucositis are impaired immune status, intestinal damage, high endogenous levels of proinflammatory cytokines, and the presence of pathogens or opportunistic infections.[223]

The delayed damage is the result of repetitive epithelial, stromal, and vascular injury. Epithelial lesions include epithelial atrophy, one of the most consistent delayed effects of therapeutic irradiation; delayed necrosis generally resulting from ischemia; and atypia of epithelial cells, which may affect either the nucleus or the cytoplasm or both and may be a source of confusion with neoplasia. Stromal alterations include fibrosis, atypical fibroblasts, necrosis, lack or paucity of cellular inflammatory reaction, and rarely neoplasia. Vascular lesions are seen in a variety of blood vessels and summarized in Table 2-9. The capillaries are the most radiosensitive vascular elements. Lesions that are apparent by light microscopy are dilatation, asymmetry with the irregularity of the wall, focally prominent endothelial cells, and rarely thrombosis. Electron microscopy reveals detachment of endothelial cells from the basal lamina, rupture of capillary wall, loss of entire capillary segments, and, sometimes, regrowth of vessels. Small-sized arteries and arterioles show subendothelial, intimal, or adventitial fibrosis; hyalinization of the media (dense, acellular, acidophilic collagenous material); and accumulation of lipid-laden macrophages in the intima. Intimal or medial fibrosis and even thrombosis can also be seen in the veins in the wall of the intestine, as often or more often than similar arterial lesions.[224]

Acute radiation injury. The precision of modern radiotherapy means that it is now rare to see the early acute mucositis in patients treated for cancer elsewhere. However, with the recent advent of short- and long-term preoperative radiotherapy for esophageal and rectal cancer, the diagnostic pathologist is now not uncommonly exposed to this type of pathology in esophageal and rectal specimens.

Table 2-9 Vascular Changes in Radiation-Induced Injury

Capillaries
- Damage to endothelial cells
- Ectasia
- Thrombosis
- Rupture
- Loss

Arterioles
- Necrosis, thrombosis
- Fibrosis of media, adventitia, or both
- Delayed acute vasculitis
- Neointima with or without lipids

Arteries
- Neointima with or without lipids
- Fibrosis of media, adventitia, or both
- Thrombosis

Veins
- Neointima
- Thrombosis
- Venoocclusive lesions (small veins)

Esophagus Radiation and chemotherapy may induce considerable alterations of the squamous epithelium. The incidence of severe acute esophagitis in patients with standard radiotherapy alone is 1.3%. In contrast, a strong radiosensitizing effect of chemotherapy given concurrently with standard thoracic radiotherapy is associated with an incidence of severe esophagitis of 14% to 49%. Acute esophagitis may be severe and disabling. The exact nature, duration, and severity depend on treatment and host factors and thus may vary greatly from patient to patient.[225] In general, there is a loss of epithelial integrity in 1 to 2 weeks after the initial treatment. The epithelium usually retains the general organization with smaller, basal-like cells and larger superficial cells, but these cells tend to be variable in shape and size in all layers. The nuclei are strangely shaped and may vary from normal to hyperchromatic, with sometimes large eosinophilic nucleoli. Mitoses are usually not present. Ulceration may develop. Repopulation of the epithelium initiates generally around 3 to 5 days after the start of the treatment. Despite this, epithelial denudation may persist for 2 to 4 weeks after the cessation of radiotherapy. There may also be changes in the submucosal glands, which may be distended with secretions and show degeneration and atrophy. Some of the glands may be lost.

Stomach In the 1950s, gastric irradiation with 500 to 2,000 rads was used as a treatment for peptic ulceration, which produced achlorhydria for periods ranging from months to years. Initial changes consisted

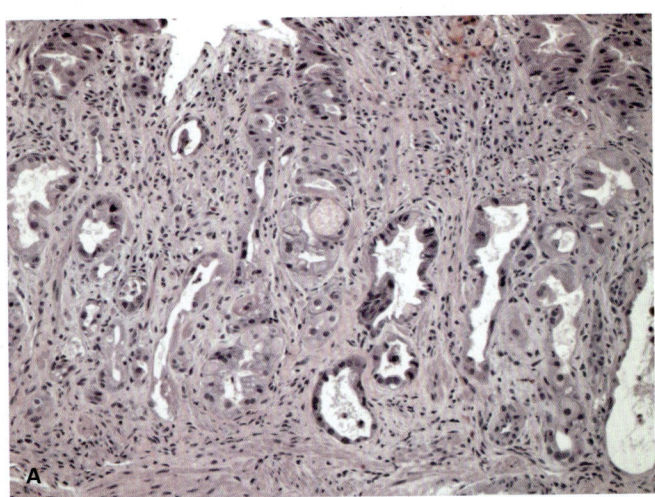 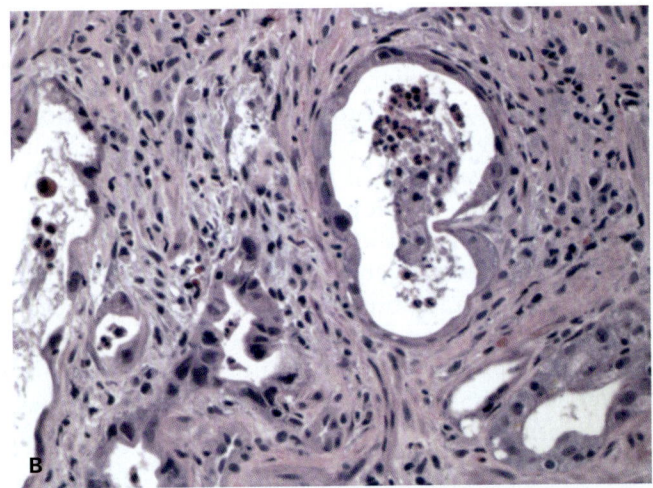

Figure 2-36. Effects of radiation as seen in a gastric biopsy. **A:** There is extensive atypia in the glandular epithelium along with lamina propria fibrosis, scant inflammation, crypt drop out and sloughed cell in the gland lumen or the surface. **B:** Higher magnification showing the atypia comprising of large hyperchromatic and pleomorphic nuclei that have smudged chromatic and are irregularly distributed. Many apoptotic cells sloughed off in the glandular lumen are also present. There are hardly any mitosis commensurate with the degree of atypia that also helps this to be differentiated from a true neoplastic change.

of degeneration and necrosis of both superficial and specialized cells, the latter becoming more eosinophilic, rounded up, and shed into the pits and the lumen (Fig. 2-36A,B).[226] Superficial foveolar cells were affected after the specialized cells, but their destruction was often quite focal. Regeneration was usually well under way within 2 to 3 weeks of cessation of irradiation, and the mucosa often appeared quite hyperplastic and mucin depleted.

With high levels of radiation the same changes progress much faster, and with complete loss of superficial epithelium to the point of ulceration. This may occur within a week or two of irradiation, but most ulcers are found within a few months of therapy and are probably best not regarded as early acute changes.

Small Intestine Acute complications are common during treatment but usually transient. Villous surface epithelial cells are damaged and lost. The total number of epithelial cells in the crypts is decreased. Partial or total villous atrophy and cystic dilatation of the crypts occur in days or weeks. Ulceration is often absent but focal erosion may be found. Inflammation is common. Repair and recovery usually take place within 72 hours after the last radiation exposure.[218]

Colon Short-term preoperative irradiation therapy generally induces severe mucosal inflammation with crypt abnormalities. The surface epithelial cells are usually absent or attenuated. Crypts show a slit-like or slightly dilated lumen lined with flattened epithelial cells. Crypt epithelium may show bizarre nuclei. The number of apoptotic bodies is generally increased. The distance between the crypt base and the muscularis mucosae is generally increased. Decreased crypt numbers or small residual crypts are usually present in areas with severe inflammation. The inflammatory infiltrate is diffuse. It is composed of a mixture of eosinophils, lymphocytes, plasma cells and histiocytes. Eosinophils may be present in between the surface epithelial cells with cryptitis and crypt abscesses. Subcryptal plasma cells and increased intraepithelial lymphocytes are not seen. The submucosa usually shows no or only minor changes (fibrosis).[227] P-cadherin, which is not expressed in normal rectal mucosa, is aberrantly expressed by colonic epithelial cells (membranous and cytoplasmic immunoreactivity) during the acute injury and early regenerative phases. The expression of E-cadherin and of β- and γ-catenins is shifted from a membranous to a cytoplasmic localization.[228]

Complications Perforation is a rare complication of radiotherapy in the acute phase.

Chronic (late) radiation injury. The late features and complications of irradiation may occur anywhere from about 6 months to 20 or more years following therapy. The reported incidence of severe late chronic radiation injury of the small intestine varies between 0.5% and 15%. Most of the chronic injury occurs between 12 and 24 months after radiation.[229] and is usually progressive. In the months and years following irradiation, obstructive symptoms, diarrhea, often with malabsorption, bleeding, pain, and symptoms of fistula formation may ensue. Neoplasms, primarily carcinoma and sarcoma, are rare late complications.[224]

Symptoms are dictated by the area of the gut that is affected. If the midgut is within the radiation field then there is hemorrhage and protein loss from the telangiectatic capillary channels within the mucosa, fibrosis-causing strictures (Fig. 2-37A–C), radionecrotic ulcers, vascular occlusion, or obstruction. A rare complication is intestinal pseudo-obstruction, which is likely secondary to adhesions or to vascular, muscular, and neural damage. More commonly the patients may develop a segment or segments of hypomotile or immotile bowel, which can lead to stasis and bacterial overgrowth. When the rectum is affected by the radiation field as in prostate or cervical radiation, then symptoms of large bowel disease tend to predominate, including blood loss, pain, diarrhea, incontinence, constipation, and sometimes both diarrhea and constipation. Sometimes the bleeding is quite apparent and can account for the reduction of serum hemoglobin. Other times the bleeding seems minor, but the anemia that develops is marked. Stenosis of the colon is common with serosal fibrosis and adhesions. Perforation is also a common presentation.

In the small bowel, a fistula can occur between adjacent organs, including the inferior vena cava. Fistulas tend to occur within the first few years following irradiation, may be multiple, and occur in patients with severe injury to the adjacent mucosa.

The most common clinical presentation of chronic radiation changes is radiation proctitis (see Fig. 2-39). This can be a very difficult condition to treat. Most therapeutic enemas such as 5-aminosalicylates, corticosteroids, sucralfate, and short-chain fatty acids fail.[230] Gastroenterologists typically treat the bleeding with thermal therapy in the form of argon plasma laser, or bipolar elctrocautery, often requiring repeated sessions. Formalin enema formulations have been tried with some success. Often the bleeding stops spontaneously without any therapy. Regarding radiation proctitis, when the lesion is identified endoscopically (usually there is an abrupt cutoff between the radiation proctitis and the normal rectum), the endoscopist should avoid biopsy because this may lead to fistulization and the endoscopic lesion is so typical that pathology adds little to the ultimate diagnosis.

Gross and endoscopic appearance: One of the characteristic features of radiation-induced changes is that they tend to be limited to the immediate field of irradiation, so that disease tends to be relatively focal, often involving one loop or portion of bowel. However, where loops of bowel are adherent to each other, disease may be present in immediately adjacent bowel loops and be quite widespread. With pelvic irradiation, it is common endoscopically to see changes limited to the rectum with an abrupt change to normal-appearing mucosa.

In patients undergoing resection, the mucosa shows a mottled red and gray appearance. The redness is rarely due to inflammation adjacent to a radionecrotic ulcer but due to numerous telangiectatic vessels in the mucosa and submucosa. A purulent exudate may be present, particularly in the vicinity of ulcers. The bowel is rather rigid and much less pliable than usual. The serosal surface is rough with varying amounts of fibrin and fibrinous adhesions. Long segments of the small intestine may be diffusely narrowed, or a short segment may develop zones of concentric constriction. Endoscopically, in symptomatic patients, changes are best documented in the rectosigmoid following colorectal irradiation. In one study, luminal narrowing was present in 80% of symptomatic patients, telangiectasia in 55%; in 27% there was mucosal friability; ulceration was present in 47%, 29% being solitary and 18% diffuse. Fistula was present in 19%.[231]

Esophagus The epithelium may become irregular with acanthotic areas and very thin zones. The capillaries may become telangiectatic and can be seen through the epithelium. The lamina propria tends to be fibrotic. The muscularis mucosae may become highly irregular with zones of thickening and areas of smooth muscle loss. Submucosal fibrosis may also extend into the muscularis propria. Mild inflammation and iron-laden macrophages may be present. Foreign body granulomatous reactions and calcifications can be noted in samples from patients treated for primary esophageal cancer. Vascular abnormalities are common, especially in patients treated for primary esophageal cancer. They include fibrosis of the intima, hypertrophy of the media, fibrinoid necrosis, thrombosis, and vasculitis (Fig. 2-38). Veins seem less damaged. Over the ensuing years, these changes may become more marked and may result in the late breakdown of overlying epithelium, including the formation of a chronic, nonhealing ulcer. This may ultimately produce a stricture, which may ulcerate and never become fully reepithelialized.

Stomach The late changes include mucosal regeneration with focal loss of pits, progressive atrophy, cyst formation, and intestinal metaplasia. Submucosal fibrosis may be quite marked. Telangiectasia of capillaries and intimal proliferation are common and progressive. Interestingly, in patients that were treated with relatively low-dose radiation (≤2,000 rads) for ulcer disease, the initial period of hypo- or achlorhydra was followed by a gradual return toward normal acid output; parietal cells appear to recover faster than the chief cell population. However, there is often a functional deficit even when the morphologic appearances have returned largely to normal. In some patients receiving successful irradiation for

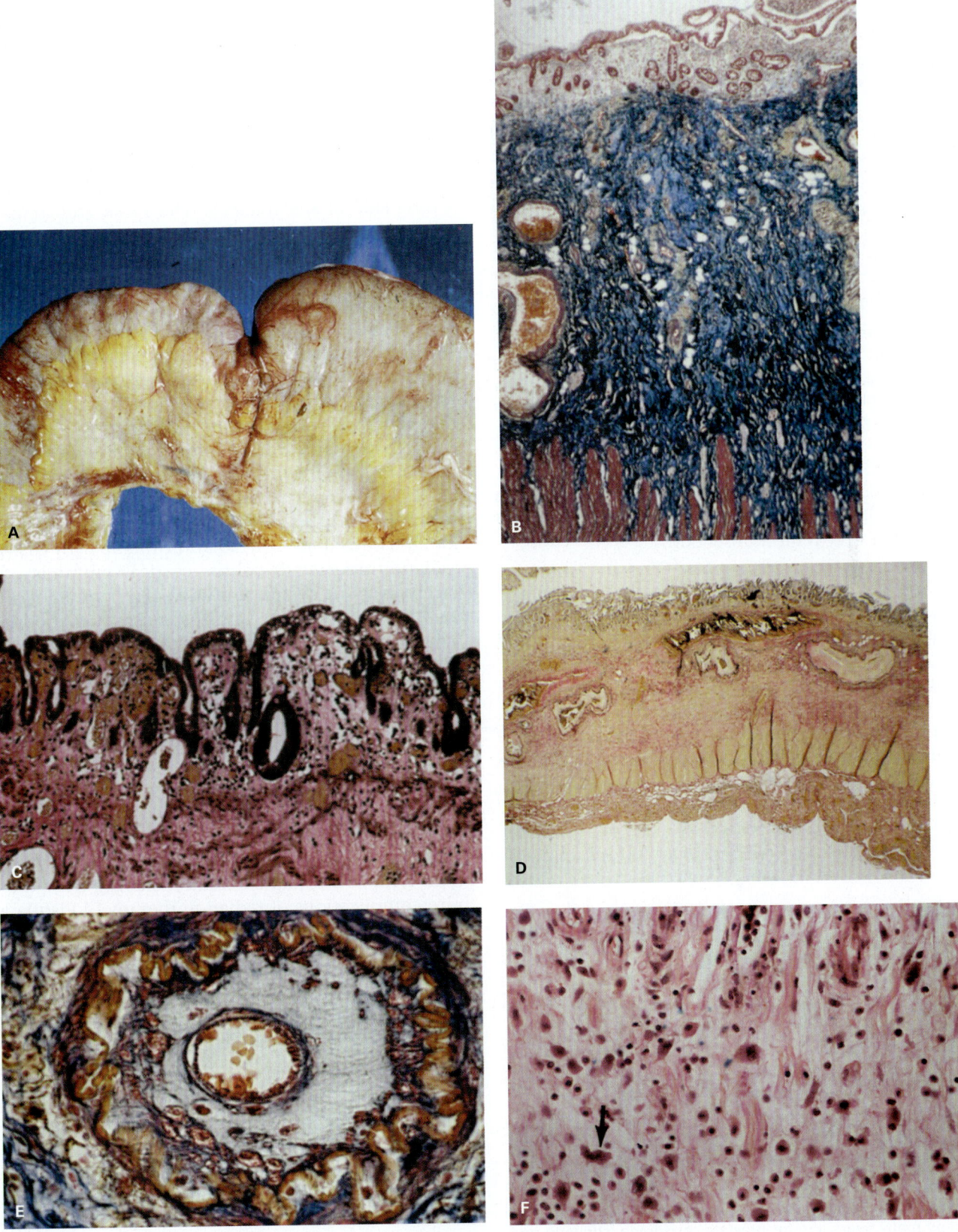

Figure 2-37. **A:** Chronic radiation enteritis showing stricture formation. Histologic features of chronic radiation enteritis. **B:** With marked submucosal fibrosis and mucosal atrophy. **C:** Higher-power magnification of part showing mucosal flattening due to loss of intestinal villi and telangiectasia of vessels. **D:** Full-thickness section of small intestine showing extensive obliterative endarteritis of submucosal vessels. **E:** Higher-power magnification showing endarteritis proliferation of a small artery. **F:** Radiation enteritis showing inflammatory fibrous tissue infiltrated with atypical fibroblasts (*arrow*).

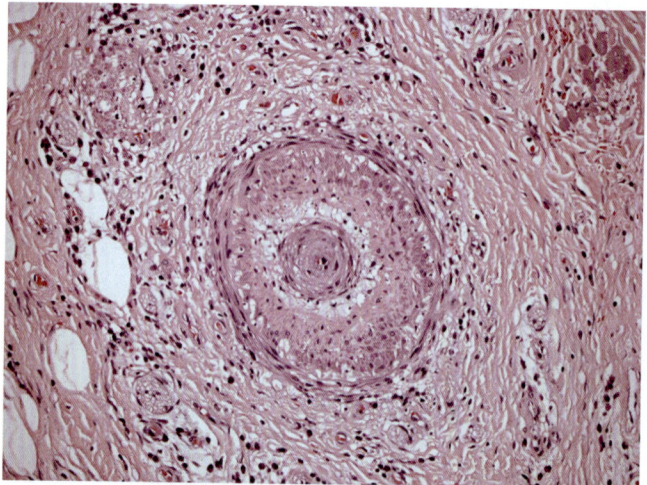

Figure 2-38. Long-term vascular changes in medium-sized artery secondary to radiation showing fibrointimal hyperplasia and almost obliterated lumen. In addition focal myxoid changes and few foamy macrophages are also seen.

diffuse tumors, the stomach may be converted into an aperistaltic organ because of marked transmural fibrosis that may require resection.[226]

Small and Large Intestines Endoscopic biopsies of the colon show a combination of mucosal atrophy and telangiectatic thick-walled capillaries (which should have at least the diameter of a normal crypt) (Fig. 2-39). The capillaries may be separated from the lumen by only one layer of columnar epithelium. Rarely platelet thrombi may be present within them. Atypical fibroblasts may be present. The remaining crypts are distorted and frequently show budding. Paneth cell metaplasia can be present in the large bowel. Mucin depletion tends to be moderate or marked and is reflected by a reduction in the number of goblet cells, although this tends to be variable even within the same specimen. Nuclei are often larger than normal, and nuclear stratification may be present. In addition, both Paneth and argentaffin cells may have an excess number of granules, and they may be present on the wrong side of the nucleus. The loose areolar tissue of the lamina propria and submucosa is replaced and thickened by homogeneous masses of collagen and fibroblasts. Fibroblasts are characteristically enlarged, and nuclei and nucleoli become enlarged and prominent. The cytoplasm tends to be basophilic. The most spectacular changes are usually seen in arterioles, small arteries, and veins, particularly those in the submucosa. Arterioles frequently show intimal proliferation and fibrosis, sometimes with "foamy" endothelial cells, particularly relatively early in the disease; the media may be hyalinized. The lumen may be thrombosed, often with recanalization, particularly in the region of an ulcer. Submucosal glands can rarely be found as a sequel to irradiation therapy. In cases of radiation-associated colitis cystica profunda, and rarely in colitis cystica profunda of other etiology, the glands may penetrate into the muscularis propria.[224] In view of the atypical nuclei that can be seen in colitis cystica profunda, it needs to be distinguished from a well-differentiated adenocarcinoma. Preservation of the lobular architecture and lack of associated tumor type desmolasia helps to differentiate it from a true adenocarcinoma.

Complications Bleeding, obstruction, fistula formation, perforation, and malignancies are all possible complications of radiation therapy. Carcinoma, malignant lymphoma, and sarcoma including GIST are all rare complications of radiation therapy.[224] Fistula formation can complicate biopsies.

VASCULAR ABNORMALITIES OF THE GASTROINTESTINAL TRACT

Vascular malformations are aberrations in the normal vascular architecture, affecting arterial, venous, capillary, and sometimes lymphatic vessels. Many of these are congenital, but some are acquired. The incidence of these lesions is estimated to be 1 in 14,000 individuals. The lesions are usually classified in a descriptive system, which combines size and type of the vessel affected and presence or absence of other somatic features (Table 2-10). Many different terms are in use, which results in confusion. Vascular ectasia simply

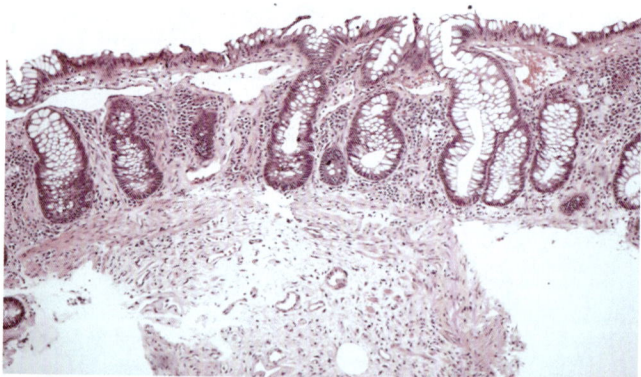

Figure 2-39. Rectal biopsy in a patient who received radiation therapy many years ago for prostate carcinoma, showing multiple dilated ectatic vessels in the lamina propria. The mucosa otherwise shows mild crypt distortion and scarring, but usually inflammation is minimal or absent. No radiation associated atypia is usually seen in this setting.

refers to dilatation of vessels (arteries or veins), and is generally applied to dilatation of preexisting small- or medium-sized vessels. These conditions can be congenital, or, more commonly, acquired. Telangiectasias generally refer to dilatation of smaller vessels that are superficial and easily seen through skin or mucosa. Some of them do have a component of arteriovenous shunting, and some have characteristic endoscopic appearances. These are more often congenital but can also be acquired. Arteriovenous malformations (AVMs) represent structurally abnormal vessels that are medium sized or larger and consist of arteries, veins, and vessels that are difficult to classify as either veins or arteries. These are present in submucosa or deeper in the wall and can be congenital or acquired. Despite an attempt to make these distinctions, it should be realized that there is considerable overlap between these entities, and since strict definitional criteria are lacking, differentiation is sometimes arbitrary.

Vascular anomalies are clinically most relevant in the small and large intestines. Clinical presentation ranges from asymptomatic to iron deficiency anemia to life-threatening bleeding. If the vascular anomaly is tumorous, it may lead to obstruction or intussusception. Rarely they are associated with hemodynamic problems (high flow—cardiac failure). Vascular anomalies are responsible for 2% to 5% of all episodes of acute upper GI bleeding and for up to 35% of cases of acute lower GI bleeding. The diagnosis can be made with endoscopy, but in certain settings angiography, video capsule endoscopy, double balloon endoscopy, intra-operative enteroscopy, tagged red blood cell scan, and MRI scan offer additional information. Video capsule endoscopy may increase the diagnostic yield, but double balloon endoscopy offers the advantage of therapy as well. Treatment can be symptomatic, including iron supplements and transfusion of blood, or directed to the vascular lesion including therapeutic endoscopy (using argon plasma laser or bipolar electrocautery), therapeutic angiography, and surgery. If these treatments are not possible, pharmacological therapy may be tried. Beneficial results have been reported with somatostatin analogues, estrogen–progesterone preparations, interferon-α, and serotonin antagonists, but these treatments have not been tested in large trials.[232]

Table 2-10 Classification of Vascular Anomalies of the GI Tract

1: Primary vascular lesions
  Nonneoplastic
  • Vascular ectasia
    • Gastric antral vascular ectasia
    • Portal hypertensive gastropathy
    • Chronic renal failure associated vascular ectasia
  • Dieulafoy malformation
  • Telangiectasia in association with congenital syndromes
    – Hereditary hemorrhagic telangiectasia (Rendu–Osler–Weber disease)
    – Turner's syndrome
  • Arteriovenous malformation
  Venous ectasia
    – Multiple phlebectasia
    – Hemorrhoids
  Neoplastic
  • Hemangioma
    – Capillary hemangioma
    – Cavernous hemangioma
    – Mixed type
    – Diffuse intestinal hemangiomatosis
    – Hereditary syndromes
      – Klippel–Trenaunay syndrome
      – Blue rubber-bleb nevus syndrome
  • Hemangiopericytoma
  • Angiosarcoma
  • Kaposi sarcoma
2: Diseases affecting blood vessels
  • Portal hypertension
    – Varices
    – Portal hypertensive gastropathy
    – Portal hypertensive colopathy
  • Renal failure
  • Connective tissue diseases
    – Ehlers–Danlos syndrome
    – Pseudoxanthoma elasticum
  • Systemic sclerosis (CREST, scleroderma)

Vascular Ectasia (Angiodysplasia)

Vascular ectasia, originally named angiodysplasia, is a distinct clinicopathologic entity, mainly occurring in elderly people. Over the years, different definitions and names have been proposed including AVM, angioma, and teleangiectasia, reflecting the uncertainty about the origin of the lesion. Moreover, the term "angiodysplasia" is confusing because this vascular anomaly is an acquired disorder and has no relation to neoplasia. As stated above, we would like to reserve the term vascular ectasia for dilatation of preexisting submucosal medium-sized vessels and overlying mucosal capillaries.[233,234] The lesions consist of irregular clusters of dilated and thin-walled vessels (veins and arteries) located in the submucosa but may expand toward the mucosa where capillaries also become dilated as a result of increased retrograde pressure. In the mucosa, a single layer of endothelium and the surface epithelium may separate the vessels from the lumen, which explains the high susceptibility for bleeding. The mucosa may show focal hemorrhages, but usually a specific bleeding point cannot be identified. Generally inflammation, fibrosis, or erosions are lacking.

Vascular ectasias are multiple, rather than single, and usually <5 mm in diameter. The pathogenesis is unclear, but it has been suggested that chronic obstruction of the submucosal veins leads to capillary dilatation and loss of competence of the precapillary sphincter. They are more common with increasing age, most often being diagnosed in those over 70 years of age. Although vascular ectasia may be found in all parts of the GI tract, such as the jejunum (10.5%), ileum (5.8%), duodenum (2.3%), or stomach (1.4%), it is most frequently situated in the right colon (77.5%). The predilection for the right colon can be explained by the high wall tension as a result of the large diameter of the colon in this area. In contrast to vascular ectasia of the colon, vascular ectasia of the small intestine is more common in young adults, suggesting possibly a congenital origin.

The prevalence in asymptomatic individuals is around 0.83%, and the incidence rates in asymptomatic and symptomatic patients are estimated to be around 0.3 and 6% to 12%, respectively. Approximately 11% to 22% of the patients with colonic lesions will have concomitant lesions in the small bowel.[235] Vascular ectasias are not associated with angiomatous lesions of the skin or other viscera. They can be found in association with other diseases such as chronic renal failure, von Willebrand's disease, or aortic valve stenosis. The lesions are identified at colonoscopy or angiography. Angiographic diagnosis depends on a blush of vessels and an early filling vein. A "microscopic variant" without lesions detected by routine endoscopy has been described. In this variant, the vascular lesions are mainly submucosal.[236]

Histologic examination of endoscopic biopsies is not a diagnostic tool in vascular ectasia, as mucosal lesions appear only in an advanced stage of the disease. The low diagnostic yield of endoscopic mucosal biopsies (50%) and the risk of inducing hemorrhage do not justify the sampling of biopsies during endoscopy.[237-239]

Gastric Antral Vascular Ectasia

Gastric antral vascular ectasia (GAVE) is a rare condition (prevalence ~3/10,000 upper endoscopies), characterized by red spots in linear array in the antrum of the stomach. Based on the striped features emanating from the antrum at endoscopy, the disorder has been called the "watermelon stomach." The pathogenesis is unknown. Hypotheses include an abnormal response to antral mechanical stress/motility problem or to vasoactive hormones.[240,241] Vasodilatatory neuropeptides such as VIP and 5-hydroxytryptamine, which are associated with the friability of the blood vessels, are present in high concentrations. The classic patient is a middle-aged female with an autoimmune or connective tissue diseases (CTD), but it may also occur in persons with chronic liver disease/cirrhosis in about 30% patients. It appears that portal hypertension probably plays no role in the pathogenesis as its reduction does not reverse GAVE; however, GAVE disappears after liver transplantation, suggesting altered liver function may be a contributory factor in some patients.[242]

Two different endoscopic patterns have been recognized: the striped pattern and the diffuse pattern.[243,244] The striped pattern is the more classical pattern that is referred to as "watermelon stomach" and is due to thickening of the antral mucosa with linear erythema radiating outward from the pylorus (Fig. 2-40A). The diffuse pattern corresponds to an advanced stage of the disease characterized by diffuse erythema with several red spots.

The histologic lesion consists of numerous dilated vessels in the mucosa, often with microthrombi, fibromuscular hyperplasia, and fibrohyalinosis of the perivascular lamina propria (Fig. 2-41A,B). Smooth muscle fibers can be seen in the lamina propria running parallel to the crypts. Fibrin thrombi are often present and can be highlighted with platelet markers (CD61). The mucosa shows no or mild chronic inflammation, and glandular atrophy with intestinal metaplasia. There are usually marked reactive epithelial changes with marked mucin depletion as described in Chapter 13. In the mucosal glands, the number of endocrine cells appears increased.[245] Dilated blood vessels can also be found in the submucosa. Based on the presence of vascular anomalies and spindle cells in the mucosa, a specific diagnostic endoscopic and histology score has been proposed.[246]

GAVE must be distinguished from portal hypertensive gastropathy (PHG), lesions, which occur in patients with portal hypertension. The distinction is important as the treatment differs. PHG responds to reduction in portal hypertension with medical or surgical therapy, while this is ineffective in GAVE, even in cases associated with cirrhosis. Treatment of GAVE requires treatment of any associated disease (autoimmune or connective tissue disorder), endoscopic ablation of the vessels (contact methods for destruction of the vessels such as heat probe and bipolar coagulation or noncontact thermal methods such as argon plasma laser therapy), or rarely antrectomy. The differentiation is easy in cases with typical endoscopic appearance and lack of portal hypertension in most cases of GAVE. PHG has a reddened and edematous mosaic-like pattern with or without red spots. Endoscopically, PHG looks like "blood under plastic wrap" (Fig. 2-40B). PHG occurs mainly in the proximal stomach, while GAVE involves the antrum. However, in some cases with portal hypertension, the endoscopic appearances are not typical, and clinical

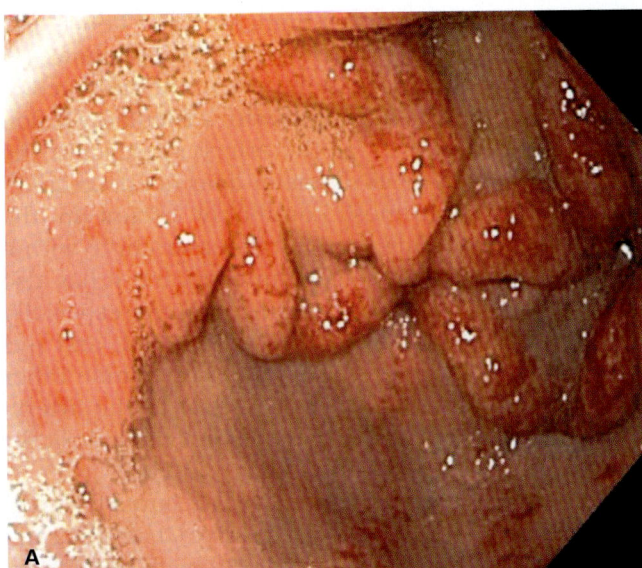
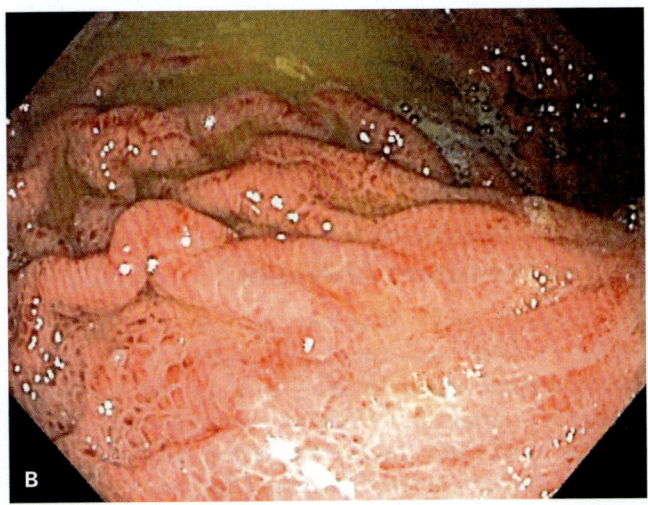

Figure 2-40. **A:** Gastric antral vascular ectasia (watermelon stomach). Endoscopic appearance showing the characteristic linear erythematous streaks on the thick mucosal folds. **B:** Endoscopic appearance of portal gastropathy showing "snake-skin"–like mosaic pattern.

overlap occurs. Presence of platelet thrombi and relatively increased vascularity has been suggested to differentiate between these conditions when other features overlap. In one study using the platelet marker (CD61) and endothelial markers (CD31 and CD34) on gastric biopsies (n = 49; GAVE = 11, PHG = 11, suspected GAVE = 15, suspected PHG = 12) identification of platelet thrombi was very helpful in correctly diagnosing GAVE in all cases.[247] In this study, staining with CD61 antibodies identified platelet thrombi in 26% of cases originally signed out as PHG, suggesting a diagnosis of GAVE that was

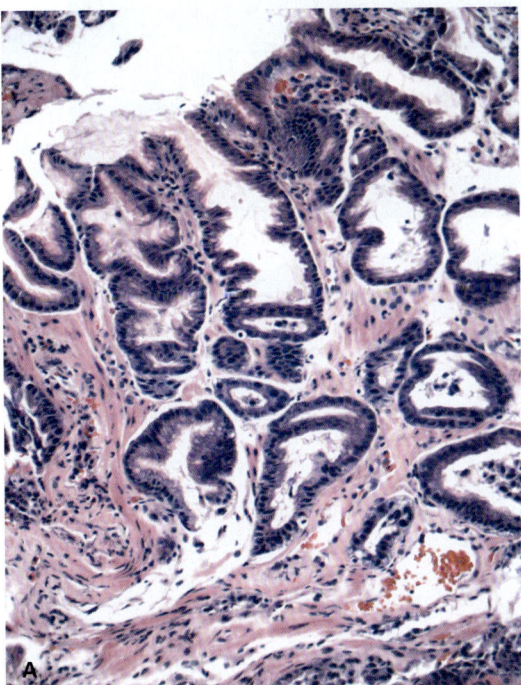
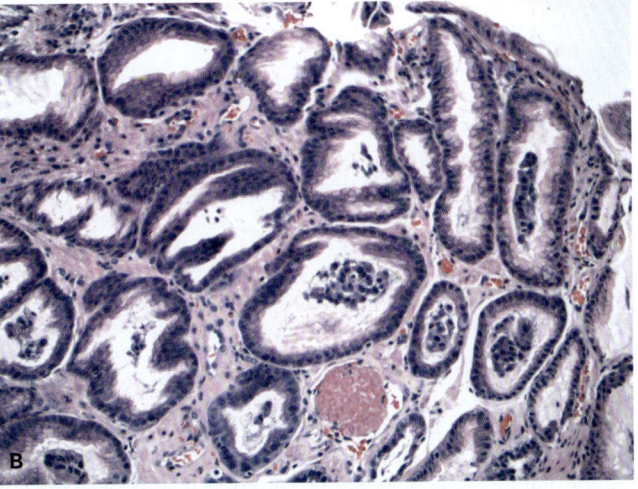

Figure 2-41. Gastric antral vascular ectasia. **A:** Prominent fibromuscular bundles lying perpendicular to the surface and parallel to the gastric pits along with few dilated vessels in the lamina propria. The crypts often show features similar to reactive gastropathy with corkscrew appearance and mucin depletion. **B:** Dilated mucosal blood vessels with occasional fibrin thrombi.

retrospectively confirmed based on clinicopathologic correlation. The vascular markers showed increased vascular density in GAVE compared to PHG based on morphometry and image analysis. However, in practice its utility seems limited. The presence of fibrohyalinosis and smooth muscle proliferation also seems to favor GAVE over PHG.[248]

Dieulafoy Malformation (Caliber-Persistent Arteriole)

The Dieulafoy lesion was actually first described by Gallard in 1884, but Dieulafoy, a French surgeon, described three cases in 1898, and got the glory. It consists of a large caliber tortuous submucosal artery, which is most often recognized when major hemorrhage occurs from a small erosion (Fig. 2-42A–C).[249,250] The pathogenesis is not precisely known. It has been proposed that the diameter of the large submucosal artery, which remains constant even after passing through the muscularis propria, is likely due to a failure of normal arterial branching and hence also called "caliber persistent artery."[251] There is however no significant difference in the size of the submucosal blood vessels between patients with a Dieulafoy lesion and controls; however, as the artery approaches the muscularis mucosae its diameter does not decrease.[251] Dieulafoy's lesion most commonly occurs in the proximal stomach high up on the lesser curve within 6 cm of the gastroesophageal junction, but it has also been described in the duodenum, jejunum (especially just distal to the ligament of Treitz), colon, and rectum. Injury to the overlying mucosa by some other means (e.g., NSAID) results in injury to the artery, and the vessel by itself is probably not the culprit for initiating the hemorrhage.

Hemorrhage from these lesions accounts for up to 15% of all cases presenting with massive GI bleeding and 1% to 2% of all upper GI bleeds. Although the disease is more common in the fifth to seventh decade, the age distribution is wide.[252] Diagnosis can be difficult because of the small size of the lesion. The endoscopic diagnosis is based on three criteria: active arterial spurting from a

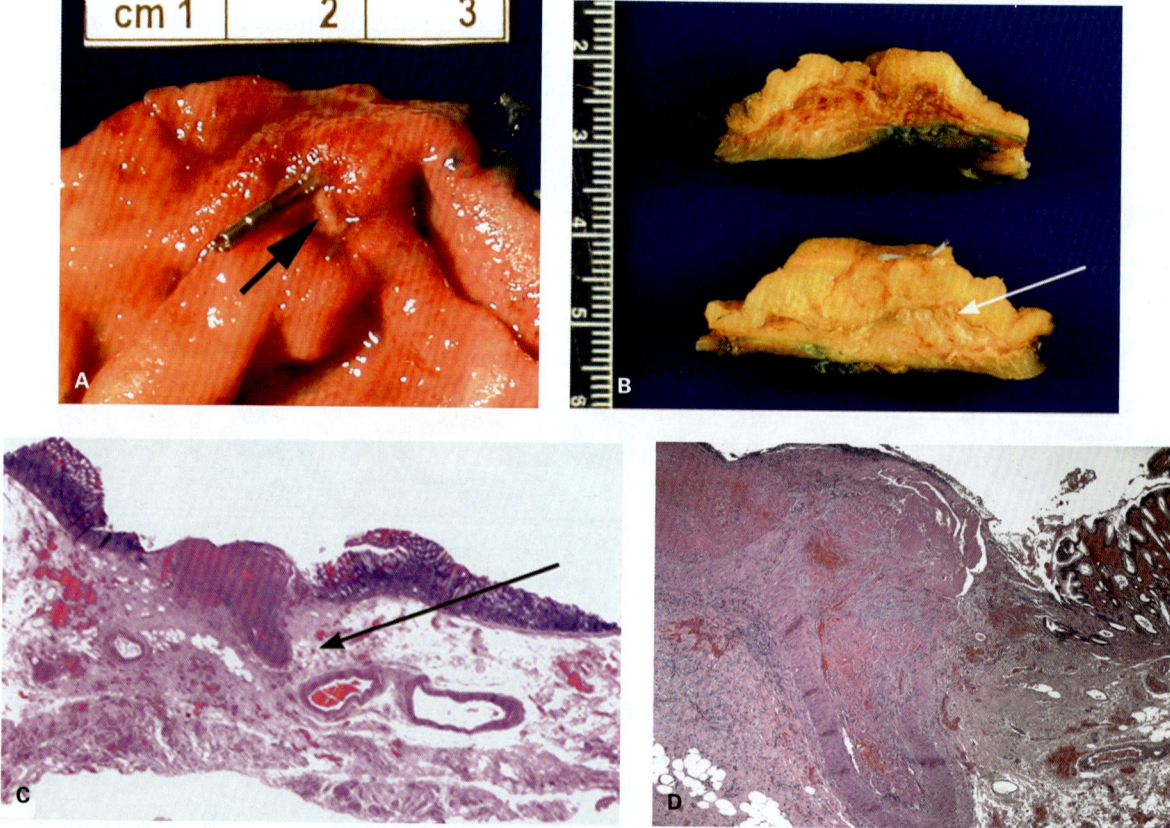

Figure 2-42. Dieulafoy's vascular malformation. **A:** Gross specimen of a proximal gastrectomy with the bleeding artery that has been clipped. The artery is visible near the surface through the mucosa (*arrow*). **B:** The cut surface shows the artery in the submucosa (*arrow*) coming close to the mucosa in the areas of ulceration, and corresponding **(C)** low magnification of the same areas to show the submucosal "caliber persistent" artery that is seen exposed to the surface in area of the ulcer (*arrow*). **D:** Closer view to show the thick artery with an organized thrombus at the base of this ulcer that led to the bleeding.

minute mucosal defect, <3 mm large; visualization of a protruding vessel with or without active bleeding within a small mucosal defect, surrounded by normal mucosa; and presence of an adherent clot attached to a small mucosal defect or a normal appearing mucosa.[253,254] Histologically, the artery appears structurally normal and is accompanied by a vein. At the site of ulceration it often undergoes thrombosis, sclerotic changes, and luminal obliteration secondarily (Fig 2-42D). Usually urgent treatment is needed because of massive bleeding. If endoscopic treatment such as sclerotherapy, ligation, or electrocoagulation fails, surgery is indicated. In preendoscopic era the mortality used to be very high up to 80%, but now this is rare.

Telangiectasias

Use of the terms vascular ectasia and telangiectasia interchangeably in the literature has resulted in a lot of confusion as to their associations and descriptions. Telangiectasias are also localized dilatations of preexisting capillaries and venules. They involve superficial small-sized vessels and hence are easily visible on the skin or mucosal surfaces. They may have a component of arteriovenous shunting; however, this is morphologically not evident on gross or microscopy and hence cannot be reliably differentiated from vascular ectasia on histology. Arterioles are only occasionally involved.[255] In contrast to vascular ectasias, which are the most often acquired condition, telangiectasias are more commonly inherited and congenital in origin. They can occur sporadically or in a syndromic setting. Telangiectasias of the whole GI tract are observed in CTDs, including scleroderma or as a part of CREST syndrome. In Turner syndrome (45XO karyotype), they may occur throughout the GI tract, but most commonly occur in the small intestine. Telangiectasias are an important component of hereditary hemorrhagic telangiectasia (HHT).

Hereditary hemorrhagic telangiectasia (Rendu–Osler–Weber Syndrome).
It is an autosomal dominant disorder associated with cutaneous and mucosal telangiectasia, mostly small in size, which increase in number and propensity to bleed with advancing age. The prevalence varies between 1 in 2,531 and 1 in 39,000. Anatomically the lesions are direct arteriovenous shunts. Molecular genetic analysis has identified several mutations in two genes, endoglin on chromosome 9 (HHT-type 1) and activin-like receptor kinase (ALK-1) on chromosome 12 (HHT-type 2).[256] Endoglin and ALK-1 are normally present on vascular endothelium and play an important role in vascular development and repair. GI involvement is more common with HHT-1 mutations. Epistaxis in childhood, repeated upper and lower GI tract bleeding, and chronic iron deficiency anemia are presenting symptoms. Telangiectasias are seen in small intestine and colon in

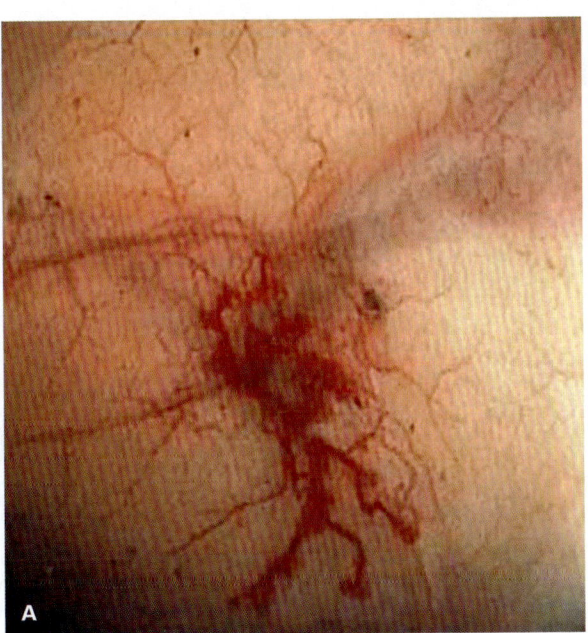 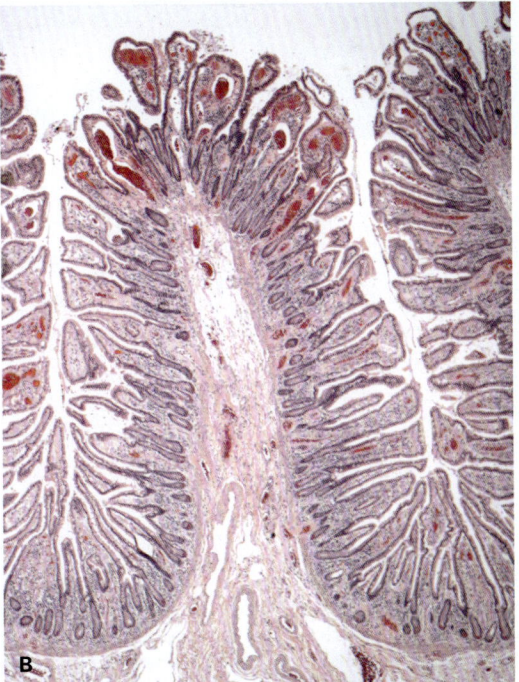

Figure 2-43. **A:** Vascular ectasia of the colon: endoscopic appearance. Note the characteristic solitary flat red spot in the mucosa. **B:** Vascular ectasia of the small intestine showing a mucosal fold with a large number of dilated, thin-walled vessels that extend in submucosa as well as mucosa.

about 15% to 25% of patients and result in acute or chronic blood loss.[256] Presentation with GI bleeding is uncommon before the age of 30. Clinical recognition depends on high degree of suspicion, a family history, and recognition of the skin lesions. The GI lesions can be identified on endoscopy (Fig. 2-43A). The lesions may regress with age.[235,236,257,258] Histologically, the lesions may be simply dilatation of mucosal and submucosal vessels, telangiectasias, or AVMs (Fig. 2-43B).

Arteriovenous Malformation

Arteriovenous malformations can be solitary or multiple and can be congenital or acquired. Congenital AVMs are found throughout the entire GI tract, but especially in the sigmoid. These are persistent communications between small- or medium-sized arteries and veins, usually located in the submucosa but may lead to capillary dilation in the mucosa and hemorrhages (Fig. 2-44A–C). Elastic tissue stains reveal vessels that clearly look like arteries or veins and some that defy precise classification. Once they bleed, secondary changes in the mucosa with scarring may result in a mucosal bump or a polypoid appearance, resulting in biopsies during a screening colonoscopy. Once hemorrhage has occurred, the lesions may undergo sclerosis and thrombosis, and aggregates of elastic fibers and scar may be seen in its place. The adjacent crypts may be distorted, and the reactive changes in the epithelium in a polypoid lesion may lead to a wrong diagnosis of an adenomatous polyp. Since the main lesions are largely submucosal, the mucosal biopsies tend to be nondiagnostic. Presence of dilated capillaries, hemosiderin-laden macrophages, and localized aggregates of elastic fibers may suggest an underlying arteriovenous malformation. Sometimes the polypoid nature of the lesions allows enough submucosa to be present in the biopsy for their correct identification.

Phlebectasia

Phlebectasia refers to a dilatation of veins, usually in the submucosa, or of the mesenteric vessels. The endothelial lining of the vessels may be abnormal. The condition is thought to be congenital in origin

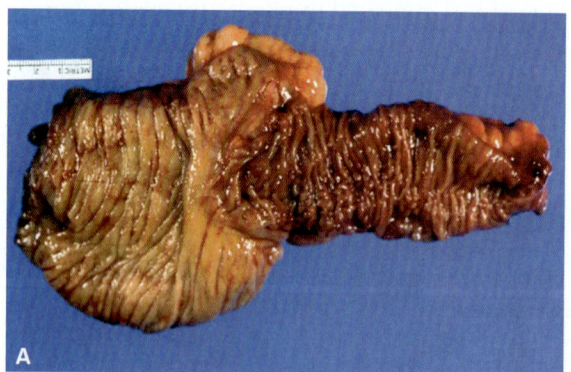
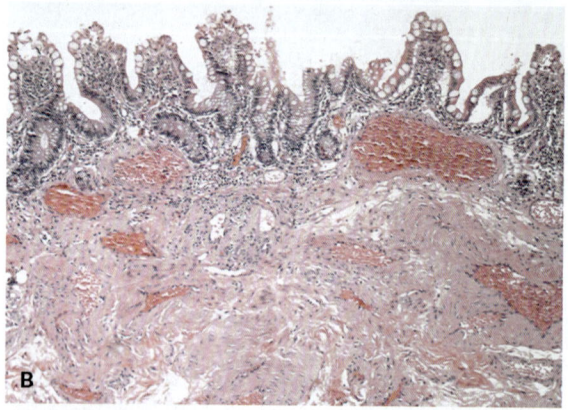
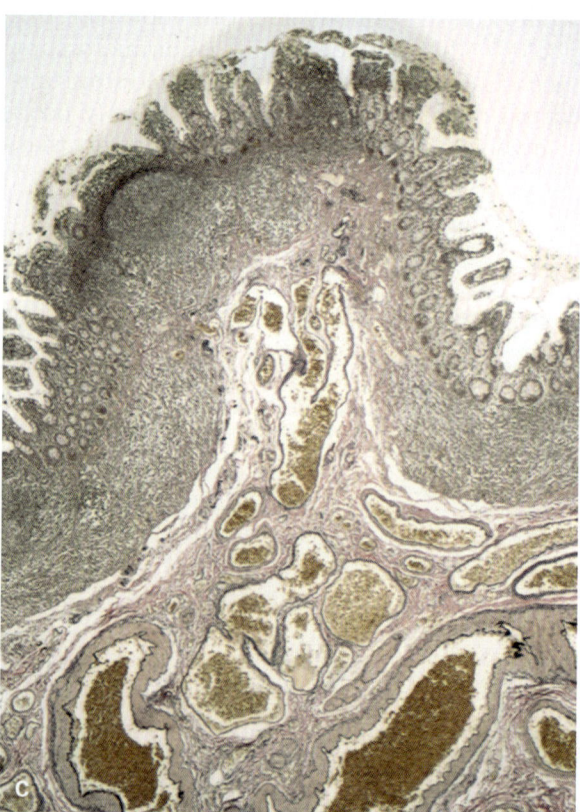

Figure 2-44. **A:** An ileocecal resection in a case with multiple AVMs grossly seen as tiny nodules on the mucosal surface that vary from grey white due to scarring and erythematous secondary to recent hemorrhages. **B:** Hematoxylin- and eosin-stained section showing an aggregate of abnormal thick- and thin-walled vessels located in the submucosa and extend into the mucosa. The true nature of the vascular lesion is difficult to appreciate in mucosal biopsies as the characteristic lesions are deeper in the submucosa. **C:** Elastic Van Giesson's stain shows the aggregates of abnormal dilated vessels in the submucosa that consist of arteries and veins. Even at this magnification, many vessels are seen that defy precise classification.

but most often presents in the middle-aged and the elderly, with signs of chronic or acute bleeding. The jejunum is the most common site involved. The abnormality may extend over several centimeters as compressible, blue-red nodules. It can be difficult to visualize on angiography.[259]

Diseases Affecting Blood Vessels

Portal hypertension, which is defined as an increase in portal venous pressure over 5 mm Hg, induces a dilatation of the venous system in the portal system, with development of collaterals between portal and systemic circulation. Dilatation of these collaterals manifests as esophageal and gastric varices. The presence of several portosystemic collaterals may also give rise to extensively dilated venules in other parts of the digestive tract, such as the duodenum (portal duodenopathy) and colon (portal colopathy). The prevalence of mucosal vascular abnormalities is up to 67% in the duodenum and even up to 84% in the colon, although on average they are more typically seen in the stomach.[23-28] PHG is more common in patients with cirrhosis (65%), but is also observed in patients with noncirrhotic portal hypertension.

In PHG endoscopy reveals four different patterns: mosaic (snake-skin) pattern, red-point lesions, cherry-red spots, and black-brown spots (Fig 2-40B). The first pattern is observed in mild degree of PHG. Histologically the lesions are characterized by dilatation of venules and capillaries at the level of the mucosa and submucosa. The lamina propria shows variable amount of inflammation, and sometimes intestinal metaplasia.[241,260-264] Lamina propria fibrohyalinosis with smooth muscle proliferation and platelet thrombi are typically absent, which help to differentiate it from GAVE (see GAVE). *Endocrine tumors* (*carcinoid*) in the ileum can cause fibrosis of the mesentery, resulting in kinking of the small bowel, intestinal obstruction, or intussusception and vascular involvement causing gut infarction. Tumoral or peritumoral secretion products (such as platelet-derived growth factor) may enhance ischemic lesions. Mesenteric arteries and veins located near the tumor, or away from it, may be thickened, and their lumen may be narrowed or occluded by elastic (perivascular) sclerosis.[265-267]

Disorders of Connective Tissue Affecting Blood Vessels

Pseudoxanthoma elasticum. This is usually an autosomal recessive condition and has been mapped to the p13.1 region of chromosome 16. It is occasionally dominantly inherited and has a prevalence of between 1/160,000 and 1/70,000. It is characterized by a defective elastin metabolism, which results in lax skin, retinal problems (angioid streaks), and degeneration of medium-sized vessels throughout the body. Abnormal vessels calcify and fail to contract normally following erosion, resulting in massive hemorrhage, particularly within the GI tract.

Patients may have a family history of the condition and usually present in their second or third decade with intestinal bleeding. Following an episode of bleeding, the gastric mucosa typically appears nodular at endoscopy, with "yellow cobblestone plaques" often surrounded by friable mucosa. The colonic mucosa also has yellowish plaques adherent. Submucosal arterioles may show degeneration of the elastica and calcification.[268]

Ehlers–Danlos syndrome. Ehlers–Danlos syndrome is a collective term for several disorders of collagen synthesis, and at least 10 subtypes are recognized.[269] Patients present with a wide variety of symptoms, such as hyperextensible joints, easy bruising, skin fragility, poor scar formation, and cardiac complaints due to valvular incompetence. Multiple modes of inheritance are described including autosomal dominant, autosomal recessive, or X-linked dominant, and precise defects have been identified in many subtypes.

GI involvement is seen with type IV, which is the most life-threatening form due to its association with spontaneous arterial rupture or visceral perforation.[270,271] It is characterized by mutations in the *COL3A1* gene, which results in defective type III collagen synthesis. Mode of transmission is autosomal dominant although many cases are sporadic. The clinical features include characteristic facial features (emaciated face, prominent cheek bones, sunken cheeks, bulging or sunken eyes, thin pinched nose, telangiectasias on eyelids), easy bruising, and a translucent skin. These signs are less obvious than the hyperflexibility of skin and joints seen in other types of Ehlers–Danlos syndrome; therefore, diagnosis of Ehlers–Danlos syndrome type IV is usually not considered until complications have occurred.[272] Complications are rare during infancy but occur in up to 25% individuals before the age of 20, and in 80% before 40 years. GI complications are relatively common and include hemorrhage from spontaneous arterial rupture, colonic perforation, diverticulitis, and rectal prolapse.[273-276] Bleeding from peptic ulcers, esophagitis, and diverticular disease of the colon can also occur. Bleeding often precedes the perforation. Other GI manifestations described are gastric infarction, visceroptosis, hiatus hernia, megaesophagus, and megacolon.

Histologically, specific lesions are not always found. In cases of spontaneous perforation, the bowel wall is typically thin, because of thin submucosa and muscularis propria.[272,277] The collagen in the stroma and blood vessels appears frayed and fragmented. Elastic tissue stains may show a fragmented elastic lamina in the arteries. Electron microscopy shows dilatation of granular endoplasmic reticulum of the dermal fibroblasts and abnormal structure of the collagen fibers; however, the changes are not specific.[278] The decreased collagen III can be shown by immunohistochemistry, although the diagnosis is generally established by identifying the mutation and showing decreased synthesis of collagen III by cultured fibroblasts obtained from skin biopsies. There is currently no specific treatment for the disease, and median survival is 48 years. About one-third of patients have recurrent perforations, and up to 8% die from bowel rupture and sepsis.

HANDLING OF SPECIMENS

Endoscopic Biopsies

Endoscopic biopsy samples can be processed routinely. Special stain for the identification of iron, elastic tissues, or collagen may be helpful in some cases.

Surgical Specimens

Ischemic disease. In acute mesenteric ischemia with gangrenous bowel disease, the main concern is the assessment of the viability of the bowel at the resection margins and the etiology of ischemia. For assessing the viability of the margins, frozen-section examination is of limited help. The surgeons have to rely on other signs such as restoration of color and pulsation of mesenteric vessels. It remains however important to assess the viability of the margins, extent of the lesion, status of the blood vessels, and if possible the etiology of the disease.

The gross features of the specimen (adhesions, strictures, color, thickness) should be defined before fixation whenever possible. Subsequently the bowel can be opened along the antimesenteric border and cleaned with tap water, or preferably with saline or buffered formalin, and the appearance, number of lesions, extent, and location must be determined. Sometimes, the bowel loops are matted together by adhesions. If possible, the adhesions should be dissected before the loops are disentangled and opened up.

In the mesentery, the vessels should be carefully examined for thrombosis and atherosclerosis. We prefer to cut the vessels transversely at different levels.

Following inspection and photography, the specimen should be fixed. Appropriate sections should include the full thickness of the involved bowel wall and the proximal and distal surgical margins. Also include, if possible, the interface with surrounding normal tissues and random normal appearing areas. In addition sections of the mesentery containing vessels are obtained.

Vascular malformations. It is important for the pathologist to be aware of the pitfalls of biopsy and resection specimens. Interpretation of biopsy specimens may be confusing due to traumatic or suction artifacts that induce vascular dilation and mucosal hemorrhage. On the other hand in resection specimens, the vessels may collapse, once blood drains out of them. Therefore, for the detection of vascular abnormalities, injection techniques have been proposed (Fig. 2-45A,B). There are two main methods, the silicon rubber technique and the barium–gelatin method. In the silicon rubber method, the specimens are first

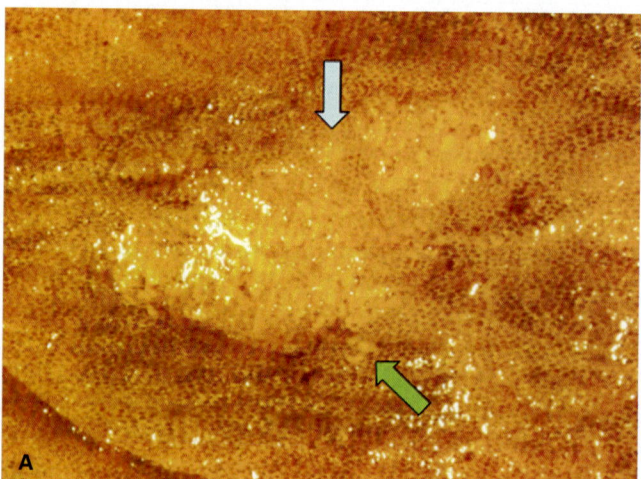
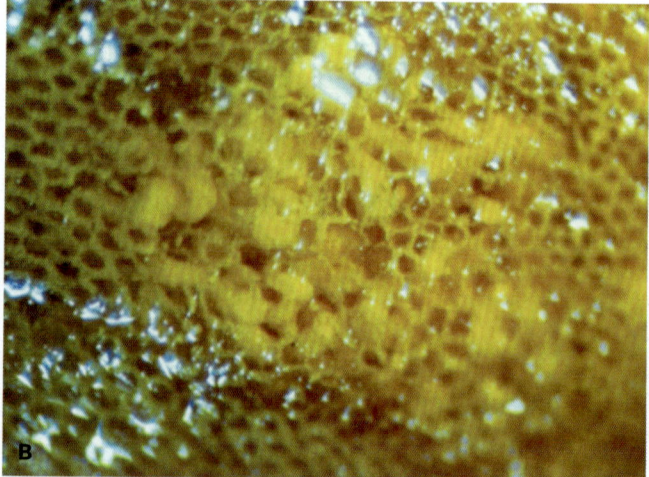

Figure 2-45. **A:** Injection study of an angiodysplastic lesion in the cecum in which the outline of the crypts can be seen together with the lesion at the center. However, this is really composed of several lesions, a larger one (**lower left**), smaller one (**upper right**), a small one between these (*blue arrow*) and a very small one (*green arrow*). **B:** A second smaller lesion in which the composite nature of the lesion, which is made up of clusters of dilated capillaries that are amalgamating. The capillaries that are ectatic are those surrounding the crypt openings. (Courtesy Roger Haggitt.)

injected with the rubber compound. Subsequently they are xerographed, cleared with methyl salicylate (oil of wintergreen), and examined with transillumination before histologic sampling. The smell of oil of wintergreen can permeate the laboratory and become quite obnoxious once the initial headiness has worn off.

The barium technique allows radiologic demonstration of the vascular abnormality and correlation with preoperative angiography. Both techniques are, however, time-consuming and expensive and hence not routinely used.[279] Extensive random sampling can also indeed reveal the lesions. Furthermore, the improvement of endoscopic detection and treatment of vascular malformations has decreased the number of surgical resections.[280] One may handle these specimens, usually operated for bleeding, differently from those obtained for ischemia. The viscus is fixed by filling up the lumen with formalin and then tying up both ends for 3 hours. This is followed by dissection of the mucosa.[281] This method could allow better identification of areas of ectatic vessels. Histologic sections taken from these areas usually show the lesions.

References

1. Pastores SM, Katz DP, Kvetan V. Splanchnic ischemia and gut mucosal injury in sepsis and the multiple organ dysfunction syndrome. *Am J Gastroenterol*. 1996;91(9):1697–1710.
2. Franssen G, Valembois P. Anatomy and embryology. In: Vantrappen G, Hellemans J, eds. *Diseases of the Esophagus*. Berlin, Germany: Springer Verlag; 1974:1–16.
3. Geboes K, Geboes KP, Maleux G. Vascular anatomy of the gastrointestinal tract. *Best Pract Res Clin Gastroenterol*. 2001;15(1):1–14.
4. Shapiro AL, Robillard GL. The esophageal arteries their configurational anatomy and variations in relation to surgery. *Ann Surg*. 1950;131(2):171–185; illust.
5. Potter SE, Holyoke EA. Observations on the intrinsic blood supply of the esophagus. *AMA Arch Surg*. 1950;61(5):944–948.
6. Butler H. The veins of the oesophagus. *Thorax*. 1951;6(3):276–296.
7. Kitano S, Terblanche J, Kahn D, Bornman PC. Venous anatomy of the lower oesophagus in portal hypertension: practical implications. *Br J Surg*. 1986;73(7):525–531.
8. Spence RA. The venous anatomy of the lower oesophagus in normal subjects and in patients with varices: an image analysis study. *Br J Surg*. 1984;71(10):739–744.
9. Noda T. Angioarchitectural study of esophageal varices. With special reference to variceal rupture. *Virchows Arch A Pathol Anat Histopathol*. 1984;404(4):381–392.
10. Kornblith PL, Boley SJ, Whitehouse BS. Anatomy of the splanchnic circulation. *Surg Clin North Am*. 1992;72(1):1–30.
11. Wenz W. *Abdominale Angiographie*. Berlin, Germany: Springer Verlag; 1972.
12. Putz R, Papst R. *Sobotta Atlas of Human Anatomy*. Munich, Germany: Urban & Schwarzenberg; 1997.
13. Gannon B. The vasculature and lymphatic drainage. In: Whitehead R, ed. *Gastrointestinal and Oesophageal Pathology*. 2nd ed. Edinburgh, UK: Churchill Livingstone; 1995:129–199.
14. Gannon B, Browning J, O'Brien P, Rogers P. Mucosal microvascular architecture of the fundus and body of human stomach. *Gastroenterology*. 1984;86(5 pt 1):866–875.
15. Piasecki C. Blood supply to the human gastroduodenal mucosa with special reference to the ulcer-bearing areas. *J Anat*. 1974;118(pt 2):295–335.
16. Ohtsuka A, Ohtani O, Murakami T. Microvascularization of the alimentary canal as studied by scanning electron microscoy of corrosion casts. In: Motta PF, Fujita H, eds. *Ultrastructure of de Digestive Tract*. Boston, MA: Martinus Nijohff Publishers; 1988:201–212.
17. Matsuura T, Yamamoto T. An electron microscope study of arteriolar branching sites in the normal gastric submucosa of rats and in experimental gastric ulcer. *Virchows Arch A Pathol Anat Histopathol*. 1988;413(2):123–131.
18. Gannon B, Rogers P, O'Brien P. Two capillary plexuses in human intestinal villi. *Micron*. 1980;11:447–448.
19. Wolfram-Gabel R, Maillot C, Koritke JG. Systematization of the angioarchitectonics of the colon in adult man. *Acta Anat (Basel)*. 1986;125(1):65–72.
20. Boley SJ, Brandt LJ, Veith FJ. Ischemic disorders of the intestines. *Curr Probl Surg*. 1978;15(4):1–85.
21. Marston A. Focal ischaemia of the small intestine. In: Marston A, ed. *Vascular Disease of the Gastrointestinal Tract: Pathophysiology, Recognition and Management*. Baltimore, MD: Williams & Wilkins; 1986:143–151.
22. Park NH, Kim JH, Choi DY, et al. Ischemic esophageal necrosis secondary to traumatic aortic transection. *Ann Thorac Surg*. 2004;78(6):2175–2178.
23. Lee KR, Stark E, Shaw FE. Esophageal infarction complicating spontaneous rupture of the thoracic aorta. *JAMA*. 1977;237(12):1233–1234.
24. Cappell MS. Esophageal necrosis and perforation associated with the anticardiolipin antibody syndrome. *Am J Gastroenterol*. 1994;89(8):1241–1245.
25. Prochaska JM, Flye MW, Johnsrude IS. Left gastric artery embolization for control of gastric bleeding: a complication. *Radiology*. 1973;107(3):521–522.
26. Bradley EL III, Goldman ML. Gastric infarction after therapeutic embolization. *Surgery*. 1976;79(4):421–424.
27. Bourdages R, Prentice RS, Beck IT, et al. Atheromatous embolization to the stomach: an unusual cause of gastrointestinal bleeding. *Am J Dig Dis*. 1976;21(10):889–894.
28. Force T, MacDonald D, Eade OE, et al. Ischemic gastritis and duodenitis. *Dig Dis Sci*. 1980;25(4):307–310.
29. Allende HD, Ona FV. Celiac artery and superior mesenteric artery insufficiency. Unusual cause of erosive gastroduodenitis. *Gastroenterology*. 1982;82(4):763–766.
30. Cherry RD, Jabbari M, Goresky CA, et al. Chronic mesenteric vascular insufficiency with gastric ulceration. *Gastroenterology*. 1986;91(6):1548–1552.
31. Talansky AL, Katz S, Naidich J. Aphthous ulcers in ischemic gastroenterocolitis: a case report. *Am J Gastroenterol*. 1985;80(4):257–259.
32. Hojgaard L, Krag E. Chronic ischemic gastritis reversed after revascularization operation. *Gastroenterology*. 1987;92(1):226–228.
33. Samama M, Gerotziafas G, Conard J, et al. Clinical aspects and laboratory problems in hereditary thrombophilia. *Haemostasis*. 1999;29(2–3):76–99.
34. Amitrano L, Brancaccio V, Guardascione MA, et al. High prevalence of thrombophilic genotypes in patients with acute mesenteric vein thrombosis. *Am J Gastroenterol*. 2001;96(1):146–149.
35. Lock G, Scholmerich J. Non-occlusive mesenteric ischemia. *Hepatogastroenterology*. 1995;42(3):234–239.
36. Trompeter M, Brazda T, Remy CT, et al. Non-occlusive mesenteric ischemia: etiology, diagnosis, and interventional therapy. *Eur Radiol*. 2002;12(5):1179–1187.
37. Haglund U, Bergqvist D. Intestinal ischemia—the basics. *Langenbecks Arch Surg*. 1999;384(3):233–238.

38. Kastin DA, Andrews J, Shah R, et al. Multiple myeloma presenting as mesenteric venous thrombosis and intestinal infarction. *Dig Dis Sci*. 2005;50(3):561-564.
39. Stoney RJ, Cunningham CG. Acute mesenteric ischemia. *Surgery*. 1993;114(3):489-490.
40. Collard CD, Gelman S. Pathophysiology, clinical manifestations, and prevention of ischemia-reperfusion injury. *Anesthesiology*. 2001;94(6):1133-1138.
41. Mansour MA. Management of acute mesenteric ischemia. *Arch Surg*. 1999;134(3):328-330; discussion 31.
42. Moawad J, Gewertz BL. Chronic mesenteric ischemia. Clinical presentation and diagnosis. *Surg Clin North Am*. 1997;77(2):357-369.
43. Cappell MS. Intestinal (mesenteric) vasculopathy. II. Ischemic colitis and chronic mesenteric ischemia. *Gastroenterol Clin North Am*. 1998;27(4):827-860, vi.
44. Connolly JE, Kwaan JH. Prophylactic revascularization of the gut. *Ann Surg*. 1979;190(4):514-522.
45. Kurland B, Brandt LJ, Delany HM. Diagnostic tests for intestinal ischemia. *Surg Clin North Am*. 1992;72(1):85-105.
46. Meaney JF, Prince MR, Nostrant TT, Stanley JC. Gadolinium-enhanced MR angiography of visceral arteries in patients with suspected chronic mesenteric ischemia. *J Magn Reson Imaging*. 1997;7(1):171-176.
47. Ming SC. Hemorrhagic necrosis of the gastrointestinal tract and its relation to cardiovascular status. *Circulation*. 1965;32(3):332-341.
48. Chiu CJ, McArdle AH, Brown R, et al. Intestinal mucosal lesion in low-flow states. I. A morphological, hemodynamic, and metabolic reappraisal. *Arch Surg*. 1970;101(4):478-483.
49. Brown RA, Chiu CJ, Scott HJ, Gurd FN. Ultrastructural changes in the canine ileal mucosal cell after mesenteric arterial occlusion. *Arch Surg*. 1970;101(2):290-297.
50. Wagner R, Gabbert H. Morphology and chronology of ischemic mucosal changes in the small intestine. A light and electron microscopic investigation. *Klin Wochenschr*. 1983;61(12):593-599.
51. Salinas-Madrigal L, Bruk A, deMello DE. Myofibrillar degeneration and necrosis of the visceral smooth musculature: an ischemic visceral myopathy. *Hum Pathol*. 1987;18(8):815-823.
52. Venance SL, Burns KL, Veinot JP, Walley VM. Contraction bands in visceral and vascular smooth muscle. *Hum Pathol*. 1996;27(10):1035-1041.
53. Guarino M, Reale D, Micoli G, et al. Smooth muscle contraction bands in intestinal infarction. *Virchows Arch A Pathol Anat Histopathol*. 1992;420(1):25-29.
54. Grendell JH, Ockner RK. Mesenteric venous thrombosis. *Gastroenterology*. 1982;82(2):358-372.
55. Mitros FA. The biopsy in evaluating patients with inflammatory bowel disease. *Med Clin North Am*. 1980;64(6):1037-1057.
56. Gandhi SK, Hanson MM, Vernava AM, et al. Ischemic colitis. *Dis Colon Rectum*. 1996;39(1):88-100.
57. Brandt LJ, Boley SJ. AGA technical review on intestinal ischemia. American Gastrointestinal Association. *Gastroenterology*. 2000;118(5):954-968.
58. Habu Y, Tahashi Y, Kiyota K, et al. Reevaluation of clinical features of ischemic colitis. Analysis of 68 consecutive cases diagnosed by early colonoscopy. *Scand J Gastroenterol*. 1996;31(9):881-886.
59. Preventza OA, Lazarides K, Sawyer MD. Ischemic colitis in young adults: a single-institution experience. *J Gastrointest Surg*. 2001;5(4):388-392.
60. Cohen DC, Winstanley A, Engledow A, et al. Marathon-induced ischemic colitis: why running is not always good for you. *Am J Emerg Med*. 2009;27(2):255 e5-e7.
61. Sanchez LD, Tracy JA, Berkoff D, Pedrosa I. Ischemic colitis in marathon runners: a case-based review. *J Emerg Med*. 2006;30(3):321-326.
62. Moses FM. Exercise-associated intestinal ischemia. *Curr Sports Med Rep*. 2005;4(2):91-95.
63. Linder JD, Monkemuller KE, Raijman I, et al. Cocaine-associated ischemic colitis. *South Med J*. 2000;93(9):909-913.
64. Lichtenstein GR, Yee NS. Ischemic colitis associated with decongestant use. *Ann Intern Med*. 2000;132(8):682.
65. Knudsen JF, Friedman B, Chen M, Goldwasser JE. Ischemic colitis and sumatriptan use. *Arch Intern Med*. 1998;158(17):1946-1948.
66. Kim HC, Park SB. Mycophenolate mofetil-induced ischemic colitis. *Transplant Proc*. 2000;32(7):1896-1897.
67. Holubar SD, Hassinger JP, Dozois EJ, Masuoka HC. Methamphetamine colitis: a rare case of ischemic colitis in a young patient. *Arch Surg*. 2009;144(8):780-782.
68. DiBaise JK. Tegaserod-associated ischemic colitis. *Pharmacotherapy*. 2005;25(4):620-625.
69. Chang L, Chey WD, Harris L, et al. Incidence of ischemic colitis and serious complications of constipation among patients using alosetron: systematic review of clinical trials and post-marketing surveillance data. *Am J Gastroenterol*. 2006;101(5):1069-1079.
70. Stillman AE, Weinberg M, Mast WC, et al. Ischemic bowel disease attributable to ergot. *Gastroenterology*. 1977;72(6):1336-1337.
71. Heyn J, Buhmann S, Ladurner R, et al. Recurrent ischemic colitis in a patient with leiden factor V mutation and systemic lupus erythematous with antiphospholipid syndrome. *Eur J Med Res*. 2008;13(4):182-184.
72. Theodoropoulou A, Sfiridaki A, Oustamanolakis P, et al. Genetic risk factors in young patients with ischemic colitis. *Clin Gastroenterol Hepatol*. 2008;6(8):907-911.
73. Wood MK, Read DR, Kraft AR, Barreta TM. A rare cause of ischemic colitis: polyarteritis nodosa. *Dis Colon Rectum*. 1979;22(6):428-433.
74. Shibata M, Nakamuta H, Abe S, et al. Ischemic colitis caused by strict dieting in an 18-year-old female: report of a case. *Dis Colon Rectum*. 2002;45(3):425-428.
75. Goumas K, Poulou A, Tyrmpas I, et al. Acute ischemic colitis during scuba diving: report of a unique case. *World J Gastroenterol*. 2008;14(20):3262-3265.
76. Arhan M, Onal IK, Odemis B, et al. Colonoscopy-induced ischemic colitis in a young patient with no risk factor. *Am J Gastroenterol*. 2009;104(1):250-251.
77. Duenas-Laita A, Mena-Martin FJ, Roquelai-Ruiz P, et al. Ischemic colitis associated with acute carbon monoxide poisoning. *Clin Toxicol (Phila)*. 2008;46(8):780-781.
78. Stewart CL, Menard GE. Sickle cell-induced ischemic colitis. *J Natl Med Assoc*. 2009;101(7):726-728.
79. Savoye G, Ben Soussan E, Hochain P, Lerebours E. How and how far to investigate ischemic colitis?. *Gastroenterol Clin Biol*. 2002;26(5 suppl):B12-B23.
80. Scowcroft CW, Sanowski RA, Kozarek RA. Colonoscopy in ischemic colitis. *Gastrointest Endosc*. 1981;27(3):156-161.
81. Brandt LJ, Katz HJ, Wolf EL, et al. Simulation of colonic carcinoma by ischemia. *Gastroenterology*. 1985;88(5 pt 1):1137-1142.
82. Brandt LJ, Boley SJ. Colonic ischemia. *Surg Clin North Am*. 1992;72(1):203-229.
83. Brandt LJ, Feuerstadt P, Blaszka MC. Anatomic patterns, patient characteristics, and clinical outcomes in ischemic colitis: a study of 313 cases supported by histology. *Am J Gastroenterol*. 2010;105(10):2245-2252.
84. Marston A, Pheils MT, Thomas ML, Morson BC. Ischaemic colitis. *Gut*. 1966;7(1):1-15.
85. Whitehead R. The pathology of ischemia of the intestines. *Pathol Annu*. 1976;11:1-52.
86. Dignan CR, Greenson JK. Can ischemic colitis be differentiated from C difficile colitis in biopsy specimens? *Am J Surg Pathol*. 1997;21(6):706-710.

87. Wang K, Weinrach D, Lal A, et al. Signet-ring cell change versus signet-ring cell carcinoma: a comparative analysis. *Am J Surg Pathol*. 2003;27(11):1429–1433.
88. Dimet S, Lazure T, Bedossa P. Signet-ring cell change in acute erosive gastropathy. *Am J Surg Pathol*. 2004;28(8): 1111–1112.
89. Whitehead R. The pathology of intestinal ischaemia. *Clin Gastroenterol*. 1972;1(3):613–637.
90. Nahon S, Dugue C, Adotti F, et al Small bowel obstruction secondary to ischemic stenosis due to cholesterol crystal embolism. *Ann Med Interne (Paris)*. 2000;151(5):417–420.
91. Ribbans WJ, Radcliffe AG. Retroperitoneal abscess following sclerotherapy for hemorrhoids. *Dis Colon Rectum*. 1985;28(3):188–189.
92. Weaver M. Atherosclerotic infarction of the rectum. *Br Med J*. 1984(288):684.
93. Nelson RL, Schuler JJ. Ischemic proctitis. *Surg Gynecol Obstet*. 1982;154(1):27–33.
94. Barnhill R, Busam K. Vascular diseases. In: Elder D, ed. *Lever's Histopathology of the Skin*. 8th ed. Philadelphia, PA: Lippincott Raven Publishers; 1997:185–208.
95. Miller LS, Barbarevech C, Friedman LS. Less frequent causes of lower gastrointestinal bleeding. *Gastroenterol Clin North Am*. 1994;23(1):21–52.
96. Tervaert JW, Kallenberg C. Neurologic manifestations of systemic vasculitides. *Rheum Dis Clin North Am*. 1993; 19(4):913–940.
97. Camilleri M, Pusey CD, Chadwick VS, et al. Gastrointestinal manifestations of systemic vasculitis. *Q J Med*. 1983;52(206):141–149.
98. Freilich BL, Bernstein CN. Vasculitis possibly confined to the small and large intestine. *West J Med*. 1995;162(1):63–65.
99. Muller-Ladner U. Vasculitides of the gastrointestinal tract. *Best Pract Res Clin Gastroenterol*. 2001;15(1):59–82.
100. Kussmaul A, Maier K. Ueber eine bisher nicht beschriebene eigenthumiliche Arterienkrankung (periarteritis Nodosa), die mit Morbus Brightii und rapid fortschreitender allgemeiner Muskellahmung einhergeht. *Dtsch Arch Klin Med*. 1866;1:484.
101. Zeek PM, Smith CC, Weeter JC. Studies on periarteritis nodosa; the differentiation between the vascular lesions of periarteritis nodosa and of hypersensitivity. *Am J Pathol*. 1948;24(4):889–917.
102. Jennette JC, Falk RJ. Small-vessel vasculitis. *N Engl J Med*. 1997;337(21):1512–1523.
103. Hunder GG, Arend WP, Bloch DA, et al. The American College of Rheumatology 1990 criteria for the classification of vasculitis. Introduction. *Arthritis Rheum*. 1990;33(8): 1065–1067.
104. Jennette JC, Falk RJ, Andrassy K, et al. Nomenclature of systemic vasculitides. Proposal of an international consensus conference. *Arthritis Rheum*. 1994;37(2):187–192.
105. Pagnoux C, Mahr A, Cohen P, Guillevin L. Presentation and outcome of gastrointestinal involvement in systemic necrotizing vasculitides: analysis of 62 patients with polyarteritis nodosa, microscopic polyangiitis, Wegener granulomatosis, Churg-Strauss syndrome, or rheumatoid arthritis-associated vasculitis. *Medicine (Baltimore)*. 2005;84(2):115–128.
106. Camilleri M, Pusey C, Chadwick V, Rees A. Vasculitis and the intestine. In: Phillips VCS, ed. *Small Intestine*. London, UK: Butterworths; 1982:227–248.
107. Langford CA. Vasculitis. *J Allergy Clin Immunol*. 2010;125(2 suppl 2):S216–S225.
108. Srigley JR, Gardiner GW. Giant cell arteritis with small bowel infarction. A case report and review of the literature. *Am J Gastroenterol*. 1980;73(2):157–161.
109. Kurata A, Nonaka T, Arimura Y, et al. Multiple ulcers with perforation of the small intestine in buerger's disease: a case report. *Gastroenterology*. 2003;125(3):911–916.
110. Edo N, Miyai K, Ogata S, et al. Thromboangiitis obliterans with multiple large vessel involvement: case report and analysis of immunophenotypes. *Cardiovasc Pathol*. 2010; 19(1):59–62.
111. Sachs IL, Klima T, Frankel NB. Thromboangiitis obliterans of the transverse colon. *JAMA*. 1977;238(4):336–337.
112. Herrington JL Jr, Grossman LA. Surgical lesions of the small and large intestine resulting from Buerger's disease. *Ann Surg*. 1968;168(6):1079–1087.
113. Lidar M, Lipschitz N, Langevitz P, et al. Infectious serologies and autoantibodies in Wegener's granulomatosis and other vasculitides: novel associations disclosed using the Rad BioPlex 2200. *Ann N Y Acad Sci*. 2009;1173:649–657.
114. Lidar M, Lipschitz N, Langevitz P, Shoenfeld Y. The infectious etiology of vasculitis. *Autoimmunity*. 2009;42(5): 432–438.
115. Matussek A, Strindhall J, Stark L, et al. Infection of human endothelial cells with *Staphylococcus aureus* induces transcription of genes encoding an innate immunity response. *Scand J Immunol*. 2005;61(6):536–544.
116. Bechah Y, Capo C, Raoult D, Mege JL. Infection of endothelial cells with virulent *Rickettsia prowazekii* increases the transmigration of leukocytes. *J Infect Dis*. 2008;197(1): 142–147.
117. Tavora F, Burke A. Review of isolated ascending aortitis: differential diagnosis, including syphilitic, Takayasu's and giant cell aortitis. *Pathology*. 2006;38(4):302–308.
118. Ferri C, Mascia MT. Cryoglobulinemic vasculitis. *Curr Opin Rheumatol*. 2006;18(1):54–63.
119. Guillevin L, Mahr A, Callard P, et al. Hepatitis B virus-associated polyarteritis nodosa: clinical characteristics, outcome, and impact of treatment in 115 patients. *Medicine (Baltimore)*. 2005;84(5):313–322.
120. Lehmann HW, von Landenberg P, Modrow S. Parvovirus B19 infection and autoimmune disease. *Autoimmun Rev*. 2003;2(4):218–223.
121. Finkel TH, Torok TJ, Ferguson PJ, et al. Chronic parvovirus B19 infection and systemic necrotising vasculitis: opportunistic infection or aetiological agent? *Lancet*. 1994;343(8908):1255–1258.
122. Meyer MF, Hellmich B, Kotterba S, Schatz H. Cytomegalovirus infection in systemic necrotizing vasculitis: causative agent or opportunistic infection? *Rheumatol Int*. 2000;20(1):35–38.
123. Fujiwara H, Hamashima Y. Pathology of the heart in Kawasaki disease. *Pediatrics*. 1978;61(1):100–107.
124. Wold LE, Baggenstoss AH. Gastrointestinal lesions of periarteritis nodosa. *Mayo Clin Proc*. 1949;24(2):28–35.
125. Lopez LR, Schocket AL, Stanford RE, et al. Gastrointestinal involvement in leukocytoclastic vasculitis and polyarteritis nodosa. *J Rheumatol*. 1980;7(5):677–684.
126. Perlemuter G, Chaussade S, Soubrane O, et al. Multifocal stenosing ulcerations of the small intestine revealing vasculitis associated with C2 deficiency. *Gastroenterology*. 1996;110(5):1628–1632.
127. Brogan P, Eleftheriou D, Dillon M. Small vessel vasculitis. *Pediatr Nephrol*. 2010;25(6):1025–1035.
128. Pinkney JH, Clarke G, Fairclough PD. Gastrointestinal involvement in Wegener's granulomatosis. *Gastrointest Endosc*. 1991;37(3):411–412.
129. Duclos B, Baumann R, Sondag D, et al. Specific gastric localization of Wegener's disease. *Gastroenterol Clin Biol*. 1987;11(2):154–157.
130. Muschen M, Warskulat U, et al. Deranged CD95 system in a case of Churg-Strauss vasculitis. *Gastroenterology*. 1998;114(6):1351–1352.
131. Churg J, Strauss L. Allergic granulomatosis, allergic angiitis, and periarteritis nodosa. *Am J Pathol*. 1951;27(2):277–301.

132. Lanham JG, Elkon KB, Pusey CD, Hughes GR. Systemic vasculitis with asthma and eosinophilia: a clinical approach to the Churg-Strauss syndrome. *Medicine (Baltimore)*. 1984;63(2):65–81.
133. Ohwada S, Yanagisawa A, Joshita T, et al. Necrotizing granulomatous vasculitis of transverse colon and gallbladder. *Hepatogastroenterology*. 1997;44(16):1090–1094.
134. Shimamoto C, Hirata I, Ohshiba S, et al. Churg-Strauss syndrome (allergic granulomatous angiitis) with peculiar multiple colonic ulcers. *Am J Gastroenterol*. 1990;85(3):316–319.
135. Gayraud M, Guillevin L, le Toumelin P, et al. Long-term followup of polyarteritis nodosa, microscopic polyangiitis, and Churg-Strauss syndrome: analysis of four prospective trials including 278 patients. *Arthritis Rheum*. 2001;44(3):666–675.
136. Lhote F, Cohen P, Guillevin L. Polyarteritis nodosa, microscopic polyangiitis and Churg-Strauss syndrome. *Lupus*. 1998;7(4):238–258.
137. Babian M, Nasef S, Soloway G. Gastrointestinal infarction as a manifestation of rheumatoid vasculitis. *Am J Gastroenterol*. 1998;93(1):119–120.
138. Marcolongo R, Bayeli PF, Montagnani M. Gastrointestinal involvement in rheumatoid arthritis: a biopsy study. *J Rheumatol*. 1979;6(2):163–173.
139. Janssen M, Dijkmans BA, Lamers CB. Upper gastrointestinal manifestations in rheumatoid arthritis patients: intrinsic or extrinsic pathogenesis? *Scand J Gastroenterol Suppl*. 1990;178:79–84.
140. Scott DG, Bacon PA, Tribe CR. Systemic rheumatoid vasculitis: a clinical and laboratory study of 50 cases. *Medicine (Baltimore)*. 1981;60(4):288–297.
141. Turner HE, Myszor MF, Bradlow A, David J. Lupus or lupoid hepatitis with mesenteric vasculitis. *Br J Rheumatol*. 1996;35(12):1309–1311.
142. Jones MP, Pandak WM, Moxley GF. Chronic diarrhea in essential mixed cryoglobulinemia: a manifestation of visceral vasculitis? *Am J Gastroenterol*. 1991;86(4):522–524.
143. Reissman P, Weiss EG, Teoh TA, et al. Gangrenous ischemic colitis of the rectum: a rare complication of systemic lupus erythematosus. *Am J Gastroenterol*. 1994;89(12):2234–2236.
144. Marshall JB, Kretschmar JM, Gerhardt DC, et al. Gastrointestinal manifestations of mixed connective tissue disease. *Gastroenterology*. 1990;98(5 pt 1):1232–1238.
145. Kagimoto S. Duodenal findings on ultrasound in children with Schonlein-Henoch purpura and gastrointestinal symptoms. *J Pediatr Gastroenterol Nutr*. 1993;16(2):178–182.
146. Powers BJ, Brown G, Williams RW, Speers W. Leukocytoclastic vasculitis, not associated with Henoch-Schonlein purpura, causing recurrent massive painless gastrointestinal hemorrhage. *Am J Gastroenterol*. 1992;87(9):1191–1193.
147. Morichau-Beauchant M, Touchard G, Maire P, et al. Jejunal IgA and C3 deposition in adult Henoch-Schonlein purpura with severe intestinal manifestations. *Gastroenterology*. 1982;82(6):1438–1442.
148. Paajanen H, Heikkinen M, Tarvainen R, et al. Anaplastic colon carcinoma associated with necrotizing vasculitis. *J Clin Gastroenterol*. 1995;21(2):168–169.
149. Saraga EP, Costa J. Idiopathic entero-colic lymphocytic phlebitis. A cause of ischemic intestinal necrosis. *Am J Surg Pathol*. 1989;13(4):303–308.
150. Lie JT. Mesenteric inflammatory veno-occlusive disease (MIVOD): an emerging and unsuspected cause of digestive tract ischemia. *Vasa*. 1997;26(2):91–96.
151. De Hertogh G, Van Eyken P, Stessens L, et al. Myointimal hyperplasia of mesenteric veins secondary to heterozygous factor V Leiden mutation. *Histopathology*. 2005;47(3):322–324.
152. Arora DS, Mahmood T, Wyatt JI. Lymphocytic venulitis: an unusual association with microscopic colitis. *J Clin Pathol*. 1999;52(4):303–304.
153. Melikoglu M, Kural-Seyahi E, Tascilar K, Yazici H. The unique features of vasculitis in Behcet's syndrome. *Clin Rev Allergy Immunol*. 2008;35(1–2):40–46.
154. Chave TA, Varma S, Patel GK, Knight AG. Malignant atrophic papulosis (Degos' disease): clinicopathological correlations. *J Eur Acad Dermatol Venereol*. 2001;15(1):43–45.
155. Tan WP, Chio MT, Ng SK. Generalized red papules with gastrointestinal complications. Diagnosis: malignant atrophic papulosis (Degos' disease). *Clin Exp Dermatol*. 2007;32(5):615–616.
156. Zhu KJ, Zhou Q, Lin AH, et al. The use of intravenous immunoglobulin in cutaneous and recurrent perforating intestinal Degos disease (malignant atrophic papulosis). *Br J Dermatol*. 2007;157(1):206–207.
157. CaseRecords. Case records of the Massachusetts General Hospital. Weekly clinicopathological exercises. Case 44–1980. *N Engl J Med*. 1980;303(19):1103–1111.
158. Hamed RM, Ghandour K. Abdominal angina and intestinal gangrene–a catastrophic presentation of arterial fibromuscular dysplasia: case report and review of the literature. *J Pediatr Surg*. 1997;32(9):1379–1380.
159. Guill CK, Benavides DC, Rees C, et al. Fatal mesenteric fibromuscular dysplasia: a case report and review of the literature. *Arch Intern Med*. 2004;164(10):1148–1153.
160. Meredith JT, Cerezo L, Alvarez M, et al. Gastrointestinal arterial fibromuscular dysplasia of childhood. *Arch Pathol Lab Med*. 1988;112(8):833–837.
161. Meacham PW, Brantley B. Familial fibromuscular dysplasia of the mesenteric arteries. *South Med J*. 1987;80(10):1311–1316.
162. Brophy CM, Frederick WG, Schlessel R, et al. Focal segmental ischemia of the terminal ileum mimicking Crohn's disease. *J Clin Gastroenterol*. 1988;10(3):343–347.
163. Hatzaras IS, Armen S, Dudrick SJ. Perforated stercoral ulcer of the sigmoid colon. *South Med J*. 2008;101(10):1072–1073.
164. deJong JL, Cohle SD, Busse F. Fatal stercoral ulcer perforation: case report. *Am J Forensic Med Pathol*. 1996;17(1):58–60.
165. Grinvalsky HT, Bowerman CI. Stercoraceous ulcers of the colon: relatively neglected medical and surgical problem. *J Am Med Assoc*. 1959;171:1941–1946.
166. Archibald SD, Jirsch DW, Bear RA. Gastrointestinal complications of renal transplantation. 2. The colon. *Can Med Assoc J*. 1978;119(11):1301–1305, 1309.
167. Bizer LS, Liebling RW, Delany HM, Gliedman ML. Small bowel obstruction: the role of nonoperative treatment in simple intestinal obstruction and predictive criteria for strangulation obstruction. *Surgery*. 1981;89(4):407–413.
168. Gutt CN, Oniu T, Schemmer P, et al. Fewer adhesions induced by laparoscopic surgery? *Surg Endosc*. 2004;18(6):898–906.
169. Majewski WD. Long-term outcome, adhesions, and quality of life after laparoscopic and open surgical therapies for acute abdomen: follow-up of a prospective trial. *Surg Endosc*. 2005;19(1):81–90.
170. Nguyen NT, Goldman C, Rosenquist CJ, et al. Laparoscopic versus open gastric bypass: a randomized study of outcomes, quality of life, and costs. *Ann Surg*. 2001;234(3):279–289; discussion 89–91.
171. Seshadri PA, Poulin EC, Schlachta CM, et al. Does a laparoscopic approach to total abdominal colectomy and proctocolectomy offer advantages? *Surg Endosc*. 2001;15(8):837–842.
172. Sosa J, Gardner B. Management of patients diagnosed as acute intestinal obstruction secondary to adhesions. *Am Surg*. 1993;59(2):125–128.

173. Frager D, Baer JW, Medwid SW, et al. Detection of intestinal ischemia in patients with acute small-bowel obstruction due to adhesions or hernia: efficacy of CT. *Am J Roentgenol.* 1996;166(1):67–71.
174. Ellis H. The cause and prevention of postoperative intraperitoneal adhesions. *Surg Gynecol Obstet.* 1971;133(3):497–511.
175. Pestieau SR, Marchettini P, Stuart OA, et al. Prevention of intraperitoneal adhesions by intraperitoneal lavage and intraperitoneal 5-fluorouracil: experimental studies. *Int Surg.* 2002;87(3):195–200.
176. Vowles K. Intestinal complications of strangulated hernia. *Br J Surg.* 1959;47:189–192.
177. Cherney LS. Intestinal stenosis following strangulated hernia; review of the literature and report of a case. *Ann Surg.* 1958;148(6):991–994.
178. Belghiti J, Rueff B, Fekele F. Umbilical hernia in cirrhotic patients with ascites. Prevalence course and management (abstract). *Gastroenterology.* 1988;84:1363.
179. Kirkpatrick S, Schubert T. Umbilical hernia rupture in cirrhotics with ascites. *Dig Dis Sci.* 1988;33(6):762–765.
180. Khan MA, Lo AY, Vande Maele DM. Paraduodenal hernia. *Am Surg.* 1998;64(12):1218–1222.
181. Gullino D, Giordano O, Gullino E. Internal hernia of the abdomen. Apropos of 14 cases. *J Chir (Paris).* 1993;130(4):179–195.
182. Tejler G, Jiborn H. Volvulus of the cecum. Report of 26 cases and review of the literature. *Dis Colon Rectum.* 1988;31(6):445–449.
183. Bhatnagar BN, Sharma CL, Gupta SN, et al. Study on the anatomical dimensions of the human sigmoid colon. *Clin Anat.* 2004;17(3):236–243.
184. Furuya Y, Yasuhara H, Yanagie H, et al. Role of ganglion cells in sigmoid volvulus. *World J Surg.* 2005;29(1):88–91.
185. Majeski J. Operative therapy for cecal volvulus combining resection with colopexy. *Am J Surg.* 2005;189(2):211–213.
186. Koffeman GI, van Gemert WG, George EK, et al. Classification, epidemiology and aetiology. *Best Pract Res Clin Gastroenterol.* 2003;17(6):879–893.
187. Fischer TK, Bihrmann K, Perch M, et al. Intussusception in early childhood: a cohort study of 1.7 million children. *Pediatrics.* 2004;114(3):782–785.
188. Treszl A, Tulassay T, Vasarhelyi B. Genetic basis for necrotizing enterocolitis–risk factors and their relations to genetic polymorphisms. *Front Biosci.* 2006;11:570–580.
189. Walker AM, Bohn RL, Cali C, et al. Risk factors for colon ischemia. *Am J Gastroenterol.* 2004;99(7):1333–1337.
190. Fishel R, Hamamoto G, Barbul A, et al. Cocaine colitis. Is this a new syndrome? *Dis Colon Rectum.* 1985;28(4):264–266.
191. Nalbandian H, Sheth N, Dietrich R, Georgiou J. Intestinal ischemia caused by cocaine ingestion: report of two cases. *Surgery.* 1985;97(3):374–376.
192. Barouk J, Doubremelle M, Faroux R, et al. Ischemic colitis after taking flutamide. *Gastroenterol Clin Biol.* 1998;22(10):841.
193. Larrey D, Lainey E, Blanc P, et al. Acute colitis associated with prolonged administration of neuroleptics. *J Clin Gastroenterol.* 1992;14(1):64–67.
194. Puspok A, Kiener HP, Oberhuber G. Clinical, endoscopic, and histologic spectrum of nonsteroidal anti-inflammatory drug-induced lesions in the colon. *Dis Colon Rectum.* 2000;43(5):685–691.
195. Cole JA, Cook SF, Sands BE, et al. Occurrence of colon ischemia in relation to irritable bowel syndrome. *Am J Gastroenterol.* 2004;99(3):486–491.
196. Hoyle M, Kennedy A, Prior AL, Thomas GE. Small bowel ischaemia and infarction in young women taking oral contraceptives and progestational agents. *Br J Surg.* 1977;64(8):533–537.
197. Lamy AL, Roy PH, Morissette JJ, Cantin R. Intimal hyperplasia and thrombosis of the visceral arteries in a young woman: possible relation with oral contraceptives and smoking. *Surgery.* 1988;103(6):706–710.
198. de Teresa E, Vera A, Ortigosa J, et al. Interaction between anticoagulants and contraceptives: an unsuspected finding. *Br Med J.* 1979;2(6200):1260–1261.
199. Abraham SC, Bhagavan BS, Lee LA, et al. Upper gastrointestinal tract injury in patients receiving kayexalate (sodium polystyrene sulfonate) in sorbitol: clinical, endoscopic, and histopathologic findings. *Am J Surg Pathol.* 2001;25(5):637–644.
200. Rashid A, Hamilton SR. Necrosis of the gastrointestinal tract in uremic patients as a result of sodium polystyrene sulfonate (Kayexalate) in sorbitol: an underrecognized condition. *Am J Surg Pathol.* 1997;21(1):60–69.
201. Chaplin AJ. The use of histological techniques for the demonstration of ion exchange resins. *J Clin Pathol.* 1999;52(10):776–779.
202. Mullick FG, McAllister HA Jr, Wagner BM, Fenoglio JJ Jr. Drug related vasculitis. Clinicopathologic correlations in 30 patients. *Hum Pathol.* 1979;10(3):313–325.
203. Fallows G, Rubinger M, Bernstein CN. Does gastroenterology consultation change management of patients receiving hematopoietic stem cell transplantation? *Bone Marrow Transplant.* 2001;28(3):289–294.
204. Yeong ML, Nicholson GI. *Clostridium septicum* infection in neutropenic enterocolitis. *Pathology.* 1988;20(2):194–197.
205. Mulholland MW, Delaney JP. Neutropenic colitis and aplastic anemia: a new association. *Ann Surg.* 1983;197(1):84–90.
206. Killian ST, Heitzman EJ. Intramural hemorrhage of small intestine due to anticoagulants. *JAMA.* 1967;200(7):591–594.
207. Birns MT, Katon RM, Keller F. Intramural hematoma of the small intestine presenting with major upper gastrointestinal hemorrhage. Case report and review of the literature. *Gastroenterology.* 1979;77(5):1094–1100.
208. Kolodny M, Mushlin AI, Baker WG Jr, et al. Intramural small intestinal hematoma. A review and a report of a new cause: uremia. *Arch Intern Med.* 1968;121(5):438–445.
209. Babb RR, Spittell JA Jr, Bartholomew LG. Gastroenterologic complications of anticoagulant therapy. *Mayo Clin Proc.* 1968;43(10):738–751.
210. Hui AJ, Wong RM, Ching JY, et al. Risk of colonoscopic polypectomy bleeding with anticoagulants and antiplatelet agents: analysis of 1657 cases. *Gastrointest Endosc.* 2004;59(1):44–48.
211. Hill H, Deppe H, Huchzermeyer H, Dormann AJ. Duodenal ileus due to an intramural duodenal haematoma. Conservative therapy using a multiple lumen intestinal probe. *Dtsch Med Wochenschr.* 2005;130(3):92–94.
212. Polat C, Dervisoglu A, Guven H, et al. Anticoagulant-induced intramural intestinal hematoma. *Am J Emerg Med.* 2003;21(3):208–211.
213. D'Abbicco D, Margari A, Amoruso M, et al. Small bowel obstruction due to intramural hematoma during anticoagulant therapy. With regard to two cases treated conservatively. *Chir Ital.* 2003;55(4):565–569.
214. Ilnyckyj A, Hosking DH, Pettigrew NM, Bernstein CN. Extracorporeal shock wave lithotripsy causing colonic injury. *Dig Dis Sci.* 1999;44(12):2485–2487.
215. Smedira N, Schecter WP. Blunt abdominal trauma. *Emerg Med Clin North Am.* 1989;7(3):631–645.

216. Schiffman MA. Nonoperative management of blunt abdominal trauma in pediatrics. *Emerg Med Clin North Am*. 1989;7(3):519–535.
217. Perez CA, Fox S, Lockett MA, et al. Impact of dose in outcome of irradiation alone in carcinoma of the uterine cervix: analysis of two different methods. *Int J Radiat Oncol Biol Phys*. 1991;21(4):885–898.
218. Kao MS. Intestinal complications of radiotherapy in gynecologic malignancy–clinical presentation and management. *Int J Gynaecol Obstet*. 1995;49(suppl):S69–S75.
219. Andreyev J. Gastrointestinal complications of pelvic radiotherapy: are they of any importance? *Gut*. 2005;54(8):1051–1054.
220. Willett CG, Ooi CJ, Zietman AL, et al. Acute and late toxicity of patients with inflammatory bowel disease undergoing irradiation for abdominal and pelvic neoplasms. *Int J Radiat Oncol Biol Phys*. 2000;46(4):995–998.
221. MacNaughton WK. Review article: new insights into the pathogenesis of radiation-induced intestinal dysfunction. *Aliment Pharmacol Ther*. 2000;14(5):523–528.
222. Beck PL, Wong JF, Li Y, et al. Chemotherapy- and radiotherapy-induced intestinal damage is regulated by intestinal trefoil factor. *Gastroenterology*. 2004;126(3):796–808.
223. Duncan M, Grant G. Oral and intestinal mucositis—causes and possible treatments. *Aliment Pharmacol Ther*. 2003;18(9):853–874.
224. Fajardo LF. The pathology of ionizing radiation as defined by morphologic patterns. *Acta Oncol*. 2005;44(1):13–22.
225. Werner-Wasik M. Treatment-related esophagitis. *Semin Oncol*. 2005;32(2 suppl 3):S60–S66.
226. Goldgraber MB, Rubin CE, Palmer WL, et al. The early gastric response to irradiation; a serial biopsy study. *Gastroenterology*. 1954;27(1):1–20.
227. Leupin N, Curschmann J, Kranzbuhler H, et al. Acute radiation colitis in patients treated with short-term preoperative radiotherapy for rectal cancer. *Am J Surg Pathol*. 2002;26(4):498–504.
228. Hardy RG, Brown RM, Miller SJ, et al. Transient P-cadherin expression in radiation proctitis; a model of mucosal injury and repair. *J Pathol*. 2002;197(2):194–200.
229. Touboul E, Balosso J, Schlienger M, Laugier A. Radiation injury of the small intestine. Radiobiological, radiopathological aspects; risk factors and prevention. *Ann Chir*. 1996;50(1):58–71.
230. Denton AS, Andreyev HJ, Forbes A, Maher EJ. Systematic review for non-surgical interventions for the management of late radiation proctitis. *Br J Cancer*. 2002;87(2):134–143.
231. den Hartog Jager FC, van Haastert M, Batterman JJ, Tytgat GN. The endoscopic spectrum of late radiation damage of the rectosigmoid colon. *Endoscopy*. 1985;17(6):214–216.
232. Camilleri M, Chadwick VS, Hodgson HJ. Vascular anomalies of the gastrointestinal tract. *Hepatogastroenterology*. 1984;31(3):149–153.
233. Foutch PG. Angiodysplasia of the gastrointestinal tract. *Am J Gastroenterol*. 1993;88(6):807–818.
234. Boley SJ, Sammartano R, Adams A, et al. On the nature and etiology of vascular ectasias of the colon. Degenerative lesions of aging. *Gastroenterology*. 1977;72(4 pt 1):650–660.
235. Meyer CT, Troncale FJ, Galloway S, Sheahan DG. Arteriovenous malformations of the bowel: an analysis of 22 cases and a review of the literature. *Medicine (Baltimore)*. 1981;60(1):36–48.
236. Weinstock LB, Larson RS, Stahl DJ, Fleshman JW. Diffuse microscopic angiodysplasia–a previously unreported variant of angiodysplasia. Report of a case. *Dis Colon Rectum*. 1995;38(4):428–432.
237. Stamm B, Heer M, Buhler H, Ammann R. Mucosal biopsy of vascular ectasia (angiodysplasia) of the large bowel detected during routine colonoscopic examination. *Histopathology*. 1985;9(6):639–646.
238. Foutch PG, Rex DK, Lieberman DA. Prevalence and natural history of colonic angiodysplasia among healthy asymptomatic people. *Am J Gastroenterol*. 1995;90(4):564–567.
239. Foutch PG. Colonic angiodysplasia. *Gastroenterologist*. 1997;5(2):148–156.
240. Selinger CP, Ang YS. Gastric antral vascular ectasia (GAVE): an update on clinical presentation, pathophysiology and treatment. *Digestion*. 2008;77(2):131–137.
241. Burak KW, Lee SS, Beck PL. Portal hypertensive gastropathy and gastric antral vascular ectasia (GAVE) syndrome. *Gut*. 2001;49(6):866–872.
242. Ward EM, Raimondo M, Rosser BG, et al. Prevalence and natural history of gastric antral vascular ectasia in patients undergoing orthotopic liver transplantation. *J Clin Gastroenterol*. 2004;38(10):898–900.
243. Jabbari M, Cherry R, Lough JO, et al. Gastric antral vascular ectasia: the watermelon stomach. *Gastroenterology*. 1984;87(5):1165–1170.
244. Gostout CJ, Viggiano TR, Ahlquist DA, et al. The clinical and endoscopic spectrum of the watermelon stomach. *J Clin Gastroenterol*. 1992;15(3):256–263.
245. Lowes J, Rode J. Neuroendocrine cell proliferations in gastric antral vascular ectasia. *Gastroenterology*. 1987;97:207–212.
246. Gilliam JH III, Geisinger KR, Wu WC, et al. Endoscopic biopsy is diagnostic in gastric antral vascular ectasia. The "watermelon stomach". *Dig Dis Sci*. 1989;34(6):885–888.
247. Westerhoff M, Tretiakova M, Hovan L, et al. CD61, CD31, and CD34 improve diagnostic accuracy in gastric antral vascular ectasia and portal hypertensive gastropathy: An immunohistochemical and digital morphometric study. *Am J Surg Pathol*. 2010;34(4):494–501.
248. Payen JL, Cales P, Voigt JJ, et al. Severe portal hypertensive gastropathy and antral vascular ectasia are distinct entities in patients with cirrhosis. *Gastroenterology*. 1995;108(1):138–144.
249. Dieulafoy G. Exulceratio simplex. L'intervention chirurigicale dans les hematemeses foudroyantes consecutives a l'exulcration simple de l'estomac. *Bull Acad Med*. 1989(49):49–84.
250. Gallard T. Aneurysmes miliaires de l'estomac, donnant lieu a des hemateneses mortelles. *Bull Soc Med Hop Paris*. 1884;1:84–91.
251. Miko TL, Thomazy VA. The caliber persistent artery of the stomach: a unifying approach to gastric aneurysm, Dieulafoy's lesion, and submucosal arterial malformation. *Hum Pathol*. 1988;19(8):914–921.
252. Veldhuyzen van Zanten SJ, Bartelsman JF, et al. Recurrent massive haematemesis from Dieulafoy vascular malformations—a review of 101 cases. *Gut*. 1986;27(2):213–222.
253. Dy NM, Gostout CJ, Balm RK. Bleeding from the endoscopically-identified Dieulafoy lesion of the proximal small intestine and colon. *Am J Gastroenterol*. 1995;90(1):108–111.
254. Reilly HF 3rd, al-Kawas FH. Dieulafoy's lesion. Diagnosis and management. *Dig Dis Sci*. 1991;36(12):1702–1707.
255. Ball NJ, Duggan MA. Hepatolithiasis in hereditary hemorrhagic telangiectasia. *Arch Pathol Lab Med*. 1990;114(4):423–425.
256. Grand'Maison A. Hereditary hemorrhagic telangiectasia. *CMAJ*. 2009;180(8):833–835.

257. Azuma H. Genetic and molecular pathogenesis of hereditary hemorrhagic telangiectasia. *J Med Invest*. 2000; 47(3-4):81-90.
258. Guttmacher AE, Marchuk DA, White RI Jr. Hereditary hemorrhagic telangiectasia. *N Engl J Med*. 1995;333(14): 918-924.
259. Mejia EM, Alvarez OA, Anderson EC, et al. Jejunal phlebectasia presenting with massive gastrointestinal hemorrhage. *J Clin Gastroenterol*. 1996;22(3):215-217.
260. Gupta R, Saraswat VA, Kumar M, et al. Frequency and factors influencing portal hypertensive gastropathy and duodenopathy in cirrhotic portal hypertension. *J Gastroenterol Hepatol*. 1996;11(8):728-733.
261. Misra V, Misra SP, Dwivedi M, Gupta SC. Histomorphometric study of portal hypertensive enteropathy. *Am J Clin Pathol*. 1997;108(6):652-657.
262. Tam TN, Ng WW, Lee SD. Colonic mucosal changes in patients with liver cirrhosis. *Gastrointest Endosc*. 1995;42(5): 408-412.
263. Geboes K, el-Deeb G, el-Haddad S, et al. Vascular alterations of the colonic mucosa in schistosomiasis and portal colopathy. *Hepatogastroenterology*. 1995;42(4):343-347.
264. Spina GP, Arcidiacono R, Bosch J, et al. Gastric endoscopic features in portal hypertension: final report of a consensus conference, Milan, Italy, September 19, 1992. *J Hepatol*. 1994;21(3):461-467.
265. Strobbe L, D'Hondt E, Ramboer C, et al. Ileal carcinoid tumors and intestinal ischemia. *Hepatogastroenterology*. 1994;41(5):499-502.
266. Bessell JR, Karatassas A, Allen PW. Intestinal ischaemia associated with carcinoid tumour: a case report with review of the pathogenesis. *J Gastroenterol Hepatol*. 1994;9(3):304-307.
267. Chaudhry A, Papanicolaou V, Oberg K, et al. Expression of platelet-derived growth factor and its receptors in neuroendocrine tumors of the digestive system. *Cancer Res*. 1992;52(4):1006-1012.
268. Fruhwirth H, Rabl H, Hauser H, et al. Endoscopic findings in pseudoxanthoma elasticum. *Endoscopy*. 1994;26(5): 507.
269. Germain D. Ehlers-Danlos syndromes. Clinical, genetic and molecular aspects. *Ann Dermatol Venereol*. 1995;122(4): 187-204.
270. Silva R, Cogbill TH, Hansbrough JF, et al. Intestinal perforation and vascular rupture in Ehlers-Danlos syndrome. *Int Surg*. 1986;71(1):48-50.
271. Germain DP. Ehlers-Danlos syndrome type IV. *Orphanet J Rare Dis*. 2007;2:32.
272. Blaker H, Funke B, Hausser I, et al. Pathology of the large intestine in patients with vascular type Ehlers-Danlos syndrome. *Virchows Arch*. 2007;450(6):713-717.
273. Habein HC. Ehlers-Danlos syndrome with spontaneous rupture of the esophagus. Report of first case. *Rocky Mt Med J*. 1977;74(2):78-80.
274. Shaikh NA, Turner DT. Ehlers-Danlos syndrome presenting with infarction of stomach. *J R Soc Med*. 1988; 81(10):611.
275. Dalle I, Geboes K. Vascular lesions of the gastrointestinal tract. *Acta Gastroenterol Belg*. 2002;65(4):213-219.
276. Solomon JA, Abrams L, Lichtenstein GR. GI manifestations of Ehlers-Danlos syndrome. *Am J Gastroenterol*. 1996;91(11):2282-2288.
277. Sykes EM, Jr. Colon perforation in Ehlers-Danlos syndrome. Report of two cases and review of the literature. *Am J Surg*. 1984;147(3):410-413.
278. Hausser I, Anton-Lamprecht I. Differential ultrastructural aberrations of collagen fibrils in Ehlers-Danlos syndrome types I-IV as a means of diagnostics and classification. *Hum Genet*. 1994;93(4):394-407.
279. Aldabagh SM, Trujillo YP, Taxy JB. Utility of specimen angiography in angiodysplasia of the colon. *Gastroenterology*. 1986;91(3):725-729.
280. Yang VX, Tang SJ, Gordon ML, et al. Endoscopic Doppler optical coherence tomography in the human GI tract: initial experience. *Gastrointest Endosc*. 2005;61(7): 879-890.
281. Thelmo WL, Vetrano JA, Wibowo A, et al. Angiodysplasia of colon revisited: pathologic demonstration without the use of intravascular injection technique. *Hum Pathol*. 1992;23(1):37-40.

3 Immunodeficiency Disorders

Chapter Outline

INTESTINAL HOST DEFENCES
FUNCTIONAL ANATOMY OF THE GI IMMUNE SYSTEM
- *Normal Distribution of Gut-associated Lymphoid Tissue*
- Humoral immune system of the gut
- Cellular immune system of the gut

IMMUNODEFICIENCY DISORDERS OF THE INTESTINAL TRACT
- Clinical features
- Histology

PRIMARY IMMUNODEFICIENCY DISORDERS
- *Predominant Antibody Defects*
- Common variable hypogammaglobulinemia (Late-onset acquired hypogammaglobulinemia, common variable immunodeficiency [CVID], Bruton's X-linked agammaglobulinemia [XLAG])
- Selective IgA deficiency
- Secretory component deficiency
- Infantile X-linked agammaglobulinemia (Bruton's agammaglobulinemia, congenital agammaglobulinemia)
- Miscellaneous B-cell disorders
- *Predominant Cell-mediated Immunodeficiency*
- Severe combined immunodeficiency disease (Swiss-type agammaglobulinemia, hereditary thymic dysplasia)
- IPEX syndrome
- Chronic mucocutaneous candidiasis

IMMUNODEFICIENCY ASSOCIATED WITH OTHER DEFECTS
- *DiGeorge's Syndrome—Third and Fourth Pouch/Arch Syndrome (Thymic Hypoplasia, Cellular Immunodeficiency with Hypoparathyroidism)*

PHAGOCYTIC AND OTHER CELL DYSFUNCTION
- *Chronic Granulomatous Disease*
- *Systemic Mastocytosis*

SECONDARY (ACQUIRED) IMMUNODEFICIENCY DISORDERS
- *Bone Marrow Transplantation*
- Transplantation regimen
- Infection
- Graft versus host disease (GVHD)
- Chronic GVHD
- *Intestinal Transplantation*
- *The Acquired Immunodeficiency Syndrome (AIDS)*
- Pathogenesis and clinical features
- GI AIDS infections
- GI neoplasms in AIDS

WORKUP OF THE IMMUNODEFICIENT PATIENT

INTESTINAL HOST DEFENCES

The gastrointestinal (GI) tract must digest and selectively absorb nutrients, while at the same time excluding large amounts of potentially harmful ingested substances such as microorganisms and toxins.[1-4] Both immune and nonimmune defense mechanisms are important for intestinal host defense.[3,5-8] This defense is provided within the lumen by secretory IgA (originating from the intestine or bile) and within the mucosa by lymphocytes (mucosal alphabeta and gammadelta T cells),[5,6,8] plasma cells, and macrophages.[9] Secretory IgA has been likened to antiseptic paint, which lines the bowel mucosa, acting as a protective layer. It has four antigen-combining sites and is very efficient at agglutinating bacteria and viruses and preventing their adherence to mucosal surfaces. In addition, IgA interferes with the absorption of many macromolecules by combining with food. This helps prevent harmful systemic immune responses. The antigens (particulate and soluble products) that do escape the action of secretory IgA and penetrate the surface epithelium may form immune complexes, which can be cleared by the liver and excreted in the bile. Alternatively, they may be cleared by locally sensitized lymphocytes, by combination with preformed antibodies, or by ingestion by macrophages.[5]

Much of the work on gut immunology has centered on the role of humoral immunity on gut defense mechanisms. However, B-cell function is often under the control of T cells.[5,10,11] Intraepithelial lymphocytes (IELs), most of which are of T-cell (CD-8) type, have an important cytotoxic action. Cell-mediated immunity appears to play an important role in fungal infections such as candidiasis, certain viral diseases, and parasitic infections, whereas humoral immunity seems more important in protecting against run-of-the-mill enteric bacterial and viral infections.[12]

A variety of nonimmunologic factors contribute to gut host defense. They include the physical integrity of the mucosa/mucosal barrier (intestinal permeability); intestinal mucus, which may impair antigen binding and allow antigen degradation by intestinal enzymes; resident microbial flora; acid and pepsin, which cause bacterial and dietary antigen degradation; bile acids, which suppress microbial proliferation; and bowel motility. The latter produces regular cleansing of the intestinal tract.[13-15]

FUNCTIONAL ANATOMY OF THE GI IMMUNE SYSTEM

Normal Distribution of Gut-associated Lymphoid Tissue

Lymphoid tissue is normally abundant throughout the GI mucosa (including IELs) with the exception of the stomach and in fact is the largest lymphoid organ in the body.[8] In the stomach, there are almost no lymphocytes and plasma cells within the gastric fundus and body and only a few within the antrum and cardia. The lymphoid tissue first appears in the lamina propria of the bowel at 10 weeks[16] and by 14 weeks lymphoid follicles develop. Plasma cells appear at birth but are very scanty.[16] The lymphoid tissue is arranged in three forms:

1. As IELs, throughout the GI tract, including the esophagus.
2. As a diffuse lymphoplasmacytic infiltrate, which is distributed evenly throughout the intestinal mucosa of the small and large intestines.
3. As lymphoid nodules. There are essentially two types:
   a. Solitary lymphoid nodules present throughout the GI tract but most numerous in the distal colon.[17]
   b. Aggregates of lymphoid nodules, which occur in the appendix and small intestine. In the small intestine, these aggregates are referred to as Peyer's patches and are most frequent in the distal ileum.[18]

The lymphoid tissue in the ileocecal valve is unique in that it is arranged circumferentially around the valve. The mesenteric lymph nodes are also usually considered part of the gut-associated lymphoid tissue (GALT). In common with the gut, mesenteric lymph nodes are exposed to considerable antigenic material via the lymphatic flow from the small and large intestines and are populated by predominantly IgA precursor B-cell lymphocytes.

The Diffuse Lymphoid Tissue This tissue is contained in two separate compartments, namely, intraepithelial and intramucosal.[19]

INTRAEPITHELIAL LYMPHOCYTES. These cells are located within the surface epithelial layer of the mucosa, the so-called IELs (Fig. 3-1A). They occur predominantly in the basal portion of the epithelial layer, between the epithelial cells and the basement membrane.[20,21]

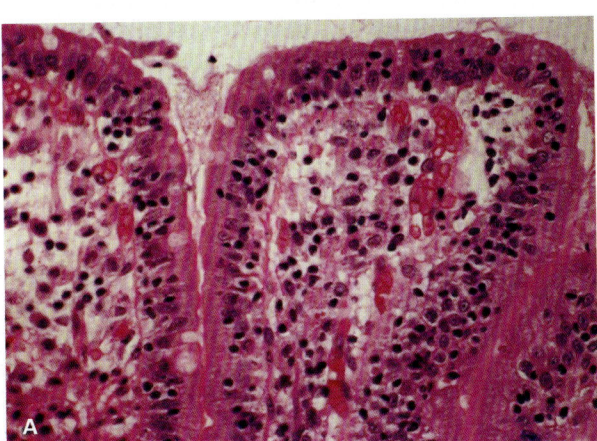 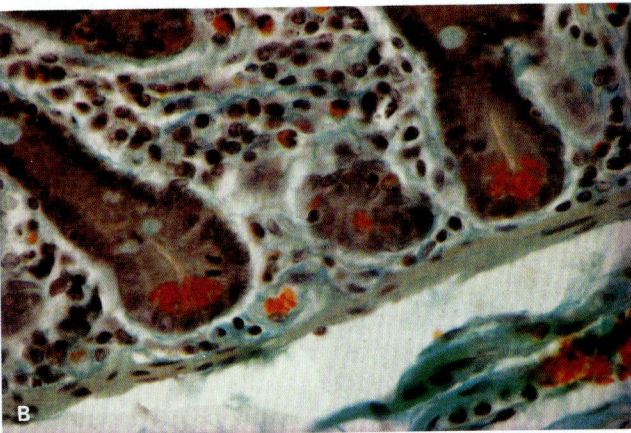

Figure 3-1. The diffuse lymphoid system of the intestinal tract. **A:** Intraepithelial lymphocytes (IELs). Mucosal biopsy specimen from a patient with tropical sprue, showing intestinal villi with an increased number of lymphocytes within the surface epithelium. **B:** Section of normal jejunal mucosa showing lymphocytes, plasma cells and eosinophils within the lamina propria between the intestinal crypts. Using this stain, Paneth cells in the crypt bases are bright orange red. (Masson's trichrome stain)

Although they appear to be few in number in any one section (at the range of 10–25 per 100 epithelial cells in the small bowel and ~5 per 100 epithelial cells in the colon),[22–24] when the entire intestine is considered, they are in fact very numerous and are said to equal in aggregate the number of lymphocytes found in the spleen. Histologically, the IELs consist of dense nuclei with minimal cytoplasm and do not have any epithelial attachment. The predominant phenotype is the cytotoxic T cell expressing $\alpha\beta$ T-cell receptors, which are CD3+, CD8+, CD103+, CD4−, and CD5−. A smaller population (10%–15%) consists of T cells expressing $\gamma\delta$ T-cell receptors that are negative for both CD4 and CD8. A third population of CD56+ IELs is also recognized that are virtually undetectable in normal mucosa. They have T-cytotoxic and natural killer (NK) properties.[20,25] The IELs overlying the lymphoid follicles consist predominantly of B cells. In addition, other intraepithelial cells such as macrophages, mast cells, neutrophils, and eosinophils may also be present.[16,23,26] IELs are greatly increased in several diseases, such as celiac sprue, tropical sprue, lymphocytic colitis, and collagenous colitis. They are typically not increased in inflammatory bowel disease.[23] In inflammatory states, neutrophils and eosinophils may also enter this compartment.[27]

Lymphocytes are also present within the esophageal squamous epithelium. They occur primarily within the suprabasal portion of the mucosa, interdigitating between the squamous cells, and phenotypically consist of CD3/CD8 cytotoxic suppressor cells.[28]

INTRAMUCOSAL CELLULAR INFILTRATE (LYMPHOCYTES, PLASMA CELLS, EOSINOPHILS, MAST CELLS, MACROPHAGES, ETC.). The cells consist primarily of numerous lymphocytes, plasma cells, and eosinophils. In addition, a heterogeneous group of other cells are also present in smaller numbers, namely, eosinophils, mast cells, macrophages, dendritic cells, rare basophils, and T lymphocytes (Fig. 3-1B). The latter consist primarily of helper inducer cells.[29]

Intramucosal lamina propria. With regard to lymphocytes, the lamina propria is the largest compartment of GI lymphocytes, the number being in the range of several thousands per square millimeter. They are located primarily in the crypt region and less frequently in the villi in the small bowel. The majority of plasma cells, many of which contain Russell bodies, consist primarily of IgA-containing cells, followed by IgM, IgG, and IgE.[25] IgD-containing plasma cells are exceedingly sparse in the normal GI tract.

Neutrophils are exceedingly rare/absent in the normal lamina propria. However, eosinophils are generally present, ranging up to 200 per mm^2.[30] The number of eosinophils in the colon is highest on the right side and lowest in the rectum. The number of eosinophils in the lamina propria also varies geographically according to latitude, as the farther north one goes in the United States, the fewer eosinophils one finds in normal colon biopsies.[31]

Mucosal mast cells. The mast cells occur predominantly in the lamina propria as well as the submucosa and appear to be more common in the ileum than the jejunum, up to about 750 cells per mm^2.[32] In the mucosa, they are primarily within the superficial half of the lamina propria. They have proved to be more numerous than was previously thought, mainly because they were previously missed in routinely prepared tissue sections. In animal studies, there is great heterogeneity among mast cells in that intestinal mast cells are morphologically and functionally distinct from peritoneal and systemic mast cells.[33] The same type of difference may also exist in man, but this remains to be proven.[34] Mast cells have physiologic regulatory effects as well as pathologic effects.[35] Their function was previously thought to be confined to IgE-mediated hypersensitivity reactions. However, recent animal studies have shown that they are also involved in the late-phase components of allergic reactions, delayed-onset hypersensitivity, and regulation of immune responses. With regard to the functional activity of the mast cells, a variety of substances are released from the cells, leading to a number of factors such as blood flow regulation, endothelial and epithelial permeability, angiogenesis, mucosal secretion, and intestinal motility.[32] Moreover, mast cells can express direct cytotoxic activity and can potentiate eosinophil and macrophage cytotoxicity.[34] In certain conditions, such as nematode infections, gastritis, celiac sprue, idiopathic inflammatory bowel disease, and irritable bowel disease, mast cell numbers may be markedly increased in concert with other inflammatory cells.[36]

Histologically, Carnoy's fixative[37] was found to be better than formalin for identifying mucosal mast cells. Recently, however, a number of immunostains have been helpful in identifying these cells such as mast cell tryptase, CD117 (C kit),[38] and CD68 (KP-1).[39] These stains seem to obviate the need for any special fixatives as they work well on formalin-fixed tissue.

Mucosal lamina propria macrophages Macrophages are present in small numbers within the lamina propria, mainly beneath the top of intestinal villi and within the surface of the large intestine. Mucosal macrophages at the base of the lamina propria are generally less numerous, occurring primarily in the stomach and small intestine. Morphologically, they may be readily missed if not deliberately searched for. However, they increase greatly in number in inflammatory conditions. Functionally, they seem to play an important role in the intestinal mucosal immune system and also in inflammatory responses.[40,41]

The Solitary and Aggregate Lymphoid Follicles (Peyer's Patch)

SOLITARY LYMPHOID FOLLICLES. These are abundant throughout the small and large bowel but are most numerous in the distal colon.[17] It has been estimated that there are several thousand follicles in the small intestine and up to 20,000 in the colon. The number of follicles within the stomach is very few. The structure and function of the lymphoid follicles appear to be similar to those of the Peyer's patches.[17,42]

PEYER'S PATCHES. *Peyer's patches* are aggregated nodules of lymphoid follicles, which are most numerous in the distal ileum,[18,43] are located on the antimesenteric border of the intestine, and measure from a few millimeters to 10 cm (Figs. 3-2 and 3-3).[18,44] The number of Peyer's patches is variable and increases with age until puberty. There are approximately 240 at puberty.[18] Thereafter, the number falls to about 100 by age 70 years.[18]

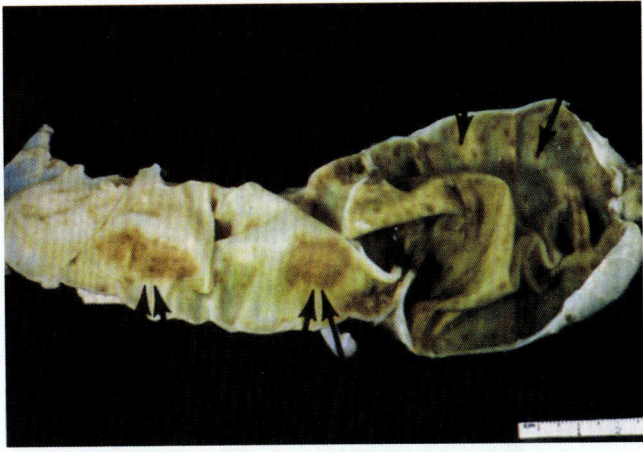

Figure 3-3. Autopsy specimen of terminal ileum and cecum. Two Peyer's patches are visible in the ileum, measuring more than 3 cm in length (*double arrows*). Solitary lymphoid follicles are discernible in the cecum as tiny brown spots (*arrow*).

Morphologically, Peyer's patches and lymphoid follicles have a distinctive structure. They are situated mainly in the mucosa but often split the muscularis mucosae and extend into the superficial submucosa. Three zones characterize them: (1) a dome region, (2) a follicular area, and (3) a parafollicular zone (Fig. 3-4).

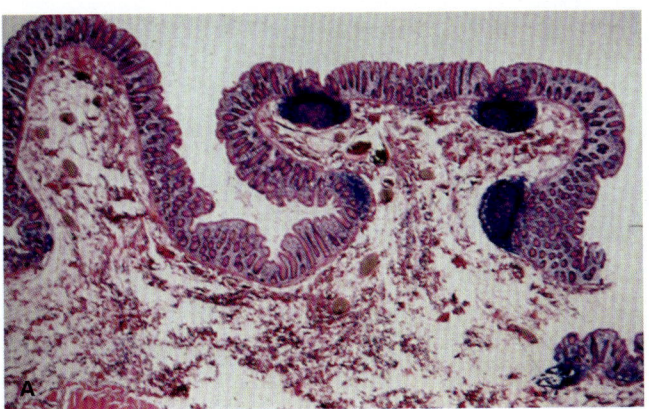

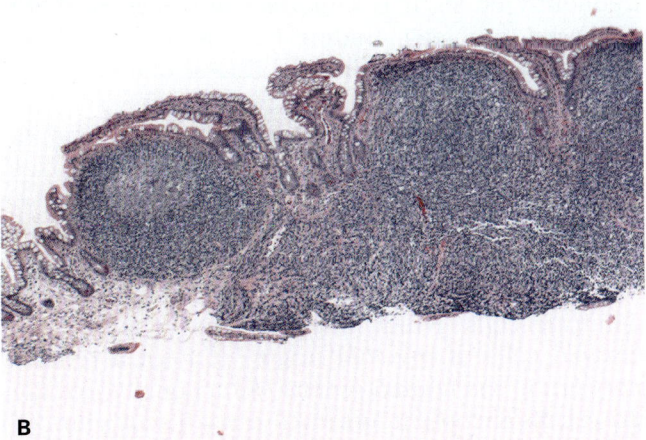

Figure 3-2. Solitary and aggregate lymphoid follicles of the human intestinal tract. **A:** Colonic mucosa and submucosa containing three solitary lymphoid follicles. The latter extend beneath the muscularis mucosae, and there is dimpling of the surface epithelium over the follicles. **B:** Peyer's patch, composed of numerous lymphoid follicles aggregated together in a linear fashion.

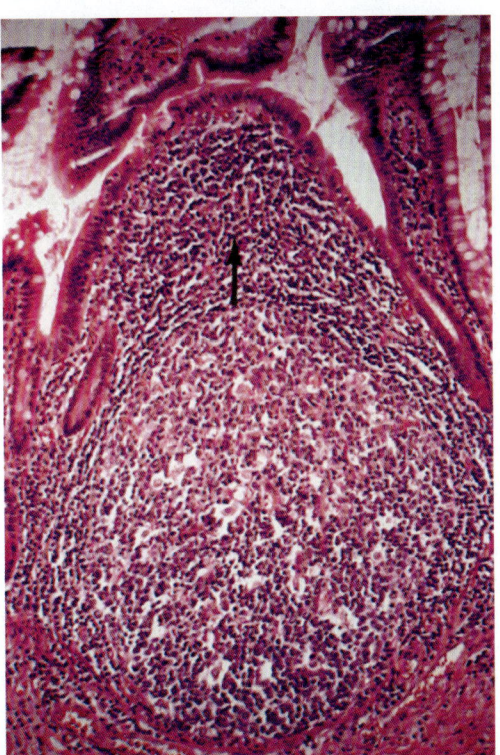

Figure 3-4. Intestinal lymphoid follicle. This is composed of a large follicular zone and the dome region, which is the area lying between the follicle and the surface epithelium (*arrow*). The mucosal surface overlying the follicle is dome shaped, devoid of villi and crypts, and lined by cuboidal epithelium.

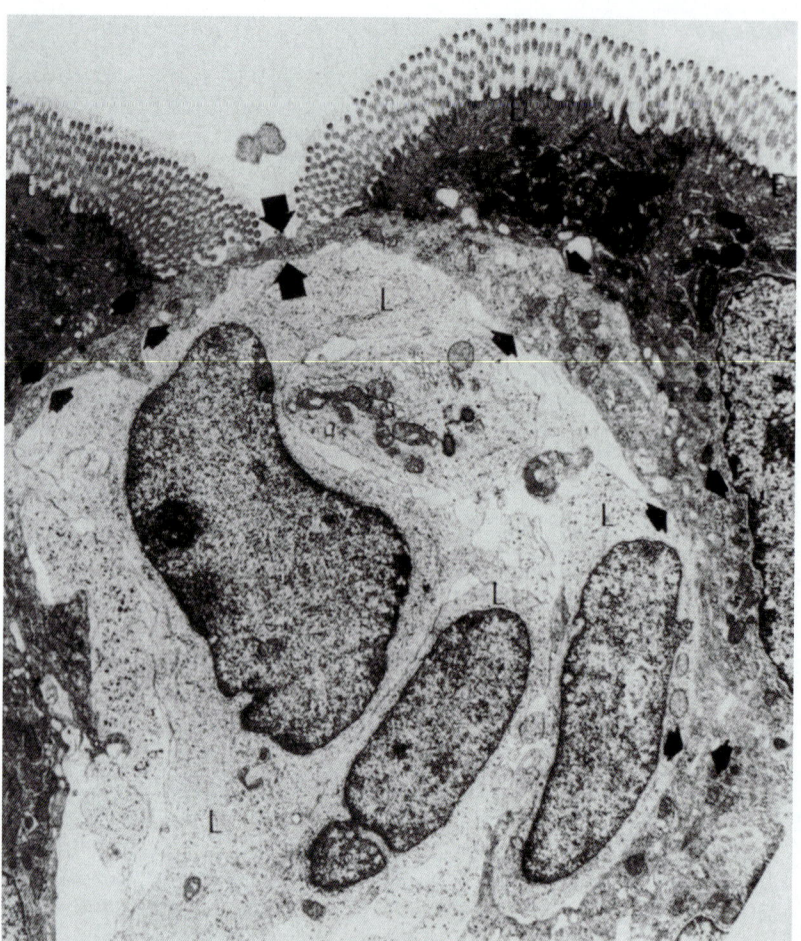

Figure 3-5. Electron micrograph of an M cell. This is a thin, membrane-like cell (*arrows*), the luminal surface of which is covered by microfolds and not microvilli. In the space below the M cell are three lymphocytes (L). (Courtesy R. L. Owen, M.D.)

The Dome Region This region lies immediately above the follicular area and is lined by a mucosal epithelium, sitting on a very porous basement membrane. This region essentially separates the lymphoid follicles from the lumen. The mucosal surface is dome shaped, relatively free of villi and crypts, and lined by a single cell layer. These cells are composed predominantly of cuboidal rather than columnar epithelial cells, a few goblet cells, the M cells (membranous or microfold epithelial cells), and occasional tuft cells.[45] The epithelial dome cells essentially consist of specialized enterocytes migrating up from a separate crypt stem cell line.[46,47] The M cells predominantly lie between the columnar cells overlying the Peyer's patches (and isolated follicles).[48,49] They are not readily visualized by light microscopy because of their size and are characterized ultrastructurally as thin membrane-like cells with luminal surface microfolds rather than microvilli (Fig. 3-5). These attenuated M cells form a latticework that allows lymphoid cells in the lamina propria to approach within 0.3 μm of the intestinal lumen while maintaining the integrity of the intestinal epithelium.[50] M cells contain multiple vesicles that suggest a transport function of luminal antigenic material to the underlying lymphoid tissue.[45,47] Lastly, it should be noted that numerous groups of IELs are also present, composed of B cells and suppressor T cells. Furthermore, lymphocytes and mononuclear cells can easily migrate through the surface epithelium and basement membrane and frequently do so. It is important to recognize this as a normal histologic finding (this is not where one should assess the numbers of IELs if one is worried about celiac disease or microscopic colitis).

The subepithelial area contains many lymphocytes, plasma cells, macrophages, and dendritic cells. The lymphocytes are large and medium sized, consisting primarily of IgM+ B cells and CD4 T cells and far fewer CD8 T cells. The macrophages not infrequently contain cellular debris and bacterial remnants. The dendritic cells, which appear to be bone marrow–derived cells of myeloid origin,[51,52] form a reticular network in the lamina propria. Functionally, the dendritic cells are potent intestinal antigen-acquiring cells with long dendritic processes that present antigens to T cells for induction of a primary T-cell response.[52,53] It has also been shown that the dendritic cells transport apoptotic intestinal epithelial cells to T-cell areas.[53] In addition, some of the dendritic cells also appear to transport antigens to lymph nodes.[52]

Tissue subjacent to the dome region contains mainly small lymphocytes and scant macrophages.

Follicular Area This lies beneath the dome region and is composed of a follicle center surrounded by the mantle and then the marginal zone. The follicular center is similar to that within lymphoid follicles and is composed predominantly of dark-staining centroblasts at its base and mainly light-staining centrocytes in the center and mucosal surface. In addition, numerous tingible body macrophages, often containing debris, are present at the center of the follicle with scattered T-cell lymphocytes.[42] The mantle zone surrounds the follicular center most prominently at the mucosal side and is composed of small B lymphocytes. Lastly, the outer portion of the follicle consists of a broad marginal zone composed of small- to intermediate-sized B lymphocytes containing a moderate amount of cytoplasm and centrocytic-type nuclei.[42]

The Parafollicular Zone This represents the thymus-dependent area and is characterized by small lymphocytes and many postcapillary venules, similar to those seen in lymph nodes. Under normal conditions, most of these lymphocytes are CD4 T-cell lymphocytes. However, in diseases such as inflammatory bowel disease, there is an increase in the number of B-cell lymphocytes with surface IgG.[27]

It should also be noted that prominent arterioles are present within the follicle and extend into the subepithelial capillary network and then to the capillary venules within the parafollicular T-cell zones. As far as lymphatics are concerned, they are prominent within the interfollicular and perifollicular areas and deal with lymphocytic migration.[54,55] Ultimately, lymphocytes migrate through the Peyer's patch and flow toward the submucosal lymphatics. From there, they exit the intestine via the afferent lymphatics into the mesenteric lymphatic vessels to mesenteric lymph nodes and ultimately to the thoracic duct and peripheral circulation.

Immunohistochemistry of Peyer's patches As far as the follicular centers are concerned, immunohistochemically they are similar to lymph node follicles and stain positively for all immunoglobulins other than IgD (primarily on the cell surface and less significantly in the cytoplasm). The follicular center cells consist of mature B cells that express CD10 antigen.[42] The surrounding mantle zone B cells stain for IgM and IgD, whereas the marginal zone B cells are IgD negative but IgM and IgA_1 positive, similar to splenic marginal zone cells. The parafollicular zone is predominantly composed of T cells, CD4 being about four times more common than CD8.

Humoral immune system of the gut. In man, five major immunoglobulins are normally synthesized and secreted by plasma cells, namely, IgG, IgA, IgM, IgD, and IgE.[56] The differences in these immunoglobulins are due to the structure of their heavy chains. In tissue, there is a close correlation between the number of specific plasma cells and the synthesis of the corresponding immunoglobulins, and specific plasma cells usually predominate in different tissues. Thus, after the neonatal period, IgA-containing plasma cells predominate in the GI tract, and the corresponding immunoglobulin is found in the intestinal secretions.[56,57] The other immunoglobulin-containing cells are also present, albeit in lesser numbers.[58] In the small intestine, it has been estimated that the ratio of IgA- to IgM- to IgG- to IgE-containing plasma cells is roughly 20:3:1:1.[56] The estimates for the large intestine and appendix are marginally different, 21:1:5:1:1.[59] IgD-containing plasma cells are exceedingly sparse in the normal GI tract.

Secretory IgA is the major immunoglobulin in the GI secretions, and most is produced by the intestinal IgA-producing plasma cells.[57] Interestingly, animal studies have shown that a significant proportion of the secretory IgA found in the intestinal juices originates from the liver.[60] The secretory IgA is elaborated within the biliary epithelium in a manner similar to that of the intestine,[60] although it is not yet clear whether most of the IgA originates from the intestinal plasma cells via the enterohepatic circulation or partially from plasma cells resident in the liver. It has been estimated that about 3 g is produced daily, with a half-life of 4 to 7 days.[61] Secretory IgA has a unique structure, which confers upon it the property of resisting degradation by intestinal enzymes. It is composed of two monomeric 7S IgA units held together by a protein, the J (joining) chain.[62] In addition, IgA also contains a nonimmunoglobulin polypeptide chain, known as the *secretory component*.[63] The dimeric IgA and the J piece are synthesized by the plasma cells of the lamina propria and are secreted into the interstitial space. They are then taken up by the intestinal epithelial cells, through the lateral cell membranes, where they acquire the secretory piece.[63] The latter may be a structural component of the lateral epithelial cell membrane. Finally, the immunoglobulin is secreted by the epithelial cell into the gut lumen, where it forms a close association with mucins and coats the apical surface of enterocytes. The secretory piece is specific for IgA and gives it a unique property, namely, protection from proteolytic degradation by the enzymes of the gut, such as trypsin and chymotrypsin.[64] There are two subclasses of IgA: IgA_1 and IgA_2. In the serum, IgA_1 accounts for approximately 90% of the IgA, whereas in secretions IgA_2 accounts for 60% of the total IgA. Other immunoglobulins are also found in small intestinal secretions and interestingly, IgM but not IgG follows a pathway similar to that of IgA.[63,65]

Immunologic Events Leading to IgA Secretion One exciting development in gut immunology is the evolving concept of the mucosa-associated immune system (MALT), of which the gut-associated lymphoid tissue (GALT) is an important component (Fig. 3-6).[7] This system confers local immunologic protection and, more importantly, is independent of the systemic immune system. The mucosa-associated immune system is present at all epithelial surfaces in contact with the external environment and is controlled by direct antigenic contact not only of the GI mucosa but also of other extraintestinal epithelial sites.[10] This system is unique in a number of ways; the antibodies produced by the plasma cells are transported to the epithelial surface and are able to function in the presence of proteolytic enzymes. Furthermore, the locally activated lymphocytes have the unique property of homing back to their site of origin and other epithelia, such as lung, breast, genitourinary tract, and female genital tract, after maturation. Thus, local antigenic stimulation at one site, such as the GI tract, elicits an immune response not only in the intestinal mucosa but also at other mucosal sites, such as the urinary tract (Fig. 3-6). The immunologic process leading to IgA secretion involves intestinal and extraintestinal events.[10] In animal studies, the first step involves sampling of antigens from the gut lumen by the M cells.[64] Macromolecules are actively transported from the lumen through the cell to lymphocytes and macrophages lying in the tissue spaces immediately beneath these thin membranes. The antigens are then delivered to the Peyer's patches where clonal proliferation of IgA precursor lymphocytes occur,[64] probably under the control of helper T lymphocytes.[11] IgA precursor lymphocytes next migrate to the mesenteric lymph nodes, thoracic duct, and systemic circulation, where they undergo maturation (possibly in the spleen) and then home back to the intestine and other mucosal sites,[64,65] where they populate the lamina propria, predominantly as IgA-synthesizing plasma cells (Fig. 3-6). Whether a similar mechanism is operative in man is uncertain.[58] The activated lymphocytes of the bowel may lodge in other secretory organs, such as salivary glands, bronchial mucosa, and the mammary glands.[64] The mammary glands are particularly important in the neonatal period in that passive transfer of IgA occurs via breast milk to confer protection to the newborn. It should be noted that the plasma cells of the GI tract develop only in response to exposure of foreign antigen within the intestinal luminal contents. Consequently, the fetal gut is devoid of plasma cells, the latter developing only after birth, following neonatal exposure to food.

Cellular immune system of the gut. The lymphocytes of the cellular immune system (T-cell system) are an important component of the gut-associated lymphoid system. They are the major component of the IELs,[6,23,26] and in the lamina propria they are distributed primarily in the interfollicular zone. The T-cell subtypes have a rather distinctive distribution, the suppressor T cells being located mainly in the epithelial compartment, while helper T cells are found in the lymphocytes of the interfollicular zone. The cellular immune system of the gut appears to be involved in the full complement of cellular immune functions, namely, recognition, processing, and destruction of antigens. Paneth cells contain a variety of substances that incude lysozyme, phospholipase, and defensins and also contribute toward innate immunity in the gut.

IMMUNODEFICIENCY DISORDERS OF THE INTESTINAL TRACT

The GI tract is frequently an important target organ in the primary as well as secondary immunodeficiency disorders[66,67] because it is constantly exposed to a heavy antigen load. Immunodeficiency is usually suspected by the clinician when patients have a history of either prolonged infections or infections caused by unusual organisms. The pathologist's role is largely to confirm and identify the frequent complications of immunodeficiency, of which infection and neoplasia are the most important. On occasion, the pathologist may be able to document the type of immunodeficiency through the

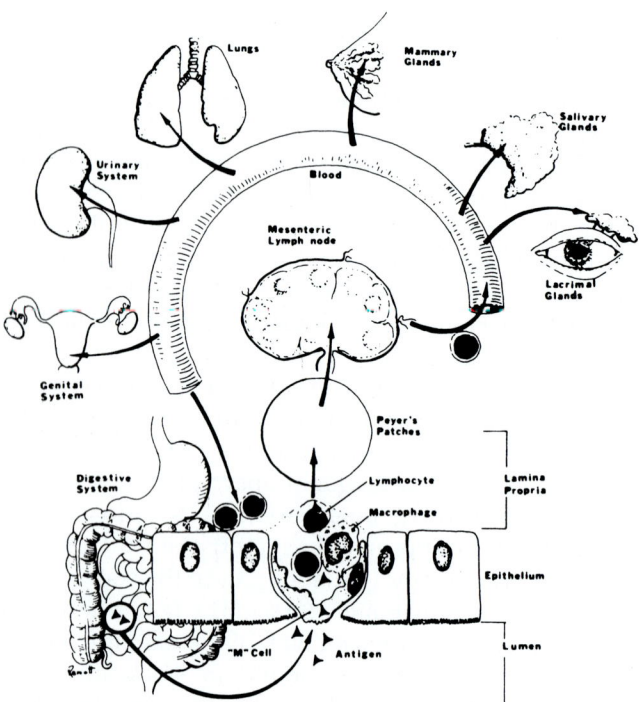

Figure 3-6. Mucosa-associated lymphoid system.

use of immunohistochemistry. Sometimes, unexpected histologic changes may be found in the gut, such as nodular lymphoid hyperplasia and giardiasis, which should lead one to suspect an immunodeficiency disorder in a clinically unsuspected case. As common variable immunodeficiency (CVID) is so common, it may sometimes be detected in relatively asymptomatic patients because of a paucity of IgA plasma cells in the lamina propria with no compensatory increase in other classes of plasma cells.

There are two major categories of immunodeficiency disorders: primary and secondary.

Primary Immunodeficiency Disorders These disorders include a large and varied group of diseases[66,67] resulting from impairment of the B- and T-cell systems, abnormalities of phagocytic function, or both. The functional interaction of B and T cells and monocytes in the expression of the immune system makes the division of immunodeficiency diseases into B- and T-cell disorders somewhat artificial.[6,68,69] Nevertheless, usually either the antibody defects or cell-mediated abnormalities predominate, allowing for a practical subdivision of the immunodeficiency disorders. In addition, genetic defects have been described in conditions such as food intolerance, in which there appear to be specific abnormalities in responsiveness to certain antigens. In these disorders, there appears to be poor antigen clearance or heightened responsiveness, leading to immune complex disease or hypersensitivity reaction.[70] In adults, common variable or late-onset immunodeficiency, and selective IgA deficiency are by far the most common immunodeficiency disorders.[15,68,71] In children, severe combined immunodeficiency disease is the most common. It usually presents soon after birth. Its diagnosis is important to prevent the sequelae of acute and chronic infection.[2]

Secondary Immunodeficiency Disorders These disorders are becoming more common. Some develop following infections, while others are iatrogenic complications of immunosuppressive therapy, radiation therapy, or bone marrow/hemopoetic stem cell transplantation (BMT/HSCT). The most important secondary immunodeficiency is acquired immunodeficiency syndrome (AIDS), which is caused by the human immunodeficiency virus (HIV).[72] There is considerable evidence to suggest that immune mechanisms are involved in the tissue injury of a number of GI disorders, such as idiopathic inflammatory bowel disease, celiac sprue, and Whipple's disease. The precise pathogenic mechanisms of these disorders remain to be elucidated and they are discussed further under each disorder.

Clinical features. Clinically, patients usually present with chronic diarrhea and malabsorption, although other symptoms may also occur based on the specific disorder (primary or secondary immunodeficiency) and its complications. The main impairment of the immune system is characterized by a decreased resistance to infection and in some cases, subsequent neoplasia.[72-74] The nature of the infection depends on the specific defect. Thus, patients with impaired B-cell function are most susceptible to bacterial and certain parasitic infections. In contrast, those with impaired T-cell function have defective cell-mediated immunity, leading to sprue-like disorders, pernicious anemia, nodular lymphoid hyperplasia, inflammatory bowel disease,[74] and an enhanced susceptibility to prolonged viral, fungal, and mycobacterial infections. The major clinical manifestations of these infections will depend on the primary site of involvement in the GI tract.[75]

The diagnosis of the primary immunodeficiency disorders is usually made readily. Patients commonly have a history of recurrent, prolonged opportunistic infections, such as pneumocystis pneumonia, giardiasis, or cryptosporidiosis. The finding of associated disorders, such as respiratory tract infections and autoimmune disorders in CVID, helps greatly in determining the precise immunologic abnormality and there is frequently a family history of immunodeficiency disease.

The categorization of the immunodeficiency disorders is based primarily on three categories of immunologic tests for humoral (B-cell) and cell-mediated (T-cell) immunity, that is, immunoglobulin concentrations, antibody formations, and cell-mediated immunity (Table 3-1).[68,69]

Histology. The pathologic changes accompanying the primary immunodeficiency disorders depend in part on the specific immunologic defect (Table 3-2). It should be stressed that in some cases there may be no significant histologic alteration. The most frequently seen histologic lesions are the results of complications, specifically infections. Intrinsic lesions of immunodeficiency are uncommon. The histologic changes fall

---

Table 3-1   Immunologic Tests for the Categorization of Primary Immunodeficiency Disease

1. Immunoglobulin concentrations in serum and mucosal secretions.
2. Assessment of antibody formation following immunization
   a. Natural antibodies such as A and B isohemagglutinins, and antistreptolysin
   b. Antibody response to immunization such as diphtheria/tetanus vaccine
   c. Quantitation of circulation B cells.
3. Cell-mediated immunity.
   a. Skin testing for delayed cutaneous hypersensitivity with antigens such as mumps, trichophyton, PPD, *Candida*, and tetanus toxoid.
   b. T-cell quantitation including helper/suppressor ratios.

Table 3-2 Pathology of the GI Tract in Primary Immunodeficiency Disorders

No change
Specific morphologic changes
Altered lymphoplasmacytic content of lamina propria
 1. Absence of lymphocytes and plasma cells
 2. Altered B- or T-cell subsets
Diffuse nodular lymphoid hyperplasia
Nonspecific morphologic changes due to bacterial overgrowth, infections, or other injury
Esophagitis
Mucosal erosions
Atrophic gastritis
Mucosal lesions (villous atrophy)
Enterocolitis
Demonstration of organisms particularly
  Candida, CMV, herpes, *Giardia*, *Trichomonas*, *Isospora belli*, *Cryptosporidium*
Neoplasia
Carcinoma
Lymphoma
Kaposi's sarcoma

containing IgM. Immunostains will show the specific cell type that is altered, for example, a diminution in number or absence of IgA-containing plasma cells.

Mucosal Lesions Resulting from Infections or Bacterial Overgrowth Infections in patients with immunodeficiency disorders tend to be more prolonged and cause more damage in the immunocompromised setting. Patients are especially prone to infections by multiple organisms, frequently of low virulence, which are not normally pathogenic to man. These include the normal commensals of the GI tract,[76] fungi such as *Candida*,[77] and viruses such as Cytomegalovirus (CMV) and herpes.[68,71,76,77] The patients are also unable to mount an effective host response to unusual organisms, not normally found in the GI microflora, such *Giardia lamblia*, *Trichomonas hominis*, *Isospora belli*, and *Cryptosporidium*.[78–81]

The histological changes in the immunocompromised patient differ from those found in the normal patient. For example, the inflammatory response may be muted in infections such as giardiasis, cryptosporidiosis, and CMV infection. By contrast, it may be exaggerated in some cases of CMV and herpetic infections such as those seen in AIDS patients. Certain histologic changes should alert the pathologist to the possibility of an unsuspected immunodeficiency disorder, for example, the finding of invasive esophageal candidiasis in AIDS or benign nodular hyperplasia in a new case of giardiasis.

The specific histologic changes in the GI tract resulting from infection will also vary somewhat with the site of involvement. In the esophagus, stomach, and large intestine, the lesions consist primarily of mucosal erosions.[75,76] In candidal infections, particu-

into four major categories as described in the paragraphs that follow.

No Change There may be no significant alteration or reduced number of inflammatory cells of the lamina propria (Fig. 3-7). For example, in late-onset immunodeficiency disease, there may be an absolute marked reduction in plasma cells. Occasionally, plasma cells are not reduced markedly. Rather, there is a reduction of IgA-containing plasma cells with a compensatory increase in the number of the other plasma cells, especially those

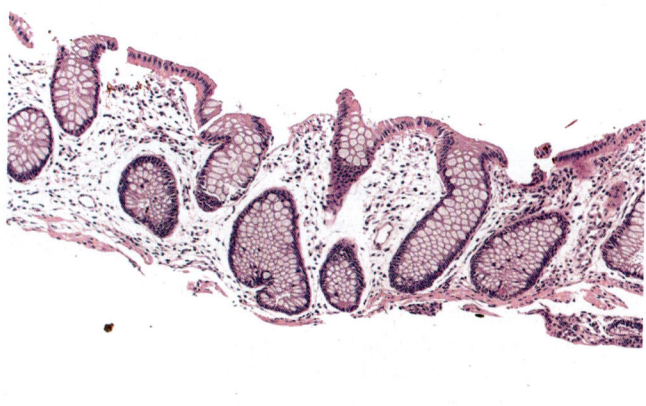
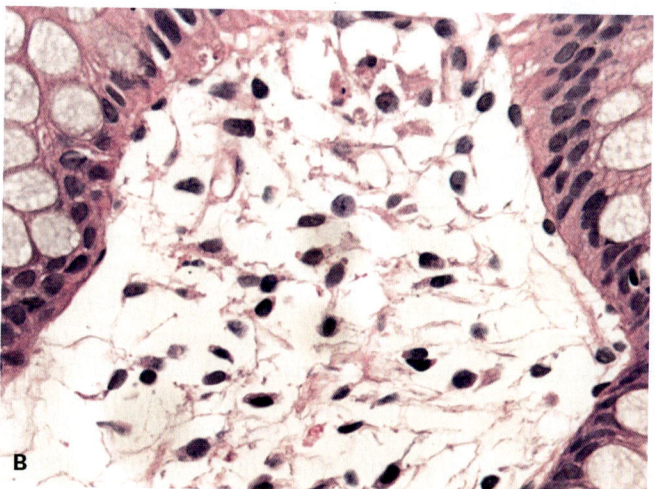

Figure 3-7. **A:** Large bowel mucosa with architectural distortion but an empty lamina propria. **B:** Detail showing almost entirely mesenchymal cells. Changes such as these can be seen in neonates and young children before the intestinal immune system has developed, in patients with immunologic disorders such as combined immunodeficiency disease, and also immediately following bone marrow transplantation before repopulation of the lamina propria has occurred. It can also be seen in some patients with inflammatory bowel disease following therapy and in remission.

larly of the esophagus, the organism is present in the superficial necrotic debris and may invade the mucosa and occasionally extend through the bowel wall. In viral infections, inclusions tend to be scant and are frequently missed unless serial sections are carefully screened. The viral inclusions are commonly associated with mucosal erosions and ulcerations, often with minimal inflammation in the early stages.[82] In AIDS, herpetic infections may be particularly intractable, especially herpetic proctitis, characterized by burrowing ulcers and destruction of the sphincter.[81]

In the small intestine, bacterial overgrowth or parasitic infections characteristically produce mucosal lesions. However, unlike celiac sprue, the mucosal lesion is often patchy and of mild or moderate severity.[71] Occasionally, crypt abscesses and a neutrophilic infiltrate of the lamina propria are seen.[75] The infections are usually due to bacterial overgrowth with aerobic and anaerobic coliforms, or protozoal infestations.[75] Giardiasis is the most common parasitic infection. The organism is found in the intestinal mucus or adherent to the epithelial microvillous surface (Fig. 3-8)[83] and, on rare occasions, within the columnar epithelial cells.[84] The only other significant protozoal infections described are the coccidial infections. Coccidia (e.g., *Cryptosporidium* and *Isospora*) are common parasites in the intestinal tracts of animals and are generally transmitted by ingestion of contaminated food or water.[80] Infections in man were once thought to be very uncommon and were usually associated with immunodeficiency states. However, recent studies of cryptosporidiosis have shown that they are a common cause of gastroenteritis in children.[85] In *Isospora* infections (*hominis* and *belli*), the parasites are found within the epithelial cell cytoplasm of the mucosa, and all stages of its life cycle have been observed. In contrast, *Cryptosporidium* (a coccidial protozoan related to *Isospora*) inhabits the striated or microvillous border of the small intestinal epithelium and, less commonly, the gastric, rectal, and billiary mucosa.[80] In general, these infections are self-limited when they occur in the normal population. However, in the immunodeficient patient, they cause prolonged illness, and in the case of cryptosporidiosis no effective therapy is available.

Intrinsic and Associated Morphologic Changes

Although the mucosal injury in the immunodeficient patient is frequently the result of superimposed infection, in certain disorders, there may be an intrinsic change independent of any recognized infection.[12] For example, a case of IgA deficiency has been described, which had a severe "flat" mucosal lesion similar to that seen in celiac sprue, but the patient did not respond to a gluten-free diet. This patient was found to have an IgG antiepithelial cell antibody.[86] In the stomach, pernicious anemia with gastric atrophy is found in some late-onset immunodeficiency syndromes. It occurs in younger patients (earlier than the usual 40–60 years

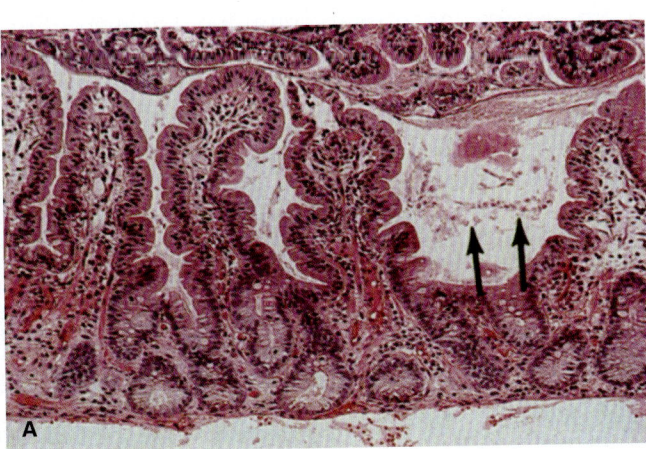
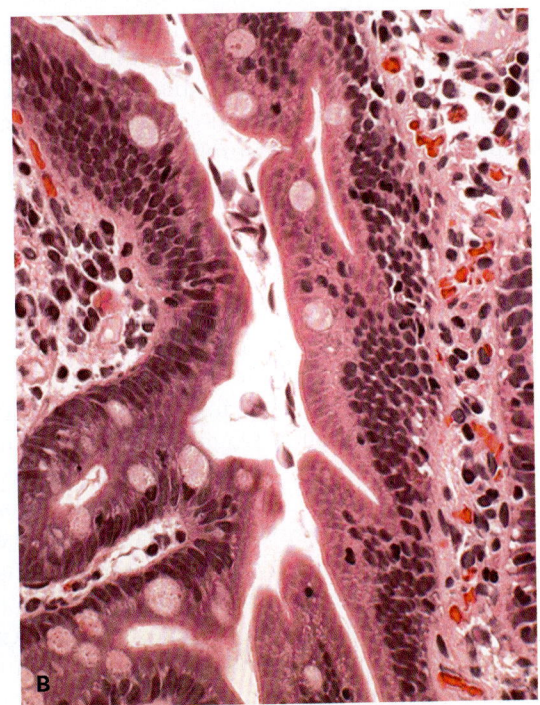

Figure 3-8. Intestinal giardiasis in a patient with common variable hypogammaglobulinemia. **A:** The jejunal mucosa is unremarkable. However, within the intestinal mucus are numerous giardial parasites (*arrows*). **B:** Detail of crypts showing numerous *Giardia* in the lumen, some probably attached to the epithelium.

Table 3-3	Incidence of Neoplasia in Immunodeficiency Disorders
Wiskott–Aldrich syndrome	15%
Ataxia telangiectasia	12%
Adult-onset common variable disease	10%
Isolated IgA deficiency	10%
Selective IgA deficiency	1%–3%
Childhood onset common variable disease	1%–3%
Severe combined immunodeficiency	1%–3%

of age), lacks plasma cells in the atrophic mucosa, and lacks antibodies to intrinsic factor and parietal cells.[76] Nodular lymphoid hyperplasia may be found in patients with CVID syndromes and selective IgA deficiency (Fig. 3-15).

Neoplasms The risk of neoplasia developing in immunodeficiency disorders is very high. In the primary immunodeficiency disorders, it has been estimated to be as high at 10,000 times that in the general age-matched population.[87] The GI tract is frequently involved in neoplasia occurring roughly 10 to 200 times that of the general age-matched population (Table 3-3).[68,87,88] The incidence of neoplasia varies with each type of immunodeficiency. The majority of malignancies are of lymphoid or hematopoietic origin (80%), the remainder being epithelial and smooth muscle.[89] However, the type of malignancy varies with the immunologic disorder.[87] Thus, in Wiskott–Aldrich syndrome, myelogenous leukemia is most common, whereas in common variable and selective IgA deficiency, epithelial tumors and lymphomas occur in approximately equal numbers. The types of neoplasms also vary with age and sex.[88] For example, children with immunodeficiency usually develop non-Hodgkin's lymphomas, whereas in adults, carcinomas and non-Hodgkin's lymphomas are found equally often. In ataxia telangiectasia, females develop epithelial malignancies more frequently than males.

Although neoplasms in the immunodeficiency disorders involve most tissues, primary tumors of the GI tract occur fairly frequently, especially in common variable deficiency.[76,88] The overall incidence of tumors in one study of CVID was 25% of patients. Approximately half of these tumors occurred in the GI tract and consisted mainly of carcinoma of the stomach and colon or lymphoma (commonly associated with diffuse nodular lymphoid hyperplasia).[87] An increased risk for neoplasia is also found in patients immunosuppressed for transplantation, or following chemotherapy for cancer.[87] The risk of neoplasia in transplant patients is approximately 100 times greater than that observed in the general population in the same age range.[87] In the transplant setting, there is about an equal incidence of developing lymphoid hyperplasia and lymphoma (posttransplant lymphoproliferative disorder, see "Lymphoma" section) and epithelial tumors, and the bowel is involved in approximately 12% of cases.[87] Finally, GI tumors, primarily lymphoma, Kaposi's sarcoma, and smooth muscle tumors,[89] can be seen in untreated AIDS patients.

PRIMARY IMMUNODEFICIENCY DISORDERS

GI diseases due to infectious, inflammatory, and malignant disorders occur in a high proportion of patients with primary immunodeficiency disorders (Table 3-3).[67,74] The functional interaction of B and T cells and monocytes makes the division of immunodeficiency disorders somewhat artificial. Nevertheless, usually either antibody defects or cell-mediated abnormalities predominate, allowing a practical subdivision.[15,68,69] This is the basis of the World Health Organization (WHO) classification of immunodeficiency disorders (Table 3-4). In addition, the WHO has included two other categories. One is characterized by the association of nonimmunologic defects. The other is characterized by a primary disorder of phagocytic function (chronic granulomatous disorder).

Predominant Antibody Defects

Common variable hypogammaglobulinemia (Late-onset acquired hypogammaglobulinemia, common variable immunodeficiency [CVID], Bruton's X-linked agammaglobulinemia [XLAG])[90–92]

Pathogenesis and Clinical Features Common variable hypogammaglobulinemia, which is a heterogeneous group of immunologic disorders, is the second most common primary immunodeficiency disorder, affecting between 1/30,000 and 1/100,000 patients.[93,94] Three major immunologic abnormalities have been described to date, namely, an intrinsic B-cell defect, an immunoregulatory T-cell abnormality, and, rarely, the production of autoantibodies to T and B cells, all of which lead to impairment of immunoglobulin secretion.[66,67,95,96] A recent study found that naive B cells from patients with CVID express much lower levels of CD70 and CD86, molecules that are critical for T- and B-cell interactions.[94] Hence, the T-cell abnormalities found in some of these patients may be secondary to an underlying B-cell defect.

In addition, this disorder is associated with celiac disease and occurs most commonly in the second to fifth decades.[78,97,98] It is often familial and sometimes autosomal dominant or recessive modes of

Table 3-4 GI Manifestations of Primary Immunodeficiency Syndromes

TYPE	POSTULATED DEFECT	MAIN GI FEATURES
A. Predominant Antibody Defects		
1. Common variable immunodeficiency	1. Predominant B-cell defect. 2. Immunoregulatory T-cell disorder. 3. Autoantibodies to B and T cells.	Intestinal infections due to *Campylobacter*, *Salmonella*, and *Strongyloides*. Sprue-like syndrome due to *Giardia* or bacterial overgrowth. Pernicious anemia, nodular lymphoid hyperplasia, nongranulomatous ulcerative jejunoileitis, and GI carcinoma and lymphoma.
2. Selective IgA deficiency	Defective IgA B-cell maturation.	Malabsorption due to bacterial overgrowth or parasite infestation, especially *Giardia*. Nodular lymphoid hyperplasia. Increased incidence of pernicious anemia, celiac disease, Crohn's disease, and ulcerative colitis.
3. Selective deficiency of other immunoglobulin isotypes, IgM, IgE, and IgD	Differentiation defect of IgM B cell to isotype-specific plasma cells.	Association with celiac disease, ulcerative colitis, Crohn's disease, and Whipple's disease.
4. Infantile X-linked agammaglobulinemia (Bruton's agammaglobulinemia)	Intrinsic defect of pre–B-cell to B-cell differentiation.	Malabsorption and chronic diarrhea due to bacterial overgrowth and persistent GI infections due to virus, *Campylobacter fetus*, *Salmonella*, and *Giardia*. Malignancy.
5. X-linked immunodeficiency with increased IgM and IgD	Defect in isotype switch prevents normal maturation of IgM B cells to IgG, IgA, and IgE cells.	Diarrhea due to *Candida* infections and cryptosporidiosis. Malignancy.
6. Transient hypogammaglobulinemia of infancy	Delayed B-cell maturation? due to defect in T-cell–dependent stimulation.	Malabsorption and diarrhea due to bacterial overgrowth, *Campylobacter fetus* and rotavirus infections, and *Giardia* infestations. Malignancy.
7. Kappa chain deficiency	Unknown.	Achlorhydria, malabsorption, and diarrhea. Cystic fibrosis.
8. Immunodeficiency with thymoma	Deficiency of pre–B cells? Defective development of stem cells.	*Salmonella* infections.
9. Secretory component deficiency		Diarrhea, *Candida* infections.
B. Predominant Defects of Cell-mediated Immunity		
1. Severe combined immunodeficiency disease (includes Nezelof's syndrome)	1. Lymphoid maturation defect. 2. T-cell defect due to adenosine deaminase deficiency. 3. Purine nucleoside phosphorylase deficiency	Malabsorption and intractable diarrhea, repeated GI viral and fungal infections (herpes, varicella, rotavirus, and *Candida*).
2. Chronic mucocutaneous candiasis	Uncertain, may be secondary to drugs.	Mouth ulcers, esophagitis, esophageal stricture, and diarrhea
C. Immunodeficiency Associated with Other Defects		
1. Wiskott–Aldrich syndrome	Cell membrane defect affecting all hemopoietic stem cell derivatives.	Recurrent bloody diarrhea and malabsorption.
2. DiGeorge's syndrome (congenital thymic aplasia)	Abnormal thymic development with resultant T-cell defects.	Malabsorption, intractable diarrhea, and severe malnutrition.
3. Ataxia telangiectasia	Defective T-cell maturation.	Nodular lymphoid hyperplasia, vitamin B_{12} malabsorption.
4. Transcobalamine deficiency	Autosomal recessive transcobalamine II deficiency.	Intractable diarrhea.
D. Phagocyte Dysfunction		
Chronic granulomatous disease	Macrophages unable to kill phagocytosed organisms.	GI obstruction, malabsorption and diarrhea.

inheritance can be discerned.[76] Patients have panhypogammaglobulinemia and tend to present in one of two ways: either with recurrent infections, especially of the respiratory tract, or with chronic diarrhea and malabsorption.[10,74,98] The intestinal symptoms are frequently due to giardiasis, although other parasites such as *Cryptosporidium* and strongyloidiasis as well as fungal overgrowth may also be responsible for the diarrhea and malabsorption.[68,69,76,80,99] Other less common causes for chronic diarrhea are bacterial infections such as *Campylobacter jejuni*.[100] These infections may sometimes be pathologically indistinguishable from ulcerative colitis or result in mucosal fissuring and necrosis resembling Crohn's disease.[92,101,102] A third of these patients develop pernicious anemia and they may also develop a variety of other maladies, such as thyrotoxicosis, myxedema, arthritis, keratoconjunctivitis, splenomegaly, sarcoidosis, and amyloidosis secondary to infection.[103] Most important, however, is the increased risk of GI tumors, especially gastric carcinoma in adults,[88,104] although lymphoma associated with nodular lymphoid hyperplasia as well as T-cell lymphoma unassociated with EBV viral infection have also been found.[105,106]

Histology The pathologic changes are found most commonly in the small intestine but may occur throughout the entire GI tract. There is a wide range of histologic findings including nonspecific mucosal lesions, features resembling acute graft versus host disease (GVHD), atrophic gastritis, hypogammaglobulinemic sprue-like features with mild to severe villous atrophy, granulomatous changes resembling Crohn's disease, histologic features resembling Whipple's, and nongranulomatous ulcerative jejunoileitis. In addition, nodular lymphoid hyperplasia and malignancy, especially gastric carcinoma, can occur.[78,87,88,92,93,102,104] The pathologic findings do not always correlate with the severity of clinical findings.

STOMACH. An atrophic gastritis similar to that of pernicious anemia but lacking the plasmacytic infiltrate is seen in some cases of CVID disease. In contrast to the usual cases of pernicious anemia, these patients do not have autoantibodies and serum gastrin levels are not elevated.[107,108] *Helicobacter pylori* appears to be an important cofactor in causing multifocal atrophic gastritis in CVID patients and probably helps explain their high incidence of gastric carcinoma.[104]

SMALL INTESTINE. Histologically, the small bowel may be unremarkable except for the decrease or absence of plasma cells, *Giardia lamblia* infestation, or both (Fig. 3-8). In patients with malabsorption, the small intestine commonly shows mucosal lesions with varying degrees of abnormalities of villous architecture,[109] even in the absence of giardiasis or bacterial overgrowth.

HYPOGAMMAGLOBULINEMIC SPRUE. The small intestinal mucosa resembles celiac sprue, in that the mucosa is flat. However, in contrast to the lesion of celiac sprue, there is usually an absence or paucity of plasma cells in the lamina propria.[76] The cause of the mucosal injury in hypogammaglobulinemic sprue appears to be multifactorial. Symptoms of diarrhea and malabsorption and the lesions improve, at least partially, with specific treatment for bacterial overgrowth or giardiasis. Some patients have been reported to improve with nonspecific therapy such as gamma globulin injections.[110] Some patients appear to develop a true, possibly transient, gluten-sensitive enteropathy.[111-113]

DIFFUSE NODULAR LYMPHOID HYPERPLASIA WITH HYPOGAMMAGLOBULINEMIA. Nodular lymphoid hyperplasia is said to occur in up to 60% of patients with common variable hypogammaglobulinemia, sometimes resulting in intestinal infection or obstruction and neoplasia.[114,115] It has also been reported in isolated IgA deficiency[116] and occasionally in patients with repeated antigenic stimuli.[117] The disorder most commonly affects the small intestine only, but occasionally colonic[118] and rarely gastric involvement may also occur. Rarely, the lesions may be confined to the colon. On gross examination, the mucosa is studded with sessile or polypoid nodules, which measure up to 5 mm in diameter[118,119] and which produce a striking radiographic finding consisting of multiple filling defects (see Chapter 4). Microscopically, the nodules are composed of one or a cluster of hyperplastic lymphoid follicles, which, when large, may produce blunting of the overlying villi. Mucosal ulceration is absent. The lymphoid nodules are confined to the lamina propria and superficial submucosa (Fig. 3-9) and differ from nodular lymphoma histologically on the basis of the presence of a polymorphous cellular infiltrate versus a monomorphous lymphomatous infiltrate. Immunohistochemistry or gene rearrangement studies may be helpful to confirm the diagnosis. A decrease or absence of plasma cells is also usually noted in the lamina propria. Some patients appear to have normal numbers of plasma cells in hematoxylin and eosin-stained sections of the jejunal mucosa. However,

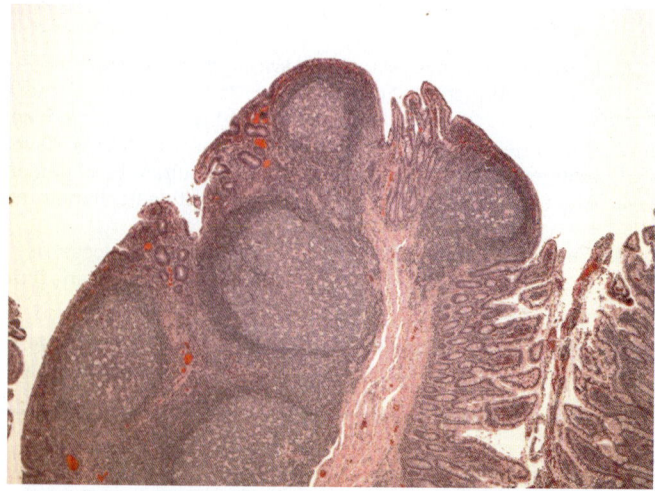

Figure 3-9. Diffuse nodular lymphoid hyperplasia in a patient with CVID. Small intestinal mucosa containing numerous prominent lymphoid nodules. The intestinal villi overlying the lymphoid nodules are stunted. The patient also had intestinal giardiasis, but this is not apparent at this magnification.

immunoperoxidase staining for specific lymphocyte isotypes reveals an absence or paucity of IgA-making cells and compensatory hyperplasia of IgM or IgG isotypes. Based on immunologic findings, it has been postulated that the lymphoid hyperplasia, which occurs in these patients, is a compensatory proliferation of lymphocytes, which are unable to undergo full maturation to immunoglobulin-secreting cells.[120,121] (For further details, see Chapter 5.)

Diffuse nodular lymphoid hyperplasia with hypogammaglobulinemia must be differentiated from the more localized nodular hyperplasia without hypogammaglobulinemia, which occurs in the colon and terminal ileum (especially in children). It is usually an incidental finding and is unassociated with any clinical manifestations. The lesion is described in further detail in the chapter on the lymphoproliferative disorders (Chapter 4).

Some patients develop a chronic inflammatory process that mimics Crohn's disease with transmural inflammation, while others may develop a granulomatous enteropathy.[122,123]

COLON. Colitis histologically similar to ulcerative colitis, but with fewer plasma cells, has been described.[101] In addition, an unusual colitis with loss of glandular elements and diffuse macrophage infiltration of the lamina propria has been described.[101]

NEOPLASMS. The reported incidence of neoplasia in CVID ranges from a low of 9% to a high of 24% of cases.[88,98] The majority occur in adults and consist of malignant epithelial neoplasms and lymphomas. A significant proportion of malignant tumors occur in the GI tract, especially in the stomach.[101] In a careful long-term study of 50 patients with idiopathic late-onset immunoglobulin deficiency, Hermans et al.[124] reported 5 patients with carcinoma of the gut (4 stomach and 1 sigmoid) and 1 with GI lymphoma out of a total of 12 patients who developed neoplasms. The other tumors consisted of thymoma (4), carcinoma of the lung (1), and agnogenic myeloid metaplasia. Nodular lymphoid hyperplasia was associated with all of the cases with GI neoplasms.

ROLE OF THE PATHOLOGIST. The role of the pathologist is twofold.

1. In established common variable disease, one should look for opportunistic infections.
2. Undiagnosed cases of common variable hypogammaglobulinemia should be suspected in the following instances:
   a. Pernicious anemia in young patients.
   b. Sporadic giardiasis in the absence of risk factors.
   c. Patients with suspected celiac sprue that fail to respond to treatment.

Although the biopsy specimens from these patients may show decreased numbers of mucosal plasma cells, one cannot rely on this finding for diagnosis; quantitative immunoglobulin tests should be performed.

Selective IgA deficiency

Pathogenesis and Clinical Features This is the most common congenital immunodeficiency syndrome,[125] with an incidence of 1 in 700 in the general population of the United States.[69,126] However, it should be noted that the incidence may vary in different countries and ethnic groups. For example, the incidence in Finland is higher than in this country, namely, 1 in 400 and lower in Japan where the incidence is 1 in 18,000.[127-129] In the United States, African Americans have an incidence of only 1 in 6,000.[128] Furthermore, in some patients, it is a secondarily acquired disorder due to infections (e.g., CMV and rubella) or drugs (phenytoin).[130] Approximately 2% of celiac patients have IgA deficiency.[95,97] It usually occurs sporadically, although rare hereditary cases have been reported.[131] The basic defect in selective IgA deficiency (which includes both the IgA_1 and IgA_2 subclasses) is not completely understood. It probably consists of a heterogeneous group of disorders, including a terminal defect in differentiation of pre–B cells to become IgA-secreting plasma cells; subtle defects in T-cell functions, such as an excess of suppressor T cells for IgA-secreting plasma cells; and, rarely, a cytoplasmic block in the ability of the cell to secrete already synthesized cytoplasmic IgA.[10,129] Most patients are asymptomatic,[76] with the IgA abnormality compensated for in part by enhanced production of secretory IgM. Patients that are symptomatic appear to have additional immunoglobulin deficiencies such as subclasses of IgG, namely, IgG_2, IgG_4, and IgE.[132,133] Only rarely do these patients develop malabsorption, sinopulmonary infections, and a variety of other disorders, such as systemic lupus erythematosus, pernicious anemia, allergic disorders, ulcerative colitis, Crohn's disease, ataxia telangiectasia (to be discussed), and neoplasia.[86,94,134-137] The malabsorption found in these patients results from infections or protozoan infestations, particularly giardiasis, or may be secondary to an associated celiac sprue.[78,138]

Histology The GI tract in most cases is unremarkable,[139] except for a paucity of IgA-containing plasma cells within the lamina propria. There may be no apparent decrease in plasma cells because of a compensatory increase in numbers of IgM- and IgG-containing plasma cells. There is a concomitant absence of secretory IgA only detectable by immunohistochemistry, but serum IgA levels are also greatly reduced (0.5 g/L).[71] Occasionally, the small intestinal mucosa is flat and resembles that of celiac sprue, but unlike the latter, there is an absence or paucity of IgA-containing plasma cells and depressed serum IgA levels.[76] The mucosa of most of these patients will improve on a gluten-free diet. When patients with celiac sprue are screened, approximately 1 in 40 are found to have IgA deficiency. However, the precise relationship of IgA deficiency to celiac sprue remains to be elucidated.[86,94] In addition, these patients are susceptible to bacterial overgrowth and opportunistic infections.

Secretory component deficiency.

The majority of these patients have a secretory component deficiency with normal serum IgA levels.[140] The clinical presentation is that of severe diarrhea, possibly due to bacterial overgrowth of jejunal contents or intestinal candidiasis. Jejunal biopsies performed in two patients were normal.[141]

Infantile X-linked agammaglobulinemia (Bruton's agammaglobulinemia, congenital agammaglobulinemia).

Infantile X-linked agammaglobulinemia is a genetic sex-linked disorder due to a maturational block in pre–B-cell to B-cell differentiation, resulting in a total lack of circulating B cells and a resultant failure to produce antibodies.[15,68,69,142,143] Cell-mediated immunity is intact. Circulating T cells and their subsets are normal in number, proportion, and function, and therefore viral infections do not occur.[144] This disorder can be definitively diagnosed by molecular genetic testing by single-stranded confirmation polymorphism in the Bruton's tyrosine kinase gene.[145]

The disorder usually presents around the sixth week of life, with recurrent pyogenic infections such as bronchitis, pneumonia, otitis media, and meningitis. This period of life coincides with the disappearance of the maternally derived IgG antibodies. GI manifestations are most uncommon and consist primarily of diarrhea[143,146] (perhaps hinting at the importance of cellular immunity in protecting the gut from infections). For example, only one of eight patients with infantile X-linked agammaglobulinemia, followed for over 15 years, developed a chronic diarrhea that was due to giardiasis.[143] In another study, which looked at GI infections in the general population caused by Campylobacter jejuni, (one of the most common causes of bacterial gastroenteritis), only two patients had X-linked agammaglobulinemia.[147] Some patients develop a Crohn's-like inflammatory process with malabsorption, ulcers, and strictures.[92,148] There is a prominent lymphocytic infiltrate, but plasma cells and granulomas are not seen.[148] Other causes of diarrhea in these patients are antibiotic-induced colitis, GVHD, and malacoplakia of the colon.[92,143,149] These patients have a virtual absence of serum immunoglobulins of all classes. The small intestine is usually normal but may show a nonspecific mucosal lesion of variable severity, with virtual absence of plasma cells and of lymphoid follicles. Crypt abscesses with neutrophilic infiltration of the lamina propria have been described in the colonic mucosa.[143] Patients with this disorder have an increased risk of malignancy, usually lymphomas and leukemias.[143]

Miscellaneous B-cell disorders.

A number of other B-cell disorders, namely, transient hypogammaglobulinemia of infancy, deficiency of kappa light chain, X-linked immunodeficiency with hyper-IgM, and selective IgM or IgD deficiency, occasionally have GI manifestations, primarily due to GI infections/parasitic infestations.[15,68,69,75,94,143,150,151] A number of other associations have also been described in some of these patients, such as celiac sprue, ulcerative colitis, Crohn's disease in selective IgM deficiency,[152,153] and cystic fibrosis in kappa light chain deficiency.[154] The specific intestinal manifestations are listed in Table 3-4. GI manifestations have not been described in the other rare immunodeficiency disorders with predominant antibody defects, such as X-linked hypogammaglobulinemia with growth hormone deficiency, autosomal recessive agammaglobulinemia, and selective IgE deficiency.[143]

Predominant Cell-mediated Immunodeficiency

Severe combined immunodeficiency disease (Swiss-type agammaglobulinemia, hereditary thymic dysplasia)

Pathogenesis and Clinical Findings This is usually a hereditary disease, transmitted either as an autosomal recessive or X-linked disorder.[93,102,155] Occasionally sporadic cases are seen.

Severe combined immunodeficiency is a heterogeneous group of disorders. Currently, there are 11 different phenotypes associated with mutations in 10 different genes.[15,68,69,156–159] Various severe deficiencies in T-, B-, and NK-cell function are seen depending on which phenotype is studied.[160]

Clinically, the disease afflicts neonates between 3 and 6 months of age, and patients rarely survive beyond 5 years unless treated with a bone marrow transplant.[94] The infants usually develop a morbilliform rash at birth, which is thought to be due to a graft versus host reaction to maternal lymphocytes. Subsequently, they suffer from repeated viral and fungal infections, especially CMV, herpes, pneumocystis, and Candida, resulting in pneumonia and encephalitis (the latter may lead to severe dementia). Ninety percent of these patients develop an irreversible enterocolitis with intractable diarrhea, which may be due to a variety of causes, such as rotavirus infection, coccidiosis, cryptosporidiosis, giardiasis, candidiasis, aspergillosis, *Salmonella*, and enteropathic *E. coli*.[94,102,143] However, the cause of the diarrhea is not always clear, since the symptoms may persist after eradication of recognizable infections. Occasionally, other causes of GI symptoms are found such as esophageal atresia, multiple intestinal atresias,[161,162] pneumatosis intestinalis, and imperforate anus.[163] Also of interest is a recent finding of gastroesophageal reflux occurring in up to 20% of patients with severe combined immunodeficiency.[164]

Although this condition was invariably fatal in the past, bone marrow transplants have been very effective, provided the diagnosis is made early (95% success rate if preformed within the first 3.5 months of life).[160]

Histology Histologically, the intestinal tract shows the usual features of immunodeficiency. Plasma cells, lymphocytes, and Peyer's patches are absent from the lamina propria, and there may be a nonspecific small intestinal mucosal lesion (Fig. 3-7), and a colitis with crypt abscesses and focal ulceration. In addition, irregularly distributed large vacuolated macrophages similar to those seen in Whipple's disease, *Mycobacterium avium* infection in AIDS, and chronic granulomatous disease may be present in the small intestine.[165] It should be noted that the vacuolated macrophages are a feature of defective phagocytic cells and per se are nondiagnostic of any specific immunologic disorder. However, as already mentioned, they do suggest a limited differential diagnosis. The final diagnosis depends on the clinical setting, which usually helps to separate the primary immunodeficiencies from Whipple's disease and AIDS, and the morphologic findings such as absence or paucity of plasma cells in the primary immunodeficiencies, the demonstration of organisms in Whipple's disease and *Mycobacterium avium* infections, and mucosal lymhangiectasis in Whipple's disease.

IPEX syndrome. The IPEX (immune dysregulation, polyendocrinopathy, enteropathy, and X-linkage) syndrome is due to a germline mutation in the forkhead box protein (*FOXP3*) gene on the X-chromosome, which in young males results in defective development of CD4+CD25+ T-regulatory cells.[166,167] This leads to a variety of autoimmune phenomena including autoimmune enteropathy, gastritis, colitis, dermatitis, thyroiditis, and type 1 diabetes. Most children have other autoimmune phenomena including Coombs' positive anemia, autoimmune thrombocytopenia, autoimmune neutropenia, and tubular nephropathy. Most of the patients have enterocyte autoantibodies against either the enterocyte brush border or goblet cells. In all patients, the antibody seems to react against a 75-kDa autoantigen. Some patients in addition may also show autoantibodies to renal proximal tubular brush border, anti–parietal cell antibodies, anti–islet cell antibodies, anti–smooth muscle antibodies, or antinuclear antibodies. Approximately 50% of males with IPEX syndrome have mutations identified in *FOXP3*. It is suggested that defects in other genes or gene products, possibly in the same pathway as *FOXP3*, may cause a similar phenotype. Like other X-linked disorders, it occurs in males, but rarely females may also be affected. Mutations in *IL2RA* (also known as *CD25*) have been identified in two patients with an IPEX syndrome–like phenotype.[168,169] The mutations were inherited in an autosomal recessive manner. Molecular genetic testing for IPEX syndrome is clinically available.

Histology Inflammatory changes of variable intensity are seen through out stomach, small bowel, and large bowel. The mucosal changes consist of lamina propria infiltration by lymphoplasmacytic cells with a variable amount of neutrophils or eosinophils, infiltration of the glandular epithelium by neutrophils or eosinophils, crypt abscesses, crypt loss, and in some cases moderate to marked increase in IELs. In small bowel and colon, gastric metaplasia may be seen. There is mucin depletion of crypts, and in some patients, there is total absence of Paneth cells, goblet cells, or endocrine cells (Figs. 3-10A and B). Apoptosis of epithelial cells can be very prominent, and some cases may show moderate to severe villous blunting. The histological changes are variable and not unique, and produce a variety of patterns that may mimic GVHD, celiac disease, or autoimmune enteropathy (Fig. 3-10).

The syndrome frequently results in death within the first 2 years of life, although a few have survived into the second or third decade. If performed early, BMT using nonmyeloablative conditioning regimens can resolve the clinical symptoms.[170,171]

Chronic mucocutaneous candidiasis. Chronic mucocutaneous candidiasis is characterized by chronic candidal infection of the skin, nails, and mucous membranes. *Candida* can normally be cultured from the mouth, sputum, and feces of healthy adults and children. It has been shown, by delayed-type hypersensitivity skin tests, that an active immune response is necessary for the body to contain *Candida* as commensals. Consequently, breakdown in the immune response can lead to local invasion and infection. Thus, chronic mucocutaneous

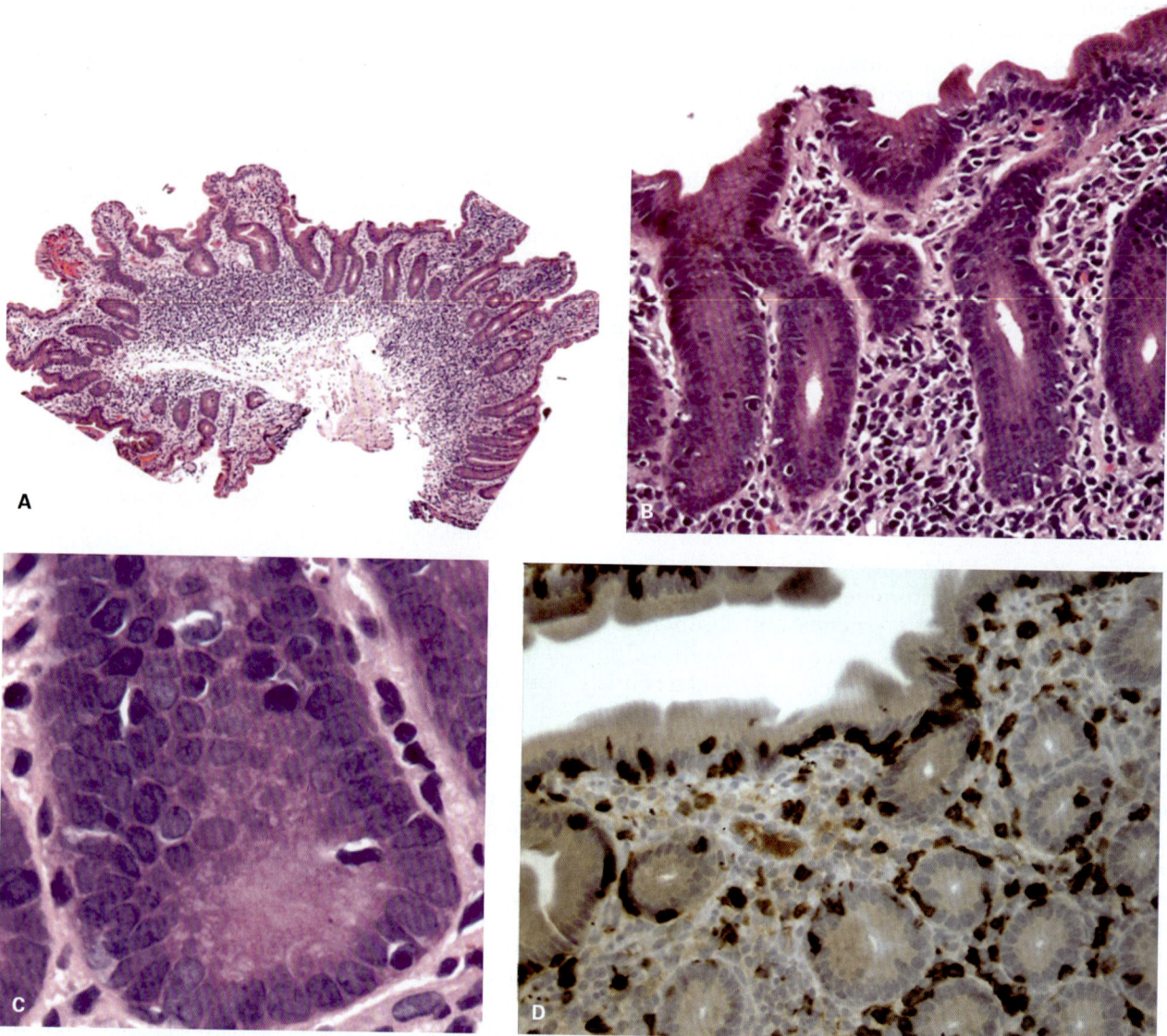

Figure 3-10. IPEX syndrome. **A:** Duodenal biopsy villi that are blunted and with increased lamina propria inflammation especially in the basal half of the mucosa. **B:** Detail of crypts with absence of goblet cells, a feature associated particularly with autoimmune enteropathies, and an intraepithelial lymphocytosis just visible in the crypt epithelium. **C:** Crypt base with absence of Paneth's and endocrine cells. In particular, no orange-red subnuclear granules typical of Kulchitsky's cells can be identified. This is also a feature of autoimmune enteropathy and IPEX syndrome. **D:** CD3 immunostain demonstrating the intraepithelial lymphocytosis. (Courtesy Dr C Streutker, St Michael's Hospital, Toronto.)

candidiasis is thought to result from a defect of the cellular immune system, either as a primary disorder, or secondary to immune suppression by drugs or other processes such as autoimmune diseases, AIDS, Addison's disease, hypothyroidism, thymomas, and interstitial keratitis.[94,172–174] In most instances, treatment is successful following cimetidine and zinc sulfate,[175] but in severe disorders allogeneic bone marrow transplant may help.[176]

In the gut, the mouth and esophagus are the main target organs, but the stomach and small intestine may occasionally be involved. Histologically, the lesions are typically superficial, consisting of mild epithelial degeneration or necrosis, with pseudohyphae growing in the necrotic epithelium (Fig. 3-11). Rarely, more extensive tissue destruction with fistula and stricture formation can be found.[94,177]

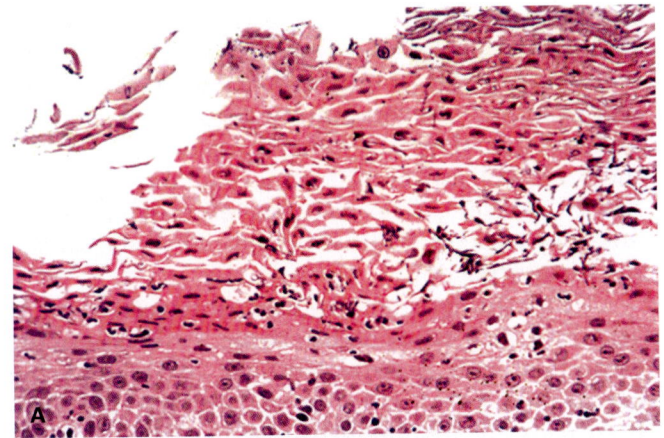
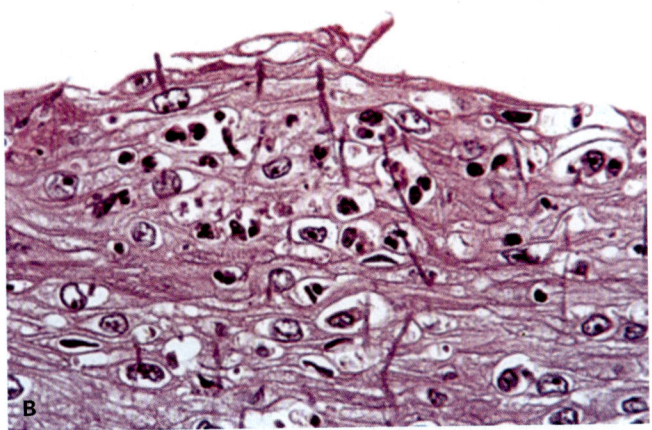
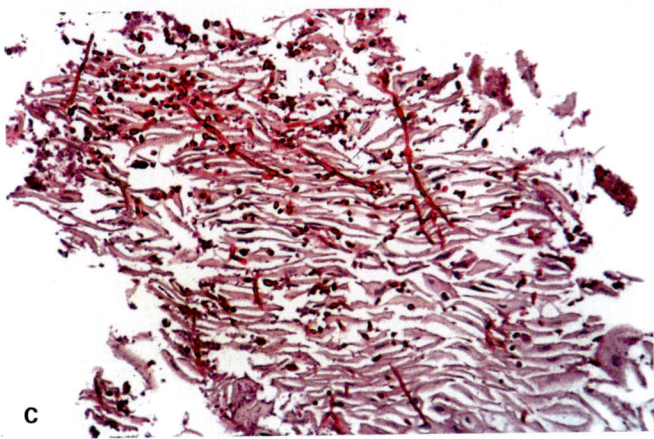

Figure 3-11. Chronic mucocutaneous candidiasis in an esophageal biopsy specimen. **A:** Low-power view of candidal esophagitis showing necrotic superficial squamous epithelium. **B:** High-power view of candidal esophagitis showing pseudohyphae growing perpendicular to the long axis of the squamous cells. **C:** PAS stain highlighting numerous yeast and pseudohyphae growing in squamous epithelium.

IMMUNODEFICIENCY ASSOCIATED WITH OTHER DEFECTS

This group of immunologic disorders is characterized by accompanying nonimmunologic defects.[15]

DiGeorge's Syndrome—Third and Fourth Pouch/Arch Syndrome (Thymic Hypoplasia, Cellular Immunodeficiency with Hypoparathyroidism)

DiGeorge's syndrome[178] is a very rare, often fatal condition characterized by thymic aplasia or hypoplasia and the absence of the parathyroid glands. Other congenital abnormalities have also been described such as nasal clefts, hypertelorism, and anomalies of the great vessels. Patients present in a number of ways such as neonatal hypocalcemia, fatal necrotizing enterocolitis, and jejunal atresia.[179,180] These patients are susceptible to a wide variety of GI tract infections. They may develop oral candidiasis and intractable diarrhea, the etiology of which is undetermined.[76,143]

Patients with DiGeorge's syndrome have been found to have 22q11 chromosomal deletion.[181,182] The T-cell defect is seldom absolute,[182] and at autopsy, remnants of thymus may be demonstrated. The humoral immune response is normal. Thymic transplantation with restoration of cell-mediated immunity has been successful in some patients.[183]

The other disorders in this group consist of the *Wiskott–Aldrich syndrome* (eczema and thrombocytopenia) due to defects of the Wiskott–Aldrich syndrome protein (WASP) gene on the X chromosome,[184] *transcobalamin II deficiency,* and *ataxia telangiectasia*[76,94] (cerebellar ataxia and telangiectasia of the conjunctivae and flexor surfaces of the arms). GI manifestations are uncommon, consisting of candidiasis, diarrhea, and GI hemorrhage.[76,94,185] In ataxia telangiectasia, there is IgA deficiency, and there may be nodular lymphoid hyperplasia. Jejunal and rectal biopsies are usually normal, however.[78,94] Patients have a 10% risk of developing neoplasia,[143] usually lymphoma, although a case of gastric carcinoma has also been reported.[186,187]

PHAGOCYTIC AND OTHER CELL DYSFUNCTION

Chronic Granulomatous Disease

This is classically an X-linked inherited congenital disorder of phagocytic leukocyte function[188] in which there is an inability to kill catalase-positive organisms, such as *Candida* and *Aspergillus*. The disease results from a deficiency of NADPH oxidase that occurs secondary to mutations in any one of four genes coding for essential subunits of the enzyme.[189]

The disorder classically involves young male children, although approximately 30% of cases are inherited in an autosomal recessive rather than an X-linked fashion.[190] The disease is characterized by recurrent infections and abscesses involving the skin, lymph nodes, and GI tract.[79,188,191–193]

Clinically, GI manifestations mimic other entities such inflammatory bowel disease and frequently cause extensive morbidity and mortality. Symptoms include fever, weight loss, abdominal pain, diarrhea, vomiting, perirectal abscess, and less commonly, steatorrhea and vitamin B_{12} malabsorption.[79,188,191] The steatorrhea is postulated to be due to interference of the enterohepatic circulation of bile salts secondary to ileal dysfunction. Because of failure of exogenous intrinsic factor to improve vitamin B_{12} absorption, it has been suggested that this malabsorption is due either to an ileal absorptive cell abnormality or to an intraluminal defect.[79] Gastric obstruction due to chronic granulomatous inflammation of the antrum may occur,[194] and most patients also have lymphadenopathy and hepatosplenomegaly.

Histology The characteristic finding in the small intestine and rectum is the presence of vacuolated brownish-yellow histiocytes in the lamina propria.[79] The histiocytes occur adjacent to the crypts and in the small intestine may extend into the villous core. They measure between 50 and 100 μm and have specific staining characteristics of glycolipid or phospholipid. The small intestinal morphology is otherwise normal, but in the rectum, granulomas with giant cells have been reported.[79] Other changes that have been reported are ulcerative stomatitis and a lesion indistinguishable from that of Crohn's disease.[192] It is unclear whether the latter represents true Crohn's disease or morphologic alterations mimicking it.[192,195]

Systemic Mastocytosis

This disorder presents classically with urticaria pigmentosa, flushing, asthma, and headaches. However, it may involve other organs such as bones, lymph nodes, and in up to 80% of patients the GI tract.[196] Clinically, the patients with GI involvement present with a variety of symptoms ranging from nausea and vomiting to severe watery diarrhea, steatorrhea, and abdominal pain.[197] The symptoms are due to increased release of histamine and prostaglandins, which induce gastric hypersecretion/peptic ulceration, increased intestinal permeability, and smooth muscle dysfunction.

Histologically, the GI changes consist of mucosal injury such as peptic ulceration,[196] villous atrophy associated with massive mucosal and submucosal edema, and mast cell infiltration. In the mucosa, the mast cells are prominent within the lamina propria but also extend into and may damage the mucosal glands. In addition to the mast cell infiltration, eosinophils may also be prominent. Special stains that help one to clearly identify mast cells include Giemsa, toluidine blue, tryptase, CD68, and CD117.[38]

SECONDARY (ACQUIRED) IMMUNODEFICIENCY DISORDERS

These are a heterogeneous group of disorders that may be acquired in a number of different ways. For example, T-cell dysfunction may develop naturally with increasing age or may complicate severe infections, such as tuberculosis, lepromatous leprosy, and viral infections such as HIV.[198,199] It may also be associated with certain malignancies such as Hodgkin's disease.[200] B-cell dysfunction with dysgammaglobulinemia may occur in malignancies such as multiple myeloma and certain lymphomas such as alpha-chain disease. Malnutrition may impair the secretory immune system, resulting in severe, prolonged gastroenteritis.[201,202] Hypogammaglobulinemia can also result from secondary loss of antibody in diseases of the kidney, the protein-losing enteropathies, intestinal lymphangiectasia,[203] Whipple's disease, and regional enteritis. Still other causes of acquired immunodeficiency are the iatrogenic complications of immunosuppressive and steroid therapy given for the treatment of autoimmune disease, neoplasia, and organ transplantation.

The pathologic manifestations in the GI tract consist primarily of infection, including disseminated parasitic infestations (strongyloidiasis),[204,205] and an increased risk of neoplasia. These morphologic changes are similar to those previously described in the primary immunodeficiency diseases. BMT and AIDS are two unique forms of acquired immunodeficiency disorders that will be described in greater detail.

Bone Marrow Transplantation

Hemopoeitic stem cell transplantation is now an established form of treatment for certain disorders, notably severe aplastic anemia, leukemias, lymphomas, carcinomas, congenital immunodeficiency syndromes, and enzyme deficiency disorders.[206-208] Long-term survival is excellent in some of these conditions, especially acute nonlymphoblastic leukemia and severe combined immunodeficiency, and approaches 50% in aplastic anemia.[209] However, injury to the GI tract is common following BMT/HSCT and results from three major causes: (1) the transplantation regimen, (2) infections complicating immunosuppression, and (3) GVHD.[209-212] Differentiating among these three major causes of injury in BMT is obviously important, since specific therapies can improve one condition but worsen another.

Transplantation regimen. This usually consists of chemotherapy plus or minus total body irradiation, which are given to immunosuppress the patient to prevent graft rejection, to create space in the marrow for the allograft, and, in the case of neoplasia, to eradicate tumor cells. In the bowel, the injury is characterized by atypia of crypt cell nuclei, decreased mitoses, degeneration, and, later, flattening of crypt epithelium, abnormal surface cells, and stunted villi in the small bowel. This may be followed by extensive necrosis of intestinal crypts and then mucosal ulceration. The mucosal injury is usually transient, lasting about 3 weeks, with complete resolution.[209]

Infection. After conditioning therapy, BMT patients are susceptible to infections such as CMV, herpes simplex virus (HSV), adenovirus, gram-positive cocci, cryptosporidiosis, and fungal organisms such as *Candida* species, *Aspergillus* species, and *Torulopsis glabrata*[198,209,210,213-215] (Table 3-5). The greatest risk for infection is at the time of acute GVHD; consequently, the mucosal changes due to infection may be compounded by the changes resulting from the graft versus host reaction.

Graft versus host disease (GVHD)

Pathogenesis Damage to the gut in patients undergoing BMT/HSCT may occur from a number of possible etiologies. GVHD is quite common and appears to be secondary to a complex reaction involving donor T lymphocytes, host antigen-presenting cells, and cytokines.[216] As we have developed techniques to decrease the number of T cells in HSCT and the amount of mucosal damage secondary to better pretransplant conditioning regimens, the incidence of GVHD has decreased. Nevertheless, GVHD becomes a chronic problem in greater than 50% of long-term survivors of HSCT.[216] In the past, GVHD was divided into acute and chronic forms based on whether the changes occurred before or after 100 days posttransplant. Evidence has shown that this arbitrary distinction can be confusing since the histologic changes of "acute GVHD" can be seen several years after transplant. An NIH consensus panel recommended using the term active GVHD to denote ongoing epithelial damage (apoptosis/necrosis) and chronic GVHD to denote scarring and scleroderma-like changes that can occur later in the posttransplant period.[216] GVHD can rarely occur in solid organ patients, most notably those who have had small bowel transplants.

Clinical Presentation Active GVHD occurs in 50% to 75% of transplant patients[217,218] and usually starts 3 to 4 weeks after HSCT (range 2–10 weeks). It is characterized by the abrupt onset of an erythematous rash, anorexia, nausea and vomiting, severe watery diarrhea, crampy abdominal pain, intestinal hemorrhage, and occasionally intestinal perforation.[210] The severity of the intestinal lesion parallels the skin involvement,[209,219,220] although the latter involvement may be more severe.[221] Untreated, death usually results from secondary infection or intestinal hemorrhage.[219,222] The histologic features are often more easily identified in the colon and small bowel versus the stomach and esophagus.[223] Also, upper GI GVHD is increasingly recognized in practice with or without accompanying colonic GVHD, and some centers frequently sample upper and lower GI at the same setting. Due to sampling issues, it is also a common practice to biopsy

Table 3-5 Common GI Infections and Parasitic Infestations in Bone Marrow Transplantation

Esophagitis
  Candida species
  Herpes simplex virus
  Cytomegalovirus
Gastroduodenal erosions and ulcers
  Candida species
  Aspergillus
Enterocolitis
  Intestinal overgrowth due to aerobic gram-negative bacteria
  Candida, Torulopsis, and *Aspergillus*
  Cytomegalovirus
Pseudomembranous colitis
  Clostridium difficile
Neutropenic colitis
  Probably due to multiple causes
Parasitic infestations
  Giardia
  Cryptosporidium
  Disseminated strongyloidiasis

multiple sites in different segments of the GI tract, especially in colon, although in most instances sigmoidoscopy without bowel preparation with biopsies from rectum and sigmoid would suffice to establish a diagnosis of GVHD. Decision to perform colonoscopy should be guided by clinical presentation and the differential diagnosis.

Gross Appearance Endoscopic changes range from normal to patchy erythema to extensive mucosal sloughing.[209] One study found that active GVHD was present in 44% of cases that were endoscopically normal, underlining the importance of taking multiple biopsies from multiple sites, even when no changes are evident grossly.[224]

Histology The early and mild histologic changes consist of mucosal edema and focal crypt cell necrosis with apoptosis.[209,225,226] The necrotic foci are characterized by apoptotic bodies, containing cellular debris lying between the crypt epithelium and its basement membrane. For this purpose, apoptotic bodies in the body or crypt bases, rather than surface, are taken into account (Figs. 3-12).[209,226] In more obvious cases, there may be extensive lamina propria lymphocytic infiltration, crypt loss, and crypt abscesses filled with apoptotic debris. Eosinophils also may be seen in variable numbers. One must be careful about diagnosing active GVHD prior to day 21 posttransplant, as the conditioning regimen can induce damage to the gut that can mimic GVHD. In more severe GVHD, the epithelial necrosis extends to involve the whole crypt, resulting in drop out of entire crypts (Fig. 3-12). At this stage, apoptotic bodies are difficult to find. Small nests of endocrine cells at the base of the mucosa may be the only epithelium one can find (Fig. 3-12). These cells seem to be more resistant to GVHD.[227] In advanced cases, there is extensive ulceration, edema, and fibrosis, and perforation may occur.[202,213,215,228] As severe GVHD heals, the architectural distortion can mimic quiescent inflammatory bowel disease; however, on careful examination, the inflammatory infiltrate is much less prominent than in IBD (Fig. 3-12).[210]

Esophageal involvement is characterized by the presence of few scattered apoptotic squamous cells in most cases.

In the stomach, the apoptotic bodies are most often seen in the neck of the glands, but can be also be seen in the deeper parts of the antral or fundic glands. Focal dilatation of the glands containing granular debris, sloughed parietal cells, or apoptotic bodies, sometimes accompanied by neutrophils, is not infrequent. Apoptotic bodies are often more subtle and smaller in gastric and small bowel biopsies, necessitating a more careful evaluation. The presence of focal areas of collections of lymphocytes or histiocytes with or without neutrophils surrounding gastric foveolae or glands, referred to as "focal active gastritis," has been suggested as a histologic marker of GVHD, especially in pediatric patients; however, this issue remains controversial.[228]

In small bowel biopsies, particularly duodenal biopsies, mild and subtle villous blunting may be seen. The apoptotic bodies are often seen in the neck and deeper parts of the crypts, rather than the villous surface.

Grading GVHD Various histologic grading systems for GVHD have been proposed; however, none has been universally accepted. Discordance in the histologic changes and clinical features is well recognized and it cannot be overemphasized that any grading system that one uses must take both clinical and histologic parameters into account. More so, histologic grading has hardly any therapeutic or prognostic implications, above and beyond clinical parameters. For these reasons, currently histologic grading of GVHD is not routinely performed in most transplant centers. If needed, a modification of the Lerner's systems can be used as follows: grade 1, isolated apoptotic epithelial cells without any crypt loss; grade 2, isolated loss of crypts; grade 3, loss of 2 or more contiguous crypts; and grade 4, extensive crypt loss with mucosal denudation.[229]

Perhaps the most challenging aspect of diagnosing GVHD in mucosal biopsy specimens is deciding what the minimal criteria for GVHD should be.

Large bowel This begs the question, what is the apoptotic count in normal colonic mucosa? While studies reporting apoptosis in normal colonic mucosa are hard to find, studies performed in asymptomatic bone marrow transplant patients, patients undergoing screening colonoscopy, or biopsies from normal mucosa in suspected functional disorders of bowel show that apoptotic bodies are present in apparently normal colonic mucosa and the counts vary depending on study design and methodology.[194–196,230–232] One study showed apoptotic counts of $1.3 \pm 0.4/10$ crypts and $0.4 \pm 0.1/10$ crypts in normal colonic mucosa with and without the prior use of bowel preparation with oral sodium phosphate, respectively.[232] Similar to the presence of inflammatory cells in colon, it has been suggested that the apoptotic bodies are more frequent in the right side of the colon compared to left side, although the issue is still controversial.[197,199,233,234] Use of specific and sensitive immunohistochemical or molecular markers obviously increases the detection rate of apoptosis; however, their use in routine clinical practice has not been validated and is not recommended. Thus currently the histologic diagnosis of GVHD is made based on assessments made on H&E sections alone.

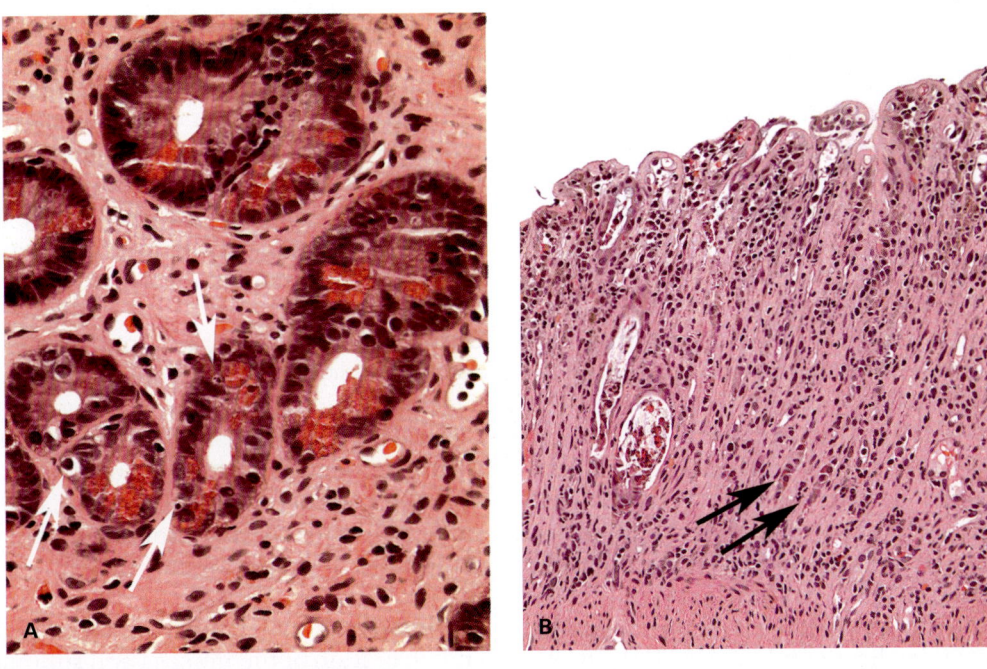
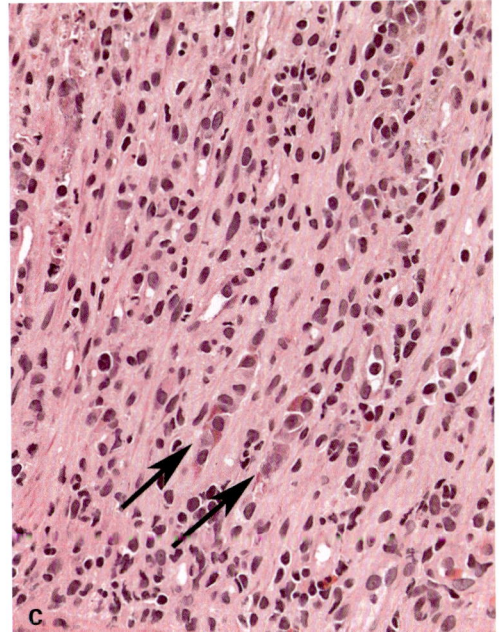
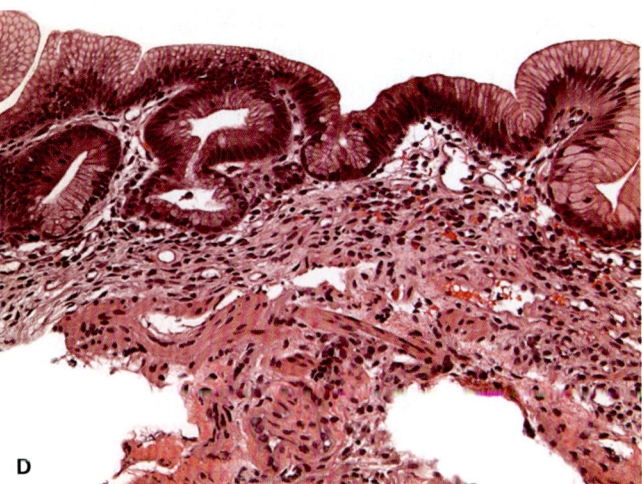
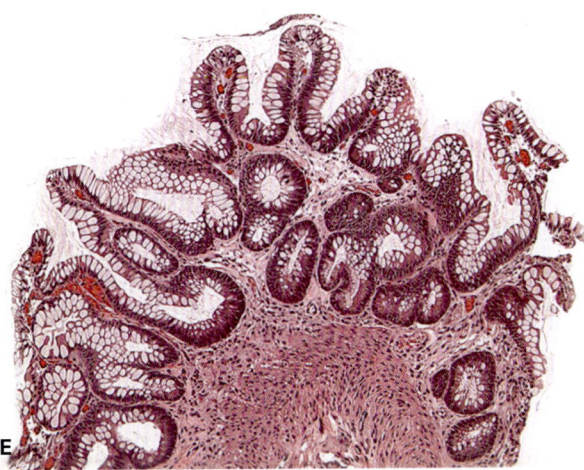

Figure 3-12. Graft versus host disease. **A:** Base of small bowel mucosa showing numerous apoptotic bodies (*arrows*). **B:** Colon with severe GVHD with necrotic crypts on the left and an empty-appearing lamina propria on the right containing a few residual endocrine cells (*arrows*). **C:** Higher-power view of (**B**) showing cords of endocrine cells (*arrows*). **D:** Gastric mucosa with marked architectural distortion secondary to GVHD (healed GVHD). **E:** Small bowel with marked architectural distortion secondary to GVHD (healed GVHD). One could easily confuse this with quiescent IBD.

This whole issue is further complicated by the fact that increase in enterocyte apoptosis may be found in a wide variety of settings besides acute GVHD. Any infection or other inflammatory disorder can induce apoptosis in the gut, as can oral sodium phosphate bowel preparations,[196,232] NSAIDs, and mycophenolate mofetil (a drug often used to treat or prophylax against GVHD).[194,198,213,215,228,230,235] Thus, it is not surprising that the minimal criteria used for making a diagnosis of GVHD vary even among institutions.

NIH consensus suggests that the minimal criterion for diagnosing GVHD in a mucosal biopsy is the presence of at least one apoptotic cell per piece of tissue.[216] This semiquantitative method depends upon the size of the biopsy forceps used, and fails to take into account varying numbers of serial sections studied, impact of commonly used medications, and bowel preparation methods. One must be careful not to overinterpret isolated apoptotic cells in the gastric antrum of patients on proton pump inhibitors, as these medications have recently been noted to induce apoptosis.[236] It needs to be realized that patients showing normal-appearing biopsies may respond to steroid therapy initiated for a presumptive clinical diagnosis of GVHD, and the presence of GVHD elsewhere is also not a conclusive evidence of GVHD in the gut. Our recommendation is that institutions need to establish their own threshold for diagnosis of minimal GVHD in the gut, and not be bullied into making this histologic diagnosis based on clinical features alone. In cases of equivocal findings in the biopsies, we generally comment in our report that "only rare apoptotic bodies identified, insufficient to make a histologic diagnosis of GVHD" or "rare apoptotic bodies seen which might represent minimal evidence of GVHD." Which phrase to choose may be a personal choice or decided following discussion with clinical colleagues.

Two other common problems encountered in this setting are making a diagnosis of GVHD in the setting of an infection (e.g., CMV or cryptosporidia) or in the presence of medication used for immunosuppresion in these patients (e.g., cellcept/mycophenolate mofetil), both of which are known to induce changes that mimic GVHD. One must search carefully for CMV inclusions and cryptosporidia prior to making a diagnosis of GHVD as the resultant immunosuppressive therapy given to treat GVHD will exacerbate such infections. In the presence of unequivocal evidence of infection in the gut, it would be wise to treat the infection first and assess for the clinical improvement, although some recommend making a concomitant diagnosis of CMV infection and GVHD when apoptosis is noted in crypts that are devoid of CMV inclusions.[216] In our opinion, the treatment for GVHD in these patients should be preferably initiated either when there is no clinical response to CMV treatment or when the response plateaus after initial few days of improvement. In the setting of mycophenolate mofetil use and GVHD-like changes, at least in the mild cases, one should contemplate altering the immunosuppresion or reducing mycophenolate mofetil dosage and watch for appropriate response. In some cases, especially with moderate to marked histological changes, one may have to initiate GVHD treatment at the same time.

Chronic GVHD. This is a multiorgan system syndrome, which resembles autoimmune disease and develops in at least 50% of long-term survivors.[216] Clinically, patients have many features in common with scleroderma patients, such as skin pigmentation and contractures, oral mucositis, oral and ocular sicca, polyserositis, and esophagitis. In addition, they sometimes develop vasculopathy.[237]

Pathology In the esophagus, there is desquamation and ulceration of the mucosa and submucosal fibrosis, which may produce stricture. The intestinal mucosa is usually spared, although rarely it may develop submucosal and subserosal fibrosis as well.[209,238] These findings are generally not diagnosable on endoscopic biopsy materials.

Intestinal Transplantation

Intestinal failure is a disorder secondary to a number of diseases such as short bowel syndrome, diffuse ischemic injury, intestinal pseudoobstruction, etc. Intestinal transplantation is now being used as an alternative treatment to chronic parenteral nutrition.[239–241] Although in the past, the majority of patients have died of rejection, sepsis, and possible GVHD within 9 days of transplantation,[242] it has now become much more successful.[239,243,244]

Histologically, rejection changes in small bowel allografts are characterized by epithelial damage and apoptosis with villus blunting, increasing mononuclear infiltrates of the lamina propria, and ultimately mucosal sloughing.[243–246] A grading scheme for acute rejection that is based on the amount of crypt apoptosis and lamina propria inflammation has been proposed (Table 3-6).

The Acquired Immunodeficiency Syndrome (AIDS)

GI complications are common in untreated AIDS patients, occurring in more than half of them and leading to disabling symptoms. The major GI manifestations are due to immunodeficiency disorders that result in malabsorption, opportunistic infections, and neoplasms.[71,247] The main role of the pathologist is to

Table 3-6 Grading Scheme for Acute Cellular Rejection in Small Bowel Allografts

GRADE	APOPTOSIS	EPITHELIAL DAMAGE	LAMINA PROPRIA
0	0	none	Normal
Indeterminate	<6/10 crypt cross sections	Mild focal crypt injury	Mild mononuclear or mixed infiltrate
Mild	6 or more/10 crypt cross sections	Diffuse crypt injury with reactive epithelial changes, villus blunting, and distortion	Mixed but primarily mononuclear infiltrate with transformed lymphs
Moderate	6 or more/10 crypt cross sections plus confluent apoptosis	More intense epithelial injury than above, erosions	As above but more intense, more transformed lymphs
Severe	May not be present due to intense epithelial damage	Diffuse erosions or ulcers, granulation tissue, and mucosal sloughing	Marked diffuse winfiltrated with transformed lymphs

From Ruiz P, Bagni A, Brown R, et al. Histological criteria for the identification of acute cellular rejection in human small bowel allografts: results of the pathology workshop at the VIII International Small Bowel Transplant Symposium. *Transplant Proc.* 2004;36(2):335–337.

identify these complications, since a number of them, for example, *Candida* infections, are readily treatable, resulting in symptomatic relief.

Pathogenesis and clinical features. AIDS is caused by HIV. The virus infects primarily the intestinal M cells and then extends to the mucosal lymphoid follicles,[248] and ultimately incapacitates the immune system, predisposing individuals to a broad range of opportunistic infections and neoplasms throughout the GI tract.[71,249-253] Infection with HIV occurs through sexual contact, most frequently via the rectal mucosa,[248] and less frequently by infected blood or blood products, and perinatally from mother to infant.[254,255] The interval between infection with HIV and the development of AIDS is long and variable.[256] The mortality of AIDS used to be 100%, yet currently a fair number of patients survive for long periods and some appear to be cured with antiviral treatment.

The major basis for the profound immunosuppression associated with HIV infection is the depletion of the helper/inducer subset of T lymphocytes, which express the CD4 phenotypic marker (the T4 cell). Almost all of the immunologic abnormalities that occur in AIDS can be attributed to the defect in the T4 subset of lymphocytes.[252,254] These cells play a crucial role in the immune response, and their impaired activity results in compromised function of a variety of other cell types, including IgA-secreting B cells.[254] Furthermore, other factors of cell-mediated immunity in AIDS patients such as zinc deficiency result from severe malnutrition due to prolonged diarrhea and steatorrhea.

In North America and Europe, approximately 90% of cases of AIDS have occurred in men.[257] Two-thirds of all cases occur in homosexual men and 17% among intravenous drug users.[256] Among the remainder are individuals who received infected blood or blood components, primarily those with hemophilia and children born to mothers with AIDS. In Africa and Haiti, the disease is more prevalent in the heterosexual population and more common among women than men.[258] Furthermore, the HIV-infected infants are underweight and often have severe life-threatening diarrhea and weight loss.[259,260]

Case definitions for AIDS surveillance have been detailed by WHO and the Centers for Disease Control.[251,261] Most patients present with opportunistic infections; *Pneumocystis carinii* pneumonia being the most common, accounting for two-thirds of cases at presentation. One-fifth of AIDS patients present with other opportunistic infections, and 15% present with Kaposi's sarcoma alone.[262]

Chronic diarrhea is the most common GI problem in HIV patients, with a cumulative incidence that ranges from 30% to 70% in industrialized nations to 100% in developing countries.[263] With the advent of highly active antiretroviral therapy (HAART) for HIV, the percentage of diarrhea caused by opportunistic infections has decreased; however, the overall prevalence of diarrhea has not changed, as many protease inhibitors (nelfinavir, ritonavir, saquinavir, and indinavir) as well as the nucleoside analog didanosine cause diarrhea.[263] Infections seen in untreated HIV patients include protozoa (*Cryptosporidium parvum*, *Isospora belli*, *Enterocytozoon bieneusi*, *Encephalitozoon intestinalis*, *Cyclospora* spp., *Entamoeba histolytica*, and *Giardia lamblia*), bacteria (*Mycobacterium avium-intracellulare*, *Clostridium difficile*, *Salmonella*, *Shigella*, and *Campylobacter jejuni*), and viruses (CMV, HSV, and adenovirus).[250,264]

The severity and duration of symptoms associated with enteric organisms are determined by the host's immunologic response to the organism, the virulence of the organism, and, most importantly, the availability of effective therapy. For example, *Giardia lamblia* may cause acute abdominal pain and diarrhea, but prolonged infections are uncommon because effective therapy is available. On the other hand, cryptosporidial infections may be severe and chronic, as there is no effective therapy for this organism.[255] A variety of nonspecific histologic abnormalities may be observed in the GI tract of patients with AIDS, and it is still unclear how many are due to the underlying immunodeficiency or due to as yet uncharacterized infections.

Esophagus A number of AIDS patients present with odynophagia and substernal pain due to single or multiple ulcerations as well as esophageal strictures.[177] While specific infections such as *Candida*, CMV, and herpes may be found (either singly or in combination), some patients develop chronic idiopathic ulcers that respond to steroid therapy.[265-268] In addition to the inflamed and ulcerative lesions, megaesophagus lesions have been found in Central and South America due to Chagas disease (a common disorder in those areas).[269]

Stomach Parietal cells are injured by HIV, resulting in reduced number of parietal cells, acid secretory failure, decrease in intrinsic factor secretion, and increase in mucus secretion. Morphologically, the parietal cells show loss of intracellular microvilli and canaliculi.[270] This leads to decreased acid secretion and bacterial overgrowth.[271] Some studies suggest that this hypoacidity increases the risk of opportunistic infections. Lastly, tumors, primarily Kaposi's sarcoma and lymphoma, also occur in the stomach (see "Gastrointestinal Tumor" section).

Small Intestine and Colon T-cell changes in the intestinal mucosa parallel those observed in the circulation of AIDS patients.[272] There is a reduction in the total T-cell population, especially CD4 T cells, resulting in a decreased helper/suppressor cell ratio and an increase in total mononuclear cells. Consequently, the immunocompromised mucosa gives rise to altered cytokine secretion leading to a breakdown of the mucosal immune barrier and secondary infections.[72] While HIV has been localized within lamina propria lymphocytes and macrophages, it is controversial whether the virus actually infects and resides in epithelial cells.[273,274]

AIDS ENTEROPATHY. The reduction in CD4 cells and the resultant immune disregulation that ensues lead to subtle abnormalities in the small bowel biopsies of HIV-positive patients, regardless of whether or not they have GI symptoms.[275-278] Greenson and colleagues found that the average villus to crypt ratio in HIV-positive patients without GI symptoms was less than 2, while HIV-negative controls had a ratio of approximately 3 (Fig. 3-13).[275] These findings are even more impressive in HIV-positive patients with diarrhea. The small bowel is the best place to biopsy when looking for occult infectious causes of diarrhea. The specific infections are discussed in Chapter 22.

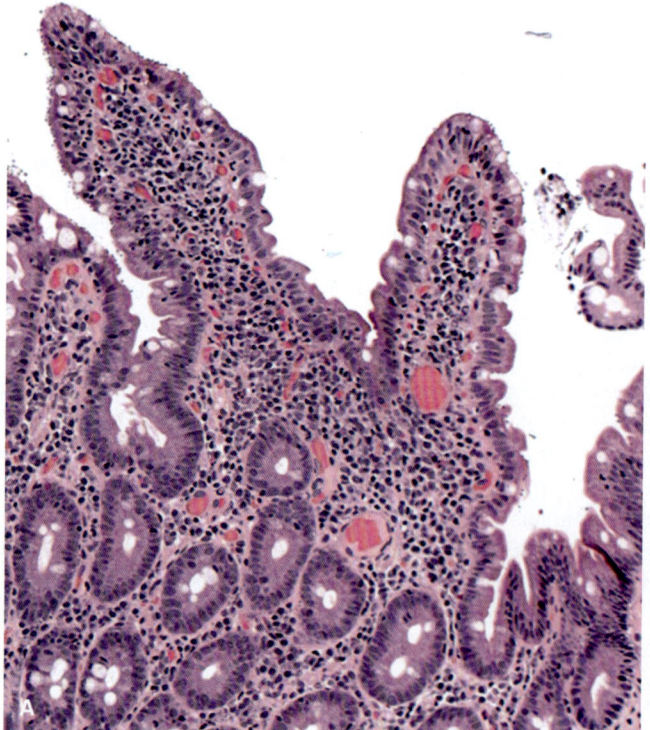 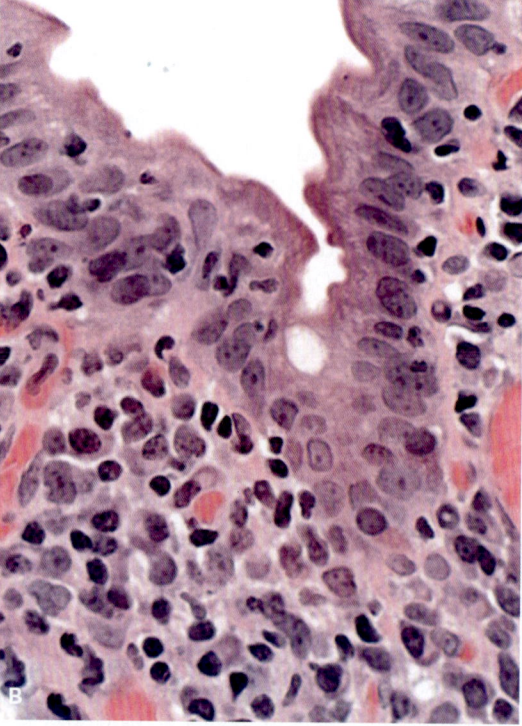

Figure 3-13. AIDS enteropathy. **A:** Villi may be blunted or focally absent with an excess of chronic inflammatory cells in the lamina propria, often with an intraepithelial lymphocytosis (**B**).

Anus/Rectum Opportunistic infections and tumors may give rise to anorectal hemorrhage, anal fissures and fistulae, perianal abscesses, and tumor masses. The latter consist primarily of Kaposi's sarcoma, condyloma acuminata/human papilloma virus (HPV)/squamous cell carcinoma, and lymphoma. Chronic herpetic infections in this area can be a debilitating problem in HIV patients. In addition, chronic ulcers can be seen for which no infection can be identified.

GI AIDS infections. The most common opportunistic infections of the GI tract in AIDS are given in Table 3-7. Patients with untreated AIDS commonly have multiple intestinal parasitic infections at any given time, namely, *Giardia lamblia, Entamoeba coli, Cryptosporidium parvum, Endolimax nana, Ascaris lumbricoides, Strongyloides stercoralis, Isospora belli,* and *Blastocystis hominis.*[279] Multiple organism infections occurred primarily among patients with < 200 per mm^3 CD4 T cells, whereas those patients with a higher number of CD4 T cells (> 200/mm^3) usually had single organism infections.[280–282] Many of the parasites, notably *Giardia lamblia, Cryptosporidium, Microsporidium,* and *Isospora belli,* are easily missed if not suspected and specifically searched for. Many of the organisms can be diagnosed more quickly and at lower cost by biopsy. Thus, it is imperative to examine the mucus adherent to the mucosa, the surface epithelium, and the crypts for these parasites before systematically examining the remainder of the histologic section. The most common symptom is diarrhea. In one study, one or more enteric pathogens were identified in 85% of patients with diarrhea.[282]

GI neoplasms in AIDS. Kaposi's sarcoma is the most common neoplasm in AIDS, followed by lymphoma and cervical cancer in women. Studies have found that the most common causes of these tumors are Herpes hominis virus 8 (HHV-8) for Kaposi's sarcoma, EBV for lymphoma (see Chapter 4), and HPV for cervical cancer in women.[253,283–286] HPV infection also appears to be responsible for an increase in anal intraepithelial neoplasia among HIV-positive men (see Chapter 22).[287]

Kaposi's Sarcoma

CLINICAL FEATURES. Prior to the AIDS epidemic, Kaposi's sarcoma was considered to be an uncommon tumor in most countries. It was recognized as an indolent cutaneous disease with a predilection for elderly men of Mediterranean descent.[288] However, Kaposi's sarcoma with visceral involvement is a much more aggressive disease in AIDS patients (and rarely organ transplant patients).[283,285,289]

Kaposi's sarcoma is the initial manifestation of AIDS in approximately 15% of patients and appears to be declining in frequency.[262] However, up to 30% of patients with advanced AIDS morbidity have been found to develop Kaposi's sarcoma.[285] It is a multisystem neoplasm in the AIDS patient, usually presenting with red to purple skin lesions. A minority of patients present with lymph node involvement, and a smaller number still with visceral involvement. Recently, it has been found that this disorder is more aggressive and life threatening in women for reasons that are currently uncertain.[290]

Kaposi's sarcoma is commonly present in the GI tract of patients with AIDS who have Kaposi's sarcoma of skin or lymph nodes. Despite the frequency of involvement, the lesions are usually silent.[253,291] However, occasionally, patients develop GI hemorrhage (both upper and lower GI) and obstruction and in a rare instance present with a rectal ulcer.[277,292]

PATHOLOGY. In one endoscopic survey, 40% of patients had lesions observed at upper endoscopy, flexible sigmoidoscopy, or both.[291] Of those with positive findings, half had involvement of upper and lower tracts; approximately one-quarter each had upper or lower involvement alone.[288] The prevalence of GI lesions appears to be independent of the numbers of skin lesions or whether there is lymph node involvement alone. Autopsy prevalence of gut lesions in those with Kaposi's sarcoma may be greater than 75%.[291]

At endoscopy, early lesions look like subepithelial hemorrhages. More advanced lesions are elevated in a dome shape, and even more advanced lesions are nodular and may contain central umbilications or ulcerations (Fig. 3-14). The lesions are located primarily in the submucosa and indent the overlying mucosa. Advanced lesions may become very large, involving all layers of the affected organ and the regional lymph nodes as well. It should be noted that especially for early lesions, endoscopic ultrasonography is helpful in determining the exact size of tumor volume.[293]

Microscopically, the lesions consist of spindle cells and vascular-appearing endothelial-lined spaces. The spindle cells may show a wide range of nuclear pleomorphism; mitoses may be numerous. Red blood

Table 3-7	Common Opportunistic GI Infections in AIDS

Parasitic
  Cryptosporidium
  Isospora belli
  Microsporidia
Bacterial
  Mycobacterium avium-intracellulare
  Salmonella
Fungal
  Candida albicans
Viral
  Cytomegalovirus
  Herpes simplex

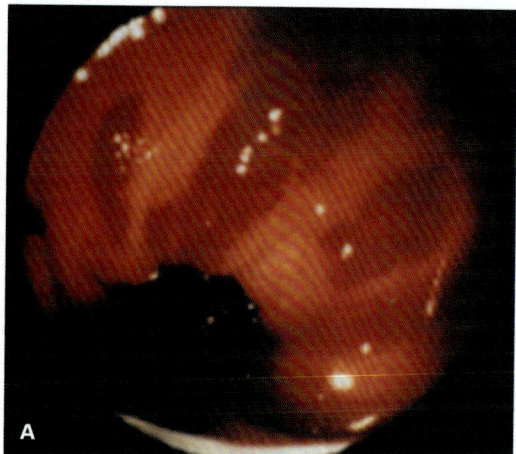 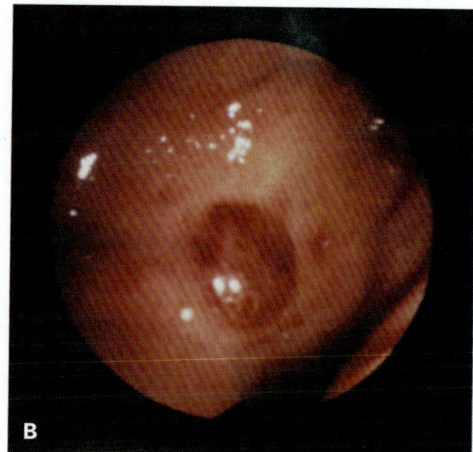

Figure 3-14. Kaposi's sarcoma of the rectum: endoscopic appearances. A: Subepithelial mucosal hemorrhages. (Courtesy K. Buch, M.D.) B: Dome-shaped red mucosal nodule.

cells fill some of the spaces between the spindle cells (Fig. 3-15). Hemosiderin may be scattered within the lesions or at their periphery.

Biopsies of obvious Kaposi's lesions are often negative[291] because of the submucosal location of the lesions. In our experience, even using larger ("jumbo") pinch biopsy forceps, a positive biopsy diagnosis is obtained in less than one-half of cases. Sometimes, the tumor infiltrate is overlooked because it is regarded as localized fibrosis or granulation tissue. On occasion, it may also be difficult to differentiate crush artifact from Kaposi's sarcoma, especially at the edges of biopsies. Infiltration of the muscularis mucosae by spindle cells is often the only clue in a mucosal biopsy specimen. An immunostain for HHV8 is very helpful in confirming the diagnosis and is vital in equivocal cases. Vascular markers such as CD 34 and CD 31 may also be helpful but are not nearly as specific for Kaposi's as HHV8. Pathologists who receive GI biopsies without clinical histories and endoscopic descriptions may mistake the spindle cells of Kaposi's for a GI stromal tumor. Kaposi's sarcoma can stain weakly for c-kit (CD117), so care must be taken in interpreting immunostains in this situation.

THERAPY. Antiretroviral therapies, in particular the protease inhibitors, appear to be changing the clinical course of Kaposi's sarcoma. It is not unusual to observe a complete resolution and control of Kaposi's sarcoma with HAART. Refractory cases may be treated with liposomal anthracylcins and interferon-alpha.[294]

Lymphoma B-cell non-Hodgkin's lymphomas are the second most common neoplasm occurring in AIDS (Fig. 3-16)[284,286,295] and usually pursue a very aggressive

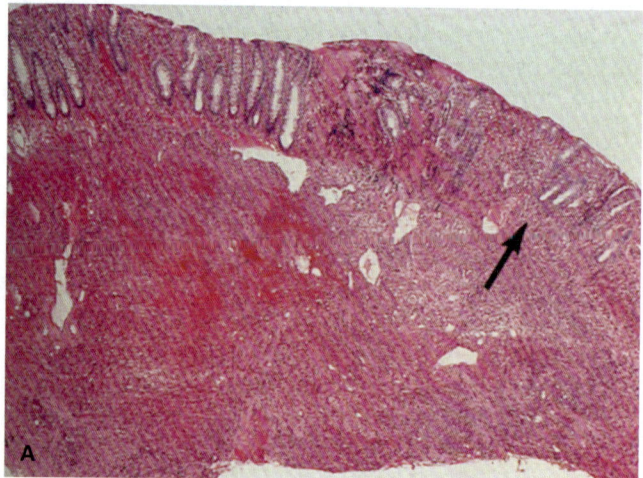 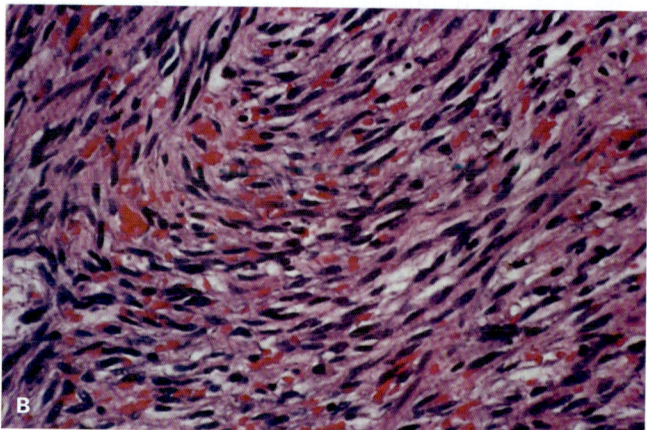

Figure 3-15. Kaposi's sarcoma of the rectum. A: Low-power view of a rectal biopsy specimen obtained with grasp forceps. The rectal mucosa is intact, although focally infiltrated by the Kaposi's sarcoma (*arrow*). However, the bulk of the lesion fills the submucosa. B: Higher-power magnification of the Kaposi's sarcoma showing the characteristic spindle cell proliferation and extravasated red blood cells.

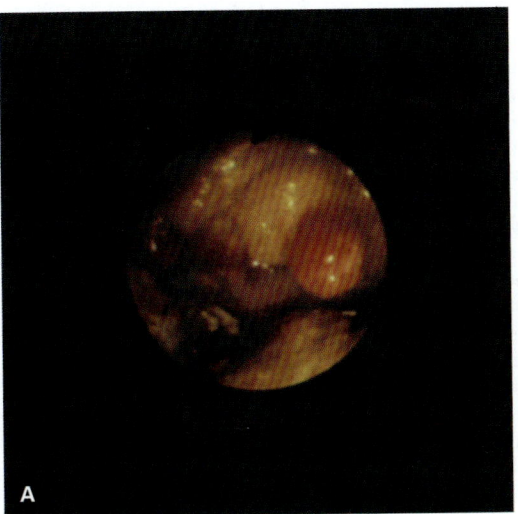
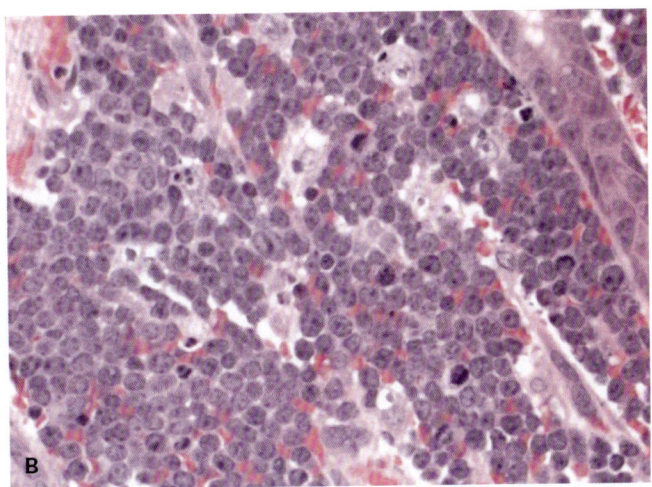

Figure 3-16. AIDS-associated non-Hodgkin's lymphoma of the rectum. **A:** Endoscopic appearance of tumorous nodules in the rectum. **B:** Detail of rectal mucosa showing diffuse infiltration of the lamina propria by a uniform population of large cell lymphoma.

course.[295,296] Hodgkin's lymphomas also occur but rather infrequently.[253] The majority of lymphomas in HIV are high-grade and about a third of patients present with acute complications. The long-term survival is poor with less than 10% 5-year survival.[297] The non-Hodgkin's lymphomas are commonly extranodal, and in one large series the GI tract was the most common extranodal site affected.[295] These lymphomas may occur anywhere in the GI tract,[298,299] and in one study were found to occur in the anorectal region in 25% of patients.[300] The lymphomas are usually high-grade B-cell lymphomas, either Burkitt's lymphoma or diffuse large-cell lymphoma, and EBV is an important cofactor.[301] The mode of presentation may be as an ulcer, a mass, a perforation, a hemorrhage, or, in the case of anorectal lymphomas, a fistula. Lymphomas of the GI tract are discussed in detail in Chapter 4.

WORKUP OF THE IMMUNODEFICIENT PATIENT

The major complication of the immunodeficiency diseases in the gut is infection, which will vary depending on the type of immunodeficiency. For example, patients with B-cell disorders are prone to gram-positive and gram-negative infections, while patients with T-cell disorders are prone to protozoal, viral, fungal, and mycobacterial infections. Patients with AIDS, by contrast, appear to be specifically prone to infections with *Candida*, CMV, herpes, *Cryptosporidium*, and *Mycobacterium avium*. Strongyloidiasis resulting from reactivation of a previous infection is an important complication in many patients who are taking steroids or who have undergone transplantation.

Thus, the full spectrum of infectious disease is seen in these immunodeficiency disorders. Consequently, knowledge of the likely infections that complicate a particular disorder would greatly aid in selecting the appropriate tests for the diagnosis of the infectious agent.

In recent years, new techniques have been developed to optimize the detection and isolation of pathogens in the GI tract. These include

1. Special concentration techniques for stool specimens for the isolation of specific pathogens, such as *Cryptosporidium*.
2. Direct swabbing of lesions seen at endoscopy.
3. Suction traps attached to endoscopes for the aspiration of selected lesions.
4. Carrier media.
5. Selective culture media.

The pathologist needs to be aware of these techniques and should work in close liaison with the endoscopist and the microbiologist in order to maximize the diagnostic yield from each specimen. For further details, see Chapter 1.

References

1. Rowlands BJ, Soong CV, Gardiner KR. The gastrointestinal tract as a barrier in sepsis. *Br Med Bull.* 1999;55(1):196–211.
2. Husby S. Normal immune responses to ingested foods. *J Pediatr Gastroenterol Nutr.* 2000;30(suppl):S13–S19.
3. Theodorou V, Fioramonti J, Bueno L. Integrative neuroimmunology of the digestive tract. *Vet Res.* 1996;27(4–5):427–442.
4. Ebrahim GJ. Immune system of the gut and the feeding of infants. *J Trop Pediatr.* 1999;45(5):256–257.
5. Simecka JW. Mucosal immunity of the gastrointestinal tract and oral tolerance. *Adv Drug Deliv Rev.* 1998;34(2–3):235–259.

6. Takahashi I, Kiyono H. Gut as the largest immunologic tissue. *J Parenter Enteral Nutr.* 1999;23(5 suppl):S7–S12.
7. Elwood CM, Garden OA. Gastrointestinal immunity in health and disease. *Vet Clin North Am Small Anim Pract.* 1999;29(2):471–500, vi–vii.
8. Mayer L. Mucosal immunity and gastrointestinal antigen processing. *J Pediatr Gastroenterol Nutr.* 2000;30(suppl):S4–S12.
9. Elson CO, Kagnoff MF, Fiocchi C, et al. Intestinal immunity and inflammation: recent progress. *Gastroenterology.* 1986;91(3):746–768.
10. Dobbins WO III. Gut immunophysiology: a gastroenterologist's view with emphasis on pathophysiology. *Am J Physiol.* 1982;242(1):G1–G8.
11. Benson EB, Strober W. Regulation of IgA secretion by T cell clones derived from the human gastrointestinal tract. *J Immunol.* 1988;140(6):1874–1882.
12. Ferguson A. Lymphocytes and cell mediated immunity in the small intestine. In: Weatherall DS, ed. *Advances in Medicine.* London, UK: Pitman Medical; 1978:14.
13. van Elburg RM, Uil JJ, de Monchy JG, Heymans HS. Intestinal permeability in pediatric gastroenterology. *Scand J Gastroenterol Suppl.* 1992;194:19–24.
14. Walker WA. Development of intestinal host defense mechanisms and the passive protective role of human milk. *Mead Johnson Symp Perinat Dev Med.* 1977(11):39–48.
15. Walker WA. Host defense mechanisms in the gastrointestinal tract. *Pediatrics.* 1976;57(6):901–916.
16. Kraft S. Intraepithelial lymphocytes revisited. In selected summaries. *Gastroenterology.* 1980;78:180–181.
17. Dukes C, Bussey HJR. The number of lymphoid follicles of the human large intestine. *J Pathol Bacteriol.* 1926;29:111–116.
18. Cornes J. Number, size and distribution of Peyer's patches in the human small intestine. Part 1. The development of Peyer's Patches. *Gut.* 1965;6:225–233.
19. Mowat A. Cellular basis of gastrointestinal immunity. In: Marsh MN, ed. *Immunopathology of the Small Intestine.* New York, NY: John Wiley; 1987.
20. Trejdosiewicz LK, Crabtree JE. Gastrointestinal intraepithelial lymphocytes in man: the saga continues. *Eur J Gastroenterol Hepatol.* 1995;7(6):537–540.
21. Trejdosiewicz LK. What is the role of human intestinal intraepithelial lymphocytes? *Clin Exp Immunol.* 1993;94(3):395–397.
22. Crowe PT, Marsh MN. Morphometric analysis of intestinal mucosa. VI—Principles in enumerating intra-epithelial lymphocytes. *Virchows Arch.* 1994;424(3):301–306.
23. Dobbins WO III. Human intestinal intraepithelial lymphocytes. *Gut.* 1986;27(8):972–985.
24. Isaacson PG. Gastric MALT lymphoma: from concept to cure. *Ann Oncol.* 1999;10(6):637–645.
25. Kunisawa J, Kiyono H. A marvel of mucosal T cells and secretory antibodies for the creation of first lines of defense. *Cell Mol Life Sci.* 2005;62(12):1308–1321.
26. Bonneville M, Janeway CA Jr, Ito K, et al. Intestinal intraepithelial lymphocytes are a distinct set of gamma delta T cells. *Nature.* 1988;336(6198):479–481.
27. Eade OE, Andre-Ukena SS, Moulton C, et al. Lymphocyte subpopulations of intestinal mucosa in inflammatory bowel disease. *Gut.* 1980;21(8):675–682.
28. Geboes K, De Wolf-Peeters C, Rutgeerts P, et al. Lymphocytes and Langerhans cells in the human oesophageal epithelium. *Virchows Arch A Pathol Anat Histopathol.* 1983;401(1):45–55.
29. Bull DM, Bookman MA. Isolation and functional characterization of human intestinal mucosal lymphoid cells. *J Clin Invest.* 1977;59(5):966–974.
30. Maluenda C, Phillips AD, Briddon A, Walker-Smith JA. Quantitative analysis of small intestinal mucosa in cow's milk-sensitive enteropathy. *J Pediatr Gastroenterol Nutr.* 1984;3(3):349–356.
31. Pascal RR, Gramlich TL, Parker KM, Gansler TS. Geographic variations in eosinophil concentration in normal colonic mucosa. *Mod Pathol.* 1997;10(4):363–365.
32. Barczyk M, Debek W, Chyczewski L. Mast cells in the gastrointestinal tract. *Rocz Akad Med Bialymst.* 1995;40(1):36–57.
33. Swieter M, Chan B, Lee T, et al. IgE receptors from rat intestinal mucosa and peritoneal mast cells subtype-specific differences. *Int Arch Allergy Appl Immunol.* 1988;88:200–202.
34. Rees PH, Hillier K, Church MK. The secretory characteristics of mast cells isolated from the human large intestinal mucosa and muscle. *Immunology.* 1988;65(3):437–442.
35. Stenton GR, Vliagoftis H, Befus AD. Role of intestinal mast cells in modulating gastrointestinal pathophysiology. *Ann Allergy Asthma Immunol.* 1998;81(1):1–11; quiz 2–5.
36. Sulik A, Kemona A, Sulik M, Oldak E. The gastrointestinal mast cell in health and disease. *Rocz Akad Med Bialymst.* 1999;44:17–23.
37. Strobel S, Miller HR, Ferguson A. Human intestinal mucosal mast cells: evaluation of fixation and staining techniques. *J Clin Pathol.* 1981;34(8):851–858.
38. Hudson NP, Pearson GT, Kitamura N, Mayhew IG. An immunohistochemical study of interstitial cells of Cajal (ICC) in the equine gastrointestinal tract. *Res Vet Sci.* 1999;66(3):265–271.
39. Li WV, Kapadia SB, Sonmez-Alpan E, Swerdlow SH. Immunohistochemical characterization of mast cell disease in paraffin sections using tryptase, CD68, myeloperoxidase, lysozyme, and CD20 antibodies. *Mod Pathol.* 1996;9(10):982–988.
40. Mahida YR. The key role of macrophages in the immunopathogenesis of inflammatory bowel disease. *Inflamm Bowel Dis.* 2000;6(1):21–33.
41. Rogler G, Hausmann M, Vogl D, et al. Isolation and phenotypic characterization of colonic macrophages. *Clin Exp Immunol.* 1998;112(2):205–215.
42. Lauffer JM, Modlin IM, Hinoue T, et al. Pituitary adenylate cyclase-activating polypeptide modulates gastric enterochromaffin-like cell proliferation in rats. *Gastroenterology.* 1999;116(3):623–635.
43. Hein WR. Organization of mucosal lymphoid tissue. *Curr Top Microbiol Immunol.* 1999;236:1–15.
44. Weiss L, Greep R. *Histology.* 4th ed. New York: NY: McGraw-Hill; 1977:663.
45. Keren D. Immunologic deficiency diseases and their effects on the gastrointestinal tract. In: Keren DF, ed. *Immunology and Immunopathology of the Gastrointestinal Tract.* Chicago, IL: American Society of Clinical Pathology; 1980:45–60.
46. Gebert A, Fassbender S, Werner K, Weissferdt A. The development of M cells in Peyer's patches is restricted to specialized dome-associated crypts. *Am J Pathol.* 1999;154(5):1573–1582.
47. Borghesi C, Taussig MJ, Nicoletti C. Rapid appearance of M cells after microbial challenge is restricted at the periphery of the follicle-associated epithelium of Peyer's patch. *Lab Invest.* 1999;79(11):1393–1401.
48. Niedergang F, Kraehenbuhl JP. Much ado about M cells. *Trends Cell Biol.* 2000;10(4):137–141.
49. Owen RL. Uptake and transport of intestinal macromolecules and microorganisms by M cells in Peyer's patches—a personal and historical perspective. *Semin Immunol.* 1999;11(3):157–163.

50. Owen RL. And now pathophysiology of M cells—good news and bad news from Peyer's patches. *Gastroenterology*. 1983;85(2):468-470.
51. Woodhead VE, Binks MH, Chain BM, Katz DR. From sentinel to messenger: an extended phenotypic analysis of the monocyte to dendritic cell transition. *Immunology*. 1998;94(4):552-559.
52. Iwasaki A, Kelsall BL. Mucosal immunity and inflammation. I. Mucosal dendritic cells: their specialized role in initiating T cell responses. *Am J Physiol*. 1999;276(5 pt 1):G1074-G1078.
53. Huang FP, Platt N, Wykes M, et al. A discrete subpopulation of dendritic cells transports apoptotic intestinal epithelial cells to T cell areas of mesenteric lymph nodes. *J Exp Med*. 2000;191(3):435-444.
54. Nagata H, Miyairi M, Sekizuka E, et al. In vivo visualization of lymphatic microvessels and lymphocyte migration through rat Peyer's patches. *Gastroenterology*. 1994;106(6):1548-1553.
55. Miura S, Tsuzuki Y, Fukumura D, et al. Intravital demonstration of sequential migration process of lymphocyte subpopulations in rat Peyer's patches. *Gastroenterology*. 1995;109(4):1113-1123.
56. Brandzaeg P, Baklein K. Immunoglobulin-producing cells in the intestine in health and disease. *Clin Gastroenterol*. 1976;5:251-269.
57. Corthesy B, Spertini F. Secretory immunoglobulin A: from mucosal protection to vaccine development. *Biol Chem*. 1999;380(11):1251-1262.
58. Spencer J, Finn T, Isaacson PG. Human Peyer's patches: an immunohistochemical study. *Gut*. 1986;27(4):405-410.
59. Bjerke K, Brandtzaeg P, Rognum TO. Distribution of immunoglobulin producing cells is different in normal human appendix and colon mucosa. *Gut*. 1986;27(6):667-674.
60. Kleinman RE, Harmatz PR, Walker WA. The liver: an integral part of the enteric mucosal immune system. *Hepatology*. 1982;2(3):379-384.
61. Mattioli CA, Tomasi TB Jr. The life span of IgA plasma cells from the mouse intestine. *J Exp Med*. 1973;138(2):452-460.
62. Hauptman SP, Tomasi TB Jr. Mechanism of immunoglobulin A polymerization. *J Biol Chem*. 1975;250(10):3891-3896.
63. Brown WR. Relationships between immunoglobulins and the intestinal epithelium. *Gastroenterology*. 1978;75(1):129-138.
64. Brown W. The gut and regulation of immune responses. *Viewpoints Digest Dis*. 1983;15:5-8.
65. Bienenstock J, Befus AD. Some thoughts on the biologic role of immunoglobulin A. *Gastroenterology*. 1983;84(1):178-185.
66. Ming JE, Stiehm ER, Graham JM Jr. Syndromes associated with immunodeficiency. *Adv Pediatr*. 1999;46:271-351.
67. Klein N, Jack D. Immunodeficiency and the gut: clues to the role of the immune system in gastrointestinal disease. *Ital J Gastroenterol Hepatol*. 1999;31(8):802-806.
68. Rosen FS, Cooper MD, Wedgwood RJ. The primary immunodeficiencies (1). *N Engl J Med*. 1984;311(4):235-242.
69. Rosen FS, Cooper MD, Wedgwood RJ. The primary immunodeficiencies. (2). *N Engl J Med*. 1984;311(5):300-310.
70. Thompson R. Immunological mechanisms. In: Asquith P, ed. *Immunology of the Gastrointestinal Tract*. New York, NY: Churchill Livingstone; 1979:14-22.
71. Bull DM, Tomasi TB. Deficiency of immunoglobulin A in intestinal disease. *Gastroenterology*. 1968;54(2):313-320.
72. Zeitz M, Ullrich R, Schneider T, et al. Mucosal immunodeficiency in HIV/SIV infection. *Pathobiology*. 1998;66(3-4):151-157.
73. Zvizdic S, Beslagic E, Kapic E, Zvizdic-Karahodzic M. Cytomegalovirus disease in immunocompromised patients. *Med Arh*. 2000;54(1):9-11.
74. Lai Ping So A, Mayer L. Gastrointestinal manifestations of primary immunodeficiency disorders. *Semin Gastrointest Dis*. 1997;8(1):22-32.
75. Ament ME. Immunodeficiency syndromes and gastrointestinal disease. *Pediatr Clin North Am*. 1975;22(4):807-825.
76. Ross I. Primary immunodeficiency and the small intestine. In: Marsh MN, ed. *Immunopathology of the Small Intestine*. New York, NY: John Wiley; 1987:283-332.
77. Wilcox CM, Schwartz DA. Endoscopic-pathologic correlates of *Candida* esophagitis in acquired immunodeficiency syndrome. *Dig Dis Sci*. 1996;41(7):1337-1345.
78. Kimura K. Gastritis and gastric cancer. Asia. *Gastroenterol Clin North Am*. 2000;29(3):609-621.
79. Ament ME, Ochs HD. Gastrointestinal manifestations of chronic granulomatous disease. *N Engl J Med*. 1973;288(8):382-387.
80. Lasser KH, Lewin KJ, Ryning FW. Cryptosporidial enteritis in a patient with congenital hypogammaglobulinemia. *Hum Pathol*. 1979;10(2):234-240.
81. Matthew M, Gottlieb J, Lewin K, Weinstein W. Gastrointestinal lesions in homosexual men with acquired cellular immunodeficiency. *Gastroenterology*. 1982;82:1126.
82. Foucar E, Mukai K, Foucar K, et al. Colon ulceration in lethal cytomegalovirus infection. *Am J Clin Pathol*. 1981;76(6):788-801.
83. Owen RL, Nemanic PC, Stevens DP. Ultrastructural observations on giardiasis in a murine model. I. Intestinal distribution, attachment, and relationship to the immune system of *Giardia muris*. *Gastroenterology*. 1979;76(4):757-769.
84. Brandborg LL, Tankersley CB, Gottieb S, et al. Histological demonstration of mucosal invasion by *Giardia lamblia* in man. *Gastroenterology*. 1967;52(2):143-150.
85. Current W, Reese N, Ernst J, et al. Human cryptosporidiosis in immunocompetent and immunodeficient persons: studies of an outbreak and experimental transmission. *N Engl J Med*. 1983;308:1253-1257.
86. McCarthy DM, Katz SI, Gazze L, et al. Selective IgA deficiency associated with total villous atrophy of the small intestine and an organ-specific anti-epithelial cell antibody. *J Immunol*. 1978;120(3):932-938.
87. Penn I. Occurrence of cancer in immune deficiencies. *Cancer*. 1974;34(3 suppl):858-866.
88. Biemer JJ. Malignant lymphomas associated with immunodeficiency states. *Ann Clin Lab Sci*. 1990;20(3):175-191.
89. Molle ZL, Moallem H, Desai N, et al. Endoscopic features of smooth muscle tumors in children with AIDS. *Gastrointest Endosc*. 2000;52(1):91-94.
90. Jones AM, Gaspar HB. Immunogenetics: changing the face of immunodeficiency. *J Clin Pathol*. 2000;53(1):60-65.
91. Petro JB, Rahman SM, Ballard DW, Khan WN. Bruton's tyrosine kinase is required for activation of IkappaB kinase and nuclear factor kappaB in response to B cell receptor engagement. *J Exp Med*. 2000;191(10):1745-1754.
92. Washington K, Stenzel TT, Buckley RH, Gottfried MR. Gastrointestinal pathology in patients with common variable immunodeficiency and X-linked agammaglobulinemia. *Am J Surg Pathol*. 1996;20(10):1240-1252.
93. Ross IN. Primary immune deficiency. In: Asquith P, ed. *Immunology of the Gastrointestinal Tract*. Vol. 9. New York, NY: Churchill Livingstone; 1979:152-182.
94. Groth C, Drager R, Warnatz K, et al. Impaired up-regulation of CD70 and CD86 in naive (CD27-) B cells from patients with common variable immunodeficiency (CVID). *Clin Exp Immunol*. 2002;129(1):133-139.
95. Prince HE, Norman GL, Binder WL. Immunoglobulin A (IgA) deficiency and alternative celiac disease-associated antibodies in sera submitted to a reference laboratory

for endomysial IgA testing. *Clin Diagn Lab Immunol.* 2000;7(2):192–196.
96. Denz A, Eibel H, Illges H, et al. Impaired up-regulation of CD86 in B cells of "type A" common variable immunodeficiency patients. *Eur J Immunol.* 2000;30(4):1069–1077.
97. Heneghan MA, Stevens FM, Cryan EM, et al. Celiac sprue and immunodeficiency states: a 25-year review. *J Clin Gastroenterol.* 1997;25(2):421–425.
98. Cunningham-Rundles C. Clinical and immunologic analyses of 103 patients with common variable immunodeficiency. *J Clin Immunol.* 1989;9(1):22–33.
99. Ament ME, Rubin CE. Relation of giardiasis to abnormal intestinal structure and function in gastrointestinal immunodeficiency syndromes. *Gastroenterology.* 1972;62(2):216–226.
100. Ahnen DJ, Brown WR. Campylobacter enteritis in immune-deficient patients. *Ann Intern Med.* 1982;96(2):187–188.
101. Strauss RG, Ghishan F, Mitros F, et al. Rectosigmoidal colitis in common variable immunodeficiency disease. *Dig Dis Sci.* 1980;25(10):798–801.
102. WHO. Primary immunodeficiency diseases. Report of a WHO Scientific Group. *Clin Exp Immunol.* 1995;99(suppl 1):1–24.
103. Sanchez-Pobre P, Casis B, Lopez Carreira M, et al. Systemic amyloidosis associated with common variable hypogammaglobulinemia and intestinal lymphoid nodular hyperplasia. *Gastroenterol Hepatol.* 1996;19(7):351–355.
104. Zullo A, Romiti A, Rinaldi V, et al. Gastric pathology in patients with common variable immunodeficiency. *Gut.* 1999;45(1):77–81.
105. Gottesman SR, Haas D, Ladanyi M, Amorosi EL. Peripheral T cell lymphoma in a patient with common variable immunodeficiency disease: case report and literature review. *Leuk Lymphoma.* 1999;32(5–6):589–595.
106. Cornelis B, Lamers M, Wagener T, et al. Jejunal lymphoma in a patient with primary adult-onset hypogammaglobulinemia and nodular lymphoid hyperplasia of the small intestine. *Digest Dis Sci.* 1980;25:553–557.
107. Hughes WS, Brooks FP, Conn HO. Serum gastrin levels in primary hypogammaglobulinemia and pernicious anemia. Studies in adults. *Ann Intern Med.* 1972;77(5):746–750.
108. James D, Asherson G, Chanarin I, et al. Cell-mediated immunity to intrinsic factor in autoimmune disorders. *Br Med J.* 1974;4(5943):494–496.
109. Eidelman S. Intestinal lesions in immune deficiency. *Hum Pathol.* 1976;7(4):427–434.
110. Binder HJ, Reynolds RD. Control of diarrhea in secondary hypogammaglobulinemia by fresh plasma infusions. *N Engl J Med.* 1967;277(15):802–803.
111. Hughes WS, Cerda JJ, Holtzapple P, Brooks FP. Primary hypogammaglobulinemia and malabsorption. *Ann Intern Med.* 1971;74(6):903–910.
112. Editorial: temporary gluten intolerance. *Lancet.* 1976;2:555.
113. Bili H, Nizou C, Nizou JY, et al. Common variable immunodeficiency and total villous atrophy regressive after gluten-free diet. *Rev Med Interne.* 1997;18(9):724–726.
114. Rebrov VG, Miskin LI, Zhuravlev AP. Nodular lymphoid hyperplasia of the small intestine in chronic enteritis and immunodeficiency. *Klin Med (Mosk).* 1990;68(3):120–125.
115. Brotzu C, Bosu C, Pisano G, Pomata M. A case of nodular lymphoid hyperplasia of the small bowel in a patient with intestinal obstruction. *G Chir.* 1997;18(6–7):355–358.
116. Gryboski JD, Self TW, Clemett A, Herskovic T. Selective immunoglobulin A deficiency and intestinal nodular lymphoid hyperplasia: correction of diarrhea with antibiotics and plasma. *Pediatrics.* 1968;42(5):833–837.
117. Persic M, Lenac T, Rubinic M, et al. Nodular lymphoid hyperplasia of the colon and terminal ileum. Case report. *Lijec Vjesn.* 1998;120(3–4):62–64.
118. Ranchod M, Lewin KJ, Dorfman RF. Lymphoid hyperplasia of the gastrointestinal tract. A study of 26 cases and review of the literature. *Am J Surg Pathol.* 1978;2(4):383–400.
119. Penny R. Nodular lymphoid hyperplasia of the small intestine and hypogammaglobulinemia. *Gastroenterology.* 1969;56(5):982–985.
120. Waldmann T, Stober W, Glaese R. Immunodeficiency diseases and malignancy. Various immunologic deficiencies of man and the role of immune processes in the control of malignant disease. *Ann Intern Med.* 1972;77:605–628.
121. Van den Brande P, Geboes K, Vantrappen G, et al. Intestinal nodular lymphoid hyperplasia in patients with common variable immunodeficiency: local accumulation of B and CD8(+) lymphocytes. *J Clin Immunol.* 1988;8(4):296–306.
122. Hermaszewski RA, Webster AD. Primary hypogammaglobulinaemia: a survey of clinical manifestations and complications. *Q J Med.* 1993;86(1):31–42.
123. Mike N, Hansel TT, Newman J, Asquith P. Granulomatous enteropathy in common variable immunodeficiency: a cause of chronic diarrhoea. *Postgrad Med J.* 1991;67(787):446–449.
124. Hermans PE, Diaz-Bubo JA, Stobo JD. Idiopathic late-onset immunoglobulin deficiency. Clinical observations in 50 patients. *Am J Med.* 1976;61(2):221–237.
125. Javier FC III, Moore CM, Sorensen RU. Distribution of primary immunodeficiency diseases diagnosed in a pediatric tertiary hospital. *Ann Allergy Asthma Immunol.* 2000;84(1):25–30.
126. Bachmann R. Studies on the serum gamma-A-globulin level. 3. The frequency of A-gamma-A-globulinemia. *Scand J Clin Lab Invest.* 1965;17(4):316–320.
127. Hammarstrom L, Vorechovsky I, Webster D. Selective IgA deficiency (SIgAD) and common variable immunodeficiency (CVID). *Clin Exp Immunol.* 2000;120(2):225–231.
128. Schroeder HW Jr. Genetics of IgA deficiency and common variable immunodeficiency. *Clin Rev Allergy Immunol.* 2000;19(2):127–140.
129. Cunningham-Rundles C. Selective IgA deficiency. *J Pediatr Gastroenterol Nutr.* 1988;7(4):482–484.
130. Gleeson M, Clancy RL, Cripps AW, et al. Acquired IgA deficiency. *Pediatr Allergy Immunol.* 1994;5(3):157–161.
131. Koistinen J. Familial clustering of selective IgA deficiency. *Vox Sang.* 1976;30(3):181–190.
132. Ochs H, Wedgwood R. Disorder of the B-cell system. In: Steihm ER, Fulginiti VA, eds. *Immunological Disorders in Infants and Children.* Philadelphia, PA: WB Saunders; 1980:239–259.
133. Buckley RH, Fiscus SA. Serum IgD and IgE concentrations in immunodeficiency diseases. *J Clin Invest.* 1975;55(1):157–165.
134. Zenone T, Souillet G. Cancer and primary humoral immunodeficiency. *Bull Cancer.* 1997;84(8):813–821.
135. Ott MM, Ott G, Klinker H, et al. Abdominal T-cell non-Hodgkin's lymphoma of the gamma/delta type in a patient with selective immunoglobulin A deficiency. *Am J Surg Pathol.* 1998;22(4):500–506.
136. Niwa Y, Kanoh T. Immune deficiency states and immune imbalance in systemic lupus erythematosus and other autoimmune diseases. *Clin Immunol Immunopathol.* 1979;12(3):289–300.
137. Falchuk KR, Falchuk ZM. Selective immunoglobulin a deficiency, ulcerative colitis, and gluten-sensitive enteropathy—a unique association. *Gastroenterology.* 1975;69(2):503–506.
138. Hoskins L, Winawer S, Broitman S, et al. Clinical giardiasis and intestinal malabsorption. *Gastroenterology.* 1967;28:81–83.
139. Lock RJ, Unsworth DJ. Identifying immunoglobulin-A–deficient children and adults does not necessarily help the

serologic diagnosis of coeliac disease. *J Pediatr Gastroenterol Nutr.* 1999;28(1):81–83.
140. Chandra RK. Nutrition and the immune system: an introduction. *Am J Clin Nutr.* 1997;66(2):460S–463S.
141. Strober W, Krakauer R, Klaeveman HL, et al. Secretory component deficiency. A disorder of the IgA immune system. *N Engl J Med.* 1976;294(7):351–356.
142. Nomura K, Kanegane H, Karasuyama H, et al. Genetic defect in human X-linked agammaglobulinemia impedes a maturational evolution of pro-B cells into a later stage of pre-B cells in the B-cell differentiation pathway. *Blood.* 2000;96(2):610–617.
143. Kirkpatrick CH. Cancer and immunodeficiency diseases. *Birth Defects Orig Artic Ser.* 1976;12(1):61–78.
144. Mohamed AJ, Nore BF, Christensson B, Smith CI. Signalling of Bruton's tyrosine kinase, Btk. *Scand J Immunol.* 1999;49(2):113–118.
145. Holinski-Feder E, Weiss M, Brandau O, et al. Mutation screening of the BTK gene in 56 families with X-linked agammaglobulinemia (XLA): 47 unique mutations without correlation to clinical course. *Pediatrics.* 1998;101(2):276–284.
146. Ochs HD, Ament ME, Davis SD. Giardiasis with malabsorption in X-linked agammaglobulinemia. *N Engl J Med.* 1972;287(7):341–342.
147. Melamed I, Bujanover Y, Igra YS, et al. Campylobacter enteritis in normal and immunodeficient children. *Am J Dis Child.* 1983;137(8):752–753.
148. Abramowsky CR, Sorensen RU. Regional enteritis-like enteropathy in a patient with agammaglobulinemia: histologic and immunocytologic studies. *Hum Pathol.* 1988;19(4):483–486.
149. Cellier C, Foray S, Hermine O. Regional enteritis associated with enterovirus in a patient with X-linked agammaglobulinemia. *N Engl J Med.* 2000;342(21):1611–1612.
150. Borisova AM, Setdikova N, Kaliazina VA, et al. Common variable immunodeficiency in adults and problems of its immunotherapy. *Ter Arkh.* 1998;70(5):14–20.
151. Bachmeyer C, Monge M, Cazier A, et al. Gastric adenocarcinoma in a patient with X-linked agammaglobulinaemia. *Eur J Gastroenterol Hepatol.* 2000;12(9):1033–1035.
152. Ferguson A, Arranz E, O'Mahony S. Spectrum of expression of intestinal cellular immunity: proposal for a change in diagnostic criteria of celiac disease. *Ann Allergy.* 1993;71(1):29–32.
153. Ross IN, Thompson RA. Severe selective IgM deficiency. *J Clin Pathol.* 1976;29(9):773–777.
154. Zegers BJ, Maertzdorf WJ, Van Loghem E, et al. Kappa-chain deficiency. An immunoglobulin disorder. *N Engl J Med.* 1976;294(19):1026–1030.
155. Puck JM, Nussbaum RL, Smead DL, Conley ME. X-linked severe combined immunodeficiency: localization within the region Xq13.1-q21.1 by linkage and deletion analysis. *Am J Hum Genet.* 1989;44(5):724–730.
156. de Moesdijk D, Weel-Sipman M. An infant with severe combined immunodeficiency syndrome, an alpha-thalassemia trait and renal Fanconi syndrome. *Bone Marrow Transplant.* 2000;26:97–99.
157. Vihinen M, Villa A, Mella P, et al. Molecular modeling of the Jak3 kinase domains and structural basis for severe combined immunodeficiency. *Clin Immunol.* 2000;96(2):108–118.
158. Puel A, Leonard WJ. Mutations in the gene for the IL-7 receptor result in T(-)B(+)NK(+) severe combined immunodeficiency disease. *Curr Opin Immunol.* 2000;12(4):468–473.
159. Cavazzana-Calvo M, Lagresle C, Hacein-Bey-Abina S, Fischer A. Gene therapy for severe combined immunodeficiency. *Annu Rev Med.* 2005;56:585–602.
160. Buckley RH. Advances in the understanding and treatment of human severe combined immunodeficiency. *Immunol Res.* 2000;22(2–3):237–251.
161. Lambrecht W, Kluth D. Hereditary multiple atresias of the gastrointestinal tract: report of a case and review of the literature. *J Pediatr Surg.* 1998;33(5):794–797.
162. Rothenberg ME, White FV, Chilmonczyk B, Chatila T. A syndrome involving immunodeficiency and multiple intestinal atresias. *Immunodeficiency.* 1995;5(3):171–178.
163. Tang ML, Williams LW. Pneumatosis intestinale in children with primary combined immunodeficiency. *J Pediatr.* 1998;132(3 pt 1):546–549.
164. Boeck A, Buckley RH, Schiff RI. Gastroesophageal reflux and severe combined immunodeficiency. *J Allergy Clin Immunol.* 1997;99(3):420–424.
165. Horowitz S, Lorenzsonn VW, Olsen WA, et al. Small intestinal disease in T cell deficiency. *J Pediatr.* 1974;85(4):457–462.
166. Bennett CL, Christie J, Ramsdell F, et al. The immune dysregulation, polyendocrinopathy, enteropathy, X-linked syndrome (IPEX) is caused by mutations of FOXP3. *Nat Genet.* 2001;27(1):20–21.
167. Patey-Mariaud de Serre N, Canioni D, Ganousse S, et al. Digestive histopathological presentation of IPEX syndrome. *Mod Pathol.* 2009;22(1):95–102.
168. Caudy AA, Reddy ST, Chatila T, et al. CD25 deficiency causes an immune dysregulation, polyendocrinopathy, enteropathy, X-linked-like syndrome, and defective IL-10 expression from CD4 lymphocytes. *J Allergy Clin Immunol.* 2007;119(2):482–487.
169. Roifman CM. Human IL-2 receptor alpha chain deficiency. *Pediatr Res.* 2000;48(1):6–11.
170. Baud O, Goulet O, Canioni D, et al. Treatment of the immune dysregulation, polyendocrinopathy, enteropathy, X-linked syndrome (IPEX) by allogeneic bone marrow transplantation. *N Engl J Med.* 2001;344(23):1758–1762.
171. Rao A, Kamani N, Filipovich A, et al. Successful bone marrow transplantation for IPEX syndrome after reduced-intensity conditioning. *Blood.* 2007;109(1):383–385.
172. Kirkpatrick CH. Chronic mucocutaneous candidiasis. *J Am Acad Dermatol.* 1994;31(3 pt 2):S14–S17.
173. Vazquez JA. Options for the management of mucosal candidiasis in patients with AIDS and HIV infection. *Pharmacotherapy.* 1999;19(1):76–87.
174. Kirkpatrick CH, Smith TK. Chronic mucocutaneous candidiasis: immunologic and antibiotic therapy. *Ann Intern Med.* 1974;80(3):310–320.
175. Polizzi B, Origgi L, Zuccaro G, et al. Case report: successful treatment with cimetidine and zinc sulphate in chronic mucocutaneous candidiasis. *Am J Med Sci.* 1996;311(4):189–190.
176. Hoh MC, Lin HP, Chan LL, Lam SK. Successful allogeneic bone marrow transplantation in severe chronic mucocutaneous candidiasis syndrome. *Bone Marrow Transplant.* 1996;18(4):797–800.
177. Wilcox CM. Esophageal strictures complicating ulcerative esophagitis in patients with AIDS. *Am J Gastroenterol.* 1999;94(2):339–343.
178. DiGeorge A. Congenital absence of the thymus and its immunologic consequences: concurrence with congenital hypoparathyroidism. In: Good RA, Bergsma D, eds. *Immunologic Deficiency Diseases in Man Birth Defects: Original Article Series.* Vol. 4. New York, NY: New York National Foundation Press; 1968:116–121.
179. Yamanaka S, Tanaka Y, Kawataki M, et al. Chromosome 22q11 deletion complicated by dissecting pulmonary arterial aneurysm and jejunal atresia in an infant. *Arch Pathol Lab Med.* 2000;124(6):880–882.

180. Agger WA, Glasser JE, Abellera RM. Fatal necrotizing enterocolitis in a neonate with DiGeorge syndrome. *Wis Med J.* 1984;83(9):16–18.
181. Maeda J, Yamagishi H, Matsuoka R, et al. Frequent association of 22q11.2 deletion with tetralogy of Fallot. *Am J Med Genet.* 2000;92(4):269–272.
182. Pierdominici M, Marziali M, Giovannetti A, et al. T cell receptor repertoire and function in patients with DiGeorge syndrome and velocardiofacial syndrome. *Clin Exp Immunol.* 2000;121(1):127–132.
183. Pahwa R, Pahwa S, O'Reilly R. Treatment of the immunodeficiiency diseases: progress towards replacement therapy emphasizing cellular macrommolecular enging. *Springer Semin Immunopath (Berlin).* 1978;1:355–404.
184. Yamada M, Ariga T, Kawamura N, et al. Determination of carrier status for the Wiskott-Aldrich syndrome by flow cytometric analysis of Wiskott-Aldrich syndrome protein expression in peripheral blood mononuclear cells. *J Immunol.* 2000;165(2):1119–1122.
185. Lau YL, Jones BM, Low LC, et al. Defective B-cell and regulatory T-cell function in Wiskott-Aldrich syndrome. *Eur J Pediatr.* 1992;151(9):680–683.
186. Haerer AF, Jackson JF, Evers CG. Ataxia-telangiectasia with gastric adenocarcinoma. *JAMA.* 1969;210(10):1884–1887.
187. Murphy RC, Berdon WE, Ruzal-Shapiro C, et al. Malignancies in pediatric patients with ataxia telangiectasia. *Pediatr Radiol.* 1999;29(4):225–230.
188. Barton LL, Moussa SL, Villar RG, Hulett RL. Gastrointestinal complications of chronic granulomatous disease: case report and literature review. *Clin Pediatr (Phila).* 1998;37(4):231–236.
189. Goebel WS, Dinauer MC. Gene therapy for chronic granulomatous disease. *Acta Haematol.* 2003;110(2–3):86–92.
190. Levine S, Smith VV, Malone M, Sebire NJ. Histopathological features of chronic granulomatous disease (CGD) in childhood. *Histopathology.* 2005;47(5):508–516.
191. Foster CB, Lehrnbecher T, Mol F, et al. Host defense molecule polymorphisms influence the risk for immune-mediated complications in chronic granulomatous disease. *J Clin Invest.* 1998;102(12):2146–2155.
192. Segal AW. The molecular and cellular pathology of chronic granulomatous disease. *Eur J Clin Invest.* 1988;18(5):433–443.
193. Barbouche M, Sighiri R, Mellouli F, et al. Chronic septic granulomatous diease. 14 cases. *Presse Med.* 1999;28:2034–2036.
194. Eckert JW, Abramson SL, Starke J, Brandt ML. The surgical implications of chronic granulomatous disease. *Am J Surg.* 1995;169(3):320–323.
195. Werlin SL, Chusid MJ, Caya J, Oechler HW. Colitis in chronic granulomatous disease. *Gastroenterology.* 1982;82(2):328–331.
196. Jensen RT. Gastrointestinal abnormalities and involvement in systemic mastocytosis. *Hematol Oncol Clin North Am.* 2000;14(3):579–623.
197. Horan RF, Austen KF. Systemic mastocytosis: retrospective review of a decade's clinical experience at the Brigham and Women's Hospital. *J Invest Dermatol.* 1991;96(3 suppl):5S–13S; discussion 13S–14S, 60S–65S.
198. Woodruff J, Woodruff J. The effect of viral infections on the functions of the immune system. In: Notkins AL, ed. *Viral Immunology and Immunopathology.* New York, NY: Academic Press; 1975:393–418.
199. Cloyd MW, Chen JJ, Wang I. How does HIV cause AIDS? The homing theory. *Mol Med Today.* 2000;6(3):108–111.
200. Twomey JJ, Laughter AH, Farrow S, Douglass CC. Hodgkin's disease. An immunodepleting and immunosuppressive disorder. *J Clin Invest.* 1975;56(2):467–475.
201. Alvarez H. Nutrition in AIDS. *Nutr Hosp.* 1999;14 (suppl 2):53S–61S.
202. Chandra R, Puri S, Vyas D. Malnutrition and intestinal immunity. In: Marsh MN, ed. *Immunopathology of the Small Intestine.* New York, NY: Wiley; 1987:105–119.
203. Strober W, Wochner RD, Carbone PP, Waldmann TA. Intestinal lymphangiectasia: a protein-losing enteropathy with hypogammaglobulinemia, lymphocytopenia and impaired homograft rejection. *J Clin Invest.* 1967;46(10):1643–1656.
204. Pernet P, Vittecoq D, Kodjo A, et al. Intestinal absorption and permeability in human immunodeficiency virus-infected patients. *Scand J Gastroenterol.* 1999;34(1):29–34.
205. Genta RM, Miles P, Fields K. Opportunistic *Strongyloides stercoralis* infection in lymphoma patients. Report of a case and review of the literature. *Cancer.* 1989;63(7):1407–1411.
206. Storb R, Thomas ED, Buckner CD, et al. Marrow transplantation in thirty "untransfused" patients with severe aplastic anemia. *Ann Intern Med.* 1980;92(1):30–36.
207. Porta F, Friedrich W. Bone marrow transplantation in congenital immunodeficiency diseases. *Bone Marrow Transplant.* 1998;21(suppl 2):S21–S23.
208. Williams M. Gastrointestinal manifestations of graft-versus-host disease: diagnosis and management. *AACN Clin Issues.* 1999;10(4):500–506.
209. McDonald GB, Shulman HM, Sullivan KM, Spencer GD. Intestinal and hepatic complications of human bone marrow transplantation. Part I. *Gastroenterology.* 1986;90(2):460–477.
210. Spencer GD, Shulman HM, Myerson D, et al. Diffuse intestinal ulceration after marrow transplantation: a clinicopathologic study of 13 patients. *Hum Pathol.* 1986;17(6):621–633.
211. Proujansky R. Fixing the intestinal mucosa in the bone marrow transplant patient: lessons from other intestinal immunodeficiencies and inflammatory disorders. *Pediatr Transplant.* 1999;3(suppl 1):9–13.
212. Hiscott A, McLellan DS. Graft-versus-host disease in allogeneic bone marrow transplantation: the role of monoclonal antibodies in prevention and treatment. *Br J Biomed Sci.* 2000;57(2):163–169.
213. Ferrara JL, Levy R, Chao NJ. Pathophysiologic mechanisms of acute graft-vs.-host disease. *Biol Blood Marrow Transplant.* 1999;5(6):347–356.
214. Manivel C, Filipovich A, Snover DC. Cryptosporidiosis as a cause of diarrhea following bone marrow transplantation. *Dis Colon Rectum.* 1985;28(10):741–742.
215. Beuzen F, Dubois S, Flejou JF. Chromosomal numerical aberrations are frequent in oesophageal and gastric adenocarcinomas: a study using in-situ hybridization. *Histopathology.* 2000;37(3):241–249.
216. Shulman HM, Kleiner D, Lee SJ, et al. Histopathologic diagnosis of chronic graft-versus-host disease: National Institutes of Health Consensus Development Project on Criteria for Clinical Trials in Chronic Graft-versus-Host Disease: II. Pathology Working Group Report. *Biol Blood Marrow Transplant.* 2006;12(1):31–47.
217. Kraus MD, Shahsafaei A, Antin J, Odze RD. Relationship of Bcl-2 expression with apoptosis and proliferation in colonic graft versus host disease. *Hum Pathol.* 1998;29(8):869–875.
218. Chirletti P, Caronna R, Arcese W, et al. Gastrointestinal emergencies in patients with acute intestinal graft-versus-host disease. *Leuk Lymphoma.* 1998;29(1–2):129–137.
219. Wu D, Hockenberry DM, Brentnall TA, et al. Persistent nausea and anorexia after marrow transplantation: a prospective study of 78 patients. *Transplantation.* 1998;66(10):1319–1324.
220. Asplund S, Gramlich TL. Chronic mucosal changes of the colon in graft-versus-host disease. *Mod Pathol.* 1998;11(6):513–515.
221. Sviland L, Pearson AD, Eastham EJ, et al. Histological features of skin and rectal biopsy specimens after autologous

and allogeneic bone marrow transplantation. *J Clin Pathol.* 1988;41(2):148–154.
222. Kingreen D, Nitsche A, Beyer J, Siegert W. Herpes simplex infection of the jejunum occurring in the early post-transplantation period. *Bone Marrow Transplant.* 1997;20: 89–991.
223. Snover DC, Weisdorf SA, Vercellotti GM, et al. A histopathologic study of gastric and small intestinal graft-versus-host disease following allogeneic bone marrow transplantation. *Hum Pathol.* 1985;16(4):387–392.
224. Thompson B, Salzman D, Steinhauer J, et al. Prospective endoscopic evaluation for gastrointestinal graft-versus-host disease: determination of the best diagnostic approach. *Bone Marrow Transplant.* 2006;38(5):371–376.
225. Washington K, Bentley RC, Green A, et al. Gastric graft-versus-host disease: a blinded histologic study. *Am J Surg Pathol.* 1997;21(9):1037–1046.
226. Epstein RJ, McDonald GB, Sale GE, et al. The diagnostic accuracy of the rectal biopsy in acute graft-versus-host disease: a prospective study of thirteen patients. *Gastroenterology.* 1980;78(4):764–771.
227. Valdez R, Giordano T, Greenson J. Endocrine cell (EC) hyperplasia of the stomach in graft-versus-host disease (GVHD). *Mod Pathol.* 2000;13:90A.
228. Xin W, Greenson JK. The clinical significance of focally enhanced gastritis. *Am J Surg Pathol.* 2004;28(10):1347–1351.
229. Lerner KG, Kao GF, Storb R, et al. Histopathology of graft-vs.-host reaction (GvHR) in human recipients of marrow from HL-A-matched sibling donors. *Transplant Proc.* 1974;6(4):367–371.
230. Selbst MK, Ahrens WA, Robert ME, et al. Spectrum of histologic changes in colonic biopsies in patients treated with mycophenolate mofetil. *Mod Pathol.* 2009;22(6):737–743.
231. Strater J, Koretz K, Gunthert AR, Moller P. In situ detection of enterocytic apoptosis in normal colonic mucosa and in familial adenomatous polyposis. *Gut.* 1995;37(6):819–825.
232. Driman DK, Preiksaitis HG. Colorectal inflammation and increased cell proliferation associated with oral sodium phosphate bowel preparation solution. *Hum Pathol.* 1998;29(9):972–978.
233. Liu LU, Holt PR, Krivosheyev V, Moss SF. Human right and left colon differ in epithelial cell apoptosis and in expression of Bak, a pro-apoptotic Bcl-2 homologue. *Gut.* 1999;45(1):45–50.
234. Anti M, Armuzzi A, Morini S, et al. Severe imbalance of cell proliferation and apoptosis in the left colon and in the rectosigmoid tract in subjects with a history of large adenomas. *Gut.* 2001;48(2):238–246.
235. Phatak UP, Seo-Mayer P, Jain D, et al. Mycophenolate Mofetil-induced colitis in children. *J Clin Gastroenterol.* 2009;43(10):907–969.
236. Welch DC, Wirth PS, Goldenring JR, et al. Gastric graft-versus-host disease revisited: does proton pump inhibitor therapy affect endoscopic gastric biopsy interpretation? *Am J Surg Pathol.* 2006;30(4):444–449.
237. Kusne S, Schwartz M, Breinig MK, et al. Herpes simplex virus hepatitis after solid organ transplantation in adults. *J Infect Dis.* 1991;163(5):1001–1007.
238. Shulman HM, Sullivan KM, Weiden PL, et al. Chronic graft-versus-host syndrome in man. A long-term clinicopathologic study of 20 Seattle patients. *Am J Med.* 1980;69(2):204–217.
239. Goulet O. Intestinal transplantation. *Curr Opin Clin Nutr Metab Care.* 1999;2(4):315–321.
240. Vennarecci G, Kato T, Misiakos EP, et al. Intestinal transplantation for short gut syndrome attributable to necrotizing enterocolitis. *Pediatrics.* 2000;105(2):E25.
241. Sigurdsson L, Reyes J, Kocoshis SA, et al. Intestinal transplantation in children with chronic intestinal pseudo-obstruction. *Gut.* 1999;45(4):570–574.
242. Grant D. Intestinal transplantation: current status. *Transplantation.* 1989;2:2868–2871.
243. Atkison P, Chatzipetrou M, Tsaroucha A, et al. Small bowel transplantation in children. *Pediatr Transplant.* 1997;1:111–118.
244. Sigurdsson L, Reyes J, Putnam PE, et al. Endoscopies in pediatric small intestinal transplant recipients: five years experience. *Am J Gastroenterol.* 1998;93(2):207–211.
245. Teitelbaum DH, Wise WE, Sonnino RE, et al. Monitoring of intestinal transplant rejection. *Am J Surg.* 1989;157(3):318–322.
246. Ruiz P, Bagni A, Brown R, et al. Histological criteria for the identification of acute cellular rejection in human small bowel allografts: results of the pathology workshop at the VIII International Small Bowel Transplant Symposium. *Transplant Proc.* 2004;36(2):335–337.
247. Sakamoto M, Adachi T, Sagara H, Yoshikawa K. Gastrointestinal diseases associated with HIV infection. *Kansenshogaku Zasshi.* 2000;74(1):57–63.
248. Schneider T, Ullrich R, Zeitz M. The immunologic aspects of human immunodeficiency virus infection in the gastrointestinal tract. *Semin Gastrointest Dis.* 1996;7(1):19–29.
249. Schwartlander B, Garnett G, Walker N, Anderson R. AIDS in a new millennium. *Science.* 2000;289(5476):64–66.
250. Chui DW, Owen RL. AIDS and the gut. *J Gastroenterol Hepatol.* 1994;9(3):291–303.
251. WHO. World Health Organization. Acquired immunodeficiency syndrome (AIDS). WHO/CDC case definition for AIDS. *Wkly Epidemiol Rec (Geneva).* 1986;61:69–73.
252. Fauci AS. The human immunodeficiency virus: infectivity and mechanisms of pathogenesis. *Science.* 1988;239(4840):617–622.
253. Friedman SL. Gastrointestinal and hepatobiliary neoplasms in AIDS. *Gastroenterol Clin North Am.* 1988;17(3):465–486.
254. Seligmann M, Pinching AJ, Rosen FS, et al. Immunology of human immunodeficiency virus infection and the acquired immunodeficiency syndrome. An update. *Ann Intern Med.* 1987;107(2):234–242.
255. Janoff EN, Smith PD. Perspectives on gastrointestinal infections in AIDS. *Gastroenterol Clin North Am.* 1988;17(3):451–463.
256. Curran JW, Jaffe HW, Hardy AM, et al. Epidemiology of HIV infection and AIDS in the United States. *Science.* 1988;239(4840):610–616.
257. Dutta SC, Simons AJ, Levine AM, et al. Surgical outcome in acquired immunodeficiency syndrome patients with non-Hodgkin's lymphoma of the gastrointestinal tract. *Dis Colon Rectum.* 1996;39(2)):167–170.
258. Chin J. Current and future dimensions of the HIV/AIDS pandemic in women and children. *Lancet.* 1990;336(8709):221–224.
259. Blanche S, Tardieu M, Duliege A, et al. Longitudinal study of 94 symptomatic infants with perinatally acquired human immunodeficiency virus infection. Evidence for a bimodal expression of clinical and biological symptoms. *Am J Dis Child.* 1990;144(11):1210–1215.
260. Guarino A, Albano F, Berni Canani R. Acute infectious diarrhea in children. *Ann Ist Super Sanita.* 1998;34(4):495–512.
261. CDC CfDC. Revision of the CDC surveillance case definition for acquired immunodeficiency syndrome. *Morb Mortal Wkly Rep.* 1987;36(suppl 1):3S–14S.
262. CDC CfDCU. Acquired immunodeficiency syndrome—United States. *Morb Mortal Wkly Rep.* 1986;35:757–766.
263. Call S, Heudebert G, Saag M, Wilcox C. The changing etiology of chronic diarrhea in HIV-infected patents with CD4 cell counts less than 200 cells/mm^3. *Am J Gastroenterol.* 2000;95:3142–3146.
264. Bonacini M, Skodras G, Quiason S, Kragel P. Prevalence of enteric pathogens in HIV-related diarrhea in the midwest. *AIDS Patient Care STDS.* 1999;13(3):179–184.

265. Laine L, Bonacini M. Esophageal disease in human immunodeficiency virus infection. *Arch Intern Med.* 1994;154(14):1577–1582.
266. Genereau T, Lortholary O, Bouchaud O, et al. Herpes simplex esophagitis in patients with AIDS: report of 34 cases. The Cooperative Study Group on Herpetic Esophagitis in HIV Infection. *Clin Infect Dis.* 1996;22(6):926–931.
267. Monkemuller KE, Wilcox CM. Diagnosis of esophageal ulcers in acquired immunodeficiency syndrome. *Semin Gastrointest Dis.* 1999;10(3):85–92.
268. Ehrenpreis ED, Bober DI. Idiopathic ulcerations of the oesophagus in HIV-infected patients: a review. *Int J STD AIDS.* 1996;7(2):77–81.
269. Oelemann WM, Teixeira MD, Verissimo Da Costa GC, et al. Evaluation of three commercial enzyme-linked immunosorbent assays for diagnosis of Chagas" disease. *J Clin Microbiol.* 1998;36(9):2423–2427.
270. Lake-Bakaar G, Elsakr M, Hagag N, et al. Changes in parietal cell structure and function in HIV disease. *Dig Dis Sci.* 1996;41(7):1398–1408.
271. Belitsos PC, Greenson JK, Yardley JH, et al. Association of gastric hypoacidity with opportunistic enteric infections in patients with AIDS. *J Infect Dis.* 1992;166(2):277–284.
272. Rodgers VD, Fassett R, Kagnoff MF. Abnormalities in intestinal mucosal T cells in homosexual populations including those with the lymphadenopathy syndrome and acquired immunodeficiency syndrome. *Gastroenterology.* 1986;90(3):552–558.
273. Nelson JA, Wiley CA, Reynolds-Kohler C, et al. Human immunodeficiency virus detected in bowel epithelium from patients with gastrointestinal symptoms. *Lancet.* 1988;1(8580):259–262.
274. Jarry A, Brousse N, Rene E. Infected cells and immune cells in the gastrointestinal tract of AIDS patients. *Gastroenterology.* 1988;94:A207.
275. Greenson JK, Belitsos PC, Yardley JH, Bartlett JG. AIDS enteropathy: occult enteric infections and duodenal mucosal alterations in chronic diarrhea. *Ann Intern Med.* 1991;114(5):366–372.
276. Batman PA, Miller AR, Forster SM, et al. Jejunal enteropathy associated with human immunodeficiency virus infection: quantitative histology. *J Clin Pathol.* 1989;42(3):275–281.
277. Chalasani N, Wilcox CM. Etiology and outcome of lower gastrointestinal bleeding in patients with AIDS. *Am J Gastroenterol.* 1998;93(2):175–178.
278. Becker K, Lindner C, Frieling T, et al. Intestinal protein leakage in the acquired immunodeficiency syndrome. *J Clin Gastroenterol.* 1997;25(2):426–428.
279. Cimerman S, Cimerman B, Lewi DS. Prevalence of intestinal parasitic infections in patients with acquired immunodeficiency syndrome in Brazil. *Int J Infect Dis.* 1999;3(4):203–206.
280. Amenta M, Dalle Nogare ER, Colomba C, et al. Intestinal protozoa in HIV-infected patients: effect of rifaximin in *Cryptosporidium parvum* and *Blastocystis hominis* infections. *J Chemother.* 1999;11(5):391–395.
281. Kotler DP. Intestinal and hepatic manifestations of AIDS. *Adv Intern Med.* 1989;34:43–71.
282. Smith PD, Lane HC, Gill VJ, et al. Intestinal infections in patients with the acquired immunodeficiency syndrome (AIDS). Etiology and response to therapy. *Ann Intern Med.* 1988;108(3):328–333.
283. Ascoli V, Scalzo CC, Danese C, et al. Human herpes virus-8 associated primary effusion lymphoma of the pleural cavity in HIV-negative elderly men. *Eur Respir J.* 1999;14(5):1231–1234.
284. Feigal EG. AIDS-associated malignancies: research perspectives. *Biochim Biophys Acta.* 1999;1423(1):C1–C9.
285. Hermans P. Epidemiology, etiology and pathogenesis, clinical presentations and therapeutic approaches in Kaposi's sarcoma: 15-year lessons from AIDS. *Biomed Pharmacother.* 1998;52(10):440–446.
286. Klassen MK, Lewin-Smith M, Frankel SS, Nelson AM. Pathology of human immunodeficiency virus infection: noninfectious conditions. *Ann Diagn Pathol.* 1997;1(1):57–64.
287. Chin-Hong PV, Palefsky JM. Human papillomavirus anogenital disease in HIV-infected individuals. *Dermatol Ther.* 2005;18(1):67–76.
288. DiGiovanna JJ, Safai B. Kaposi's sarcoma. Retrospective study of 90 cases with particular emphasis on the familial occurrence, ethnic background and prevalence of other diseases. *Am J Med.* 1981;71(5):779–783.
289. Penn I. Kaposi's sarcoma in organ transplant recipients: report of 20 cases. *Transplantation.* 1979;27(1):8–11.
290. Nasti G, Serraino D, Ridolfo A, et al. AIDS-associated Kaposi's sarcoma is more aggressive in women: a study of 54 patients. *J Acquir Immune Defic Syndr Hum Retrovirol.* 1999;20(4):337–341.
291. Friedman SL, Wright TL, Altman DF. Gastrointestinal Kaposi's sarcoma in patients with acquired immunodeficiency syndrome. Endoscopic and autopsy findings. *Gastroenterology.* 1985;89(1):102–108.
292. Bini EJ, Micale PL, Weinshel EH. Risk factors for rebleeding and mortality from acute upper gastrointestinal hemorrhage in human immunodeficiency virus infection. *Am J Gastroenterol.* 1999;94(2):358–363.
293. Zoller WG, Bogner JR, Liess H, et al. Diagnosis and therapy of gastrointestinal Kaposi's sarcoma in AIDS. *Bildgebung.* 1994;61(suppl 1):46–52.
294. Aversa SM, Cattelan AM, Salvagno L, et al. Treatments of AIDS-related Kaposi's sarcoma. *Crit Rev Oncol Hematol.* 2005;53(3):253–265.
295. Knowles DM, Chamulak GA, Subar M, et al. Lymphoid neoplasia associated with the acquired immunodeficiency syndrome (AIDS). The New York University Medical Center experience with 105 patients (1981–1986). *Ann Intern Med.* 1988;108(5):744–753.
296. Knowles DM. Immunodeficiency-associated lymphoproliferative disorders. *Mod Pathol.* 1999;12(2):200–217.
297. Whooley BP, Bernik S, Sarkis AY, Wallack MK. Primary gastrointestinal non-Hodgkin's lymphoma: increasingly AIDS-related. *Am Surg.* 1998;64(2):137–143.
298. Steinberg JJ, Bridges N, Feiner HD, Valensi Q. Small intestinal lymphoma in three patients with acquired immune deficiency syndrome. *Am J Gastroenterol.* 1985;80(1):21–26.
299. Ioachim HL, Weinstein MA, Robbins RD, et al. Primary anorectal lymphoma. A new manifestation of the acquired immune deficiency syndrome (AIDS). *Cancer.* 1987;60(7):1449–1453.
300. Ioachim HL, Antonescu C, Giancotti F, et al. EBV-associated anorectal lymphomas in patients with acquired immune deficiency syndrome. *Am J Surg Pathol.* 1997;21(9):997–1006.
301. Carbone A, Gloghini A. AIDS-related lymphomas: from pathogenesis to pathology. *Br J Haematol.* 2005;130(5):662–670.

Lymphoproliferative Disorders of the Gastrointestinal Tract

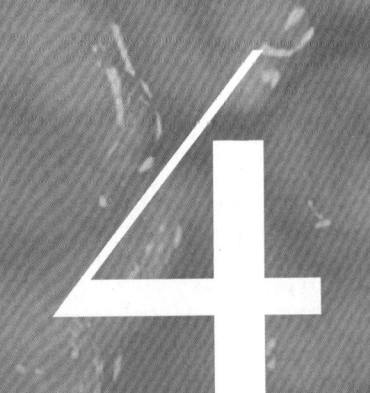

Chapter Outline

- OVERVIEW
  - Introduction
  - Definition
  - Incidence
  - Pathogenesis of GI Lymphoma
  - Classification of GI Lymphomas
  - Clinical Presentation and Other Practical Diagnostic Issues
  - Role of Molecular Diagnosis in GI Tract Lymphomas
  - Workup of Lymphoproliferative Disorders of the GI Tract
- LYMPHOID HYPERPLASIA OF THE GASTROINTESTINAL TRACT
  - Localized Lymphoid Hyperplasia of the Stomach—Gastric Lymphoid Hyperplasia (Pseudolymphoma)
    - Pathology
  - Angiofollicular Hyperplasia (Lymphoid Hyperplasia with "Castleman-like" Features)
    - Immunohistochemical features and molecular genetics
  - Localized Lymphoid Hyperplasia of the Small Intestine
    - Localized (lymphoid) hyperplasia of the terminal ileum and appendix
    - Localized lymphoid hyperplasia of the duodenum and small intestine excluding the terminal ileum
  - Localized Lymphoid Hyperplasia of the Rectum
  - Diffuse Nodular Lymphoid Hyperplasia of the Intestine
    - Diffuse nodular lymphoid hyperplasia with hypogammaglobulinemia
    - Diffuse nodular lymphoid hyperplasia without hypogammaglobulinemia
- LYMPHOPROLIFERATIVE DISORDERS OF THE ESOPHAGUS
- LYMPHOPROLIFERATIVE DISORDERS OF THE STOMACH
  - Malt Lymphoma (Extra Nodal Marginal Zone Lymphoma)
    - Pathogenesis
    - Clinical features
    - Pathology
    - Immunophenotype and molecular genetics
    - Treatment and prognosis
    - Reporting MALT lymphomas
    - Follow-up of patients with treated MALT lymphoma
    - Role of the pathologist
    - Differential diagnosis and practical approach to the difficult diagnosis
  - Diffuse Large B-cell Lymphoma of the Stomach
  - Primary Gastric T-cell Lymphoma
    - Pathology
  - Other Miscellaneous Lymphoproliferative Disorders
- LYMPHOPROLIFERATIVE DISORDERS OF THE SMALL INTESTINE
  - MALT Lymphoma (Extranodal Marginal Zone Lymphoma) and Diffuse Large B-cell Lymphoma of the Small Intestine (Western-type Lymphoma)
  - Immunoproliferative Small Intestinal Disease (Mediterranean Lymphoma, α-Chain Disease)
    - Etiopathogenesis
    - Clinical features
    - Pathology
    - Immunophenotype and molecular genetics
    - Diagnosis and differential diagnosis
    - Treatment and prognosis
  - Burkitt's and Burkitt's-like Lymphoma (Malignant Lymphoma of the Small, Noncleaved Type)
    - Clinical presentation
    - Pathology
    - Immunophenotype and molecular genetics
    - Prognosis and treatment
  - Enteropathy-type T-cell Lymphoma
    - Pathogenesis
    - Clinical presentation
    - Pathology
    - Immunophenotype and molecular genetics
    - Treatment and prognosis
  - CD4 Positive Small Intestinal T-cell Lymphoma
  - Other Miscellaneous Lymphoproliferative Disorders
- LYMPHOPROLIFERATIVE DISORDERS OF THE APPENDIX, COLON, AND ANAL CANAL
  - MALT Lymphomas of the Colon
  - Mantle Cell Lymphoma
  - Multiple Lymphomatous Polyposis
- MISCELLANEOUS LYMPHOPROLIFERATIVE DISORDERS OF THE GI TRACT
  - Follicular Lymphomas (Follicular and Diffuse Types)
    - Clinical features
    - Pathology
    - Immunophenotype and molecular genetics
    - Differential diagnosis
    - Treatment and prognosis
  - Lymphoplasmacytic Lymphoma/Waldenström's Macroglobulinemia
  - Immunodeficiency-Associated Lymphoproliferative Disorders
    - Primary immunodeficiency-associated lymphoproliferative disorders
    - Acquired immunodeficiency-associated lymphoproliferative disorders
  - Solitary Plasmacytomas of the Gastrointestinal Tract
  - Lymphomatoid Granulomatosis (Angiocentric Lymphoproliferative Lesion)
  - Mycosis Fungoides Involving the Gastrointestinal Tract

Anaplastic Large-cell Lymphoma
(Ki-1 Lymphoma)
Extranasal NK Cell or NK-like T-cell
Lymphoma
  NK cell enteropathy

Hodgkin's Lymphoma of the
Gastrointestinal Tract
True Histiocytic Lymphomas (Histiocytic
Sarcoma) of the GI Tract
Langerhans Cell Histiocytosis
(LCH, Histiocytosis X) of the GI Tract

Other Miscellaneous Lymphomas
of the GI Tract
Angioimmunoblastic Lymphadenopathy
Involving GI Tract
The Gastrointestinal Tract in Leukemia
and Granulocytic Sarcoma

OVERVIEW

Introduction

The gastrointestinal (GI) tract contains the largest aggregate of lymphoid tissue aside from lymph nodes, and it is the most frequent site of extranodal lymphoma.[1,2] Surprisingly, the most common site of lymphoma in the GI tract is the stomach, which normally has only rudimentarily organized lymphoid tissue. Advances in molecular genetics have led to a better understanding of the pathogenesis of GI lymphoproliferative disorders and have had a great impact on how we approach these lesions in clinical practice today.

Understanding the organization of normal lymphoid tissue in the gut is essential to understanding its lymphoproliferative disorders. A detailed description of GI lymphoid tissue and its functions is provided in Chapter 5, and only a brief discussion is presented here.[3] Aside from the mesenteric lymph nodes, the GI lymphoid tissue is represented by organized mucosa-associated lymphoid tissue (MALT), intraepithelial lymphocytes (IELs), and lamina propria lymphoid cells. Of these, MALT and IELs are unique in many ways.

MALT in the GI tract refers to unencapsulated lymphoid aggregates associated with specialized epithelium, best represented by Peyer's patches in the terminal ileum and lymphoid tissue of the appendix. However, they are widely distributed throughout the GI tract and vary in size and numbers considerably, not only among different individuals but also in the same individual over time. Similar to lymph nodes, these aggregates have organized B- and T-cell zones along with many accessory cells. The B-cell zone consists of lymphoid aggregates, which may develop germinal centers when stimulated, each of which is surrounded by an outer mantle and an outermost marginal zone similar to lymph nodes. The marginal zone is a broad area populated by small- to intermediate-sized cells that morphologically resemble germinal center cells (centrocyte-like cells [CLC]) or monocytes (monocytoid B cells). The marginal zone cells extend toward the epithelium and can be seen entering the overlying epithelium constituting "lymphoepithelium," which is the defining feature of MALT. These lymphocytes are IgM-positive and IgD-negative or weakly positive, as compared to mantle zone cells that are positive for both IgM and IgD. The follicles are flanked on the lateral as well as the basal aspects by a T-cell area similar to the paracortical T-cell zone of the lymph nodes.

The lamina propria throughout the gut is populated by a mixture of plasma cells, lymphocytes (B and T cells), mast cells, eosinophils, and macrophages. The composition and the density of this population vary between different GI segments among individuals and even within an individual over a period of time. The plasma cells secrete predominantly IgA but also IgM, IgG, and IgE. The CD4:CD8 ratio of the T-cell population is approximately 4:1. About 50% of these cells express CD103, which represents integrin $\alpha 4\beta 7$ that plays a role in the adhesion of these cells to the epithelium and lymphocyte homing to the gut.

IELs away from MALT areas are largely T cells of a heterogeneous phenotype. They are widely present throughout the GI tract, including the squamous mucosa. The predominant phenotype is the cytotoxic T-cell expressing $\alpha\beta$ T-cell receptors (TCRs), which are CD3+, CD8+, CD103+, CD4−, and CD5−. A smaller population (10%–15%) consists of T cells expressing $\gamma\delta$ TCRs that are negative for both CD4 and CD8. A third population of CD56+ IELs is also recognized that are virtually undetectable in normal mucosa. They T-cytotoxic and natural killer (NK) properties.

Studies, largely from experimental animals, show that lymphocytes from MALT have receptors that recognize specific cellular adhesion molecules on high endothelial venules that regulate their circulation and homing. This applies to both B and T cells. The MALT obviously functions as the host's immune response to various luminal organisms and allergens. IELs are known to increase in response to infections or food-induced enteropathies and are also likely to be an important component of the host's immune response; however, their specific function is poorly understood, although as predominantly CD8+ cells they likely downregulate any immune response.

Definition

Primary GI lymphomas have been defined as those lymphomas that are present in the GI tract with no evidence of liver, spleen, peripheral lymph nodes, or bone marrow involvement at the time of presentation or when the bulk of the disease is in the gut.[4] Also included are those lymphomas originating in the mesenteric lymph nodes. This is because of their similarity in clinical presentation and causal relationship to the prelymphomatous intestinal diseases, such as celiac disease and immunoproliferative small intestinal disease (IPSID) in some cases. However, this definition is somewhat restrictive. Problems arise in those cases that present with GI manifestations but on workup are found to be disseminated. For example, it is now well recognized that about 10% of gastric MALT lymphomas have bone marrow involvement at presentation, and secondary dissemination occurs in roughly 50% of patients.[5] Using sensitive techniques, it is possible to detect circulating lymphoma cells in about 21% of cases,[6] although the clinical implications of this apparent dissemination are unclear as most of these tumors remain localized. However, these should still be regarded as primary GI lymphomas with dissemination, although it is possible that some cases may represent dissemination of nodal lymphomas. This question should be easily resolved in the near future as advances in the molecular diagnostics may provide tools that could help in better classification and subtyping of lymphoma despite clinical, morphologic, and immunophenotypic overlaps. For example, the presence of t(11;18)(q21;q21) can help to differentiate low-grade B-cell gastric MALT lymphomas from their nodal counterparts (marginal zone lymphomas) that are otherwise identical in their morphology and immunophenotype.[7] Such a differentiation is currently not possible with regard to many other forms of GI lymphomas, for example, diffuse large B-cell gastric lymphoma from a nodal diffuse large B-cell lymphoma (DLBCL). From a practical point of view, the question is somewhat moot, as the management of these tumors currently depends on the histologic subtype.

Incidence

The GI tract accounts for about 50% of all primary extranodal lymphomas. In addition, GI involvement occurs in up to 50% of patients with disseminated nodal lymphomas or lymphocytic leukemias, in autopsy studies.[8,9] Nevertheless, in the United States, GI lymphomas are still relatively uncommon compared to other GI tumors, primarily adenocarcinomas. Thus, although more than half of all primary and secondary GI lymphomas in the United States are of gastric origin, they represent only about 5% of all gastric tumors.

It should also be noted that there is a marked geographic variation in the types and the site predilection of GI lymphomas (see Table 4-2). In the United States and Europe, the most frequent site of GI lymphomatous involvement is stomach (50%), followed by the small intestine (37%) (primarily the ileum and the ileocecal region) and anorectal region (3%).[2,10-13] Involvement of the remainder of the intestinal tract, such as duodenum and mesentery, is uncommon.[14] In contrast, in the Middle East and South Africa, the incidence of intestinal lymphomas is much more common than that of gastric lymphomas, ranging from 35% to 75% of all GI lymphomas, due to a relatively higher incidence of Mediterranean lymphoma and α-chain disease.[15] Interestingly, the duodenal lymphomas occur most frequently around the ampulla of Vater and consist primarily of follicular lymphomas, which are exceedingly rare in other portions of the GI tract.[16]

Pathogenesis of GI Lymphoma

The predisposing conditions for GI lymphoma are varied and include infections such as *Helicobacter pylori* (*H. pylori*) celiac disease, diffuse and nodular lymphoid hyperplasia (which themselves are likely secondary), immunodeficiency disorders (primary or acquired), and occasionally familial tendency. Lymphoma has also been described in association with ulcerative colitis, Crohn's disease, and epithelial neoplasms.

Details of the pathogenesis of the common GI lymphomas are unraveling a number of interesting associations.[3] While the pathogenesis of the nodal lymphomas remains unclear, primary GI lymphomas have led the way in understanding the "genesis" of lymphoma. The key theme of chronic antigenic stimulation (infectious or noninfectious) and immune dysregulation leading to benign proliferations that may eventually lead to a malignant disease is exemplified by many primary GI lymphomas. This process is in a way similar to the "hyperplasia–adenoma–carcinoma" sequence of epithelial neoplasms, although it is currently difficult to define the concept of "prelymphoma" or "lymphocytic dysplasia." Understanding the pathogenic mechanisms has had a great impact not only on the understanding of these disorders but on their management as well. A leading example of this is *H. pylori*–related gastric MALT lymphoma, where treatment of *H. pylori* results in disappearance of the lymphoma. As our understanding of *H. pylori*–induced gastric MALT lymphoma continues to evolve, the search for infectious etiologies of other types of lymphomas has already begun to show promising results. Infectious agents that have been implicated in the etiopathogenesis of other lymphomas include *Campylobacter jejuni*, *Clamydia psittaci*, *Borrelia burgdoferi*, Epstein Barr virus (EBV), and hepatitis B and C viruses.[17-20] Of these, EBV has already been a subject of interest for many years.

Classification of GI Lymphomas

The accurate classification of GI lymphomas is important for identifying specific disease entities and also for determining treatment protocols and assessing prognostic factors. The literature on GI lymphoma suffers from the use of nonuniform classification systems, making it difficult to compare results.

Until fairly recently, the major lymphoma classifications used were the Working Formulation, Rappaport's classification, WHO modification of the Working Formulation, and Kiel classification, all of which were based primarily on morphologic and immunophenotypic features.[21-24] The problem with the Working Formulation was that the classification was originally developed for the nodal lymphomas, and it was found that many extranodal lymphomas were not variants of nodal lymphomas but were histologically and clinically distinctive. For example, MALT lymphoma, IPSID, and enteropathy-associated T-cell lymphoma (EATL) have histologic features quite distinct from the nodal lymphomas. The Kiel classification was also morphologic based and divided lymphomas primarily into two broad categories, namely, B and T cells, and then classified them on the basis of cytologic morphology and grading. Although the grading frequently predicted the clinical outcome, lymphomas like the mantle cell lymphomas that were morphologically considered low grade are actually aggressive. Other lymphomas, such as the anaplastic large-cell lymphomas, that were considered high grade and to have an aggressive natural history show excellent response to chemotherapy with prolonged disease-free survival.[25]

To address these issues, in 1994 a new lymphoma classification was introduced by the International-American Lymphoma Study Group, labeled as the Revised European American Lymphoma (REAL) classification.[26] This classification subdivided lymphomas into distinctive entities, based on multiple parameters, including clinical presentation, site of the primary lesion, natural history and clinical course, morphologic appearance, and immunophenotypic and genetic factors. The site of the primary lesion

Table 4-1 Tumor Site of Gastrointestinal Lymphomas

TUMOR TYPE	TUMOR SITE USUAL	LESS FREQUENT SITES
B-CELL TYPE		
GUT TYPE		
MALT lymphoma	Stomach	Esophagus, small intestine, and large intestine
IPSID and α-chain disease (Mediterranean lymphoma)	Small intestine	Stomach, colon
NODAL TYPE (primary or secondary)		
Mantle-cell lymphoma	Ileocecal region and stomach	
Follicular center cell lymphoma	Ileocecal region	Colon and stomach
Diffuse large B- cell lymphoma	Small intestine	Colon and stomach
Burkitt's and Burkitt's-like type	Ileocecal region	Throughout the gastrointestine
AIDS-associated lymphoma	Stomach	Colon, ileum, esophagus, and duodenum
Miscellaneous B-cell TYPE		
PTLD	Throughout the GI tract	
Plasmacytoma	Stomach and small intestine	
T-CELL TYPE		
GUT TYPE		
Enteropathy associated T-cell (EATL)	Jejunum	Remainder small intestine and stomach
		Mesenteric lymph nodes
NODAL TYPE (Primary or secondary)		
Nonenteropathy associated lymphoma	Throughout the GI tract	
Angiocentric lymphoproliferative lesion	Throughout the GI tract and mesentery	
Mycosis fungoides	Throughout the GI tract and mesentery	

MALT, mucosa-associated lymphoid tissue; IPSID, immunoproliferative small intestinal disease; PTLD, posttransplant and other iatrogenic lymphoproliferative disorders.

is important for most extranodal tumors, including many GI lymphomas. This REAL classification was upgraded in 1999 and has now been adopted by the WHO classification.[27-29] While the lymphoma classifications will continue to evolve, disease-specific rather than morphology-centered classification is likely to remain a central theme.

The classification of GI lymphomas suggested here is based on the REAL and WHO classifications (Table 4-1). A fair number of distinctive lymphomas occur in the GI tract, although the frequency of the specific types varies greatly from one site to another (Table 4-2).

The vast majority (85%) of GI lymphomas are of B-cell origin, of which most are MALT lymphomas. T-cell lymphomas are rare and occur most often in the small intestine accounting for 34% of cases in one study. The latter are often associated with celiac disease. Since the advent of AIDS and organ transplantation, several new types of lymphomas have been recognized that can involve the GI tract. Only a handful of patients with Hodgkin's disease and other tumors, such as solitary plasmacytoma, large-cell anaplastic lymphoma, and true histiocytic neoplasms, have been described in the GI tract. The GI tract is also commonly involved secondarily in advanced stages of nodal lymphomas and leukemia. Lastly, a number of lymphomas are impossible to subclassify beyond their lymphoid derivation and are designated as unclassified.

Clinical Presentation and Other Practical Diagnostic Issues

The clinical presentation, radiologic findings, and endoscopic appearances of the lymphoproliferative disorders of the GI tract are frequently indistinguishable from other tumors and sometimes from benign ulcers or inflammatory lesions. Because of improving endoscopic techniques and advancing knowledge in

Table 4-2 Classification of GI Lymphomas

B CELL	T CELL	MISCELLANEOUS

GUT TYPE
1. MALToma (extranodal marginal zone B-cell lymphoma)
2. IPSID and α-chain disease (Mediterranean lymphoma)
    i. Stage A
    ii. Stage B
    iii. Stage C/DLBCL
NODAL TYPE (PRIMARY OR SECONDARY)
1. Follicular lymphoma
2. Mantle-cell lymphoma
3. Burkitt's and Burkitt's-like lymphoma
4. DLBCL
5. SLL
6. Lymphoplasmacytic lympoma
7. Anaplastic large-cell lymphoma B-cell type
8. Plasma cell myeloma/plasmacytoma
9. Plasmablastic lymphoma
10. T-cell rich B-cell lymphoma
11. Angiocentric lymphoproliferative lesion (lymphomatoid granulomatosis)
MISCELLANEOUS B-CELL LYMPHOMAS
1. Primary immunodeficiency-associated lymphoma
2. HIV-associated lymphoma
3. PTLD
    i. Plasma cell hyperplasia (polyclonal)
    ii. Polymorphous—usually monoclonal
    iii. Lymphoma/myeloma (plasmacytoma)
4. Other iatrogenic and mediation-associated lymphomas
	GUT TYPE
	Enteropathy associated T-cell lymphoma (EATL)
	Small intestinal CD4 positive lymhoma
	NODAL TYPE (PRIMARY OR SECONDARY)
	1. Peripheral T-cell lymphoma, not otherwise categorized
	2. Mycosis fungoides/Sezary's syndrome
	3. Angioimmunoblastic T-cell lymphoma
	4. Anaplastic large-cell lymphoma T-cell type
	MISCELLANEOUS T-CELL LYMPHOMAS
	PTLD
	   Monomorphic T/NK-cell type
		1. Hodgkin's disease
		2. PTLD
		    Hodgkin's type
		3. Histiocytic lymphoma (Histiocytic sarcoma)
		4. Langerhans cell histiocytosis
		5. Mastocytosis
		6. Unclassified lymphoma
		7. Leukemic involvement of the GI tract. (Granulocytic sarcoma)
		8. Composite lymphoma
		    Mixed type lymphoma
		    Carcinoma/lymphoma

MALT, mucosa-associated lymphoid tissue; IPSID, immunoproliferative small intestinal disease; PTLD, posttransplant and other iatrogenic lymphoproliferative disorders

related fields, GI lymphoma is increasingly recognized at an early stage. Particularly with regard to gastric lymphoma, presentation with a large mass lesion is a rarity these days in developed countries. With the increasing use of video capsule endoscopy, one could expect similar changes with regard to intestinal lymphomas. As increasingly early lesions are diagnosed, the role of the pathologist has shifted from merely subtyping or grading the lymphoma or both to differentiating it from benign and reactive disorders. It should also be recognized that traditional staging systems are poor in predicting the prognosis of primary GI lymphomas, particularly MALT lymphomas. Alternate staging systems have been developed, of which modified Ann-Arbor system is most widely used in practice (Table 4-3).[30] Distinguishing benign from malignant lymphoproliferative lesions of the gut can be difficult due to small biopsy size, tissue artifacts, limited tissue to assess the architectural pattern, confounding presence of lymphoid follicles that can be seen in both benign and malignant lesions, or because lymphoid markers may not be either readily available or easy to carry out in biopsies. In such situations, application of advanced molecular diagnostics could be of immense help.

Role of Molecular Diagnosis in GI Tract Lymphomas

Molecular diagnostics has made significant advances in the recent years, and the utility of various techniques has been well established.[31,32] Diagnosis and proper classification of lymphoma in current practice is based on a multidisciplinary approach, in which clinical features, morphology, immunophenotype, and cytogenetic and molecular characteristics are all important to varying extent in a given case. In practice, the diagnosis of lymphoma can be established with morphology and immunohistochemical analysis in most cases, while in some cases additional evidence of monoclonality may be essential in establishing a definitive diagnosis. In addition to clonality assessment, molecular techniques also help in some cases to establish the cell lineage, correctly classify the lymphoma, differentiate Hodgkin's from non-Hodgkin's lymphoma, and detect minimal residual disease.

The targets for molecular diagnosis of lymphoma in routine practice are (a) rearrangement of immunoglobulin (Ig) and TCR genes, (b) specific chromosomal translocations, and (c) viral infection (e.g., EBV) in certain situations.[32]

The commonly used molecular techniques in clinical practice include (a) southern blot analysis, (b) polymerase chain reaction (PCR) and reverse transcription PCR (RT-PCR), and (c) fluorescence in situ hybridization (FISH) or RNA in situ hybridization. Other evolving technologies that may find a significant role in the clinical practice in future include spectral karyotyping and gene expression profiling by cDNA microarray. Southern blot analysis remains the gold standard in clonality testing. However, it requires fresh tissue for obtaining large amounts of high-quality DNA, is labor-intensive, requires longer time, uses radioactive materials in the detection system, and has a low analytical sensitivity. In most labs, PCR-based assays have replaced southern blot assays for molecular diagnostics and are the preferred first-line approach. They have the following advantages: they require less tissue, they can use DNA or RNA as templates, DNA quality is less critical allowing fixed and archival material to be used, they have rapid turnaround time and superior sensitivity, and they do not require radioactive detection systems and can be automated. The electrophoretic systems that allow discrimination of PCR products have also evolved over time, and the newer systems, for example, capillary electrophoresis, have higher resolution allowing greater sensitivity of the assays. While this is extremely helpful in detection of minimal residual disease where neoplastic cells are expected to be scanty, they carry a disadvantage of identifying small clonal populations in benign reactive

Table 4-3 Modified Ann-Arbor Staging System for Primary Gastrointestinal Lymphomas

Stage	Description
IE	Localized involvement without lymph node metastases
IE-1	Early lymphoma. Tumor confined to the mucosa and submucosa
IE-2	Lymphoma extends beyond the submucosa
IIE	Lymphoma of any depth of infiltration with lymph node metastases
IIE-1	Lymphoma with contiguous regional node metastases
IIE-2	Lymphoma with lymph node metastases beyond contiguous regional nodes
IIIE	Localized lymphomatous involvement with lymph nodes on both sides of the diaphragm (from a practical point almost never applies to the stomach)
IVE	GI lymphoma with or without associated lymph node metastases with diffuse lymphomatous dissemination beyond the GI tract

The suffix E denotes extranodal.

conditions. Using sensitive techniques, about 10% to 15% cases of *H. pylori*–related chronic gastritis without any histologic evidence of lymphoma may show clonal B-cell populations. The choice of the molecular technique in a given situation depends upon the clinical setting, target to be assayed and the test availability. Further discussion of the technical aspects of molecular tests and their limitations are beyond the scope of this book.

The key role of molecular testing lies in the demonstration of monoclonality in difficult cases. The detection of Ig heavy chain gene rearrangement is the most commonly used assay for establishing B-cell clonality in most labs, although assays for Ig light chains are also available. The qualitative sensitivities of these assays vary widely from < 50% to virtually 100% and depend upon assay design, primer selection, detection system, and case type. False-negative results are more likely to occur in follicular lymphomas, marginal zone lymphomas, and DLBCLs largely due to V-region somatic hypermutations, which affect primer annealing in complementary-determining region 3 assays.[32] For assessment of T-cell clonality, the TCRγ gene is preferentially used in most labs due to simplicity of its genomic structure and requirement of relatively few Vγ and Jγ primers to detect all possible rearrangements.[32] TCRγ rearranges fairly early in both αβ+ and γδ+ T cells and provides a suitable molecular target irrespective of the nature of the ultimate surface receptor expression. TCRβ gene rearrangement assays are also available but are less frequently used in practice.

Detection of specific lymphoma-associated translocations forms an important component of molecular tests and is used for diagnostic purposes, proper classification, detection of minimal residual disease, and follow-up. The translocations not only provide supportive evidence for clonal expansion of lymphocytes but also point toward specific pathogenic events in the lymphoma development. They may be detected by a variety of techniques including southern blot, DNA-PCR, RT-PCR, conventional cytogenetics, and FISH. The most commonly assessed translocation in this regard are t(14;18)(q32;q21) for follicular lymphoma, t(11;14)(q12;q32) for mantle lymphoma, and t(2;5)(q23;351) for anaplastic large-cell lymphoma.

Viral infections have been implicated in the development of many lymphomas, of which EBV is the most important from an etiologic as well as diagnostic stand point. The Demonstration of EBV is important in posttransplant lymphoproliferative disease and primary effusion lymphoma among many other conditions. EBV can be demonstrated in a number of ways using immunohistochemical, southern blot and PCR-based techniques, although the method of choice is in situ hybridization for EBER.[32] This is relatively inexpensive and can be easily applied to paraffin sections with high sensitivity and specificity.

Among evolving newer technologies from a diagnostic clinical application stand point, gene expression profiling using cDNA microarray technology remains the most promising.[32] The technique allows for genomic-scale gene expression profiling of tumors. It offers opportunity for refining existing lymphoma classification, provides data regarding expression of novel markers, and helps in development of targeted therapies and prognostication. cDNA chips are commercially available and can also be custom designed. The current technique requires undegraded mRNA from the tissue samples, and it is of utmost importance that laboratories harvest fresh tissue for any future use in this regard.

It cannot be overstated that clonality does not equate to malignancy, nor does its absence exclude malignancy. For example, a number of clonal but benign lymphocytic proliferations have been described at other sites, such as benign monoclonal gammopathy, cutaneous lymphoid hyperplasia, drug-induced dermatoses, myoepithelial sialadenitis, and idiopathic cold hemagglutinin disease, all of which have an increased but not absolute risk of malignant transformation.[32] In many cases that eventually transform to malignancy, clonal identity can be shown between the clone detected at the initial reactive stage and the subsequent malignancy.[33,34] This would suggest that monoclonality might be an intermediate stage in the evolution of lymphoma, requiring additional steps before malignant transformation, very similar to the multistep carcinogenesis of epithelial tumors. It should also be recognized that well-defined cases of lymphoma fail to show IgH rearrangement by PCR in about 10% to 30% of cases.[32] Possible reasons include poor DNA preservation, chromosomal abnormalities involving the immunoglobulin locus, or poor primer binding associated with ongoing mutations within the gene.

Clonal B-cell proliferations have also been detected in cases of follicular chronic gastritis, the rates varying greatly among studies.[33,35,36] It has been shown that the clones fluctuate and may disappear or evolve over a period of time.[37] In a prospective study of chronic gastritis with monoclonality and without any histologic suspicion of lymphoma, it has been shown that some cases evolve over time into definite lymphomas while some do not.[37,38] PCR performed retrospectively on prior benign biopsies in cases that eventually developed lymphoma has shown identical clonal B-cell populations in the absence of histologic evidence of lymphoma.[33] While more studies are needed to clearly define the clinical significance of monoclonality in this setting and its long-term outcome, in routine practice, presence of clonal B-cell proliferation in absence of histologic evidence of lymphoma cannot be totally disregarded.[39]

False-negative and false-positive results have been recognized in the literature with each molecular technique in use, and the rates tend to vary with techniques and among laboratories.[32] The sensitivity and the specificity of currently used various molecular techniques in experienced laboratories generally exceeds 90%. However, tremendous interlaboratory variability exists and there is a lack of standardization of techniques. For the practicing pathologist it is important to realize the utility and limitations of each technique and know the sensitivity and the specificity of the assays used. It cannot be overemphasized that diagnosis of lymphoma should never be made in isolation entirely based on molecular assays, but should be interpreted in light of clinical context, histology, and other laboratory data.

Workup of Lymphoproliferative Disorders of the GI Tract

First, if the endoscopist suspects he or she is dealing with a case of GI lymphoma, the pathology lab should be alerted that the tissue is coming so it can be processed immediately, and some of the biopsies should be placed in saline or culture medium for flow cytometry and some in formalin. Many institutions have a "lymphoma protocol" that caters to all of these needs. In practice the pathologic diagnosis of lymphoma is made under two circumstances: (a) in clinically unsuspected cases where examination of the biopsy or resection specimen is the first indication of lymphoma or (b) lymphoma is either known or suspected prior to the biopsy or resection. In the first circumstance, there is often no choice. However, in the second situation care must be taken to appropriately triage tissues for lymphoma workup. Most of the common antibodies for immunohistochemical analysis needed for the diagnostic workup of lymphoproliferative disorders, gene rearrangement studies, in situ hybridization, and FISH for molecular genetic analysis can be performed on formalin-fixed paraffin-embedded tissues. Fresh tissues in appropriate media are needed for flow cytometry, conventional cytogenetics, and tissue cultures. Need for these additional studies is based on the complexity of a case and the academic and research interests at an institution.

Flow cytometry is an invaluable adjunct to diagnostic workup of lymphoproliferative disorders as it provides superior immunophenotyping opportunities and clonality assays based on unique immunophenotype and light chain restriction and provides very fast results. Flow cytometry is of somewhat limited use in the workup of T-cell lymphomas and more so for Hodgkin's lymphomas. Nucleic acid extraction and PCR-based assays while often performed on paraffin-embedded tissues provide better yield with frozen tissue samples. Touch/imprint smears made from fresh tissues often provide better cytologic details while compromising architectural pattern recognition. They are invaluable not only in the immediate assessment of tissues with a suspected diagnosis of a lymphoproliferative disorder often for intraoperative consultation but could also help in deciding proper tissue triage for diagnostic workup. Based on the resources available and the needs, each laboratory must design a lymphoma protocol to be applied to suspected cases of lymphoma. In many laboratories, the tissues are initially handled by individuals in training or technicians, and the opportunity to adequately work up complex cases is inadvertently lost in some cases. It is of utmost importance to have a strong suspicion based on the clinical circumstances to appropriately triage tissues for a lymphoma workup. Pathologists, especially trainees, should not hesitate to consult the seniors or contact their clinical counterparts whenever the need arises. Often frozen sections and touch preparations prepared just to properly triage tissue specimens pay rich dividends.

LYMPHOID HYPERPLASIA OF THE GASTROINTESTINAL TRACT

Lymphoid hyperplasia occurs in virtually all parts of the GI tract. Its frequency is difficult to assess, as it is often physiologic, asymptomatic, and seldom biopsied.[40] Diagnostic criteria to differentiate it from normal are lacking so the diagnosis of lymphoid hyperplasia is entirely subjective. In general, lymphoid nodules in a quiescent gut are not visible to naked eye, other than those in the terminal ileum. Visibility on naked eye examination or endoscopy that roughly corresponds to nodules >0.2 mm is an indirect and arbitrary criteria of hyperplastic lymphoid follicles. The situation is more complex when dealing with lymphoid hyperplasia at sites that normally contain abundant lymphoid tissues like terminal ileum and appendix. Unlike appendix, terminal ileal mucosa is accessible to visual examination to both gastroenterologists and pathologists, and everyone intuitively develops a sense of what is normal and what is not especially once normal Peyer's patches can be identified. Regarding the appendix, its size is so variable that it cannot even be used for defining lymphoid hyperplasia.

There are several situations where lymphoid tissue may be recognized clinically including *Helicobacter* gastritis especially in children; in the duodenum where it is a cause of nodularity; when appendiceal lymphoid tissue can be seen during endoscopic screening of mucosa at the appendiceal orifice and is biopsied as a "mucosal polyp"; in resected appendices, mostly for acute appendicitis, when obliteration of its lumen could be used as indirect evidence of lymphoid hyperplasia; in children in whom it may form the apex of an intussusception, often associated with adenovirus infection, and in diversion colitis/proctitis when the lymphoid hyperplasia can be seen grossly. Histologically, it is even more difficult to define lymphoid hyperplasia. The presence of lymphoid follicles with large secondary germinal center often correlates with grossly enlarged lymphoid nodules. The challenge is often to ensure that there are plasma cells present and that this is not a manifestation of common variable immunodeficiency (CVID) disease, and, if it is, that organisms such as *Giardia* are not present.

Lymphoid hyperplasia can be either localized or diffuse and can be assigned to one of five distinct clinicopathologic groups:

1. Localized lymphoid hyperplasia of the stomach: gastric lymphoid hyperplasia.
2. Localized lymphoid hyperplasia of the small intestine (excluding terminal ileum).
3. Localized nodular lymphoid hyperplasia of the terminal ileum and appendix.
4. Localized lymphoid hyperplasia of the rectum (benign lymphoid polyp, rectal tonsil).
5. Diffuse nodular lymphoid hyperplasia.

On rare occasions lymphoid hyperplasias have also been described in unusual locations such as esophagus and colon.[41-44]

Familiarity with various forms of GI lymphoid hyperplasia is important, particularly for its distinction from malignant lymphoma of the GI tract. Lymphoid hyperplasia may also occur as a secondary component in a number of disorders, which include nonerosive gastritis, immunodeficiency disorders, Crohn's disease, ulcerative colitis, and diversion colitis, and may sometimes cause difficulty in diagnosis. However, in primary lymphoid hyperplasia, the proliferation of lymphoid tissue is the predominant or the only pathologic feature, which is responsible for producing topographic and structural changes.

Localized Lymphoid Hyperplasia of the Stomach—Gastric Lymphoid Hyperplasia (Pseudolymphoma)

The evolution of this entity and the term "pseudolymphoma" is very interesting. This concept was first suggested by Smith and Helwig in 1958.[45] After reviewing all their cases of gastric lymphoma, they suggested that many cases actually represented benign reactive hyperplasia and that gastric lymphoma was overdiagnosed. This was based on the reactive-looking histology and excellent prognosis of these cases. The term pseudolymphoma was coined by Jacobs in 1963 for such lesions.[46] Subsequently, the term gastric pseudolymphoma was widely used and understandably so.[47-50] After MALT lymphomas of the stomach were described by Isaacson in 1983, gastric pseudolymphomas became uncommon.[51] In 1997 Abbondanzo and Sobin reviewed all their cases of gastric "pseudolymphoma," and based on histology and immunostains they concluded that 77 of the 93 cases diagnosed as pseudolymphoma represented true lymphomas (51 MALT lymphomas, 10 mantle cell lymphomas, 9 DLBCLs, and 7 follicular lymphomas).[52] Five cases were considered as atypical lymphoid infiltrate and only five were considered truly benign chronic follicular gastritis. Gene rearrangement and cytogenetic studies were not performed in this study and the follow-up was limited. The authors concluded that the majority of pseudolymphoma cases represent true lymphomas, and the term should be abandoned. Indeed, cases that represent extreme hyperplasia of gastric lymphoid tissue in current practice are extremely rare, and search of current literature fails to reveal any such convincing cases. The term gastric lymphoid hyperplasia, if used at all, should be confined to cases of chronic nonspecific gastric inflammation, in which the proliferation of lymphoid tissue presents as a tumorous mass, and the possibility of a lymphoma, especially of the MALT-type, has been excluded.

However, a diffuse fine nodularity is most commonly associated with *H. pylori* and tends to regress following its eradication.[48,53,54] Patients usually present with symptoms suggestive of peptic ulcer disease or chronic gastritis, although occasionally they have gastric outlet obstruction.[55]

Pathology. Morphologically, these lesions consist of either fine gastric mucosal nodularity, primarily in children, or small nodular or microscopic lesions in adults.[56] In these cases, the lymphoid infiltrate, often with germinal centers, produces mucosal thickening, which may be accompanied by either an ulcer with raised margins or a localized plaque-like thickening of the rugal folds without a recognizable ulcer (Fig. 4-1).

The lesions are usually solitary and small. Mucosal ulceration, when present, is superficial. In most instances, these lesions seem to represent less advanced examples of gastric lymphoid hyperplasia in current practice, because of early recognition and treatment of *H. pylori* infection.

The typical gastric lymphoid hyperplasia is associated with a dense polymorphous inflammatory infiltrate,

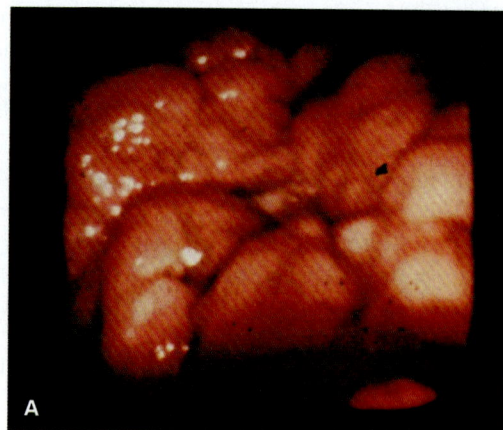
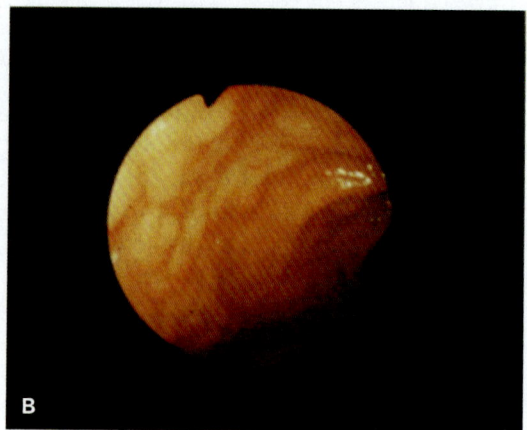

Figure 4-1. Endoscopic appearances of gastric lymphoid hyperplasia. **A:** Central ulceration surrounded by severe mucosal nodularity. **B:** Plaque-like thickening of rugal folds without ulceration.

admixed with lymphoid follicles with germinal centers and fibrosis (Fig. 4-2). Since reactive lymphoid follicles may also be found within gastric lymphomas, one cannot rely on these follicles for distinguishing lymphoid hyperplasia from lymphoma. Clumps of IELs mimicking lymphoepithelial lesions of MALT lymphomas may also occasionally be found, but they differ from the latter in that they consist of mature lymphocytes, mostly T cells, usually have less than three cells, and do not cause epithelial destruction or degeneration.

Angiofollicular Hyperplasia (Lymphoid Hyperplasia with "Castleman-like" Features)

On very rare occasions, these variants of lymphoid hyperplasia have been reported in the stomach and small intestine.[47,57] Angiofollicular lymphoid hyperplasia of the GI tract is morphologically similar to its nodal counterpart, showing a lymphoid infiltrate with numerous lymphoid follicles containing hyalinized germinal centers and vascular structures.[47] Unlike the usual gastric lymphoid hyperplasias, these lesions are not associated with ulceration or fibrosis. It is unclear if they have any significant clinical implication or just represent a histologic variation of reactive lymphoid hyperplasia. Its relationship to HIV infection has not been studied to date.

Immunohistochemical features and molecular genetics. Immunohistochemistry of the lymphoid infiltrate is expected to show a typical polyclonal pattern of the immunoglobulin light chains. (In addition, there is a marked T-cell reaction occurring in a perivascular location in the mucosa and in submucosal nodules.[58]) Sometimes, it may be extremely difficult to differentiate between a lymphoid hyperplasia and a low-grade lymphoma on a small biopsy specimen, especially, in suboptimally fixed or distorted specimens. In such a situation, repeat biopsy with optimum fixation, immunohistochemistry, and gene rearrangement studies could be helpful (see also section on

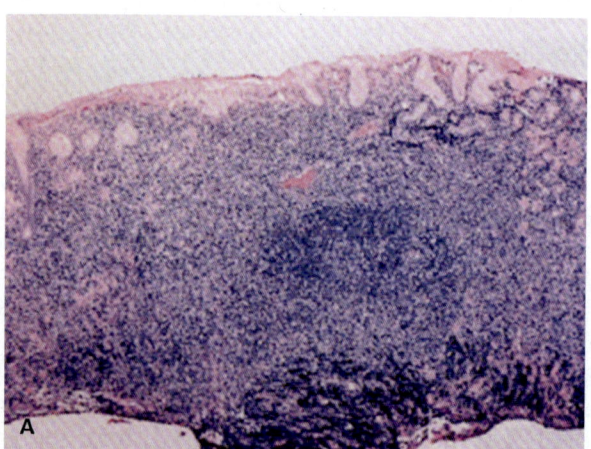
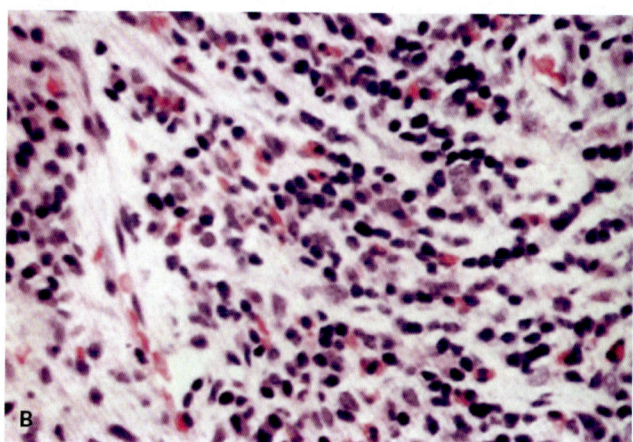

Figure 4-2. Endoscopic biopsy specimen of gastric lymphoid hyperplasia. **A:** Low-power view showing a dense mucosal inflammatory infiltrate. **B:** Detail of part **(A)** showing a polymorphous infiltrate composed of mature lymphocytes, plasma cells, eosinophils, and histiocytes.

differential diagnosis of MALT lymphoma).[59] Presence of a clonally rearranged Ig gene detected by PCR in this setting is likely to represent a lymphoma, and the histology needs to be interpreted with extreme caution.[59,60]

Localized Lymphoid Hyperplasia of the Small Intestine

Localized lymphoid hyperplasia may occur anywhere along the length of small intestine from duodenum to the terminal ileum. There appear to be two distinct clinicopathologic groups.

Localized (lymphoid) hyperplasia of the terminal ileum and appendix.
Lymphoid tissue is normally abundant in the terminal ileum, and it is not surprising that lymphoid hyperplasia has often been reported at this location.[61] Lymphoid hyperplasias can cause problems in younger patients undergoing colectomy for familial adenomatous polyposis (FAP), as the inexperienced surgeon may interpret the physiological lymphoid nodularity in the terminal ileum as FAP involving the ileum. While this can happen, the density of the lymphoid nodules is apparent and a frozen section can readily resolve the issue. In contrast, lymphoid hyperplasia of the appendix (where lymphoid tissue is also abundant) is rarely documented in the literature.[62] The reason for the rarity of the diagnosis of appendiceal lymphoid hyperplasia is probably because the appendix in childhood normally has abundant active lymphoid tissue, and as discussed earlier reliable diagnostic criteria for lymphoid hyperplasia are lacking. Pathologic features that have the potential for producing symptoms, such as thickening and swelling of the appendix with luminal narrowing, should be seen before a diagnosis of focal lymphoid hyperplasia is made. However, in most instances these cases come to attention due to acute appendicitis, which by itself is capable of mucosal swelling and luminal narrowing.

Lymphoid hyperplasia of the small intestine and appendix may occur either together or separately and is usually found in children or young adults.[61–64] Patients usually present with ileocecal intussusception or a clinical syndrome, which simulates acute appendicitis.[65,66] Less frequently, hematochezia may be the major complaint.[66] Patients with lymphoid hyperplasia of the terminal ileum, who develop ileocecal intussusception, are usually infants.[65] The reason for this propensity in infants is not clear. However, not all infants who develop ileocecal intussusception have an ileocecal mass due to lymphoid hyperplasia. The strategic circumferential distribution of the lymphoid tissue at the ileocecal valve may be important in providing the stimulus for intussusception.[67] The older patients suffering from focal lymphoid hyperplasia usually present with abdominal pain often associated with a mass-like lesion in the right iliac fossa, raising a concern for malignancy.

The isolation of various adenovirus strains from patients with ileocecal intussusception, the occasional demonstration of adenovirus in intussuscepted tissue, suggests that at least some cases may have an infective etiology.[66,68] Intranuclear inclusions can be seen in the attenuated epithelium overlying the hyperplastic lymphoid tissue (Fig. 4-3A–D). Unlike diffuse nodular lymphoid hyperplasia, those with lymphoid hyperplasia confined to the terminal ileum and appendix do not have hypogammaglobulinemia.

Pathology Roentgenograms show variable luminal narrowing of the terminal ileum, and in patients with intussusception a filling defect may be present in the cecal area. On gross examination, the mucosa of the terminal ileum is thickened and may have a cobblestone appearance (Fig. 4-4). A more distinct mass lesion due to lymphoid hyperplasia has been described in patients who present with intussusception, and on occasion this may have a papillary appearance. Marked swelling and thickening of the mucosa and submucosa and luminal obliteration characterizes lymphoid hyperplasia of the appendix.

Both the terminal ileum and the appendix show marked hyperplasia of the lymphoid tissue in the mucosa and superficial submucosa, with many lymphoid follicles containing conspicuous germinal centers (Figs. 4-5 and 4-6). In some cases the germinal centers are so large, distorted, and covered by only a thin mantle of mature lymphocytes that they may be confused with follicular lymphoma. In these cases, lack of BCL-2 expression or determination of the clonality of the infiltrate resolves the issue.

The rarer adult lesion, found in older patients, often has a diffuse interfollicular lymphoplasmacytic infiltrate frequently with numerous eosinophils, in addition to the lymphoid hyperplasia. Furthermore, it frequently appears to extend beyond the submucosa through the muscularis propria to serosa, raising a suspicion of a low-grade lymphoma.[69] It should, however, be stressed that lymphoid follicles in the terminal ileum in young adults and children are often labeled as "hyperplasia" by the endoscopist, while they are actually normal and of no clinical relevance.

Localized lymphoid hyperplasia of the duodenum and small intestine excluding the terminal ileum.
Prominent lymphoid nodules in the proximal duodenum and bulb are frequently encountered, and biopsied to exclude an underlying neoplasm. These are likely physiologic and clinically inconsequential. Larger lesions that may be symptomatic or produce a worrisome endoscopic or radiologic appearance are exceedingly uncommon, with only few cases described

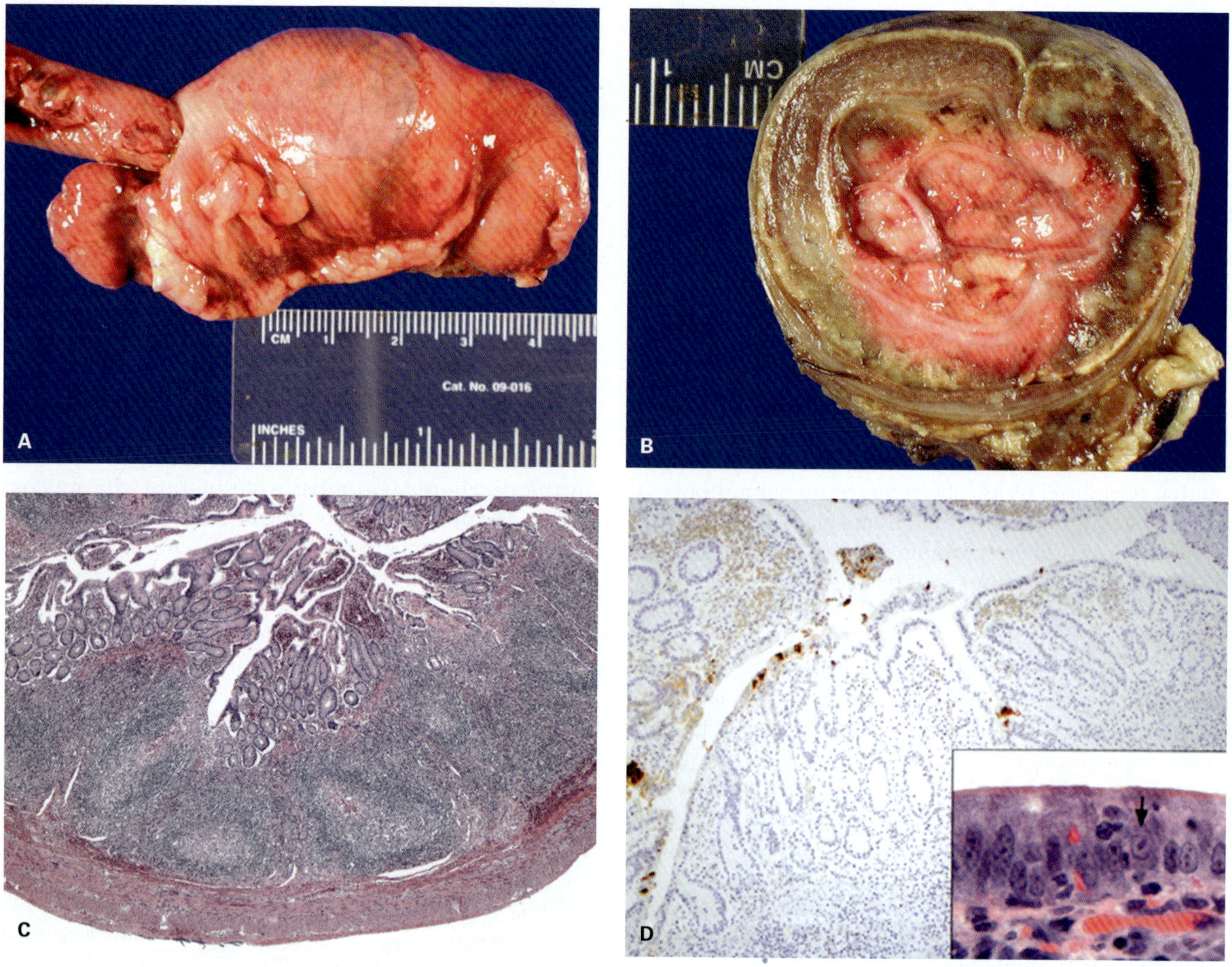

Figure 4-3. Lymphoid hyperplasia in small bowel and colon leading to intussusception of terminal ileum into the colon **(A)**. The transverse section showing fleshy tissue in the invaginated segment representing lymphoid hyperplasia **(B)**. Histology of the lymphoid hyperplasia in the colonic segment from the same case showing numerous lymphoid follicles with reactive germinal centers **(C)**. The immunostain for adenovirus shows strong positivity in the overlying epithelium **(D)**. Note the adenovirus nuclear inclusions (*arrow*) in the overlying epithelium (**inset**).

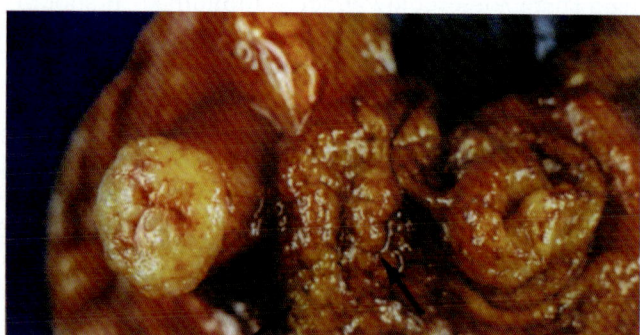

Figure 4-4. Focal lymphoid hyperplasia of the terminal ileum and appendix from a patient with symptoms of acute appendicitis. Gross appearances showing cobble stoning of ileal mucosa (*arrow*) and marked thickening of the appendix with luminal obliteration.

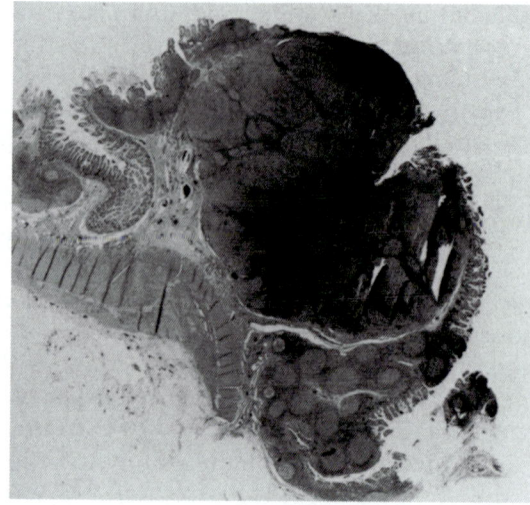

Figure 4-5. Focal lymphoid hyperplasia of the terminal ileum and appendix. Note the follicular hyperplasia of Peyer's patch in the terminal ileum, on the right, extending into the appendix.

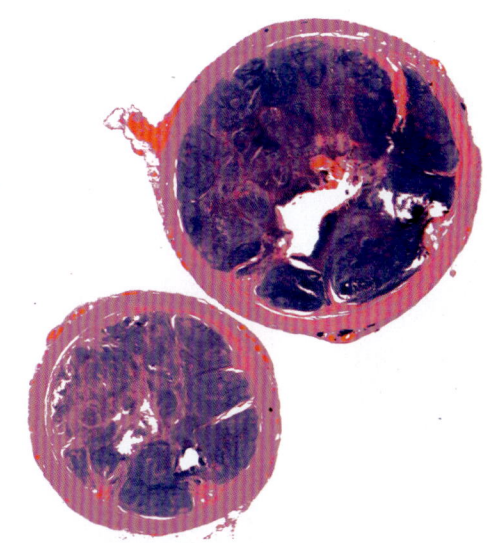

Figure 4-6. Focal lymphoid hyperplasia of the appendix. Lower-power photomicrograph of a cross-sectional cut demonstrating marked mucosal thickening, follicular hyperplasia, and luminal obliteration.

in the literature that were clearly distinguished from a lymphoma.[49,70] Patients usually present with recurrent abdominal pain. Radiologic examination may show a focal constricting lesion. Grossly, there is nodular thickening of the mucosa, which may be circumferential (Fig. 4-7). Microscopically, the lymphoid infiltrate may involve only the mucosa and submucosa or, less frequently, the full thickness of the intestinal wall. The differential diagnosis is not a problem because of the mature, bland nature of the lymphoid infiltrate and the presence of follicles with germinal centers throughout the lesion.[49] The lamina propria should be examined to ensure that adequate numbers of plasma cells are present, and that this is not secondary to a B-cell lymphoma. If there is any doubt, immunohistochemistry can be performed to ensure particularly that most of the plasma cells are IgA and that this is not part of IgA deficiency or CVID syndrome. Confirmation can be obtained from serum immunoglobulins.

Localized Lymphoid Hyperplasia of the Rectum

Localized lymphoid hyperplasia of the large intestine, other than in the ileocecal area, appears to be located almost exclusively in the rectum.[71,72] This lesion is also known as benign lymphoid polyp or rectal (anal) tonsil.[73] It may occur in all age groups but is most common in the second to fifth decades. The lesion has also been described in children.[49,74] Patients with benign lymphoid hyperplasia have a variety of symptoms, which include rectal bleeding, altered bowel habits, anal discomfort, and prolapse of a rectal mass. Many patients have associated anorectal lesions, such as hemorrhoids, anal fissures, and colonic carcinoma, which may contribute to their symptoms. Most patients have no evidence of nodular lymphoid hyperplasia elsewhere in the colon.

Pathology Localized lymphoid hyperplasia of the rectum usually affects its lowermost portion.[49] About 60% to 80% of the lesions present as single polyp, and when multiple they are usually fewer than six. However, the polyps may be numerous on occasion and may impart a cobblestone appearance to the rectal mucosa.[73] They are most commonly sessile, have a smooth surface, and have a pale yellow or white surface on endoscopy. They range from a few millimeters to 5 cm in diameter.[49,71,73]

A heavy lymphoid infiltrate is present in the lamina propria and submucosa. Large follicles with prominent germinal centers are always present, although they may be difficult to identify in poorly prepared tissue (Figs. 4-8 and 4-9). Eosinophils and plasma cells are not prominent. The majority of polyps are covered by intact, although at times attenuated, colonic epithelium.[49,71,73] Low-lying polyps may be covered by anal squamous epithelium. The lymphoid nodules straddle the mucosa and submucosa and are therefore in a location similar to the solitary lymphoid nodules found in the normal colon. The muscularis mucosae show irregular proliferation and may be focally

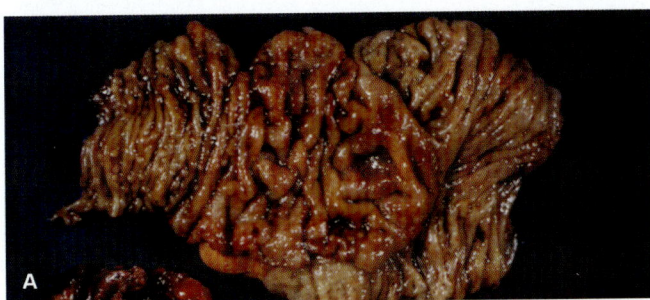

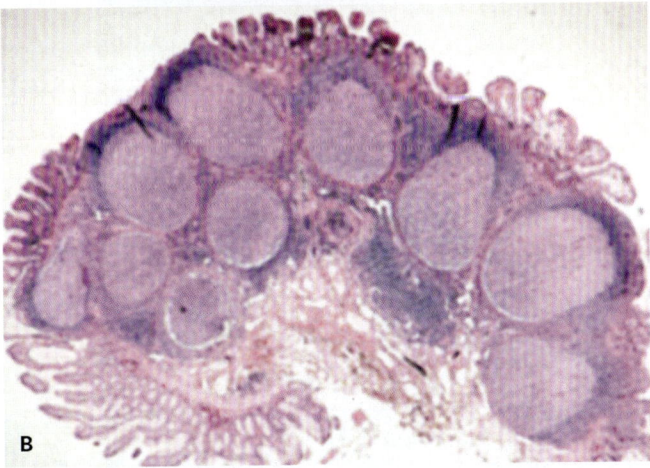

Figure 4-7. Focal lymphoid hyperplasia of the duodenum. **A:** The mucosal folds are focally thickened and edematous. Additionally, there are numerous nodules in both the edematous and nonedematous mucosa. **B:** Low-power photomicrograph of part **(A)** illustrating hyperplastic lymphoid follicles in the mucosa and submucosa. (Courtesy M. Ranchod, M.D.)

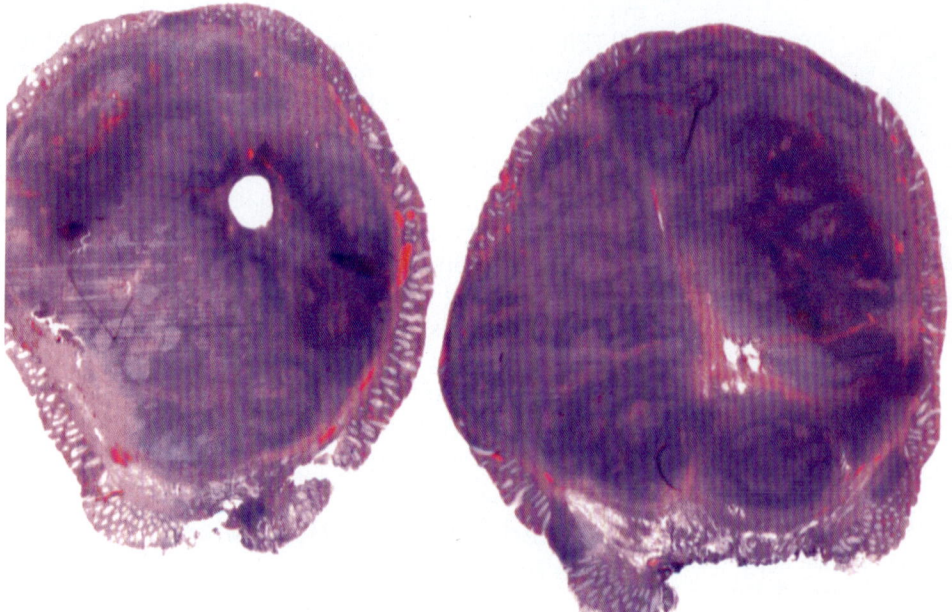

Figure 4-8. Focal lymphoid hyperplasia of the rectum (lymphoid polyp) demonstrating the polypoid appearance of the lesion. The lesion is covered by intact, focally attenuated colonic epithelium and contains large lymphoid follicles with prominent germinal centers.

absent. Focal lymphoid hyperplasia of the rectum is readily differentiated from malignant lymphoma (see the discussion of lymphoid hyperplasia of terminal ileum). It should also be kept in mind that malignant lymphoma is exceedingly rare at this site.[13] As discussed in the preceding section, an immunodeficiency syndrome should be excluded.

Lymphoid polyps of the rectum should be well sampled for diagnostic purposes. If the lesions are multiple and the patient is asymptomatic, complete excision is not necessary, since the lesions may regress spontaneously. The incidence of local recurrence is low even after incomplete excision.[49,73]

Diffuse Nodular Lymphoid Hyperplasia of the Intestine

Diffuse lymphoid hyperplasia in the small intestine can be either associated with or without hypogammaglobulinemia.

Diffuse nodular lymphoid hyperplasia with hypogammaglobulinemia. This disorder occurs primarily in patients with underlying congenital or acquired

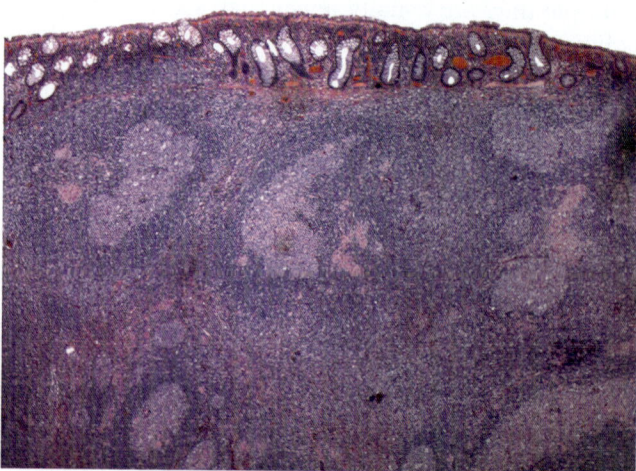

Figure 4-9. Microscopic appearance of rectal lymphoid hyperplasia showing numerous lymphoid follicles with germinal centers. Note that the infiltrate tends to push the crypts apart.

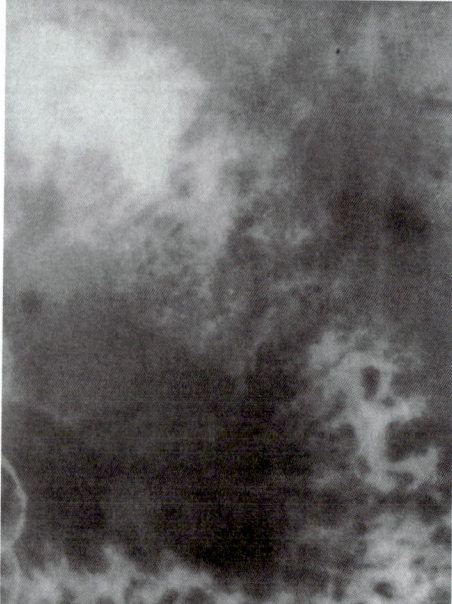

Figure 4-10. Nodular lymphoid hyperplasia with hypogammaglobulinemia: x-ray appearances. The barium radiograph is characterized by numerous nodular translucencies representing the mucosal lymphoid nodules.

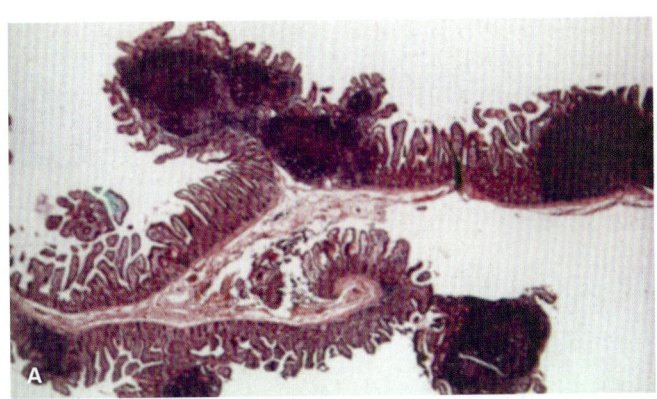
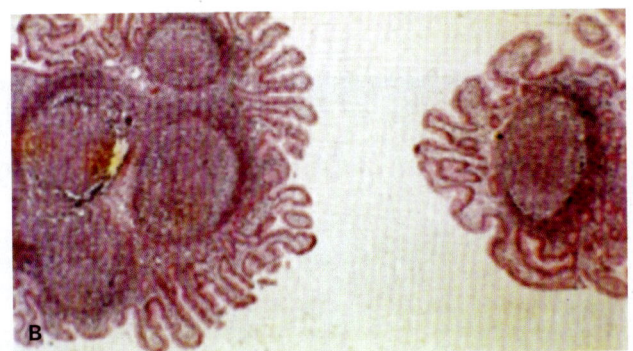

Figure 4-11. Low-power view showing hyperplastic mucosal lymphoid follicles. The mucosal nodules are composed of either (A) single or (B) clusters of hyperplastic lymphoid nodules.

immunodeficiency syndromes (see also Chapter 5). Commonly associated immune disorders are CVID (late-onset hypogammaglobulinemia), selective IgA deficiency, and X-linked immunoproliferative disorder.[76–78]

Pathology The mucosa of the small intestine is studded with closely packed sessile or polypoid nodules measuring < 5 mm in diameter. On x-ray, this produces a very striking picture characterized by numerous filling defects (Fig. 4-10). Rarely gastric and colonic involvement may occur.[49,79]

The lesions consist of one or a cluster of hyperplastic lymphoid nodules, which are confined to the lamina propria and superficial submucosa (Fig. 4-11). They often produce shortening and blunting of the overlying intestinal villi. A decrease or absence of plasma cells is often noted in the lamina propria throughout the GI tract in CVID. Patients with selective IgA deficiency show absence of IgA immunoreactive plasma cells in the lamina propria in the background of normal IgG- and IgM-positive plasma cells. Untreated patients frequently have a superimposed parasitic infection, especially giardiasis. In rare instances, lymphoma has supervened.[80,81] (For a more detailed discussion, see the description of "Immunoeficiency Disorders" in Chapter 3.)

Diffuse nodular lymphoid hyperplasia without hypogammaglobulinemia. Diffuse nodular lymphoid hyperplasia of the intestine can occur in the absence of hypogammaglobulinemia and may be more frequent than that associated with late-onset hypogammaglobulinemia.[82–85] In a study of 1,000 consecutive autopsies, Robinson et al.[85] found 30 cases of nodular lymphoid hyperplasia. The small intestine alone was involved in 13% of the cases, the large intestine alone in 40%, and both in 47%. The patients died of a variety of causes; none had GI symptom, giardiasis, or hypogammaglobulimia.

Nodular lymphoid hyperplasia of the colon has been observed in children undergoing barium enemas for a variety of GI complaints. It is clearly a common incidental finding that is unrelated to the patient's symptoms.[82,84,86] Serum immunoglobulin levels and T- and B-cell function studies found to be normal.[82,84,85]

It is likely that the lymphoid nodules represent hyperplasia of the solitary lymphoid follicles normally present in large numbers in the GI tract resulting in the characteristic radiologic and gross findings.[82,86,87] Radiologically the lesions show umbilication of the nodules, which is a helpful diagnostic clue.[82] One or more of the crypts overlying the lymphoid follicle are widened and elongated, allowing them to trap barium and produce the umbilication seen radiologically.

Pathology The lesions are grossly visible as pale yellow or white mucosal nodules and normally measure up to 0.4 cm in diameter, although rarely they may be as large as 2 cm (Figs. 4-12 and 4-13). Histologically, the mucosal nodules are similar to those seen in nodular lymphoid hyperplasia with hypogammaglobulinemia except that the lamina propria contains normal or increased numbers of plasma cells.

Clinical Implications and Differential Diagnosis of Diffuse Nodular Lymphoid Hyperplasia The clinical importance of diffuse lymphoid nodular hyperplasia lies in the recognition of the underlying immune disorder, differentiation from lymphoma, and increased risk of developing GI neoplasms, primarily lymphoma and carcinoma.[81,88] It is also clear that diffuse nodular lymphoid hyperplasia may also occur in the small and large intestines in patients without associated hypogammaglobulinemia and giardiasis. In some cases, it may represent underlying food allergy.[89,90] It may be found incidentally during the radiologic examination of the GI tract or at autopsy and should not be immediately incriminated for any GI symptoms the patient may have.

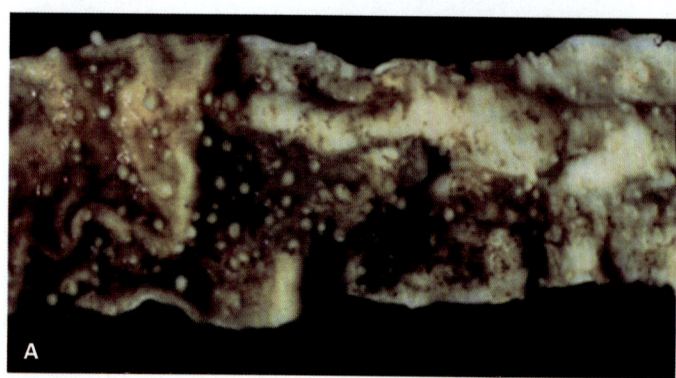
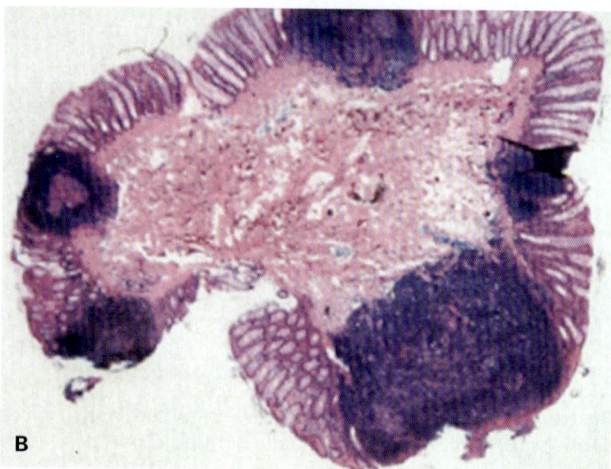

Figure 4-12. Nodular lymphoid hyperplasia of the large intestine. **A:** Showing mucosa studded with small, sessile nodules. **B:** Showing hyperplastic mucosal lymphoid follicles.

Nodular lymphoid hyperplasia of the ileum has also been described in patients with familial adenomatosis coli and Gardner's syndrome, where it may give rise to multiple filling defects in the colon and occasionally in the ileum. This possibility should be considered with the usual small white bumps of the terminal ileum that represent normal lymphoid follicles and are routinely seen at endoscopy. Occasionally, this finding has resulted in colectomy with first-degree relatives of patients with familial adenomatosis coli as the polyps were presumed to be adenomatous without a biopsy.[91] This also becomes important in youngsters as the surgeon may raise the question of ileal involvement and consider resecting affected small bowel.[92,93] Since patients with nodular lymphoid hyperplasia without hypogammaglobulinemia are asymptomatic and may undergo spontaneous regression, treatment of these lesions is unnecessary.[82,86] Most importantly, diffuse nodular lymphoid hyperplasia needs to be distinguished from various lymphomas that may present as multiple lymphomatous polyposis of the GI tract (see later).[94] However, patients with diffuse nodular lymphoid hyperplasia without hypogammaglobulinemia only rarely develop lymphoma. Kahn and Novis reported a patient with multifocal "histiocytic" lymphoma of the GI tract.[95] Matuchansky et al. reported a patient with nodular lymphoid hyperplasia who developed a jejunal lymphoma.[96] Their case is of interest because they demonstrated immunohistochemically a transition from a hyperplastic lymphoid follicle to a neoplastic one. It is of interest that on many occasions when intestinal follicular or marginal zone lymphoma cases are examined, one can find hyperplastic lymphoid follicles immediately adjacent to the lymphoma and sometimes they even show same B-cell clones by molecular genetic analysis.

LYMPHOPROLIFERATIVE DISORDERS OF THE ESOPHAGUS

Primary lymphomas of the esophagus are extremely rare and account for <1% of all GI lymphomas.[97–101] Many of these have been reported in the setting of immunodeficiency, particularly HIV infection.[100,102–107] Secondary involvement of the esophagus from a mediastinal or gastric lymphoma is more frequently encountered in practice than a primary esophageal tumor. Clinically the patients present with symptoms that simulate carcinoma such as dysphagia, especially when the mass involves the distal esophagus.[100,108] The lesions tend to present as polypoid masses, prominent rugae, ulcers, or strictures.[100,104,106,109,110] Multiplicity of lesions in this setting favors a lymphoma over a carcinoma. The majority of the lymphomas are of B-cell type. MALT lymphomas similar to those found elsewhere are also known to arise and tend to show similar histology (see the section on gastric MALT lymphoma).[111] Histology reveals lymphoid follicles that are

Figure 4-13. Nodular lymphoid hyperplasia of the large intestine: endoscopic appearance. The mucosa is studded with numerous pearly white nodules. (Courtesy S. Weiss, M.D.)

surrounded by a diffuse infiltrate of CLC and a variable degree of plasma cell differentiation. Tumor cells infiltrating the overlying squamous epithelium are often present, suggesting epitheliotropism similar to lymphoepithelial lesions of gastric MALT lymphomas. Due to rarity of these lesions, it is unknown if the molecular genetics of these tumors is similar to MALT lymphomas at other sites. DLBCLs similar to their nodal counterparts are also known to arise in esophagus. Primary esophageal lymphomas including T-cell lymphoma, large-cell anaplastic Ki-1 lymphoma, Hodgkin's lymphoma, and plasmacytoma have been reported in the literature and are exceedingly rare.[97,98,106,110,112,113]

LYMPHOPROLIFERATIVE DISORDERS OF THE STOMACH

More than half of all primary and secondary GI lymphomas in the United States are of gastric origin. However, they represent only about 4% to 10% of all gastric tumors.[114]

MALT Lymphoma (Extra Nodal Marginal Zone Lymphoma)

Among the extranodal non-Hodgkin's lymphomas, the stomach is the most commonly involved site in the Western countries, of which MALT-type lymphomas (MALTomas or MALT lymphomas) are the most frequent.[1,2]

Pathogenesis. Understanding the pathogenesis of gastric lymphoma has been one of the major triumphs of this past century and continues to lead the way in our understanding of lymphomagenesis (Fig. 4-14). The association of H. pylori infection in patients with MALT lymphoma is currently well established.[8,115–119] Initial studies showed that H. pylori is associated with MALT lymphomas in 92% to 97% of the cases—a finding that is similar to gastric carcinoma—80% to 90% of which are also associated with H. pylori infection.[119,120] The prevalence of H. pylori infection in the general population in Western countries is about 30% but is much higher in developing countries where, in contrast to developed countries, children still tend to become infected early in life. Studies of archived gastric biopsies and sequential serological studies have shown that H. pylori infection precedes the development of gastric MALT lymphomas.[33,34,119] With disease progression, the tumor growth tends to become independent of the organisms. At later stages, it is likely that the gastric environment becomes atrophic and no longer conducive to the survival of H. pylori, and either the organisms disappear or become too sparse to be visualized in biopsies. Thus, it is not surprising that the association of H. pylori with transformed

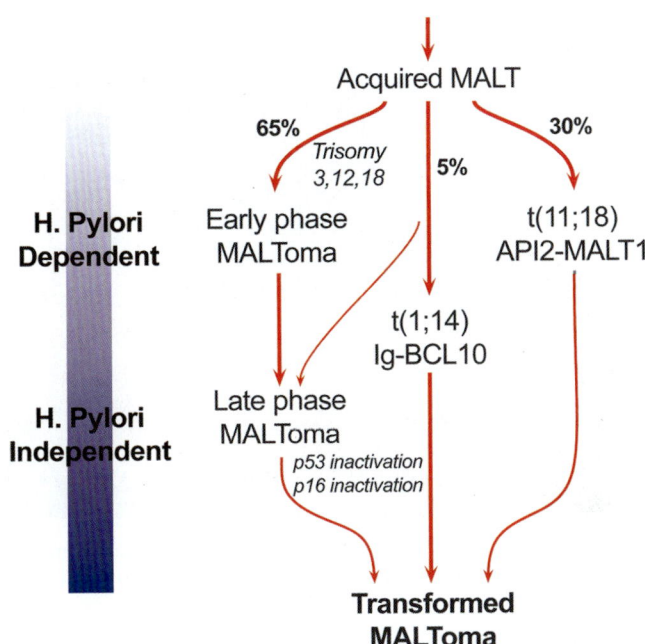

Figure 4-14. Schematic diagram showing the progression of H. pylori–driven B-cell proliferation leading to lymphoma.

MALT lymphomas (MALT lymphoma with a large B-cell component) is only 52% to 71%, while with purely DLBCLs (formerly high-grade MALToma) it is only 25% to 38%.[121–123] Similarly, H. pylori can be demonstrated in 90% of cases when the tumor is limited to mucosa and submucosa, but in only 76% of the cases with submucosal spread of the tumor, and 48% of the cases when the tumor extends beyond submucosa.[124]

The notion that the gastric mucosa (unlike small and large bowels) normally lacks organized lymphoid tissue is belied by experience in which small lymphoid aggregates can be found immediately above the muscularis mucosae even in children who have no indication of ever having had Helicobacter. However, the lamina propria shows only scattered lymphocytes and plasma cells. It has been hypothesized that H. pylori induces a lymphoid infiltrate associated with lymphoid follicles that is similar to the MALT of intestines and provides the background for the development of lymphoma.[120] It has been shown in vitro that the tumor cells from a MALT lymphoma proliferate when incubated with heat-killed H. pylori, but die rapidly in the absence of H. pylori or when only chemical mitogens are used.[125] This proliferative response also disappears when the T cells are removed from the culture.[126] Addition of supernatant from another culture of unseparated tumor cells fails to restore cell proliferation, suggesting direct contact with T cells rather than secreted cytokines is important.[126] This proliferative response to H. pylori not only appears to be strain specific for a given tumor, but varies among tumors from different patients. These observations suggest that the tumor is at least in part antigen dependent

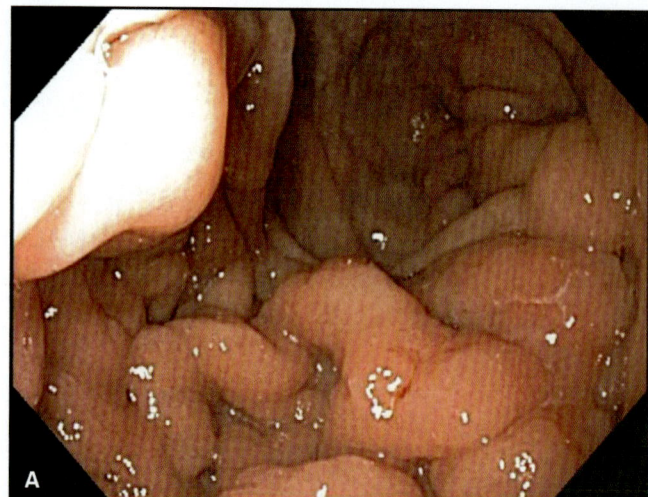 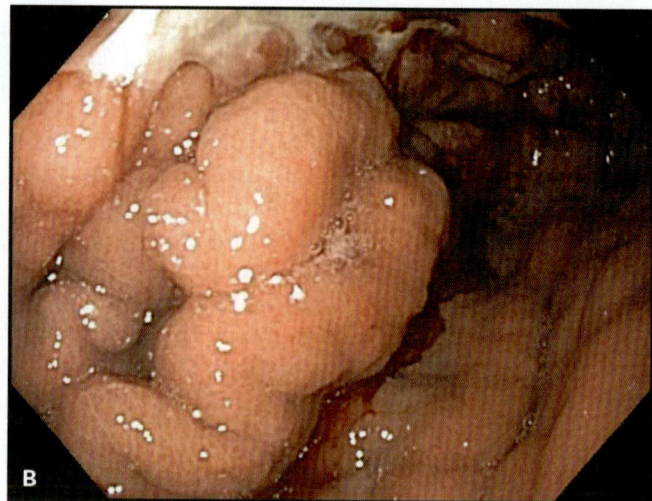

Figure 4-15. Lymphoma of the stomach: endoscopic appearances. **A:** Showing nodular mucosal lesions. **B:** Showing irregular mucosal masses, which may be indistinguishable from carcinoma. (Courtesy J. Nord, M.D.)

and that *H. pylori* is the most likely antigen. It is also clear from these experiments that T cells play a vital role in the B-cell proliferation and that the B cells themselves are not *H. pylori* specific but make antibodies to a variety of autoantigens, including parietal cells and the proton pump that can result in gradual atrophy of specialized gastric mucosa. While the initial B-cell proliferation is *H. pylori* driven and polyclonal, subsequent molecular and genetic alterations lead to clonal expansion and autonomous growth. Whether *H. pylori*–specific factors play a role in the development of lymphoma is still somewhat controversial.[127–129] The *H. pylori* strains, which accelerate the tumor growth, include the Cag A strain, a gene found in approximately 60% of *H. pylori* organisms, and the vac A (vacuolating cytotoxin) genotype.[129–131] MALT lymphomas associated with *H. heilmanni* infection have also been reported.[132] The cell of origin of MALT lymphomas is a B-cell that is identical to lymphocytes of the marginal zone of lymphoid follicles. These represent postfollicular B cells, and antigen selection occurs in some cases.[133–135]

Clinical features. MALT lymphomas occur predominantly in the stomach in middle-aged or older patients although on rare occasions they have been reported in younger patients, as young as 7 years of age.[136,137] The tumor occurs more commonly in males (M:F = 1.5:1), the mean age being around 60 for males and 65 for females. The majority of the patients present with nonspecific symptoms that include epigastric pain, nausea, vomiting, or dyspepsia, similar to peptic ulcer disease. Patients with advanced disease or high-grade lymphomas tend to have signs and symptoms that mimic gastric carcinoma, such as early satiety, weight loss, hemorrhage, and anemia. Some cases may have a frank obstruction accompanied by a palpable mass.

Endoscopically, the tumors often have a varied and nondiagnostic appearance that includes severe thickened folds, superficial erosions, or deep ulcers (Fig. 4-15). In some instances the mucosa may show only minimal hyperemia or even appear normal. The lesions may be multifocal as shown by the microscopic involvement of apparently normally appearing mucosa in some cases. These findings are also reflected in the imaging studies, either CT scan or ultrasound-based evaluations. Endoscopic ultrasound (EUS) is a valuable imaging modality in evaluating the extent of involvement by lymphoma.[138]

Pathology. The gross appearance of the tumor is highly varied and includes flat, granular, or nodular mucosa; minimal to mild surface erosions; thickened folds; and ulcers or ill-defined diffusely infiltrative lesions (Fig. 4-16). However, the most common presentation resembles chronic active gastritis or gastric ulcers. Polypoid masses or ugly ulceroproliferative lesions are most commonly associated with advanced disease or high-grade tumors where the lesions could easily reach 8 cm in diameter. Typically, the lesions are localized to the mucosa and submucosa, and the infiltrative growth results in either uniform or localized thickening of the wall. In some cases tumors are associated with the destruction of the full thickness of the gastric wall without an associated desmoplastic reaction and may lead to perforation. On cut section they have a characteristic white homogeneous fish-flesh appearance. As most of the lymphomas are low grade, detected early, and treated medically, fewer gastric resections with large lesions are encountered in current practice.

The most common site at presentation is the antrum. However, subsequently the tumor may spread throughout the stomach. Frequently it is multifocal,

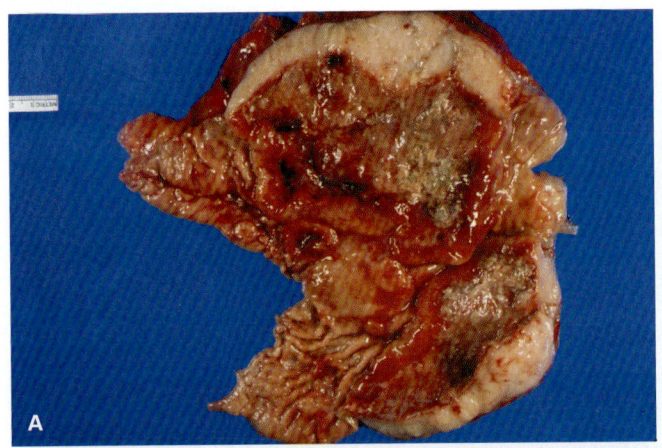
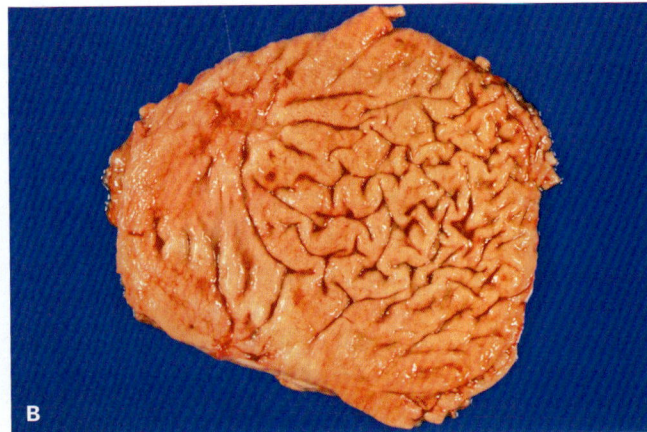
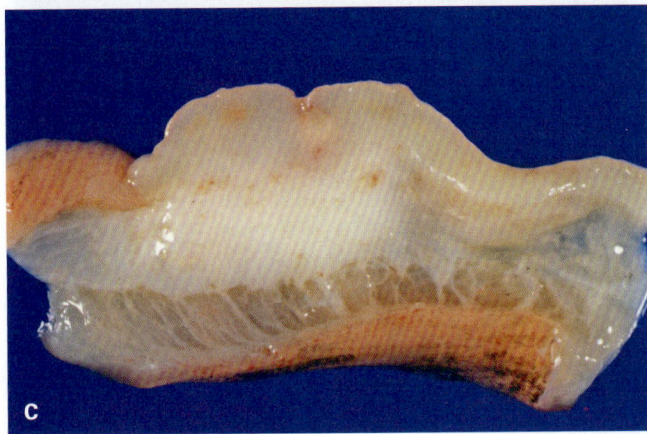

Figure 4-16. **A:** Gross photograph of a resection specimen of stomach showing large ulcerating lesion with marked thickening of the stomach wall. The cut section shows fleshy grey-white tumor diffusely involving the wall without any well-defined borders. **B:** Another specimen of stomach showing smaller ulcerating lesion with thickening of the mucosal folds around it. **C:** The cut section shows fleshy grey-white tumor infiltrating into the submucosa and muscularis propria without any well-defined borders.

although many foci may be microscopic in size. Once the infiltrate extends into the submucosa, it tends to separate the muscle fibers of the muscularis mucosae and either grows in a band-like manner, with a pushing border, or invades with an irregularly infiltrating margin. Eventually, the muscle undergoes atrophy, resulting in the marked weakening of the viscus and a propensity to perforation. The regional lymph node involvement is distinctly uncommon with superficial lesions and is seen once the tumor spreads to the muscularis propria or undergoes transformation to high grade.

The microscopic findings in MALT lymphomas are also varied and range from chronic active gastritis-like to typical nodal marginal zone lymphomas (Fig. 4-17). The majority of MALT lymphomas are limited to the mucosa and superficial submucosa, resulting in thickening of the mucosa with separation or gradual replacement of the glandular component. Initially, the crypts or glands are pushed apart from one another and upward from the underlying muscularis mucosae by the lymphoid infiltrate. Morphologically, the MALT lymphomas characteristically have histologic features that mimic normal MALT and are most commonly associated with a background of chronic active gastritis, but in which the monomorphous lymphoma appears to push aside the *Helicobacter* gastritis. The tumor cells tend to form monomorphous sheets of lymphocytes and infiltrate into the gastric pits, glands, or surface epithelium. The latter create the lymphoepithelial lesions, which are characterized by clusters of at least three or more atypical B cells infiltrating and destroying the foveolar or glandular epithelium (see Figs. 4-17 and 4-19). As normal IELs are usually T cells and therefore CD3 immunoreactive, the presence of these cells as B cells also aids with the diagnosis. However, if T-cell stains are carried out, MALT lymphomas appear to be T-cell driven so that the number of T cells is invariably as frequent as B cells to the point that a dearth of T cells should cast doubt on the diagnosis. The damaged epithelial cells often assume an eosinophilic/oncocytic appearance and may not be readily appreciable on H&E sections. In such situations, keratin stains are very useful to highlight the lymphoepithelial lesions. Occasionally, benign-appearing clusters of lymphocytes are found in the surface and crypt epithelium that represent the normal transmigrating lymphocytes. They differ from the lymphoepithelial lesions in that phenotypically they are T cells and they do not destroy the epithelium.[139,140]

Lymphoid follicles are almost invariably present in MALT lymphomas and are frequently partially or totally surrounded by a sheath of atypical lymphocytes and plasma cells, which may be reactive or monotypic, occupying the mantle or marginal zones. These cells

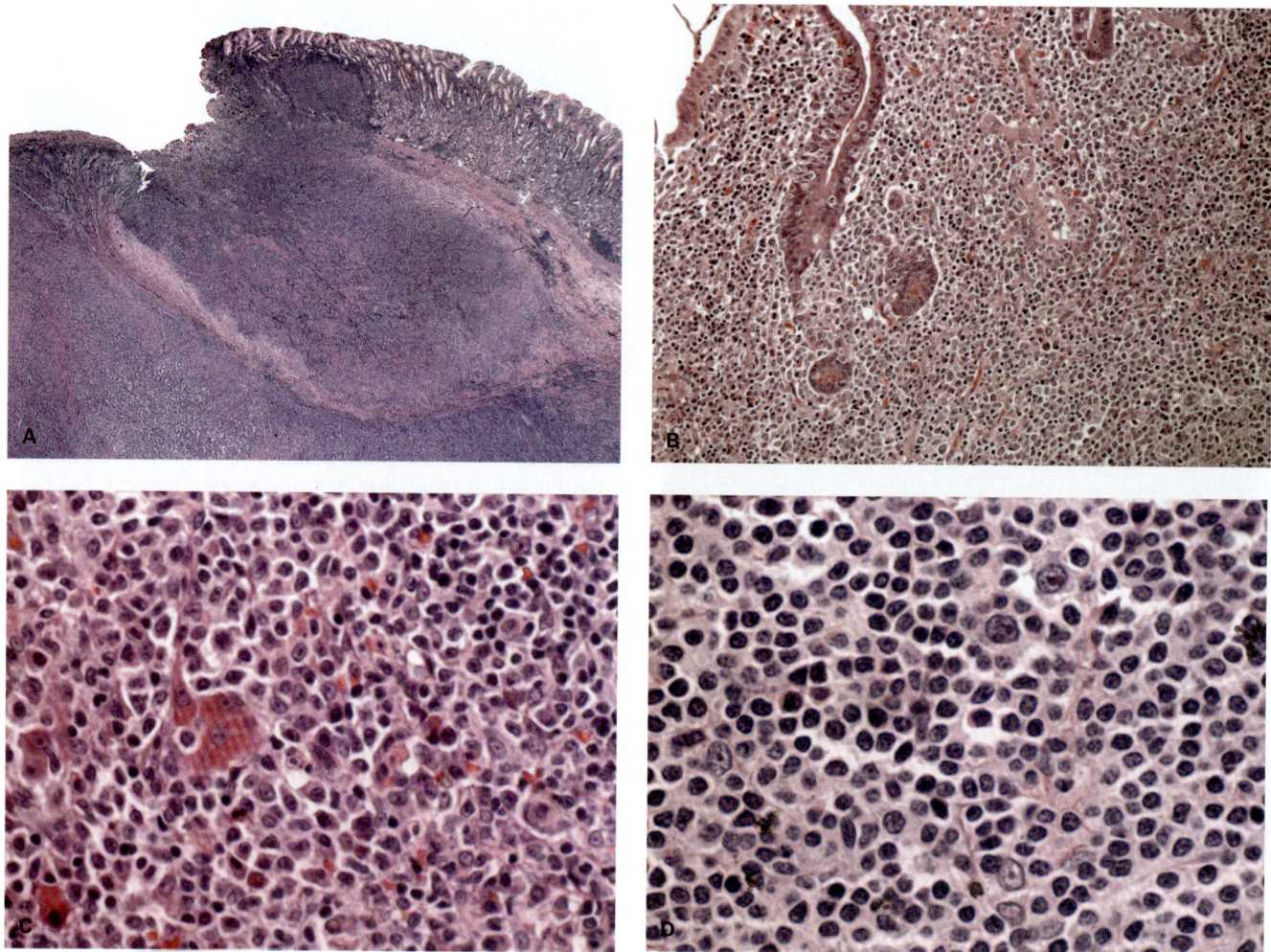

Figure 4-17. Microscopic appearance of gastric malt lymphoma. **A:** Low power showing extensive lymphocytic infiltrate with ulceration of mucosa and extension into the wall of the stomach. **B:** Lymphoepithelial lesions showing clusters of monocytoid B-cell infiltrating the glands. **C:** High power showing mixture of cells with many small lymphocyte-like cells, centrocyte-like cells, and plasma cells. **D:** High power showing large centroblasts/immunoblast-like cells interspersed among small lymphocyte-like cells.

tend to spread out from the marginal zone of the follicle to infiltrate the interfollicular zone and destroy the glands. Occasionally, these cells may also infiltrate the center of the follicle (follicular colonization), producing a vague nodular architecture (Fig. 4-18).[141] This can be easily demonstrated by dendritic cell markers (CD21, CD23, or CD35) that highlight the background of dendritic reticulum cells in the colonized follicle. Another invariable finding in over 90% of these patients is the presence of *H. pylori* infection.

Cytologically, the MALT lymphomas frequently consist of an admixture of various lymphocytic cell types, although one cell type may predominate in a given case. The commonly found types of lymphocytes are the following:

1. Small lymphocytes resembling normal mature lymphocytes but differing slightly in that they have somewhat enlarged irregular or wrinkled nuclei with less dense chromatin. MALT lymphomas with predominantly these types of cells may be difficult to distinguish from disseminated nodal small lymphocytic lymphoma/chronic lymphocytic leukemia (SLL/CLL) or occasionally a mantle cell lymphoma.
2. Lymphoplasmacytoid cells often containing intracytoplasmic immunoglobulin, commonly of the IgM class, with light chain restriction and Dutcher bodies (intranuclear periodic acid Schiff [PAS] positive inclusions). The presence of lymphoplasmacytoid cells in MALT lymphomas needs to be differentiated from the rare pure "small lymphocytic or plasmacytoid lymphomas" (immunocytomas of the Kiel classification), which are found in lymph nodes, spleen, bone marrow, and less frequently extranodal sites. Some of these cases may be associated with Waldenström's macroglobulinemia. Some authorities consider this tumor to be distinct from MALT lymphomas.

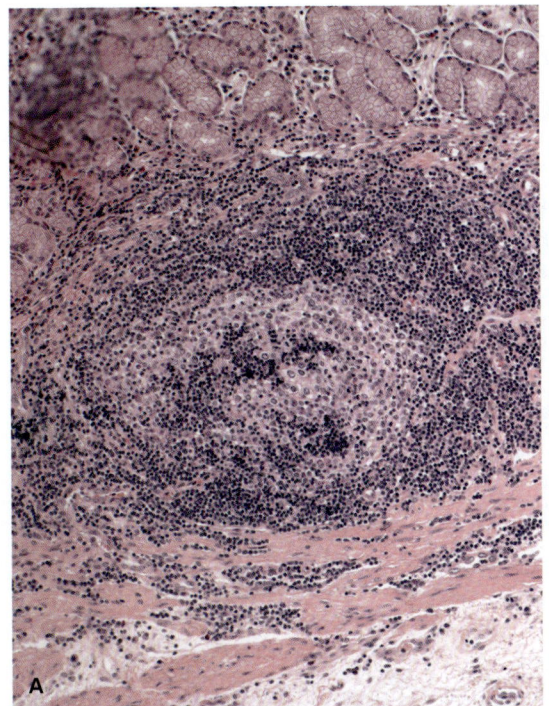

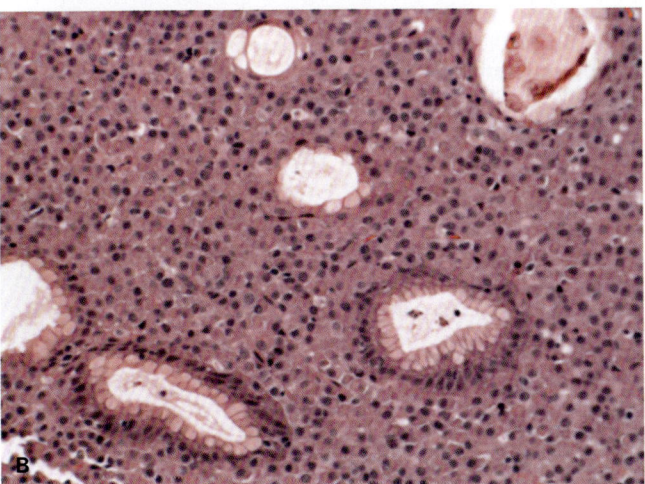

Figure 4-18. **A:** Microscopic appearance of follicular invasion by the marginal bone cells in a case of malt lymphoma of the stomach. **B:** Malt lymphoma of the stomach showing a predominant population of plasma cells. Often the plasma cells are localized in the superficial lamina propria.

3. CCLs are lymphocytes intermediate between small lymphocytic and small cleaved cell lymphomas, which have dense nuclei that are irregular in shape but are not as cleaved as the classical cleaved cell lymphoma. Variants of these cells, which have more abundant clear cytoplasm and well-defined cell margins, resembling *monocytoid B cells*, are frequently found.

In addition, large noncleaved lymphoblasts or immunoblasts may be scattered in between the small lymphocytes and do not imply high-grade transformation (Fig. 4-17C). Frequently there are large numbers of interspersed reactive T cells. Mature plasma cells are also frequently present and are most commonly distributed below the surface epithelium. The plasma cell component can be very prominent in some cases and may mimic a primary plasma cell disorder (see Fig. 4-18B). The cytoplasmic immunoglobulin in the lymphoplasmacytic cells has a perinuclear distribution and may be so abundant that it produces a "signet-ring"–like appearance mimicking a carcinoma.[142] Since the immunoglobulin is preserved in formalin-fixed tissues and is PAS positive, it may cause further confusion with signet-ring cell carcinoma to the unwary, especially in small biopsies. On rare occasions metaplastic goblet cells from the surface or glandular epithelium may become pinched off by the lymphoid infiltrate and appear to lie isolated in the stroma, simulating signet-ring cell carcinoma.

Immunophenotype and molecular genetics. Immunohistochemically, the lymphomatous cells express surface and to a lesser extent cytoplasmic immunoglobulin, primarily IgM, which shows light chain restriction and rarely IgG or IgA. In addition, they are characteristically CD5, CD10, BCL1, and CD23 negative, but positive for the other B-cell markers (CD20, CD21, CD22, CD35, BCL2, CD79a, and CD23) and often CD43.[8] In small biopsies, it may not be possible to perform all the markers, and one has to wisely choose a small panel that helps to differentiate MALT lymphoma from its mimics in a given case (see Table 4-5).

Many genetic and epigenetic abnormalities have been described in MALT lymphomas. However, most MALT lymphomas (about 70%–85%) do not have a specific translocation, yet there are four translocations that are specifically associated with MALT lymphomas and at the molecular level share a physiological role for BCL10 and MALT1 in antigen receptor–mediated NFkB activation.[143] These include chromosomal translocations: t(11;18)(q21;q21), important because it predicts lack of response to *Helicobacter* eradication therapy, and t(1;14)(p22;q32) and t(14;18)(q32;q21) that seem to be specific for MALT lymphomas and have diagnostic and prognostic importance.[144-146] Another more recently recognized translocation with MALT lymphomas is t(3;14)(p14.1q32) and suggests a role of FOXP-1. The proposed molecular mechanisms and pathogenesis of *H. pylori*–associated MALT lymphomas are shown in Figure 4-14. Other abnormalities include trisomies 3, 12, 18; *p53* mutation/LOH; *p15* and *p16* promoter methylation; and *fas* mutation.[147-154]

Translocation t(11;18)(q21;q21) In most of the translocation positive cases, t(11;18)(q21;q21) is the sole chromosomal abnormality.[144,145] This translocation causes reciprocal fusion of the API2 and MALT1

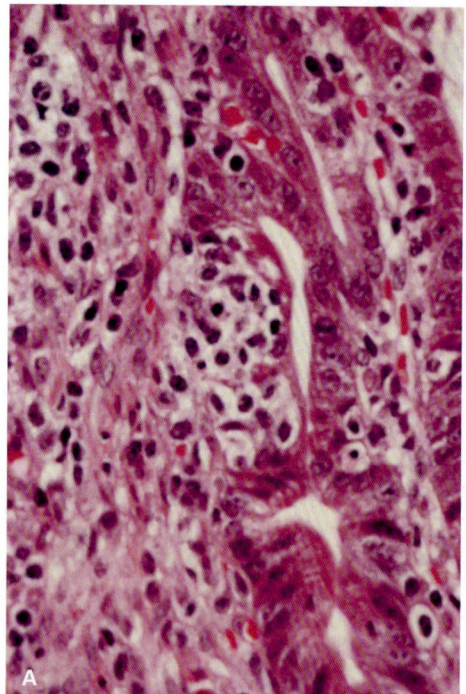
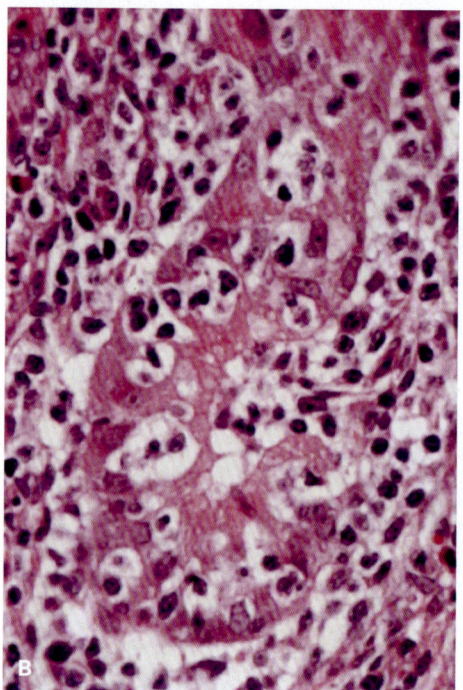
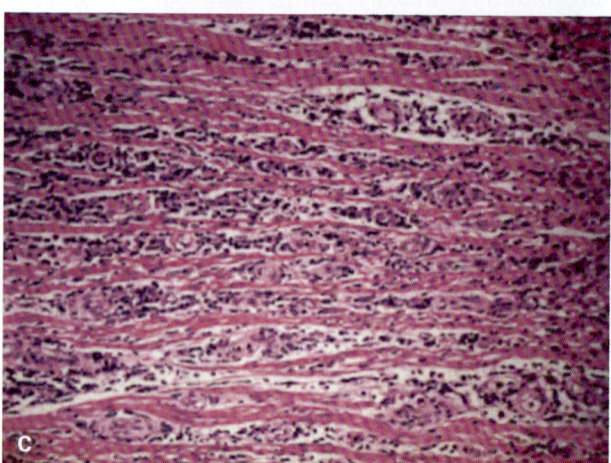

Figure 4-19. MALT lymphoma of the stomach. **A,B:** Medium-power photomicrographs showing infiltration of glands by the atypical lymphocytes. **C:** Lymphoma showing separation of the muscle fibers of the muscularis propria by the lymphomatous infiltrate.

genes.[155–157] The API2 is an apoptosis inhibitor, whereas MALT1 is involved in antigen receptor–mediated NFkB activation. The fusion transcript is consistently expressed in these cases and is believed to be oncogenic. Unlike wild-type API2 and MALT1, API2–MALT1 fusion product is a potent activator of NFkB. NFkB activation in turn leads to activation of other cytokine and growth factor genes that are important for cellular activation, proliferation, and survival, thus contributing to tumor development.[158–160] This translocation is seen in about 15% to 30% of gastric MALT lymphomas.[161] The same translocation has also been described in MALT lymphomas of other sites including skin and lungs. However, it is absent in nodal and splenic marginal zone lymphomas.[162–165] Cases of *H. pylori* gastritis also do not show this translocation. MALT lymphomas with this translocation do *not* respond to *H. pylori* eradication and more often spread to distant sites including regional lymph nodes.[166] An initial report suggested that despite the association of t(11;18)(q21;q21) with adverse clinical features, the translocation is uncommonly found in cases with DLBCLs or so-called transformed MALT lymphomas, that is, low-grade MALT lymphomas with a large-cell component.[167,168] A subsequent study however shows that this translocation is seen with almost equal frequency in transformed MALT lymphomas or DLBCLs of the stomach.[169] Even if found, *H. pylori* eradication treatment is undertaken together with other lymphoma therapy.

Translocation t(1;14)(p22;q32) The second common MALT lymphoma associated translocation is t(1;14)(p22;q32). Cases positive for this translocation are often associated with trisomies 3, 12, and 18, unlike t(11;18)(q21;q21).[146] The translocation brings the entire BCL10 gene under the regulatory control of the Ig gene and deregulates its expression.[143,170] Earlier studies showed that although BCL10 activates NFkB, it is weakly pro-apoptotic.[171,172] However, subsequent studies have shown that BCL10 does not have proapoptotic activity in vivo.[173,174] It is essential for the development of B- and T-cell functions and specifically links the antigen receptor signaling to NFkB pathway.[175-177] In response to the surface antigen receptor stimulation, BCL10 oligomerizes and binds to MALT1, leading to MALT1 oligomerizartion that in turn activates NFkB. In line with the physiological role of BCL10 in normal B cells, the protein is expressed predominantly in the cytoplasm of germinal center B cells.[178] BCL10 is strongly expressed in the nuclei of MALT lymphomas with t(1;14)(p22;q32) or its variants.[178] However, moderate nuclear BCL10 expression is also seen in about 50% of cases negative for this translocation and in almost all t(11;18)(q21;q21)-positive cases.[161,165,179] Studies using BCL10 immunostains and interphase FISH analysis show that t(1;14)(p22;q32) is specifically associated with MALT lymphomas and not with other lymphoma subtypes.[165] This translocation occurs in about 5% of gastric MALT lymphomas and has also been associated with MALT lymphomas of lungs.[165] Gastric MALT lymphomas with this translocation are typically at advanced stages and unlikely to respond to H. pylori eradication.

Translocation t(14;18)(p32;q21) The third MALT lymphoma associated translocation t(14;18)(p32;q21) is different from the similar translocation seen in follicular lymphomas. In follicular lymphomas this translocation brings BCL2 at 18q21 in proximity to Ig heavy chain (IgH) locus. The same breakpoint in MALT lymphomas involves MALT1 instead of BCL2.[180] It is proposed that IgH-MALT1 fusion results in activation of MALT1 that somehow stabilizes BCL10 in the cytoplasm. BCL10 in turn then leads to aberrant activation of NFkB pathway. This translocation has so far been shown to be associated with MALT lymphomas of the lungs and ocular adenxae, but not stomach.[164,180,181]

Translocation t(3;14)(p14;1q32) This is the more recently recognized MALT lymphoma–associated translocation that brings FOXP1 gene in proximity to Ig heavy chain gene and results in its deregulation.[182] FOXP1 belongs to the Forkhead box family of winged-helix transcription factors that have diverse function in different cell types and plays an important role in B-cell development. This translocation was detected in a single case (1.7%, n = 59) of MALT lymphoma studied and seems to correlate with poor outcome and transformation to DLBCL.[182,183] This translocation has also been reported in isolated cases of gastric DLBCL.

Treatment and prognosis. These are typically slow-growing lesions that remain localized to the stomach for long periods (stage 1E), often more than 7 to 10 years.[138,184,185] The majority of gastric MALT lymphomas at the time of presentation are confined to the mucosa and submucosa. There is a low incidence of mesenteric node involvement and extraintestinal dissemination, although in one study bone marrow involvement was found in 10% of the patients.[5] Recurrence of these low-grade tumors occurs primarily in patients with an increased number of transformed lymphocytes (5%–10%) and involves the original site or other parts of the GI tract, mesenteric lymph nodes, or Waldeyer ring, rather than widespread extraintestinal dissemination.

The overall prognosis of these patients is excellent. As has been discussed earlier, remission of the majority of MALT lymphomas (67%–90%) occurs following the treatment of H. pylori.[186-188] This is largely applicable to tumors that do not have a high-grade component and are localized to mucosa or superficial submucosa. Advanced tumors or those with a high-grade component have also been reported to respond to H. pylori eradication, but infrequently. In several large studies, 90% of patients survived for 5 years and 65% to 75% of patients for 10 years. Whether the patients are truly cured still remains to be determined. Relapses have been shown to occur in about 10% of patients.[189] In some patients, the relapses have been associated with reinfection with H. pylori and successful remission following eradication of the infection again.

It is increasingly becoming clear that molecular genetics has an important role in predicting the behavior of gastric MALT lymphomas. Tumors with t(11;18)(q21;q21) translocation generally do not respond to H. pylori eradication, even though they are rarely associated with large-cell transformation. Chemotherapy (sometimes with radiation) and occasionally surgery are the options for cases that do not respond to H. pylori eradication. Surgical resection on its own has been associated with prolonged survival in some studies.[190] Involvement of the resection margin and advanced stage are poor prognostic factors, but not when adjuvant chemotherapy is also used.[191] These tumors invariably express CD20, and resistant cases or those with large-cell component have been successfully treated with rituximab; however, long-term outcome of such cases is still unknown.[192] Irrespective of the treatment modality, the only independent prognostic variables are stage and tumor grade.[191,193-196]

Reporting MALT lymphomas. There is considerable variation in how pathologists report gastric MALT lymphomas in biopsies. When the biopsies are adequate and the morphology and immunohistochemistry are typical, many are comfortable making the diagnosis, while some always hedge by stating "consistent with". One of the problems with MALT lymphomas is the lack of a distinct immunohistochemical profile, and stains are largely used to exclude other lymphoma types (mantle, follicular, CLL etc). Presence of one of the MALT associated translocation should certainly help one in making a definitive diagnosis however, these are present only in a small proportion of cases and are still not readily available in all labs. Nevertheless, pathologists should still be comfortable making this diagnosis in the presence of appropriate histology with the knowledge that the first line of therapy is *Helicobacter* eradication followed by re-endoscopy and biopsy a few months later. If the morphology and immunohistochemistry are all correct, but *Helicobacter* cannot be demonstrated or the biopsies are too small, reporting them as "atypical lymphoid infiltrate" and suggest follow-up biopsies for a full lymphoma work-up with flow-cytometry, molecular assays and serology for *Helicobacter*.

Follow-up of patients with treated MALT lymphoma. Follow-up of these patients after therapy involves periodic endoscopic and EUS examinations and biopsies.[197] It should be remembered that where there has been an endoscopically visible lesion associated with *Helicobacter*, following its eradication the primary purpose of the endoscopy is to ensure that the lymphoma is regressing or at least not increasing in size. The latter would suggest incomplete eradication of *Helicobacter*, a translocation associated with lack of response to *Helicobacter* therapy or a large-cell component. Biopsies would therefore be *expected* to contain residual MALT lymphoma, and the demonstration that this is the case is unnecessary.

Role of the pathologist. The role of the pathologist is therefore not to just confirm the presence of residual lymphoma, which is a given as these cells are long-lived and may persist for long periods of time following the withdrawal of the antigenic stimulus, but to also

1. Identify the presence of a large-cell component when present.
2. Identify *Helicobacter* if present (coccoid forms are not acceptable and are much more likely to be oral or enteric in origin). It should also be recalled that patients on long-term PPIs may allow oral organisms to grow in their stomachs. These are usually polymorphous and can include fungi. *Helicobacter* therefore have to be photographable (stand up in court) but are important to identify as the lymphoma will not regress until eradication is complete.
3. A useful stain is Mib-1 to evaluate the proportion of cells in non-G0 phase of cell cycle, especially if this can be compared with a pretreatment biopsy, as the proliferation usually falls off markedly once the antigenic stimulus is withdrawn. In the absence of a large-cell component, a persistently high Mib-1 rate suggests persistent *Helicobacter*, but if these are really absent, one needs to carry out translocation studies. Although monoclonal antibodies to one of the translocation products and also BCL10, which has been suggested as a surrogate marker, are helpful, at the time of writing these are not reliable enough to be part of routine practice. However, in some centers it is thought that there is an economic advantage in looking for the translocations, especially the t(11;14), as it can be predicted that these will not respond to *Helicobacter* eradication, so the patients will need chemotherapy (which does not preclude *Helicobacter* eradication).

The long-term follow-up biopsies from patients continuing to respond to *Helicobacter* eradication therapy ultimately show that the number of biopsies with MALT tend to diminish and disappear over time. At this stage biopsies often show an empty-looking lamina propria with rare B cells or plasma cells.[198] Sometimes small aggregates of normal-appearing small lymphocytic B cells and scattered T cells are also evident and do not imply residual/recurrent lymphoma. Studies using PCR and Ig gene rearrangement have shown that residual clones can be identified in many cases without any histologic evidence of residual disease.[197,199] It has been shown that histologic remission may take many months or years (median 33, range 0–65 months), while molecular remission takes longer.[198,200–202] At present, the significance of the persistent molecular abnormality in the setting of clinical and histologic remission remains unclear. However, current data also do not justify further treatment of persistent monoclonality by molecular assays in the absence of histologic or clinical disease.

Lastly, it should be noted that the patients with MALT lymphomas also seem to have an increased incidence of gastric adenocarcinoma.[203] This often arises in the distal stomach and appears to occur irrespective of the type of therapy for the lymphoma.

Differential diagnosis and practical approach to the difficult diagnosis. Whenever there is dense lymphocytic infiltrate in the gastric mucosal biopsies, the differential diagnosis includes a lymphoma. The problems often one faces in this situation are as follows:

1. When the infiltrate is polymorphous, the issue is to differentiate between *H. pylori*–associated chronic active gastritis and MALT lymphoma.

2. When only a small focus of B lymphocytes invading a crypt forming an isolated lymphoepithelial lesion is identified (mini-MALT lymphoma).
3. When the lymphocytic infiltrate is clearly neoplastic, the issue is the correct subclassification of the lymphoma.

Chronic Gastritis versus Malt Lymphoma This situation is frequently encountered in routine practice. The lymphocytic infiltrate in lymphoma tends to be more destructive and expansible, with extensive permeation between the glands. The presence of significant numbers of small cleaved cells (CLC or monocytoid B cells) also supports the diagnosis; however, in some cases these features are not readily evident. The presence of convincing lymphoepithelial lesions strongly favors the diagnosis of MALT lymphoma, although one needs to be careful as they can also be seen in florid *H. pylori* gastritis (usually single, consist of <3 cells and rarely destructive) as well as other types of lymphomas. The presence of Dutcher bodies or intranuclear inclusions in more than a few plasma cells is also suggestive of lymphoma; however, similar to other sites mere presence of these inclusions by itself is not diagnostic. In reactive lymphoid infiltrate the B cells are typically organized in nodules even though the lymphoid follicles may not be easily evident, and the T cells reside in the interfollicular zones. This pattern can be easily appreciated with CD20 and CD3 immunostains. If CD20 stain shows a diffuse densely packed infiltrate of B cells with limited number of interspersed T cells, this pattern supports a diagnosis of lymphoma. Light chain restriction using immunostains for κ and λ light chains may be helpful in demonstrating a monotypic Ig supporting the diagnosis of lymphoma. However, interpretation of these immunostains performed on paraffin sections is not always straightforward unless overtly plasmacytic. In addition, a polyclonal infiltrate of chronic gastritis often coexists in the background, and one needs to carefully interpret the stain in the atypical cells. Coexpression of CD43 by CD20-positive B cells also supports the diagnosis of lymphoma, although a normal immunophenotype does not exclude this possibility. Detection of a clonally rearranged Ig gene by PCR in the presence of atypical infiltrate is diagnostic of lymphoma. However, a diagnosis of lymphoma should never be based solely based on this finding. Demonstration of any of the MALT lymphoma–associated translocations as discussed above using RT-PCR or FISH is also diagnostic of lymphoma. This not only provides an evidence of a clonal B-cell expansion but represents a MALT-specific abnormality that also has a prognostic significance. If the studies are inconclusive or equivocal, and the biopsy shows an evidence of *H. pylori* gastritis, repeat biopsies can be suggested following the treatment for *H. pylori*. In such a setting, it would be appropriate to use the designation "atypical lymphocytic infiltrate of uncertain nature or significance." If in a similar setting *H. pylori* is negative, repeat biopsy with more sampling should be suggested sooner than later. If biopsies are performed for confirming a diagnosis of lymphoma, it is advantageous to have additional samples for flow cytometry and molecular studies obtained at the outset.

Mini-MALT Lymphomas In *Helicobacter*-positive patients, one sometimes comes across a focus of monotonous lymphoid cells surrounding one or two pits that contrasts with the plasma cell rich polymorphous infiltrate of the background gastritis. Further, there may be a focus of IELs mimicking a lymphoepithelial lesion, although these are rarely destructive. In our experience, some of them even show B-cell clonality based on immunoglobulin gene rearrangement studies. These likely represent the earliest stages of MALT lymphoma and likely disappear following *H. pylori* eradication. Since prospective studies looking at the natural history of such lesions are lacking, a cautious approach is warranted. We do not report these as MALT lymphomas but do not ignore them completely either, stating that a lymphoepithelial-like lesion is present associated with the *Helicobacter* gastritis and that this will likely disappear following *Helicobacter* eradication therapy. While calling such lesions as outright MALT lymphoma in the absence of any supportive molecular evidence may be an overkill, a suggestion in the report that *Helicobacter* eradication therapy should be considered to ensure these lesions do not progress is justified. Given the frequency of these lesions if carefully looked for and the rarity of MALT lymphomas, it is likely that progression of these lesions to overt MALT lymphoma is extremely rare.

Subtyping of a Small Lymphocytic Lymphoma In some cases, the lymphomatous nature of the infiltrate is obvious on histology due to the monotonous appearance of the infiltrate, its destructive nature, or cellular anaplasia. However, not all lymphomas of the stomach are MALT lymphomas, and proper subtyping of the lymphoma is essential as the clinical outcome of similar-appearing lesions is vastly different. The difficulties often arise due to small sample size or crush artifacts that obscure the histologic details and pattern. The entities that often come into the differential diagnosis include SLL/CLL, follicular lymphoma, and mantle cell lymphoma. The presence of lymphoepithelial lesions, though helpful, is not diagnostic in this situation as they have been described with a variety of other primary or secondary lymphomas of the stomach. Immunophenotyping and demonstration of specific translocations are extremely valuable in this setting. However, if the sample is small and the findings are inconclusive, additional biopsies for diagnostic workup should be requested. CLL/SLLs have often involvement of peripheral blood, and knowledge of the peripheral blood findings could be helpful.

One of the most difficult and controversial issues is the recognition of DLBCL or, as formerly called, "large-cell/high-grade transformation" of MALT lymphomas (also see later). As defined in the WHO classification, the presence of sheets of large B cells is required to make this diagnosis; however, what constitutes a "sheet" is unclear.[29] Scattered centroblasts and immunoblasts intermingled with the infiltrate are not uncommon in MALT lymphomas, and it has been suggested that more than 10% of large cells should prompt a diagnosis of DLBCL. More than 30% staining with Ki67 has also been suggested to support the diagnosis of DLBCL.

Diffuse Large B-cell Lymphoma of the Stomach

This group comprises MALT lymphomas with high-grade transformation and primary de novo large B-cell lymphomas of the stomach.[8,204] It had been lumped under high-grade MALT lymphomas in the past. The recommendation of the WHO classification is not to use the term high-grade MALT lymphoma,[28] although if one of the recognized MALT translocations or other appropriate molecular abnormalities is present or the patient had a previous low-grade gastric MALT lymphoma, it is difficult to come to any other conclusion. DLBCL can be divided into the following categories:

1. Low-grade MALT lymphoma with a minor DLBCL component comprised of only occasional clusters of large cells.
2. Equal admixture of DLBCL and MALT lymphoma components.
3. DLBCL with a small component of MALT lymphoma.
4. DLBCL without a MALT lymphoma component.

The relative proportion of each group varies in different studies largely due to lack of uniform diagnostic criteria and variation in classification.[205–207] The presence of identical Ig heavy chain rearrangement in both components strongly suggests transformation of the low-grade MALT lymphoma to the large-cell component in many cases.[208,209] Occasionally, genetic difference between the two components suggests an independent evolution or dedifferentiation. Cases of purely DLBCL may represent cases of MALT lymphomas, where the large-cell component may have completely overgrown the low-grade tumor or a de novo large B-cell lymphoma (Fig. 4-20).[194] Nevertheless, an increasing large-cell component is associated with a reduced positivity for *H. pylori*, increasing non-responsiveness to *H. pylori* eradication, and higher stage, and hence the rationale to lump them together as DLBCL seems justified.

What is the minimum requirement to classify a case as DLBCL is unclear. Scattered large cells represented by centroblasts or immunoblasts are often seen admixed with the small lymphocytic infiltrate in MALT lymphomas. Studies have shown that diffusely scattered large cells when not forming clusters or sheets do not adversely affect the prognosis, even if they constitute about 20% of the cell population.[195,205] However, others have reported that the presence of up to 10% of scattered large cells, some of which form small clusters, have a worse outcome after a long-term follow-up.[195] What is a small cluster or a sheet to qualify for a large-cell transformation also remains

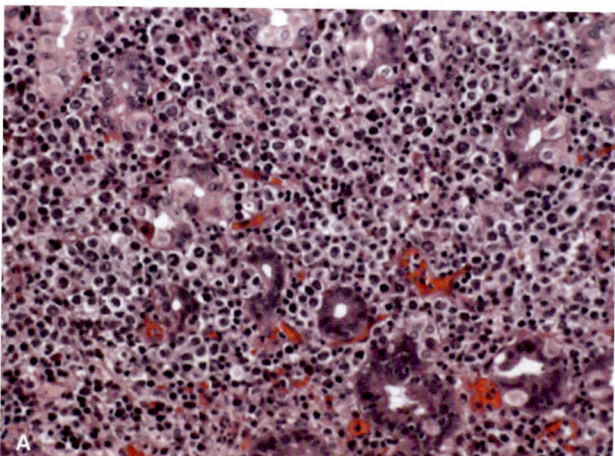
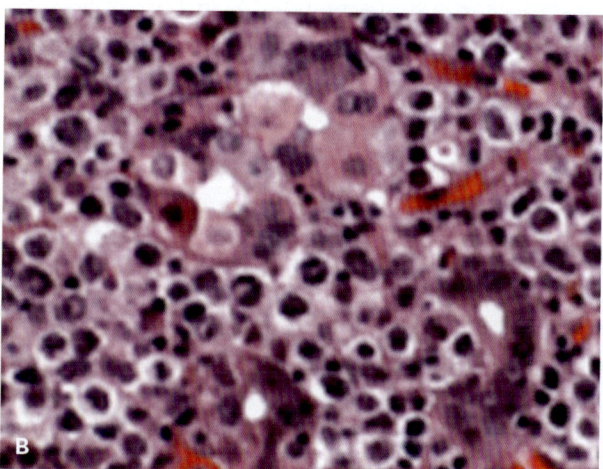

Figure 4-20. A: Appearance of DLBCL of the stomach. The morphology resembles that of an extranodal DLBCL of the stomach. **B:** There are numerous large cells in a background of *H. pylori*–positive MALT-type lymphomas and lymphoepithelial lesions are still clearly visible.

unclear; however, most authorities require the presence of at least 20 large cells.[195,205] In practice, counting such large cells is not practical, and most people simply eyeball the large-cell component, and despite the lack of any consensus in literature, most cases do not pose any problems in practice (Fig 4-20A).

The DLBCL tend to occur in older individuals (mean seventh decade) as compared to MALT lymphomas, and there is a slight male predominance.[205,206] The clinical presentation and symptoms more frequently mimic gastric carcinoma compared to MALT lymphomas.

The immunophenotype of DLBCL as expected shows considerable overlap with low-grade MALT lymphoma. Although most of the cases are CD10 and BCL6 negative, a subset may express CD10, BCL6, or BCL2.[206,210,211] In some cases, the phenotype (CD10−, BCL6+) is suggestive of a germinal center cell differentiation. Ig heavy and light chains are clonally rearranged, while some cases may also show BCL6 rearrangement. Although initial studies showed MALT-associated t(11;18) was uncommon in DLBCL, a subsequent study shows that this translocation is seen with almost equal frequency in transformed MALT lymphomas or DLBCLs of the stomach.[169]

The molecular events underlying the transformation of MALT lymphoma are complex and not fully understood.[212] Various molecular genetic events that have been associated with large-cell transformation include inactivation of tumor suppressor gene *p53* by allelic deletion and mutation, LOH of *APC* gene, homologous deletion of the *p16* gene, which is an inhibitor of the cyclin-dependent kinase Cdk4 and Cdk6, chromosomal translocation involving the *c-myc* and *BCL6* genes, and mutations in the *fas* gene.[3] Amplification of genomic material in the BCL6 location and mixed lineage leukemia (MLL) gene has been found in some cases. However, in general, currently no reliable genetic abnormality differentiates transformed MALT lymphomas from de novo DLBCL.[3]

Changing nomenclature and classification systems make it very difficult to compare long-term outcome of DLBCL. However, it is clear from many studies that as the high-grade component increases, the response to *H. pylori* eradication decreases and long-term outcome becomes poor. While the overall 5-year survival appears to be about 65%, differences exist between subtypes of DLBCL.[213] The 5-year survival rate for DLBCL with low-grade MALT lymphoma component varies between 84% and 92%, while 5-year survival for a DLBCL without a low-grade MALT lymphoma component in a study was estimated to be only 30%.[205,206] In another study, 5-year survival of a de novo DLBCL was estimated to be 64%. Some transformed MALT lymphomas do respond to *H. pylori* eradication, and even spontaneous remission has been reported rarely with nonspecific therapy.[214–216] Thus, recognizing a background of low-grade MALT lymphoma and *H. pylori* positivity is important when making a diagnosis of DLBCL and needs to be mentioned in the pathology reports. This can potentially save more toxic chemotherapy in a subgroup of DLBCL patients. In this group of patients, the outcome of long-term studies and better ways to differentiate different biologic and prognostic groups are still awaited.

Primary Gastric T-cell Lymphoma

These are rare gastric lymphomas.[217–222] However, the reports underestimate the true incidence, as they do not include some lymphomas with distinctive morphology, such as the anaplastic large-cell lymphomas, some of which are phenotypically T-cell lymphomas (see later Ki-1 lymphomas). In addition, the stomach may be secondarily involved in rare cases of EATL and node-based adult T-cell leukemia/lymphoma.

Clinically, there have been too few cases in the stomach to be certain about the predictability of the clinical behavior of these lymphomas. In one report of four cases, one patient died within 6 months of diagnosis, but the others were in remission—two patients at 3 years and one at 4 years after surgical resection.[217] Overall, more than half the patients reported to date were in remission following treatment. However, the length of the follow-up period in some cases was fairly short, and furthermore the tumor stage was not always clear.

Pathology. Grossly, the primary gastric T-cell lymphomas can present as multiple polypoid lesions or as a localized protuberant, polypoid, or deeply ulcerated masses.

Histologically, these tumors may resemble lymph node–based peripheral T-cell lymphomas, with a polymorphous infiltrate of lymphocytes admixed with histiocytes, eosinophils, clusters of epithelioid histiocytes, and occasionally stromal fibrosis.[217,219,222] The polymorphous lymphocytic infiltrate consists of an admixture of small lymphocytes with somewhat wrinkled nuclei; plasmacytoid-type cells containing peripherally located cerebriform vesicular nuclei with prominent eosinophilic nucleoli, resembling the immunoblastic-type T-cell lymphoma; or lymphocytic blast cells with deeply indented or gyriform vesicular nuclei, indistinct nucleoli, and abundant clear cytoplasm. Occasionally, multinucleated giant cells can also be seen.[219,220] Immunohistochemically, the majority of the T-cell lymphomas are phenotypically CD3+ and CD4+ although occasional CD3+ and CD8+ phenotypes have also been described.[217] Some cases may show phenotypes similar to IELs, with expression of human mucosal lymphocyte antigen1 and CD103, similar to intestinal T-cell lymphomas.[223] Rearrangement of the TCR can be demonstrated in these cases and is very helpful in the diagnosis, especially when dealing with small biopsies.

Other Miscellaneous Lymphoproliferative Disorders

Various other nodal types of non-Hodgkin's lymphomas, Hodgkin's lymphomas, and immunodeficiency-associated lymphomas that may involve stomach primarily or secondarily are discussed in the subsequent sections of this chapter.

LYMPHOPROLIFERATIVE DISORDERS OF THE SMALL INTESTINE

Despite being the longest segment of the GI tract, small bowel tumors account for only about 2% of all GI malignancies. However, lymphomas constitute about 30% to 50% of all malignancies at this site as epithelial and mesenchymal neoplasms are even less common. In Western countries, small intestinal lymphomas constitute about 10% to 12% of all extranodal lymphomas and 15% to 30% of all GI lymphomas.[224] In the Middle East, they constitute about 50% of all extranodal lymphomas, largely due to the high incidence of IPSID in this region. In the small intestine, lymphomas occur throughout its length (duodenum 11%, jejunum 9%, ileum and ileocecum 80%). The majority are B-cell lymphomas (85%), and fewer cases represent T-cell lymphomas (15%). Of the B-cell neoplasms, about 69% are DLBCL, while 18% are marginal zone lymphomas of the MALT-type. The nature of DLBCL remains somewhat controversial, although many believe they also arise from MALT. IPSID is considered a special subtype of MALT lymphoma under the new WHO classification.

MALT Lymphoma (Extranodal Marginal Zone Lymphoma) and Diffuse Large B-cell Lymphoma of the Small Intestine (Western-type Lymphoma)

These lymphomas are often referred to as Western-type lymphoma to differentiate them from Mediterranean lymphoma, which is a unique type of MALT lymphoma (discussed later). Small intestinal MALT-type lymphomas and DLBCL are very similar to their gastric counterparts. They are discussed here together as many feel intestinal DLBCLs also arise from MALT and share many features. Molecular genetics also show that when DLBCL is seen in the background of a low-grade marginal zone lymphoma, they are clonally related. Unlike gastric MALT lymphomas, no causative organism similar to H. pylori has been identified so far, and the majority (85%) of cases are transformed to high-grade MALT lymphomas or DLBCL, and hence the outcome is less favorable.[1,225,226] This is largely due to the fact that diagnosis is often delayed till they become symptomatic, which in most cases is due to obstruction, perforation, bleeding, or a mass lesion.

They arise in older adults and have slight male preponderance.[227] DLBCL may also be seen in young children, mostly in boys in whom it almost exclusively involves the ileocecal region.[228,229] A serum IgM component can be seen in some cases. Gross appearance varies and includes thickened and nodular folds, multiple raised erosive lesions, and polypoid or ulcerated masses (Fig. 4-21).[227] DLBCL generally tends to present with larger obstructive mass lesions, sometimes with perforation. The histology and immunophenotype is similar to their gastric counterparts, although lymphoepithelial lesions are less frequent (Fig. 4-22).[225] The DLBCL shows large noncleaved centroblasts, often with an admixture of immunoblasts or multilobated large B cells. In 10% to 50% cases, a low-grade component is evident in the background. The low-grade lesions are mostly confined to mucosa without nodal involvement and rarely show distant involvement. In contrast, the disease is widespread in >50% of high-grade lesions (transformed MALT lymphomas and DLBCL) at presentation. Rare examples that possibly represent multifocal involvement of gastric MALT lymphoma have been reported to respond to H. pylori eradication. A study showed the presence of t(11;18)(q21;q21) in 2 of 16 intestinal MALT-type lymphomas. It is unclear if the study group included both low-grade MALT lymphomas and DLBCL.[180] However, subsequent studies of primary small intestinal MALT lymphomas have shown higher frequency (12.5%) of this translocation.[230] This study also showed that trisomy 3 (12.5%) and 18 (81%) are detected more frequently in primary small intestinal MALT lymphoma compared to its gastric counterpart.[230] Translocations involving IgH (27%), BCL6 (23%–35%), BCL2 (0–21%), and C-MYC (7%) are seen in DLBCL suggesting it is a heterogenous group.[231]

In the low-grade lesions, the prognosis is good, with a 5-year survival reported to be about 44% to 75%.[8,227,232] The DLBCLs are more aggressive, with a 5-year survival reported to be about 25% to 67%.[8,213,232] The criteria for defining large-cell lymphoma of the MALT-type and high-grade transformation are lacking. While lymphomas without any low-grade component should be classified as DLBCL, the significance of finding small clusters or admixed large cells/

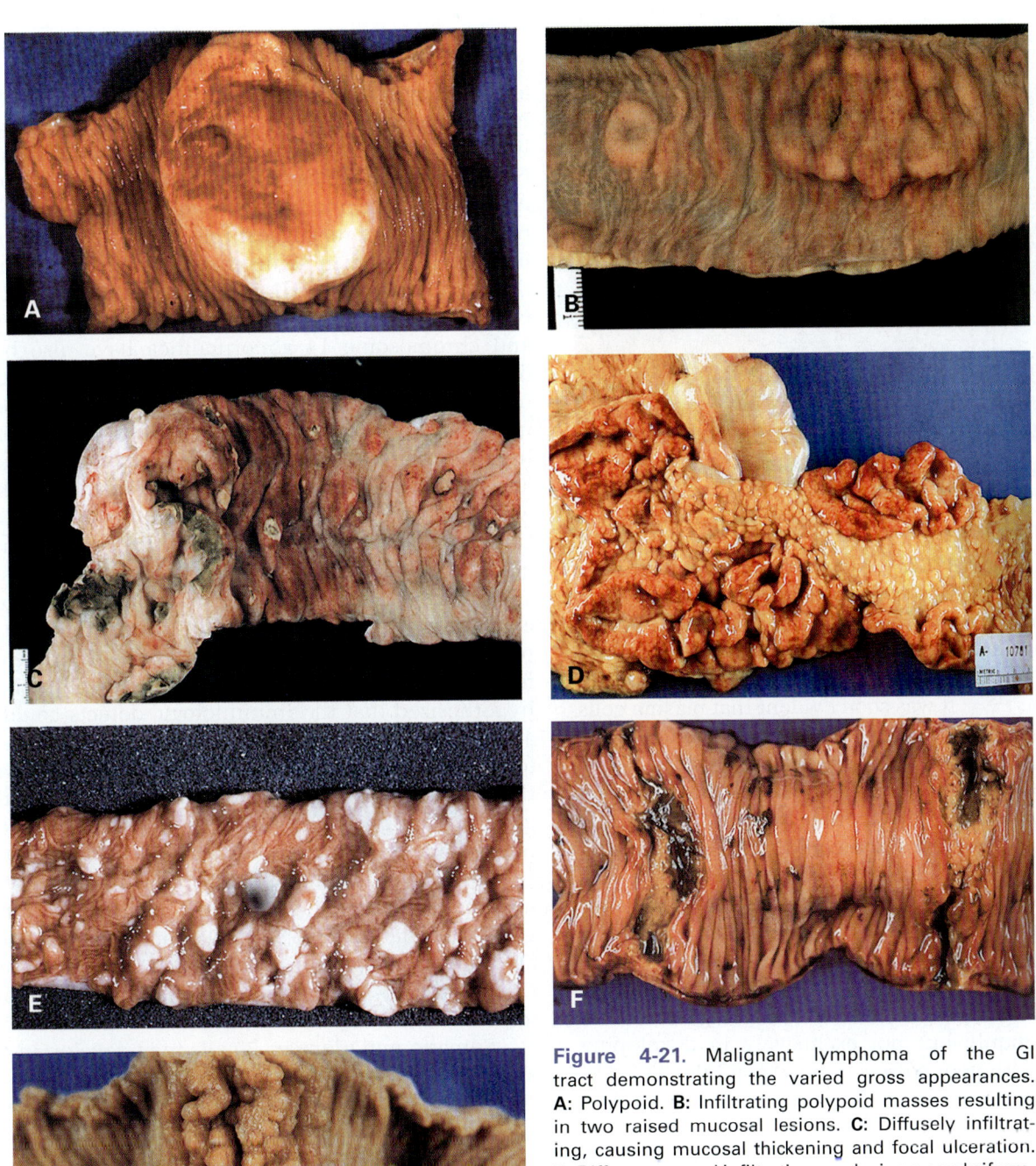

Figure 4-21. Malignant lymphoma of the GI tract demonstrating the varied gross appearances. **A:** Polypoid. **B:** Infiltrating polypoid masses resulting in two raised mucosal lesions. **C:** Diffusely infiltrating, causing mucosal thickening and focal ulceration. **D:** Diffuse mucosal infiltration producing a cerebriform-like appearance. There is also a diffuse mucosal nodularity. **E:** Lymphomatous polyposis. **F:** Ulcerating. This segment of ileum shows two areas of mucosal ulceration with bile staining. Grossly the bowel beneath the ulcers was not thickened, but histologically it was diffusely infiltrated by lymphoma. **G:** Circumferential nodular infiltrate.

immunoblasts in the background of low-grade lesion remains unclear. In one series DLBCL cases with a background of low-grade lymphoma had a slightly favorable outcome compared to pure DLBCL. In view of this it has been suggested that such cases be designated as composite marginal zone and DLBCL.

Immunoproliferative Small Intestinal Disease (Mediterranean Lymphoma, α-Chain Disease)

An increased incidence of primary small intestinal lymphoma in the Mediterranean countries was first

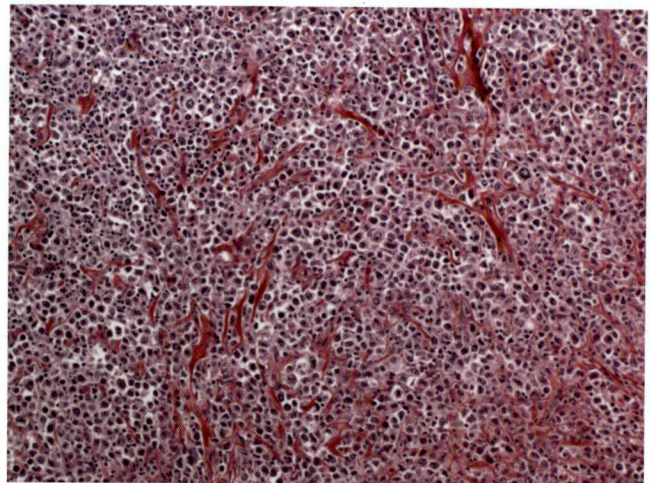

Figure 4-22. Microscopic appearance of a DLBCL of the small intestine (Western-type lymphoma).

noted by Azar in 1962.[233] A subsequent report in 1965 characterized this as a disease of young adults that manifested with diarrhea and malabsorption.[234] The majority of such cases came from Mediterranean countries, and it soon became known as "Mediterranean lymphoma."[235-239] It was soon evident that plasma cells of this lesion make a partial immunoglobulin composed of only α-heavy chains, and the term "α-heavy chain disease" was coined.[237] It was also realized that the disease had an early benign phase that could be treated with antibiotics and could progress to a frank lymphoma with an adverse outcome. The term "IPSID" was coined by the WHO to encompass this spectrum of disease in 1976. In 2008, WHO lymphoma classification this is now considered a variant of marginal zone lymphoma of the MALT-type (MALT lymphoma).[29]

IPSID has a distinctive epidemiology. It occurs most commonly but not exclusively in developing countries with poor socioeconomic conditions.[236,240,241] The disorder was originally reported in a group of Sephardic Jews, Arabs, and South Africans from the Cape Region. It is endemic in Mediterranean Basin, with a higher incidence at the shores compared to the other areas of the same country.[236,241-244] The few cases reported from Italy, Spain, and France were also from the southern Mediterranean shores of these countries. The disease is now recognized worldwide, including Far East, Africa, and Latin America. Rare cases of this disorder have been described in the United States.[2,236,245] Over the last three decades, there has been a decline in the incidence of IPSID in the Middle East, a phenomenon that cannot be fully explained by improved socioeconomic and hygienic conditions.[246]

Etiopathogenesis. The etiology and pathogenesis of IPSID are unclear. They are multifactorial and probably vary from one area to another. Most cases have been reported in patients with a low socioeconomic status, poor hygiene, malnutrition, and a high degree of intestinal infections.[236,241] Interestingly, biopsies from apparently healthy individuals living in the same geographic area show increased lymphocytes and plasma cells in the lamina propria. Although no specific infectious agent has been identified, recent reports suggest that *Campylobacter jejuni* may be involved in some cases.[18,247,248] A number of these patients are of HLA-A9, HLA-AW19, and HLA-B12 types.[236,244,249] An association with blood group B and chromosome 14 abnormalities have also been described. Increased intestinal alkaline phosphatase in healthy relatives of IPSID patients and increased incidence of IPSID in relatives, even living apart, have been reported.[249] Occult defects of the cellular and humoral immunity have been detected in otherwise healthy relatives of some patients with IPSID.[250] IPSID patients generally have lower serum immunoglobulin levels, show low response to recall and sensitizing antigens, and have low proportion of T-cell compared to matched controls. It is of interest that reports on IPSID started to appear in these areas a few years after the Eltor cholera epidemic. It has been hypothesized that the immunologic defects could be attributed to the modulatory effects of *Vibrio cholerae* toxin acquired during the 1960s epidemic that swept these geographic areas.[246] These findings indicate that genetic, immunologic, and environmental factors may be operative in the etiopathogenesis of IPSID.

It has been postulated that in the presence of an acquired immunodeficiency state, a continuous antigenic stimulation (e.g., *C. jejuni* or other infectious agent) leads to proliferative plasma cell response.[246] *C. jejuni* and its cytolethal distending toxin are known to produce breaks in double stranded DNA.[251]

Somatic mutations in B cells may develop in this situation that lead to aberrant plasma cells that make truncated α-heavy chain proteins (αHCP). These heavy chains are 29,000 to 34,000 molecular weight proteins that have deletions of VH and CH-1 regions and are devoid of light chains.[246] In the early stages, the neoplastic lymphoid cells retain the function of their normal counterparts, namely, response to antigenic stimulation by undergoing plasma cell differentiation, resulting in massive plasma cell infiltration of the lamina propria. Later, as the neoplasm dedifferentiates and becomes autonomous, the cells gradually lose this characteristic and become replaced by atypical lymphoid cells. However, they still retain their ability to circulate via the lymphatic and vascular systems and to home back to the gut mucosa.

Clinical features. IPSID affects mainly older children and young adults in the 10 to 35 age range of low socioeconomic status. It is uncommon in very young children and older adults. The disease has equal sex distribution. The patients reported from the United States have been somewhat older, and some had other underlying problems, such as bone marrow transplantation in one case and celiac disease in another.[2,236] Patients present with intermittent abdominal pain, diarrhea, and features of malabsorption. Anorexia, low-grade fever, and clubbing of fingers may be seen in some cases. The majority of IPSID patients (87%) show the presence of αHCP in the serum.[246] Besides serum, αHCP can also be detected in intestinal juice, urine, and saliva. Rare cases that show γ-heavy chains instead of α-chains have been reported.[252] The serum levels of IgG and IgM are variable. However, cases making αHCP have low IgA. Bence Jones protein is typically absent. Parasitic infections particularly *Giardia lamblia* are frequently seen. A rare nonsecretory variant of IPSID has also been described that is characterized by the absence of αHCP in the serum, but demonstrable by immunohistochemistry of IgA alone in the plasma cells.[253] It has been suggested that this variant occurs in older individuals and is probably more responsive to therapy. This variant is usually associated with diffuse follicular hyperplasia rather than dense plasma cell infiltrate that is typical of IPSID.[254] The endoscopic appearance depends on the stage of the disease. Early stages may show a normal appearance. As the infiltrate increases in later stages, mucosal folds appear thickened and nodular masses or strictures may be seen with advanced stages. Conventional radiology and nuclear imaging often show nonspecific findings, and their role in diagnosis and staging remains undefined. Radionucleotide imaging with ⁶⁷Ga citrate demonstrates activity over the entire abdomen.[246] Currently laparotomy/laparoscopic examination remains the best method for staging.

Pathology. IPSID is characterized by a dense mucosal band like infiltrate that involves the entire length of at least the proximal small bowel. The infiltrate is composed of variable admixture of plasma cells and CLCs. The disease shows a histologic spectrum from a benign-appearing infiltrate to a frank lymphoma and has been morphologically divided into three stages (Table 4-4).[255]

Gross findings in the early stages are minimal and may even appear normal. With increasing infiltrate erythema, nodularity and thickening of the mucosal folds may be seen (Fig. 4-23A). Malignant lymphoma complicating IPSID representing advanced stage is characterized by diffuse thickening of the viscus and may be multifocal. Ulcerated lesions, some with raised margins, as well as multiple polypoid lesions may also be seen.

Stage A is characterized by benign-appearing, diffuse plasmacytic infiltrate of the lamina propria (Fig. 4-23B). There is involvement of the jejunum, with frequent extension to the ileum. If the jejunum is not involved, the disease is most unlikely to be IPSID. Gastric and large bowel involvement is rare. The plasmacytic infiltrate is confined to the lamina propria and is composed of mature-appearing plasma cells with smaller numbers of marginal zone B cells (CLCs). The crypts are widely separated and frequently displaced upward and away from the muscularis mucosae by the infiltrate. There is a variable villous lesion ranging from mild blunting to a totally flat mucosa. Lymphoepithelial lesions may also be found. Occasionally a diffuse mucosal infiltrate is composed predominantly of mature lymphocytes rather than plasma cells.[236,256-258] Whether these cases represent variants of IPSID is presently unknown. In some cases especially nonsecretory variants, lymphoid follicles rather than plasma cells are prominent resulting in polypoid nodules.[254] The lymph nodes are also involved by plasmacytic infiltrate without effacement of the nodal architecture.

Stage B is characterized by atypical plasmacytoid cells and immunoblasts scattered singly or in small clusters between the plasmacytic infiltrate that is otherwise similar to stage A and extension of the infiltrate beyond the mucularis mucosae. A moderate to severe mucosal lesion with total to subtotal villous blunting is present. Follicular colonization of the lymphoid follicles by marginal zone cells may impart a nodular appearance to the infiltrate. The lymph nodes may show subtotal to total effacement of the architecture due to atypical lymphoplasmacytic infiltrate.

Stage C is characterized by the development of high-grade lymphoma. Most cases are of the diffuse large

Table 4-4 Galian Staging System for IPSID

STAGE	SMALL INTESTINAL HISTOLOGY	LYMPH NODES HISTOLOGY
A.	Lymphoplasmacytic or plasmacytic infiltration of the lamina propria, variable villous atrophy	Plasmacytic infiltration, nodal architecture generally preserved
B.	Atypical lymphoplasmacytic or plasma cells with immunoblast-like cells with extension to at least submucosal, subtotal, or total villous atrophy	Atypical plasmscytic infiltrate with immunoblast-like cells, subtotal or total effacement of nodal architecture
C.	Frankly malignant invasion through entire intestinal wall	Malignant effacement of entire lymph node

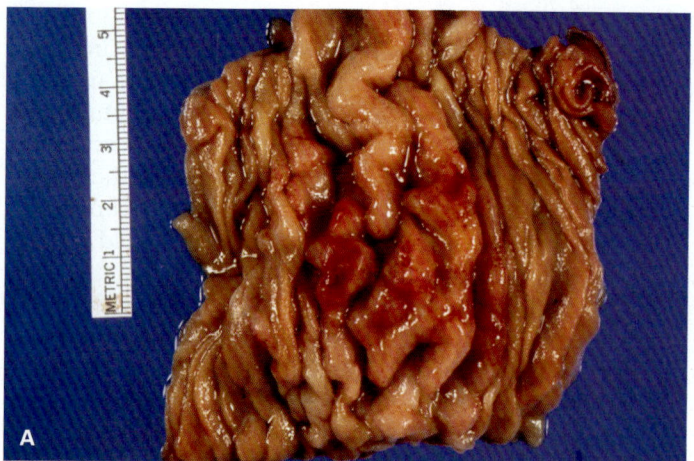
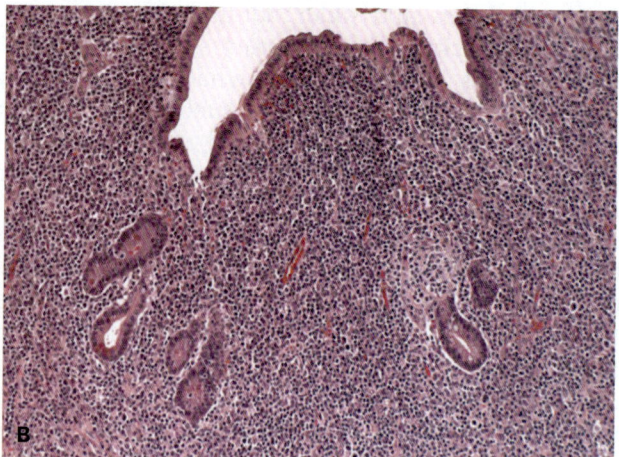

Figure 4-23. **A:** Gross appearance of small intestine in a case of IPSID showing thickening of the mucosal folds without a well demarcated mass. **B:** Microscopic appearance of a case of IPSID showing polymorphic cell population consisting of an admixture of lymphocytes, plasma cells, immunoblasts, and occasional eosinophils. There is some villous blunting. This would constitute stage A IPSID.

B-cell immunoblastic-type and have a characteristic polymorphous appearance consisting of cells ranging from atypical, small, often wrinkled lymphocytes to large noncleaved cells, plasmacytoid cells, and Reed–Sternberg-like cells. In some cases the cells are bizarre and markedly pleomorphic. Some cases are monomorphous, resembling a DLBCL.

Stage A does not invariably progress to later stages; in fact, many cases do not progress, and some even regress with antibiotic therapy.[259] The rate of evolution from a low grade to high grade is unknown. However, most patients with lymphomatous transformation are generally about 6 years older than the patients with early-stage IPSID.[260] Also, patients presenting with lymphomatous transformation often have a history of preceding IPSID-like symptoms for 5 to 10 years.[260]

Although the lymphoma usually involves the jejunum, it sometimes spares the small intestine and involves only the mesenteric lymph nodes.[236] In these cases, the pattern of nodal infiltration is unusual in that there is follicular and marginal zone colonization, with preservation of the medullary sinuses.

Immunophenotype and molecular genetics. The cases of IPSID with α-heavy chain disease have cytoplasmic α-heavy chain predominantly of the subclass α-1 but occasionally α-2, and an absence of demonstrable light chain, IgG and IgM within the plasmacytic infiltrate.[261] The mature plasma cells, especially those associated with lymphoepithelial lesions, stain with anti-CD20 and anti-CD22 antibody, but are negative with CD5 and CD10. In addition, molecular genetic studies have shown clonal heavy and light chain rearrangements, even in the antibiotic responsive early stages.[262,263] When lymphoma supervenes, with rare exceptions, the abnormal cytoplasmic immunoglobulins are no longer demonstrable, and the serum αHCP also tends to decrease or disappear. Occasionally cytogenetic changes have been identified that include t(9;14) and t(2;14); however, no consistent abnormality has been associated with IPSID.[264] In a study none of the 22 IPSID cases showed any of the MALT-type translocations.[165]

Diagnosis and differential diagnosis. There may be considerable histologic overlap with celiac sprue, and differentiation could be difficult especially in small biopsies. However, the clinical setting, patient demographics, and serologic finding are so different from celiac disease that it is not a practical issue. The differentiation from other causes of a nonspecific flat or variably blunted mucosa poses little problem, since in IPSID the dominant feature is the dense plasma cell infiltration, often causing expansion of the subcryptal region, in contrast to the other conditions, including celiac disease or infectious gastroenteritis, where the infiltrate is a secondary feature and not nearly as massive (see Chapter 20). Also, although it is tempting to run κ- and λ-immunohistochemistry, these will be negative and need heavy chains to be run to show that the plasma cells are producing only IgA (rarely IgG), to the virtual exclusion of other immunoglobulins.

When lymphoma supervenes in IPSID, it is important to demonstrate the massive plasmacytic infiltration in the adjacent mucosa in order to sustain the diagnosis. Once IPSID is confirmed, it should be determined whether the patient has α-chain disease. The paraprotein should be sought in the serum, urine (and jejunal juices if possible), as well as by immunohistochemistry in tissue sections. It should be noted that in many cases the abnormality is not detected by routine immunoelectrophoresis with polyvalent antiserum; thus monospecific antiserum to IgA is essential.[265]

The small intestinal lymphomas seen in North America and Europe, the so-called "Western-type" lymphomas, differ in many respects from the IPSID-associated lymphomas.[236] They are located mainly in the stomach and ileum, in contrast to the jejunum, and lack the massive plasma cell infiltrate in the lamina propria adjacent to the tumor. Occasionally, these tumors have been reported to produce α-heavy chain, but they lack the other clinicopathologic features of Mediterranean lymphomas.

IPSID-associated lymphoma may also be confused with Hodgkin's lymphoma because of the finding of Reed–Sternberg-like cells. However, Hodgkin's lymphoma of the bowel is very uncommon, does not have atypical lymphocytes, and has a different immunophenotype.

Treatment and prognosis. Similar to gastric MALT lymphomas, conventional lymphoma staging systems are of little use in IPSID. IPSID rarely involves extra-abdominal sites and involvement of spleen, peripheral lymph nodes, or bone marrow is rare.[266] The prognosis depends upon histology and anatomic spread of the disease, and the therapeutic strategies have been designed accordingly.

To date there have been no large therapeutic trials, and the long-term outcome of IPSID remains unclear. However, it is becoming apparent that stage A of this disorder may persist for years without progression to lymphoma.[245] Some cases achieve remission spontaneously or with antibiotic therapy.[263,267-269] For early stage disease most agree that antibiotics are the treatment of choice. Complete remission sustained for >5 years have been reported in 33% to 70% of the patients.[15] Some cases of low-grade IPSID may relapse and still be responsive to antibiotics. Higher stage and failure to respond to antibiotics are indications for chemotherapy.[267] Once high-grade lymphoma develops, the prognosis is generally poor, although sometimes long periods of survival occur.[270] Various regimens including CHOP with or without radiation have been used, and the best 2- and 3-year survival rates have been 90% and 67%, respectively. Since the outlook for patients with this disorder is generally poor once lymphoma has developed, it has been recommended that a staging laparotomy be performed once a diagnosis of IPSID has been made in order to determine accurately the extent of disease.[259] Surgery has limited role in the treatment and is reserved for palliation or when there is obstruction. Unresponsive disease progresses relentlessly with a variable pace, and most patients die of malnutrition, sepsis, intestinal obstruction, or other disabling complications due to massive abdominal involvement. Results of newer therapies like anti-CD20 (rituximab) and intensive chemotherapy with stem cell transplantation are still awaited.

Burkitt's and Burkitt's-like Lymphoma (Malignant Lymphoma of the Small, Noncleaved Type)

Burkitt's lymphoma is an aggressive B-cell neoplasm. It can present with nodal or extra-nodal disease and lymphomatous or leukemic presentation. It has a strong association with EBV and characterized by translocation involving C-myc oncogene. Three forms are recognized: endemic, sporadic, and immunodeficiency associated. The endemic form is seen in equatorial Africa and Papua, New Guinea, and is almost always associated with EBV.[271,272] It is seen mostly in children, with peak incidence between 4 and 7 years, and is twice as common in boys as girls. In this form, the predominant presentation is with involvement of the facial and jaw bones; however, involvement of other sites including GI tract can also be seen. The sporadic form has a worldwide distribution. It occurs in children and young adults, with a median age of 30 years, and is about two to three times more common in males. EBV is demonstrated in only a third of the sporadic cases. The predominant presentation is with abdominal masses, and ileocecal region is the most frequently involved site. The immunodeficiency-associated cases are mostly seen with HIV infection, and 25% to 40% of the cases are EBV associated. This form frequently presents with nodal disease and bone marrow involvement.

Clinical presentation. Although they can occur anywhere in the bowel, they are found most commonly around the ileocecal region, presenting with obstruction and intussusception (Fig. 4-24A).[225] They are usually advanced at the time of diagnosis, often involving large lengths of the intestine and mesenteric nodes. Local recurrence with widespread peritoneal dissemination is common following treatment.

Pathology. Grossly, the tumors are often bulky and fleshy and may form polypoid or ulceroproliferative masses. Morphologically, they characteristically have a "starry sky" pattern and consist of medium-sized (12–15 μm) lymphoid cells with scant basophilic cytoplasm, regular round nuclei, finely dispersed chromatin, and multiple small nucleoli (Fig. 4-24B–D). Cytologic features of the tumor cells are best appreciated on touch preparations or imprint smears. The starry sky pattern is produced by the presence of lightly stained macrophages, often containing multiple tingible bodies in a background of darkly staining dense population of lymphoma cells. The mitotic activity is very high. Some cases show plasmacytic differentiation, with cells having basophilic cytoplasm, eccentric nucleus, single prominent nucleolus, and sometimes pleomorphic

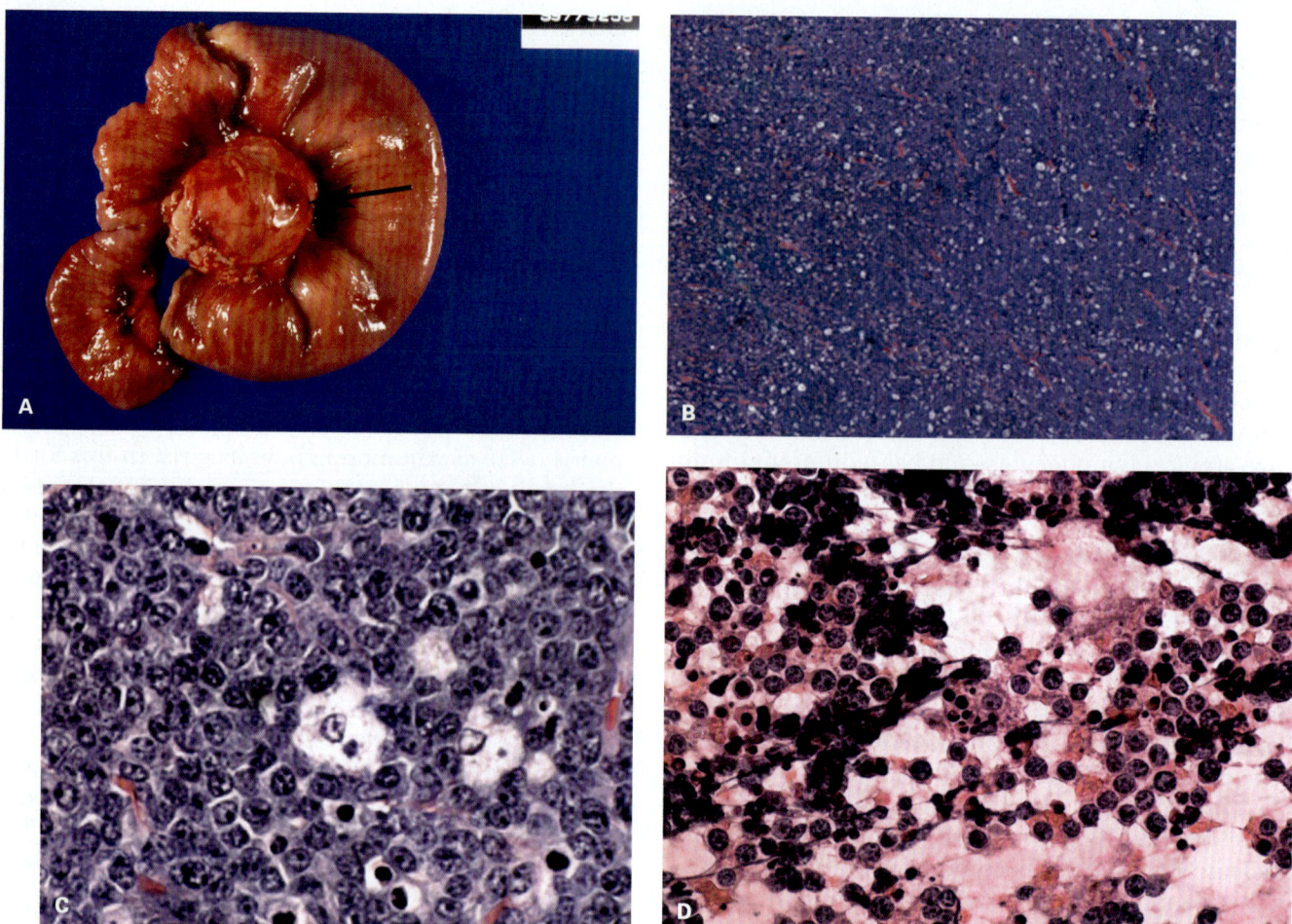

Figure 4-24. A: Burkitt's lymphoma in a 7-year-old child who presented with intussusception. The specimen of small intestine shows in addition a large mesenteric lymph node involved by Burkitt's lymphoma (to add new). **B:** Microscopy of a case of Burkitt's lymphoma showing classic "starry sky" pattern. The empty holes (*stars*) in the deep blue background of tumor cells (*sky*) are represented by pale staining tingible-body macrophages. **C:** High power of Burkitt's lymphoma showing intermediate-size cells with speckled chromatin, few nucleoli, and thin rim of cytoplasm. **D:** Touch preparation from a case of Burkitt's lymphoma showing the cytology of the tumor cells.

nuclei. This variant is most often seen in immunodeficiency-associated cases. The Burkitt's-like variant tends to show more nuclear pleomorphism and fewer but larger nucleoli. Occasionally, Burkitt's lymphoma has a nodular pattern and may selectively involve B-cell areas such as Peyer's patches and solitary lymphoid follicles.

Immunophenotype and molecular genetics. The tumors cells have a mature B-cell phenotype and suggest a germinal center cell origin. They express SIgM+ with light chain restriction—CD19, CD20, CD22, CD79A, CD10, and BCL6. They do not express CD23, TdT (terminal deoxynucleotidyl transferase), and BCL2. Endemic forms may show positivity for CD21—the receptor for C3d. Clonal gene rearrangements of Ig heavy and light chains are seen. The proliferative index is very high, and Ki67 staining shows virtually 100% positivity. All cases exhibit characteristic translocation of MYC on chromosome 8 to Ig heavy chain loci on chromosome 14 or less commonly to light chain loci on chromosome 2 or 22. In addition, inactivating mutations of *p53* can be seen in about 30% of the endemic and sporadic cases. As discussed above, EBV genome can be demonstrated in varying proportion of cases.

Prognosis and treatment. These are aggressive tumors with rapid doubling time; however, many cases respond well to intensive chemotherapy and cure can be achieved in some. The cure rates with low stage approach 90% and high stage disease about 60% to 80%. The children have a more favorable outcome compared to adults. Cases presenting with intussusception or perforation may necessitate surgery. The majority of the relapses tend to occur within a year, and cases without relapse for more than 2 years are regarded as cured.

Enteropathy-type T-cell Lymphoma

T-cell lymphomas constitute only about 5% of all GI lymphomas, and their association with celiac disease has been recognized for a long time.[273] Initially in 1937 when an association between lymphoma and malabsorption was reported, it was believed that lymphoma was somehow responsible for the malabsorption; however, subsequently it became clear that there was an associated malabsorptive disorder. It was soon realized that patients with celiac disease, with or without dermatitis herpetiformis, have an increased risk of developing GI lymphoma or carcinoma, and this complication is a major cause of death in these patients.[274-279] Subsequently, it was found that most lymphomas were of T-cell origin, and O'Farrelly et al.[280] coined the term EATL. It also became clear that many cases presented with lymphoma, and a definite diagnosis of celiac disease could not be established. In some of these cases, the uninvolved intestine showed villous atrophy similar to celiac disease, while in some cases the histology appeared normal. Hence, in the 2001 WHO classification, the designation "enteropathy-associated" T-cell lymphoma has been changed to "enteropathy-type" T-cell lymphoma (ETL).

It has now become clear that while some patients with ETL have a preceding long-standing history of celiac disease, in about 50% of patients who present with T-cell lymphoma, a diagnosis of celiac disease is made simultaneously or later. The cases of ETL can be divided into the following categories:

1. Patients with a long-standing history of celiac disease that often become resistant to gluten-free diet and develop overt T-cell lymphoma.
2. Patients that present with T-cell lymphoma and a diagnosis of celiac sprue is established simultaneously based on histology and celiac sprue serology.
3. Patients that present with T-cell lymphoma and the adjacent nonneoplastic small bowel mucosa shows histologic features similar to celiac sprue, but patients are gluten resistant and the celiac sprue serology is negative.
4. Patients that present with T-cell lymphoma and the histology of the nonneoplastic small bowel mucosa is normal, and there is no clinical or serologic evidence of celiac sprue.

Patients with celiac disease who respond poorly, or do not adhere strictly to a gluten-free diet appear to be more liable to develop malignancy, although this is somewhat controvertial.[275,281,282] Its incidence follows the incidence of celiac disease. It should be noted that celiac disease is most common in Northern Europe and uncommon in other countries such as Japan. As a result these lymphomas are rare in the latter countries, although occasional cases have been reported.[277] A small series of Mexican patients reported a younger age of (median 24 years) presentation of T-cell lymphomas, and EBV infection has been suspected to play a role in these cases.[283,284]

The true incidence and the relative risk of developing lymphoma in celiac disease is difficult to estimate.[285] As more sensitive and specific serologic tests have evolved, it has become apparent that many patients with celiac disease are clinically asymptomatic and have near-normal or patchy histologic changes and never come to clinical attention. Initial studies indicated a strong relative risk of 40- to 100-fold of lymphoma in patients with celiac disease, although more recent studies show that the risk is substantially lower at < 5.[285] This possibly reflects the fact that a significant group of patients have a milder/asymptomatic disease and may have a lower risk of developing lymphoma.[285]

Pathogenesis. The association of celiac disease with T-cell lymphoma clearly suggests a role for persistent antigenic stimulation of T cells (usually intraepithelial) that leads to proliferation and eventually a clonal expansion, resulting in lymphoma.[286] In a subset of cases, a role for EBV has also been suggested. In this multistep process the key genetic events are yet unidentified. However, it is clear that in many cases a T-cell clone develops in the IEL compartment that marks the development of gluten resistance and represents an intermediate step before the development of overt lymphoma.[287] Studies have also shown that these clones are not stationary, and evolution of newer clones with disappearance of the older ones is common. At this stage, T cells may also show loss of CD8.[288] The intestinal epithelium has been shown to overexpress IL15 in celiac disease that can preferentially stimulate the expansion and survival of the T-cell clones.[289] The pathogenesis of evolution of this abnormal phenotype and its relationship to gluten resistance remain unclear. Subsequent events in the development of a lymphoma from a stage of cryptic lymphoma are also unclear.

Clinical presentation. Clinically, the majority of patients with celiac disease and lymphoma are in their 60s, and there is a male predominance.[227,290] Some patients have a history of long-standing malabsorption or celiac disease averaging 8 to 10 years. In some cases, the preceding history of malabsorption is short or both disorders are discovered simultaneously.[291] Only few patients have childhood onset celiac disease, and the lymphoma typically doesn't occur in children. It should be stressed that in some patients with intestinal lymphoma, the association with celiac sprue may not be obvious. Thus, the small bowel mucosa away from the tumor should be carefully examined for changes of celiac disease. In addition, if feasible, serologic tests for celiac disease should be carried out. Small bowel biopsies in patients who develop primary intestinal lymphoma with no apparent predisposing cause may also be helpful in establishing a link with celiac disease.[276] Clinically, patients developing lymphoma usually present with recurrence of one or all of the following in the face of a strict gluten-free diet: malabsorption, weight loss, or prominent abdominal pain. The latter is particularly important, as pain is not a prominent feature of uncomplicated celiac disease. About 40% to 50% of patients present as an emergency with severe abdominal pain, GI hemorrhage, obstruction, or perforation.[227,290] In rare instances, celiac disease complicated with lymphoma may present with multiple lymphomatous gastric ulcers unresponsive to therapy.[279] Ulcerative jejunitis, a complication of celiac disease may also develop or, much more likely, be part of early T-cell lymphoma.[8,292] However, careful search of multiple blocks and immunohistochemistry for T cells (CD3) may be necessary to highlight both the atypical cells that can be very subtle in the base of the ulcer and to demonstrate their T-cell nature to confirm this diagnosis. The majority of cases with ulcerative jeunoileitis show T-cell monoclonality and aberrant IEL population. While some cases have obvious T-cell lymphoma at presentation, some are considered "cryptic lymphomas" that over a period of time may progress to overt disease. Patients with celiac disease are also prone to a number of other neoplastic complications such as B-cell non-Hodgkin's lymphoma and carcinomas, especially in the oropharynx, esophagus, as well as the small bowel.[282]

Pathology. It is interesting that while histologic changes of celiac disease are most prominent in the duodenum, the most commonly involved segment by lymphoma is jejunum followed by ileum.[290] Grossly, the majority of lesions are single and found in the jejunum but may sometimes be multiple or diffuse and involve other portions of the intestine and stomach. Occasionally, the mesenteric nodes alone are involved, with sparing of the small intestine. The diseased bowel is usually thickened and may show ulceration or strictures. These ulcers may be circumferential and may be mistakenly diagnosed as benign (ulcerative jejunoileitis) (Fig. 4-25A).[293] Rarely, they may form large protuberant or polypoid masses sometimes associated with extensive necrosis. In fact an isolated segment of jejunitis on imaging warrants consideration of a lymphoma diagnosis and even a segmental resection to be sure this is not the diagnosis.

Lymphomas complicating celiac sprue have a variable appearance. Some are monomorphous of the diffuse large-cell type, while the majority are pleomorphic resembling node-based peripheral T-cell lymphomas.[290,294] The majority of the pleomorphic lymphomas are high-grade, consisting of a diffuse infiltration of atypical lymphocytes admixed with histiocytes, eosinophils, epithelioid histiocytes, and occasionally stromal fibrosis. The lymphocytic infiltration is typically polymorphous, consisting of small lymphocytes with somewhat wrinkled nuclei; lymphocytes with features of large-cell immunoblastic T-cell lymphoma, characterized by plasmacytoid cells containing peripherally located cerebriform vesicular nuclei with prominent eosinophilic nucleoli; or blast cells with deeply indented or gyriform vesicular nuclei, indistinct nucleoli, and abundant clear cytoplasm. The presence of multinucleated giant cells (Reed–Sternberg-like cells) has also been described. Sometimes, these tumors are overshadowed by extensive necrosis or accompanying inflammatory cells and may be misdiagnosed as benign ulcerative jejunoileitis (Fig. 4-25).[220,293,295] It should be stressed that the previously described histologic features may not be distinctive of T-cell lymphoma and that a definitive diagnosis can be made only with the help of immunohistochemistry and T-cell gene rearrangement studies.[296-298] Microscopic tumor foci are not uncommonly present in the liver, spleen, and bone marrow. An easy pointer to the diagnosis is the presence of numerous large IELs with a cytoplasmic halo, in the adjacent villi, which typically does not have the flattened cuboidal epithelium seen in untreated celiac disease but instead are lined by tall columnar cells. This feature is rarely present in duodenal biopsies but when present does allow the diagnosis to be considered.

The early lymphomatous lesions may be patchy and difficult to diagnose, especially in mucosal biopsy material and because of the polymorphous nature of the infiltrate.[274,299] There are a number of histologic features, which should alert one to the possibility of lymphomatous change in celiac sprue. One is the replacement of plasma cells by lymphocytes as the predominant inflammatory cell component. A second is a biopsy resembling a Marsh 1 lesion of celiac disease with well-formed villi, but with tall columnar epithelium (unlike the cuboidal epithelium seen in celiac disease) containing numerous large IELs with a prominent perinuclear halo. This is reminiscent of the changes frequently seen adjacent to overt lymphomatous lesions, but rarely can be seen in duodenal biopsies. Another is the finding of a dense inflammatory infiltrate, which permeates the crypts, separates the base of the crypts from the muscularis mucosae, and extends beyond the muscularis mucosae into the submucosa. The presence of scattered, atypical large lymphoid cells within the inflammatory infiltrate is more definitive evidence of a malignant

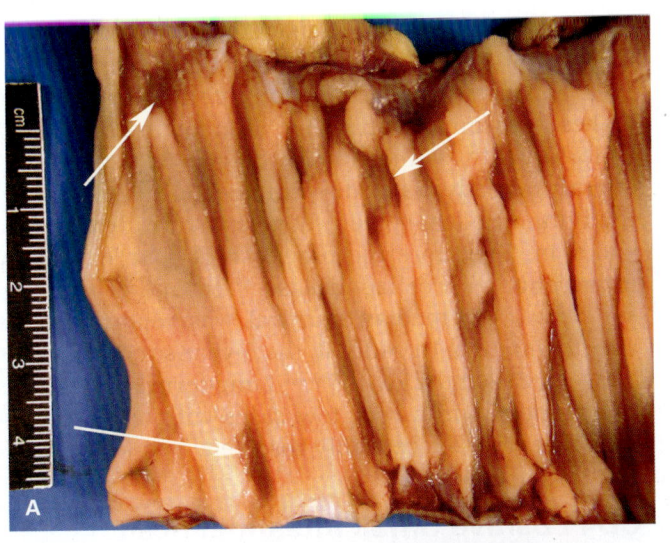
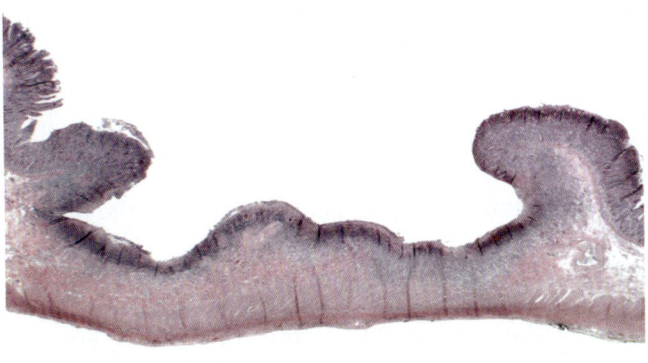
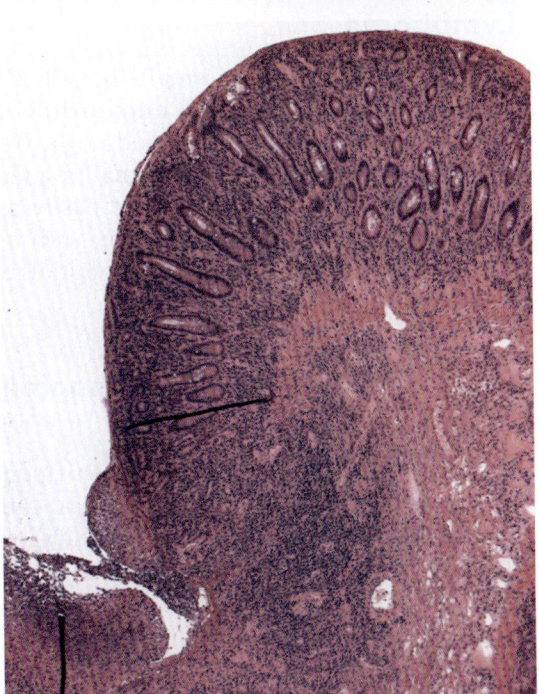
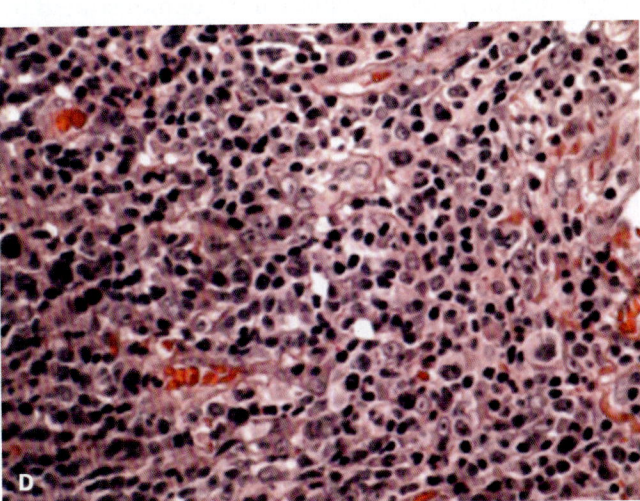
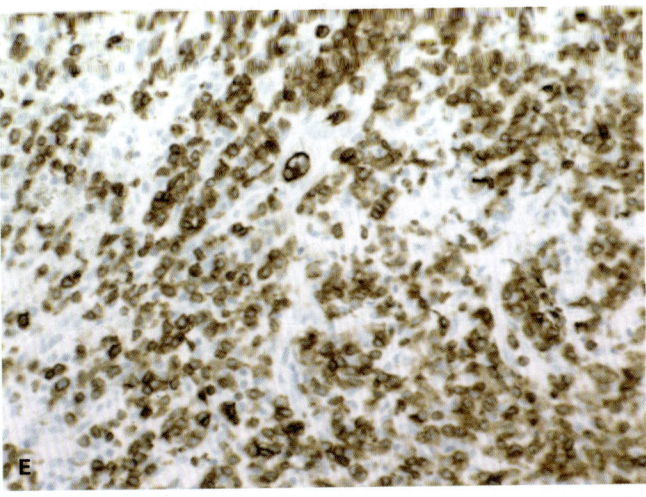

Figure 4-25. A: EATL lymphoma showing multiple benign-appearing ulcers (*arrows*) in a segment of jejunum. No mass-forming lesion is evident. **B:** EATL presenting as ulcerative jejunoileitis. There is moderate infiltrate at the base of the ulcer. The low-power view appears benign without any obvious mass-like lesion. **C:** Enteropathy-type changes in the adjacent mucosa and a polymorphous infiltrate in the lamina propria and the ulcer base. **D:** Detail of the infiltrate showing scattered atypical large cells admixed with a population composed of small- and intermediate-sized lymphocyte and plasma cells. **E:** The large cells as well as the majority of the background cells are CD3-positive T cells. The TCR in this case was clonally rearranged, confirming the diagnosis of an EATL.

change. In cases of ulcerative jejunoileitis, it is important to take multiple histologic samples especially from the margins of ulcers and examine serial sections, especially in small biopsies. Lastly, immunohistochemistry and molecular genetics may be necessary to confirm the diagnosis of a lymphoma.

Immunophenotype and molecular genetics. Similar to the histology there is some variability in the immunophenotype of EATL. In most cases the phenotype of the tumor cells is CD3+, CD4−, CD8−, CD7+ and CD103+, although many retain their C8 immunoreactivity. Cytotoxic T-cell–associated markers, T-cell intracellular antigen (TIA-1) and granzyme B, are also expressed.[3,294] These tumor cells are derived from α/β T-cells, rather than γ/δ T-cells as initially thought. Rearrangement of γ- and β-chains can be demonstrated by PCR in almost all cases.[297,298] Interestingly, in many cases associated with celiac disease the intraepithelial lymphocytes in the adjacent nonneoplastic mucosa show a similar T-cell population that is negative for CD8 and shows an identical TCR rearrangement supporting their role in the disease evolution (see also section on refractory celiac disease).[281,298] It should however be recognized that IELs may normally show oligoclonal pattern, and clonal expansion should be interpreted with caution.[123,300] Some cases are negative for CD3 while some may express CD8. The cases showing an anaplastic large-cell component are usually positive for CD30 (Ki-1); however, they do not express ALK. The subset composed of monomorphic small lymphoid cells has often a distinctive phenotype represented by CD3+, CD8+, CD56+, and granzyme B+.

The genetic and epigenetic phenomena associated with evolution of T-cell clones and eventually T-cell lymphoma in celiac disease are poorly understood. No specific cytogenetic abnormality has been recognized. Partial trisomy of 1q region is strongly associated with gluten resistance in celiac disease and is possibly an early event associated with evolution of T-cell clones. Recurrent gains at 9q33-34, 7q, 5q34-35, and 1q21-23 and recurrent loss at 8p, 13q, and 9p21 have been shown by comparative genomic hybridization, of which gain of 9q33-34 is the most frequent abnormality seen in about 58% of EATL cases.[301] It has been shown that this abnormality is associated with amplification of ABL1 and NOTCH1—important genes in regulation of hematopoiesis.[302] It has been postulated that synergistic activation of ABL1 and NOTCH1 results in PI3-kinase activation that inhibits apoptosis and facilitates cell cycle dysregulation. Frequent deletion of 9p21 accompanied by inactivation of the tumor suppressor gene *p16* has also been demonstrated.[303] Almost all cases of EATL show accumulation of *p53*; however, the underlying mechanisms are unclear.[303]

Treatment and prognosis. Treatment modalities include surgery and multiagent chemotherapy. However, concurrent malabsorption due to celiac disease makes it extremely difficult to tolerate any therapy.[304] Unfortunately, at the time of diagnosis, patients frequently already have disseminated diseases involving lymph nodes, spleen, bone marrow, liver, lungs, and skin. Therefore the prognosis is poor, especially in patients with celiac disease.[277] In one of the largest series, the median survival was reported to be about 3 months. In general, the 5-year survival ranges between 8% and 25%.[227,290,304] Long-term survival has been reported in a very few cases with localized disease that were successfully resected.[290,304]

CD4 Positive Small Intestinal T-cell Lymphoma

These are rare types of small intestinal lymphoma that are not associated with enteropathy and characterized by CD4+ phenotype, and negative CD8, CD7, CD56 and EBER. The cells are small to medium sized, and lymphoepithelial lesions are easily seen. These have a relatively better prognosis with slow relentless course, with some showing initial response to corticosteroids.[304a]

Other Miscellaneous Lymphoproliferative Disorders

Various other nodal types of non-Hodgkin's lymphomas, Hodgkin's lymphomas, and immunodeficiency-associated lymphomas that may involve small intestine primarily or secondarily are discussed in the subsequent sections of this chapter.

LYMPHOPROLIFERATIVE DISORDERS OF THE APPENDIX, COLON, AND ANAL CANAL

Lymphoma of the colon is uncommon and constitutes about 0.2% of all colonic malignancies, 3% of all extranodal lymphomas, and 10% to 20% of all GI lymphomas.[225,305] The most common sites of involvement are the cecum and rectum. There is a predilection for the rectum and anal canal in the setting of HIV infection and homosexual men.[306,307] Known risk factors include inflammatory bowel disease (IBD), in particular ulcerative colitis and immunodeficiency.[228] The clinical presentation is often similar to colonic carcinoma, with abdominal pain and bleeding being the most common symptoms. Other manifestations include weight loss, anemia, diarrhea, an abdominal mass, or change in bowel habits. Ulcerative colitis may present with worsening of symptoms once lymphoma develops, while some cases are found incidentally. Growth patterns and gross appearances are varied and include polypoid or protuberant masses, infiltrative growth, strictures, or ulcers. The clinical behavior and prognosis are similar to their small bowel counterparts. Involvement of other sites in the GI tract including small intestine and stomach is not uncommon. All histologic types are known to occur, of which lymphomas of the MALT-type are the most common.[228] Follicular lymphomas, mantle cell lymphoma, and Burkitt's lymphoma are also known to arise in the colon and are similar in their immunophenotype and molecular genetics to their nodal counterparts.

The primary lymphomas of the appendix are uncommon and seen in 0.015% to 0.022% of all appendectomies.[308,309] They tend to occur in younger individuals (mean age 25.7 years), and the majority present with acute appendicitis. DLBCL and Burkitt's lymphoma are the most common histologic types. Other less common and rare types reported include mantle cell lymphoma, marginal zone lymphoma, and T-cell lymphoma.[310–312]

MALT Lymphomas of the Colon

MALT lymphomas are similar to their small bowel counterparts, except that IPSID does not involve colon. MALT-type translocations have also been described in the colonic tumors. A recent study of 16 intestinal MALT lymphomas (5 small intestine, 11 colorectal cases) showed t(11;18)(q21;q21) in 2 colorectal cases. Trisomy 3 and 18 was also detected in all cases.[180] The lesions may present as discrete single protuberant/polypoid mass or as diffusely infiltrative lesions.[313] The other gross appearances included multiple sessile polyps (multiple lymphomatoid polyposis) and nodular or granular mucosa.[228,314] Rare examples presenting as mucosal erythema but with no obvious mass have also been reported,[315] and occasionally lesions indistinguishable from MALT lymphomas elsewhere are found in random biopsies. Colonic MALT lymphomas unlike their gastric and small bowel counterparts have not been well studied. So far, they have not been associated with or any infectious organism. Rare cases of colonic involvement in gastric MALT lymphomas have been described, of which some cases have responded to *H. pylori* eradication.[185] Their prognosis seems favorable and depends on the extent of the disease. Surgery has been suggested as the treatment of choice for localized disease. However, chemotherapy has also been employed with good results. With chemotherapy, remission rates of 100% have been attained, with projected 5-year survival, and disease-free survival rates of 100% and 85% have been reported.[316]

Mantle Cell Lymphoma

Mantle cell lymphoma comprises 2.5% to 7% of all non-Hodgkin's lymphomas, and the GI tract has been suggested to be involved in about 10% to 30% of the cases.[228,317,318] However, one study of mucosal biopsies obtained from patients without any GI symptoms and with normal enodoscopic findings revealed microscopic GI involvement in 45% (10/22) and 84% (26/31) of upper GI and colonic biopsies, respectively.[319] The majority of the patients with GI symptoms, however, present with multiple polyps (multiple lymphomatous polyposis). Invariably when the GI disease is diagnosed, the lymphoma is widespread, and in cases of primary nodal disease GI involvement is very common.[319] It is still unclear whether mantle cell lymphoma could be a primary disorder of the GI in cases of multiple lymphomatous polyposis or is almost always representative of a disseminated disease, where the nodal involvement may not initially be obvious. Terminally widespread dissemination with involvement of the liver, spleen, bone marrow, and lymph nodes is usual.

Clinical Features Mantle cell lymphoma is a disease of the middle-aged and elderly (mean 60 years) and is more common in males.[228,317] Patients usually present with nonspecific features such as iron-deficiency anemia, weight loss, fatigue, abdominal pain, diarrhea, and malena, and no differences are apparent among patients presenting with or without multiple lymphomatous polyposis. Any part of the GI tract may be involved including the stomach; howeverm the ileocecal region is the most common site.

Pathology Grossly, the disease commonly tends to present as multiple polyps (Fig. 4-21E). Other gross presentations include inflamed mucosa, nodular mucosa, ulcers, thickened folds, or a solitary mass.[318–320] In patients presenting with nodal disease, the grossly normal mucosa also shows frequent microscopic involvement. Microscopically, the polyps straddle the muscularis mucosae involving the mucosa and superficial submucosa causing displacement and disruption of the epithelium, but lymphoepithelial lesions are not found (Fig. 4-26). Morphologically the mantle cell lymphoma lesions consist of nodular aggregates of intermediate-type lymphocytes (intermediate between small lymphocytic and large cleaved cell lymphomas). The cells show scant pale cytoplasm and nuclei that are round or moderately irregular with dispersed chromatin and inconspicuous nucleoli, resembling mantle zone lymphocytes. Occasionally, the lymphocytes are transformed into large blastoid cells with smooth euchromatic nuclear chromatin. These cases tend to have a more aggressive clinical

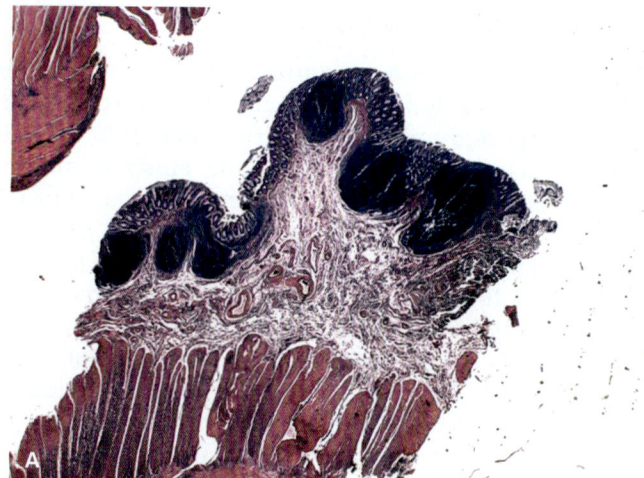
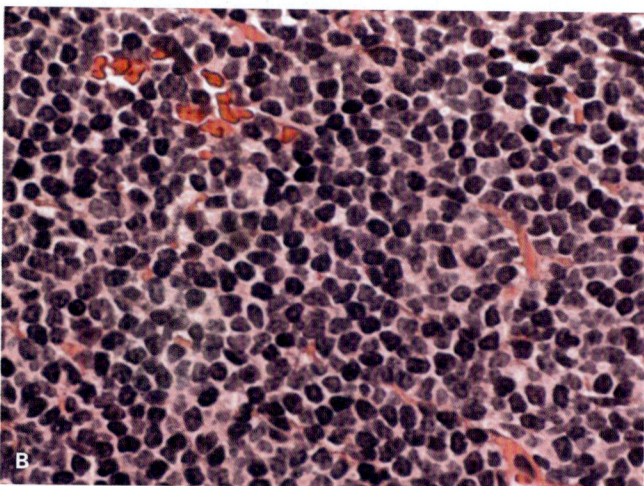

Figure 4-26. Mantle cell lymphoma. **A:** Lymphoid nodules straddling the muscularis mucosae and expanding the mucosa. **B:** Small lymphocytic cells with cytologic features typical of a mantle cell lymphoma. Tumor cells were CD5+ and cyclinD1+.

evolution. The tumor cells sometime surround and infiltrate lymphoid follicles and show intermingled follicular dendritic cells.

Immunophenotype and Molecular Genetics The immunophenotype and molecular genetics is identical to the nodal disease.[317] The tumor cells have features typical of mature B cells and show surface IgM and IgD. Light chain restriction is often seen, and predominance of λ light chains has been reported. The tumor cells express B-cell markers CD19, CD20, CD22, CD24, and CD35 and PAX5, and characteristically also coexpress T cell markers—CD5 and CD43. Virtually all cases express nuclear BCL1 (cyclin D1). CD10, CD11c, and CD23 are negative. Interestingly, cases that involve the gut seem to express the α4β7 integrin (CD103) similar to MALT lymphomas, which may be responsible for their GI localization. In addition, the cytogenetic and molecular studies show the translocation of the cyclin-D1 gene on chromosome 11 to chromosome 14 or close to IgH gene, BCL1 gene rearrangement, or both.[321-323]

Differential Diagnosis Morphologically, the tumor cells of mantle cell lymphoma per se, as well as the perifollicular growth pattern, especially in biopsies, may closely resemble MALT lymphomas. In these cases the only definitive way of differentiating one from the other is by demonstrating the presence of CD5 and cyclin-D1, which are present in the mantle cell lymphomas and not in the MALT lymphomas. With regard to the polypoid nature of the lesions, they may be confused with nodular lymphoid hyperplasia and follicular lymphoma. However, the diffuse nature of the infiltrate versus true nodular lymphomatous proliferation, the distinctive cytology and the characteristic immunophenotype as noted above, should help in the differential diagnosis.

Treatment and Prognosis Mantle cell lymphomas show widespread dissemination (stage IV) at the time of diagnosis. The clinical course is aggressive and not curable by currently available therapy. Response to chemotherapy is seen in only half of the patients, and the median survival time is around 2 to 5 years.[321,323] Recently, somewhat better remission rates have been reported with anti-CD20 (rituximab) used in combination chemotherapy.

Multiple Lymphomatous Polyposis

The entity of multiple lymphomatous polyposis was first introduced by Cornes in 1961 to describe an intestinal lymphoma that presented as multiple polyps affecting long segments of the GI tract.[94] The term in the past was restricted to involvement of GI tract with mantle cell lymphoma. However, it is now recognized that although most cases represent mantle cell lymphoma, overall it is a heterogeneous group comprised of other lymphomas, including follicular lymphomas and occasionally MALT lymphomas.[313,324-327] It commonly involves the colon, but can involve the small bowel and rarely the stomach. In a study from Japan of 35 cases presenting as multiple lymphomatous polypsis, mantle cell lymphomas ($n = 12$), follicular lymphomas ($n = 14$), and MALT lymphomas ($n = 9$) were identified (314). Of these 35 cases, 14 (40%) cases showed involvement of multiple sites in the GI tract. In 10 (28.5%) cases, polyps were limited to colon, and in 11(31.4%) cases, only small bowel and/or stomach was involved. Among the cases with colonic and extracolonic GI tract involvement, mantle cell lymphoma (8/14) was the most common type, followed by follicular lymphoma (4/14) and MALT lymphoma (2/14). Among cases of purely colonic involvement, MALT lymphoma (7/10) was the most common type, followed by follicular lymphoma (2/10) and mantle cell lymphoma (1/10). Grossly, the lesions are numerous, tiny, tan colored, mucosal nodules, about 2 to 3 mm in diameter (Fig. 4-21E). Occasionally the polyps may be larger measuring up to 2 cm. There may be a myriad of lesions producing a mucosal studding or a cobblestone appearance of the mucosa, or the lesions may be more widely spaced. It should be stressed that secondary involvement of the GI tract by leukemia and other nodal lymphomas may also result in multiple intestinal polyps and in fact occurs more commonly than multiple lymphomatous polyposis.

The lymphomatous polyps due to secondary involvement by nodal lymphomas are usually much larger (often >5 mm in diameter) than those found in multiple lymphomatous polyposis. The leukemic lesions, which are commonly a terminal event, on the other hand, consist of usually multiple, small, bluish mucosal nodules. The prognosis and treatment depends upon the subtype of lymphoma and extent of the disease.

MISCELLANEOUS LYMPHO-PROLIFERATIVE DISORDERS OF THE GI TRACT

Follicular Lymphomas (Follicular and Diffuse Types)

Involvement of the GI tract by follicular lymphomas can be either primary or secondary and constitutes 1% to 3.6% of all primary GI tract lymphomas.[328,329] While it shares many features with its nodal counterpart, it has some unique features as well. In contrast to nodal follicular lymphoma, which has a similar worldwide distribution, primary GI follicular lymphoma shows a higher incidence in Japan, and about half of all cases reported are from Japan.[328] The median age at presentation is 56 years (range 26–81 years). While few studies show a slight female preponderance, overall it appears to have no gender predilection similar to nodal follicular lymphomas.[329,330] Primary GI follicular lymphomas have also been shown to express α4β7 integrin/CD103 (GI homing receptor) unlike their nodal counterparts, very similar to other non-Hodgkin's lymphomas that localize to the gut.[331] They seem to remain localized to GI tract for long period, and it is speculated that chronic antigenic stimulation may play a role in their development. Although no *H. pylori*–type infectious etiology has been identified so far, treatment with antibiotics has been attempted without any consistent response.[328]

Clinical features. It appears that many patients (43.3%) remain asymptomatic, and the lesions are detected incidentally during routine endoscopy.[328] The most common clinical presentation among symptomatic patients is pain abdomen. Other presenting symptoms include intestinal obstruction, GI bleeding, anemia, or vague abdominal symptoms. Rarely they may present with diarrhea or protein-losing enteropathy with hypoalbuminemia.

Pathology. The most common sites involved in the GI tract are the ileocecal region and duodenum.[16] The disease can be unifocal or multifocal in the GI tract. As the use of videocapsule endoscopy and double balloon enteroscopy has increased, it appears that the disease is more often multifocal (70%) than previously realized.[328,329,332] The tumors most commonly present as multiple mucosal nodules and sometimes as solitary masses (Fig. 4-27A). It may occasionally also present as multiple lymphomatous polyposis.[79,330] Histologically and phenotypically the lymphoma resembles its nodal counterpart, that is, consists of centrocytes and centroblasts with nodular, diffuse, or mixed patterns (Fig. 4-27B–D). They are graded similar to nodal follicular lymphomas based on the proportion (G1 < 5%, G2 = 5%–15%, G3 > 15%) of the large cells (centroblasts). The follicles in follicular lymphomas have a pale center composed of centrocytes and centroblasts similar to a reactive follicle. However, they generally lack a starry-sky appearance due to the paucity of tingible body macrophages and a mantle zone. The follicles are generally of the same size as reactive follicles but tend to be more uniform. The tumors generally lack lymphoepithelial lesions and a superficial plasma cell-rich infiltrate, although rarely presence of lymphoepithelial lesions can create confusion with a MALT lymphoma.[2]

Immunophenotype and molecular genetics. The GI follicular lymphomas are similar in their immunophenotype to their nodal counterparts and express B-cell differentiation markers (CD19, CD20 CD22, CD10, Pax5, and BCL2) and are negative for CD5 and BCL1. Similar to its nodal counterpart GI follicular lymphomas show t(14;18)(q32;q21) in 70% to 95% of cases.[328] The translocation causes fusion of *BCL2* gene with the immunoglobulin heavy chain–joining region (IgH), which prevents normal switching off of *BCL2*. The translocation can be demonstrated by Southern blotting, PCR, or FISH assays, of which FISH seems to be the most sensitive method.

Differential diagnosis. The differential diagnosis of follicular lymphomas often includes reactive follicular hyperplasia, MALT lymphoma, and mantle cell lymphoma. CD10 and bcl-2 are helpful in differentiating follicular lymphoma from reactive follicles and its other mimics. In follicular lymphoma the germinal centers diffusely express BCL2, and in more than

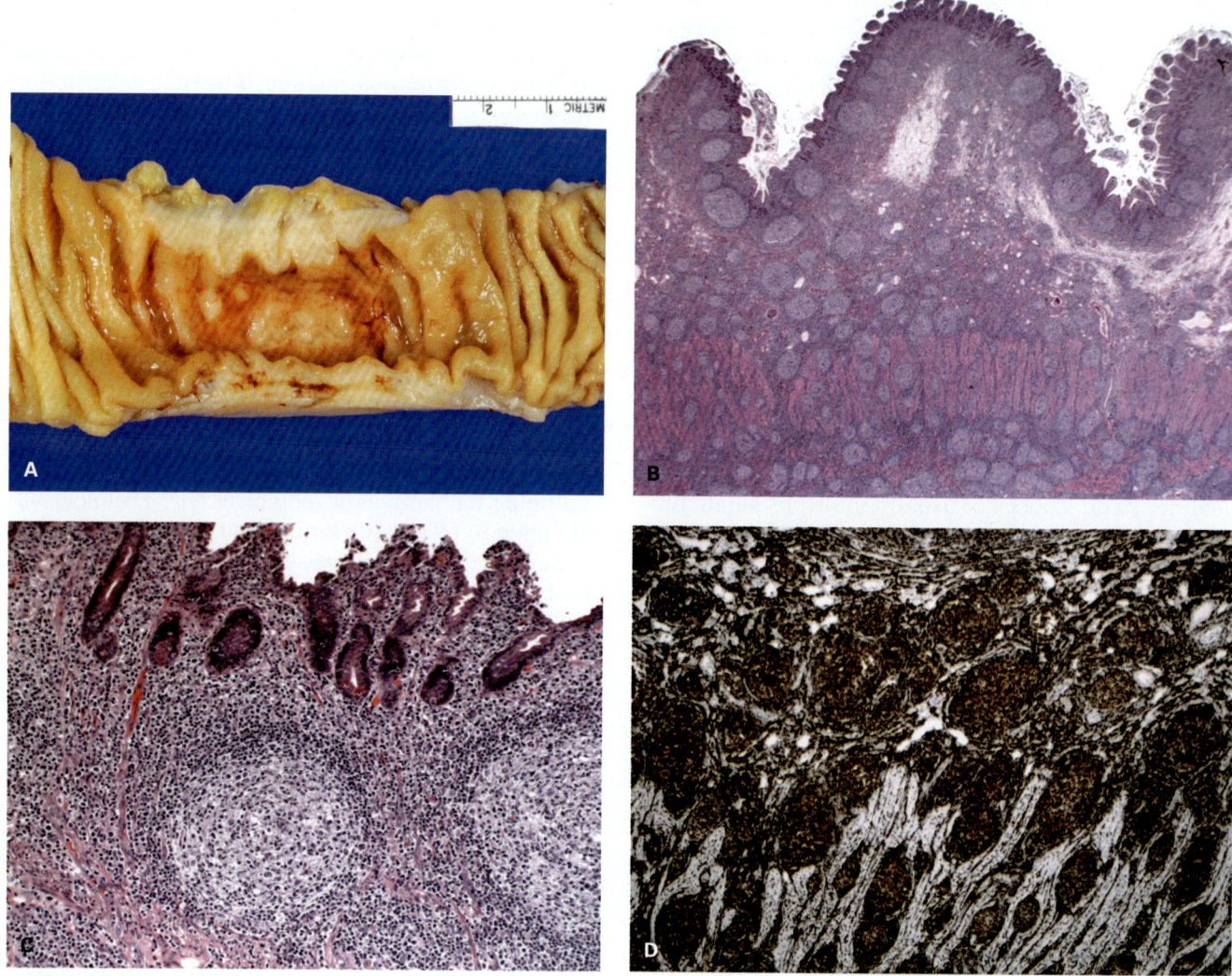

Figure 4-27. **A:** Gross photographs of a follicular lymphoma in a 71-year-old man involving the small intestine. The involved area shows thickening of the wall and of the overlying mucosal folds. **B:** Follicular lymphoma involving the small intestine. The infiltrate is seen extending transmurally and preserved follicles are easily visible even at low magnification. **C:** Higher magnification of the follicles. **D:** Immunostain for Bcl2 shows diffuse staining of the follicles and the surrounding infiltrate.

90% cases also CD10. Reactive follicles express only CD10, mantle cell lymphomas are negative for both CD10 and BCL2, and MALT lymphoma is negative for CD10 but may sometimes express BCL2. Immunophenotyping (Table 4-5) and the presence of characteristic translocation helps in establishing the correct diagnosis.[141,333]

Treatment and prognosis. The long-term outcome of primary GI follicular lymphomas is unclear as cases in the literature are few and long-term outcome data are lacking. Primary GI follicular lymphoma tends to remain localized for long time unlike its nodal counterpart, which is often a disseminated disease at presentation.[334] In a study of 193 GI follicular lymphomas patients where the staging data were available, 128 (66.3%) were at stage I and 52 (26.9%) were at stage II.[328] In general, GI follicular lymphomas are more indolent and have a better prognosis than their nodal counterparts. However, this may be an artifact as patients with disseminated disease at presentation (stages 3 and 4) are often excluded from the studies on primary follicular GI lymphomas, as by definition they don't qualify as primary GI lymphomas.[329,330] There is no standard therapy for follicular lymphomas, and various combinations of surgery, conventional chemotherapy, radiation, and rituximab are used, and remission is achieved in about 42% of patients.[328] The median relapse-free time ranges from 31 to 45 months based on few series with long-term outcome data.[328] The disease is indolent, and in patients without any treatment the median time to disease progression is about 37.5 months, which is very similar to median time to relapse following remission.[328] The disease can show waxing and waning course and sometimes even spontaneous remission.[335] Due to its indolent course

Table 4-5	Immunohistochemical Differentiation of Small Lymphocytic Gastrointestinal Lymphomas				
	MALTOMA	IPSID	MANTLE CELL	FOLLICULAR CENTER	CLL
Ig	M+, G&A RARELY+	IgA-α HEAVY CHAIN (LIGHT CHAIN NEGATIVE)	D, M+	G, M+	D, M+
CD5	−	−	+	−	+
CD10	−	−	±	+	−
CD20	+	+	+	+	+
CD23	−	−	−	±	+
CD43	±	±	+	−	NA
BCL2	±	NA	±	+	NA
Cyclin D1	−	NA	+	−	−

NA, studies not available.

and lack of any definite survival benefit from therapy, many advocate wait-and-watch policy for asymptomatic patients, at least for the early stage disease.[328]

Lymphoplasmacytic Lymphoma/ Waldenström's Macroglobulinemia

Rarely, lymphoplasmacytic lymphomas may arise as a primary tumor in the GI tract.[336–338] The lymphoma is characterized by the presence of a diffuse proliferation of small mature B lymphocytes, plasmacytoid lymphocytes, and plasma cells. A typical case shows B-cell–associated antigens (CD19, CD20, CD22, CD79a, Pax5) and plasmacytic markers (CD138) and lacks CD5, CD10, CD103, and CD23. Some cases express CD5. It is one of the tumors that readily shows light-chain restriction immunohistochemically. Most cells express surface Ig, usually IgM, but sometimes IgA, especially in the GI tract. The plasma cells present express cytoplasmic Ig of the same type. It shares overlapping histologic and immunophenotypic features with extranodal marginal zone lymphomas/MALT lymphoma and SLL/CLL. Differentiation in some cases requires correlation with serum/urine electrophoresis findings and bone marrow involvement.[336] Rare cases with gastric involvement have been reported to show lymphoepithelial lesions (Fig. 4-28) and have been mistaken for MALT-type lymphoma.[338] We have seen a rare example in the stomach that did not show obvious plasmacytic differentiation. This case lacked the usual B-cell–associated antigens, lacked the presence of interspersed T cells that are invariably seen with B-cell lymphomas of the GI tract, and was even negative for pan-leukocyte marker (CD45). This case was strongly and diffusely CD138 positive (see Fig. 4-28). Rare cases of small bowel tumors have presented with diarrhea.[337] In small bowel, biopsy chunks of IgM deposited in the lamina propria may be mistaken for amyloid, although the lesion is virtually diagnostic provided one is aware of the appearance.

When associated with Waldenström's macroglobulinemia the cells characteristically express surface IgM and have elevated serum IgM paraprotein. A minority has both IgM and IgG or some other paraprotein. The t(9;14) chromosomal translocation has been found in 50% of all lymphoplasmacytic lymphoma cases. Bone marrow is invariably involved; however, the clinical course is usually indolent. While thinking of mimics of lymphomas (e.g., some leukemias), one should also think of lymphoplasmacytic lymphoma. Careful examination does provide the hint of plasmacytoid differentiation (Fig 4-28A–F) that may trigger CD138 stain and lead to the correct diagnosis.

Immunodeficiency-Associated Lymphoproliferative Disorders

Immunodeficiency disorders have not only increased the risk of developing infections but also a variety of lymphoproliferative disorders. Although some variations occur with respect to the type of immunodeficiency, many similarities exist. In general, a range of lymphoproliferative diseases arise in this setting that include reactive hyperplasias to intermediate polymorphous polyclonal disorders to frank clonal lymphomas. Many of these are often associated with EBV. The treatment and prognosis varies and depends on the underlying primary disorder as well as the nature of lymphoproliferative disease.

Primary immunodeficiency-associated lymphoproliferative disorders. There is a well-documented increase in lymphoproliferative disease developing in primary immunodeficiency disorders (see also Chapter 5) that include Ataxia telangiectasia, Wiskott–Aldrich syndrome, CVID syndrome, severe combined immunodeficiency syndrome, X-linked lymphoproliferative disorder, Nijmegen breakage syndrome, hyper IgM syndrome, and autoimmune lymphoproliferative syndrome.[339] Extranodal involvement is frequent and

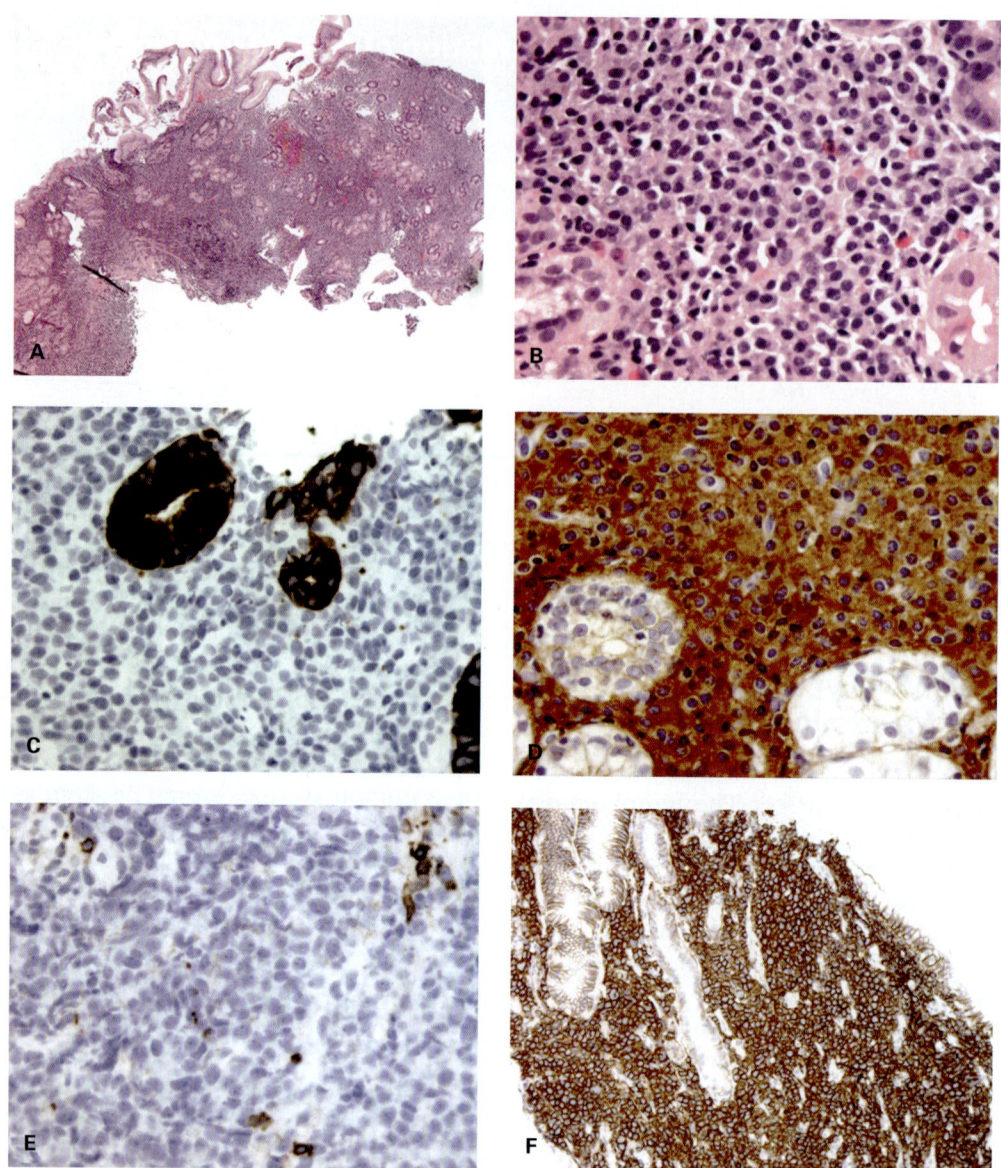

Figure 4-28. **A:** *H. pylroi*–negative gastric lymphoma that shows diffuse infiltration of the lamina propria by mononuclear cells. **B:** Detail shows focal plasmacytic differentiation Keratin stain highlights a lymphoepithelial lesion **(C)**. The tumor cells show strong positivity for IgA **(D)**. The tumor was negative for CD45 **(E)**, and strongly and diffusely positive for CD138 **(F)**. This was designated as lymphoplasmacytic lymphoma.

includes the GI tract and the central nervous system. The clinical manifestations vary from infection-like presentation to an obvious mass. In some conditions like CVID, autoimmune lymphoproliferative disorder or Wiskott–Aldrich syndrome, chronic antigenic stimulation leads to lymphoid hyperplasia in the GI tract that may progress to frank lymphoma in some cases.[340] In others, defective T-cell function leads to EBV-driven B-cell proliferations and lymphoma.[341] Intestinal lymphangiectasia and protein-losing enteropathies lead to hypogammaglobulinemia and lymphoma, where treatment of the lymphoma in some cases results in the cure of the primary defect.[342] In hyper-IgM syndrome the peripheral blood B cells bear only IgM and IgD, germinal centers are absent in lymph nodes, and patients develop marked proliferations of IgM-containing plasma cells, frequently at extranodal sites that include GI tract, gall bladder, and liver. These lesions may be extensive and fatal without ever progressing to frank lymphoma. The type of lymphoproliferative disease is somewhat dependent on the nature of the primary immune defect.[339] Overall DLBCL is the most common lymphoproliferative disease in the setting of primary immunodeficiency disorders, although any other nodal type of lymphoma and polymorphous PTLD-type lesions can occur. Immunoblastic variant is more frequent than the centroblastic variant. Fatal infectious mononucleosis with systemic B-cell proliferation tends to occur in patients with X-linked lymphoproliferative disease and SCID. The lesion is characterized by proliferation of plasmacytoid cells and immunoblasts, sometimes containing admixed Reed–Sternberg-like cells. Hemophagocytosis is often present and may lead to pancytopenia and further infectious complications. In the GI tract the terminal ileum is the most frequently involved site. Lymphomatoid granulomatosis is seen in some cases of Wiskott–Aldrich syndrome and is characterized by angiocentric and angiodestructive lymphoid proliferation that tends to respond to immunomodulatory therapy (e.g., interferon α2b) in some cases. In some cases it may progress to frank DLBCL. Unlike other primary immunodeficiency disorders, in ataxia telangiectasia, T-cell neoplasms are more frequently seen than B-cell neoplasms. Peripheral T-cell lymphomas have also been reported in CVID and autoimmune lymphoproliferative disease. Hodgkin's lymphoma and Hodgkin's-like lymphomas are also known to occur in the setting of primary immunodeficiency syndromes. Prognosis and treatment depend on the underlying primary disorder as well as the type of lymphoproliferative disease. Bone marrow transplantation used in some conditions as a treatment of the primary immunodeficiency disease has been associated with reduction in the risk of developing a subsequent lymphoproliferative disorder.[343,344]

Acquired immunodeficiency-associated lymphoproliferative disorders

AIDS-associated Lymphoma AIDS patients are prone to quite a number of neoplasms.[345–347] The two most common tumors are Kaposi's sarcoma (Herpes virus-8 associated) and lymphoma, which are also designated as AIDS defining illnesses. The incidence of lymphoma is estimated to be increased 60 to 200-fold in AIDS patients.[347] Since the availability of highly active antiretroviral therapy (HAART), there has been a marked improvement in the survival of patients with HIV infection with a reduction in the infectious complications and decrease in the incidence of Kaposi's sarcoma and primary CNS lymphoma.[348] The reduction in the incidence of other lymphomas in comparison has been less dramatic. The lymphomas are frequently extranodal and most frequently involve the GI tract. In addition a fair number of other tumors can also occur in AIDS patients, namely, anal cancer, cervical cancer, leiomyoma, leiomyosarcoma, brain tumors, and conjunctival cancer. Similar to other immunodeficiency-associated lymphomas, AIDS-related lymphomas have also been associated with oncogenic viruses. Overall, EBV has been associated with about 60% of lymphomas seen with HIV infection, although the association varies markedly with the lymphoma subtype.[349] While about 80% of the DLBCL of the immunoblastic-type are associated with EBV, only 30% to 50% of Burkitt's lymphomas are associated with EBV. There appears to be a slight increase in the incidence of Hodgkin's lymphoma with HIV infection, and almost all cases are associated with EBV. Human herpes virus 8 (HHV8), also known as Kaposi's sarcoma herpes virus (KSHV), has been associated with primary effusion lymphoma, multicentric Castleman's disease, and Kaposi's sarcoma.[349]

The most frequent site of involvement in GI tract is the anorectal region, followed by the small intestine and stomach. The signs and symptoms and gross appearances are similar to their counterparts in immunocompetent hosts. A wide range of lymphoma subtypes occur in AIDS, and the classification of common sub-types is shown in Table 4-6. Almost all are of B-cell phenotype, although rare T-cell types have also been reported. Histologically, the majority of

Table 4-6 Lymphomas Associated with HIV Infection

1. Lymphomas also occurring in immunocompetent patients
    - Burkitt's lymphoma
        - Classical
        - With plasmacytoid differentiation
        - Atypical
    - Diffuse large B-cell lymphoma
        - Centroblastic
        - Immunoblastic
    - Extranodal marginal zone B-cell lymphoma of mucosa-associated lymphoid tissue type (MALT lymphoma) (rare)
    - Peripheral T-cell lymphoma (rare)
    - Classical Hodgkin's lymphoma
2. Lymphomas occurring more specifically in HIV+ patients
    - Primary effusion lymphoma
    - Plasmablastic lymphoma of the oral cavity
3. Lymphomas also occurring in other immunodeficiency states
    - Polymorphic B-cell lymphoma (PTLD-like)

AIDS-associated lymphomas are composed of either DLBCL (immunoblastic or centroblastic variants) or Burkitt's/Burkitt's-like lymphoma. Their histologic features, immunophenotype and genotype are similar to those seen outside the AIDS setting. Many of the lymphomas are multifocal and show extraintestinal spread at the time of diagnosis.

A unique type of lymphoma seen predominantly in AIDS patients is primary effusion lymphoma that tends to involve the peritoneal, pleural, or pericardial cavities.[350,351] In most cases, a solid mass is lacking and the tumor cells are initially detected in the cytologic preparations of effusion fluids. Rare examples of solid tumors, most commonly involving the GI tract or soft tissues, have also been described.[352,353] In some of these cases, the effusions appear later. The tumor cells are large with abundant cytoplasm and appear immunoblastic, plasmablastic, or anaplastic in appearance. They are positive for CD45 (LCA) and often express several plasma cell markers that include CD138, VS38c, and MUM-1/IRF4.[351,354] Activation-associated markers CD30, CD38, CD71, and EMA are also generally positive.[352] They lack expression of B- and T-cell markers but invariably show Ig gene rearrangement by PCR suggestive of a B-cell derivation.[355] They are invariably associated with HHV8/KSHV, which can be demonstrated by PCR or immunohistochemical methods.[350] The primary effusion lymphomas can be easily differentiated from other high-grade B-cell lymphomas that may secondarily involve the serosal cavities. DLBCL and Burkitt's lymphoma that represent the most common differential diagnosis are always associated with a solid tumor mass, express B-cell markers, and are invariably negative for HHV8/KSHV.

The prognosis of these lymphomas has been poor with all therapies before the HAART era, mean survival being 3.6 ± 2.2 months.[356] Patients with early stages and those with surgically resectable disease tend to do better. In advanced stages patients often develop peripheral lymphadenopathy, cachexia, and hepatosplenomegaly, and often succumb to opportunistic infections, therapy-related toxicity, or direct complications of the lymphoma. Since the availability of HAART, many patients are now able to tolerate the chemotherapy better, and recent studies suggest an improvement in the prognosis.[345] Long-term outcomes of newer therapies in this setting are still awaited.

Posttransplant Lymphoproliferative Disorders Posttransplant lymphoproliferative disorder (PTLD) consists of a group of lymphoproliferative disorders that occurs in solid organ and bone marrow transplant recipients.[357-359] Since its initial description in 1969, it has been recognized as one of the most serious complications of transplantation. The incidence varies depending on the type of organ transplant, age of the patient, and immunosuppressive regimen, being about 1% to 5% in renal and liver transplants, 5% to 15% in heart and heart–lung transplants, and 10% to 15% in intestinal transplants.[358,360-364] The incidence in bone marrow transplants is 0.5% after HLA-matched and noncomplicated transplants, and 25% after HLA-mismatched, T-cell depleted and highly immunosuppressed patients.[358] The incidence is also higher in pediatric transplant patients and has been attributed to the development of primary EBV infection after transplantation. The majority (85%) of PTLDs are associated with EBV and represent B-cell tumors.[365] T-cell lymphomas are less common, and other types are even rarer.

ETIOLOGY AND PATHOGENESIS. Strong association of PTLD with EBV suggests an important role for the virus in lymphomagenesis. EBV is a ubiquitous virus, and >90% of the general population develops EBV infection, especially during the early years of life. The virus can stay in a latent phase in memory B cells. During immunosuppression, reactivation of the virus with active replication occurs. The early changes of PTLD represent a spectrum of EBV-driven polyclonal B-cell proliferations. These subsequently may progress to a monoclonal monomorphous B-cell lymphoma.

In some instances the involved B lymphocytes are of donor origin, apparently originating from "passenger" lymphocytes within the donor organ.[366-369] PTLD can also sometimes occur in nonimmunosuppressed individuals.

CLINICAL PRESENTATION. PTLD may manifest with a variety of symptoms and must be suspected in any patient who undergoes solid organ transplantation. The clinical features depend upon the type of immunosuppression and type of organ transplant. Patients who receive cyclosporine as the immunosuppressant tend to present earlier (median 15 months) as compared to those who get azathioprine (median 48 months).[370] PTLD can occur as early as 4 to 6 weeks posttransplantation, but usually develops within 6 months of transplantation. In general, EBV-positive cases tend to present earlier compared to EBV-negative cases, and cases presenting 5 years after transplantation are often EBV negative.[371-373] In azathioprine-based regimens the sites of involvement are often extranodal. In cases receiving cyclosporine or tacrolimus-based regimens, lymph nodes and GI tract are frequently involved.[365,374] With bone marrow transplants the disease is often widespread. Clinical presentation is variable and includes GI bleeding, weight loss, protein-losing enteropathy, bacteremia, lymphadenopathy, infectious mononucleosis-like symptoms, or a mass lesion. Presentation as a mass occurs most frequently in extranodal locations such as the GI tract, the allograft itself, or the brain. The fulminant form of PTLD is characterized by a combination of peripheral lymphadenopathy, severe metabolic acidosis, organ failure, or allograft dysfunction.

PATHOLOGY. Gross presentation of PTLDs involving the GI tract resembles other primary GI lymphomas such as a nodular mass or an infiltrative lesion. The lesions are commonly ulcerated and covered with a greenish-yellow fibrinous exudate. On cut section they characteristically have a grayish color and soft consistency and may extend to the serosa, which sometimes leads to necrosis and perforation.

The GI tract is one of the common sites of extranodal involvement of PTLD, and its histologic features in the GI tract are no different from those described at other sites. Initially, the infiltrate is confined to the mucosa and submucosa and subsequently extends into the muscularis propria and beyond, similar to the other lymphomas. Morphologically, PTLD is characterized by a dense mononuclear infiltrate, with a histologic spectrum ranging from that commonly found in infectious mononucleosis to that of a lymphoma.[358] As a result they are either polymorphous or monomorphous and may be associated with extensive necrosis. Morphologically, there are three major patterns.[358]

Plasma cell–rich or infectious mononucleosis-like lesion These lesions involve primarily the lymphoid tissue of the oropharynx and lymph nodes.[375] The infiltrate is plasma cells rich with scattered immunoblasts. The underlying architecture of the tissue or the organ is preserved. The lymph nodes tend to show plasma cell–rich pattern while the extranodal sites tend to show infectious mononucleosis-type infiltrate. In addition, there is evidence of EBV infection. Oncogene and tumor suppressor gene alterations are lacking. The Ig gene rearrangement studies may show a small clonal, oligoclonal, or polyclonal pattern.[376]

Polymorphous B-cell hyperplasia and lymphoma These lesions consist of a dense polymorphous infiltrate composed of B and T cells, which range from small and mature cells to small and large cleaved or noncleaved cells, plasma cells, and plasmacytoid cells, as well as immunoblasts, some of which may be atypical (Fig. 4-29A,B). Scattered multinucleated or pleomorphic bizarre cells may also be present. The infiltrate is destructive and results in the effacement of the tissue architecture of the organ involved.[377,378] Mitotic figures are commonly present. There may be extensive necrosis, and in these cases numerous neutrophils and histiocytes are commonly seen. The cells express normal B-cell markers and may express surface or cytoplasmic Ig that could be polytypic or monotypic. The majority of these polymorphous lesions have been shown to be monoclonal using gene rearrangement studies and contain a single form of EBV, but lack evidence of oncogene (c-MYC and RAS) and tumor suppressor gene (p53) alterations.[376–378] Mutations of BCL-6 have been reported in one study to occur in about 40% cases.[379]

The monomorphous monoclonal lymphomatous infiltrate These tend to resemble various nodal type lymphomas and should be classified as such.[358,380] Almost all cases are of B-cell origin, although rare instances of T-cell proliferations have been reported. Most often this variant consists of large atypical lymphocytes and represents a DLBCL, frequently of the immunoblastic type. Some cases resemble centroblastic and less commonly anaplastic-type DLBCL. Despite the designation "monomorphic," they may show some pleomorphism and variation in the cells with plasmacytic cells but lack the degree of polymorphism

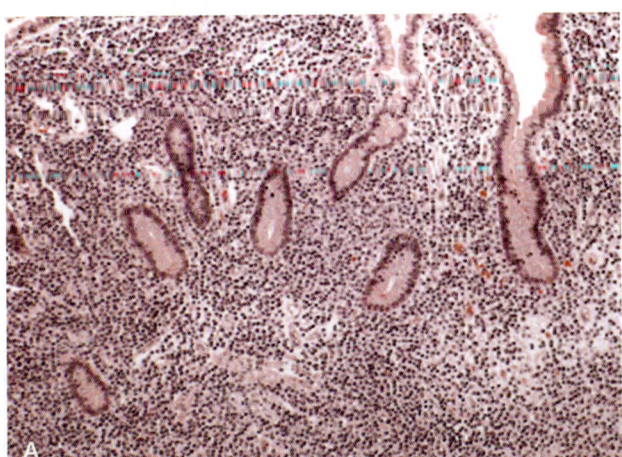
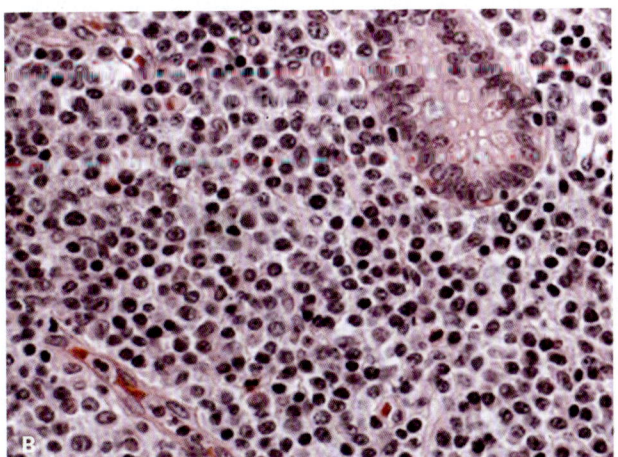

Figure 4-29. Posttransplant lymphoproliferative involving the small bowel disorder in a 17-year-old girl who received liver transplant. **A:** Low power shows transmural infiltrate. **B:** Higher magnification shows a polymorphous population composed of lymphocytes, plasma cells, immunoblasts, and few eosinophils. The PTLD in this case resolved on withdrawal of immuosuppression only to recur 1 year later as monomorphic DLBCL requiring chemotherapy.

and full range of differentiation seen in the polymorphic PTLD. These lesions are also destructive and result in the effacement of tissue architecture of the involved organ. Immunophenotypically they express B-cell markers similar to their nodal counterparts. In addition, some also express T-cell markers, CD43 and CD45RO. Many cases express CD30 with or without anaplastic histology. Ig gene rearrangement studies show clonal pattern in virtually all cases, and majority of the cases express EBV-associated antigens (EBV-LMP1 and EBNA).[381-383] Abnormalities of MYC, RAS, and p53 are seen frequently similar to de novo DLBCL. Mutations of BCL6 have been reported in a study to occur in all cases of monomorphic PTLD.[379]

Rare miscellaneous PTLD patterns These include Hodgkin's lymphoma, Hodgkin's-like PTLD, T/NK cell, multiple myeloma, and plasmacytoma-like histology.[358]

Treatment and prognosis Reduction of immunosuppression is the primary treatment of choice, although as stated above, some tumors are unresponsive to this regimen and there is obvious risk of loss of the transplanted organ, which in many instances may itself either be fatal or necessitate dialysis.[375,376,384] This therapy is usually coupled with the administration of acyclovir and surgery for lesions such as intestinal perforation and obstruction. The early plasma cell hyperplasia or infectious mononucleosis-like lesions tend to respond very well to withdrawal or reduction in immunosuppression. Some cases recur and may progress to polymorphic or monomorphic PTLD. The polymorphic and less often monomorphic PTLD may also respond to reduction in immunosupression.[358] Tumor regression within 1 to 2 weeks is not unusual and in some instances appears to be accompanied by maturation of the clonal PTLD cells into mature plasma cells concurrent with a reduction in their numbers. In other instances progressively more malignant clones develop, leading to disease progression and mortality. Tumors that do not respond to reduction of immunosuppression are treated similar to high grade nodal lymphomas.

Unfortunately, it is difficult to reliably predict the behavior of PTLD in individual patients. For example, some polymorphous polyclonal PTLDs developing shortly after transplantation may have a fulminant and fatal course, while some monoclonal PTLDs have regressed completely following discontinuation of all immunosuppressive therapy, but often with the inevitable consequences for the transplanted organ, so the decision-making process is not easy. However, generally monoclonal PTLDs especially those involving multiple sites, have a worse prognosis, and do not respond to immunosuppression reduction alone. In one study, the presence of a BCL6 mutation in PTLD seems to predict poor response to immunosuppression reduction. The mortality of PTLD in solid organ allograft recipients and stem cell transplants is 60% and 80%, respectively.

Differential diagnosis The monomorphous lymphoproliferative lesions occurring in posttransplant patients are easily diagnosed as lymphomas, and the only issues in this situation may be demonstration of association with EBV and proper subtyping. The diagnostic difficulties arise in the early and polymorphic lesions, which may be difficult to differentiate from other inflammatory lesions such as transplant rejection, infections, and rare disorders such as HIV-associated lymphadenopathy and systemic Castleman's disease. The clinical setting (posttransplantation) and demonstration of EBV markers either by immunohistochemistry or in situ hybridization are very helpful in supporting the diagnosis of PTLD. Identifying EBV is possibly the most useful adjunct in the diagnosis of early PTLD. Demonstration of clonal expansion by gene rearrangement studies is also very helpful in differentiating PTLD from reactive or inflammatory conditions, including transplant rejection in the later stages of the disease.

Inflammatory Bowel Disease–associated Lymphomas

There is a reported increase in the incidence of lymphoma in the setting of IBD particularly ulcerative colitis, although the overall risk appears low and somewhat controversial.[385,386] The exact etiopathogenesis is unknown. However, underlying immune dysregulation in IBD, chronic inflammation, infections, and chronic immune stimulation are likely to play a role. About 3% to 15% of all colorectal lymphomas occur in patients with ulcerative colitis.[228,387] The mean interval to develop lymphoma has been suggested to be about 12 years.[388] With the use of more potent immunosuppressive drugs, the risk seems to increase and the mean interval to develop lymphomas appears to be 3.1 years, which is substantially less.[386] Since azathioprine and 6-mercaptopurine have been in use for the treatment of IBD, there appears to have been an increase in the number of IBD-associated lymphomas, many of which are associated with EBV.[389-392] However, large-scale population-based studies have failed to validate this finding.[393] The long-term effect of newer therapies that include Remicade (Infliximab) is still unknown, although some recent reports suggest an increase in the incidence of lymphoma with its use.[385,394,395]

A wide range of lymphoma subtypes have been described. However, the majority are high-grade B-cell lymphomas. Follicular lymphoma, marginal zone lymphoma, Hodgkin's lymphoma, and PTLD-type polymorphous lymphoma are also known to occur, although less frequently.[2,228,324,386,388] The lymphomas are often multifocal, most frequently involve the distal colon, and almost always occur in the actively inflamed segments of the bowel.[388] The prognosis and the long-term outcome depend on the types of lymphoma and stage at diagnosis. Especially in younger male patients on TNFα antagonists there is a very small risk of γδ T-cell lymphoma. However this does not affect the GI tract.

Methotrexate-associated Lymphoproliferative Disorders These are extremely uncommon and about 100 cases have been reported to date. The majority of the patients have rheumatoid arthritis who have been treated with methotrexate.[396-399] It is still somewhat unclear if the increased risk of lymphoma is related to rheumatoid arthritis itself or is secondary to methotrexate.[400,401] The time to develop lymphoma is about 15 years from the time of initiation of therapy, and it is estimated that about 0.8 g of cumulative dose of methotrexate is required.[397,402] Various histologic types similar to other immunodeficiency-associated lymphoproliferative disorders are known to occur and about 50% are associated with EBV.[399] A polymorphous lymphoplasmacytic-type similar to PTLD is also described. In about 40% cases, the lesions are extranodal including GI tract. Some cases show at least partial response to methotrexate withdrawal.[399]

Solitary Plasmacytomas of the Gastrointestinal Tract

Solitary plasmacytomas of the GI tract are uncommon, accounting for approximately 4% to 12% of all extramedullary cases.[403-407] Clinically, they have many of the features of myeloma, being more common in middle-aged and elderly men, and sometimes presence of a monoclonal protein spike in the serum or urine.[405,407,408] The gastric plasmacytomas commonly present with ulcer symptoms, whereas the less common intestinal tumors present with obstructive features. Occasionally, they present with other features such as massive GI hemorrhage or vitamin B_{12} deficiency.[409]

The majority of the tumors are located in the stomach and small bowel and rarely in the colon.[405,410,411] At endoscopy the lesions grossly resemble other lymphomas. They commonly present as ulcerated masses, but may also occur as single or multiple polypoid lesions.[412,413] Grossly, the tumors may be large, measuring as large as 15 cm in diameter, and extend from the mucosa to serosa. On cut section they have a rubbery consistency and a gray-white or pinkish coloration, similar to that of lymphomas.

The lesions are composed of a monomorphous infiltrate of plasma cells, which may appear mature or pleomorphic (Fig. 4-30). Extracellular amyloid deposition is seen in some cases. GI plasmacytomas must be differentiated from localized extramedullary manifestations of multiple myeloma, inflammatory pseudotumors (plasma cell granulomas), and plasma cell–rich MALT lymphomas/IPSID.[236,407,411] Histologically, plasmacytomas are differentiated from pseudotumors by demonstrating a monomorphic population of plasma cells, with little admixture of inflammatory cells or granulomatous change (in contrast to

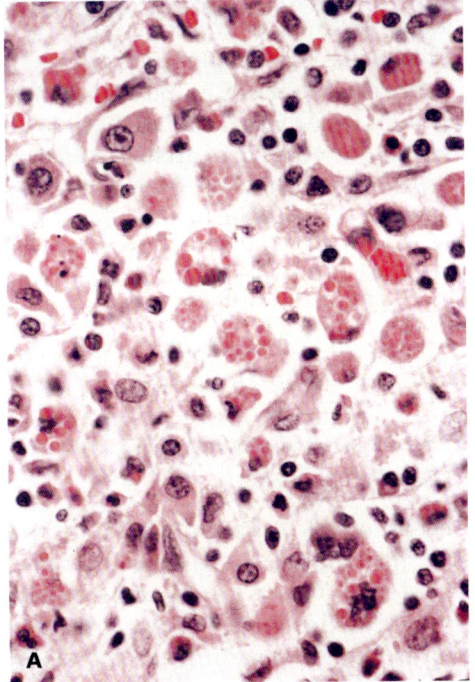
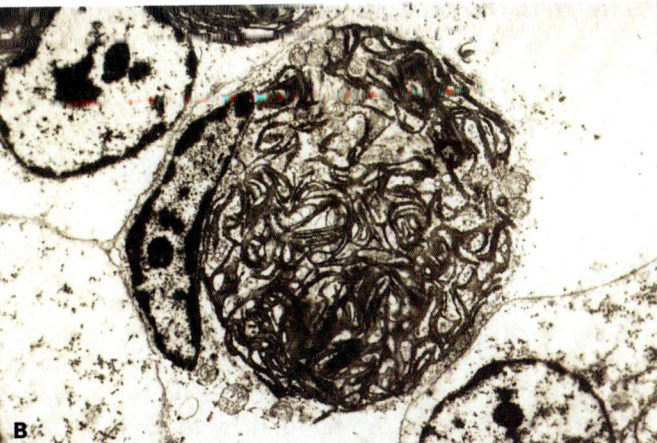

Figure 4-30. Atypical gastric plasmacytoma. **A:** Higher-power magnification showing an infiltrate composed of mature and immature plasma cells. Many plasma cells contain numerous bizarre Russell bodies. **B:** Electron micrographs of the Russell bodies illustrated in part **(A)**. These consist of aggregate of membranes. (Courtesy M. Janssen, M.D.)

the polymorphous infiltrate seen in the inflammatory pseudotumors). The plasma cells may contain crystalline inclusions, and in rare cases may contain numerous bizarre Russell bodies. These cases are invariably associated with a dysproteinemia. In addition, the neoplastic nature of the lesion can be shown immunohistochemically by the demonstration of a single immunoglobulin in the plasma cells. Multiple myeloma should be excluded by demonstrating the lack of bone marrow involvement. Bone marrow aspirates from several sites and a reasonable period of follow-up is needed to differentiate localized plasmacytoma from multiple myeloma.[407,413] The cases should also be differentiated from MALT lymphomas with extensive plasmacytic differentiation, especially in small bowel biopsies, as some reported cases of gastric plamacytomas seem to respond to *H. pylori* eradication and possibly represent a variation of MALT lymphoma. IPSID has no kappa or lambda but does have IgA heavy chain only by immunohistochemistry.

Surgery, with or without local radiotherapy, appears to be the treatment of choice for solitary GI lesions, although some authorities have advocated chemotherapy. Although the survival time in the literature varies from 2 to 26 years, the prognosis is generally good for extramedullary plasmacytomas, with only few patients progressing to multiple myeloma. In one study, four of five cases of primary gastric plasmacytoma consisted of early lesions confined to the mucosa and submucosa, and following surgery no tumor recurred in the 12 year of follow-up.[404]

Lymphomatoid Granulomatosis (Angiocentric Lymphoproliferative Lesion)

Lymphomatoid granulomatosis is an angiocentric and angiodestructive lymphoproliferative disorder that primarily affects the lungs, but extrapulmonary disease has also been described in up to 83% of cases, primarily in the kidney, skin, central nervous system, and liver.[414-418] GI tract involvement is uncommon.[416,417] Although it was initially thought to be a T-cell disorder, now it has been identified as an EBV-driven B-cell lymphoproliferative disorder that is rich in reactive T cells.[415,418,419] Patients with underlying immunodeficiency are at an increased risk of developing lymphomatoid granulomatosis.

The gross appearance varies depending on the site of involvement. Gastric lesions range from superficial erosions to deep serpiginous ulcers. Involvement of the intestines usually results in matted loops of bowel. Hemorrhage with hematoma formation, necrosis, and perforation are common. Sometimes there are multiple intestinal strictures.[417] The process often extends to the mesentery and retroperitoneal tissues.

Only rare reports describe features of lymphomatoid granulomatosis as seen on mucosal biopsies, which tend to show only nondiagnostic inflammation and necrosis. Characteristic necrotizing granulomatous process centered on vessels is seen on autopsy or resection specimens. There is an intense vasculitis, involving both arteries and veins, frequently with marked coagulative necrosis and a dense transmural angiodestructive polymorphous infiltrate composed of atypical lymphocytes (small and or large cleaved), histiocytes, plasma cells, and neutrophils. The disease has a histologic spectrum, and clinical aggressiveness depends on the proportion of the neoplastic B cells.[418] Grade 1 lesions are polymorphous with few B cells that lack cytologic atypia and scanty or no necrosis. Grade 2 lesions are similar but tend to show few admixed large atypical B cells with increasing necrosis. Grade 3 lesions show easily identifiable large atypical B cells, while the inflammatory background may still be appreciable. Grade 3 lesions are easily identified as a lymphoma, and in fact represent variants of a DLBCL. The atypical cells express CD20 and sometimes CD30 but are negative for CD15. The T-cell population appears to be a mix of CD4+ and CD8+ cells. EBV positivity can be demonstrated by positivity for LMP1 or in situ hybridization in most of the cases. Clonal Ig gene rearrangement can be shown by molecular techniques in almost all cases of grade 2 and 3 lesions. The clonality results are inconsistent in grade 1 lesions.

The differential diagnosis consists of polyarteritis nodosa and lymphoma, especially Hodgkin's lymphoma.[417] Polyarteritis nodosa differs from lymphomatoid granulomatosis in that it lacks the atypical histiocyte-like cells and usually spares the veins. Gene rearrangement studies and EBV positivity may further help to differentiate these lesions. Most of the other lymphomas do not normally produce a vasculitis.

The response to treatment is variable. The grade 1 and 2 lesions may respond to interferon α2b, while grade 3 lesions seem to respond to chemotherapy similar to high grade B-cell lymphomas.[418] GI involvement when present indicates an ominous prognosis, with most reported patients dying of GI hemorrhage, gastric ulceration, and perforation.

Mycosis Fungoides Involving the Gastrointestinal Tract

Mycosis fungoides is a distinctive T-cell lymphoma of the skin, usually of the helper/inducer phenotype (CD3+ and CD4+) that subsequently may involve lymph nodes and viscera. Involvement of the GI tract is most often clinically silent. However, occasionally these lymphomas may present with malabsorption, hemorrhage, and perforation from lymphomatous infiltration and lead to mortality.[420-424]

Autopsy studies show that up to 40% of patients with disseminated mycosis fungoides have GI involvement, which may occur anywhere from the esophagus to the colon.[420]

On gross examination, there is tumor nodule formation, often with ulceration, hemorrhage, and perforation.[420,424] There is infiltration of the bowel wall by a dense monomorphous infiltrate of large, atypical mononuclear cells, many of which retain the features of the mycosis cell, with its characteristic cerebriform nucleus and scanty cytoplasm. The infiltrate tends to become more pleomorphic with systemic spread of the disease. Histologically, mycosis fungoides may be confused with other lymphomas, especially immunoblastic lymphoma and Hodgkin's lymphoma, because of the admixed eosinophils, plasma cells, and lymphocytes. A previous history of mycosis fungoides usually aids in the diagnosis. Furthermore, the mycosis cells are not found in immunoblastic lymphoma and Hodgkin's lymphoma.

Most cases express T-cell antigens, namely, CD2, CD3, CD4, and CD5. About a third of cases express CD7. Rare cases are positive for CD8 and CD25. In addition, interdigitating and Langerhans cell can be demonstrated in the background by positivity for S-100 and CD1a.

Anaplastic Large-cell Lymphoma (Ki-1 Lymphoma)

This is a rare heterogeneous group of lymphoma that involves lymph nodes as well as other organs, such as the GI tract.[425,426] Histologically, the lymphoma is characterized by sheets of large noncleaved lymphocytes, immunoblasts, and undifferentiated lymphocytes resembling Reed–Sternberg cells.[427–430] There are relatively few admixed inflammatory cells. Because of their immunoreactivity with the monoclonal anti-Ki-1 antibody, they have also been called Ki-1 lymphomas. Phenotypically, these tumors may be of B-T-or null-cell type, although those that express B-cell phenotype are now grouped with DLBCL.[431] The tumors typically express CD30 and EMA. Expression of T-cell markers is variable, and CD2 and CD4 are more frequently seen compared to CD3, CD5, and CD7. Majority of the T- or null-cell type are characterized by t(2:5)(p23:q35), which brings novel anaplastic leukemia kinase and nucleophosmin genes together. The translocation generates a fusion protein called ALK that can be demonstrated immunohistochemically in about 60% to 85% of cases, and imparts a better prognosis.[431] Histologically, these tumors may be confused with Hodgkin's lymphoma (see the discussion under Hodgkin's Lymphoma) and also other undifferentiated tumors (Fig. 4-31). The clinical presentation of these GI tumors is similar to the other large-cell lymphomas of the GI tract.[427] Untreated the tumors have an aggressive course; however, tumors expressing ALK seem to show an excellent response to therapy.[431]

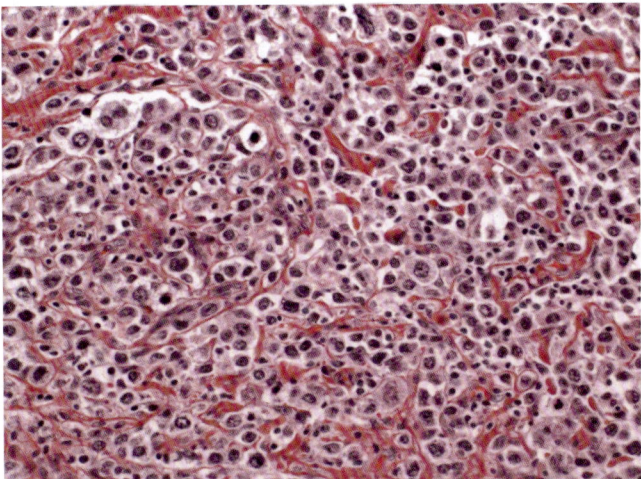

Figure 4-31. Microscopy from an anaplastic large-cell lymphoma showing cells with moderate amount of cytoplasm and resemblance to a poorly differentiated carcinoma.

Extranasal NK Cell or NK-like T-cell Lymphoma

These are rare type of highly aggressive tumors that most commonly involve mucosa of the head and neck regions.[432–434] GI tract appears to be the next common site of involvement.[434] It is more frequently seen in Asians, and the common presenting GI symptoms are abdominal pain, rectal bleeding, and perforation. The median age of presentation is 47.5 years (range 30–77). In the GI tract any site can be involved, although the colon appears to be the most common. In some cases of small intestinal involvement, enteropathy-type features may be seen without any evidence of Celiac disease.[435] The tumor cells may be small, medium sized, or sometimes very pleomorphic and anaplastic. Cytotoxic granules may be seen on Giemsa-stained cytologic smears or electron microscopy. Angiocentricity and tumor necrosis are frequently seen. The tumor cells express NK cell marker CD56/NCAM (neuronal cell-adhesion molecule) and cytoplasmic CD3ε and CD2. Typical cases do not express surface CD3, and the TCR remains in the germline configuration.[434] Cytotoxic granules–associated proteins—granzyme B, perforin, and TIA—are often also positive. Some cases do have a T-cell phenotype with surface CD3 positivity and TCR rearrangement, and rare cases can be negative for CD56. EBV positivity is seen in most cases. Despite histologic and immunophenotypic heterogeneity the tumors are invariably fatal with a median survival of 14 months despite therapy.[434] These tumors need to be differentiated from NK cell enteropathy which is largely benign (see Chapter 18).

NK cell enteropathy. Some patients with mucosal infiltration by atypical lymphoid infiltrate consisting of primarily NK cells and mimicking a NK cell lymphoma that has a benign outcome has been reported as "NK cell enteropathy" (see Chapter 18).

Hodgkin's Lymphoma of the Gastrointestinal Tract

Extranodal Hodgkin's lymphoma is very rare. When it does occur the GI tract is the most common site.[2,436-439] The majority of the cases in the GI tract are probably secondary to nodal involvement. Primary GI tumors are rare and most commonly occur in the stomach. Rare cases have also been reported in duodenum, small intestine, ileocecal region, as well as colon.[2,436,438-441] Some of the primary tumors have been associated with other GI disorders such as Crohn's disease.[437] Metastatic involvement of the GI tract secondary to the typical nodal Hodgkin's disease is relatively uncommon, having been reported in < 10% of autopsy cases.[442] There is also a reported composite lymphoma, comprising of DLBCL and Hodgkin's lymphoma, in a case of Crohn's disease.[443]

Clinically, most of the patients reported to date have been in their 50s or 60s, with equal involvement of both sexes, although in one study of gastric Hodgkin's lymphoma, there was a slight male predominance.[441,444] The modes of presentation are similar to those of other GI lymphomas as described earlier.

The gross appearance is often of an ulcerating lesion or a tumorous mass. The tumor may be confined to the mucosa and submucosa or extend into the muscularis propria, serosa, and the regional lymph nodes.

On histologic examination, there is frequent mucosal ulceration. In the stomach the tumor may focally infiltrate between the gastric glands or replace them. The microscopic features are similar to those of nodal disease, namely, Reed–Sternberg and atypical mononuclear cells in a background of inflammatory cells composed of small mature lymphocytes, prominent eosinophils, plasma cells, and histiocytes. The common subtypes include mixed cellularity, nodular sclerosis, or lymphocyte predominant type. Lymphocyte-depleted Hodgkin's disease of the GI tract is rare, and most of the reported cases were probably large-cell lymphomas.[441,445] In the stomach mucosa adjacent to the lymphoma frequently shows chronic gastritis and intestinal metaplasia.[441]

Hodgkin's lymphoma needs to be differentiated from inflammatory conditions and other lymphomas. The reactive inflammatory processes include Crohn's disease, eosinophilic gastritis, and inflammatory fibroid polyp. In these conditions confusion may arise because of the polymorphous infiltrate containing numerous eosinophils and large lymphocytes or immunoblasts. One should be aware that large lymphoid cells or immunoblasts with prominent nucleoli may be seen in reactive processes and should not be confused with Reed–Sternberg cells. In problematic cases careful examination of the clinical setting, the background histologic features, and immunohistochemical studies are usually helpful in the differential diagnosis.

Differentiation from Langerhans cell histiocytosis, immunoblastic lymphoma, true histiocytic neoplasms, and other DLBCL may be more difficult, since they may all have a polymorphous infiltrate and contain Reed–Sternberg-like cells. Careful study of the background lymphocytes is usually very helpful. In Hodgkin's disease the lymphocytes are typically small whereas in non-Hodgkin's lymphomas there is usually a broader spectrum in the size of lymphocytes ranging from small to large.[441] The histiocytes of Langerhans cell histiocytosis have a distinctive morphology and immunophenotype and in practice generally do not pose a problem. Lymphocyte-depleted Hodgkin's lymphoma may be difficult to differentiate from Ki-1 (CD30)–positive anaplastic large-cell lymphoma as the latter frequently contains large bizarre cells with huge nucleoli, which mimic Reed–Sternberg cells. The large atypical mononuclear and typical Reed–Sternberg cells are CD15 (Leu-M 1) positive and CD45 negative. In contrast anaplastic large-cell lymphomas are CD15 negative and CD45 positive.[441,444,446] However, there may be overlap and some cases of Hodgkin's lymphoma have been shown to be CD30 positive, while some cases of anaplastic large-cells lymphoma may be CD45 negative. In summary, because of the rarity of Hodgkin's lymphoma and the frequent confusion with other large-cell non-Hodgkin's lymphomas, it is recommended that the diagnosis of Hodgkin's lymphoma be based on adequate histology and confirmed by immunohistochemistry.

True Histiocytic Lymphomas (Histiocytic Sarcoma) of the GI Tract

The histiocytic lymphomas reported prior to widespread use of immunohistochemical and molecular techniques largely represented B-cell, T-cell, or anaplastic large-cell lymphomas.[447,448] True histiocytic neoplasms are rare and have been designated as histiocytic sarcomas in the 2001 WHO classification. The diagnosis of histiocytic neoplasms depends not only on the demonstration of histiocyte-associated markers, but also on exclusion of its mimics that include other non-Hodgkin's lymphomas, poorly differentiated carcinoma, melanoma, and other specific sarcomas. The disease frequently involves extranodal sites, and besides skin, GI tract is commonly involved.[447-449] It occurs in a wide age range, but is more common in middle age and elderly individuals. Almost any site in the GI tract can be involved. The clinical signs and symptoms and gross appearances of the lesions are similar to any other high-grade lymphomas. The tumor cells tend to grow in diffuse noncohesive pattern, although some cases may deceptively appear cohesive mimicking a carcinoma or melanoma. The tumor cells are large ranging from normal histiocyte-like to large pleomorphic cells with abundant eosinophilic cytoplasm, prominent nucleoli, and numerous mitoses.[447-449] Phagocytosis by the tumor cells, once thought to be the histologic hallmark of histiocytic neoplasms, is seen only infrequently. Sometimes cells with foamy or vacuolated cytoplasm, bizarre-shaped multilobulated nuclei, or sarcomatoid spindle cell morphology are also seen. Variable numbers of benign lymphocytes, histiocytes, and eosinophils are seen in the background, and the overall histologic appearance of the tumors could be monomorphic or polymorphic. The tumor cells by definition express at least one or more histiocyte markers including CD68, lysozyme, CD11c, and CD14. They are also positive for CD45 (LCA), HLA-DR, and CD45RO.[447-449] CD4 positivity is frequently seen, while variable and weak expression of CD31, CD30, CD1a, and S100 is seen in some cases. Because of the immunohistochemical overlap with B- and T-cell neoplasms, correlation with other immunohistochemical markers and Ig and TCR gene rearrangement studies is required to make a definitive diagnosis. Because of the rarity of these tumors, their outcome is still somewhat unclear. Generally they have been regarded as aggressive neoplasms with poor response to therapy and fatal outcome.[449] A subset of cases, however, has been reported to respond to multidrug chemotherapy, and in some cases of localized disease, surgery has resulted in a favorable outcome.

Langerhans Cell Histiocytosis (LCH, Histiocytosis X) of the GI Tract

These are rare disorders that are most commonly seen in children, and GI tract is reported to be involved in about 2% to 13% of cases with disseminated disease.[450-455] Most, but not all, cases tend to have skin involvement. Rare examples of primary involvement of the GI tract have also been reported.[456] A few gastric cases in middle-aged patients presenting as a focal ulcerated mass or mucosal nodularity of the stomach have been described. The manifestations of GI involvement include failure to thrive, abdominal pain, vomiting, constipation, intractable diarrhea, malabsorption, bloody stools, protein-losing enteropathy, and intestinal perforation.[453-455] While in many cases the GI involvement clinically and pathologically mimics IBD, rare examples of Langerhans cells histiocytosis complicating Crohn's disease are reported.[456]

The involved mucosa may appear normal or show mucosal nodularity or granularity. The histology of the lesions is similar to the Langerhans cell histiocytosis involvement elsewhere, and the key is to demonstrating Langerhans cells in a polymorphic inflammatory background. The Langerhans cells can be easily identified by CD1a and S100 positivity. Electron microscopy to demonstrate characteristic Birbeck granules is seldom required in routine practice. The clinical outcome is highly variable with complete remission in some cases, and rapid downhill course with fatal outcome in others.[455]

Other Miscellaneous Lymphomas of the GI Tract

As in nodal lymphomas, unusual varieties of GI lymphomas are sometimes encountered. Rare examples include signet-ring cell lymphoma and T-cell lymphoma mimicking lymphocytic gastritis.[457-460] Rare cases of primary GI follicular dendritic cell tumor have also been reported.[461] In addition there are reports of lymphomas associated with other tumors, such as adenocarcinomas.[462] A number of lymphomas are unclassifiable. In some cases this is because of poor histology or an inability to perform immunophenotyping and molecular genetic analysis. Many of these specimens are large and fixed en masse resulting in considerable variation in cytological preservation. Preservation is usually best near the mucosal or serosal surfaces, where the tissue is most rapidly exposed to the fixative. Some of the difficulties can be circumvented by promptly triaging tissues when lymphoma is suspected.

The clinical features of disseminated lymphoma with secondary GI involvement do not differ significantly from those of primary GI lymphomas.[438,463] About 20% of patients have palpable abdominal masses. The sites of involvement by tumor are also similar to those of patients with primary intestinal lymphoma: 56% gastric, 25% small intestine, and 10% colon. Pathologically, the secondary lymphomas tend to produce punched out ulcers in the stomach and frequently involve multiple GI sites.

Angioimmunoblastic Lymphadenopathy Involving GI Tract

This entity involves primarily lymph nodes and other extranodal sites, such as the liver, spleen, skin, and bone marrow.[464] A rare case has also been described involving the GI tract producing multiple mucosal polyps resembling GI lymphomatous polyposis.[465] Microscopically, these lesions are characterized by distortion of the mucosal architecture, blood vessel proliferation, and dense infiltration of lymphocytes, plasma cells, and immunoblasts. The case reported with predominant GI involvement presented with fever, diarrhea, abdominal mass, ascites, and generalized lymphadenopathy. The patient initially responded to chemotherapy, but subsequently died of infections.

The Gastrointestinal Tract in Leukemia and Granulocytic Sarcoma

GI involvement can occur in any form of leukemia—acute or chronic; lymphoid or myeloid. GI complications of leukemia are common, occurring in up to 25% of acute leukemia cases, but not so common with chronic leukemia.[466–470] They are more frequent in the acute leukemias, especially during the inductive phase of therapy and also following stem cell transplant.[471] Most of the reports in the literature date from the 1960s and 1970s. Whether this is a reflection of a decrease in the incidence of GI complications of leukemia. Any segment of the GI tract may be involved, and often multiple sites are involved. The leukemic infiltrates may ulcerate, bleed, or give rise to intussusception.[472,473] Ulceration may result in neutropenic enterocolitis, septicemic shock, and pneumatosis coli. Massive hemorrhage may be associated with thrombocytopenia and may occur from gastric "stress" erosions or ulcerated leukemic infiltrates. Sometimes, no obvious source of bleeding can be found. Other GI symptoms include proctologic problems resulting from stercoral ulceration and anal or perineal abscesses.[467] Opportunistic infections and nonspecific ulceration are other complications.[474] Candidiasis, usually localized to the esophagus, cecum, or occasionally stomach, is common and may sometimes become disseminated. Neutropenic patients are also prone to a form of enterocolitis, which may result in multifocal ulceration, necrosis, perforation, and gram-negative sepsis[469] (see Chapter 19).

The GI biopsies in leukemia cases are most often performed to evaluate complications like opportunistic infections and graft versus host disease that are associated with the leukemia or its treatment. Rarely the leukemic involvement of the GI tract is the first presentation of the disease, mostly in the form of a mass lesion and associated complications.

The majority of the lesions found in leukemia occur in the intestines; however, the stomach and esophagus are not spared. The lesions mirror the complications of leukemia, generally consisting of leukemic infiltration resulting in mucosal ulceration, bowel obstruction, opportunistic infections, and GI hemorrhage, and together are found in up to 75% of patients with leukemia at autopsy.[467,470,475–477]

Grossly, leukemic infiltration of the GI tract is characterized by four types of lesions (Fig. 4-32).

1. Multiple bluish nodules of the mucosa, which may be superficially ulcerated, resulting from leukemic infiltration of the solitary lymphoid follicles and Peyer's patches.
2. Leukemic plaques, which are mainly submucosal but may infiltrate the muscle coats.
3. Diffuse leukemic infiltrates of the mucosa, especially the stomach, which produce a characteristic convoluted "brain-like" appearance.
4. Multiple leukemic polyposis.

Histological features and immunophenotype of the infiltrate are typical of the particular leukemia in question. Cases that present with GI mass lesions mostly represent myeloid leukemia (granulocytic sarcoma), although this could occur with any other form of leukemia. The cells of granulocytic sarcoma resemble similar lesions elsewhere. The cells show somewhat plasmacytoid appearance with some cells showing eosinophilic granules (eosniophilic myelocytes) and occasionally a polymorphic population suggestive of

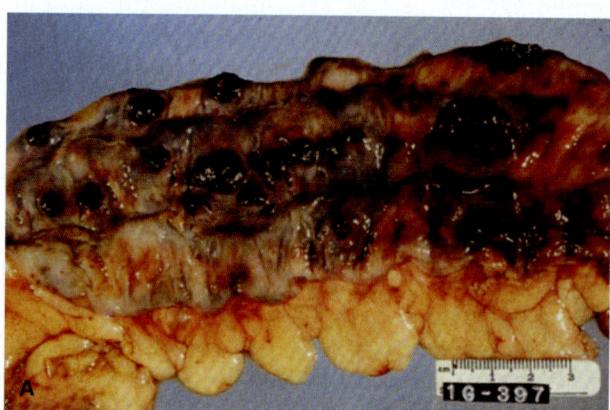
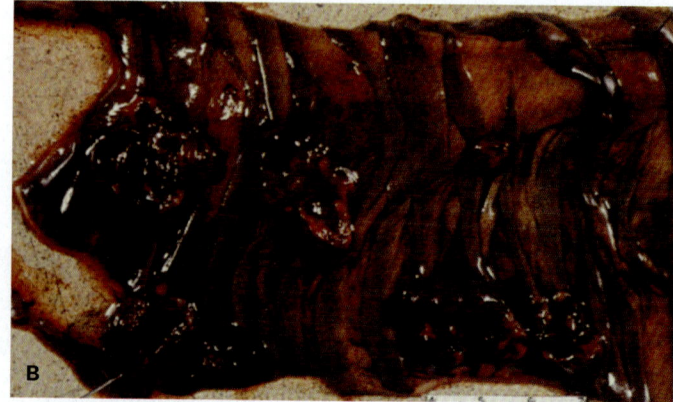

Figure 4-32. Colon from a patient with acute leukemia. **A:** Submucosal infiltration resulting in mucosal nodulation and surface ulceration. **B:** Multiple bluish mucosal nodules resulting from leukemic infiltration.

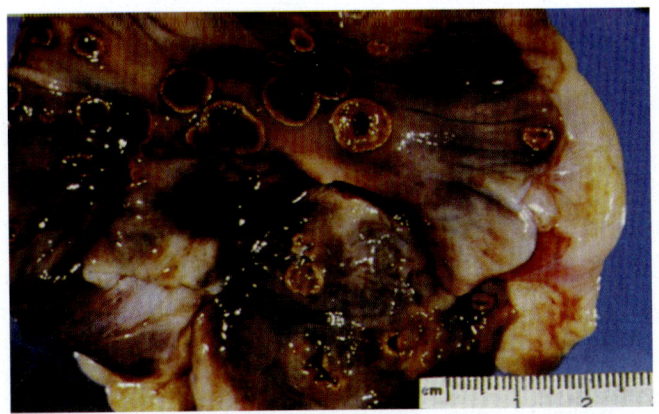

Figure 4-33. Colon from a patient who died of acute leukemia. This patient had extensive candidiasis of the GI tract. The cecum shows plaques of fungus growing on the mucosa in a manner resembling a culture plate.

myeloid maturation. Myeloid differentiation can be easily shown using the chloracetate esterase stain or immunostain for myeloperoxidase. Examination of blood smears and bone marrow will usually confirm the diagnosis of leukemia. In most cases the bone marrow is involved; however, in some cases the disease is confined to the bowel. Opportunistic infections consist primarily of candidiasis, which may become disseminated (Fig. 4-33). It results in irregular small ulcers covered by a fibrino-hemorrhagic exudate. Sometimes other fungi such as *Aspergillus* or *Zygomycosis* may also occur.

In most cases, the diagnosis of leukemia is known and the biopsies are performed to evaluate various GI complication associated with the disease. Thus in most cases the diagnosis of the leukemic infiltration when present does not pose a diagnostic challenge (provided the history is known). CLL sometimes needs to be differentiated from low-grade MALT lymphomas and chronic inflammation. Difficulty arises as the CLL cells tend to resemble small mature lymphocytes in sections. The monomorphic nature of the infiltrate and distinctive immunophenotype help to differentiate it from a chronic inflammatory lesion as well as a MALT lymphoma. The differential diagnosis of granulocytic sarcoma in a given case may include plasmacytic tumors, other lymphomas, melanoma, or tumors considered in the category of "small blue round cell tumors." Immunostains are frequently helpful in differentiating various lesions and establishing the correct diagnosis in difficult cases.

References

1. Isaacson PG. Gastrointestinal lymphomas of T- and B-cell types. *Mod Pathol*. 1999;12(2):151–158.
2. Lewin KJ, Ranchod M, Dorfman RF. Lymphomas of the gastrointestinal tract: a study of 117 cases presenting with gastrointestinal disease. *Cancer*. 1978;42(2):693–707.
3. Isaacson PG, Du MQ. Gastrointestinal lymphoma: where morphology meets molecular biology. *J Pathol*. 2005;205(2):255–274.
4. Dawson IM, Cornes JS, Morson BC. Primary malignant lymphoid tumours of the intestinal tract. Report of 37 cases with a study of factors influencing prognosis. *Br J Surg*. 1961;49:80–809.
5. Thieblemont C, Berger F, Dumontet C, et al. Mucosa-associated lymphoid tissue lymphoma is a disseminated disease in one third of 158 patients analyzed. *Blood*. 2000;95(3):802–806.
6. Bertoni F, Gisi M, Roggero E, et al. Molecular detection of circulating neoplastic cells in patients with clinically localised gastric and non-gastric mucosa-associated lymphoid tissue lymphoma. *Dig Liver Dis*. 2000;32(3):188–191.
7. Rosenwald A, Ott G, Stilgenbauer S, et al. Exclusive detection of the t(11;18)(q21;q21) in extranodal marginal zone B cell lymphomas (MZBL) of MALT type in contrast to other MZBL and extranodal large B cell lymphomas. *Am J Pathol*. 1999;155(6):1817–1821.
8. Isaacson PG. Gastrointestinal lymphoma. *Hum Pathol*. 1994;25(10):1020–1029.
9. Lewin KJ, Riddell RH, Weinstein WM. Lymphoproliferative disorders. In: Lewin KJ, Riddell, RH, Weinstein WM, eds. *Gastrointestinal Pathology and Its Clinical Implications*. New York, NY: Igaku-Shoin; 1992:151–196.
10. Ioachim HL, Weinstein MA, Robbins RD, et al. Primary anorectal lymphoma. A new manifestation of the acquired immune deficiency syndrome (AIDS). *Cancer*. 1987;60(7):1449–1453.
11. Auger MJ, Allan NC. Primary ileocecal lymphoma. A study of 22 patients. *Cancer*. 1990;65(2):358–361.
12. Foss HD, Stein H. Pathology of intestinal lymphomas. *Recent Results Cancer Res*. 2000;156:33–41.
13. Vanden Heule B, Taylor CR, Terry R, Lukes RJ. Presentation of malignant lymphoma in the rectum. *Cancer*. 1982;49(12):2602–2607.
14. Hande KR, Fisher RI, DeVita VT, et al. Diffuse histiocytic lymphoma involving the gastrointestinal tract. *Cancer*. 1978;41(5):1984–1989.
15. Salem P, el-Hashimi L, Anaissie E, et al. Primary small intestinal lymphoma in adults. A comparative study of IPSID versus non-IPSID in the Middle East. *Cancer*. 1987;59(9):1670–1676.
16. Yoshino T, Miyake K, Ichimura K, et al. Increased incidence of follicular lymphoma in the duodenum. *Am J Surg Pathol*. 2000;24(5):688–693.
17. Okano M. Haematological associations of Epstein-Barr virus infection. *Baillieres Best Pract Res Clin Haematol*. 2000;13(2):199–214.
18. Petersen MC. Immunoproliferative small intestinal disease associated with Campylobacter jejuni. *N Engl J Med*. 2004;350(16):1685–1686; author reply -6.
19. de la Fouchardiere A, Vandenesch F, Berger F. Borrelia-associated primary cutaneous MALT lymphoma in a non-endemic region. *Am J Surg Pathol*. 2003;27(5):702–703.
20. Chanudet E, Zhou Y, Bacon CM, et al. Chlamydia psittaci is variably associated with ocular adnexal MALT lymphoma in different geographical regions. *J Pathol*. 2006;209(3):344–351.
21. Lennert K, Feller A. *Histopathology of Non-Hodgkin's Lymphomas*. 2nd ed. New York, NY: Springer-Verlag; 1992.
22. Rappaport H. Tumors of the hematopoietic system. (3). 1966. washington DC, Armed Forces Institute of Pathology. Atlas of Tumor Patholoy (Report). 1966.
23. Rosenberg SA, Berard CW, Brown BW. National Cancer Institute sponsored study of classifications of non-Hodgkin's lymphomas: summary and description of a working formulation for clinical usage. The non-Hodgkin s lymphoma pathologic classification project. *Cancer*. 1982;49:2112–2135.

24. Stansfeld AG, Diebold J, Noel H, et al. Updated Kiel classification for lymphomas [letter] [published erratum appears in Lancet 1988; 1(8581):372]. *Lancet*. 1988;1:292–293.
25. Jaffe ES. Hematopathology: integration of morphologic features and biologic markers for diagnosis. *Mod Pathol*. 1999;12(2):109–115.
26. Harris NL, Jaffe ES, Stein H, et al. A revised European-American classification of lymphoid neoplasms: a proposal from the International Lymphoma Study Group. *Blood*. 1994;84(5):1361–1392.
27. Harris NL, Jaffe ES, Diebold J, et al. Lymphoma classification—from controversy to consensus: the R.E.A.L. and WHO Classification of lymphoid neoplasms. *Ann Oncol*. 2000;11(suppl 1):3–10.
28. Harris NL, Jaffe ES, Diebold J, et al. The World Health Organization classification of hematological malignancies report of the Clinical Advisory Committee Meeting, Airlie House, Virginia, November 1997. *Mod Pathol*. 2000;13(2):193–207.
29. Swerdlow SH, Campo E, Harris NL, et al. *WHO classification of tumors of haematopoetic and lymphoid tissues* (4th ed.). Lyon, France: IARC Press; 2008.
30. Compton CC, Sobin LH. Protocol for the examination of specimens removed from patients with gastrointestinal lymphoma. A basis for checklists. The Cancer Committee, College of American Pathologists, and the Task Force for Protocols on the Examination of Specimens From Patients With Gastrointestinal Lymphoma. *Arch Pathol Lab Med*. 1997;121(10):1042–1047.
31. Heerema NA, Bernheim A, Lim MS, et al. State of the art and future needs in cytogenetic/molecular genetics/arrays in childhood lymphoma: summary report of workshop at the First International Symposium on childhood and adolescent non-Hodgkin lymphoma, April 9, 2003, New York City, NY. *Pediatr Blood Cancer*. 2005;45(5):616–622.
32. Spagnolo DV, Ellis DW, Juneja S, et al. The role of molecular studies in lymphoma diagnosis: a review. *Pathology*. 2004;36(1):19–44.
33. Nakamura S, Aoyagi K, Furuse M, et al. B-cell monoclonality precedes the development of gastric MALT lymphoma in *Helicobacter pylori*-associated chronic gastritis. *Am J Pathol*. 1998;152(5):1271–1279.
34. Zucca E, Bertoni F, Roggero E, et al. Molecular analysis of the progression from *Helicobacter pylori*-associated chronic gastritis to mucosa-associated lymphoid-tissue lymphoma of the stomach. *N Engl J Med*. 1998;338(12):804–810.
35. Wundisch T, Neubauer A, Stolte M, et al. B-cell monoclonality is associated with lymphoid follicles in gastritis. *Am J Surg Pathol*. 2003;27(7):882–887.
36. de Mascarel A, Dubus P, Belleannee G, et al. Low prevalence of monoclonal B cells in *Helicobacter pylori* gastritis patients with duodenal ulcer. *Hum Pathol*. 1998;29(8):784–790.
37. Lo WY, Li JY, Chan YK, et al. Instability of clonality in gastric lymphoid infiltrates: a study with emphasis on serial biopsies. *Am J Surg Pathol*. 2005;29(12):1582–1592.
38. Yamauchi A, Tomita Y, Miwa H, et al. Clonal evolution of gastric lymphoma of mucosa-associated lymphoid tissue type. *Mod Pathol*. 2001;14(10):957–962.
39. Savio A, Franzin G, Wotherspoon AC, et al. Diagnosis and posttreatment follow-up of *Helicobacter pylori*-positive gastric lymphoma of mucosa-associated lymphoid tissue: histology, polymerase chain reaction, or both? *Blood*. 1996;87(4):1255–1260.
40. Platz CE. Lymphoid proliferations of the stomach. In: Appleman HD. *Pathology of the Esophagus, Stomach and Duodenum*. New York, NY: Churchill Livingstone; 1984:243–287.
41. Sheahan DG, West AB. Focal lymphoid hyperplasia (pseudolymphoma) of the esophagus. *Am J Surg Pathol*. 1985;9(2):141–147.
42. Gervaz E, Potet F, Mahe R, Lemasson G. Focal lymphoid hyperplasia of the oesophagus: report of a case. *Histopathology*. 1992;21(2):187–189.
43. Schwartz DC, Cole CE, Sun Y, Jacoby RF. Diffuse nodular lymphoid hyperplasia of the colon: polyposis syndrome or normal variant? *Gastrointest Endosc*. 2003;58(4):630–632.
44. Nagaoka S, Bandoh T, Takemura T. Lymphoid hyperplasia of the large intestine: a case report with immunohistochemical and gene analysis. *Pathol Int*. 2000;50(9):750–753.
45. Smith J, Helwig EB. Malignant lymphoma of the stomach:its diagnosis, distinction and biologic behavior [Abstract]. *Am J Clin Pathol*. 1958;34:553.
46. Jacobs DS. Primary Gastric Malignant Lymphoma and Pseudolymphoma. *Am J Clin Pathol*. 1963;40:379–394.
47. Brooks JJ, Enterline HT. Gastric pseudolymphoma. Its three subtypes and relation to lymphoma. *Cancer*. 1983;51(3):476–486.
48. Matsumoto S, Kohda K, Koike K, et al. Diagnosis and prognosis of reactive lymphoreticular hyperplasia of the stomach. *Jpn J Cancer Res*. 1998;83:288–293.
49. Ranchod M, Lewin KJ, Dorfman RF. Lymphoid hyperplasia of the gastrointestinal tract. A study of 26 cases and review of the literature. *Am J Surg Pathol*. 1978;2(4):383–400.
50. Takano Y, Kato Y, Sugano H. Histopathological and immunohistochemical study of atypical lymphoid hyperplasia and benign lymphoid hyperplasia of the stomach. *Jpn J Cancer Res*. 1992;83(3):288–293.
51. Isaacson P, Wright DH. Malignant lymphoma of mucosa-associated lymphoid tissue. A distinctive type of B-cell lymphoma. *Cancer*. 1983;52(8):1410–1416.
52. Abbondanzo SL, Sobin LH. Gastric "pseudolymphoma": a retrospective morphologic and immunophenotypic study of 97 cases. *Cancer*. 1997;79(9):1656–1663.
53. Chen XY, Liu WZ, Shi Y, et al. *Helicobacter pylori* associated gastric diseases and lymphoid tissue hyperplasia in gastric antral mucosa. *J Clin Pathol*. 2002;55(2):133–137.
54. Weston AP, Campbell DR, McGregor DH, Cherian R. Endoscopic and histologic resolution of gastric pseudolymphoma (reactive lymphoid hyperplasia) following treatment with bismuth and oral antibiotics. *Dig Dis Sci*. 1994;39(12):2567–2574.
55. Misra SP, Misra V, Dwivedi M, Singh PA. *Helicobacter pylori*-induced lymphonodular hyperplasia: a new cause of gastric outlet obstruction. *J Gastroenterol Hepatol*. 1998;13(12):1191–1194.
56. Hassall E, Dimmick JE. Unique features of *Helicobacter pylori* disease in children. *Dig Dis Sci*. 1991;36(4):417–423.
57. Moss SF, Thomas DM, Mulnier C, et al. Intestinal lymphangiectasia associated with angiofollicular lymph node hyperplasia (Castleman's disease). *Gut*. 1992;33(1):135–137.
58. Jarry A, Brousse N, Souque A, et al. Lymphoid stromal reaction in gastrointestinal lymphomas: immunohistochemical study of 14 cases. *J Clin Pathol*. 1987;40(7):760–765.
59. Saraga P, Hurlimann J, Ozzello L. Lymphomas and pseudolymphomas of the alimentary tract. An immunohistochemical study with clinicopathologic correlations. *Hum Pathol*. 1981;12(8):713–723.
60. Saxena A, Moshynska O, Kanthan R, et al. Distinct B-cell clonal bands in *Helicobacter pylori* gastritis with lymphoid hyperplasia. *J Pathol*. 2000;190(1):47–54.
61. Molas G, Potet R, Nogig P. Hyperplasie lymphoide focale (pseudolymphome) de l'ileon terminal chez l'adulte. *Gastroenterologic Clinique et Biologique (Paris)*. 1985;9:630.
62. Nathans AA, Merenstein H, Brown SS. Lymphoid hyperplasia of the appendix; clinical study. *Pediatrics*. 1953;12(5):516–524.
63. Selke AC Jr, Jona JZ, Belin RP. Massive enlargement of the ileocecal valve due to lymphoid hyperplasia. *Am J Roentgenol*. 1976;127(3):518–520.

64. Cornes JS, Dawson IM. Papillary lymphoid hyperplasia at the ileocaecal valve as a cause of acute intussusception in infancy. *Arch Dis Child.* 1963;38:89–91.
65. Sarason EL, Prior JT, Prowda RL. Recurrent intussusception associated with hypertrophy of Peyer's patches. *N Engl J Med.* 1955;253(21):905–908.
66. Swartley RN, Stayman JW Jr. Lymphoid hyperplasia of the intestinal tract requiring surgical intervention. *Ann Surg.* 1962;155:238–240.
67. Perrin WS, Lindsay EC. Intussusception: a monograph based on 400 cases. *Br J Surg.* 1921;9:46–71.
68. Yunis EJ, Hashida Y. Electron microscopic demonstration of adenovirus in appendix vermiformis in a case of ileocecal intussusception. *Pediatrics.* 1973;51(3):566–570.
69. Rubin A, Isaacson PG. Florid reactive lymphoid hyperplasia of the terminal ileum in adults: a condition bearing a close resemblance to low-grade malignant lymphoma. *Histopathology.* 1990;17(1):19–26.
70. Gudjonsson H, Jones M, Krawitt EL, Kaye MD. Pseudolymphoma of the jejunum. *Dig Dis Sci.* 1987;32(11):1314–1318.
71. Helwig EB, Hansen J. Lymphoid polyps (benign lymphoma) and malignant lymphoma of the rectum and anus. *Surg Gynecol Obstet.* 1951;92(2):233–243.
72. Holtz F, Schmidt LA III. Lymphoid polyps (benign lymphoma) of the rectum and anus. *Surg Gynecol Obstet.* 1958;106(6):639–642.
73. Cornes JS, Wallace MH, Morson BC. Benign lymphomas of the rectum and anal canal: a study of 100 cases. *J Pathol Bacteriol.* 1961;82:371–382.
74. Rittmeyer C, Nakayama D, Ulshen MH. Lymphoid hyperplasia causing recurrent rectal prolapse. *J Pediatr.* 1997;131(3):487–488.
75. Meissner WW. Benign lymphoma of the rectum; review of the literature and report of fifteen additional cases. *J Int Coll Surg.* 1956;26(6):739–749.
76. Brotzu C, Bosu C, Pisano G, Pomata M. A case of nodular lymphoid hyperplasia of the small bowel in a patient with intestinal obstruction. *G Chir.* 1997;18(6–7):355–358.
77. Hermans PE, Diaz-Buxo JA, Stobo JD. Idiopathic late-onset immunoglobulin deficiency. Clinical observations in 50 patients. *Am J Med.* 1976;61(2):221–237.
78. Vayre-Oundjian L, Boruchowicz A, Bloget F, Triboulet JP, Gosselin B, Colombel JF. Pseudotumor nodular lymphoid hyperplasia of the ileum. *Gastroenterol Clin Biol.* 1997;21(12):990–993.
79. Moynihan MJ, Bast MA, Chan WC, et al. Lymphomatous polyposis. A neoplasm of either follicular mantle or germinal center cell origin. *Am J Surg Pathol.* 1996;20(4):442–452.
80. Lamers CB, Wagener T, Assmann KJ, van Tongeren JH. Jejunal lymphoma in a patient with primary adult-onset hypogammaglobulinemia and nodular lymphoid hyperplasia of the small intestine. *Dig Dis Sci.* 1980;25(7):553–557.
81. Matuchansky C, Touchard G, Lemaire M, et al. Malignant lymphoma of the small bowel associated with diffuse nodular lymphoid hyperplasia. *N Engl J Med.* 1985;313(3):166–171.
82. Capitanio MA, Kirkpatrick JA. Lymphoid hyperplasia of the colon in children. Roentgen observations. *Radiology.* 1970;94(2):323–327.
83. Persic M, Lenac T, Rubinic M, et al. Nodular lymphoid hyperplasia of the colon and terminal ileum. Case report. *Lijec Vjesn.* 1998;120(3–4):62–64.
84. Riddlesberger MM Jr, Lebenthal E. Nodular colonic mucosa of childhood: normal or pathologic? *Gastroenterology.* 1980;79(2):265–270.
85. Robinson MJ, Padron S, Rywlin AM. Enterocolitis lymphofollicularis. Morphologic, pathologic, and serum immunoglobulin patterns. *Arch Pathol.* 1973;96(5):311–315.
86. Theander C, Tragardh B. Lymphoid hyperplasia of the colon in childhood. *Acta Radiol Diagn (Stockh).* 1976;17(5A):631–640.
87. Louw JH. Polypoid lesions of the large bowel in children with particular reference to benign lymphoid polyposis. *J Pediatr Surg.* 1968;3(2):195–209.
88. Aguilar FP, Alfonso V, Rivas S, et al. Jejunal malignant lymphoma in a patient with adult-onset hypo-gamma-globulinemia and nodular lymphoid hyperplasia of the small bowel. *Am J Gastroenterol.* 1987;82(5):472–475.
89. Kokkonen J, Ruuska T, Karttunen TJ, Maki M. Lymphonodular hyperplasia of the terminal ileum associated with colitis shows an increase gammadelta+ t-cell density in children. *Am J Gastroenterol.* 2002;97(3):667–672.
90. Kokkonen J, Karttunen TJ. Lymphonodular hyperplasia on the mucosa of the lower gastrointestinal tract in children: an indication of enhanced immune response? *J Pediatr Gastroenterol Nutr.* 2002;34(1):42–46.
91. Venkitachalam PS, Hirsch E, Elguezabal A, Littman L. Multiple lymphoid polyposis and familial polyposis of the colon: a genetic relationship. *Dis Colon Rectum.* 1978;21(5):336–341.
92. Dorazio RA, Whelan TJ Jr. Lymphoid hyperplasia of the terminal ileum associated with familial polyposis coli. *Ann Surg.* 1970;171(2):300–302.
93. Gruenberg J, Mackman S. Multiple lymphoid polyps in familial polyposis. *Ann Surg.* 1972;175(4):552–554.
94. Cornes JS. Multiple lymphomatous polyposis of the gastrointestinal tract. *Cancer.* 1961;14:249–257.
95. Kahn LB, Novis BH. Nodular lymphoid hyperplasia of the small bowel associated with primary small bowel reticulum cell lymphoma. *Cancer.* 1974;33(3):837–844.
96. Matuchansky C, Morichau-Beauchant M, Touchard G, et al. Nodular lymphoid hyperplasia of the small bowel associated with primary jejunal malignant lymphoma. Evidence favoring a cytogenetic relationship. *Gastroenterology.* 1980;78(6):1587–1592.
97. Ahmed N, Ramos S, Sika J, et al. Primary extramedullary esophageal plasmacytoma: First case report. *Cancer.* 1976;38(2):943–947.
98. Bolondi L, De Giorgio R, Santi V, et al. Primary non-Hodgkin's T-cell lymphoma of the esophagus. A case with peculiar endoscopic ultrasonographic pattern. *Dig Dis Sci.* 1990;35(11):1426–1430.
99. Doki T, Hamada S, Murayama H, et al. Primary malignant lymphoma of the esophagus. A case report. *Endoscopy.* 1984;16(5):189–192.
100. Weeratunge CN, Bolivar HH, Anstead GM, Lu DH. Primary esophageal lymphoma: a diagnostic challenge in acquired immunodeficiency syndrome—two case reports and review. *South Med J.* 2004;97(4):383–387.
101. Soon MS, Yen HH, Soon A, et al. Primary esophageal B-cell lymphoma: evaluation by EUS. *Gastrointest Endosc.* 2005;61(7):901–903.
102. Bernal A, del Junco GW. Endoscopic and pathologic features of esophageal lymphoma: a report of four cases in patients with acquired immune deficiency syndrome. *Gastrointest Endosc.* 1986;32(2):96–99.
103. Matsuura H, Saito R, Nakajima S, et al. Non-Hodgkin's lymphoma of the esophagus. *Am J Gastroenterol.* 1985;80(12):941–946.
104. Nagrani M, Lavigne BC, Siskind BN, et al. Primary non-Hodgkin's lymphoma of the esophagus. *Arch Intern Med.* 1989;149(1):193–195.
105. Okerbloom JA, Armitage JO, Zetterman R, Linder J. Esophageal involvement by non-Hodgkin's lymphoma. *Am J Med.* 1984;77(2):359–361.

106. Pearson JM, Borg-Grech A. Primary Ki-1 (CD 30)-positive, large cell, anaplastic lymphoma of the esophagus. *Cancer.* 1991;68(2):418–421.
107. Tsukada T, Ohno T, Kihira H, et al. Primary esophageal non-Hodgkin's lymphoma. *Intern Med.* 1992;31(4):569–572.
108. Gupta NM, Goenka MK, Jindal A, et al. Primary lymphoma of the esophagus. *J Clin Gastroenterol.* 1996;23(3):203–206.
109. Berman MD, Falchuk KR, Trey C, Gramm HF. Primary histiocytic lymphoma of the esophagus. *Dig Dis Sci.* 1979;24(11):883–886.
110. Stein HA, Murray D, Warner HA. Primary Hodgkin's disease of the esophagus. *Dig Dis Sci.* 1981;26(5):457–461.
111. Soweid AM, Zachary PE Jr. Mucosa-associated lymphoid tissue lymphoma of the oesophagus. *Lancet.* 1996;348(9022):268.
112. Fujisawa S, Motomura S, Fujimaki K, et al. Primary esophageal T cell lymphoma. *Leuk Lymphoma.* 1999;33(1–2):199–202.
113. George MK, Ramachandran V, Ramanan SG, et al. Primary esophageal T-cell non-Hodgkin's lymphoma. *Indian J Gastroenterol.* 2005;24(3):119–120.
114. Hamilton SR, Aaltonen AL, eds. *Pathology and Genetics of Tumors of the Digestive System.* Lyon, France: IARC Press; 2000.
115. Genta RM, Hamner HW, Graham DY. Gastric lymphoid follicles in *Helicobacter pylori* infection: frequency, distribution, and response to triple therapy. *Hum Pathol.* 1993;24(6):577–583.
116. Go MF, Smoot DT. *Helicobacter pylori*, gastric MALT lymphoma, and adenocarcinoma of the stomach. *Semin Gastrointest Dis.* 2000;11(3):134–141.
117. Heise W. Gastric lymphomas: aspects of follow-up and after-care. *Recent Results Cancer Res.* 2000;156:69–77.
118. Isaacson PG. Gastric lymphoma and *Helicobacter pylori*. *N Engl J Med.* 1994;330(18):1310–1311.
119. Parsonnet J, Hansen S, Rodriguez L, et al. *Helicobacter pylori* infection and gastric lymphoma. *N Engl J Med.* 1994;330(18):1267–1271.
120. Wotherspoon AC, Ortiz-Hidalgo C, Falzon MR, Isaacson PG. *Helicobacter pylori*-associated gastritis and primary B-cell gastric lymphoma. *Lancet.* 1991;338(8776):1175–1176.
121. Gisbertz IA, Jonkers DM, Arends JW, et al. Specific detection of *Helicobacter pylori* and non-*Helicobacter pylori* flora in small- and large-cell primary gastric B-cell non-Hodgkin's lymphoma. *Ann Oncol.* 1997;8(suppl 2):33–36.
122. Karat D, O'Hanlon DM, Hayes N, et al. Prospective study of *Helicobacter pylori* infection in primary gastric lymphoma. *Br J Surg.* 1995;82(10):1369–1370.
123. Bouzourene H, Haefliger T, Delacretaz F, Saraga E. The role of *Helicobacter pylori* in primary gastric MALT lymphoma. *Histopathology.* 1999;34(2):118–123.
124. Nakamura S, Yao T, Aoyagi K, et al. *Helicobacter pylori* and primary gastric lymphoma. A histopathologic and immunohistochemical analysis of 237 patients. *Cancer.* 1997;79(1):3–11.
125. Hussell T, Isaacson PG, Crabtree JE, Spencer J. The response of cells from low-grade B-cell gastric lymphomas of mucosa-associated lymphoid tissue to *Helicobacter pylori*. *Lancet.* 1993;342(8871):571–574.
126. Hussell T, Isaacson PG, Crabtree JE, Spencer J. *Helicobacter pylori*-specific tumour-infiltrating T cells provide contact dependent help for the growth of malignant B cells in low-grade gastric lymphoma of mucosa-associated lymphoid tissue. *J Pathol.* 1996;178(2):122–127.
127. de Jong D, van der Hulst RW, Pals G, et al. Gastric non-Hodgkin lymphomas of mucosa-associated lymphoid tissue are not associated with more aggressive *Helicobacter pylori* strains as identified by CagA. *Am J Clin Pathol.* 1996;106(5):670–675.
128. Eck M, Schmausser B, Haas R, et al. MALT-type lymphoma of the stomach is associated with *Helicobacter pylori* strains expressing the CagA protein. *Gastroenterology.* 1997;112(5):1482–1486.
129. Peng H, Ranaldi R, Diss TC, et al. High frequency of CagA+ *Helicobacter pylori* infection in high-grade gastric MALT B-cell lymphomas. *J Pathol.* 1998;185(4):409–412.
130. Blaser MJ. *Helicobacter pylori* phenotypes associated with peptic ulceration. *Scand J Gastroenterol Suppl.* 1994;205:1–5.
131. Cover TL, Tummuru MK, Cao P, et al. Divergence of genetic sequences for the vacuolating cytotoxin among *Helicobacter pylori* strains. *J Biol Chem.* 1994;269(14):10566–10573.
132. Stolte M, Kroher G, Meining A, et al. A comparison of *Helicobacter pylori* and *H. heilmannii* gastritis. A matched control study involving 404 patients. *Scand J Gastroenterol.* 1997;32(1):28–33.
133. Banks PM, Isaacson PG. MALT lymphomas in 1997. Where do we stand? *Am J Clin Pathol.* 1999;111(1 suppl 1):S75–S83.
134. Du M, Diss TC, Xu C, et al. Ongoing mutation in MALT lymphoma immunoglobulin gene suggests that antigen stimulation plays a role in the clonal expansion. *Leukemia.* 1996;10(7):1190–1197.
135. Qin Y, Greiner A, Trunk MJ, et al. Somatic hypermutation in low-grade mucosa-associated lymphoid tissue-type B-cell lymphoma. *Blood.* 1995;86(9):3528–3534.
136. Radaszkiewicz T, Dragosics B, Bauer P. Gastrointestinal malignant lymphomas of the mucosa-associated lymphoid tissue: factors relevant to prognosis. *Gastroenterology.* 1992;102(5):1628–1638.
137. Sharon N, Kenet G, Toren A, et al. *Helicobacter pylori*-associated gastric lymphoma in a girl. *Pediatr Hematol Oncol.* 1997;14(2):177–180.
138. Nakamura S, Matsumoto T, Suekane H, et al. Predictive value of endoscopic ultrasonography for regression of gastric low grade and high grade MALT lymphomas after eradication of *Helicobacter pylori*. *Gut.* 2001;48(4):454–460.
139. Zukerberg LR, Ferry JA, Southern JF, Harris NL. Lymphoid infiltrates of the stomach. Evaluation of histologic criteria for the diagnosis of low-grade gastric lymphoma on endoscopic biopsy specimens. *Am J Surg Pathol.* 1990;14(12):1087–1099.
140. Arista-Nasr J, Jimenez A, Keirns C, et al. The role of the endoscopic biopsy in the diagnosis of gastric lymphoma: a morphologic and immunohistochemical reappraisal. *Hum Pathol.* 1991;22(4):339–348.
141. Isaacson PG, Wotherspoon AC, Diss T, Pan LX. Follicular colonization in B-cell lymphoma of mucosa-associated lymphoid tissue. *Am J Surg Pathol.* 1991;15(9):819–828.
142. Zamboni G, Franzin G, Scarpa A, et al. Carcinoma-like signet-ring cells in gastric mucosa-associated lymphoid tissue (MALT) lymphoma. *Am J Surg Pathol.* 1996;20(5):588–598.
143. Willis TG, Jadayel DM, Du MQ, et al. Bcl10 is involved in t(1;14)(p22;q32) of MALT B cell lymphoma and mutated in multiple tumor types. *Cell.* 1999;96(1):35–45.
144. Ott G, Katzenberger T, Greiner A, et al. The t(11;18)(q21;q21) chromosome translocation is a frequent and specific aberration in low-grade but not high-grade malignant non-Hodgkin's lymphomas of the mucosa-associated lymphoid tissue (MALT-) type. *Cancer Res.* 1997;57(18):3944–3948.
145. Auer IA, Gascoyne RD, Connors JM, et al. t(11;18)(q21;q21) is the most common translocation in MALT lymphomas. *Ann Oncol.* 1997;8(10):979–985.

146. Wotherspoon AC, Soosay GN, Diss TC, Isaacson PG. Low-grade primary B-cell lymphoma of the lung. An immunohistochemical, molecular, and cytogenetic study of a single case. Am J Clin Pathol. 1990;94(5):655–660.
147. Chan WY, Wong N, Chan AB, et al. Consistent copy number gain in chromosome 12 in primary diffuse large cell lymphomas of the stomach. Am J Pathol. 1998;152(1):11–16.
148. Du M, Peng H, Singh N, et al. The accumulation of p53 abnormalities is associated with progression of mucosa-associated lymphoid tissue lymphoma. i. 1995;86(12):4587–4593.
149. Wotherspoon AC, Finn TM, Isaacson PG. Trisomy 3 in low-grade B-cell lymphomas of mucosa-associated lymphoid tissue. Blood. 1995;85(8):2000–2004.
150. Wotherspoon AC, Pan LX, Diss TC, Isaacson PG. Cytogenetic study of B-cell lymphoma of mucosa-associated lymphoid tissue. Cancer Genet Cytogenet. 1992;58(1):35–38.
151. Peng H, Chen G, Du M, et al. Replication error phenotype and p53 gene mutation in lymphomas of mucosa-associated lymphoid tissue. Am J Pathol. 1996;148(2):643–648.
152. Neumeister P, Hoefler G, Beham-Schmid C, et al. Deletion analysis of the p16 tumor suppressor gene in gastrointestinal mucosa-associated lymphoid tissue lymphomas. Gastroenterology. 1997;112(6):1871–1875.
153. Peng H, Diss T, Isaacson PG, et al. c-myc gene abnormalities in mucosa-associated lymphoid tissue (MALT) lymphomas. J Pathol. 1997;181(4):381–386.
154. Van Krieken JH, Medeiros LJ, Pals ST, et al. Diffuse aggressive B-cell lymphomas of the gastrointestinal tract. An immunophenotypic and gene rearrangement analysis of 22 cases. Am J Clin Pathol. 1992;97(2):170–178.
155. Akagi T, Motegi M, Tamura A, et al. A novel gene, MALT1 at 18q21, is involved in t(11;18) (q21;q21) found in low-grade B-cell lymphoma of mucosa-associated lymphoid tissue. Oncogene. 1999;18(42):5785–5794.
156. Dierlamm J, Baens M, Wlodarska I, et al. The apoptosis inhibitor gene API2 and a novel 18q gene, MLT, are recurrently rearranged in the t(11;18)(q21;q21)p6ssociated with mucosa-associated lymphoid tissue lymphomas. Blood. 1999;93(11):3601–3609.
157. Morgan JA, Yin Y, Borowsky AD, et al. Breakpoints of the t(11;18)(q21;q21) in mucosa-associated lymphoid tissue (MALT) lymphoma lie within or near the previously undescribed gene MALT1 in chromosome 18. Cancer Res. 1999;59(24):6205–6213.
158. Uren AG, O'Rourke K, Aravind LA, et al. Identification of paracaspases and metacaspases: two ancient families of caspase-like proteins, one of which plays a key role in MALT lymphoma. Mol Cell. 2000;6(4):961–967.
159. Lucas PC, Yonezumi M, Inohara N, et al. Bcl10 and MALT1, independent targets of chromosomal translocation in malt lymphoma, cooperate in a novel NF-kappa B signaling pathway. J Biol Chem. 2001;276(22):19012–19019.
160. McAllister-Lucas LM, Inohara N, Lucas PC, et al. Bimp1, a MAGUK family member linking protein kinase C activation to Bcl10-mediated NF-kappaB induction. J Biol Chem. 2001;276(33):30589–30597.
161. Liu H, Ye H, Dogan A, et al. T(11;18)(q21;q21) is associated with advanced mucosa-associated lymphoid tissue lymphoma that expresses nuclear BCL10. Blood. 2001;98(4):1182–1187.
162. Kalla J, Stilgenbauer S, Schaffner C, et al. Heterogeneity of the API2-MALT1 gene rearrangement in MALT-type lymphoma. Leukemia. 2000;14(11):1967–1974.
163. Motegi M, Yonezumi M, Suzuki H, et al. API2-MALT1 chimeric transcripts involved in mucosa-associated lymphoid tissue type lymphoma predict heterogeneous products. Am J Pathol. 2000;156(3):807–812.
164. Remstein ED, Kurtin PJ, Einerson RR, et al. Primary pulmonary MALT lymphomas show frequent and heterogeneous cytogenetic abnormalities, including aneuploidy and translocations involving API2 and MALT1 and IGH and MALT1. Leukemia. 2004;18(1):156–160.
165. Ye H, Liu H, Attygalle A, et al. Variable frequencies of t(11;18)(q21;q21) in MALT lymphomas of different sites: significant association with CagA strains of H pylori in gastric MALT lymphoma. Blood. 2003;102(3):1012–1018.
166. Liu H, Ye H, Ruskone-Fourmestraux A, et al. T(11;18) is a marker for all stage gastric MALT lymphomas that will not respond to H. pylori eradication. Gastroenterology. 2002;122(5):1286–1294.
167. Chuang SS, Lee C, Hamoudi RA, et al. High frequency of t(11;18) in gastric mucosa-associated lymphoid tissue lymphomas in Taiwan, including one patient with high-grade transformation. Br J Haematol. 2003;120(1):97–100.
168. Remstein ED, Kurtin PJ, James CD, et al. Mucosa-associated lymphoid tissue lymphomas with t(11;18)(q21;q21) and mucosa-associated lymphoid tissue lymphomas with aneuploidy develop along different pathogenetic pathways. Am J Pathol. 2002;161(1):63–71.
169. Toracchio S, Ota H, de Jong D, et al. Translocation t(11;18)(q21;q21) in gastric B-cell lymphomas. Cancer Sci. 2009;100(5):881–887.
170. Zhang Q, Siebert R, Yan M, et al. Inactivating mutations and overexpression of BCL10, a caspase recruitment domain-containing gene, in MALT lymphoma with t(1;14)(p22;q32). Nat Genet. 1999;22(1):63–68.
171. Koseki T, Inohara N, Chen S, et al. CIPER, a novel NF kappaB-activating protein containing a caspase recruitment domain with homology to Herpesvirus-2 protein E10. J Biol Chem. 1999;274(15):9955–9961.
172. Yan M, Lee J, Schilbach S, et al. mE10, a novel caspase recruitment domain-containing proapoptotic molecule. J Biol Chem. 1999;274(15):10287–10292.
173. Yoneda T, Imaizumi K, Maeda M, et al. Regulatory mechanisms of TRAF2-mediated signal transduction by Bcl10, a MALT lymphoma-associated protein. J Biol Chem. 2000;275(15):11114–11120.
174. Ruland J, Duncan GS, Elia A, et al. Bcl10 is a positive regulator of antigen receptor-induced activation of NF-kappaB and neural tube closure. Cell. 2001;104(1):33–42.
175. Thome M, Martinon F, Hofmann K, et al. Equine herpesvirus-2 E10 gene product, but not its cellular homologue, activates NF-kappaB transcription factor and c-Jun N-terminal kinase. J Biol Chem. 1999;274(15):9962–9968.
176. Zhou H, Wertz I, O'Rourke K, et al. Bcl10 activates the NF-kappaB pathway through ubiquitination of NEMO. Nature. 2004;427(6970):167–171.
177. Sun L, Deng L, Ea CK, et al. The TRAF6 ubiquitin ligase and TAK1 kinase mediate IKK activation by BCL10 and MALT1 in T lymphocytes. Mol Cell. 2004;14(3):289–301.
178. Ye H, Dogan A, Karran L, et al. BCL10 expression in normal and neoplastic lymphoid tissue. Nuclear localization in MALT lymphoma. Am J Pathol. 2000;157(6):1147–1154.
179. Maes B, Demunter A, Peeters B, De Wolf-Peeters C. BCL10 mutation does not represent an important pathogenic mechanism in gastric MALT-type lymphoma, and the presence of the API2-MLT fusion is associated with aberrant nuclear BCL10 expression. Blood. 2002;99(4):1398–1404.
180. Streubel B, Lamprecht A, Dierlamm J, et al. T(14;18)(q32;q21) involving IGH and MALT1 is a frequent chromosomal aberration in MALT lymphoma. Blood. 2003;101(6):2335–2339.

181. Murga Penas EM, Hinz K, Roser K, et al. Translocations t(11;18)(q21;q21) and t(14;18)(q32;q21) are the main chromosomal abnormalities involving MLT/MALT1 in MALT lymphomas. *Leukemia.* 2003;17(11):2225-2229.

182. Nakamura S, Ye H, Bacon CM, et al. Clinical impact of genetic aberrations in gastric MALT lymphoma: a comprehensive analysis using interphase fluorescence in situ hybridisation. *Gut.* 2007;56(10):1358-1363.

183. Sagaert X, de Paepe P, Libbrecht L, et al. Forkhead box protein P1 expression in mucosa-associated lymphoid tissue lymphomas predicts poor prognosis and transformation to diffuse large B-cell lymphoma. *J Clin Oncol.* 2006;24(16):2490-2497.

184. Ruskone-Fourmestraux A, Lavergne A, Aegerter PH, et al. Predictive factors for regression of gastric MALT lymphoma after anti-*Helicobacter pylori* treatment. *Gut.* 2001;48(3):297-303.

185. Sackmann M, Morgner A, Rudolph B, et al. Regression of gastric MALT lymphoma after eradication of *Helicobacter pylori* is predicted by endosonographic staging. MALT Lymphoma Study Group. *Gastroenterology.* 1997;113(4):1087-1090.

186. Thiede C, Morgner A, Alpen B, et al. What role does *Helicobacter pylori* eradication play in gastric MALT and gastric MALT lymphoma? *Gastroenterology.* 1997;113(6 suppl):S61-S64.

187. Pinotti G, Zucca E, Roggero E, et al. Clinical features, treatment and outcome in a series of 93 patients with low-grade gastric MALT lymphoma. *Leuk Lymphoma.* 1997;26(5-6):527-537.

188. Wotherspoon AC, Doglioni C, Diss TC, et al. Regression of primary low-grade B-cell gastric lymphoma of mucosa-associated lymphoid tissue type after eradication of *Helicobacter pylori*. *Lancet.* 1993;342(8871):575-577.

189. Neubauer A, Thiede C, Morgner A, et al. Cure of *Helicobacter pylori* infection and duration of remission of low-grade gastric mucosa-associated lymphoid tissue lymphoma. *J Natl Cancer Inst.* 1997;89(18):1350-1355.

190. Fung CY, Grossbard ML, Linggood RM, et al. Mucosa-associated lymphoid tissue lymphoma of the stomach: long term outcome after local treatment. *Cancer.* 1999;85(1):9-17.

191. Montalban C, Castrillo JM, Abraira V, et al. Gastric B-cell mucosa-associated lymphoid tissue (MALT) lymphoma. Clinicopathological study and evaluation of the prognostic factors in 143 patients. *Ann Oncol.* 1995;6(4):355-362.

192. Martinelli G, Laszlo D, Ferreri AJ, et al. Clinical activity of rituximab in gastric marginal zone non-Hodgkin's lymphoma resistant to or not eligible for anti-*Helicobacter pylori* therapy [see comment]. *J Clin Oncol.* 2005;23(9):1979-1983.

193. Castrillo JM, Montalban C, Abraira V, et al. Evaluation of the international index in the prognosis of high grade gastric malt lymphoma. *Leuk Lymphoma.* 1996;24(1-2):159-163.

194. Cogliatti SB, Schmid U, Schumacher U, et al. Primary B-cell gastric lymphoma: a clinicopathological study of 145 patients. *Gastroenterology.* 1991;101(5):1159-1170.

195. de Jong D, Boot H, van Heerde P, et al. Histological grading in gastric lymphoma: pretreatment criteria and clinical relevance. *Gastroenterology.* 1997;112(5):1466-1474.

196. Sanchez-Bueno F, Garcia-Marcilla JA, Alonso JD, et al. Prognostic factors in primary gastrointestinal non-Hodgkin's lymphoma: a multivariate analysis of 76 cases. *Eur J Surg.* 1998;164(5):385-392.

197. Yamashita H, Watanabe H, Ajioka Y, et al. When can complete regression of low-grade gastric lymphoma of mucosa-associated lymphoid tissue be predicted after *helicobacter pylori* eradication? *Histopathology.* 2000;37(2):131-140.

198. Begum S, Sano T, Endo H, et al. Mucosal change of the stomach with low-grade mucosa-associated lymphoid tissue lymphoma after eradication of *Helicobacter pylori*: follow-up study of 48 cases. *J Med Invest.* 2000;47(1-2):36-46.

199. Fischbach W, Goebeler-Kolve ME, Dragosics B, et al. Long term outcome of patients with gastric marginal zone B cell lymphoma of mucosa associated lymphoid tissue (MALT) following exclusive *Helicobacter pylori* eradication therapy: experience from a large prospective series. *Gut.* 2004;53(1):34-37.

200. de Mascarel A, Ruskone-Fourmestraux A, Lavergne-Slove A, et al. Clinical, histological and molecular follow-up of 60 patients with gastric marginal zone lymphoma of mucosa-associated lymphoid tissue. *Virchows Archiv.* 2005;446(3):219-224.

201. Raderer M, Streubel B, Woehrer S, et al. High relapse rate in patients with MALT lymphoma warrants lifelong follow-up. *Clin Cancer Res.* 2005;11(9):3349-3352.

202. Montalban C, Santon A, Boixeda D, et al. Treatment of low grade gastric mucosa-associated lymphoid tissue lymphoma in stage I with *Helicobacter pylori* eradication. Long-term results after sequential histologic and molecular follow-up. *Haematologica.* 2001;86(6):609-617.

203. Morgner A, Miehlke S, Stolte M, et al. Development of early gastric cancer 4 and 5 years after complete remission of *Helicobacter pylori* associated gastric low grade marginal zone B cell lymphoma of MALT type. *World J Gastroenterol.* 2001;7(2):248-253.

204. Chan JK, Ng CS, Isaacson PG. Relationship between high-grade lymphoma and low-grade B-cell mucosa-associated lymphoid tissue lymphoma (MALToma) of the stomach. *Am J Pathol.* 1990;136(5):1153-1164.

205. Ferreri AJ, Freschi M, Dell'Oro S, et al. Prognostic significance of the histopathologic recognition of low- and high-grade components in stage I-II B-cell gastric lymphomas. *Am J Surg Pathol.* 2001;25(1):95-102.

206. Takeshita M, Iwashita A, Kurihara K, et al. Histologic and immunohistologic findings and prognosis of 40 cases of gastric large B-cell lymphoma. *Am J Surg Pathol.* 2000;24(12):1641-1649.

207. Raderer M, Valencak J, Osterreicher C, et al. Chemotherapy for the treatment of patients with primary high grade gastric B-cell lymphoma of modified Ann Arbor Stages IE and IIE. *Cancer.* 2000;88(9):1979-1985.

208. Montalban C, Manzanal A, Castrillo JM, et al. Low grade gastric B-cell MALT lymphoma progressing into high grade lymphoma. Clonal identity of the two stages of the tumour, unusual bone involvement and leukemic dissemination. *Histopathology.* 1995;27(1):89-91.

209. Peng H, Du M, Diss TC, et al. Genetic evidence for a clonal link between low and high-grade components in gastric MALT B-cell lymphoma. *Histopathology.* 1997;30(5):425-429.

210. Villuendas R, Piris MA, Orradre JL, et al. Different bcl-2 protein expression in high-grade B-cell lymphomas derived from lymph node or mucosa-associated lymphoid tissue. *Am J Pathol.* 1991;139(5):989-993.

211. Omonishi K, Yoshino T, Sakuma I, et al. bcl-6 protein is identified in high-grade but not low-grade mucosa-associated lymphoid tissue lymphomas of the stomach. *Mod Pathol.* 1998;11(2):181-185.

212. Starostik P, Greiner A, Schultz A, et al. Genetic aberrations common in gastric high-grade large B-cell lymphoma. *Blood.* 2000;95(4):1180-1187.

213. Chan JK. Gastrointestinal lymphomas: an overview with emphasis on new findings and diagnostic problems. *Semin Diagn Pathol*. 1996;13(4):260–296.
214. Chen LT, Lin JT, Tai JJ, et al. Long-term results of anti-*Helicobacter pylori* therapy in early-stage gastric high-grade transformed MALT lymphoma. *J Natl Cancer Inst*. 2005;97(18):1345–1353.
215. Sugimoto M, Kajimura M, Sato Y, et al. Regression of primary gastric diffuse large B-cell lymphoma after eradication of *Helicobacter pylori*. *Gastrointest Endosc*. 2001;54(5):643–645.
216. Watari J, Saitoh Y, Fujiya M, et al. Spontaneous remission of primary diffuse large B-cell gastric lymphoma. *J Gastroenterol*. 2005;40(4):414–420.
217. Banerjee D, Walton JC, Jory TA, et al. Primary gastric T-cell lymphoma of suppressor-cytotoxic (CD8+) phenotype: discordant expression of T-cell receptor subunit beta F1, CD7, and CD3 antigens. *Hum Pathol*. 1990;21(8):872–874.
218. Foss HD, Coupland SE, Stein H. Clinico-pathologic forms of peripheral T-and NK-cell lymphomas. *Pathologe*. 2000;21(2):137–146.
219. Kurihara K, Mizuseki K, Ichikawa M, et al. Primary gastric T-cell lymphoma with manifold histologic appearances. *Acta Pathol Jpn*. 1991;41(11):824–828.
220. Shepherd NA, Blackshaw AJ, Hall PA, et al. Malignant lymphoma with eosinophilia of the gastrointestinal tract. *Histopathology*. 1987;11(2):115–130.
221. Shimada-Hiratsuka M, Fukayama M, Hayashi Y, et al. Primary gastric T-cell lymphoma with and without human T-lymphotropic virus type 1. *Cancer*. 1997;80(2):292–303.
222. Yatabe Y, Mori N, Oka K, et al. Primary gastric T-cell lymphoma. Morphological and immunohistochemical studies of two cases. *Arch Pathol Lab Med*. 1994;118(5):547–550.
223. Foss HD, Schmitt-Graff A, Daum S, et al. Origin of primary gastric T-cell lymphomas from intraepithelial T-lymphocytes: report of two cases. *Histopathology*. 1999;34(1):9–15.
224. Yoshida N, Wakabayashi N, Nomura K, et al. Ileal mucosa-associated lymphoid tissue lymphoma showing several ulcer scars detected using double-balloon endoscopy. *Endoscopy*. 2004;36(11):1022–1024.
225. Isaacson PG, Norton AJ. *Extrnodal Lymphomas*. Edinburgh, UK: Churchill Livingstone; 1994.
226. Isaacson PG, Spencer J. Malignant lymphoma of mucosa-associated lymphoid tissue. *Histopathology*. 1987;11(5):445–462.
227. Domizio P, Owen RA, Shepherd NA, et al. Primary lymphoma of the small intestine. A clinicopathological study of 119 cases. *Am J Surg Pathol*. 1993;17(5):429–442.
228. Shepherd NA, Hall PA, Coates PJ, Levison DA. Primary malignant lymphoma of the colon and rectum. A histopathological and immunohistochemical analysis of 45 cases with clinicopathological correlations. *Histopathology*. 1988;12(3):235–252.
229. Kojima M, Nakamura S, Kurabayashi Y, et al. Primary malignant lymphoma of the intestine: clinicopathologic and immunohistochemical studies of 39 cases. *Pathol Int*. 1995;45(2):123–130.
230. Streubel B, Seitz G, Stolte M, et al. MALT lymphoma associated genetic aberrations occur at different frequencies in primary and secondary intestinal MALT lymphomas. *Gut*. 2006;55(11):1581–1585.
231. Yoshida N, Nomura K, Wakabayashi N, et al. Cytogenetic and clinicopathological characterization by fluorescence in situ hybridization on paraffin-embedded tissue sections of twenty-six cases with malignant lymphoma of small intestine. *Scand J Gastroenterol*. 2006;41(2):212–222.
232. Nakamura S, Matsumoto T, Takeshita M, et al. A clinicopathologic study of primary small intestine lymphoma: prognostic significance of mucosa-associated lymphoid tissue-derived lymphoma. *Cancer*. 2000;88(2):286–294.
233. Azar HA. Cancer in Lebanon and the Near East. *Cancer*. 1962;15:66–78.
234. Ramot B, Shahin N, Bubis JJ. Malabsorption syndrome in lymphoma of small intestine. A Study of 13 Cases. *Isr J Med Sci*. 1965;1:221–226.
235. Isaacson P, Al-Dewachi HS, Mason DY. Middle Eastern intestinal lymphoma: a morphological and immunohistochemical study. *J Clin Pathol*. 1983;36(5):489–498.
236. Lewin KJ, Kahn LB, Novis BH. Primary intestinal lymphoma of "Western" and "Mediterranean" type, alpha chain disease and massive plasma cell infiltration: a comparative study of 37 cases. *Cancer*. 1976;38(6):2511–2528.
237. Rambaud JC, Matuchansky C. Alpha-chain disease. Pathogenesis and relation to Mediterranean lymphoma. *Lancet*. 1973;1(7817):1430–1432.
238. Seligmann M. Immunochemical, clical, and pathological features of alpha-chain disease. *Arch Intern Med*. 1975;135(1):78–82.
239. Shahid MJ, Alami SY, Nassar VH, et al. Primary intestinal lymphoma with paraproteinemia. *Cancer*. 1975;35(3):848–858.
240. Fine KD, Stone MJ. Alpha-heavy chain disease, Mediterranean lymphoma, and immunoproliferative small intestinal disease: a review of clinicopathological features, pathogenesis, and differential diagnosis. *Am J Gastroenterol*. 1999;94(5):1139–1152.
241. Trotman BW, Pavlick AC, Igwegbe IC, Goldstein MM. Immunoproliferative small intestinal disease: case report and literature review. *J Assoc Acad Minor Phys*. 1999;10(4):88–93.
242. Malik IA, Shamsi Z, Shafquat A, et al. Clinicopathological features and management of immunoproliferative small intestinal disease and primary small intestinal lymphoma in Pakistan. *Med Pediatr Oncol*. 1995;25(5):400–406.
243. Nasr K, Haghighi P, Bakhshandeh K, Haghshenas M. Primary lymphoma of the upper small intestine. *Gut*. 1970;11(8):673–678.
244. Novis BH, Bank S, Marks IN, et al. Abdominal lymphoma presenting with malabsorption. *Q J Med*. 1971;40(160):521–540.
245. Lin OS, Gray GM. Immunoproliferative small intestinal disease: prolonged 30-year course without development of lymphoma. *Am J Gastroenterol*. 2001;96(9):2769–2774.
246. Salem PA, Estephan FF. Immunoproliferative small intestinal disease: current concepts. *Cancer J*. 2005;11(5):374–382.
247. Lecuit M, Abachin E, Martin A, et al. Immunoproliferative small intestinal disease associated with Campylobacter jejuni. *N Engl J Med*. 2004;350(3):239–248.
248. Suarez F, Lortholary O, Hormine O, Lecuit M. Infection-associated lymphomas derived from marginal zone B cells: a model of antigen-driven lymphoproliferation. *Blood*. 2006;107(8):3034–3044.
249. Nikbin B, Banisadre M, Ala F, Mojtabai A. HLA AW19, B12 in immunoproliferative small intestinal disease. *Gut*. 1979;20(3):226–228.
250. Khojasteh A, Haghighi P. Immunoproliferative small intestinal disease: portrait of a potentially preventable cancer from the Third World. *Am J Med*. 1990;89(4):483–490.
251. Hassane DC, Lee RB, Pickett CL. Campylobacter jejuni cytolethal distending toxin promotes DNA repair responses in normal human cells. *Infect Immun*. 2003;71(1):541–545.
252. Bender SW, Danon F, Preud'homme JL, et al. Gamma heavy chain disease simulating alpha chain disease. *Gut*. 1978;19(12):1148–1152.

253. Matuchansky C, Cogne M, Lemaire M, et al. Nonsecretory alpha-chain disease with immunoproliferative small-intestinal disease. *N Engl J Med.* 1989;320(23):1534–1539.
254. Nassar VH, Salem PA, Shahid MJ, et al. "Mediterranean abdominal lymphoma" or immunoproliferative small intestinal disease. Part II: pathological aspects. *Cancer.* 1978;41(4):1340–1354.
255. Galian A, Lecestre MJ, Scotto J, et al. Pathological study of alpha-chain disease, with special emphasis on evolution. *Cancer.* 1977;39(5):2081–2101.
256. Cammoun M, Jaafoura H, Tabbane F, Halphen M. Immunoproliferative small intestinal disease without alpha-chain disease: a pathological study. *Gastroenterology.* 1989;96(3):750–763.
257. Gilinsky NH, Novis BH, Mee AS, et al. Immunoproliferative small-intestinal disease: follow-up of an alpha-chain negative, lymphoma-free group. *J Clin Gastroenterol.* 1983;5(5):421–428.
258. Price SK. Immunoproliferative small intestinal disease: a study of 13 cases with alpha heavy-chain disease. *Histopathology.* 1990;17(1):7–17.
259. Gilinsky NH, Chaimowitz G, Van Staden MC. Immunoproliferative small-intestinal disease with lymphoma—diagnostic difficulties and pitfalls. Case reports. *S Afr Med J.* 1986;69(4):260–262.
260. Al-Saleem T, Zardawi IM. Primary lymphomas of the small intestine in Iraq: a pathological study of 145 cases. *Histopathology.* 1979;3(2):89–106.
261. Isaacson PG, Dogan A, Price SK, Spencer J. Immunoproliferative small-intestinal disease. An immunohistochemical study. *Am J Surg Pathol.* 1989;13(12):1023–1033.
262. Isaacson PG, Price SK. Light chains in Mediterranean lymphoma. *J Clin Pathol.* 1985;38(6):601–607.
263. Smith WJ, Price SK, Isaacson PG. Immunoglobulin gene rearrangement in immunoproliferative small intestinal disease (IPSID). *J Clin Pathol.* 1987;40:1290–1297.
264. Berger R, Bernheim A, Tsapis A, et al. Cytogenetic studies in four cases of alpha chain disease. *Cancer Genet Cytogenet.* 1986;22(3):219–223.
265. Organization WH. Alpha-chain disease and related small intestinal lymphoma: report of a WHO meeting of investigators. *Arch Fr Mal App Dig.* 1976;65:591–607.
266. Chang CS, Lin SF, Chen TP, et al. Leukemic manifestation in a case of alpha-chain disease with multiple polypoid intestinal lymphocytic lymphoma. *Am J Hematol.* 1992;41(3):209–214.
267. Akbulut H, Soykan I, Yakaryilmaz F, et al. Five-year results of the treatment of 23 patients with immunoproliferative small intestinal disease: a Turkish experience. *Cancer.* 1997;80(1):8–14.
268. Ben-Ayed F, Halphen M, Najjar T, et al. Treatment of alpha chain disease. Results of a prospective study in 21 Tunisian patients by the Tunisian-French intestinal Lymphoma Study Group. *Cancer.* 1989;63(7):1251–1256.
269. Gilinsky NH, Novis BH, Wright JP, et al. Immunoproliferative small-intestinal disease: clinical features and outcome in 30 cases. *Medicine (Baltimore).* 1987;66(6):438–446.
270. Novis BH, King HS, Gilinsky NH, et al. Long survival in a patient with alpha-chain disease. *Cancer.* 1984;53(4):970–973.
271. Anaissie E, Geha S, Allam C, et al. Burkitt's lymphoma in the Middle East. A study of 34 cases. *Cancer.* 1985;56(10):2539–2543.
272. Carbone A, Canzonieri V, Gloghini A, et al. Burkitt's lymphoma: historical background and recent insights into classification and pathogenesis. *Ann Otol Rhinol Laryngol.* 2000;109(7):693–702.
273. Gough KR, Read AE, Naish JM. Intestinal reticulosis as a complication of idiopathic steatorrhoea. *Gut.* 1962;3:232–239.
274. Baer AN, Bayless TM, Yardley JH. Intestinal ulceration and malabsorption syndromes. *Gastroenterology.* 1980;79(4):754–765.
275. Cooper BT, Holmes GK, Ferguson R, Cooke WT. Celiac disease and malignancy. *Medicine (Baltimore).* 1980;59(4):249–261.
276. Freeman HJ, Weinstein WM, Shnitka TK, et al. Primary abdominal lymphoma. Presenting manifestation of celiac sprue or complicating dermatitis herpetiformis. *Am J Med.* 1977;63(4):585–594.
277. Katoh A, Ohshima K, Kanda M, et al. Gastrointestinal T cell lymphoma: predominant cytotoxic phenotypes, including alpha/beta, gamma/delta T cell and natural killer cells. *Leuk Lymphoma.* 2000;39(1–2):97–111.
278. Pricolo VE, Mangi AA, Aswad B, Bland KI. Gastrointestinal malignancies in patients with celiac sprue. *Am J Surg.* 1998;176(4):344–347.
279. Roehrkasse RL, Roberts IM, Wald A, et al. Celiac sprue complicated by lymphoma presenting with multiple gastric ulcers. *Gastroenterology.* 1986;91(3):740–745.
280. O'Farrelly C, Feighery C, O'Briain DS, et al. Humoral response to wheat protein in patients with coeliac disease and enteropathy associated T cell lymphoma. *Br Med J (Clin Res Ed).* 1986;293(6552):908–910.
281. Carbonnel F, Grollet-Bioul L, Brouet JC, et al. Are complicated forms of celiac disease cryptic T-cell lymphomas? *Blood.* 1998;92(10):3879–3886.
282. Holmes GK, Prior P, Lane MR, et al. Malignancy in coeliac disease—effect of a gluten free diet. *Gut.* 1989;30(3):333–338.
283. Quintanilla-Martinez L, Lome-Maldonado C, Ott G, et al. Primary non-Hodgkin's lymphoma of the intestine: high prevalence of Epstein-Barr virus in Mexican lymphomas as compared with European cases. *Blood.* 1997;89(2):644–651.
284. Isaacson PG. Intestinal lymphoma and enteropathy. *J Pathol.* 1995;177(2):111–113.
285. Kumar P. Coeliac disease and lymphoma. *Eur J Gastroenterol Hepatol.* 2006;18(2):131–132.
286. Isaacson PG, Du MQ. MALT lymphoma: from morphology to molecules. *Nat Rev Cancer.* 2004;4(8):644–653.
287. Cellier C, Patey N, Mauvieux L, et al. Abnormal intestinal intraepithelial lymphocytes in refractory sprue. *Gastroenterology.* 1998;114(3):471–481.
288. Bagdi E, Diss TC, Munson P, Isaacson PG. Mucosal intra-epithelial lymphocytes in enteropathy-associated T-cell lymphoma, ulcerative jejunitis, and refractory celiac disease constitute a neoplastic population. *Blood.* 1999;94(1):260–264.
289. Mention JJ, Ben Ahmed M, Begue B, et al. Interleukin 15: a key to disrupted intraepithelial lymphocyte homeostasis and lymphomagenesis in celiac disease. *Gastroenterology.* 2003;125(3):730–745.
290. Chott A, Haedicke W, Mosberger I, et al. Most CD56+ intestinal lymphomas are CD8+CD5-T-cell lymphomas of monomorphic small to medium size histology. *Am J Pathol.* 1998;153(5):1483–1490.
291. Mathus-Vliegen EM, Van Halteren H, Tytgat GN. Malignant lymphoma in coeliac disease: various manifestations with distinct symptomatology and prognosis? *J Intern Med.* 1994;236(1):43–49.
292. Ashton-Key M, Diss TC, Pan L, et al. Molecular analysis of T-cell clonality in ulcerative jejunitis and enteropathy-associated T-cell lymphoma. *Am J Pathol.* 1997;151(2):493–498.
293. Biagi F, Lorenzini P, Corazza GR. Literature review on the clinical relationship between ulcerative jejunoileitis, coeliac disease, and enteropathy-associated T-cell. *Scand J Gastroenterol.* 2000;35(8):785–790.

294. Chott A, Vesely M, Simonitsch I, et al. Classification of intestinal T-cell neoplasms and their differential diagnosis. *Am J Clin Pathol.* 1999;111(1 suppl 1):S68–S74.
295. Isaacson P. Primary gastrointestinal lymphoma. *Virchows Arch A Pathol Anat Histol.* 1981;391(1):1–8.
296. Tallini G, West AB, Buckley PJ. Diagnosis of gastrointestinal T-cell lymphomas in routinely processed tissues. *J Clin Gastroenterol.* 1993;17(1):57–66.
297. Alfsen GC, Beiske K, Bell H, Marton PF. Low-grade intestinal lymphoma of intraepithelial T lymphocytes with concomitant enteropathy-associated T cell lymphoma: case report suggesting a possible histogenetic relationship. *Hum Pathol.* 1989;20(9):909–913.
298. Murray A, Cuevas EC, Jones DB, Wright DH. Study of the immunohistochemistry and T cell clonality of enteropathy-associated T cell lymphoma. *Am J Pathol.* 1995;146(2):509–519.
299. Corlin RF, Pops MA. Nongranulomatous ulcerative jejunoileitis with hypogammaglobulinemia. Clinical remission after treatment with gamma-globulin. *Gastroenterology.* 1972;62(3):473–478.
300. Barrett MT, Sanchez CA, Prevo LJ, et al. Evolution of neoplastic cell lineages in Barrett oesophagus. *Nat Genet.* 1999;22(1):106–109.
301. Zettl A, Ott G, Makulik A, et al. Chromosomal gains at 9q characterize enteropathy-type T-cell lymphoma. *Am J Pathol.* 2002;161(5):1635–1645.
302. Cejkova P, Zettl A, Baumgartner AK, et al. Amplification of NOTCH1 and ABL1 gene loci is a frequent aberration in enteropathy-type T-cell lymphoma. *Virchows Arch.* 2005;446(4):416–420.
303. Obermann EC, Diss TC, Hamoudi RA, et al. Loss of heterozygosity at chromosome 9p21 is a frequent finding in enteropathy-type T-cell lymphoma. *J Pathol.* 2004;202(2):252–262.
304. Egan LJ, Walsh SV, Stevens FM, et al. Celiac-associated lymphoma. A single institution experience of 30 cases in the combination chemotherapy era. *J Clin Gastroenterol.* 1995;21(2):123–129.
304a. Svrcek M, Garderet L, Sebbagh V, et al. Small intestinal CD4+ T-cell lymphoma: a rare distinctive clinicopathological entity associated with prolonged survival. *Virchows Arch.* 2007;451(6):1091–1093.
305. Romaguera J, Hagemeister FB. Lymphoma of the colon. *Curr Opin Gastroenterol.* 2005;21(1):80–84.
306. Ioachim HL, Dorsett B, Cronin W, et al. Acquired immunodeficiency syndrome associated lymphomas: clinical, pathologic, immunologic, and viral characteristics of 111 cases. *Hum Pathol.* 1991;22(7):659–673.
307. Levine AM. Acquired immunodeficiency syndrome related lymphoma. *Blood.* 1992;80(1):8–20.
308. Muller G, Dargent JL, Duwel V, et al. Leukaemia and lymphoma of the appendix presenting as acute appendicitis or acute abdomen. Four case reports with a review of the literature. *J Cancer Res Clin Oncol.* 1997;123(10):560–564.
309. Sin IC, Ling ET, Prentice RS. Burkitt's lymphoma of the appendix: report of two cases. *Hum Pathol.* 1980;11(5):465–470.
310. Kitamura Y, Ohta T, Terada T. Primary T-cell non-Hodgkin's malignant lymphoma of the appendix. *Pathol Int.* 2000;50(4):313–317.
311. Karabulut R, Sonmez K, Turkyilmaz Z, et al. Mucosa-associated lymphoid tissue lymphoma in the appendix, a lead point for intussusception. *J Pediatr Surg.* 2005;40(5):872–874.
312. Tan KB, Tan LH, Soo R, et al. Involvement of the appendix and palate by pleomorphic variant mantle cell lymphoma. *Leuk Lymphoma.* 2006;47(8):1704–1707.
313. Esteban JM, Gutierrez del Olmo A, Baki W, et al. Colonic mucosa-associated lymphoid tissue lymphoma presenting as multiple polyposis. *Gastrointest Endosc.* 2005;61(7):928–930.
314. Kodama T, Ohshima K, Nomura K, et al. Lymphomatous polyposis of the gastrointestinal tract, including mantle cell lymphoma, follicular lymphoma and mucosa-associated lymphoid tissue lymphoma. *Histopathology.* 2005;47(5):467–478.
315. Lee YG, Lee S, Han SW, Lee JS. A case of multiple mucosa-associated lymphoid tissue (MALT) lymphoma of the colon identified as simple mucosal discoloration. *J Korean Med Sci.* 2005;20(2):325–328.
316. Zinzani PL, Pulsoni A, Gentilini P, et al. Effectiveness of fludarabine, idarubicin and cyclophosphamide (FLUIC) combination regimen for young patients with untreated non-follicular low-grade non-Hodgkin's lymphoma. *Leuk Lymphoma.* 2004;45(9):1815–1819.
317. Banks PM, Chan J, Cleary ML, et al. Mantle cell lymphoma. A proposal for unification of morphologic, immunologic, and molecular data. *Am J Surg Pathol.* 1992;16(7):637–640.
318. Okazaki K. Multiple lymphomatous polyposis form is common but not specific for mantle cell lymphoma in the gastrointestinal tract. *J Gastroenterol.* 2004;39(10):1023–1024.
319. Romaguera JE, Medeiros LJ, Hagemeister FB, et al. Frequency of gastrointestinal involvement and its clinical significance in mantle cell lymphoma. *Cancer.* 2003;97(3):586–591.
320. Tamura S, Ohkawauchi K, Yokoyama Y, et al. Non-multiple lymphomatous polyposis form of mantle cell lymphoma in the gastrointestinal tract. *J Gastroenterol.* 2004;39(10):995–1000.
321. Campo E, Raffeld M, Jaffe ES. Mantle-cell lymphoma. *Semin Hematol.* 1999;36(2):115–127.
322. Kumar S, Krenacs L, Otsuki T, et al. bcl-1 rearrangement and cyclin D1 protein expression in multiple lymphomatous polyposis. *Am J Clin Pathol.* 1996;105(6):737–743.
323. O'Briain DS, Kennedy MJ, Daly PA, et al. Multiple lymphomatous polyposis of the gastrointestinal tract. A clinicopathologically distinctive form of non-Hodgkin's lymphoma of B-cell centrocytic type. *Am J Surg Pathol.* 1989;13(8):691–699.
324. Breslin NP, Urbanski SJ, Shaffer EA. Mucosa-associated lymphoid tissue (MALT) lymphoma manifesting as multiple lymphomatosis polyposis of the gastrointestinal tract. *Am J Gastroenterol.* 1999;94(9):2540–2545.
325. Endoh M, Hiraishi H, Terano A. Gastrointestinal: multiple lymphomatous polyposis. *J Gastroenterol Hepatol.* 1999;14(9):937.
326. Hashimoto Y, Nakamura N, Kuze T, et al. Multiple lymphomatous polyposis of the gastrointestinal tract is a heterogenous group that includes mantle cell lymphoma and follicular lymphoma: analysis of somatic mutation of immunoglobulin heavy chain gene variable region. *Hum Pathol.* 1999;30(5):581–587.
327. Ohtsuka T, Kodama K, Nishikata F, et al. Mucosa-associated lymphoid tissue lymphoma of the duodenum forming multiple polypoid lesions: report of a case. *Surg Today.* 1999;29(6):557–559.
328. Yamamoto S, Nakase H, Yamashita K, et al. Gastrointestinal follicular lymphoma: review of the literature. *J Gastroenterol.* 2010;45(4):370–388.
329. Shia J, Teruya-Feldstein J, Pan D, et al. Primary follicular lymphoma of the gastrointestinal tract: a clinical and pathologic study of 26 cases. *Am J Surg Pathol.* 2002;26(2):216–224.

330. Damaj G, Verkarre V, Delmer A, et al. Primary follicular lymphoma of the gastrointestinal tract: a study of 25 cases and a literature review. *Ann Oncol*. 2003;14(4): 623-629.
331. Bende RJ, Smit LA, Bossenbroek JG, et al. Primary follicular lymphoma of the small intestine: alpha4beta7 expression and immunoglobulin configuration suggest an origin from local antigen-experienced B cells. *Am J Pathol*. 2003;162(1):105-113.
332. Nakamura S, Matsumoto T, Umeno J, et al. Endoscopic features of intestinal follicular lymphoma: the value of double-balloon enteroscopy. *Endoscopy*. 2007;39(suppl 1): E26-E27.
333. LeBrun DP, Kamel OW, Cleary ML, et al. Follicular lymphomas of the gastrointestinal tract. Pathologic features in 31 cases and bcl-2 oncogenic protein expression. *Am J Pathol*. 1992;140(6):1327-1335.
334. The Non-Hodgkin's Lymphoma Classification Project. A clinical evaluation of the International Lymphoma Study Group classification of non-Hodgkin's lymphoma. *Blood*. 1997;89(11):3909-3918.
335. Mori M, Kobayashi Y, Maeshima AM, et al. The indolent course and high incidence of t(14;18) in primary duodenal follicular lymphoma. *Ann Oncol*. 2010;21(7):1500-1505.
336. Lin P, Bueso-Ramos C, Wilson CS, et al. Waldenstrom macroglobulinemia involving extramedullary sites: morphologic and immunophenotypic findings in 44 patients. *Am J Surg Pathol*. 2003;27(8):1104-1113.
337. Veloso FT, Fraga J, Saleiro JV. Macroglobulinemia and small intestinal disease. A case report with review of the literature. *J Clin Gastroenterol*. 1988;10(5):546-550.
338. Okada Y, Mori H, Maeda T, et al. Autopsy case of lymphoplasmacytic lymphoma with a large submucosal tumor in the stomach. *Pathol Int*. 2001;51(10):802-806.
339. Borisch B, Raphael M, Swerdlow SH, Jaffe ES. Lymphoproliferative disease associated with primary immune disorders. In: Jaffe EHN, Stein H, Vardiman JW, eds. *Pathology & genetics: tumours of haematopoietic and lymphoid tissues*. Lyon, France: IARC Press; 2001.
340. Sander CA, Medeiros LJ, Weiss LM, et al. Lymphoproliferative lesions in patients with common variable immunodeficiency syndrome. *Am J Surg Pathol*. 1992;16(12):1170-1182.
341. Purtilo DT, Strobach RS, Okano M, Davis JR. Epstein-Barr virus-associated lymphoproliferative disorders. *Lab Invest*. 1992;67(1):5-23.
342. Broder S, Callihan TR, Jaffe ES, et al. Resolution of long-standing protein-losing enteropathy in a patient with intestinal lymphangiectasia after treatment for malignant lymphoma. *Gastroenterology*. 1981;80(1):166-168.
343. Duplantier JE, Seyama K, Day NK, et al. Immunologic reconstitution following bone marrow transplantation for X-linked hyper IgM syndrome. *Clin Immunol*. 2001;98(3): 313-318.
344. Hadzic N, Pagliuca A, Rela M, et al. Correction of the hyper-IgM syndrome after liver and bone marrow transplantation. *N Engl J Med*. 2000;342(5):320-324.
345. Lim ST, Levine AM. Recent advances in acquired immunodeficiency syndrome (AIDS)-related lymphoma. *CA Cancer J Clin*. 2005;55(4):229-241; 60-61, 64.
346. Carbone A, Gloghini A. AIDS-related lymphomas: from pathogenesis to pathology. *Br J Haematol*. 2005;130(5): 662-670.
347. Raphael M, Borisch B, Jaffe ES. In: Jaffe EHN, Stein H, Vardiman JW, eds. *Pathology & genetics: tumours of haematopoietic and lymphoid tissues*. Lyon, France: IARC Press; 2001.
348. Matthews GV, Bower M, Mandalia S, et al. Changes in acquired immunodeficiency syndrome-related lymphoma since the introduction of highly active antiretroviral therapy. *Blood*. 2000;96(8):2730-2734.
349. Raphael M, Borisch B, Jaffe ES. Lymphomas associated with infection by the human immune deficiency virus (HIV). In: Jaffe EHN, Stein H, Vardiman JW, eds. *Pathology & genetics: tumours of haematopoietic and lymphoid tissues*. Lyon, France: IARC Press; 2001.
350. Said W, Chien K, Takeuchi S, et al. Kaposi's sarcoma-associated herpesvirus (KSHV or HHV8) in primary effusion lymphoma: ultrastructural demonstration of herpesvirus in lymphoma cells. *Blood*. 1996;87(12):4937-4943.
351. Nador RG, Cesarman E, Chadburn A, et al. Primary effusion lymphoma: a distinct clinicopathologic entity associated with the Kaposi's sarcoma-associated herpes virus. *Blood*. 1996;88(2):645-656.
352. Beaty MW, Kumar S, Sorbara L, et al. A biophenotypic human herpesvirus 8-associated primary bowel lymphoma. *Am J Surg Pathol*. 1999;23(8):992-994.
353. DePond W, Said JW, Tasaka T, et al. Kaposi's sarcoma-associated herpesvirus and human herpesvirus 8 (KSHV/HHV8)-associated lymphoma of the bowel. Report of two cases in HIV-positive men with secondary effusion lymphomas. *Am J Surg Pathol*. 1997;21(6):719-724.
354. Knowles DM, Inghirami G, Ubriaco A, et al. Molecular genetic analysis of three AIDS-associated neoplasms of uncertain lineage demonstrates their B-cell derivation and the possible pathogenetic role of the Epstein-Barr virus. *Blood*. 1989;73(3):792-799.
355. Matolcsy A, Nador RG, Cesarman E, Knowles DM. Immunoglobulin VH gene mutational analysis suggests that primary effusion lymphomas derive from different stages of B cell maturation. *Am J Pathol*. 1998;153(5):1609-1614.
356. Levine AM, Sullivan-Halley J, Pike MC, et al. Human immunodeficiency virus-related lymphoma. Prognostic factors predictive of survival. *Cancer*. 1991;68(11):2466-2472.
357. Harris NL, Ferry JA, Swerdlow SH. Posttransplant lymphoproliferative disorders: summary of Society for Hematopathology Workshop. *Semin Diagn Pathol*. 1997;14(1):8-14.
358. Harris NL, Swerdlow SH, Frizzera G, Knowles DM. Post-transplant lymphoproliferative disorders. In: Jaffe EHN, Stein H, Vardiman JW, eds. *Pathology & genetics: tumours of haematopoietic and lymphoid tissues*. Lyon, France: IARC Press; 2001.
359. Gottschalk S, Rooney CM, Heslop HE. Post-transplant lymphoproliferative disorders. *Annu Rev Med*. 2005;56: 29-44.
360. Sivaraman P, Lye WC. Epstein-Barr virus-associated T-cell lymphoma in solid organ transplant recipients. *Biomed Pharmacother*. 2001;55(7):366-368.
361. Jain M, Badwal S, Pandey R, et al. Post-transplant lymphoproliferative disorders after live donor renal transplantation. *Clin Transplant*. 2005;19(5):668-673.
362. Taylor AL, Marcus R, Bradley JA. Post-transplant lymphoproliferative disorders (PTLD) after solid organ transplantation. *Crit Rev Oncol Hematol*. 2005;56(1):155-167.
363. Caillard S, Dharnidharka V, Agodoa L, et al. Posttransplant lymphoproliferative disorders after renal transplantation in the United States in Era of modern immunosuppression. *Transplantation*. 2005;80(9):1233-1243.
364. Faye A, Vilmer E. Post-transplant lymphoproliferative disorder in children: incidence, prognosis, and treatment options. *Paediatr Drugs*. 2005;7(1):55-65.
365. Ferry JA, Jacobson JO, Conti D, et al. Lymphoproliferative disorders and hematologic malignancies following organ transplantation. *Mod Pathol*. 1989;2(6):583-592.

366. Spiro IJ, Yandell DW, Li C, et al. Brief report: lymphoma of donor origin occurring in the porta hepatis of a transplanted liver. *N Engl J Med.* 1993;329(1):27–29.
367. Armes JE, Angus P, Southey MC, et al. Lymphoproliferative disease of donor origin arising in patients after orthotopic liver transplantation. *Cancer.* 1994;74(9):2436–2441.
368. Larson RS, Scott MA, McCurley TL, Vnencak-Jones CL. Microsatellite analysis of posttransplant lymphoproliferative disorders: determination of donor/recipient origin and identification of putative lymphomagenic mechanism. *Cancer Res.* 1996;56(19):4378–4381.
369. Weissmann DJ, Ferry JA, Harris NL, et al. Posttransplantation lymphoproliferative disorders in solid organ recipients are predominantly aggressive tumors of host origin. *Am J Clin Pathol.* 1995;103(6):748–755.
370. Penn I. The changing pattern of posttransplant malignancies. *Transplant Proc.* 1991;23(1 pt 2):1101–1103.
371. Leblond V, Davi F, Charlotte F, et al. Posttransplant lymphoproliferative disorders not associated with Epstein-Barr virus: a distinct entity? *J Clin Oncol.* 1998;16(6):2052–2059.
372. Nelson BP, Nalesnik MA, Bahler DW, et al. Epstein-Barr virus-negative post-transplant lymphoproliferative disorders: a distinct entity? *Am J Surg Pathol.* 2000;24(3):375–385.
373. Ghobrial IM, Habermann TM, Macon WR, et al. Differences between early and late posttransplant lymphoproliferative disorders in solid organ transplant patients: are they two different diseases? *Transplantation.* 2005;79(2):244–247.
374. Nalesnik MA, Jaffe R, Starzl TE, et al. The pathology of posttransplant lymphoproliferative disorders occurring in the setting of cyclosporine A-prednisone immunosuppression. *Am J Pathol.* 1988;133(1):173–192.
375. Lones MA, Mishalani S, Shintaku IP, et al. Changes in tonsils and adenoids in children with posttransplant lymphoproliferative disorder: report of three cases with early involvement of Waldeyer's ring. *Hum Pathol.* 1995;26(5):525–530.
376. Knowles DM, Cesarman E, Chadburn A, et al. Correlative morphologic and molecular genetic analysis demonstrates three distinct categories of posttransplantation lymphoproliferative disorders. *Blood.* 1995;85(2):552–565.
377. Frizzera G, Hanto DW, Gajl-Peczalska KJ, et al. Polymorphic diffuse B-cell hyperplasias and lymphomas in renal transplant recipients. *Cancer Res.* 1981;41(11 pt 1):4262–4279.
378. Hanto DW, Gajl-Peczalska KJ, Frizzera G, et al. Epstein-Barr virus (EBV) induced polyclonal and monoclonal B-cell lymphoproliferative diseases occurring after renal transplantation. Clinical, pathologic, and virologic findings and implications for therapy. *Ann Surg.* 1983;198(3):356–369.
379. Cesarman E, Chadburn A, Liu YF, et al. BCL 6 gene mutations in posttransplantation lymphoproliferative disorders predict response to therapy and clinical outcome. *Blood.* 1998;92(7):2294–2302.
380. Hsi ED, Singleton TP, Swinnen L, et al. Mucosa-associated lymphoid tissue-type lymphomas occurring in post-transplantation patients. *Am J Surg Pathol.* 2000;24(1):100–106.
381. Cleary ML, Warnke R, Sklar J. Monoclonality of lymphoproliferative lesions in cardiac-transplant recipients. Clonal analysis based on immunoglobulin-gene rearrangements. *N Engl J Med.* 1984;310(8):477–482.
382. Cleary ML, Nalesnik MA, Shearer WT, Sklar J. Clonal analysis of transplant-associated lymphoproliferations based on the structure of the genomic termini of the Epstein-Barr virus. *Blood.* 1988;72(1):349–352.
383. Kaplan MA, Ferry JA, Harris NL, Jacobson JO. Clonal analysis of posttransplant lymphoproliferative disorders, using both episomal Epstein-Barr virus and immunoglobulin genes as markers. *Am J Clin Pathol.* 1994;101(5):590–596.
384. Starzl TE, Nalesnik MA, Porter KA, et al. Reversibility of lymphomas and lymphoproliferative lesions developing under cyclosporin-steroid therapy. *Lancet.* 1984;1(8377):583–587.
385. Kwon JH, Farrell RJ. The risk of lymphoma in the treatment of inflammatory bowel disease with immunosuppressive agents. *Crit Rev Oncol Hematol.* 2005;56(1):169–178.
386. Farrell RJ, Ang Y, Kileen P, et al. Increased incidence of non-Hodgkin's lymphoma in inflammatory bowel disease patients on immunosuppressive therapy but overall risk is low. *Gut.* 2000;47(4):514–519.
387. Fan CW, Changchien CR, Wang JY, et al. Primary colorectal lymphoma. *Dis Colon Rectum.* 2000;43(9):1277–1282.
388. Lenzen R, Borchard F, Lubke H, Strohmeyer G. Colitis ulcerosa complicated by malignant lymphoma: case report and analysis of published works. *Gut.* 1995;36(2):306–310.
389. Korelitz BI, Mirsky FJ, Fleisher MR, et al. Malignant neoplasms subsequent to treatment of inflammatory bowel disease with 6-mercaptopurine. *Am J Gastroenterol.* 1999;94(11):3248–3253.
390. Kandiel A, Fraser AG, Korelitz BI, et al. Increased risk of lymphoma among inflammatory bowel disease patients treated with azathioprine and 6-mercaptopurine. *Gut.* 2005;54(8):1121–1125.
391. Dayharsh GA, Loftus EV Jr, Sandborn WJ, et al. Epstein-Barr virus-positive lymphoma in patients with inflammatory bowel disease treated with azathioprine or 6-mercaptopurine. *Gastroenterology.* 2002;122(1):72–77.
392. Kumar S, Fend F, Quintanilla-Martinez L, et al. Epstein-Barr virus-positive primary gastrointestinal Hodgkin's disease: association with inflammatory bowel disease and immunosuppression. *Am J Surg Pathol.* 2000;24(1):66–73.
393. Bernstein CN, Blanchard JF, Kliewer E, Wajda A. Cancer risk in patients with inflammatory bowel disease: a population-based study. *Cancer.* 2001;91(4):854–862.
394. Thayu M, Markowitz JE, Mamula P, et al. Hepatosplenic T-cell lymphoma in an adolescent patient after immunomodulator and biologic therapy for Crohn disease. *J Pediatr Gastroenterol Nutr.* 2005;40(2):220–222.
395. Bucher C, Degen L, Dirnhofer S, et al. Biologics in inflammatory disease: infliximab associated risk of lymphoma development. *Gut.* 2005;54(5):732–733.
396. Bachman TR, Sawitzke AD, Perkins SL, et al. Methotrexate-associated lymphoma in patients with rheumatoid arthritis: report of two cases. *Arthritis Rheum.* 1996;39(2):325–329.
397. Kamel OW, van de Rijn M, LeBrun DP, et al. Lymphoid neoplasms in patients with rheumatoid arthritis and dermatomyositis: frequency of Epstein-Barr virus and other features associated with immunosuppression. *Hum Pathol.* 1994;25(7):638–643.
398. Paul C, Le Tourneau A, Cayuela JM, et al. Epstein-Barr virus-associated lymphoproliferative disease during methotrexate therapy for psoriasis. *Arch Dermatol.* 1997;133(7):867–871.
399. Salloum E, Cooper DL, Howe G, et al. Spontaneous regression of lymphoproliferative disorders in patients treated with methotrexate for rheumatoid arthritis and other rheumatic diseases. *J Clin Oncol.* 1996;14(6):1943–1949.
400. Isomaki HA, Hakulinen T, Joutsenlahti U. Excess risk of lymphomas, leukemia and myeloma in patients with rheumatoid arthritis. *J Chronic Dis.* 1978;31(11):691–696.
401. Symmons DP. Neoplasms of the immune system in rheumatoid arthritis. *Am J Med.* 1985;78(1A):22–28.
402. Menke DM, Griesser H, Moder KG, et al. Lymphomas in patients with connective tissue disease. Comparison of p53 protein expression and latent EBV infection in patients immunosuppressed and not immunosuppressed with methotrexate. *Am J Clin Pathol.* 2000;113(2):212–218.

403. Griffiths AP, Shepherd NA, Beddall A, Williams JG. Gastrointestinal tumour masses due to multiple myeloma: a pathological mimic of malignant lymphoma. *Histopathology*. 1997;31(4):318–323.
404. Ishido T, Mori N. Primary gastric plasmacytoma: a morphological and immunohistochemical study of five cases. *Am J Gastroenterol*. 1992;87(7):875–878.
405. Nakanishi I, Kajikawa K, Migita S, et al. Gastric plasmacytoma: an immunologic and immunohistochemical study. *Cancer*. 1982;49(10):2025–2028.
406. Wendum D, Vissuzaine C, Bellanger J, et al. A case of polypoid solitary colonic plasmocytoma. *Ann Pathol*. 1994;14(4):248–250.
407. Wiltshaw E. The natural history of extramedullary plasmacytoma and its relation to solitary myeloma of bone and myelomatosis. *Medicine (Baltimore)*. 1976;55(3):217–238.
408. Homma K, Ihzumi T, Nemoto K, Ohnishi Y. Primary extramedullary plasmacytoma of the small intestine. *Int J Hematol*. 1992;56(2):179–184.
409. Doberauer C, Sanner B, Henning B. Multiple myeloma involving the stomach with vitamin B_{12} deficiency. *Eur J Gastroenterol Hepatol*. 1999;11(2):205–207.
410. Rygaard-Olsen C, Boedker A, Emus HC, Olsen HA. Extramedullary plasmacytoma of the small intestine: a case report studied with electron microscopy and immunoperoxidase technique. *Cancer*. 1982;50(3):573–576.
411. Gleason TH, Hammar SP. Plasmacytoma of the colon: case report with lambda light chain, demonstrated by immunoperoxidase studies. *Cancer*. 1982;50(1):130–133.
412. Goeggel-Lamping C, Kahn SB. Gastrointestinal polyposis in multiple myeloma. *JAMA*. 1978;239(17):1786–1787.
413. Line DH, Lewis RH. Gastric plasmacytoma. *Gut*. 1969;10(3):230–233.
414. Homma K, Umezu H, Nemoto K, et al. Angiocentric immunoproliferative lesion of the stomach. *Virchows Arch A Pathol Anat Histopathol*. 1991;418(3):267–270.
415. Jaffe ES, Wilson WH. Lymphomatoid granulomatosis: pathogenesis, pathology and clinical implications. *Cancer Surv*. 1997;30:233–248.
416. Rattinger MD, Dunn TL, Christian CD Jr, et al. Gastrointestinal involvement in lymphomatoid granulomatosis. Report of a case review of the literature. *Cancer*. 1983;51(4):694–700.
417. Rubin LA, Little AH, Kolin A, Keystone EC. Lymphomatoid granulomatosis involving the gastrointestinal tract. Two case reports and a review of the literature. *Gastroenterology*. 1983;84(4):829–833.
418. Jaffe ES, Wilson WH. Lymphomatoid granulomatosis. In: Jaffe EHN, Stein H, Vardiman JW, eds. *Pathology & genetics: tumours of haematopoietic and lymphoid tissues*. Lyon, France: IARC Press; 2001.
419. Nicholson AG, Wotherspoon AC, Diss TC, et al. Lymphomatoid granulomatosis: evidence that some cases represent Epstein-Barr virus-associated B-cell lymphoma. *Histopathology*. 1996;29(4):317–324.
420. Camisa C, Goldstein A. Mycosis fungoides. Small-bowel involvement complicated by perforation and peritonitis. *Arch Dermatol*. 1981;117(4):234–237.
421. Chen KR, Tanaka M, Miyakawa S. Granulomatous mycosis fungoides with small intestinal involvement and a fatal outcome. *Br J Dermatol*. 1998;138(3):522–525.
422. Ganz R, Olinger E, Variakojis D, Gordon L. Mycosis fungoides with gastrointestinal involvement. *Gastrointest Endosc*. 1988;34(6):478–481.
423. Rappaport H, Thomas LB. Mycosis fungoides: the pathology of extracutaneous involvement. *Cancer*. 1974;34(4):1198–1229.
424. Slater DN, Bleehen SS, Beck S. Gastrointestinal complications of mycosis fungoides. *J R Soc Med*. 1984;77(2):114–119.
425. Kadin ME. Primary Ki-1-positive anaplastic large-cell lymphoma: a distinct clinicopathologic entity. *Ann Oncol*. 1994;5(suppl 1):25–30.
426. Griesser H, Henry M, Boie C, Banerjee D. Large-cell anaplastic lymphoma of the gastrointestinal tract: an immuno- and genotypic study on archival material. *Hematol Pathol*. 1994;8(4):121–134.
427. Paulli M, Rosso R, Kindl S, et al. Primary gastric CD30 (Ki-1)-positive large cell non-Hodgkin's lymphomas. A clinicopathologic analysis of six cases. *Cancer*. 1994;73(3):541–549.
428. Ross CW, Hanson CA, Schnitzer B. CD30 (Ki-1)-positive, anaplastic large cell lymphoma mimicking gastrointestinal carcinoma. *Cancer*. 1992;70(10):2517–2523.
429. Matsumoto H, Koga H, Honda K, et al. Characterization of secondary GI lesions with anaplastic large-cell (Ki-1) lymphoma: a first report of two cases. *Gastrointest Endosc*. 2005;61(4):607–609.
430. Nakamura S, Aoyagi K, Ohkuni A, et al. Rapidly growing primary gastric CD30 (Ki-1)-positive anaplastic large cell lymphoma. *Dig Dis Sci*. 1998;43(2):300–305.
431. Delsol G, Ralfkiaer E, Stein H, et al. Anaplastic large cell lymphoma. In: Jaffe EHN, Stein H, Vardiman JW, eds. *Pathology & genetics: tumours of haematopoietic and lymphoid tissues*. Lyon, France: IARC Press; 2001.
432. Chim CS, Au WY, Shek TW, et al. Primary CD56 positive lymphomas of the gastrointestinal tract. *Cancer*. 2001;91(3):525–533.
433. Ko YH, Cho EY, Kim JE, et al. NK and NK-like T-cell lymphoma in extranasal sites: a comparative clinicopathological study according to site and EBV status. *Histopathology*. 2004;44(5):480–489.
434. Chan JKC, Jaffe ES, Ralfkiaer E. Extranodal NK/T-cell lymphoma, nasal type. In: Jaffe EHN, Stein H, Vardiman JW, eds. *Pathology & genetics: tumours of haematopoietic and lymphoid tissues*. Lyon, France: IARC Press; 2001.
435. Chuang SS, Jung YC. Natural killer cell lymphoma of small intestine with features of enteropathy but lack of association with celiac disease. *Hum Pathol*. 2004;35(5): 639–642.
436. Julka PK, Singhal RM, Mukhopadhaya S, Dawar R. Primary Hodgkin's disease of small intestine: a report of two cases. *Indian J Gastroenterol*. 1993;12(4):152–153.
437. Kelly MD, Stuart M, Tschuchnigg M, et al. Primary intestinal Hodgkin's disease complicating ileal Crohn's disease. *Aust N Z J Surg*. 1997;67(7):485–489.
438. Libson E, Mapp E, Dachman AH. Hodgkin's disease of the gastrointestinal tract. *Clin Radiol*. 1994;49(3):166–169.
439. Vadmal MS, LaValle GP, DeYoung BR, et al. Primary localized extranodal hodgkin disease of the transverse colon. *Arch Pathol Lab Med*. 2000;124(12):1824–1827.
440. Chang KL, Kamel OW, Arber DA, et al. Pathologic features of nodular lymphocyte predominance Hodgkin's disease in extranodal sites. *Am J Surg Pathol*. 1995;19(11):1313–1324.
441. Devaney K, Jaffe ES. The surgical pathology of gastrointestinal Hodgkin's disease. *Am J Clin Pathol*. 1991;95(6):794–801.
442. Grogan TM, Berard CW, Steinhorn SC, et al. Changing patterns of Hodgkin's disease at autopsy: a 25-year experience at the National Cancer Institute, 1953–1978. *Cancer Treat Rep*. 1982;66(4):653–665.
443. Vanbockrijck M, Cabooter M, Casselman J, et al. Primary Hodgkin disease of the ileum complicating Crohn disease. *Cancer*. 1993;72(5):1784–1789.
444. Soderstrom KO, Joensuu H. Primary Hodgkin's disease of the stomach. *Am J Clin Pathol*. 1988;89(6):806–809.

445. Colucci G, Giotta F, Maiello E, et al. Primary Hodgkin's disease of the stomach. A case report. *Tumori*. 1992;78(4):280–282.
446. Leoncini L, Del Vecchio MT, Kraft R, et al. Hodgkin's disease and CD30-positive anaplastic large cell lymphomas—a continuous spectrum of malignant disorders. A quantitative morphometric and immunohistologic study. *Am J Pathol*. 1990;137(5):1047–1057.
447. Hornick JL, Jaffe ES, Fletcher CD. Extranodal histiocytic sarcoma: clinicopathologic analysis of 14 cases of a rare epithelioid malignancy. *Am J Surg Pathol*. 2004;28(9):1133–1144.
448. Copie-Bergman C, Wotherspoon AC, Norton AJ, et al. True histiocytic lymphoma: a morphologic, immunohistochemical, and molecular genetic study of 13 cases. *Am J Surg Pathol*. 1998;22(11):1386–1392.
449. Weiss LM, Grogan TM, Muller-Hermelink HK, Stein H. Histiocytic sarcoma. In: Jaffe EHN, Stein H, Vardiman JW, eds. *Pathology & genetics: tumours of haematopoietic and lymphoid tissues*. Lyon, France: IARC Press; 2001.
450. Viollet L, Commare-Nordmann MC, Langlais J, et al. Basedow's disease in an adolescent with histiocytosis X. *Arch Pediatr*. 1997;4(7):656–658.
451. Iwafuchi M, Watanabe H, Shiratsuka M. Primary benign histiocytosis X of the stomach. A report of a case showing spontaneous remission after 5 1/2 years. *Am J Surg Pathol*. 1990;14(5):489–496.
452. Groisman GM, Rosh JR, Harpaz N. Langerhans cell histiocytosis of the stomach. A cause of granulomatous gastritis and gastric polyposis. *Arch Pathol Lab Med*. 1994;118(12):1232–1235.
453. Geissmann F, Thomas C, Emile JF, et al. Digestive tract involvement in Langerhans cell histiocytosis. The French Langerhans Cell Histiocytosis Study Group. *J Pediatr*. 1996;129(6):836–845.
454. Damry N, Hottat N, Azzi N, et al. Unusual findings in two cases of Langerhans' cell histiocytosis. *Pediatr Radiol*. 2000;30(3):196–199.
455. Nanduri VR, Kelly K, Malone M, et al. Colon involvement in Langerhans' cell histiocytosis. *J Pediatr Gastroenterol Nutr*. 1999;29(4):462–466.
456. Lee-Elliott C, Alexander J, Gould A, et al. Langerhan's cell histiocytosis complicating small bowel Crohn's disease. *Gut*. 1996;38(2):296–298.
457. Chim CS, Ma SK, Lam CK, Liang R. Two uncommon lymphomas. Case 2: signet ring lymphoma of the bone marrow. *J Clin Oncol*. 1999;17(2):728–729.
458. Hernandez JA, Sheehan WW. Lymphomas of the mucosa-associated lymphoid tissue. Signet ring cell lymphomas presenting in mucosal lymphoid organs. *Cancer*. 1985;55(3):592–597.
459. Miyazaki K, Shimizu Y, Oiwa T, et al. Gastric signet ring cell lymphoma. *Nippon Naika Gakkai Zasshi*. 2000;89(4):760–761.
460. Tungekar MF. Gastric signet-ring cell lymphoma with alpha heavy chains. *Histopathology*. 1986;10(7):725–733.
461. Agaimy A, Wunsch PH. Follicular dendritic cell tumor of the gastrointestinal tract: Report of a rare neoplasm and literature review. *Pathol Res Pract*. 2006;202(7):541–540.
462. Takenaga T, Sakano T, Kitahara T, et al. Five cases of malignant lymphoma associated with early gastric cancer. *Jpn J Clin Oncol*. 1978;8:209–218.
463. Gray GM, Rosenberg SA, Cooper AD, et al. Lymphomas involving the gastrointestinal tract. *Gastroenterology*. 1982;82(1):143–152.
464. Nathwani BN, Winberg CD, Bearman RM. Angioimmunoblastic lymphadenopathy with dysproteinemia and its progression to malignant lymphoma. In: Jaffe ES, ed. *Surgical Pathology of the Lymph Nodes and Related Organs*. Philadelphia, PA: WB Saunders Co.; 1985.
465. Goenka MK, Vaiphei K, Nagi B, et al. Angioimmunoblastic lymphadenopathy: an etiology for gastrointestinal lymphomatous polyposis. *Am J Gastroenterol*. 1996;91(6):1236–1238.
466. Ahsan N, Sun CC, Di John D. Acute ileotyphlitis as presenting manifestation of acute myelogenous leukemia. *Am J Clin Pathol*. 1988;89(3):407–409.
467. Cornes JS, Jones TG. Leukaemic lesions of the gastrointestinal tract. *J Clin Pathol*. 1962;15:305–313.
468. Kuse R, Lueb H. Gastrointestinal involvement in patients with chronic lymphocytic leukemia. *Leukemia*. 1997;11(suppl 2):S50–S51.
469. Moir DH, Bale PM. Necropsy findings in childhood leukaemia, emphasizing neutropenic enterocolitis and cerebral calcification. *Pathology*. 1976;8(3):247–258.
470. Prolla JC, Kirsner JB. The gastrointestinal lesions and complications of the leukemias. *Ann Intern Med*. 1964;61:1084–1103.
471. Kletzel M, Meitar D, El-Youssef M, Cohn SL. Gastrointestinal relapse of leukemia, mimicking acute graft vs. host disease, following a stem cell transplant. *Med Pediatr Oncol*. 2000;34(4):287–289.
472. Manglani MV, Rosenthal J, Rosenthal NF, et al. Intussusception in an infant with acute lymphoblastic leukemia: a case report and review of the literature. *J Pediatr Hematol Oncol*. 1998;20(5):467–468.
473. McCarthy D, Holland I, Lavender JP, Catovsky D. Pneumatosis coli in adult acute myeloid leukaemia. *Clin Radiol*. 1979;30(2):175–178.
474. Sherman NJ, Williams K, Woolley MM. Surgical complications in the patient with leukemia. *J Pediatr Surg*. 1973;8(2):235–244.
475. Brugo EA, Marshall RB, Riberi AM, Pautasso OE. Preleukemic granulocytic sarcomas of the gastrointestinal tract. Report of two cases. *Am J Clin Pathol*. 1977;68(5):616–621.
476. Sasaki A, Tsukaguchi M, Takayasu K, Hanai T. Myelodysplastic syndrome developing acute myelocytic leukemia with gastric mucormycosis. *Rinsho Byori*. 1993;11(9):1054–1058.
477. Takeuchi M, Uno H, Matsuoka H, et al. Acute necrotizing gastritis associated with adult T-cell leukemia in the course of chemotherapy. *Gan To Kagaku Ryoho*. 1995;22(2):289–292.

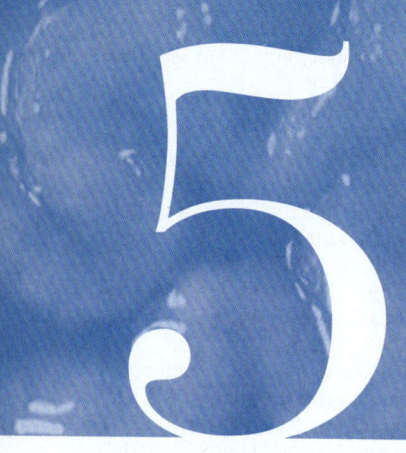

Disorders of Endocrine Cells

Chapter Outline

INTRODUCTION AND HISTORICAL PERSPECTIVE
From the APUD System (Amine Precursor Uptake and Decarboxylation) and on
THE NORMAL ENDOCRINE CELLS AT SPECIFIC GASTROINTESTINAL SITES: WHERE THEY ARE AND WHAT THEY DO
THE DISEASES: PERSPECTIVES BASED ON CLINICAL IMPLICATIONS
GENETICS OF ENDOCRINE TUMORS AND ENDOCRINE SYNDROMES INVOLVING THE GUT
CARCINOID TUMORS (WELL-DIFFERENTIATED ENDOCRINE TUMORS)
General Information
Gross Examination
    Gross appearance
    Gross dissection recommendations
Staging and Grading
CARCINOID TUMORS (NETs) IN SPECIFIC SITES
Carcinoid Tumors (NETs) of the Esophagus

Carcinoid Tumors (NETs) of the Stomach
    Type I carcinoid tumors
    Type II carcinoid tumors
    Type III carcinoid tumors
    Potential type IV carcinoid tumors
Carcinoid Tumors of the Duodenum
    Gastrinomas
    Somatostatinomas
    Gangliocytic paraganglioma
Carcinoid Tumors of the Jejunum and Ileum (Midgut Carcinoids, NETs)
    Incidental finding of carcinoid in biopsies of the cecum or terminal ileum
Carcinoid Tumors of the Appendix
Carcinoid Tumors of the Abdominal Colon
Carcinoid Tumors of the Rectum
POORLY DIFFERENTIATED ENDOCRINE NEOPLASMS (NEUROENDOCRINE OR ENDOCRINE CARCINOMAS)
General Information
Esophageal Tumors
Colonic and Rectal Tumors

ADENOMAS AND ADENOCARCINOMAS WITH BOTH EPITHELIAL AND ENDOCRINE DIFFERENTIATION
Tumors in Which Endocrine and Columnar Cells are Mixed
Tumors with Separate Components (Composite Tumors)
ENDOCRINE TUMORS ASSOCIATED WITH ULCERATIVE COLITIS AND CROHN'S DISEASE
HYPERPLASIAS
ENTEROENDOCRINE CELL DYSGENESIS
METASTATIC ENDOCRINE TUMORS WITH AN UNKNOWN PRIMARY
PRACTICAL APPROACHES TO GASTROINTESTINAL ENDOCRINE ABNORMALITIES
General Information
Tumors

INTRODUCTION AND HISTORICAL PERSPECTIVE

The gastrointestinal (GI) tract is loaded with endocrine cells that vary from one site to the other based on the functional necessities of each site. They have been recognized for more than a century. One type was originally described by Nicholas in 1891 and Kultschitzky in 1897[1,2] as basigranulated cells situated in the intestinal crypts that were characterized by having small infranuclear eosinophilic granules (Fig. 5-1). The enterochromaffin (EC) cells in the base of the intestinal crypts are the role models for this cell. Subsequently, other observers discovered a second cell, the *clear cell*, which was characterized by a diffusely pale or vacuolated cytoplasm[3] (Fig. 5-2). The gastrin-producing or G cell of the gastric antrum is a typical example of this cell type. A variety of names were given to these two cell types, which reflected their histologic or histochemical properties, for example, *yellow* or *enterochromaffin cells*,[4,5] attributed to the yellow staining of the granules with chromium salts, and *argentaffin* and *argyrophil cells*[6] to describe their silver-reducing power. The gastrointestinal endocrine cells were postulated to arise from either endoderm or neuroectoderm. As early as 1924, Masson[7] suggested that there was a neuroectodermal origin for argentaffin cells based on his observation of the association of appendiceal carcinoid tumors with submucosal nerve fiber hyperplasia. In 1938, Feyrter[3] suggested that the gastrointestinal endocrine cells formed an integral part of a diffuse endocrine system, the constituent cells of which were diffusely scattered throughout the tissues of the body, either singly or in

Chapter 5 Disorders of Endocrine Cells

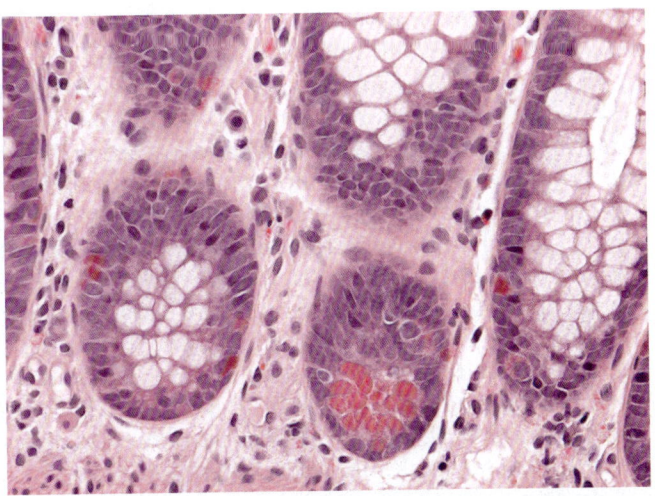

Figure 5-1. Normal endocrine cells with subnuclear red granules in all crypts, but especially that lower left center. These contrast with the larger supranuclear granules of the Paneth cells in the crypt lower right center.

small groups. He postulated that they arose from the epithelium in which they were found, which in the case of the GI tract was the endoderm.

From the APUD System (Amine Precursor Uptake and Decarboxylation) and on

Between 1966 and 1968, Pearse[8,9] described a group of widely dispersed endocrine cells whose products appeared to be amines and peptide hormones that were linked together by their possession of a common set of cytochemical characteristics. These included nonspecific esterase and cholinesterase, alpha-glycerophosphate dehydrogenase in the cytoplasm, and the ability to produce certain biogenic amines such as adrenalin, dopamine, and 5-hydroxytryptamine (serotonin).[10] Pearse coined the term APUD

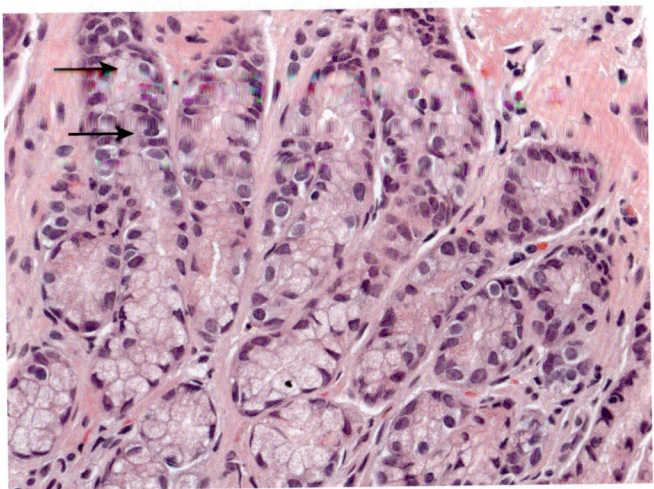

Figure 5-2. Endocrine cells with clear cytoplasms (*arrows*) surrounding the nuclei along the sides of the gastric glands and necks.

system for this group of dispersed endocrine cells, an acronym for their common ability to engage in Amine Precursor Uptake and Decarboxylation. The APUD system was expanded to include most endocrine cells producing polypeptide hormones, carotid body type I cells, melanoblasts, and the clear cells of the urogenital tract.[11-14] The common cytochemical features of the APUD cells were interpreted by Pearse to reflect a common embryologic origin, which he postulated was the neural crest. Subsequently, Pearse concluded that his APUD system corresponded to Feyrter's earlier description of the diffuse endocrine system.[3] Pearse's hypothesis did not hold up in experimental studies. Thus, while allograft studies of the neural crest conclusively showed the C cells of the thyroid, the parathyroids, the adrenal medulla, and the ganglion cells of the myenteric plexus were derived from the neural crest, they were equally conclusive in showing that the gastric and pancreatic endocrine cells originated from endoderm.[15,16] Other studies by Andrew[17] and Pictet et al.[18] showed that removing the neural crest from developing rabbit embryos does not prevent the development of insulin-producing B cells, which appeared to have a common endodermal precursor with pancreatic exocrine cells. Furthermore, cell turnover data pointed to the crypt base as the site of origin for all epithelial cell types, including the endocrine cells.[19] Finally, studies on gastrointestinal tumors demonstrated an increasing number with mixed epithelial and endocrine cell components and rare tumors in which dense core granules and zymogenic granules were found within the same cells, while cell line cultures suggested that there are common endoderm precursor cells for both gut epithelial and endocrine cells.

The Pearse hypothesis linking all endocrine cells and neural cells presumably led to the designation of the endocrine cells as "neuroendocrine cells" and to the designation of the neoplasms containing such cells as "neuroendocrine neoplasms." This seems cumbersome and even pedantic, since the cells of these tumors in the gut have no neural features. They look like endocrine cells. So, we will drop the neuro part of the adjective, and, in this chapter, we will refer to the cells as endocrine cells and to the neoplasms containing endocrine cells as endocrine neoplasms. After all, this is five letters shorter and takes nothing away from the subject. In the 200 World Health Organization book covering tumors of the digestive system, all the tumors containing these cells are included in chapter entitled "Endocrine tumors," rather than "Neuroendocrine tumors," so a precedent for this shorter name has already been established. However, the seventh edition of AJCC cancer staging manual has retained the term "neuroendocrine" and the newest WHO classification does the same, thus the saga continues.

Over the years, the gut endocrine cells have been characterized using different techniques which looked at them from different perspectives. First, there were the light microscopic basigranulated and clear cells. Later, as mentioned above, they were separated by the reactions of their granules with silver stains into argentaffin and argyrophil types. Next, they were analyzed by the electron microscopic appearances of their secretory granules which tended to be distinctive, resulting in an alphabet soup of cells called D, G, L, M, N, P, and S cells and there were also cells designated by various combinations of two or more letters. More recently, they have been characterized by the specific substances their granules contain based upon immunocytochemical techniques that employ antibodies directed against each of these substances. From a practical point of view, at this stage in our analyses, we rarely use the silver staining techniques, nor do we use the electron microscope. We have enormous amounts of data based on these analyses, but when we really want to find out what the cells are doing, that is, what they are making and possibly secreting, we have specific antibodies with which to stain them. Some cells communicate with the lumen of the glands or crypts or pits, while others are buried deep in these structures with no such communication.

THE NORMAL ENDOCRINE CELLS AT SPECIFIC GASTROINTESTINAL SITES: WHERE THEY ARE AND WHAT THEY DO

In the esophagus, there are too few endocrine cells to discuss, probably because there is nothing there for them to do.

In the stomach, in contrast, the endocrine cells are critical for gastric acid secretion. Here, there are mainly three cell types. The antrum contains the gastrin-producing cells or G cells. Gastrin is a direct stimulus for parietal cell acid production and it also stimulates the second gastric endocrine cell, the enterochromaffin-like cell, or ECL cell in the body mucosa to produce histamine, which in turn stimulates acid secretion by parietal cells. The G cells appear as round to oval cells with pale finely granular cytoplasm and central nuclei, and they are found at the base of the mucus neck cells and the superficial mucus gland cells. The ECL cells are found diffusely throughout the glands in the body mucosa and do not stand out in H and E-stained sections. The third type of endocrine cell, the D cell, also located mainly in the antrum, but also in the body mucosa, produces somatostatin which inhibits gastrin production by the G cells. These cells are also not obvious in H and E-stained sections (see Chapter 13).

In the small intestine from the duodenum through the ileum, in the appendix, and in the colon and rectum, the endocrine cells are located at the base of the crypts, although sometimes found higher up in the crypts. The EC cells have very fine red basal granules. They are more difficult to find in the small intestine than in the colon, because they are in about the same location as the much more numerous Paneth cells which also have red granules that are larger and coarser than those in the endocrine cells and that are situated on the luminal side of the cell.

In the normal duodenum, there are a variety of endocrine cells that affect function. These cells include a scattering of G cells in the duodenum, D cells that produce somatostatin, and cells that produce a number of other peptide hormones, such as secretin, cholecystokinin, and enteroglucagon.

In the normal small intestine, the jejunum and ileum, the important endocrine cell is the enterochromaffin cell or EC cell, which produces serotonin (Kulchitsky cells). Some cells produce substance P. Both seratonin and substance P are important mediators of motility of the gut.

In the appendix, the endocrine cells are found in the base of the crypts and as single cells in the lamina propria. They include serotonin-producing EC (argentaffin) cells and L cells producing peptide YY (PYY), which is said to be involved in appetite suppression.[20]

In the normal colon and rectum, there are some EC cells that produce serotonin or substance P, and some cells that produce a number of other substances, including pancreatic polypeptide, but it is not clear exactly what the function of many of these substances are. There must be a reason why a substance with the name of pancreatic polypeptide is produced not just in the pancreas but also in the colon. Also, PYY-containing cells are found in the colon and rectum as are cells producing glucagon-like immunoreactive peptides, one of which may be glicentin.[21]

Endocrine cells, all of which are serotonin producing, have also been identified in the anal canal, predominantly in the anal ducts and in the transitional zone epithelium, but not in the more distal squamous epithelium.[22]

THE DISEASES: PERSPECTIVES BASED ON CLINICAL IMPLICATIONS

Considering the richness of the endocrine cell population and the hormonal complexities of the gastrointestinal endocrine system, it is surprising that the diseases of that system are so limited. The most important gastrointestinal endocrine diseases are tumors. There is a tendency to group all the endocrine tumors, both the carcinoid tumors and the carcinomas, into the generic name of "neuroendocrine tumor"/neoplasm and then

Table 5-1 Classification of Endocrine Tumors in the Gastrointestinal Tract

OUR PREFERRED TERMINOLOGY	COMMONLY USED EQUIVALENTS	WHO/AJCC TERMINOLOGY
Well-differentiated endocrine neoplasm	Carcinoid	Well-differentiated neuroendocrine tumor
Moderately differentiated endocrine neoplasm	Atypical carcinoid	Well-differentiated neuroendocrine carcinoma
Poorly differentiated endocrine neoplasm 1. Small cell carcinoma 2. Large cell endocrine carcinoma/non–small cell endocrine carcinoma	Small cell carcinoma Large cell endocrine carcinoma Neuroendocrine carcinoma	Poorly differentiated neuroendocrine carcinoma 1. Small cell carcinoma 2. Large cell endocrine carcinoma

subdivide them based on the degree of differentiation (Table 5-1).[23] Table 5-2 lists the tumors described in the endocrine tumor chapters in the various sites. The more common of the endocrine tumors by far is the low-grade, highly differentiated neoplasm, generically referred to as a carcinoid tumor. Then, there are a variety of gastrointestinal carcinomas that contain different amounts of an endocrine cell component, which varies from single cells scattered about to large areas of endocrine differentiation. These have been given different names but are best considered adenocarcinomas with variable endocrine differentiation. The carcinoid tumors differ by site, by their products, and by their prognosis. In contrast, the small and large cell endocrine carcinomas have little site-dependent variability, and prognostically they are much the same regardless of site.

What is the origin of tumors composed of endocrine cells, regardless of differentiation? In the literature, there are statements about the cells of origin and that these tumors can be classified based on the cell of origin.[24] In fact, although we know the site of origin, we do not know the cell of origin of any endocrine tumor, except perhaps for the carcinoid tumors that arise in a field of endocrine cell hyperplasia, such as occurs in the gastric body mucosa in autoimmune gastritis or associated with the duodenal gastrinomas in multiple endocrine neoplasia type I (MEN-I). For solitary spontaneous endocrine tumors, we have no candidate cell of origin and no pretumorous endocrine cell dysplasia, comparable to that for GI tract adenocarcinomas. However, we can tell how the tumor cells have differentiated, that is, what they are making and secreting using immunohistochemical reagents directed against the various products, including peptide hormones and bioactive amines. Unfortunately, all too often in the medical literature, the word "origin" is used synonymously with the word "differentiation."

Table 5-2 Endocrine Tumors in the Gastrointestinal Tract and Their Distribution

TUMOR TYPE	ESOPHAGUS	STOMACH	DUODENUM-PROXIMAL JEJUNUM	JEJUNUM–ILEUM	APPENDIX	COLON AND RECTUM
Carcinoid tumor (well-differentiated endocrine neoplasm)	xxx	xxx	xxx	xxx	xxx	xxx
Small cell carcinoma	xxx	xxx				xxx
Large cell endocrine carcinoma						xxx
Gastrin cell tumor		xxx	xxx			
Somatostatin cell tumor			xxx			
ECL-cell carcinoid tumor		xxx				
EC-cell, serotonin producing carcinoid tumor		xxx	xxx	xxx	xxx	xxx
L-cell, glucagon-like peptide and PP/PY producing carcinoid tumor			xxx		xxx	xxx

GENETICS OF ENDOCRINE TUMORS AND ENDOCRINE SYNDROMES INVOLVING THE GUT

Are there specific genetic abnormalities that are common to all the endocrine tumors or that separate them by site or product? The most common genetic syndrome involving endocrine diseases of the GI tract is MEN-I, an autosomal dominant hereditary disorder characterized mainly by tumors in the parathyroids, pituitary, and endocrine pancreas, but there are also gastrointestinal endocrine tumors, almost all of which are gastrinomas in the duodenum. This syndrome results from a germ line mutation in the MEN-I tumor suppressor gene that is situated on the 11q13 chromosome.[25] Over 200 specific mutations have been identified in different MEN-I patients. Mutations in this gene or loss of heterozygosity of the 11q13 chromosome is also found in sporadic endocrine tumors that are comparable to those in MEN-I. This suggests that this gene or potential tumor suppressor genes distal to it on the same chromosome are important in the development of sporadic tumors. In one study analyzing sporadic tumors, it was found that in a little over half of the foregut tumors, all of which were pancreatic, there were abnormalities in the gene, chromosome, or both, whereas this rarely occurred in mid- and hindgut tumors. Therefore, the gene seemed to be important only in sporadic foregut tumors. In contrast, mid- and hindgut carcinoids frequently have loss of 18q.

In neurofibromatosis, type I, rare somatostatin-producing duodenal periampullary carcinoid tumors occur with microscopic peculiarities, which will be discussed later. The syndrome is due to abnormalities in the NF-1 tumor suppressor gene on chromosome 17. However, abnormalities in this gene have not yet been associated with sporadic gut endocrine tumors. Gastrointestinal stromal tumors, often multiple, can also be found (see Chapter 7).

As with tumors throughout the body, gut endocrine tumors have been analyzed for numerous genetic changes and for cell proteins encoded by specific genes. Some of these genetic changes and changes in protein expression correlate with prognosis or with supposed tumor evolution. The list of such genes and proteins is already exhaustive, and is likely to expand quickly as new antibodies are produced and new technology becomes available. So far, gut endocrine tumors have been analyzed for AP-1 transcription factor, epidermal growth factor receptor, p27, thyroid transcription factor-1, neuroendocrine secretory protein-55, ghrelin, transforming growth factor-beta type II receptor, Survivin, TPHi, VMAT1, notch signaling for endocrine marker expression, allelic loss on the X-chromosome, hepatocyte growth factor, human achaete-scute homolog gene-I, K-ras mutations, p53 mutations, changes in chromosome 18, RASSFIA promoter methylation, 3p21.3 loss of heterozygosity, lumican, CDX-2 homeobox gene product, 11q allelic losses, methylation of RAS-association domain family-1, isoform A, and p16, just to name a few. We are eagerly awaiting the study that analyzes all of these at the same time and subject the results to multivariate analysis to see which of these genes and proteins really is independently important.

CARCINOID TUMORS (WELL-DIFFERENTIATED ENDOCRINE TUMORS)

General Information

Carcinoid tumor is a name from pathology antiquity coined in German by Oberndorfer in 1907 in a study of intestinal endocrine tumors as "karzinoide," which meant carcinoma like.[26] Later, similar tumors in other sites in the gut and elsewhere, such as the lung, were given the same name. The classic carcinoid tumors were in the terminal ileum and appendix and produced serotonin. The term "carcinoid tumor" remains popular in spite of the attempt to replace it with the designation "well-differentiated endocrine tumor/neoplasm," and published reports of these tumors continue to refer to them as carcinoid tumors, not by the more cumbersome and less catchy name. We know that carcinoid tumors are usually harmless, but we also know that some metastasize, so, the use of the carcinoma-like designation is as acceptable as is the term "adenocarcinoma" for pleomorphic, proliferating, often extensive, necrotic epithelial tumors that commonly metastasize, although many do not. Therefore, in this chapter, the term "carcinoid tumor" is used without synonyms and without apology. In fact, often they will be referred to simply as "carcinoids," dropping the "tumor" word.

There is a certain lack of uniformity among clinicians and pathologists regarding the use of the term "carcinoid tumor." Is this a specific type of endocrine tumor that is defined by its product, namely serotonin, or is it a generic type of tumor, based only on the low-grade cell type, regardless of the secretory product? The use of the term is clearly site related, since we use it for low-grade endocrine tumors of the gut, the lung, the thymus, and a few other sites, but very similar tumors in the endocrine pancreas have different names. Carcinoid tumors of the gut are among the most histologically uniform tumors anywhere in the body and they are comparable to low-grade tumors that arise in other endocrine organs, such as

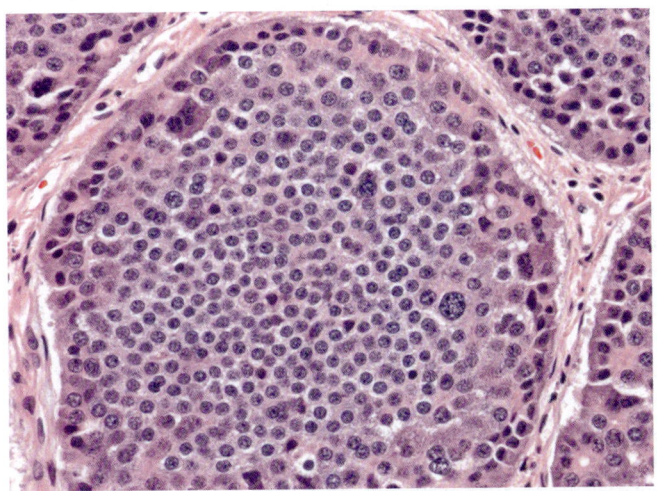

Figure 5-3. Carcinoid tumor (well differentiated NET) with a large nest containing mostly uniform cells except for occasional cells with larger nuclei.

the pituitary, the parathyroid glands, and the islets of Langerhans. Regardless of the sites in which they arise, they are composed of much the same type of bland-appearing cuboidal cells or short columnar cells that are, in general, remarkably uniform, except for a few nuclei that may be slightly bigger than their neighbors, or occasional cells that may have more fine cytoplasmic granules than do other cells (Fig. 5-3). Mitoses are usually infrequent. Most tumors have little or no necrosis. The only histologically interesting aspect is that these uniform cells are arranged in several patterns, including in large nests referred to as the insular pattern, in ribbons of cells that often interconnect; and in tubules or glands in which the cells are arranged around small lumens (Fig. 5-4). Certain growth patterns are more common in certain tumor locations, although there is considerable overlap among sites. Thus, although ileal tumors usually have the nest or insular pattern, every so often the cells are arranged in ribbons or tubules. Most textbooks and published papers also spend a lot of words describing the growth patterns of carcinoid tumors in different sites, with trabecular, glandular, or insular patterns occurring in this or that site, but these differences are not important in clinical practice. If we see a carcinoid tumor of the small intestine that has a trabecular growth pattern when the literature tells

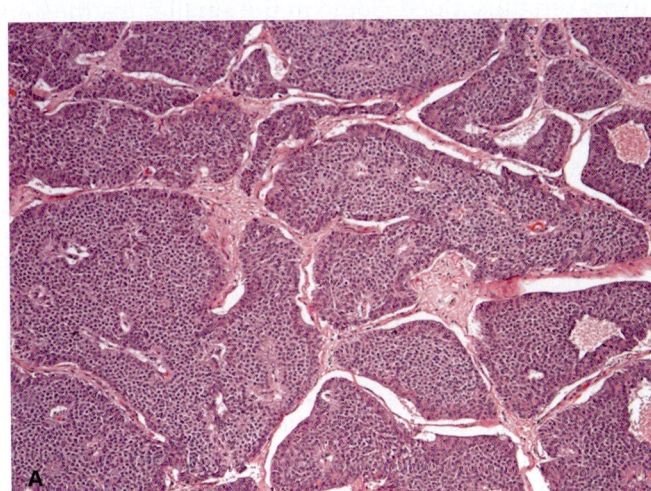

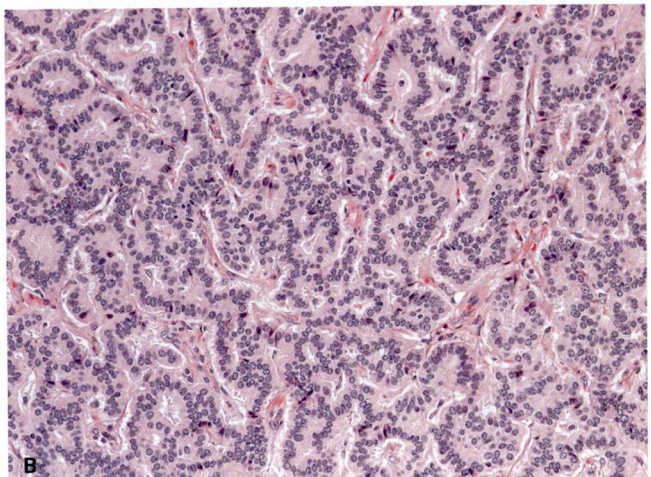

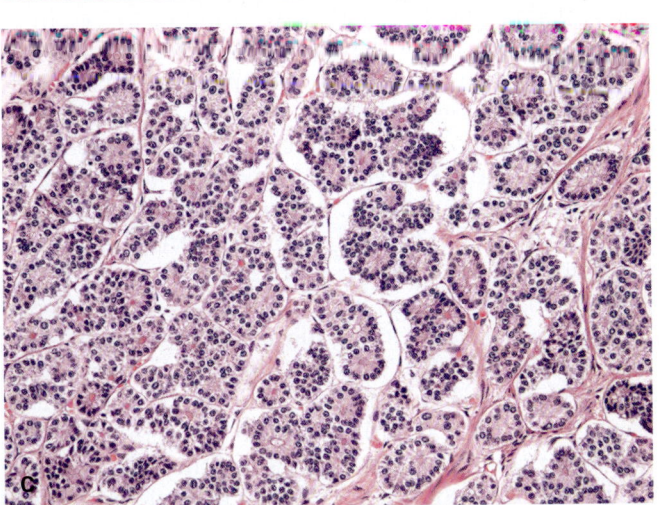

Figure 5-4. Common growth patterns of carcinoid tumors. **A:** Insular growth pattern: Large tumor nests separated by fibrovascular stroma. **B:** Interconnecting ribbons of cells. **C:** Tubular or glandular pattern in which the tumor cells surround tiny lumens.

us it is supposed to have an insular pattern, will we panic or deny its existence because it is growing the wrong way? Of course not! We will accept this aberrant growth pattern and wonder what it means in terms of behavior or treatment, or if it is an unusual cell type. In this chapter, we will spend few words about growth patterns. The carcinoid tumors differ from one site to another in the background mucosa in which they arise, in their relation to other hormones on which their constituent cells are dependent, and in the substances they produce.

After an exhaustive literature review of reported carcinoid tumors, Modlin and colleagues concluded that 38% of the carcinoid tumors occurred in the small intestine, 18% in the appendix, 21% in the rectum, 12% in the colon, and 6% in the stomach.[27] A subsequent Japanese study of 6,799 gastrointestnal carcinoid showed the distribution to be 24.5% in rectum, 18.4% in stomach, 13.6% in duodenum, 19.4% in jejunum and ileum, 15.5% in appendix, 4% in colon, and 0.7% in esophagus.[28] This kind of information gives us a rough estimate or location, but these numbers are likely to change with greater use of upper endoscopy with detection of small carcinoid tumors complicating autoimmune gastritis and lower endoscopy with detection of small rectal carcinoid tumors. The often quoted demographic information on asymptomatic tumors is useless. What difference does it make if appendiceal carcinoids are more common in males or females, or if they occur at one age or another? They are often incidental findings in appendectomies, which are usually performed for the clinical features of acute appendicitis, especially since incidental appendectomies performed during other abdominal operations are becoming less common.

The carcinoid tumors differ from one site to another in terms of the types of mucosa in which they arise, in their relation to other hormones on which their constituent cells are dependent, and in the substances they produce. In fact, many contain multiple substances including hormones and amines such as serotonin.

Almost all carcinoids in the appendix and rectum are asymptomatic as are most of the gastrin-induced tumors in the stomach that accompany both autoimmune atrophic gastritis and the Zollinger-Ellison syndrome (ZES), although there are a few exceptional larger metastasizing tumors in these settings. Symptoms caused by carcinoid tumors are the results of their bioactive products, an uncommon situation, or structural changes that the products induce.

Prognostically, metastatic risk for carcinoid tumors at all sites is size, site, and product dependent. This probably explains the differences in metastases between ileal and appendiceal or rectal tumors. At the time of diagnosis, ileal carcinoids as a group are larger than those at other sites, presumably because they are found when they produce symptoms, and in order to produce symptoms, they need to grow large enough to either metastasize or kink the bowel and cause obstruction. In contrast, appendiceal and rectal tumors are discovered by accident when they are small. Of course, this may also indicate inherent differences in growth capabilities. Ileal carcinoid tumors may have more growth potential than those in the other two sites. With regard to site and product, duodenal carcinoids producing gastrin (gastrinomas) are more likely to metastasize when they are much smaller than carcinoids at other sites producing other substances, and the same situation holds, although less so, for somatostatin-producing duodenal carcinoids. There is little information on the prognostic importance of other parameters such as the number of mitoses, nuclear pleomorphism, and vascular invasion.

Gross Examination

Gross appearance.
Many carcinoids are so small that they are not recognized grossly. As they enlarge, they form firm intramural nodules that often look deceptively circumscribed. Some in the small intestine and appendix are yellow because of the lipid content of the tumor cells. Larger ones tend to be half-moon–shaped masses with a convexity facing the outside of the bowel, while there is often a depression on the mucosal aspect (Fig. 5-5). This depression is probably due to the dense desmoplasia in the center of the tumors and contraction of the constituent myofibroblasts, similar to what happens in a scar.

Gross dissection recommendations.
For resected carcinoid tumors: These resections should be handled like resections for carcinomas. The tumor should be measured, the depth of invasion ascertained, the status of the margins evaluated, and the regional lymph nodes resected and submitted. There do not seem to be any grossing issues that are unique to carcinoid tumors. When cut, the muscularis propria frequently appears greatly thickened, yet intact, despite being completely infiltrated.

For carcinoids found incidentally in appendectomy specimens: These are unlikely to be recognized in the gross examination. Be prepared to submit more sections of the appendix, often the entire appendix, to determine the extent of the tumor and the status of the resection margin at the base (cecal aspect) of the appendix. Besides submitting the distal 2 cm of the bivalved tip, which allows measurement of tumors that are <20 mm accurately on the slide, a size that is critical with regard to carcinoids and the tip being the most common site of these tumors, we routinely also submit a cross section of the base of

Chapter 5 Disorders of Endocrine Cells

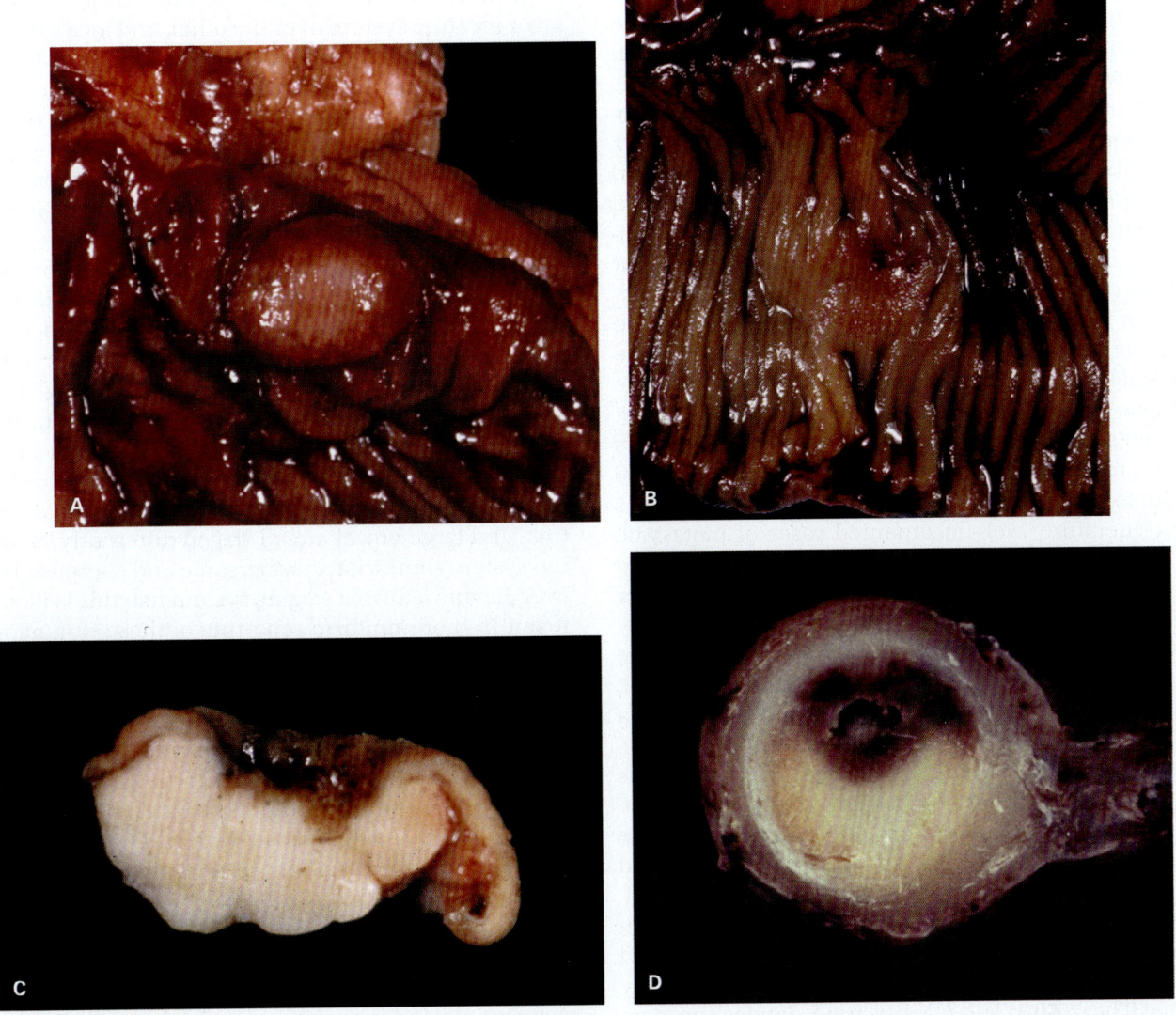

Figure 5-5. Common gross appearances of carcinoid tumors. **A:** A smooth nodule projecting into the lumen. **B:** Less circumscribed mucosal expansion with central depression. **C:** Cross section of an expansile lesion which has circumscribed borders and a central depression. **D:** Cross section of half-moon–shaped yellow appendiceal carcinoid with central depression.

the appendix identified by marking with ink as the surgical margin in every appendectomy. Submitting the margin is helpful in making important immediate recommendation for further resection when a tumor is unexpectedly identified. This is especially important if the tumor is identified on retrospective review of slides and the gross specimen has already been discarded. Spread into the mesoappendix, which is also potentially a resection margin, infrequently occurs, although this is more likely to be relevant in the goblet cell carcinoids, which are covered in the appendix chapter.

For carcinoid tumors found during polypectomies: These specimens will be handled exactly like other polypectomy specimens, because the tumor will not be recognized grossly. Don't worry, this is the best that can be done!

Staging and Grading

There is an overwhelming desire among clinicians and pathologist alike to designate tumors as benign or malignant for good reasons; however, we have learnt from many situations in other organ systems and certain tumor types that this is not always possible, and this also holds true for endocrine tumors of the GI tract. For example, size and site are probably the most reliable criteria in predicting outcome. However, it is interesting that most texts, reviews, staging manuals, or studies on endocrine tumors do not even mention the practical problems associated with measurement of size of endocrine tumors. For example, most of the appendeceal or rectal carcinoids are detected incidentally and the size of the tumor is evaluated by measuring it on the slides. Every pathologist recognizes that while measuring the two dimensions of a lesion on the slide is not problematic, constructing the three dimensions of a tumor is inaccurate, especially when dealing with measurements in millimeter range. This almost implies that the entire appendix has to be submitted for histology, the cross sections of the appendix have to be submitted in some form of sequence, and tissue blocks have to be exactly of the same thickness.

The issue with the rectal carcinoids detected incidentally in polyps is that when the tumor is present at the base of the excision biopsy, there is no way of knowing what is left behind. The only solace one can derive from this is that most of the data in the literature come from such inaccurate measurements! The other issue with size is that while carcinoids smaller than 1 cm at most sites behave in a benign fashion, identical tumors in the small intestine even when less that 1 cm are known to metastasize. In our own experience as well as in the literature, well-documented cases of metastatic carcinoids are described where extensive search failed to reveal a primary site. This raises a suspicion of either a very small primary or difficult-to-evaluate primary sites, including appendix. For these reasons, despite the fact that most carcinoids behave in a benign manner, they should be considered potentially malignant as a group and hence the need for a staging system.

The other confounding factor with these tumors is that histologically identical tumors have widely variable outcomes depending on site, location, and the nature of background disease. While less differentiated tumors have generally more aggressive behavior, well-differentiated histology does not guarantee a benign behavior. Thus histologic grading is also an issue and many different classification schemes are currently in use. The 2010 WHO classification divides the neuroendocrine neoplasms into two groups: (a) Well-differentiated neuroendocrine tumors that include the conventional carcinoids (well-differentiated neuroendocrine neoplasm), and (b) neuroendocrine carcinomas that include the atypical carcinoid/moderately differentiated endocrine neoplasms and poorly differentiated neuroendocrine carcinomas (small cell and large cell type). The idea appears to be that by using the term "tumor" as opposed to "carcinoma," one can imply a more benign behavior, a concept that all may not agree with. The American Joint Committee on Cancer (AJCC, 2010) grading system further puts well-differentiated neuroendocrine tumors (carcinoids) in three grades (G1–G3) taking mitotic activity and proliferative index (ki67 index) into account, even though there are (currently) no data to support these of being of value outside of the pancreas.[29] Other systems have used histologic differentiation, mitotic activity, and tumor necrosis in classifying the endocrine tumors into well-, moderately, and poorly differentiated categories. In the absence of overwhelming data specific to gastrointestinal endocrine tumors, it is difficult to favor any one system over the other, and local/regional requirements may guide the reporting of these tumors.

The other problem with staging of endocrine tumors is that progressively increasing depth of invasion in the bowel wall does not necessarily imply a progressively poor outcome unlike adenocarcinomas. Despite many studies that show some trends, it is not clear whether some of the histologic features that in other cancers imply an aggressive behavior for example, angioinvasion, perineural invasion, or infiltrative growth pattern, indicate a poor outcome in endocrine tumors of the GI tract and would benefit from a more aggressive therapy. Thus formulating a staging system for these endocrine tumors has been difficult, but at last the AJCC has published a staging system in 2010 that takes the site, size, and extent of tumor spread into account.[29] Tumors from appendix, stomach, small intestine, and large bowel are all staged differently, making the system somewhat cumbersome and complex. However, having a formal staging system like this is likely to result in more uniform reporting of these tumors with better comparison of data across geographical borders, and one cannot argue against its utility.

The seventh edition of the cancer staging manual from the AJCC (2010) includes staging protocols for all endocrine (neuroendocrine) tumors of stomach, small intestine, colon and rectum, and appendix.[29] The definition of the T stages is site specific and is mainly based on size, involvement of muscularis propria and serosa, and involvement of adjacent structures. There is only a single N designation, meaning involvement of regional nodes is considered N1 regardless of the total number of nodes. This should be emphasized that this staging is applied only for the well-differentiated endocrine tumors/carcinoids, atypical carcinoids (well-differentiated neuroendocrine carcinoma), and gangliocytic paragangliomas. Moderately to poorly differentiated endocrine carcinomas (small cell and large cell endocrine carcinomas) and mixed tumors are staged just like carcinomas at that site. It still remains to be seen whether this staging system would have any practical implications in guiding treatment strategies, beyond what is achieved by accounting for site-specific management guidelines.

CARCINOID TUMORS (NETs) IN SPECIFIC SITES

Carcinoid Tumors (NETs) of the Esophagus

The esophagus is a rare site for carcinoid tumors. In fact, esophageal carcinoid tumors are so rare that there are many more small cell carcinomas in comparison.

As a result, there is little important information that has accumulated about esophageal carcinoid tumors.[30,31] The few that have been reported are in the lamina propria and deeper, and they look like carcinoid tumors elsewhere, although some of them have been reported as atypical or malignant carcinoid tumors. They tend to produce single lumps or masses, but some of them have been found in association with Barrett's mucosa, even as separate foci adjacent to invasive Barrett's adenocarcinomas. In fact, it is possible that the Barrett's setting is more common than the sporadic setting. It appears that some of the reported cases are not typical carcinoid tumors with uniform cells and nuclei, but atypical forms or even small cell carcinomas. So the esophageal carcinoid literature may be contaminated with other tumors. There is little long-term follow-up information, so it is impossible to get hard data about metastases, survival, and features of the tumors that correlate with adverse outcome. However, the limited published data suggest that esophageal carcinoid tumors are likely to have a favorable outcome, but survival seems to be stage related and possibly also related to whether they are histologically typical carcinoids or if they have atypical features, such a pleomorphism, mitoses, or necrosis. They do not make anything that results in any clinical syndrome.

Carcinoid Tumors (NETs) of the Stomach

The stomach is a rich source of carcinoid tumors, but most, by far, are clinically insignificant in terms of long-term patient survival. Gastric carcinoid tumors occur in three well-established different settings, with a potential fourth, all of which are described below[32] (Table 5-3).

Type I carcinoid tumors. These arise in the body or fundic mucosa that has been ravaged by (autoimmune) atrophic gastritis, or simply "autoimmune gastritis," since atrophy is simply one of several microscopic characteristics. All patients with pernicious anemia (PA) have this form of atrophic gastritis, but so do a lot of other patients, almost certainly resulting from "creeping atrophy" secondary to Helicobacter gastritis that extends by direct extension from the antrum with age in Hp+ patients.

PA is a macrocytic anemia that is caused by vitamin B_{12} deficiency, as a result of intrinsic factor deficiency. Patients with autoimmune gastritis also commonly have autoantibodies to parietal cells, an intrinsic factor, or both. Increasingly it appears that many of these occur on a background of long-standing *H. pylori* gastritis, in whom parietal cell antibodies are relatively common. Indeed, it is now unclear whether the "typical" variant of PA seen in patients, e.g., in patients of Scandinavian decent, really needs *H. pylori* as a triggering or potentiating agent. However, there appear to be genuine hereditary forms of the disease, such as that associated with autoimmune polyendocrine syndrome type 1, or the X-linked polyendocrinopathies that include the immune dysfunction, polyendocrinopathy, and enteropathy, X-linked (IPEX) syndrome that do not require *H. pylori*.

Autoimmune gastritis is a condition in which parietal cells are destroyed, leading to lack of acid production, which, in turn, leads to loss of acid inhibition of gastrin production by the antral G cells, leading to hypergastrinemia (the pathology of this is described further in Chapter 13). Normally, the EC-like cells or ECL cells on the basement membrane of the glands are stimulated by gastrin to secrete histamine, but hypergastrinemia also leads to proliferation of these cells, especially when there are no parietal cells which are also targets of gastrin. This proliferation takes several patterns, but the most obvious is the nodular pattern in which tiny nodules of ECL cells develop at the base of the mucosa (Fig. 5-6). Other changes also occur in autoimmune gastritis, including glandular atrophy; pyloric, pancreatic, and intestinal metaplasias; and inflammation, which can direct the observer to look for the ECL-cell nodules. It is thought that such nodules progressively enlarge and eventually develop neoplastic features, including infiltration of mucosa and submucosa. The type I gastric carcinoid tumors account for at least three-fourths of all gastric

Table 5-3 Gastric Enterochromaffin-like Cell (ECL-Cell) Carcinoid Tumors Subtypes

TYPE	PROPORTION (OR %)	ADJACENT MUCOSA	GASTRIN-CELL HYPERPLASIA	HYPERGASTRINEMIA	GASTRIC ACID SECRETION	METASTASIS	5-YR SURVIVAL
I	80%–90%	Autoimmune gastritis	+++	+++	Low to absent	1%–3%	100%
II	5%–7%	Parietal cell hypertrophy/hyperplasia	ooo	+++	High	10%–30%	60%–90%
III	10%–15%	Normal	ooo	ooo	Normal	50%	<50%
IV (not in WHO system)	Rare	Parietal cell hypertrophy/hyperplasia	+++	+++	Low to absent	Unknown	Unknown

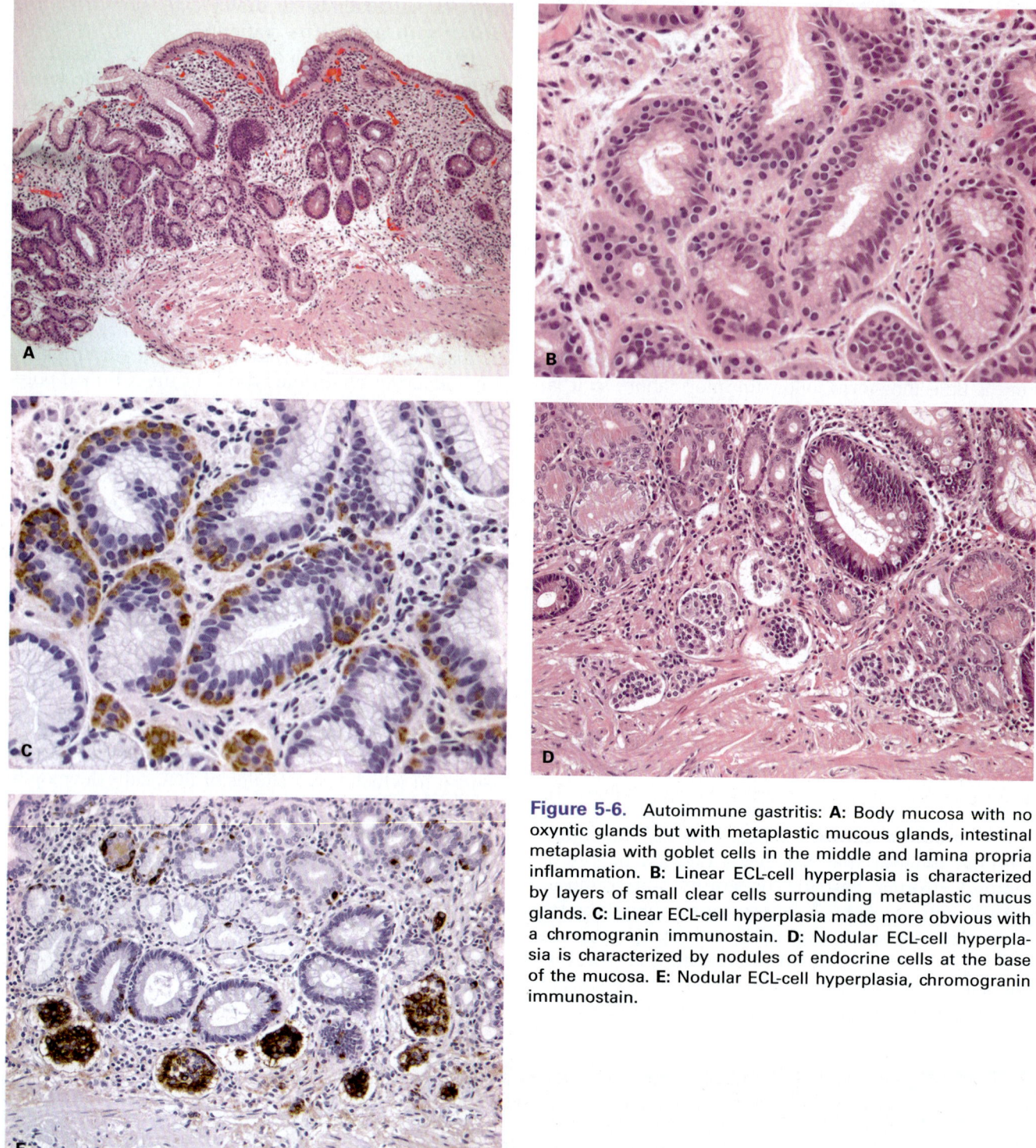

Figure 5-6. Autoimmune gastritis: **A:** Body mucosa with no oxyntic glands but with metaplastic mucous glands, intestinal metaplasia with goblet cells in the middle and lamina propria inflammation. **B:** Linear ECL-cell hyperplasia is characterized by layers of small clear cells surrounding metaplastic mucus glands. **C:** Linear ECL-cell hyperplasia made more obvious with a chromogranin immunostain. **D:** Nodular ECL-cell hyperplasia is characterized by nodules of endocrine cells at the base of the mucosa. **E:** Nodular ECL-cell hyperplasia, chromogranin immunostain.

carcinoids. Thus any generic discussion of gastric carcinoid tumors is likely to be heavily weighted toward these type I tumors. This number is likely to increase as more cases of unsuspected autoimmune gastritis are uncovered as a result of increasing upper endoscopy. At what point is an ECL-cell proliferation considered to be a carcinoid tumor? There are some seemingly arbitrary definitions that simplify this issue, which are listed in the WHO book on tumors of the digestive system.[33] First, there is a phase referred to as "dysplasia" in which the cells become relatively atypical and the nodule enlarge and fuse with micro-invasion of newly formed stroma (Fig. 5-7). Then, when the nodules reach a size larger than 1/2 of a millimeter or

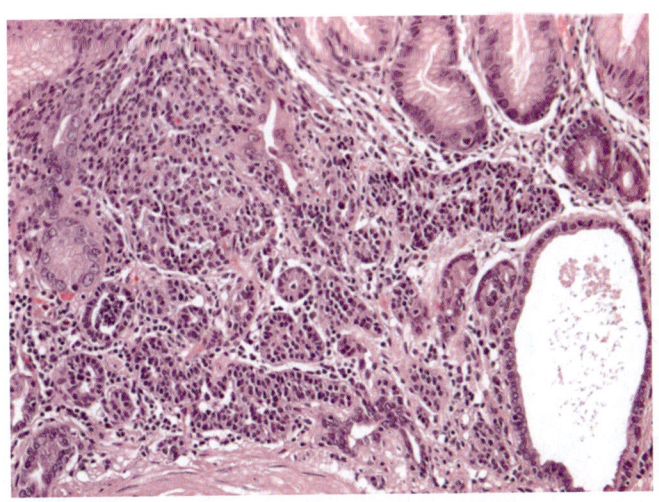

Figure 5-7. ECL-cell dysplasia: Multiple nodules, some fused, and apparently invading lamina propria.

invade into the submucosa, they are classified as carcinoid tumors/NETs (Figs. 5-8 and 5-9). Type I tumors are invariably asymptomatic, commonly multiple, and small and often microscopic. These tumors tend to be easily treatable by local endoscopic excision if large or forming an endoscopic polyp, or by simple follow-up to ensure tumors are not enlarging, which is rarely seen, with a generally excellent outcome. They rarely metastasize, probably because they are not large enough when we find them. Only when a tumor reaches about 2 cm across, is metastasis a concern and type I tumors of this size are rare. Lymph node metastases from these tumors are rare, and deaths almost unrecorded.

Any time a gastric carcinoid/NET is biopsied incidentally, usually as the result of the finding of a small endoscopic nodule or polyp in the body or fundus, the chances are at least 3 to 1 that it is a type I tumor, and almost all these patients need no additional therapy. Periodic surveillance endoscopy is advisable in patients with autoimmune gastritis primarily to screen for dysplasia or carcinomas, for which the risk is increased by about a factor of 7. We have seen several cases in which total gastrectomies were performed for type I carcinoid tumors, which was unnecessary and a therapeutic overkill. Therefore, whenever a gastric carcinoid tumor/NET is found in a biopsy, it is critical that the flat body mucosa be

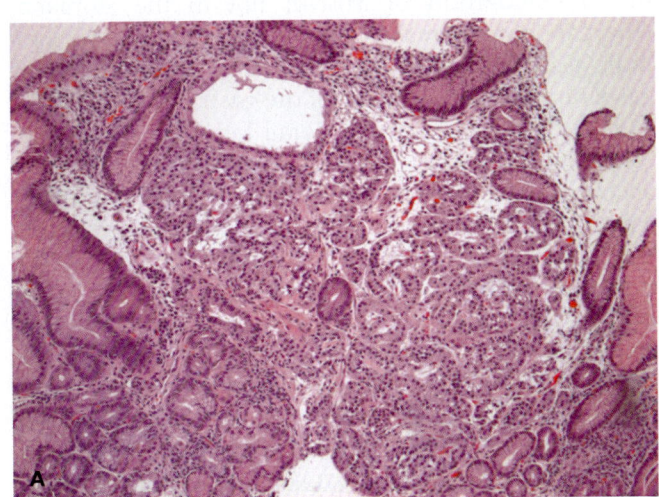

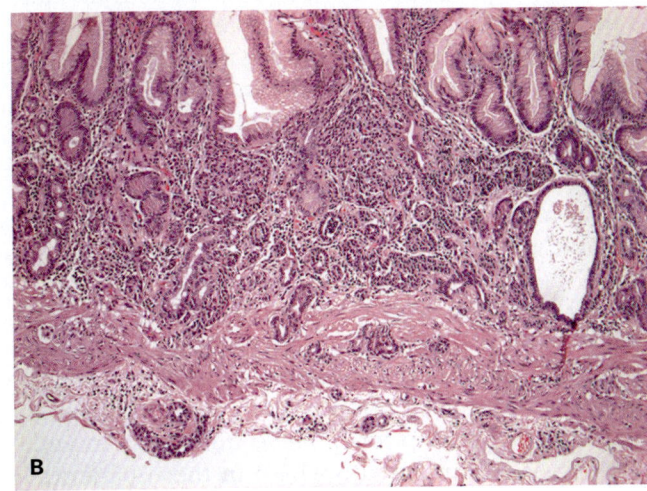

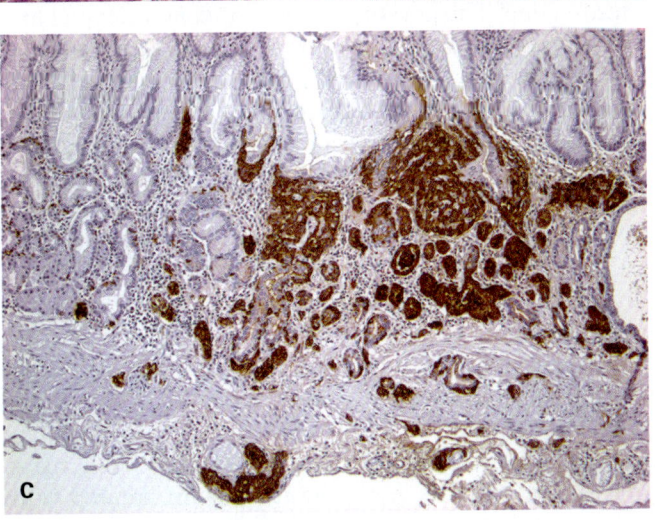

Figure 5-8. Type I carcinoid tumors. **A:** A small carcinoid tumor fills the lamina propria and surrounds a few residual tubules. This tumor reached the minimal size of 0.5 mm required for the carcinoid tumor designation. **B:** A small carcinoid tumor that has barely invaded the superficial submucosa at the lower left. This tumor was <0.5 mm, but the submucosal invasion satisfied the carcinoid tumor designation. **C:** The same tumor stained for chromogranin makes the submucosal invasion easier to see at the bottom, and it also brings out the nodular and linear hyperplasia in the autoimmune gastritis peripherally to the tumor.

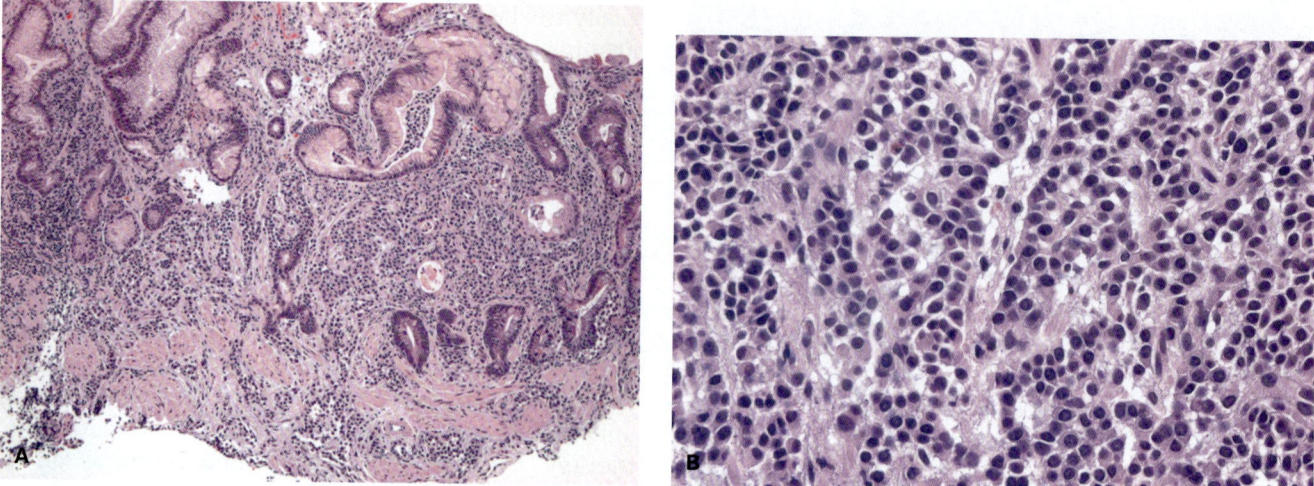

Figure 5-9. A: A larger type I carcinoid tumor, easily seen endoscopically, fills the lamina propria surrounds intestinalized tubules and invades the muscularis mucosae at the bottom. **B:** The cells of this tumor are uniform, have a plasmacytoid appearance with eccentric nuclei, and are arranged in interconnecting cords.

examined for autoimmune gastritis. Unfortunately, in most such situations, the endoscopists usually only biopsy the small polyp and the status of the adjacent mucosa remains unknown. In such cases, the pathology report should discuss this issue that there is insufficient adjacent mucosa to tell if the carcinoid is arising in autoimmune gastritis, and that this determination is critical for patient management. Often, a repeat upper endoscopy is required to sample the flat body mucosa from greater curvature, lesser curvature, and incisura. Surprisingly, antral biopsies can also be of value in showing a G-cell hyperplasia in atrophic gastritis, but usually no G-cell hyperplasia when there is a gastrinoma; however, antral biopsies alone in the absence of sampling from the body mucosa are insufficient to render a diagnosis of autoimmune gastritis. The presence of Helicobacter or extensive multifocal atrophy with metaplasia might indicate current or prior *H. pylori* infection. An ancillary test is serum gastrin, which in these patients is very high, excluding the diagnosis of sporadic (type III) carcinoids; however, one should ensure that the patient is off any proton pump inhibitors for sufficient time before measuring serum gastrin levels.

Type II carcinoid tumors. These arise as a result of excessive gastrin production by gastrin-producing endocrine tumors, known as gastrinomas, resulting in the ZES. Presumably, they evolve much the way the type I carcinoids evolve, through a hyperplasia–neoplasia sequence of ECL cells. However, the background body mucosa is not atrophic, but thicker than normal due to hypertrophy of the parietal cells, also caused by the hypergastrinemia. Although the ZES occurs both sporadically and as a consequence of MEN-I, virtually all of the patients with type II carcinoid tumors have MEN-I. Gastric carcinoids arising in the sporadic ZES are extremely rare.

Although the bulk of G cells are in the gastric antrum, peculiarly, the gastrinomas are almost always in the duodenum in MEN-I, not in the stomach, whereas the pancreas is a more common site for sporadic gastrinomas. Very rarely, the cause of the hypergastrinemia is hyperplasia of the gastric antral G cells. This is discussed in more detail later in this chapter under hyperplasias. Type II carcinoid tumors only account for about 5% of all gastric carcinoid tumors. The type II ECL tumors, those that arise secondary to the gastrinomas in the MEN-I syndrome, are like the type I tumors, small and multiple, and usually occur in the body and fundus, but a few have been found in the antrum.[34–36] In contrast to the type I tumors, they are likely to be more aggressive and metastasize more often to lymph nodes and liver, so they may need more aggressive therapy. Possibly this is due to some effect of the somatic defect due to abnormalities in the Menin gene. The combined data concerning type I and II tumors suggest that hypergastrinemia by itself can cause ECL-cell hyperplasia, but not neoplastic transformation and the development of carcinoid tumors. This additional step to neoplasia apparently requires other genetic defects. In addition to the MEN-I genetic change, Bcl2, p53, and MMP9 have been implicated.[32]

There is clinical evidence that decreasing the gastrin levels to normal in both the autoimmune gastritis and MEN-I Zollinger–Ellison settings results in regression or stabilization of the ECL carcinoid tumors. Since antral G-cell hyperproduction of gastrin is the stimulus for ECL-cell carcinoids in autoimmune gastritis, normalization of gastrin can be achieved by antrectomy with removal of the entire G-cell mass, and some patients have actually been treated with this procedure.[37-39] However, this is rarely used, since the small type 1 carcinoids are easily handled by simple endoscopic removal. Since gastrinomas are the stimulus for ECL-cell carcinoids in MEN-I ZES, normalization of gastrin is achieved by removal of all gastrin-producing tumors that are mainly in the duodenum.[39] This situation is so rare that we have hardly any data on the proper approach to these tumors. In the past, they were all removed because of the ulcers, not because of the carcinoid tumors. There is little information on the approach to these tumors in the current age of super proton pump inhibitors which effectively suppress acid production and thus prevent the ulcers.

The finding of ECL hyperplasia and neoplasia with hypertrophied vacuolated parietal cells diffusely throughout the oxyntic mucosa implies marked hypergastrinemia in nonatrophic mucosa, which should be confirmed. Usually, there is a history of ulcer disease that may have been treated with PPIs. Nevertheless, if this is not the case, the possibility of type IV ECL hyperplasia/neoplasia (see below) should be considered, and a gastric pH of <7 excludes this. If there is the usual history of peptic acid disease, then a search for duodenal carcinoid is required as it excision is curative, if there is no metastatic disease. Antral biopsies should be normal except that the number of antral G cells should be decreased in untreated ZES as the result of ectopic gastrin tumor secretion; however, if patients have been treated with long-term PPIs, it is possible that this may be lost. However, there are no data that confirm this.

Type III carcinoid tumors. These are sporadic, meaning that there is no known underlying precursor condition. About 20% of gastric carcinoids are type III. The type III carcinoid tumors are solitary, are likely to grow to metastasizable size, and present much like gastric carcinomas (Fig. 5-10). Thus they are targets for much more aggressive therapy, generally some type of gastrectomy. Unlike type I and II carcinoids, these tend to be aggressive, have overt mitotic activity, often have metastatic disease at presentation, and have a much worse prognosis. This is the only situation where mib-1 (along with p53) shows marked differences from other gastric endocrine tumors, but immunohistochemistry is not required for the diagnosis or to determine that it is an aggressive tumor.

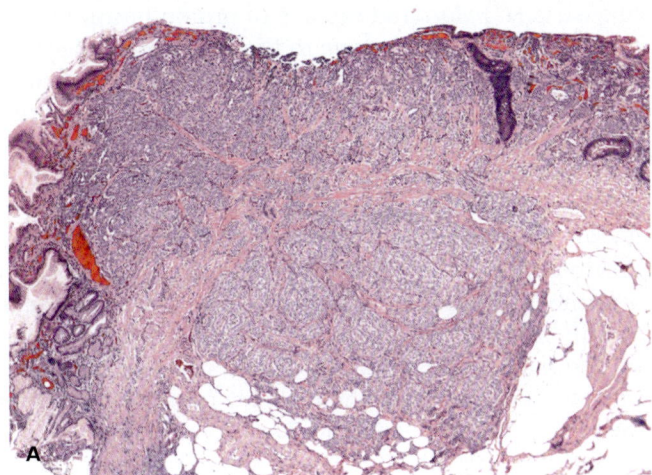
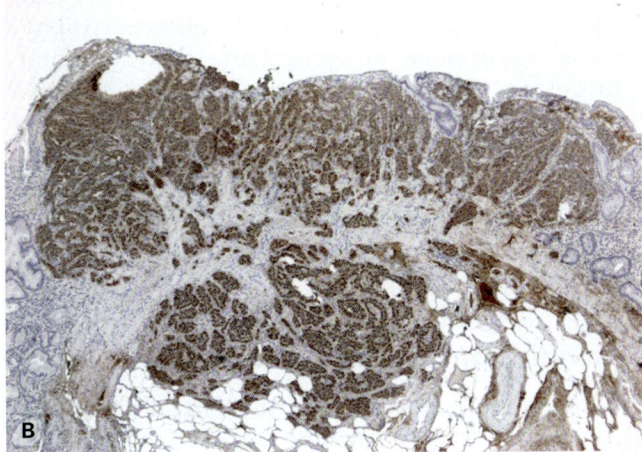
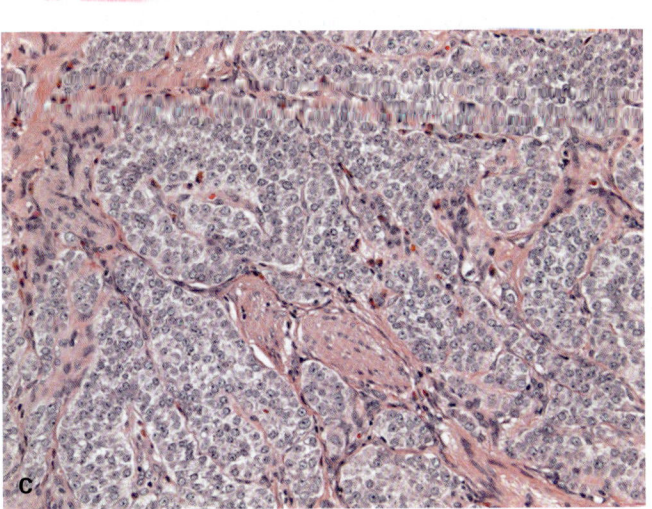

Figure 5-10. A: A sporadic (type III) carcinoid extends deeply into the submucosa. **B:** The true extent of this tumor is brought out by the chromogranin stain. **C:** The tumor is composed of small nests and cords of uniform endocrine cells separated by fibrovascular septa.

Potential type IV carcinoid tumors. Two patients have been described who had the combination of achlorhydria, parietal cell hyperplasia, and multiple gastric carcinoid tumors, who also had very high serum gastrin levels.[40] In the most detailed case, there was also G-cell hyperplasia in the antrum, presumably a secondary response to the achlorhydria. The fundamental defect has been postulated to be an inability by the parietal cells to secrete acid, essentially a spontaneous alteration identical to the gastric changes in patients on long-term protein pump inhibitor therapy. The lack of acid results in G-cell hyperplasia and continual severe hypergastrinemia, and subsequent marked parietal cell hypertrophy and hyperplasia, and ECL hyperplasia and carcinoids. The morphologic changes in the body mucosa are therefore identical to the changes in the body mucosa in the ZES. However, in the ZES, there is pronounced hyperacidity with low pH of the gastric contents, even in those on long-term PPI therapy, while in this newly described syndrome, there is no acid secretion, so the pH of the gastric contents is always 7. From a histologic standpoint, the combination of changes in these two patients is also similar to that seen in patients on long-term proton pump inhibitors, including decreased gastric acid production, hypergastrinemia, although not the very high levels in these patients, and parietal cell hypertrophy.

The importance of recognizing this syndrome is to ensure that it is not misdiagnosed as ZES, so that there is no hunt for duodenal gastrinoma, and the diagnostic test is the pH of the gastric contents. However, since only two patients have been described with this syndrome, it is not clear if these carcinoid tumors should be designated as a fourth type of gastric carcinoid tumor.

Carcinoid Tumors of the Duodenum

The duodenum, despite being so short, is an unusually fertile ground for carcinoid tumors.[41-47] This is the same for stromal tumors and adenomas. About 20% of duodenal carcinoids occur in the ampullary region, where they commonly lead to obstructive jaundice, but only rarely to acute pancreatitis.

Some duodenal carcinoids produce gastrin, and many of these cause the ZES. These are also known as gastrinomas, which is much shorter than "gastrin-producing carcinoid tumors (or NETs)," so it is an acceptable name. Others produce somatostatin and are known as somatostatinomas for the same reason. Duodenal somatostatinomas do not cause a syndrome, although some that arise in the pancreas do produce the somatostatinoma syndrome. The somatostatinomas are far less common than the gastrinomas. Many duodenal carcinoids contain multiple substances (somatostain, gastrin, secretin, pancreatic polypeptide, adrenocorticotropic hormone); however, most by far are clinically nonfunctional.

Gastrinomas. Gastrinomas occur both as part of MEN-I and sporadically, although most sporadic gastrinomas occur in the pancreas. In MEN-I, the duodenal tumors, including gastrinomas, are often multiple and arise in a field of G-cell hyperplasias that is comparable to the ECL-cell hyperplasia in autoimmune gastritis, with diffuse, linear, and nodular patterns, and microtumors with and without invasion of the adjacent tissue[41] (Fig. 5-11). In contrast, in patients with duodenal gastrinomas who do not have MEN-I, these G-cell proliferations may or may not occur. G-cell hyperplasia in the antrum is not an integral part of MEN-I; however, patients with MEN-I with peptic ulcers due to duodenal gastrinomas are likely to be treated with PPIs, and a secondary effect of long-term PPI therapy is G-cell hyperplasia in the antrum. As a result, an MEN-I patient with a duodenal gastrinoma is likely to have G-cell hyperplasia in both the duodenum and the gastric antrum. Patients with solitary gastrinomas of the duodenal bulb have also been reported to be accompanied by G-cell hyperplasia, which seems to be associated with the presence of gastric *H. pylori* and the use of proton pump inhibitors.[48] However, analogous to the hyperplasia seen in the gastric body, they seem to be without evidence of metastasizing potential and had no evidence of clinical hypergastrinemia.

Duodenal gastrinomas may metastasize, and it is common for those measuring 2 cm or more across to do so. However, some metastasize, even when they are much smaller, 1 cm or even less. We have seen a number of cases in which the bulk of the tumor is within nodal metastases, and it takes perseverance on the part of the surgeons to find the tiny duodenal primary; occasionally, the primary remains unknown despite extensive search. Rarely gastrinomas are found in other sites such as the gallbaldder, biliary tree, liver, ovary and even the heart.

Somatostatinomas. Some of the somatostatin-producing tumors also have an unusual growth pattern in which the tumor cells form glands or tubules in which calcospherites (psammoma bodies) are often found (Fig. 5-12). These duodenal glandular and psammomatous somatostatinomas are usually found in the periampullary regions in patients with multiple neurofibromatosis (von Recklinghausen's syndrome), especially black patients with the syndrome. Some somatostatinomas accompany MEN-I, but appear to be without metastasizing potential. Those we have seen have had a very low mib-1 index ($<1/\times 40$ hpf); several nodules can be present.

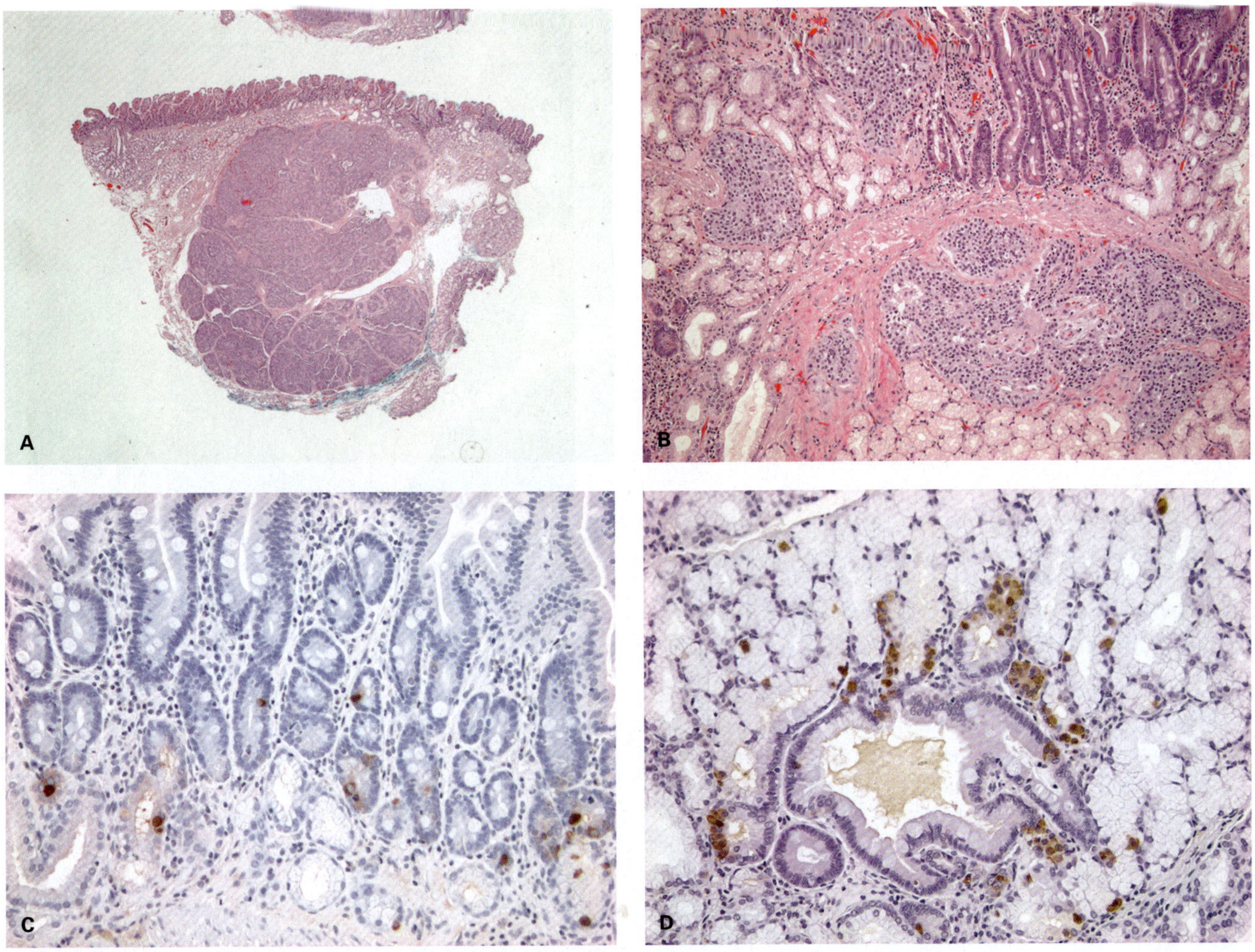

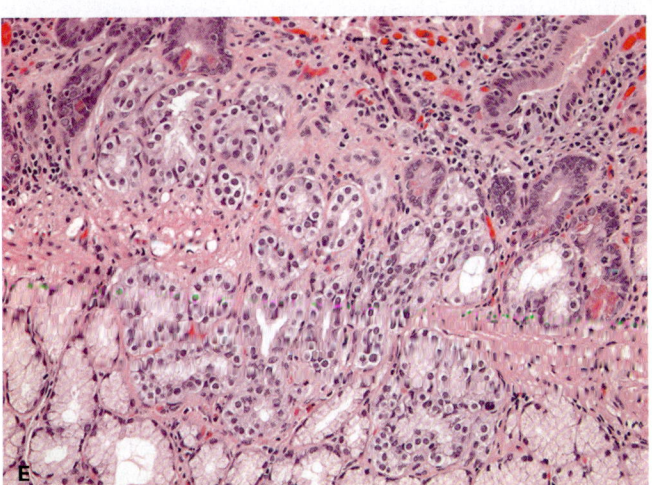

Figure 5-11. **A:** A large duodenal carcinoid tumor fills the submucosa. Even at this low magnification, the insular growth pattern can be seen. **B:** Three tiny duodenal carcinoids, two in the base of the mucosa and the third in the superficial submucosa. Tumors this small sometimes metastasize, especially if they are gastrinomas. **C:** Normal distribution of G cells in the duodenal bulb: Scattered cells in the crypts and Brunner's glands. **D:** Linear and nodular G-cell hyperplasia in a patient with MEN-I. **E:** Linear and nodular G-cell hyperplasia at the base of the mucosa in an MEN-I patient. This looks almost identical to the ECL-cell hyperplasia in autoimmune gastritis in Figure 5-6B. (**A, B, E:** H&E. **C and D:** Gastrin immunostains.)

Gangliocytic paraganglioma. These are unique triphasic tumors that are composed of admixture of endocrine cells, Schwann-like cells, and ganglion cells. These are discussed in more detail in Chapter 7. The three components can be intimately admixed or be separate. The endocrine cells are arranged in trabeculae, nests, or pseudo-glandular structures, often with psammomatous calcifications, mimicking somatostatinomas.[49,50] These tumors may be confused with ampullary adenocarcinoma by the unwary, especially in cases where the overlying mucosa shows atypia mimicking dysplasia, a situation very similar to that of granular cell tumors. While most tumors are benign, few cases with local nodal metastasis have been reported.

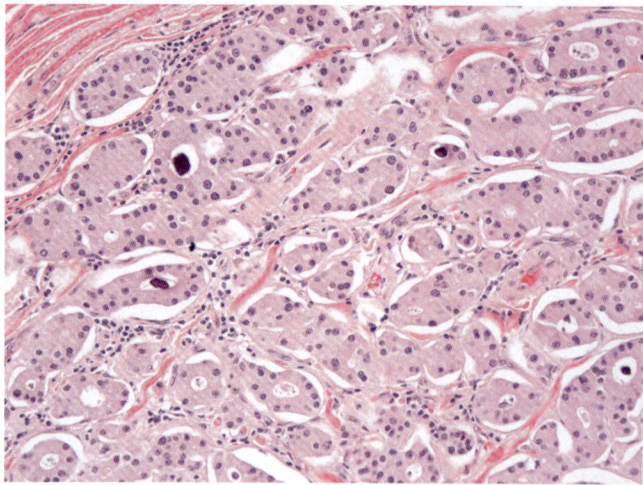

Figure 5-12. Glandular carcinoid tumor with psammoma bodies. Many tumors with this appearance produce somatostatin.

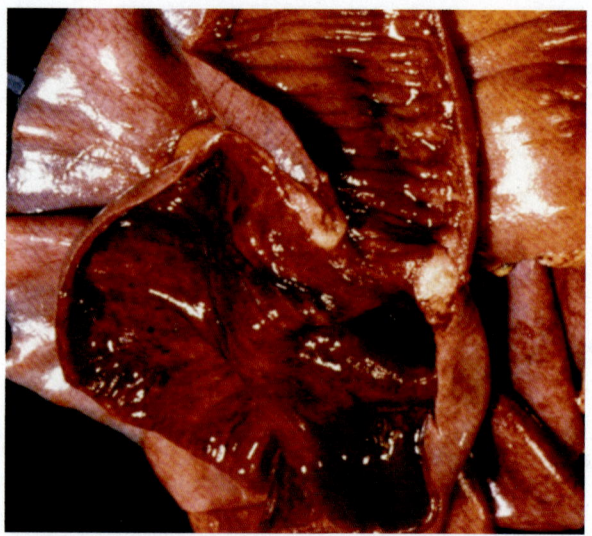

Figure 5-13. Small intestinal carcinoid tumor at the center right produced a kink in the bowel leading to obstruction.

Carcinoid Tumors of the Jejunum and Ileum (Midgut Carcinoids, NETs)

The small intestine, especially the terminal ileum, is the site of the most common clinically significant carcinoid tumors. Actually, there is virtually no information that deals with jejunal carcinoids specifically, but when they are compared to those in the ileum, they are numerically insignificant. In a report from the Armed Forces Institute of Pathology covering jejunoileal carcinoid tumors retrieved from their files over 14 years, 118 were ileal and only 18 were jejunal.[51] Of course, this might not reflect the true distribution in the general population, since this is a referral center database, but it might not be too much different. Because so little is known about the jejunal tumors, this discussion will focus on those in the ileum.

Ileal carcinoids are the classic EC cell tumors that were the subject of the original descriptions. They generally have the microscopic insular growth pattern, produce serotonin, and can grow large enough to metastasize even before they are discovered. Once they metastasize, especially to the liver, their active products can reach the systemic circulation and can cause the carcinoid syndrome. Furthermore, these are the carcinoid tumors that promote dense collagenous desmoplasia that kinks the bowel and causes obstructions (Fig. 5-13). A small subset of them also cause vascular changes in the mesenteric vessels, especially perivascular elastosis, also known as mesenteric angiopathy, that lead to ischemic necrosis and ulcers[52] (Fig. 5-14). Such patients tend to present with acute abdomens. Midgut carcinoid tumors associated

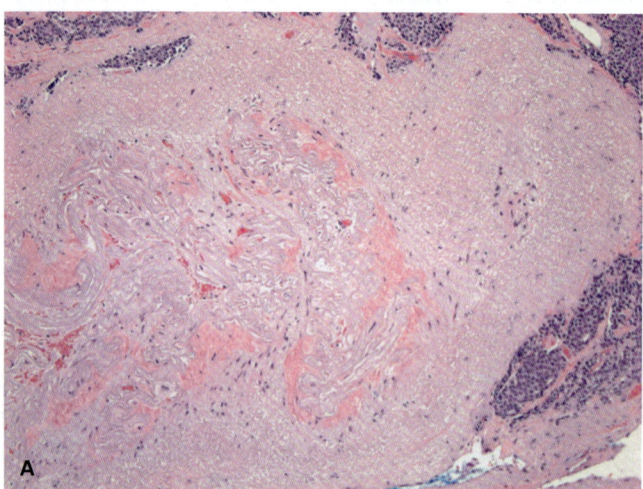
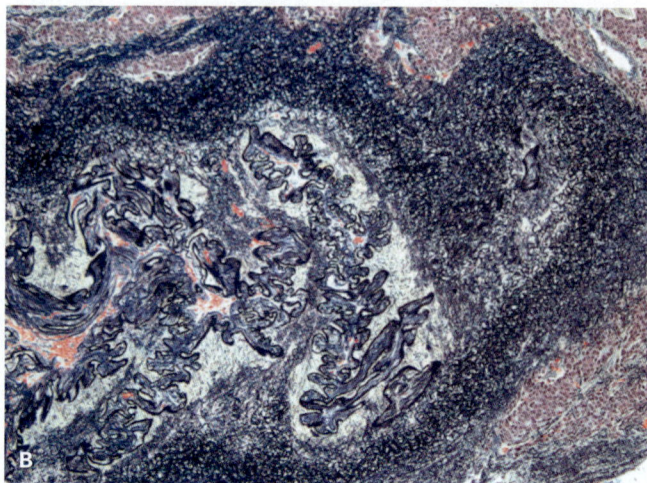

Figure 5-14. Mesenteric angiopathy caused by a small intestinal carcinoid tumor. **A:** On H&E, the central collapsed vessel identified by its elastic lamina is surrounded by a dense mat of elastic fibers. **B:** This is more obvious on an elastic stain (Movat pentachrome).

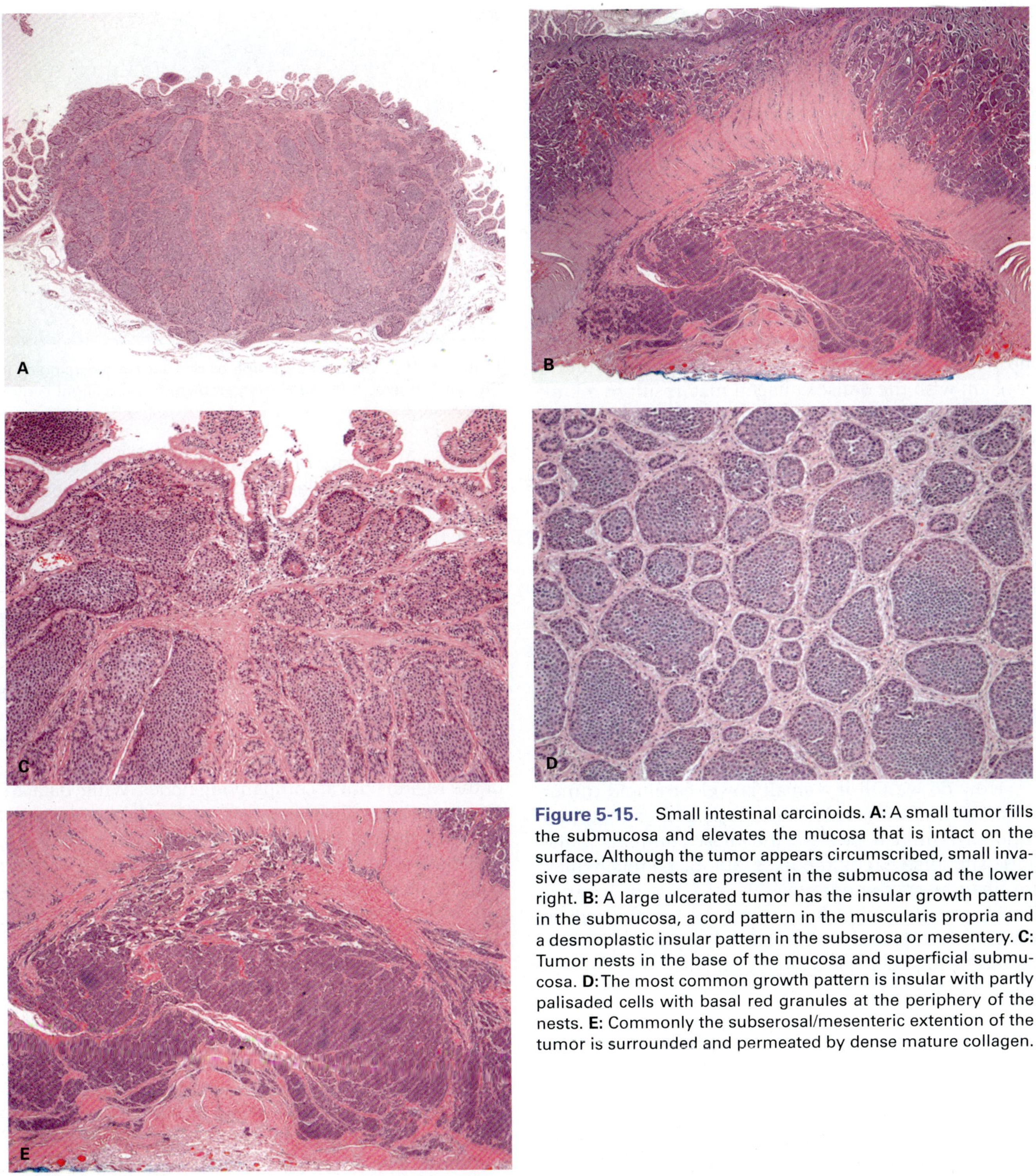

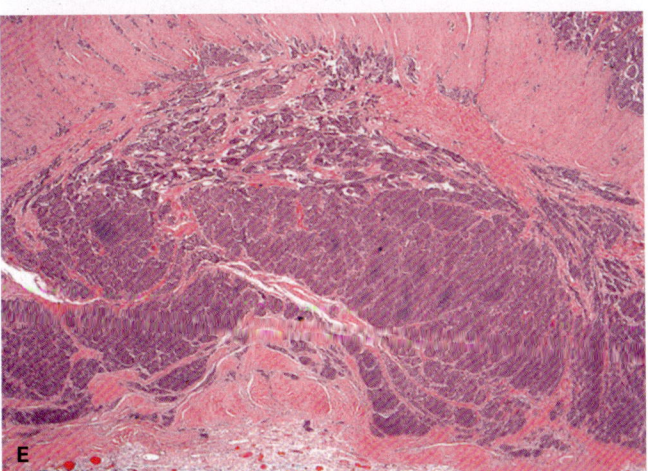

Figure 5-15. Small intestinal carcinoids. **A:** A small tumor fills the submucosa and elevates the mucosa that is intact on the surface. Although the tumor appears circumscribed, small invasive separate nests are present in the submucosa ad the lower right. **B:** A large ulcerated tumor has the insular growth pattern in the submucosa, a cord pattern in the muscularis propria and a desmoplastic insular pattern in the subserosa or mesentery. **C:** Tumor nests in the base of the mucosa and superficial submucosa. **D:** The most common growth pattern is insular with partly palisaded cells with basal red granules at the periphery of the nests. **E:** Commonly the subserosal/mesenteric extention of the tumor is surrounded and permeated by dense mature collagen.

with mesenteric angiopathy, when compared with those without angiopathy, tended to have higher levels of BMP4, a substance important in regulating cell growth and matrix production, including bone formation, and lower levels of NGF, which has regulatory functions in angiogenesis.[53]

Several cases of granulation tissue-like polyps in the same segment as the carcinoid tumors have been reported.[54,55] The explanation for these polyps is not known, but in one study, they were felt to be similar to prolapsed mucosa.

The tumors form small nests in the lamina propria, but they have no intraepithelial component. The bulk of these tumors occurs typically in the submucosa, even when they have invaded transmurally into the mesentery (Fig. 5-15). The pattern is predominantly insular with large nests of tumor cells surrounded by dense collagenous stroma. Artifactual retraction spaces are commonly found between the nests and the thick collagen bundles mimicking lymphovascular spread. The cells at the periphery of the nests are sometimes palisaded and often have fine basal red granules, while the cells deeper in the nests have less obvious granules. This feature can be very useful when metastases are biopsied to suggest the small bowel as the primary site. In the bowel, as the tumors invade the muscularis propria, the insular pattern is often lost, and scattered small tumor nests with little collagen may be all that is found in this layer. As they invade the mesentery, the dense collagenous desmoplasia reappears, but often the insular pattern does not, and the tumor cells are found in small nests, in short cords, or even in tiny tubules. This transmural invasion with the dense collagen may result in a kink in the bowel wall. In the mucosa, the tumor cells form small nests at the base, but there is no indication as to the type of mucosal involvement that is the initial focus. Every so often, a mucosal biopsy of the terminal ileum will enable the diagnosis of carcinoid tumor to be made. Close to 90% of ileal carcinoids are serotonin makers, positive with the appropriate antibody. There are a number of other substances that can be found in these tumors, and surprisingly, 20% of the tumors tested contained prostatic acid phosphatase, less than the rate in rectal carcinoids, while none contained prostate-specific antigen.[51] However, there is generally no need to stain them for anything, unless the diagnosis of carcinoid tumor is in doubt, in which case the stain for chromogranin A should be positive.

How do we tell if a small bowel carcinoid tumor is malignant? Obviously, metastasis proves that, and regional lymph nodes are the most common metastatic site followed by the liver. Mitotic counts, which are likely not to be reproducible, and size of 1 cm or more correlated with distant, but not nodal metastases in the AFIP study.[51] Tumors < 1 cm across metastasized to regional nodes about one-fifth of the time, and tumors as small as < 2 mm can metastasize. Nodal metastases increased with increasing size to 35% for tumors 2 cm or larger. It is not surprising that survival is stage dependent.

In about a quarter of resection specimens for ileal carcinoid tumors, there is more than one tumor[55,56] (Fig. 5-16). In one study, when compared with patients with solitary tumors, patients with multiple tumors were slightly younger, they were more likely to have the carcinoid syndrome, and they were more likely either to be alive with residual tumor or to have died with their tumor. There is an historical debate about whether these represent multiple independent primaries, or retrograde mucosal spread from nodal metastases. While there is evidence to support both views, the issue is unresolved, but clinically largely irrelevant.

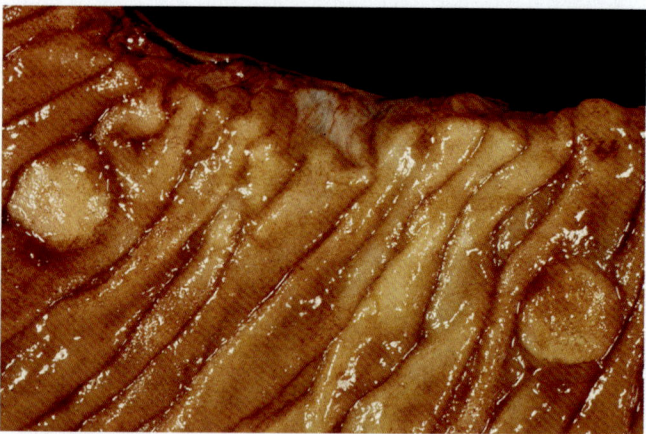

Figure 5-16. Gross photograph of two separate carcinoids in the small bowel, both appearing as plaques with slight central depressions.

Incidental finding of carcinoid in biopsies of the cecum or terminal ileum. Occasionally, biopsies with incidental typical midgut carcinoids are encountered from the distal embryonic midgut, mainly terminal ileum, but also cecum; these are usually biopsies of small nodules but may also be completely incidental findings, sometimes in patients with underlying inflammatory bowel disease. These patients are at risk for nodal metastasis, and ultimately liver metastases and carcinoid syndrome. If these are of a size that has metastatic potential (1 cm or more, but tumors < 5 mm can still metastasize), then assuming that patients have a normal life expectancy, they need to undergo excision of the region with accompanying nodes. While data are scarce, in a small series of six incidental ileal tumors, all three tumors 1 cm or more had nodal metastases, while those smaller than this did not.[57] There were no comments about multifocality, which is an issue as one has no desire to find other more proximal carcinoids of metastasizing size subsequently. Despite their low mitotic rate and mib-1 index, it is difficult to know if there are ever circumstances when surgical excision including local nodes is not the treatment of choice in an otherwise healthy patient, for even if only a few millimeter in size, one cannot take the chance of them recurring and being of a size where they can metastasize. Endoscopic follow-up, and chromogranin or serotonin levels can theoretically be used, but increase in serotonin levels usually indicates hepatic metastases. Treatment of all of these lesions should, therefore, be surgical, including excision of nodes, unless there are very good contraindications.

Carcinoid Tumors of the Appendix

The appendix is a common site for carcinoid tumors, but almost all appendiceal carcinoid tumors are found by accident in appendectomy specimens performed for symptoms of acute appendicitis or in incidental appendectomies performed during other abdominal surgical procedures, such as hysterectomies or colectomies, but these are less common than in the past. It has been estimated that a carcinoid tumor is found only in one in 100 to 300 appendectomies, so even this relatively common tumor is actually not so common. Because they are so often discovered in appendices removed for acute appendicitis, they may be hidden by the intense inflammation. We wonder how many of these tumors we have overlooked over the years because of this inflammation or because the part of the appendix containing the tumor was never sampled.

There are unique appendiceal tumors that are composed mainly of mature goblet cells arranged in cords and nests in which there are scattered endocrine cells and even occasional Paneth cells. This tumor has been designated as the "goblet cell carcinoid tumor," although endocrine cells are only a minor component. In most chapters and texts that discuss appendiceal endocrine tumors, goblet cell carcinoid tumors are included.[33] Some goblet cell carcinoids contain an additional adenocarcinoma component, making them even less endocrine and are best designated "goblet cell carcinomas." These are discussed further in the section on epithelial appendiceal neoplasms (Chapter 15).

The most common site for carcinoids is at the tip. There are two microscopic types. The more common is the insular type that resembles that in the terminal ileum (Fig. 5-17). The insular type is a serotonin-producing, EC cell tumor, much like the tumors in the terminal ileum. Like its ileal counterparts, it often forms small nests in the deep lamina propria. This corresponds to the location of a population of endocrine cells that are found in the appendiceal lamina propria, separate from the epithelial structures.[58] Some tumors have no mucosal component and are entirely within the submucosa and deeper. Some tumors have different cell types and patterns with pale cells, excessively granulated cells, and cord and small nest patterns, but these are included in the insular group. Also, this is the only GI tract carcinoid in which the nests of tumor cells are partly surrounded by S-100 spindle cells, presumably Schwann cells, presumably some hint of the

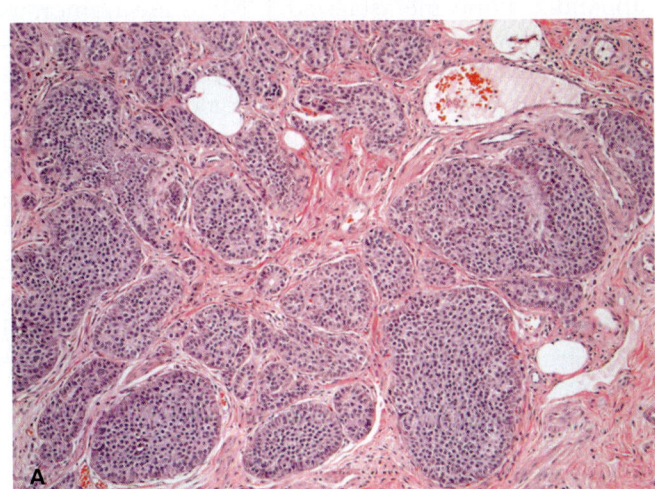

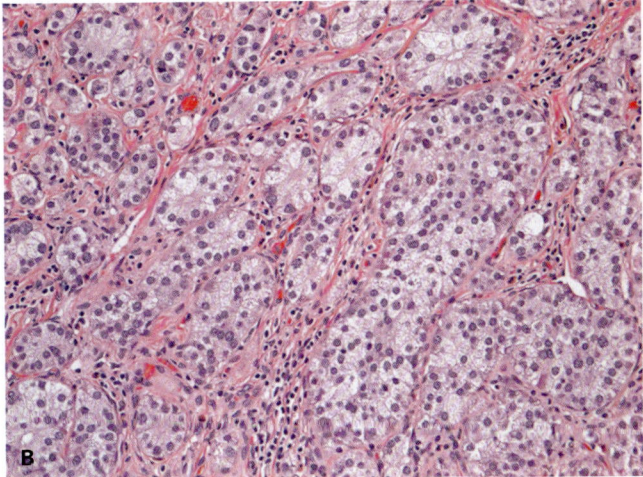

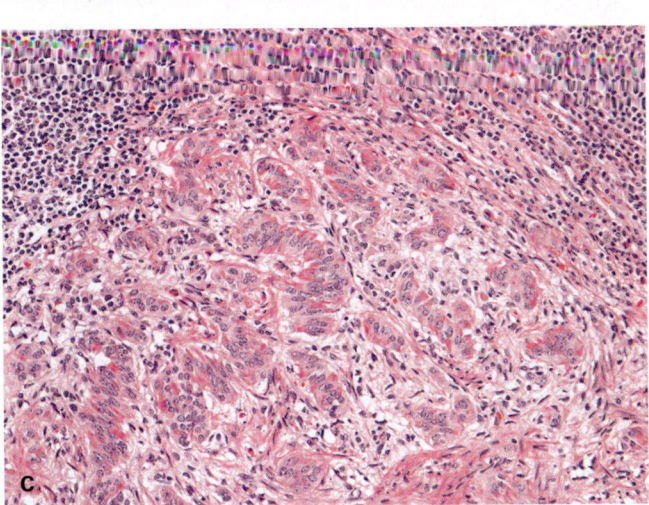

Figure 5-17. Appendiceal carcinoid tumors. A: Insular pattern with the granular cells identical to the small intestinal carcinoid tumors. B: An unusual pale cell type without granules. C: Another unusual type with cords of columnar cells full of red granules.

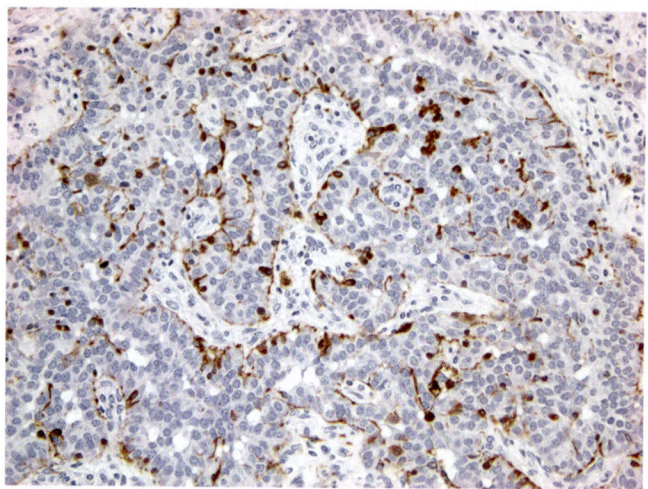

Figure 5-18. S-100 positive spindle cells, presumably Schwann cells, wrap around the carcinoid tumor nests, a phenomenon that seems to be limited to appendiceal tumors.

close relationship between appendiceal carcinoids and nerves, a phenomenon described by Masson over 80 years ago (Fig. 5-18).

The second type is the tubular carcinoid that is unique to the appendix.[59] These tumors are virtually always tiny, no more than a few millimeters across, and are confined to the appendiceal tip, sometimes next to an obliterated lumen, where they grow in short cords, some of which contain lumens (Fig. 5-19). These structures are separated by abundant collagen-rich stroma that seems to be a mature type of desmoplasia, as opposed to the looser, immature desmoplastic stroma of adenocarcinoma. However, because of the cords and tubules that seem to have a desmoplastic stroma, they are often confused with metastatic carcinomas. In our experience, they tend to occur mainly in young women. Some of these do not stain for chromogranin A, but they will usually stain for synaptophysin. Some or all of these are presumably L-cell tumors, similar to those in the rectum, in which the cells produce enteroglucagons and peptide YY, so they are likely to stain for glucagon.[33] If tumors containing these cells were functioning, then the patients might be expected to be anorexic and lose weight (or increase weight once removed). However, we know of no reports of such functioning tumors.

Metastases are really unusual for appendiceal carcinoids. It has been said that tumors 2 cm or more are at risk for metastases, whereas those 1 cm or less hardly ever metastasize. This is fortunate, since up to three quarters of appendiceal carcinoid tumors are 1 cm or less when they are discovered. The problem ones are those between 1 and 2 cm, the size range of metastatic unpredictability; although in a large series from the Mayo Clinic, no tumor <2 cm across metastasized.[60] Depth of invasion of small tumors does not seem to correlate with metastases. In a study of 15 tumors <2 cm across that had invaded the mesoappendix, none metastasized.[61] There are numerous papers on when right hemicolectomy should be carried out, but most are based on opinion, older papers to which genuflexion is made, and good data to justify this are conspicuously absent. Involvement of the serosal surface does not predispose to local or peritoneal recurrence, neither (with incredibly rare exceptions worthy of case reports) does involvement of the mesoappendix, and there are no data that lymphovascular invasion, rare as it is, carries a worse prognosis to justify right hemicolectomy. However, transection of a carcinoid, whether in the mesoappendix or base

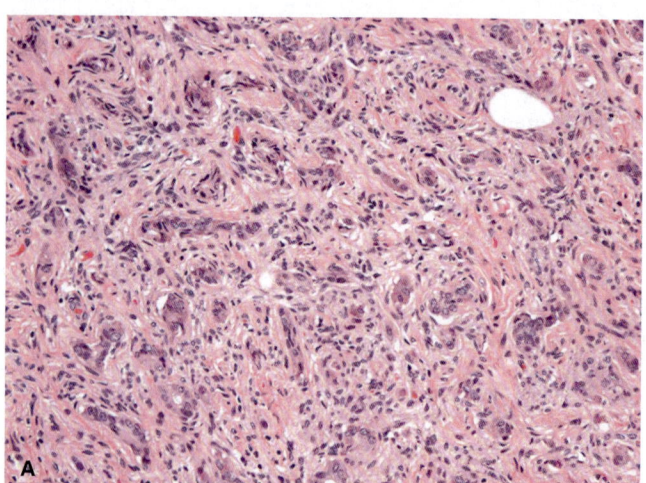 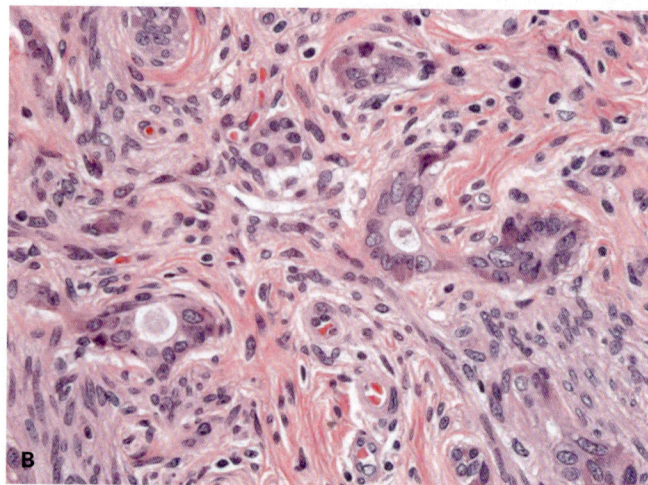

Figure 5-19. The tubular pattern of appendiceal carcinoid tumor. **A:** The tumor forms small discrete nests and cords. **B:** Some of the cords and nests contain well-formed lumens.

of the appendix, could be used as an argument to perform right hemicolectomy or partial cecal resection, but even then older patients or those that are at poor operative risk may have a better survival if nothing further is done.

Carcinoid Tumors of the Abdominal Colon

The abdominal colon is the second least common site for carcinoid tumors, following the esophagus, and this is comparable to the situation with stromal tumors. For instance, in a study from the Armed Forces Institute of Pathology covering 84 rectal and colonic carcinoids submitted to this gigantic referral center between 1982 and 1988, only three cases of colonic carcinoid tumor were included, and these were in the distal sigmoid colon.[62] The other 81 were in the rectum. Telling the distal sigmoid colon from the proximal rectum is not always easy, so it is possible that these three sigmoid tumors might have been in the rectum. Therefore, there is little published information about colonic carcinoid tumors, including where they occur, what types of cells they contain, their growth patterns, and their prognosis.[62] There is a cancer registry based report from Connecticut covering the 1976 to 1986 period in which 54 patients with colonic carcinoids were analyzed.[63] About half were in the cecum, with an additional sixth in the ascending colon. Most tumors were large when they were discovered, and about three-fourths of those larger than 2 cm metastasized, so these data are comparable to those for small bowel tumors. However, such cancer registry data are not controlled histologically, so it never is clear exactly what tumors are included in such analyses.

Carcinoid Tumors of the Rectum

The rectum is a relatively common site for carcinoid tumors. In this site, they are mostly asymptomatic and are found by accident during endoscopic exams for a variety of reasons, including adenoma and cancer screening. Endoscopically they look like polyps. In our experience, almost all of them are small enough when they are discovered that the endoscopists do not suspect that they are any different than the myriad of other polyps, such as adenomas and hyperplastic polyps, that they see every day. We have rarely seen carcinoids in random biopsies when no mucosal lesion or polyp was obvious, especially in the deeper parts of the biopsy. So they are often a surprise for the clinicians, who then must decide what to do about them. Microscopically, they tend to have a growth pattern of interconnecting ribbons of uniform endocrine cells (Fig. 5-20).

Since the tumors are removed by polypectomy, that is, gross total endoscopic resection, it is critical that we know what the indications are for further treatment, such as local resection of the polypectomy site or even rectal resection. The usual problem is that when the patient is reexamined, there is no sign of the site of the lesion, and its site has not been accurately recorded. If a scar is present this can be biopsied and tattooed, but, if not, the patient is just followed occasionally to ensure the tumor does not recur.

In a study of rectal carcinoids from the AFIP published in 1990, 4 of 35 tumors with follow-up metastasized.[62] All were larger than 2 cm across and were ulcerated, and 3 had more than 2 mitoses per 10 high power fields. Therefore, in this study, size and, to a lesser extent, mitoses correlated with metastases. In a similar study from MD Anderson published in 1997, there were no metastases in all patients with tumors <1 cm across, tumors from 1 to 2 cm across metastasized one-quarter of the time, and tumors >2 cm across metastasized three quarters of the time.[64] Tumors with atypical histologic features were associated with an aggressive clinical course, but these atypical features were not defined in detail, possibly because none of the authors of this study was a pathologist. In a study from Japan of 66 rectal carcinoid tumors, the authors found that tumors 1 cm or less did not invade the muscularis propria and did not metastasize. Invasion of the muscularis propria and metastases began to occur at the 11-mm size. The study concluded that polypectomy was an adequate treatment if the tumor was <11 mm across, if there was no invasion of the muscularis propria, and if there was no depression or ulcer on the surface. Vascular invasion did not seem to correlate with metastasis as long as the tumor was small.[65] Of course, a major concern with such data is how perfectly a given tumor is measured, since there are significant differences in behavior of tumors between 10 and 11 mm. In polyps with tumors that are smaller than 10 mm with tumor present at the base of the biopsy ("resection margin" in this case), we end up reporting that the tumor likely measures "at least" 10 mm. We also suggest further investigations with various imaging modalities (endoscopic ultrasound or PET scans), repeat examination with colonoscopy and biopsies, and serum chromogranin A (CGA) assays to ensure that no tumor is left behind. A similar approach can be undertaken for lesions larger than 10 mm in size; although once the tumor exceeds 20 mm, the point is moot. The utility of this approach in ensuring that metastatic risk is appropriately evaluated has largely been untested in scientific studies; however, it seems to be logical and practical.

In a 1990 study of 81 rectal carcinoids and 3 in the distal sigmoid colon, probably equivalent to the

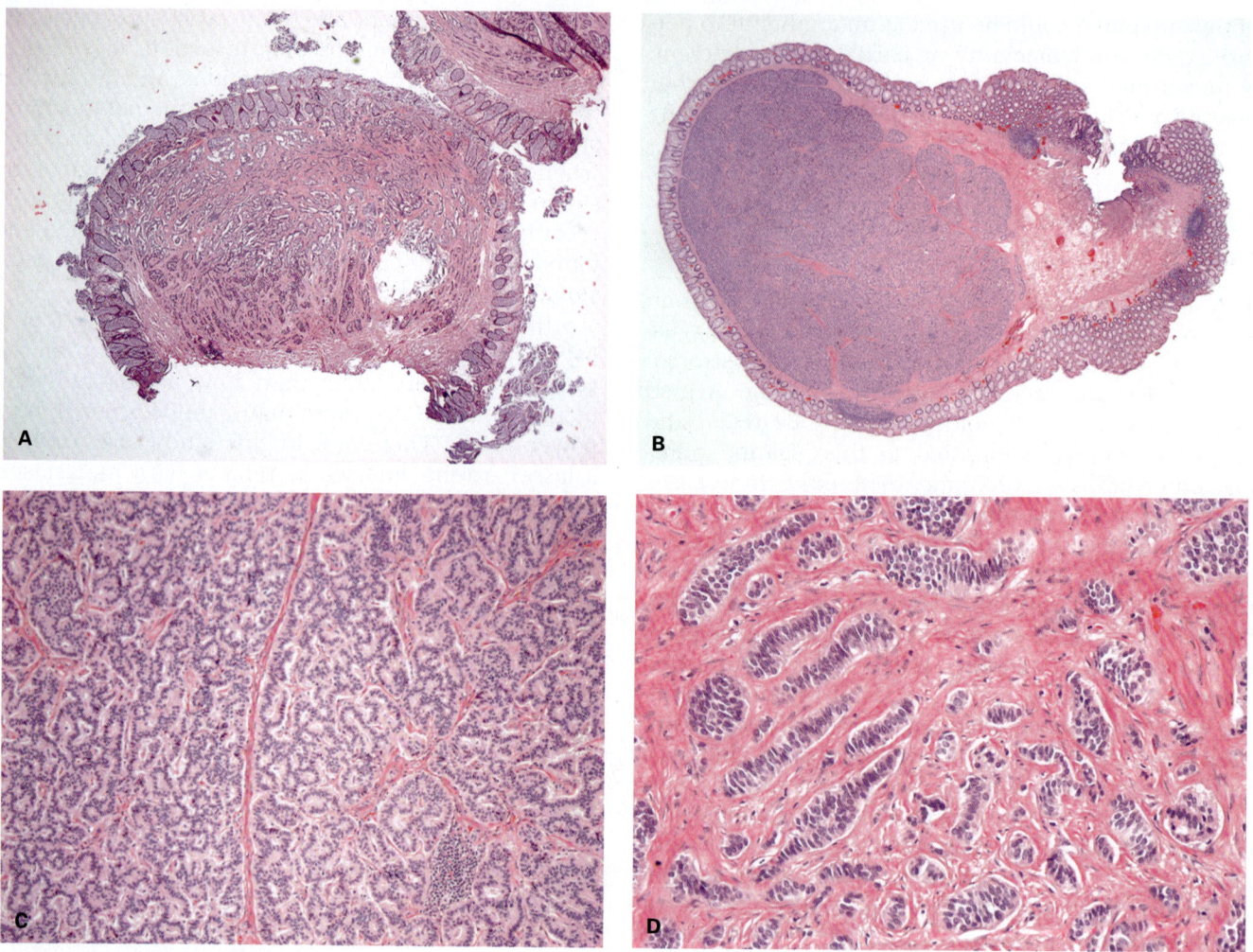

Figure 5-20. Rectal carcinoid tumors. **A:** A common specimen, a polypectomy with the tumor at the deep margin. **B:** A more substantial polypectomy specimen with the tumor well away from the cauterized amputation site in the upper right. **C:** One of the common patterns of rectal carcinoid tumors is interconnecting ribbons of uniform cells. **D:** Another pattern is short cords embedded in a dense collagenous stroma.

rectum, only 58% were positive for chromogranin, but synaptophysin was not tested. This group also had 45% positivity for serotonin, 46% positivity for pancreatic polypeptide, and 10% or less positivity for glucagon, gastrin, somatostatin, and ACTH. However, these were 1990 antibodies, and maybe current antibodies will give a different profile.[62] Most of these tumors may actually be L-cell tumors, and they may not stain for chromogranin A, but they will for synaptophysin.

In some rectal carcinoids, the tumor cells contain prostatic acid phosphatase, as do some in the small bowel. The published studies indicate that three quarters or even more are positive for this marker.[66,67] Of course, this is an annoying finding for the cases in which the differential diagnosis includes carcinoid tumor and direct extension into the rectum of a prostatic carcinoma, which can at times look like a well-differentiated endocrine tumor. The prostate-specific antigen stain should solve this potential dilemma, because it is negative in carcinoid tumors.

In summary, the vast majority of rectal carcinoids need no further treatment. If it is clear that local excision may have been incomplete, completion of the excision endoscopically is all that is required for most tumors. Should they recur, endoscopic or transanal excision ensuring a clear margin may be considered. It is only tumors exceeding 10 mm in size that pose any risk of metastases, and even in these, it may be possible just to excise the tumor and follow with endoscopic ultrasound or serum CGA assays. The more tumors exceed 10 mm, the more likely they are to metastasize, and the risks and benefits of resection, which may even involve a colostomy, need to be weighed against the risks and benefits of doing nothing. All one is treating is local lesion and regional lymph nodes; the tumor either has or has not already escaped to the liver.

POORLY DIFFERENTIATED ENDOCRINE NEOPLASMS (NEUROENDOCRINE OR ENDOCRINE CARCINOMAS)

General Information

The most common of the poorly differentiated endocrine neoplasms in the gut is the **small cell carcinoma**. This is a dead ringer for the neoplasm of the same name that arises in the lung in smokers. In fact, the histologic criteria for inclusion of a tumor into the small cell category are often stated to be the same as those for the pulmonary small cell carcinomas, namely, a diffuse growth of small cells with hyperchromatic round or spindle-shaped nuclei, fine granular chromatin, inconspicuous nucleoli, thin nuclear membranes, scanty cytoplasm, and ill-defined cell borders[68–70] (Fig. 5-21). The most common sites are the esophagus and the colorectum, where enough of these tumors have been described in the literature for us to draw some conclusions on what they look like, how they behave, and if they can be treated. The possibility that those in the esophagus are derived from Merkel cells (see Chapter 9) has, to our knowledge, never been investigated. In contrast, there are so few reported cases of small cell carcinomas in the stomach and small bowel that we do not have much information about them that can be useful or helpful. A few such tumors have been reported to occur in the anal canal.

There are also a much smaller group of primary gastrointestinal large cell or non–small cell endocrine or neuroendocrine carcinomas as well as some endocrine carcinomas that have cells that seem to be intermediate between small and non–small cell types. Some of these are buried in reports of neuroendocrine carcinomas which also include small cell carcinomas, so prying out the data on these non–small cell tumors is a challenge and a chore. The histologic criteria for the diagnosis of *large cell endocrine carcinoma* have been very difficult to find. In a 2006 paper from Japan, the morphologic criteria for large cell endocrine carcinomas, in this case limited to the stomach, were detailed at long last. They were characterized as having kind of specific architectural and cytologic features. The architectural features included organoid architecture defined as solid nests, sheets, and broad trabeculae with peripheral palisading and rosettes (Fig. 5-22). The cytologic features included hyperchromatic nuclei with finely to coarsely granular but evenly distributed chromatin; thin and smooth nuclear membranes; generally uniform polygonal, oval, and cuboidal cell shapes; eosinophilic and finely granular cytoplasm; indistinct cytoplasmic membranes; and ill-defined cellular boundaries.[71] In a more recent paper from USA, the authors borrowed the criteria for pulmonary endocrine tumors from the WHO/International Association for the Study of Lung Cancer. They defined the histologic characteristics of large cell neuroendocrine carcinoma as having a diffuse growth pattern or "neuroendocrine architecture," which included organoid, palisading, rosettes, or trabecular, monotonous round to oval cells with moderate amounts of cytoplasm and granular to vesicular nuclei, with or without nuclei. They also demanded some immunohistochemical proof of epithelial and endocrine differentiation, including positivity for AE1/AE3 for epithelium and positivity in over 20% of the cells for any one of three endocrine markers, including chromogranin, synaptophysin, and CD56.[72] They also suggested that classifying all high-grade endocrine

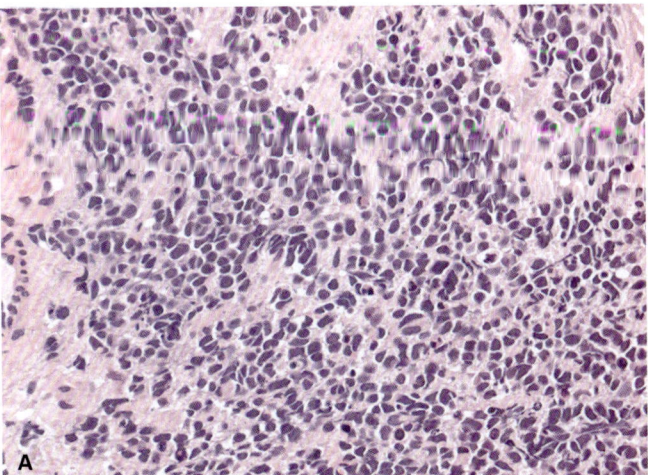
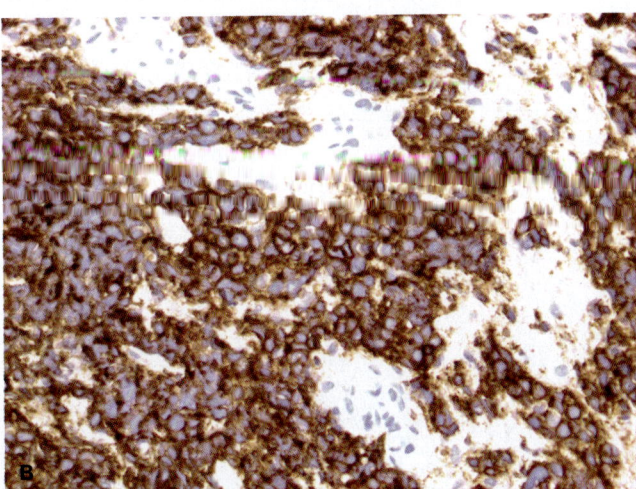

Figure 5-21. Small cell carcinoma of the esophagus. **A:** The tumor cells resemble those in the comparable small cell carcinomas of the lung. There is a diffuse growth of small cells with hyperchromatic round or spindle-shaped nuclei, fine granular chromatin, inconspicuous nucleoli, thin nuclear membranes, scanty cytoplasm, and ill-defined cell borders. **B:** The cells stained with the antibody to CD56, one of the endocrine markers.

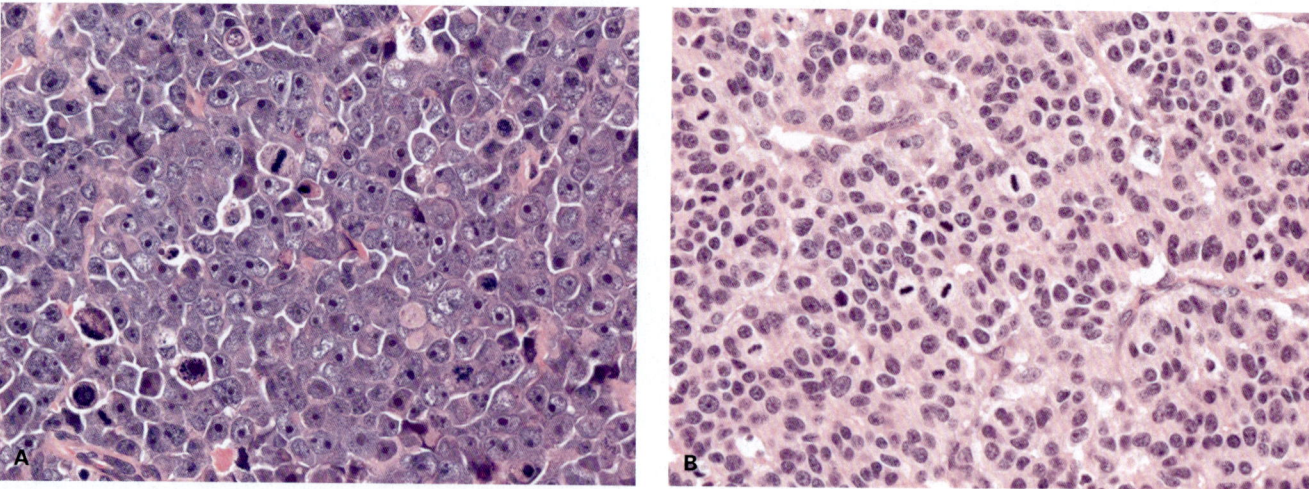

Figure 5-22. Two different large cell endocrine or neuroendocrine carcinomas, both of which stained strongly for endocrine markers. **A:** This tumor looks anaplastic with sheets of cells with large nuclei, prominent nuclei (unusual for most such tumors), frequent mitoses, necrotic single cells, and pale cytoplasm. **B:** This tumor has a nested pattern, so it looks more endocrine. The cells also have large nuclei, pale cytoplasm, and many mitoses.

tumors of the gut into small cell and non–small cell types made sense. Some of these large cell carcinomas, regardless of site, also have areas of squamous or adenocarcinomatous differentiation (Fig. 5-23). In this study, gastric large cell carcinomas had a significantly worse prognosis than did usual gastric adenocarcinomas.

Esophageal Tumors

Reports of small cell carcinomas in the esophagus are not consistent in exactly what tumors are included. In some reports, the authors adhere rigidly to the diagnostic criteria listed above. In others, somewhat different cells often with round nuclei are included. Some reports include only tumors that are pure small cell, while other reports include both pure tumors and those in which there are differentiated components that are described as squamous cell carcinoma, adenocarcinoma, and even mucoepidermoid carcinoma. Several reported cases had in situ squamous cell carcinoma in the overlying epithelium.[73]

In some reports, there is at least one pathologist among the authors, suggesting that the tumors were subject to pathologist review. However, in many reports, there is no pathologist, but the tumors were included based solely on the diagnoses in the institutions' archives, so in such reports, it is not clear if the authors included small cell carcinomas or if other carcinomas were mixed in based on misdiagnoses.[74–78] Nevertheless, this is the literature with which we have to deal with. Based on these studies, it seems that the location parallels that for squamous cell carcinoma, with almost all occurring in the middle and lower thirds, probably in fairly equal proportions. Some of them grossly look like standard esophageal carcinomas, but the reported cases suggest that many are long segment tumors producing strictures. They occur more in males and when they are detected, like squamous and adenocarcinomas, they are commonly in high stage. Almost all have invaded the muscularis propria (T2), while about half have invaded beyond the muscularis (T3 and T4), and nodal metastases have already occurred in most cases by the time of diagnosis. They have been treated with a combination of resection and chemo/radiation therapy, much like small cell carcinomas of the lung. The survival is measured in months, with some minor variations that are stage related. In one study, the median survival of four patients with disease confined to the esophagus with or without regional node involvement was 18.5 months, while that for more widely metastatic disease was only 11 months.[74]

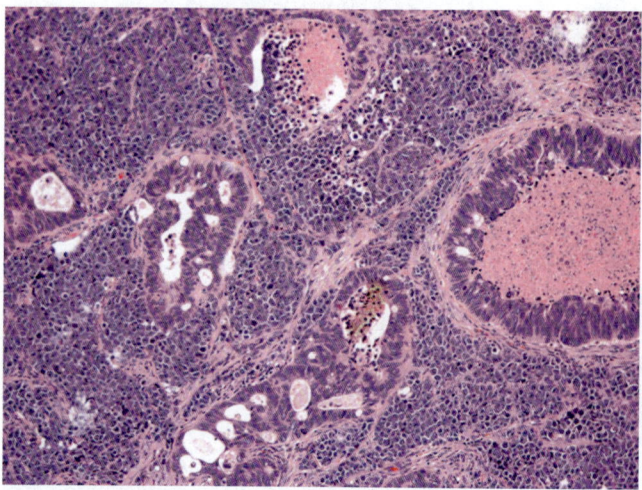

Figure 5-23. This large cell carcinoma has areas of adenocarcinoma differentiation, not unusual for these tumors.

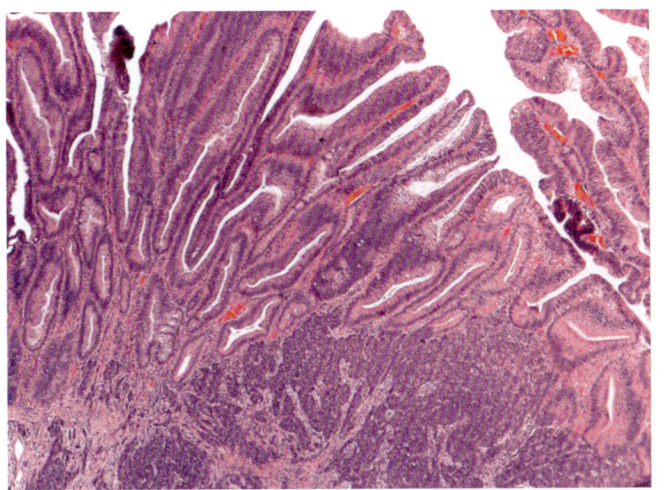

Figure 5-24. Small cell carcinoma of the colon arising from the base of a sessile adenoma.

Colonic and Rectal Tumors

Primary small cell carcinomas of the colon and rectum arise mainly at the two ends: the cecum and proximal right colon, and the sigmoid-rectum.[79-84] They often are found at the base of large sessile adenomas, which may have a prominent villous component (Fig. 5-24). They also often have foci of squamous or adenocarcinomatous differentiation (Fig. 5-25). Up to half of the tumors express an endocrine marker, such as chromogranin or synaptophysin, but more are likely to have endocrine granules when they are studied by electron microscopy. CD56 is also a potentially useful diagnostic marker. A survey of case reports and small series indicates that the age, sex, and gross appearance are like those for colorectal carcinomas. About 90% have metastasized to nodes and about 70% to liver at the time of diagnosis, and tumors as small as 3 mm across have metastasized. The median survival is generally less than a year. In one study, there was no difference in survival between small cell and large cell carcinomas.[79] In another study, small cell carcinomas that expressed endocrine markers were much more aggressive than those that did not have such markers. The markers included synaptophysin, chromogranin, and SNAP25.[82] There is much less published data on the behavior of colorectal large cell carcinomas, but the limited information suggests that their prognosis is much the same as that for small cell carcinomas.[72]

ADENOMAS AND ADENOCARCINOMAS WITH BOTH EPITHELIAL AND ENDOCRINE DIFFERENTIATION

Tumors in Which Endocrine and Columnar Cells are Mixed

Adenomas and adenocarcinomas throughout the gut commonly have a variety of cell types. These include differentiated mucin-containing cells, some of which look like goblet cells, while others are columnar with apical mucin vacuoles. Other cells are differentiated Paneth cells with coarse eosinophilic granules. In some adenomas and adenocarcinomas, most of the cells are primitive columnar or cuboidal cells with neither mucin content nor Paneth cell granules. Since endocrine cells seem to derive from the glandular or tubular epithelium of the gut, there is every reason to expect that adenomas and adenocarcinomas of the gut will contain differentiated endocrine cells, with their differentiation proven by their positive staining with antibodies to chromogranin, synaptophysin or other

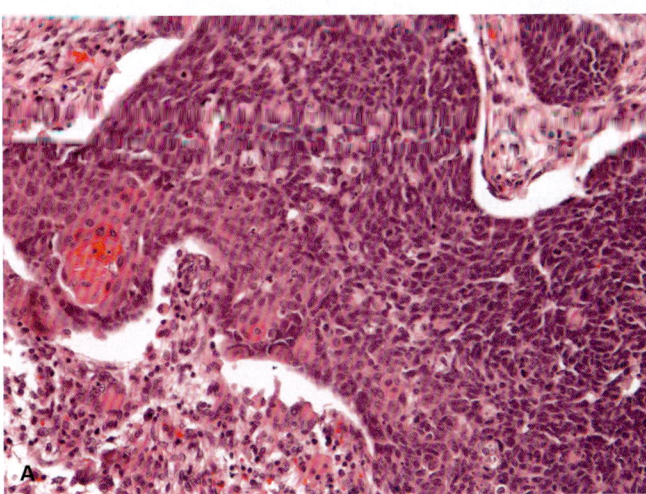
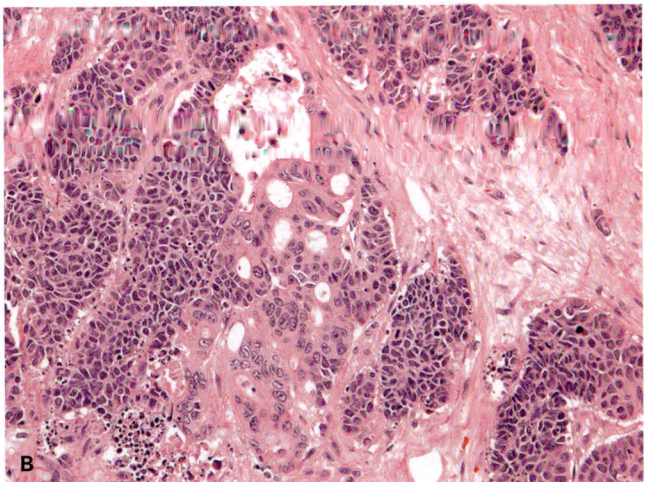

Figure 5-25. Small cell carcinoma of the colon with **(A)** squamous differentiation on the left and **(B)** adenocarcinoma differentiation in the center.

endocrine markers, such as CD56 and CD57. And that is exactly the case. If we stain a thousand adenocarcinomas and adenomas of the gut in every site, the chances are great that there will be some endocrine cells among the other types of cells that commonly populate these neoplasms (Fig. 5-26). Studies documenting this go back to the days of silver staining.[85] The amount of endocrine differentiation varies from scattered cells here and there to larger areas of the adenomas or carcinoma that are purely endocrine. In one study of adenomas, endocrine cells were more likely to be present and to occur in greater numbers in those adenomas that were more tubular and had lower degrees of dysplasia.[86] In the stomach, the diffuse pattern of carcinoma was more likely to contain endocrine cells than the intestinal or tubular pattern.[87] There has been a lot of literary discussion concerning the proper classification of these tumors based on the extent of endocrine differentiation.[88] However, we really want to know if these endocrine cells are clinically important, that is, what degree of endocrine differentiation changes the behavior and management of a carcinoma. Does it require 1% or 50% endocrine differentiation or any per cent in between to make an adenocarcinoma something different in terms of behavior or response to therapy than were it a standard brand adenocarcinoma? The following is a small sample of the published data. In one study from Japan,[89] colonic adenocarcinomas with more than 1 cell staining positively for chromogranin A per square millimeter had a significantly worse prognosis than those with fewer positive cells. However, in a study from the United States, about 40% of 48 stage III colon carcinomas had chromogranin positive endocrine cells, and those tumor behaved no differently than did those without positive cells.[90] Finally, endocrine cell differentiation is occasionally prominent in colorectal hyperplastic polyps. The significance of this finding is unknown (Fig. 5-26).

Tumors with Separate Components (Composite Tumors)

In addition to adenomas and carcinomas with scattered endocrine cells, there are also adenomas and carcinomas with distinct hyperplasia of enodocrine

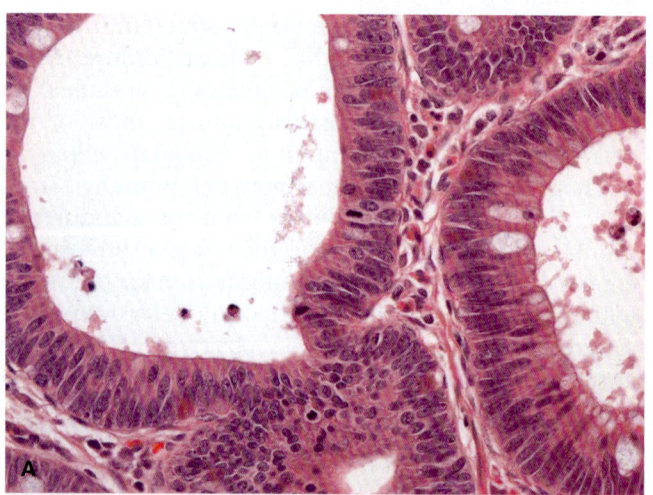

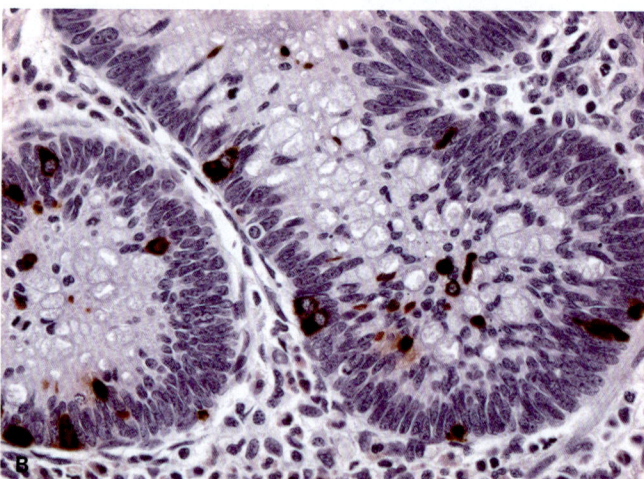

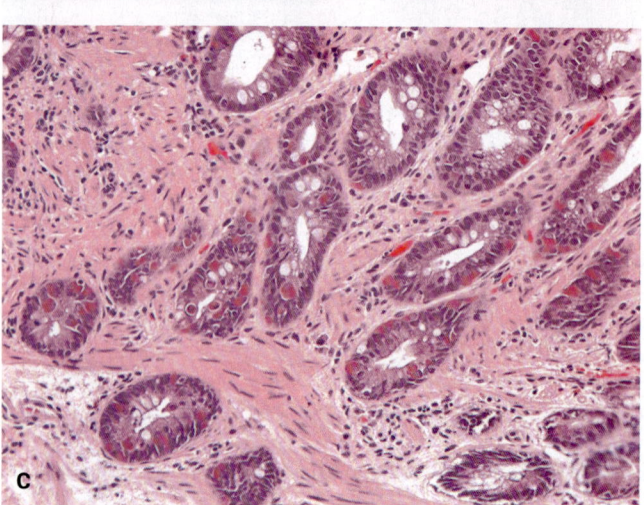

Figure 5-26. Endocrine cells in colorectal polyps. **A:** Scattered endocrine cells with basal red granules in an adenoma. **B:** Chromogranin stain of an adenoma brings out the endocrine cells, many more than are seen by H&E. **C:** Many endocrine cells with basal red granules (serotonin-producing Kulchitsky cells) at the base of a hyperplastic polyp.

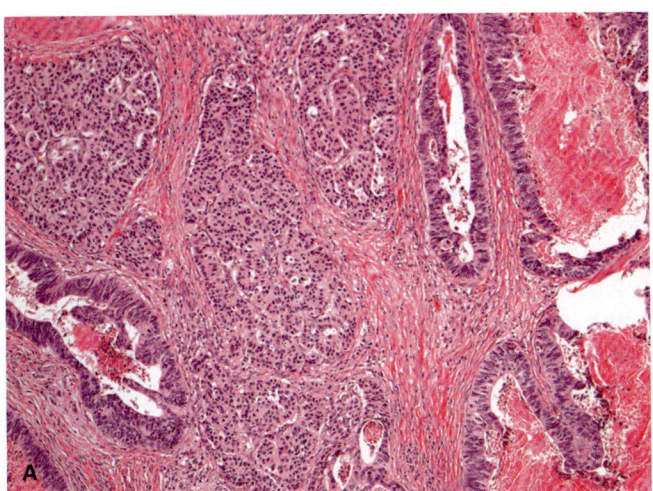 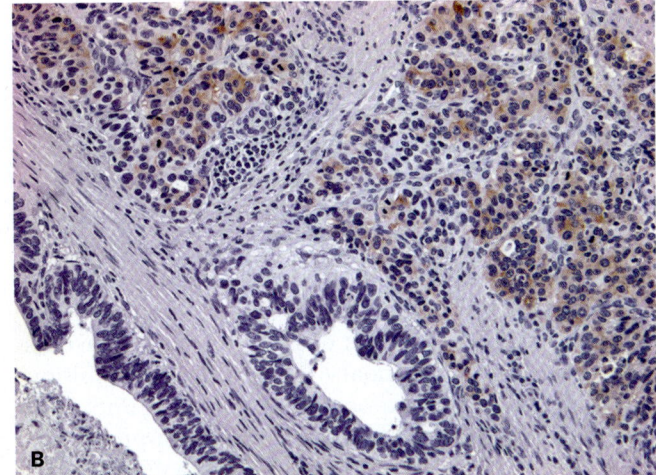

Figure 5-27. Composite carcinoma, in this case a Barrett's carcinoma with differentiated adenocarcinoma mixed with islands of large cell endocrine carcinoma. **A:** H&E. **B:** The synaptophysin immunostain colors the endocrine component but not the adenocarcinoma.

cells or microcarcinoids that sometimes can mimic invasive carcinoma.[91] In addition, adenomas and carcinomas with discrete foci of well-formed endocrine tumor, including carcinoid tumor and endocrine carcinoma are also reported. Then there are the composite tumors with two distinct components one of which is endocrine and can involve any site in the GI tract[92-96] (Fig. 5-27). Some reports seem to include goblet cell carcinoid tumors, just to confuse the issue. It is not clear whether these composite tumors behave differently than the usual adenocarcinomas, because there are so few of them for meaningful data to have accumulated.

In one study of rectal carcinomas that were treated with neoadjuvant radiation, some also with chemotherapy, increased endocrine cells were found in residual tumor compared to the pretreatment biopsies, following resection in about two thirds of the cases, and over half of these residual carcinomas had chromogranin positivity in 20% or more of the cells.[97] The authors postulated that this increase in endocrine cells may be an induction of endocrine differentiation by the treatment. We have observed similar endocrine cells in treated Barrett's carcinomas.

ENDOCRINE TUMORS ASSOCIATED WITH ULCERATIVE COLITIS AND CROHN'S DISEASE

There are a few reported cases of colonic carcinoid tumors in ulcerative colitis.[98-102] Most of these were in the rectum, and some occurred in mucosae that had endocrine cell hyperplasia in the crypts. This has been documented in a number of case reports and small published series, so it is possible that these rectal carcinoids were the result of endocrine cell hyperplasia secondary to the chronic colitis, perhaps a similar situation to autoimmune gastritis where carcinoids are postulated to arise in fields of ECL-cell hyperplasia. We have seen a few cases of ulcerative colitis in which the endocrine cell hyperplasia was spectacular. We have no idea why this occurs. This is discussed in more detail below in the section on Hyperplasias. In some reports, the carcinoid tumors that occurred in ulcerative colitis patients were in the appendix and they were identical to the tiny incidental carcinoid tumors that are so often found in appendectomy specimens removed for the clinical features of acute appendicitis. Since there is no reason to suspect that such tiny appendiceal carcinoid tumors have anything to do with the acute appendicitis, there is no reason to suspect that they have anything to do with ulcerative colitis either. Similarly in Crohn's disease, there are reports of endocrine tumors, four of which were small appendiceal carcinoids and two of which were small tumors found incidentally in the small bowel at the time of resection.[102] Also there is a report of three high grade endocrine tumors mixed with adenocarcinomas in both UC and Crohn's colitis with adjacent high-grade dysplasia. These are undoubtedly adenocarcinomas with foci of endocrine cell differentiation, comparable to identical tumors that occur without precursor inflammatory diseases.[102] A small cell carcinoma arising in a colitic colon has also been reported, but many more cases are needed before we can make any association between the tumor and the colitis.[103]

HYPERPLASIAS

In the stomach, there are hyperplasias of ECL cells and G cells, but as far as we know, there is no D-cell hyperplasia. ECL hyperplasia is almost always a secondary phenomenon, the result of excess gastrin stimulation (hypergastrinemia) caused by two established abnormalities and a proposed third one as mentioned in the section on gastric carcinoid tumors. The first established cause of ECL-cell hyperplasia is hypergastrinemia secondary to loss of acid inhibition of gastrin secretion, as occurs in autoimmune atrophic gastritis. The second cause is a gastrin-producing carcinoid tumor (gastrinoma), which usually is in the duodenum and is part of the ZES. The postulated third cause is inability to make acid resulting in neutral gastric pH leading to permanent hypergastrinemia. The gastrin producing tumor and the acid secretory defect both result in marked parietal cell hypertrophy and hyperplasia. Of these three causes, the most common cause by far is autoimmune gastritis, a disease that destroys the parietal cells, leading to increased pH in the antrum and lack of inhibition of the G cells. This has been discussed in detail earlier in this chapter.

In regard to hyperplasia of gastrin cells (G cells), in current practice, the most common cause of by far is long-term proton pump inhibitor therapy. Prolonged inhibition of acid secretion by medications, mainly proton pump inhibitors, less often by H2 blockers, leads to G-cell hyperplasia, and there is evidence that there is an increase in the numbers of ECL cells as well, but not to the extent found in autoimmune gastritis. In patients on long-term protein pump inhibitors, G-cell hyperplasia is usually obvious even on H and E stained sections of gastric antrum. The G cells line up in large numbers from the tops of the mucus glands to the lower pits (Fig. 5-28).

There is also a primary G-cell hyperplasia, an extraordinarily rare condition that is associated with severe peptic ulcer disease, much like in the ZES.[104] In fact, it has even been designated as the "pseudo-ZES." The diagnosis requires proof that there is no gastrin producing tumor, and then fastidious counting of G cells is required with a bunch of normal antrums to serve as controls. There are too few cases of this primary hyperplasia for us to know if it affects the ECL cells.

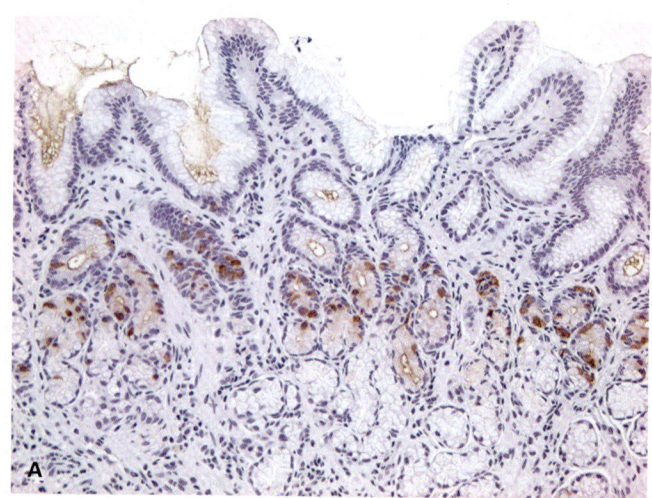

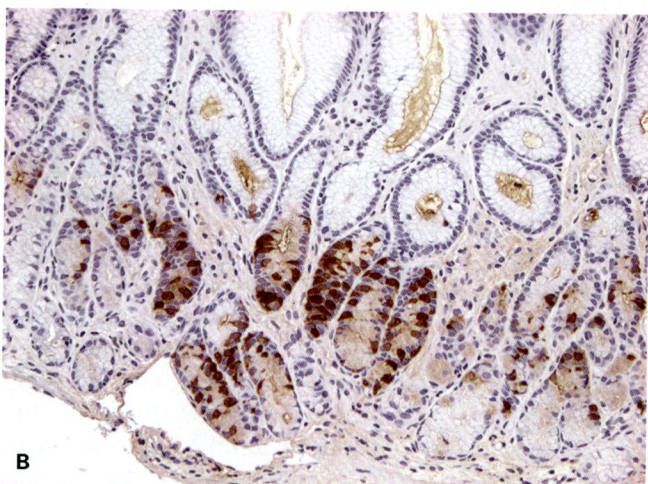

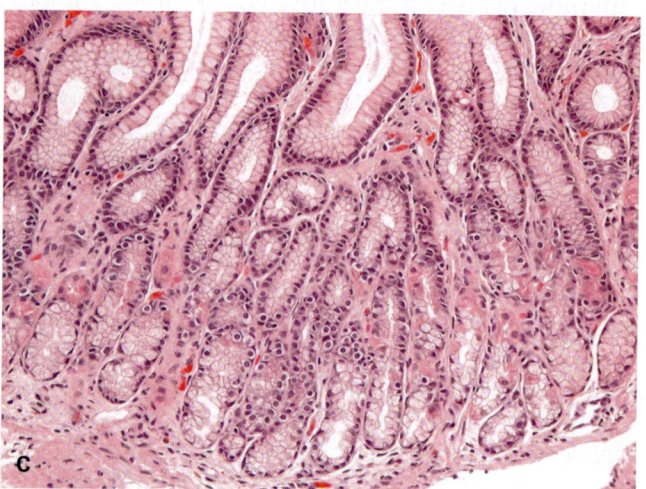

Figure 5-28. Antral gastrin producing cells (G cells). **A:** Gastrin immunostains of normal antrum. The G cells are in the middle of the mucosa in the necks and tops of the glands. **B:** Antrum in a patient on chronic proton pump inhibitor treatment. The G cells are much more numerous than in the normal antrum and they cover more of the glands. **C:** In florid cases of PPI effect, the increase in G cells is also obvious in the H&E sections as the many small cells with perinuclear halos on the outsides of the glands.

Hyperplasia of G cells in the duodenum occurs in MEN-I as discussed in the section on duodenal carcinoid tumors, and rarely in patients on long term PPIs or having Helicobacter.[48]

Hyperplasia of endocrine cells in the small intestine of patients with celiac sprue has been reported. These are predominantly the serotonin-producing cells or EC cells.[105] The reason for and importance of this hyperplasia is unknown.

Apparent hyperplasia of colonic endocrine cells seems to occur in some cases of ulcerative colitis (Fig. 5-29). We have seen a number of biopsies and resections of ulcerative colitis in its severely distorted phases when there are unusually large numbers of endocrine cells in the crypt bases. Perhaps it is comparable to the Paneth cell metaplasia and hyperplasia that is so common in long standing ulcerative colitis. Or perhaps it has something to do with the resistance of endocrine cells to destruction that seems to occur in a number of situations, including graft versus host disease (GVHD) and radiation injury. This may relate to the same things that cause the endocrine cells of the pancreas to persist

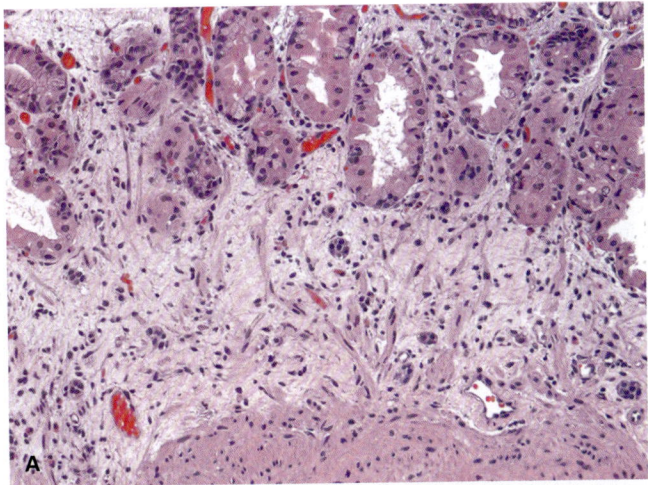
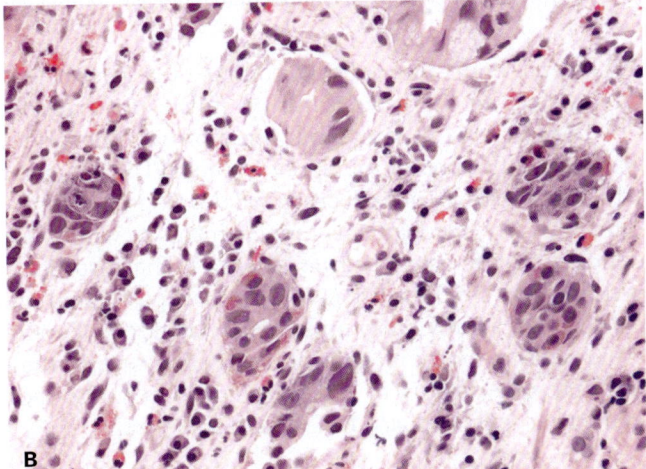

Figure 5-30. Persistent endocrine cells after severe mucosa injuries. **A:** Nests of endocrine cells in the base of the gastric mucosa in a patient with graft versus host disease. Note the marked parietal cell hypertrophy indicative of hypergasatrinemia. All of these changes could be associated with long-term PPI ingestion. **B:** Similar nests of endocrine cells at the base of the rectal mucosa following irradiation.

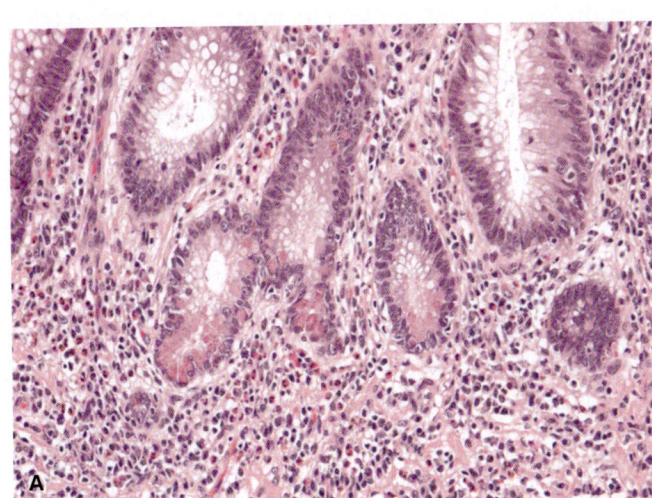
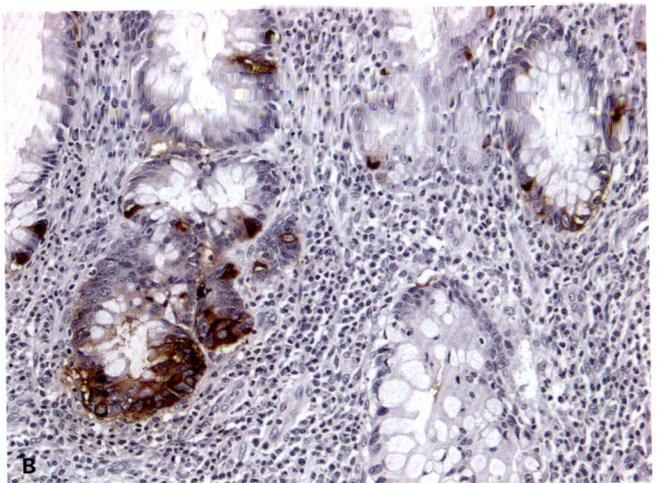

Figure 5-29. Striking increase in basally granulated endocrine cells in ulcerative colitis. **A:** H&E. **B:** Chromogranin immunostain.

and seem to increase in chronic pancreatitis. In GVHD and radiation injury, the crypts or glands at the base of the mucosa may be totally wiped out, but there may be clusters of residual endocrine cells (Fig. 5-30). The presence of too many endocrine cells in these injurious situations may not really be hyperplasias, but they may simply be persistent endocrine cells that were not destroyed by the injuries during their active phases.

ENTEROENDOCRINE CELL DYSGENESIS

Three male infants with severe congenital malabsorption for all nutrients except for water were reported to have almost total absence of endocrine cells in the small bowel and colon.[106] The endocrine cells that were still present had fewer chromogranin positive granules than

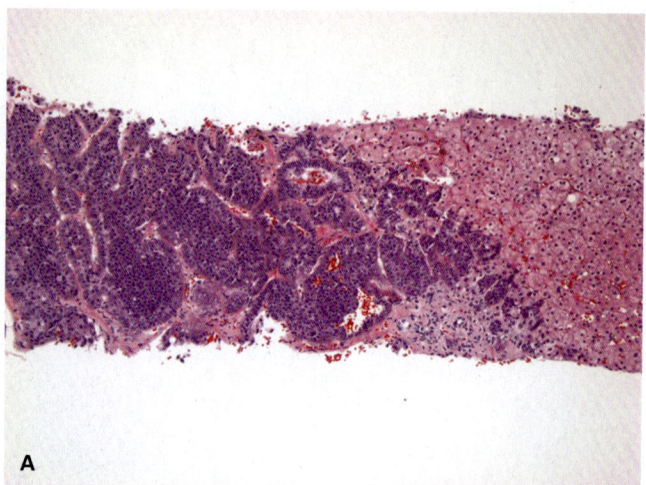
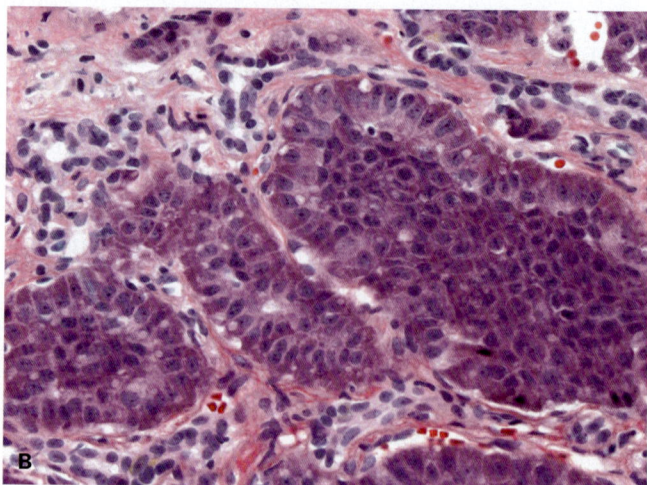

Figure 5-31. Metastatic endocrine neoplasm in the liver. **A:** Low power view. **B:** Nests of cells with granular cytoplasm.

did normal endocrine cells. In contrast, the gastrin producing cells in the gastric antrum in the two patients in whom they were evaluated were normal. The defect was the result of point mutations in the NEUROG3 gene which led to arrest of endocrine cell development in the intestines. The mechanism or mechanisms by which this deficiency of enteroendocrine cells led to malabsorption is not known, so the authors of the report postulated the existence of a "previously underappreciated role of endocrine cells in nutrient absorption." Patients with autoimmune enteropathy or IPEX syndrome may also lack endocrine cells, and also Paneth and goblet cells.

METASTATIC ENDOCRINE TUMORS WITH AN UNKNOWN PRIMARY

On occasions, a biopsy of a liver or a lymph node, or, much less commonly, other tissues, will contain a metastatic endocrine tumor. The obvious issue is determining the primary site. Primary hepatic endocrine tumors have been described, but such primary tumors are so rare that when an endocrine tumor is found in a liver biopsy, a metastasis is the overwhelming first option. In our experience, most of the time, our clinical colleagues have already performed all the requisite imaging studies in an attempt to find the primary, and in many cases they already know where it is, and it is usually the pancreas. Therefore, it has been our practice to find out if our clinical friends already know the primary site. In those cases in which they do not, the pancreas remains the most likely site for metastatic well-differentiated endocrine tumors that do not have cells with basal granules. However, for those tumors that do have basal granulated cells, the small bowel is the common site (Fig. 5-31). This has been supported by a study of 143 carcinoid tumors of unknown site presenting with their metastases.[107] If the clinicians want our help in finding the primary site, there are limited things that we pathologists can do. For the well-differentiated tumors, staining for various pancreatic and carinoid type hormones (such as insulin, gastrin, serotonin, glucagon, etc.) is often tried but is rarely useful. Intense positive staining for serotonin may be helpful, since it points to the small bowel as the likely source. Some studies have shown staining with TTF-1, PDX, CDX2, and NESP-55 may be helpful in differentiating metastatic carcinoids from various sites.[108,109] CDX2, an intestinal differentiation marker in nuclei, has been found to be strongly positive in small intestinal and appendiceal carcinoid tumors, but, peculiarly, it was only weakly positive in duodenal or rectal tumors, although they are also intestinal tumors[110] (Fig. 5-32). Weak positivity was also present in nonfunctioning pancreatic and gastric tumors. TTF-1 similarly

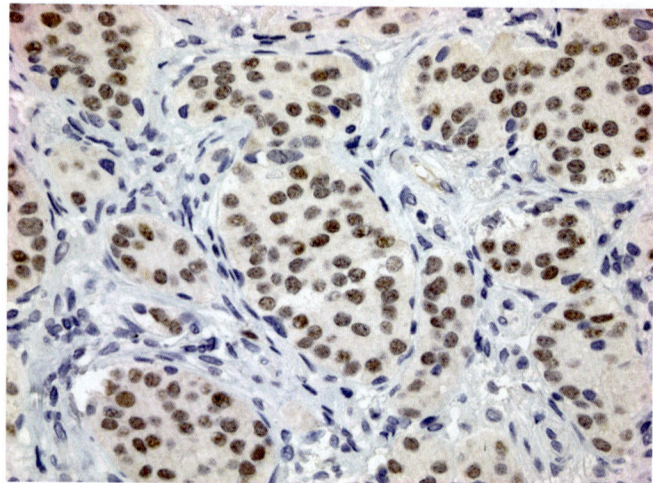

Figure 5-32. Positive nuclear staining of a metastatic endocrine tumor in the liver for CDX2, an intestinal differentiation marker, strongly suggests that the primary tumor is in the gut, most commonly the small intestine.

stains mostly pulmonary carcinoids, while PDX-1 is a marker for gastric, duodenal, and pancreatic endocrine tumors. NESP-55 is neurosecretory protein in the chromogranin family and shows granular cytoplasmic positivity in predominantly pancreatic endocrine tumors and tumors of adrenal medulla (pheochromocytomas).[109] So staining for these differentiation markers could be potentially helpful in the workup of metastatic endocrine tumors of unknown primary.

What about metastatic small cell carcinoma in a liver or lymph node? For small cell carcinomas, the odds overwhelmingly favor a primary in the lung, since the lung has more primary small cell carcinomas than all the other sites combined. If the primary is not in the lung, then everywhere else is a possibility, since small cell carcinomas arise virtually in every site in the body. As mentioned previously, the esophagus and colon are the most common GI sites. On rare occasions, such tumors present with metastases when they are small and clinically occult. At present, there do not seem to be any markers that separate pulmonary from extrapulmonary small cell carcinomas. For instance, thyroid transcription factor-1 (TTF1) was found to be positive in about 80% of both pulmonary and extrapulmonary small cell cancers.[111]

PRACTICAL APPROACHES TO GASTROINTESTINAL ENDOCRINE ABNORMALITIES

General Information

The endocrine tumors of stomach, duodenum, and rectum are usually first identified in endoscopic biopsies as are the occasional carcinoid tumors that arise in the distal-most terminal ileum. The large ileal tumors that produce symptoms, such as intestinal obstruction or the carcinoid syndrome, are found at the time of laparotomy. Virtually all appendiceal carcinoid tumors are incidental findings in appendectomies that are performed for the clinical syndrome of acute appendicitis. The various endocrine cell hyperplasias in the stomach are readily detected in biopsies.

Tumors

Since the most common endocrine abnormalities in the gut are the tumors, we need a systematic approach to them. The following are our recommendations and the justifications for those recommendations.

1. **What are the circumstances that allow us to suspect that a tumor is an endocrine tumor?**
   Carcinoids have the typical morphologic features mentioned in the text above. Usually, the growth patterns and cell type are so characteristic that they are readily detected by light microscopy. There is a limited light microscopic differential diagnosis. In our experience, the situation in which carcinoid tumors are most commonly misdiagnosed is in the rectum, where they are more likely to have a ribbon-like or a glandular growth pattern that is less typical for carcinoid tumors and may be confused with adenocarcinoma. Or, if a rectal carcinoid has an insular growth pattern, it may resemble the basaloid variant of anal transitional carcinoma which invades the distal rectum. Less experienced pathologists may not recognize these as carcinoid tumors. If a carcinoid tumor is not part of a pathologist's differential diagnosis of a submucosal tumor in the gut, then that tumor is not likely to be stained with endocrine markers. On the other hand, the endocrine markers (chromogranin and synaptophysin) are easily available in most labs and it does not harm to confirm the diagnosis in any suspected case of endocrine neoplasm. Further, chromogranin immunoreactivity may allow follow-up, with serum CGA measurements as a gauge to response to therapy.

   Gastrointestinal small cell carcinomas look much like their counterparts in the lung, so the same histologic features are applicable to them as they are to those in the lung. Since these tumors are so primitive and they mimic other primitive tumors such as large cell lymphomas, small cell melanomas, and anaplastic carcinomas of other types, it is sometimes helpful to stain them for a variety of tumor markers useful for evaluating undifferentiated neoplasms. These include lymphoma and melanoma markers, cytokeratins, and endocrine markers to prove their endocrine differentiation, so that the appropriate therapy will be given. However, many of these tumors do not express endocrine markers, so it may be necessary to make the diagnosis based on the histologic appearance coupled with negative lymphocyte, carcinoma, and melanoma markers. Electron microscopy may be useful in some cases; however, it is available only in limited centers.

   Large cell endocrine carcinomas are as much a diagnostic problem in the gut as they are in the lung. They appear mainly as anaplastic or undifferentiated carcinomas with subtle features of endocrine differentiation, such as the lack of any other kind of differentiation, their growth pattern with nests and occasional peripheral palisades, and the cytologic feature of nuclear molding in which one nucleus in indented by the nucleus of its neighbor. They may not express endocrine markers or only a few cells may stain positively, so this diagnosis is sometimes made with best intentions but with little substantiation.

2. **What is the preferred antibody for proving that a cell has endocrine differentiation?** Currently, there are four general endocrine antibodies: Chromogranin A, synaptophysin, CD56, and CD57 (Leu7). For the carcinoid tumors, chromogranin and synaptophysin antibodies are the most commonly used. We often use both, since some carcinoid tumors, particularly those in the rectum and the tubular carcinoids in the appendix, do not stain with one or the other. For the small cell carcinomas, CD56 stains most of them, whereas chromogranin and synaptophysin are much less predictable. CD56 also stains other nonendocrine tumor and tissues including lymphocytes and lymphomas that are sometimes part of the differential diagnosis of small cell carcinomas, and one should be cautious in using this as a sole evidence of endocrine differentiation. Small cell carcinomas can be easily differentiated from lymphomas when positive for CD56 as they are negative for other lymphocytic markers. CD57 stains some endocrine cells and tumors, but it is less predictable than the other three markers. Also noteworthy is that virtually all arise from an associated adenoma or carcinoma, and pure small cell endocrine carcinomas are virtually undescribed. Under these circumstances, one does well to consider metastases from lung primaries.

3. **Is it necessary to stain every carcinoid tumor to substantiate the fact that the cells are endocrine cells?** We do not believe that it is necessary to stain a tumor that is an obvious carcinoid tumor on H and E-stained sections. However, different pathologists may disagree on this point. Many pathologists choose to prove that suspected carcinoid tumors are just that by easily available endocrine markers, because positive staining adds to the comfort of making the diagnosis.

   For carcinoid tumors that are functional, the clinicians, rather than the pathologists, may want immunohistochemical confirmation that the resected tumor is the one producing the excessive hormone, peptide, or amine. In such cases, when we are asked to stain for the appropriate substance because the information is clinically important, we should do so.

4. **Don't forget to check the background or surrounding mucosa in every gastric carcinoid tumor. For almost all gastric carcinoids, this involves looking for changes in autoimmune atrophic gastritis**. These changes include not just glandular atrophy and intestinal or mucus gland metaplasia, or both, but also hyperplasia of the ECL cells at the base of the mucosa that may form small cellular balls or nodules. In fact, this nodular ECL-cell hyperplasia is probably the best hint of autoimmune gastritis, since it really does not occur in any other atrophic gastritis. This is a situation where we have found chromogranin staining to be useful. It brings out the ECL cells in all their glory and helps in determining if the ECL-cell nodules are big enough and infiltrative enough to qualify as carcinoid tumors according to current guidelines. These proliferations, as they expand, insinuate among the basal glands which are invariably metaplastic mucus glands, and the distinction between glands and endocrine cell clusters may be difficult. Chromogranin staining makes this distinction easy. In addition, if the carcinoid tumor is occurring in a background not of atrophy but of parietal cell hypertrophy and hyperplasia, then this may be a type II tumor or the recently described type IV tumor.

References

1. Nicholas A. Recherches sur l'epithelium de l'intestine. *Int Monatschr Anat Physiol.* 1891;8:1–62.
2. Kultschitzky N. Zur (rage unber den Bau des Darmkanals). *Arch Mikrosk Anat.* 1897;49(7):35.
3. Feyrter I. Uber diffuse endokrine epitheliale Organe. *Zentralbl Innere Med.* 1938;29:545–556.
4. Ciaccio C. Ricerche istologiche e citologiche sul timo degli uccelli. *Anat Anz.* 1906;29(597):600.
5. Schmidt JE. Beitrage zur normalen and pathologischen Histologic einiger Zellarten der Schleimhaut des menschilken Darmkanales. *Arch Mikrosk Anat.* 1905;36(12):40.
6. Masson P. La glande endocrine de l'intestine chez l'homme. *C R Acad Sci Paris.* 1914;158:59–61.
7. Masson P. Appendcite neurogene et carcinoides. *Ann Anat Pathol Medicochir.* 1924;1:3.
8. Pearse AG. Common cytochemical properties of cells producing polypeptide hormones, with particular reference to calcitonin and the thyroid C cells. *Vet Rec.* 1966;79(21):587–590.
9. Pearse AG. Common cytochemical and ultrastructural characteristics of cells producing polypeptide hormones (the APUD series) and their relevance to thyroid and ultimobranchial C cells and calcitonin. *Proc Roy Soc London B Biol Sci.* 1968;170(18):71–80.
10. Pearse AG, Chey WY, Brooks FP. Cytochemical and ultrastructural characteristics of cells producing polypeptide hormones and their relevance to gut hormones. *Endocrinol of the Gut.* Thorofare, NJ: Slack; 1974:24–34.
11. Pearse AG, Polak JM, Bloom SR. The diffuse neuroendocrine system and the APUD concept. *Gut Hormones.* Edinburgh, UK: Churchill Livingstone; 1978:33–39.
12. Pearse AG. The cytochemistry and ultrastructure of polypeptide hormone-producing cells of the APUD series and the embryologic, physiologic and pathologic implications of the concept [Review] [39 refs]. *J Histochem Cytochem.* 1969;17(5):303–313.
13. Pearse AG, Grossman MI, Brazier MA, Lechago J. The diffuse neuroendocrine system: falsification and verification of a concept. In: Grossman MI, Brazier MAB, Lechago J, eds. *Cellular Basis of Chemical Messengers in the Digestive System.* New York, NY: Academic Press; 1981:13–19.
14. Pearse AG, Polak JM. Neural crest origin of the endocrine polypeptide (APUD) cells of the gastrointestinal tract and pancreas. *Gut.* 1971;12(10):783–788.

15. LeDouarin N, Lelievre C. Sur l'origine des cellules a calcitonine du corps ultimobranchial de l'embryon d'Oiseau. *C R Assoc Anat.* 1971;152:558–586.
16. LeDouarin N, Bloom SR. The embryological origin of the endocrine cells associated with the digestive tract: experimental analysis based on the use of a stable cell marking technique. *Gut Hormones.* Edinburgh, UK: Churchill Livingstone; 1978:49–56.
17. Andrew A. Further evidence that enterochromaffin cells are not derived from the neural crest. *J Embryol Exp Morphol.* 1974;31(3):589–598.
18. Pictet RL, Rall LB, Phelps P, Rutter WJ. The neural crest and the origin of the insulin-producing and other gastrointestinal hormone-producing cells. *Science.* 1976;191(4223):191–192.
19. Leblond CP, Cheng H, Cairnie AB, et al. Identification of stem cells in the small intestine of the mouse. *Stem Cells of Renewing Cell Population.* New York, NY: Academic Press; 1976:7–31.
20. le Roux CW, Bloom SR. Peptide YY. Appetite and food intake [Review] [49 refs]. *Proc Nutr Soc.* 2005;64(2):213–216.
21. Fiocca R, Capella C, Buffa R, Fontana R, Solcia E, Hage E, et al. Glucagon-, glicentin-, and pancreatic polypeptide-like immunoreactivities in rectal carcinoids and related colorectal cells. *Am J Pathol.* 1980;100(1):81–92.
22. Fetissof F, Dubois MP, Assan R, et al. Endocrine cells in the anal canal. *Virchows Arch A Pathol Anat Histopathol.* 1984;404(1):39–47.
23. Kloppel G, Anlauf M. Epidemiology, tumour biology and histopathological classification of neuroendocrine tumours of the gastrointestinal tract [Review] [43 refs]. *Best Pract Res Clin Gastroenterol.* 2005;19(4):507–517.
24. Modlin IM, Kidd M, Latich I, et al. Current status of gastrointestinal carcinoids [Review] [331 refs]. *Gastroenterology.* 2005;128(6):1717–1751.
25. D'Adda T, Pizzi S, Azzoni C, et al. Different patterns of 11q allelic losses in digestive endocrine tumors. *Hum Pathol.* 2002;33(3):322–329.
26. Oberndorfer S. Karzinoide tumoren des Dunndarms. *Frankf Z Pathol.* 1907(1):426–432.
27. Modlin IM, Lye KD, Kidd M. A 5-decade analysis of 13,715 carcinoid tumors. *Cancer.* 2003;97(4):934–959.
28. Soga J. Early-stage carcinoids of the gastrointestinal tract: an analysis of 1914 reported cases. *Cancer.* 2005;103(8):1587–1595.
29. Edge SB, Byrd DR, Compton CC, Fritz AG, et al. *American Joint Committee on Cancer Cancer Staging Manual.* 7th ed. New York, NY: Spinger; 2010.
30. Lindberg GM, Molberg KH, Vuitch MF, Bores-Saavedra J. Atypical carcinoid of the esophagus: a case report and review of the literature [Review] [21 refs]. *Cancer.* 1997;79(8):1476–1481.
31. Hoang MP, Hobbs CM, Sobin LH, Bores-Saavedra J. Carcinoid tumor of the esophagus: a clinicopathologic study of four cases [Review] [22 refs]. *Am J Surg Pathol.* 2002;26(4):517–522.
32. Delle FG, Capurso G, Milione M, Panzuto F. Endocrine tumours of the stomach [Review] [63 refs]. *Best Pract Res Clin Gastroenterol.* 2005;19(5):659–673.
33. Capella C, Solcia E, Sobin L, Arnold R, et al. Endocrine tumours of the appendix. *Pathology and Genetics Tumours of the Digestive System, World Health Organization Classification of Tumours.* Lyon, France: IARC Press; 2000:53–57.
34. Norton JA, Melcher ML, Gibril F, Jensen RT. Gastric carcinoid tumors in multiple endocrine neoplasia-1 patients with Zollinger–Ellison syndrome can be symptomatic, demonstrate aggressive growth, and require surgical treatment. *Surgery.* 2004;136(6):1267–1274.
35. Bordi C, Corleto VD, Azzoni C, et al. The antral mucosa as a new site for endocrine tumors in multiple endocrine neoplasia type 1 and Zollinger–Ellison syndromes. *J Clin Endocrinol Metab.* 2001;86(5):2236–2242.
36. Hirschowitz BI, Griffith J, Pellegrin D, Cummings OW. Rapid regression of enterochromaffinlike cell gastric carcinoids in pernicious anemia after antrectomy. *Gastroenterology.* 1992;102(4:Pt 1):1409–1418.
37. Eckhauser FE, Lloyd RV, Thompson NW, et al. Antrectomy for multicentric, argyrophil gastric carcinoids: a preliminary report. *Surgery.* 1988;104(6):1046–1053.
38. Richards ML, Gauger P, Thompson NW, Giordano TJ. Regression of type II gastric carcinoids in multiple endocrine neoplasia type 1 patients with Zollinger–Ellison syndrome after surgical excision of all gastrinomas. *World J Surg.* 2004;28(7):652–658.
39. Abraham SC, Carney JA, Ooi A, et al. Achlorhydria, parietal cell hyperplasia, and multiple gastric carcinoids: a new disorder [see comment]. *Am J Surg Pathol.* 2005;29(7):969–975.
40. Bordi C, Falchetti A, Azzoni C, et al. Aggressive forms of gastric neuroendocrine tumors in multiple endocrine neoplasia type I. *Am J Surg Pathol.* 1997;21(9):1075–1082.
41. Anlauf M, Perren A, Meyer CL, et al. Precursor lesions in patients with multiple endocrine neoplasia type 1-associated duodenal gastrinomas. *Gastroenterology.* 2005;128(5):1187–1198.
42. Dayal Y, Doos WG, O'Brien MJ, et al. Psammomatous somatostatinomas of the duodenum. *Am J Surg Pathol.* 1983;7(7):653–665.
43. Dayal Y, Tallberg KA, Nunnemacher G, et al. Duodenal carcinoids in patients with and without neurofibromatosis. A comparative study. *Am J Surg Pathol.* 1986;10(5):348–357.
44. Burke AP, Federspiel BH, Sobin LH, et al. Carcinoids of the duodenum. A histologic and immunohistochemical study of 65 tumors. *Am J Surg Pathol.* 1989;13(10):828–837.
45. Burke AP, Sobin LH, Shekitka KM, et al. Somatostatin-producing duodenal carcinoids in patients with von Recklinghausen's neurofibromatosis. A predilection for black patients. *Cancer.* 1990;65(7):1591–1595.
46. Burke AP, Sobin LH, Federspiel BH, et al. Carcinoid tumors of the duodenum. A clinicopathologic study of 99 cases. *Arch Pathol Lab Med.* 1990;114(7):700–704.
47. Heymann MF, Hamy A, Triau S, et al. Endocrine tumors of the duodenum. A study of 55 cases relative to clinicopathological features and hormone content. *Hepato-Gastroenterology.* 2004;51(59):1367–1371.
48. Merchant SH, VanderJagt T, Lathrop S, Amin MB. Sporadic duodenal bulb gastrin-cell tumors: association with *Helicobacter pylori* gastritis and long-term use of proton pump inhibitors. *Am J Surg Pathol.* 2006;30(12):1581–1587.
49. Scholthauer BW, Nora FE, Lechago J, et al. Duodenal gangliocytic paraganglioma. Clinicopathologic and immunocytochemical study of 11 cases. *Am J Clin Pathol.* 1986;86(5):559–565.
50. Burke AP, Helwig EB. Gangliocytic paraganglioma. *Am J Clin Pathol.* 1989;92(1):1–9.
51. Burke AP, Thomas RM, Elsayed AM, Sobin LH. Carcinoids of the jejunum and ileum: an immunohistochemical and clinicopathologic study of 167 cases. *Cancer.* 1997;79(6):1086–1093.
52. Eckhauser FE, Argenta LC, Strodel WE, et al. Mesenteric angiopathy, intestinal gangrene, and midgut carcinoids. *Surgery.* 1981;90(4):720–728.
53. Zhang PJ, Furth EE, Cai X, et al. The role of beta-catenin, TGF beta 3, NGF2, FGF2, IGFR2, and BMP4 in the

pathogenesis of mesenteric sclerosis and angiopathy in midgut carcinoids. *Hum Pathol.* 2004;35(6):670–674.
54. Allibone RO, Hoffman J, Gosney JR, Helliwell TR. Granulation tissue polyposis associated with carcinoid tumours of the small intestine. *Histopathology.* 1993;22(5): 475–480.
55. Abrahams NA, Vesoulis Z, Petras RE. Angiogenic polypoid proliferation adjacent to ileal carcinoid tumors: a nonspecific finding related to mucosal prolapse. *Mod Pathol.* 2001;14(9):821–827.
56. Yantiss RK, Odze RD, Farraye FA, Rosenberg AE. Solitary versus multiple carcinoid tumors of the ileum: a clinical and pathologic review of 68 cases [see comment]. *Am J Surg Pathol.* 2003;27(6):811–817.
57. Yarze JC, Herlihy KJ, Coombes JM, et al. Detection of asymptomatic ileal carcinoid tumors during ileal intubation at screening colonoscopy: a case series. *Am J Gastroenterol.* 2009;104(12):3114–3115.
58. Stinner B, Rothmund M. Neuroendocrine tumours (carcinoids) of the appendix [Review] [32 refs]. *Best Pract Res Clin Gastroenterol.* 2005;19(5):729–738.
59. Burke AP, Sobin LH, Federspiel BH, et al. Goblet cell carcinoids and related tumors of the vermiform appendix. *Am J Clin Pathol.* 1990;94(1):27–35.
60. Moertel CG, Weiland LH, Nagorney DM, Dockerty MB. Carcinoid tumor of the appendix: treatment and prognosis. *N Engl J Med.* 1987;317(27):1699–1701.
61. Rossi G, Valli R, Bertolini F, et al. Does mesoappendix infiltration predict a worse prognosis in incidental neuroendocrine tumors of the appendix? A clinicopathologic and immunohistochemical study of 15 cases. *Am J Clin Pathol.* 2003;120(5):706–711.
62. Federspiel BH, Burke AP, Sobin LH, Shekitka KM. Rectal and colonic carcinoids. A clinicopathologic study of 84 cases. *Cancer.* 1990;65(1):135–140.
63. Ballantyne GH, Savoca PE, Flannery JT, et al. Incidence and mortality of carcinoids of the colon. Data from the Connecticut Tumor Registry. *Cancer.* 1992;69(10):2400–2405.
64. Koura AN, Giacco GG, Curley SA, et al. Carcinoid tumors of the rectum: effect of size, histopathology, and surgical treatment on metastasis free survival. *Cancer.* 1997;79(7):1294–1298.
65. Kobayashi K, Katsumata T, Yoshizawa S, et al. Indications of endoscopic polypectomy for rectal carcinoid tumors and clinical usefulness of endoscopic ultrasonography [see comment]. *Dis Colon Rectum.* 2005;48(2):285–291.
66. Azumi N, Traweek ST, Battifora H. Prostatic acid phosphatase in carcinoid tumors. Immunohistochemical and immunoblot studies [see comment]. *Am J Surg Pathol.* 1991;15(8):785–790.
67. Kimura N, Sasano N. Prostate-specific acid phosphatase in carcinoid tumors. *Virchows Arch A Pathol Anat Histopathol.* 1986;410(3):247–251.
68. Japanese Society for Esophageal D. *Guidelines for Clinical and Pathologic Studies on Carcinoma of the Esophagus.* Tokyo, Japan: Kanehara & Co; 2001.
69. Law SY, Fok M, Lam KY, et al. Small cell carcinoma of the esophagus. *Cancer.* 1994;73(12):2894–2899.
70. Casas F, Ferrer F, Farrus B, et al. Primary small cell carcinoma of the esophagus: a review of the literature with emphasis on therapy and prognosis [Review] [78 refs]. *Cancer.* 1997;80(8):1366–1372.
71. Jiang SX, Mikami T, Umezawa A, et al. Gastric large cell neuroendocrine carcinomas: a distinct clinicopathologic entity. *Am J Surg Pathol.* 2006;30(8):945–953.
72. Shia J, Tang LH, Weiser MR, et al. Is nonsmall cell type high-grade neuroendocrine carcinoma of the tubular gastrointestinal tract a distinct disease entity? *Am J Surg Pathol.* 2008;32(5):719–731.
73. Takubo K. Undiffrentiated carcinoma. In: Takubo K, ed. *Pathology of the Esophagus (An Atlas & Textbook).* 2nd ed. Hongkong: Spinger; 2007:224–234.
74. Bennouna J, Bardet E, Deguiral P, Douillard JY. Small cell carcinoma of the esophagus: analysis of 10 cases and review of the published data [Review] [29 refs]. *Am J Clin Oncol.* 2000;23(5):455–459.
75. Hosokawa A, Shimada Y, Matsumura Y, et al. Small cell carcinoma of the esophagus. Analysis of 14 cases and literature review [Review] [16 refs]. *Hepato-Gastroenterology.* 2005;52(66):1738–1741.
76. Medgyesy DC, Wolff TA, Putnam JB Jr, Ajani JA. Small cell carcinoma of the esophagus. The University of Texas MD Anderson Cancer Center experience and the literature review. *Cancer.* 1999;88:262–267.
77. Takubo K, Nakamura K, Sawabe M, et al. Primary undifferentiated small cell carcinoma of the esophagus. *Hum Pathol.* 1999;30(2):216–221.
78. Wu A, Ma JY, Yand JJ, et al. Primary small cell carcinoma of the esophagus: report of 9 cases. *World J Gastroenterol.* 2004;10:3680–3682.
79. Bernick PE, Klimstra DS, Shia J, et al. Neuroendocrine carcinomas of the colon and rectum. *Dis Colon Rectum.* 2004;47(2):163–169.
80. Burke AB, Shekitka KM, Sobin LH. Small cell carcinomas of the large intestine. *Am J Clin Pathol.* 1991;95(3):315–321.
81. Gaffey MJ, Mills SE, Lack EE. Neuroendocrine carcinoma of the colon and rectum. A clinicopathologic, ultrastructural, and immunohistochemical study of 24 cases. *Am J Surg Pathol.* 1990;14(11):1010–1023.
82. Grabowski P, Schonfelder J, hnert-Hilger G, et al. Expression of neuroendocrine markers: a signature of human undifferentiated carcinoma of the colon and rectum. *Virchows Arch.* 2002;441(3):256–263.
83. Mills SE, Allen MS Jr, Cohen AR. Small-cell undifferentiated carcinoma of the colon. A clinicopathological study of five cases and their association with colonic adenomas. *Am J Surg Pathol.* 1983;7(7):643–651.
84. Wick MR, Weatherby RP, Weiland LH. Small cell neuroendocrine carcinoma of the colon and rectum: clinical, histologic, and ultrastructural study and immunohistochemical comparison with cloacogenic carcinoma. *Hum Pathol.* 1987;18(1):9–21.
85. Gibbs NM. Incidence and significance of argentaffin and paneth cells in some tumours of the large intestine. *J Clin Pathol.* 1967;20(6):826–831.
86. Van den Ingh HF, Van den Broek LJ, Verhofstad AA, Bosman FT. Neuroendocrine cells in colorectal adenomas. *J Pathol.* 1986;148(3):231–237.
87. Waldum HL, Aase S, Kvetnoi I, et al. Neuroendocrine differentiation in human gastric carcinoma. *Cancer.* 1998;83(3):435–444.
88. Lewin K. Carcinoid tumors and the mixed (composite) glandular-endocrine cell carcinomas. *Am J Surg Pathol.* 1987;11(suppl 1):71–86.
89. Hamada Y, Oishi A, Shoji T, et al. Endocrine cells and prognosis in patients with colorectal carcinoma. *Cancer.* 1992;69(11):2641–2646.
90. Foley EF, Gaffey MJ, Frierson HF Jr. The frequency and clinical significance of neuroendocrine cells within stage III adenocarcinomas of the colon. *Arch Pathol Lab Med.* 1998;122(10):912–914.
91. Pulitzer M, Xu R, Suriawinata AA, et al. Microcarcinoids in large intestinal adenomas. *Am J Surg Pathol.* 2006;30(12):1531–1536.

92. Jain D, Eslami-Varzaneh F, Takano AM, et al. Composite glandular and endocrine tumors of the stomach with pancreatic acinar differentiation. *Am J Surg Pathol.* 2005;29(11):1524–1529.
93. Hernandez FJ, Reid JD. Mixed carcinoid and mucus-secreting intestinal tumors. *Arch Pathol Lab Med.* 1969;88(5):489–496.
94. Toker C. Observations on the composition of certain colonic tumors. *Cancer.* 1969;24(2):256–260.
95. Klappenbach RS, Kurman RJ, Sinclair CF, James LP. Composite carcinoma-carcinoid tumors of the gastrointestinal tract. A morphologic, histochemical, and immunocytochemical study. *Am J Clin Pathol.* 1985;84(2):137–143.
96. Moyana TN, Qizilbash AH, Murphy F. Composite glandular-carcinoid tumors of the colon and rectum. Report of two cases. *Am J Surg Pathol.* 1988;12(8):607–611.
97. Shia J, Tickoo SK, Guillem JG, et al. Increased endocrine cells in treated rectal adenocarcinomas: a possible reflection of endocrine differentiation in tumor cells induced by chemotherapy and radiotherapy [erratum appears in Am J Surg Pathol. 2002 Sep;26(9):1241]. *Am J Surg Pathol.* 2002;26(7):863–872.
98. Aoki S, Watanabe M, Hasegawa H, et al. Rectal carcinoid arising in ulcerative colitis associated with rectal adenocarcinoma. *J Gastroenterol.* 2004;39(7):697–698.
99. Quinn P, Platell CF. Resolving microcarcinoids in ulcerative colitis: report of a case. *Dis Colon Rectum.* 2004;47(3):387–391.
100. Stewart CJ, Matsumoto T, Jo Y, et al. Multifocal microcarcinoid tumours in ulcerative colitis [comment]. *J Clin Pathol.* 2005;58(1):111–112.
101. Greenstein AJ, Balasubramanian S, Harpaz N, et al. Carcinoid tumor and inflammatory bowel disease: a study of eleven cases and review of the literature [Review] [37 refs]. *Am J Gastroenterol.* 1997;92(4):682–685.
102. Sigel JE, Goldblum JR. Neuroendocrine neoplasms arising in inflammatory bowel disease: a report of 14 cases. *Mod Pathol.* 1998;11(6):537–542.
103. Yaziji H, Broghamer WL Jr. Primary small cell undifferentiated carcinoma of the rectum associated with ulcerative colitis. *South Med J.* 1996;89(9):921–924.
104. Tomaszewska R, Kedra B, Stachura J. Hypertrophic gastritis, primary diffuse G-cell hyperplasia and pancreatic metaplasia of the gastric mucosa (pseudo-Zollinger-Ellison syndrome)—case report. *Pol J Pathol.* 2000;51(1):51–54.
105. Moyana TN, Shukoor S. Gastrointestinal endocrine cell hyperplasia in celiac disease: a selective proliferative process of serotonergic cells. *Mod Pathol.* 1991;4(4):419–423.
106. Cortina G, Smart CN, Farmer DG, et al. Enteroendocrine cell dysgenesis and malabsorption, a histopathologic and immunohistochemical characterization. *Hum Pathol.* 2007;38(4):570–580.
107. Kirshbom PM, Kherani AR, Onaitis MW, et al. Carcinoids of unknown origin: comparative analysis with foregut, midgut, and hindgut carcinoids. *Surgery.* 1998;124(6):1063–1070.
108. Srivastava A, Hornick JL. Immunohistochemical staining for CDX-2, PDX-1, NESP-55, and TTF-1 can help distinguish gastrointestinal carcinoid tumors from pancreatic endocrine and pulmonary carcinoid tumors. *Am J Surg Pathol.* 2009;33(4):626–632.
109. Srivastava A, Padilla O, Fischer-Colbrie R, et al. Neuroendocrine secretory protein-55 (NESP-55) expression discriminates pancreatic endocrine tumors and pheochromocytomas from gastrointestinal and pulmonary carcinoids. *Am J Surg Pathol.* 2004;28(10):1371–1378.
110. Barbareschi M, Roldo C, Zamboni G, et al. CDX-2 homeobox gene product expression in neuroendocrine tumors: its role as a marker of intestinal neuroendocrine tumors. *Am J Surg Pathol.* 2004;28(9):1169–1176.
111. Kaufmann O, Dietel M. Expression of thyroid transcription factor-1 in pulmonary and extrapulmonary small cell carcinomas and other neuroendocrine carcinomas of various primary sites. *Histopathology.* 2000;36(5):415–420.

6 Motility Disorders

Chapter Outline

DIVERTICULAR DISEASE OF THE SMALL AND LARGE INTESTINES
- Definition
- Terminology

LARGE BOWEL DIVERTICULAR DISEASE (DIVERTICULOSIS OF THE COLON)
- Definitions
- Pathogenesis
- Clinical Features
- Endoscopy
- Imaging
- Gross Pathology
  - Prediverticular disease
  - Handling of specimens
- Histology
  - Defining diverticulitis

POLYPS AND NEOPLASMS ASSOCIATED WITH AND WITHIN DIVERTICULA
- Diverticular Polyps
  - Inverted diverticulum
- Other Polyps
  - Carcinoma in diverticular disease

DIVERTICULAR DISEASE AND ENDOMETRIOSIS

DIVERTICULAR DISEASE AND IBD
- Differential Diagnosis and Clinical Implications

DIVERTICULOSIS OF THE CECUM AND PROXIMAL COLON (RIGHT-SIDED DIVERTICULOSIS)
- Pathogenesis
- Clinical Features
- Pathology

DIVERTICULOSIS OF THE DUODENUM AND SMALL INTESTINE
- Pathogenesis
- Duodenal Diverticula (Single or Isolated)
  - Extraluminal diverticula
  - Intraluminal duodenal diverticulum (prolapsed diaphragm)
- Jejunoileal Diverticula
  - Pathogenesis and clinical features
  - Gross appearance
  - Histology
- Meckel's Diverticulum

GASTROINTESTINAL MOTILITY DISORDERS
- The Normal Motility Apparatus of the Gut
- Musculature of the Gut
- Demonstration of Smooth Muscle in Motility Disorders

ENTERIC NERVOUS SYSTEM
- Interstitial Cells of Cajal

MOTILITY DISORDERS

ESOPHAGEAL DISORDERS
- Achalasia (Cardiospasm)
  - Gross appearance
  - Histology
- Secondary Achalasia

OTHER MOTOR DISORDERS OF THE ESOPHAGUS

MOTOR DISORDERS OF THE STOMACH
- Pyloric Stenosis
  - Infantile pyloric stenosis (congenital hypertrophic pyloric stenosis)
  - Adult pyloric stenosis
- Gastroparesis

INTESTINAL PSEUDOOBSTRUCTION
- Definition
  - Acute intestinal pseudoobstruction
  - Ogilvie's syndrome
- Pathogenesis and Clinical Presentation of Chronic Pseudoobstruction
  - Chronic intestinal pseudoobstruction

CHRONIC IDIOPATHIC (PRIMARY) INTESTINAL PSEUDOOBSTRUCTION
- Examining Resections for CIIP
- Familial or Sporadic Visceral Myopathy
  - Pathology
  - Gross appearance
  - Histology
- α-Smooth Muscle Actin Deficiency
- Familial Visceral Myopathy with α-SMA–Positive Inclusion Bodies
  - Differential diagnosis
- Desmin Myopathy
- African Visceral Myopathy
- Issues Reporting Motility Disorders

PRIMARY VISCERAL NEUROPATHIES
- Familial Visceral Neuropathy
- Paraneoplastic Syndromes
- Sporadic Visceral Neuropathy
  - Differential diagnosis
- Abnormalities of Interstitial Cells of Cajal
  - Hyperplasia of ICCs
  - Prognosis and therapy of CIIP
- Diffuse Lymphoid Infiltration
- Diffuse Eosinophilic Infiltrate
- Slow Transit Constipation: Severe Idiopathic Constipation

HIRSCHSPRUNG'S DISEASE
- Clinical Presentation and Features
- Etiology and Pathogenesis
- Gross Appearance
- Histology
- Diagnosis of Hirschsprung's Disease
  - Types of biopsy
  - Intraoperative frozen section
- Variants of Hirschsprung's Disease

INTESTINAL NEURONAL DYSPLASIA

INTERNAL SPHINCTER ACHALASIA (ULTRASHORT HIRSCHSPRUNG'S DISEASE)

MEGACYSTIS MICROCOLON INTESTINAL HYPOPERISTALSIS
- Diagnosis
- Immature Ganglia
- Mural Eosinophils in Hirschsprung's Disease

IDIOPATHIC MEGACOLON

SEVERE IDIOPATHIC CONSTIPATION

ACQUIRED VISCERAL NEUROPATHIES
- Toxic or Drug-Induced Visceral Neuropathy

Inflammatory Visceral Neuropathy
  (Acquired Aganglionosis)
Chagas' Disease (American
  Trypanosomiasis)
  Gross appearance
  Histology
  Differential diagnosis
Paraneoplastic Neuropathy
Miscellaneous Visceral Neuropathies
GI Manifestations Secondary to
  Neurologic Disorders of the Brain and
  Spinal Cord

CHRONIC INTESTINAL
PSEUDOOBSTRUCTION ASSOCIATED
WITH GENERALIZED DISEASE AND THE
MUSCULAR DYSTROPHIES
Myotonic Muscular Dystrophy
  Histology
Progressive Muscular Dystrophy
Acquired Jejunal Diverticulosis
SOLITARY RECTAL ULCER SYNDROME
OF THE RECTUM AND INFLAMMATORY
CLOACOGENIC POLYP (MUCOSAL
PROLAPSE SYNDROMES)
Gross and Endoscopic Appearances

Histology
Differential Diagnosis
Proctitis (localized colitis) cystica
  profunda (hamartomatous inverted
  polyp of the rectum)
  Gross and endoscopic appearances
  Pathogenesis and histology
  Nuclear atypicality, dysplasia, and carcinoma
  Inflammatory cloacogenic polyp
Irritable Bowel Syndrome
  Pathology of irritable bowel syndrome
  Mastocytic enterocolitis
  Role of the pathologist

DIVERTICULAR DISEASE OF THE SMALL AND LARGE INTESTINES

Definition

Intestinal diverticula are outpouchings, herniations, or protrusions (all tend to be sued as synonyms) of mucosa and submucosa through areas of relative weakness in the bowel wall, usually immediately adjacent to the arterioles that penetrate the bowel wall. Less commonly, they consist of herniations of all layers of the intestine, sometimes referred to as "congenital," which is usually correct. Pseudodiverticulosis refers to apparent diverticula, especially seen on imaging, which are the result of eccentricity, often fibrosis in the bowel wall that resemble diverticula, being outpouchings of the bowel wall, but retain all layers of the bowel.

Terminology

The singular is diverticulum and the plural diverticula.

Note: The frequently used plurals of diverticulae and diverticuli are both incorrect and should therefore not be used, especially by pathologists and clinicians purporting to have a gastrointestinal (GI) interest or expertise! We all have too many areas of relative ignorance to make overt errors over simple things. Diverticular disease is fine as, of course, is diverticulitis and diverticulosis.

Diverticula occur in all parts of the GI tract, specifically the duodenum, jejunum, the ileum including Meckel's diverticulum, in the appendix, and large bowel. Meckel's diverticulum is described in Chapter 16 and diverticula of the appendix in Chapter 15.

LARGE BOWEL DIVERTICULAR DISEASE (DIVERTICULOSIS OF THE COLON)

This is a very common acquired disorder of the colon, most prevalent in the Western Hemisphere.[1] It is characterized by a markedly thickened muscularis propria, through which herniations of the mucosa and submucosa pass through the muscularis propria into the subserosal connective tissue. The diverticula are distributed predominantly in the sigmoid and descending colon, although they may be found throughout the colon.

Clinically, the condition may be symptomatic or asymptomatic. There is not a good correlation between symptoms and pathologic findings unless there are inflammatory complications such as diverticulitis, abscess formation, or perforation. Diverticula may be the site of polyps or tumor, both within it and at their opening, although these are rare.

Definitions

The term *diverticular disease* has been used in two ways in the large bowel: (1) generically, to refer to all colons with diverticula, irrespective of whether there is an accompanying inflammation or not, and (2) specifically to refer to colonic diverticula with complications, such as inflammation and hemorrhage. We prefer the former definition and have used *diverticular disease* in a generic sense in this chapter.

Diverticulosis refers to a colon with uncomplicated diverticula, and *diverticulitis* is that condition in which diverticula are associated with inflammation and its complications. In the large bowel there are two forms of diverticular disease, namely, (1) the more common *left-sided diverticula*, which predominate in the sigmoid colon but may also be diffuse involving the entire colon, and (2) *right-sided diverticula,* which are rare in North America and Europe but common in other parts of the world, such as Asia where it is the predominant form of the disease.[2-4] These can also extend to the left colon. Thus, there appear to be two distinct conditions, one being primary right-sided diverticular disease that sometimes extends to the left colon and the other, left-sided disease that sometimes extends to the right colon. When the disease is pancolonic, recognition of the underlying type may become problematic.

Several clinical situations or syndromes are generally recognized and can occur in all diverticula irrespective of location:

1. Diverticulosis—the asymptomatic presence of multiple colonic diverticula
2. Painful diverticula—symptoms associated with uncomplicated diverticula
3. Diverticulitis—associated with inflammation in one or more of the diverticula. This may result in perforation with abscess or fistula formation.
4. Hemorrhage—often associated with right-sided diverticula but also occurs in the left colon and is often arterial, so associated with bright red blood
5. Diverticular colitis—which is a form of inflammatory bowel disease (IBD) affecting the region of the diverticula. The condition and its differential diagnosis are discussed later and in more detail with IBD chapter (see Chapter 18).

Pathogenesis

The *prevalence* of diverticulosis varies greatly in different geographic areas of the world. It is most common in the Western Hemisphere and rare in Africa, Asia, and many parts of South America. In the Western Hemisphere, diverticular disease has an overall frequency of 15% to 35% using barium studies and is primarily left sided[5,6] and up to 50% to 70% by age 75. In the West, about 95% of patients have disease involving the sigmoid and left colon, but with age, they occur progressively more proximally. Right-sided diverticular disease is therefore found in older patients with pan-diverticular disease.[7]

In Southeast Asia, right sided diverticular disease is the most frequent form of diverticular disease and has a barium enema frequency of 8% to 22% and affects the right side of the colon in 70% to 98% of patients.[8,9] In sub-Saharan Africa, diverticular disease is uncommon and affects mostly the right colon.[10-12]

Interestingly, the risk of diverticular disease in black Africans living in Western countries is higher than that in their indigenous counterparts.[4] The risk of diverticular disease is related to a patient's age and ethnicity.[4] Men and women are equally affected.[4]

In Western countries, diverticulosis is uncommon before the age of 40. Diverticular disease incidence increases progressively,[4] so that by age 90 about 50% of the population have it. Men and women are equally affected.

The *pathogenesis* of diverticulosis is not well understood and is likely multifactorial. Evidence suggests dietary fiber may be protective as one of the major differences between the populations of areas of low and high incidence is diet. In the Western Hemisphere, diets tend to be highly refined and fiber deficient, compared with those of African countries, which have a diet high in vegetable fiber and low in refined carbohydrates.[13] The incidence of diverticula increases when people migrate from low-prevalence areas to Westernized communities, for example, among Japanese migrants to Hawaii.[2,4] Also it has been found that the prevalence of diverticulosis in vegetarians is three times less than in nonvegetarians.[14] Even rats fed with low-fiber diet seem to develop diverticulosis more frequently compared to controls.[15,16] The question is: How does a low-residue diet result in diverticulosis? For diverticula to develop, two requirements are necessary: (1) increased intraluminal pressure of the colon and (2) points of relative weakness in the bowel wall through which the bowel mucosa protrudes to form diverticula:

1. It has been postulated that people with high-fiber diets have increased stool bulk, which increases the tone of the bowel wall, resulting in faster intestinal transit with more frequent stools and less fecal stasis. In contrast, lack of dietary residue (i.e., fecal bulk) has been postulated to produce irregular and uncoordinated peristalsis, which converts the colon into a series of saccules sealed off from one another by a valvular mechanism produced by alternating and overlapping semicircular arcs of thickened circular muscle. This is thought to result in a markedly increased intraluminal pressure, hypertrophy of the muscularis propria, and consequent diverticular outpouchings.[17] Another interesting hypothesis put forward for increased intraluminal pressure is related to the posture during defecation. It has been suggested that the natural position for defecation for human is squatting, where the rectum and sigmoid are more aligned in a straight line requiring less intraluminal pressure for the passage of stools from sigmoid to rectum. In contrast, in the sitting position, the rectosigmoid angle is close to 90 degrees requiring higher intraluminal pressure for defecation. This would also explain the lower rates of diverticulosis in parts of the world where defecation in sitting position is still the preferred mode, while diverticulosis is far more common in Western societies or

in populations in developing countries who have been increasingly adopting Western lifestyle.[18-20] Muscular thickening of the bowel wall usually accompanies diverticulosis, but it is still unclear whether this is a secondary phenomenon resulting from a need for increased intraluminal pressure or is a primary pathology.

2. The points of diminished resistance of the bowel wall occur at those sites where the nutrient arteries pass through the muscularis propria into the submucosa, between the mesenteric and antimesenteric tenia. These areas are covered by connective tissue. It has been suggested that the collagen in these areas gradually loses its flexibility and tensile strength with age, resulting in weakening of the bowel wall and a predisposition to diverticula formation. This mechanism may help to explain the presence of diverticula in those cases of left-sided diverticulosis in which increased luminal pressure, reduced fecal weight, and prolonged intestinal transit are not found.[21] What is less clear is the role that veins play as these accompany the arterioles or whether the outpouchings are really along the tracts created by the veins. And if so, does this create local congestion? Which shows how little we know about this disease.

The importance of an intact connective tissue in maintaining the structural integrity of the colon is further attested to by the following observations:

a. Cases of diverticulosis occurring primarily in the cecum and right colon with luminal pressures that are lower than normal and do not show muscular thickening

b. The finding of diverticulosis in young patients with connective tissue disorders, such as *Marfan's disease*[22,23] and *Ehlers–Danlos syndrome*[24]

c. Acromegaly is also associated with an increased prevalence of diverticular disease.[25]

However, the notion that interplay between muscle fibers, nerves, interstitial cells of Cajal (ICC), neurotransmitters, and possibly inflammatory cells plays a part in the development of diverticula is increasingly recognized. In one study, ICC and glial cells were decreased in colonic diverticular disease, whereas enteric neurons appear to be normally represented.[26] Mast cells have also shown to be increased,[27] but how these all fit together is not entirely clear and many of the histologic changes in the neuromuscular apparatus reported are likely secondary in nature.

Diverticulitis has been attributed to trapped fecaliths in diverticula.[28] Since these have at most a muscularis mucosae, impacted feces cannot be ejected so become hard and they cannot pass back into the lumen. Subsequently, edema and inflammation may further narrow the diverticula necks and impede the outflow of feces from diverticula.[28] Mucosal inflammation can readily extend to the submucosa of the diverticula, which is directly subjacent to either the peritoneal cavity or the retroperitoneum where further extension of the inflammation admixed with fecal contents may occur, and can result in fistula tracts.

Clinical Features

Diverticular disease increases with age and is found in approximately one-third to one-half of the patients over 60. Men and women are equally affected.[29,30] Though presumed to be a rare entity, diverticulitis in patients younger than 40 years old has gradually risen.[31,32] Uncomplicated diverticular disease (diverticulosis) is often asymptomatic[33] but may be associated with crampy abdominal pain and diarrhea alternating with constipation.[33] In this setting, symptoms may be attributed to diverticula, but this is usually difficult to prove.[33-35]

Diverticulosis may be present for months or years before complications ensue. Complications in diverticulosis occur in only about 20% to 25% of patients,[36] and only a small minority develop severe or life-threatening complications.[2]

Diverticulitis or its complications may be confined to a single attack with permanent remission or may consist of repeated episodes over many years. The symptoms and signs of diverticulitis are left lower abdominal pain, fever and, commonly, a palpable, tender, rope-like mass. Acute diverticulitis almost invariably results from perforations that are often quite small at the tip of the diverticulum. This area usually becomes walled off, with local abscess formation, fever, and abdominal tenderness. Generalized peritonitis is very uncommon.[37] Sometimes adjacent structures, such as the bladder, intestinal loops, vagina, anterior abdominal wall, and, rarely, adjacent vascular structures, become adherent to the inflamed colon, resulting in fistula formation. In 5% to 10% of cases, resolution of diverticulitis results in severe scar formation with large bowel obstruction, which may mimic carcinoma clinically.[30]

Hemorrhage is an uncommon complication of diverticular disease and is not usually associated with acute diverticulitis clinically,[38] although necrosis of arteriolar walls must occur, which presumably results from inflammation. Interestingly, often arterioles adjacent to the diverticula have marked luminal obliteration resulting from reactive intimal proliferation, even in the absence of active inflammation. Vascular injection studies have shown a close relation between blood vessels and diverticula, as well as features of vascular ectasia.[39] It has been estimated that diverticular hemorrhage accounts for between 20% and 48% of lower GI bleeding,[40,41] but these figures are likely erroneous, since endoscopic experience has shown that many patients with GI hemorrhage previously thought to be due to diverticular disease on clinical and radiologic grounds are due to other patients such as vascular ectasia. Clinically, bleeding from diverticula is usually abrupt and painless but, in some patients may be massive and life threatening. The blood is usually bright red and arteriolar, being most overt if the hemorrhage occurs from disease in the sigmoid colon.[38] The site of origin of hemorrhage can be difficult to localize. Selective arteriography may be helpful, especially in those patients with persistent, life-threatening hemorrhage in whom surgery is contemplated.[42]

Some patients develop inflammation indistinguishable from IBD in the segment of colon with diverticula, also referred to as diverticular colitis or segmental colitis associated with diverticular disease (SCAD). Prolapse-type polyps may also develop at the orifices of diverticula. Its differential diagnosis is Crohn's disease especially if the rectum is spared and ulcerative colitis when the disease extends into the rectum. Thus, demonstration of a normal rectal biopsy is intrinsic in the diagnosis, as is the presence of proximal lack of involvement.

Endoscopy

At colonoscopy, diverticula are characterized by 3- to 5-mm-wide orifices lying in shallow haustral pouches commonly separated by ridgelike elevations (Fig. 6-1).[43] The mucosa around the mouths of the diverticula may be inflamed, with patchy erythema, and may sometimes be raised above adjacent mucosa mimicking polyps. Only rarely is blood or purulent material seen extruding from the diverticulum. In diverticular strictures, the lumen becomes quite distorted and narrowed, but overlying mucosa is intact, and the valvulae appear symmetrical and regular, in contrast to their appearance with carcinoma.

Imaging

Imaging is important diagnostically, and ultrasound, barium enema, computed tomography (CT), and magnetic resonance imaging are all used. CT has largely replaced barium enema primarily because of its ability to identify extracolonic disease and its extent, and CT is also the procedure of choice in acute disease. If barium enema is used, the presence of extraluminal barium pockets, which persist on the postevacuation film (Fig. 6-2), remains useful in some settings. Other findings include the demonstration of mucosal ridges and sacculations, mirroring the gross appearances. CT can also demonstrate diverticulosis, inflamed diverticula, and abscess both intra- and extramural, as well as less common complications such as hepatic abscesses (Fig. 6-3).

Gross Pathology

The vast majority of diverticula occur in the sigmoid colon, but they can extend proximally to the cecum and do so to some extent in about 15% of patients.[44] Externally, they typically appear in two rows on either side of the colon between the mesenteric and antimesenteric (lateral) teniae at points of entry of the nutrient arteries within the pericolic fat, especially the appendices epiploicae, and have a globular or fusiform configuration. They measure around 1 cm in diameter, although this may vary from a barely perceptible bump to sacs 2 cm or larger (Fig. 6-4). Internally, there are one or more rows of diverticula that are visible to varying extent but are enhanced if the bowel is inflated with formalin overnight. When the disease is severe, there are invariably mucosal ridges longitudinally marking the position of the taeniae coli between which diverticula can be seen to be protruding but also numerous transverse ridges that appear either circumferential (Fig. 6-5) or interdigitating (Fig. 6-6). The ridges do not usually extend around the circumference of the bowel wall but tend to consist of overlapping semilunar arcs of thickened circular muscle confined to

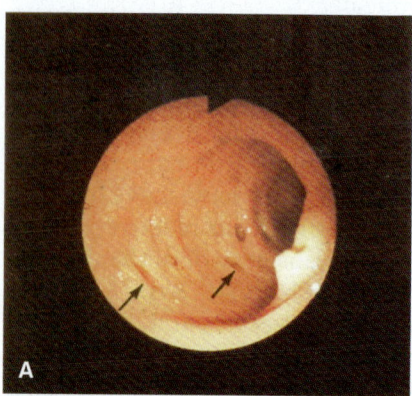
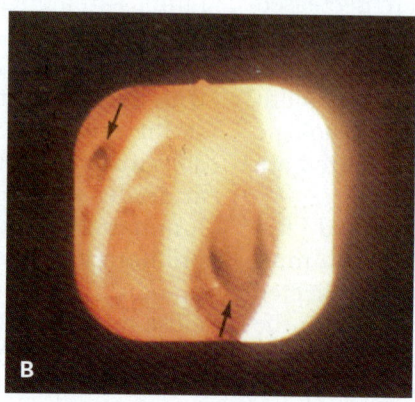

Figure 6-1. Left-sided diverticulosis: colonoscopic appearances. **A:** The orifices of diverticula are seen adjacent to the mucosal ridges (*arrows*). The raised, whitish mucosa at the right margin is the site of a polypectomy. (Courtesy M. Derezin, MD.) **B:** In this colon, there are prominent mucosal ridges. The openings of the diverticula can be seen within the sacculations (*arrows*).

the zone between the mesenteric and antimesenteric teniae.[44,45] Between the ridges, the colon shows saccular dilatation, and this is where the orifices of the diverticula lie. The latter vary in size from 3 to 5 mm in diameter, may contain impacted fecaliths, and are connected to the diverticula by necks of varying lengths (Figs. 6-4 and 6-5). Invariably, the muscularis propria is markedly thickened, often to over 5 mm when it appears shiny white to the point of looking almost cartilaginous; this is invariably a prominent feature of the disease (Fig. 6-7). The affected bowel is shortened ("myochosis") with exaggerated mucosal folds, which appear almost redundant. Polyps either on the redundant mucosal folds or around ostia of the diverticula can form, which show many of the features of mucosal prolapse (see later).

Prediverticular disease. In some patients, the muscle abnormality of diverticular disease is present in the absence of true diverticula, although outpouchings of what looks like excess mucosa and submucosa are present that initially resemble diverticula but which do not actually pass through the muscularis propria

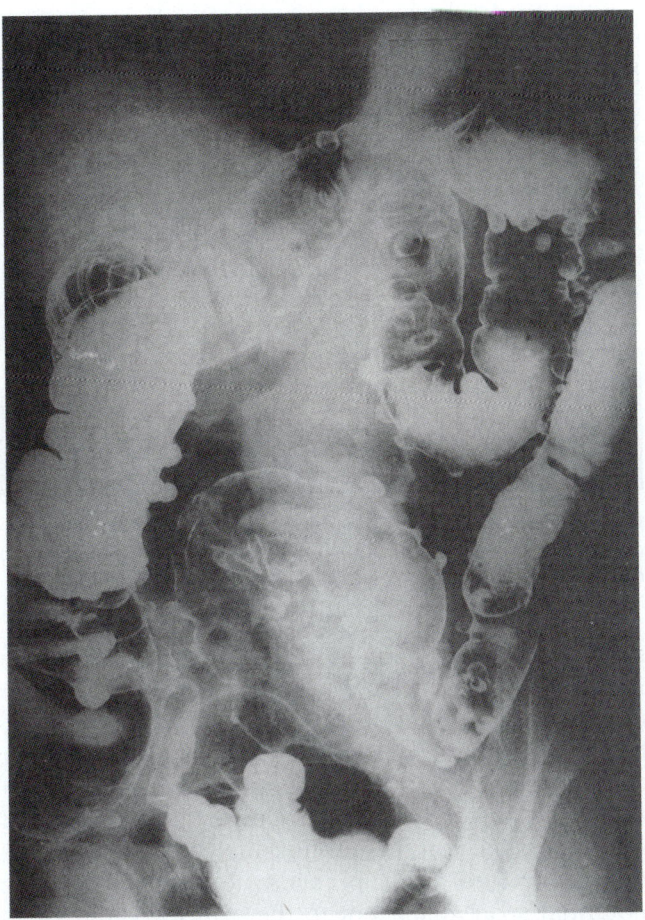

Figure 6-2. X-ray appearance of colonic diverticulosis demonstrating numerous extraluminal sacculations, some of which are filled with barium. (Courtesy M. Weiner, MD.)

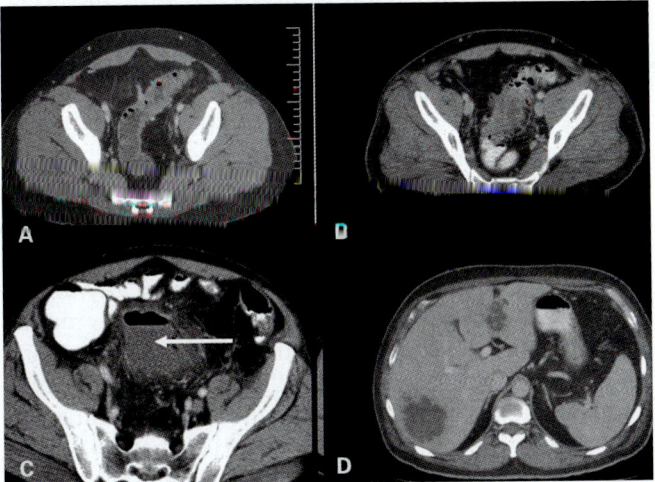

Figure 6-3. CT images of diverticular disease and its complications. **A:** Diverticulosis with a single inflamed diverticulum. **B:** Patient with diverticular disease with an intramural abscess. **C:** Abscess around sigmoid colon (*arrow*) **D:** Liver with multiple abscesses following an episode of diverticulitis. (Images courtesy of Dr. Nasir Jaffer, Mt. Sinai Hospital, Toronto, ON.)

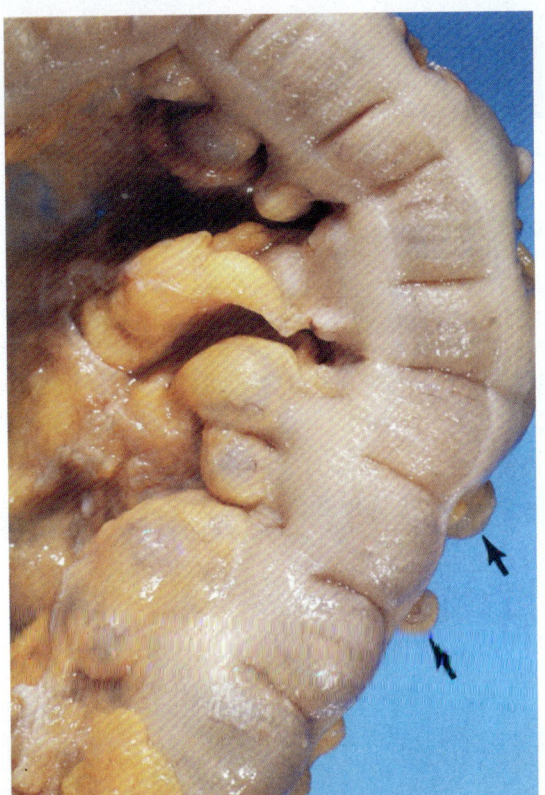

Figure 6-4. Diverticulosis of the colon: external appearance. The two antimesenteric taeniae are readily visible at the top of the specimen, and there are no diverticula between these in this patient, although numerous haustrations are visible between the taenia, which are the external counterpart of those seen internally (see subsequent figures). However, numerous diverticula are apparent adjacent to the left taenia protruding toward the mesentery and involving the appendices epiploicae. A second row of diverticula is just visible on the right side (*arrows*).

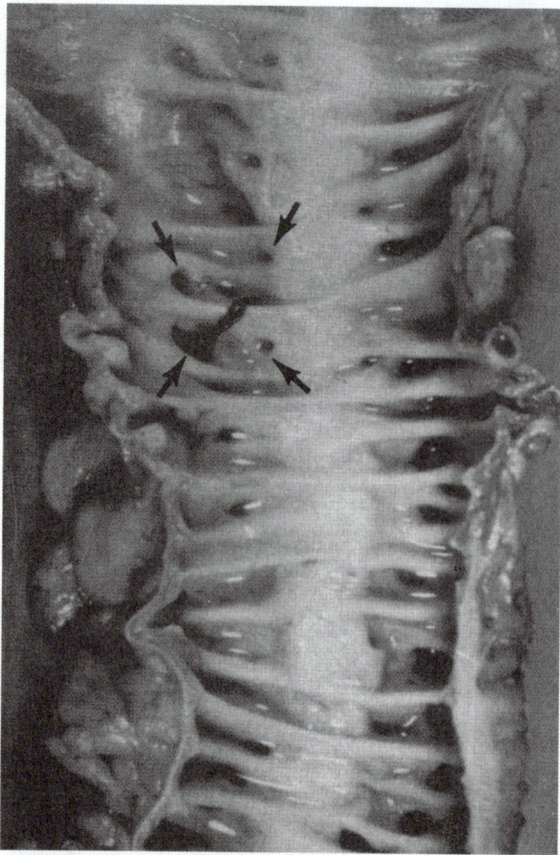

Figure 6-5. Diverticulosis of the colon showing the prominent mucosal ridges and intervening saccular dilatations. Within the saccular dilatations, the orifices of the diverticula can be seen, sometimes forming two rows on either side of the taenia (*arrows*).

(Figs. 6-7 and 6-8). This is presumably because of persistent contraction of both circular and longitudinal muscle of the muscularis propria. Since radiologic follow-up of some patients with this type of thickening

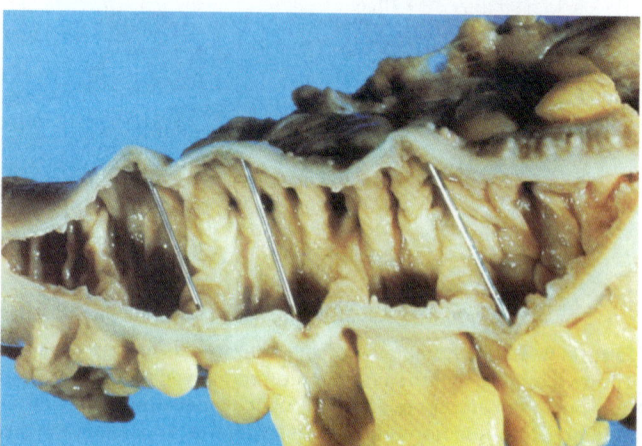

Figure 6-6. Diverticulosis of the colon demonstrating numerous mucosal ridges protruding into the lumen. Note that those arising in the lower part of the specimen tend to interdigitate with those from the upper part producing a concertina-like appearance. Note also the diffuse thickening of the muscularis propria.

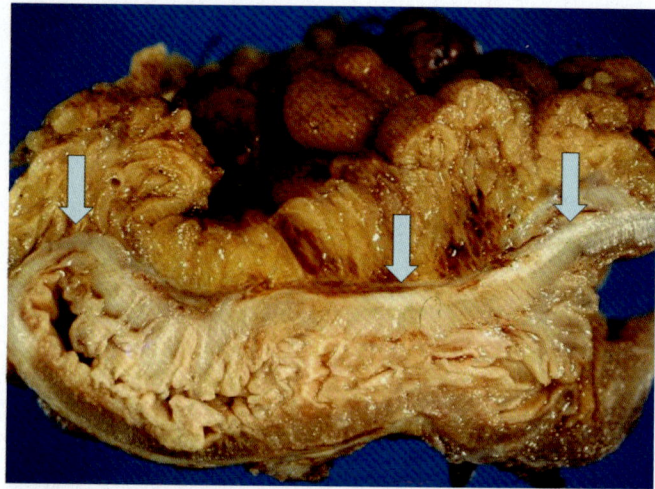

Figure 6-7. Diverticular disease showing the thickened muscularis propria (*arrows*) and concertina-like infoldings of the mucosa and submucosa.

showed development of diverticula later (hardly a controlled trial), this does suggest this may be an early stage of the disease.[46,47] The same changes may be seen in patients with typical diverticulosis in other areas of the colon, so it is generally believed that it represents the earliest phase of diverticular disease. It is also possible that the intraluminal pressure required for the mucosa and submucosa to pass through the potential spaces adjacent to the arterioles and veins never occurs in some of these patients.

Handling of specimens. There are two ways in which the specimens can be handled on receipt from the operating room. The first is to insufflate the segment of colon with formalin, after first rinsing out the intestinal contents with saline, and fix it overnight. It can then be opened either longitudinally or transversely. This demonstrates virtually all diverticula so that those that are inflamed can be more readily identified. This method has the advantage of distending all the diverticula and making their examination easier. The second method is to open the colon immediately on receipt and then, after gross examination, to pin it out for fixation. One can insert a little finger in the lumen prior to making any cuts to avoid cutting through any unsuspected lesions such as large adenomas or a carcinoma. This method thus has the advantage of identifying any unexpected pathology that rarely may alter the immediate intraoperative management of the patient and also allows detection of abnormalities that are sometimes difficult to find in the fixed state, such as the points of origin of diverticular hemorrhage. It should be stressed that the mere finding of hemorrhage in a diverticulum does not prove that it originated from that site, since it may well have filled with blood from the lumen. To prove that blood has originated from a given diverticulum, it is necessary to demonstrate a

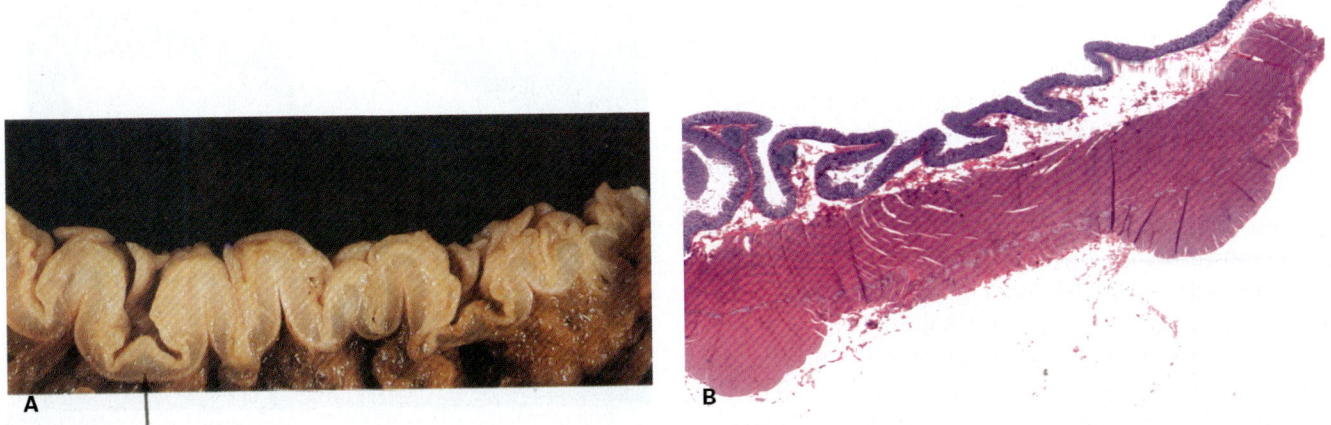

Figure 6-8. **A:** Longitudinal section of a colon demonstrating early diverticular disease. The bowel wall is thrown into numerous folds and ridges, and the thickened muscle coat can be clearly seen as a tan translucent tissue (*arrow*). **B:** Histologic section of Figure 6-8A showing mucosal folds and ridges in the absence of diverticula.

bleeding point histologically. This can be impractical if it requires examining every diverticulum, which are often numerous; however, examining most or all of them grossly is not too onerous. Many of the changes of diverticular disease may not be clearly visualized if the opened colon is examined in random transverse cuts unless these are done every few millimeters. In fixed specimens, abnormalities are also well demonstrated using serial longitudinal cuts parallel to the length of bowel wall through the rows of diverticula.

Histology

Diverticula consist of mucosa and muscularis mucosae and covered by pericolic adipose tissue, serosa, and, occasionally, a few fascicles of longitudinal muscle (Fig. 6-9). The necks of the diverticula lie between the hypertrophied fascicles of circular muscle between the taeniae coli. The muscularis propria is often hugely thickened and the neural plexi similarly hypertrophied.

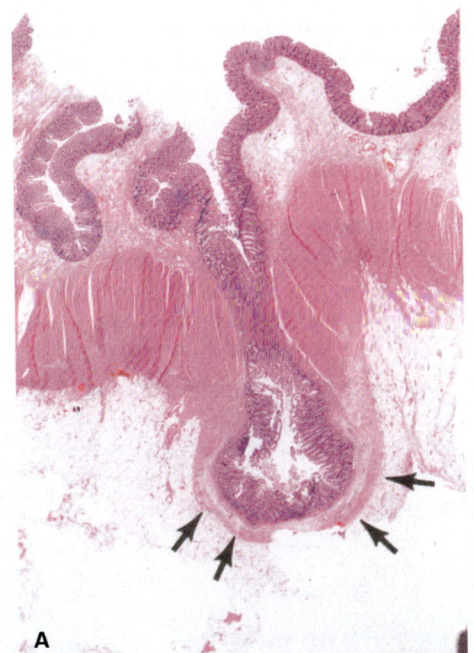
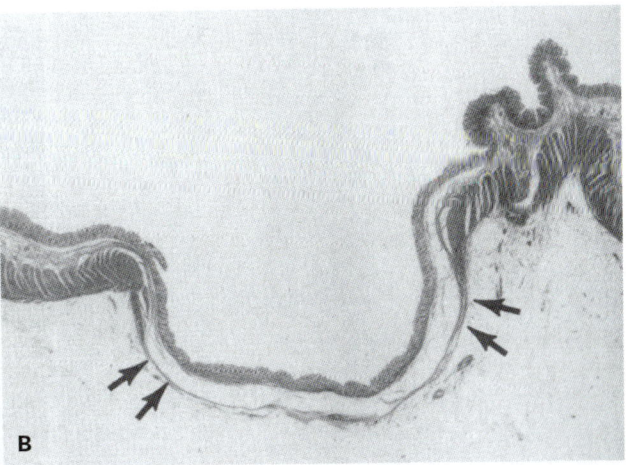

Figure 6-9. Low-power magnification of diverticulosis showing herniations of mucosa between the muscle coat. Diverticulum with a long, narrow neck **(A)** and diverticulum with a wide-mouthed opening **(B)**. Both diverticula are lined by mucosa and covered by pericolonic connective tissue, a few fascicles of longitudinal muscle (*arrows*), suggesting that the loss of muscularis is slow and acquired, and finally pericolic fat or serosa.

The inflammation in diverticulitis invariably has a chronic lymphoplasmacytic component and can mimic diversion disease, infection, and IBD. There can therefore be lymphoid aggregates often with germinal centers, similar to that seen with diversion colitis or bacterial overgrowth, which may spill into the pericolonic fat. Cryptitis and crypt abscesses can mimic infectious/self-limited colitis, while crypt architectural distortion, and rarely even granulomas can mimick IBD. Diverticular colitis can have all of the histologic features of IBD (see Chapter 18).

Usually, one or at most a few diverticula are affected, and these commonly contain fecaliths. Rarely, all diverticula are acutely inflamed. The inflammation usually involves the apical region of the diverticulum where it is frequently associated with a fecalith but may begin as a focus of acute inflammation and then an erosion and finally an ulcer. It can also start in the neck of the diverticulum (Fig. 6-10). This results initially in microperforations and so may form peridiverticular inflammation and abscess (Fig. 6-11). Sometimes, there is a foreign body giant cell reaction and occasionally genuine granulomas to the inspissated feces. The inflammation is often restricted to the diverticulum, and spread to the mucosa around the diverticular orifices and beyond (diverticular colitis) is uncommon (Fig. 6-12).

In most instances, diverticulitis remains localized, being contained by the appendices epiploicae, pericolic fat, mesentery, or adjacent organs. In severe diverticulitis, inflammation may spread along the outside of the bowel wall, ensheathing it in fibrous tissue to produce a large mass around the colon. Occasionally, the abscess

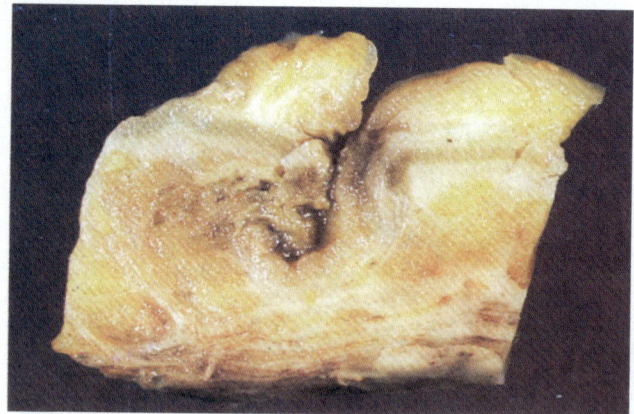

Figure 6-11. Longitudinal section of colon in diverticulitis demonstrating perforation and peridiverticular inflammation and fibrosis.

dissects along the serosa parallel to the outer aspect of the deep muscle layers. Consequently, inflammation from one diverticulum may spread widely up and down the bowel wall, ensheathing it with inflammatory tissue and producing a large mass around the colon.[17] However, inflammation rarely spreads within the bowel itself, and the luminal mucosa usually remains uninvolved (Fig. 6-12), but its presence in the absence of diverticulitis represents diverticular colitis/SCAD segmental colitis associated with diverticular disease— (see Chapter 18). Rarely, perforation occurs into the peritoneal cavity resulting in peritonitis, and occasionally, the perforation is unaccompanied by inflammation, but the ruptured diverticulum exudes mucin forming a peridiverticular mucin lake (Fig. 6-13).

Resolution of the inflammation results in fibrosis leading to a thickened and stenotic colon with marked distortion of the lumen. A variable mononuclear infiltrate can be present, which may include numerous submucosal and serosal lymphoid aggregates, mimicking Crohn's

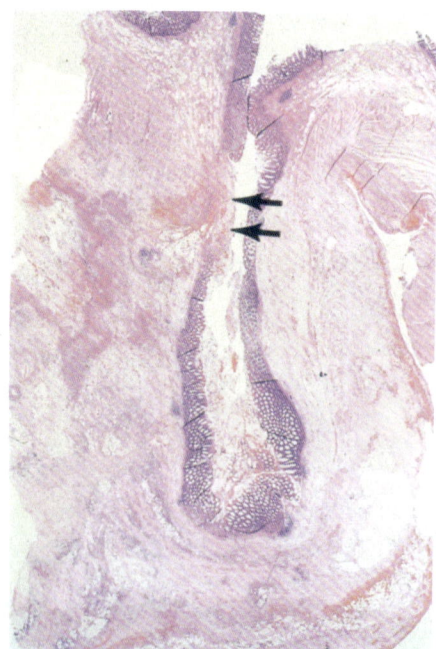

Figure 6-10. Diverticulitis showing focal mucosal erosion (*arrows*) and diffuse inflammation with marked edema and focal necrosis.

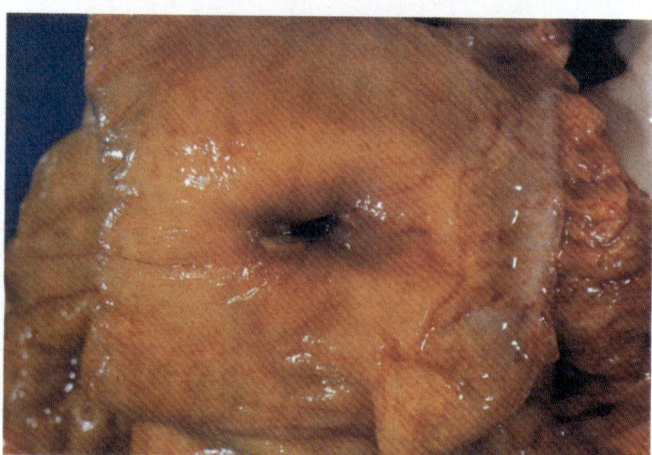

Figure 6-12. Colonic mucosa overlying inflamed diverticulum. Although there is a mild redness/inflammation of the mucosa around the orifice of the diverticulum, it has not spread to the mucosa beyond grossly.

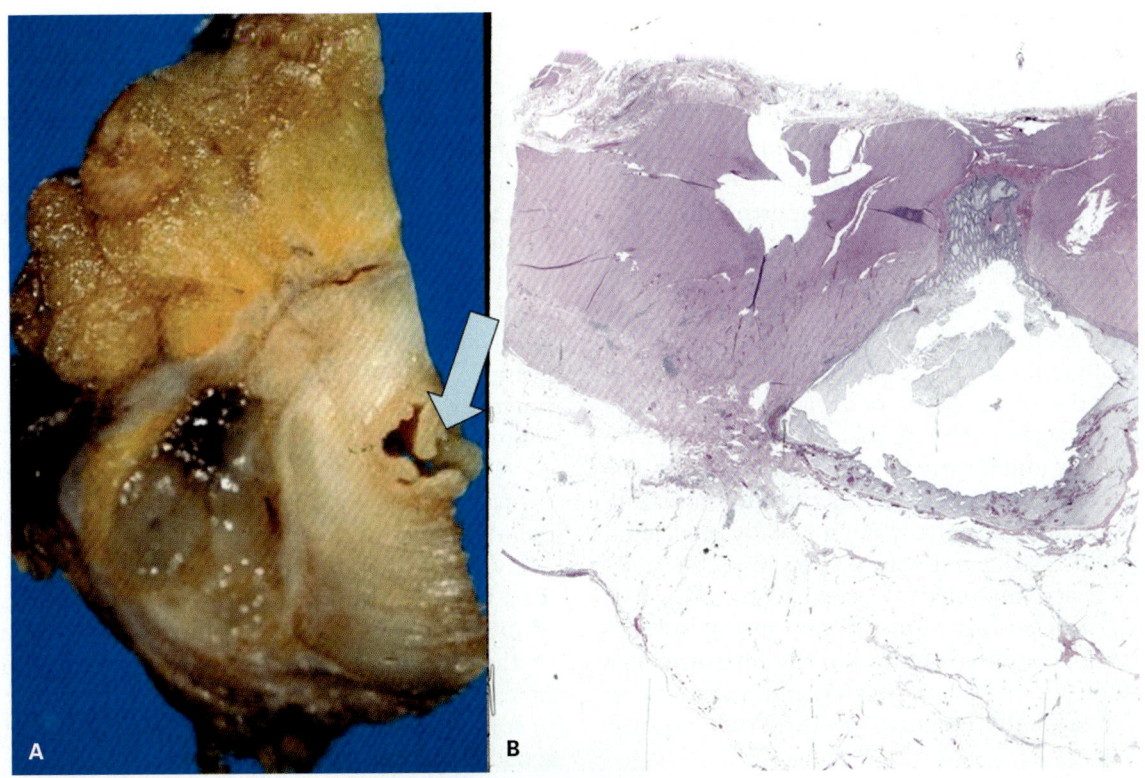

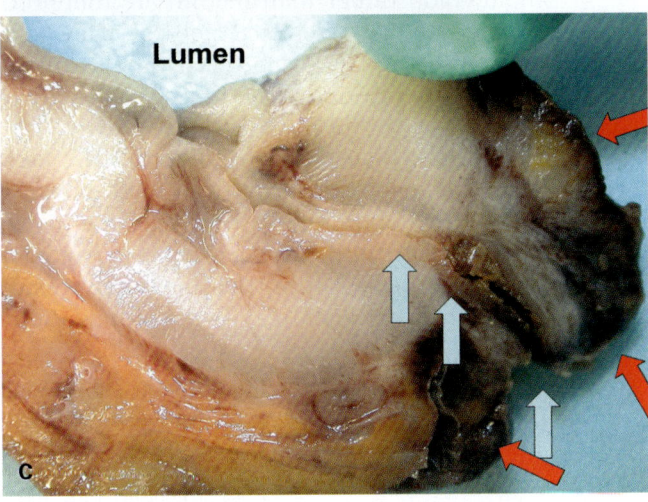

Figure 6-13. Perforated diverticulum. Diverticulum with perforation but mucous extrusion. **A:** Same specimen as Figure 6-7 showing a cross section of the bowel wall in which the lumen is right (*arrow*) and a thickened muscularis propria is present between the lumen and the diverticulum that is full of mucin. **B:** Section of diverticulum showing mucous extravasation without inflammation. (Courtesy Dr. Jorge Albores-Saavedra.) **C:** Perforated diverticulum in which the lumen is top left and the tract of the diverticulum (*blue arrows*) courses through the hypertrophied muscle into an abscess cavity, outlined by the *brown discoloration*. The serosa is shown by *red arrows*.

disease[28] (see subsequent discussion). Involvement of adjacent structures such as the bladder wall, other intestinal loops, vagina, and the anterior abdominal wall is also rare and may result in fistula formation and massive hemorrhage if vessels are involved. Occasionally, rupture occurs and mucus is extravasated into the surrounding tissue (Fig. 6-13). This is similar to nonneoplastic mucoceles of the appendix and carries no increased risk of pseudomyxoma. Whether "chronic diverticulitis" is a true clinicopathologic entity is debatable. However, when symptoms persist, one must consider the diagnosis of pericolic abscesses.

Since most resections in patients with diverticulosis are performed for diverticulitis or their complications, clinicians hope the pathologic examination can confirm the cause, while pathologists also want the same result with reasonable sampling not requiring submission of every diverticulum. Sometimes, this does requires going back to the specimen more than once for additional sections.

Defining diverticulitis. This becomes an issue when the question is whether the patient's symptoms can be attributed to the inflammation present. In some ways this duplicates the same issue with appendicitis and mucosal inflammation. There are no established guidelines for minimal criteria. There is frequently more inflammation in and around the diverticula than the adjacent mucosa, but it is unclear if it is of any significance. Traditionally, the presence of neutrophils and extension of the inflammatory infiltrate beyond the muscularis mucosae have been used as pathologic definitions for diverticulitis. If carefully examined, most diverticula even in asymptomatic individuals show at least some increase in lamina propria inflammation with lymphoid follicles, indicative of bacterial stasis; however, it is the presence of neutrophils in the inflammatory infiltrate that seems to correlate clinically with acute diverticulitis.[48]

Hemorrhage Hemorrhage in diverticular disease is traditionally said to be associated with erosions of arterioles on the necks of the diverticula as it is often bright red. However, it may also be associated with vascular ectasia and/or erosion into submucosal vessels (Fig. 6-14), but this is often difficult to demonstrate grossly and microscopically. It is not usually associated with symptoms associated with diverticulitis. As most arterioles are accompanied by at least one vein, it is unclear why the walls of veins are not just as susceptible as arterioles to involvement in the inflammatory process. Medications such as NSAIDs and ASA increase the risk of diverticular hemorrhage, (and perforation).

POLYPS AND NEOPLASMS ASSOCIATED WITH AND WITHIN DIVERTICULA

Diverticular Polyps

A variety of polyps occur around diverticula. These can include inflammatory polyps following localized ulcers, but the most frequent are prolapse-type polyps that can be found at the orifices of diverticula.

First described as polypoid prolapsing mucosal folds in 1991,[49] these polyps have been described under a variety of other synonyms,[50-52] all of which refer to their location or appearance. These include myoglandular polyps,[53-57] which are regarded as a variant of inflammatory polyps with features of prolapse. They can occur both in association with colonic diverticula or, like inflammatory polyps, anywhere secondary to local inflammation and erosion or ulceration. Terms such as mucosubmucosal polyps, long pedunculated polyp and colonic mucosubmucosal elongated polyp,[50,52] and filiform polyposis have also been used; however, these are distinct lesions and discussed more in detail elsewhere (see Chapters 18 and 20).[51]

Grossly, the polyps occur around the orifices of diverticula and are usually red or brown from the vascularity including thrombi or hemosiderin within them. They have a combination of all of the features associated with inflammatory polyps together with features of prolapse, which include fibromuscular proliferation in the lamina propria. Either component may dominate, but prolapse-type features are invariably present to some extent. Polyps with the appearance of solitary rectal ulcer syndrome (SRUS) but being from the sigmoid colon rather than rectum are therefore likely to be diverticular associated polyps. They can ulcerate and subsequently develop crypt architectural distortion and focal serrations in the mucosa close to the surface.

Inverted diverticulum. Diverticula occasionally spontaneously invert into the large bowel and form a smooth polyp, where they are not recognized for what they are and polypectomy is carried out. If there is surface peritoneum, this inevitably results in free air in the peritoneal cavity with or without signs of

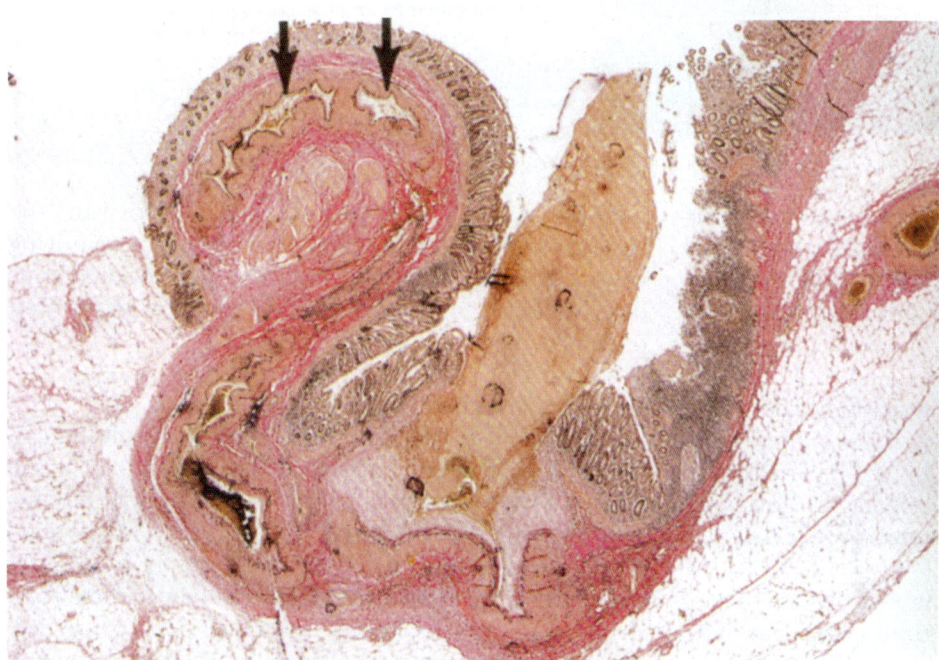

Figure 6-14. Hemorrhage in diverticular disease of the colon. This section of colon shows erosion of a large vessel with an adherent thrombus projecting into the lumen. Its base arises from a dilated vessel and indicates why these lesions can bleed briskly. In addition, there are many prominent blood vessels in the submucosa (*arrows*) (Elastic stain).

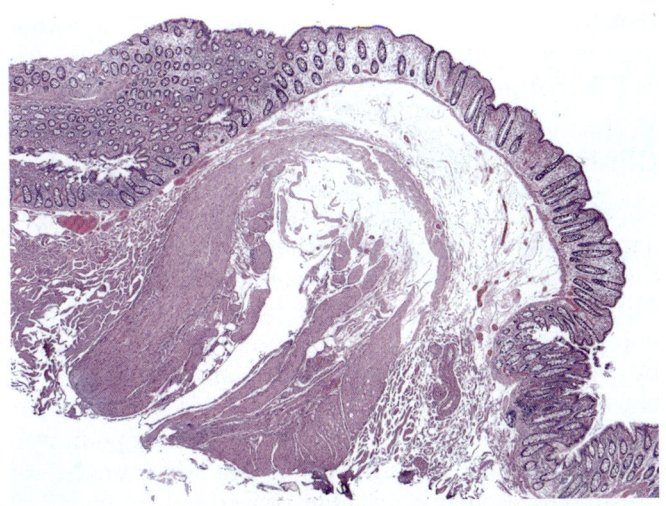

Figure 6-15. Inverted diverticulum that was removed as a polyp. Note that the muscularis propria is thick at the base of the polyp but thin superficially, recapitulating the same appearance seen in a typical diverticulum (see Fig. 6-8), but inverted. As there is clearly serosa present, inevitably, it resulted in perforation that required closing.

peritonitis, and either endoscopic or surgical repair is required[58-60] (Fig. 6-15). If resected, the clue is the thinned muscularis propria.

Other Polyps

Diverticula are not immune to the usual range of epithelial polyps,[61] and there is likely an increased risk of polyps of all types.[62] The main issue with polyps within the diverticulum is that if attempts are made to excise them colonoscopically, there is risk of perforation as these are covered only by a muscularis mucosae.[63] Provided it is recognized that polyp is actually extending in to the diverticulum (they may be inverted), they need to be either followed or resected with the adjacent portion of bowel.

Carcinoma in diverticular disease. This is rare, and reported cases are barely in double digits, many being from Japan and are "early" and likely include intramucosal carcinomas. Truly invasive carcinomas arising in diverticula therefore remain vanishingly rare. The major issue is that any infiltrating carcinoma developing in a fully formed diverticulum beyond the bowel wall is by definition a T3 lesion the moment it invades, although that does not mean it carries the same prognosis as all T3 lesions, but data are obviously lacking.[64]

One study looking at the risk of colon cancer in diverticulosis found that it did not increase the risk of colon cancer in the long term and that a history of diverticular disease does not affect colon cancer mortality; however, there was an apparent increased risk of colon cancer within the first 12 months after diagnosing diverticular disease that was thought most likely due to increased surveillance.[65]

DIVERTICULAR DISEASE AND ENDOMETRIOSIS

It is surprising that while the large bowel is a frequent site for endometriosis, an association with a diverticular disease seems not to be described (other than Meckel's and urethral diverticula, in which endometriosis is well described), possibly because of the differences in age in both groups.

DIVERTICULAR DISEASE AND IBD

While there is no reason that these two diseases should not coexist,[66,67] it should also be recognized that resolving diverticulitis can exhibit many of the features of Crohn's disease. These include focal mucosal ulcerations and inflammation, transmural inflammation in the form of numerous submucosal and serosal lymphoid aggregates (Fig. 6-16), and rarely even granulomas. Interpretation of these changes is clearly subjective. It has been shown that most of these patients do not represent Crohn's disease unless they already have it.[68] In one review of 50 patients with Crohn's-like features in diverticular disease, only 2 patients recurred with Crohn's disease following resection.[69] Similarly, of the 77 cases with ulcerative colitis–like diverticular colitis, only 8 developed classical ulcerative colitis on follow-up.[69] A diagnosis of diverticulitis *and* IBD should therefore *not* be made unless there is other clinical evidence of IBD elsewhere. In some cases, even though the findings of diverticulitis are absolutely indistinguishable from IBD, it is wise to wait for the latter to reveal itself in due course of time and

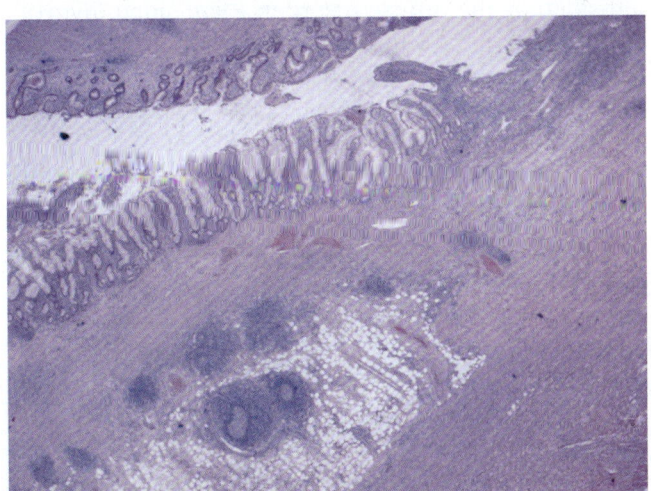

Figure 6-16. Ulcerated diverticulum that is partially reepithelialized with epithelium showing typical architectural distortion. However, note the "rosary-bead" Crohn's-like nodules of lymphoid tissue.

not generate an extensive clinical workup except possibly for a full colonoscopy (if not performed recently) or start presumptive treatment. The finding of diverticula that are incidentally involved with contiguous inflammatory disease occurs but is surprisingly rare.

Differential Diagnosis and Clinical Implications

Because diverticulosis is such a prevalent disorder in the Western Hemisphere, it is not surprising that other intra-abdominal disorders may occur concurrently. The presence of diverticula should not blind one to the possibility of other, possibly more serious lesions elsewhere. As discussed above, diverticular disease does not increase the risk of colon cancer,[65] although diverticula may hinder the endoscopic or radiologic detection of adenomas and carcinomas. Clinically, both conditions may produce intestinal obstruction. Colonoscopy and imaging studies are helpful in differentiating between them.

Other fibrosing constrictive lesions of the colon, such as Crohn's disease, ischemic colitis, and radiation colitis, may also be confused clinically with diverticulitis and, on occasion, occur concurrently. The problem is usually clinical, since the pathologic features of the resected specimen are usually fairly distinctive. In patients with IBD-like colitis involving the luminal mucosa, a possibility of diverticular colitis needs to be considered.

DIVERTICULOSIS OF THE CECUM AND PROXIMAL COLON (RIGHT-SIDED DIVERTICULOSIS)

Diverticulosis of the cecum and the proximal colon appears to be an entirely different disease from the left-sided or the diffuse disorder. Right-sided diverticular disease is rare in the Western Hemisphere[70] but is the predominant disorder in Hawaii, Japan, and many other countries in Asia.[71,72] For unexplained reasons, it is rapidly increasing in incidence.[4]

Pathogenesis

The pathogenesis of right-sided diverticulosis remains obscure. It has been attributed to environmental factors, probably dietary, superimposed upon a genetically predisposed population.[73,74] However, although population studies in Japan have indicated a higher level of dietary fiber intake than in the Western Hemisphere, there is no proof that these factors are related.[75] Right-sided diverticula may be "true congenital diverticula"[76] in the sense that they are composed of all layers of the bowel wall as opposed to outpouchings of mucosa and submucosa through the muscularis propria. However, others have not substantiated this,[7,77] and some think that "congenital cecal diverticula are largely a pathologic myth."[7] Some are clearly secondary to motility disorders (see those sections subsequently descriptions).

Clinical Features

Right-sided diverticular disease occurs in a younger age group (~10 years younger) than left-sided diverticular disease[78] and shows a 3:1 male:female predominance.[79] Clinically, up to two-thirds of patients are symptomatic. The disease commonly mimics acute appendicitis.[72] Other modes of presentation are disturbance in bowel habits, abdominal distention, and melena.[80] We have seen several instances where a bleeding point was demonstrated in the right colon that was resected as presumed vascular ectasia but proved to be a bleeding diverticulum and even produced frank rectal bleeding. On rare occasions, a single diverticulum is the cause of solitary ulceration of the cecum.[81] Right-sided diverticular disease may be found in association with other disorders, such as vascular diseases including hypertension and extracolonic malignancies.[79] It should be noted that while right-sided diverticular disease is the most prevalent diverticular disorder in this high-risk population, left-sided disease can also occur, usually in older people, and is found in about one-third of patients.[79] As many patients routinely take aspirin or nonsteroidal anti-inflammatory drugs (NSAIDs), the possibility that inflammation and ulceration in right-sided diverticular disease may be medication associated always needs to be considered.

Pathology

In about 20% of patients, the lesions are solitary, 60% contain up to 10 diverticula, and 20% contain more than 10. The solitary lesions frequently occur close to the ileocecal junction and may be quite large (Fig. 6-17), while the multiple lesions may be found more distally in the cecum and ascending colon.

Histologically, diverticula have a variable appearance. In the West, the majority of them are similar to left-sided diverticula, consisting of outpouchings of mucosa and submucosa devoid of a muscle coat, but in parts of the world where left-sided diverticula are uncommon, they may have all layers of the bowel wall, and these have been considered congenital or true diverticula.[2,3,28,82] We have noted that many of these have fibrosis of the muscularis propria raising the possibility of potential motility disorders. Both types are prone to the same complications as left-sided diverticulosis.

Occasionally, diverticulosis of the diffuse type extends to involve the right side of the colon, and the lesions have the typical features of the diffuse disorder, that is, they are multiple, are usually associated with lesions on the left side, and are devoid of muscle coats in their wall.

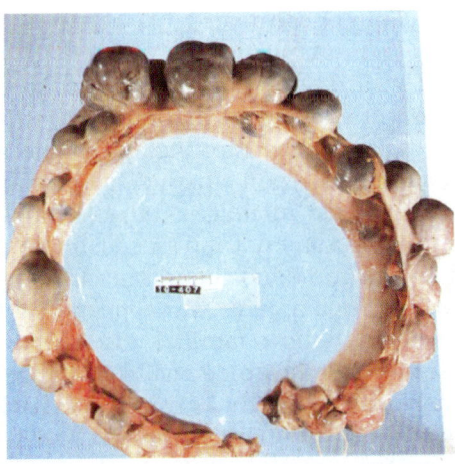

Figure 6-17. Jejunal diverticulosis characterized by numerous large diverticula situated along the mesenteric border.

DIVERTICULOSIS OF THE DUODENUM AND SMALL INTESTINE

Small intestinal diverticula occur most frequently in the duodenum with fewer cases in the jejunum and ileum.[83] They are surprisingly common, may be single or multiple, and are usually asymptomatic. Most busy radiology departments will probably encounter one of these daily as an incidental finding in upper GI studies.[84]

Pathogenesis

Small intestinal diverticula may be congenital or acquired. Though familial aggregation has been described in some cases,[85] for the most part, pathogenesis appears to be multifactorial. Herniation appears to occur where paired blood vessels penetrate the mesentery into the bowel wall. Diverticula are most readily identified in the duodenum, proximal jejunum, and distal ileum, where vasa recti are of greatest diameter.[86,87] Diverticula are also frequently associated with intestinal motility disorders, such as progressive systemic sclerosis, visceral neuropathies, myopathies, and sometimes mitochondriopathies where abnormal contractions and fibrosis of the muscularis propria can result in the formation of diverticula.[88,89] The pathology is that associated with motility disorders (vide supra).

Duodenal Diverticula (Single or Isolated)

These are by far the most common diverticula of the small bowel.[90] The number decreases distally with nearly 80% of the remaining in the jejunum and 15% in the ileum.[91] Duodenal diverticula can be either extraluminal or rarely intraluminal.

Extraluminal diverticula. The vast majority of duodenal diverticula are extraluminal. They usually occur in the medial portion of the second part of the duodenum within 2 cm of the papilla of Vater.[90] Most are asymptomatic and found incidentally on imaging (Fig. 6-18). Thus, prophylactic removal is not necessary. Only rarely do they cause symptoms resulting from bleeding, perforation, obstruction, or malabsorption secondary to bacterial overgrowth.[92-94] In addition, there is an association between periampullary duodenal diverticula and choledocholithiasis that has been ascribed to papillary dysfunction.[95] In contrast to their frequent detection using imaging studies, they are rarely recognized at endoscopy because the orifice communicating with the duodenal lumen is typically a mere slit and is obscured by the mucosal folds. Duodenal diverticula consist of mucosal and submucosal outpouchings into the serosa and lack a muscle coat, appearances similar to those of left-sided colonic diverticular disease.

Intraluminal duodenal diverticulum (prolapsed diaphragm). This is an uncommon congenital anomaly characterized by an intraluminal mucosal pouch, usually located in the second portion of the duodenum adjacent to the papilla of Vater. The anomaly is thought to be part of the spectrum of failure of recanalization of the duodenum in embryonic life. Depending on its severity, lesions may range from atresia to stenosis, diaphragm formation, and intraluminal diverticulum.[96] There may be an association with other congenital defects, such as Down's syndrome, cardiovascular lesions, intestinal malrotation, and omphalocele.[97,98] In adults, intraluminal diverticula usually presents between the third and fifth decades with symptoms of partial obstruction. Rarely, pancreatitis and hemorrhage secondary to ulceration have been reported.[99,100] Resection is the usual form of treatment for symptomatic diverticula, although therapeutic endoscopy with

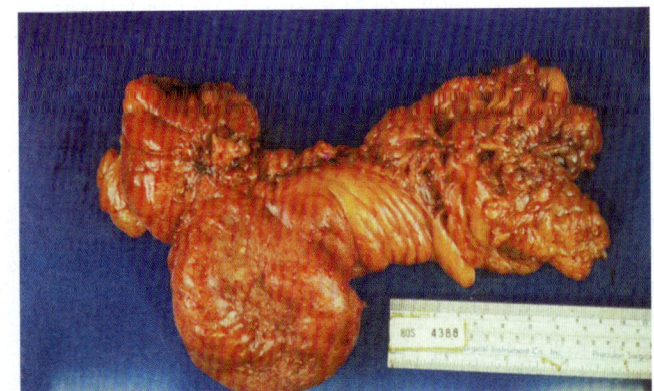

Figure 6-18. A solitary giant diverticulum of the colon, measuring approximately 10 cm in diameter.

incision or excision of the membrane may be indicated in selected patients.[101]

Gross Appearance Endoscopically, these lesions may resemble polyps,[96] up to 12 cm in length and 6 cm in width, usually attached to part of the bowel wall, and material such as stones and foreign bodies may become trapped in the pouch.

Histologic Examination This shows duodenal mucosa lining both sides of the pouch with submucosa but no muscle.

Jejunoileal Diverticula

Pathogenesis and clinical features. The most common location of diverticulosis is in the proximal jejunum; ileal diverticula are rare. Most cases are asymptomatic and found incidentally on imaging. Sometimes they cause symptoms due to bleeding, perforation, obstruction, or malabsorption secondary to stagnation of intestinal contents.[82,102–104]

This is a rare heterogeneous group of conditions with a reported incidence in the general population of <0.1%.[82] They may be congenital or acquired; the congenital ones are exceeding rare and are often associated with enteric duplications and defects in the spinal column[105] as well as motility disorders. Intestinal diverticula of the acquired type result from mucosal herniation through the muscle layer along the mesenteric border in relation to the perforating arteries. Concurrent colonic diverticula have been reported in up to 40% of cases, but this is approximately the prevalence in the general population.[91] Most cases of acquired small intestinal diverticulosis occur in older patients, and many are associated with intestinal pseudoobstructions, such as *familial visceral myopathy or neuropathy, mitochondriopathies, scleroderma, and Fabry's disease,*[89,106] or have local pathology indistinguishable from that of these disorders. Indeed, at any age, the battery of special stains carried out in intestinal pseudoobstruction should be carried out, or these changes are readily missed. If the muscle has disappeared, they are interpreted as "western type" rather than considering the possibility that the muscle has been lost from disease associated with motility disorders.

Gross appearance. *Acquired small intestinal diverticula* are usually multiple, wide-mouthed, paper-thin mucosal herniations situated along the mesenteric border of the bowel, measuring up to 4 cm in diameter (Fig. 6-17). Rarely, obstructing phytobezoar may be lodged within the diverticula.[104] The "congenital" diverticula are usually solitary and present on the antimesenteric border (Fig. 6-18).[84]

Histology. Jejunoileal diverticula may be composed of mucosa and submucosa only or of all layers of the jejunal wall. In the congenital diverticula, there is protrusion of all coats of the intestinal wall, which is greatly thinned. The morphology of the acquired diverticula depends upon whether the primary lesion is neural or muscle related, so adjacent and remote muscle in the specimen always needs to be carefully sampled and examined for neuromuscular disorders.

Some diverticula have an appearance indistinguishable from hollow/familial visceral myopathy lesions, some have scleroderma-like changes, while mitochondriopathies such as familial mitochondrial neurogastrointestinal encephalopathy (MNGIE) also have them (see section on mitochondriopathies). However, in "congenital" diverticula, there is invariably a degree of atrophy of the muscularis propria that gives rise to diverticular outpouchings made up of remaining layers of the bowel wall. All are covered by serosa, so it is necessary to find where the muscle stops and then identify the associated lesion (see section on intestinal pseudoobstruction). The trap is that if the muscularis propria is completely fibrosed, the appearance may at first glance resemble an acquired diverticulum as only the muscularis mucosae is visible. Careful examination of a trichrome stain usually reveals the fibrosis that is all that remains of the thickened muscularis propria, but examination away from the diverticula invariably reveals focal or complete loss of muscularis propria indicative of the underlying disease. The usual panel of histochemical and immunostains is therefore desirable to demonstrate muscle layers, nerves, ICCs, fibrosis, etc., as discussed later.

Diverticulitis and its complications, such as perforation, hemorrhage, inflammation, and obstruction, may occur but are rare. Those cases secondary to pseudoobstruction will show histologic features of the underlying disorder, namely, either a myopathy or a neuropathy.

Meckel's Diverticulum

See Chapter 16.

GASTROINTESTINAL MOTILITY DISORDERS

The Normal Motility Apparatus of the Gut

Normal intestinal motility depends on the coordinated activity and interplay of intestinal smooth muscle, the extrinsic and intrinsic nervous system and their neurotransmitters, the ICCs, and the GI hormones. Abnormalities in any of these result in abnormal intestinal motility and potentially failure of sphincteric function. Luminal contents also modify motility either by using and modifying the intrinsic apparatus. The clinical manifestations depend on the location and extent of the abnormalities and may be localized, as is usually the case in Hirschsprung's disease, or diffuse, as in visceral myopathy and degenerative neural diseases. Lesions in the esophagus can result in achalasia; in the stomach, they can result in gastroparesis, in the small intestine lead to pseudoobstruction, and in the colon lead to severe constipation and/or pseudoobstruction.

Musculature of the Gut

This is covered in detail in each chapter on the respective organ or site. To summarize here, there are two major muscle coats within the intestines, the muscularis mucosae and muscularis propria. Both have two layers, although that in the muscularis mucosae can be more difficult to see, but especially when hypertrophied, both are readily visible and are oriented in the same directions as the muscularis propria. While in some conditions with myopathies similar changes occur in the muscularis mucosae however, these tend to be subtle and diagnostically unhelpful.

With the exception of the stomach, the external muscle coats of the GI tract are organized into two layers, an inner circular and an outer longitudinal coat (Fig. 6-19). The circular layer is complete throughout the intestines. While the longitudinal muscle is complete in the small intestine, in the large intestine, it is focally condensed to form three taeniae coli, one on the mesenteric border, and two antimesenteric taeniae. They all fuse in the appendix proximally and splay out distally in the rectum again to form a complete muscularis propria.

All layers of the muscularis are richly innervated; indeed, all of the small "holes" seen on hematoxylin and eosin (H&E) sections are nerves. The ICCs are limited to the muscularis propria and myenteric plexus. This becomes important when assessing innervation.

The musculature of the upper third of the *esophagus* consists of striated muscle, and the remainder consists of smooth muscle, although there is a mixture of the two where they merge.

The musculature of the *stomach* is more complex. It consists of three layers, namely, an outer longitudinal coat, a middle circular coat, and an inner oblique coat. The outer longitudinal coat is continuous with the corresponding muscle of the esophagus and duodenum. It is relatively sparse anteriorly and posteriorly, except at the pylorus, where the musculature of the greater and lesser curvatures converges to form a circumferential sheet. The middle circular muscle coat is continuous with the esophagus and surrounds the whole stomach. However, at the pyloric sphincter, it bends on itself to form a muscular thickening and is not continuous with the circular muscle coat of the duodenum. The inner oblique coat courses from the cardia to the greater curvature, gradually merging with the circular muscle coat. Absence of this layer in the lesser curvature creates a depression, the so-called magenstrasse.

The cardiac, or lower esophageal sphincter, is poorly defined anatomically.

The pyloric sphincter consists of a thick band of muscle at the distal end of the stomach, which forms the gastroduodenal junction. The muscle bundle of the sphincter is composed of the circular muscle coat of the stomach, which is bent on itself and separated from the circular muscle coat of the duodenum by a thin band of fibroconnective tissue.[107] In cross section, smooth muscle fibers have a dense pink cytoplasm with round to irregular borders, depending on the state of contractility at the time of fixation. With autolysis, the cytoplasm may become swollen and stain poorly.[108] In H&E-stained sections, it may sometimes be difficult to distinguish poorly stained normal muscle fibers from atrophic fibers or collagen; thus, a trichrome stain is very useful for the interpretation of the intestinal musculature. The myenteric plexus lies between the longitudinal and circular muscle coats.

Demonstration of Smooth Muscle in Motility Disorders

Although demonstrable on H&E stains, fibrosis can be difficult to appreciate. Trichrome stains help considerably, enhancing not only fibrosis of the muscle, but whether it is occurring predominantly in the

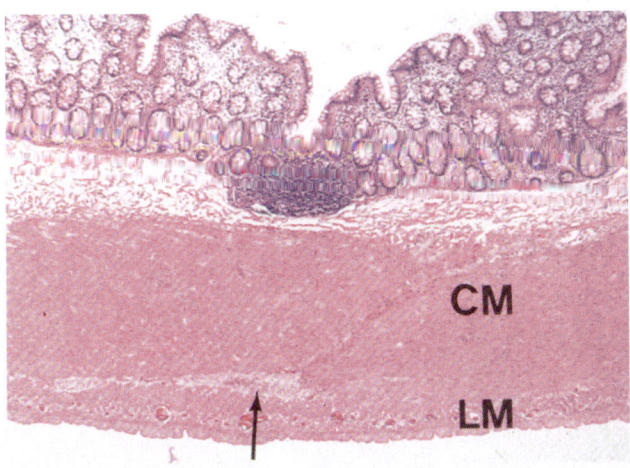

Figure 6-19. Longitudinal section of normal colon demonstrating the inner circular (CM) and the thinner outer longitudinal (LM) muscle coats of the muscularis propria. The intermyenteric nerve plexus (Auerbach's) lies between the two muscle coats (*arrow*).

circular, longitudinal, or both layers and also demonstrates the pattern that could be delicate interstitial or broad zones of fibrosis that frequently encases the muscularis propria on both internal and external aspects. It can also bring out additional layers of muscle that may be either in the submucosa or subserosa but can be subtle, especially the latter. Any marker for smooth muscle also enhances these changes.

ENTERIC NERVOUS SYSTEM

This system has two components, an extrinsic nerve supply and an intrinsic system. The intrinsic system is analogous to a microprocessor in close proximity to the effector system that initiates and programs the behavior of effector systems and automatically makes adjustments in behavior. The extrinsic system can be likened to a main computer that monitors sensory information from the gut and issues commands appropriate for the digestive tract.[109] The extrinsic nerves reach the gut via the vagus, mesenteric, and pelvic nerves and consist of sympathetic and parasympathetic nerve fibers, which mesh with the fibrillary network of the submucosal and myenteric plexuses and also interface with muscle fibers of the muscularis mucosae and muscularis propria.[108,110-116] The sympathetic system originates from cells in the prevertebral ganglia and synapses directly with the enteric ganglion cells. It exerts an inhibitory effect on the motor activity of the entire gut, with the exception of the sphincters, and decreases blood flow during physical activity and enhances it after feeding. It does not appear to influence GI secretions. The parasympathetic cholinergic fibers consist of the vagal and pelvic outflow tracts and innervate primarily the esophagus, stomach, rectum, and anus.[3,11] They control esophageal peristalsis, the esophageal sphincter, gastric emptying, and the internal sphincter of the anus.

The intrinsic (enteric) nervous system, in concert with ICC and gut hormones, is important in controlling intestinal motility and contributes to GI secretion. It is a complex but orderly system containing many chemically distinct types of nerves. Each type of nerve appears to have a characteristic cell shape and a precise projection pattern, sending processes in specific directions to specific targets.[12] Numerous different groups of chemically distinct peptides are found in the enteric nerves. These include substance P, vasoactive intestinal polypeptide (VIP), opioid peptides, somatostatin, cholecystokinin (CCK), neurotensin, and gastrin-releasing peptide.[12]

Histologically, the enteric nervous system consists of two nerve plexuses:

1. Auerbach's myenteric plexus, situated between the circular and longitudinal muscle coats
2. The submucosal plexus, which has superficial, mid, and deep parts[117]
   i. Meissner's submucosal plexus is the superficial component close to the muscularis mucosae (Fig. 6-20).
   ii. Henle's plexus, which is the deep component and situated immediately superficial to the circular layer of the muscularis propria
   iii. There is a less well-defined plexus between these two that tends to be in the superficial part of the muscularis mucosae and so, closer to the muscularis mucosae than the muscularis propria.

Microscopically, the plexuses consist of a meshwork of neurons aggregated into ganglia, axons,

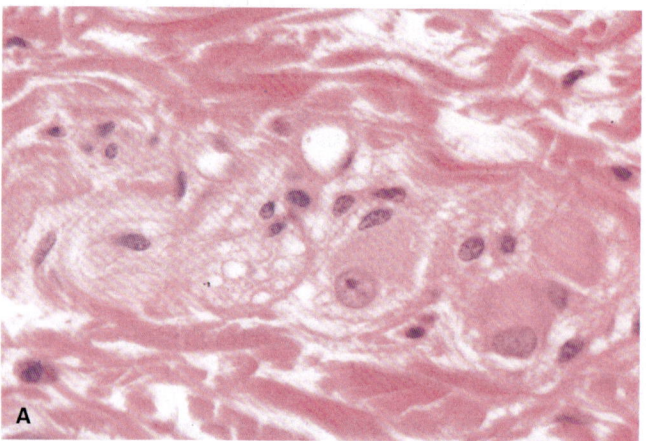 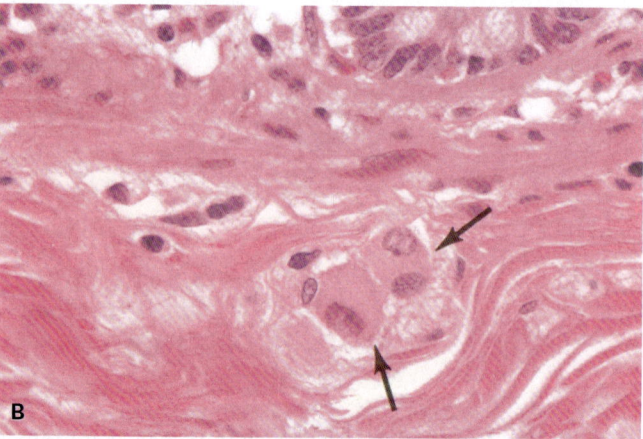

Figure 6-20. Nerve plexuses of the intestinal tract. **A:** Auerbach's myenteric plexus showing the bundles of nerve fibers and the ganglion cells with their characteristic ample basophilic cytoplasm. **B:** Meissner's submucosal nerve plexus. Note the submucosal ganglion cells (*arrows*) lying immediately beneath the muscularis mucosae.

dendrites, and nerve fibers. The latter communicate between the ganglia, muscle fibers, and mucosa. In the myenteric plexus, there are also numerous ICC that extend into the muscularis propria (see subsequent section). By conventional histology in perpendicularly cut sections, only a tiny amount of the plexus is visualized because the primary plane of the plexus lies in a horizontal direction. Furthermore, neuronal processes and nerve fibers remain unstained by H&E. Neurons can be demonstrated using neural strains but also stain strongly with Bcl2 and mismatch repair gene proteins. A subpopulation of ganglion cells are immunoreactive with calretinin, and calretinin immunoreactive nerves are also present. In the mucosa, these are markedly enhanced in Hirschsprung's disease.

Historically, the plexi were visualized in thick sections taken from between the muscle coats, cut parallel to the surface, and stained by a silver method[110] to produce a black stain in neurons, axons, dendrites, and nerve fibers (Fig. 6-21). The intensity of staining varies from intense black for the so-called argyrophilic neurons to pale tan for argyrophobic neurons.

Interpretation of these thick (up to 50 μm) silver-stained sections requires both specialized equipment and considerable experience with what is normal. However, there has been little correlation of silver studies using this method with either immunohistochemical or other histochemical techniques such that the interpretation of these stains in practice is fraught with many difficulties. However, there was much good work carried out that may therefore pass into obscurity.

The second component of the neural plexi is the massive innervation of the muscle layers, and both components need to be examined. An immunohistochemical nerve stain is mandatory in evaluating motility problems and depends on what is working well in your lab. Protein gene product 9.5 (PGP9.5), glial fibrillary acidic protein (GFAP), and potentially CD56, neuron-specific enolase (NSE), etc., can all be used, while S100 that stains the supporting glia can usually be used as a substitute (Fig. 6-22). Sometimes, they stain differently, so specialized centers may wish to do a specific neural stain as well as S100; however, there are few data on the correlations when these differ or

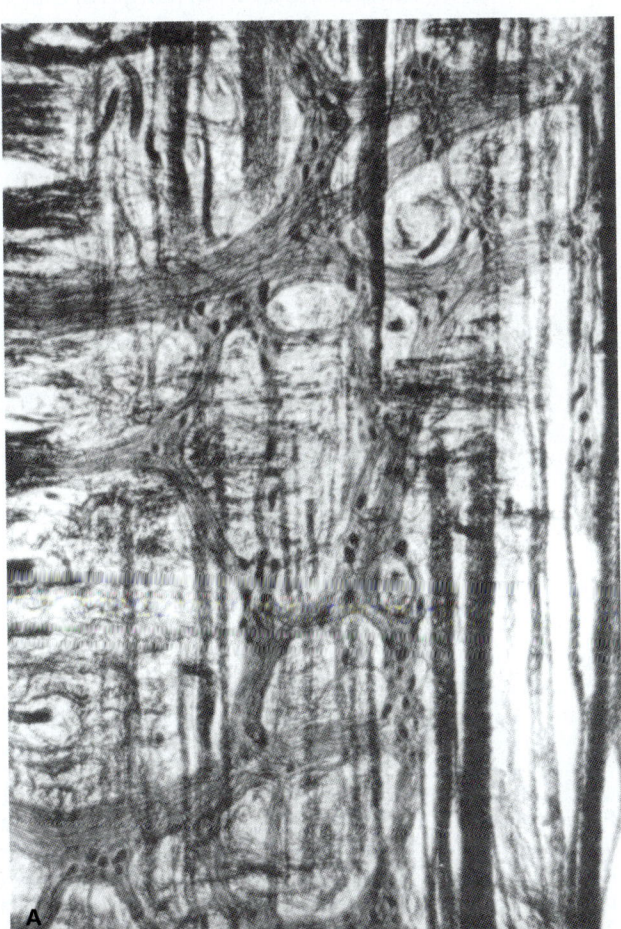
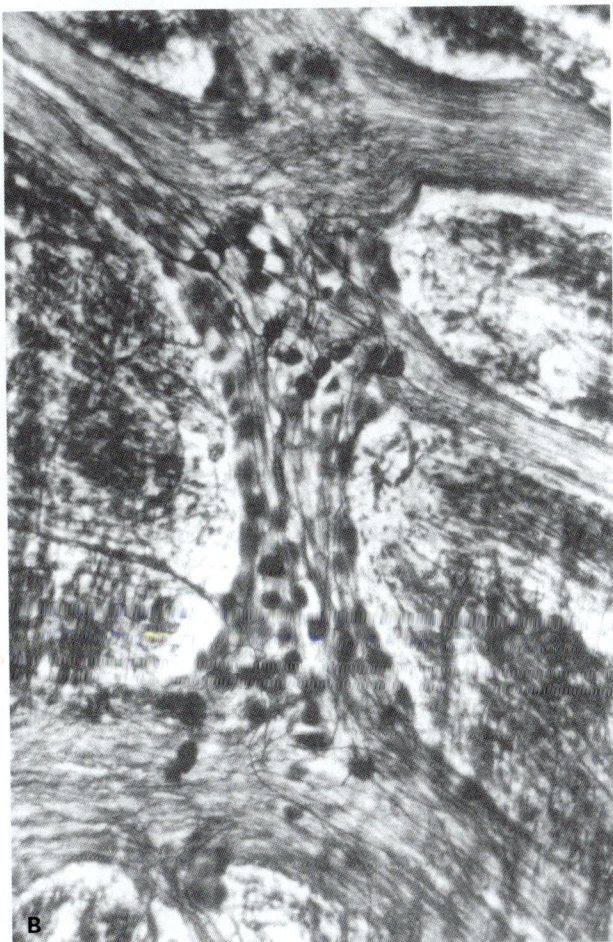

Figure 6-21. Myenteric plexus of the small intestine. **A:** The plexus consists of a mesh-like structure with neurons aggregated in ganglia near the intersections of the mesh (50-μm silver stain). (Courtesy M. Schuffler, MD.) **B:** Higher-power magnification of a ganglion showing numerous neurons and intervening thin nerve fibers. (Courtesy M. Schuffler, MD.)

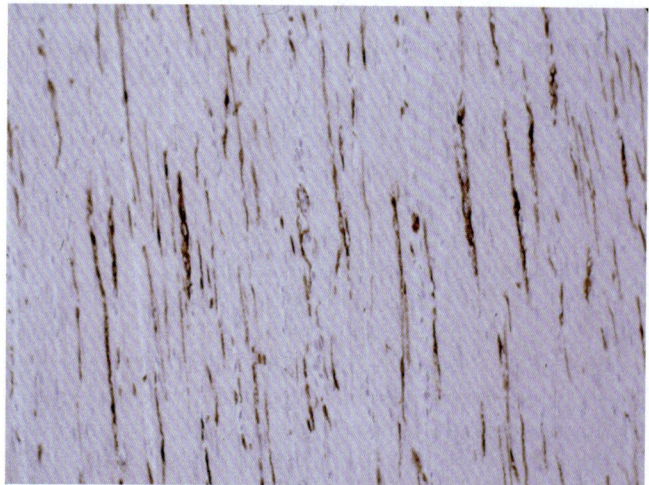

Figure 6-22. Neural innervation in normal bowel (S100 immunostain) in longitudinal section. These fibers are not visible on H&E stains and appear as very small round holes that are often interpreted as being artifactual as they are so numerous. When evaluating nerves, or their loss, it is imperative to have a normal control from the same region. It is also ideal to take sections both transversely and longitudinally so that nerves can be observed in the plane illustrated in both the circular and longitudinal layers of the muscularis propria. It also allows ICCs to be visualized in both planes.

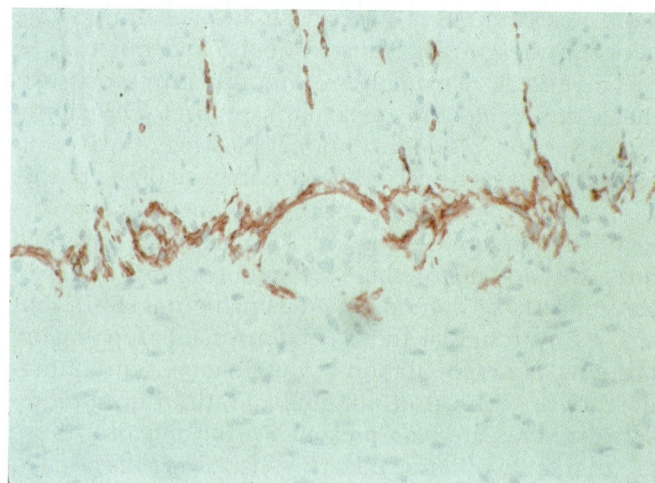

Figure 6-23. ICCs in the normal small intestine (CD117 immunostain). In the center, these form an almost complete sheath but one that tends to be deficient externally (longitudinal muscle side). In the large bowel, they are much less numerous, which is why it is always wise to compare with a normal control. In the top half, numerous intramuscular ICCs can be seen passing toward (or from) the internal surface of the circular muscle.

their significance. However, it is necessary to know what normal looks like in the part of the bowel being examined to interpret abnormal, so centers doing few cases should consider using normal controls if at all possible. Increasingly, the role of loss of nitric oxide synthase (NOS) producing nerves in motility disorders is being appreciated, and this may become a standard practice to evaluate this in motility disorders. Calretinin immunoreactive nerves are described in the previous section. There may be an argument for using this in motility disorders but it has to be regarded as experimental and controls are essential.

Interstitial Cells of Cajal

Interstitial cells of Cajal are thought to be the pacemaker cells of the gut initiating and maintaining its rhythmical contractions. They form from embryonic mesenchyme when cells differentiate into ICCs, likely as a result of sonic Hedgehog activation, and form a network that is found throughout the human GI tract and, when displayed appropriately, have numerous processes extending out akin to nerves. They are found

a) Primarily in and around the myenteric plexus (Fig. 6-23).
b) Within the muscularis propria, especially in the circular muscle. When examining ICCs, both major components need to be considered even though their interpretation is still in its infancy (Fig. 6-23).
c) Immediately beneath the internal margin of the circular margin, the deep submuscular plexus (Fig. 6-24).

ICCs have processes similar to neurons that can sometimes be observed (Fig. 6-25). To date, ICCs have not been identified in the mucosa or submucosa in man.

In patients with motility problems, most of the attention focuses on the myenteric plexus as that is where abnormalities are most easily recognized, but

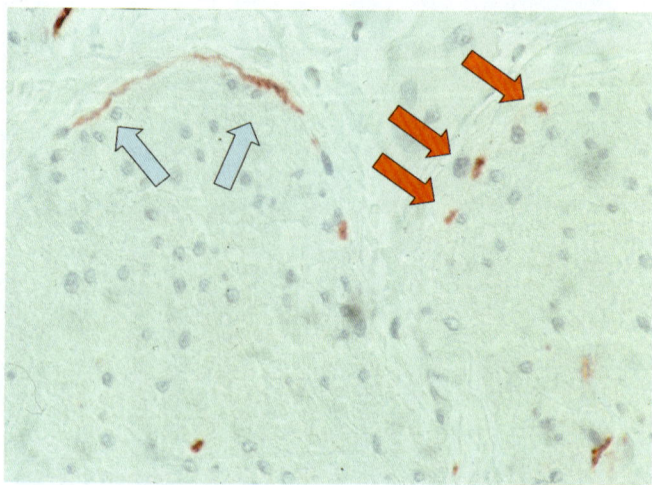

Figure 6-24. Submuscular (deep muscular) plexus that is immediately beneath the internal surface of the circular muscle immediately deep to the submucosa. These are thought by some to be the site of origin of contractions in the gut. Occasional mast cells can also be seen (a good reason to use DOG1 as the routine antibody for staining ICCs). ICCs are rarely "caught" lengthwise as seen on the left (*blue arrows*) but can frequently be identified as dots as seen on the right (*orange arrows*) (CD117). They are difficult or impossible to assess, and to date, disease caused by their isolated loss is scant.

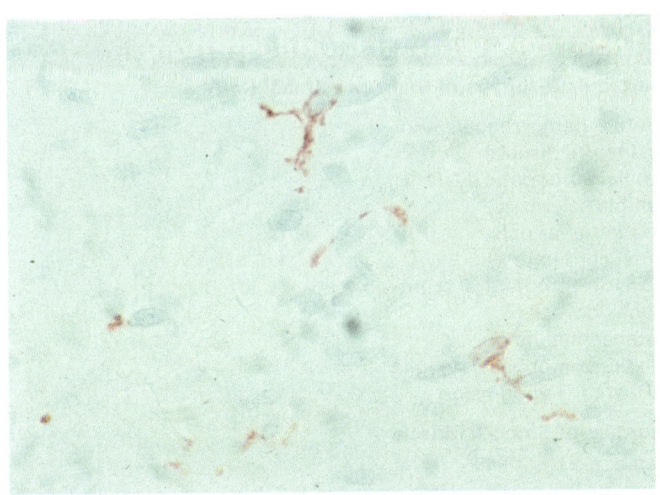

Figure 6-25. ICCs have processes similar to those seen in neurons, which are sometimes identified (CD117).

loss of ICCs in this location is invariably accompanied by their loss within the muscle layers and loss of nerves. It is also unclear whether just one component of the ICC network can be affected in isolation. Many other aspects of ICC related to possible hypertrophy, their regulation, and development remain poorly understood.

ICCs are accompanied by a specialized fibroblast network of cells, that is CD34, and possibly PDGFRα, immunoreactive, but unreactive with CD117 or DOG1; they are thought to express small-conductance Ca(2+)-activated K(+) channels (SK3). ICCs are thought to be the cells of origin of GI stromal tumors, but it is unclear if the fibroblasts have any role in these tumors. A complex consisting of the cholinergic and nitric oxide (NO)–containing nerves with neural vesicle, ICCs, and the fibroblast-like cells form a network that interplays with adjacent smooth muscle cells, forming a cooperating mechanism that controls motility, and loss of any of the components can result in motility disorders. Further, loss of one component may result in degeneration of another part of the network, so that loss of nerves may result in loss of ICCs and muscle and fibrosis (denervation atrophy) and vice versa. It can therefore be difficult to determine the initial insult in motility disorders, as by the time they are examined several components may be abnormal.

The number and distribution of ICCs vary from organ to organ.

In the esophagus, ICCs are present within both muscle layers but appear not to be present in Auerbach's plexus.

In the stomach, they are also present in the circular and longitudinal muscle of the corpus, but in the antrum, they are also present in Auerbach's plexus but are more frequent in antrum and corpus than in the fundus.

In the human small intestine, they are numerous in both longitudinal and circular muscle and abundant in around the Auerbach's plexus where they form almost a complete sling (Fig. 6-23).

In the large bowel, their distribution is similar to small bowel, but ICCs are much fewer around the Auerbach's plexus. In the appendix, they are distributed diffusely throughout both muscle layers (as are the ganglion cells).

Whenever the motility apparatus is being examined, it is worth running normal controls from the same organ for comparison. ICCs are immunoreactive with CD117 (Kit) and DOG1. Increasingly, we use DOG1 in motility disorders as the possibility of misinterpreting mast cell fragments as ICCs is abolished. Although there are (to date) no papers on using DOG1 in this manner, we have found that both antibodies stain ICC virtually identically other than there being no mast cell staining with DOG1. We do not use CD34 as there are too many cells other than ICC that stain.

MOTILITY DISORDERS

The etiology, pathogenesis, and pathology of motility disorders are something of a moving target, such that these are continually evolving and a long-lasting classification becomes difficult to achieve. Simplistically, it is easy to subdivide these into disorders of muscle, ICCs, nerves (intrinsic and extrinsic), and hormonal/neurotransmitter modulation, but there is considerable overlap. For example, some that are inflammatory disorders primarily target nerves but may also cause abnormalities of ICCs. Similarly, mitochondriopathies that are increasingly recognized to play a role in myopathies likely affect many other components of the motility apparatus as well.

The neurogenic disorders may be limited to the GI tract or may be part of a generalized neurologic illness. Similarly, damage to the intestinal musculature may be limited to the GI tract or may be part of a systemic illness, such as scleroderma, polymyositis, or myotonic dystrophy (Table 6-1). Currently, the most useful classification is the London classification[110] (Table 6-2), but the multiple components of this exemplify the difficulty in readily classifying many of them. These fall into the same basic groups making up its function, namely, disorders of muscle, nerve, and ICCs. What is less clear is how these relate, as disorders in one are often accompanied by disorders in the others, making it difficult to determine the primary cause. Most of these are rare, but some disorders, such as diverticular disease, are common and readily included within motility disorders, hence included in this chapter. Practically, while it is possible to follow the London

Table 6-1 Classification of Neuromuscular Disorders with GI Manifestations

Neurologic Disorders

Primary Visceral Neuropathies
Achalasia
Visceral neuropathy (degenerative noninflammatory)
    Familial
    Sporadic
Developmental abnormalities
    Hirschsprung's disease
    Maturation arrest of myenteric plexus
    Gangliocytic dysplasia
    Idiopathic megacolon
Jejunal diverticulosis
Severe idiopathic constipation

Secondary Visceral Neuropathies
Acute
    Postoperative ileus
    Ogilvie's (acute colonic pseudoobstruction)
Degenerative inflammatory
    Chagas' disease
    Paraneoplastic syndromes
Amyloid
Diabetes
Drug-induced/toxins (e.g., anthraquinones)
Jejunal diverticulosis (multiple causes)

Neurologic Disorders of Brain and Spinal Cord

Cerebral hemorrhage/stroke
Parkinson's disease
Familial autonomic dysfunction
Multiple sclerosis
Pseudobulbar palsy
Spinal cord injury
    Amyotrophic lateral sclerosis
    Tabes dorsalis
Postencephalitis
Calcification of basal ganglia
Orthostatic hypotension

Disorders of Smooth Muscle

Primary
Diffuse esophageal spasm
Pyloric stenosis
    Congenital
    Adult
Visceral myopathies
    Familial
    Sporadic
    Diffuse lymphoid infiltration (often muscle and nerve)
    Diffuse eosinophilic infiltration (often muscle and nerve)

Secondary
Progressive systemic sclerosis
Amyloidosis
Hypothyroidism
Myotonic dystrophy
Progressive muscular dystrophy

---

classification, it is easier to discuss the more traditional diseases by anatomical sites of involvement, and we have chosen to do it this way.

ESOPHAGEAL DISORDERS

Achalasia (Cardiospasm)

Achalasia is an uncommon disorder of unknown cause in which there is absence of peristalsis of the lower esophageal musculature and failure of the esophagogastric sphincter to relax normally with swallowing. This results in chronic stasis, with esophageal dilatation and hypertrophy. The prevalence has been estimated to be <1/100.000 of the population[119] and affects elderly Caucasian adults of both sexes equally. There is loss of innervation of the esophagus, with loss of ganglion cells and degeneration of neurons. There is also a reduction in the number of fibers containing the relaxant neurotransmitter, VIP. These findings may explain the incomplete relaxation and the increased resting tone of the lower esophageal sphincter characteristic of achalasia.[120] First-degree family members are sometimes affected, and an association has been found with class II histocompatibility antigen (HLA) DQw1, at least in white patients.[121] There is almost certainly an autoimmune component. Case report of an association with both Sjögren's and sicca syndromes, with identification of antimyenteric neuronal antibodies in some patients, lends support to an autoimmune mechanism.[121,122]

Patients typically present in adulthood with dysphagia for solids and liquids. In advanced disease, patients suffer from aspiration into the tracheobronchial tree.[123] A diagnosis is usually suspected by the characteristic symptoms and confirmed by x-ray, which shows a characteristic proximal distention with distal beak-like tapering (Fig. 6-26A).[17] Manometry reveals abnormal peristalsis, increased pressure, and delayed and incomplete relaxation of the lower esophageal sphincter. Endoscopy and endoscopic ultrasonography are complementary procedures to manometry and x-ray and help differentiate achalasia from pseudoachalasia due to tumor infiltration.[17,18] Treatment consists of rupture of the muscle of the lower esophageal sphincter, either with pneumatic

Table 6-2 London Classification of GI Neuromuscular Pathology

1. Neuropathies
    1.1 Absent neurons
        1.1.1 Aganglionosis[a]
    1.2 Decreased numbers of neurons
        1.2.1 Hypoganglionosis
    1.3 Increased numbers of neurons
        1.3.1 Ganglioneuromatosis[b]
        1.3.2 IND, type B[c]
    1.4 Degenerative neuropathy[d]
    1.5 Inflammatory neuropathies
        1.5.1 Lymphocytic ganglionitis[e]
        1.5.2 Eosinophilic ganglionitis
    1.6 Abnormal content in neurons
        1.6.1 Intraneuronal nuclear inclusions
        1.6.2 Megamitochondria
    1.7 Abnormal neurochemical coding[f]
    1.8 Relative immaturity of neurons
    1.9 Abnormal enteric glia
        1.9.1 Increased numbers of enteric glia
2. Myopathies
    2.1 Muscularis propria malformations[g]
    2.2 Muscle cell degeneration
        2.2.1 Degenerative leiomyopathy[h]
        2.2.2 Inflammatory leiomyopathy
            2.2.2.1 Lymphocytic leiomyositis
            2.2.2.2 Eosinophilic leiomyositis
    2.3 Muscle hyperplasia/hypertrophy
        2.3.1 Muscularis mucosae hyperplasia
    2.4 Abnormal content in myocytes
        2.4.1 Filament protein abnormalities
            2.4.1.1 Alpha-actin myopathy[i]
            2.4.1.2 Desmin myopathy
        2.4.2 Inclusion bodies
            2.4.2.1 Polyglucosan bodies
            2.4.2.2 Amphophilic
            2.4.2.3 Megamitochondria[j]
    2.5 Abnormal supportive tissue
        2.5.1 Atrophic desmosis[k]
3. ICC abnormalities (enteric mesenchymopathy)
    3.1 Abnormal ICC networks[l]

[a]Can include rare cases of non-Hirschsprung's disease severe hypoplastic hypoganglionosis with long interganglionic intervals (zonal aganglionosis).
[b]Although neurons have not been formally quantified, gross increases of disorganized neurons are evident.
[c]Can include retarded neuronal maturation.
[d]May occur with or without neuronal loss but is best regarded as a separate entity.
[e]May occur with neuronal degeneration and/or loss; lymphocytic epithelioganglionitis is a variant.
[f]Includes neurotransmitter loss (e.g., reduced or absent expression) or loss of a neurochemically defined functional subset of nerves (see text).
[g]Includes absence, fusion, or additional muscle coats.
[h]Hollow visceral myopathy may be diagnosed in familial cases with other characteristic phenotypic features; myopathy with autophagic activity and pink blush myopathy with nuclear crowding are rare variants in which degenerative findings are less overt.
[i]α-Smooth muscle actin deficiency is best described, although deficiencies of other proteins related to the contractile apparatus of myocytes have been reported.
[j]MNGIE causes a degenerative appearance predominantly in the longitudinal muscle.
[k]Absent connective tissue scaffold has been almost exclusively described in the colon.
[l]Generally reduced or absent ICC, although abnormal morphology also reported.
ICC, interstitial cells of Cajal; IND, intestinal neuronal dysplasia.
From Knowles CH, De Giorgio R, Kapur RP, et al. The London classification of gastrointestinal neuromuscular pathology: report on behalf of the Gastro 2009 International Working Group. *Gut.* 2010;59(7):882-887.

dilatation or at surgery with myotomy. Occasionally, esophagectomy is necessary in those patients who do not respond to esophagomyotomy.[19]

Gross appearance. The degree of esophageal dilatation varies with the duration and stage of disease (Fig. 6-26B). In advanced cases of achalasia, the esophagus is tortuous, enormously dilated (megaesophagus), and filled with stagnant, foul-smelling fluid and partially digested food. By endoscopy, the lower esophageal sphincter is closed and does not open during the procedure. However, gentle pressure allows the instrument to pass through the sphincter into the stomach, in contrast to a true stricture.

Histology. A variety of abnormalities have been described. In the majority, there is thickening and redundancy of the squamous epithelium, mucosal inflammation, and hypertrophy of the circular muscle of the lower esophagus (Fig. 6-26C). However, the major abnormality affects the nerve plexuses. There is degeneration, marked reduction, or complete absence of neurons. The glia may also be lost or proliferate. Frequently, there is an accompanying lymphocytic, and occasionally eosinophilic, inflammation and ganglionitis.[124-126] All areas of the esophagus are involved, although the dilated segment tends to be more severely affected, often with complete loss of ganglion cells.[20] The axonal and dendritic processes frequently show degenerative changes, such as swelling and irregular, club-shaped processes using special stains or electron microscopy (EM). One can also demonstrate loss of NOS producing neurons using immunostains.[124]

There may be an accompanying ganglionitis of the residual ganglia, but whether this represents a primary inflammatory disorder of the myenteric plexus (likely) or secondary change is unclear. Occasionally, lymphocytes may be observed infiltrating the cytoplasm of ganglion cells. Most chronic inflammatory

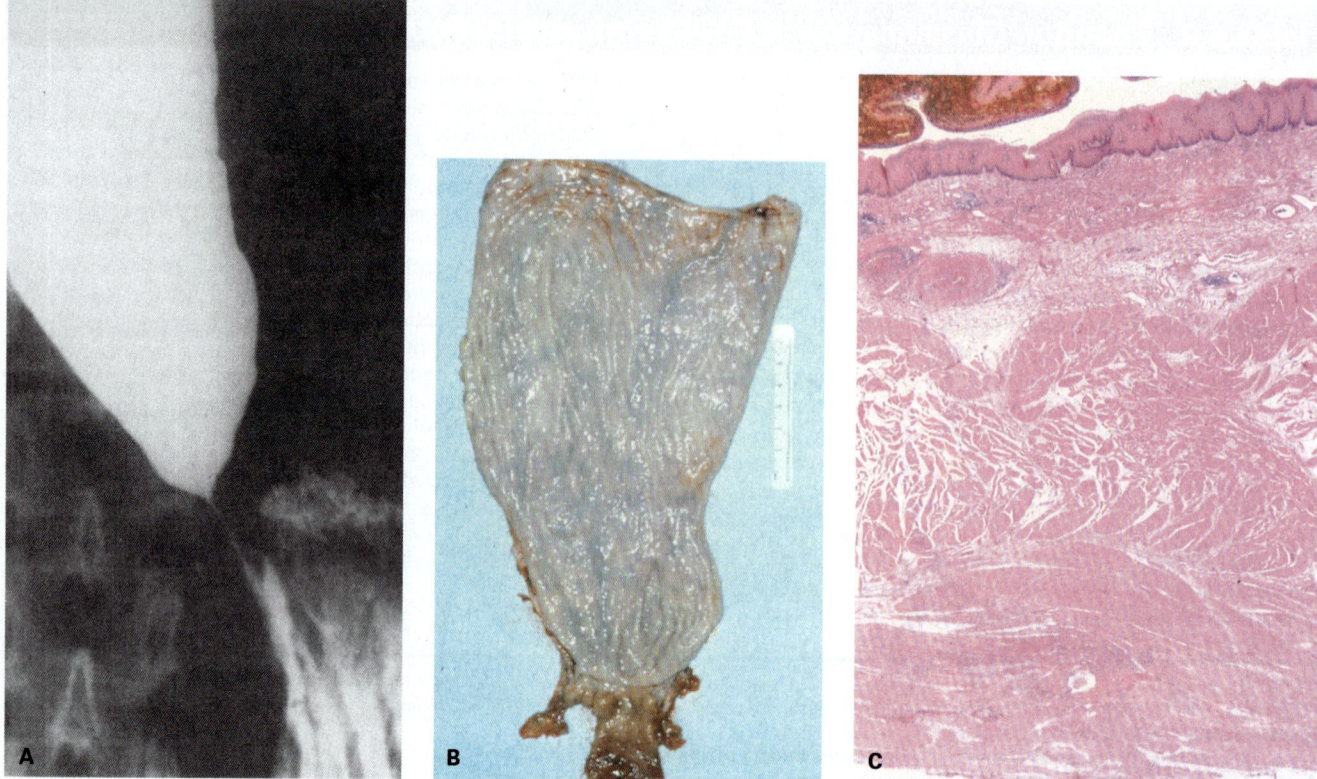

Figure 6-26. Achalasia of the esophagus. **A:** Barium examination demonstrating proximal distention and the beak-like tapering distally. **B:** Gross appearance of the esophagus showing marked distention. **C:** Low-power view of esophagus demonstrating marked hypertrophy of muscularis propria. (Courtesy F. Mitros, MD.)

cells are CD3+CD8+ T cells, but these cells decrease with disease progression.[127–129] Activated cytotoxic cells are also prominent.

Some cases of achalasia show a primary degeneration of dorsal motor nuclei of the vagus or the vagus itself, but these changes are inconsistent.[130] Hypertrophied muscle may show degenerative changes, including cytoplasmic vacuolation and liquefactive necrosis. The mucosa is invariably thickened with diffuse squamous hyperplasia, papillomatosis, basal cell hyperplasia, and lamina propria inflammation.[131] There may also be an increase in intraepithelial lymphocytes (lymphocytic esophagitis). Some of these changes mimic reflux esophagitis, although the sustained lower esophageal pressure prevents reflux of gastric contents into the esophagus. Patients with achalasia have been reported to have an increased risk of developing squamous carcinoma of the esophagus (in the range of 2% to 14%)[132,133]; however, in our experience, this is very rare. One study by Chuong et al.[134] failed to substantiate this increased risk, although another retrospective study from Sweden showed increased risk for both squamous and adenocarcinoma.[135] Carcinomas mimicking achalasia (pseudoachalasia) continue to be described.[136]

The pathologist does not commonly examine the esophagus of patients with achalasia, except at autopsy. However, in the evaluation of these patients, biopsy specimens may be submitted from the gastroesophageal region to exclude other pathologies, such as infiltrating cancer.

Secondary Achalasia

Tumor involvement of the esophagus can give rise to clinical, radiographic, and manometric manifestations identical to those of idiopathic achalasia. The tumor may be at the gastroesophageal junction or in close proximity, for example, small cell carcinoma of the lung or metastatic carcinoma.[21–24] Small cell carcinoma can also produce a paraneoplastic neuropathy of the myenteric plexus, with its esophageal involvement manifesting as achalasia.[137,138] Patients with secondary achalasia are usually older than those with the idiopathic form, have a short history, and have usually lost weight.

Esophageal leiomyomatosis and also sarcoidosis have been reported to present with achalasia.[139–141] The latter was associated with inflammation around myenteric plexus, but granulomas were not identified in biopsies. One patient had symptom resolution with steroids.[139]

Chagas' disease. This relatively rare cause of achalasia results from infection with the protozoan

Trypanosoma cruzi,[142,143] which is acquired through the bite of blood-sucking reduviid bugs. The disease is limited to parts of the world, such as South or Central America and Africa, but is uncommon in the United States and is seen almost exclusively in immigrants from endemic countries especially Brazil. Any part of the GI tract may be affected, but the esophagus and the sigmoid colon are the most frequently involved sites. This causes dysmotility and often massive dilatation (e.g., megaesophagus, megacolon). Esophageal symptoms closely resemble those of idiopathic achalasia, while colonic involvement results in constipation and intestinal pseudoobstruction. These features are all seen in the chronic phase of the disease, so that by the time symptoms occur, the organisms cannot be demonstrated in the myenteric plexus. Histologically, cases of Chagas' disease are indistinguishable from other causes of motility-associated neuropathy.

OTHER MOTOR DISORDERS OF THE ESOPHAGUS

A variety of poorly understood motor disorders of the esophagus have been the subject of recent interest because they may be associated with chest pain that mimics angina or, more rarely, dysphagia.[144] They are all likely associated with increased intraesophageal pressure and affect adults of all ages and both sexes. Many also have diabetes, raising the question of a possible associated neuropathy. Rare cases with possibly autosomal dominant inheritance have been reported associated with an Alport-like nephropathy and bilateral cataracts.[145] Squamous cell carcinoma has also been described in some cases.[146]

Idiopathic muscular hypertrophy of esophagus. Pathologically, the muscularis propria appears markedly thickened, particularly toward the lower end[147] (Fig. 6-27). Some have a mild lymphocytic infiltrate in the myenteric plexus, but usually lack evidence of muscle degeneration or fibrosis, and show no neural or ganglion cell abnormality.

Diffuse esophageal spasm is the best studied of them. It is a rare condition of unknown etiology seen predominantly in males over 40 and characterized by dysphagia and retrosternal pain, sometimes mimicking that of angina.[148,149] It is characterized by simultaneous esophageal contractions, which can be demonstrated manometrically and sometimes radiographically on barium swallow as segmental spasm (corkscrew esophagus) (Fig. 6-28). Not all patients are symptomatic; often the manometric and radiologic esophageal abnormalities can be demonstrated in the absence of pain and dysphagia. The pathology has not been described, but many patients have uncontrolled gastroesophageal reflux, so proton pump inhibitors are often used.

Idiopathic hypertrophy of the lower esophageal muscle has been found at autopsy in apparently asymptomatic patients.[150] A few patients have been

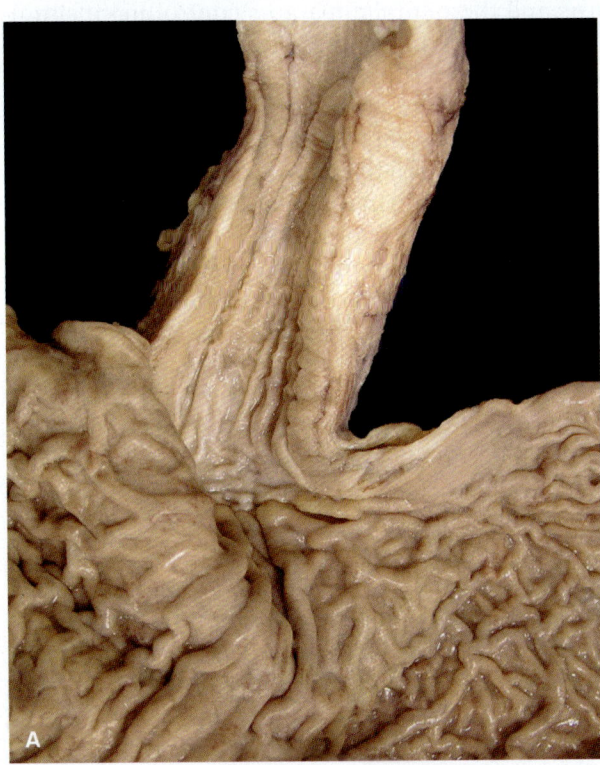
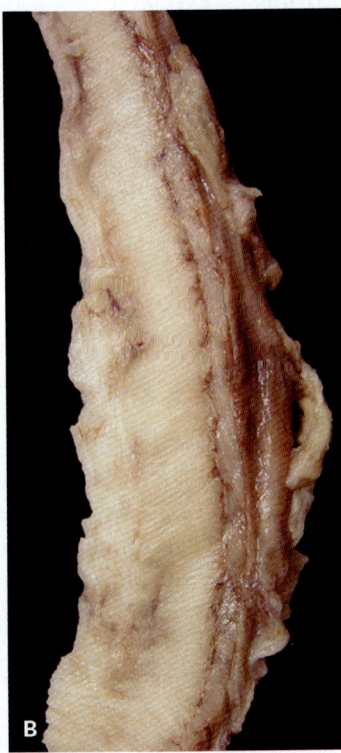

Figure 6-27. Idiopathic muscular hypertrophy of esophagus. **A:** Gross specimen showing marked thickening of the muscularis propria of the esophagus that is more prominent distally toward the gastroesophageal junction. Compare this with normal wall thickness of the stomach and lack of any gross mucosal abnormalities. **B:** A cross section of hypertrophic muscle from this case compared to a normal esophagus side by side.

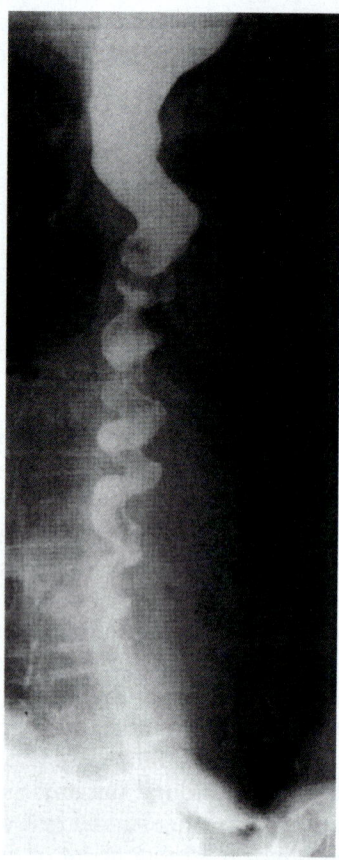

Figure 6-28. Diffuse esophageal spasm. Barium swallow showing typical segmental spasm (corkscrew esophagus). (Courtesy M. Weiner, MD.)

described who have progressed to achalasia, leading some to believe that the two entities are related[151]; however, the majority do not progress.

MOTOR DISORDERS OF THE STOMACH

Pyloric Stenosis

There are two types, an infantile type and a rare adult form.

Infantile pyloric stenosis (congenital hypertrophic pyloric stenosis)

Pathogenesis and Clinical Features Infantile pyloric stenosis (IPS) is a relatively common disorder with a high familial incidence as well as a marked male predominance. It causes severe, often projectile and nonbilious, vomiting in the first few weeks or months of life. The vomitus is nonbilious as there is no duodenogastric reflux as seen in most other forms of vomiting. The danger is from dehydration and electrolyte disturbance, which can be fatal. The treatment is surgical pyloromyotomy, an operation first introduced by Wilhelm Conrad Ramstedt in 1911, although the condition was first described by Harald Hirschsprung in 1888. It is caused by failure of relaxation and normal peristalsis of the pyloric sphincter, which can often be palpated as an olive-shaped mass in the middle upper part or right upper quadrant.

The prevalence is about 3/1,000 live births, with males being affected about four times as frequently as females. While the etiology is debated, it seems very likely that IPS is due to an inherited predisposition that results in delayed innervation of the pylorus, which includes nerves and their neurotransmitters, especially NO, ICC, and supporting cells. As these elements grow in after birth in these infants, the symptoms gradually resolve, explaining why this condition resolves spontaneously in those patients able to avoid pyloromyotomy. Gut motility does not occur until late gestation and after birth[152] indicating that there is a significant time lag between the appearance of neurons within the gut and the establishment of neural control of gut motility. There is a strong hereditary predisposition, and the risk is higher in both sexes if the mother, rather than the father, was the affected parent.[153]

The complete pathogenesis of congenital hypertrophic pyloric stenosis remains unclear, although the pieces are starting to fall into place. A variety of chromosomal links have been demonstrated including those controlling NO and carbon monoxide.[154] While it would make more sense if symptoms were present at birth, presumably the pylorus develops postnatally in response to feeding and food in the stomach, with the gradual development of both the pylorus and the neural apparatus controlling it simultaneously. The changes in the pyloric muscle are predominantly hypertrophic and therefore develop after birth, explaining the postnatal onset of symptoms.[155] In IPS, the innervation seems to lag behind the development of the muscle (which of course could also be prodigious), resulting in unopposed contraction of the smooth muscle, which produces both the symptoms and the muscular lump that may be felt clinically.

Grossly, the pylorus has a fusiform appearance with a greatly thickened, firm, pale muscle coat 3 to 5 cm in length. The thickening comes to an abrupt end distally, and proximally, the stomach is dilated.[156]

Histologically, the circular muscle of the pylorus is up to four times thicker than normal, shows disorganization of muscle fibers and an increase in connective tissue, and generally resembles a leiomyoma.[156] Desmin staining is strong, whereas in fetal and normal pylorus at this age, it is absent or weak.[157] The longitudinal muscle layer is frequently attenuated. Secondary mucosal edema and ulceration may occur in patients with a prolonged history.

Ganglion cells have variously been reported as normal or immature. The enteric nerve plexuses show hypertrophy of nerves, a relative increase in the number of Schwann cell nuclei, and degeneration of glial cells characterized by pyknosis and vacuolation.[156] Remaining nerves within the circular muscle are thickened/hypertrophied.[158]

Nerve and glial immunostains such as PGP9.5, CD56, and S100 are either absent or weak within the hypertrophied muscle layers as opposed to strong immunostaining in controls.[159,160] However, the remaining nerves are thickened/hypertrophied.[158]

Additionally, there is a loss of peptide immunoreactivity in nerve fibers in the circular muscle, while the reactivity is retained in the fibers and in nerve cell bodies of the myenteric plexus[161] NO is produced by neural nitric oxide synthase enzyme (nNOS) and is a transmitter of inhibitory neurons supplying the muscle of the GI tract, which are necessary for sphincter relaxation, thereby allowing the passage of gut contents.

ICC and their neurotransmitters, especially CO and NO, are markedly reduced in IPS. Further, mice lacking the nNOS gene had marked enlargement of the stomach with hypertrophy of the pyloric sphincter and the circular muscle layer, and is the best model of IPS.[162] However, ICCs both depend on NOS for their formation and produce NOS as the major source of NO for interacting with smooth muscle. Thus, the reduction and interrelationship between NOS and ICCs in IPS may be one of codependence.[163] In children who have undergone pyloromyotomy for IPS but in whom it was possible to examine the pylorus subsequently, the muscular hypertrophy and all other abnormalities returned to normal.[164] All of these data support delayed innervation of the sphincter as the underlying pathology of IPS, which reverts to normal with time. Although the background genetics that must underlie this condition are still unclear, there is a familial tendency, high concordance rate in twins that is higher in monozygotic twins than dizygotic twins.[165] Multiple genetic loci (IHPS1-5) have been associated with IPS, the strongest being with IHPS-1, which regulates the NOS1 gene.[166] nNOS is the critical enzyme that leads to the production of NO that mediates relaxation of pyloric smooth muscle. In addition, several RET variants have also been identified, but their role is unclear and likely not major.[167] Linkage studies have found loci on chromosomes 2, 6, 7, 11, 12, 16, and X to be associated with the disease, suggesting multiple pathways. However, within a single family, the disease may be linked to a single locus or gene.[168,169]

Adult pyloric stenosis. The adult form of pyloric stenosis is usually secondary and often a complication of peptic ulcer disease affecting the pylorus causing gastric outlet obstructions. A variety of other less common causes include neoplasms and other inflammatory disorders (e.g., Crohn's disease, eosinophilic gastroenteritis). However, apparent idiopathic cases may represent persistence of infantile stenosis.[10] Why the patients remain asymptomatic until they present in adulthood is unexplained. The pathologic features of the idiopathic form resemble those of the infantile disorder from the point of view of circular muscle, but the neural and ICCs changes have yet to be reported.[170,171]

Gastroparesis

Most gastroparesis is diabetes associated, but some patients have gastroparesis without diabetes, and rarely, it may be part of a paraneoplastic syndrome. Most present with intractable vomiting. There have been few studies on the morphology. One study in patients undergoing gastrectomy found smooth muscle degeneration and fibrosis, with eosinophilic inclusion bodies (M-bodies) that were thought to be specific.[172] A second patent with idiopathic gastroparesis undergoing subtotal gastrectomy was found to have hypoganglionosis, neuronal dysplasia, and a marked reduction in both myenteric and intramuscular ICC.[173] One study looked at the fibroblast-like cells (CD34+, PDGFRα+) in patients with both idiopathic and diabetic gastroparesis but found no difference from controls.[174] It is therefore currently difficult to justify gastric biopsy, which would need to be full thickness. The diagnosis is made by measuring gastric emptying, invariably endoscopy to exclude other gastric pathology as well as seeing the typical features associated with failure to empty. Management may require diet modification, prokinetics, antiemetics, neuromodulators, and ultimately may require jejunal feeding. The role of gastrectomy is not established.

INTESTINAL PSEUDOOBSTRUCTION

Definition

Intestinal pseudoobstruction consists of a group of propulsive disorders in which there are no gross lesions causing mechanical obstruction of the intestinal lumen.[44-50] It should be stressed that there is nothing "pseudo" about the intestinal obstruction, as in most patients an abnormality can be demonstrated in the propulsive mechanism of the gut even if it cannot be demonstrated by traditional imaging or endoscopy, although its motility consequences are readily apparent. The term therefore refers to the absence of a lesion usually associated with mechanical obstruction.

It can be *acute* or *chronic* and either *idiopathic (primary)* or *secondary* to *local or systemic disease*. The primary form of chronic pseudoobstruction is usually referred to as *chronic idiopathic intestinal pseudoobstruction (CIIP)* and may affect any part of the intestinal tract. It can often be further divided into *familial* and *nonfamilial* types, bearing in mind that autosomal recessive forms may not have a family history. *Colonic pseudoobstruction* refers to a form of pseudoobstruction that is limited to the colon and can be acute or chronic. Colonic forms may be amenable to colonic resection.

Acute intestinal pseudoobstruction. This disorder consists of paralytic ileus and may follow abdominal surgery, peritonitis, and a variety of intra-abdominal disorders.[45] Clinically, it is usually self-limited and is not discussed further.

Ogilvie's syndrome. This term is used synonymously with severe acute *colonic pseudoobstruction*, often in the postoperative period, especially following coronary artery bypass surgery and joint replacement. It can also be seen in patients with serious infections, cardiorespiratory insufficiency, neurologic disorders, and metabolic disturbances. However, drugs modifying colonic motility, such as anticholinergics or opioids, can contribute to its development. By definition, it excludes mechanical causes of colonic dilatation, such as tumor or volvulus. There is often massive dilatation of the cecum with a diameter >10 cm and right colon on abdominal x-ray. While most patients resolve, the mortality may still be as high as 30%, although the underlying disease clearly contributes to this.[52,53] Changes tend to be related to stercoral ulceration and associated ischemia, but (as yet) there is no specific described pathology. It is named after the British surgeon Sir William Heneage Ogilvie, who first reported it in 1948.

Pathogenesis and Clinical Presentation of Chronic Pseudoobstruction

GI motility is controlled by four main factors:

1. GI smooth muscle
2. Intrinsic and extrinsic nerves
3. Interstitial cells of Cajal
4. GI hormones, both local and circulating substances, such as prostaglandins. Therefore, abnormality of any of these factors can theoretically cause abnormal GI motility and pseudoobstruction.[51]

Chronic intestinal pseudoobstruction. This may be primary or secondary, the latter being part of widespread systemic disease. The diseases causing pseudoobstruction are listed in Table 6-3. Primary intestinal pseudoobstruction, also known as *chronic idiopathic intestinal pseudoobstruction (CIIP)*, consists of a rare group of propulsive disorders without widespread

Table 6-3 Chronic Idiopathic Intestinal Pseudoobstruction

TYPES	CLINICAL MANIFESTATIONS (OTHER THAN INTESTINAL OBSTRUCTION)	PATHOLOGY
A. Disorders of smooth muscle		
1. Familial visceral myopathy		Familial and sporadic forms all show thinning of bowel wall, vacuolar degeneration and dropout of smooth muscle, and variable fibrosis.
a. Autosomal dominant	Megaduodenum, megacolon, megacystis	
b. Autosomal recessive	Ptosis and external ophthalmoplegia Gastroparesis	
2. Sporadic visceral myopathy	Similar to dominant variant of familial visceral myopathy	
B. Disorders of myenteric plexus		
1. Familial visceral neuropathy		Degeneration of neurons and reduction throughout GI tract. Intranuclear inclusions in some cases of recessive type
a. Autosomal dominant		
b. Autosomal recessive	Mental retardation and calcification of basal ganglia in some cases	Argyrophilic and argyrophobic neurons degenerated and swollen
2. Sporadic visceral neuropathy	Some cases associated with small cell carcinoma of the lung	Glial cell proliferation. Chronic inflammation in some cases
3. Arrested development	With or without mental retardation or other neurologic abnormalities	Varies with stage of maturation arrest, from rudimentary ganglia and neurons to reduced number of fully developed neurons
4. Hirschsprung's disease	Constipation, abdominal distention; rarely, intestinal malrotation and ophthalmologic defects	Spastic (contracted) aganglionic segment, hypertrophied nerves
C. Jejunal diverticulosis		Variable pathology; may show changes of familial visceral myopathy, neuropathy. Sometimes secondary to scleroderma or Fabry's disease, mitochondriopathies (e.g., MNGIIE syndrome)

extraintestinal systemic diseases. Morphologically, chronic intestinal pseudoobstruction is characterized by abnormalities of nerves, ICC, or smooth muscle and often a combination of these so that it may be unclear which is the primary cause. However, the pathogenesis of many of these disorders is unknown.

Clinical Features The clinical presentation varies greatly and is often intermittent for unexplained reasons; the first attack may even occur in childhood. The symptoms are mainly those of intestinal obstruction with abdominal pain, distention, nausea, and vomiting. Occasionally, dysphagia signals accompanying esophageal involvement. Constipation is present with colonic involvement, often associated with colonic dilatation and abdominal distension, and bouts of diarrhea may also occur. Thus, the symptoms depend on the site of involvement (Table 6-3). Some patients may have malabsorption due to bacterial overgrowth in distended loops of small bowel. Chronic malnutrition is a major cause of morbidity of long-standing pseudoobstruction. It occurs most commonly because patients are unable to eat enough, since symptoms are provoked by eating. Management is difficult because of the lack of efficacious medications and extension of the disease to other regions, and some patients still undergo laparotomy looking for a cause of obstruction such as adhesions. This may make matters worse as once any form of exploratory procedure has been carried out, there is a subsequent risk of genuine adhesions, which may make the diagnosis more difficult. Biopsy of affected areas (thin or thick wall) may be undertaken and is discussed subsequently. The goals of treatment are the restoration of normal gut peristalsis if this is possible and the correction of nutritional deficiencies.[45]

Clinicopathologic Implications In adults, the diagnosis is now made commonly without resorting to surgery, which is sometimes done in adults but more commonly in children to rule out mechanical causes of obstruction and delayed-onset (or recognition of) Hirschsprung's disease. If that is ruled out, tissue may then be submitted to the pathologist to confirm the presence and type of CIIP or the presence of ganglion cells.

OBTAINING TISSUE. The key to the diagnosis of intestinal pseudoobstruction lies in obtaining good-sized (ideally 1 cm²) full-thickness biopsies of the muscularis propria, orientated so that the submucosal and serosal sides of muscularis propria, together with the intervening myenteric plexus, are all clearly visible in the plane of the section. Mucosal biopsies are of no value in the diagnosis of these disorders. It is also important to remember that lesions are frequently distributed irregularly and not diffuse. Thus, the specimen may confirm but does not exclude a diagnosis of neuromuscular disorder. The surgeon can help by selecting tissue from areas most likely to yield positive histology, namely, the dilated thin segments of bowel wall showing abnormal contractility. Some like a control biopsy from unaffected bowel for comparison. For the pathologist, it is important to remember that

i) The changes may be located in either the muscularis propria or the myenteric plexus including ICCs and are easily missed in conventional H&E-stained sections.
ii) Most biopsies tend to be taken longitudinally so that the circular muscle is seen in cross section, which is good for estimating loss of neural tissue, while the longitudinal muscle is not, so nerves are long but their number more difficult to assess. Ideally, if a square of muscularis propria is taken, it is worth taking a transverse section from both ends across the longitudinal muscle and then cutting the rest longitudinally so that both muscle coats can be assessed with ease.

Abnormalities such as fibrosis may be apparent only with special stains, such as trichrome. The tissues are best fixed in the usual fixative of the department so that any immunohistochemistry is reliable and reproducible. Frozen tissues can be kept, if possible as they may allow histochemical stains for mitochondriopathies to be performed and are better for any advanced molecular studies (nucleic acid or mRNA extraction), if needed. EM may help in a few so a few 1-mm cubes in glutaraldehyde can be helpful.

For routine examination, one needs a minimum of an

Hematoxylin and eosin
Trichrome to demonstrate fibrosis
Congo red for amyloidosis if suggested by the morphology. If present, immunohistochemistry may be required to determine subtype (see Chapter 8).
PAS—polyglucosan bodies and other inclusions

IMMUNOSTAINS. *A nerve stain* (e.g., PGP9.5, GFAP)—these sometimes differ from S100 that stains glia (Schwann cells), while PGP9.5, CD56, and CD57 stain nerves, although the latter two tend to be more promiscuous so not a first choice, so we tend to use S100, usually with PGP9.5, but there are virtually no description of abnormalities in one without the other.

A ganglion cell stain is sometimes useful, although these are stained by neural stains, but Bcl2, calretinin, or a mismatch repair gene stain (e.g., MLH1) can be useful. However, they tend to add little and so are optional and to some extent still experimental.

A ***Smooth muscle stain*** such as α-smooth muscle actin (SMA), muscle-specific actin, or caldesmon, but any would suffice and tend to complement or enhance findings present in the trichrome. The muscle markers highlight the fibrosis as negatively stained areas. If SMA is used, the issues around the existence of possible α-SMA deficiency and the controversies surrounding it need to be appreciated (see later).[175] We carry it out to gain experience with the variations of immunostaining but always include another smooth muscle stain when unusual staining patterns are encountered.

A ***stain for ICCs*** is required. We find that DOG1 is better than CD117 as it does not stain the mast cells, which can cause difficulties in interpretation when present in between the muscle fibers. We have stopped using CD34 as a part of this panel as it seems to add nothing and can be difficult to interpret as it stains many other cells types. Also, there are no data (as yet) on whether abnormalities of the CD34 and PDGFRα+ immunoreactive fibroblasts that accompany ICCs are responsible for any motility disturbances.

Specific neurotransmitters are optional and used for research or occasionally to answer specific questions, for example, especially NOS, but could include serotonin, VIP, calcitonin gene-related peptide, neuropeptide Y, substance P, CCK, CO, and possibly tyrosine hydroxylase as a marker of extrinsic innervation. However, these are largely experimental/research, and there is no reason to carry these out.

Inflammation. This can be quite subtle, and an argument can be made for routine staining with CD45 to detect all leucocytes and then CD3 to detect T cells more specifically. Interpretation can be difficult without experience of normal when scant inflammatory cells are present within the plexi, especially the myenteric plexus.

ELECTRON MICROSCOPY. It is worth considering taking a couple of 1-mm pieces of tissue and fixing them in glutaraldehyde in case EM is needed. Usually, this is to confirm abnormal mitochondria. In addition, abnormalities of myofilaments can be detected ultrastructurally in cases of visceral myopathies. Although EM can also show abnormalities of ICCs, the ease of using immunostains for this purpose combined with the difficulty of EM interpretation has made EM obsolete for this purpose in clinical practice.

SPECIFIC ENZYMES. This may require freezing of a piece of tissue for specific enzyme activity analysis.

MOLECULAR AND GENETIC STUDIES. These can be carried out on resected tissue or peripheral blood lymphocytes as deemed necessary.

CHRONIC IDIOPATHIC (PRIMARY) INTESTINAL PSEUDOOBSTRUCTION

CIIP consists of a heterogeneous group of disorders, which produce ineffective intestinal propulsion and which are not (obviously) secondary to other causes and especially to multisystem disorders such as scleroderma[108,176,177]. However, there are numerous other causes of CIIP that need to be considered as shown in Table 6-4.

CIIP also encompasses a group of disorders previously reported under the designations of *idiopathic megaduodenum, megajejunum,* and *megacolon* and is also implicated in jejunal diverticulosis in those disorders associated with loss of jejunal propulsion (visceral myopathy, mitochondriopathies such as MNGIE). CIIP may therefore sometimes be a familial disorder. CIIP is seen in adults and children and is being increasingly recognized in the pediatric population.

Examining Resections for CIIP

A spectrum of changes are seen, some of which can be seen in CIIP of almost any cause. These include

a) Diffuse thickening of the muscularis propria—usually readily visible just looking at the slide (Fig. 6-29). Although the longitudinal layer of the muscular propria is diffuse in the small bowel, on the large bowel, the non-taenia longitudinal muscle is also markedly thickened. This represents the inevitable secondary hypertrophy and possible hyperplasia in an attempt to keep the bowel moving. It is clear that muscle can regenerate and proliferate, for example,

Table 6-4 Major Secondary Causes of CIIP

Extrinsic (sympathetic and parasympathetic) nervous system
Stroke, diabetes, encephalitis, orthostatic hypotension, calcification of basal ganglia
Intrinsic (enteric) nervous system
Paraneoplastic syndromes, viral infections, medications (anthraquinones, clonidine, antidepressants, phenothiazines, antineoplastic agents, antiparkinsonians, bronchodilators), Chagas' disease, von Recklinghausen's disease
Disorders affecting intestinal smooth muscle
Myotonic dystrophies, progressive systemic sclerosis, amyloidosis, Ehlers–Danlos syndrome
Endocrine abnormalities
Hypothyroidism, hypoparathyroidism, pheochromocytoma

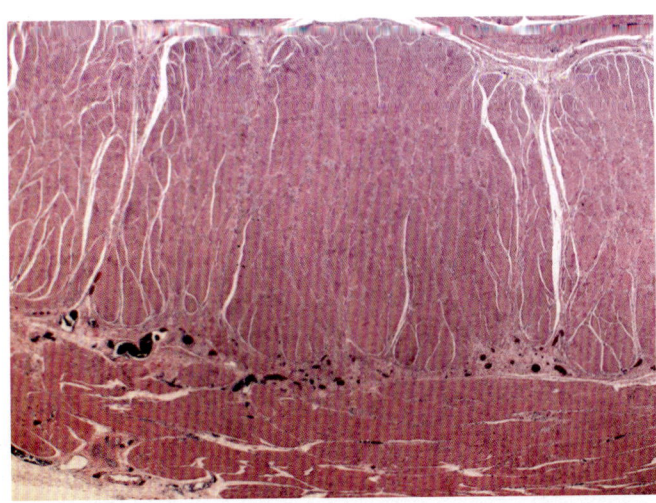

Figure 6-29. Hypertrophied muscularis propria in pseudoobstruction. H&E showing thickening of both elements of the muscularis propria.

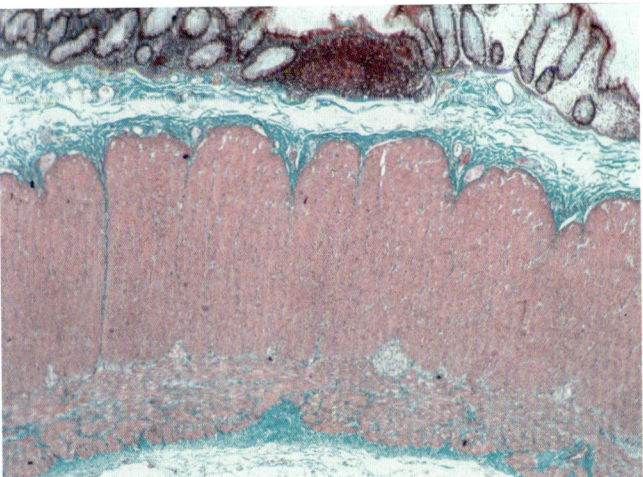

Figure 6-30. Trichrome stain of large bowel in CIIP demonstrating the markedly thickened muscularis propria (*red/brown*) and the *green* cocoon-like bands of fibrosis on both its internal and external surfaces, ensheathing the muscle and likely physically inhibiting contractions. The fibrosis can focally extend into the muscle.

beneath ulcers, so the notion of "terminally differentiated cells" completely losing any regenerative power is clearly erroneous.

b) The muscularis is often ensheathed in a layer of fibrosis, almost cocoon-like (Fig. 6-30). While readily visible on the H&E stain, it is also easily missed, and readily brought out in a trichrome stain.

c) There may be fibrosis of one or both muscle layers of the muscularis propria (Fig. 6-31).

d) There may be additional muscle layers, seen best on the trichrome stain or one of the muscle immunostains, although again visible on the H&E if looked for. These are usually external to the muscularis propria (Figs. 6-32 and 6-33) or less commonly in the submucosa (Figs. 6-34 and 6-35).

e) Loss of ICCs (needs CD117 or DOG1 immunostain) (Fig. 6-36)

f) Loss of nerves (needs S100 stain), often with varicose residual nerves (Fig. 6-37). Ganglion cells are not usually lost unless large areas of the entire plexus are also lost.

g) It is always necessary to examine the serosa, especially for adhesions that may potentiate the disease but adhesions alone cannot give rise to most of these changes. However, ischemia can cause fibrosis of the muscularis propria in the region of the ulcer, which can mimic the muscle fibrosis seen in scleroderma-like changes.

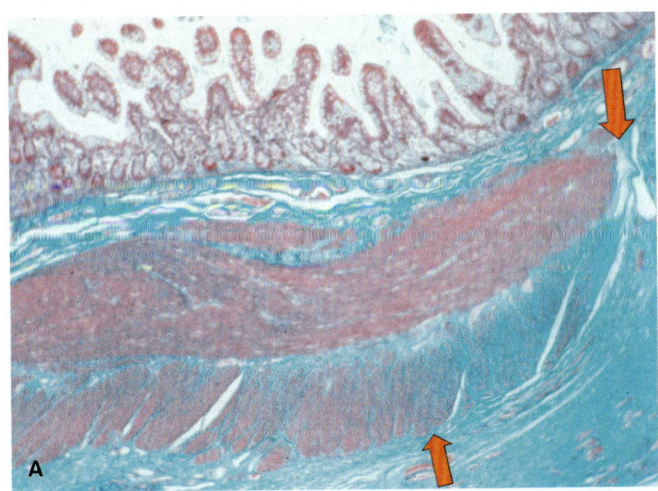
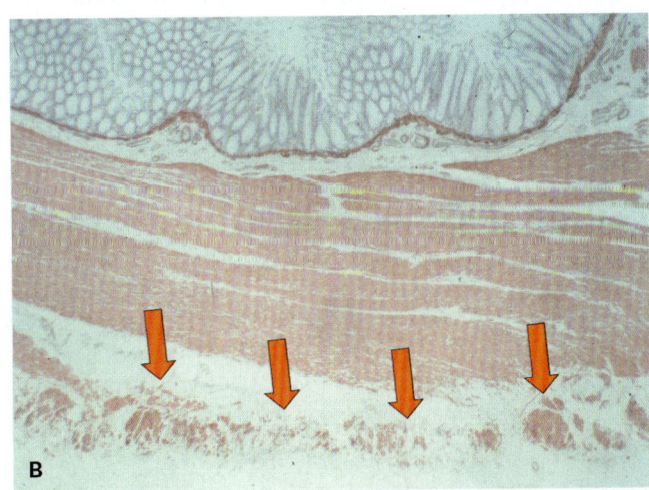

Figure 6-31. **A:** Trichrome stain of small intestine with fibrosis of both layers of the muscularis propria. In this section, the external layer appears to be more severely affected than the circular muscle, stopping (*lower arrow*) before the similar changes in the circular muscle (*upper arrow*), although to the right there is ultimately complete fibrosis of the entire muscularis propria that stops abruptly (*right of upper arrow*). **B:** Large bowel in which the outer longitudinal layer is largely destroyed, while the circular muscle is hypertrophied but not fibrosed (*arrows*). These changes are often called scleroderma-like, although very few patients with them have scleroderma or any other related disease (desmin immunostain).

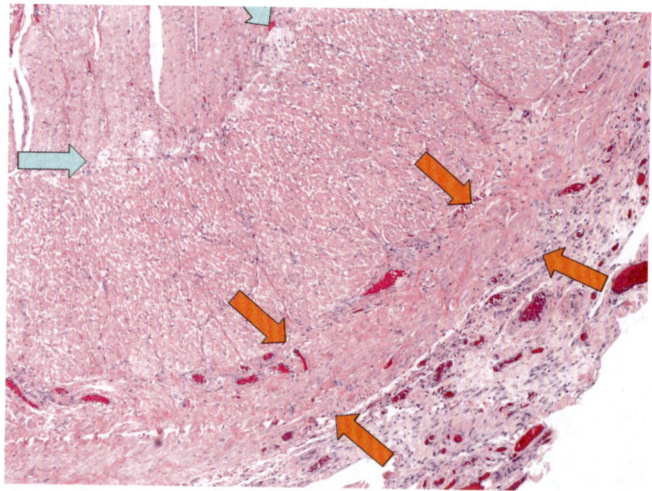

Figure 6-32. Additional external layer of the muscularis propria presumably acquired. The myenteric plexus (*blue arrows*) marks the junction between very thickened circular muscle above and longitudinal muscle beneath. However, demarcated by the *orange arrows* is an additional layer of muscle that is readily missed.

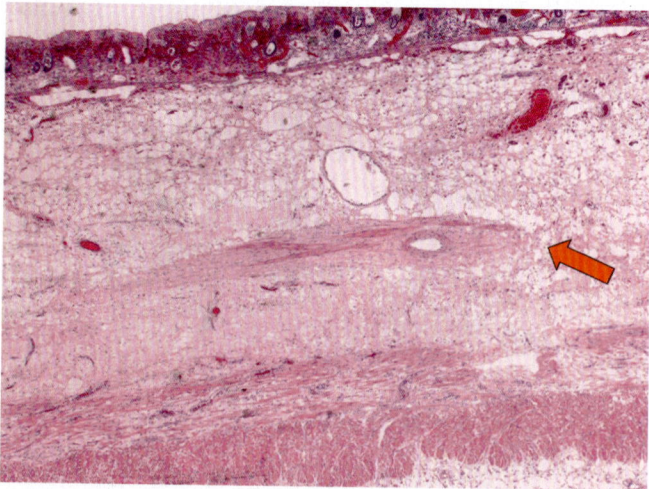

Figure 6-34. Large bowel with partial formation of an additional rudimentary muscle layer in the submucosa (*arrow*).

Interestingly, the most internal layer of the circular layer often remains in ischemic bowel for reasons that are totally obscure. There is therefore a thin layer of innermost circular layer, the remainder of the circular muscle being fibrotic, and a relatively normal longitudinal layer. It is unclear why this innermost layer of the circular muscle is spared.

Familial or Sporadic Visceral Myopathy

This condition, formerly known as *hollow visceral myopathy*, is a common cause of CIIP and is often familial. Apart from the GI tract involvement, there may be megacystis with muscle atrophy and fibrosis of the bladder wall. An autosomal recessive form has also been described, characterized by gastroparesis, jejunal diverticulosis, and external ophthalmoplegia.[56,178]

Pathology. Depending upon the particular subgroup, this entity may involve either the whole GI tract or localized areas.[44,46,57]

Gross appearance. Multiple sites of the bowel may be involved, showing diffuse or segmental dilatation (Fig. 6-38), thickening, or thinning, depending on whether the muscle is atrophic or thickened, and sometimes diverticular mucosal outpouchings. Megaduodenum[44] is common, and sometimes there is dilatation of the entire GI tract.[56] In the atrophic areas, the characteristic tan-colored, glistening muscle coat

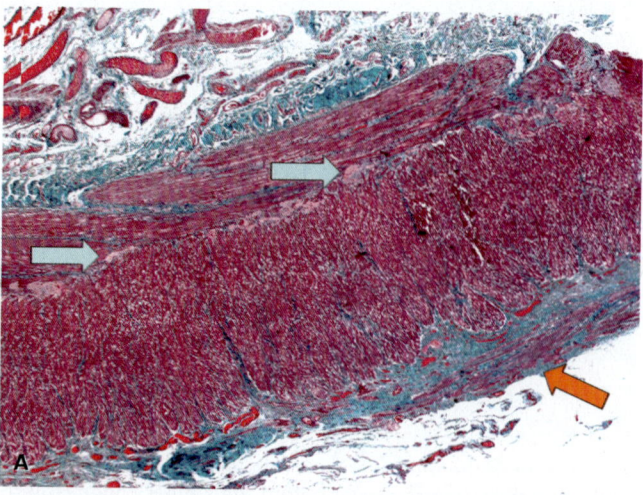
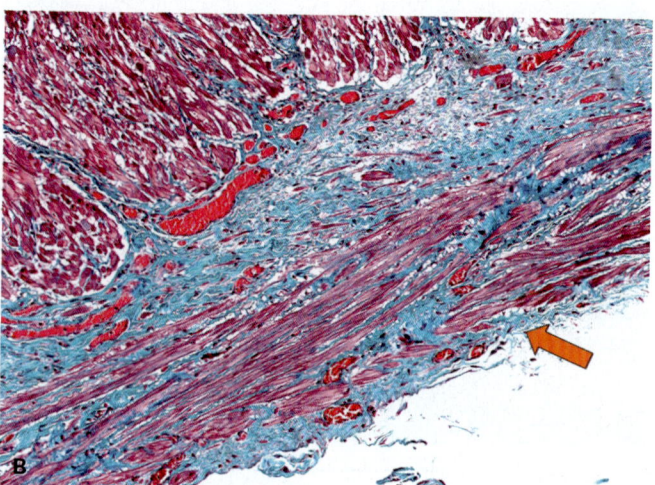

Figure 6-33. A,B: More subtle external layer of muscularis propria. The myenteric plexus (*blue arrows*) separates the circular and longitudinal muscle layers, but an additional partially developed compensatory external muscle layer can also be seen (*orange arrow*) that is orientated in the same plane as the circular muscle and opposite in direction to the fibers of the longitudinal muscle immediately above (**top left**).

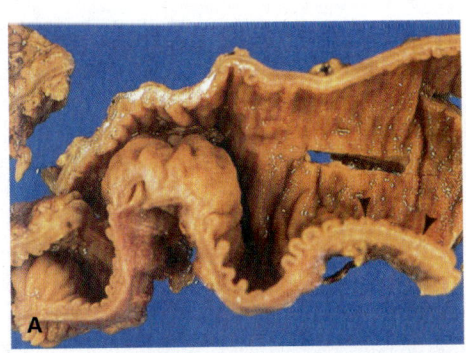
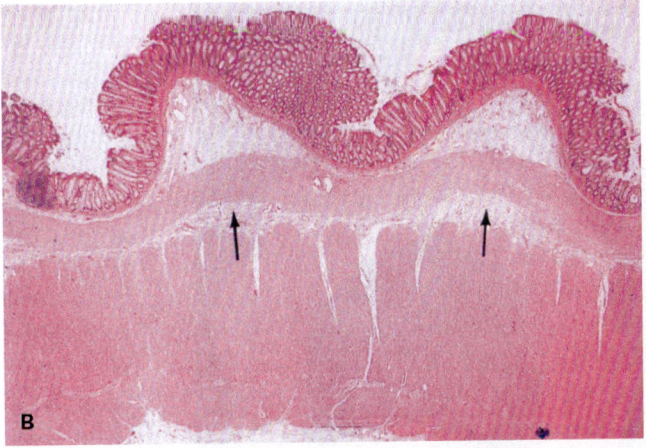

Figure 6-35. A complete additional submucosal muscle layer is present in a patient undergoing colectomy for severe constipation. **A:** Large bowel in which foci of ulceration are present in some areas, but a *white* submucosal band can be seen that is not usually present on the cross section of the muscle. **B:** Microscopically, this consists of a thick additional layer of muscle immediately above the circular layer of the markedly hypertrophied muscularis propria. Note that the overlying mucosa, including the muscularis mucosae, is architecturally and structurally normal and that the submucosa is not fibrosed, strongly suggesting that this part of the bowel was not previously ulcerated. It is assumed that this represents a further attempt at compensatory hypertrophy.

is frequently not visible or is obscured by gray-white tissue in transverse section. As indicated, the bladder may also be involved, with the gross findings of megacystis.

Histology. Visceral myopathy has several forms but is characterized by degeneration of the muscularis propria and fibrosis in the absence of inflammation and of vascular and neural abnormalities. The outer longitudinal muscle appears to be preferentially involved but either can be affected. The most characteristic change is vacuolar degeneration of muscle fibers, which may be encircled by collagen fibers (Figs. 6-39 and 6-40). In severe cases, muscle cells drop out, leaving a clear space surrounded by acellular collagen (Fig. 6-40). By EM, muscle cells show degenerative changes. They become electrolucent due to variable loss of myofilaments and mitochondrial swelling. In later stages, cells lyse and the cellular debris is surrounded by collagen.[44,58,59] In H&E section, the degenerative changes may appear pale and difficult to visualize (Fig. 6-39). However, the histologic changes are readily visualized, even at low power, by trichrome stains (Fig. 6-40). The degenerative muscular changes are confined to the smooth musculature of the muscularis propria, and the muscularis mucosa and musculature of the blood vessels remain normal.[58] In Figure 6-41, the outer layer of the

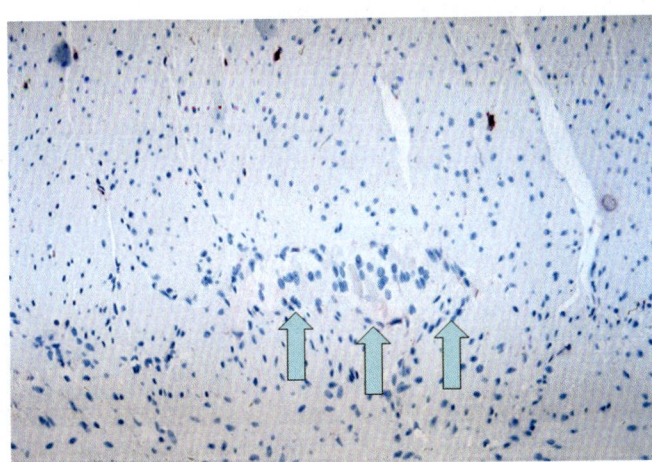

Figure 6-36. CIIP—complete loss of ICCs with occasional mast cells (CD117). The plexus is indicated by the *arrows*.

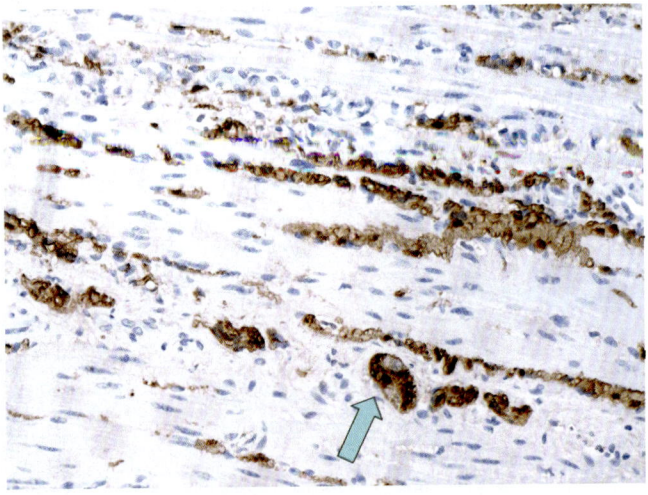

Figure 6-37. Residual nerves in the muscularis propria that are thickened and varicose (compare with the normal in Figure 6-21). Ganglion cells in the myenteric plexus *arrowed*.

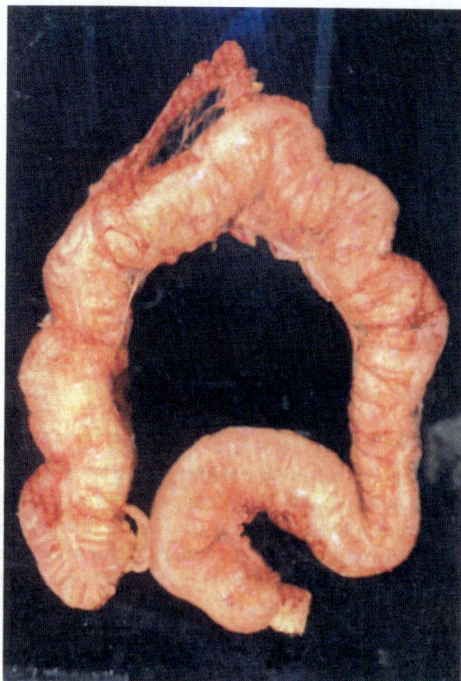

Figure 6-38. Sporadic visceral myopathy of the colon showing generalized dilatation.

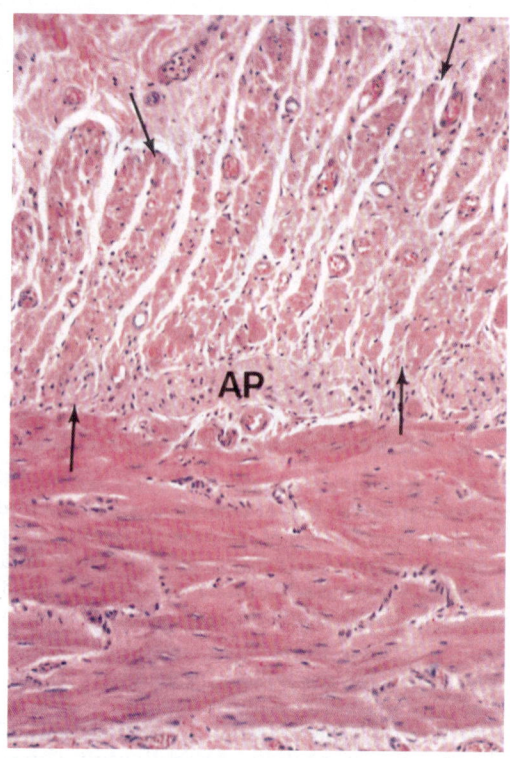

Figure 6-39. Familial visceral myopathy. The muscularis propria shows a rather indistinct vacuolar degeneration of the inner circular muscle layer in this hematoxylin and eosin–stained section (*arrows*). Auerbach's intermyenteric plexus (AP) appears to be normal.

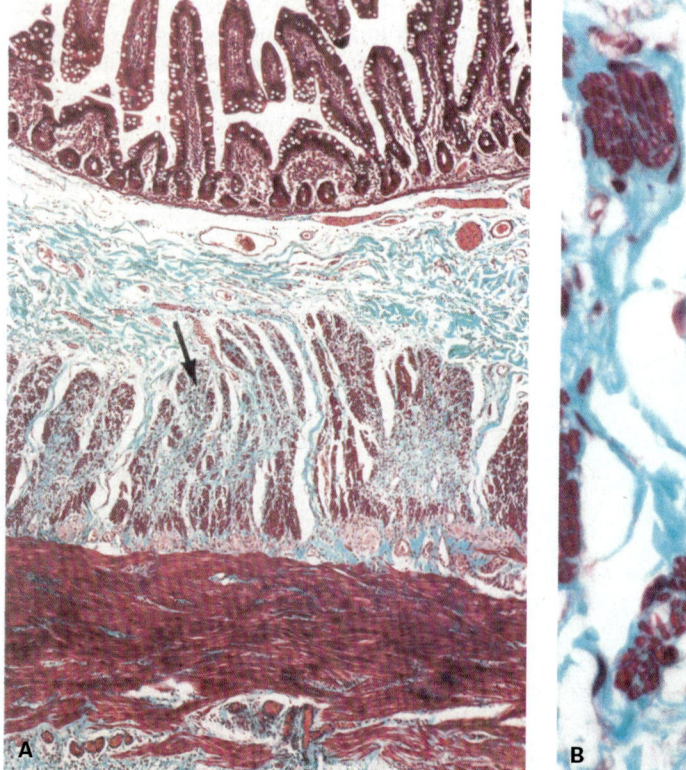
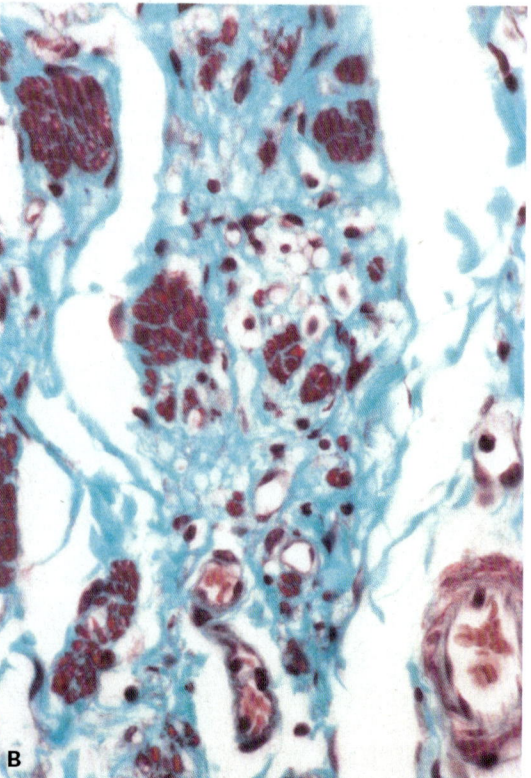

Figure 6-40. *Familial* visceral myopathy. **A:** In this section, stained with Masson's trichrome, the degeneration of the inner muscle layer is more readily visualized (*arrow*). **B:** Higher-power magnification of A showing the vacuolar degeneration of muscle fibers. Note the clear spaces resulting from the dropout of muscle fibers surrounded by acellular collagen.

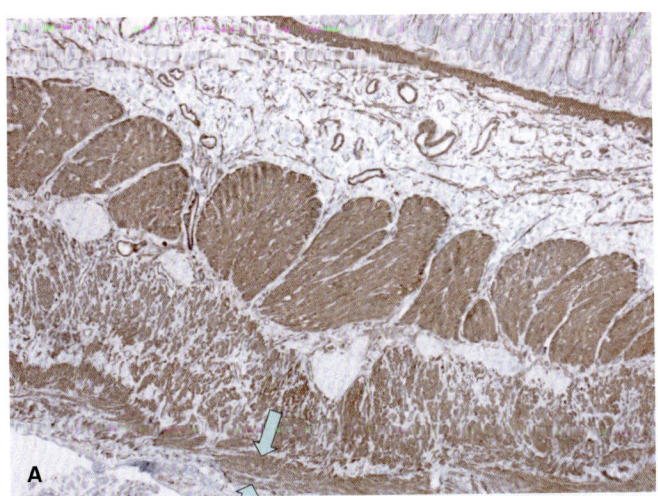 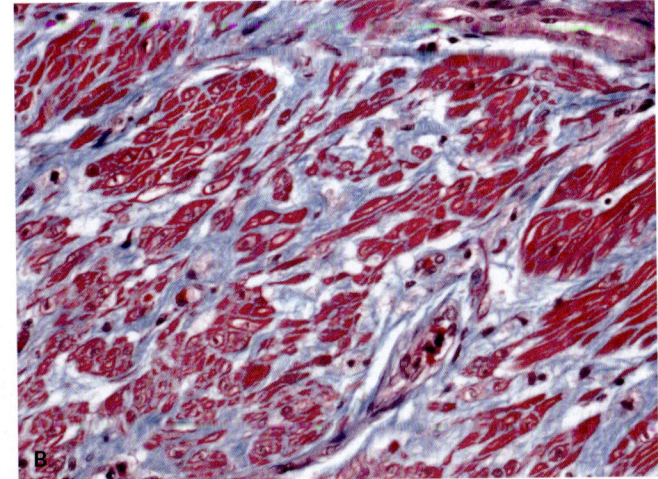

Figure 6-41. Visceral myopathy-like changes in the longitudinal layer of the muscularis propria. **A:** Actin stain showing the thickened muscularis propria and additional third layer of the muscularis propria (*arrowed*) orientated in the same plane as the circular muscle. **B:** Trichrome stain showing isolation and fibrosis of individual muscle fibers with focal vacuolar changes showing as white holes in the red muscle fibers.

myenteric plexus is preferentially affected. Note the additional layer of muscle external to the longitudinal muscle oriented in the same plane as the circular muscle.

While both sporadic and familial myopathic forms are recognized,[108] the familial form may be difficult to diagnose as involved family members may be asymptomatic. Other organs such as the urinary bladder and biliary tract may also be involved.[179,180] Subtypes include the following:

- Type I is the most common and can involve multiple organs including a dilated redundant colon, esophageal dilatation, megaduodenum, megacystis, and sometimes uterine inertia.
- Type II usually has gastric dilatation, occasionally a degree of small intestinal dilatation, and may include diverticula. Ptosis and ophthalmoplegia may also be present.
- Type III may involve the entire GI tract, from esophagus to rectum, which may all be markedly dilated.
- Type IV typically has gastroparesis, a narrowed tubular small intestine, but the esophagus and colon are usually normal.[181]

Other rare forms, partially resembling type I and III, with autosomal recessive mode of transmission, and esophageal and cardiac abnormalities have also been described.[182]

Sporadic cases are virtually indistinguishable from their familial counterparts, especially type III.

Although smooth muscle degeneration is thought to be responsible for bowel dysmotility, the etiopathogenesis for most of these cases remains obscure. Rare cases with actin or desmin abnormalities have been described.[183,184]

α-Smooth Muscle Actin Deficiency

This is a difficult entity to evaluate. In some patients with motility disorders, immunohistochemistry for α-SMA shows loss of immunoreactivity in all of the circular muscle of the small intestine except for a thin band on its innermost aspect (Fig. 6-42). Some reports suggest a relative decrease in staining in the circular compared to the longitudinal muscle, which may also occur in controls and has not been associated with any disease. It is also unclear whether, when these changes are present, they affect only the small bowel or other parts of the intestinal tract. The issue is with these changes is whether this is a variant of normal or whether it has clinical significance. It is included in the London Classification,[118] but it remains a confusing entity. Alpha and gamma smooth muscles are the two isoforms of actin (there are six) occurring in the intestines. It is interesting that when there is intestinal ischemia, the same immunoreactive internal layer is often spared when the rest of the circular muscle is fibrosed.

Following a single case report of complete loss of α-SMA,[184] a further study using SMA antibody immunohistochemically found it reduced or absent in 24% of 115 patients with pseudoobstruction undergoing full-thickness jejunal biopsies, being complete in three-fourths and partial in the remainder. However, there were only 20 controls, while identical changes were found in 10% of control ileal biopsies. Further CD117 immunostaining was not carried out in any of these patients, so this finding is

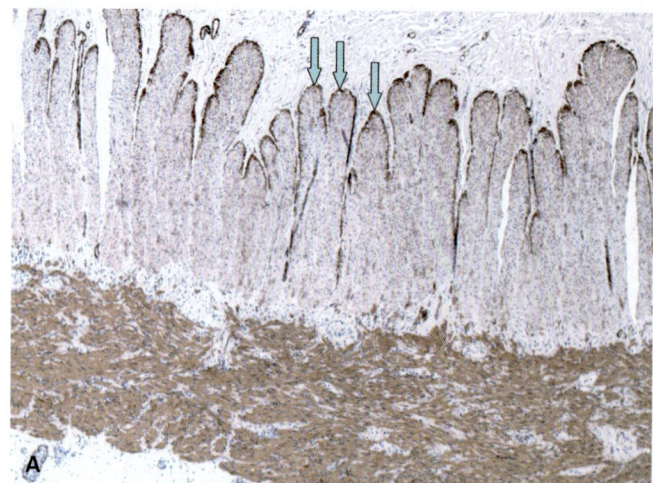
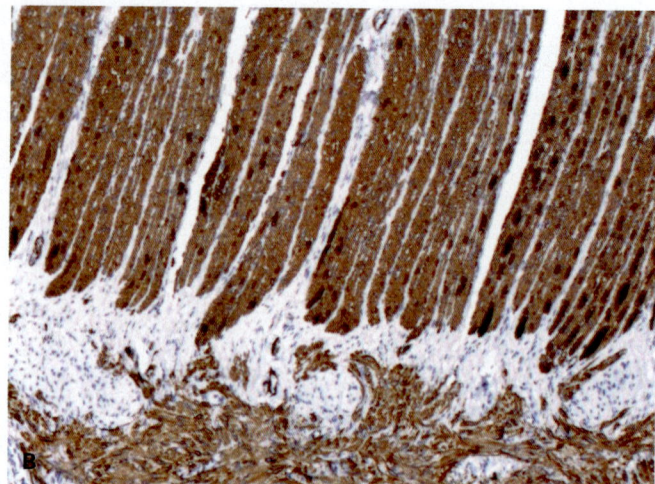

Figure 6-42. **A:** α-SMA immunostain of small bowel (this only affects small bowel) showing the characteristic loss of staining of the circular muscle only except for a rim of staining on its innermost surface (*arrows*). This also corresponds to the location of the deep muscular/submuscular plexus (see Fig. 6-24). This layer tends to persist when the rest of the circular muscle has been fibrosed. **B:** Caldesmon stain of an adjacent section that stains smooth muscle showing the usual pattern of staining.

a little suspect.[185] A second study showed the same changes to be present in 11/15 controls, and in those in whom large bowel was included the staining was normal.[186]

We have also noted similar loss of SMA staining in the inner circular muscle of the terminal ileum only, in right hemicolectomy specimens performed for carcinomas and no clinical evidence of motility disorder, and we believe that, at least in some patients, and possibly all, this is an artifact of unclear nature.

In an uncontrolled study of a family with visceral myopathy, the inner circular layer of the muscularis propria contained alpha-SMA–positive and, in more advanced disease, also periodic acid-Schiff–positive inclusion bodies. The inclusions were invisible in routine H&E-stained sections but were visible in immunohistochemical stainings for alpha-SMA.[175] However, anecdotally, we have seen these in patients without CIIP so that controlled studies are required to understand their true significance.

To complicate things further, a patient with *megacystis-microcolon-intestinal hypoperistalsis syndrome (MMIHS)* in which molecular observations have linked the disease to the neuronal nicotinic acetylcholine receptor (etaAChR), specifically with absence of its functional alpha3 subunit, was found to have a deletion of the proximal long arm of chromosome 15 (15q11.2). Histologic evaluation revealed an appropriate light microscopic appearance of both the circular and longitudinal layers of the small bowel muscularis propria, but immunohistochemical staining for SMA, however, was selectively absent in the circular layer, in a manner virtually identical to alpha-SMA deficiency discussed earlier.[187]

Familial Visceral Myopathy with α-SMA–Positive Inclusion Bodies

This has been reported in three generations of one family, involved members having degeneration and fibrosis of the muscularis propria. In addition, the inner circular layer of the muscularis propria has alpha-SMA–positive inclusion bodies giving an almost checkerboard-like appearance to the circular muscle. In more advanced disease, periodic acid-Schiff–positive inclusion bodies could also be seen. All inclusions were invisible in routine H&E-stained sections. The main problem with the study is the lack of controls subjects.

Differential diagnosis. Visceral myopathy must be differentiated from the secondary causes of pseudoobstruction such as scleroderma, the muscular dystrophies, amyloidosis, and sclerosing mesenteritis. Most of these entities can be excluded clinically with the demonstration of extraintestinal manifestations, although in some diseases, for example, muscular dystrophy, GI involvement may precede systemic disease. Histologically, idiopathic visceral myopathy can usually be differentiated from the secondary disorders by the absence of inflammation, neural changes, and vascular changes. *Scleroderma* is the most important and difficult lesion to differentiate histologically, since it is also characterized by muscle atrophy and fibrosis. Vacuolar degeneration is not seen, the remaining muscle cells are normal or atrophied, and the fibrosis is much denser, replacing all muscle fibers.[2,46,47] In contrast to idiopathic visceral myopathy, scleroderma damages predominantly the inner circular muscle coats rather than the outer longitudinal coat. It also involves the esophagus most commonly and shows more patchy involvement. The *muscular dystrophies* involve skeletal muscle, including the striated muscle of the esophagus, in addition to the smooth muscle coats of the small intestine and colon. They are characterized by coagulative necrosis (pink hyaline cytoplasmic change), atrophy, and fatty infiltration of striated muscle. *Sclerosing mesenteritis* is a condition that primarily involves the mesentery, producing fibrous thickening and chronic inflammation. In some cases, the inflamed fibrous tissue extends into the bowel to produce fibrosis of the muscularis propria

Desmin Myopathy

Rare cases with desmin abnormalities (desmin myopathy) have been described that as well as the intestines also involve systemic skeletal and cardiac muscle.[183,184]

African Visceral Myopathy

A distinct form of nonfamilial visceral myopathy has been described in children primarily from the Western Cape region of South Africa. The mean age at presentation was 9.5 years (range 6 months to 16 years). Clinical features included a chronic, insidious history of repeated attacks of abdominal distension, abdominal pain, and vomiting; marked gaseous distension with atony; and pseudoobstruction. Megacolon was the most common radiologic feature, but pseudoobstruction extended proximally into the small intestine in some patients with advanced disease. In the majority, the condition was progressive and eventually affected the entire GI tract.[188]

Issues Reporting Motility Disorders

While the majority of resections for severe constipation of small bowel motility tend to fall into the "end stage," often scleroderma-like changes, the changes can also be complex and difficult to evaluate, especially where the bowel is dilated and thinned so that it is difficult to come to a definitive conclusion. An example occurring in jejunal diverticulosis is shown in Figure 6-43. The diverticula expand and thin the muscularis propria, so it is difficult to know whether changes in muscle are reactive and whether reduction of ICCs or nerves is genuine or secondary to the dilatation present. In this instance, because there were changes in the longitudinal muscle resembling visceral myopathy, the possibility that this was the underlying disease was suggested. However, notice that nerves are also markedly reduced and ICCs variable.

PRIMARY VISCERAL NEUROPATHIES

In common with the visceral myopathies, *familial* and *sporadic* cases are described. It may be the result of abnormalities of the intrinsic or extrinsic neural network of the bowel.[108,189]

Many neuropathies cannot be readily diagnosed in conventionally stained sections of bowel because, neural networks (neurons) within the muscle are difficult to visualize in conventionally stained H&E sections. Stains for nerve and ICCs are therefore required, but the major problem is that both are frequently lost

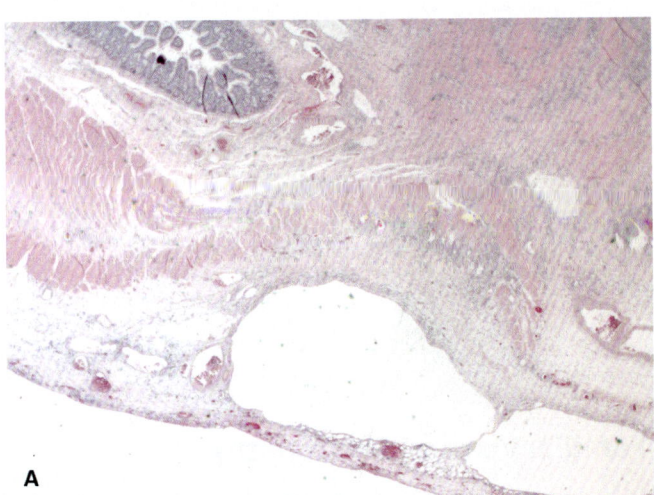
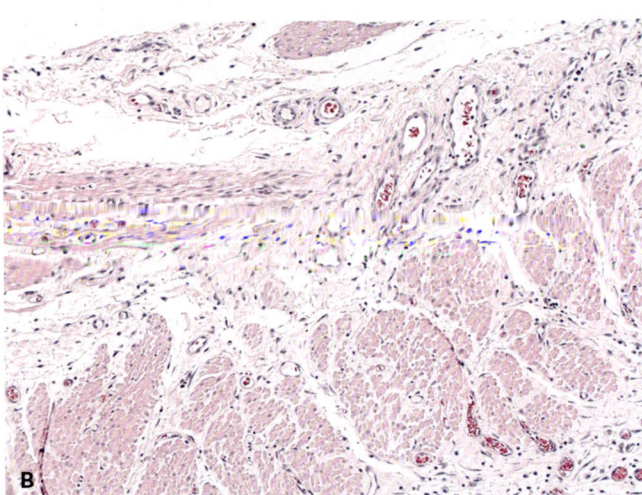

Figure 6-43. Jejunal diverticulum with thinning of muscle, loss of neurons and ICCs, and visceral myopathy-like changes in the longitudinal muscle. **A:** Overview showing mucosa with villi that are shortened and inflamed, likely from bacterial overgrowth. The diverticulum is pushing out the muscle, which therefore retains all of its muscle coats and so is readily considered to be "congenital." **B:** Muscle is thinned, and the fibers of the circular muscle are splayed with a little fibrosis (**C**—trichrome stain), while the longitudinal muscle (**bottom**) shows pericellular fibrosis suggestive of visceral myopathy (detail in **D**).

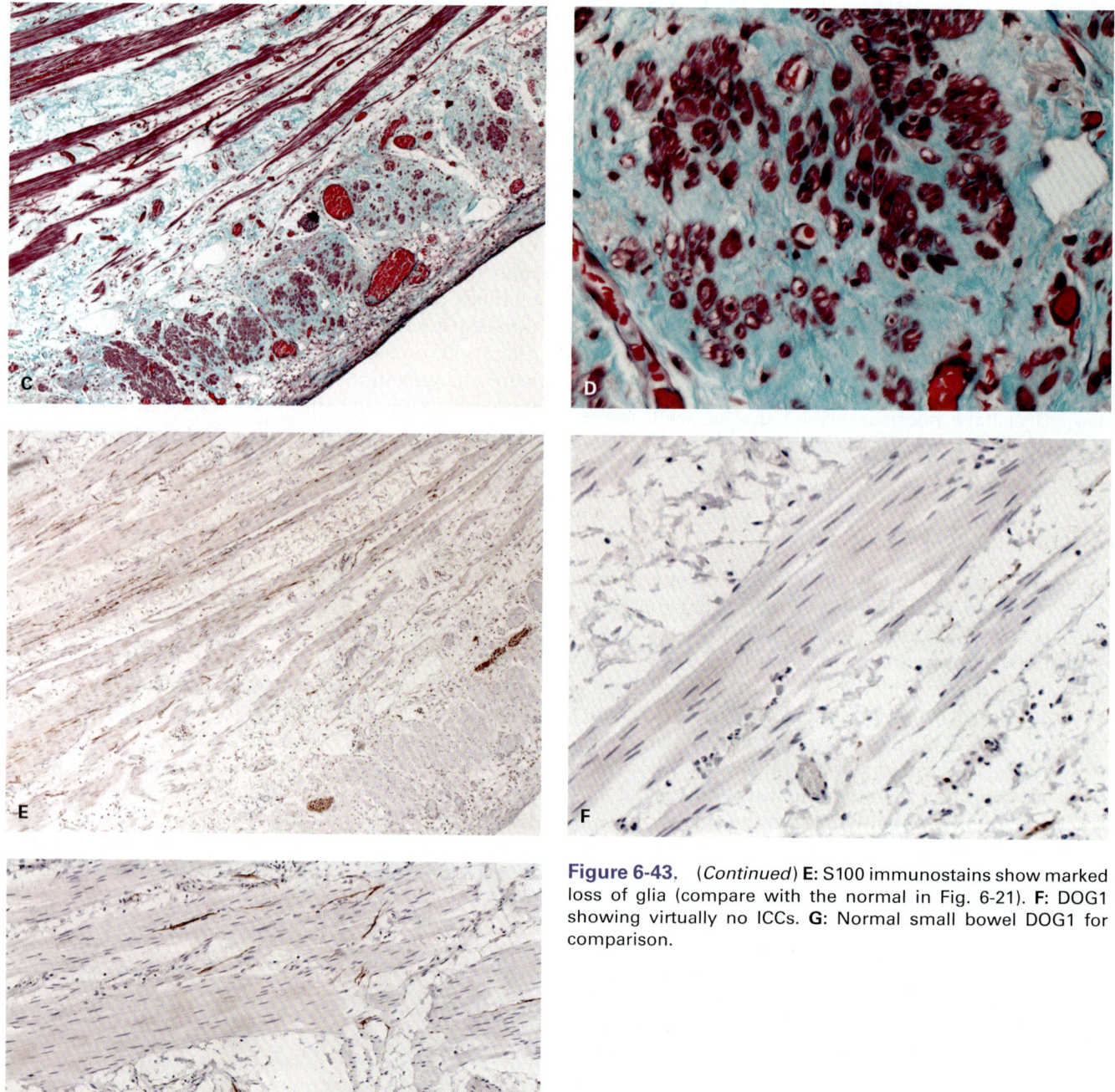

Figure 6-43. (*Continued*) **E:** S100 immunostains show marked loss of glia (compare with the normal in Fig. 6-21). **F:** DOG1 showing virtually no ICCs. **G:** Normal small bowel DOG1 for comparison.

so that it is impossible to know which came first. The spaces that nerves occupy are readily visualized as minute holes in the smooth muscle, especially the inner circular muscle. What cannot be detected on H&E stains is whether they are still present or have been lost; hence the need for immunohistochemical stains.

Familial Visceral Neuropathy

Inheritance can be autosomal dominant, autosomal recessive, or, rarely, X-linked, but it is the autosomal recessive cases that tend to have the intranuclear inclusions in ganglion cells that are visible in H&E-stained sections. Some have mental retardation and

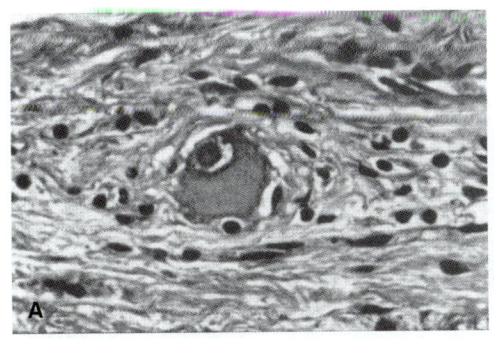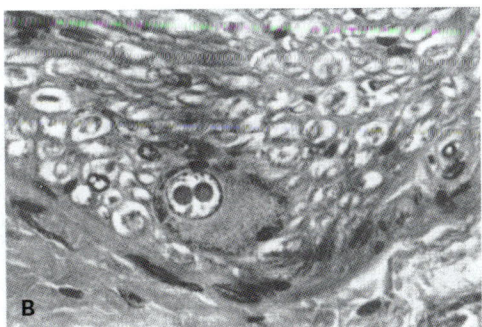

Figure 6-44. Familial visceral neuropathy showing a neuronal intranuclear inclusion in **(A)** and two intranuclear inclusions in **(B)**. The sections came from two siblings. (Courtesy M. Schuffler, MD.)

basal ganglia calcification, but the autosomal dominant variant does not have extraintestinal manifestations. The X-linked form is associated with malrotation, short small intestine, and pyloric hypertrophy.[190]

The major histologic changes of the familial type consist of patchy degeneration of the myenteric plexus with neuronal degeneration and dropout (Fig. 6-44). Neurons, when present, show degenerative changes, such as abnormal shapes and club-shaped dendrites. A number of subtypes have now been described, characterized clinically by calcification of basal ganglia, external ophthalmoplegia, ptosis and peripheral neuropathy in one type, and histologically by *intranuclear neuronal inclusions,* which can be identified in regular H&E-stained sections in a second type[2,46,53,60-63] (Table 6-3). The intranuclear neuronal inclusions are large, round, and eosinophilic, with a surrounding halo, and resemble cytomegalovirus (CMV) inclusions (Fig. 6-44). Histochemically, however, they are devoid of DNA. By EM they are composed of curving filaments, which do not look like virus.[2] CMV can be easily excluded by immunostain.

The causes of the neurodegenerative changes in the gut remain relatively obscure. Several mechanisms are likely involved including alterations in calcium signaling, mitochondrial dysfunction, and free radical injury.[191] Some autosomal recessive patients present with a progressive multisystem neurodegenerative disorder and are reflected by abnormalities in mitochondrial DNA.[192] A variety of genes have been linked to syndromic forms of CIIP including thymidine phosphorylase (also known as endothelial cell growth factor-1 or [ECGF-1]), mutations of which appear to be the cause of *familial mitochondrial neurogastrointestinal encephalomyopathy (MNGIE),* a disorder characterized by intestinal pseudoobstruction, progressive external ophthalmoplegia, ptosis, polyneuropathy, and leukoencephalopathy.[193,194] This disorder is characterized by fibrosis of the external longitudinal layer of the muscularis propria, which may be complete so that the myenteric plexus has only fibrosis beyond it. However, this may be followed by loss of circular muscle, so that the entire muscle layer stops abruptly, with formation of diverticula. A cursory look at these could be interpreted as a typical large bowel–type diverticulum as the diverticulum appears to go through the muscularis propria when the latter is in fact completely lost. The diverticula can become infected and form abscesses or perforate (the latter was the case with this patient) (Fig. 6-45). Decreased ganglion cell survival may be a factor in some cases, as suggested by decreased *Bcl-2* gene product in the enteric ganglion cells.[195]

Paraneoplastic Syndromes

Some cases reveal inflammatory neuronal degeneration, which suggests an autoimmune or infectious etiology[196]; neuronal autoantibodies are detected in some patients.[197] Some of these cases represent a paraneoplastic manifestation, while some remain idiopathic.[198] DNA polymerase gamma gene and SOX10[199] that acts as a transcription factor may also be involved (Fig. 6-46).

Sporadic Visceral Neuropathy

This type of neuropathy also shows loss and degeneration of neurons and/or nerve tracts and often secondary glial cell proliferation. In addition, there may be an accompanying lymphocytic and plasma cell infiltrate in rare cases (degenerative inflammatory).[64]

Differential diagnosis. An inflammatory visceral neuropathy has been described in cases of paraneoplastic syndrome associated with small cell carcinoma (Fig. 6-46).[61,65] The neuropathy, however, may not be confined to the bowel and may involve other sites, such as the peripheral and central nervous system.[66] Since the myenteric plexus is part of the nervous system, it is not surprising that the bowel can be involved in numerous neuropathies. These are listed in Table 6-2.

Abnormalities of Interstitial Cells of Cajal

It is common to find a decreased number of ICCs in patients undergoing resection for pseudoobstruction, and it is often associated with loss of neurons and

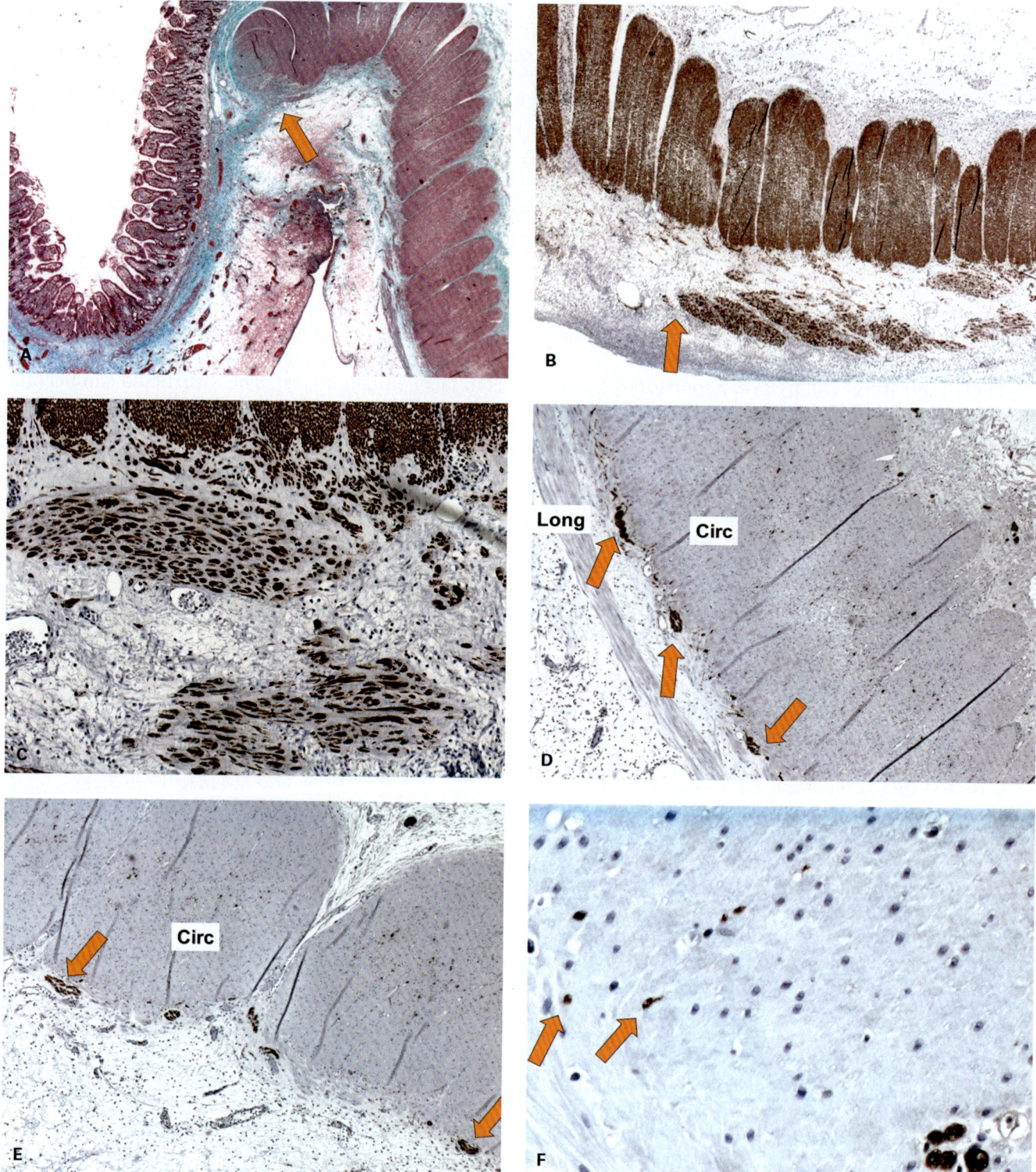

Figure 6-45. Changes in jejunum in MNGIE. **A:** Jejunum with perforation of diverticulum through the muscularis propria thereby resembling an acquired diverticulum. The muscularis propria stops at the *arrow* denoting the beginning of the diverticulum. **B:** Desmin highlights the muscularis propria illustrating the focal complete loss of the muscularis propria (*arrow*). **C:** Focally, this loss has visceral myopathy-like changes with pericellular fibrosis. **D:** S100 shows the myenteric plexus (*arrows*) and an extremely thinned muscularis propria external (**left**) to it. **E:** The location of the myenteric plexus (*arrows*) now shows that the longitudinal muscle has been lost. **F:** S100 shows marked loss of neurons/glia with almost total denervation. Residual processes are *arrowed*. A cluster of ganglion cells is present bottom right representing part of the myenteric plexus.

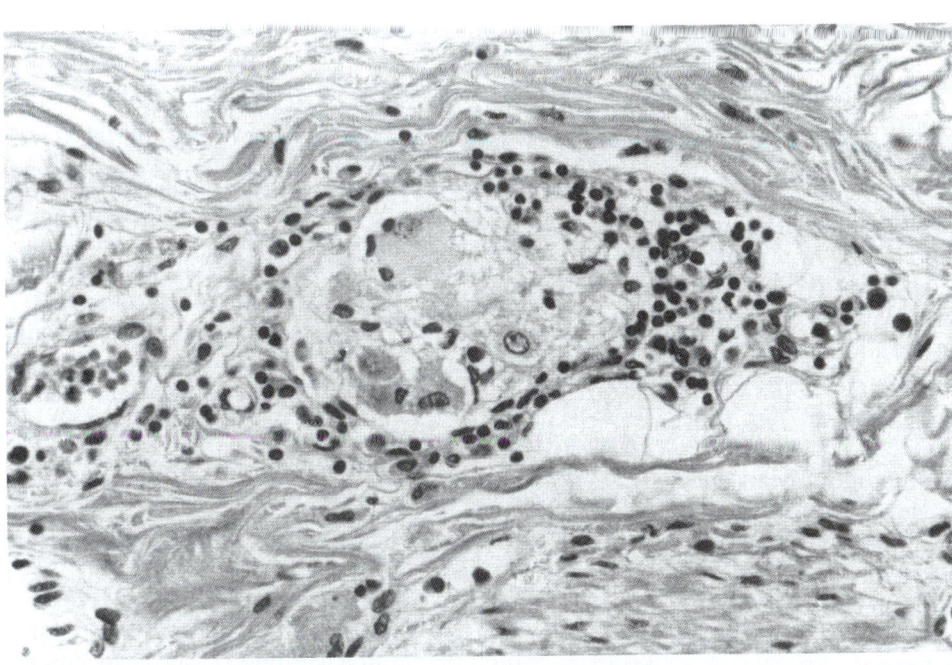

Figure 6-46. Paraneoplastic visceral neuropathy showing infiltration of the myenteric plexus with lymphocytes and plasma cells. (Courtesy M. Schuffler, MD.)

fibrosis of the muscularis propria. The loss of ICCs may involve the myenteric plexus and often the intramuscular ICCs. It is not usually appreciated that ICCs are dynamic with occasional cells undergoing apoptosis and presumably others proliferating. This raises numerous issues about why and how they become depleted if they have regenerative potential. Morphologically, ICCs are elongated and have occasional processes, but in some conditions, the number of processes seems hugely increased so that almost every ICC has them. It is unclear if this is a reactive hyperplasia but may well be the case (Fig. 6-47). However, it is also clear that in some patients, there appears to be a degree of hyperplasia, although whether primary lesions affect only ICCs or their accompanying fibroblasts in addition, is unclear. However the latter is, certainly implied in the London Classification of motility disorders.[118]

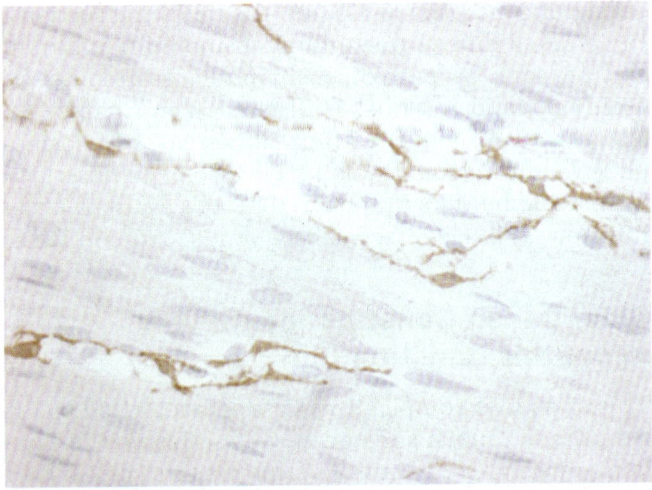

Hyperplasia of ICCs. This is described in patients with germline mutations of the kit gene. Affected patients have a markedly thickened band of ICCs occupying the position of the myenteric plexus but occupy about 25% of the thickness of the muscularis propria. The findings are diagnostic of this condition and are invariably found in resections for gastrointestinal stromal tumors (GISTs); indeed, all resections for GISTs should include examination of the myenteric plexus region for such hyperplasia as it predicts increased likelihood of further GISTs (see Chapter 7). An infant with congenital hyperplasia of ICCs had a motility disturbance interpreted as intestinal neuronal dysplasia (IND)[200]:

i) There is a case report of focal massive hyperplasia of ICCs that virtually replaced the muscularis propria resulting in a diverticulum and with a somatic, not germline, mutation in the kit gene.[201]

ii) Patients with small bowel motility disorders having what was called intestinal lymphocytic epithelioganglionitis, a combination of intraepithelial lymphocytosis and myenteric ganglioneuritis accompanied by hyperplasia and hypertrophy of the ICC in the small intestinal wall. This was reported in a study of 28 patients with intestinal motor dysfunction.[202] All patients had full-thickness jejunal biopsies, but the diagnosis required quantitation. The mean number of intraepithelial CD3+ lymphocytes was 36 per 100 epithelial cells (range 27 to 68) where the upper limit of normal was 25 (but still readily visible as it is the same sort of figure as that seen in celiac disease).

Figure 6-47. DOG1 immunostain showing probable hyperplasia of ICCs. Note the numerous processes anastomosing to adjacent ICCs forming a network.

The myenteric ganglionitis was of variable severity (mean 4.6 myenteric lymphocytes per ganglion—upper normal limit 2). Myenteric neurons showed signs of degeneration and an abnormal immunohistologic pattern.

Hyperplasia and hypertrophy of Cajal cells were observed, ICC nuclei per 1 mm length of the myenteric plexus and ICC nuclei per 1 mm² circular muscle being counted. Control values (SD) of the ICC-AP in the controls was 16.1 (2.8) and that of the ICC-CM was 9.4 (2.2). The upper normal limit was set at mean + 2 SD, that is, 22 ICC-AP nuclei and 16 ICC-CM nuclei per mm². The lower normal limit was set at mean) 2 SD, that is, 11 ICC-AP and five ICC-CM. The longitudinal muscle layer was thickened in many cases. Nevertheless, some patients presenting with CIIP have numerous readily visible ICCs that exhibit numerous dendrite-like process and represent a form of hyperplasia (Fig. 6-47).

Prognosis and therapy of CIIP. CIIP usually has a prolonged course lasting for decades, while infants and children tend to have a poorer prognosis and may die at a young age[203] depending to some extent on the underlying pathology, which part of the gut is involved and its extent. Treatment is symptomatic, but medication, surgery, and sometimes biofeedback therapy are used with varying success. Surgical resection, especially colectomy, may be undertaken in resistant cases and do well especially if pathology is limited to the large bowel. The cuff of terminal ileum in subtotal colectomies is therefore critical in determining if it is involved. Favorable outcome is expected in cases with limited bowel involvement. However, in some, substantial resection of small bowel may be required, resulting in dependence on total parenteral nutrition. Not surprisingly, intestinal transplantation is gradually emerging as a possible treatment option in intractable cases.[204] Death may be related to surgery, total parenteral nutrition or posttransplant complications,[203] especially infections.

The underlying condition also plays a role in prognosis, as those with systemic diseases such as progressive systemic sclerosis, systemic lupus erythematosus, or amyloidosis generally follow the course of the underlying disease so many die of renal, cardiac, or pulmonary complications, usually within a decade. Those with paraneoplastic syndromes usually die within a year of the underlying disease. Those associated with viral infection are generally self-limited.

Diffuse Lymphoid Infiltration

This is a rare and unusual variant of visceral myopathy. It has the same clinical manifestations as visceral myopathy, such as diarrhea, malabsorption, and pseudoobstruction, but unlike the latter, it is characterized

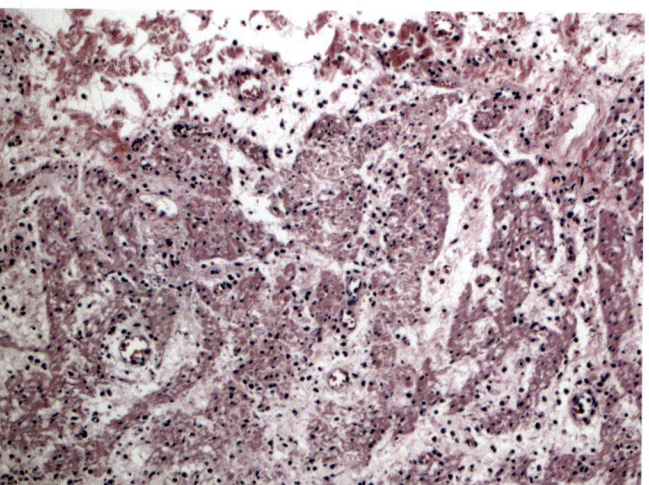

Figure 6-48. CIIP with diffuse lymphocytic infiltrate.

by a dense lymphocytic infiltrate of the muscularis propria, which separates individual muscle fibers. However, the muscle fibers appear to be morphologically intact. There is a dense lymphocytic infiltrate affecting the entire muscularis propria (Fig. 6-48); but the lymphocytic infiltrate can also involve the other layers of the intestine. Immunohistochemical staining of the lymphoid infiltrate shows polyclonality of lymphocytes, thus excluding malignancy. The myenteric plexus shows no abnormality of neurons or axons.[2]

Whether this disorder represents another still undefined smooth muscle disorder or is secondary to some possibly autoimmune disorder remains to be determined.

Diffuse Eosinophilic Infiltrate

This is described primarily as a complication of Hirschsprung's disease and seems to be of no clinical significance (Fig. 6-49) (see the following section). In adults, a diffuse transmural eosinophilic infiltrate can be seen as part of eosinophilic gastroenteritis (Fig. 6-50; and see further discussion in Chapter 8), allergies, parasites, etc. Minimal increases in eosinophils requiring quantitation have also been described in irritable bowel syndrome (IBS), but again, the significance is unclear (see subsequent section on IBS).

Slow Transit Constipation: Severe Idiopathic Constipation

This symptom complex was first characterized by Sir Arbuthnot Lane, a surgeon at Guy's Hospital in London whose greater claim to fame was the first use of silver wire, then steel screws, and then plates and screws for internal fixation of fractures, for which he was initially derided. Slow transit constipation

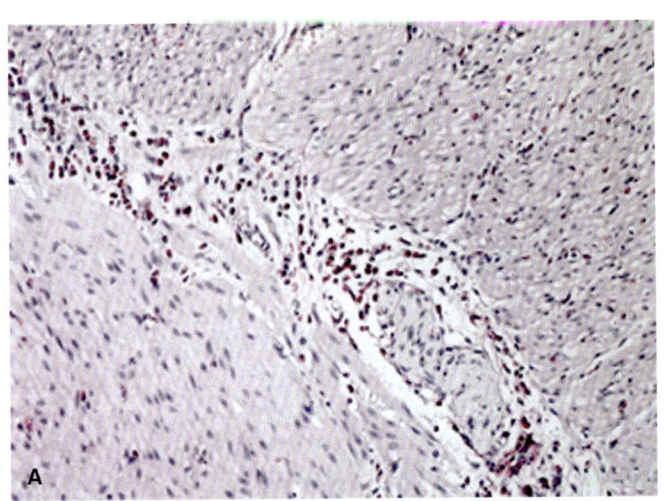
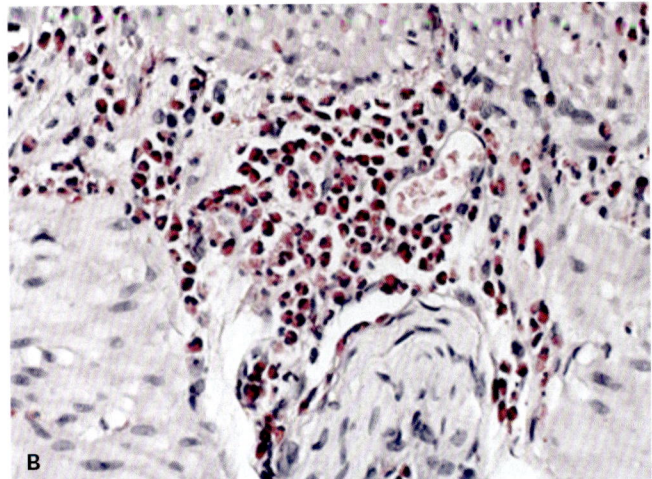

Figure 6-49. A,B: Hirschsprung's disease with a diffuse eosinophilic infiltrate. While initially disconcerting, this appears to be of no clinical significance. (Courtesy of Dr. Gabriel Becheanu, Bucharest, Rome.)

(STC) is characterized by reduced colonic propulsion resulting in chronic constipation, often with overflow incontinence.[205,206] It usually affects young women, sometimes even in childhood, but occasionally in older women. Since many patients end up taking laxatives daily, associated melanosis coli is common, and in some, this may play a role in increasing symptoms (cathartic colon), the obvious problem being knowing whether increasing symptoms are the result of disease progression or laxative use. In severe and resistant cases, colectomy may have to be performed, which is exactly what Arbuthnot Lane did as well as using high-residue diets. What is far less clear is whether this is a separate condition to intestinal pseudoobstruction or whether this can be one of the clinical manifestations of those diseases. This likely explains the variety of pathologies that have been described and that both may ultimately be treated by resection.

STC therefore likely represents a group of disorders possibly having a similar spectrum of pathology to CIIP. Abnormalities have been shown in the number of ICC, which have been found to be reduced, along with reduced numbers of ganglion cells and intraganglionic neurofilaments.[205,207,208] While it is said that the disease may be characterized by amphophilic, hyaline round to ovoid (4 to 22 μm) cytoplasmic inclusions, in smooth muscle cells,[209] they can be identified in normal colon, or small bowel, as well as in Chagas' disease and so are likely of no diagnostic importance.

However, the relationship with females raises the issue of overexpression of receptors or undue sensitivity to estrogen or progestogen, the latter particularly as it is associated with relaxation of smooth muscle, and that the condition invariably gets worse during pregnancy, and possibly even during the luteal phase of the cycle.[210] This may be mediated by the serotonin pathway, which regulates progesterone receptors, which in turn causes smooth muscle relaxation. The COX pathway is also involved, as signal transduction pathways are associated with impaired basal motility due to down-regulation of COX-1 resulting in decreased levels of thromboxane A2 and PGF2a. These are prostaglandins that contract circular muscle cells, while upregulation of COX-2 proteins results in increased PGE2 that relaxes circular muscle cells.[210]

HIRSCHSPRUNG'S DISEASE

Hirschsprung's disease is a congenital severe motility disorder of the large bowel, primarily involving the rectum and sigmoid colon but sometimes extending proximally, usually but not always in continuity with distal disease, and may involve the whole of the

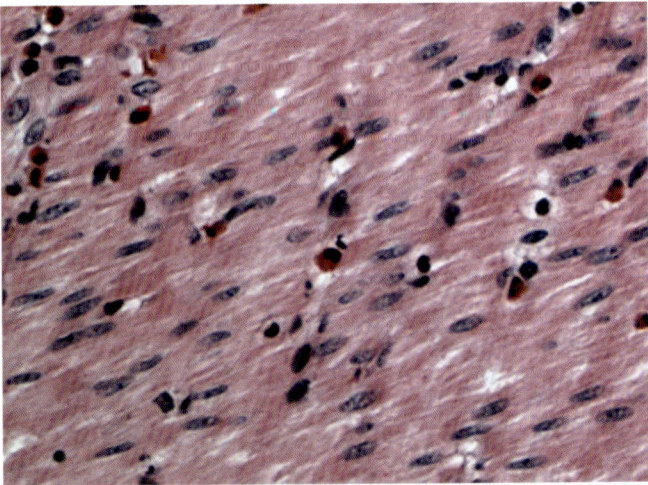

Figure 6-50. Transmural eosinophilic infiltrate seen as part of eosinophilic gastroenteritis.

large and rarely the small bowel. It is characterized by the absence of ganglion cells and the presence of numerous hypertrophied nerves in both plexi and the mucosa. In the latter, they are characteristically enhanced with cholinesterase on frozen sections section but are immunonegative with calretinin antibodies in formalin-fixed paraffin-embedded tissue. Both of these stains can therefore be used in making the diagnosis. The disorder results in severe constipation or other manifestations of obstruction.

Clinical Presentation and Features

The vast majority of cases (over 90%) occur in the neonatal period with delayed passage of meconium beyond 48 hours, but rare cases have been described in adults, some of whom have had symptoms since childhood. Others have presented later in infancy through to adulthood,[72–75] usually with chronic constipation often with abdominal distention and sometimes vomiting. Clinical symptoms are due to a contracted, spastic, aganglionic segment, and most patients present with constipation. Diagnosis is facilitated with imaging studies, sometimes rectal manometry, but is established by suction mucosal biopsy. There may be an accompanying severe colitis or enterocolitis, which is more commonly seen in patients with Down's syndrome and leads to perforation (Fig. 6-51). The etiology of this remains unclear,[211,212] and while *Clostridium difficile* may be cultured, neonatal bowel has no receptors for the toxin and so is almost certainly incidental.

The incidence of HD is about 1/5,000 live births, and there is a marked male preponderance of between 3 and 4.5:1. Some cases present in adult life, presumably those missed in the neonatal period and not severe enough to result in death, but still causing severe constipation. Acquired loss of ganglion cells can also result from destruction of ganglion cells by Chagas' disease resulting in a similar syndrome.[213] Long-segment disease and total bowel aganglionosis show familial aggregation, suggesting a specific genetic defect. Familial forms of long- and short-segment disease are autosomal dominant with incomplete penetrance. However, variants associated with other congenital malformations are mostly autosomal recessive. Sporadic cases are thought to have variable patterns of inheritance.

A variety of associated conditions have been reported. About 10% occur in children with trisomy 21 or Down's syndrome, and about 5% are associated with other congenital abnormalities such as ophthalmologic defects, intestinal malrotation, and duodenal stenosis.[68,71] Neurofibromatosis, Down's syndrome, cardiovascular malformations, Laurence–Moon–Bardet–Biedl syndrome, Waardenburg syndrome, Haddad syndrome, multiple endocrine neoplasia (MEN), and neuroblastoma, many of them belonging to the group of neural crest disorders ("neurocrestopathies").[214] Imperforate anus, usually associated with long-segment disease, has also been reported.[215]

Etiology and Pathogenesis

The aganglionic segment in Hirschsprung's disease results from the failure in utero of nerve plexus development, especially ganglion cells that fail to migrate from the neural crest in their most caudal part. In about 5% of patients, this is more extensive and involves the entire large bowel, occasionally going into the ileum, and rarely, it affects the entire small and large intestine. This is accompanied by what is likely a compensatory hypertrophy of residual nerves in all layers of the bowel. These are seen predominantly in the submucosa but also extend into the mucosa and may be demonstrated by stains for acetylcholinesterase (ACh) in frozen sections or PGP9.5 in paraffin sections.[69,70] More reliably, the mucosal nerves are entirely calretinin immunonegative. The aganglionic zone is spastic and acts as a barrier to the coordinated forward propulsion of intestinal contents. The spasm appears to result from unopposed extrinsic parasympathetic activity, but adrenergic hyperactivity may also contribute.[70]

As ganglion cells are known to migrate from the neural crest during embryogenesis, genes controlling this are likely implicated, as they control migration, colonization, and survival of ganglion cells in the bowel during embryogenesis. Numerous genes play a role in this process[214,216–222] including *RET, EDNRB, EDN3, GDNF, SOX10, ECE1, NTN, ZEB2, PHOX2B, L1CAM, KIAA1279, TCF4, NRG1, RELN, GAL, GAP43, NRSN1*, and *GABRG2*.[223–225] These genes are involved in neuronal migration, growth, stimulation, neurotransmitter receptors, or smooth muscle relaxation.[225] If searched

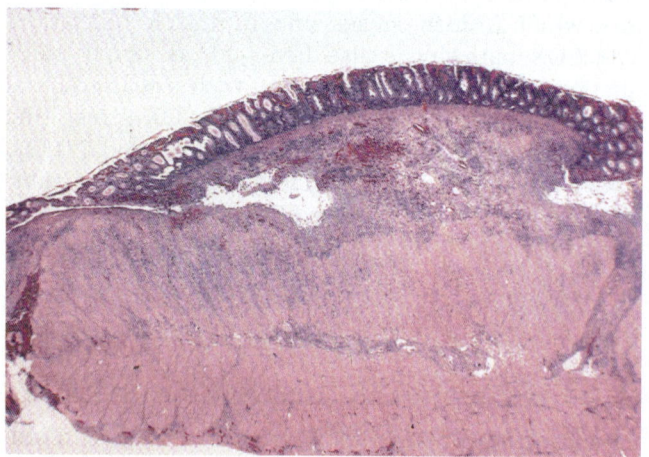

Figure 6-51. Necrotizing enterocolitis secondary to Hirschsprung's disease. There is mucosal ulceration, hemorrhage, and inflammation extending into the muscularis propria. The mononuclear cells with cytoplasmic halos are mast cells.

for, about one-half of patients with Hirschsprung's disease are found to have specific genetic abnormalities, the remainder being unknown.[224] The most frequent are mutations of the RET protooncogene, which are present in 20% to 25% patients with short-segment disease but 40% to 70% of long-segment disease. Other genetic mutations are found in <10%. Genetic polymorphisms in genes such as *RET* or *NRG1* almost certainly result in an increased risk for Hirschsprung's disease.[226,227] The mode of inheritance is variable.

Gross Appearance

Hirschsprung's disease is characterized by a distal contracted segment of bowel, a short distal narrow aperistaltic hypertonic segment with an immediately proximal intermediate funnel-shaped zone, and a proximally dilated region (Fig. 6-52). The proximal normally innervated region is barely dilated in the early stages of the disease but becomes massively distended with time. The length of the contracted segment varies. In over 90% of cases, it is short (short-segment Hirschsprung's disease) and is present in the rectum and distal sigmoid colon.[68,76] In about 5% of patients, the aganglionic segment is long, often involving the entire large bowel and rarely extending into the small bowel up to the duodenum.

Histology

The histology reflects the gross description with a distal narrow aganglionic aperistaltic hypertonic segment of large bowel immediately proximal to the anus with an immediately proximal intermediate funnel-

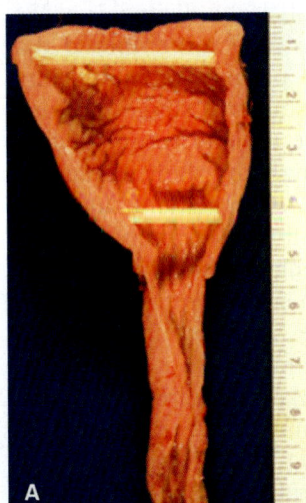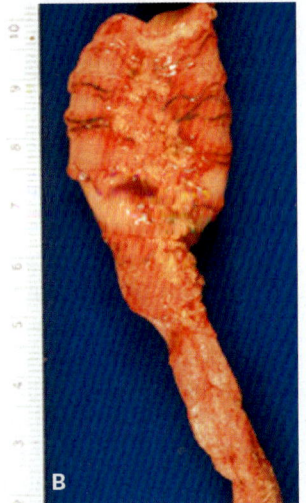

Figure 6-52. Hirschsprung's disease. Resection showing a short-segment (classic) Hirschsprung's disease. **A:** The proximal normally innervated dilated part leads into the tightly constricted aganglionic segment with a transitional zone in between. **B:** External appearance.

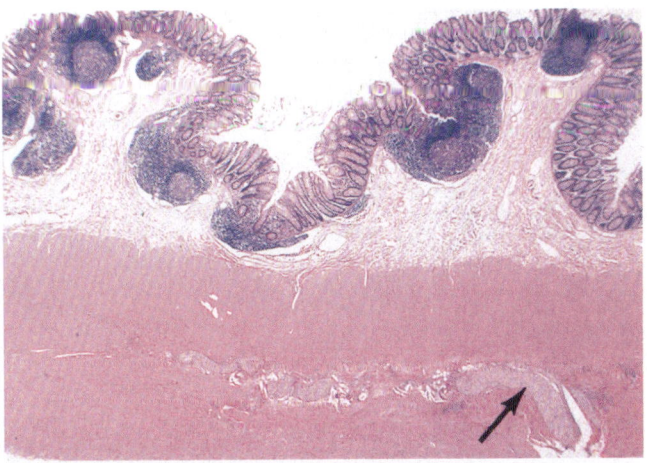

Figure 6-53. Hirschsprung's disease. Longitudinal section of an aganglionic segment of colon showing hypertrophied intermyenteric nerve (*arrow*).

shaped zone and a proximal dilatation. Hypertrophied extrinsic nerve bundles, containing numerous Schwann cells, are present together with a thickened muscularis propria (Figs. 6-53 and 6-54). The major abnormality is found in the contracted distal segment. In the funnel-shaped segment proximal to the contracted zone, there may be hypoganglionosis. The proximal segment shows a thickened muscularis propria but contains normal nerve plexuses.[77] The plexus abnormalities involve both the submucosal and myenteric plexuses. Ganglion cells are absent, but the dense, non–myelinated nerve bundles and Schwann cells are coarse, wavy, and hypertrophied (Figs. 6-54 and 6-55).

Hypertrophied nerve bundles are prominent in the submucosa, and an increased number extend into the mucosa where they can be demonstrated with stains for ACh on frozen section (Fig. 6-56), which shows a plethora of neurons in the muscularis mucosae and mucosa. In addition, the same nerves show loss of the normal calretinin immunoreactivity in paraffin sections (Figs. 6-57).[69,78-83] As with all immunodiagnoses that require demonstration of lack of immunoreactivity, it is therefore important to have an appropriate positive (and ideally, but less importantly a negative) control on the same slide to ensure that if there is total lack of immunoreactivity, it represents a true negative stain.

Diagnosis of Hirschsprung's Disease

In clinically suspected cases, the diagnosis of Hirschsprung's disease can be strongly suspected from imaging that may include barium enema and rectal manometry.[68] However, it must be confirmed by biopsy because occasionally other conditions, such as idiopathic megacolon, can be confused clinically.

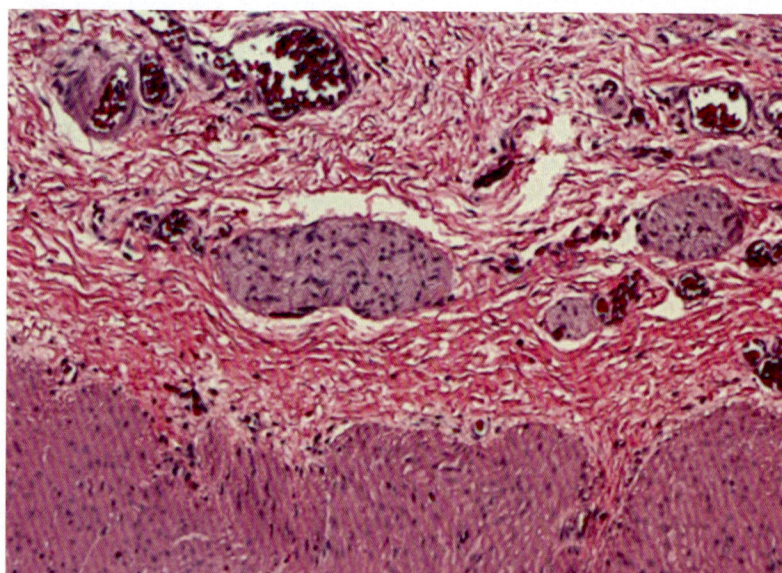

Figure 6-54. Detail showing a hypertrophied myenteric nerve and absence of ganglion cells.

Furthermore, it can be useful to take multiple biopsy specimens from the suspected segment and above in order to establish the upper limit of the aganglionic zone. Diagnosis can be facilitated using ACh stains that require frozen section or loss of the normal calretinin immunoreactivity as shown in Figures 6-56 and 6-57.

The only exception to preoperative biopsy confirmation is in those infants with acute obstruction in whom decompression is necessary as an emergency. In these cases, intraoperative biopsy specimens are usually obtained.

Immunohistochemical staining of paraffin sections for calretinin is very helpful in identifying ganglia and is becoming the ancillary method of choice, possibly being superior and more reliable than Ach staining of frozen sections.[228–232]

On H&E sections, the most diagnostic findings are those of absent ganglia and hypertrophied nerve bundles in the submucosal plexus, if mucosal biopsies taken include submucosa, and in the myenteric plexus on those occasions when full thickness biopsies have been taken to establish the diagnosis at laparotomy. However, it needs to be remembered that immature ganglion cells in premature infants and neonates are smaller and frequently single and may not have an open chromatin, so may resemble lymphocytes, but can be recognized by their vacuolated cytoplasm and garland-like arrangement in small nerve plexuses.[83] It is important to examine enough sections (50 or more serial cuts) in order not to miss them when truly present. On both calretinin and ACh stains, normally some nerve fibers are found in the muscularis mucosae, with fine nerve twigs extending up into the lamina propria parallel to the crypts. About one nerve twig is normal between every three to four crypts on ACh staining. On the other hand, in Hirschsprung's disease, several coarse nerve twigs are usually found between each crypt, and an increased number are also found within the muscularis mucosae. Despite some reports of 100% success in the diagnosis of Hirschsprung's disease with ACh staining, in about 10% of cases, there is only a minimal increase

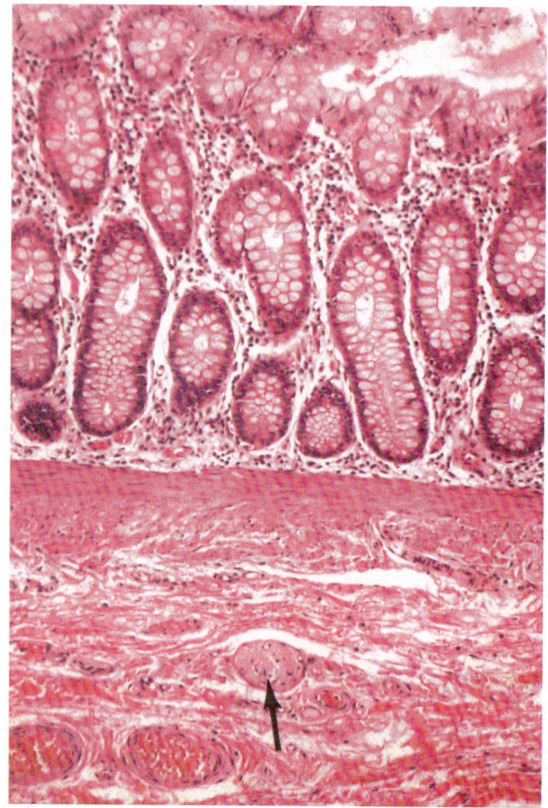

Figure 6-55. Hirschsprung's disease. Section of mucosa and submucosa showing a small nerve bundle (*arrow*) but no ganglion cells.

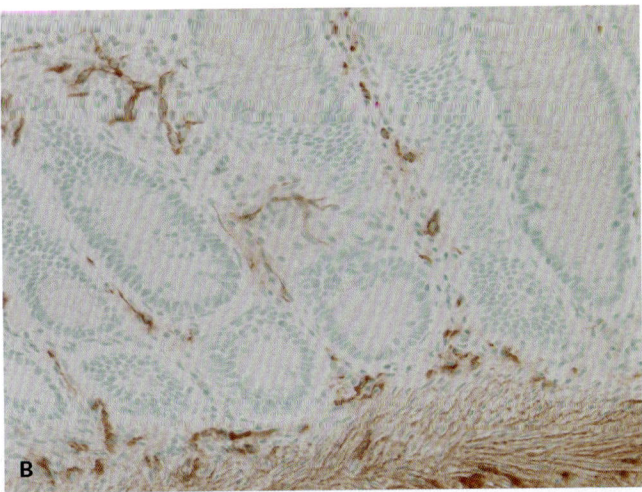

Figure 6-56. Acetyl cholinesterase stains on frozen section. **A:** Normal cholinesterase on frozen section showing scant fibers in both the muscularis mucosae and between the crypts of the mucosa. **B:** Hirschsprung's disease—thickened nerve fibers are present both in the muscularis mucosae but especially between the crypts in the mucosa. (Courtesy of Dr. Catherine Chung, HSC, Toronto, ON.)

in nerve fibers. These may represent hypoganglionosis but, more likely, represent biopsy specimens taken from within 2 cm of the pectinate line.

Types of biopsy. Full-thickness biopsy under anesthesia used to be the standard procedure for the diagnosis of Hirschsprung's disease, and in some institutions, this remains the case but now it is largely used intraoperatively to establish the proximal limit of disease. However, they have the advantage that the myenteric plexus and its nerves are readily visualized and lack of ganglion cells and lack of calretinin immunoreactive nerves can also be readily established. There is a hypoganglionic zone in the 1 to 2 cm above the dentate line, so biopsies are usually taken at least 2 cm proximal to this.

Mucosal biopsies are much less invasive and ideally include the submucosa so that the submucosal plexus and its ganglion cells or the hypertrophied nerves are visible. It should not include the anal transition zone, which cannot be seen endoscopically, so biopsies are taken at least 2 cm proximal to the dentate line to avoid this. Should anal transitional mucosal be present in the biopsy, the presence of ganglion cells can be used to exclude Hirschsprung's disease, but as the zone is often hypoganglionic, it should not be used to make a diagnosis of Hirschsprung's disease. Since Hirschsprung's disease involves both submucosal and myenteric nerve plexuses, mucosal suction or other biopsies developed to include submucosa (rather than grasp forceps biopsies, which are usually too shallow) are usually adequate to demonstrate the aganglionosis

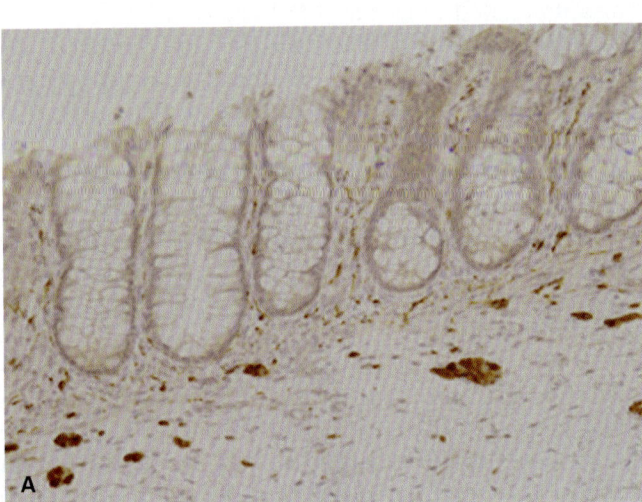
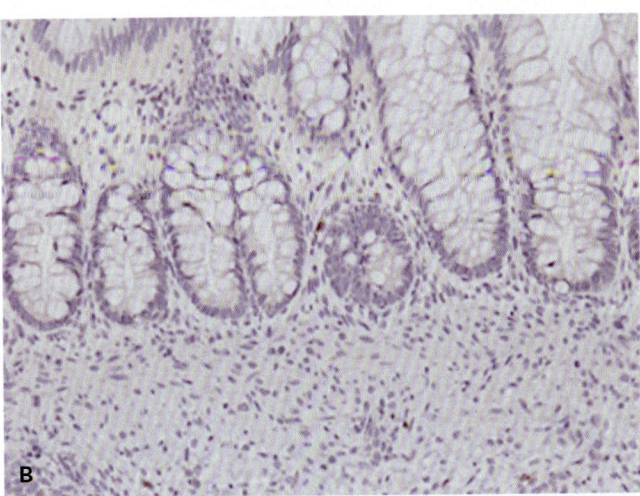

Figure 6-57. Hirschsprung's disease. **A:** Rectum—Normal calretinin immunostaining showing clusters of ganglion cells in the superficial submucosa and fibers passing into the lamina propria. **B:** Hirschsprung's disease—calretinin staining showing virtual absence of ganglion cells or nerve twigs between the crypts, appearances. (Courtesy of Dr. Catherine Chung, HSC, Toronto, ON.)

and hypertrophy of nerves, which commonly extend into the mucosa.[83,85,86] Mucosal biopsy (ideally including submucosa) has therefore become the standard procedure for diagnosis of Hirschsprung's disease.

Theoretically, one should not need submucosa as the mucosal plexus is well demonstrated using acetyl cholinesterase stains on frozen sections or lack of calretinin fibers in formalin-fixed paraffin-embedded sections. Whether we have reached the point of not requiring submucosa is an institutional decision based on the level of comfort with the procedure used and its perceived sensitivity, specificity, and ability to handle those patients with disease that does not fit classical morphology. Most centers still prefer ensuring the presence of submucosa along with calretinin and/or cholinesterase stains to maximize the chances of a correct diagnosis.

Intraoperative frozen section. Frozen sections at the time of surgery have a well-defined role, firstly in the selection of the proximal end of resection to determine whether ganglion cells are present and to avoid the rare cases of skip section and secondly in rare life-threatening situations, such as enterocolitis, in which Hirschsprung's disease is suspected. The finding of ganglion cells at surgery may prevent unnecessary resections. From a practical standpoint, the following need to be emphasized:

1. As in routine biopsies, if no ganglion cells are found in the first frozen section, multiple levels should be examined before being satisfied that ganglion cells are indeed absent and suggesting a diagnosis of Hirschsprung's disease.
2. Care should be taken to orient the biopsy specimen properly before freezing the tissue, so that the muscularis propria and Auerbach's plexus are seen. If the plexus is not found, serial sections or rotation of the block may be necessary.
3. If Hirschsprung's disease appears to involve the entire colon, some surgeons sometimes opt merely to take out the appendix for examination for ganglion cells. Pathologists need to be aware that in the neonatal appendix, ganglion cells normally can be found almost randomly throughout the muscularis propria; this does not indicate neuronal dysplasia. Because special stains such as the cholinesterase or calretinin may be very helpful in the diagnosis, adequate samples need to be taken, and if ACh staining is to be carried out, then tissues need to be kept frozen. Remaining tissue or an additional biopsy form the same site should be put into formalin.

Variants of Hirschsprung's Disease

These are conditions that clinically resemble Hirschsprung's disease, despite the presence of ganglion cells, and have been described under numerous terms such as pseudo-Hirschsprung's disease, neonatal intestinal pseudoobstruction, intestinal hypoperistalsis, and even CIIP. The diagnosis is made on biopsies using histology, immunohistochemistry, and sometimes EM. One group has examined a large series of these and found the conditions shown in Table 6-5.[233]; this also gives an idea of their approximate frequency.[233]

Table 6-5 Variants of Hirschsprung's Disease and Approximate Frequency

VARIANTS OF HIRSCHSPRUNG'S DISEASE	APPROXIMATE FREQUENCY
IND	43% (76)
Internal sphincter achalasia	26% (46)
MMIHS	14% (25)
Hypoganglionosis	10% (18)
Immature ganglia	6% (10)
Absence of argyrophil plexus	2% (3)

Modified from Mundt E, Bates MD. Genetics of Hirschsprung disease and anorectal malformations. [Review]. *Semin Pediatr Surg*. 2010;19(2):107–117.

INTESTINAL NEURONAL DYSPLASIA

This is an entity whose definition has changed with time, even to the point that it was thought to be so irreproducible that there were calls for it to be abandoned. However, there do appear to be at least two variants (called IND-A and IND-B).

IND-A is rare and has aplasia or hypoplasia of the sympathetic nerves with enhanced parasympathetic activity that is reflected by increased ACh activity in the lamina propria mucosae, which is why it comes into the differential diagnosis of Hirschsprung's disease but also involves eye muscles. One variant involves the submucosal plexus with large groups of ganglion cells and Schwann's cells reflected by lack of motility and megacolon. It usually presents at about 6th months of life.[234]

IND-B is also controversial, mainly due to changing criteria for its diagnosis and its reproducibility. The most commonly used diagnostic criteria to date are the findings of hyperganglionosis and >20% of giant ganglia with >8 ganglion cells in the submucosa of 30 serial sections in addition to hyperganglionosis.[235-237] However, in the first year of life, giant ganglia may be misinterpreted because immature ganglia often have an incomplete differentiation in nerve cells.[233] At least 25 submucosal ganglia should be evaluated, and a diagnosis of IND-B should be made only in children older than 1 and less than 4 years of age.[238] An increase or decrease in number of ganglions may be seen secondary to mechanical obstruction, so caution is required as to the precise location of the biopsy. IND-B now usually does not require surgical treatment.

INTERNAL SPHINCTER ACHALASIA (ULTRASHORT HIRSCHSPRUNG'S DISEASE)

Rarely, the contracted segment is ultrashort but better called internal anal sphincter achalasia or anal outlet obstruction.[239,240] Like pyloric stenosis, it is associated with lack of NO neurons,[241] while ganglion cells are normal, but it causes severe constipation, and while it responds in the short term to botulinum toxin injections, internal anal sphincter myotomy works better in the long term.[239] Pathology has no role in this diagnosis other than to confirm that ganglion cells are present, thereby excluding the diagnosis of Hirschsprung's disease. The most reliable way may be by rectal manometry.

Hypoganglionosis is poorly documented but consists of a reduced number of ganglia with a decreased number of ganglion cells per ganglion and smaller size of ganglia[242] causing intestinal pseudoobstruction. It may coexist in variable lengths with Hirschsprung's disease or as an isolated primary condition. Criteria have always been the problem, but it has been suggested that < 10 ganglion cells/mm and/or < 2 ganglions/mm constitute hypoganglionosis.[242] There may also be absent or low mucosal ACh activity and hypertrophy of the muscularis mucosae and circular muscle.[243] A seminal study found about 40% of patients had decreased numbers of nerve cells and double the normal distance between ganglia, together with a plexus area only one third the area of normal.[242] The problem is that criteria have been established from either ACh staining or 15-μm-thick frozen sections stained with lactate dehydrogenase and so cannot readily be applied to paraffin-embedded sections with a different neuronal marker or H&E stains.[242] A full-thickness biopsy is necessary for the diagnosis of these rare variants of Hirschsprung's disease to be able to quantitate a sufficient ganglion cells. Rarely, in *zonal aganglionosis* (skip-segment Hirschsprung's disease),[77,81,90,91] there may be a zone of hypoganglionic or aganglionic colon between areas of normal colon.[77] This may be especially important in the placing of colostomies but is entirely dependent on detecting the proximal aganglionic segment.

Hyperganglionosis has an increased number of ganglion cells or ectopic ganglia in the lamina and is primarily associated with IND type B (IND-B) as described previously. It may also be associated with nodular proliferation of ganglion cells (ganglioneuroma) that may occur as either a localized lesion or diffusely in ganglioneuromatosis. Although isolated ganglion cells are not infrequent in IBD where submucosal ganglion cells get incorporated into the lamina propria following deep ulceration, they are rare in normal biopsies, although one study did find ganglion cells in 15% of biopsies from females and 5% in males. So by these criteria the changes of hyperganglionosis would not be considered pathological.[244]

Diffuse ganglioneuromatosis is invariably part of MEN type IIb (MEN IIB) and its associated mutation in the *RET* protooncogene.

MEGACYSTIS MICROCOLON INTESTINAL HYPOPERISTALSIS

MMIHS is rare, almost certainly inherited as an autosomal recessive condition, and produces a severe form of neonatal intestinal obstruction. The syndrome causes massive abdominal distension caused by a microcolon, decreased or absent intestinal peristalsis, and a dilated but nonobstructed bladder. A possible clue to the etiology is a case report in which the large bowel showed deficiency of α-SMA in the internal circular muscle similar to that seen in the so-called congenital α-SMA deficiency, which is not usually associated with MMIHS. However, there was also a chromosomal abnormality with a deletion in the chromosome 15q11; this is usually associated not only with the Prader–Willi or Angelman syndromes, autism, and schizophrenia but also with AChR abnormalities, and thus may influence the expression of the AChR.[187]

Diagnosis

The diagnosis of MMIHS is based primarily on prenatal ultrasound findings and the clinical presentation. The myenteric and submucosal plexuses usually are unremarkable with normal ganglion cells and ICCs in about three-fourths of patients. However, the rest have a variety of abnormalities including hypoganglionosis, hyperganglionosis, and immature ganglia.[245] Now, α-SMA immunoreactivity needs to be included as mentioned previously, and there are data to support the same changes in bladder muscle in α-SMA and also desmin and dystrophin of MMHIS patients compared with controls.[246] Some have vacuolar degeneration in smooth muscle cells of bowel and bladder as well as thinning of the longitudinal muscle.[233]

Immature Ganglia

This is a tough primary diagnosis because in the first year of life, immature ganglia often have an incomplete differentiation, so giant ganglia may be misinterpreted as immature ganglia[235] and may be missed in Hirschsprung's disease. They are also part of the MMHIS syndrome seen in the preceding section.

Mural Eosinophils in Hirschsprung's Disease

A small proportion of patients with Hirschsprung's disease have an accompanying eosinophilia that dominates the muscularis propria and myenteric plexus.[247] Its significance is unclear, but it may well be related to a similar eosinophilia sometimes found in patients with chronic pseudoobstruction[248,249] (see Fig. 6-49).

IDIOPATHIC MEGACOLON

This condition is characterized by constipation and colonic dilatation and may be confused with Hirschsprung's disease; however, unlike the latter, the colon is histologically normal and does not have a narrowed, aganglionic segment. It usually presents later than most cases of Hirschsprung's disease, and rather than having absolute constipation, these patients often exhibit fecal soiling of the perineum. The etiology of this disorder is unclear, but unless the typical workup for pseudoobstruction is carried out as outlined and illustrated above, the question always remains as to whether it really represents one of these disorders. It is therefore a diagnosis of exclusion, but the exclusion needs to be more than looking at the H&E slides as many of the potential changes found are either subtle and readily overlooked or not visible on H&E sections.

SEVERE IDIOPATHIC CONSTIPATION

This is a rare form of severe constipation found almost exclusively in females in the absence of any recognized underlying causes. Many of these patients require colectomies for relief of their constipation.[74,95] On histology, the colon appears unremarkable in H&E-stained sections, so all of the caveats from the previous section apply. However, with silver stains, the argyrophilic neurons are reduced in number and are small and irregular but with prominent, active-looking nuclei,[95] but the correlation with current immunohistochemical abnormalities will likely never be carried out, and it likely overlaps with the pervious section.

ACQUIRED VISCERAL NEUROPATHIES

Since the myenteric plexus is part of the autonomic nervous system, it is not surprising that primary and secondary disorders of the brain, spinal cord, and peripheral nervous system can involve the gut. Lesions of the peripheral nervous system can be further divided into those primarily affecting the *intrinsic* innervation of the bowel and those involving the *extrinsic* nerves. The major GI manifestations of these disorders are listed in Table 6-4.

Toxic or Drug-Induced Visceral Neuropathy

Chronic ingestion of certain laxatives, such as the anthraquinones, has been found to be associated with loss of argyrophilic neurons, marked axonal fragmentation, and glial cell proliferation in some patients with severe constipation.[4,95,96] Although these changes have been ascribed to the laxatives, it is possible that they represent a primary disorder of the enteric plexus, which was responsible for the ingestion of the laxatives in the first place.[95] Additional features seen more commonly in these patients are melanosis coli and rectal ulceration (cathartic ulcers).

Certain other drugs, particularly the *antineoplastic drugs* such as the *vinca alkaloids,* as well as others, such as the *phenothiazines, tricyclic antidepressants,* and *anticholinergics,* may also produce severe intestinal motor dysfunction in addition to stercoral ulceration. It is postulated that these drugs act as neurotoxins, damaging the myenteric plexus.[54,95]

Inflammatory Visceral Neuropathy (Acquired Aganglionosis)

Chagas' disease is the most important disease entity in this group. The paraneoplastic visceral neuropathies are exceedingly rare, and the pathology of the other disorders described, such as the postischemic aganglionosis, remains disputed.[61,65,81]

Chagas' Disease (American Trypanosomiasis)

This is a rare cause of secondary destruction of the myenteric plexus in the United States[97] but is much more frequent in South and Central America. It is due to *Trypanosoma cruzi,* which resides in the intestinal tract of the blood-sucking reduviid bugs. When these bugs bite a human, they also deposit contaminated feces around the bite mark.[98] The irritation of the bite results in scratching and rubbing the contaminated feces into the wound. The trypanosomes are phagocytosed by the skin histiocytes, multiply within them, and then burst out into the interstitial tissues. They then progressively disseminate, first to the lymph nodes and then widely to many organs, primarily the brain, heart, and intestines.

Clinically, there are two phases—an acute phase, which lasts for up to 2 months and is characterized by generalized symptoms, such as fever, malaise, and lymphadenopathy, and a chronic phase, the symptoms of which depends on the organ involved. The causes of the chronic injury have been variously ascribed to the release of a toxin or to an immune cross-reactivity between the Trypanosoma and the myenteric plexus.[2,99,100]

Gross appearance. Chagas' disease may involve the entire GI tract but is most frequent in the esophagus and the sigmoid colon.[101] It results in enteromegaly, "mega disease," that is, megaesophagus, megacolon and constipation, and pseudoobstruction of the small intestine. Clinically, chagasic megaesophagus is identical to idiopathic achalasia,[102] but it differs from the latter in that there is usually evidence of disease outside the esophagus.

Histology. The morphologic changes of Chagas' disease are those of an inflammatory neuropathy with destruction of the myenteric plexus.[2] The parasite is not usually found in the myenteric plexus. This injury is not uniform, being most marked in the esophagus and colon, and some areas may be spared. The degeneration is often extreme, with loss of up to 95% of all neurons in the esophagus and colon.[103,104] In the small intestine, neuronal loss is usually <50%. In H&E-stained sections, the myenteric plexus shows loss of neurons and a lymphoplasmacytic cell infiltration. Silver stains show degeneration of argyrophilic and argyrophilic neurons with irregular, swollen processes, axonal dropout, and destruction. Degeneration of the dorsal nucleus of the vagus and the hypoglossal nucleus has also been reported.[105]

Differential diagnosis. Histologically, Chagas' disease may resemble achalasia of the esophagus, as well as the primary and paraneoplastic visceral neuropathies. The primary visceral neuropathies can be differentiated by the absence of an accompanying inflammatory reaction in the myenteric plexus. Achalasia of the esophagus and the paraneoplastic lesions are morphologically similar and must be differentiated clinically. Thus, compared to achalasia of the esophagus, Chagas' disease can often be demonstrated to involve other areas of the GI tract. Furthermore, in the United States, the disease is virtually confined to individuals who have come from endemic areas such as Brazil.

Paraneoplastic Neuropathy

A paraneoplastic visceral neuropathy involving the GI tract in association with small cell carcinoma of the lung and, in one case, a carcinoid tumor has been reported.[61,65] Although these diseases are usually accompanied by extraintestinal neurologic manifestations and evidence of the primary tumor, pseudoobstruction may sometimes precede the clinical manifestations of the primary tumor.

Histologically, there is a marked reduction in the number of neurons and infiltration of the myenteric plexus with plasma cells and lymphocytes (Fig. 6-46). It has been hypothesized that the tumor antigens elicit an immune response.[2,54,65] Histologically, the inflammatory reaction of the myenteric plexus that accompanies the paraneoplastic visceral myopathies differentiates this lesion from that of the primary visceral neuropathies, which lack the inflammatory component. Chagas' disease may be indistinguishable morphologically; however, the clinical setting will normally differentiate the two entities.

Miscellaneous Visceral Neuropathies

A number of miscellaneous conditions can develop secondary visceral neuropathy. These include *amyloidosis, ischemia, ulcerative colitis (toxic megacolon), cathartic colon, cytomegalovirus infection,* and *drugs* such as antimetabolites and the phenothiazines.[2,96] In amyloidosis, there is infiltration of the myenteric plexus as well as in other sites, namely, blood vessels and lamina propria. In the cathartic colon, it is often uncertain whether degeneration of the myenteric plexus preceded laxative use.

GI Manifestations Secondary to Neurologic Disorders of the Brain and Spinal Cord

There are three major clinical manifestations: (1) upper GI hemorrhage, (2) motility disorders, and (3) abdominal pain.[106,107]

GI hemorrhage is associated with acute neurologic disease, the most noteworthy being head trauma (Cushing's ulcers), and results from an erosive gastritis.[108] These patients have an elevated serum gastrin level and increased acid output (see the discussion of stress lesions in erosive gastritis in Chapter 14).

Dysphagia and esophageal motility disorders are frequently associated with Parkinson's disease, bulbar palsy, amyotrophic lateral sclerosis, and multiple sclerosis. Frequently, no histologic change is observed in the bowel.[106,109] Rare cases of pseudoobstruction have also been described.[66]

Similarly, severe abdominal pain may accompany porphyria, tabes dorsalis, and peripheral neuropathies, without evident pathologic abnormalities in the gut. Neurofibromatosis of the GI tract may be associated with severe abdominal pain, GI hemorrhage, and intestinal obstruction. It is discussed in Chapter 8.

CHRONIC INTESTINAL PSEUDOOBSTRUCTION ASSOCIATED WITH GENERALIZED DISEASE AND THE MUSCULAR DYSTROPHIES

The GI manifestations of secondary pseudoobstruction are similar to those of the idiopathic form. Usually, the diagnosis is readily made because of the extraintestinal manifestations of the diseases. However, difficulty may arise in those occasional patients in whom the GI abnormalities antedate the generalized disorder.

Scleroderma. This, or a virtually identical disease but without the rest of the systemic manifestations of scleroderma, is likely the most common cause of pseudoobstruction. It is described under the differential diagnosis of familial visceral myopathy and in greater detail in Chapter 8.

Amyloidosis and hypothyroidism. These are other rare causes of secondary pseudoobstruction and are discussed in Chapter 9. It is usually not worth doing amyloid stains routinely in cases with pseudoobstruction if there is no other indication of amyloid clinically or histologically in the mucosa, submucosa, or vessels, as it is invariably seen in advanced disease. However, it is necessary to ensure that none of these changes are present on the H&E stain and that the patient has nothing to suggest the disease clinically.

Myotonic Muscular Dystrophy

This is a slowly progressive disorder inherited as an autosomal dominant trait and characterized by difficulty in muscular relaxation. It involves primarily the skeletal and cardiac muscles but can also involve the GI musculature from the pharynx down to the anus.[110-112] In one report, 82% of patients with myotonic dystrophy had GI involvement, which can sometimes dominate the clinical picture and may even antedate the musculoskeletal symptoms.[113-116] Clinically, symptoms result from muscle dysfunction and range from dysphagia (the most common symptom)[117-119] to cramping abdominal pain, diarrhea, and constipation.[110,111]

Histology. The pathologic changes described are limited to rare case reports. A few describe degenerative changes in the smooth muscle coats of the bowel, such as muscle atrophy with focal fiber swelling, fragmentation, destruction, and replacement by fat features similar to those found in the skeletal muscle.[111,120,121] However, in one report, abnormalities were found in the myenteric plexus, but none in the muscle coat.[122]

Progressive Muscular Dystrophy

A small number of studies have reported GI symptoms in this group of disorders.[110,111,123] The histologic changes described consist of atrophy and fibrosis of the muscularis mucosae and propria. These changes occur throughout the GI tract and are indistinguishable from those of disseminated systemic sclerosis.

Acquired Jejunal Diverticulosis

It is currently thought that most cases of acquired jejunal diverticulosis are associated with intestinal pseudoobstruction, such as familial visceral myopathy and neuropathy, scleroderma, and Fabry's disease.

SOLITARY RECTAL ULCER SYNDROME OF THE RECTUM AND INFLAMMATORY CLOACOGENIC POLYP (MUCOSAL PROLAPSE SYNDROMES)

Solitary rectal ulcer syndrome (SRUS) is a condition that results from local mucosal prolapse and probably has an underlying neural or muscular defect affecting the pelvic floor. Its name is largely a misnomer, for ulcers may or may not be present and, if present, are sometimes multiple; lesions may be rectal or anal. The histologic abnormality that characterizes this disease, while classically in the midrectum, may extend distally to the anorectal junction, where one of its less common manifestations is the so-called inflammatory cloacogenic polyp, but it may also extend proximally into the sigmoid colon, where its differential diagnosis is with diverticular polyps. Its major complication is proctitis (localized colitis) cystica profunda, which may cause a submucosal mass.

SRUS is a relatively uncommon condition that occurs in both sexes and over a wide age range including children[250] but tends to have its peak in women in the second to fourth decades. It is characterized by rectal bleeding, mucous discharge, often alteration in bowel habit, a sense of prolapse, sometimes pain, and rarely hemorrhage. In many patients, a history of marked straining during defecation can be elicited. It is an unusual disease in that, both clinically and histologically, it is usually missed when first seen, but once it has been encountered and recognized, subsequent patients are usually diagnosed with ease.

The pathogenesis of this condition is unclear. Many patients appear to have a paradoxical contraction of the levator ani part of the pelvic floor musculature on straining down, with subsequent prolapse of the rectal wall, particularly anteriorly.[251] Increased intrarectal pressure is also associated with a high external and sphincter pressure.[252] Neural damage that occurs in the distribution of the pudendal nerves is a late complication and is probably secondary.[253] In rare patients, there seems to be an association with ergot use; however, it is possible that this precipitates the final ulceration, which is almost certainly ischemic in origin, thereby drawing attention to the underlying disease.[254] There have also been suggestions of a psychological component, but it is unclear which comes first.

The natural history is variable. Some suggest that there is relatively little change and that those presenting with ulcers tend not to heal them, while those without them tend not to develop them.[255] Others suggest that some ulcers heal and that healing may be accompanied by elevated nodular margins that may ultimately replace the original ulcer bed.[256]

Ulceration may result from restriction of the blood supply at the time of prolapse, when vessels may be stretched and rupture. Mucosal fibromuscular obliteration may also help reduce blood flow. Superficial ulceration may also result from impaction of the prolapsed mucosa in the anal canal or lower rectum, with subsequent pressure necrosis. This therefore also has an ischemic component. Attempts to replace the prolapsed mucosa digitally if the patient is aware of the mass may cause further trauma (Fig. 6-58).

Gross and Endoscopic Appearances

These are quite variable. In some patients, there is only an area of redness, but this may also have a distinct nodularity or be overtly polypoid, often with multiple polyps. Ulceration may be present anywhere in the rectum and occurs in about one-half of patients, primarily on the anterior or anterolateral wall in the midrectum (Fig. 6-59).[251] The margin may be punched out and well demarcated but often are raised with a distinct nodularity; in 5% to 10% of patients, more than one ulcer is present. In some patients, there is a large polypoid mass that may also be ulcerated, and it may masquerade as a neoplasm, although considering both the chronic inflammation present and the frequency of rectal carcinoma in the population, the combination of dysplasia and carcinoma is vanishingly uncommon. The redness, ulceration, or nodularity may result in endoscopic misinterpretation as ulcerative proctitis or Crohn's disease with inflammatory polyps or a villous adenoma, while the presence of a hard polypoid mass may raise the question of carcinoma. In most patients, a request to strain down results in prolapse usually of the anterior rectal wall into the anorectum. If ulceration is present, it is frequently at the apex of this prolapse and tends to provide the best site for biopsy. It is important to establish the diagnosis for both therapeutic and prognostic reasons.

Histology

Histologic changes also vary depending upon whether the lesion is fully developed or not and where the biopsies have taken from. In biopsies taken from the most affected area, the histologic appearances are virtually diagnostic.[251,257] The mucosa is frequently thickened, and the normal architecture is usually partially or

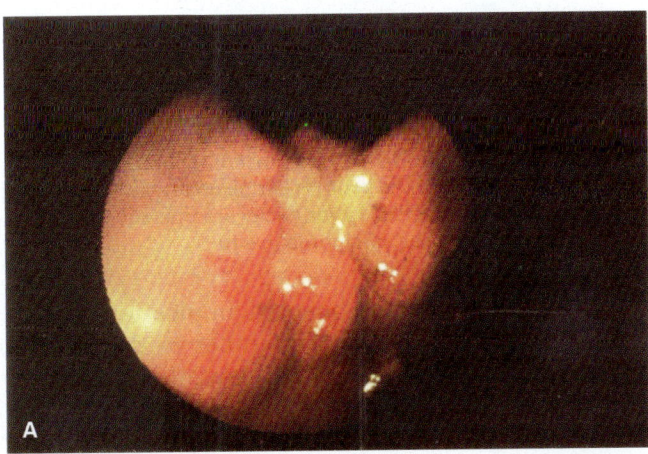
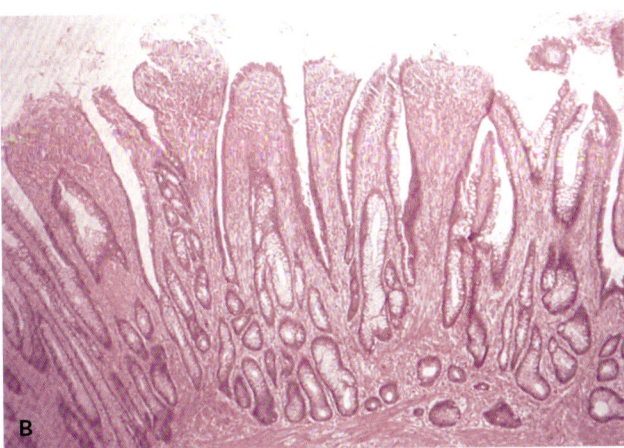

Figure 6-58. Solitary rectal ulcer syndrome. **A:** Endoscopic view showing a punched-out white ulcer base with surrounding nodules. **B:** The mucosa is usually thickened and architecturally distorted, and the normal inflammatory infiltrate in the mucosa is replaced by fibromuscular obliteration.

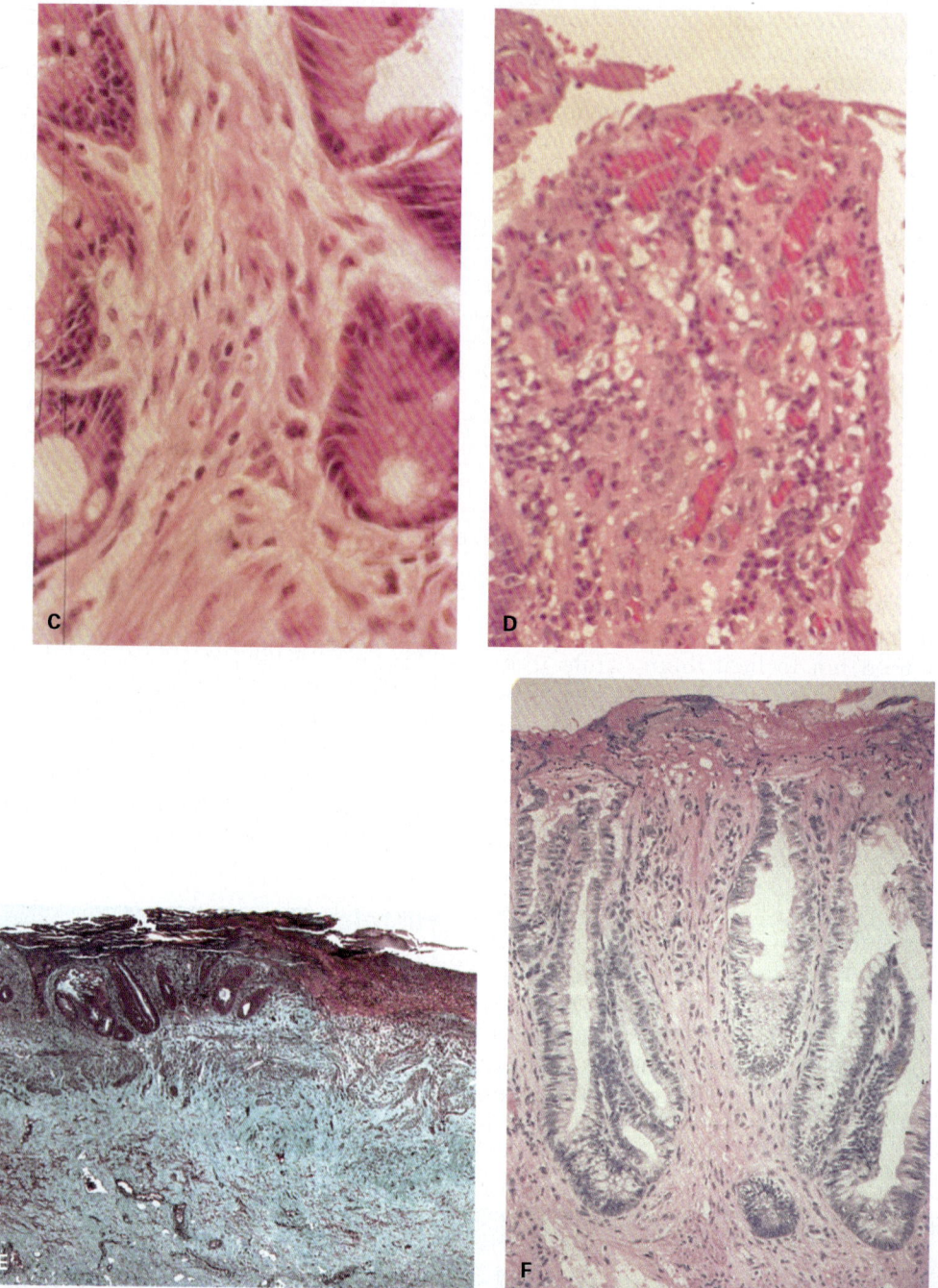

Figure 6-58. (*Continued*) **C:** Detail showing smooth muscle fibers passing up between the crypt bases. **D:** Initial surface ulceration is typically ischemic, with dilated capillaries and superficial neutrophils; a pseudomembrane may be present. **E:** Established ulceration (**right**) has marked submucosal and mucosal fibrosis, here stained green with a trichrome stain. **F:** Occasionally, there is marked nuclear hyperchromatism that may be indistinguishable from dysplasia other than the fact that fewer nuclei are present. In the presence of an architectural back-to-back appearance, it is easy to over interpret such changes as carcinoma in situ.

completely lost, with numerous bifid and distorted crypts. The crypts are tightly packed and often contain abundant mucus within the goblet cells, in contrast to the mucin depletion often seen in IBD. This may resemble the so-called transitional mucosa seen over most submucosal lesions and visible on Alcian blue high–iron diamine stain by lack of staining of the latter and the associated mucosal hyperplasia. Crypts close to or immediately beneath an ulcerated surface may have a serrated lumen similar to that seen in hyperplastic polyps (HP). However, the characteristic feature is a thickened muscularis mucosae (and muscularis propria if resection is carried out), from which muscle fibers and fibroblasts run perpendicularly up between the crypts, replacing the normal inflammatory cells of the lamina propria (Fig. 6-58).

The latter is readily demonstrated on trichrome stains and is a diffuse mucosal change, in contrast to chronic ischemia, where it is often focal.[257] This is perhaps a little surprising, as the ulceration in this condition is probably also ischemic in nature. The bundles of thickened muscularis mucosa can often press on the bases of the crypt producing indentations. The submucosa frequently shows fibrosis.

Ulceration is heralded by capillary dilatation immediately beneath the surface epithelium in which neutrophils accumulate, marginate, and pass through the endothelium into the adjacent lamina propria and epithelium (Fig. 6-58D). The surface epithelium can initially become attenuated, especially at the tip of the folds, and then lost with erosions. This is followed by a whitish-yellow pseudomembranous type of exudate and rarely full-thickness mucosal ulceration.

In patients in with unsuspected clinical diagnosis where the biopsy may not have been taken from an area of maximum pathology or if the lesion is not fully developed, the biopsy appearances may be less than typical. The most common feature is diffuse fibrosis of the lamina propria, with a reduction in the inflammatory infiltrate. Rare smooth muscle fibers may be seen extending between the crypts, but architectural changes may be minimal. Although ulceration is relatively uncommon at this stage, it does sometimes occur. If some features of the lesion are present, one should ensure that the biopsy was not taken close to the anal verge where these features of prolapse are frequently present. If the diagnosis is in question, we suggest that the patient be reexamined with a view to establishing the presence of prolapse of the rectal wall on straining and, if present, that biopsy be repeated from the anterior rectal wall at about 10 cm from the apex of the prolapse.

Differential Diagnosis

There are several features of the histology that may prove problematic. In practice, common mistake is to label some of these as serrated polyps. As discussed above, serrated crypts are not unusual in an ulcerated mucosa, one needs to see more than one to two crypts to diagnose a serrated polyp. It should be recognized that serrated polyps (sessile serrated polyp or HP) can arise in any part of the columnar mucosa down to the junction with anal squamous mucosa. Once these polyps reach a certain size, especially the more distal ones, they develop superimposed feature of prolapse. The presence of branching crypts, nuclear atypia, and extension below the muscularis mucosae can add to the diagnostic dilemma. Unlike SRUS, serrated polyps should be completely resected, and thus, the distinction becomes important. For making the diagnosis of distal serrated polyps with superimposed prolapse-type features, one should require that more than a few crypts with typical serrations (convincing ones) are present.

Some examples of SRUS may be confused with adenomatous polyps due to the presence of marked nuclear atypia with enlarged, hyperchromatic nuclei mimicking dysplasia (Fig. 6-58F). When this is present in crypts surrounded by a sheath of smooth muscle, it may even be mistaken for invasive carcinoma. Sometimes, marked regenerative features, with vesicular nuclei and prominent eosinophilic nucleoli, may be similarly misinterpreted. Accompanying proctitis cystica profunda may enhance many of these possibilities for error. In any of these situations, one needs to carefully examine the surface where in adenomas, one is likely to see dysplastic epithelium suggesting lack of maturation, while in SRUS, the changes either are restricted to the base or show some maturation to the surface. In addition, when this happens in SRUS, there are frequently surface erosions present.

The "invasion" of thickened muscle fibers up between the crypts may also cause consideration of an underlying stromal tumor (leiomyosarcoma) infiltrating the mucosa; however, in practice, this is seldom a problem.

Diffuse fibrosis of the lamina propria is relatively uncommon in other conditions, including radiation; in ischemia of any cause, it tends to be focal.[257] In collagenous colitis, fibrosis is limited to the superficial lamina propria, and sometimes the pericrypt region, and therefore does not enter into the differential diagnosis. Some patients with IBD or IBS may occasionally have wispy fibrosis of the lamina propria, but this is not sufficiently dense to cause a reduction in the inflammatory cell component of the lamina propria. If the biopsy is taken very close to the anorectal junction, some features of prolapse may be present.

Polyps in the sigmoid colon have numerous features in common with diverticular polyps, and the diagnosis may depend on the demonstration of diverticular disease and clinically the lack of prolapse features in the rectal mucosa and associated changes on rectal defecography where that is available.

Proctitis (localized colitis) cystica profunda (hamartomatous inverted polyp of the rectum)

Although traditionally called *localized colitis cystica profunda*, this is a misnomer as these should be called *proctitis cystica profunda*. When this involves both the colon and rectum, it can be designated *proctocolitis cystica profunda*.

Proctitis cystica profunda is a local complication of the SRUS, having in addition misplaced glands in

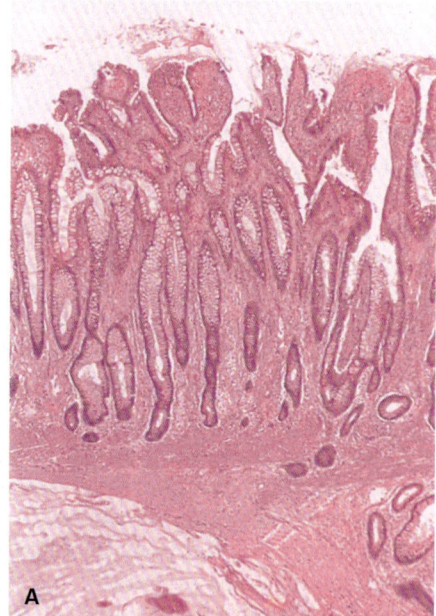 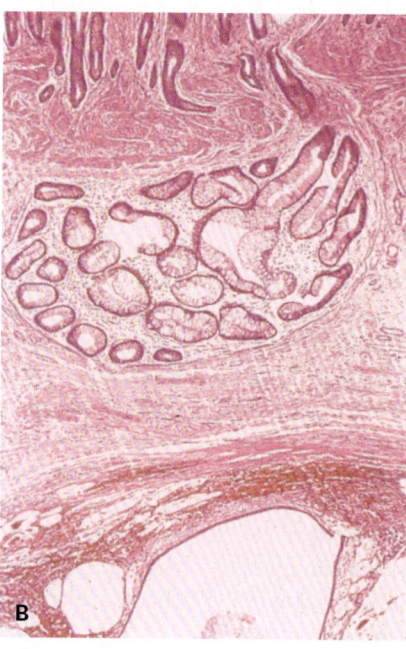

Figure 6-59. Proctitis cystica profunda in the SRUS (hamartomatous inverted polyp of the rectum). **A,B:** The overlying mucosa is that of the SRUS, but submucosal glands are present in direct continuity with the surface mucosa. These may be cystic. Residual hemorrhage may also be present along with hemosiderin-laden macrophages.

the submucosa. It has also been called *hamartomatous inverted polyp of the rectum*. It always shows the changes of SRUS in the overlying mucosa if these are looked for. The similarities, both clinically and on biopsy, between patients with the SRUS with and without this complication are becoming increasingly apparent.[258]

Gross and endoscopic appearances. This disease frequently produces a mass lesion that is readily interpreted as a benign or malignant neoplasm, sometimes with an area of ulceration enhancing the clinical interpretation. Indeed, the challenge with this disease is to recognize histologically that this is not a neoplasm, thereby preventing unnecessary resection.

Pathogenesis and histology. This lesion is almost certainly the result of rupture of one of the enlarged but thin-walled vessels in the submucosa, which causes a hematoma at the time of straining when prolapse is maximal. This may resolve by reabsorption and hemosiderin deposition; however, should the hematoma involve the mucosa and the crypt region, epithelium may gain access to the hemorrhagic cavity formed and treat it like any other ulcerated surface by relining it (Fig. 6-59).[251] This epithelium then may release mucin, thereby possibly increasing the size of the submucosal mass and producing a combination of blood and mucus in the cavity. Epithelium also traverses the sinuses of the cavity in the submucosa, initially with thin, attenuated, low cuboidal epithelium containing widely separated nuclei, although this subsequently increases in height to become tall columnar. During this phase, all the features of regeneration may be present, with open vesicular nuclei containing prominent eosinophilic nucleoli. These features persist through a stage in which the nuclei gradually return to the base of the cells, but at this point, some degree of stratification and hyperchromicity may be present. The clue that this is the nature of the underlying change is the presence of attenuated, actively regenerating epithelium with widely separated nuclei rather than the normal closely packed nuclei. However, once reepithelialization has been completed, the epithelium may also become cuboidal because of pressure from mucin secreted into the cavity, which causes pressure atrophy; however, the nuclei are small and unlikely to cause diagnostic problems. This mechanism explains the presence of epithelium giving rise to the typical lesion of proctitis cystica profunda and indicates why this lesion is so frequently accompanied by hemosiderin-laden macrophages or pools of fresh blood. A typical lamina propria may ultimately develop around the misplaced glands.

Nuclear atypicality, dysplasia, and carcinoma. Atypical nuclei may occur as part of the process of reepithelialization, as described in the preceding section. However, the overlying epithelium is sometimes atypical, and occasionally genuinely dysplastic. On occasion, we have been unable to distinguish these changes from those seen in an adenoma and have interpreted them as dysplasia; we have also seen a focus of carcinoma in situ and also one unequivocally invasive colloid carcinoma, as indicated by an invasive margin or infiltration into the muscularis propria by dysplastic epithelium. This occurred in a 46-year-old man at the site where a typical SRUS-related proctitis cystica profunda lesion had been resected 2 years earlier.

A very well-differentiated adenocarcinoma may be considered, particularly if atypical glands are found within bundles of smooth muscle, which can be variously misinterpreted either as carcinoma infiltrating muscle or as a smooth muscle tumor infiltrating mucosa. The organization of crypts and the lack of any atypical features in the muscle should prevent the latter, together with strong staining for muscle-specific actin, which is strong in ordinary smooth muscle but weak or absent in most malignant tumors. The exclusion of a very well-differentiated infiltrating adenocarcinoma usually demands recognition of the formation of a typical lamina propria around the glands, which may not always be present, as well as the lack of any other features of invasion or carcinoma in situ in the epithelium. Rarely, it may be necessary to suggest some form of rebiopsy or local excision of the lesion and the adjacent mucosa to be certain of the diagnosis.

Nevertheless, there are rare case reports of adenocarcinoma in SRUS[259,260] and squamous dysplasia and carcinoma in patients with inflammatory cloacogenic polyps.[261,262] Not surprisingly, the converse is true and neoplasia can mimic SRUS.[263–265]

Inflammatory cloacogenic polyp. This is a polypoid lesion that presents at the anorectal junction. Most, but possibly not all, cases are associated with the SRUS. Such polyps are characterized by an overlying epithelium consisting partly of the anal transition zone and partly of the mucosa overlying the lowest portion of the rectum (Fig. 6-60). Indeed, it is the partial covering by anal transitional mucosa that allows this diagnosis to be made in the absence of

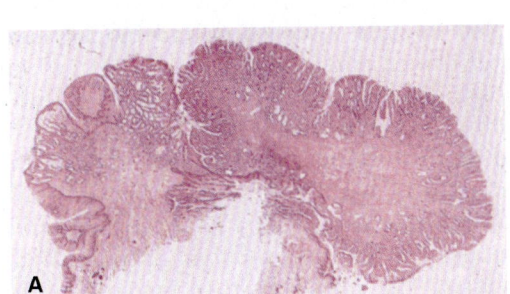
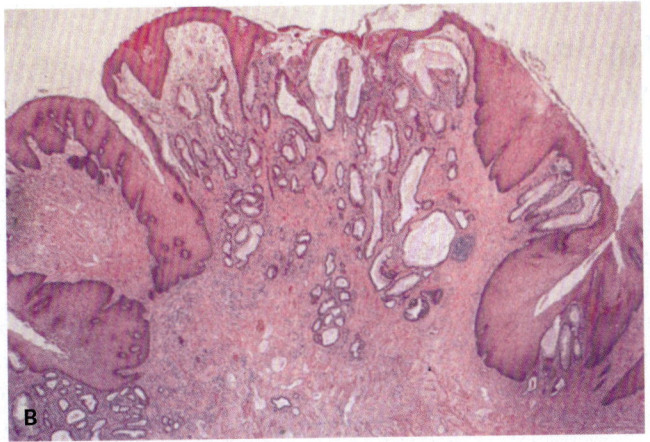
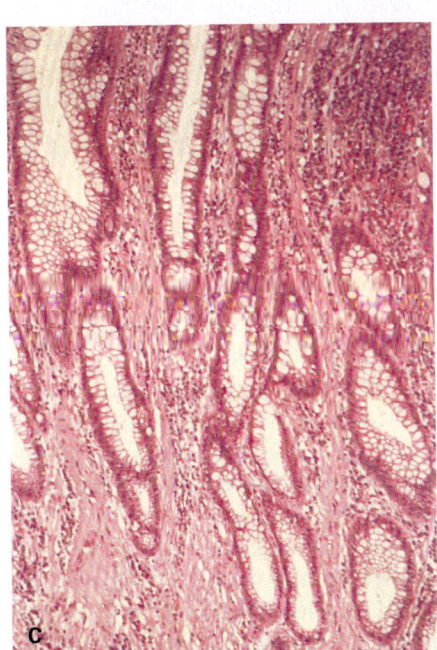
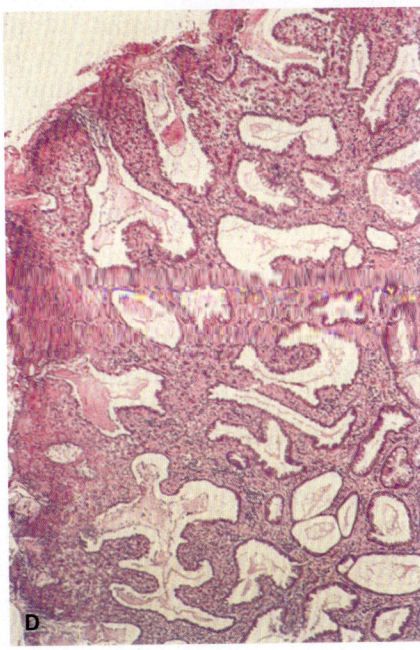
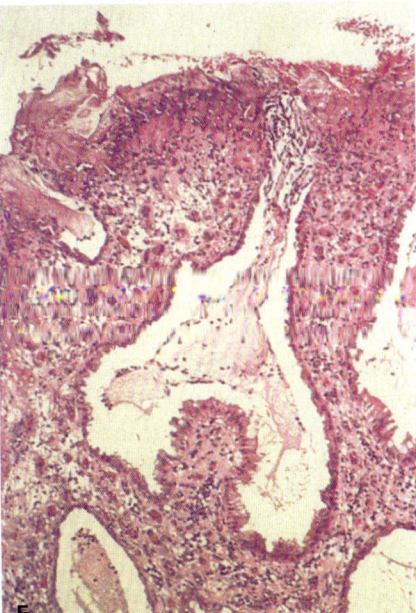

Figure 6-60. Inflammatory cloacogenic polyp, also with proctitis cystica profunda. **A:** An entire polyp in which the epithelial anorectal junction is present on the left. **B:** Detail of the junction. **C:** Detail of the remainder of the polyp, showing typical features of mucosal prolapse (see text). **D,E:** Another polyp in which there is superficial attenuation of mucosa beneath an ulcerated surface.

any clinical history. The changes in the lamina propria are identical to those described above, but they seem more likely to have superficial ulceration and florid regenerative epithelial changes, together with misplaced glands in the submucosa. Accompanying diseases include Crohn's disease, more proximal adenocarcinoma, hemorrhoids, and condyloma.[266]

While the major differential diagnosis should be with prolapsing hemorrhoids, in which the overlying mucosa can also show marked features of prolapse, this seems to be a surprisingly infrequent problem. This is presumably because the underlying hemorrhoids are usually easy to recognize. In addition, hemorrhoids characteristically contain almost atrophic-appearing rectal crypts. If the mucosal changes are marked or dominate the picture, the possibility of associated SRUS can always be suggested, with appropriate reendoscopy and biopsy at follow-up.

Irritable Bowel Syndrome

Irritable bowel syndrome is one of a number of the so-called "functional" disturbances of the GI tract and is defined as abdominal discomfort or pain associated with altered bowel habits for at least 3 days per month in the previous 3 months, with the absence of organic disease.[267] It is essentially a diagnosis of exclusion. In North America, the prevalence of IBS is about 5% to 10% although some think that 25% of patients have symptoms at some time. The peak prevalence is in the 20 to 39 years of age. Cramping abdominal pain that may be relieved by defecation is the most common symptom, but other common symptoms include diarrhea (IBS-D), constipation (IBS-C), or alternating diarrhea and constipation. It is the most frequent exit diagnosis from gastroenterology clinics, so it is inevitable that, apart from ensuring that the patient is not on medications causing this, especially NSAIDs as well cathartics, some patients are scoped to ensure that there is no treatable cause, especially for diarrhea.

There appear to be triggering factors that often include infections, so that the resulting diarrhea persists for months or years, even after the disappearance of the infection. Food allergies or intolerance may well also play a role, and some patients do get relief by avoiding gluten or dairy products. In one study, intolerance to two to five different foods was found in half of the patients studied, especially to dairy products and grains.[268,269] In diseases such as IBD, diverticular disease, and even ileoanal pouches, it can be difficult to know when symptoms are those of underlying disease or IBS. There may also be a genetic predisposition, especially affecting the tumor necrosis factor family of genes.[270] Therapy is aimed at symptom relief and improved quality of life and can include exercise, antibiotics, antispasmodics, and peppermint oil. Probiotics also appear to improve symptoms, while antidepressants and psychotherapy have also been found to be useful. Some medications, including lubiprostone (which activates chloride channel protein 2) for IBD-C, alosetron (a 5-HT3 antagonist), and tegaserod (a 5-HT4 antagonist), both of which are restricted in some countries, have been used in patients with severe symptoms where conventional therapy has failed. Indeed, there are considerable data suggesting that the serotonin/5HT pathway is involved in IBS.[271-274]

Pathology of irritable bowel syndrome. A variety of abnormalities have been described in IBS. Postinfectious IBS is characterized by an increase in both intraepithelial lymphocytes and enterochromaffin (Kulchitsky) cells in the large bowel.[272] Increases in other inflammatory cells including mast cells and eosinophils have also been described; however, all require quantitation and so are unlikely to move into "prime time" for the practicing pathologist.[275]

Investigation of patients with suspected IBS may therefore include endoscopy and biopsy, usually of the large bowel, particularly in patients in whom there is a possibility of underlying treatable organic disease including unsuspected IBD and microscopic colitis including its variants (see Chapter 18) and Brainerd-type diarrheas, which are almost certainly infectious and characterized either by changes suggestive of an infectious-type colitis or by an intraepithelial lymphocytosis. The importance in recognizing it is that it does ultimately resolve although may take many months.[276] It also needs to be recognized that prominent lamina propria eosinophils, including intraepithelial eosinophils, may indicate allergy to either food items or medications, especially NSAIDs.

Mastocytic enterocolitis. There have been suggestions that mast cells may be increased in number in some patients with IBS in all parts of the GI tact[277-283] and that examination of biopsies in patients with IBS-like symptoms is incomplete without a mast cell stain, as patients with an increased number may respond to histamine H1 or H2 receptor antagonists or a combination of both.[280] However, at the time or writing, there are insufficient data either for or against to justify routine staining for mast cells in the interpretation of biopsies with IBS.[284]

Role of the pathologist. While biopsy specimens are traditionally described as being normal, it is important for the pathologist to know that they should be looking for features that might indicate quiescent IBD, variants of microscopic colitis including Brainerd-type diarrhea, or an excess of eosinophils.

References

1. Weizman AV, Nguyen GC. Diverticular disease: epidemiology and management. [Review]. *Can J Gastroenterol.* 2011;25(7):385–389.
2. Almy TP, Howell DA. Medical progress. Diverticular disease of the colon. [Review]. *New Engl J Med.* 1980;302(6):324–331.
3. Segal I, Leibowitz B. The distributional pattern of diverticular disease. [Research Support, Non-U.S. Gov't]. *Dis Colon Rectum.* 1989;32(3):227–229.
4. Golder M, Ster IC, Babu P, et al. Demographic determinants of risk, colon distribution and density scores of diverticular disease. [Research Support, Non-U.S. Gov't]. *World J Gastroenterol.* 2011;17(8):1009–1017.
5. Blachut K, Paradowski L, Garcarek J. Prevalence and distribution of the colonic diverticulosis. [Review of 417 cases from Lower Silesia in Poland]. *Rom J Gastroenterol.* 2004;13(4):281–285.
6. Koehler R. The incidence of colonic diverticulosis in Finland and Sweden. *Acta Chir Scand.* 1963;126:148–155.
7. Hughes LE. Postmortem survey of diverticular disease of the colon. II. The muscular abnormality of the sigmoid colon. *Gut.* 1969;10(5):344–351.
8. Chan CC, Lo KK, Chung EC, et al. Colonic diverticulosis in Hong Kong: distribution pattern and clinical significance. *Clin Radiol.* 1998;53(11):842–844.
9. Miura S, Kodaira S, Shatari T, et al. Recent trends in diverticulosis of the right colon in Japan: retrospective review in a regional hospital. *Dis Colon Rectum.* 2000;43(10):1383–1389.
10. Ihekwaba FN. Diverticular disease of the colon in black Africa. *J R Coll Surg Edinb.* 1992;37(2):107–109.
11. Madiba TE, Mokoena T. Pattern of diverticular disease among Africans. *East Afr Med J.* 1994;71(10):644–646.
12. Baako BN. Diverticular disease of the colon in Accra, Ghana. *Br J Sur.* 2001;88(12):1595.
13. Burkitt DP. A deficiency of dietary fiber may be one cause of certain colonic and venous disorders. *Am J Dig Dis.* 1976;21(2):104–108.
14. Gear JS, Ware A, Fursdon P, et al. Symptomless diverticular disease and intake of dietary fibre. *Lancet.* 1979;1(8115):511–514.
15. Fisher N, Berry CS, Fearn T, et al. Cereal dietary fiber consumption and diverticular disease: a lifespan study in rats. [Research Support, Non-U.S. Gov't]. *Am J Clin Nutr.* 1985;42(5):788–804.
16. Hodgson J. An animal model for diverticular disease. *Gut.* 1972;13(10):838.
17. Morson BC, Dawson IMP. *Gastrointestinal Pathology.* Oxford, UK: Blackwell Scientific Publications; 1972.
18. Sikirov BA. Etiology and pathogenesis of diverticulosis coli: a new approach. *Med Hypotheses.* 1988;26(1):17–20.
19. Sikirov BA. Straining forces at bowel elimination. [Comparative Study]. *Isr J Med Sci.* 1989;25(1):55–56.
20. Sikirov D. Comparison of straining during defecation in three positions: results and implications for human health. [Comparative Study Research Support, Non-U.S. Gov't]. *Dig Dis Sci.* 2003;48(7):1201–1205.
21. Eastwood MA, Smith AN, Brydon WG, Pritchard J. Colonic function in patients with diverticular disease. *Lancet.* 1978;1(8075):1181–1182.
22. Suster SM, Ronnen M, Bubis JJ. Diverticulosis coli in association with Marfan's syndrome. [Case Reports Letter]. *Arch Intern Med.* 1984;144(1):203.
23. Eliashar R, Sichel JY, Biron A, Dano I. Multiple gastrointestinal complications in Marfan syndrome. [Case Reports]. *Postgrad Med J.* 1998;74(874):495–497.
24. Beighton PH, Murdoch JL, Votteler T. Gastrointestinal complications of the Ehlers-Danlos syndrome. *Gut.* 1969;10(12):1004–1008.
25. Wassenaar MJ, Cazemier M, Biermasz NR, et al. Acromegaly is associated with an increased prevalence of colonic diverticula: a case–control study. *J Clin Endocrinol Metab.* 2010;95(5):2073–2079.
26. Bassotti G, Battaglia E, Bellone G, et al. Interstitial cells of Cajal, enteric nerves, and glial cells in colonic diverticular disease. *J Clin Pathol.* 2005;58(9):973–977.
27. Bassotti G, Villanacci V, Nascimbeni R, et al. The role of colonic mast cells and myenteric plexitis in patients with diverticular disease. *Int J Colorectal Dis.* 2013;28(2):267–272.
28. West AB. The pathology of diverticulitis. [Review]. *J Clin Gastroenterol.* 2008;42(10):1137–1138.
29. Painter NS, Burkitt DP. Diverticular disease of the colon, a 20th century problem. *Clin Gastroenterol.* 1975;4(1):3–21.
30. Parra-Blanco A. Colonic diverticular disease: pathophysiology and clinical picture. [Research Support, Non-U.S. Gov't Review]. *Digestion.* 2006;73(Suppl 1):47–57.
31. McConnell EJ, Tessier DJ, Wolff BG. Population-based incidence of complicated diverticular disease of the sigmoid colon based on gender and age. *Dis Colon Rectum.* 2003;46(8):1110–1114.
32. Konvolinka CW. Acute diverticulitis under age forty. *Am J Surg.* 1994;167(6):562–565.
33. Kang JY, Firwana B, Green AE, et al. Uncomplicated diverticular disease is not a common cause of colonic symptoms. *Aliment Pharmacol Ther.* 2011;33(4):487–494.
34. Boles RS Jr, Jordan SM. The clinical significance of diverticulosis. *Gastroenterology.* 1958;35(6):579–582.
35. Connell AM. Applied physiology of the colon: factors relevant to diverticular disease. *Clin Gastroenterol.* 1975;4(1):23–36.
36. Maconi G, Barbara G, Bosetti C, et al. Treatment of diverticular disease of the colon and prevention of acute diverticulitis: a systematic review. [Review]. *Dis Colon Rectum.* 2011;54(10):1326–1338.
37. Sheth AA, Longo W, Floch MH. Diverticular disease and diverticulitis. [Review]. *Am J Gastroenterol.* 2008;103(6):1550–1556.
38. Symeonidis N, Psarras K, Lalountas M, et al. Clinical features of colonic diverticular disease. *Tech Coloproctol.* 2011;15(Suppl 1):S5–S8.
39. Heald RJ, Ray JE. Bleeding from diverticula of the colon. *Dis Colon Rectum.* 1971;14(6):420–427.
40. Longstreth GF. Epidemiology and outcome of patients hospitalized with acute lower gastrointestinal hemorrhage: a population-based study. [Research Support, Non-U.S. Gov't]. *Am J Gastroenterol.* 1997;92(3):419–424.
41. Strate LL, Ayanian JZ, Kotler G, Syngal S. Risk factors for mortality in lower intestinal bleeding. [Research Support, N.I.H., Extramural Research Support, Non-U.S. Gov't Research Support, U.S. Gov't, P.H.S.]. *Clin Gastroenterol Hepatol.* 2008;6(9):1004–1010; quiz 955.
42. Tedesco FJ, Waye JD, Raskin JB, et al. Colonoscopic evaluation of rectal bleeding: a study of 304 patients. *Ann Intern Med.* 1978;89(6):907–909.
43. Blackstone MO. *Endoscopic Interpretation: Normal and Pathologic Appearances of the Gastrointestinal Tract.* New York, NY: Raven Press; 1984.
44. Goodwin FH, Collins EN. Diverticulosis of the colon; review of 726 consecutive cases. *Cleve Clin Q.* 1948;15(4):194–201.
45. Morson BC. The muscle abnormality in diverticular disease of the colon. *Proc R Soc Med.* 1963;56:798–800.
46. Arfwidsson S, Knock NG, Lehmann L, Winberg T. Pathogenesis of multiple diverticula of the sigmoid colon in diverticular disease. *Acta Chir Scand Suppl.* 1964;63(Suppl 342):1–68.

47. Fleischner FG, Henken EM, Ming SC. Revised concepts on diverticular disease of the colon. I. Diverticulosis: emphasis on tissue derangement and its relation to the irritable colon syndrome. *Radiology.* 1964;83:859–872.
48. Tursi A, Brandimarte G, Elisei W, et al. Assessment and grading of mucosal inflammation in colonic diverticular disease. *J Clin Gastroenterol.* 2008;42(6):699–703.
49. Kelly JK. Polypoid prolapsing mucosal folds in diverticular disease. *Am J Surg Pathol.* 1991;15(9):871–878.
50. Matake H, Matsui T, Yao T, et al. Long pedunculated colonic polyp composed of mucosa and submucosa: proposal of a new entity, colonic muco-submucosal elongated polyp. *Dis Colon Rectum.* 1998;41(12):1557–1561.
51. Kim HS, Lee KY, Kim YW. Filiform polyposis associated with sigmoid diverticulitis in a patient without inflammatory bowel disease. *J Crohns Colitis.* 2010;4(6):671–673.
52. Ambrosio MR, Rocca BJ, Ginori A, et al. Long pedunculated colonic polyp with diverticulosis: case report and review of the literature. *Pathologica.* 2011;103(1):8–10.
53. Nakamura S, Kino I, Akagi T. Inflammatory myoglandular polyps of the colon and rectum. A clinicopathological study of 32 pedunculated polyps, distinct from other types of polyps. *Am J Surg Pathol.* 1992;16(8):772–779.
54. Hirasaki S, Kanzaki H, Matsubara M, Suzuki S. Inflammatory myoglandular polyps: a case series of four patients and review of the literature. *Gastroenterol Res Pract.* 2010;2010:984092.
55. Chung SH, Son BK, Park YS, et al. Inflammatory myoglandular polyps causing hematochezia. *Gut Liver.* 2010;4(1):146–148.
56. Becheanu G, Gheorghe C, Dumbrava M, et al. Inflammatory myoglandular colorectal polyps: a series of seven cases and review of literature. *Chirurgia (Bucur).* 2011;106(5):613–617.
57. Becheanu G, Stamm B. Inflammatory myoglandular polyp—a rare but distinct type of colorectal polyps. *Pathol Res Pract.* 2003;199(12):837–839.
58. D'Ovidio V, Di Camillo M, Pimpo MT, et al. An unusual complicated polypectomy and inverted colonic diverticula. *Colorectal Dis.* 2010;12(5):491–492.
59. Friedel D. Beware the inverted diverticulum! *South Med J.* 2009;102(3):235.
60. Neumann H, Vieth M, Atreya R, et al. Inverted diverticulum or adenomatous lesion? Identification using confocal laser endomicroscopy. *Gastrointest Endosc.* 2012;75(5):1102; discussion 3.
61. Donatelli G, Dhumane P, Dabo C, et al. A sessile (diminutive) polyp within a sigmoid diverticulum—EMR or observe? *Indian J Gastroenterol.* 2012;31(4):201–202.
62. Hirata T, Kawakami Y, Kinjo N, et al. Association between colonic polyps and diverticular disease. *World J Gastroenterol.* 2008;14(15):2411–2413.
63. Xu J, Yang L, Guo Y, et al. Perforation of sigmoid diverticulum following endoscopic polypectomy of an adenoma. *BMJ Case Rep.* 2010;2010; doi: 10.1136/bcr.07.2009.2077.
64. Fu KI, Hamahata Y, Tsujinaka Y. Early colon cancer within a diverticulum treated by magnifying chromoendoscopy and laparoscopy. *World J Gastroenterol.* 2010;16(12):1545–1547.
65. Granlund J, Svensson T, Granath F, et al. Diverticular disease and the risk of colon cancer—a population-based case-control study. [Research Support, Non-U.S. Gov't]. *Aliment Pharmacol Ther.* 2011;34(6):675–681.
66. Schmidt GT, Lennard-Jones JE, Morson BC, Young AC. Crohn's disease of the colon and its distinction from diverticulitis. *Gut.* 1968;9(1):7–16.
67. Peck DA, Labat R, Waite VC. Diverticular disease of the right colon. *Dis Colon Rectum.* 1968;11(1):49–54.
68. Gledhill A, Dixon MF. Crohn's-like reaction in diverticular disease. *Gut.* 1998;42(3):392–395.
69. Ludeman L, Warren BF, Shepherd NA. The pathology of diverticular disease. *Best Pract Res Clin Gastroenterol.* 2002;16(4):543–562.
70. Fischer MG, Farkas AM. Diverticulitis of the cecum and ascending colon. *Dis Colon Rectum.* 1984;27(7):454–458.
71. Sugihara K, Muto T, Morioka Y, et al. Diverticular disease of the colon in Japan. A review of 615 cases. *Dis Colon Rectum.* 1984;27(8):531–537.
72. Ngoi SS, Chia J, Goh MY, et al. Surgical management of right colon diverticulitis. *Dis Colon Rectum.* 1992;35(8):799–802.
73. Simpson J, Scholefield JH, Spiller RC. Pathogenesis of colonic diverticula. [Review]. *Br J Surg.* 2002;89(5):546–554.
74. Stollman N, Raskin JB. Diverticular disease of the colon. [Review]. *Lancet.* 2004;363(9409):631–639.
75. Ohi G, Minowa K, Oyama T, et al. Changes in dietary fiber intake among Japanese in the 20th century: a relationship to the prevalence of diverticular disease. [Research Support, Non-U.S. Gov't]. *Am J Clin Nutr.* 1983;38(1):115–121.
76. Martens T, Fierens K. Giant cecal diverticulum in a child. [Case Reports]. *J Pediatr Surg.* 2011;46(6):e23–e25.
77. Graham SM, Ballantyne GH. Cecal diverticulitis. A review of the American experience. [Review]. *Dis Colon Rectum.* 1987;30(10):821–826.
78. Shepherd NA. Diverticular disease and chronic idiopathic inflammatory bowel disease: associations and masquerades. [Review]. *Gut.* 1996;38(6):801–802.
79. Kubo A, Kagaya T, Nakagawa H. Studies on complications of diverticular disease of the colon. *Jpn J Med.* 1985;24(1):39–43.
80. Inglis FG, Hampson LG. Solitary diverticulitis of the caecum and ascending colon. *Can J Surg.* 1959;2(2):166–175.
81. Williams KL. Acute solitary ulcers and acute diverticulitis of the caecum and ascending colon. *Br J Surg.* 1960;47:351–358.
82. Maglinte DD, Chernish SM, DeWeese R, et al. Acquired jejunoileal diverticular disease: subject review. [Review]. *Radiology.* 1986;158(3):577–580.
83. Akhrass R, Yaffe MB, Fischer C, et al. Small-bowel diverticulosis: perceptions and reality. *J Am Coll Surg.* 1997;184(4):383–388.
84. Longo WE, Vernava AM III. Clinical implications of jejunoileal diverticular disease. [Review]. *Dis Colon Rectum.* 1992;35(4):381–388.
85. Koch AD, Schoon EJ. Extensive jejunal diverticulosis in a family, a matter of inheritance? [Case Reports Letter]. *Neth J Med.* 2007;65(4):154–155.
86. Mendonca HL, Vieta JO, Ling WS. Jejunal diverticulosis with massive hemorrhage. [Case Reports]. *Am J Gastroenterol.* 1978;70(6):657–659.
87. Maull KI, Nicholson BW, Mendez-Picon G. Jejunoileal diverticulosis. [Case Reports]. *South Med J.* 1981;74(7):792–795.
88. Kongara KR, Soffer EE. Intestinal motility in small bowel diverticulosis: a case report and review of the literature. [Case Reports Review]. *J Clin Gastroenterol.* 2000;30(1):84–86.
89. Krishnamurthy S, Kelly MM, Rohrmann CA, Schuffler MD. Jejunal diverticulosis. A heterogenous disorder caused by a variety of abnormalities of smooth muscle or myenteric plexus. [Research Support, U.S. Gov't, P.H.S.]. *Gastroenterology.* 1983;85(3):538–547.
90. Leivonen MK, Halttunen JA, Kivilaakso EO. Duodenal diverticulum at endoscopic retrograde cholangiopancreatography, analysis of 123 patients. *Hepatogastroenterology.* 1996;43(10):961–966.

91. Benson RE, Dixon CF, Waugh JM. Nonmeckelian diverticula of the jejunum and ileum. *Ann Surg.* 1943;118(3):377–393.
92. Manny J, Muga M, Eyal Z. The continuing clinical enigma of duodenal diverticulum. *Am J Surg.* 1981;142(5):596–600.
93. Milnerowicz S, Strutynska-Karpinska M, Nienartowicz E. Duodenal diverticulum mimicking duodenal stromal tumor. *Pol Przegl Chir.* 2011;83(1):51–54.
94. Mantas D, Kykalos S, Patsouras D, Kouraklis G. Small intestine diverticula: Is there anything new? *World J Gastrointest Surg.* 2011;3(4):49–53.
95. Kennedy RH, Thompson MH. Are duodenal diverticula associated with choledocholithiasis? *Gut.* 1988;29(7):1003–1006.
96. Karoll MP, Ghahremani GG, Port RB, Rosenberg JL. Diagnosis and management of intraluminal duodenal diverticulum. [Case Reports]. *Dig Dis Sci.* 1983;28(5):411–416.
97. Boyden EA, Cope JG, Bill AH Jr. Anatomy and embryology of congenital intrinsic obstruction of the duodenum. *Am J Surg.* 1967;114(2):190–202.
98. Fleming CR, Newcomer AD, Stephens DH, Carlson HC. Intraluminal duodenal diverticulum. Report of two cases and review of the literature. *Mayo Clin Proc.* 1975;50(5):244–248.
99. De Rai P, Castoldi L, Tiberio G. Intraluminal duodenal diverticulum causing acute pancreatitis: CT scan diagnosis and review of the literature. [Case Reports Review]. *Dig Surg.* 2000;17(3):288–292.
100. De Castro ML, Hermo JA, Pineda JR, et al. Acute bleeding and anemia associated with intraluminal duodenal diverticulum: case report and review. [Case Reports Review]. *Gastrointest Endosc.* 2003;57(7):976–979.
101. D'Alessio MJ, Rana A, Martin JA, Moser AJ. Surgical management of intraluminal duodenal diverticulum and coexisting anomalies. [Case Reports Research Support, N.I.H., Extramural Research Support, Non-U.S. Gov't Research Support, U.S. Gov't, P.H.S.]. *J Am Coll Surg.* 2005;201(1):143–148.
102. Wilcox RD, Shatney CH. Massive rectal bleeding from jejunal diverticula. [Case Reports]. *Surg Gynecol Obstet.* 1987;165(5):425–428.
103. Palder SB, Frey CB. Jejunal diverticulosis. *Arch Surg.* 1988;123(7):889–894.
104. Lough E, Richmond B, Maxwell D, Hayes JD. Obstructing phytobezoar arising from proximal jejunal diverticulum. [Case Reports]. *Am J Surg.* 2008;195(1):106–107.
105. Goldberg HM, Johnson TP. Posterior abdomino-thoracic enteric duplication. *Br J Surg.* 1963;50:445–449.
106. Friedman LS, Kirkham SE, Thistlethwaite JR, et al. Jejunal diverticula with perforation as a complication of Fabry's disease. [Case Reports Research Support, U.S. Gov't, P.H.S.]. *Gastroenterology.* 1984;86(3):558–563.
107. Dunn DH, Eisenberg MM, Berk JE. *Applied Anatomy and Anomalies of the Stomach. Bockus Gastroenterology.* Philadelphia, PA: WB Saunders; 1985:851–873.
108. Krishnamurthy S, Schuffler MD. Pathology of neuromuscular disorders of the small intestine and colon. [Review] [207 refs]. *Gastroenterology.* 1987;93(3):610–639.
109. Wood JD, Johnson LR. *Physiology of the Enteric Nervous System. Physiology of the Gastrointestinal Tract.* New York, NY: Raven Press; 1987:67–109.
110. Smith B. *The Neuropathology of the Alimentary Tract.* London, UK: Edward Arnold; 1972.
111. Andrew A. The origin of intramural ganglia. IV. The origin of enteric ganglia: a critical review and discussion of the present state of the problem. [Review] [77 refs]. *J Anat.* 1971;108(Pt 1):1–84.
112. Elliott K, Lawrensen G. *Development of the Autonomic Nervous System.* London, UK: Pitman Medical (Ciba Foundation Symposium 83); 1981.
113. Furness JB, Costa M. Types of nerves in the enteric nervous system. [Review] [137 refs]. *Neuroscience.* 1980;5(1):1–20.
114. Gershon MD, Erde SM. The nervous system of the gut. [Review] [254 refs]. *Gastroenterology.* 1981;80(6):1571–1594.
115. Cooke HJ. Neurobiology of the intestinal mucosa. [Review] [203 refs]. *Gastroenterology.* 1986;90(4):1057–1081.
116. Huizinga JD, Daniel EE. Control of human colonic motor function. [Review] [97 refs]. *Dig Dis Sci.* 1986;31(8):865–877.
117. Hoyle CH, Burnstock G. Neuronal populations in the submucous plexus of the human colon. *J Anat.* 1989;166:7–22.
118. Knowles CH, De Giorgio R, Kapur RP, et al. The London classification of gastrointestinal neuromuscular pathology: report on behalf of the Gastro 2009 International Working Group. *Gut.* 2010;59(7):882–887.
119. Peracchia A, Segalin A, Bardini R, et al. Esophageal carcinoma and achalasia: prevalence, incidence and results of treatment. *Hepatogastroenterology.* 1991;38(6):514–516.
120. Aggestrup S, Uddman R, Sundler F, et al. Lack of vasoactive intestinal polypeptide nerves in esophageal achalasia. *Gastroenterology.* 1983;84(5:Pt 1):924–927.
121. Latiano A, De Giorgio R, Volta U, et al. HLA and enteric antineuronal antibodies in patients with achalasia. *Neurogastroenterol Motil.* 2006;18(7):520–525.
122. Ruiz-de-Leon A, Mendoza J, Sevilla-Mantilla C, et al. Myenteric antiplexus antibodies and class II HLA in achalasia. *Dig Dis Sci.* 2002;47(1):15–19.
123. Clouse RE, Sleisenger MH, Fordtran JS. *Motor Disorders. Gastrointestinal Disease: Pathophysiology, Diagnosis, Management.* Philadelphia, PA: WB Saunders; 1989:559–593.
124. Smith B. The neurological lesion in achalasia of the cardia. *Gut.* 1970;11(5):388–391.
125. Lendrum FC. Anatomic features of the cardiac orifice of the stomach with special references to cardiospasm. *Arch Intern Med.* 1937;59:474–511.
126. Cassella RR, Brown AL Jr, Sayre GP, Ellis FH Jr. Achalasia of the esophagus: pathologic and etiologic considerations. *Ann Surg.* 1964;160:474–487.
127. Clark SB, Rice TW, Tubbs RR, et al. The nature of the myenteric infiltrate in achalasia: an immunohistochemical analysis. *Am J Surg Pathol.* 2000;24(8):1153–1158.
128. Gockel I, Bohl JR, Doostkam S, et al. Spectrum of histopathologic findings in patients with achalasia reflects different etiologies. *J Gastroenterol Hepatol.* 2006;21(4):727–733.
129. Villanacci V, Annese V, Cuttitta A, et al. An immunohistochemical study of the myenteric plexus in idiopathic achalasia. *J Clin Gastroenterol.* 2010;44(6):407–410.
130. Paterson WG. Etiology and pathogenesis of achalasia. *Gastrointest Endosc Clin N Am.* 2001;11(2):249–266, vi.
131. Lehman MB, Clark SB, Ormsby AH, et al. Squamous mucosal alterations in esophagectomy specimens from patients with end-stage achalasia. *Am J Surg Pathol.* 2001;25(11):1413–1418.
132. Tucker HJ, Snape WJ Jr, Cohen S. Achalasia secondary to carcinoma: manometric and clinical features. *Ann Intern Med.* 1978;89(3):315–318.
133. Hankins JR, McLaughlin JS. The association of carcinoma of the esophagus with achalasia. *J Thorac Cardiovasc Surg.* 1975;69(3):355–360.
134. Chuong JJ, DuBovik S, McCallum RW. Achalasia as a risk factor for esophageal carcinoma. A reappraisal. *Dig Dis Sci.* 1984;29(12):1105–1108.
135. Zendehdel K, Nyren O, Edberg A, Ye W. Risk of esophageal adenocarcinoma in achalasia patients, a retrospective cohort study in Sweden. *Am J Gastroenterol.* 2011;106(1):57–61.

136. Chun CL, Eisenstat S, Dormady S, et al. Esophageal adenocarcinoma presenting as pseudo-achalasia in a patient with juvenile polyposis syndrome: an enemy out of the blue. *Dig Dis Sci*. 2011;56(7):1944-1948.
137. Kahrilas PJ, Kishk SM, Helm JF, et al. Comparison of pseudoachalasia and achalasia. *Am J Med*. 1987;82(3):439-446.
138. Liu W, Fackler W, Rice TW, et al. The pathogenesis of pseudoachalasia: a clinicopathologic study of 13 cases of a rare entity. *Am J Surg Pathol*. 2002;26(6):784-788.
139. Bredenoord AJ, Jafari J, Kadri S, et al. Case report: achalasia-like dysmotility secondary to oesophageal involvement of sarcoidosis. [Case Reports]. *Gut*. 2011;60(2):153-155.
140. Katzka DA, Smyrk TC, Chial HJ, Topazian MD. Esophageal leiomyomatosis presenting as achalasia diagnosed by high-resolution manometry and endoscopic core biopsy. *Gastrointest Endosc*. 2012;76(1):216-217.
141. Dufresne CR, Jeyasingham K, Baker RR. Achalasia of the cardia associated with pulmonary sarcoidosis. [Case Reports]. *Surgery*. 1983;94(1):32-35.
142. Koberle F. Chagas' disease and Chagas' syndromes: the pathology of American trypanosomiasis. *Adv Parasitol*. 1968;6:63-116.
143. Pinotti HW, Felix VN, Zilberstein B, Cecconello I. Surgical complications of Chagas' disease: megaesophagus, achalasia of the pylorus, and cholelithiasis. *World J Surg*. 1991;15(2):198-204.
144. Katz PO, Dalton CB, Richter JE, et al. Esophageal testing of patients with noncardiac chest pain or dysphagia. Results of three years' experience with 1161 patients. *Ann Intern Med*. 1987;106(4):593-597.
145. Legius E, Proesmans W, Van Damme B, et al. Muscular hypertrophy of the oesophagus and "Alport-like" glomerular lesions in a boy. *Eur J Pediatr*. 1990;149(9):623-627.
146. Shimada H, Kise Y, Chino O, et al. A case of superficial esophageal cancer complicated with idiopathic muscular hypertrophy of the esophagus. *Tokai J Exp Clin Med*. 2003;28(3):103-108.
147. Iyer SK, Chandrasekhara KL, Sutton A. Diffuse muscular hypertrophy of esophagus. *Am J Med*. 1986;80(5):849-852.
148. Castell DO. Achalasia and diffuse esophageal spasm. [Review] [67 refs]. *Arch Intern Med*. 1976;136(5):571-579.
149. Horton ML, Goff JS. Surgical treatment of nutcracker esophagus. *Dig Dis Sci*. 1986;31(8):878-883.
150. Demian SD, Vargas-Cortes F. Idiopathic muscular hypertrophy of the esophagus. Postmortem incidental finding in six cases and review of the literature. *Chest*. 1978;73(1):28-32.
151. Vantrappen G, Janssens J, Hellemans J, Coremans G. Achalasia, diffuse esophageal spasm, and related motility disorders. *Gastroenterology*. 1979;76(3):450-457.
152. Burns AJ, Roberts RR, Bornstein JC, Young HM. Development of the enteric nervous system and its role in intestinal motility during fetal and early postnatal stages. *Semin Pediatr Surg*. 2009;18(4):196-205.
153. Carter CO, Evans KA. Inheritance of congenital pyloric stenosis. *J Med Genet*. 1969;6(3):233-254.
154. Panteli C. New insights into the pathogenesis of infantile pyloric stenosis. *Pediatr Surg Int*. 2009;25(12):1043-1052.
155. Rollins MD, Shields MD, Quinn RJ, Wooldridge MA. Pyloric stenosis: congenital or acquired? *Arch Dis Child*. 1989;64(1):138-139.
156. Spicer RD. Infantile hypertrophic pyloric stenosis: a review. [Review] [118 refs]. *Br J Surg*. 1982;69(3):128-135.
157. Guarino N, Shima H, Puri P. Structural immaturity of the pylorus muscle in infantile hypertrophic pyloric stenosis. *Pediatr Surg Int*. 2000;16(4):282-284.
158. Kobayashi H, Miyahara K, Yamataka A, et al. Pyloric stenosis: new histopathologic perspective using confocal laser scanning. *J Pediatr Surg*. 2001;36(8):1277-1279.
159. Kobayashi H, O'Briain DS, Puri P. Selective reduction in intramuscular nerve supporting cells in infantile hypertrophic pyloric stenosis. *J Pediatr Surg*. 1994;29(5):651-654.
160. Kobayashi H, O'Briain DS, Puri P. Immunochemical characterization of neural cell adhesion molecule (NCAM), nitric oxide synthase, and neurofilament protein expression in pyloric muscle of patients with pyloric stenosis. *J Pediatr Gastroenterol Nutr*. 1995;20(3):319-325.
161. Okorie NM, Dickson JA, Carver RA, Steiner GM. What happens to the pylorus after pyloromyotomy? *Arch Dis Child*. 1988;63(11):1339-1341.
162. Huang PL, Dawson TM, Bredt DS, et al. Targeted disruption of the neuronal nitric oxide synthase gene. *Cell*. 1993;75(7):1273-1286.
163. Piotrowska AP, Solari V, de Caluwe D, Puri P. Immunocolocalization of the heme oxygenase-2 and interstitial cells of Cajal in normal and aganglionic colon. *J Pediatr Surg*. 2003;38(1):73-77.
164. Vanderwinden JM, Liu H, Menu R, et al. The pathology of infantile hypertrophic pyloric stenosis after healing. *J Pediatr Surg*. 1996;31(11):1530-1534.
165. Yang G, Brisseau G, Yanchar NL. Infantile hypertrophic pyloric stenosis: an association in twins? *Paediatr Child Health*. 2008;13(5):383-385.
166. Chung E, Curtis D, Chen G, et al. Genetic evidence for the neuronal nitric oxide synthase gene (NOS1) as a susceptibility locus for infantile pyloric stenosis. [Research Support, Non-U.S. Gov't]. *Am J Hum Genet*. 1996;58(2):363-370.
167. Serra A, Schuchardt K, Genuneit J, et al. The role of RET genomic variants in infantile hypertrophic pyloric stenosis. [Comparative Study]. *Eur J Pediatr Surg*. 2011;21(6):389-394.
168. Everett KV, Capon F, Georgoula C, et al. Linkage of monogenic infantile hypertrophic pyloric stenosis to chromosome 16q24. [Research Support, Non-U.S. Gov't]. *Eur J Hum Genet*. 2008;16(9):1151-1154.
169. Everett KV, Chioza BA, Georgoula C, et al. Genome-wide high-density SNP-based linkage analysis of infantile hypertrophic pyloric stenosis identifies loci on chromosomes 11q14-q22 and Xq23. [Research Support, Non-U.S. Gov't]. *Am J Hum Genet*. 2008;82(3):756-762.
170. Zarineh A, Leon ME, Saad RS, Silverman JF. Idiopathic hypertrophic pyloric stenosis in an adult, a potential mimic of gastric carcinoma. *Patholog Res Int*. 2010;2010:614280.
171. Hellan M, Lee T, Lerner T. Diagnosis and therapy of primary hypertrophic pyloric stenosis in adults: case report and review of literature. *J Gastrointest Surg*. 2006;10(2):265-269.
172. Ejskjaer NT, Bradley JL, Buxton-Thomas MS, et al. Novel surgical treatment and gastric pathology in diabetic gastroparesis. *Diabet Med*. 1999;16(6):488-495.
173. Zarate N, Mearin F, Wang XY, et al. Severe idiopathic gastroparesis due to neuronal and interstitial cells of Cajal degeneration: pathological findings and management. *Gut*. 2003;52(7):966-970.
174. Grover M, Bernard CE, Pasricha PJ, et al. Platelet-derived growth factor receptor alpha (PDGFRalpha)-expressing "fibroblast-like cells" in diabetic and idiopathic gastroparesis of humans. *Neurogastroenterol Motil*. 2012;24(9):844-852.
175. Sipponen T, Karikoski R, Nuutinen H, et al. Three-generation familial visceral myopathy with alpha-actin-positive inclusion bodies in intestinal smooth muscle. [Case Reports]. *J Clin Gastroenterol*. 2009;43(5):437-443.

176. Colemont LJ, Camilleri M. Chronic intestinal pseudo-obstruction: diagnosis and treatment. [Review] [38 refs]. *Mayo Clin Proc.* 1989;64(1):60-70.
177. Dyer NH, Dawson AM, Smith BF, Todd IP. Obstruction of bowel due to lesion in the myenteric plexus. *Br Med J.* 1969;1(5645):686-689.
178. Anuras S, Mitros FA, Nowak TV, et al. A familial visceral myopathy with external ophthalmoplegia and autosomal recessive transmission. *Gastroenterology.* 1983;84(2):346-353.
179. Schuffler MD, Pope CE II. Studies of idiopathic intestinal pseudoobstruction. II. Hereditary hollow visceral myopathy: family studies. *Gastroenterology.* 1977;73(2):339-344.
180. Schuffler MD, Lowe MC, Bill AH. Studies of idiopathic intestinal pseudoobstruction. I. Hereditary hollow visceral myopathy: clinical and pathological studies. *Gastroenterology.* 1977;73(2):327-338.
181. Kansu A, Ensari A, Kalayci AG, Girgin N. A very rare cause of intestinal pseudoobstruction: familial visceral myopathy type IV. *Acta Paediatr.* 2000;89(6):733-736.
182. Mungan Z, Akyuz F, Bugra Z, et al. Familial visceral myopathy with pseudo-obstruction, megaduodenum, Barrett's esophagus, and cardiac abnormalities. *Am J Gastroenterol.* 2003;98(11):2556-2560.
183. Ariza A, Coll J, Fernandez-Figueras MT, et al. Desmin myopathy: a multisystem disorder involving skeletal, cardiac, and smooth muscle. *Hum Pathol.* 1995;26(9):1032-1037.
184. Smith VV, Lake BD, Kamm MA, Nicholls RJ. Intestinal pseudo-obstruction with deficient smooth muscle alpha-actin. *Histopathology.* 1992;21(6):535-542.
185. Knowles CH, Silk DB, Darzi A, et al. Deranged smooth muscle alpha-actin as a biomarker of intestinal pseudo-obstruction: a controlled multinational case series. *Gut.* 2004;53(11):1583-1589.
186. Gamba E, Carr NJ, Bateman AC. Deficient alpha smooth muscle actin expression as a cause of intestinal pseudo-obstruction: fact or fiction? *J Clin Pathol.* 2004;57(11):1168-1171.
187. Szigeti R, Chumpitazi BP, Finegold MJ, et al. Absent smooth muscle actin immunoreactivity of the small bowel muscularis propria circular layer in association with chromosome 15q11 deletion in megacystis-microcolon-intestinal hypoperistalsis syndrome. *Pediatr Dev Pathol.* 2010;13(4):322-325.
188. Moore SW, Schneider JW, Kaschula RD. Non-familial visceral myopathy: clinical and pathologic features of degenerative leiomyopathy. *Pediatr Surg Int.* 2002;18(1):6-12.
189. Roper EC, Gibson A, McAlindon ME, et al. Familial visceral neuropathy: a defined entity? *Am J Med Genet A.* 2005;137(3):249-254.
190. Auricchio A, Brancolini V, Casari G, et al. The locus for a novel syndromic form of neuronal intestinal pseudoobstruction maps to Xq28. *Am J Hum Genet.* 1996;58(4):743-748.
191. Hall KE, Wiley JW. Neural injury, repair and adaptation in the GI tract I. New insights into neuronal injury: a cautionary tail. *Am J Physiol.* 1998;274:G978-G983.
192. Haftel LT, Lev D, Barash V, et al. Familial mitochondrial intestinal pseudo-obstruction and neurogenic bladder. *J Child Neurol.* 2000;15(6):386-389.
193. Hirano M, Silvestri G, Blake DM, et al. Mitochondrial neurogastrointestinal encephalomyopathy (MNGIE): clinical, biochemical, and genetic features of an autosomal recessive mitochondrial disorder. *Neurology.* 1994;44(4):721-727.
194. Nishino I, Spinazzola A, Papadimitriou A, et al. Mitochondrial neurogastrointestinal encephalomyopathy: an autosomal recessive disorder due to thymidine phosphorylase mutations. *Ann Neurol.* 2000;47(6):792-800.
195. De Giorgio R, Santini D, Ceccarelli C. Defective expression of Bcl-2 in the enteric nervous system (ENS): a new potentially useful marker for severe functional bowel disorders (abstract). *Ital J Gastroenterol.* 1996;28:100.
196. Schobinger-Clement S, Gerber HA, Stallmach T. Autoaggressive inflammation of the myenteric plexus resulting in intestinal pseudoobstruction. *Am J Surg Pathol.* 1999;23(5):602-606.
197. Smith VV, Gregson N, Foggensteiner L, et al. Acquired intestinal aganglionosis and circulating autoantibodies without neoplasia or other neural involvement. *Gastroenterology.* 1997;112(4):1366-1371.
198. De Giorgio R, Barbara G, Stanghellini V, et al. Clinical and morphofunctional features of idiopathic myenteric ganglionitis underlying severe intestinal motor dysfunction: a study of three cases. *Am J Gastroenterol.* 2002;97(9):2454-2459.
199. De Giorgio R, Sarnelli G, Corinaldesi R, Stanghellini V. Advances in our understanding of the pathology of chronic intestinal pseudo-obstruction. *Gut.* 2004;53(11):1549-1552.
200. Jeng YM, Mao TL, Hsu WM, et al. Congenital interstitial cell of cajal hyperplasia with neuronal intestinal dysplasia. *Am J Surg Pathol.* 2000;24(11):1568-1572.
201. Agaimy A, Markl B, Arnholdt H, et al. Sporadic segmental Interstitial cell of cajal hyperplasia (microscopic GIST) with unusual diffuse longitudinal growth replacing the muscularis propria: differential diagnosis to hereditary GIST syndromes. *Int J Clin Exp Pathol.* 2010;3(5):549-556.
202. Veress B, Nyberg B, Tornblom H, Lindberg G. Intestinal lymphocytic epithelioganglionitis: a unique combination of inflammation in bowel dysmotility: a histopathological and immunohistochemical analysis of 28 cases. *Histopathology.* 2009;54(5):539-549.
203. Stanghellini V, Cogliandro RF, De Giorgio R, et al. Natural history of chronic idiopathic intestinal pseudo-obstruction in adults: a single center study. *Clin Gastroenterol Hepatol.* 2005;3(5):449-458.
204. Masetti M, Di Benedetto F, Cautero N, et al. Intestinal transplantation for chronic intestinal pseudo-obstruction in adult patients. *Am J Transplant.* 2004;4(5):826-829.
205. Krishnamurthy S, Schuffler MD, Rohrmann CA, Pope CE II. Severe idiopathic constipation is associated with a distinctive abnormality of the colonic myenteric plexus. *Gastroenterology.* 1985;88(1 Pt 1):26-34.
206. Preston DM, Hawley PR, Lennard-Jones JE, Todd IP. Results of colectomy for severe idiopathic constipation in women (Arbuthnot Lane's disease). *Br J Surg.* 1984;71(7):547-552.
207. Wedel T, Spiegler J, Soellner S, et al. Enteric nerves and interstitial cells of Cajal are altered in patients with slow-transit constipation and megacolon. *Gastroenterology.* 2002;123(5):1459-1467.
208. He CL, Burgart L, Wang L, et al. Decreased interstitial cell of cajal volume in patients with slow-transit constipation. *Gastroenterology.* 2000;118(1):14-21.
209. Knowles CH, Nickols CD, Scott SM, et al. Smooth muscle inclusion bodies in slow transit constipation. *J Pathol.* 2001;193(3):390-397.
210. Guarino M, Cheng L, Cicala M, et al. Progesterone receptors and serotonin levels in colon epithelial cells from females with slow transit constipation. *Neurogastroenterol Motil.* 2011;23(6):575-e210.
211. Austin KM. The pathogenesis of Hirschsprung's disease-associated enterocolitis. *Semin Pediatr Surg.* 2012;21(4):319-327.
212. Frykman PK, Short SS. Hirschsprung-associated enterocolitis: prevention and therapy. *Semin Pediatr Surg.* 2012;21(4):328-335.

213. Barnes PR, Lennard-Jones JE, Hawley PR, Todd IP. Hirschsprung's disease and idiopathic megacolon in adults and adolescents. *Gut*. 1986;27(5):534–541.
214. Reyes-Mugica M. Hirschsprung disease. *Path Case Rev*. 2000;5:51–59.
215. Zundel S, Obermayr F, Schaefer JF, Fuchs J. Hirschsprung disease associated with total colonic agenesis and imperforate anus—case report and review of the literature. [Case Reports Review]. *J Pediatr Surg*. 2010;45(1):252–254.
216. Kapur RP. Hirschsprung disease and other enteric dysganglionoses. *Crit Rev Clin Lab Sci*. 1999;36(3):225–273.
217. Angrist M, Jing S, Bolk S, et al. Human GFRA1: cloning, mapping, genomic structure, and evaluation as a candidate gene for Hirschsprung disease susceptibility. *Genomics*. 1998;48(3):354–362.
218. Doray B, Salomon R, Amiel J, et al. Mutation of the RET ligand, neurturin, supports multigenic inheritance in Hirschsprung disease. *Hum Mol Genet*. 1998;7(9):1449–1452.
219. Hofstra R, Valenaire O, Arch E. A loss of function mutation in the endothelin converting enzyme 1 (ECE-1) associated with Hirschsprung disease. *Am J Hum Genet*. 1998;64:304–308.
220. Myers SM, Salomon R, Goessling A, et al. Investigation of germline GFR alpha-1 mutations in Hirschsprung disease. *J Med Genet*. 1999;36(3):217–220.
221. Gath R, Goessling A, Keller KM, et al. Analysis of the RET, GDNF, EDN3, and EDNRB genes in patients with intestinal neuronal dysplasia and Hirschsprung disease. *Gut*. 2001;48(5):671–675.
222. Chakravarti A. Endothelin receptor-mediated signaling in Hirschsprung disease. *Hum Mol Genet*. 1996;5:503–507.
223. Panza E, Knowles CH, Graziano C, et al. Genetics of human enteric neuropathies. *Prog Neurobiol*. 2012;96(2):176–189.
224. Mundt E, Bates MD. Genetics of Hirschsprung disease and anorectal malformations. [Review]. *Semin Pediatr Surg*. 2010;19(2):107–117.
225. Saeed A, Barreto L, Neogii SG, et al. Identification of novel genes in Hirschsprung disease pathway using whole genome expression study. *J Pediatr Surg*. 2012;47(2):303–307.
226. Phusantisampan T, Sangkhathat S, Phongdara A, et al. Association of genetic polymorphisms in the RET-protooncogene and NRG1 with Hirschsprung disease in Thai patients. *J Hum Genet*. 2012;57(5):286–293.
227. Wu TT, Tsai TW, Chang H, et al. Polymorphisms of the RET gene in Hirschsprung disease, anorectal malformation and intestinal pseudo-obstruction in Taiwan. [Comparative Study Research Support, Non-U.S. Gov't]. *J Formos Med Assoc*. 2010;109(1):32–38.
228. Barshack I, Fridman E, Goldberg I, et al. The loss of calretinin expression indicates aganglionosis in Hirschsprung's disease. *J Clin Pathol*. 2004;57(7):712–716.
229. Guinard-Samuel V, Bonnard A, De Lagausie P, et al. Calretinin immunohistochemistry: a simple and efficient tool to diagnose Hirschsprung disease. *Mod Pathol*. 2009;22(10):1379–1384.
230. Holland SK, Ramalingam P, Podolsky RH, et al. Calretinin immunostaining as an adjunct in the diagnosis of Hirschsprung disease. *Ann Diagn Pathol*. 2011;15(5):323–328.
231. Kapur RP, Reed RC, Finn LS, et al. Calretinin immunohistochemistry versus acetylcholinesterase histochemistry in the evaluation of suction rectal biopsies for Hirschsprung Disease. *Pediatr Dev Pathol*. 2009;12(1):6–15.
232. Yin H, Boyd T, Pacheco MC, et al. Rectal biopsy in children with Down syndrome and chronic constipation: Hirschsprung disease vs non-Hirschsprung disease. *Pediatr Dev Pathol*. 2012;15(2):87–95.
233. Puri P, Gosemann JH. Variants of Hirschsprung disease. *Semin Pediatr Surg*. 2012;21(4):310–318.
234. Fadda B, Maier WA, Meier-Ruge W, et al. [Neuronal intestinal dysplasia. Critical 10-years' analysis of clinical and biopsy diagnosis]. *Z Kinderchir*. 1983;38(5):305–311.
235. Meier-Ruge WA, Ammann K, Bruder E, et al. Updated results on intestinal neuronal dysplasia (IND B). *Eur J Pediatr Surg*. 2004;14(6):384–391.
236. Montedonico S, Caceres P, Munoz N, et al. Histochemical staining for intestinal dysganglionosis: over 30 years experience with more than 1,500 biopsies. *Pediatr Surg Int*. 2011;27(5):479–486.
237. Pini Prato A, Rossi V, Fiore M, et al. Megacystis, megacolon, and malrotation: a new syndromic association? *Am J Med Genet A*. 2011;155A(8):1798–1802.
238. Meier-Ruge WA, Bruder E, Kapur RP. Intestinal neuronal dysplasia type B: one giant ganglion is not good enough. *Pediatr Dev Pathol*. 2006;9(6):444–452.
239. Friedmacher F, Puri P. Comparison of posterior internal anal sphincter myectomy and intrasphincteric botulinum toxin injection for treatment of internal anal sphincter achalasia: a meta-analysis. *Pediatr Surg Int*. 2012;28(8):765–771.
240. Koivusalo AI, Pakarinen MP, Rintala RJ. Botox injection treatment for anal outlet obstruction in patients with internal anal sphincter achalasia and Hirschsprung's disease. *Pediatr Surg Int*. 2009;25(10):873–876.
241. Moore BG, Singaram C, Eckhoff DE, et al. Immunohistochemical evaluations of ultrashort-segment Hirschsprung's disease. Report of three cases. *Dis Colon Rectum*. 1996;39(7):817–822.
242. Meier-Ruge WA, Brunner LA, Engert J, et al. A correlative morphometric and clinical investigation of hypoganglionosis of the colon in children. *Eur J Pediatr Surg*. 1999;9(2):67–74.
243. Dingemann J, Puri P. Isolated hypoganglionosis: systematic review of a rare intestinal innervation defect. *Pediatr Surg Int*. 2010;26(11):1111–1115.
244. Tunru-Dinh V, Wu ML. Intramucosal ganglion cells in normal adult colorectal mucosa. *Int J Surg Pathol*. 2007;15(1):31–37.
245. Gosemann JH, Puri P. Megacystis microcolon intestinal hypoperistalsis syndrome: systematic review of outcome. *Pediatr Surg Int*. 2011;27(10):1041–1046.
246. Rolle U, Puri P. Structural basis of voiding dysfunction in megacystis microcolon intestinal hypoperistalsis syndrome. *J Pediatr Urol*. 2006;2(4):277–284.
247. Lowichik A, Weinberg AG. Eosinophilic infiltration of the enteric neural plexuses in Hirschsprung's disease. *Pediatr Pathol Lab Med*. 1997;17(6):885–891.
248. Chander B, Fiedler P, Jain D. Eosinophilic myenteric ganglionitis: a case of intestinal pseudo-obstruction in a 93-year-old female. [Case Reports]. *J Clin Gastroenterol*. 2011;45(4):314–316.
249. Ooms AH, Verheij J, Hulst JM, et al. Eosinophilic myenteric ganglionitis as a cause of chronic intestinal pseudo-obstruction. [Case Reports]. *Virchows Arch*. 2012;460(1):123–127.
250. Dehghani SM, Malekpour A, Haghighat M. Solitary rectal ulcer syndrome in children: a literature review. *World J Gastroenterol*. 2012;18(45):6541–6545.
251. Rutter KR, Riddell RH. The solitary ulcer syndrome of the rectum. [Case Reports Comparative Study]. *Clin Gastroenterol*. 1975;4(3):505–530.
252. Womack NR, Williams NS, Holmfield JH, Morrison JF. Pressure and prolapse—the cause of solitary rectal ulceration. [Research Support, Non-U.S. Gov't]. *Gut*. 1987;28(10):1228–1233.

253. Snooks SJ, Henry MM, Swash M. Anorectal incontinence and rectal prolapse: differential assessment of the innervation to puborectalis and external anal sphincter muscles. [Research Support, Non U.S. Gov't] *Gut* 1985;26(5):470–476.
254. Eckardt VF, Kanzler G, Remmele W. Anorectal ergotism: another cause of solitary rectal ulcers. [Case Reports Research Support, Non-U.S. Gov't]. *Gastroenterology*. 1986;91(5):1123–1127.
255. Ford MJ, Anderson JR, Gilmour HM, et al. Clinical spectrum of "solitary ulcer" of the rectum. *Gastroenterology*. 1983;84(6):1533–1540.
256. Franzin G, Dina R, Scarpa A, Fratton A. "The evolution of the solitary ulcer of the rectum"—an endoscopic and histopathological study. *Endoscopy*. 1982;14(4):131–134.
257. Levine DS, Surawicz CM, Ajer TN, et al. Diffuse excess mucosal collagen in rectal biopsies facilitates differential diagnosis of solitary rectal ulcer syndrome from other inflammatory bowel diseases. [Research Support, U.S. Gov't, P.H.S.]. *Dig Dis Sci*. 1988;33(11):1345–1352.
258. Levine DS. "Solitary" rectal ulcer syndrome. Are "solitary" rectal ulcer syndrome and "localized" colitis cystica profunda analogous syndromes caused by rectal prolapse? [Research Support, U.S. Gov't, P.H.S. Review]. *Gastroenterology*. 1987;92(1):243–253.
259. Tsuchida K, Okayama N, Miyata M, et al. Solitary rectal ulcer syndrome accompanied by submucosal invasive carcinoma. *Am J Gastroenterol*. 1998;93(11):2235–2238.
260. Nonaka T, Inamori M, Kessoku T, et al. A case of rectal cancer arising from long-standing prolapsed mucosa of the rectum. *Intern Med*. 2011;50(21):2569–2573.
261. Jaworski RC, Biankin SA, Baird PJ. Squamous cell carcinoma in situ arising in inflammatory cloacogenic polyps: report of two cases with PCR analysis for HPV DNA. *Pathology*. 2001;33(3):312–314.
262. Hanson IM, Armstrong GR. Anal intraepithelial neoplasia in an inflammatory cloacogenic polyp. *J Clin Pathol*. 1999;52(5):393–394.
263. Rodriguez-Leal GA, Moran Villota S, Milke Garcia P, Vargas Rodriguez A. Inflammatory cloacogenic polyp and solitary rectal ulcer syndrome resemble rectal adenocarcinoma. *Am J Gastroenterol*. 1995;90(8):1362–1363.
264. Li SC, Hamilton SR. Malignant tumors in the rectum simulating solitary rectal ulcer syndrome in endoscopic biopsy specimens. *Am J Surg Pathol*. 1998;22(1):106–112.
265. Amaechi I, Papagrigoriadis S, Hizbullah S, Ryan SM. Solitary rectal ulcer syndrome mimicking rectal neoplasm on MRI. *Br J Radiol*. 2010;83(995):e221–e224.
266. Saul SH. Inflammatory cloacogenic polyp: relationship to solitary rectal ulcer syndrome/mucosal prolapse and other bowel disorders. *Hum Pathol*. 1987;18(11):1120–1125.
267. Brandt LJ, Chey WD, Foxx-Orenstein AE, et al. An evidence-based position statement on the management of irritable bowel syndrome. *Am J Gastroenterol*. 2009;104(Suppl 1):S1–S35.
268. Nanda R, James R, Smith H, et al. Food intolerance and the irritable bowel syndrome. *Gut*. 1989;30(8):1099–1104.
269. Carroccio A, Brusca I, Mansucto P, et al. A comparison between two different in vitro basophil activation tests for gluten- and cow's milk protein sensitivity in irritable bowel syndrome (IBS)-like patients. *Clin Chem Lab Med*. 2012:1–7.
270. Swan C, Duroudier NP, Campbell E, et al. Identifying and testing candidate genetic polymorphisms in the irritable bowel syndrome (IBS): association with TNFSF15 and TNFalpha. *Gut*. 2013;62(7):985–994.
271. Foley S, Garsed K, Singh G, et al. Impaired uptake of serotonin by platelets from patients with irritable bowel syndrome correlates with duodenal immune activation. *Gastroenterology*. 2011;140(5):1434–1443.e1.
272. Spiller RC, Jenkins D, Thornley JP, et al. Increased rectal mucosal enteroendocrine cells, T lymphocytes, and increased gut permeability following acute *Campylobacter* enteritis and in post-dysenteric irritable bowel syndrome. *Gut*. 2000;47(6):804–811.
273. Dunlop SP, Jenkins D, Neal KR, Spiller RC. Relative importance of enterochromaffin cell hyperplasia, anxiety, and depression in postinfectious IBS. *Gastroenterology*. 2003;125(6):1651–1659.
274. Dunlop SP, Coleman NS, Blackshaw E, et al. Abnormalities of 5-hydroxytryptamine metabolism in irritable bowel syndrome. *Clin Gastroenterol Hepatol*. 2005;3(4):349–357.
275. Kirsch R, Riddell RH. Histopathological alterations in irritable bowel syndrome. *Mod Pathol*. 2006;19(12):1638–1645.
276. Bryant DA, Mintz ED, Puhr ND, et al. Colonic epithelial lymphocytosis associated with an epidemic of chronic diarrhea. *Am J Surg Pathol*. 1996;20(9):1102–1109.
277. Bassotti G, Villanacci V, Nascimbeni R, et al. Increase of colonic mast cells in obstructed defecation and their relationship with enteric glia. *Dig Dis Sci*. 2012;57(1):65–71.
278. Bassotti G, Villanacci V. Mast cells in intestinal motility disorders: please also look beyond IBS. *Dig Dis Sci*. 2012;57(9):2475–2476; author reply 6.
279. Ogilvie-McDaniel C, Blaiss M, Osborn FD, Carpenter J. Mastocytic enterocolitis: a newly described mast cell entity. *Ann Allergy Asthma Immunol*. 2008;101(6):645–646.
280. Jakate S, Demeo M, John R, et al. Mastocytic enterocolitis: increased mucosal mast cells in chronic intractable diarrhea. *Arch Pathol Lab Med*. 2006;130(3):362–367.
281. Akhavein MA, Patel NR, Muniyappa PK, Glover SC. Allergic mastocytic gastroenteritis and colitis: an unexplained etiology in chronic abdominal pain and gastrointestinal dysmotility. *Gastroenterol Res Pract*. 2012;2012:950582.
282. Ramsay DB, Stephen S, Borum M, et al. Mast cells in gastrointestinal disease. *Gastroenterol Hepatol (N Y)*. 2010;6(12):772–777.
283. Thonhofer R, Siegel C, Trummer M, Langner C. Mastocytic enterocolitis as a rare cause of chronic diarrhea in a patient with rheumatoid arthritis. *Wien Klin Wochenschr*. 2011;123(9–10):297–298.
284. Schaeffer DF, Kirsch R, Riddell RH. Mast cells and intestinal motility disorders (mastocytic enteritis/colitis). *Dig Dis Sci*. 2012;57(5):1118–1121.

7. MESENCHYMAL TUMORS

Chapter Outline

INTRODUCTION
GASTROINTESTINAL STROMAL TUMORS
- *Histogenesis*
- *Demography and Clinical Aspects*
- *Diagnostic Procedures*
- *Targeted Therapy with Imatinib*
- *Surgery for GIST*
- *Frozen Section Diagnosis*
- *Gross Examination and Appearances*
- *Microscopic Appearances*
  - Unusual morphologic variants
  - Posttreatment changes
- *Immunohistochemistry*
  - False-positive immunoreactivity
  - CD117-negative GISTs
- *CD117- and DOG1-Positive Tumors Other Than GISTs*
- *Molecular Features and Mutational Analysis*
  - Succinyl dehydrogenase subunit B (SDHB) expression, NF1 mutations, and BRAF mutations
  - SDHB-deficient GISTs
  - Chromosomal alterations
- *Predicting Behavior*
- *GIST Syndromes*
  - Familial GIST syndrome
  - Neurofibromatosis type 1 (von Recklinghausen's disease)
  - Carney's triad
  - GIST-paraganglioma syndrome (Carney–Stratakis syndrome)
  - Sporadic multiple GIST
  - Pediatric GIST
  - Small GIST
- *Differential Diagnosis*
- *Reporting GIST*

SMOOTH MUSCLE TUMORS
- *Leiomyomas*
- *Epstein–Barr Virus–Associated Smooth Muscle Tumors*
- *Leiomyomatosis*
- *Smooth Muscle Hamartoma*
- *Leiomyomatosis Peritonealis Disseminata*
- *Glomus Tumor*
- *Leiomyosarcoma*

NEUROGENIC TUMORS
- *Schwannoma*
- *Neurofibroma*
- *Ganglioneuroma*
  - Polypoid ganglioneuromas
  - Ganglioneuromatous polyposis
  - Diffuse ganglioneuromatosis
- *Mucosal Neuroma/Schwann Cell "Hamartoma"*
- *Perineurioma and Fibroblastic Polyp*
  - Perineurioma
  - Fibroblastic polyps
- *Biopsy Diagnosis of Polypoid Neural Lesions*
- *Paraganglioma*
- *Granular Cell Tumor*
- *Malignant Peripheral Nerve Sheath Tumor*
- *Mixed Neuronal Glial Tumor*

FIBROBLASTIC/MYOFIBROBLASTIC TUMORS
- *Desmoid Tumor (Intraabdominal Fibromatosis)*
- *Inflammatory Fibroid Polyp*
- *Plexiform Fibromyxoma of the Gastric Antrum*
- *Inflammatory Myofibroblastic Tumor*
- *Solitary Fibrous Tumor/Hemangiopericytoma*
- *Calcifying Fibrous Tumor*
- *Elastofibroma*

ADIPOCYTIC LESIONS
- *Lipohyperplasia of the Ileocecal Valve*
- *Submucosal Lipoma*
- *Atypical Lipoma*
- *Angiolipoma*
- *Lipomatous Polyposis and Epiploic Lipomatosis*
- *Liposarcoma*
- *Differential Diagnosis of Fatty Tumors*

ENDOTHELIAL AND VASCULAR TUMORS
- *Hemangioma*
- *Angiosarcoma*
- *Kaposi's Sarcoma*
- *Lymphangioma*
- *Intestinal Vascular Lesions Associated with Clinical Syndromes*

STRIATED MUSCLE TUMORS
- *Rhabdomyoma*
- *Rhabdomyosarcoma*

MISCELLANEOUS SARCOMAS
- *Clear Cell Sarcoma*
- *Malignant Gastrointestinal Neuroectodermal Tumor (GINECT)*
- *Endometrial Stromal Sarcoma*
- *Undifferentiated High Grade Pleomorphic Sarcoma/Malignant Fibrous Histiocytoma*
- *Undifferentiated Sarcoma*

PERIVASCULAR EPITHELIOID CELL TUMORS
- *PEComa*
- *Angiomyolipoma*

BIPHASIC EPITHELIAL–MESENCHYMAL LESIONS
- *Synovial Sarcoma*
- *Spindle Cell Carcinoma/Carcinosarcoma*
- *Gastroblastoma (Epithelial Biphasic Tumor of Young Adults)*

NONMESENCHYMAL TUMORS THAT MAY MIMIC MESENCHYMAL NEOPLASMS
- *Melanoma*
- *Follicular Dendritic Cell Sarcoma*
- *Lymphoma*
- *Sarcomatoid Adult Granulosa Cell Tumor*

FIBROSING LESIONS OF THE MESENTERY, PERITONEUM, AND RETROPERITONEUM
- *Sclerosing Mesenteritis*
- *Sclerosing Peritonitis*
- *Idiopathic Retroperitoneal Fibrosis*
- *Weber–Christian Disease*

NONNEOPLASTIC LESIONS THAT MAY MIMIC MESENCHYMAL NEOPLASMS
- *Reactive Nodular Fibrous Pseudotumor*
- *Pseudosarcomatous Granulation Tissue*
- *Heterotopic Mesenteric Ossification*
- *Xanthogranulomatous Pseudotumor*
- *Mycobacterial Spindle Cell Pseudotumor*

INTRODUCTION

Mesenchymal tumors of the gastrointestinal (GI) tract can be classified as shown in Table 7-1. Some are unique to the GI tract (e.g., gastrointestinal stromal tumor [GIST], inflammatory fibroid polyp [IFP], etc.), but most have identical counterparts in soft tissues. GIST, the most common of the GI mesenchymal tumors, has been in the spotlight since the "*KIT* revolution" provided a firm framework for its diagnosis and treatment. Advances in diagnostic, molecular, prognostic, and therapeutic aspects of these tumors have been exponential. Meanwhile, the list of other mesenchymal tumors involving the GI tract continues to expand.

The increase in screening colonoscopy has seen the emergence of several new mesenchymal polypoid lesions including benign fibroblastic polyp, perineurioma, benign epithelioid peripheral nerve sheath tumor, and Schwann cell "hamartoma." In addition, reactive nodular fibrous proliferation and heterotopic mesenteric ossification have emerged as new reactive entities.

A number of rare mesenchymal tumors are starting to be seen as GI primaries (e.g., PEComa, clear cell sarcoma, and calcifying fibrous tumor) sometimes mimicking GISTs. Molecular testing has revealed some "CD117-negative GISTs" to be synovial sarcomas and some "metastatic melanomas" to be clear cell sarcomas. The ever-changing landscape of mesenchymal tumors and the rarity of most lesions pose significant challenges to surgical pathologist. This chapter aims to provide a current view of mesenchymal tumors, offering practical approaches to diagnostic challenges and highlighting their clinical implications.

Table 7-1 Classification of Gastrointestinal Mesenchymal Tumors

Gastrointestinal stromal tumor
Spindled, epithelioid, mixed, pleomorphic

Smooth muscle tumors
Leiomyoma
Epstein–Barr virus–associated smooth muscle tumors
Leiomyomatosis
Smooth muscle hamartoma
Leiomyomatosis perionealis disseminata
Glomus tumors
Leiomyosarcoma

Neural tumors
Schwannoma, neurofibroma, neuroma, perineurioma, Schwann cell hamartoma
Ganglioneuroma (polypoid ganglioneuroma, ganglineuromatous polyposis, diffuse ganglioneuromatosis)
Paraganglioma
Granular cell tumor
Malignant peripheral nerve sheath tumor

Fibroblastic/myofibroblastic proliferations
Intraabdominal fibromatosis (desmoid tumor)
Inflammatory fibroid polyp
Inflammatory myofibroblastic tumor
Plexiform fibromyxoma of the gastric antrum
Solitary fibrous tumor (hemangiopericytoma)
Benign fibroblastic polyp
Calcifying fibrous tumor
Elastofibroma

Adipocytic tumors
Lipohyperplasia
Submucosal lipomas
Lipomatosis
Liposarcomas

Endothelial and vascular tumors
Hemangioma
Angiosarcoma
Lymphangioma

Striated muscle tumors
Rhabdomyoma
Rhabdomyosarcoma

Biphasic epithelial-mesenchymal tumors
Gastroblastoma
Synovial sarcoma

Miscellaneous sarcomas
Clear cell sarcoma
Malignant gastrointestinal neuroectodermal tumor (GINECT)
Endometrial stromal sarcoma
Malignant fibrous histiocytoma/pleomorphic undifferentiated sarcoma
Undifferentiated sarcoma

Perivascular epithelioid tumors
PEComa
Angiomyolipoma

Mesenteric fibrosing lesions
Sclerosing mesenteritis
Sclerosing peritonitis
Retroperitoneal fibrosis
Weber–Christian disease

Nonmesenchymal tumors that mimic mesenchymal neoplasms
Spindle cell carcinoma (sarcomatoid carcinoma)
Melanoma
Follicular dendritic cell sarcoma
Lymphoma
Adult granulosa cell tumor (diffuse, sarcomatoid)

Nonneoplastic lesions that mimic mesenchymal neoplasms
Reactive nodular fibrous pseudotumor
Pseudosarcomatous proliferations
Heterotopic mesenteric ossification
Xanthogranulomatous pseudotumor
Mycobacterial spindle cell tumor

GASTROINTESTINAL STROMAL TUMORS

GISTs have evolved from poorly defined, histogenetically obscure GI mesenchymal tumors to well-defined oncogenic entities with distinctive clinical, morphologic, ultrastructural, histiogenetic, and molecular features, for which targeted therapy is available.

Histogenesis

Many tumors currently defined as GISTs were, in the past, thought to be smooth muscle or neural tumors due to their morphologic resemblance to these lesions.[1-4] When immunohistochemistry became available, substantial proportions were found to have neither typical smooth muscle nor neural differentiation. The noncommittal term "GI stromal tumor" to accommodate this group of tumors was coined.[5] The major conceptual breakthrough came in 1998 with the discovery of activating mutations in the receptor tyrosine kinase c-kit gene[6] and overexpression of its product CD117[7,8] in the vast majority of these tumors. GISTs are currently believed to arise from or differentiate along the lines of interstitial cells of Cajal (ICC) (the "pacemaker" cells of the GI tract), which they resemble at a morphologic, ultrastructural, and immunohistochemical (CD117+, DOG1+) level.[7,8]

Demography and Clinical Aspects

Although rare, GISTs are the most common mesenchymal tumor of the GI tract. Population-based studies from the United States, Sweden, Iceland, the Netherlands, and Spain indicate that GIST has an annual incidence in the range of 6.5–14.5/million.[9-13] Up to 4,500 to 6,000 new cases are diagnosed per year in the United States.[4] GISTs occur mainly in adults with a median age of 55 to 60 years (over 90% occur after 40 years). The age-adjusted incidence for blacks is almost twice that of whites. GISTs show a slight male predominance in adults, while in the pediatric population females are more frequently affected.[12,14] GISTs arise most commonly in the stomach (60%) and jejunum and ileum (30%) and less frequently in the duodenum (5%), colorectum (<5%), and esophagus (<1%). Rare sites include the omentum, mesentery, and retroperitoneum.[15] Case reports of GIST involving the gallbladder, liver, pancreas, and urinary bladder are on record.[16-19]

GI bleeding (acute or insidious) is the most common presentation but GISTs may also present with bloating, early satiety, abdominal pain, palpable mass, obstructive symptoms, tumor rupture (rare), or incidentally at endoscopy or surgery. Most symptomatic patients present with GISTs that are larger than 5 cm in maximum dimension.

Approximately, 20% to 25% of gastric GISTs and 40% to 50% of small intestinal GISTs behave in a clinically malignant fashion. Metastases usually involve the abdominal cavity and liver. Rarely, the musculoskeletal system or skin may be involved, while metastasis to lymph nodes or lungs is extremely rare. Since metastasis can occur 10–15 years after initial presentation, long-term follow-up is required.

Complete surgical excision is the treatment of choice, but patients with unresectable or metastatic disease are treated with c-kit/PDGFRA tyrosine kinase inhibitors such as imatinib. Most patients show a partial or complete remission, but the development of resistance (due to secondary mutations or clonal selection) has limited the long-term efficacy of this therapy. In such cases, second-line tyrosine kinase inhibitors such as sunatinib may be used.[15,20]

Diagnostic Procedures

The majority of GISTs are diagnosed only after pathologic examination of the resected specimen. However, most gastric, duodenal, and colonic GISTs undergo endosocopy and barium studies as initial investigations.[21,22] Endoscopically, GISTs may vary from dome-shaped, submucosal tumors to large, fungating or annular tumors. Some show one or more deep central ulcers, which may be the site of hemorrhage[23] (Fig. 7-1). Since the overlying mucosa is intact in most cases, endoscopy is usually nondiagnostic. Ulcerated lesions may have a higher diagnostic yield. In the latter, biopsies should be taken from the margins of the ulcer and from the surface of depressed lesions.[22] Exuberant fibroblastic and granulation tissue may be sampled and should not be misinterpreted as a stromal tumor (occasional CD34 and CD117 immunoreactivity presents a potential pitfall). All endoscopic lesions should be biopsied since carcinoid tumors, and even carcinomas, may endoscopically resemble GIST if they have a prominent submucosal component. Endoscopic ultrasound (EUS) is emerging as a useful diagnostic modality.[21,22]

Mesenchymal tumors display similar echogenicity to the surrounding muscle layer, which helps to narrow the differential diagnosis. EUS features of GIST including size >4 cm, irregular extraluminal borders, echogenic foci >3 mm, and cystic spaces >4 mm were identified as factors that correlated with its malignant behavior.[24] EUS-guided fine-needle aspiration biopsy is a safe and reliable method for obtaining tissue for cytologic assessment (immunostains can be performed on cytologic material or cell blocks). However, this procedure is currently available only in a few specialized centers and is not practical in most clinical settings. Also, GIST lesions can be highly vascularized and this may present an unacceptable risk for biopsy.

Preoperative computed tomography (CT) scan is performed to assess the resectability of large tumors.

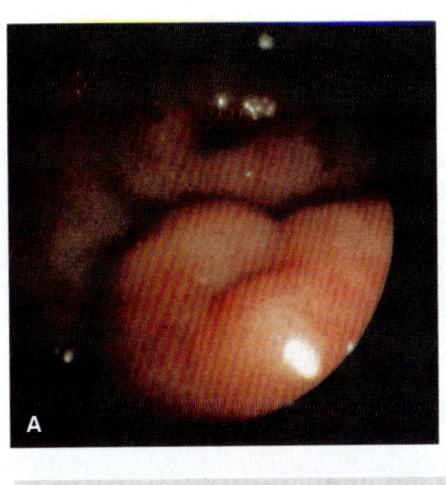
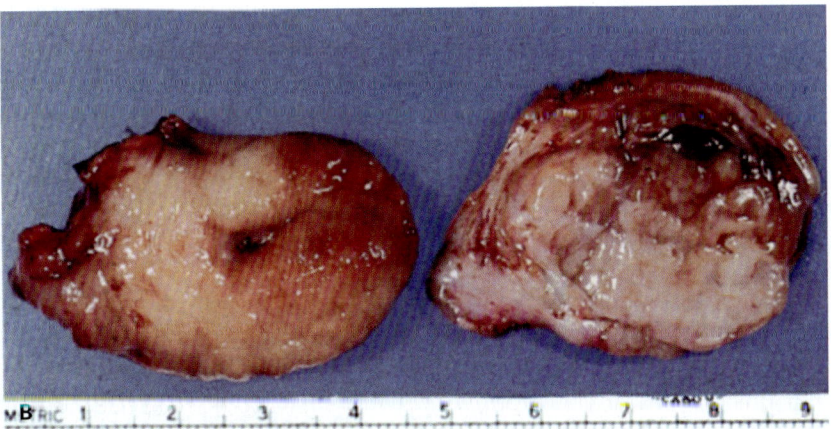
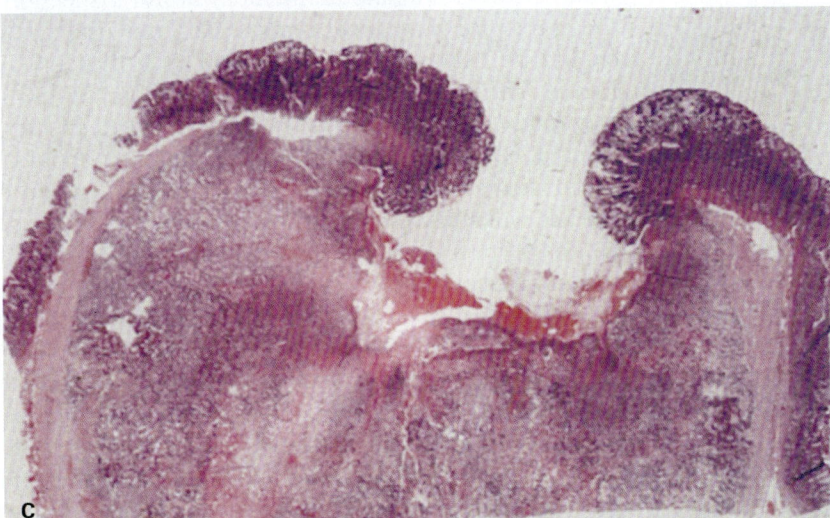
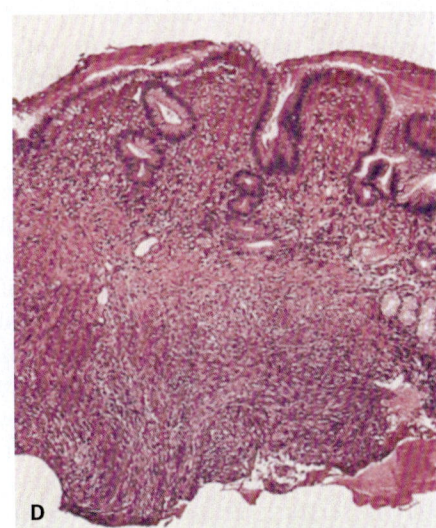

Figure 7-1. Gastric GIST. **A:** Endoscopic appearance of the GIST (foreground) largely covered by intact mucosa but showing a central ulcer from which it may bleed. A normal pylorus is in the background. **B:** Superficial ulcerated part of the stromal tumor **(left)** with its cut surface **(right). C:** Whole-mount section of a gastric GIST showing the central ulcer. Tumor in the ulcer base is probably the most accessible to biopsy for the bold. The margin of the ulcer may also yield diagnostic material. **D:** In GIST with an intact mucosa, deep biopsies can occasionally demonstrate these tumors especially if they infiltrate the lamina propria (but in many cases the biopsy is negative unless other techniques [needle/core biopsies] are used).

Tumor size, adjacent organ involvement, metastatic spread to the liver omentum or peritoneum, and ascites are also determined. Contrast CT shows peripheral enhancement in most GISTs, often with central areas of low attenuation representing hemorrhage, necrosis, or cystic degeneration.[21] Magnetic resonance imaging (MRI) is inferior to CT for visualizing gastric GIST but is useful in the assessment of hepatic metastases. If available, fluorine-18 deoxyglucose positron emission tomography (^{18}FDG-PET), in combination with CT scan, may help to delineate lesions more precisely, especially in earlier stage disease and also smaller lesions (< 1 cm in size). GIST lesions are quite FDG-avid, and this type of functional imaging is currently used to monitor response to therapy in these patients. Percutaneous or laparoscopic biopsies of localized tumors should be avoided due to the risk of tumor spillage and dissemination.[22] However, metastatic tumors are frequently subjected to this procedure.

Targeted Therapy with Imatinib

With the advent of molecularly targeted therapies and detailed identification of molecular signatures in GIST, a group of investigators from academia and industry developed and characterized signal transduction inhibitor (STI-571) or imatinib mesylate as a potent tyrosine kinase inhibitor of both c-kit and PDGF receptor (PDGFR).[24a] Since then, there has been an extraordinary expansion in the clinical development of imatinib and similar class of inhibitors for molecularly targeted therapy of GIST.

Imatinib significantly improves clinical outcomes in patients with metastatic disease and in the postsurgical adjuvant setting. In addition, imatinib is often used in the preoperative setting to reduce tumor bulk to improve resectability and/or to avoid a more extensive surgical procedure with associated morbidity.[24b] *KIT* and *PDGFRA* mutational status is helpful in predicting response to imatinib and determining the optimal dose of therapy (see Molecular Features). Primary resistance to imatinib is observed in about 15% GIST patients, but more than 80% will ultimately develop secondary resistance driven by additional KIT mutations.[24c] Sunitinib maleate has been used as a second-line agent in imatinib-resistant patients. Sunitinib has also been used as first-line treatment in GISTs that are wild type for KIT and PDGFRA or that have mutations that are known to confer imatinib resistance. Although imatinib is quite well tolerated, long-term intake of sunitinib is complicated by significant adverse effects (fatigue, diarrhea, hand-foot syndrome, hypertension, and myelosuppression) in nearly 20% of patients.[24d] Several other drugs are being tested for patients progressing on imatinib and sunitinib (e.g., regorafenib, sorafenib, dasatinib, nilotinib),[24c,24d] with regorafenib showing significant survival benefit in a randomized, placebo-controlled phase 3 trial.[24c]

Surgery for GIST

Surgery remains the primary mode of therapy for GISTs. Its goal is complete resection with negative gross and microscopic margins avoiding breach of the pseudocapsule/serosa.[20] Surgical specimens include gastric wedge resections, segmental resections of small or large bowel, or en-bloc resections. The latter procedure is performed when tumor is adherent to surrounding organs, tissues, or both to avoid disruption of the tumor with associated intraabdominal spillage and peritoneal seeding. Laparoscopic surgery for tumors < 5 cm appears to be safe in skilled hands if care is taken to avoid tumor spillage. Enucleation surgery is not recommended. Total gastrectomy and formal lymph node dissections offer no apparent survival benefit and are generally not performed.[21,22] Should small polypoid GISTs ever be removed by endoscopic polypectomy, further surgical resection of the appropriate area is required as it is impossible to include the muscularis propria and associated myenteric plexus, from where these tumors arise, in the polypectomy short of perforating the bowel.

Frozen Section Diagnosis

Frozen sections are usually not requested for suspected GISTs that are resectable. However, when the radiology is inconclusive or the disease advanced, the surgeon may want to know the tumor type intraoperatively. Frozen sections are also frequently requested on small, serosal GISTs incidentally found during surgery for other reasons. The diagnosis of "spindle cell tumor" can usually be made and is not a major diagnostic problem. On frozen sections, it is sometimes very difficult to distinguish sheets of adenocarcinoma cells from those of epithelioid stromal tumors, large noncleaved lymphomas, and even carcinoid tumors. Tumors should not be shelled out because of the risk of local recurrence. The differential diagnosis of tumors that have an organoid pattern and form definite nests excludes lymphomas and most carcinomas. It includes epithelioid GISTs, glomus tumors, carcinoids, paragangliomas, ectopic pancreas, rarely metastases, and, in theory, pyloric gland tumors, although the last are unlikely to cause problems. Fortunately, all of these tumors require primary resection. However, gastric carcinomas will require total or partial gastrectomy with regional lymph node dissection compared to the more conservative surgery performed on GIST (see above), while in lymphoma sampling of periaortic lymph nodes may be performed.

Gross Examination and Appearances

Gross examination should include careful inspection of the serosa for peritoneal breach. The mucosal surface should be examined for ulceration or tumor involvement. The maximum tumor dimension should be accurately recorded as this is a critical prognostic determinant. The serosa and resection margins should be inked and adequately sampled. Inspection of the cut surface will show most GISTs to be centered in the muscularis propria although they may extend inward toward the submucosa, outward toward the serosa, or both (Fig. 7-2). A few have a characteristic dumbbell shape with tumor on either side of the muscularis propria. Some project into the lumen while others hang off the serosal surface. GISTs occasionally appear as omental or mesenteric nodules. GISTs vary in size from < 1 cm to over 35 cm, with a median size of approximately 5 cm.

Small incidental GISTs have a predilection for the proximal stomach and gastroesophageal junction. Most GISTs are well circumscribed and nonencapsulated (Fig. 7-2) but some compress surrounding muscle and connective tissue creating the impression of a capsule. GISTs generally lack the whorled appearance of leiomyomas and have a more homogenous, often lobulated, cut surface (Fig. 7-2B). They vary from tan to red to brown. Cystic degeneration and hemorrhage are frequent (particularly in large tumors, Fig. 7-2D–G), and necrosis may be present. Degenerative features do not indicate malignancy but are seen primarily in larger tumors, which are more likely to behave aggressively.

Most GISTs are solitary, but multifocal GISTs may be seen in association with tumor syndromes (see GIST syndromes) or sporadically.[2–4,15,23] At the time of gross examination of a suspected GIST, it is useful to freeze some fresh tissue in case PDGFRA/KIT mutational studies or molecular studies (to rule out certain GIST mimics—see later) are needed (see later); however, paraffin sections suffice in most cases.

Microscopic Appearances

Histologically, GISTs may display spindle (70%), epithelioid (20%), mixed spindle and epithelioid (10%), and rarely pleomorphic morphology.[1–4,25–27] Detail of each morphologic subtype is provided in Figures 7-3 to 7-5.

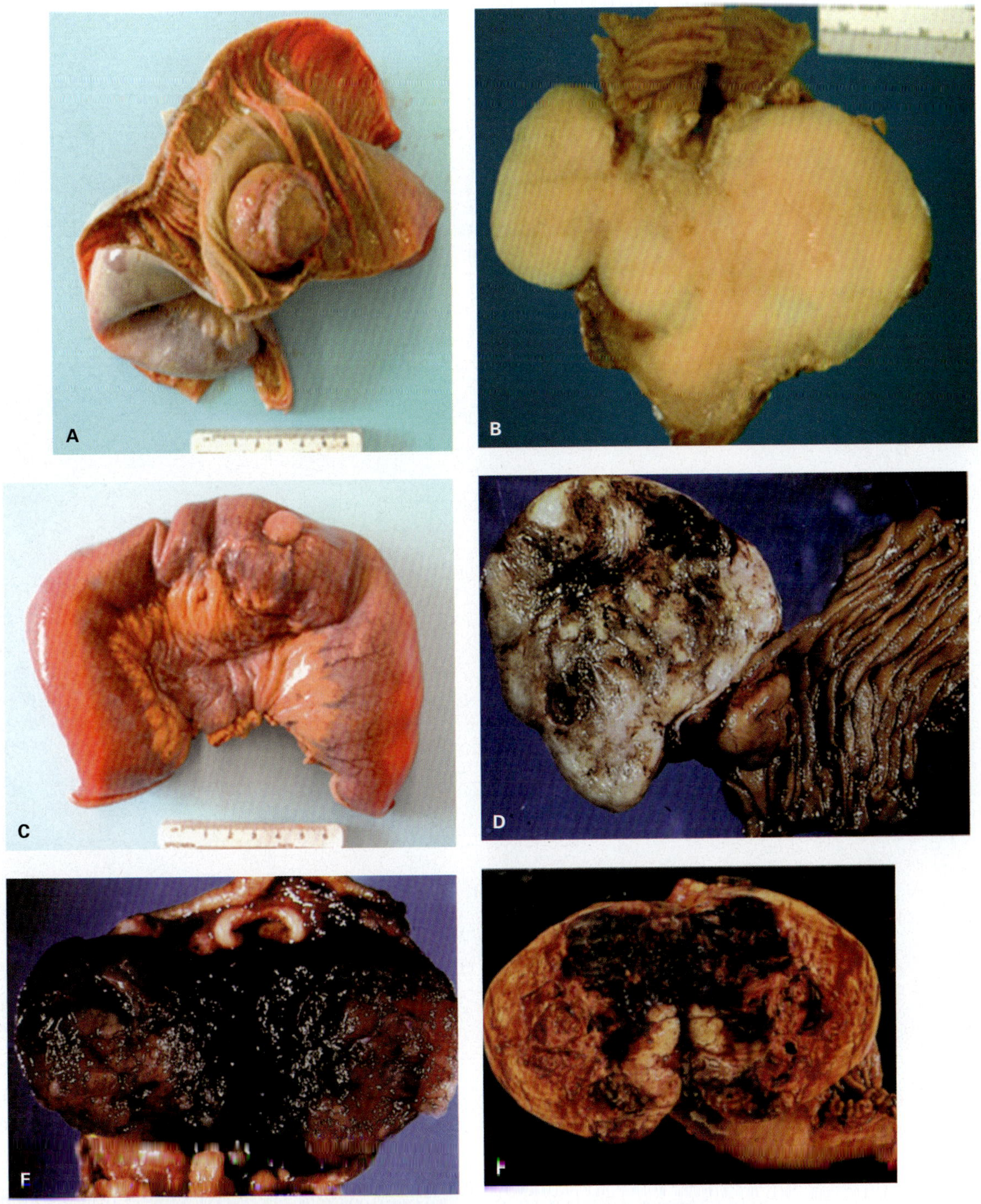

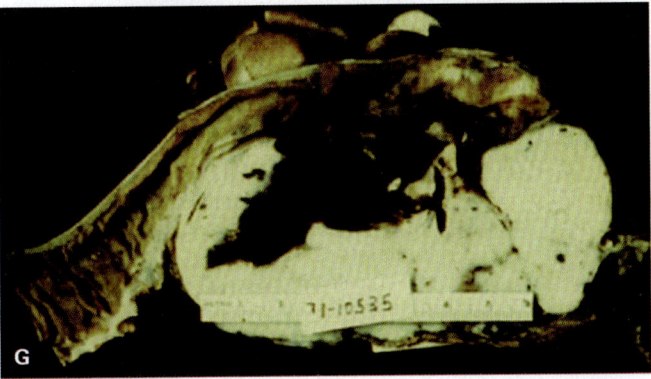

Figure 7-2. Gross appearances of GIST. **A:** Polypoid small intestinal GIST with central ulceration. **B:** Lobulated, homogenous cut surface of a small intestinal GIST. **C:** Small subserosal GIST of the small bowel. **D:** Foci of hemorrhage in a polypoid small bowel tumor. **E:** Gastric epithelioid GIST with diffuse hemorrhage. **F:** Focal areas of hemorrhage and necrosis in a jejunal stromal tumor. **G:** Cavitation in a small bowel stromal tumor with extension well beyond the muscularis propria.

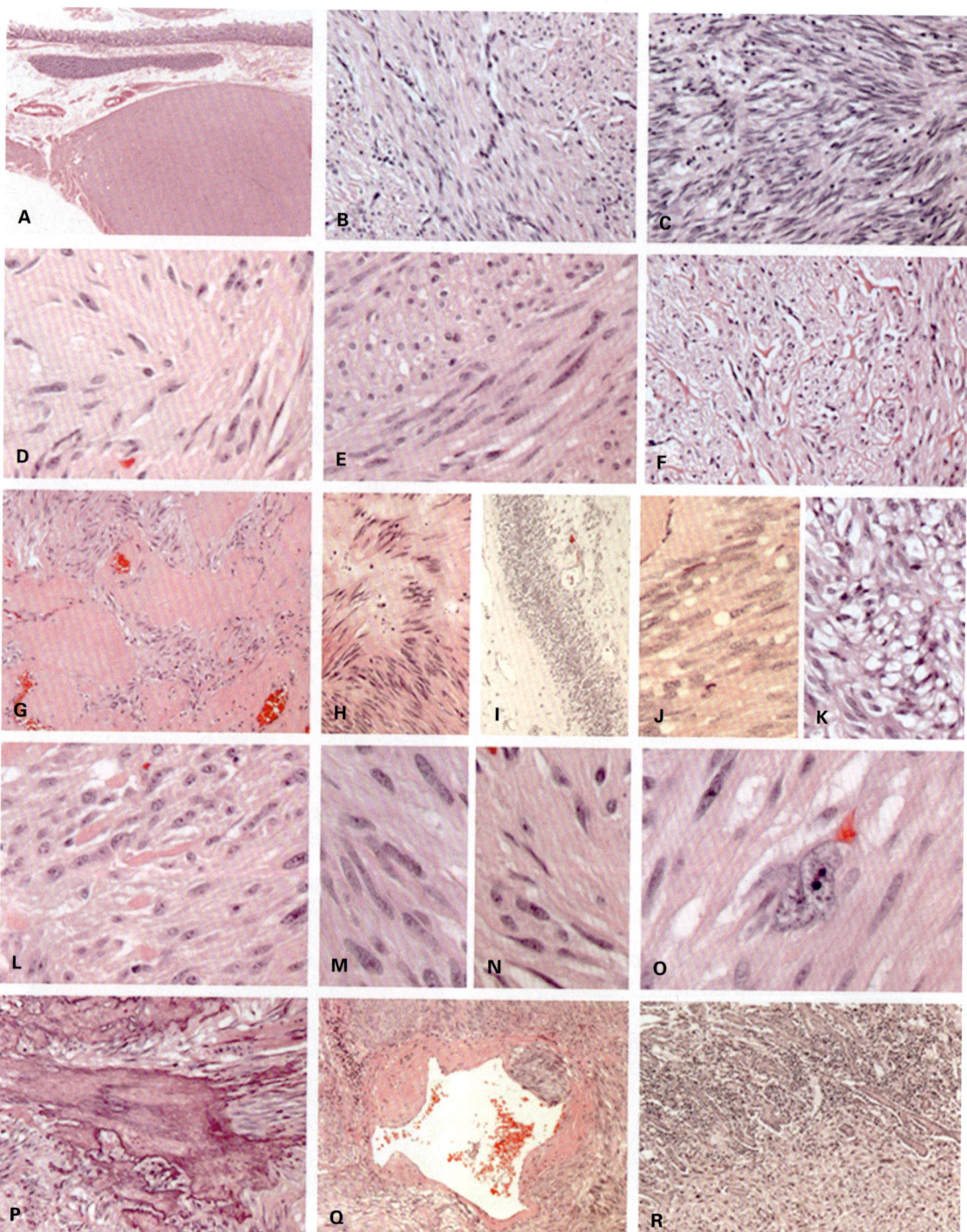

Figure 7-3. Spindle cell GIST. **A:** GISTs are generally well circumscribed and mostly centered in the muscularis propria. Cellularity varies from moderate **(B)**, to marked **(C)**, to low **(D)**. The tumor cells are often arranged in fascicles or bundles **(E,F)** separated by delicate fibrous septa **(F)** or a collagenous **(G)** to myxoid stroma. Nuclear pallisading can be striking **(H,I)**—such prominent pallisading is rarely seen in gastrointestinal schwannomas and when present favors a GIST. **J,K:** Cytoplasmic vacuolation is a frequent finding. **L:** Distinctive extracellular aggregates of hyaline collagen, named skenoid fibers due to their ultrastructural lamellar concentric appearance, are seen almost exclusively in small intestinal GISTs and appear to be a favorable prognostic feature. They may also occasionally be seen in other tumors such as fibromatosis and inflammatory myofibroblastic tumors (see Fig. 7-22). **M,N:** The tumor cells have uniform elongated nuclei with blunt **(M)** or pointed **(N)** ends, delicate chromatin and inconspicuous nucleoli. The cytoplasm is eosinophilic, fibrillary, and generally paler than that of smooth muscle cells. The mitotic rate is variable but is low most tumors. **O:** Focal nuclear pleomorphism is not uncommon. **P:** Some cases show prominent dystrophic calcification. **Q:** Blood vessels can be prominent, resembling those of solitary fibrous tumor, and often hyalinized. **R:** Infiltration of surrounding tissues or lamina propria infiltration may indicate aggressive behavior.

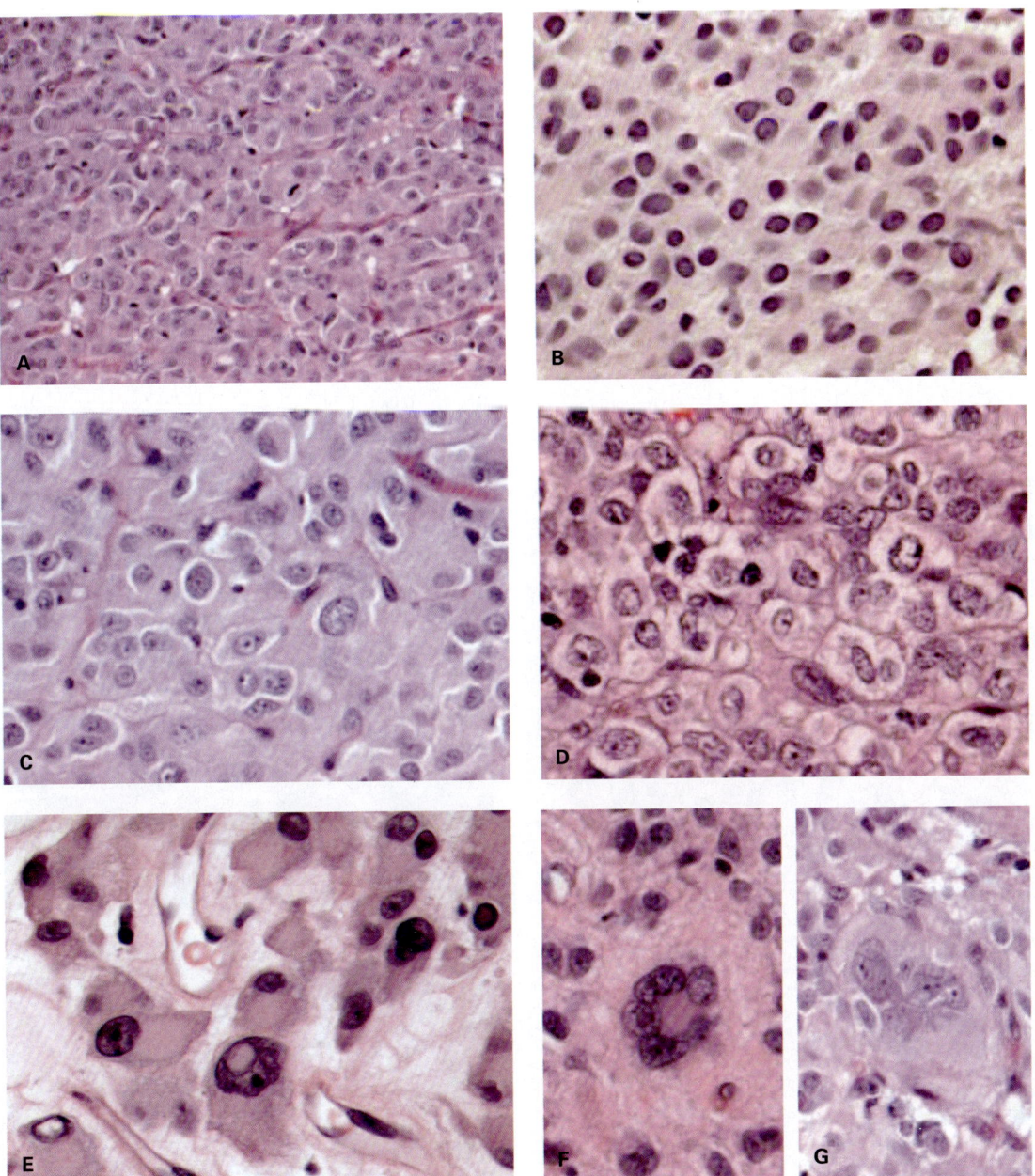

Figure 7-4. Epithelioid GIST. Most have nested (**A**) or diffuse (**B**) arrangements of closely packed, round to polygonal cells with abundant eosinophilic (**C**) or clear (**D**) cytoplasm and round central nuclei. Cell borders may be prominent (**D**). Some are diffusely pleomorphic and dyshesive (**E**). Florel-type multinucleated giant cells (**F**) and focal nuclear pleomorphism (**G**) are frequently encountered in gastric epithelioid GIST and have no prognostic significance.

Epithelioid morphology is seen in 40% of gastric GISTs but is rare in small intestinal GISTs (5%). Most GISTs are cytologically bland although focal cytologic atypia is not uncommon. Diffuse pleomorphism is distinctly unusual and should prompt consideration of alternative diagnoses (e.g., sarcoma, melanoma, or sarcomatoid carcinoma). Examples of pleomorphic GIST are shown in Figure 7-5. The Armed Forces Institute of Pathology (AFIP) series of 1,765 gastric GISTs, the largest single site series to date, described eight distinctive histologic variants (four spindled and four epithelioid) with consistent and reproducible morphology[3] (Fig. 7-6). Small intestinal GISTs could not be similarly subclassified.[2]

Unusual morphologic variants. GISTs may rarely display unusual features that can lead to diagnostic confusion (Fig. 7-7). GISTs may rarely show epithelioid differentiation to the point of gland formation,[28] prominent signet ring cell morphology (often merging with areas of more conventional GIST),[29] rhabdoid morphology including paranuclear whorls of vimentin filaments and often PDGFRA mutations[30]

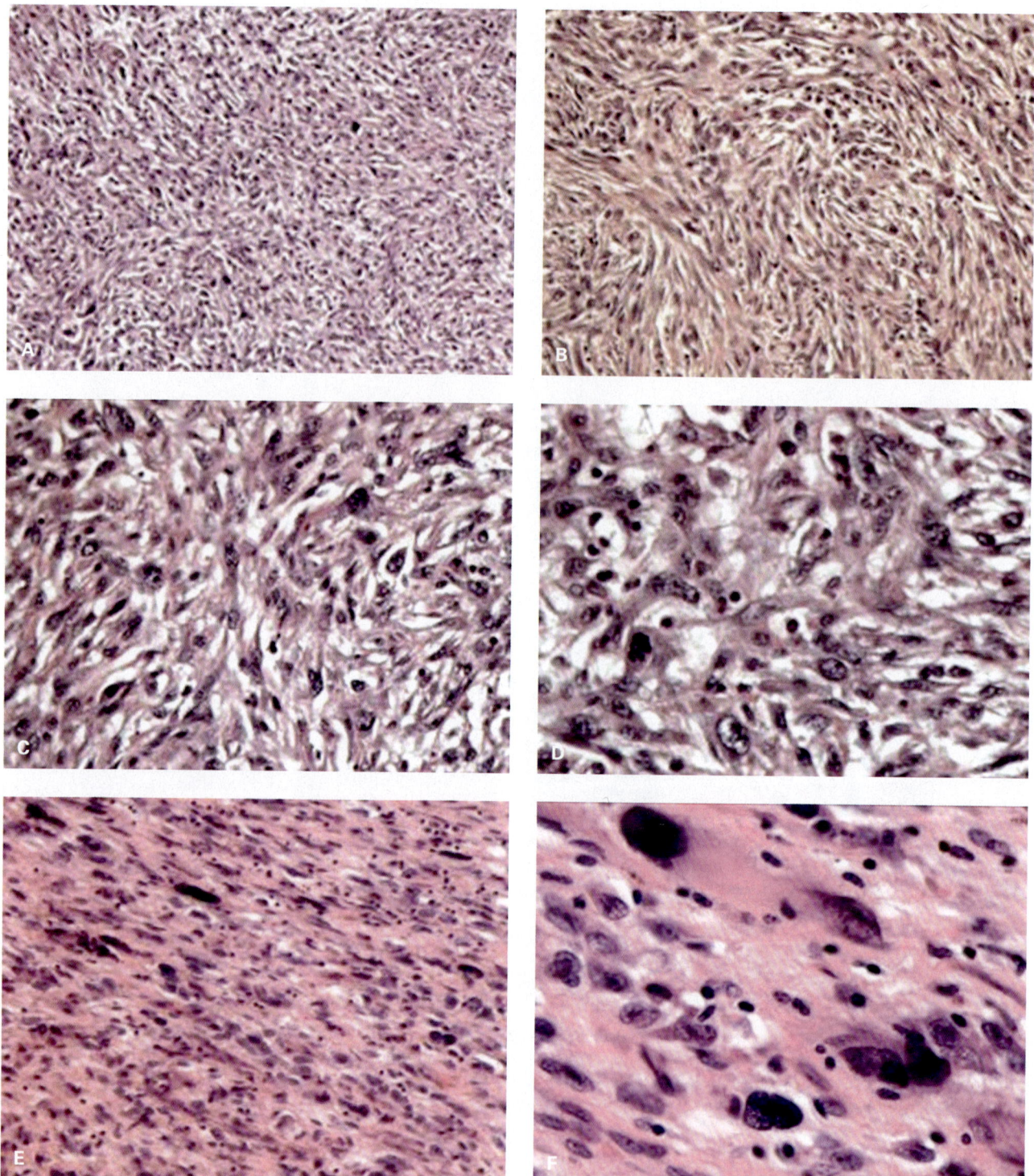

Figure 7-5. Pleomorphic GIST. Diffuse pleomorphism is uncommon in GIST. **A–D:** This pleomorphic, CD117-negative, gastric GIST could be mistaken for a storiform malignant fibrous histiocytoma/pleomorphic undifferentiated sarcoma. The demonstration of an exon 18 *PDGFRA* mutation (D809V) allowed for the correct diagnosis. **E,F:** A second sarcomatoid CD117-negative GIST associated with a PDGFRA mutation.

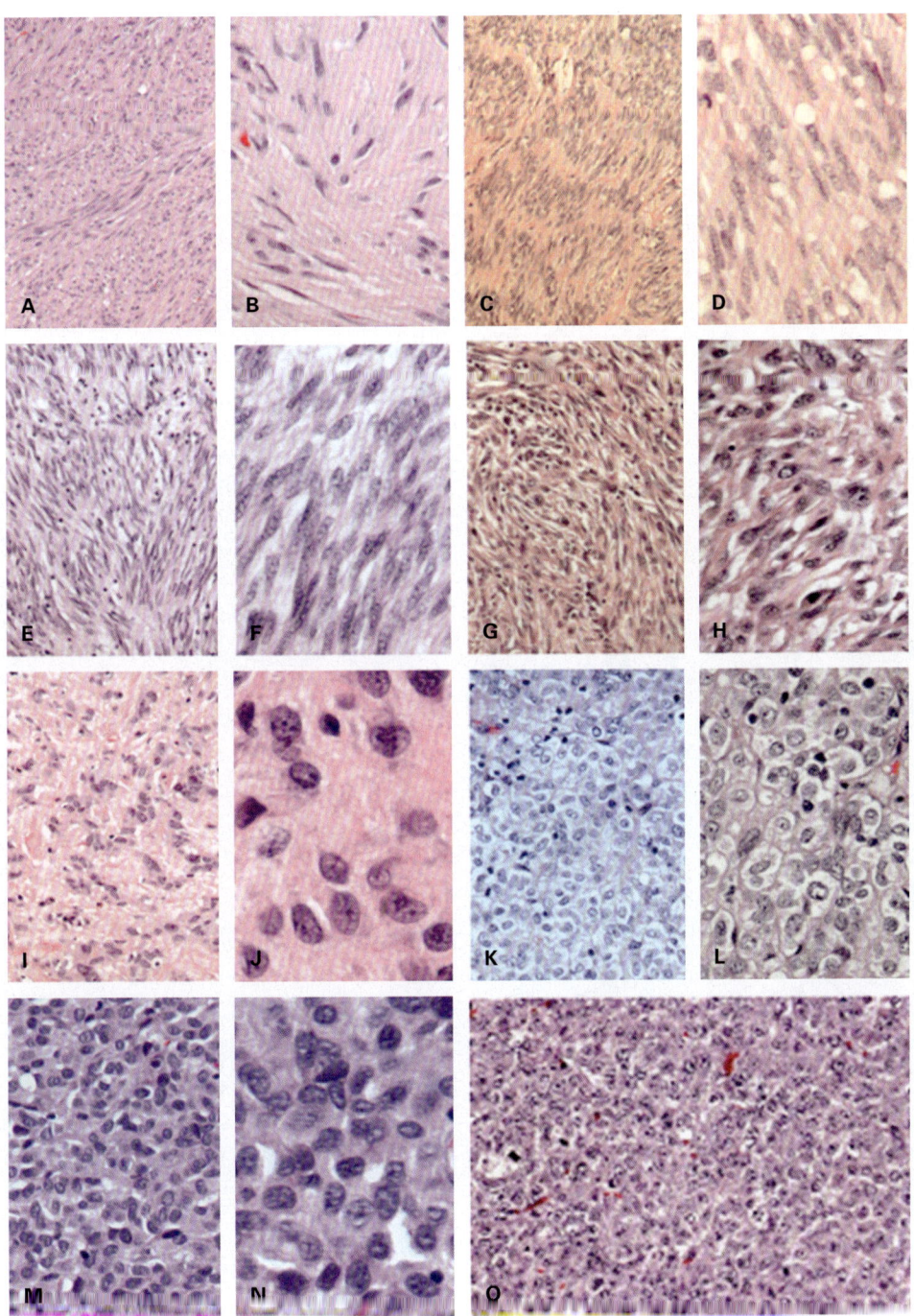

Figure 7-6. Morphologic spectrum of gastric GIST. In the AFIP series of 1765 gastric GISTs, 70% could be classified into one of the eight histologic subtypes (four spindle and four epithelioid), the remainder contained mixtures. The subtypes were as follows: **A,B:** Sclerosing spindle cell GIST, which is paucicellular with abundant extracellular collagen and shows no nuclear atypia and low mitotic activity. **C,D:** Pallisading vacuolated spindle cell GIST, which is more cellular with plump, often vacuolated spindle cells with nuclear pallisading, limited atypia, and low mitotic activity. **E,F:** Hypercellular spindle cell GIST with densely packed spindle cells in sheets with limited atypia, pallisading, perinuclear vacuolation, and a mitotic rate rarely exceeding 15/50 HPF. **G,H:** Sarcomatous spindle cell GIST with spindled to oval cells showing diffuse atypia often in bundles separated by a myxoid stroma and with a mitotic rate of >20/50 HPF. **I,J:** Sclerosing epithelioid GIST with a syncytial pattern composed of cohesive, uniform cells with indistinct cell borders, a low mitotic rate, and a collagenous stroma. **K,L:** Epithelioid GIST with a dyscohesive pattern featuring large polygonal cells with abundant cytoplasm, distinct borders, scant stroma, occasional focal atypia, and a low mitotic rate. **M,N:** Hypercellular epithelioid GIST with diffuse sheets of small epithelioid cells, with a higher nuclear to cytoplasmic ratio than the above, and a mitotic rate, which rarely exceeds 10/50 HPF. **O:** Sarcomatous epithelioid GIST with back-to-back cells, a high nuclear to cytoplasmic ratio, moderate diffuse atypia, prominent nucleoli, and a high mitotic rate.

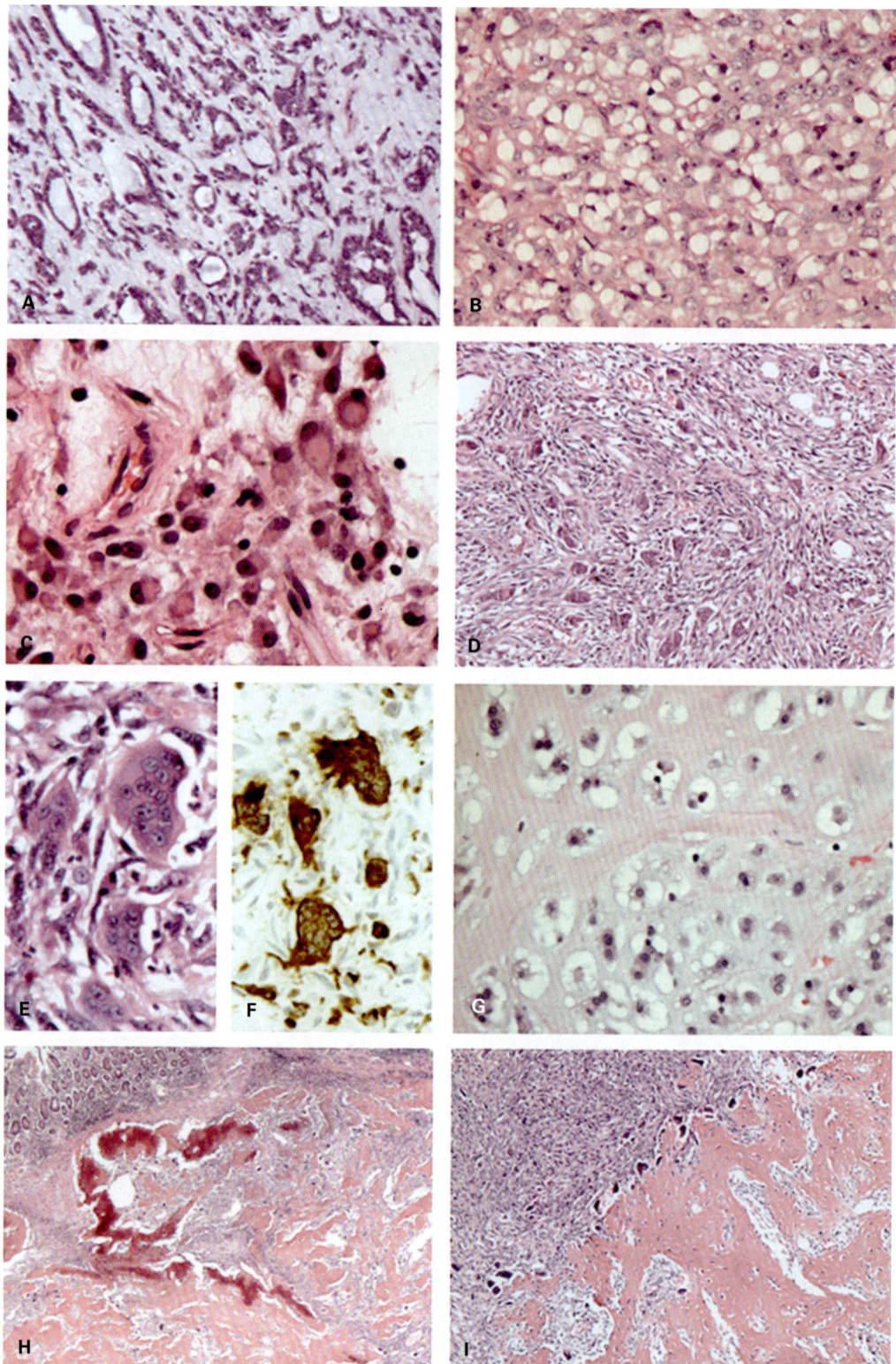

Figure 7-7. Unusual morphologic variants of GIST. **A:** Gastric GIST with epithelioid differentiation to the point of gland formation. Elsewhere this tumor showed more conventional spindled and epithelioid morphology. All components were immunoreactive for CD117. **B:** GIST with signet ring cell morphology due to prominent cytoplasmic vacuolation. **C:** Epithelioid GIST with rhabdoid morphology associated with a D842V exon 18 *PDGFRA* mutation. **D–F:** GIST with osteoclast-like giant cells. The latter were immunoreactive for CD68 **(F)** and negative for CD117 indicating their reactive nature. **G:** GIST with a prominent osteochondromatous matrix associated with a novel exon 14 *PDGFRA* mutation (K646E). **H,I:** GIST with prominent osteoid production with areas of mineralization.

and rhabdomyomatous morphology.[17] Other variants include paraganglioma-like GISTs,[3] GISTs with prominent osetoclastic-like giant cells,[31] mesothelioma-like GIST (with epithelioid cord-like areas and pseudoglandular formations in a myxoid stroma), oncocytic variants (with abundant mitochondria), small cell variants (with crowded angulated nuclei), and cytotoxic T-lymphocyte–rich GIST (infiltrated by cytotoxic T cells).

Posttreatment changes. Histologic changes described postimatinib include those associated with tumor cell necrosis as well as phenotypic changes in residual tumor cells. Most GISTs show some histopathologic response to imatinib, but this is usually incomplete and does not correlate with clinical or radiologic response. Even tumors with a very good histologic response (i.e., >90% necrosis or hyalinization or both) show focal residual viable tumor in most cases if carefully looked for. Immunohistochemistry for CD117 or DOG1 may help to highlight such foci, although CD117 immunoreactivity, in particular, may be lost. DOG1 immunoreactivity tends to be better retained.[32]

The histologic response often varies between and within individual nodules. Some tumors have a distinctive myxohyaline stroma, while others show extensive cystic change or hemorrhage. A small minority of tumors may show phenotypic alterations in residual tumor including switch from a spindled to epithelioid phenotype, small cell phenotype, acquisition of myoid phenotype (including desmin expression and ultrastructural features), and loss of CD117 and CD34 immunoreactivity.

Diagnostic problems may arise when secondary tumors with unusual morphology and unexpected immunohistochemical profiles arise at new locations. Mutational analysis may be extremely helpful in such circumstances.[33-35] The pathology report should include an estimate of the proportion of necrotic/hyalinized tumor as an indication of pathologic response. A grading system for pathologic response has been proposed, but this is not widely used outside the research setting.[36]

Immunohistochemistry

Approximately, 95% of GISTs are immunoreactive for CD117. Staining is usually strong and diffuse, most often cytoplasmic but can also be membranous or may involve the paranuclear "Golgi zone" with dot-like immunoreactivity (Fig. 7-8A–D). Membrane staining is more often appreciated in epithelioid GISTs, while staining in spindle cell GISTs is typically pancytoplasmic; membrane staining may difficult to appreciate in spindled cells due to their narrower width. Epithelioid GISTs often show less uniform staining and are sometimes only weakly positive or negative (Fig. 7-8E).[2,3]

DOG1 (discovered on GIST 1) is a highly sensitive GIST marker, staining approximately 95% of these tumors. Originally identified in gene expression profiling studies, DOG1 is a calcium-activated chloride channel protein, also known as anoctamin 1 or TMEM16A. DOG1 shows a cytoplasmic and/or membranous pattern of staining similar to that seen with CD117.[37,38] DOG1 appears to be a more specific marker of GIST than is CD117, although a handful of tumors other than GIST may occasionally express this protein (see below).

A number of alternative immunohistochemical markers for GIST have been evaluated, including nestin, protein kinase C theta, and PDGFRA. While nestin and protein kinase C theta have a high sensitivity, their expression by a wide range of histologic mimics of GIST limits their utility.[32] PDGFRA has been reported by some to be highly sensitive and generally specific for CD117-negative GISTs.[39,40] However, the unpublished experience of most large GIST centers (including our own) is that reliability and reproducibility of commercial sources of this antibody are poor and therefore not suitable in the diagnostic setting.[41]

Other commonly expressed but nonspecific markers include CD34, nestin, Bcl2, and h-caldesmon. Smooth muscle actin (SMA) is expressed in a minority of cases (30%–40%), while S100 immunoreactivity is rare (5%–10%).[1,4,42-46] GISTs may occasionally show immunoreactivity for CK18 (4%–8%)[25,47] and to a lesser extent CK8,[15] but are nonreactive for AE1/AE3.[48,49] Expression of desmin is uncommon (<2%) and usually encountered in gastric epithelioid GISTs where expression is focal. Desmin may also be expressed following treatment with imatinib.[35] While interpretation of CD117 immunoreactivity is usually straightforward, significant challenges may arise particularly in small biopsy specimens. These challenges are outlined below together with practical measures to overcome them.

False-positive immunoreactivity. Overdiagnosis of GIST through misinterpretation of CD117 immunohistochemistry is more frequent than underdiagnosis due to failure to perform or correctly interpret CD117 immunohistochemistry. False-positive immunoreactivity is largely related to technical factors such as antibody dilutions, particular sources of commercial antibodies, and overvigorous antigen retrieval techniques, in particular heat-induced epitope retrieval (HIER).[1,42,50-52] A prime example is the early report of CD117 immunoreactivity (antibody source and dilution related) in desmoid tumors,[53] which under optimum technical conditions are CD117-negative tumors.

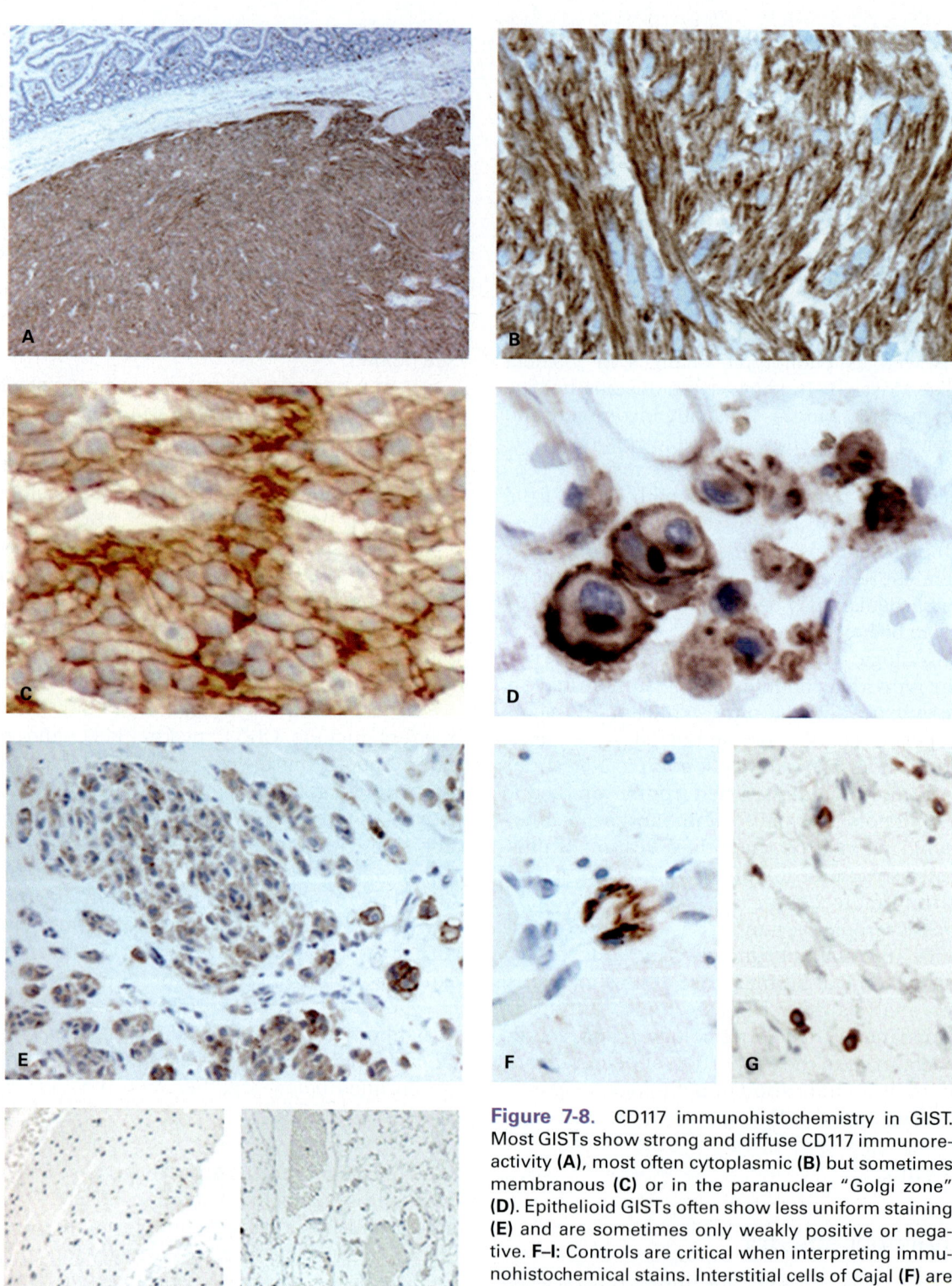

Figure 7-8. CD117 immunohistochemistry in GIST. Most GISTs show strong and diffuse CD117 immunoreactivity (A), most often cytoplasmic (B) but sometimes membranous (C) or in the paranuclear "Golgi zone" (D). Epithelioid GISTs often show less uniform staining (E) and are sometimes only weakly positive or negative. F–I: Controls are critical when interpreting immunohistochemical stains. Interstitial cells of Cajal (F) are good controls but mast cells less good as they are so immunoreactive and mast cells (G) serve as good positive controls, while smooth muscle (H) and fibroblasts (I) serve as negative controls. These are generally present in blocks containing muscularis propria.

The use of HIER in CD117 immunohistochemistry is controversial and conflicting recommendations have been made regarding its use.[3,10,54] Irrespective of the method used, careful attention to positive controls (particularly ICC but also mast cells) and negative controls (especially smooth muscle and fibroblasts) is critical when establishing immunohistochemistry protocols (Fig. 7-8F–I). For this purpose, we select blocks, wherever possible, that include muscularis propria and myenteric plexus and titrate out until any smooth muscle or fibroblast immunoreactivity has been quenched.

In practice, false-positive immunoreactivity is rarely a problem with resected tumors, where blocks containing in-built controls can be selected. The greatest difficulties arise with limited biopsy specimens, usually from metastatic sites. Here, the pattern of CD117 staining within cells, the distribution of staining in the biopsy, and profile of other markers (e.g., DOG1) need to be taken into account. Non-GISTs rarely show either membranous staining or paranuclear membrane accentuation. Rather, the staining is typically cytoplasmic and granular and usually focal and weak. If present, the staining of control material (usually mast cells) is much stronger. Nonspecific staining toward the edge of the biopsy specimen (fringe artifact) should be ignored and not interpreted as focal positive staining.[55] Other factors that weigh into the interpretation include tumor location, morphology, and the results of other immunostains (see above). If doubt regarding CD117 immunoreactivity persists, referral to a center with special expertise and/or mutational analyses and/or rebiopsy may help to resolve the diagnosis.[20,55,56]

CD117-negative GISTs. A small subset of tumors (approximately 5%) qualify as GISTs by all other criteria (including demographics, clinical presentation, anatomic location, morphology and immunohistochemical profile) but are negative for CD117 on immunohistochemistry. Lack of immunoreactivity may be due to technical factors (suboptimal fixation, excessive heat during section drying, or very prolonged storage of slides), sampling error (small biopsies from GISTs with only focal CD117 overexpression), loss of KIT overexpression following clonal evolution (e.g., after imatinib therapy), or genuine lack of CD117 overexpression.[56] Up to 50% of CD117-negative GISTs are immunoreactive for DOG1. A study of 1,040 GIST cases found only 2.6% of GISTs to be both CD117 and DOG1 negative. The true figure is likely to be even lower since two-thirds of CD117/DOG1– GIST that were tested for *KIT* and *PDGFRA* mutations were negative, challenging the original diagnosis. Two other studies have reported CD117–/DOG1– cases to comprise 0.9% and 1.6% of all GISTs.[57,58]

Up to 90% of CD117-negative tumors have mutations in either *PDGFRA* (35%–80%) or *KIT* (15%–20%).[4,12,59-61] Mutational analysis is therefore advocated where feasible in all CD117 tumors that otherwise have the typical features of GISTs.[4,61] Turnaround time for this has improved dramatically beyond the point where it was easier to determine clinical response to imatinib than to wait for mutational analysis reports in overtly malignant tumors.

CD117- and DOG1-Positive Tumors Other Than GISTs

A number of tumors other than GISTs can express CD117 (Table 7-2). Fortunately, most do not overlap morphologically with GISTs.[52] Those may include melanoma,[62] angiosarcoma,[63] endometrial stromal sarcoma,[64] PEComa,[65] and Kaposi's sarcoma.[63] A small percentage (2%–4%) of colorectal adenocarcinomas may overexpress CD117[66-68]. The figure of CD117 positivity is higher (10%–15%) for non–small cell carcinomas of the lung.[69] As melanoma can occur as both primary and polypoid metastases throughout the GI tract, this is the main issue with CD117 immunoreactive tumors. At least one melanoma marker (e.g., S100) should always be in a panel, and any immunoreactivity should lead to staining for additional markers, for example, HMB-45, MART-1, or tyrosinase.

Table 7-2	Potential GIST Mimics that May Express CD117 and/or DOG1
CD117	
Angiosarcoma	
De-differentiated liposarcoma	
Ewing's sarcoma	
Endometrial stromal sarcoma	
Kaposi's sarcoma	
Melanoma	
PEComa	
Phyllodes tumor	
Seminoma/dysgerminoma	
Spindle cell carcinoma	
Synovial sarcoma	
DOG1	
Angiosarcoma	
Ewing's sarcoma	
Glomus tumor	
Peritoneal leiomyomatosis	
Synovial sarcoma	
Uterine-type retroperitoneal leiomyoma	
Melanoma	
CD117 and DOG1	
Angiosarcoma	
Ewing's sarcoma	
Synovial sarcoma	
Melanoma	

Potential histologic mimics of GIST that may express DOG1 include Ewing's sarcoma, glomus tumor, synovial sarcoma, angiosarcoma, leiomyosarcoma, peritoneal leiomyomatosis, uterine-type retroperitoneal leiomyoma, and desmoplastic melanoma. To date, there are only four GIST mimics that can express both CD117 and DOG1 (namely angiosarcoma, synovial sarcoma, Ewing's sarcoma, and melanoma). In all four tumors, staining is focal with at least one of the markers. Thus, GIST remains the only mesenchymal neoplasm that can show diffuse immunoreactivity for both markers.[32] Therefore, in a morphologically typical GIST that shows diffuse immunoreactivity for CD117 and DOG1, no further immunohistochemical stains should be necessary.

Molecular Features and Mutational Analysis

Approximately, 80% of GISTs have mutations in *KIT*, while about 5% to 7% have *PDGFRA* mutations; *KIT* and *PDGFRA* mutations are mutually exclusive. *KIT* mutations lead to constitutive upregulation of the protein tyrosine kinase, through ligand independent dimerization.[15,70,71] Most *KIT* mutations occur in exon 11 (60%–70%), followed by exon 9 (10%–15%; almost exclusively small intestinal GIST), exon 13 (1%–4%), and exon 17 (<1%).[4,42,72] Very rarely, mutations have been identified in exons 8, 12, 14, and 18 in primary GIST.[73,74] Exon 11 and 9 mutations cause dysregulation through alterations of the juxtamembrane autoinhibitory region of c-kit, while exon 13 and 17 mutations activate c-kit's enzyme pocket directly. *PDGFRA* mutations are strongly associated with gastric location and epithelioid phenotype.[2,3,59,60,75,76] The most common is the D842V point mutation on occurring on exon 18, which comprises over 80% *PDGFRA* mutations.[73]

The nature and site of *KIT* and *PDGFRA* mutations predict response to imatinib mesylate. *KIT* mutations involving exon 11 are associated with a far better response to imatinib mesylate therapy than those involving exon 9.[42] The *PDGFRA* exon 18 mutation (D842V) is associated with a poor response to imatinib, while GISTs with other *PDGFRA* mutations are potentially imatinib sensitive.[61,73,75] GISTs lacking either *KIT* or *PDGFRA* are poorly responsive.[42] The occasional presence of *KIT* mutations in melanoma[77] may represent a potential diagnostic pitfall. *KIT* mutations may also be found in seminomas and systemic mastocytosis, they fortunately do not occur in tumors overlapping morphologically with GIST. Mutational studies performed on frozen tumor provide the best diagnostic yield. Although reasonable yields may also be obtained from DNA extracted from paraffin sections, this diminishes considerably with old archival material.[71] Areas of the slide containing tumor should be selected (using microdissection if necessary) to ensure a high proportion of tumor cells in the sample. Failure to do so may result in a false-negative result due to a high background of wild-type DNA.

Mutational analysis has considerable utility in a number of situations. It is particularly useful in the workup of suspected GISTs that are CD117 negative, since the vast majority have mutations in either *KIT* or *PDGFRA* genes.[4,42,61] It may also be helpful in predicting response to imatinib (see above) and determining the optimal dose of therapy. For example, *KIT* exon 9 mutations are associated with a significantly longer disease-free survival when GISTs are treated with high-dose imatinib compared to standard dosages; such benefits are not observed in GISTs with other mutations.[78] Mutational status may also predict response to the second-line agent sunitinib as those harboring *KIT* exon 9 mutations appear to be more sensitive to this agent than those harboring exon 11 mutations. The clinical benefit of sunitinib in wild-type cases has also been reported.[71] The type of mutation may also have prognostic implications. For example, gastric GISTs with *missense* mutations in exon 11 seem to have a better prognosis than those with exon 11 *deletions* (no such association is found for small intestinal GISTs). Earlier reports of an unfavorable outcome for exon 9 mutations seem to be related to the poorer prognosis in small intestinal GISTs where these mutations are markedly overrepresented. At present, there are insufficient data for incorporation of mutational status into risk stratification schemes.[15,71] Mutational analysis facilitates the diagnosis of familial GIST syndromes associated with germline mutations in *KIT* or *PDGFRA*. Here, both tumor and surrounding nontumorous tissue exhibit the same mutation. The demonstration of wild-type *KIT* and *PDGFRA* may provide indirect support for the diagnosis of neurofibromatosis 1 (NF1) or Carney's-associated GISTs in the right clinical setting (see below). Mutational studies can demonstrate secondary *KIT* mutations associated with the onset of secondary resistance to imatinib. Finally, mutational analysis can distinguish multiple sporadic GISTs (showing distinct *KIT* mutations in different tumors) from metastases or multiple familial GIST, which share a common mutation (see Sporadic multiple GIST below).

There are differing views as to whether mutational analysis should be a part of the routine diagnostic workup of all GISTs.[41] Most would argue that this is not justified at present and should be reserved for specific situations such as those outlined above, or when contemplating neoadjuvant therapy in unresectable tumors. However, mutational studies should continue to be performed in the research setting particularly in studies evaluating new therapies.

Succinyl dehydrogenase subunit B (SDHB) expression, NF1 mutations, and BRAF mutations. Of the 10% to 15% of GISTs that are wild type for *KIT* or *PDGFRA*, a proportion will show other molecular abnormalities, including loss of succinyl dehydrogenase subunit B (SDHB) expression, NF1 mutations, and occasionally BRAF mutations (the latter reported in 7%–11% of wild-type GIST).[32,79-82] Mutations in any one of the SDH subunits A to D can result in loss of immunohistochemical expression of SDHB.[83]

SDHB-deficient GISTs. SDHB-deficient GISTs have distinctive clinicopathologic features. They are seen almost exclusively in children or young adults, have a female predominance, have a gastric location, are frequently multicentric and/or multinodular (often with a plexiform growth pattern), have epithelioid morphology, and frequently display lymphovascular invasion (Fig. 7-9F,G). Despite a high frequency of liver and lymph node metastasis, survival is disproportionately long compared to unselected metastatic GISTs, and clinical behavior is *not* predicted by size and mitotic rate.[81,83,84] SDHB-deficient GISTs are resistant to imatinib but may show a greater sensitivity to the second-line agent sunitinib than do *KIT*- and *PDGFRA*-mutated GISTs.[81]

Four clinical subgroups are strongly associated with SDHB-deficient GISTs, namely Carney's triad, Carney-Stratakis syndrome, pediatric GIST (see below), and a proportion of sporadic GIST in young adults. In an unselected series of 746 gastric GISTs, 7.5% were found to be SDHB deficient.[81] SDHB-deficient GISTs have been shown to overexpress insulin-like growth factor receptor 1 (IGFR1).[84] Thus, it could be argued that GISTs with classical clinicopathologic features and an SDHB–/IGFR1+ immunoprofile do not require the more costly *KIT* and *PDGFRA* mutational analysis.

Chromosomal alterations. While *KIT* and *PDGFA* mutations are the earliest genetic changes in most GISTs, chromosomal losses (and gains) accumulate with progression to more aggressive phenotypes. Most low/very low malignant potential GISTs have a normal karyotype or loss of 14q (the latter occurs in 2/3 of GISTs overall). Intermediate malignant potential GISTs may show further loss of 22q (present in 1/2 of GISTs overall) and/or loss of 1p. Overtly malignant GISTs usually show further chromosomal loss (such as 9p, 11p, 13, 15, or 18) or gains (such as 5p, 8q, 17q, or 20q). Of interest, chromosome 9p21 contains the tumor suppressor gene *CDKN2A*, which encodes the cell cycle inhibitors p16^{INK4A} and p14^{ARF}. Immunohistochemical and comparative genomic hybridization studies have shown p16 loss in GIST to be associated with a poor prognosis.[70,71,85]

Predicting Behavior

The presence of histologically confirmed metastases clearly indicates a malignant tumor. It is good practice to histologically confirm the nature of suspected metastases found at surgery by biopsy; rarely these prove to be from a different tumor that demands different therapy. Such "metastases" may occasionally prove to be unrelated benign lesions (e.g., focal nodular hyperplasia in the liver, granulomata, or Von-Meyenburg complexes). Biopsy eliminates such uncertainties. Stromal tumors are also lethal by virtue of their local recurrence and invasion of other organs. Incomplete resection clearly indicates an increased likelihood of local recurrence even in the absence of metastases.[23] Tumor rupture at presentation or at surgery is independently associated with a poor outcome; fortunately, this complication occurs in <5% of patients.[86,87]

A variety of prognostic factors have been evaluated in localized, surgically resectable GIST. These including tumor size, mitotic rate, site, tumor rupture, serosal involvement, mucosal ulceration, histologic type or pattern, lamina propria infiltration, coagulative necrosis, cellularity, degree of atypia, Ki67/MIB-1 index, p53, p16, ploidy, and others. Of these, tumor size and mitotic rate have consistently emerged as important independent prognostic factors. The significance of other factors has been difficult to ascertain due to small cohort size, selection bias, and association with other high-risk factors.[87] The NIH consensus classification system—based on a GIST workshop in 2001—stratified risk of aggressive behavior on the basis of size and mitotic rate (Table 7-3).[88] This system was based on consensus opinion rather than distinct data sets but accumulating evidence has confirmed its prognostic utility. Two very large studies from the

Table 7-3	The NIH 2001 Consensus Classification Scheme for Risk Stratification in GIST	
RISK OF AGGRESSIVE BEHAVIOR	SIZE (cm)	MITOTIC COUNT (/50 hpf)
Very low	<2	<5
Low	2–5	<5
Intermediate	<5	6–10
	5–10	<5
High	>5	>5
	>10	Any
	Any	>10

Reference: 88.

AFIP including 1,765 gastric GISTs (1,074 with full long-term follow-up data; 48% alive and disease free at a median of 14.1 years) and 906 small intestinal GISTs (629 with full long-term follow-up data; 34% alive and disease free at median of 15.5 years) have shown tumor site to be an important independent predictor of prognosis,[2,3] confirming the findings of previous smaller studies.[89-91]

Failure to account for site may result in significant overestimation of the risk of aggressive behavior in gastric GIST using the NIH 2001 risk stratification scheme. For example, while NIH scheme would place gastric GISTs >10 cm in size and with <5 mitoses/HPF into the high risk category, the AFIP study found that only 11% of these patients died of their GISTs during long-term follow-up. Other adverse prognostic features in the AFIP series included coagulative necrosis, mucosal invasion, and ulceration (gastric and small intestinal GISTs); proximal location in stomach versus antrum and exon 11 deletions versus point mutations (gastric GISTs); and diffuse cytologic atypia and epithelioid cytology (small intestinal GISTs). The authors have proposed a new set of guidelines with separate criteria for gastric and small intestinal GISTs (modified in Table 7-4). The currently available data on GISTs at uncommon sites such as esophagus, colon, and rectum, although limited, suggest that these should be stratified similar to small intestinal GISTs.[15] Proliferation markers might be useful in assessing the proliferative rate but have not proved superior to mitotic rate in predicting aggressive behavior. As noted earlier, the behavior of SDHB-deficient GIST (which are exclusively gastric) is *not* predicted by size and mitotic rate.

Mitotic rate counting may be subject to number of influences including interobserver variability, specimen fixation, section thickness, size of fields examined, variation in tumor cellularity and tumor cell size, and fastidiousness of the pathologist, all of which may affect reproducibility. If modern wide-field eyepieces are used, the mitotic rate should be adjusted to correspond to the same total area examined in the largest (AFIP) studies on which prognostic data are based (i.e., 5 mm²). Counts should be performed in the most mitotically active area and should proceed until either 50 fields are viewed or 100 mitoses have been counted.[2,3] Tissue should be adequately fixed and sections should not exceed 4 to 5 μm in thickness. Care should be taken not to count pyknotic nuclei or nuclear debris as mitotic figures. Two studies have stratified GISTs into high- and low-risk groups based on gene expression profiles and chromosome complexity, both outperforming the AFIP grading system.[92,93] It is therefore possible that morphology-based risk stratification schemes might ultimately be replaced by risk stratification based on a molecular profiling.

GIST Syndromes

Four GIST syndromes have been described: (1) familial GIST syndrome, (2) neurofibromatosis type 1 (von Recklinghausen's disease), (3) Carney's triad, and (4) GIST paraganglioma syndrome (Table 7-5).

Familial GIST syndrome. Familial GIST syndrome, associated with germline mutations in *KIT*[94-100] or *PDGFRA*[101] genes, is extremely rare with at least 25 kindreds reported.[102,103] Those affected have several family members who develop multiple primary

Table 7-4 Risk Stratification Scheme Based on Long-term Follow-up Data from >1,600 Patients from the Armed Forces Institute of Pathology Prior to the Era of Imatinib Therapy

RISK CATEGORY	SIZE (CM)	MITOTIC RATE (/5 mm²)*	SITE	RISK OF PROGRESSIVE DISEASE OR MORTALITY (%)
Probably benign	≤2	≤5	Any	0
Low	>2 but ≤5	≤5	Any	1.9 (stomach), 4.3 (small intestine)
	>5 but ≤10	≤5	Stomach	3.6
Intermediate	>5 but ≤10	≤5	Small intestine	24
	>10	≤5	Stomach	12
	>2 but ≤5	>5	Stomach	16
High	>10	≤5	Small intestine	52
	>2 but ≤5	>5	Small intestine	73
	>5 but ≤10	>5	Any	55 (stomach), 85 (small intestine)
	>10	>5	Any	86 (stomach), 90 (small intestine)
	Any[a]	Any[a]	Tumor rupture[a]	>80[a]

Note: Rare tumors ≤2 cm in size and with >5 mitoses/5 mm² cannot be assigned a risk category due to the paucity of cases in these categories.
Modified from references: 2,3,15
*5 mm² is equivalent to 50 HPF in the original AFIP studies, but in many microscopes is 17–20 HPF so calibration is required.
[a]Inclusion of tumor rupture in the high-risk category is based on the findings of Takahashi et al.[86]

Table 7-5 Molecular Classification of Gastrointestinal Stromal Tumors

GIST TYPE	COMMENTS
KIT or PDGFRA MUTATED (85%–90%)	
SPORADIC	
KIT mutation	
Exon 11 (60%–70%)	85% respond to imatinib
Exon 9 (10%–15%)	45% respond to imatinib; better at a higher dose
Exon 11 (1%–4%)	Some respond to imatinib (few cases)
Exon 17 (<1%)	Some respond to imatinib (few cases)
Exons 8 and 14 (<0.5%)	
PDGFRA mutation	
Exon 18 (4%–5%)	Poor response to imatinib
Exons 12 and 14 (1%)	Some respond to imatinib (few cases)
SYNDROMIC	
Familial GIST syndrome (n = 24)[a]	
Exon 11 (n = 16)	Skin pigmentation, variable mastocytosis, and dysphagia
Exon 13 (n = 3)	No mastocytosis or dysphagia; variable skin hyperpigmentation (mostly absent)
Exon 17 (n = 4)	Variable dysphagia
Exon 8 (n = 1)	Mastocytosis and dysphagia
PDGFRA mutation (n = 3)[a]	
Exon 18 (n = 1)	Large hands
Exon 12 (n = 2)	V561D: Multiple fibrous polyps and lipomas; Y555C: Multicentric intestinal (CD117–)
WILD-TYPE KIT/PDGFRA (10%–15%)	
SPORADIC	
SDHB deficient	Include almost all pediatric GISTs and some GIST in young adults; imatinib resistant
BRAF mutation (V600E)	7%–13% of wild-type GIST; possible predilection for small bowel
SYNDROMIC	
Neurofibromatosis 1	Multicentric, predilection for jejunum, usually low malignant potential
Carney's triad	Multicentric, gastric epithelioid GIST, paraganglioma, and pulmonary chondroma
Carney-Stratakis syndrome	GIST and paraganglioma. Germline mutation in succinyl dehydrogenase subunit genes SDHB, SDHC, and SDHD; endocrinopathy

References: 42, 74, 79, 80, 81, 101, 103, 106.
[a]At time of going to press.

GISTs at early age (on average two decades earlier than sporadic GISTs) (Fig. 7-9A–E). GISTs typically develop in a background of diffuse ICC hyperplasia. Depending on the mutation involved, patients may develop a variety of cutaneous lesions (including hyperpigmentation of per oral, axillary, perineal regions and hands, lentigines, café au lait macules, benign nevi, urticaria pigmentosa, and melanoma), hematologic malignancies, or dysphagia (presumably due to dysmotility associated with ICC hyperplasia) (Table 7-5). There is an autosomal dominant pattern of inheritance.[42,94-101] In this setting, multiple primary GISTs are distinguished from metastases on the basis of their small size, lack of mitotic activity, and uneventful follow-up (unless associated with a concurrent malignant tumor).[2]

Neurofibromatosis type 1 (von Recklinghausen's disease). Patients with NF1 are at increased risk of the development of GISTs. A Swedish study found the incidence of clinically apparent GISTs to be approximately 7% in NF1 patients and 33% in an autopsy series.[104] NF1 is overrepresented by 50- to 150-fold among patients with GISTs.[10,105,106] GISTs associated with NF1 are frequently multicentric (60%) and often accompanied by ICC hyperplasia. The vast majority occurs in the small intestine (usually jejunum) with the stomach infrequently involved.[105-108] On average, NF1-associated GISTs present approximately 10 years earlier than sporadic GISTs.[106] Most GISTs occurring in the setting of NF1 have low-grade morphology, low mitotic rates, abundant skenoid fibers, and a good clinical outcome,[4,105,106,109] but a minority may show more aggressive behavior.[106,108] Despite CD117 overexpression, almost all lack *KIT* or *PDGFRA* mutations.[105-107] NF1-associated GISTs show diffuse S100 immunoreactivity in up to 40% to 60% of cases.[106,109] Occasionally, GISTs may be the first presentation in clinically unrecognized NF1.[110] The pathologist should be alert to this possibility when confronted with multiple GIST, ICC hyperplasia, strong S100 immunoreactivity, and absence of *KIT* or *PDGFRA* mutations.

Carney's triad. Carney's triad is a tumor syndrome characterized by multicentric, functioning extraintestinal paraganglioma, pulmonary chondroma, and

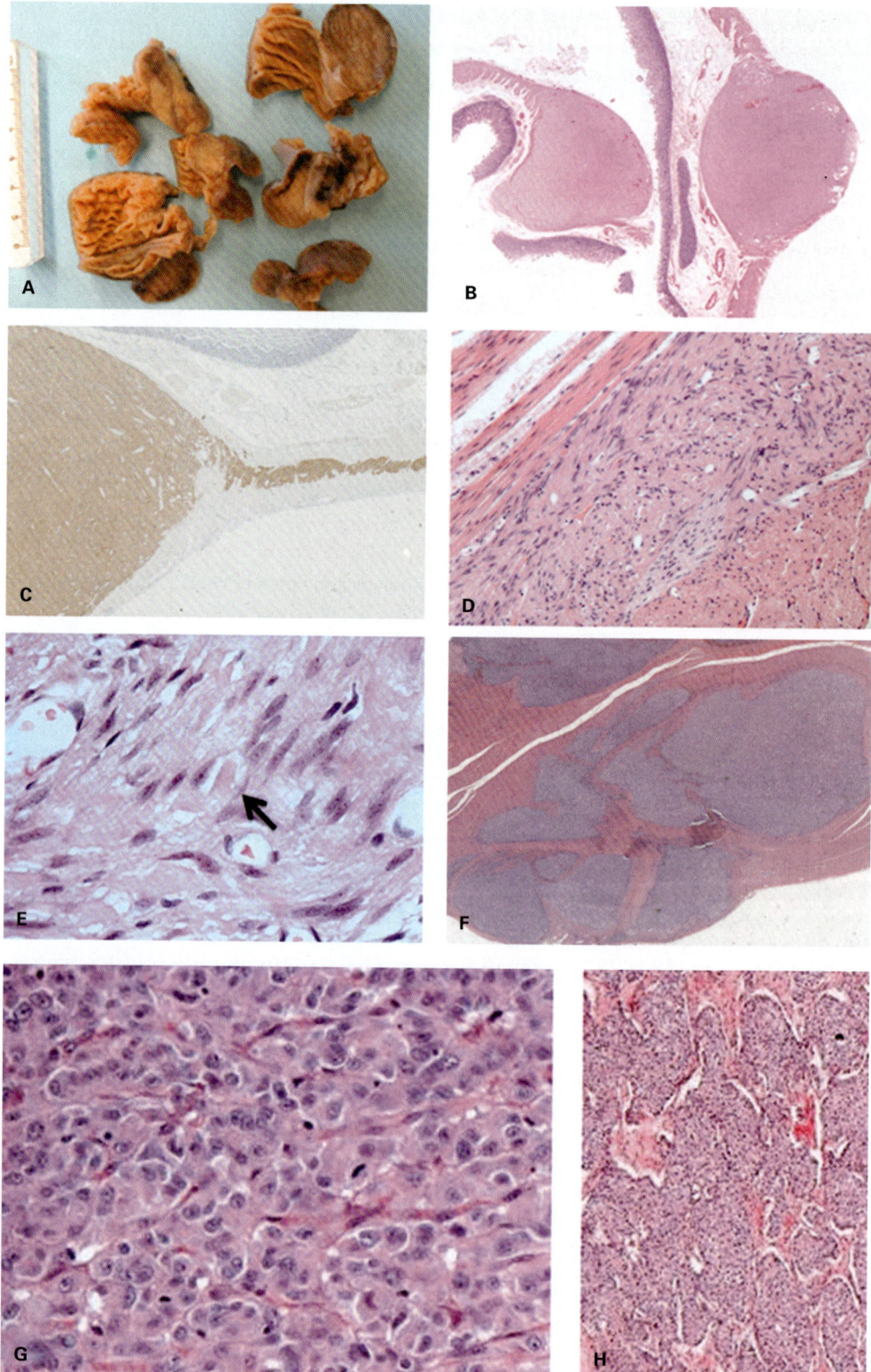

Figure 7-9. GIST syndromes. **A–E:** A 33-year-old female with multiple GISTs associated with a germline, exon 13 *KIT* mutation. **A:** The gross specimen received in consultation was fragmented due to prior sampling but several GISTs can still be appreciated. **B:** Scanning view of two of the GISTs centered in the muscularis propria. **C:** CD117 immunohistochemistry highlights massive ICC hyperplasia adjacent to a GIST. ICC hyperplasia is characteristic of germline *KIT/PDGFRA* mutations but can also be seen in NF1. ICC hyperplasia is readily appreciated on H&E **(D)** shows an identical morphologic appearance to the adjacent GIST, complete with skenoid fibers (**E**, *arrow*). **F,G:** Gastric epithelioid GIST associated with wild type *KIT/PDGFRA* in a 22-year-old female patient. The young age, female gender, gastric location, multinodular and plexiform growth pattern, and epithelioid morphology are highly suggestive of a succinyl dehydrogenase subunit B (SDHB)-deficient GIST. Such GISTs may be associated with Carney's triad or GIST–paraganglioma syndrome. No history of prior paraganglioma **(H)** or

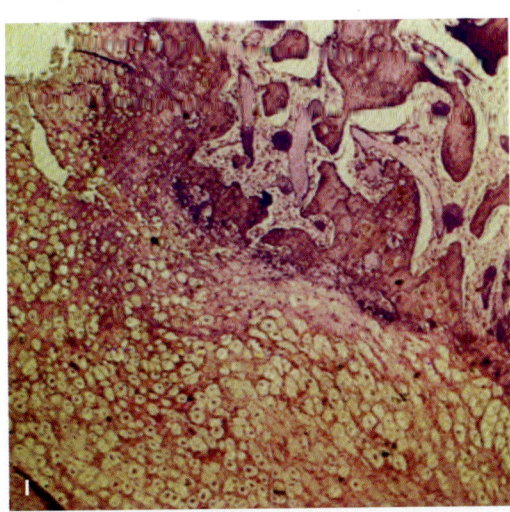

Figure 7-9. (*Continued*) pulmonary chondroma (**I**) was forthcoming, but GISTs may be the initial presentation in such patients.

gastric epitheliod GIST (Fig. 7-9F–I). Gastric GIST may precede the other tumors by several years. About 80 cases have been reported in the literature to date.[111–113] Most are sporadic. Distinctive clinicopathologic features include a striking female predominance (>85% of cases), young age at presentation (>80% of patients <30 years), frequent multifocality, consistent epithelioid morphology, and a relatively indolent course despite a high rate of local recurrence and metastases (41% and 55% respectively).[111,112] These GISTs also lack *KIT/PDGFRA* mutations as well as the nonrandom loss of 14q and 22q, characteristic of sporadic GIST. The response to imatinib in this setting is generally considered to be poor.[114]

GIST-paraganglioma syndrome (Carney–Stratakis syndrome). This novel familial GIST syndrome (involving 12 patients from 7 families) overlaps with Carney's triad in that patients develop both paragangliomas and GISTs at a young age.[115,116] However, it differs from Carney's triad in that there is an equal sex predilection, an absence of pulmonary chondromas, and an autosomal dominant pattern of inheritance with incomplete penetrance.[115] The majority of patients with this syndrome have germline loss-of-function mutations in the succinyl dehydrogenase subunit genes *SDHB*, *SDHC*, and *SDHD*,[116] leading to loss of SDHB expression and overexpression of IGF1R.

Sporadic multiple GIST. Multiple primary GISTs were thought to occur only in the clinical syndromes described above. However, a total of 21 patients with multiple primary sporadic GISTs (with differing *KIT* or *PDGFRA* mutations in each lesion) have been described in four studies.[117–120] In 19 patients, the tumors arose in the same organ (16 stomach, 3 small intestine), while in 2 cases they involved different organs (stomach and small intestine, small intestine and peritoneum). Most were situated within 3 cm of one another. The mean age at presentation was 72.4 years. In about half of the cases, at least one of the lesions was under 1 cm in size. However, in one study five patients had two separate lesions >1.5 cm size (mean of 4.3 cm).[118] Sporadic multiple GISTs differ from those associated with GIST syndromes in that patients are older, have fewer GISTs (usually 2–3), lack ICC hyperplasia, often have smaller tumors, show a predilection for the proximal stomach (versus small bowel for familial and NF1-associated GISTs), are usually closely approximated (<3 cm), and show different *KIT* or *PDGFRA* mutations in each tumor. The existence of multiple sporadic GISTs has important clinical implications. Patients presenting with multiple GISTs in the absence of clinicopathologic features of GIST syndromes may be misdiagnosed as having metastatic disease (as occurred in 2/6 patients in one study) and treated with imatinib.[118] Molecular testing of each tumor is therefore recommended in this setting.

Pediatric GIST. Very occasionally, GISTs may present in children or young adults. Pediatric GISTs display a number of characteristic clinicopathologic features including a striking female predominance, a predominantly gastric location, a strong tendency for multifocality, a frequent epithelioid morphology, and high rate of local recurrence and lymph node metastasis.[81,121–123] Almost all reported pediatric GISTs so far are negative for *KIT* or *PDGFRA* mutations,[122–124] although an isolated case with a novel exon 9 *KIT* mutation was reported.[124]

Small GIST. Small, clinically silent GISTs are being detected with increasing frequency,[125] raising questions as to their clinical significance and management. Several studies suggest a high prevalence in the general population. Agaimy et al. detected small GIST in 22.5% of 98 consecutive autopsy cases by gross examination (this included only grossly recognizable lesions).[126] Kawanowa et al. detected microscopic GIST in 35 out of 100 gastrectomies (performed for unrelated tumors) when sectioned at 5 mm intervals.[127] Two studies of esophagogastrectomy specimens found microscopic GIST or minute lesions (≤1 mm) termed "ICC hyperplasia" in approximately 10% of patients[128,129]; good criteria for separating focal ICC hyperplasia and microscopic GIST do not exist. Small GISTs show a predilection for the proximal stomach and gastroesophageal junction. Most are solitary but up to 30% may be multiple. Reported cases have ranged from GISTs range from 0.2 mm in size to up to 10 mm. The lesions frequently show hyalinization and calcification leading to the suggestion that many may regress/involute.[126] The reported rates of *KIT* and *PDGFRA* mutations vary but they occur in up to 85% of GISTs ≤10 mm in size.[130] Variable terminology has been applied to these lesions (microscopic GIST, minimal GIST, minute GISTs, GIST tumorlets, ICC hyperplasia, etc.), and there is no consensus on terminology. The simplest approach might be to regard all GIST-like lesions ≤10 mm in size as "small, incidental GIST" given their uniformly indolent behavior. The vast majority either involute or remain asymptomatic. A small minority may accrue additional genetic alterations and evolve into clinically significant GIST.

Differential Diagnosis

In our experience, overdiagnosis of GIST is more frequent an occurrence than underdiagnosis. This is likely due to the increased awareness of GIST that has followed the advent of targeted therapy. The differential diagnosis is best considered in the context of six broad morphologic patterns of GIST (Table 7-6). The majority of lesions entering the differential diagnosis fall into the "spindled, cytologically bland" category with desmoid tumor, leiomyomas, schwannoma, and IFP, the most frequent mimics. Salient anatomical, morphologic, and immunohistochemical features separating these lesions are summarized in Table 7-7.

Table 7-6 Differential Diagnosis Based on Morphologic Subgroup

SPINDLED BLAND	SPINDLED MALIGNANT	EPITHELIOID BLAND	EPITHELIOID MALIGNANT	MIXED SPINDLED AND EPITHELIOID (OR BIPHASIC)	PLEOMORPHIC
Fibromatosis	Spindle cell carcinoma	Glomus tumor	Melanoma	Melanoma	Melanoma
Leiomyoma	Melanoma	Neuroendocrine tumor	Carcinoma	Carcinoma	Carcinoma
Inflammatory fibroid polyp	Leiomyosarcoma	Benign epithelial peripheral nerve sheath tumor	Epithelioid leiomyosarcoma	Clear cell sarcoma	Leiomyosarcoma
Schwannoma	Malignant peripheral nerve sheath tumor	Paraganglioma	Epithelioid angiosarcoma	PEComa	Pleomorphic undifferentiated sarcoma (malignant fibrous histiocytoma)
Inflammatory myofibroblastic tumor	Synovial sarcoma	Mesothelioma	Neuroendocrine tumor (poorly differentiated)	Gastroblastoma	Pleomorphic liposarcoma
Reactive nodular fibrous proliferation	Endometrial stromal sarcoma		Mesothelioma	Synovial sarcoma	
Solitary fibrous tumor	Clear cell sarcoma		PEComa	Follicular dendritic cell sarcoma	
Mesenteric/peritoneal fibrosing lesions	De-differentiated liposarcoma		Malignant gastrointestinal neuroectodermal tumor (GINECT)		
Perineurioma/ benign fibroblastic polyp	Malignant gastrointestinal neuroectodermal tumor (GINECT)				
Calcifying fibrous tumor	PEComa				
Plexiform fibromyxoma	Unclassified sarcoma				
	Follicular dendritic cell sarcoma				
	Angiosarcoma				
	Kaposi sarcoma				
	Mesothellioma				
	Adult granulosa cell tumor				
	Sclerosing lymphoma				

Chapter 7 Mesenchymal Tumors 311

Table 7-7 Key Anatomic, Morphologic, and Immunohistochemical Features of Lesions to Be Considered in the Differential Diagnosis of Spindled, Cytologically Bland GIST

TUMOR	SIZE MEAN (RANGE)	ANATOMICAL SITE MOST FREQUENTLY INVOLVED	LAYER OF GUT MOST FREQUENTLY INVOLVED	KEY HISTOLOGIC FEATURES	IMMUNOHISTOCHEMISTRY (MAIN FINDINGS)
GIST	5 cm (<1–35 cm)	1. Stomach (60%) 2. Small bowel (30%)	Muscularis propria	Pushing margins, moderate cellularity, fascicles/bundles, uniform nuclei, frequent pallisading, vacuolation, skenoid fibers, usually few mitoses	CD117 positive (95%) and DOG1 positive (95%)
Fibromatosis	11 cm (3–45 cm)	Mesentery (most frequent mesenteric tumor)	Serosa and muscularis propria	Infiltrative margins, low cellularity, long broad fascicles, collagenous to myxoid matrix, bland wavy nuclei, collagenous matrix, muscularized arteries, few mitoses	Nuclear β-catenin (90%), patchy SMA (most), CD34, keratin and S100 negative, CD117 and DOG1 negative
Leiomyoma	Esophagus: 5 cm (1–18 cm) Colorectum: 0.4 cm (0.1–2.2 cm)	1. Esophagus 2. Colorectum	Esophagus: Muscularis propria Rectum: Muscularis mucosae	Circumscribed, low to moderate cellularity, intersecting bundles, myoid cells, abundant eosinophilic cytoplasm, bland blunt ended nuclei, few mitoses	SMA, desmin positive CD117 and DOG1 negative
Inflammatory myofibroblastic tumor	8 cm (0.3–20 cm)	Mesentery and omentum	Muscularis propria and serosa (when involving tubular gut)	Three patterns: (1) myxoid vascular, (2) compact spindled cell and (3) hypocellular sclerotic. Spindled, fusiform or plump cells, focal atypia (50%), lymphocytes/plasma cells, few mitoses	Patchy SMA (most), ALK-1 protein (40%–60%), CD34, CD117 and DOG1 negative
Inflammatory fibroid polyp	3.5 cm (0.2–30 cm)	1. Gastric antrum 2. Small bowel	1. Gastric: Submucosa 2. Small bowel: Transmural	Often infiltrative, low cellularity, bland spindled and stellate cells, loose edematous, collagenous matrix, perivascular "onion skinning," inflammatory cells (eosinophils)	CD34 positive, focal SMA (minority positive), CD117 and DOG1 negative
Schwannoma	4.5 cm (1–12 cm)	Stomach	Muscularis propria	Circumscribed nonencapsulated, peripheral lymphoid cuff, elongated nuclei with tapered ends, variation in size and shape, infrequent pallisading, absent, mitoses rare	S100 positive, GFAP positive, CD34 minority positive, CD117 and DOG1 negative
Reactive nodular fibroblastic pseudotumor	6 cm (<1–10 cm)	Small and large bowel	Serosa (may extend transmurally)	Hypocellular, bland spindled and stellate cells in short fascicles or haphazardly, collagenous, myxoid or fibromyxoid stroma, few intralesional mononuclear cells, mitoses rare or absent	SMA (most), AE1/AE3 and CD117 conflicting data (see text)

(Continued)

Table 7-7 Key Anatomic, Morphologic, and Immunohistochemical Features of Lesions to Be Considered in the Differential Diagnosis of Spindled, Cytologically Bland GIST *(Continued)*

TUMOR	SIZE MEAN (RANGE)	ANATOMICAL SITE MOST FREQUENTLY INVOLVED	LAYER OF GUT MOST FREQUENTLY INVOLVED	KEY HISTOLOGIC FEATURES	IMMUNOHISTOCHEMISTRY (MAIN FINDINGS)
Solitary fibrous tumor	8 cm (2–20 cm)	Peritoneum, retroperitoneum	Serosa	Circumscribed (± pseudocapsule), bland oval, fusiform or spindled cells in short fascicles, whorls or patternless pattern, alternating cellularity, keloidal collagen, hemangiopericytoma-like vessels.	CD34 positive (80%–90%), SMA minority positive, CD117 and S100 negative
Perineurioma	Colorectal polyps: (0.2–0.6 mm) Mass lesions: (1.5–4.5 cm)	Colorectum Occasionally mass lesion at other sites	1. Colorectal polyps: Lamina propria 2. Mass lesions: Submucosa	Variably circumscribed, whorls, interwoven fascicles and storiform arrangements, bland, spindled cells, collagenous to myxoid stroma, tapered, wavy bland nuclei, pale cytoplasm, indistinct cell borders, infiltrate between crypts, mitoses rare or absent	EMA positive, CD34 occasionally positive, S100, keratin and CD117 negative
Calcifying fibrous tumor	(<1–10 cm)	1. Mesentery and omentum 2. Visceral	Subperitoneal (but occasionally intramural)	Circumscribed, hypocellullar, uniform, bland spindled cells, hyalinized stroma with extensive dystrophic and psammomatous calcification, patchy, perivascular lymphoplasmacytic infiltrate	Factor XIIIa positive, CD34, CD117, SMA negative
Plexiform fibromyxoma	3–15 cm (median 5.5 cm)	Gastric antrum	Centered in muscularis propria; often involves submucosa and subserosa	Characteristic plexiform growth pattern; dissects through muscularis propria; myxoid to collagenized stroma; prominent arborizing thin walled vascularity; low to focally moderate cellularity; uniform oval to spindled nuclei; mitoses rare or absent; focal pseudovascuolar lacunar spaces	SMA positive; usually desmin and caldesmon negative; CD117 and DOG1 negative

In the spindled, cytologically malignant category, the most important considerations include spindle cell carcinoma, melanoma, and sarcomas. Bland epithelioid tumors should be distinguished from glomus tumor, carcinoid, and paraganglioma, while melanoma and carcinoma should be excluded when confronted with malignant epithelioid tumors. Both may also show mixed spindled and epithelioid morphology. Pleomorphic morphology is highly unusual for GIST and should prompt consideration of alternative diagnoses including carcinoma, melanoma, or sarcoma. A variety of less common lesions also enter the differential diagnosis from time to time (Table 7-6). Demographic, anatomic, gross, morphologic, and immunohistochemical features can all provide useful clues to the diagnosis and are outlined in the text that follows. Practical approaches to the differential diagnosis of GIST have been the subject of numerous reviews.[131,132] It should be emphasized that small mesenchymal polyps confined to the mucosa and/or submucosa cannot be GISTs, as the latter originate in the muscularis propria and only involve the submucosa or mucosa by extension from a larger mural mass.

Reporting GIST

The pathologist should ensure that at a minimum, all information required to accurately prognosticate is included in the pathology report. Synoptic reports are gaining in popularity and we prefer this form of reporting for GISTs; an example of our GIST synoptic report is illustrated in Table 7-8. The minimum information necessary includes site of tumor, extent of disease (i.e., localized or invasion surrounding tissues), tumor size, resection margins, perforation or serosal involvement, and mitotic rate. Along with the diagnosis, the pathologist should convey the risk of aggressive behavior based on the above observations. Metastatic, unresectable, or locally advanced disease will by definition be associated with a high risk of aggressive behavior. In localized, surgically resected GISTs, we take into account size, mitotic rate, site, and serosal involvement (perforation) and favor risk stratification schemes that include these factors (see Table 7-4). Since more than one risk stratification scheme now exists, it is important to document which scheme has been used for risk stratification.

SMOOTH MUSCLE TUMORS

Leiomyomas

In the era of CD117 immunohistochemistry, true smooth muscle tumors of the GI tract are rare and substantially outnumbered by GISTs. Two notable exceptions include leiomyomas of the esophagus and the colorectal muscularis mucosae, which remain the most common mesenchymal tumors at their respective sites. In the esophagus, leiomyomas outnumber GISTs by two- to threefold, occur in younger patients (mean 35 years), show a mild male predominance, and have a predilection for the distal esophagus and esophagogastric junction. They are often discovered incidentally but can present with dysphagia, retrosternal or epigastric pain or bleeding. In one large series, esophageal leiomyomas ranged from 1 to 18 cm in size (mean 5 cm).[26] Clinically occult "seedling" tumors are common. In a study of 150 esophagogastrectomy specimens for gastric or esophageal carcinoma, careful examination revealed incidental esophageal leiomyomas in 47% of patients. These had a mean size of 1.7 mm (range 1–13 mm) with a mean of 3 leiomyomas per patient (range 1–13).[128] The main differential diagnosis includes a small

Table 7-8 Example of GIST Synoptic Report

Synoptic report:
Tumor location:
Maximal tumor dimension:
Perforation:
Local spread:
Resection margins:
Solitary/multifocal:
Metastatic tumor deposits (specify site):
Morphology (spindle/epithelioid/mixed/pleomorphic):
Mitotic count (per 50 HPF, per 5 mm^2):
Cellularity (low/moderate/high):
Cellular atypia (minimal/moderate/marked):
Tumor necrosis:
Invasion of lamina propria/mucosa
Serosal involvement:
Lymphovascular invasion:
ICC hyperplasia:
MIB-1 index (optional):
Additional comments:

Immunohistochemistry:
CD117:
DOG1:
Additional stains:
KIT and PDGFRA mutation analysis:

Risk stratification:
The tumor is considered _____ risk for malignant behavior based on tumor size, mitotic rate and site (and, in applicable perforation).[2,3,85,86]

Diagnosis:
Stomach, wedge resection:
– Gastrointestinal stromal tumor, CD117/DOG1 immunoreactive
– _____ risk of malignant behavior

GIST (see above). Grossly, esophageal leiomyomas generally arise from the muscularis propria and are usually well demarcated and spherical to oval shaped. Larger tumors may be elongated with sausage, dumbell or horseshoe shapes. They may form polypoid lesions, which project into the lumen. The cut surface is firm, white to gray-tan, whorled, and often lobulated resembling leiomyomas of the myometrium. Focal hemorrhage may be present. Histologically, the tumors are of low to moderate cellularity and composed of intersecting fascicles of bland spindled cells with abundant eosinophilic cytoplasm, which is often fibrillary or clumped. The nuclei are elongated, usually with blunt ended, and may be indented by a paranuclear vacuole. The arrangement of tumor cells is more haphazard than in the surrounding muscle layers with which it may merge at the periphery. Occasionally, the tumors may show epithelioid morphology. Rarely, leiomyomas may have a plexiform appearance similar to that seen in neural tumors.[26,133] Areas of hyalinization may be seen. Mitotic figures are rare or absent.[26,131,134] In the colon, leiomyomas are usually found incidentally as small polyps at screening colonoscopy or in resection specimens (Fig. 7-10A–C).[135] They arise almost exclusively from the muscularis mucosae and, because of their superficial location, are usually amenable to endoscopic removal by snare resection. Grossly, they are white, firm, circumscribed nodules. Most are < 5 mm in size but examples of up to 2.2 cm are described. Histologically, they often exhibit a storiform rather than herringbone pattern. Older tumors may be heavily collagenized (Fig. 7-10C). They typically merge with the surrounding muscularis mucosae. Some display prominent eosinophilic hyaline globules with immunohistochemical and ultrastructural features of actin and desmin filaments (Fig. 7-10B, inset). Skenoid fibers are absent.[136] Rarely, colorectal leiomyomas display marked atypia resembling that seen in symplastic uterine leiomyomas but mitotic figures are rare or absent.[135] Leiomyomas occur uncommonly in the small intestine, stomach, appendix, or intramural within the anorectum. At all sites, leiomyomas behave in a clinically benign manner with little tendency for recurrence; morbidity, if any, is related to local effects of the lesions.

The major issue with leiomyomas is to avoid misdiagnosis as other tumors, especially GIST. Leiomyomas are generally less cellular than GISTs, have plumper cells with more abundant and more eosinophilic cytoplasm, and in the case of colorectal leiomyomas, their origin from the muscularis mucosae is an important clue to their diagnosis. Leiomyomas are immunoreactive for smooth muscle markers and, more importantly, negative for CD117 and DOG1. Some apparently typical GI leiomyomas contain abundant admixed CD117+/DOG1+ ICC (or occasionally S100+ fibers) throughout the tumor (Fig. 7-10G,H). Such tumors may represent a form of nodular hyperplasia or hamartoma rather than a true leiomyoma.[32] They behave identically to leiomyomas, and the key issue here is not to misinterpret the admixed CD117+/DOG1+ cells as evidence of a GIST. In addition, care should also be taken not to interpret intralesional mast cells as focal CD117 immunoreactivity. The storiform arrangement often seen in colorectal leiomyomas may lead to confusion with a small, fibrous histiocytoma, but the merging of the tumor with the muscularis mucosae should suggest the correct diagnosis. The distinction between leiomyomas (low to moderate cellularity, mitotically inactive, and clinically benign) and leiomyosarcomas (high grade, highly cellular, mitotically active, and clinically aggressive—see below) is usually easily made. Thus, unlike GISTs, the problem of predicting the behavior of paucicellular, well-differentiated tumors is not commonly encountered.[26,27] Finally, smooth muscle pseudotumors may be created artificially if part of the muscularis propria (or the muscularis mucosae in the esophagus) is sampled in deep biopsies. These are more likely to be obtained when punch or basket rather than flat surgical biopsy forceps are used.[23]

Epstein–Barr Virus–associated Smooth Muscle Tumors

Distinctive smooth muscle tumors associated with Epstein–Barr virus (EBV) infection may arise in immunocompromised patients including those with HIV infection (predominantly children or young adults), organ transplant recipients, or children with congenital immunodeficient states.[137,138] The GI tract is one of the most common sites involved (after lung and liver). Endoscopically, these tumors often have a centrally ulcerated, nodular appearance. They are usually multiple. Histologically, they resemble typical smooth muscle tumors but show a spectrum of features, which range from paucicellular, uniform, mitotically inactive tumors resembling leiomyomas to densely cellular, pleomorphic, and mitotically active tumors resembling leiomyosarcomas. Small lesions often show a close relationship with the walls of blood vessels. Many contain foci of primitive round cells with irregular contours, which are actin positive. Such foci may be extensive and do not appear to have a prognostic significance. A minority contains a prominent T-cell infiltrate.[137] The lesional cells are immunoreactive for SMA and variably reactive for desmin, CD21 (EBV receptor), and EBV nuclear antigen 2. EBV latent membrane protein is usually negative. In situ

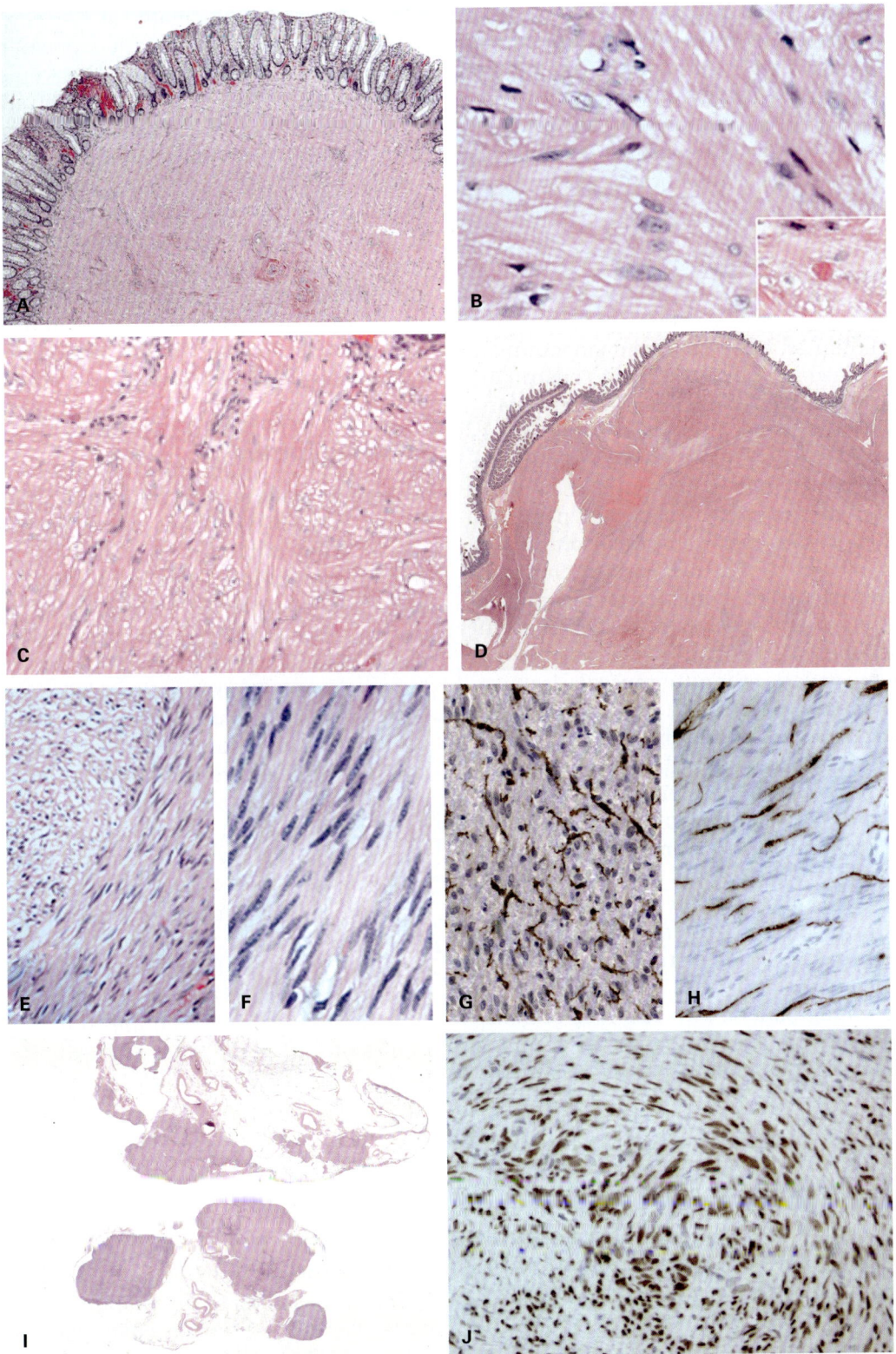

Figure 7-10. Leiomyomas. Submucosal leiomyomas of the colon (**A–C**). Note the intimate association with the muscularis mucosae, which is no longer readily identifiable. **Inset B**: Distinctive hyaline globules frequently described in these tumors. (**C**) In some tumors, a storiform pattern is readily apparent but much of the tumor consists of collagen. Leiomyoma arising in the muscularis propria of the small intestine (**D–H**) showing features typical of leiomyomas elsewhere, but with immunohistochemical evidence of admixed CD117– (and DOG1–) positive ICC (**G**), suggesting that this lesion might represent some form of nodular hyperplasia or hamartoma. Such staining should not be interpreted as evidence of a GIST. Rarely, a similar distribution of admixed S100-positive neural cells (**H**) may also be encountered. Leiomyomatosis disseminata peritonealis in a 43-year-old female (**I**). The patient had innumerable peritoneal nodules at laparotomy and was thought to have disseminated malignancy. These tumors are generally positive for both estrogen (**J**) and progesterone receptors.

hybridization for EBV early RNA (EBER) showing nuclear staining is the most helpful test to confirm the association with EBV.[138] Although many tumors would meet the criteria for leiomyosarcoma as proposed by Billings, these patients have an excellent prognosis and very few die of their disease.[137] Distinction from GISTs and true leiomyosarcomas is therefore important.

Leiomyomatosis

Esophageal leiomyomatosis is a rare condition characterized by multifocal, often confluent smooth muscle proliferations, which can form linear constricting lesions. Most patients are young (mean age 25.6 years) and present with dysphagia and achalasia-like manometric findings. Over 2/3 have Alport's syndrome. Other associations include gastroesophageal-vulvar leiomyomatosis and multiple endocrine neoplasia type 1 (MEN 1). The stomach and tracheobronchial tree may be involved.[139-141] The diagnosis is often difficult and patients may have symptoms for many years before the correct diagnosis is made. EUS is a useful diagnostic modality. Histologically, the lesions can arise from the muscularis propria or muscularis mucosae and are composed of well-differentiated smooth muscle cells arranged in fascicles, bundles, or whorls. Adjacent lesions may become confluent. Cellularity is low and cytologic atypia, and mitotic activity is absent or minimal. The vast majority of patients require esophagectomy with reconstruction due to intractable symptoms. About 5% of patients are asymptomatic and can be followed conservatively.[139] Rarely, leiomyomatosis may involve the colon or small intestine.[142] A leiomyomatosis-like lesion termed "leiomyomatosis-like lymphangiomatosis" has been described in the colon of a young patient with tuberous sclerosis and renal angiomyolipoma. Although overlapping morphologically with leiomyomatosis, it was distinguished by a component of epithelioid cells that were HMB-45 positive.[143]

Smooth Muscle Hamartoma

Smooth muscle hamartomas have rarely been reported in the setting of tuberous sclerosis. In these lesions, proliferating bundles of mature smooth muscle obliterate the lamina propria and surround crypts or glands.[144]

Leiomyomatosis Peritonealis Disseminata

This rare condition is characterized by diffuse peritoneal and omental leiomyomas (Fig. 7-10I,J). It is often detected incidentally at surgery and may be alarming to the surgeon as its appearance mimics a disseminated malignancy. Leiomyomatosis peritonealis disseminata (LPD) generally affects females of the reproductive age group with a strong relationship to endogenous or exogenous excess of female sex steroid hormones.[145-147] Histologically, the tumors are identical to conventional leiomyomas. LPD generally pursues a benign course and leiomyomas may even involute after pregnancy or removal of the source of excess estrogen; rare malignant transformation has been reported.[148] Cases of disseminated GIST[149,150] and reactive nodular fibrous pseudotumor (RNFP)[151] grossly mimicking LPD have been reported.

Glomus Tumor

Although they are primarily tumors of skin and soft tissue, over 100 GI glomus tumors have been reported to date. They occur almost exclusively in the stomach (mainly antrum)[152,153] but occasionally in the small and large intestine.[154,155] The median age is 55 with a wide range, and there is a strong female predominance. Grossly, they are usually small (median size 2 cm, range 1–7 cm), multinodular, and intramural with variable serosal or mucosal involvement and sometimes ulceration.[150] Histologically, they are composed of solid sheets of epithelioid cells with central, round uniform nuclei, delicate chromatin, clear to deeply eosinophilic cytoplasm, and distinct cell borders (Fig. 7-11). Varying numbers of dilated or hemangiopericytoma-like vessels are present.[152,153] Vascular invasion is not uncommon and does not seem to influence outcome. The mitotic rate is usually very low (<1/50 HPF) but can rarely reach 4/50 HPF. Focal hemorrhage is frequent but coagulative necrosis does not occur.[153] Glomus tumors are diffusely immunoreactive for SMA and exhibit characteristic pericellular staining for collagen IV. Focal CD34 staining is seen in up to 25% of cases. The tumor cells are negative for CD117, S100 protein, desmin, and keratin.[153] The vast majority behave in a benign manner, but rarely they can metastasize and have a fatal outcome.[152,153,156] Histology has not been reliable in predicting the malignant behavior in gastric glomus tumors. Criteria for malignancy in glomus tumors of deep soft tissue do seem to apply to gastric counterparts. The only tumor to metastasize in Miettenen's series of 32 GI glomus tumors was the largest gastric tumor (size 6.5 cm) that appeared histologically bland. It has been suggested that larger GI glomus tumors may have a low but unpredictable malignant potential. Glomus tumors should be differentiated from epithelioid GISTs (which have less rounded, more polygonal/oval tumor cells, less prominent

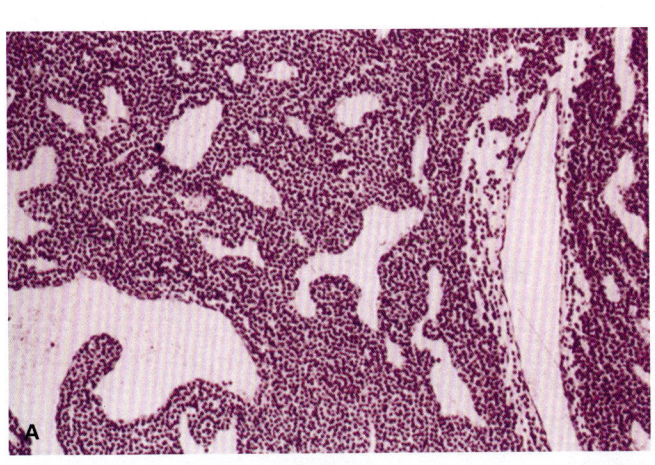
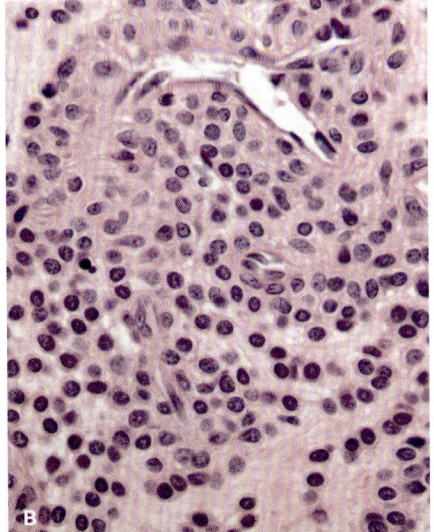
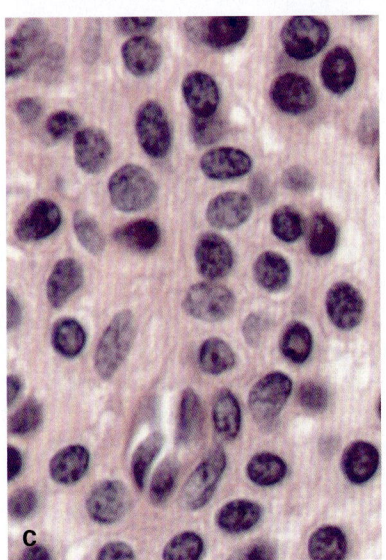
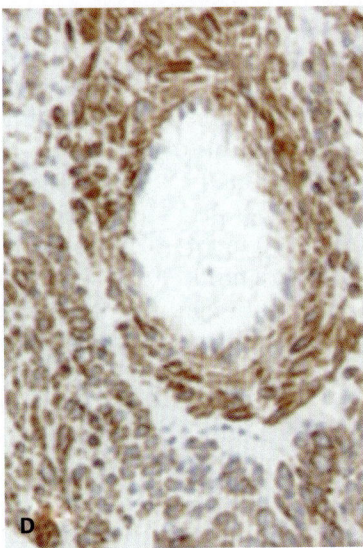

Figure 7-11. Gastric glomus tumor. **A:** Characteristic dilated vascular channels with intervening cellular tumor. **B,C:** Detail of round, uniform perivascular tumor cells with distinct cell borders. **D:** The tumor cells are immunoreactive for smooth muscle markers (in this case, caldesmon).

dilated capillaries and veins, and CD117 immunoreactivity), paraganglioma (which are chromogranin and synaptophysin positive and actin negative), carcinoid tumors (which have less defined cell borders, coarser chromatin, and neuroendocrine marker expression), hemangiopericytoma (which have oval to spindled cells with less-defined cell borders and exceptional actin immunoreactivity), and vascular leiomyoma (which have oval to spindled cells resembling mature smooth muscle).[153,157]

Leiomyosarcoma

Leiomyosarcomas of the GI tract are rare with just over 50 cases reported to date.[25–27,47,158] Infantile GI leiomyosarcomas have also been reported. The small intestine is the most frequent site followed by the colon, anorectum, esophagus, and stomach. There is a wide age range (16–80 years), but most cases present in middle or older age; gastric leiomyosarcomas appear to be the exception with the few reported cases occurring mostly in young adults. Patients may present with bleeding, abdominal pain, obstructive symptoms, or a mass lesion. Leiomyosarcomas of the small bowel are usually large, bulky tumors (average size >10 cm), while those of the colon and rectum are smaller (average size 6.3 and 3.1 cm, respectively). The predominantly polypoid growth in rectal leiomyosarcomas may explain their smaller size at presentation. Ulceration of the overlying mucosa is common.

Histologically, they usually show recognizable smooth muscle differentiation (intersecting bundles, elongated blunt ended nuclei, eosinophilic cytoplasm), focal or diffuse nuclear pleomorphism, and a high mitotic rate (Fig. 7-12). In the AFIP series, over 75%

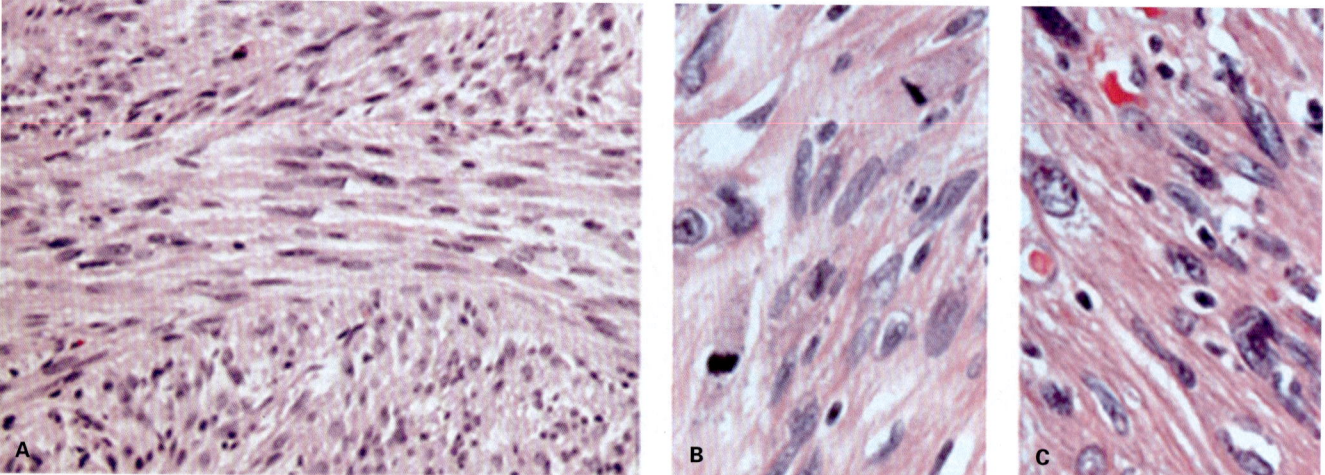

Figure 7-12. Leiomyosarcoma showing characteristic right-angled intersection of fascicles **(A)** composed of tumor cells with pleomorphic often blunt-ended nuclei and abundant eosinophilic cytoplasm **(B,C)**.

had a mitotic rate of >10/10 HPF, all recorded rates were >5/10 HPF. Only rare cases with mitotic rates of <5/10HPF have been reported elsewhere.[158] Leiomyosarcomas are immunoreactive for SMA (usually global but sometimes focal) and caldesmon, are variably immunoreactive for desmin, and are negative for CD117 and DOG1.[25-27,47,158] Leiomyosarcomas are clinically aggressive with approximately 50% of patients dying of disease during follow-up. Rectal tumors have a lower mortality rate, likely related to their smaller size at presentation.

NEUROGENIC TUMORS

Schwannoma

GI schwannomas comprise approximately 3% to 6% of GI mesenchymal tumors (Fig. 7-13). The stomach is by far the most frequent GI site, but schwannomas have also been reported in the colorectum, and rarely in the esophagus and small bowel. They occur mostly in middle-aged and elderly patients (median 60 years), with a female predominance, and have a uniformly benign clinical course.[159-163] Most are centered in the muscularis propria, but they may arise in the submucosa or serosa. The size ranges from <1 to >10 cm (median 4.5 cm). Patients may be asymptomatic or present with bleeding, abdominal pain, or both. The clinical and radiologic features are often indistinguishable from GIST. Grossly, GI schwannomas are well circumscribed, nonencapsulated tumors that may merge with surrounding smooth muscle layers.[162] Hemorrhage, necrosis, and cystic degeneration are typically absent. Histologically, gastric schwannomas are characterized by a peripheral cuff of lymphoid tissue, often with germinal centers, that is almost invariably present and a useful indicator of the diagnosis. Tumor cells are usually arranged in a so-called microtrabecular pattern with cohesive groups of tumor cells separated by a loose or collagenized stroma, but sheet-like arrangements may also be seen. Diffuse intratumoral lymphocytic infiltration, with or without plasma cells, is present in all cases (Fig. 7-13). The cellularity is usually moderate, and almost all cases show focal areas of nuclear atypia. The nuclei are elongated with tapered ends, are often wavy, and show considerable variation in size and shape. Mitoses are usually absent or infrequent, but occasionally may exceed 5/50 HPF. Although a high mitotic rate has not been associated with aggressive behavior, those with a mitotic rate >10/50 HPF should be reported with a degree of caution given the limited experience on their long term follow-up.[163]

GI schwannomas differ from their soft tissue counterparts in several respects. They are nonencapsulated, have a characteristic peripheral lymphoid cuff and typically lack the hemorrhage, cystic degeneration, pronounced pallisading (focal or vague pallisading may be present), Verocay bodies, vascular hyalinization, and xanthoma cells frequently seen in soft tissue schwannomas. Most GI schwannomas exhibit GFAP immunoreactivity, which is not a feature of their soft tissue counterparts.[159-162] Moreover, they lack the NF2 gene alterations seen in many soft tissue schwannomas. Thus, GI schwannomas may represent a distinctive group of peripheral nerve sheath tumors.[160] Schwannomas show morphologic overlap with GISTs, from which they need to be distinguished. The characteristic peripheral lymphoid cuff of schwannoma is rarely seen in GIST. Conversely, prominent pallisading is far more likely

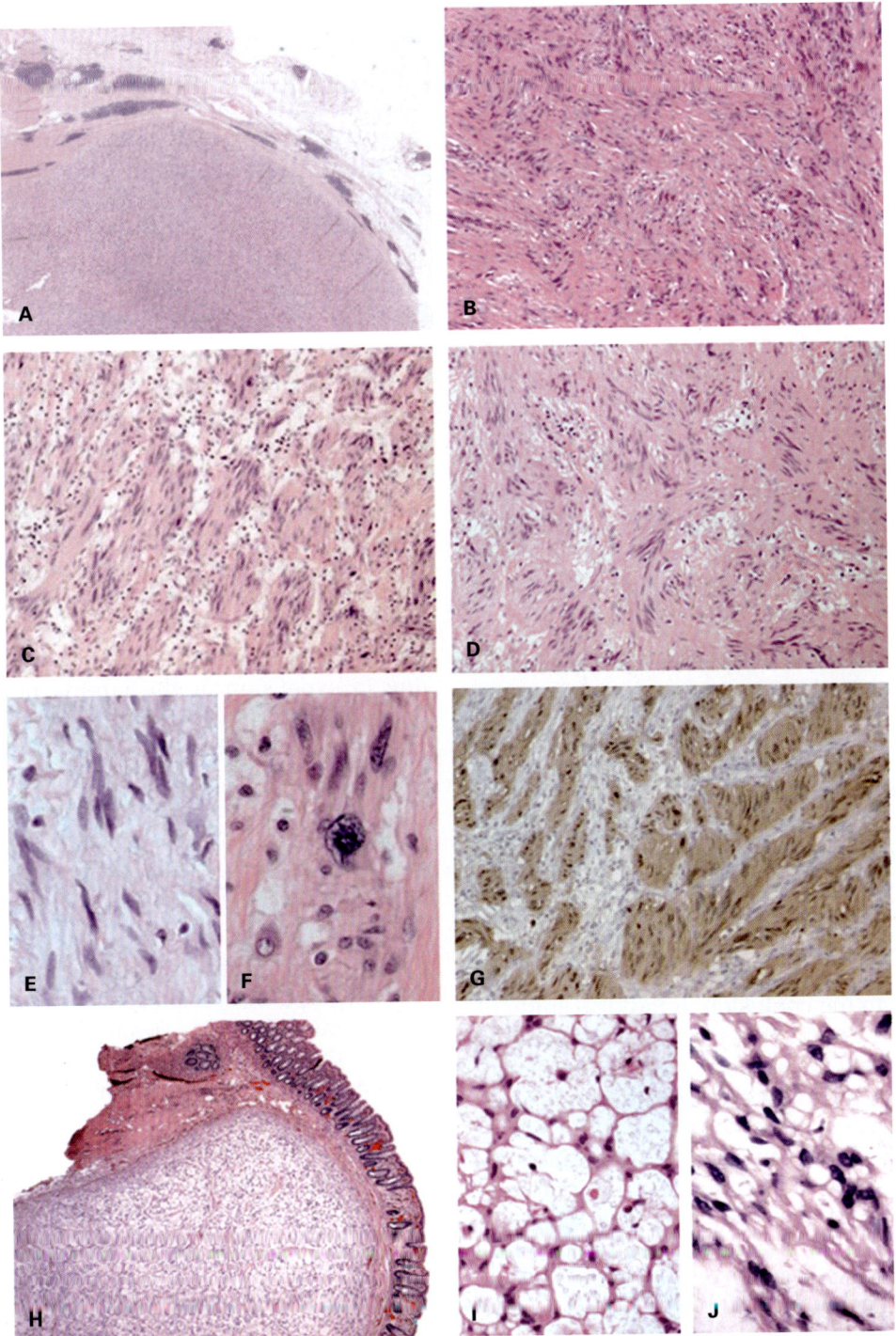

Figure 7-13. Schwannoma showing characteristic peripheral lymphoid cuff **(A)**, sheet-like and trabecular growth patterns **(B and C,** respectively). Nuclear pallisading **(D)** is usually not prominent in gastrointestinal schwannomas and seen more frequently in GISTs. Higher magnification shows the typical wavy tapered nuclei **(E)** and focal cytologic atypia **(F)** characteristic of these tumors. The diagnosis is confirmed by strong and diffuse S100 immunoreactivity **(F)** and negative CD117. Reticular/microcystic schwannoma in the colon **(G–I)**. This well-circumscribed submucosal lesion is composed of spindle cells in a microcystic ("sponge-like") pattern within a myxoid stroma **(J)**. At higher magnification, fairly uniform spindled cells with tapered, hyperchromatic nuclei can be appreciated. The tumor was mitotically inactive and diffusely immunoreactive for S100.

to be associated with GIST than schwannoma. Ultimately, the diagnosis depends on immunohistochemistry—strong and diffuse S100 immunoreactivity and lack of CD117 immunoreactivity. A small minority of schwannomas are immunoreactive for CD34.[159-162] Unusual morphologic variants of GI schwannoma include epithelioid, plexiform,[161,164] melanocytic,[165] microcytic/reticular (Fig. 7-13H–J), and psammomatous melanotic schwannomas,[166] the latter often associated with Carney's complex.

Epithelioid schwannoma (benign epithelioid peripheral nerve sheath tumor) is a rare, benign, often incidental lesion of the lamina propria or submucosa with a predilection for the colorectum. They are usually <10 mm in size and composed predominantly of epithelioid cells sometimes with a smaller spindled component. The tumor cells are arranged in nests and whorls, often with infiltrative borders. The nuclei are uniform, bland, and mitotically inactive. The immunohistochemical profile is similar to that of conventional schwannomas.[161,167]

Neurofibroma

GI neurofibromas are rare and usually occur in the setting of NF1, although isolated sporadic cases are reported. In the pre-CD117 era, neurofibromas were considered among the most common GI lesions in NF1.[168] However, many were probably GISTs based on their reported predilection for the jejunum, multiplicity, and associated with "myenteric plexus" hyperplasia (features of NF1-associated GISTs).[169] S100 immunoreactivity in a proportion of NF1-associated GISTs[109] may add to the confusion. A Swedish study of 70 patients with NF1 found that 7% had GISTs but not a single patient had a microscopically confirmed neurofibroma.[104] Genuine neurofibromas are often small polypoid tumors arising in the submucosa (presumably in the submucosal plexus) but may be larger, intramural lesions intimately related to the myenteric plexus. They have a heterogeneous cell population including bland Schwann cells, fibroblasts, perineurial-like cells and axons in a variably myxoid to collagenous matrix. Those occurring in the setting of NF1 are frequently plexiform and associated with mesenteric or subserosal nerves.[170] The most important differential diagnosis includes a GIST (neurofibromas are CD117 and DOG1 negative). The report of neurofibroma-like submucosal gastric GIST (CD117 positive, S100 negative) associated with a novel PDGFRA mutation on exon 18 highlights the potential overlap between these lesions.[171]

Ganglioneuroma

GI ganglioneuromas can be divided into three groups: (1) polypoid ganglioneuroma (Fig. 7-14), (2) diffuse ganglioneuromatosis, and (3) ganglioneuromatous polyposis. All are primarily colorectal in location unlike neurofibromas and GISTs, which mainly affect the small intestine and stomach. *Diffuse ganglioneuromatosis* has a strong association with MEN 2b (Fig. 7-15) and NF1 and may also be seen association with Cowden's (Fig. 7-16) and Ruvalcaba–Myhre–Smith syndromes. These associations are not observed with either polypoid ganglioneuroma or ganglioneuromatous polyposis.

Polypoid ganglioneuromas. *Polypoid ganglioneuromas* are small, mucosal or submucosal, sessile or pedunculated polyps, which are usually discovered incidentally. They occur at any age but most frequently under the age of 20. They are usually solitary or few in number. Histologically, they are composed of spindle cells in a fibrillar matrix together with ganglion cells in irregular groups or nests (Fig. 7-14). The spindle cells often merge imperceptibly with the surrounding lamina propria. Polypoid ganglioneuromas frequently resemble juvenile polyps at low power due to expansion of the lamina propria and dilatation and distortion of entrapped crypts. Others may resemble neurofibromas with nodular expansions in the lamina propria or submucosa, sometimes in continuity, and with plexiform arrangements of the neural elements. Others infiltrate the lamina propria without significant disturbance of the underlying architecture.[23,172,173]

Ganglioneuromatous polyposis. *Ganglioneuromatous polyposis* is associated with multiple polyps (>20 to innumerable) with a similar endoscopic appearance to that of polypoid ganglioneuromas (i.e., sessile or pedunculated, mucosal or submucosal or both, 1 mm to 2.2 cm in size). They are seen primarily in the colon and terminal ileum but can occur elsewhere (e.g., stomach and appendix). Compared to polypoid ganglioneuromas, ganglioneuromatous polyposis shows a greater variation in relative proportions of ganglion, neural and supportive cell elements but may be indistinguishable from the former. Some form small filiform projections containing clusters of ganglion cells with little or no evident neural component.[172,173] *Ganglioneuromatous polyposis* is frequently associated with extraintestinal manifestations such as lipomas and acrochordons, possibly representing a distinct syndrome for which the underlying genetic abnormality is as yet undetermined.[23,172,173]

Diffuse ganglioneuromatosis. *Diffuse ganglioneuromatosis* is a disseminated, nodular or diffuse, intramural or transmural neural proliferation, which can involve any site from the lips to the anus. The lesions

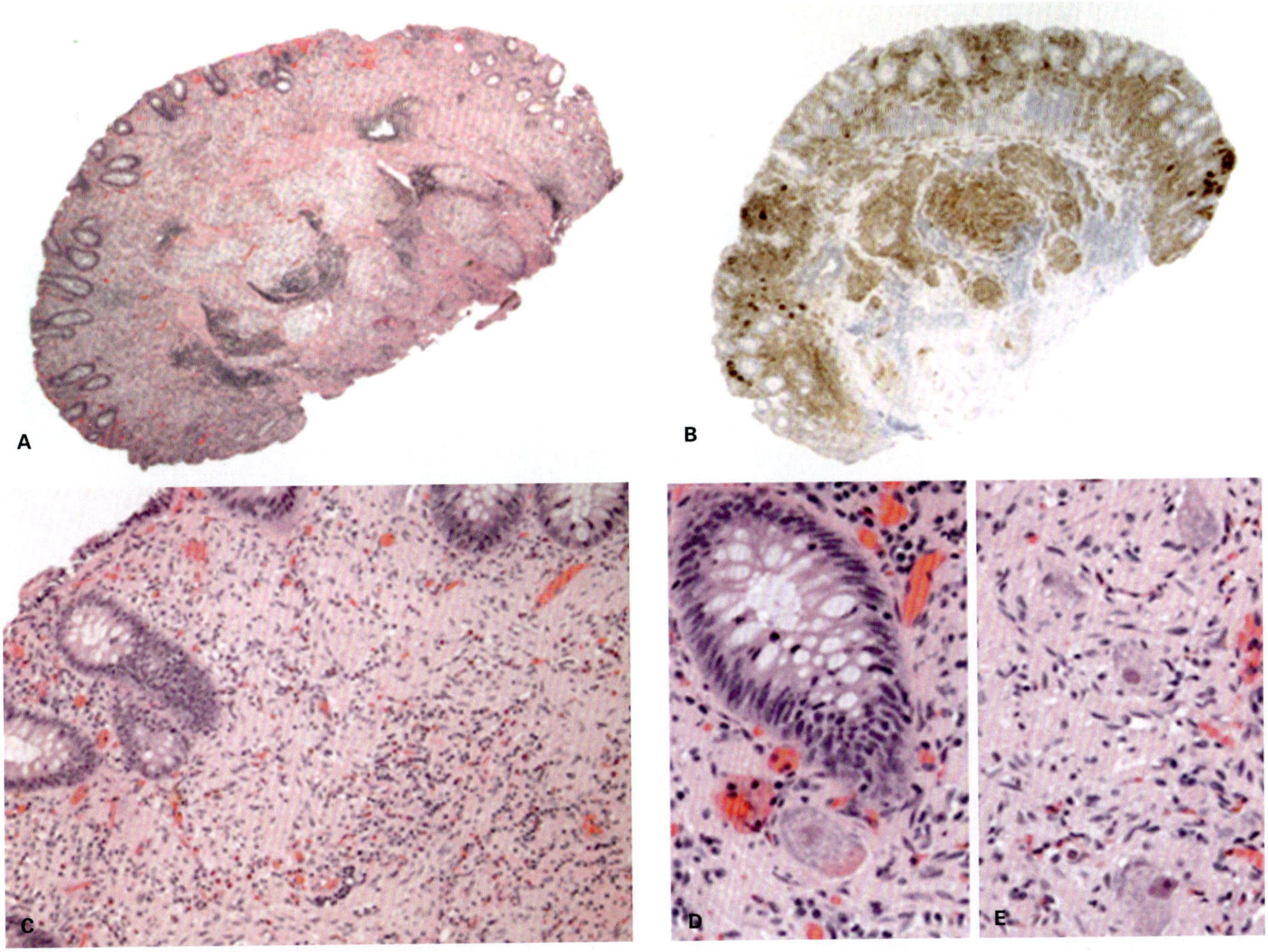

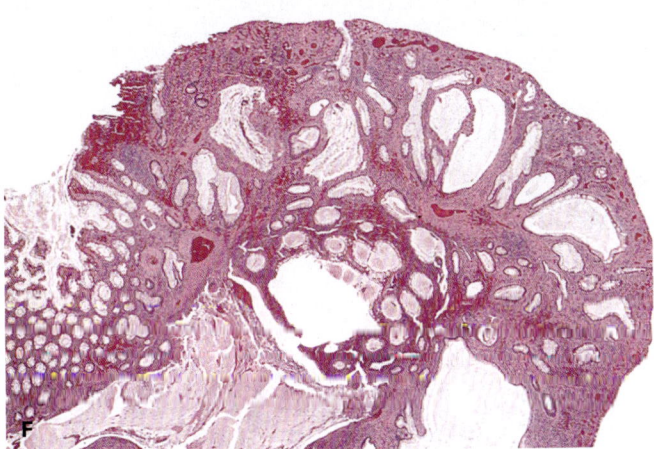

Figure 7-14. Polypoid ganglioneuroma of the colon shown at low magnification (A) with corresponding S100 immunohistochemistry (B). The lamina propria is expanded by a diffuse neural proliferation (C) with scattered large, cytologically abnormal ganglia. D,E: A second polypoid ganglioneuroma of the colon with an expanded lamina propria, dilated glands, and eroded surface imparting a low power appearance of juvenile polyp. Ganglion cells are present but not visible at this magnification. F: Colonic ganglioneuroma. The expanded stroma, dilated glands, and eroded surface resemble a juvenile polyp. Although the ganglion cells are not visible at this magnification, they were as shown in (E). (Part F reprinted from Riddell RH, Petras RE, Williams GT, et al. Atlas of Tumor Pathology: Tumors of the Intestines. Washington, DC: Armed Forces Institute of Pathology; 2003, with permission.)

range from a few millimeters to 17 cm in size, are poorly circumscribed, and can involve all layers of the bowel although the muscularis propria is commonly the epicenter. Grossly, the lesions may appear as irregular nodular mucosal lesions or as more diffuse constricting lesions mimicking malignancies. Larger lesions may ulcerate.[172,173] Ganglioneuromatous proliferations are usually readily diagnosed on mucosal biopsy specimens by the presence of focal aggregates of loose, often myxoid neural tissue partly replacing the lamina propria. Ganglion cells are invariably present but may be focal, so that multiple levels may be needed to identify them or they may be absent altogether in a particular biopsy specimen. Therefore, a negative biopsy does not exclude ganglioneuromatosis.[23] In resection specimens, the histology

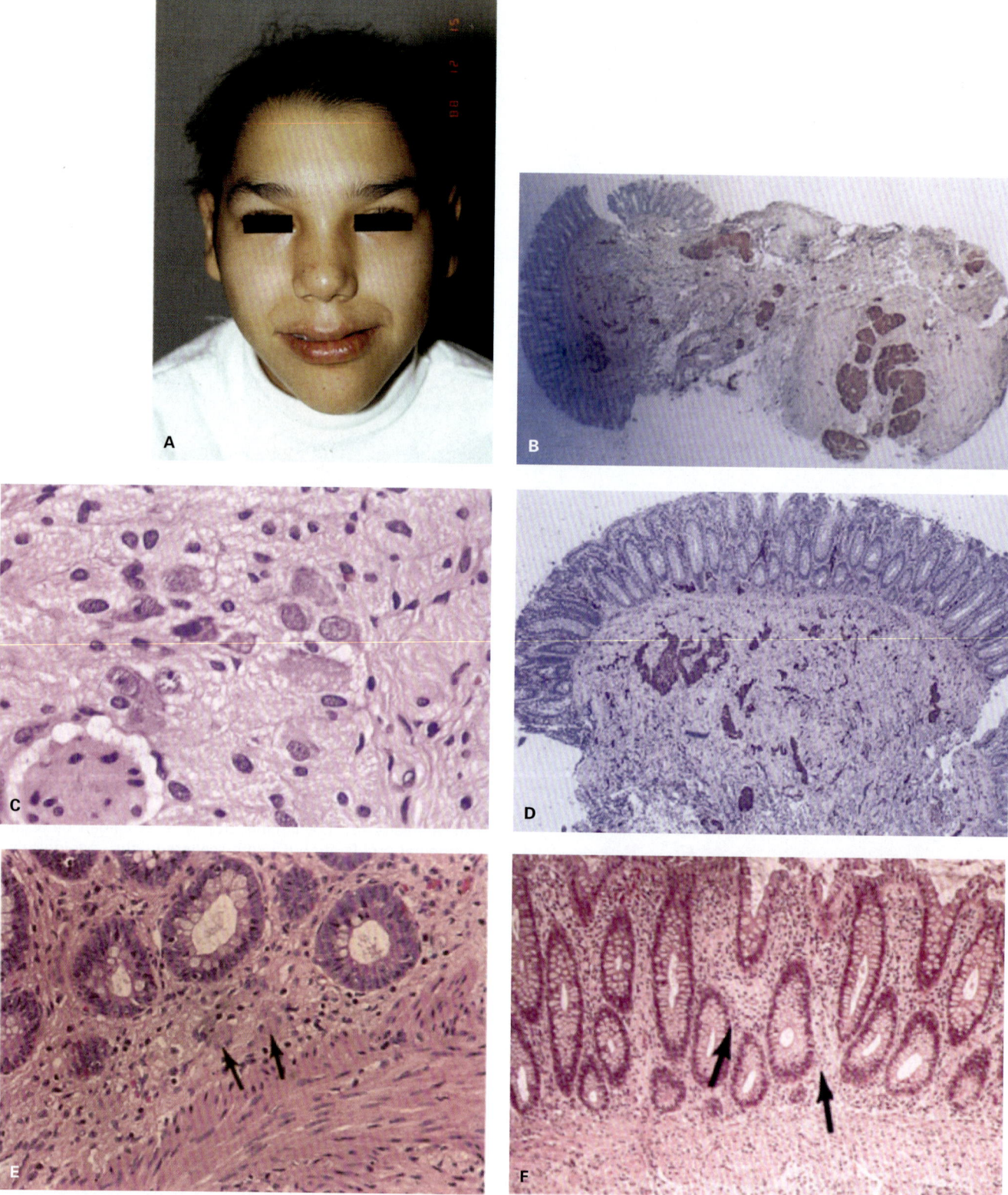

Figure 7-15. Multiple endocrine neoplasia IIB. **A:** A 13-year-old girl showing enlargement of the lips, nose, and ears resulting from subcutaneous neural proliferation. **B:** Part of a full thickness colonic biopsy showing marked proliferation of the plexi (PGP 9.5 immunostain). **C:** Detail of the myenteric plexus showing myriad ganglion cells. **D:** Mucosal and submucosal nerves demonstrated by PGP 9.5. **E:** Neural proliferation with ganglion cells unusually situated immediately above the muscularis mucosae (*arrows*). **F:** Mucosa with focal myxoid expansions between some of the crypts, pushing them apart (*arrows*).

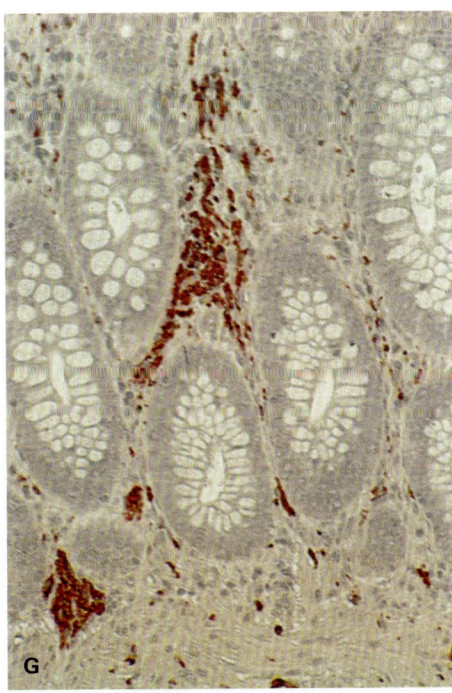

Figure 7-15. (*Continued*) **G:** PGP 9.5 demonstrates these to be abnormal bundles of nerves. Note the numerous smaller twiglets in addition to the large bundles.

ranges from diffuse myenteric plexus hyperplasia to transmural ganglioneuromatosis, which includes nerve fibers, ganglion cells, and supporting cells. One study suggested that transmural gangliomatous neural hyperplasia in all layers of the bowel wall with predominant involvement of the myenteric plexus was found in patients affected by MEN 2b, in contrast to the predominantly mucosal form that tended to be associated with NF1.[174] In addition in MEN 2b (in which ganglioneuromatosis is invariably present if looked for) and NF1, diffuse ganglioneuromatosis may occur in a number of settings including Hirschsprung' disease, tuberous sclerosis, Cowden's syndrome, other polyposis syndromes such as familial adenomatosis coli and juvenile polyposis. In patients with MEN 2b and diffuse ganglioneuromatosis, intestinal dysmotility and constipation often dominate the clinical picture but patients may also present with diarrhea. Immunohistochemical stains for S100 protein, neuron-specific enolase, and synaptophysin highlight the neural hyperplasia in the various intestinal layers.[23]

Mucosal Neuroma/Schwann Cell "Hamartoma"

Not infrequently one encounters benign-appearing neural (S100+) proliferations lacking ganglion cells in the colorectal lamina propria. While the lesions are not uncommon in clinical practice, there is no recognized uniformly used terminology, although most

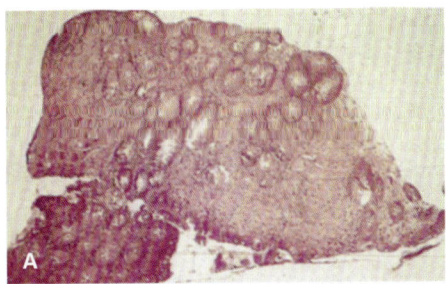
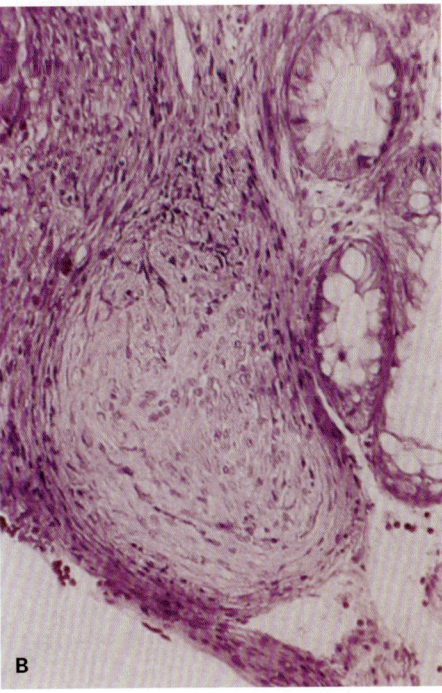

Figure 7-16. **A,B:** Neuromatous proliferation in a mucosal biopsy from the colon in a patient with Cowden's disease.

pathologists recognize them as benign and clinically inconsequential. We would like to lump these lesions under the noncommittal term mucosal neuromas, although one study described 26 such lesions in the colorectal lamina propria as "Schwann cell hamartoma."[175] These small sessile polypoid lesions (1–6 mm) are found mostly in the distal colon as incidental findings at screening colonoscopy, often in older people. Most of the patients do not show either additional neural lesions or features of NF1.

Histologically, these lesions are characterized by a diffuse, cellular proliferation of spindle cells in the lamina propria, which entrap crypts (Fig. 7-17). The lesional cells have bland elongated tapering nuclei and dense eosinophilic cytoplasm. Atypia, mitotic activity, and ganglion cells are absent. The cells are not arranged in obvious fascicles, whorls, or palisades. The lesions are confined to the mucosa, have ill-defined borders, and are not associated with a peripheral lymphoid cuff. Few rare examples that are entirely composed of structures resembling Wagner–Meissner corpuscles have been

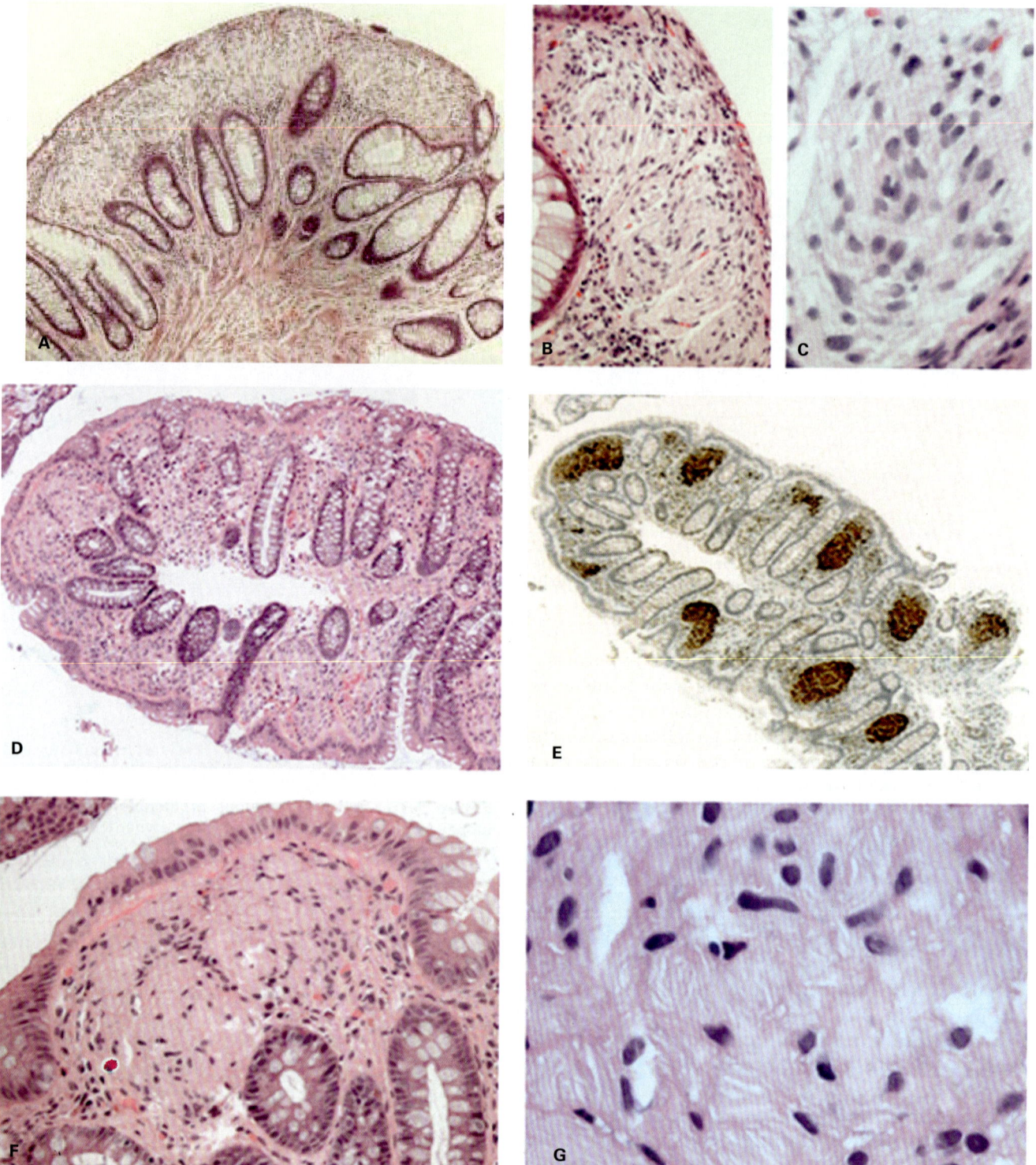

Figure 7-17. Mucosal neuronal proliferations without ganglion cells presenting as incidental colonic polyps—more termed Schwann cell "hamartoma." The first polyp (**A–C**) shows diffuse expansion of the lamina propria by a neural proliferation. The second polyp (**D–G**) shows a distinctly nodular neural proliferation, highlighted by S100 immunostain. **D:** This differs from the reported diffuse infiltrate of Schwann cell "hamartomas" but still seems to fit best in to this category. (**E**) shows typical S100 immunoreactivity between crypts. **F,G:** Note the low cellularity and bland appearance of the spindle cells.

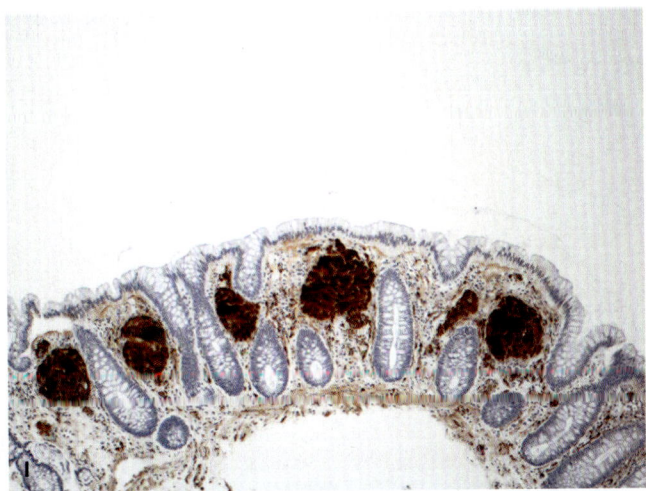

Figure 7-17. (*Continued*) **H,I:** Another lesion that is composed of S100-positive nodular spindle cell structures that resemble Wagner–Meissner corpuscles **(H)** and also appears to be in the same category. S100 stain shows multiple such structures in the lamina propria **(I)**.

described that were not associated with any hereditary conditions or neural lesions elsewhere and likely represent variation of the same theme (Fig. 7-17H,I). These lesions display diffuse and strong immunoreactivity for S100. Compared to neurofibromas, mucosal neuromas are generally more cellular, homogeneous, show more diffuse S100 immunoreactivity, and lack neurofilament positive axons. However, distinction between these lesions may be difficult on H&E and often relies on exclusion of a submucosal mass at endoscopy and immunohistochemistry for S100 and neurofilament. It is important to differentiate these lesions from GI schwannomas, neurofibromas, and ganglioneuromas, as these are not associated with any hereditary conditions.[175] Whether these lesions represent true hamartomas or benign neoplasms is debatable. These days even the concept of hamartoma itself is questionable, and we prefer the term mucosal neuroma.

Neural proliferations of various types can also be seen in the appendix, not uncommonly and some of them do resemble mucosal neuromas elsewhere in the GI tract.[176] Other forms of mucosal neural proliferation are very rare and seen mostly in MEN 2b, mainly on the lips and tongue, and also called mucosal neuromas. These are characterized by hyperplastic bundles of nerve fibers including frequent axons, which can be highlighted by neurofilament stain.[175] Traumatic neuromas may occur at anastomosis sites or in areas of bowel damage, whereas marked neuronal hyperplasia may be seen in Crohn's disease and other obstructing disorders.

Perineurioma and Fibroblastic Polyp

These are two similar, and likely identical, lesions, but as at the time of writing this is not fully resolved, we will consider them here separately.

Perineurioma. These are rare benign peripheral nerve sheath tumors occurring mainly in soft tissues but are also described in the GI tract. They form submucosal mass lesions (1.5–4.5 cm in size) in the stomach, jejunum, and colon.[177,178] Mass lesions show variable circumscription and focal infiltration of the muscularis propria and mucosa. They are composed of bland spindled cells in whorls, interwoven fascicles, and storiform arrangements in a collagenous to myxoid stroma. The tumor cells have tapered, wavy nuclei without atypia, and pale to clear elongated cytoplasm with indistinct cell borders (Fig. 7-18). Electronmicroscopy performed in one of the tumors in this study showed widely spaced spindle cells in a collagenous background, long bipolar cytoplasmic processes, prominent pinocytic vesicles, and sparse organelles, suggestion of a wispy basal lamina, consistent with perineurial fibroblasts. The mitotic rate does not exceed 1/10 HPF.[177,178] Perineuriomas are immunoreactive for EMA (sometimes quite weakly) and negative for keratin, S100, CD117, DOG1, SMA, and caldesmon. A small minority is positive for CD34.[177,178] Based on the limited number of such cases described, these lesions appear to be benign; however, resection would be indicated in most cases to exclude other more aggressive lesions, particularly GISTs.

Fibroblastic polyps. These are benign lesions that consist of bland fibroblast-type cells in the distal large bowel and are mostly incidental findings.[179] Most are <5 mm in diameter, but some may be as large as 15 mm. Histologically, they are composed of bland, plump, spindled cells with pale eosinophilic cytoplasm that infiltrate the lamina propria separating crypts. They are typically located within the mucosa and often seem to split the muscularis mucosae in a manner that one can see a thin layer

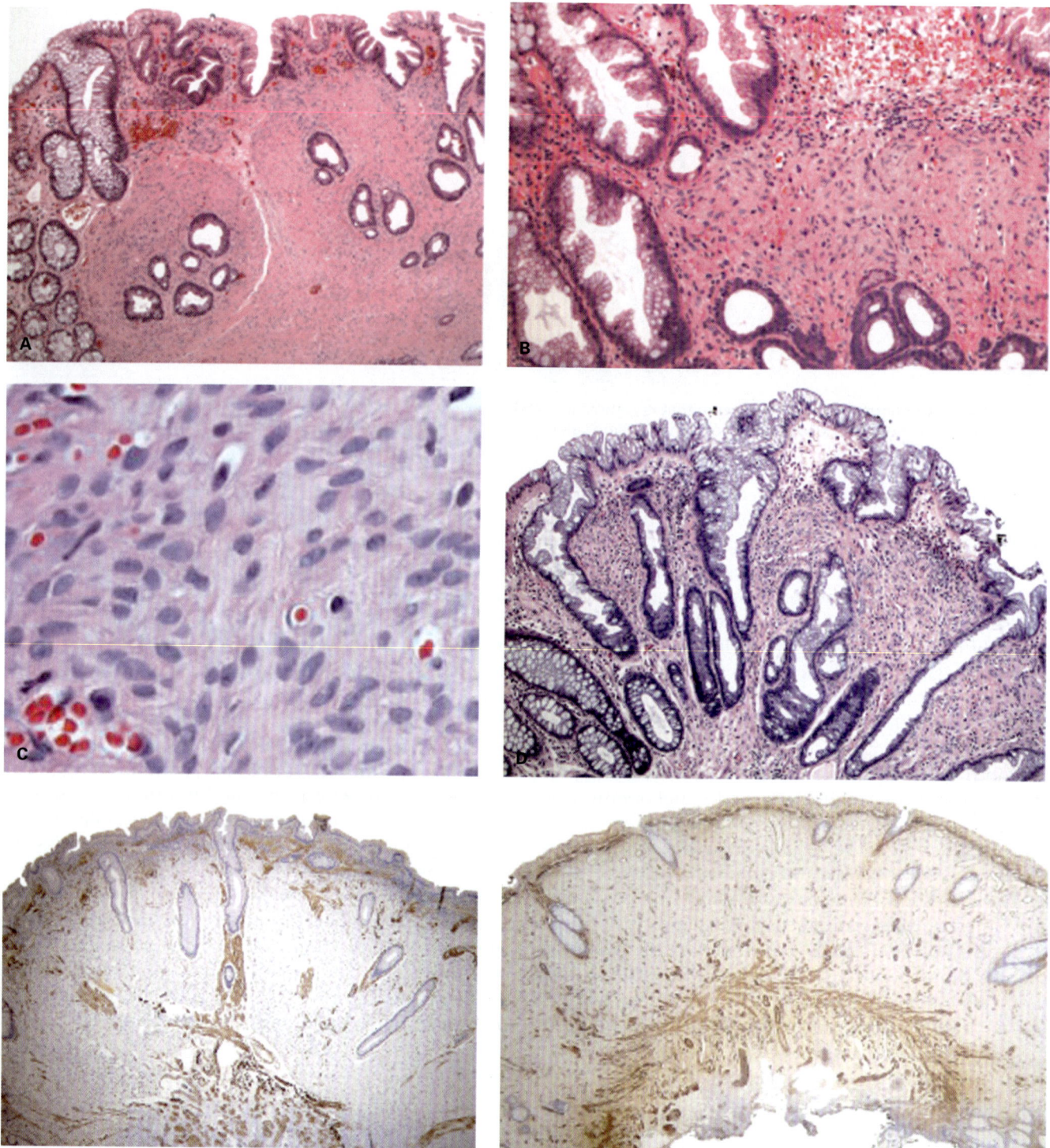

Figure 7-18. Colonic mucosal perineurioma (formerly "benign fibroblastic polyp") showing expansion of the lamina propria and separation of crypts, a fairly well-demarcated lateral border **(A,B)**. Detail of the lesion shows plump, spindled cells with bland nuclei and abundant pale cytoplasm **(C,D)**.

of smooth muscle on each side of the lesion, especially with smooth muscle markers. These often disrupt the underlying muscularis mucosae, but rarely ever extend into the submucosa. Margins are pushing rather than infiltrative (Fig. 7-18). They are frequently associated with or admixed with a hyperplastic polyp or a serrated sessile polyp that frequently harbors BRAF mutations.[180,181] This association is interesting and suggests an unrecognized etiopathogenetic link. Subsequent studies have suggested some evidence of perineural differentiation both ultrastructurally and immunohistochemically (EMA, Glut1, claudin 1, and collagen type IV positivity).[178,182,183] Positivity for these makers have been inconsistent in our hands, especially for EMA, and positivity is seen only in a subset when higher antibody concentrations and prolonged incubation times are used. However, these findings suggest that these may arise from perineurial fibroblastic sheath, and hence some have suggested that these should be called perineuriomas. Considering their close association with serrated polyps, the other putative cell of origin remains the pericryptal fibroblast. Although the exact cell of origin remains unclear, there is general agreement that mucosal perineurioma and benign fibroblastic polyp reported in the literature represent the same entity and are likely derived from some specialized fibrobast.[182–184] These lesions are almost exclusively mucosal, have so far no recognized potential malignant or recurrence risk, have a strong association with serrated polyps, and seem distinct from the submucosal perineuriomas. Hence, we prefer the term fibroblastic polyp to differentiate these lesions from the submucosal perineurioma, or at least suggest using the term "mucosal perineurioma." The main differential diagnosis is from a mucosal neuroma (Schwann cell hamartoma), and a S100 stain is often sufficient to differentiate them. Sometimes scarring in the lamina propria may mimic a fibroblastic polyp, especially when associated with a serrated polyp. However, the expansile nature of the fibroblastic polyp and relatively higher cellularity of the lesion can help in their differentiation. Their histology is fairly distinctive, and in clinical practice besides occasionally demonstrating a negative S100 stain, elaborate IHC workup is not required.

Biopsy Diagnosis of Polypoid Neural Lesions

With the increase in screening colonoscopy programs, the above-mentioned benign polypoid neural lesions are increasingly encountered. Accurate diagnosis is important given the association of certain lesions with neuroproliferative syndromes (see below). These lesions all have in common the presence of S100-positive spindle cells in the lamina propria. Such lesions should be carefully examined for ganglion cells, which often requires multiple levels and immunostains. Occasionally, ganglion cells predominate and the neural component is quite subtle. Before diagnosing a ganglioneuroma, consideration should be given to other possibilities including normal entrapped ganglia in unrelated spindle cell lesions (e.g., GIST), ectopic ganglion cells from incorporation of the submucosal plexus into newly regenerated mucosa postulceration, gangliocytic and paraganglioma. Careful attention to the distribution and cytologic appearance of the ganglion cells is helpful. The presence of either immature ganglion cells or clusters of ganglion cells in the lamina propria points to ganglioneuroma since neither are seen with normal entrapped ganglia. In addition, the myxoid nature of the lesion, frequent absence of a large mass, and immunohistochemical profile distinguish it from a GIST. Ectopic ganglion cells associated with repair lack an accompanying S100-positive spindle cell proliferation. Like ganglioneuroma, gangliocytic paraganglioma contain both ganglion cells and spindled cells. However, gangliocytic paraganglioma typically occurs in the duodenum or proximal jejunum and often contains epithelioid cells with an endocrine pattern. Isolated polypoid ganglioneuromas lack clinical associations and therefore need to be distinguished from ganglioneuromatous polyposis (associated with Cowden's syndrome) and diffuse ganglioneuromatosis (associated with NF1 and MEN 2b). It is therefore essential to know whether the lesion was isolated or part of a more diffuse process (gross/endoscopic findings described above).

The differential diagnosis for S100-positive proliferations *without ganglia* includes neurofibroma, mucosal neuroma/Schwann cell "hamartoma," schwannoma, and benign epithelioid peripheral nerve sheath tumor. It should be kept in mind that a small biopsy of a ganglioneuroma may not contain identifiable ganglion cells. Neurofibromas are distinguished by their cytologic variability (they are a mixture of Schwann cells, fibroblasts, axons, and perineurial cells), corresponding *patchy* S100 immunoreactivity and scattered neurofilament positive axons. Their diagnosis raises the clinical suspicion for NF1 (especially if plexiform) since sporadic GI neurofibromas are exceedingly rare. Mucosal neuromas are characterized by hyperplastic bundles of nerve fibers including frequent axons, which can be highlighted by neurofilament stain. They are strongly associated with MEN 2b (see above). Schwannomas may present an intraluminal polypoid mass in the colon and are distinguished by their mural involvement, characteristic peripheral lymphoid cuff, and circumscription. Infiltration of the lamina propria is not a feature. Schwann cell "hamartomas" are pure Schwann cell proliferations limited to the lamina propria—S100 immunoreactivity is diffuse. Benign epithelioid peripheral nerve sheath tumors are also diffuse S100-positive lamina propria infiltrates but are distinguished on the basis of their epithelioid appearance. They may form a morphologic continuum with Schwann cell "hamartomas." Schwannoma, Schwann cell "hamartoma," and benign epithelioid peripheral nerve sheath tumor have not been associated with any clinical syndromes. Perineurioma/benign fibroblastic polyp enters the morphologic differential diagnosis of mucosal neural proliferations but lacks S100 immunoreactivity.

Paraganglioma

The vast majority of GI paragangliomas occur in the duodenum but have also been described in the esophagus, stomach, and elsewhere in the small intestine.[185] Most occur sporadically but there are familial forms associated with germline loss-of-function mutations in the succinyl dehydrogenase subunit genes *SDHB*, *SDHC*, and *SDHD* (recognized to underlie the GIST-paraganglioma syndrome).[116] Other associations include NF-1, MEN 2, von Hippel–Lindau disease, and Carney's triad. Morphologically, they can be of the usual type (i.e., nests or "zelballen" of polygonal epithelioid cells separated by rich vasculature) (Fig. 7-19) or, in the duodenum in particular, the gangliocytic type. The latter show a combination of three cell types namely epithelioid (typically forming a carcinoid pattern), ganglion-like cells, and spindle cells.[186,187] The relative proportions of these cell types vary, and one cell type usually predominates. While most tumors show an admixture of these components, in some the components may be separated to the point where the lesion resembles a collision tumor. Immunohistochemically, somatostatin stains the ganglion cells as well as the carcinoid component; the latter is variably

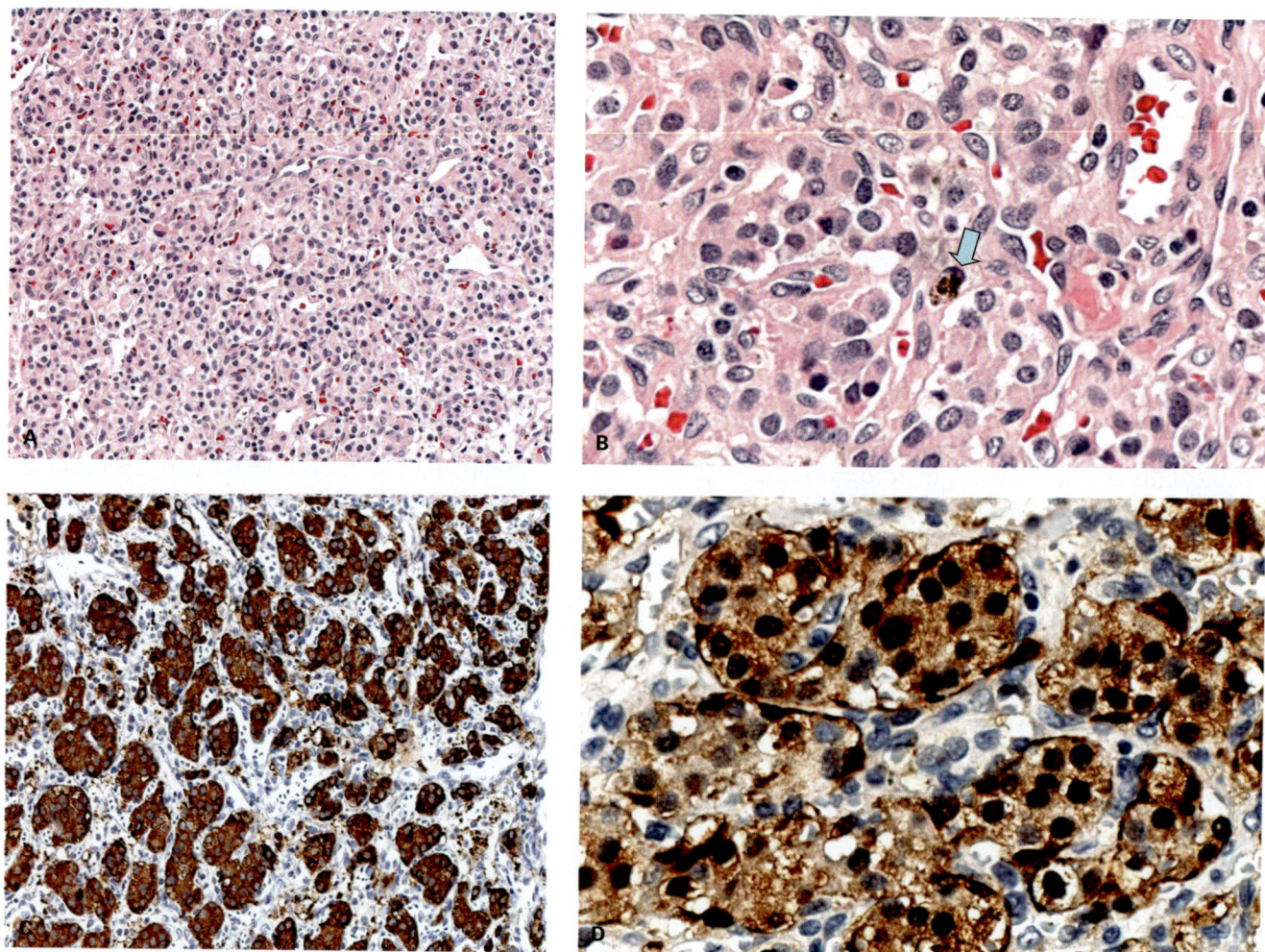

Figure 7-19. Duodenal paraganglioma. **A,B:** Vascular poorly formed nests of cells focally forming irregular nests. Focal hemosiderin is present (*arrow*). **C:** Synaptophysin showing both the irregularly diffuse staining often seen in these tumors, but also the nesting and abundant vascular stroma that is negatively stained. **D:** S100 outlining the nests, but at their periphery, the more spindly sustentacular cells can be seen.

immunoreactive for somatostatin and chromogranin. The neuroid spindle cell component stains with a variety of neural markers, including neurofilaments, neuron-specific enolase, S100, glial fibrillary acidic protein, and PGP 9.5. Generally, these tumors pursue a benign clinical course but uncommonly they may recur or spread to regional lymph nodes; distant metastases are exceedingly rare. Conventional paragangliomas often arise from the external surface of the bowel, extending inward, whereas gangliocytic paragangliomas are usually centered in the submucosa. The former should be distinguished from epithelioid GIST (paraganglioma-like GIST variants are described). In morphologically challenging cases, immunohistochemistry for neuron-specific enolase, GFAP (strong and diffuse), chromogranin and synaptophysin (more heterogeneous), and CD117 (negative) confirms the diagnosis of paraganglioma. The distinction between gangliocytic paraganglioma and polypoid ganglioneuroma has been discussed earlier.

Granular Cell Tumor

These uncommon tumors, probably of Schwann cell origin, can be found throughout the GI tract, most commonly in the esophagus followed by the colon and anal canal and duodenum (Fig. 7-20). They occur at any age with a peak in the fifth decade. They are usually asymptomatic and detected during endoscopy for unrelated symptoms. Large lesions may cause dysphagia. Endoscopically, esophageal lesions are grayish yellow, firm to hard, sessile lesions often described as having a "submucosal pill" like appearance.[188] Anal lesions may present as nodules, masses, or polyps, and may sometimes be confused with hemorrhoids.[189] Most are solitary but multiple tumors do occur, particularly

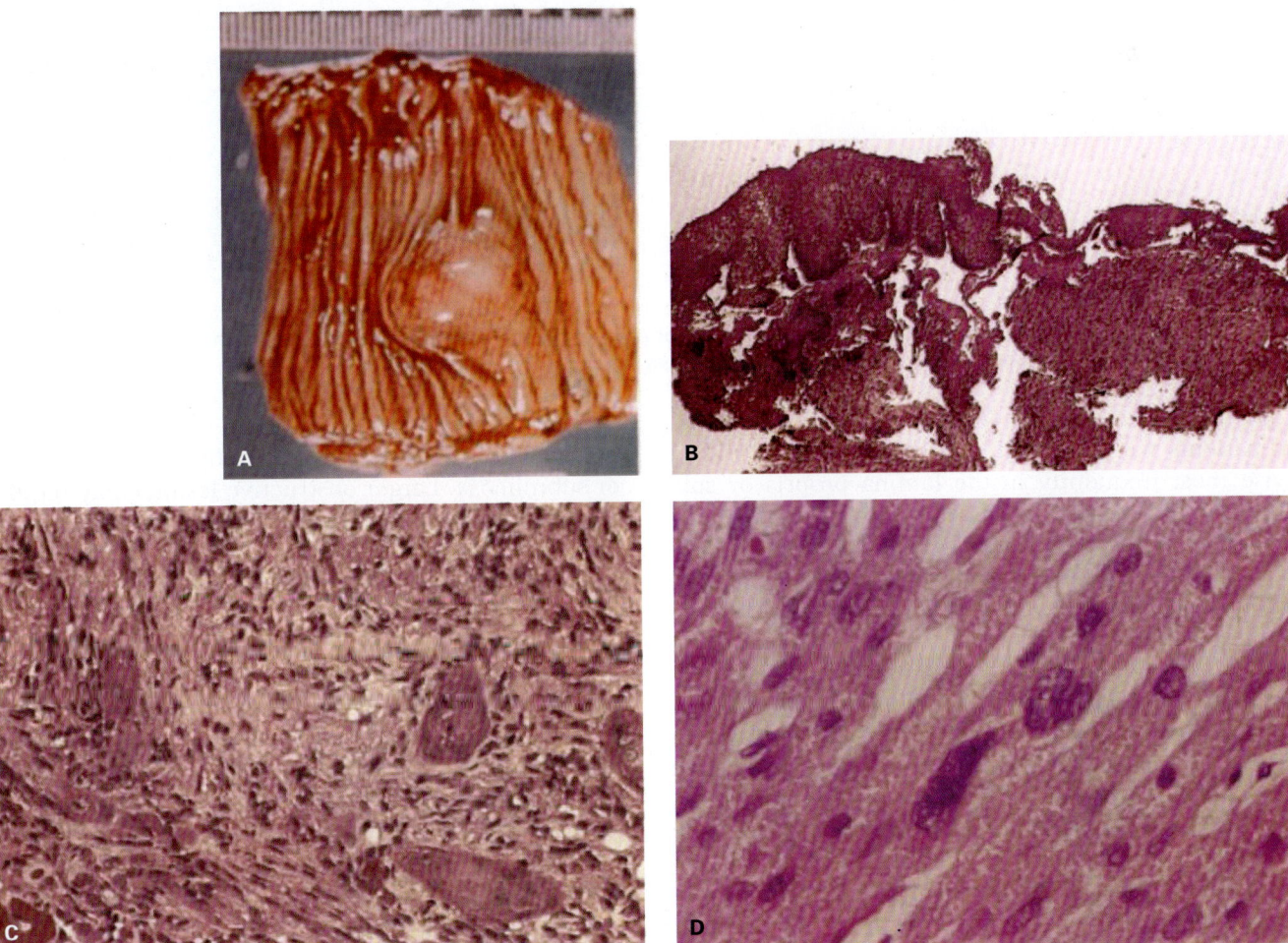

Figure 7-20. Granular cell tumors. **A:** Jejunal granular cell tumor showing the characteristics of a typical polypoid submucosal tumor. **B,C:** Esophageal granular cell tumor. **B:** Biopsy showing hyperplastic squamous epithelium **(left)** and tumor **(right)**. **C:** Detail of the tumor showing pseudoepitheliomatous hyperplasia, which can be misinterpreted as infiltrating carcinoma. **D:** Patient with multiple esophageal and gastric granular cell tumors, some of which showed the nuclear pleomorphism, said to be associated with aggressiveness but which rarely metastasizes or behave aggressively.

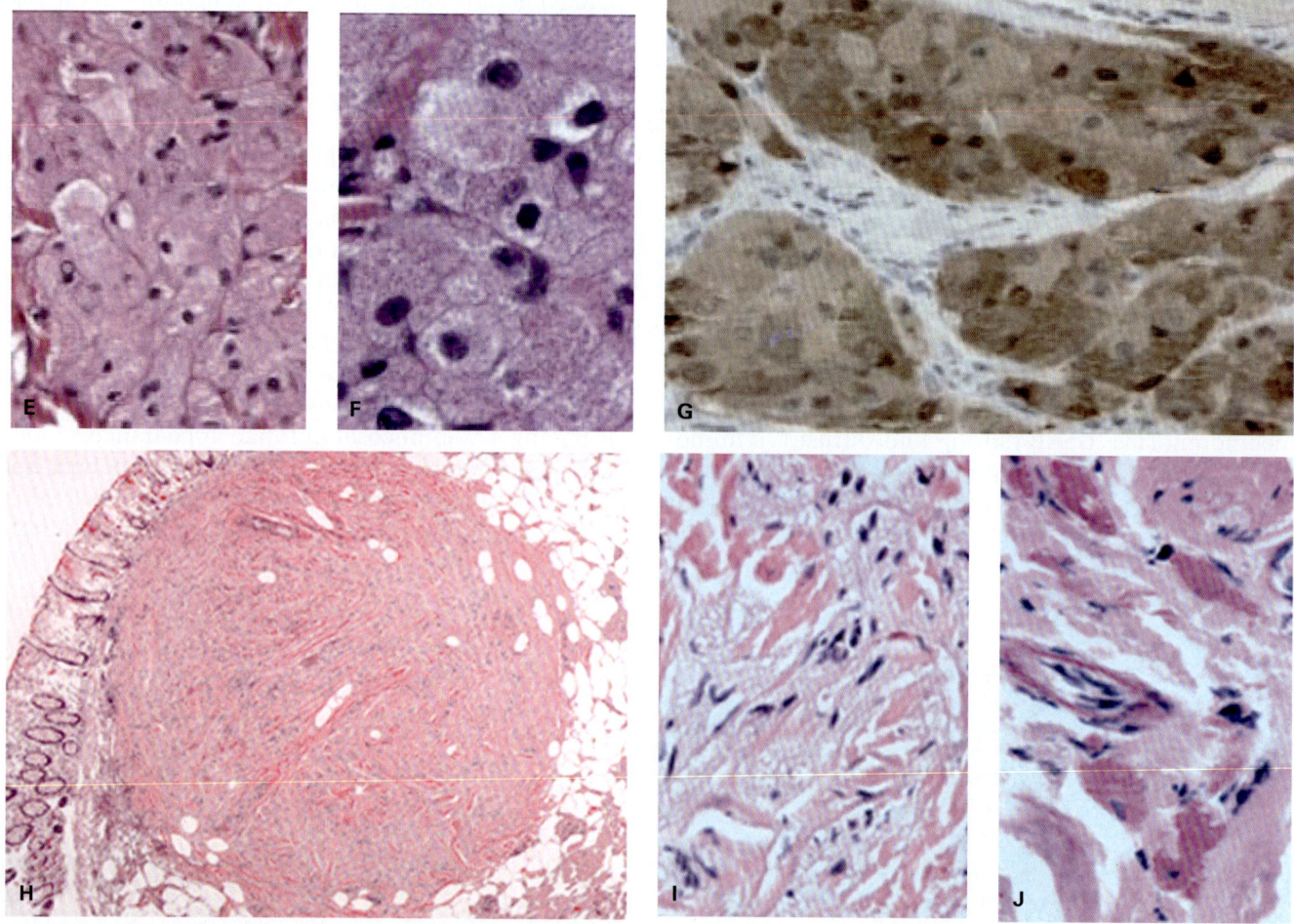

Figure 7-20. (*Continued*) **E,F:** Detail of a more typical granular cell tumor with small pyknotic nuclei. **G:** Diffuse S100 immunoreactivity is a feature of these tumors. **H:** Colonic granular cell tumor presenting as a small polyp. **I,J:** Detail of the lesion showing more spindled morphology and digested periodic acid-Schiff positive cytoplasm (**J**).

in patients with these tumors at other sites.[190] They arise most frequently in the lamina propria or submucosa, and consist of masses of histiocyte-like cells with fine granular, eosinophilic, or amphophilic cytoplasm. In the esophagus, overlying squamous epithelium frequently shows florid pseudoepitheliomatous hyperplasia (Fig. 7-20B and C), which can divert attention from the tumor and occasionally lead to a misdiagnosis of squamous carcinoma. The diagnosis can be confirmed by the presence of the strong, relatively coarse periodic acid-Schiff (PAS)-diastase-positive cytoplasmic granules, which are of lysosomal origin, and also by their S100 immunoreactivity. Malignancy is extremely rare and diagnosis requires demonstration of metastases. Features reported more commonly in malignant tumors include necrosis, spindling of the tumor cells, vesicular nuclei with large nucleoli, increased mitotic rate, a high nuclear-to-cytoplasmic ratio, and pleomorphism.[191] Small asymptomatic lesions may be managed conservatively with endoscopic follow-up. Endoscopic mucosal resection can be performed in lesions < 2 cm confined to the mucosa or submucosa. Larger obstructive lesions may require surgical resection.[188]

Malignant Peripheral Nerve Sheath Tumor

Malignant peripheral nerve sheath tumor (MPNST) may arise in the retroperitoneum[192] and rarely the GI tract.[193,194] They can arise from neurofibromas or de novo from peripheral nerves. There is a strong association with NF1. MPNSTs may show considerable morphologic heterogeneity but most are highly cellular tumors composed of fascicles of spindled cells showing marked nuclear atypia and hyperchromasia (Fig. 7-21). A variety of morphologic patterns may be seen including fibrosarcoma-like (dense fascicles with herringbone pattern), neurofibroma-like (like neurofibromas but with mitotic activity, cellularity, or necrosis), malignant fibrous histiocytoma (MFH)-like (markedly pleomorphic with bizarre giant tumor cells), and epithelioid. The mitotic rate is generally high and necrosis

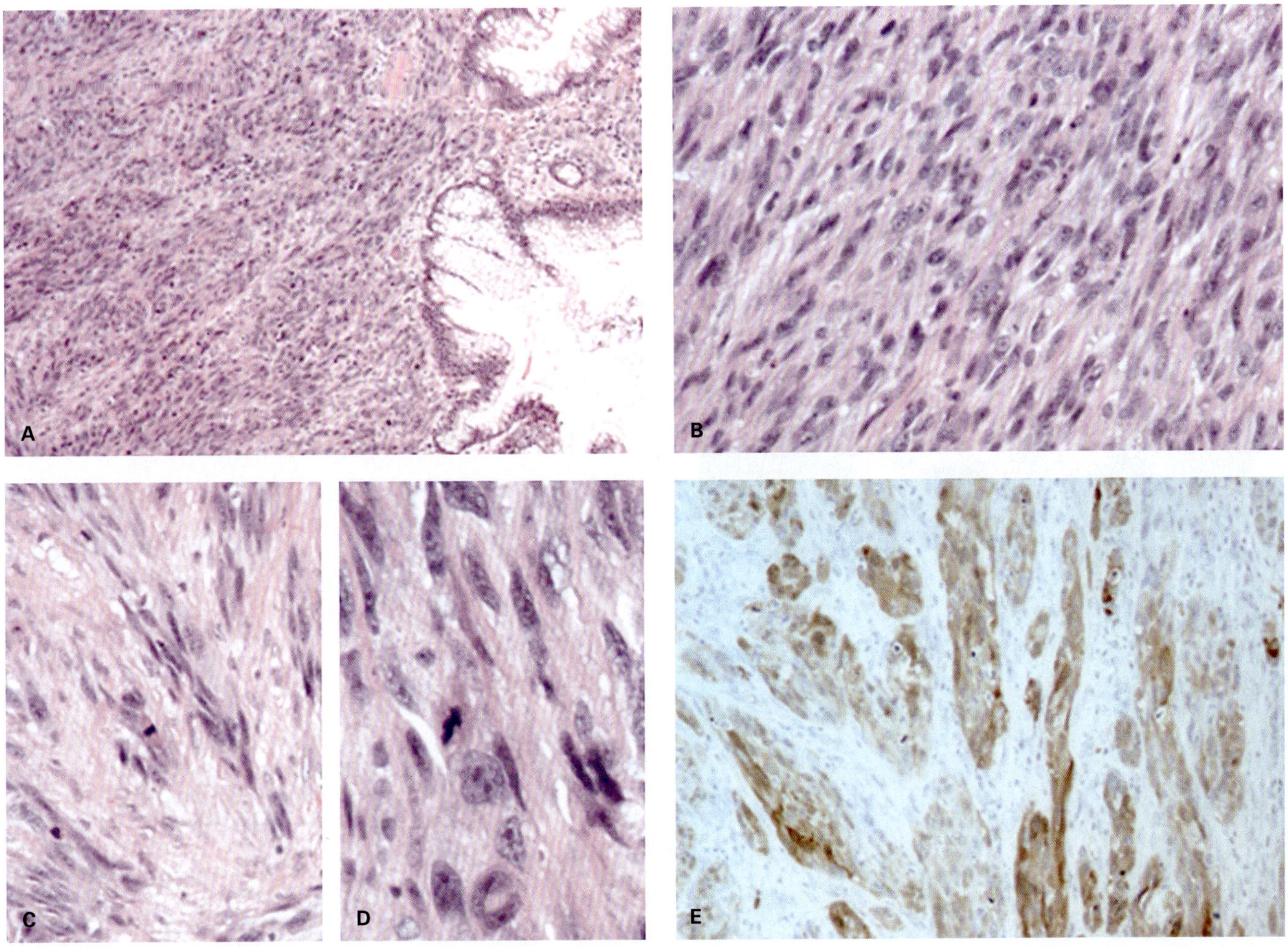

Figure 7-21. Malignant peripheral nerve sheath tumor of the rectum. Cellular spindle cell lesion with fascicular growth pattern **(A,B)**, areas of alternating cellularity **(C)**, hyperchromatic, tapering or curved, mitotically active nuclei, **(D)** and patchy S100 immunoreactivity **(E)**. The main issue here is distinction from melanoma. The immunohistochemical panel should therefore include additional melanoma markers (HMB-45, tyrosinase, MART-1, etc.) and electron microscopy should be performed looking for features of neural differentiation and melanosomes/premelanosomes.

is frequent.[193,194] A mitotic rate of >1/20 HPF indicates potential for malignant behavior. Morphologic clues to the diagnosis (not always present) include alternating areas of hyper- and hypocellularity, comma shaped or pointed nuclei, and formation of structures resembling nerves or Meissner corpuscles. MPNSTs usually show focal or patchy S100 immunoreactivity (50%–75% of tumors) and are negative for CD117. Since melanoma can be sarcomatoid and S100 positive, the panel should always include additional melanoma markers such as HMB-45, MART-1, and tyrosinase. Electron microscopy can be helpful in some cases.

Mixed Neuronal Glial Tumor

An ileal tumor with morphologic and immunohistochemical and ultrastructural features of glial and neural differentiation has been described. Additional cases are as yet described.[195]

FIBROBLASTIC/MYOFIBROBLASTIC TUMORS

Desmoid Tumor (Intraabdominal Fibromatosis)

Although rare, desmoid tumor is the most common primary tumor of the mesentery. It is usually seen in association with FAP but may occur sporadically often following trauma or surgery (including patients with Crohn's disease), with a possible role for estrogenic stimulation.[23,196,197] Most patients are in their fourth and fifth decades but pediatric and elderly populations can also be affected. Desmoid tumors occur in approximately 10% of patients with FAP (relative risk of 852 times the general population). About 2/3 have a history of intraabdominal surgery and most tumors develop within 5 years of surgery. Desmoid tumors are a leading cause of morbidity and mortality in FAP patients who have undergone colectomy. Although often locally aggressive, they lack the capacity to metastasize. Local complications include intestinal obstruction, mucosal ischemia, intestinal fistulae, and ureteral obstruction.[23] Grossly, they usually have ill-defined margins, a typical whorled appearance on cut section, and occasionally foci of myxoid degeneration (Fig. 7-22). If resection is attempted for cure, it has to extend well beyond the obvious macroscopic limits of

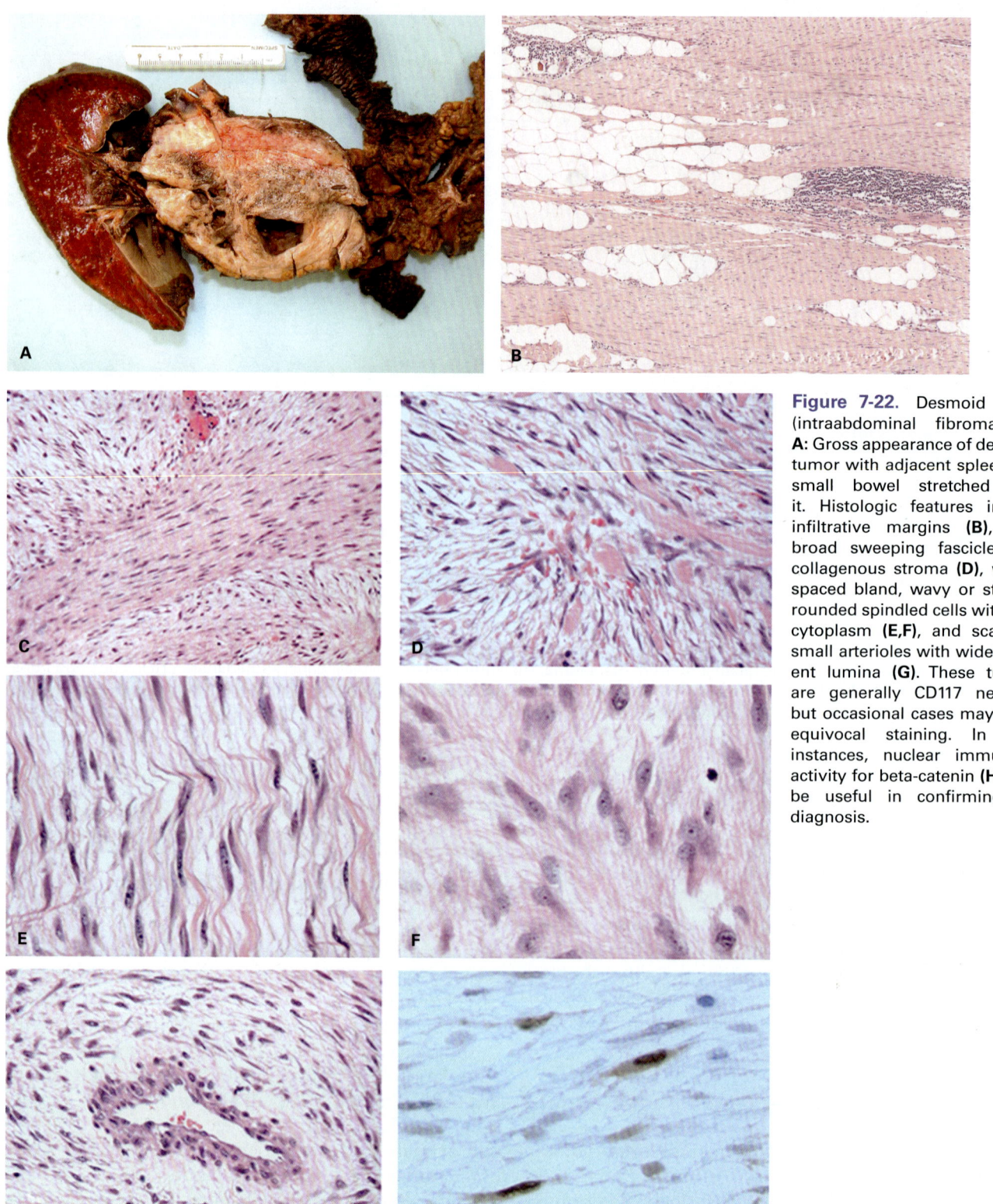

Figure 7-22. Desmoid tumor (intraabdominal fibromatosis). **A:** Gross appearance of desmoid tumor with adjacent spleen and small bowel stretched over it. Histologic features include infiltrative margins **(B)**, long broad sweeping fascicles **(C)**, collagenous stroma **(D)**, widely spaced bland, wavy or stellate, rounded spindled cells with pale cytoplasm **(E,F)**, and scattered small arterioles with widely patent lumina **(G)**. These tumors are generally CD117 negative but occasional cases may show equivocal staining. In such instances, nuclear immunoreactivity for beta-catenin **(H)** may be useful in confirming the diagnosis.

the tumor because, like all aggressive fibromatoses, it infiltrates with numerous finger-like extensions which, if not removed, serve as a source of subsequent recurrence. Death usually results from obstruction caused as much by tumor bulk compressing loops of bowel as by direct infiltration of the bowel wall.

Histologically, fibromatoses/desmoids are paucicellular spindled cell tumors with infiltrative margins (Fig. 7-22). The tumor cells are arranged in long and broad sweeping fascicles and evenly distributed within a collagenous matrix showing variable hyalinization and myxoid change. They have wavy with pale tapering cytoplasm and uniform elongated nuclei without atypia. Extracellular keloidal-type collagen is present in most cases and may merge imperceptibly with the cytoplasm of neighboring cells. Prominent muscular arteries with wide lumens and ectatic thin walled veins surrounded by extravasated erythrocytes are characteristic. Tumors may demonstrate a focal increase in cellularity usually in the form of stellate or rounded fibroblasts with plump nuclei and more abundant cytoplasm. The mitotic rate is generally low (<1/10 HPF.) and rarely exceeds 2/10 HPF. Scattered foci of perivascular chronic inflammation are usually present and scattered mast cells are a constant feature. Atypical mitoses, necrosis, and cystic degeneration are absent.[198,199]

Although desmoid tumor primarily affects the anterior abdominal wall and mesentery, it may occasionally encroach onto, infiltrate or arise from the wall of the stomach or intestine,[199] leading to potential confusion with a GIST. Most are readily distinguishable from GISTs on morphological grounds but our experience suggests that problems with this differential diagnosis persist. Similar experience has been reported elsewhere with up to 35% to 50% of mesenteric desmoid tumors seen in consultation practice originally diagnosed as GIST.[198,199] Attention to the infiltrative margins, low cellularity, long broad sweeping fascicles, and keloidal collagen should facilitate the correct diagnosis in most cases.

Most desmoids show patchy immunoreactivity for SMA and MSA and are negative for S100, CD34, and keratin. There have been conflicting reports regarding CD117 immunoreactivity with some investigators reporting cytoplasmic staining[49,199] and others not.[50,200] These inconsistencies appear to relate to the commercial source of the antibody used as well as variations in the use of antigen retrieval techniques,[53,198] and under optimum technical conditions, desmoid is a CD117-negative tumor.[53] Nuclear immunoreactivity for β-catenin in desmoids has been reported to be useful in differentiating these tumors from GISTs, which are nonreactive.[49] Overexpression of β-catenin is the result of somatic mutations in adenomatous polyposis coli (APC) or β-catenin genes. Ultrastructurally, desmoid tumors demonstrate features of fibroblastic and myofibroblastic differentiation. Surgical excision with clear margins is the mainstay of therapy; local recurrences in incompletely excised tumors are often well controlled by radiation therapy.[199]

Inflammatory Fibroid Polyp

IFP, previously also called Vanek tumor, is a rare, clinically benign, mesenchymal lesion seen mostly in the gastric antrum but also in the small and large bowel and esophagus.[201] The peak incidence is in the sixth to seventh decade. Most are polypoid lesions smaller than 5 cm but examples up to 20 cm have been described. Gastric IFP tends to form single smooth, broad-based or sessile polyps confined to the submucosa and amenable to endoscopic removal. Surgically resected specimens are more frequently ileal (Fig. 7-23), and these often show transmural infiltration sometimes destroying the muscularis propria and often extending into the serosa (Fig. 7-24A,B).[132,202] Small polyps are often incidental but larger polyps (generally ileal) may cause symptoms, particularly abdominal pain related to obstruction or intussusception.[203,204] In this situation, IFPs form potato-shaped and potato-sized masses that may be rather pedunculated (Fig. 7-23A), often with surface ulceration (Fig. 7-23B). Early lesions are invariably sessile and only later become pedunculated and frankly polypoid. Histologically, IFP is a circumscribed, predominantly

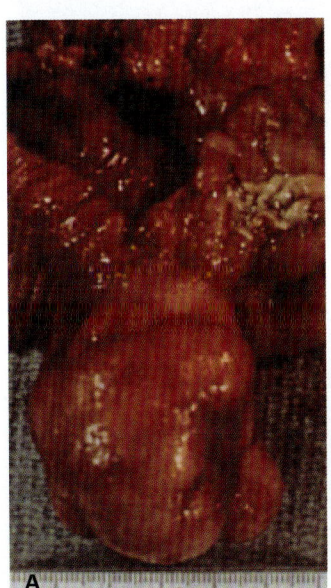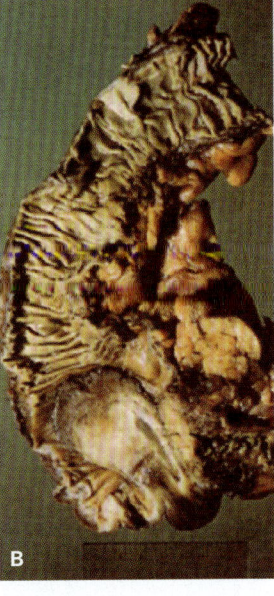

Figure 7-23. Gross appearances of inflammatory fibroid polyps. A: Irregular, multilobated inflammatory tumor from the ileum. B: Polypoid tumor with superficial ulceration at the apex of an intussusception at the ileocecal valve.

submucosal proliferation of spindled and stellate mesenchymal cells in a loose and edematous to collagenous stroma (Fig. 7-24C–J). There is a network of capillary channels and a variety of inflammatory cells scattered throughout the stroma. Eosinophils are usually prominent and lymphocytes, plasma cells, mast cells, and rarely multinucleated giant cells are also seen. Arteries, veins, and lymphatics may be present. Vessels are often surrounded by a characteristic cuff of spindled cells in an edematous stroma ("onion-skinning") (Fig. 7-24G,H). The latter is less prominent in small intestinal IFPs.[201,205] Larger tumors tend to acquire more fibrous tissue and collagen and become more sclerotic, at which time they have relatively

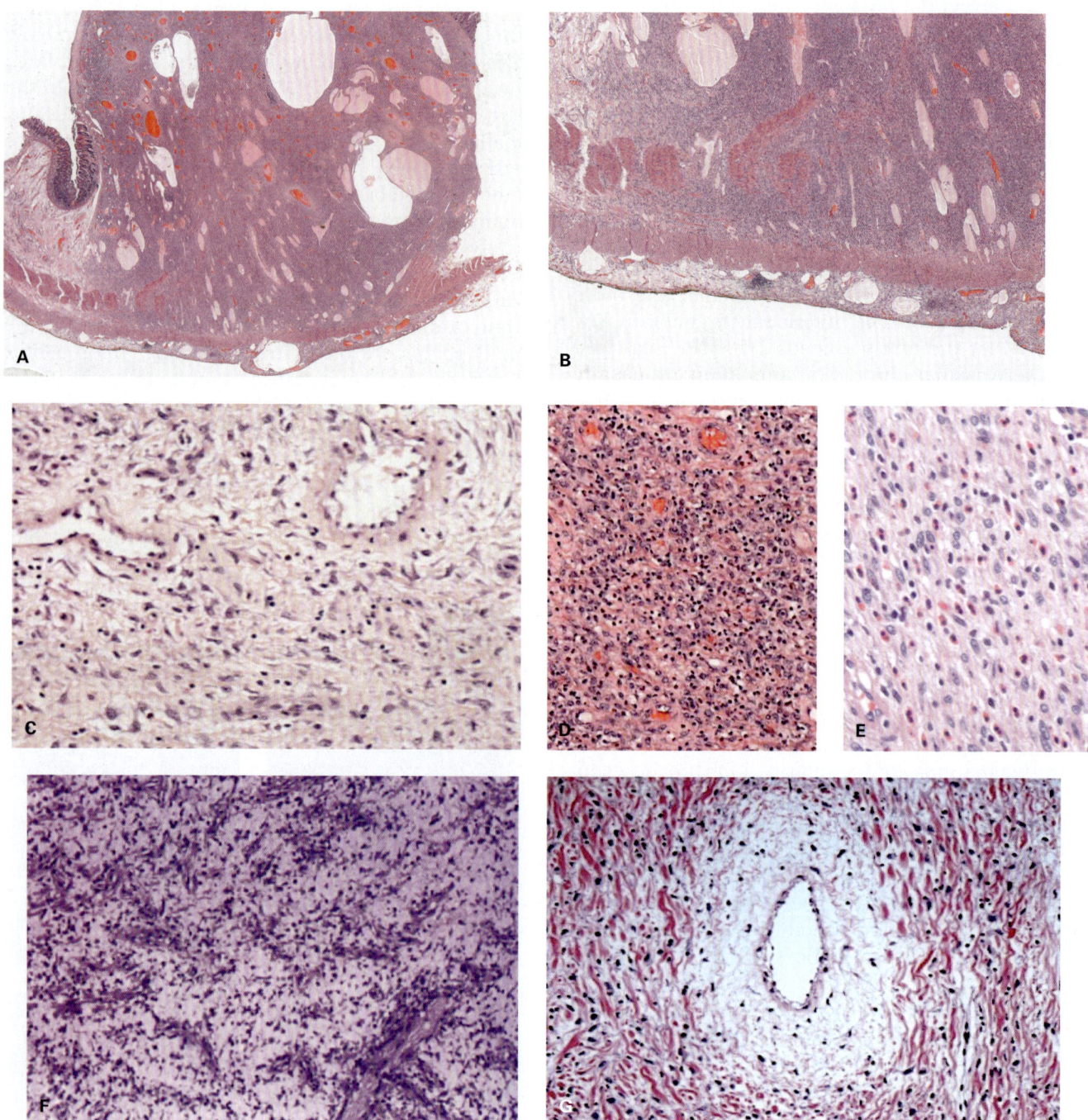

Figure 7-24. Inflammatory fibroid polyp. **A:** Whole-mount section of a small intestinal inflammatory fibroid polyp showing transmural extension, which is not uncommon in these tumors. **B:** Detail of infiltration through the muscularis propria to involve the subserosa (**right bottom**). **C–E:** Most lesions have a loose, myxoid stroma often with a chronic inflammatory infiltrate rich in eosinophils (**D,E**). **F:** Prominent, often interlacing, vascular channels are frequently present. **G:** Perivascular edema and

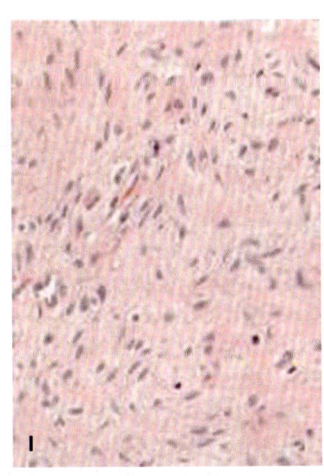
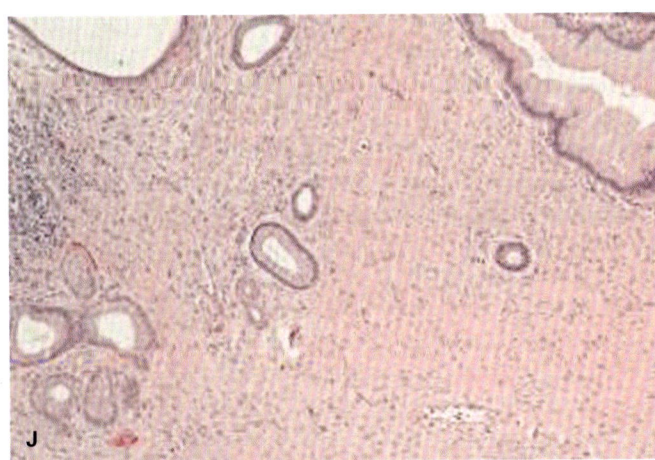

Figure 7-24. (*Continued*) (**H**) onion-skinning of the spindled cells are characteristic features of this tumor. **I,J:** Some tumors have a more fibrous stroma and a less inflammatory background. Because they can percolate into the lamina propria in a relative nondestructive manner, inflammatory fibroid polyps are often amenable to biopsy. They are one of the few tumors that infiltrate the lamina propria and muscularis propria and yet are entirely benign.

little myxoid tissue or vascularity (Fig. 7-24I,J). It is these tumors that can be fibroid-like. Some parts of the tumor may be quite cellular, and mitotic activity may be conspicuous and disconcerting. Despite these features, which in certain areas may mimic an MFH, with infiltration through the wall of the bowel and large subserosal component, these tumors are benign and metastases have not been reported. In some tumors, the overlying glands may dip into the tumor; rarely, a genuine enteritis cystica profunda is a part of the tumor. Although confusion with eosinophilic gastroenteritis rarely occurs, as the latter is diffuse, frequently accompanied by a peripheral eosinophilia, and is steroid responsive, occasional examples of this disease can also be polypoid.

The histogenesis of IFP remains undetermined although fibroblastic, fibrohistiocytic, myofibroblastic, vascular, and dendritic cell origins have all been proposed.[132,206] Approximately 50% to 60% of IFPs harbor mutations in the PDGFRA gene,[202,207,208] including identical mutations to those seen in GIST. Exon 12 mutations appear to predominate in small intestinal IFP, while exon 18 mutations predominate in gastric IFP. Rare exon 14 mutations have also been described.[207] Although once considered a reactive process, the finding of activating PDGFRA mutations now favors a neoplastic process. This is further supported by rare familial occurrence of IFP[209] and rare reports of multiple IFPs associated with PDGFRA germline mutations.[210,211] Some IFPs are immunoreactive for CD34 and a minority show focal immunoreactivity for SMA.[201,206,212] Vascular markers including CD34 tend to highlight numerous small capillary-sized vessels in the stroma mimicking a vascular neoplasm. Although initially suggested to be immunoreactive for CD117, this has not been confirmed in subsequent studies.

A subset of IFPs lack the classical onion-skin pattern and CD34 immunoreactivity. It has been speculated that these may represent a distinctive lesion perhaps more closely related to inflammatory myofibroblastic tumor (IMT).[201] When an IFP shows transmural or lamina propria infiltration, it can resemble an aggressive GIST. This may be compounded by CD34 immunoreactivity and the presence of scattered CD117 immunoreactive mast cells, which may be interpreted as focal CD117 expression by the tumor. The presence of *PDGFRA* mutations in most IFP represents a further potential pitfall. Careful morphologic examination with attention to its submucosal location, relative hypocellularity, loose edematous stroma, characteristic "onion skin" arrangement of spindled cells around vessels, and inflammatory infiltrate rich in eosinophils should facilitate the correct diagnosis. As only malignant GISTs infiltrate the lamina propria, a mistaken diagnosis of GIST may have important consequences. Other tumors that may enter the differential diagnosis include IMT, perineurioma, schwannoma, and inflamed granulation tissue.

Plexiform Fibromyxoma of the Gastric Antrum

These are distinctive mesenchymal neoplasms that occur in the gastric antrum, which may be confused with inflammatory fibroid polyps (IFPs) or myxoid GISTs.[213,214] A series of 12 cases from AFIP occurred in both men and women (7–75 years, median age 41 years) exclusively in the gastric antrum. Clinical presentation is similar to GISTs or IFPs. The tumor size ranges from 3 to 15 cm (median 5.5 cm), and they are located in the muscularis propria with infiltrative margins to the mucosa. The tumor size ranges from 3 to 15 cm (median 5.5 cm). Plexiform fibromyxomas are typically centered in the muscularis propria, have infiltrative margins, and often extend into the submucosa, but only rarely the mucosa and/or subserosa, extragastric soft tissue, and the duodenal bulb. Grossly, the tumors appear pale tan, mucoid, gelatinous or hemorrhagic mural or partly extramural masses, or occasionally grape-like nodules with mucoid consistency.

Histologically they are composed of plexiform nodules of scattered ovoid cells in a myxoid or fibromyxoid matrix. A prominent arborizing capillary network is present (Fig. 7-25A–E). Intravascular involvement in some cases is seen in veins and lymphatics (Fig. 7-25F). Cellularity is generally low, but some cases show focally increased cellularity or a more collagenized stroma. Necrosis is not described. Nuclei are bland and uniform, and the mitotic count is low (<1/50 HPF). Sometimes the tumor cells are surrounded by a pseudovacuolar lacunar space limited by a network of fibrous matrix (Fig. 7-25G). Most of the tumors show immunoreactivity for SMA (Fig. 7-25H) consistent with myofibroblastic differentiation and are negative for desmin, CD34, DOG1, c-Kit, and S100. No specific molecular or cytogenetic abnormalities have yet been identified in these tumors as yet. None of the tumors with adequate follow-up in this study recurred or was associated with myxomas at other sites or any other syndrome. The differential diagnosis includes GIST, IFP, plexiform neurofibroma, myxoid leiomyoma, and desmoid. Characteristic histology combined with lack of specific markers for other tumors should help in establishing the correct diagnosis. Interestingly, extensive review of AFIP files for similar tumors at other sites in GI tract failed to show any.

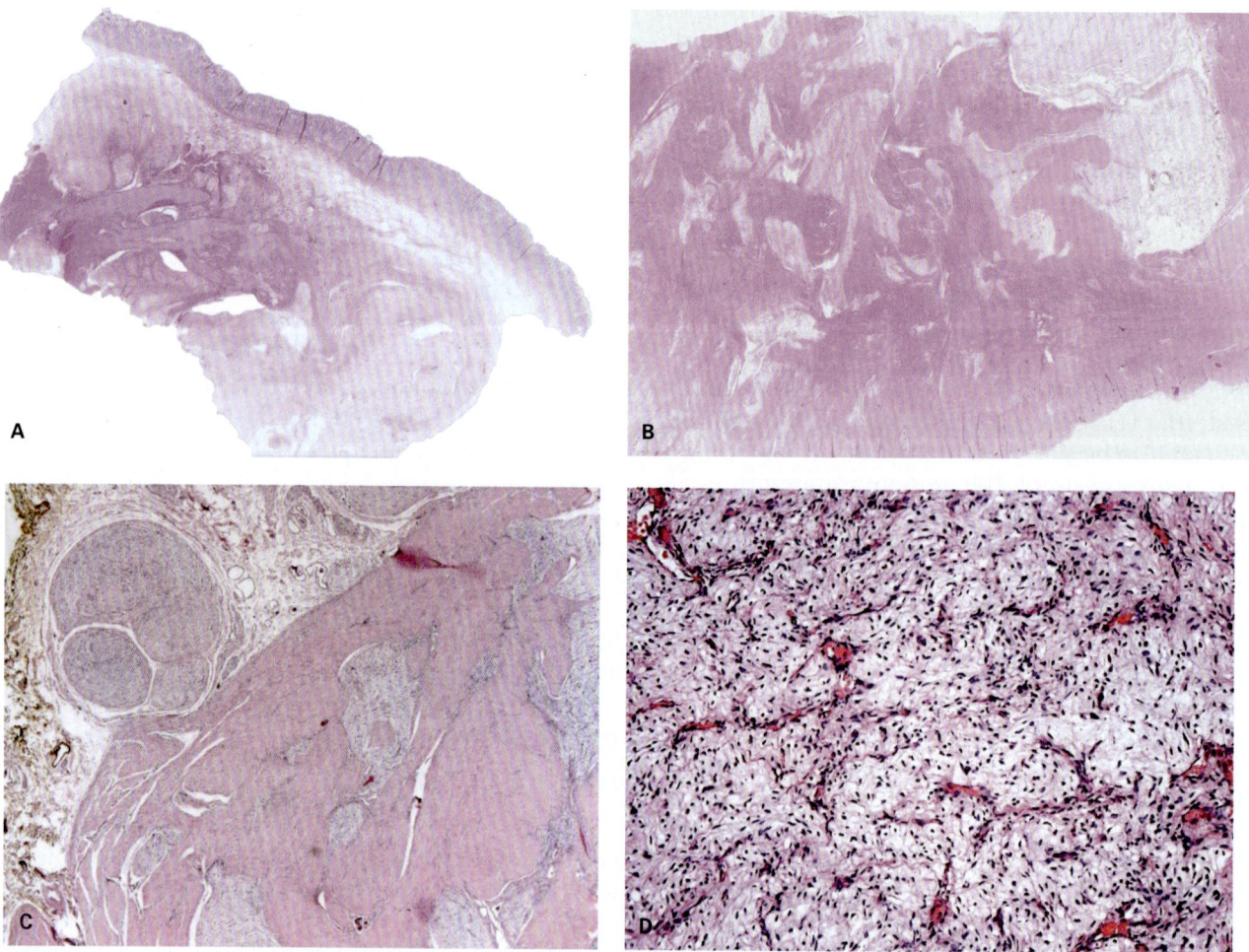

Figure 7-25. Plexiform fibromyxoma of the gastric antrum. The tumor has a characteristic multinodular plexiform pattern at low power, infiltrating the muscularis propria and often extending into the submucosa and/or subserosa (A–C). Cellularity is generally low with scattered ovoid cells dispersed in a myxoid or fibromyxoid matrix (D,E).

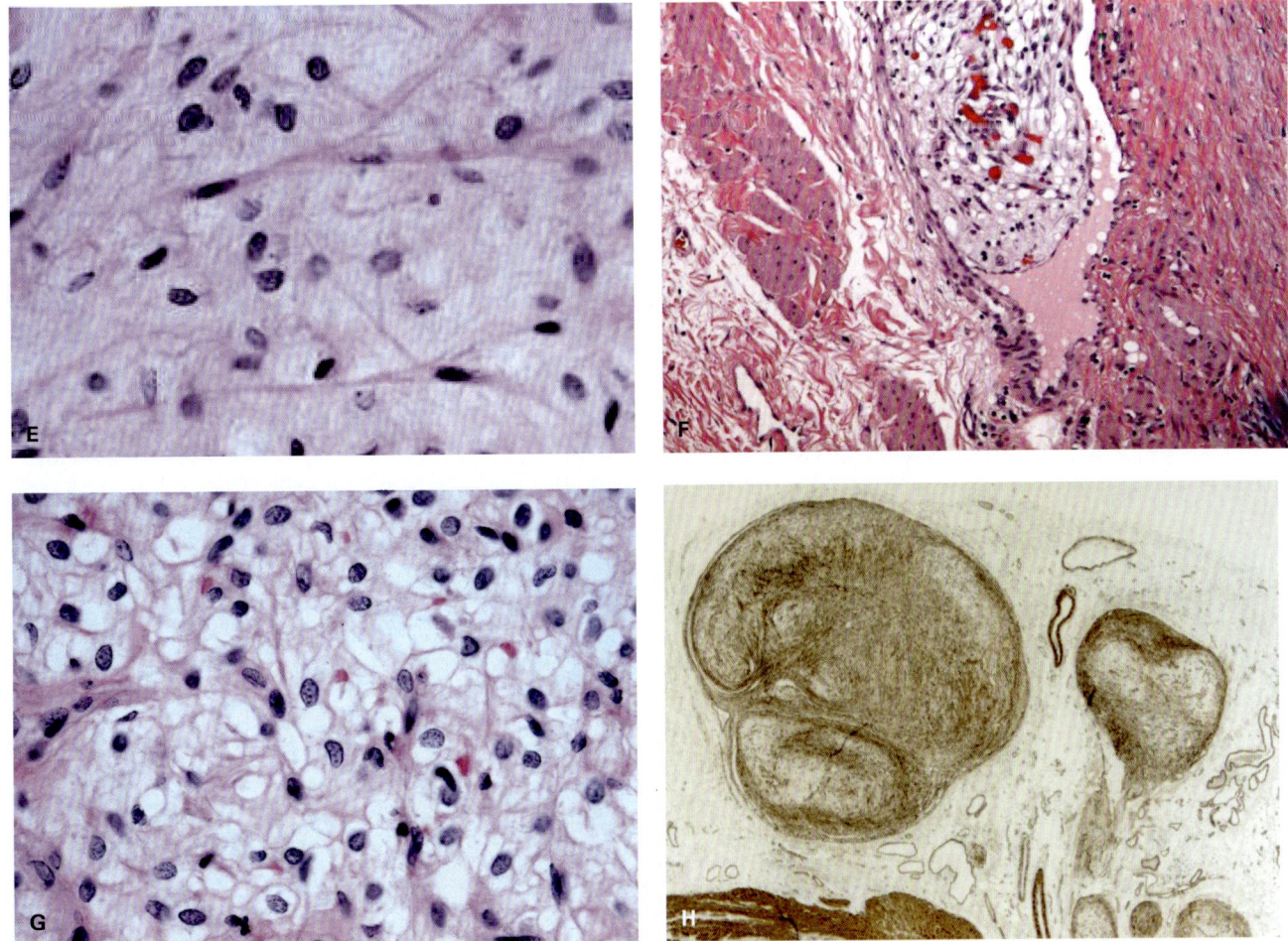

Figure 7-25. (*Continued*) A prominent arborizing capillary network is usually present (**D**). Intravascular involvement or veins and/or lymphatics are seen in some cases (**F**). Most tumors contain foci in which tumor cells are surrounded by a pseudovacuolar lacunar space limited by a meshwork of collagen fibers (**G**). The majority of tumors are immunoreactive for SMA (**H**).

Inflammatory Myofibroblastic Tumor

IMT is an uncommon mesenchymal neoplasm composed of myofibroblasts and a mixed inflammatory infiltrate in which plasma cells and lymphocytes are prominent, but in which neutrophils, eosinophils, and mast cells can also be found. IMT mainly affects children and young adults but occurs over a wide age range. The lung is the most frequently involved visceral site. The majority of extrapulmonary IMTs are intraabdominal, mostly involving the mesentery, omentum, and liver.[212,215-217] Rarely, IMT arises in the wall of the stomach, small intestine, appendix, colon, or rectum.[212,215] Patients may present with abdominal pain, or with constitutional symptoms such as fever, night sweats, and weight loss. A minority of patients show laboratory abnormalities including anemia, leukocytosis, thrombocytosis, hypergammaglobulinemia, and an elevated erythrocyte sedimentation rate (ESR), which often resolve postresection.[212,215,218]

Grossly, IMTs are usually well circumscribed and vary in size (<1 cm to >35 cm) with larger tumors usually situated within the mesentery or abdominal cavity, where they may impinge on, or infiltrate them (Fig. 7-26A,B). Cut section shows them to be white-tan-yellow, fleshy, lobulated, or whorled. Some are polypoid or pedunculated. Histologically, those involving the wall of the gut are poorly defined and frequently infiltrate the muscularis propria, where they sometimes cause a peculiar splitting of the muscle layer (Fig. 7-26B).[212] Three histologic patterns of IMT are described: (1) The myxoid/vascular pattern shows widely separated stellate to plump spindle cells in an edematous, myxoid, or loose fibrous stroma accompanied by inflammatory cells and fairly evenly distributed vascularity. (2) The compact spindled cell pattern shows cells arranged in fascicles, storiform arrangements or haphazardly, intralesional inflammatory cells, often in a prominent regular vascular network (Fig. 7-26C,D). (3) The hypocellular sclerotic pattern resembles a scar or fibromatosis.[212,215] The lesional cells are spindled, fusiform, or plump and resemble fibroblasts/myofibroblasts morphologically, immunohistochemically, and ultrastructurally.

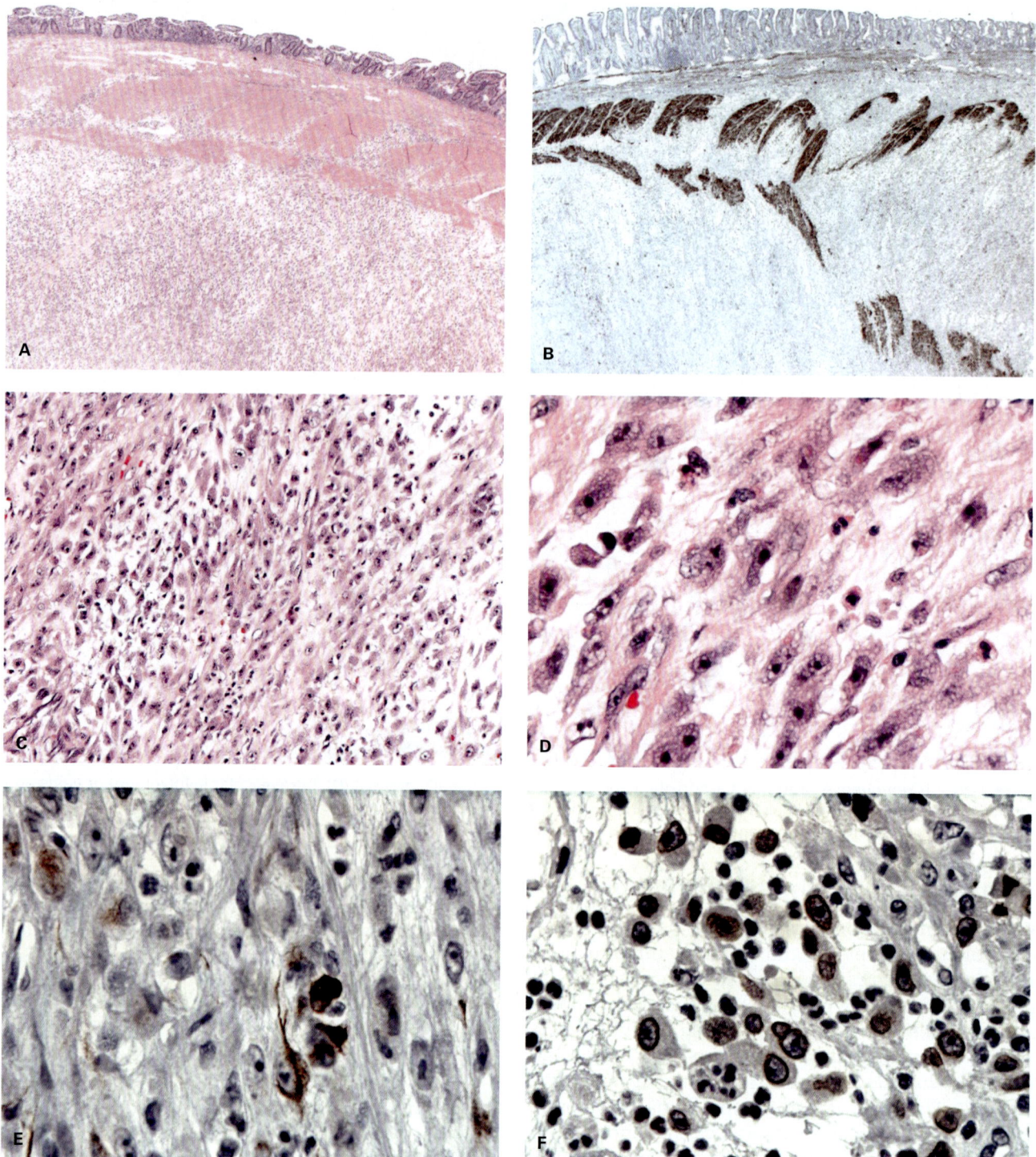

Figure 7-26. Inflammatory myofibroblastic tumor **(A)**. Overview of tumor impinging on the jejunum and **(B)** infiltrating into the muscularis propria, separating it into two parts (desmin). **C,D**: Fascicles of spindled cells with occasional rounded more epithelioid cells together with a smattering of eosinophils and neutrophils. **E**: Alk1 showing the nuclear membrane staining that portends a poor prognosis and may justify tumors of this type being called "sarcomas." **F**: Desmin stain showing occasional immunoreactive cells and their processes.

Moderate to marked cytologic atypia is seen in about 50% of cases (Fig. 7-26D). The mitotic rate rarely exceeds 1–2/10 HPF. The inflammatory infiltrate is usually dominated by plasma cells and may include lymphoid follicles, sometimes with reactive germinal centers (Fig. 7-24F and H).[212] Round to polygonal cells with large vesicular nuclei, prominent nucleoli, and abundant eosinophilic or amphophillic cytoplasm are admixed with the spindled cells (Fig. 7-26D). They may predominate in clinically more aggressive tumors (round cell transformation).[212,216] Most IMTs are at least focally immunoreactive for SMA and sometimes desmin (Fig. 7-26F) and about a third are positive for keratin, usually diffusely, but are negative for CD34, S100, CD117, and DOG1. About 40% to 60% of IMTs are immunoreactive for the anaplastic lymphoma kinase (ALK) protein,[216,219] and a subgroup harbors clonal chromosomal rearrangements involving chromosome band 2p23, the site of the *ALK* gene.[219] Some believe this warrants a change of suffix to "sarcoma" from "tumor" in view of the poor prognosis of these tumors. It also appears to be linked to the RANBP2-ALK fusion product.[220] An example with this fusion product is shown in Figure 7-26E.

The differential diagnosis depends on the morphologic pattern. *Myxoid/vascular* lesions overlap with IFP, *compact spindle cell* lesions with GIST, fibrohistiocytic lesions, lymphoma (Hodgkin's and non-Hodgkin's), follicular and interdigitating dendritic cell sarcoma, histiocytic sarcoma and metastatic carcinoma, and *hypocellular, sclerotic* lesions with fibromatosis, sclerosing mesenteritis, and sclerosing lymphomas. Clues to the diagnosis include clinical (young age, constitutional symptoms, abnormal laboratory findings) and morphologic (spindled or fusiform tumor with inflammatory infiltrate rich in plasma cells). The morphologic pattern will dictate the immunohistochemical panel required to rule out the abovementioned possibilities.

Most tumors are clinically benign but about 25% may recur locally and rare examples of malignant transformation and metastasis are reported.[212,215] Histology does not reliably predict outcome although some have found poorer outcome to correlate with marked cytologic atypia[212,221,222] and the compact cellular pattern.[212] Surgical resection is the mainstay of treatment.

Solitary Fibrous Tumor/Hemangiopericytoma

Solitary fibrous tumor is a rare, predominantly pleural-based tumor,[223] which may also arise in the peritoneum or retroperitoneum.[224,225] When adherent to the visceral peritoneum, it may present clinically as GI tumor.[226,227] Grossly, solitary fibrous tumors are well circumscribed, often pseudoencapsulated, and frequently distinctly lobulated.[223,224,228] Histologically, they feature ovoid to fusiform, spindled cells arranged in short fascicles, whorls or a "patternless pattern." The tumor cells have bland, uniform nuclei, inconspicuous nucleoli, and fairly scant eosinophilic cytoplasm that often merges with the surrounding collagen (Fig. 7-27). Other typical features include alternating areas of hypo- and hypercellularity, ropy keloidal collagen, hyalinized areas, and "hemangiopericytoma-like" vessels[223,224,229] (Fig. 7-27). Most are immunoreactive for CD34 (80%–90%) and CD99 (70%) while a minority express BCl-2, EMA, and SMA. They are negative for CD117, cytokeratin, desmin, and S100.[224,229,230] Ultrastructurally, they show fibroblastic or occasional myofibroblastic differentiation.[224] Most solitary fibrous tumors are cured by complete local excision but roughly 10% to 15% of extrapleural tumors recur or metastasize.[230] Histology is unreliable in predicting clinical behavior but large tumor size, infiltrative margins, high cellularity, nuclear pleomorphism, tumor necrosis, and high mitotic activity (>4/10 HPF) are associated with an increased risk of malignant behavior.[230]

A few cases of GI hemangiopericytoma have been reported in the older literature.[231,232] Most would likely be reclassified today as solitary fibrous tumor or as other tumors with hemangiopericytomatous vasculature. Given the major histologic and immunohistochemical overlap between hemangiopericytoma and solitary fibrous tumor and lack of clear distinguishing criteria, pathologists are gradually abandoning of the term hemangiopericytoma in favor of solitary fibrous tumor.[230]

Calcifying Fibrous Tumor

This rare soft tissue tumor of young adults may arise in the mesentery, omentum, stomach, or small intestine, with over 30 intraabdominal cases reported to date.[233–240] They may be multifocal.[234,238,241] Most gastric and small intestinal lesions arise beneath the peritoneum, but mural lesions also occur. They are well circumscribed, paucicellular lesions composed of bland spindled cells in a hyalinized collagenous stroma with a patchy perivascular lymphoplasmacytic infiltrate. Extensive dystrophic or psammomatous calcification is a defining feature (Fig. 7-28).[233,235,236,238,239] Most cases should be readily diagnosed on the basis of their classic morphology. However, if not recognized as such, the potential for confusion with GIST, desmoid tumor, IMT, and solitary fibrous tumor exist. Although long-term follow-up data are limited, recurrences have not been reported to date. A conservative approach therefore seems reasonable with radiologic follow-up for lesions removed by enucleation.

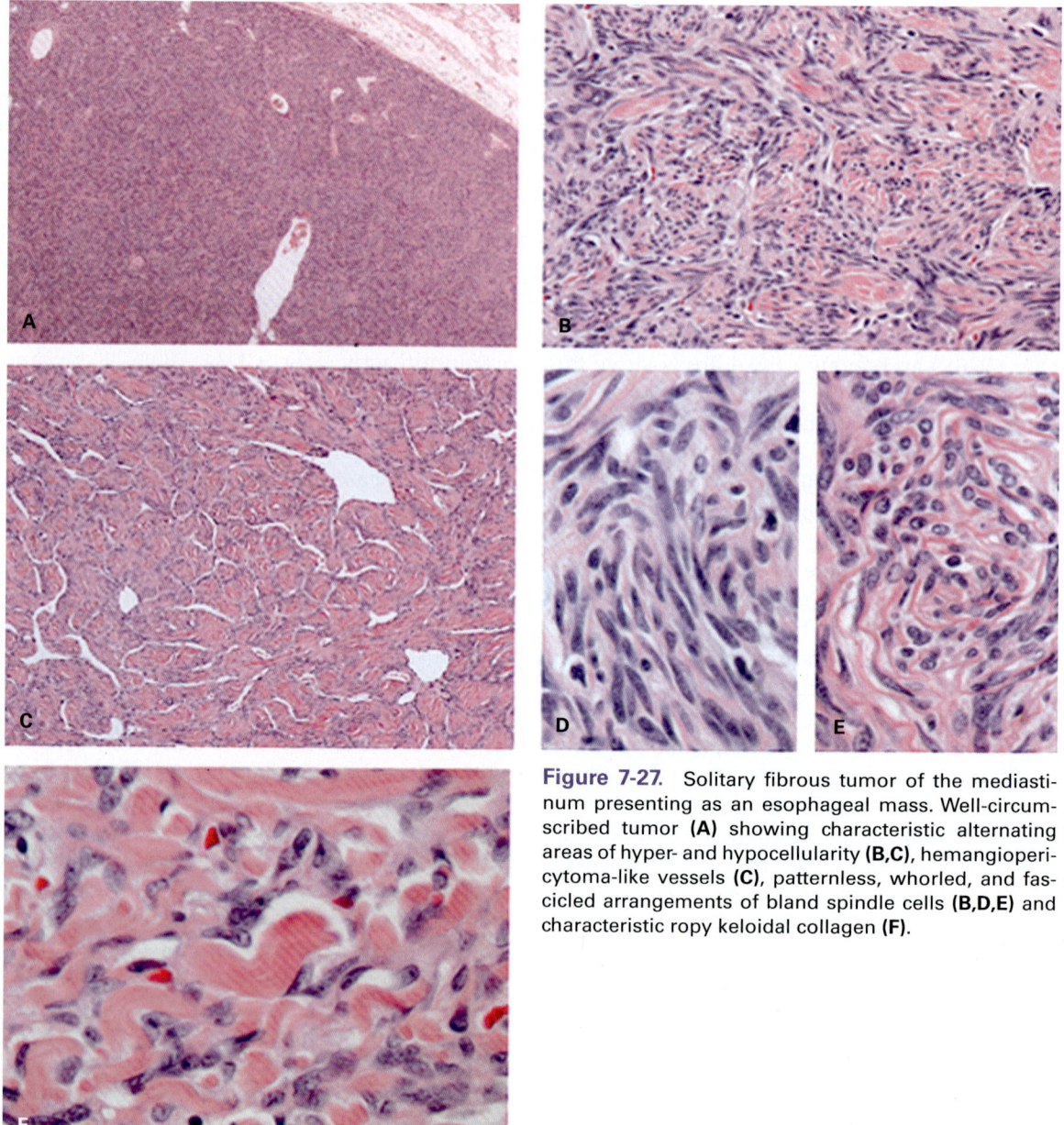

Figure 7-27. Solitary fibrous tumor of the mediastinum presenting as an esophageal mass. Well-circumscribed tumor **(A)** showing characteristic alternating areas of hyper- and hypocellularity **(B,C)**, hemangiopericytoma-like vessels **(C)**, patternless, whorled, and fascicled arrangements of bland spindle cells **(B,D,E)** and characteristic ropy keloidal collagen **(F)**.

Elastofibroma

There are rare reports of elastofibroma-like lesions in the GI tract. Two occurred in the stomach[242,243] and two in the sigmoid colon (both polyps).[244,245] One of the gastric elastofibromas was associated with elastofibromas in the subscapular region.[242] One of sigmoid elastofibromas occurred at a polypectomy site (for adenomatous polyp), suggesting a reactive process.[244] Elastofibromatous change and elastosis in the GI tract are described, mostly presenting as mucosal polyps. These do not form distinct mass lesions. Whether some of them represent residual of sclerosed vessels, especially arteriovenous malformations remains a speculation. They may mimic amyloid on H&E but lack congophilia.[246,247]

ADIPOCYTIC LESIONS

Lipohyperplasia of the Ileocecal Valve

This is by far the most common lipomatous lesion in the GI tract and is strongly associated with obesity. In an autopsy series, over 50% of all cases had moderate or marked lipohyperplasia. The degree of lipohyperplasia correlated with body weight and the

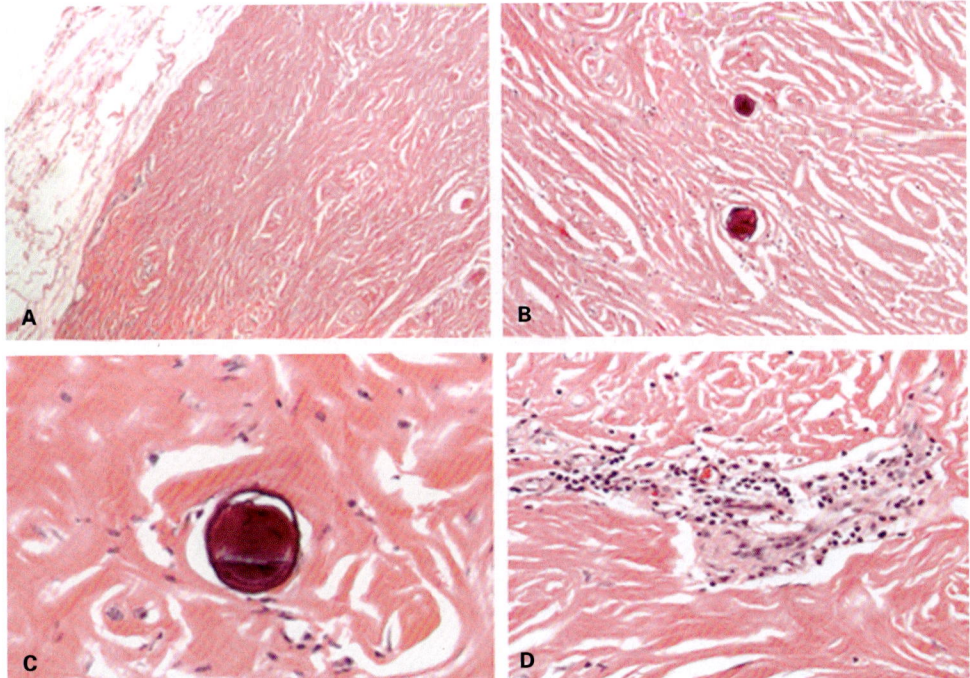

Figure 7-28. Calcifying fibrous tumor with characteristic circumscribed border (A), low cellularity and hyalinized collagenous stroma (A-C), psammomatous calcification (D,C), and patchy perivascular chronic inflammation (D).

degree of right ventricular fatty infiltration.[248] Grossly, the ileocecal valve appears patulous due to submucosal fat deposition (Fig. 7-29) but may also produce a tumor-like lesion resembling a lipoma. Occasionally, this is biopsied due to concern over the possibility of a neoplasm. Its characteristic structure, namely an inner "spine" of muscularis propria (Fig. 7-29), may not be evident on biopsy. It is usually asymptomatic, but larger examples may produce clinical and radiologic signs and symptoms of a tumor, for example, obstruction and intussusception.[248]

Submucosal Lipoma

These are among the most frequently encountered mesenchymal tumors in the large bowel at colonoscopy[249] and are found, albeit rarely, in all other parts of the GI tract, including the small bowel (Fig. 7-30).[250] They are usually recognized endoscopically because of their yellow color and pliability, although they may be quite firm. They frequently have a smooth surface, but may have unusual shapes resulting from peristalsis (squeeze sign). The overlying mucosa is often

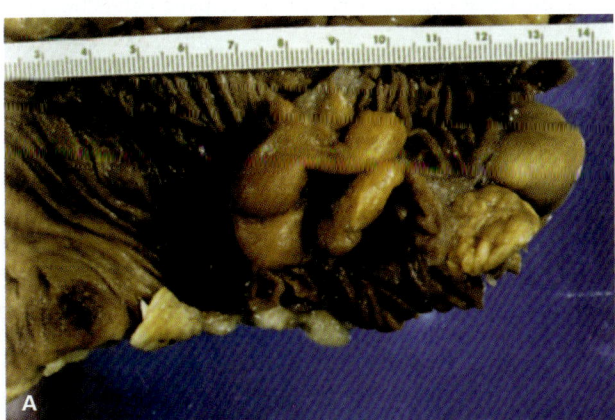
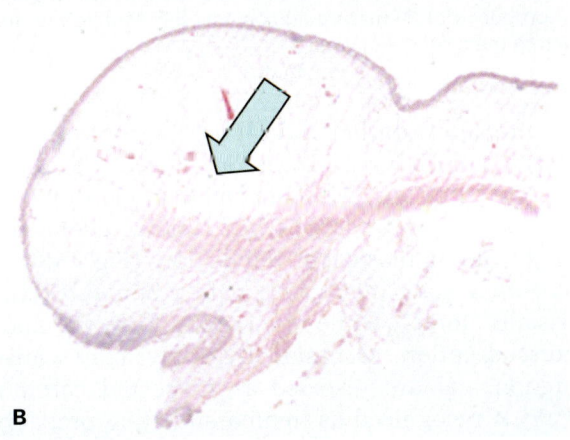

Figure 7-29. Lipohyperplasia of the ileocecal valve. A: Gross specimen showing the typical pouted lips of lipohyperplasia. B: Section through the ileocecal valve demonstrating the marked submucosal fat deposition and inner "spine" of the muscularis propria (arrow) going toward the mucosal junction of the ileum (lower left) and large bowel (top right). Abundant fat is also seen beyond the muscularis propria.

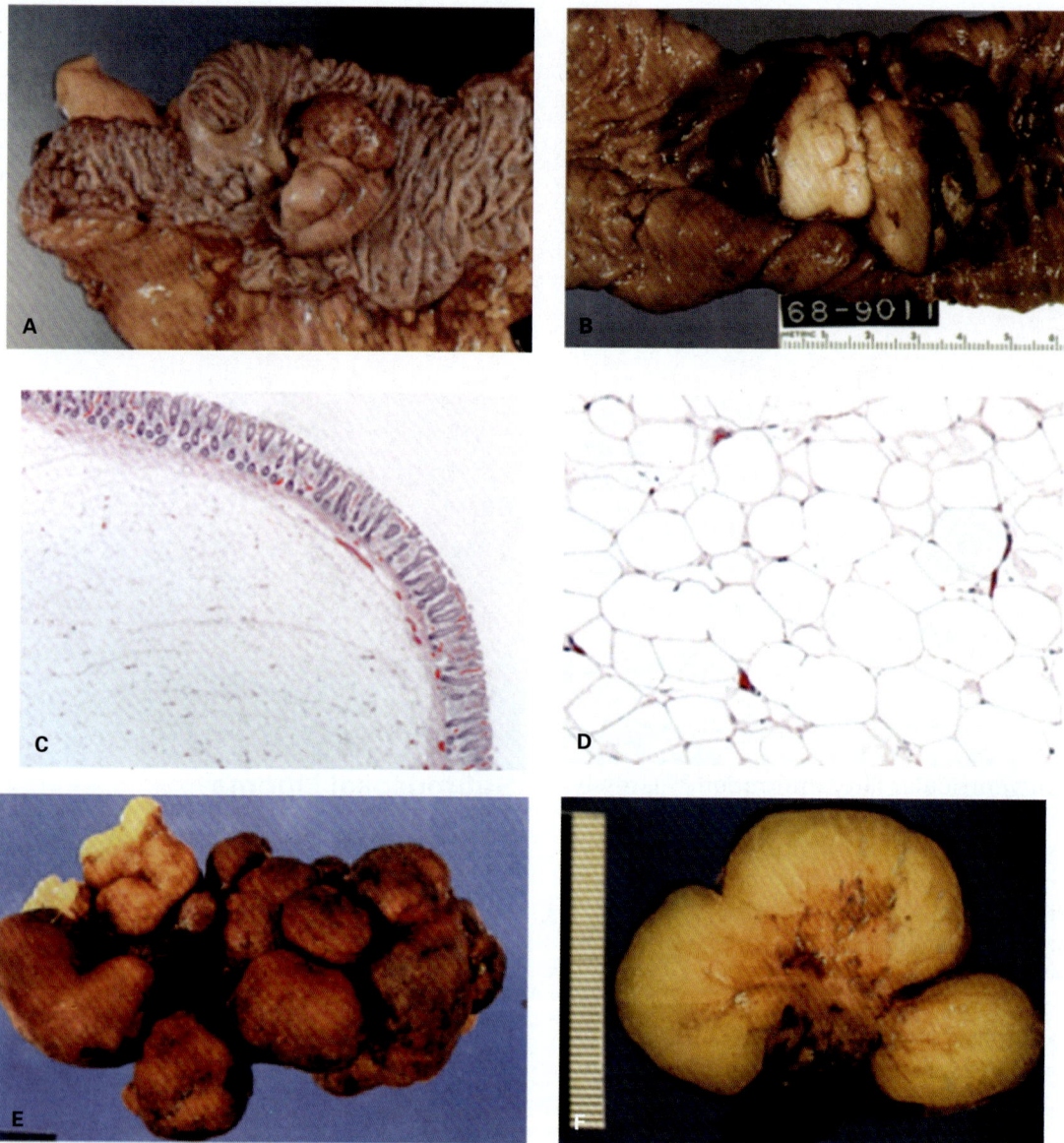

Figure 7-30. Submucosal lipomas. **A:** Typical multilobated submucosal lipoma, here in the ascending colon, with overlying mucosa covering the tumor. **B:** Superficial ulceration and hemorrhage in the mucosa overlying a lipoma. **C,D:** Histology shows a submucosal tumor composed of 30 mature adipocytes. **E,F:** Multilobed duodenal lipoma that caused recurrent acute pancreatitis by repeatedly obstructing the ampulla of Vater.

easily retracted from the underlying fat (tenting) and if biopsied can give the impression of pushing into a sponge (cushion sign). Most are small and asymptomatic but rarely can be large, with central ulceration, bleeding, and hemosiderin deposition (Fig. 7-30B). Those with a stalk may cause pain when subjected to peristaltic forces, while others may form the apex of intussusception. Occasionally, they may cause obstruction and are resected as suspected carcinomas.[251,252] If recognized as lipomatous, they probably best left untouched unless there is an indication to do otherwise. As with all submucosal tumors, simple forceps biopsy is usually not deep enough to obtain diagnostic material. However, a biopsy may be submitted to prove that the overlying mucosa is indeed normal, and, by inference, that the tumor is submucosal. Electrocautery snare polypectomy is usually avoided because of the significant risk of bleeding from the stalk. In instances where these tumors are resected endoscopically or surgically, they are well circumscribed, often encapsulated and limited to the submucosa, consisting of mature lipocytes (Fig. 7-30).

Atypical Lipoma

Rarely, atypical features are found in large bowel lipomas, including increased cellularity and fibrosis, atypical hyperchromatic nuclei, and increased mitotic activity, with occasional atypical forms associated with ulceration. They do not indicate malignancy.[253]

Angiolipoma

Rare reports of angiolipoma, identical to those occurring in soft tissue, have been described in the stomach, duodenum, and colon. These tumors contain focal proliferations of capillaries often with luminal fibrin thrombi.[254–256]

Lipomatous Polyposis and Epiploic Lipomatosis

Lipomatous polyposis is a rare condition characterized by tens to hundreds of polypoid submucosal lipomas of the colon, which may be massive (Fig. 7-31), and with fatty masses elsewhere in the abdomen. Sometimes there is massive hypertrophy of the appendices epiploicae of the colon (epiploic lipomatosis). The small intestine may also be involved,[257] and myriads of submucosal lipomas may be present (Fig. 7-31).[258,259] In general, these polyps do not undergo malignant transformation,[260] although an isolated case of a mesenteric liposarcoma occurring in the setting of sigmoid lipomatosis is on record.[261] They are sometimes associated with volvulus, small intestinal antimesenteric diverticula,[262] and ileal intussusception.[263] It is not uncommon to see changes of a hyperplastic polyp or sessile serrated polyp overlying a submucosal lipoma.

Liposarcoma

Most cases represent secondary GI involvement by a retroperitoneal or mesenteric liposarcoma. Primary GI liposarcoma is very rare and tends to be gastric. Isolated cases in the small and large intestine are described. Primary GI liposarcomas are clinically aggressive. Dedifferentiated liposarcoma frequently expresses CD34 and smooth muscle actin, and less commonly CD117; however, dedifferentiated liposarcomas do not express DOG1, thereby mitigating confusion with GIST. Further, GIST-type kit mutations are absent, although some have been shown to contain single-nucleotide polymorphisms in codon 7.[264] Dedifferentiated liposarcoma typically shows MDM2 amplification and/or overexpression. This is present in a minority of other neoplasms, including

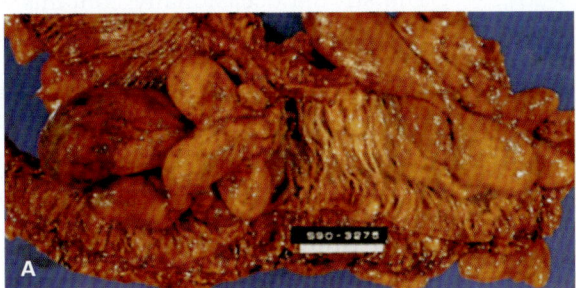
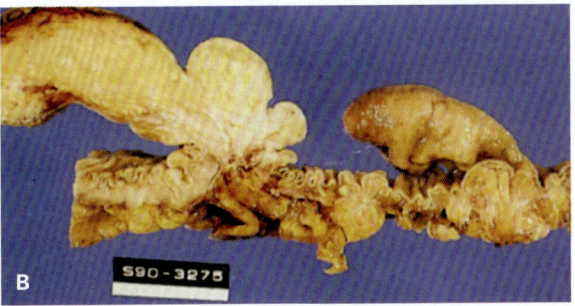
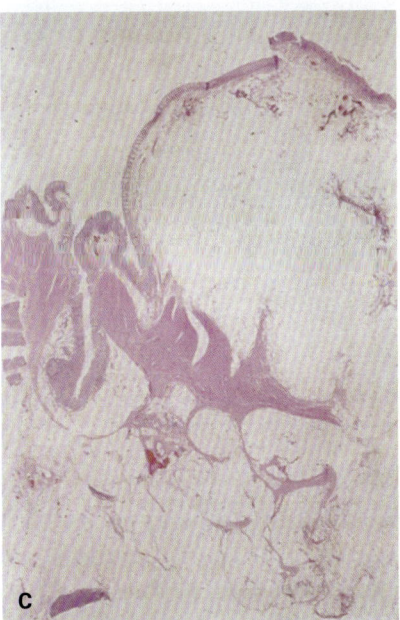

Figure 7-31. Massive submucosal lipomatosis of the sigmoid colon, which presented with features of obstruction and bleeding. An intussusception was found but could not be completely reduced. **A:** Resected specimen showing numerous lipomas, the largest of the most distal group being superficially ulcerated. **B:** Sections through the distal tumors displaying the fat. **C:** Part of one tumor showing extension through the muscularis propria.

3% to 5% of GISTs; therefore, interpretation in the appropriate clinical–radiologic and pathologic context is necessary.[265,266]

Differential Diagnosis of Fatty Tumors

While this comment may seem a little fatuous (groan), it should be remembered that gas penetrating the wall of the large bowel at colonoscopy (pseudolipomatosis)[253] and the injection of fatty substances (oleogranuloma) can both cause lesions resembling fat cells (see Chapter 20). In both of these cases, there is usually a mucosal and a submucosal component, the latter containing spaces too large for fat cells. Apart from the fairly characteristic endoscopic features described above, CT provides a good method of distinguishing fat from other tissue.[267]

ENDOTHELIAL AND VASCULAR TUMORS

Angiodysplasia and other vascular malformations are described in Chapter 2. Kaposi's sarcoma involving the GI tract is reviewed in Chapter 3 but is discussed briefly.

Hemangioma

Hemangiomas of the GI tract may be classified on the basis of the predominant vessel type as capillary, cavernous, venous, arteriovenous, or other mixtures.[268] They occur most commonly in the small intestine with the colon, the second most common site.[269] Capillary hemangiomas are very rare, typically small (although can exceed 10 cm), usually solitary, generally submucosal lesions composed of small closely packed capillaries often surrounded by a thin fibrous capsule. Endoscopically, they appear as bluish-red polypoid or ill-defined nodular lesions. Some lesions reported as capillary hemangiomas may, in fact, be vascular ectasias. Capillary hemangiomas rarely cause clinical symptoms. Cavernous, venous, arteriovenous, and other mixed hemangiomas can occur in a localized or diffuse form[270-272] and have a similar distribution and clinical significance regardless of histologic vessel type.[273] Patients may present at any age with symptoms of a mass or with rectal bleeding, which may be massive and life threatening. Endoscopically, the lesions appear as red or blue, compressible mucosal papules, nodules, or cysts. Diffuse forms may contiguously involve large segments of intestine (up to 30 cm). In resection specimens, hemangiomas vary in appearance from red to purple nodular, localized (often submucosal) lesions sometimes with discernable cysts or vascular spaces, to grossly ectatic vascular channels traversing the intestinal wall or involving the subserosal connective tissues (Fig. 7-32). Histologically, cavernous hemangiomas are composed of blood-filled, sinus-like spaces supported by connective tissue (Fig. 7-33).[270,273]. The stroma occasionally contains smooth muscle. Fibrin thrombi often organizing, hyalinization and calcification may be present. A lesion composed of an abnormal proliferation of veins and arteries with evidence of arteriovenous shunting is referred to as an arteriovenous hemangioma. Venous hemangiomas are characterized by large thick-walled vessels resembling normal veins but occasionally having more disorganized smooth muscle in their walls.[268] There

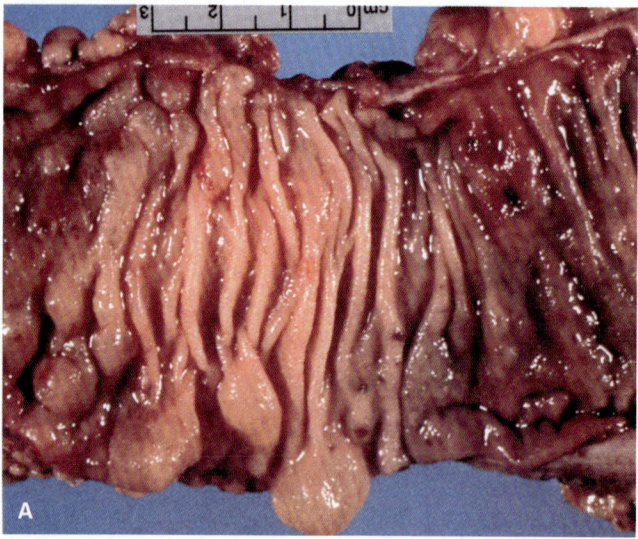
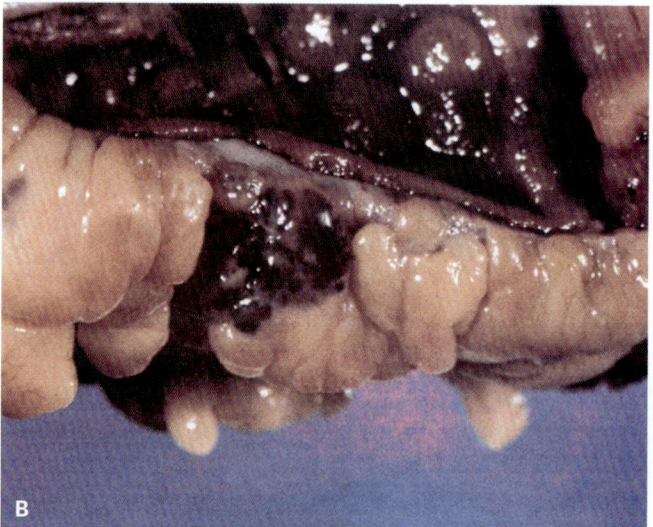

Figure 7-32. Cavernous hemangioma gross. **A:** Opened colonic specimen demonstrates mucosal polypoid systs. **B:** Abnormal vascular structure in the subserosa of a colonic cavernous hemangioma. (Reprinted from Riddell RH, Petras RE, Williams GT, et al. *Atlas of Tumor Pathology: Tumors of the Intestines.* Washington, DC: Armed Forces Institute of Pathology, 2003, with permission.)

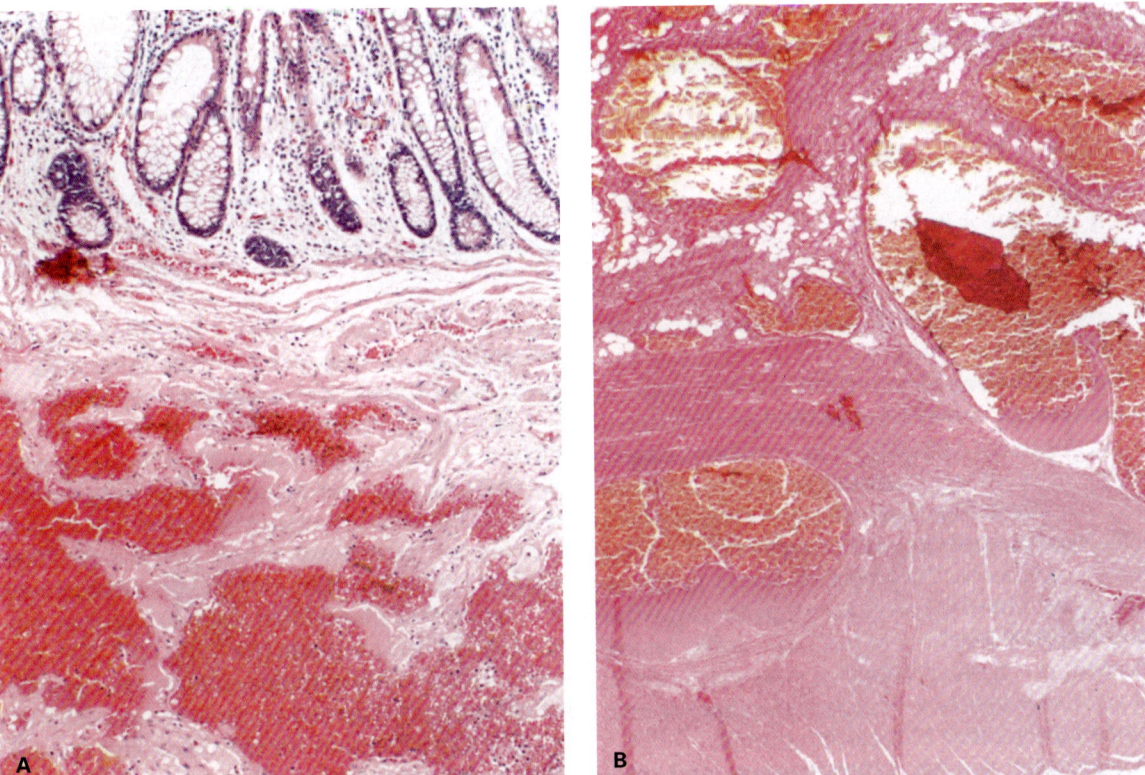

Figure 7-33. Cavernous hemangioma micro. **A:** The Hemangioma is composed of blood-filled sinus-like spaces that are supported by connective tissue in the submucosa. **B:** The lesion involves the submucosa and muscularis propria. (Reprinted from Riddell RH, Petras RE, Williams GT, et al. *Atlas of Tumor Pathology: Tumors of the Intestines.* Washington, DC: Armed Forces Institute of Pathology, 2003, with permission.)

are extremely rare reports of tumors composed of a mixture of dilated vascular channels and lymphatics. These can be referred to as hemangiolymphangiomas, mixed hemangioma and lymphangioma, or lymphaticovenous malformations.[23,269] Localized hemangiomas can be treated by fulguration, excision, or sometimes radiation therapy, whereas diffuse forms may require surgical resection where possible. In unresectable lesions, treatment should be directed toward controlling complications (e.g., sclerotherapy or embolization).[23,269]

Angiosarcoma

Angiosarcoma only rarely arises in the GI tract, usually in the small or large intestine (Fig. 7-34A–C).[274] It is a highly aggressive tumor with a poor prognosis. The median age at presentation is 65 and most present with bleeding or anemia. The varied histologic spectrum of angiosarcoma, ranging from well-formed vascular structures to sheets of malignant epithelioid or spindle cells, encompasses a wide histologic differential diagnosis, which includes poorly differentiated adenocarcinoma, Kaposi's sarcoma, melanoma, other sarcomas with epithelioid morphology and GIST. Grossly, angiosarcoma may be solitary or multifocal and typically forms red-gray polypoid masses or mural nodules[23] (Fig. 7-32A). As with most deep-seated angiosarcomas, those arising in the GI tract usually have epithelioid morphology. Interestingly, those associated with prior radiation or foreign material have a propensity for classical well-differentiated vasoformative morphology.[274]

The poorly differentiated epithelioid variant, which is characterized by sheets of malignant polygonal cells and only rare vasoformative structures or intracytoplasmic lumens, may be confused with an adenocarcinoma. This problem is compounded by their frequent immunoreactivity for the pankeratin AE1/AE3, CAM5.2, and CK19[274] and the absence of ultrastructural features of endothelial differentiation in some poorly differentiated tumors. Cytokeratins should, therefore, not be used in isolation when working up an undifferentiated epithelioid neoplasm. The panel should include endothelial markers (CD31, CD34, and factor VIII), of which CD31 is the most reliable. A careful search for subtle clefting or occasional intracytoplasmic lumina containing erythrocytes should be performed. The frequent immunoreactivity of angiosarcoma for both CD117 and CD34, occasional immunoreactivity for DOG1, may lead to confusion with a GIST, particularly in those with a sheet-like architecture; a panel of endothelial markers can prevent this pitfall.

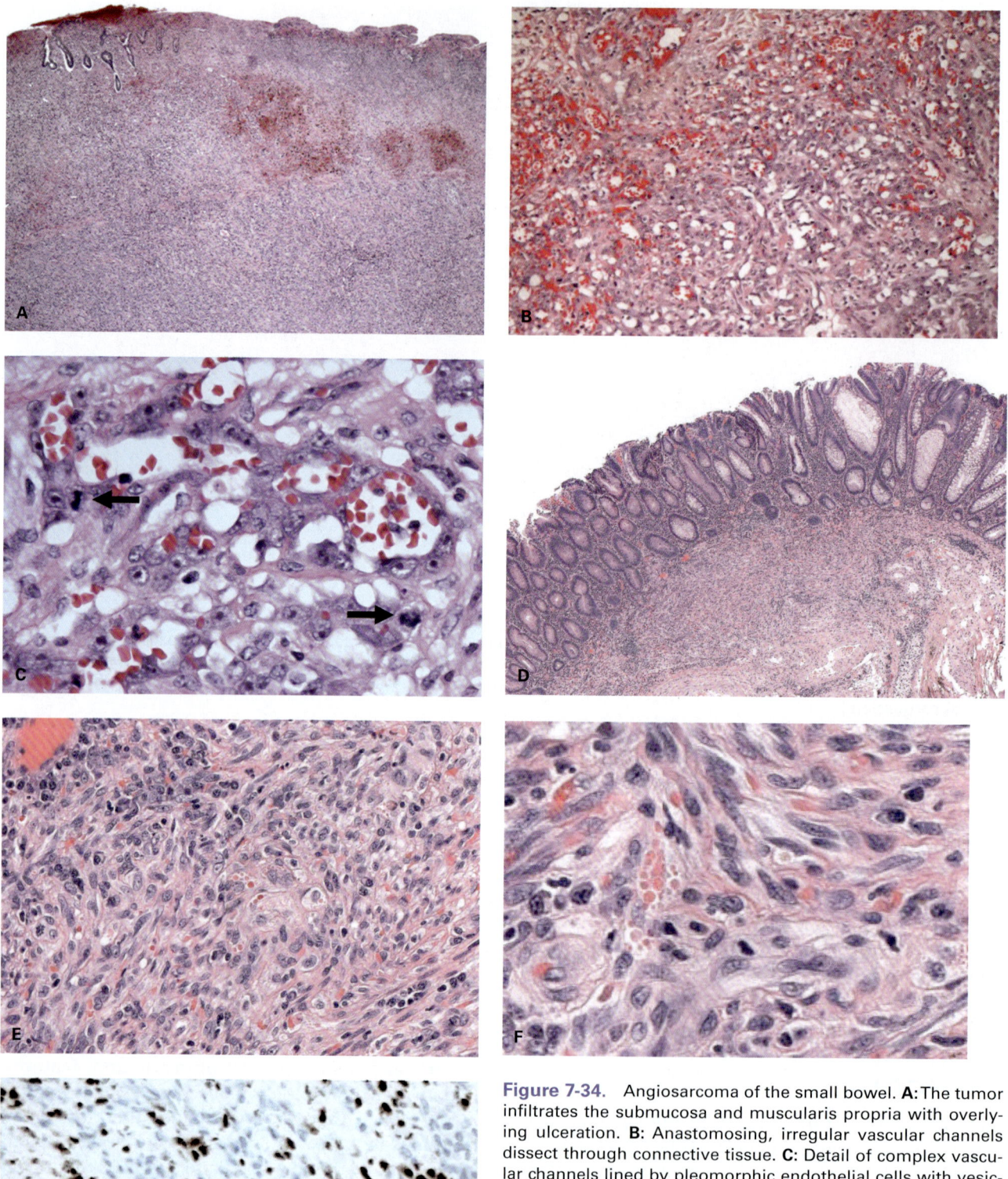

Figure 7-34. Angiosarcoma of the small bowel. A: The tumor infiltrates the submucosa and muscularis propria with overlying ulceration. B: Anastomosing, irregular vascular channels dissect through connective tissue. C: Detail of complex vascular channels lined by pleomorphic endothelial cells with vesicular nuclei, prominent nucleoli, and frequent mitotic figures (arrows). D–G: Kaposi's sarcoma arising in a tubular adenoma. E,F: Spindle cells line slit-like vascular spaces containing erythrocytes. F: Eosinophilic hyaline globules and plasma cells are typically present. G: The tumor shows immunoreactivity for HHV-8. (Courtesy of Dr David Driman, London, Ontario.).

Angiosarcoma may be mimicked by a florid but benign vascular proliferation occurring in the setting of mucosal prolapse or intussusception.[275] These lesions are characterized by a proliferation of small vessels that may extend throughout the full thickness of the bowel as seen with angiosarcoma. Clues to the diagnosis include the presence of lobular architecture, benign cytologic features, and infrequent mitoses and absence of abnormal forms, features of mucosal prolapse or intussusception, and benign clinical course. This benign entity should be considered before diagnosing angiosarcoma in the setting of mucosal prolapse or intussusception.[275]

Kaposi's Sarcoma

Kaposi's sarcoma can usually be distinguished based on the clinical history of immunosuppression, morphology, and immunoreactivity for human herpes virus 8 (see Chapter 3). The well-differentiated forms can be difficult to distinguish from a hemangioma. However, dissection of vascular channels through connective tissues, formation of interanastomosing sinusoids, hyperchromatic nuclei, frequent mitoses figures, and cellular "piling up," usually help to correctly identify angiosarcoma (Fig. 7-34D–G).

Lymphangioma

These rare localized small tumors occur most frequently in the duodenum and colon, and histologically can initially be confused with intestinal lymphangiectasia. Lymphangiomas invariably have numerous dilated lymphatic channels but are localized (Figs. 7-35 and 7-36); conversely, in intestinal malabsorption, lymphangiectasia tends to be variable, ranging from single dilated lymphatic channels in only occasional villi to numerous dilated channels. However, malabsorption and more generalized lymphedema (Milroy's disease) is invariably present. Rarely, a single dilated lymphatic can be found in a villus as an isolated microscopic finding in the absence of lipid vacuoles in enterocytes that might indicate a possible postprandial effect (Fig. 7-35E). Small submucosal lymphatic cysts are quite common in the small intestine if searched for; one study found them in 35/150 consecutive autopsies, all <1 cm in diameter

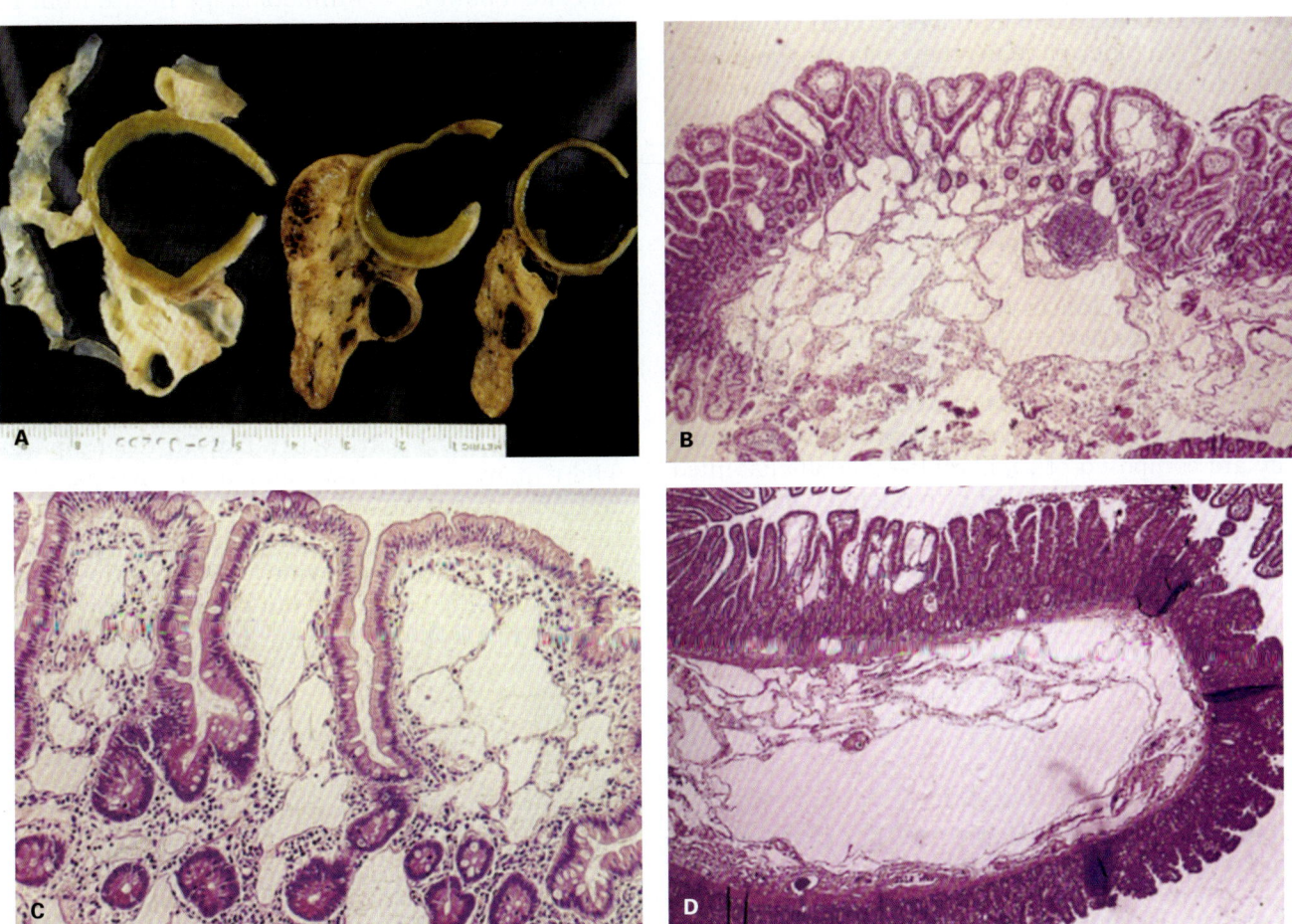

Figure 7-35. Localized lymphangioma. **A:** Gross appearance of a sectioned lymphangioma involving the small bowel. **B,C:** Localized lymphangioma in the duodenum with numerous dilated lymphatic channels in the mucosa and submucosa. **D:** Jejunal tumor in which most of the lesion is submucosa, with focal extension into the mucosa.

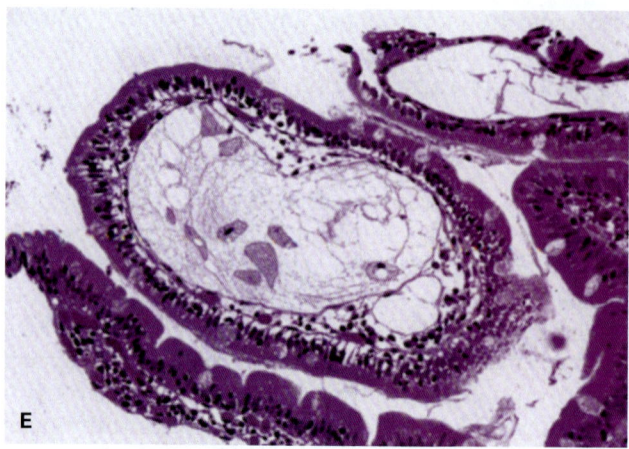

Figure 7-35. (*Continued*) **E:** An isolated group of villi biopsied incidentally. No lesion was visible endoscopically.

and all in patients 55 years old or more.[276] We have also found them in patients undergoing resection for Crohn's disease; we suspect that it may represent pre-existing lymphatic dilatation potentiated by the lymphangiectasia seen in Crohn's disease.

Most lymphangiomas are asymptomatic and incidental. However, larger mass lesions may sometimes present with rectal bleeding and pain, often in younger patients[277]; in older patients, they may also be associated with diarrhea. Exophytic lesions may result in intussusception or obstruction. Most are solitary but multiple lesions may occur (intestinal lymphangiomatosis). There is a wide age range but no particular sex preference. They vary from 1 to 8 cm in diameter and appear to occur anywhere in the small or large bowel or in the mesentery.[277] Rarely, large submucosal lymphatic channels occur that may be cystically dilated (chylous cyst)[278]; however, extension into the mucosa is not a prominent feature. Endoscopically, they appear as translucent, broad-based lesions with a smooth overlying mucosal surface. Histologically, they are composed of capillary-like endothelial-lined channels varying from few to numerous and in any or all parts of the bowel wall. They frequently contain eosinophilically staining lymph, which may contain lymphocytes but do not contain red cells (Fig. 7-35 and 7-36). The lining cells are immunoreactive for D2-40 but generally do not express factor VIII-related antigen. Sometimes, tumors occur that are a combination of hemangioma and lymphangioma (hemangiolymphangioma).

Intestinal Vascular Lesions Associated with Clinical Syndromes

Intestinal vascular lesions can be associated with a number of recognized clinical syndromes including hereditary hemorrhagic telangiectasia (Osler–Weber–Rendu disease), progressive systemic sclerosis, blue rubber bleb nevus syndrome, Turner's syndrome, Klippel–Trenaunay syndrome, pseudoxanthoma elasticum, Ehlers–Danlos syndrome, and multifocal lymphangio-endotheliomatosis with thrombocytopenia. These are discussed in Chapters 2 and 8.

STRIATED MUSCLE TUMORS

Rhabdomyoma

There are isolated reports of rhabdomyoma occurring in the esophagus, stomach, and perianal regions including both adult and fetal types.[279–281]

Rhabdomyosarcoma

These tumors primarily involve the head and neck and the urogenital sinus region in children, but rarely arise in the GI tract, mostly the perianal region (about 2% of all rhabdomyosarcomas).[282] Isolated cases are reported in the esophagus, stomach, ampulla of Vater, and small bowel.[283–286] Tumors range in size from 1 to 20 cm (median 4 cm) and have infiltrating margins. Botryoid lesions are polypoid. Histologically, they may resemble either alveolar or embryonal (botryoid) rhabdomyosarcomas (Fig. 7-37).[282] The major issue is differentiating them from other small cell tumors such as lymphomas or even chronic inflammatory tissue. The diagnosis can usually be confirmed using a panel of immunohistochemical markers including myo-D1, myogenin, muscle-specific actin, and desmin. Rhabdomyosarcomas are extremely rare in adults. Therefore, identification of rhabdomyosarcomatous elements in biopsies should prompt consideration of rhabdomyomatous differentiation in a carcinosarcoma. This is particularly true in the esophagus where many so-called rhabdomyosarcomas have been described as having an additional invasive squamous carcinoma, dysplasia, or carcinoma in situ in the adjacent mucosa. A careful search for such epithelial components should be carried out before an unequivocal diagnosis of esophageal rhabdomyosarcoma is made.

MISCELLANEOUS SARCOMAS

Clear Cell Sarcoma

This rare malignant tumor primarily affects tendon sheaths and aponeuroses of the distal extremities in adolescents and young adults[287,288] but rarely arises in the GI tract.[289–295] It can be morphologically,

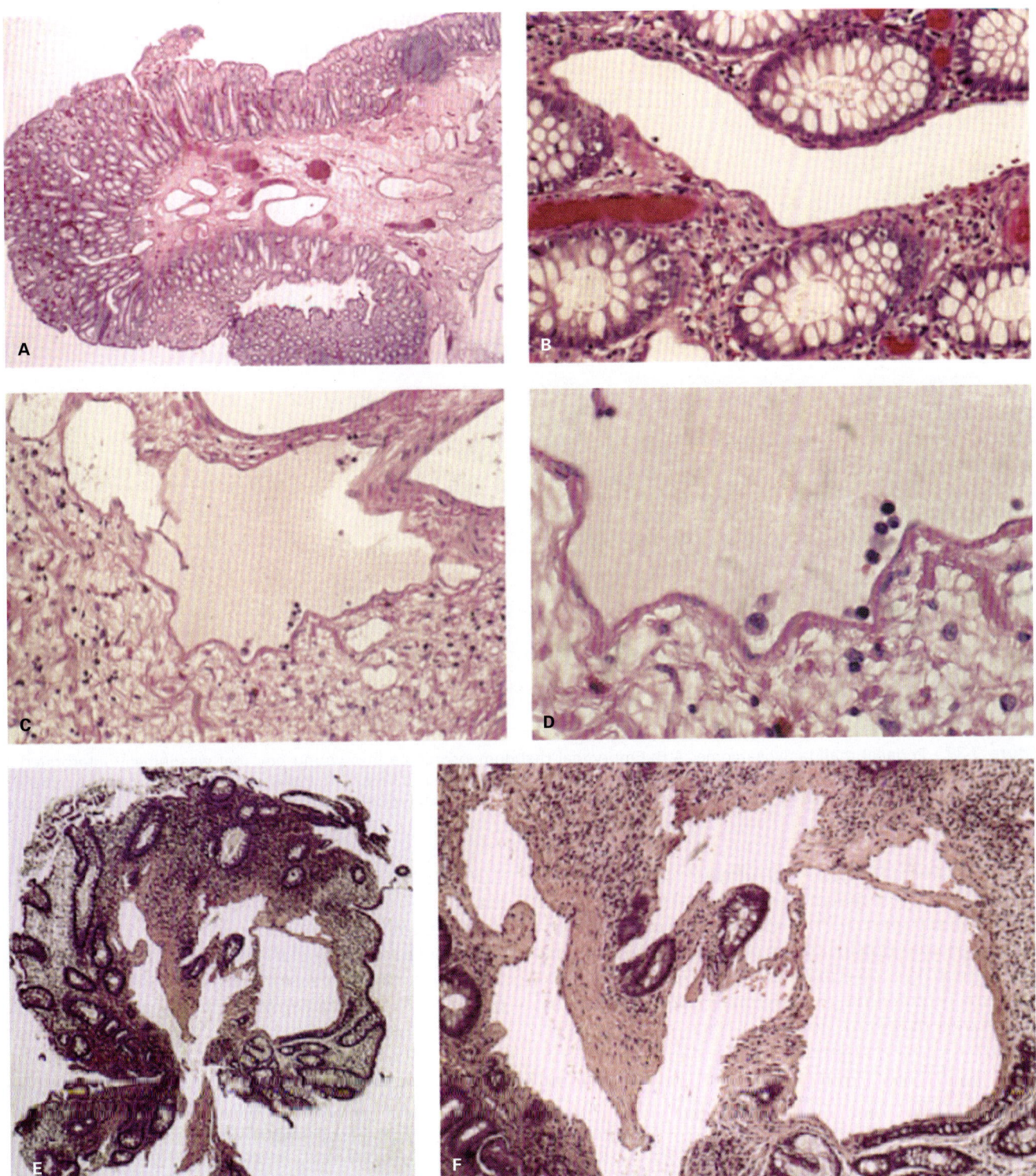

Figure 7-36. Lymphangioma of the large bowel. **A:** Polypoid configuration. **B:** Dilated, endothelium-lined channels penetrating the lamina propria. **C:** Submucosal component of a tumor showing dilated channels containing eosinophilic material without red cells. **D:** Detail showing lymphocytes within the channels. **E,F:** Differential diagnosis is with a localized hemangioma, such as this one in a child with the blue rubber bleb nevus syndrome (see Chapter 2).

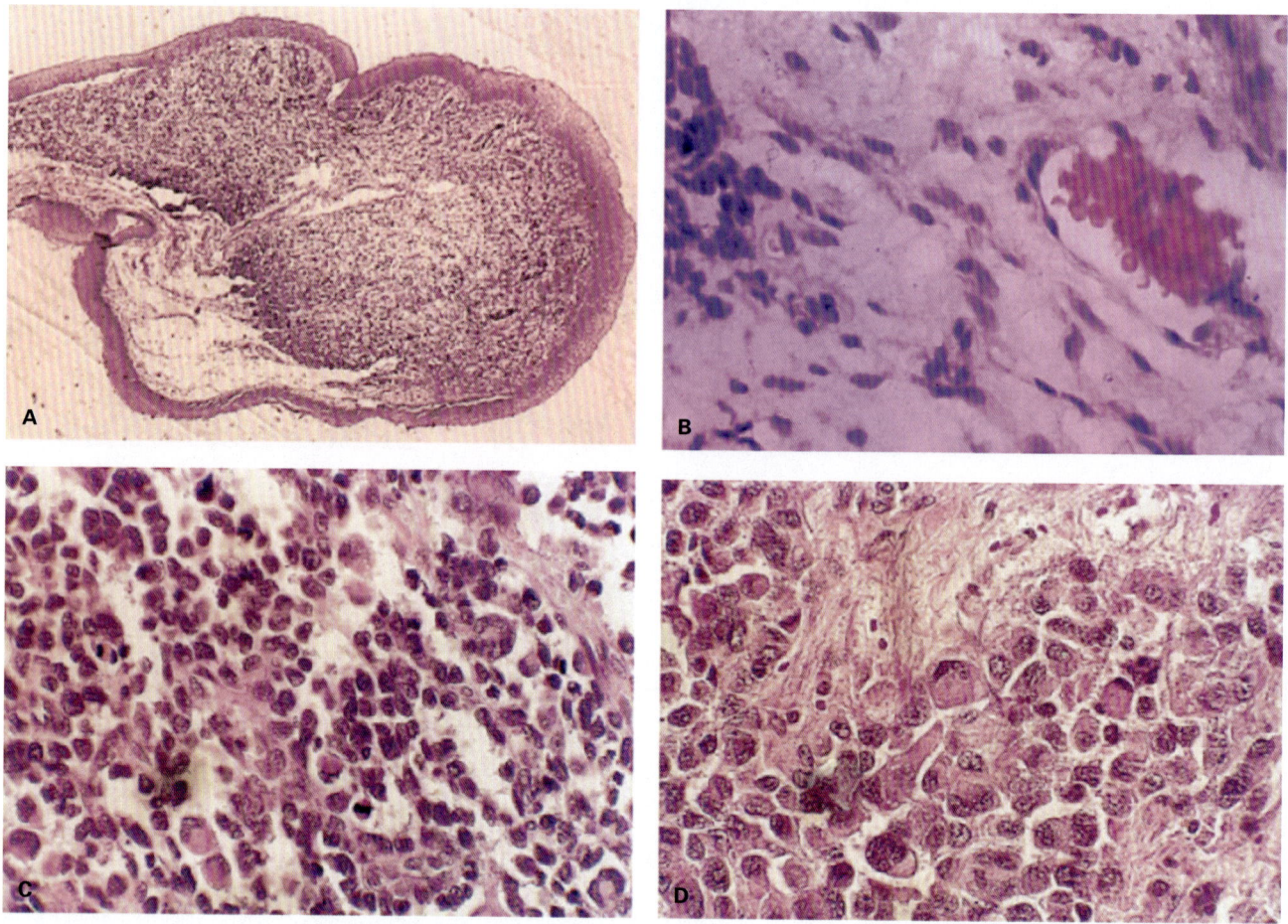

Figure 7-37. Perianal rhabdomyosarcoma. **A,B:** Embryonal rhabdomyosarcoma in a young boy that was initially interpreted as being inflammatory because of the presence of numerous small, lymphocyte-like cells. **C,D:** Perianal alveolar rhabdomyosarcoma in which the more typical alveolar pattern can be appreciated at lower power, with typical rhabdomyoblasts containing eccentric nuclei.

immunohistochemically, and ultrastructurally indistinguishable from melanoma (hence the term "melanoma of soft parts").[289,296] Most clear cell sarcomas have a specific translocation t (12;22) (q13;q12) creating a chimeric *EWS-ATF1* fusion transcript, which is not seen in cutaneous melanoma.[289] Some apparent melanomas metastatic to the GI tract may represent primary clear cell sarcomas. In one study, 2/20 cases originally diagnosed as metastatic melanoma harbored the t (12;22) (q13;q12) translocation.[289] A subsequent study found this translocation in 4/7 cases originally diagnosed as GI melanoma in patients without a history of cutaneous melanoma.[297] Histologically, clear cell sarcomas are composed of cells arranged in nests and short fascicles separated by fibrous septa (Fig. 7-38A–C). The tumor cells are polygonal or spindled with fairly monomorphic nuclei, vesicular chromatin, prominent nucleoli, and clear to eosinophilic cytoplasm (Fig. 7-38D). The mitotic rate is variable but may be low. They show diffuse immunoreactivity for S100, variable immunoreactivity for HMB-45, Melan-A and tyrosinase, and are negative for CD117, CD34, EMA, keratins, MSA, and SMA.[289–293] Ultrastructurally, most show melanosomes at varying stages of development.[292] A possible variant with prominent CD68-positive osteoclast-like giant cells has been described.[290,291,294] It resembles clear cell sarcoma morphologically, is diffusely immunoreactive for S100, and often harbors the t (12;22) (q13;q12) translocation. It is usually HMB-45 and Melan-A negative. Whether this represents a morphologic variant of clear cell sarcoma or a distinct tumor is a matter of debate.[290] Melanoma is the major consideration in the differential diagnosis. Consideration should be given to molecular studies (see above) in apparent metastatic melanomas with no documented cutaneous lesion. GIST, PEComa, leiomyosarcoma, and carcinoma also enter the differential diagnosis.

Malignant Gastrointestinal Neuroectodermal Tumor (GINECT)

A series of 16 cases of this distinctive aggressive mesenchymal tumor was reported in 2012.[298] The tumors

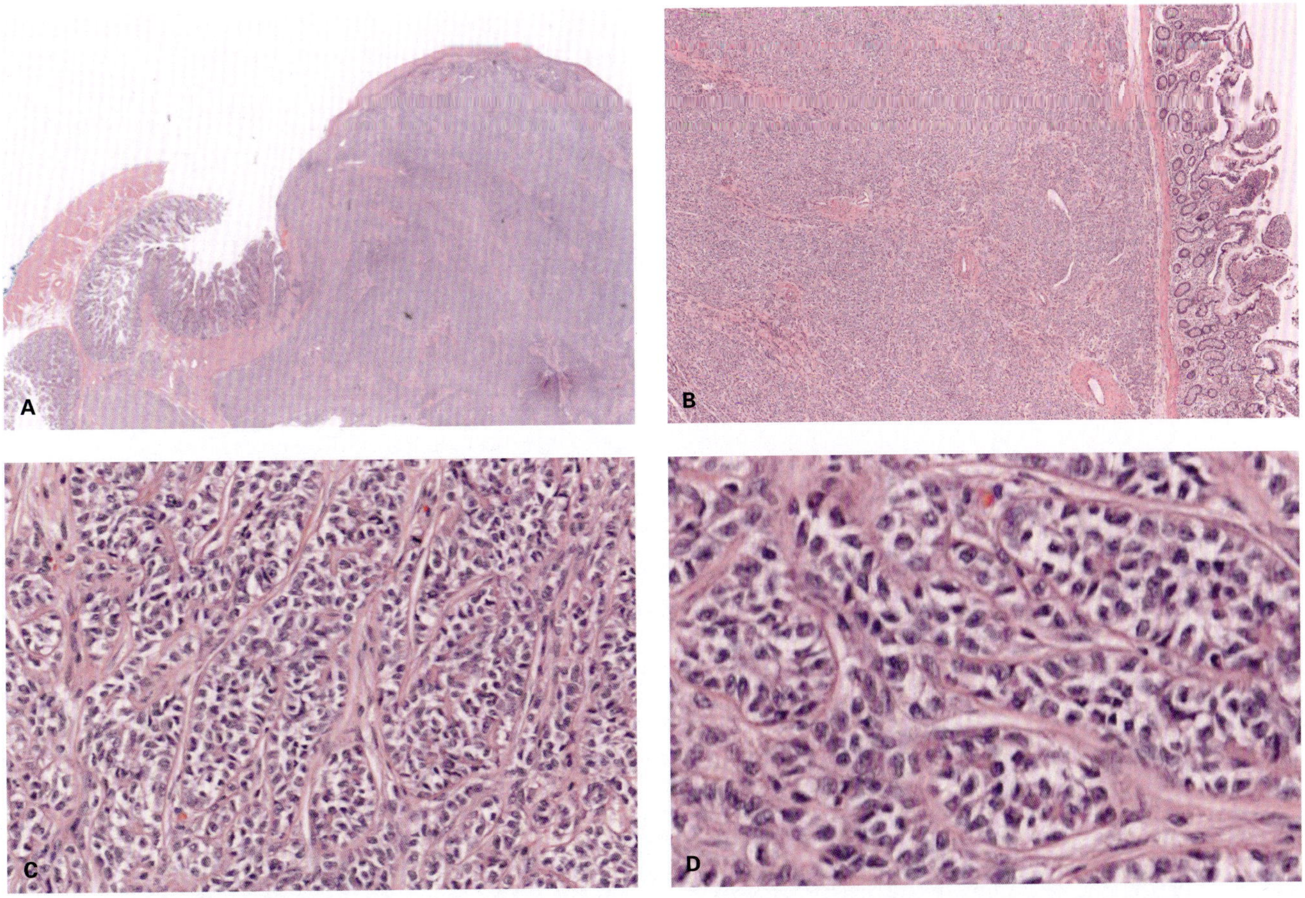

Figure 7-38. Clear cell sarcoma presenting as a polyp in the small bowel. **A:** At scanning power, the tumor is centered in the submucosa **(A,B).** The tumor cells are arranged in nests and short fascicles separated by fibrous septa **(C,D)** and are polygonal or spindled with fairly monomorphic nuclei, vesicular chromatin, prominent nucleoli, and clear to eosinophilic cytoplasm **(D).**

arose mainly in the small bowel but also in the stomach and colon. They were characterized histologically by a sheet-like or nested proliferation of epithelioid or oval-to-spindled cells with small nucleoli and scattered mitoses (Fig. 7-39). One-third showed focal clearing of the cytoplasm. Scattered osteoclast-like giant cells were present in half of the cases. The tumors were all diffusely immunoreactive for S100 and SOX10, were variably immunoreactive for synaptophysin, NB84, and neuron-specific enolase, and were negative for CD117, DOG1, keratins, MiTF-1, Melan A, HMB45, tyrosinase, desmin, and SMA. Some showed ultrastructural features of primitive neuroectodermal cells, but all lacked evidence of melanocytic differentiation. Twelve out of 14 cases tested (86%) showed evidence of a chromosomal translocation involving the EWSR1 gene (six demonstrating rearrangement of the partner gene ATF1 and three with rearrangement of CREB1). These tumors have very similar morphologic, immunohistochemical, ultrastructural, and molecular features to a tumor previously designated "clear cell sarcoma–like tumors of the GI tract"[290,291,294] and likely represents the same entity. These are highly malignant tumors with a poor prognosis.[298]

Endometrial Stromal Sarcoma

Endometrial stromal sarcoma rarely involves the GI tract either as a metastasis[299,300] (sometimes decades after hysterectomy) or as a primary tumor arising from endometriotic foci, usually in the rectovaginal septum, rectum, or sigmoid colon.[301-304] Diagnosis is often challenging since they are usually not considered at this site, particularly if a history of hysterectomy for fibroids, for example, is not forthcoming. They are often initially mistaken for GIST, especially since up to 40% are immunoreactive for CD117. Clues to the diagnosis include multinodularity, tongue-like infiltrative growth, venous invasion and at least focal prominence of spiral arterioles around which the monomorphous oval to plump spindled cells form characteristic perivascular whorls (Fig. 7-40). In areas a fascicular pattern may predominate. High-grade tumors are characterized by marked nuclear enlargement and atypia and a high mitotic rate.[305] The diagnosis can be confirmed by immunoreactivity for CD10. Most tumors are immunoreactive for estrogen and progesterone receptors and Bcl-2 and are negative for CD34. SMA expression is variable.[299,302-304]

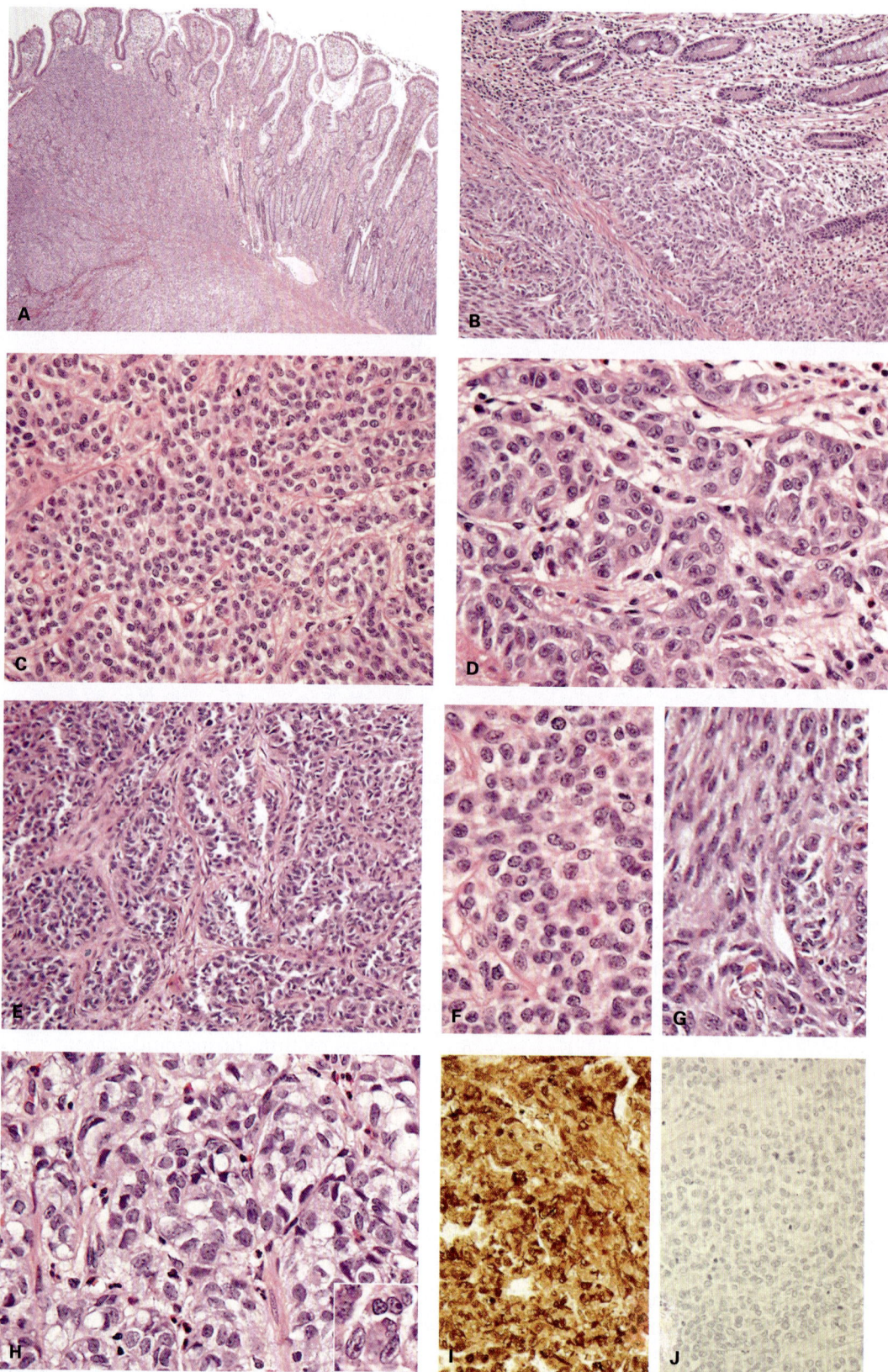

Figure 7-39. Malignant gastrointestinal neuroectodermal tumor (GINECT) involving the small bowel **(A,B)**. The tumor infiltrates the submucosa and overlying lamina propria. Tumor cells arranged in solid sheets **(C)** or nests **(D)** with a focal pseudoalveolar pattern **(E)**. Morphology is predominantly epithelioid **(F)**, but focal spindled areas are also present **(G)** (some tumors may be purely or predominantly spindled). Focal clearing of the cytoplasm **(H)** can be seen in one-third of cases. The tumor cells have vesicular nuclei, and nucleoli are usually indistinct although occasionally prominent (inset). GINECTs are diffusely immunoreactive for S100 **(I)** and negative for all melanoma markers, including Melan-A **(J)**. (Courtesy: Dr. Jason Hornick, Brigham and Women's Hospital Department of Pathology, Boston, MA.)

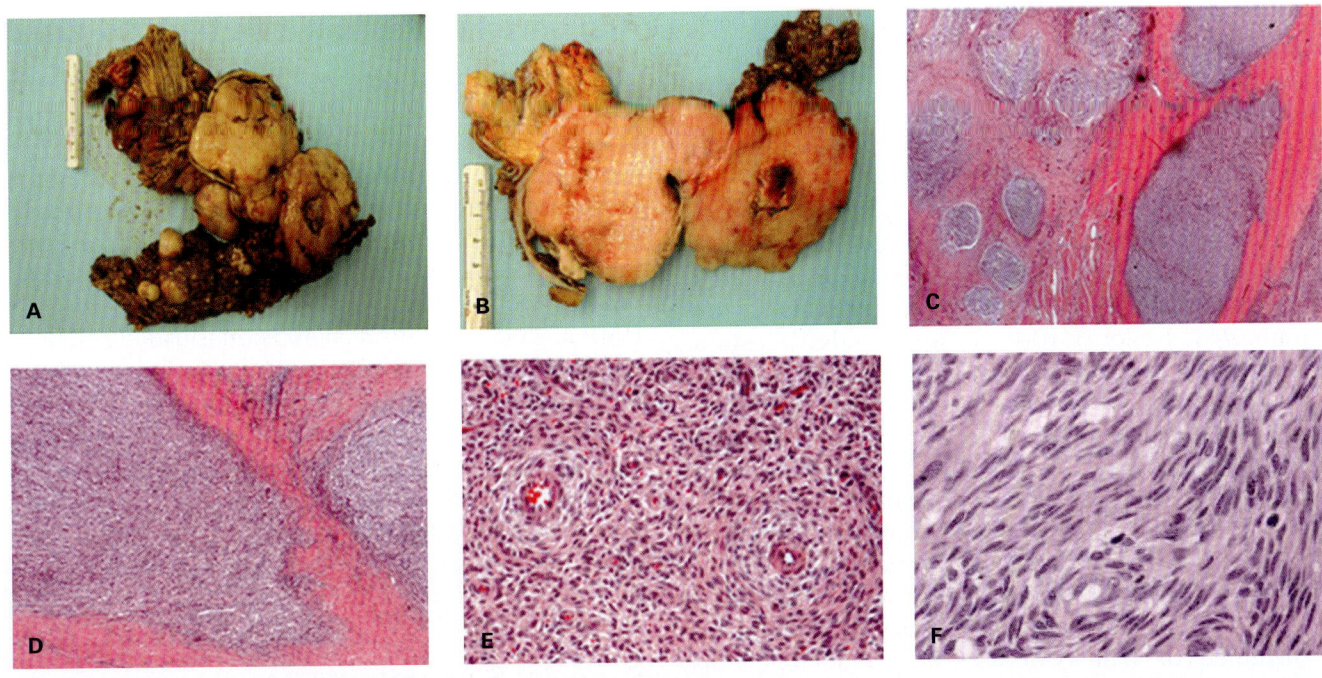
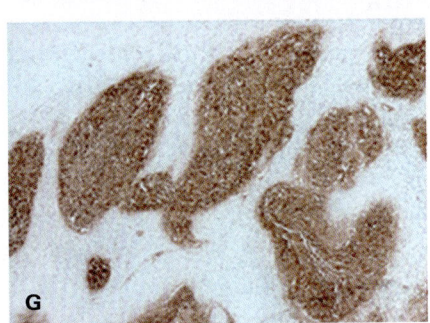

Figure 7-40. Endometrial stromal sarcoma metastatic to small bowel in a patient with a remote (forgotten) hysterectomy. **A:** Large, multicentric tumor involving the mesentery and wall of the small bowel. **B:** Cut section through the dominant mass shows a solid, fleshy tumor with central necrosis. **C:** Scanning power shows a multinodular growth pattern typical of this tumor. **D:** A tongue-like pattern of invasion is characteristic. **E:** Perivascular whorls of tumor cells around prominent spiral arterioles are often striking and a useful diagnostic clue when present. **F:** A more fascicular pattern in some cases may lead to confusion with GIST, particularly when focal CD117 immunoreactivity is present (as in this case). **G:** Strong immunoreactivity for CD10 (as well as estrogen and progesterone receptor) facilitates the correct diagnosis.

Undifferentiated High Grade Pleomorphic Sarcoma/Malignant Fibrous Histiocytoma

Primary and metastatic MFHs of the GI tract are rare. Approximately 50 primary and fewer than 10 metastatic cases have been reported in the literature.[306] Term "undifferentiated high grade pleomorphic sarcoma/MFH" is preferred in the latest WHO classification since these tumors lack true fibrohistiocytic differentiation. Histologically, MFH is characterized by large highly pleomorphic, plump spindled or epithelioid, mitotically active cells arranged in sheets, storiform patterns or fascicles with a variable inflammatory background. Similar features may be seen in a wide variety of other tumors including sarcomatoid carcinoma, melanoma, pleomorphic leiomyosarcoma, dedifferentiated liposarcoma, dedifferentiated pleomorphic GISTs, malignant PEComa, follicular dendritic cell sarcoma, and others. Many cases of apparent MFH are reclassified as other tumors when extensively sampled or appropriate ancillary studies are performed.[306,307] Therefore, before rendering a diagnosis of primary GI MFH, it is essential that (1) previous or concurrent tumors be excluded by appropriate clinical and imaging studies, (2) the tumor be extensively sampled to exclude a better differentiated component of mimics (see above), (3) a wide panel of immunohistochemical markers to exclude the above mimics, and (4) consideration be given to molecular studies to exclude a pleomorphic GIST (Fig. 7-5).

Undifferentiated Sarcoma

This group of undifferentiated sarcomatous tumors cannot be histogenetically defined on the basis of immunohistochemical markers. Grossly, they may simulate GISTs but histologically tend to show greater nuclear pleomorphism.[1]

PERIVASCULAR EPITHELIOID CELL TUMORS

PEComa

PEComas are a rare family of tumors that show perivascular epithelioid cell differentiation. They occur in both pediatric and adult populations with a strong female predominance. Over 20 gastrointestinal PEComas have been reported.[308-311] They may present as mucosal or submucosal polyps, usually in the rectum or cecum (Fig. 7-41A,B), or as mass lesions involving the serosa or bowel wall.[310] Histologically, most feature epithelioid cells (less commonly spindled cells) with clear to granular eosinophilic cytoplasm, arranged in nests or sheets (Fig. 7-41C,D) with at least a focal close association with blood vessel walls. Short-fascicular or storiform patterns may also be seen.[65,308,309] The vast majority are immunoreactive for HMB-45, melan-A, and SMA (often focal).[309] The differential diagnosis includes clear cell sarcoma, melanoma, epithelioid GIST, leiomyosarcoma, and alveolar soft part sarcoma.[310] The occasional immunoreactivity of PEComa for CD117 presents a potential diagnostic pitfall.[65,312] To avoid this, myomelanocytic markers be included in the GIST panel in atypical cases.[65,312] Criteria for malignancy have been proposed for soft tissue and gynecologic PEComas,[313] but their applicability to GI PEComas remains to be determined (the paucity of cases and limited follow-up data preclude this). Nonetheless, tumor size of >5 cm and coagulative tumor necrosis seem to be associated with early tumor recurrence.[310]

Angiomyolipoma

There are isolated reports of angiomyolipoma arising in the GI tract, mostly the colon[314,315] and small bowel.[314,315] Most present as small polyps, but may form larger obstructing lesions mimicking carcinoma. Most cases are not associated with tuberous sclerosis. Like angiomyolipomas elsewhere, one element may predominate, especially the smooth muscle component, which shows variable immunoreactivity for HMB-45 and SMA. Surgical excision is usually curative and local recurrence is rare. These lesions represent the other spectrum of PEComas and many consider them synonymous.

BIPHASIC EPITHELIAL–MESENCHYMAL LESIONS

Synovial Sarcoma

Primary GI synovial sarcoma is rare with around 30 reported cases. Most involve the stomach and

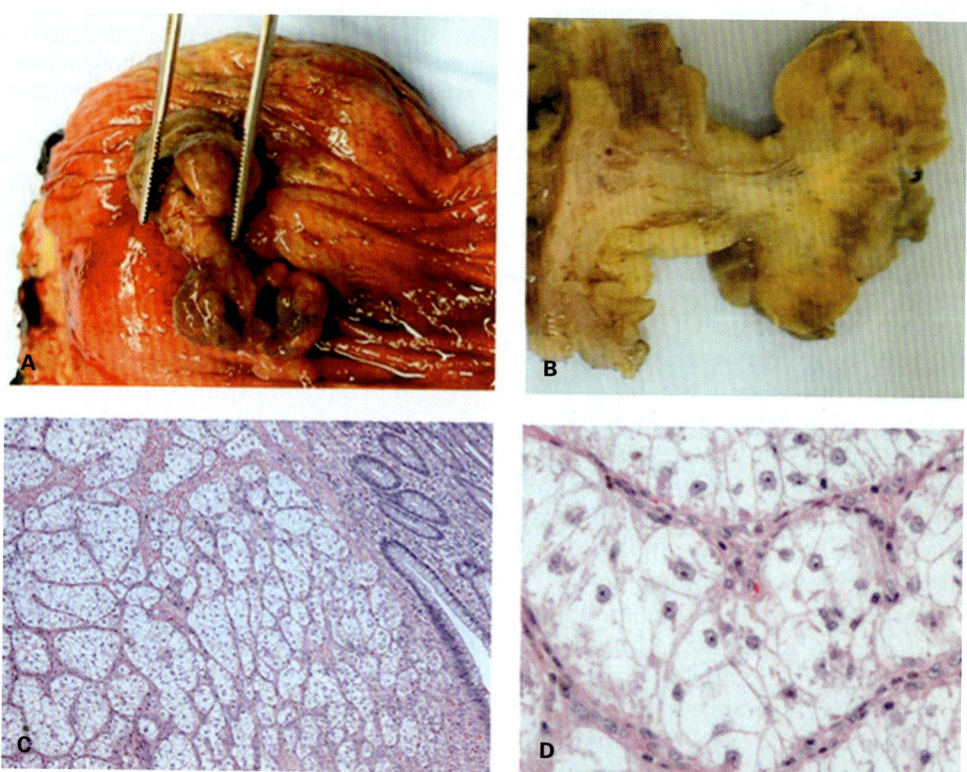

Figure 7-41. PEComa of the rectum in a 15-year-old girl. **A,B:** Gross specimen shows a pedunculated polyp without gross involvement of the muscularis propria. **C,D:** Histology shows a predominantly submucosal tumor with a distinct nested pattern and intervening delicate fibrovascular septa. The tumor cells have abundant clear cytoplasm and well-defined cell borders. Diagnosis was confirmed by immunoreactivity for HMB-45 and demonstration of melanosomes and premelanosomes on electron microscopy. The tumor cells were negative for S100, MART-1, and the EWS/AFT-1 fusion gene product of clear cell sarcoma. Despite the relatively small size and superficial location of the tumor, metastatic deposits were identified in two regional lymph nodes. (Images courtesy Dr. Paul Ryan.)

esophagus with isolated cases in the duodenum and colon.³¹⁶⁻³²⁰ Gastric synovial sarcomas are mainly monophasic, while those in the esophagus are biphasic. Grossly, gastric tumors tend to be ulcerated, cup-shaped, plaque-like, or oval lesions predominantly on the luminal aspect with variable extension into the muscularis propria (occasionally transmural), while esophageal tumors are endophytic. The median age at presentation is 52 for gastric and 25 for esophageal tumors. Histology is identical to their soft tissue counterparts (Fig. 7-42). Synovial sarcomas need to be distinguished from CD117-negative GISTs (sarcomatous

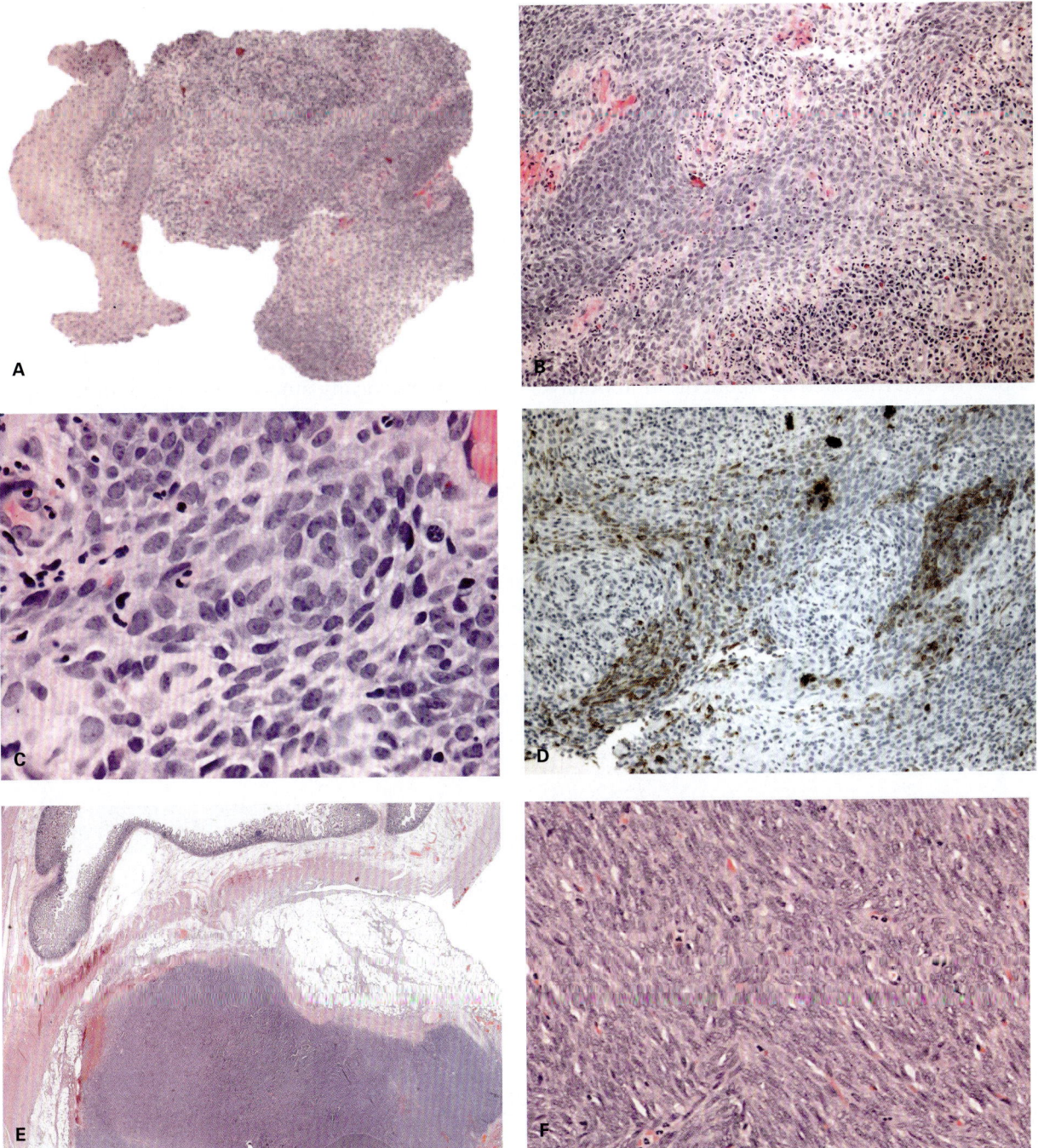

Figure 7-42. Synovial sarcoma. **A–D:** Monophasic synovial sarcoma of the esophagus. **A,B:** The tumor is densely cellular with cells arranged in vague nests or fascicles. **C:** Detail of the tumor showing ovoid cells with hyperchromatic, mildly pleomorphic nuclei with small nucleoli. **D:** Patchy immunoreactivity for the pankeratin AE1/AE3, which led to an initial mistaken diagnosis of poorly differentiated carcinoma. However, the diagnosis of synovial sarcoma was later confirmed by demonstrating the characteristic SYT-SXX fusion transcript. **E,F:** Monophasic synovial sarcoma involving the mesentery of the small bowel. **E:** At scanning power, the tumor appears relatively well circumscribed. **F:** Detail of the tumor showing densely cellular, hyperchromatic, relatively uniform spindle cells with frequent nuclear overlap and a high mitotic rate.

spindled cell variant) and spindle cell sarcomatoid carcinomas. GISTs are typically centered in the muscularis propria in contrast to most synovial sarcomas (see above). Synovial sarcomas are one of the few GIST mimics with the potential to coexpress CD117 and DOG1[36]; however, such coexpression would be uncommon and typically focal with at least one marker (see GIST immunohistochemistry). Cytokeratin 7, AE1/AE3, and EMA are focally positive in most synovial sarcomas but not in GISTs (although exceptional EMA immunoreactivity may occur). GISTs may be reactive for CK18 and less frequently CK8, so that antibodies to these keratins (e.g., CAM5.2) are unhelpful in this setting. In difficult cases, molecular studies for the SYT-SXX fusion transcript and *KIT/PDGFRA* mutations may prove helpful. Careful inspection for a frank carcinomatous component or dysplasia in the overlying epithelium should be performed in all cases. The prognosis appears variable. Small gastric tumors lacking a poorly differentiated component tend to have a better prognosis, while large tumors and those with a poorly differentiated component often behave more aggressively.[318]

Spindle Cell Carcinoma/Carcinosarcoma

Carcinomas in virtually any organ, irrespective of the epithelial type of tumor (e.g., adenosquamous, squamous, transitional) can transform into a spindle cell variant of carcinoma that may mimic mesenchymal tumors. They may retain markers of epithelial differentiation by electron microscopy or immunocytochemistry. However, these markers may be lost (Fig. 7-43), and the tumor may acquire true evidence of mesenchymal proliferation, with differentiation along traditional sarcomatous lines (smooth muscle, rhabdomyosarcoma, chondrosarcoma, osteosarcoma, etc.). In the GI tract, this tends to occur primarily, but rarely, in the esophagus (see Chapter 12), but it can also occur in other sites such as the stomach, small bowel (see Chapter 14) or large bowel (see Chapter 21).[321-326]

Occasionally, tumors display multiple patterns of epithelial differentiation—for instance, an adenosquamous carcinoma with a sarcomatous element showing osseous and cartilaginous differentiation. Some spindle cell carcinomas may resemble GISTs, although the degree of nuclear pleomorphism usually exceeds that of GIST. About 2% to 4% of colorectal carcinomas are CD117 positive, representing a potential pitfall (Fig. 7-43). Conversely, GIST may occasionally show immunoreactivity for CK18 (4%–8%)[25,47] and to a lesser extent CK8,[15] but not AE1/AE3.[48,49] Mesenchymal differentiation in esophageal tumors may be unequivocally smooth muscle, with the squamous component sometimes only evident in metastases. We therefore treat all apparent leiomyosarcomas of the esophagus with considerable caution. In any apparent mesenchymal tumor in the GI tract, it is essential to sample extensively both tumor and adjacent and overlying epithelium for evidence of carcinomatous or dysplastic features that would imply epithelial origin. Carcinomatous elements are found most readily at the infiltrating margin. Sarcomatoid carcinomas are generally aggressive but a peculiar variant in the

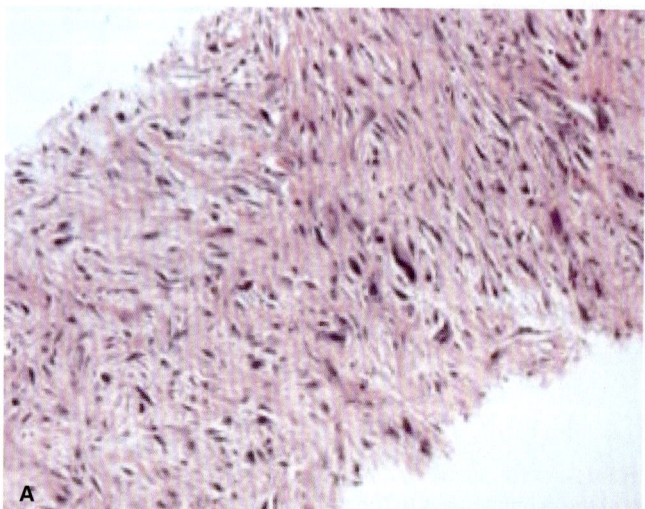
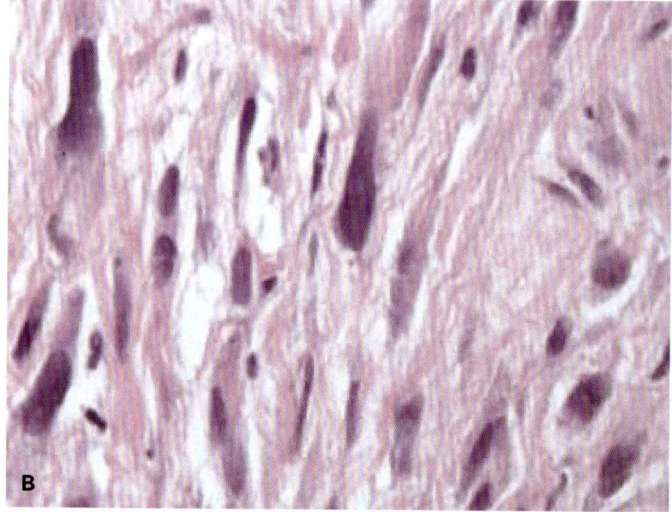

Figure 7-43. Spindle cell carcinoma of the colon **(A–E).** The spindled morphology may lead to confusion with mesenchymal tumors including GIST **(A).** Compared to GIST, spindled cell carcinomas are generally more pleomorphic **(A,B)** and have overtly infiltrating margins.

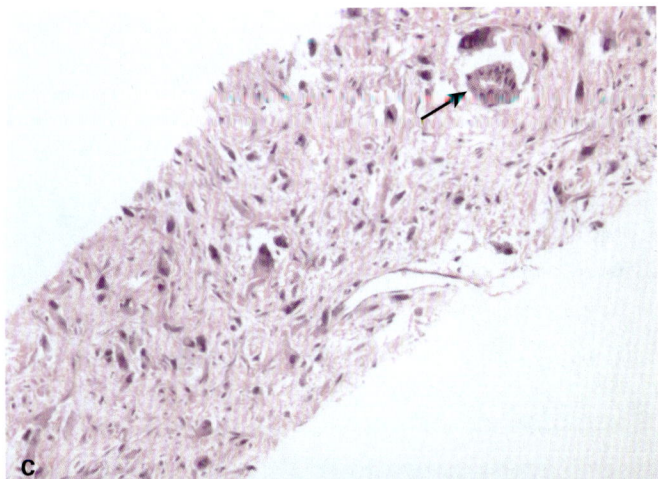
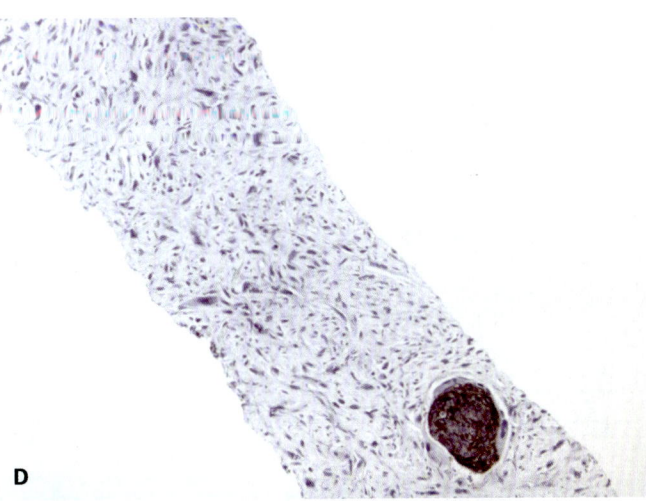
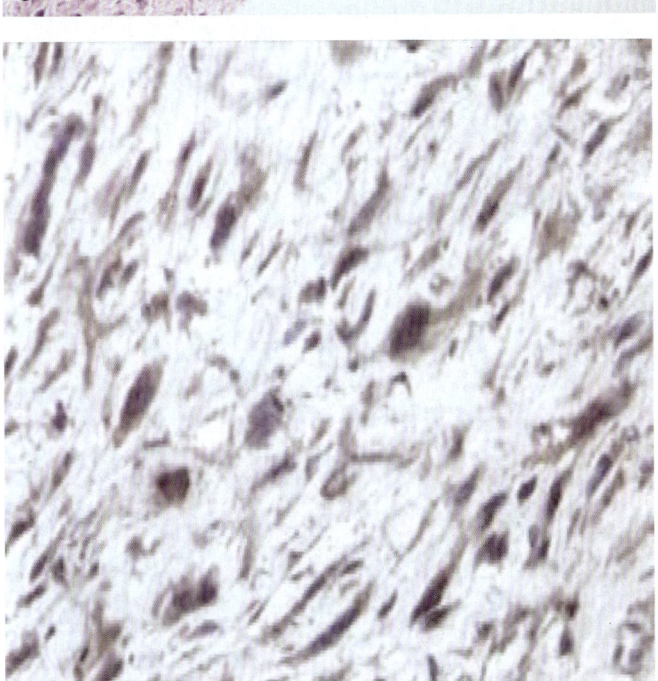

Figure 7-43. *(Continued)* The advancing edge tends to be where glandular differentiation is identified (**C**, *arrow*). The spindled component may lack immunoreactivity for cytokeratin—note the reactivity in the glandular component (**D**). CD117 immunoreactivity in the spindled component is uncommon (**E**) and represents a potential diagnostic pitfall.

esophagus (variously termed spindle cell squamous carcinoma, pseudosarcomatous squamous carcinoma, polypoid carcinoma, and carcinosarcoma) has a better prognosis than conventional squamous carcinomas of comparable size, probably due to its propensity for intraluminal rather than transmural growth.[321,327]

Gastroblastoma (Epithelial Biphasic Tumor of Young Adults)

This is quite a characteristic biphasic tumor showing both mesenchymal and glandular differentiation.[328,329] So far such tumors have only been described in the stomach. The tumors occur in young adults in their late teens to thirties, and they present with pain, bleeding, or symptoms of anemia. Tumors occur in any part of the stomach and the clinical diagnosis is usually a GIST that is resected. Tumors can be up to 15 cm in diameter and are multinodular or polypoid, and well circumscribed with much of the tumor being submucosal (Fig. 7-44).

Histologically, tumors have a background diffuse mesenchymal pattern that has a dominant ovoid, slightly spindled component with minimal atypicality (Fig. 7-45A,B). However within this, and intimately

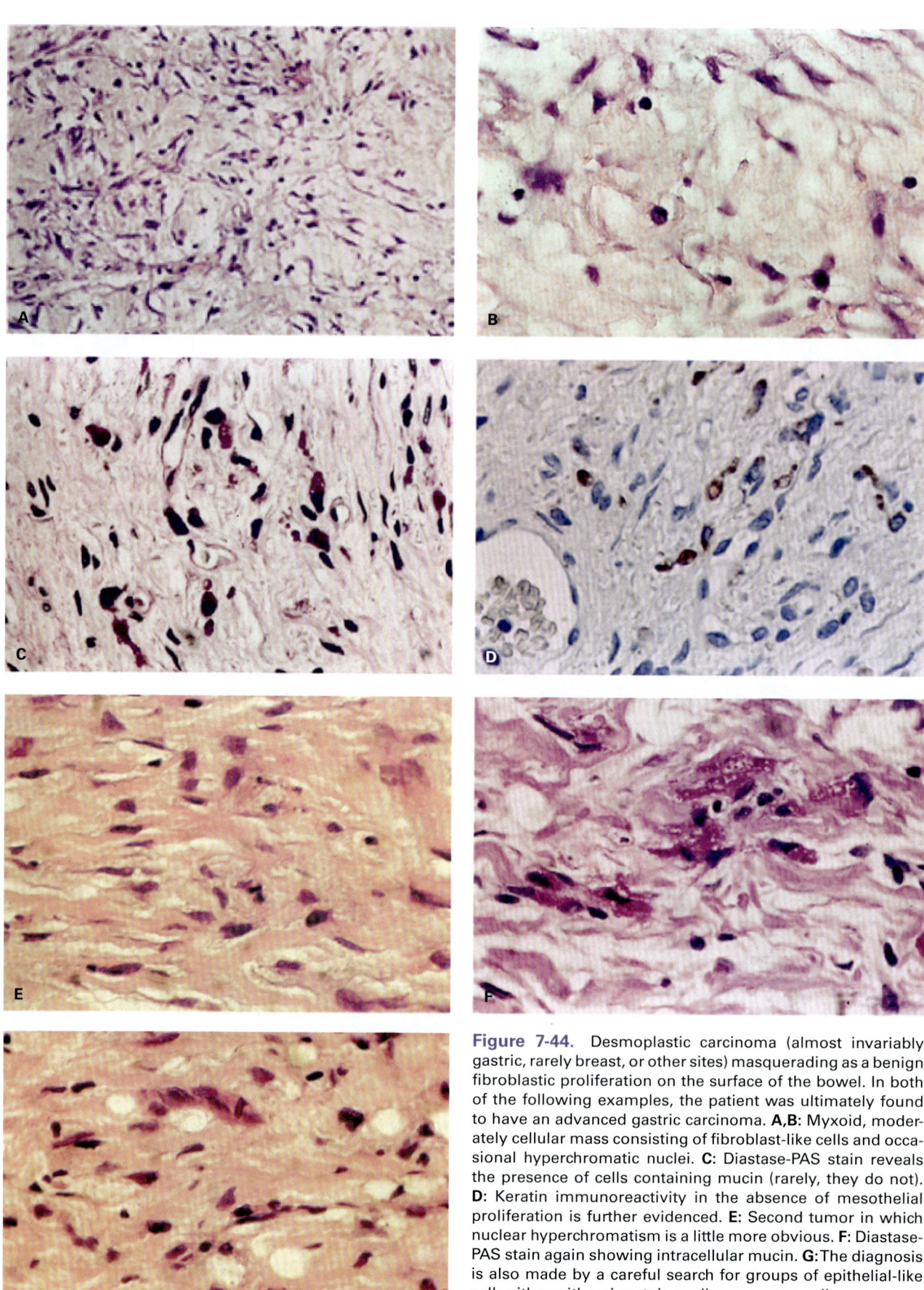

Figure 7-44. Desmoplastic carcinoma (almost invariably gastric, rarely breast, or other sites) masquerading as a benign fibroblastic proliferation on the surface of the bowel. In both of the following examples, the patient was ultimately found to have an advanced gastric carcinoma. **A,B:** Myxoid, moderately cellular mass consisting of fibroblast-like cells and occasional hyperchromatic nuclei. **C:** Diastase-PAS stain reveals the presence of cells containing mucin (rarely, they do not). **D:** Keratin immunoreactivity in the absence of mesothelial proliferation is further evidenced. **E:** Second tumor in which nuclear hyperchromatism is a little more obvious. **F:** Diastase-PAS stain again showing intracellular mucin. **G:** The diagnosis is also made by a careful search for groups of epithelial-like cells either with a signet ring cell appearance, adherent to one another, arranged in single file or attempting to form glands.

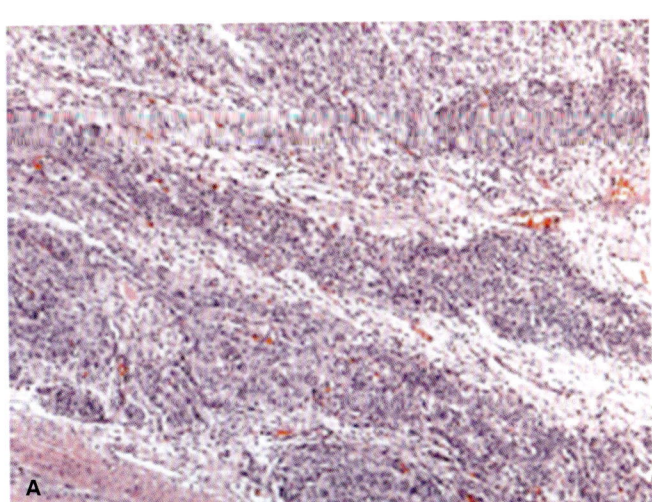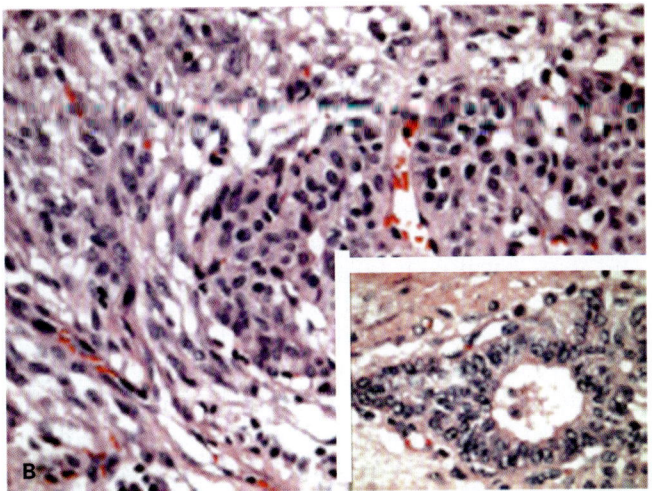

Figure 7-45. **A:** Overview of a gastroblastoma showing the biphasic nature of the tumor with sharply demarcated epithelial islands with a background of mesenchymal spindle cells. The mesenchymal elements are positive for vimentin and CD10, and negative for c-kit and smooth muscle markers. **B:** Detail showing the spindle cell component with minimal nuclear atypia and no mitotic figures. The epithelial component shows mild nuclear pleomorphism and few mitotic figures. Other areas of the tumor showed glandular differentiation as well (**inset**). The epitheliomesenchymal demarcation may not be as sharp in some cases, and the epithelial component can show significant atypia and mitotic activity.

mingled with it are more overt islands of epithelioid and spindled cells, that stain more intensely so are readily visible at low power. Within these islands, some of the cells form glands, which vary from just visible to overt. The mitotic rate and Mib-1 rate are low. Immunohistochemically, the mesenchymal component stains with vimentin and CD10 only, but the spindle/epithelial component also stains for Pan CK, CK7, CK19, CK20, and EMA, but not CK5 or CK18. GIST markers CD117 and DOG1 may exhibit weak immunoreactivity, but CD34 is negative. Apart from weak SMA or NSE immunoreactivity, other markers are negative.[328] Four of the five cases reported to date had an indolent clinical behavior with no recurrence or metastasis, but the most recently reported case had widespread nodal liver and peritoneal metastasis, indicating that these neoplasms have malignant potential.[329]

Differential diagnosis includes other biphasic tumors that can occur in the stomach like synovial sarcoma, teratoma, carcinosarcoma, and mesothelioma. Synovial sarcoma in stomach tends to be monophasic and the epithelial component when recognizable forms syncytia that merge with the mesenchymal elements rather than forming distinct glandular structures seen in gastroblastoma. Translocation studies for synovial sarcoma may be needed to definitively exclude this possibility. Carcinosarcomas in the stomach are also rare; however, they tend to occur in older individuals, show marked atypia in the epithelial as well as mesenchymal elements, and have a more aggressive behavior. Gastric teratomas are primarily seen in infants and show a wider histologic diversity with neural, neuroepithelial, cystic, and cartilaginous components. Gastroblastomas also need to be differentiated from GISTs, especially if weak immunoreactivity for CD117 or DOG1 is found, and because of this, mutational analysis for GISTs may be necessary. The other tumors that may be considered in the differential diagnosis include carcinoid, melanoma, and PEComa. The possibility of involvement by tumors from outside the stomach that can be biphasic may also be considered, such as pancreatic solid/pseudopapillary tumor, mesothelioma, endometrial or ovarian tumors.[328] Provided the diagnosis of gastroblastoma is considered, the histologic features are virtually pathognomonic despite the long list of differential diagnoses, and may require only select immunhistochemical markers to differentiate from its mimics.

NONMESENCHYMAL TUMORS THAT MAY MIMIC MESENCHYMAL NEOPLASMS

Mesenchymal tumors may be mimicked by a variety of nonmesenchymal neoplasms including metaplastic spindle cell carcinoma, melanoma, histiocytic neoplasms, follicular dendritic cell sarcoma, and metastatic adult granulosa cell tumors.

Melanoma

Melanoma is the most common tumor metastatic to the GI tract, usually the small intestine.[330,331] It may also arise a primary tumor in the anorectum and esophagus.[62,332,333] Melanomas are composed of epithelioid cells, spindled cells, or mixtures of both and amelanotic variants are not uncommon (Fig. 7-46).[334] Amelanotic spindled cell melanomas, especially when accompanied by a desmoplastic stroma, may mimic mesenchymal tumors.[335] Both spindled and epithelioid melanomas may overlap morphologically with GIST and up to 75% of melanomas may be immunoreactive for CD117.[62] We therefore always include at least one melanoma marker (e.g., S100) in our GIST panel, and any immunoreactivity will lead to additional markers (e.g., HMB-45, Melan-A, and tyrosinase). In equivocal cases, the demonstration of melanosomes by electron microscopy may be helpful in obtaining a diagnosis.

Follicular Dendritic Cell Sarcoma

This uncommon neoplasm arises from follicular dendritic cells of lymph nodes or extranodal tissues.[336,337] There have been isolated reports of follicular dendritic cell sarcomas involving the stomach,[338] small bowel,[339] colon,[336] and mesentery.[337,339] Histology features fascicles, whorls, storiform, and sometimes sheet-like arrangements of spindled, oval, and polygonal cells with round to oval nuclei, moderate, pale eosinophilic cytoplasm, and indistinct cell borders imparting a characteristic syncytial appearance (Fig. 7-47). Nuclei have delicate, smooth membranes, clear chromatin and distinct, usually single, small- to medium-sized nucleoli. Nuclear atypia is usually mild although pleomorphic cells can be found in some

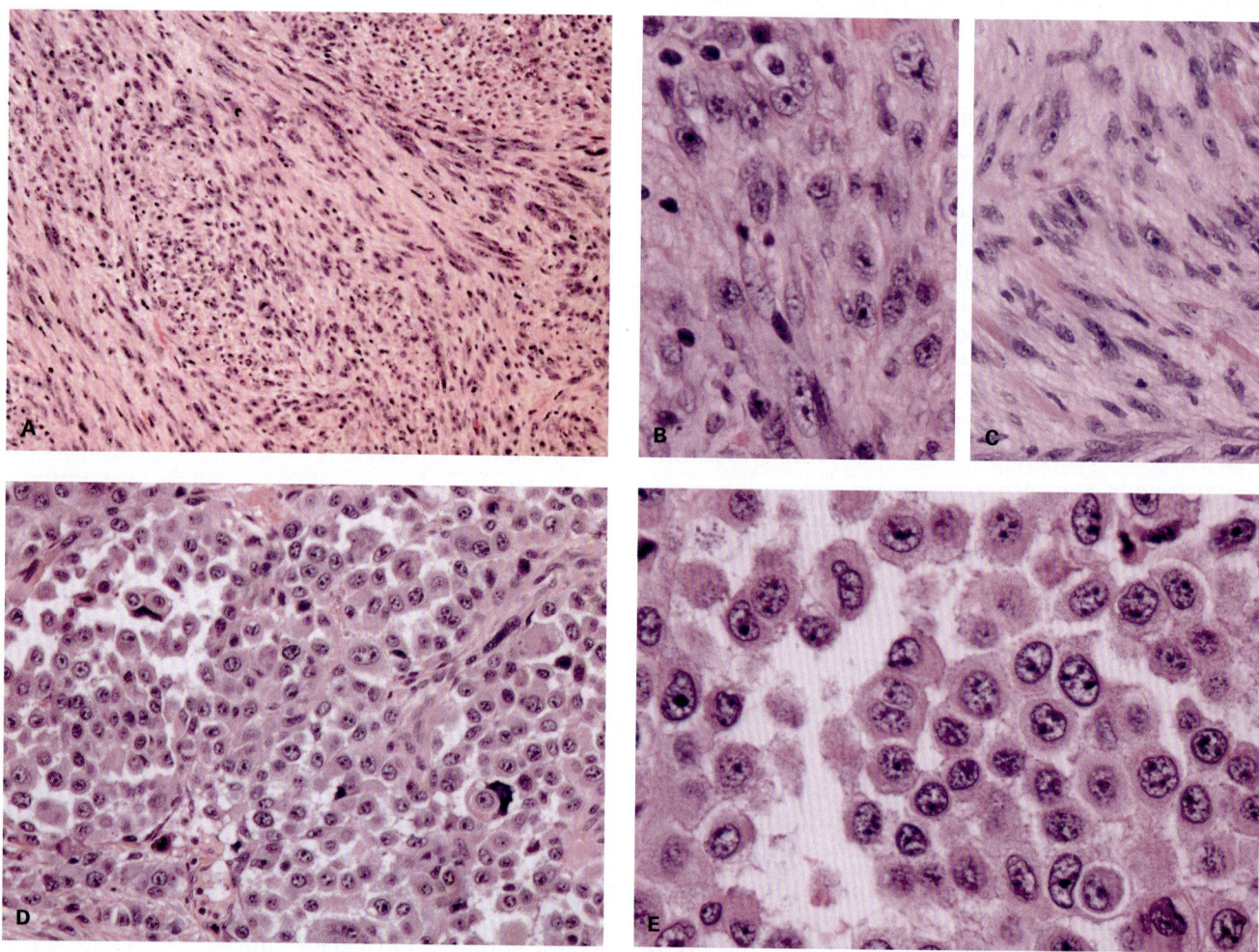

Figure 7-46. Melanoma. A–C: Primary anorectal (amelanotic) melanoma in a 35-year-old female. This case was initially thought to represent a sarcoma due to its fascicular growth pattern and pleomorphic spindled morphology **(A,B).** The tumor was diffusely immunoreactive for S100 and focally reactive for MART-1 and HMB-45. Identification of melanosomes/premelanosomes and absence of neural differentiation may be helpful in separating this tumor from malignant peripheral nerve sheath tumor (S100 immunoreactivity in the latter tends to be patchy). **D,E:** Metastatic (amelanotic) melanoma to small intestine showing epithelioid morphology. These tumors overlap morphologically with poorly differentiated carcinoma, epithelioid GIST and lymphoma.

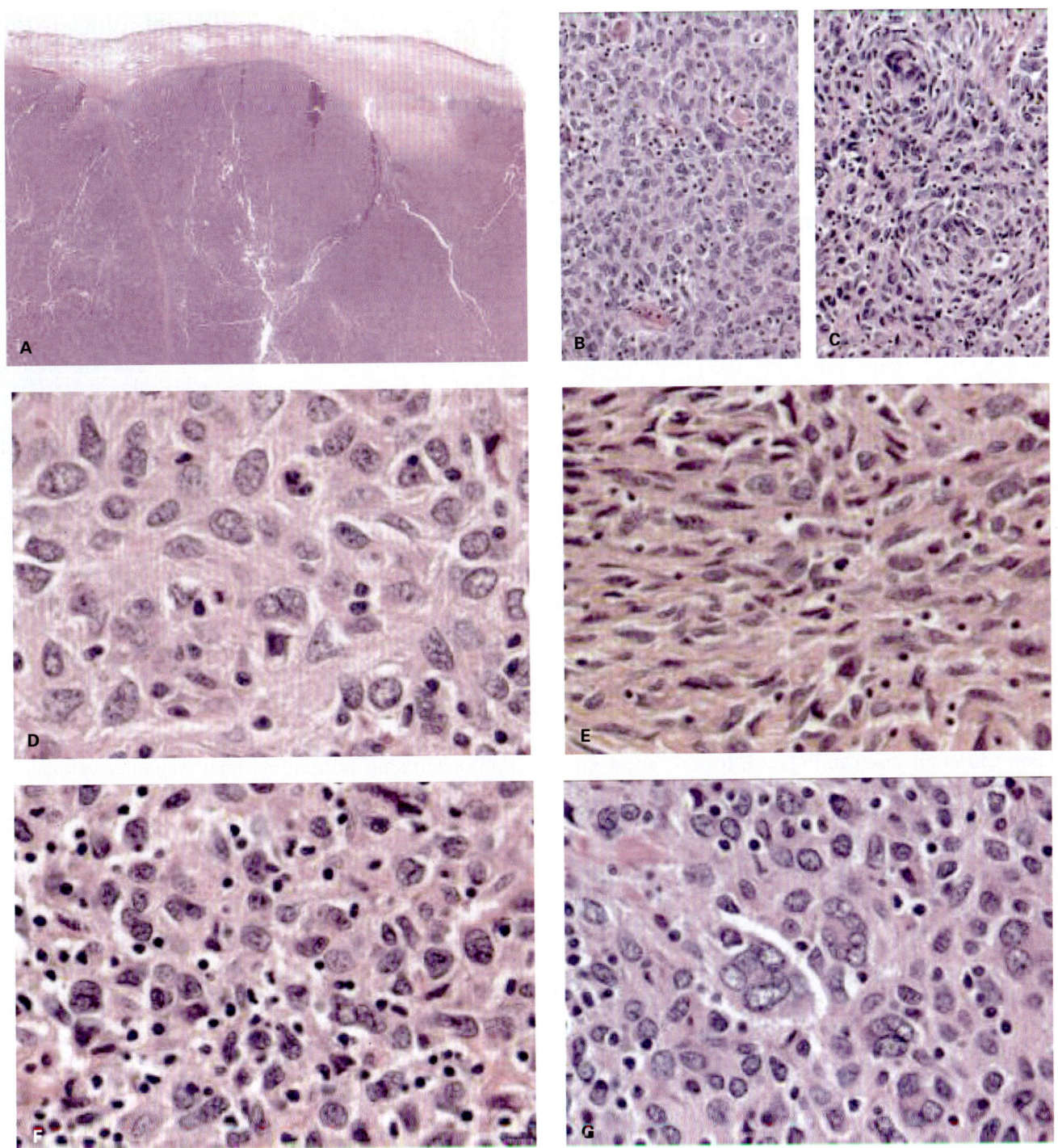

Figure 7-47. Follicular dendritic cell sarcoma of the stomach. **A:** Scanning power shows a fairly circumscribed, cellular tumor arranged in sheets **(B)** and whorls **(C)**. Indistinct cell borders impart a characteristic syncytial appearance **(D)**. The tumor cells may be epithelioid **(C)** or spindled **(D)**. Admixed lymphocytes are typically prominent **(E,F)**. Nuclear pleomorphism may be seen some resembling giant cells **(G)**.

cases. Mature lymphocytes scattered throughout the tumor is a characteristic feature. The mitotic rate is variable. Margins are typically pushing. They are immunoreactive for at least one follicular dendritic cell marker (CD21, CD23, and CD35), show variable EMA, S100, and CD68 expression, and are negative for CD117 and CD34.[336,337,339] Ultrastructurally, the tumor cells show long and thin interdigitating cytoplasmic processes and desmosomal cell junctions between adjacent cell processes.[337,340] They may be confused with mesenchymal tumors especially GIST. Recognition of their distinctive morphologic features (Fig. 7-44) should guide selection of appropriate immunohistochemical stains.

Lymphoma

Non-Hodgkin's lymphomas may be occasionally associated with prominent sclerosis resulting in compression and compartmentalization of tumor cells. This together with a prominent fibrous matrix may lead to misdiagnosis as a spindle cell neoplasm.[192]

Sarcomatoid Adult Granulosa Cell Tumor

Adult granulosa cell tumors of the ovary are characterized by delayed recurrences and metastases. When these occur intraabdominally (particularly sarcomatoid or diffuse variants), they may mimic a variety of mesenchymal tumors including GIST,[192,341] leiomyosarcoma, and hemangiopericytoma.[342] Immunoreactivity for alpha-inhibin may be helpful.[341]

FIBROSING LESIONS OF THE MESENTERY, PERITONEUM, AND RETROPERITONEUM

This group of mesenteric, peritoneal, or retroperitoneal lesions, characterized by fibrosis and variable chronic inflammation, includes sclerosing mesenteritis (idiopathic retractile mesenteritis), sclerosing peritonitis, idiopathic retroperitoneal fibrosis, and Weber–Christian disease.[192] These lesions show considerable histologic overlap and are therefore best separated on the basis of clinical features and the gross appearances of the lesions.

Sclerosing Mesenteritis

Sclerosing mesenteritis is a rare idiopathic condition characterized by thickening and shortening of the mesentery. It occurs mainly in middle-aged and elderly adults (average age 60 years) with a male:female ratio of 2:1. Patients usually present with abdominal pain, a palpable mass, or small bowel obstruction. Grossly, hard nodules result in thickening and shortening of the mesentery with narrowing of the adjacent bowel lumen. The bowel may become kinked and fixed causing obstruction or a tumor-like mass (Fig. 7-48). Histologically, there is dense fibrosis associated with variable chronic inflammation, occasional lymphoid aggregates, and often fat necrosis (Fig. 7-49). Some lesions show extensive hyalinization (Fig. 7-49C). More cellular lesions may show spindled cells arranged in fascicles or in storiform patterns (Fig. 7-49D). Some cases have been shown to contain IgG4-positive plasma cells and the condition has been included under the ever-expanding list of IgG4-associated autoimmune disorders.[343] The main considerations in the differential diagnosis include mesenteric fibromatosis, IMT, sclerosing lymphoma (see *idiopathic retroperitoneal fibrosis*), and Whipple's disease.

Sclerosing mesenteritis can be distinguished from mesenteric fibromatosis by the fact that it stops abruptly at the bowel wall unlike the latter which usually infiltrates the muscularis propria. IMT typically occurs in younger patients, usually as a grossly circumscribed mass lesion, and is often more cellular (although sometimes sclerotic) with a prominence of plasma cells; about 40% are immunoreactive for ALK-1. The possibility of Whipple's disease should always be considered when evaluating mesenteric and retroperitoneal lesions with fibrosis and lipogranulomatous inflammation as this condition responds well to antibiotics but usually fatal if untreated. Whipple's disease is characterized by lipogranulomatous inflammation associated with empty round spaces mainly due to lymphatic dilatation and bright, coarsely granular PAS-positive diastase-resistant inclusions within macrophages. All biopsies from the mesentery and retroperitoneum showing fat necrosis and foamy histiocytes should therefore be subjected to digested PAS stain. The causative bacillus may be verified by electron microscopy or polymerase chain reaction (PCR). Sclerosing mesenteritis generally has a favorable prognosis and may be self-limiting. Asymptomatic patients are often left untreated and observed.

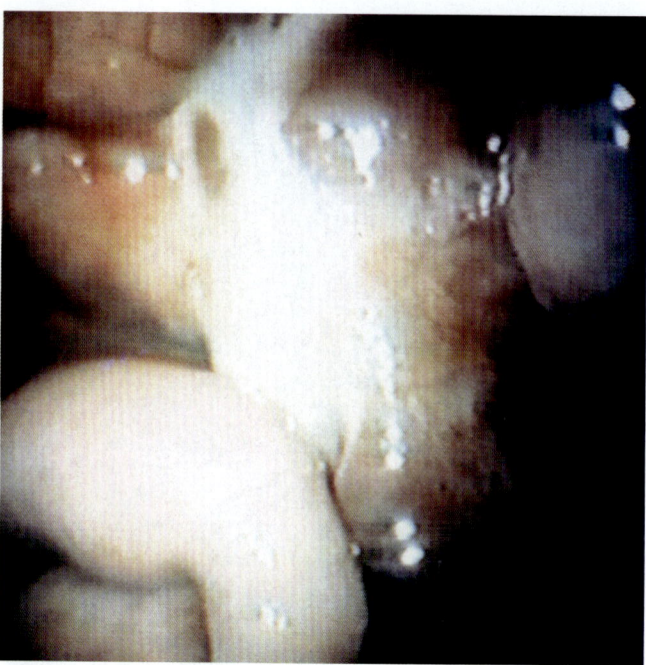

Figure 7-48. Sclerosing mesenteritis. Laparoscopic view of sclerosing mesenteritis forming a sclerosing mass lesion that thickens and shortens the mesentery. (Reprinted from Riddell RH, Petras RE, Williams GT, et al. *Atlas of Tumor Pathology: Tumors of the Intestines*. Washington, DC: Armed Forces Institute of Pathology, 2003, with permission.)

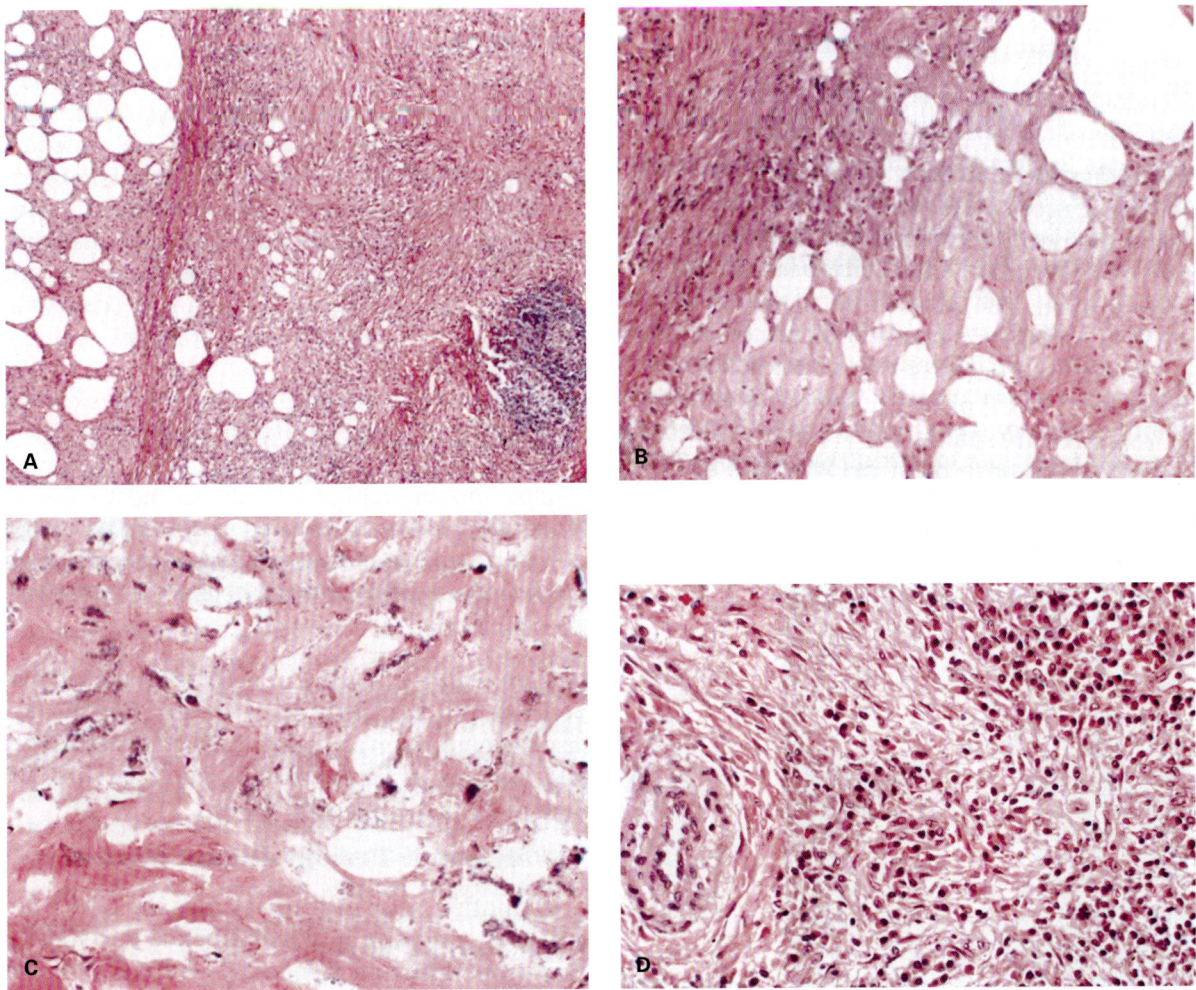

Figure 7-49. Sclerosing mesenteritis. **A–C:** Fat necrosis, sclerosing fibrosis, chronic inflammation with scattered germinal centers, and focal areas of calcification. Polymorphonuclear leukocytes are rare and the vascularity meager. The spindle cells lack nuclear atypia. **D:** There are numerous chronic inflammatory cells and fibrosis. (Reprinted from Riddell RH, Petras RE, Williams GT, et al. *Atlas of Tumor Pathology: Tumors of the Intestines.* Washington, DC: Armed Forces Institute of Pathology, 2003, with permission.)

However, some patients respond to hormonal therapy, while some respond to aggressive immunosuppressive therapy.[344–346] Surgery is reserved for cases that develop complications such as bowel obstruction or perforation.[23,192,347]

Sclerosing Peritonitis

This sclerosing condition of the visceral peritoneum mostly affects young girls but may be seen in older patients and in men. There is a strong association with chronic peritoneal dialysis and the use of β-blockers, but some cases may be idiopathic. Patients usually present with small bowel obstruction, an abdominal mass, or both. The gross appearance may be dramatic with dense fibrous tissue encasing a segment of small bowel ("cocooning peritonitis," "peritonitis fibroplasia encapsulatum"). Histology features fibrotic thickening of the visceral peritoneum with focal chronic inflammation and fibrin deposition and reactive mesothelial hyperplasia. Spindled cells may display fascicular or storiform patterns. Treatment of choice is surgical removal of the thickened peritoneum, lysis of adhesions and in some instances resection of the affected segment of small bowel.[23,192]

Idiopathic Retroperitoneal Fibrosis

This fibrosing/sclerosing condition is usually centered in the lower lumber region, surrounding the aorta and iliac vessels, and extending into the retroperitoneum often enveloping the ureters. Occasionally, it may present at atypical locations such as periduodenal, peripancreatic, or pelvic regions. Patients may present with lower back pain, hydronephrosis, or a pelvic mass. Most cases are idiopathic but can occur secondary to certain drugs (particularly ergot alkaloid derivatives), malignancy, infections (Whipple's disease, tuberculosis), previous surgery, and radiation.[348] Up to 15% of idiopathic cases are associated with other fibroinflammatory conditions including Reidel's thryroiditis, sclerosing mediastinitis, sclerosis of large bile duct, and inflammatory orbital pseudotumor.[23,192] The etiology is uncertain but an autoimmune process is favored.

Grossly, the lesions appear as white, hard, poorly circumscribed, retroperitoneal plaques of variable thickness. Those associated with malignancy are usually more irregular and often occur in atypical locations.[348] Histologically, retroperitoneal fibrosis is characterized by sclerotic tissue infiltrated by a mixture of inflammatory cells including lymphocytes, plasma cells, histiocytes, and eosinophils (Fig. 7-50). Occasionally, a mononuclear cell "vasculitis" may be seen. Early lesions tend to be edematous, vascular, and inflammatory, while older lesions are often densely sclerotic and paucicellular with scattered foci of calcification.[23,192,348] A careful search for an underlying neoplasm should be performed in all retroperitoneal fibrosing lesions. Non-Hodgkin's lymphoma of the retroperitoneum is frequently associated with dense sclerosis and the diagnosis may be missed due to sampling error or difficulty in recognizing extranodal lymphoma on routine stains unless specifically looked for. Immunohistochemistry and gene rearrangement studies are helpful in confirming a suspected diagnosis. Metastatic carcinoma can be associated with inflammation and fat necrosis or may elicit a desmoplastic response to the point where underlying neoplastic infiltrate is obscured and the lesion mimics a benign fibroblastic proliferation (Fig 7-42).

Careful examination of the H&E slide will reveal suspicious or malignant cells in most cases and the diagnosis can be confirmed by mucin stains and cytokeratin immunohistochemistry. Sarcomas of the retroperitoneum may mimic fat necrosis (e.g., liposarcoma)

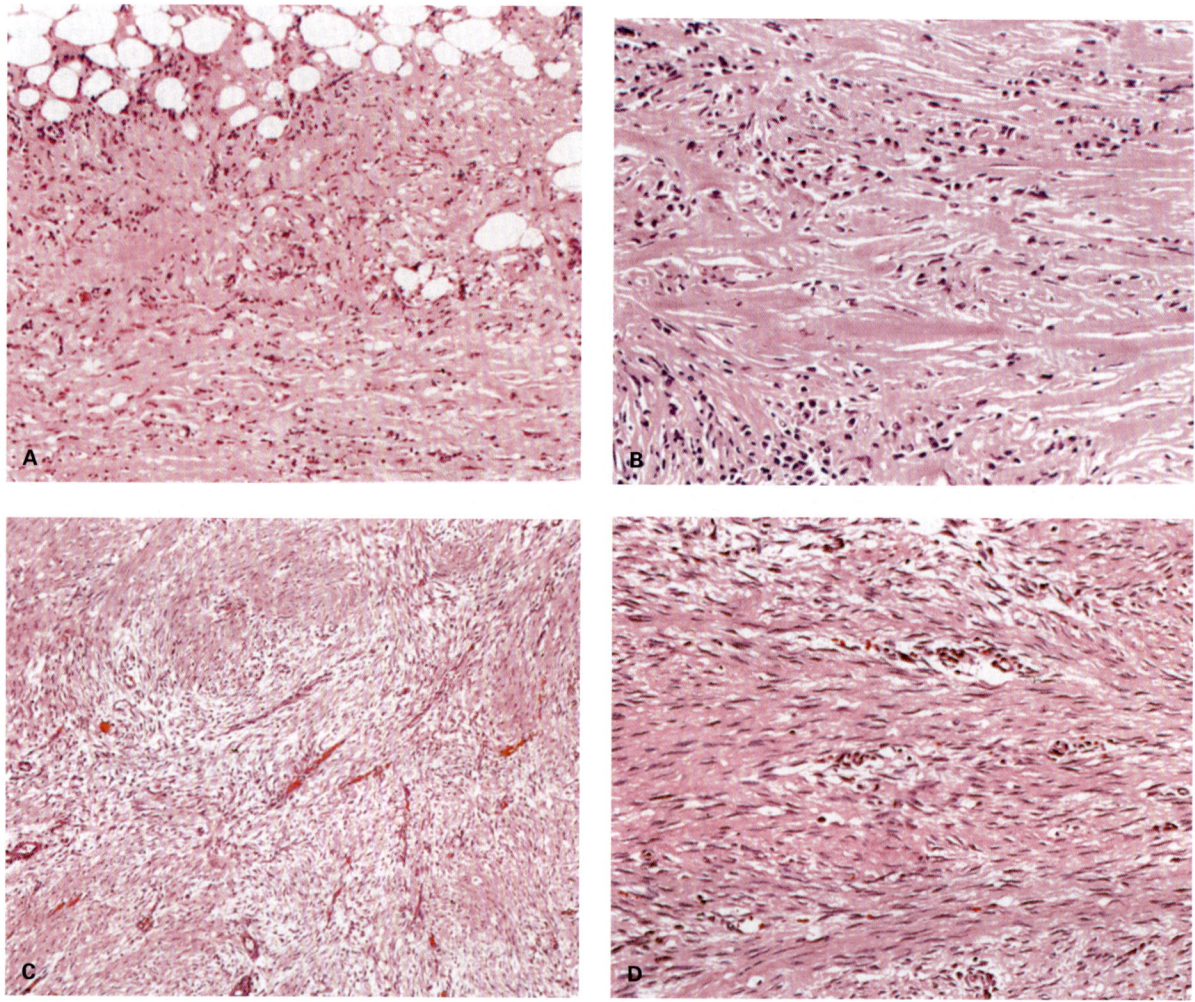

Figure 7-50. Retroperitoneal fibrosis. A: Fat necrosis, dense fibrosis, and infiltration of fibrosis into adipose tissue. B: Note the similarity to mesenteric fibromatosis. C: There is a uniform fibroblastic proliferation with areas of increased cellularity. D: The spindle cells are arranged into interlacing bundles. (Reprinted from Riddell RH, Petras RE, Williams GT, et al. *Atlas of Tumor Pathology: Tumors of the Intestines*. Washington, DC: Armed Forces Institute of Pathology, 2003, with permission.)

or have an associated inflammatory component (e.g., inflammatory MFH, GIST, smooth muscle tumors) leading to confusion with retroperitoneal fibrosis. Sarcomas usually exhibit increased cellularity, prominent atypia, and increased mitotic activity. However, in inflammatory MFH the atypical cells may be quite sparse and sometimes obscured by the inflammation requiring careful inspection of inflamed areas.[23]

Retroperitoneal fibromatosis is characterized by uniform cells in long broad sweeping fascicles and infiltrative margins and most cases are associated with Gardner's syndrome. IMT of the retroperitoneum usually presents as a huge mass lesion in children and young adults. Infective conditions including Whipple's disease (see above) and tuberculosis may result in retroperitoneal fibrosis and inflammation and should always be considered in the differential diagnosis.[23,348] Steroids are the mainstay of treatment for idiopathic retroperitoneal fibrosis and the prognosis is generally favorable. Untreated patients may develop severe local complications including obstructive end-stage renal failure. Surgical therapy is reserved for relief of ureteral obstruction and does not prevent disease progression or recurrence.[348]

Weber–Christian Disease

This rare systemic inflammatory disorder of fat affects mainly young women. Patients typically present with multiple, tender skin nodules on lower extremities, relapsing fever, and other systemic symptoms. Histologically, the skin lesions show subcutaneous inflammation and fat necrosis (i.e., panniculitis). Similar lesions may be seen in the pericardium, bone marrow, retroperitoneum, and mesentery. Differentiation from sclerosing mesenteritis depends on the presence of clinical picture described above.[23,347]

NONNEOPLASTIC LESIONS THAT MAY MIMIC MESENCHYMAL NEOPLASMS

Reactive Nodular Fibrous Pseudotumor

RNFP was first described as a series of five cases by Yantiss et al. in 2003 with a further 11 cases subsequently reported.[151,349-352] It occurs mostly in adults but the age range is wide (1–72 years). Most cases are associated with previous surgery, trauma, or underlying pathology (e.g., diverticulum, ulcer, or endometriosis). Most arise in the outer layer of the bowel wall but transmural extension can occur. Histologically, they are hypocellular lesions composed of bland spindled and stellate cells in collagenous, fibromyxoid, or myxoid stroma (Fig. 7-51). Cells are arranged either in short intersecting fascicles or haphazardly. Mitoses are absent or sparse. Scattered intralesional mononuclear cells and occasional lymphoid aggregates are often present. Margins may be circumscribed or infiltrative.[151,349-352] There have been conflicting reports with respect to their immunohistochemical profile. CD117 immunoreactivity was initially reported in 80% of cases,[349] but this was not confirmed by a subsequent study.[351] Similarly, AE1/AE3 expression varied from absent[349] to present in over 80% of cases,[351] likely relating different sources of antibody used. Most tumors show focal immunoreactivity for actin and ultrastructural features of myofibroblastic differentiation. To date, all have behaved in a benign manner.[151,349-352]

Pseudosarcomatous Granulation Tissue

Pseudosarcomatous change can be seen in granulation tissue of GI ulcers and polyps, particularly in the esophagus but also in the stomach and colon. The inflamed granulation tissue contains bizarre stromal cells with large nuclei, prominent nucleoli, and amphophilic cytoplasm. Cytologic atypia can be extreme and can lead to misdiagnosis of malignancy[353] (Fig. 7-52). Atypia is usually most marked immediately below the fibrin exudate. Useful clues to the reactive nature of the lesion are the lack of marked cellularity, the prominent inflammatory component, and corresponding reactive atypia in endothelial cells and adjacent epithelium.

Heterotopic Mesenteric Ossification

This is a rare reactive process analogous to myositis ossificans in soft tissue. To date, 19 cases have been reported, all but one occurring in men, mostly in mid adulthood and almost invariably following trauma or intraabdominal surgery. The vast majority present with small bowel obstruction. Histologically, the lesions show distinct zonation with a central zone of exuberant fibroblastic proliferation and fat necrosis surrounded by a cartilaginous zone with peripheral ossification. Lace-like osteoid may be present. These tumors may be mistaken for osteosarcoma. Clues to the diagnosis include the history of surgery/trauma and the distinct pattern of zonation which is the reverse of that seen in osteosarcoma. Heterotopic mesenteric ossification is a reactive process which rarely recurs and has no metastatic potential. Treatment is therefore conservative and confined to simple removal of involved segments and lysis of adhesions.[192,354]

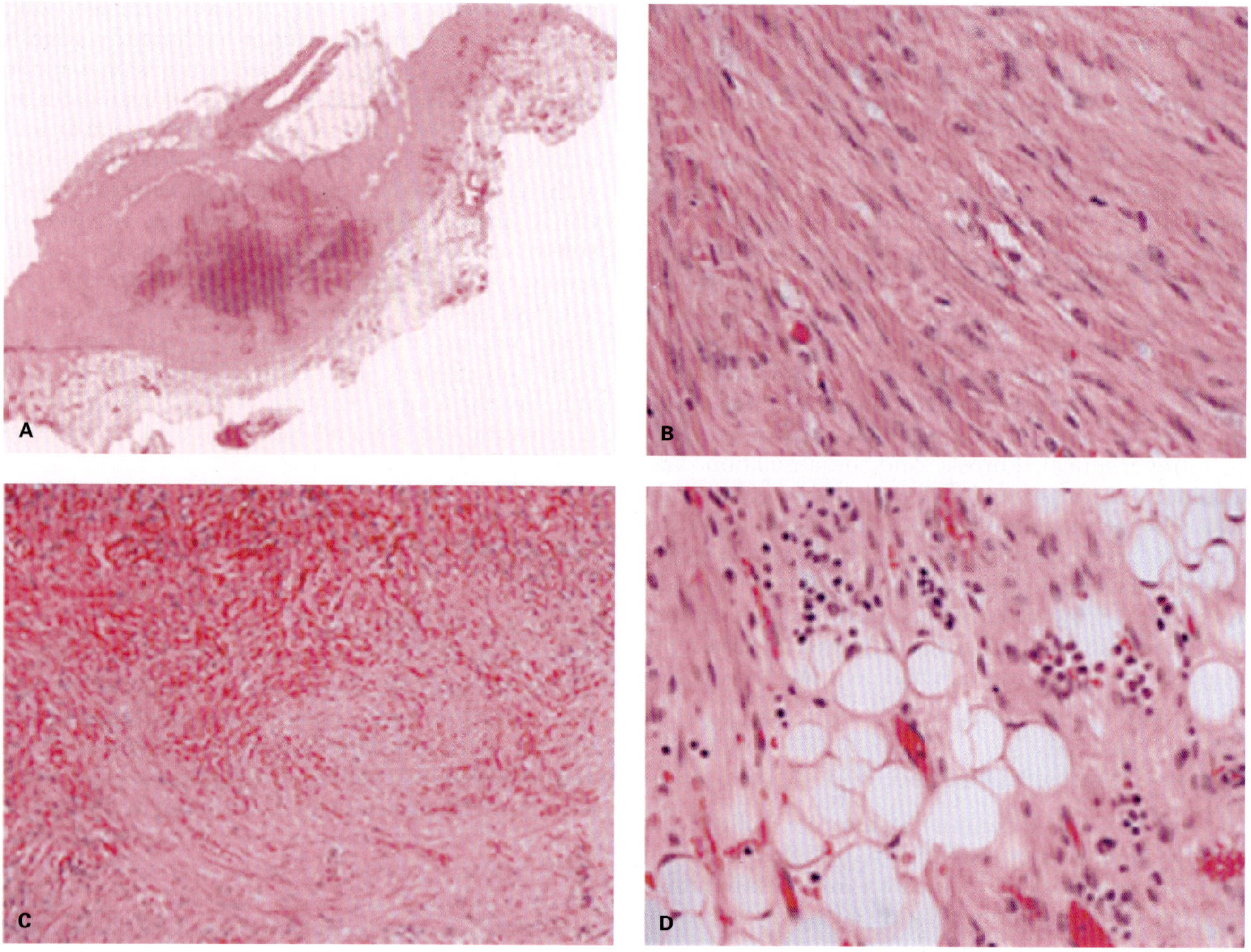

Figure 7-51. Reactive fibrous nodular pseudotumor. Serosal nodule (one of several) **(A)** consisting of an admixture of bland spindled cells, areas of hypocellularity and collagen **(B)**, but also hemorrhage **(C)**, and focally an infiltrating margin with patchy chronic inflammation **(D)**.

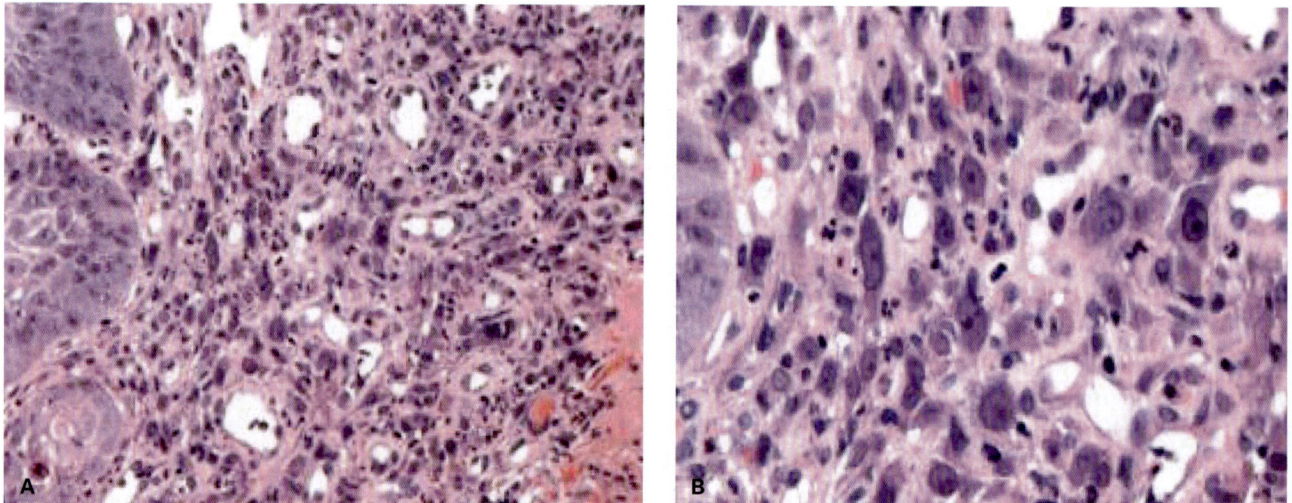

Figure 7-52. Pseudosarcomatous spindle cell proliferations. **A–C:** Biopsy of an ulcerated esophageal polyp (squamous mucosa is left) showing extreme cytologic atypia of stromal cells **(B)**, with similar reactive changes in endothelial cells **(C)** providing a clue to the reactive nature of this lesion.

Figure 7-52. (*Continued*) **D:** This is a different highly cellular reactive spindle cell proliferation that occurred at the site of a polypectomy for an adenomatous polyp. Its mild, focal CD117 immunoreactivity prompted consideration of a GIST.

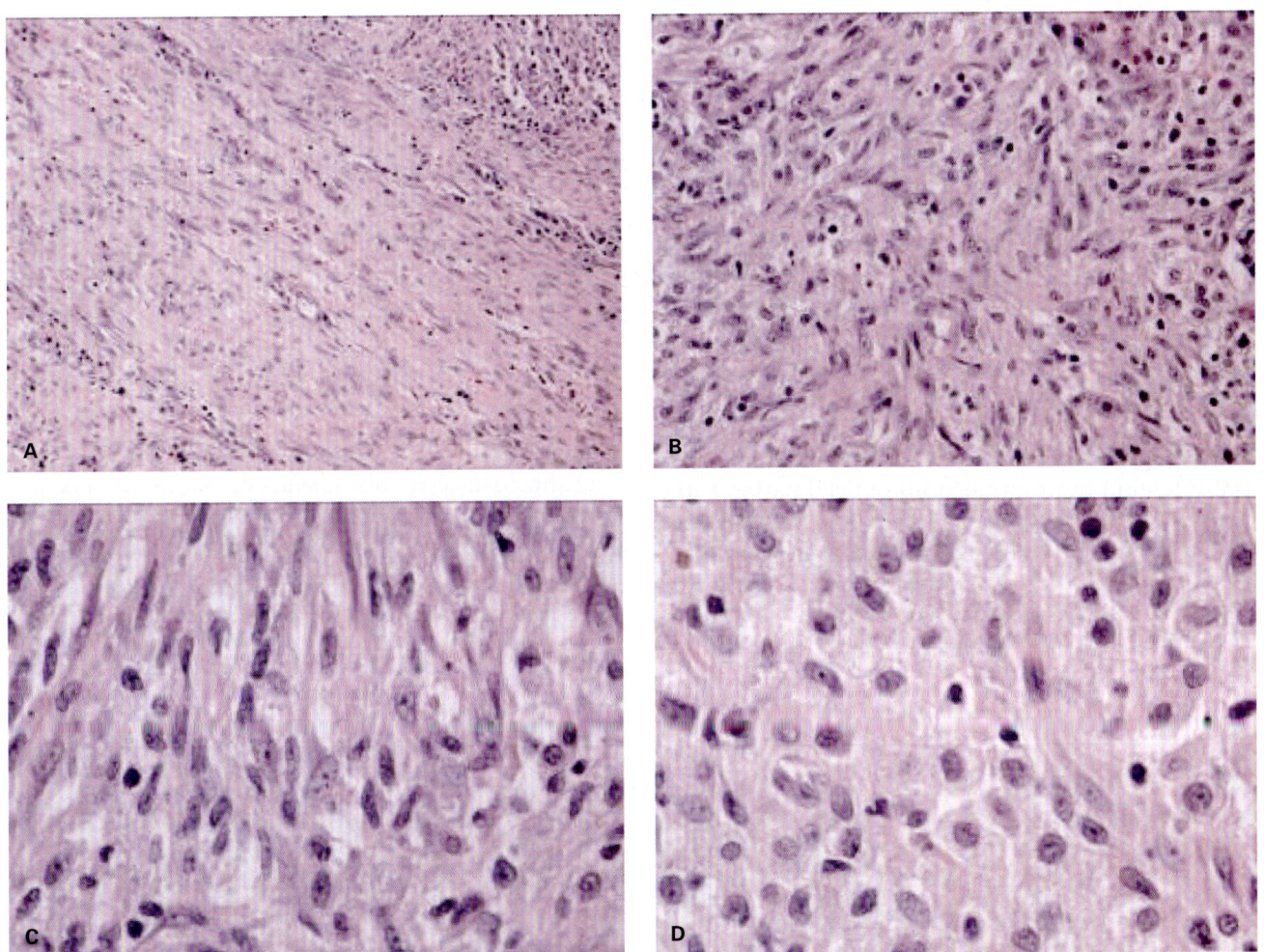

Figure 7-53. Xanthogranulomatous pseudotumor presenting as a mesenteric mass in Crohn's disease. **A–C:** Some areas show sheets of spindled cells in fascicles or haphazardly, raising the possibility of a mesenchymal tumor. **D:** However, other areas are clearly xanthogranulomatous with lipid laden macrophages and admixed inflammatory cells.

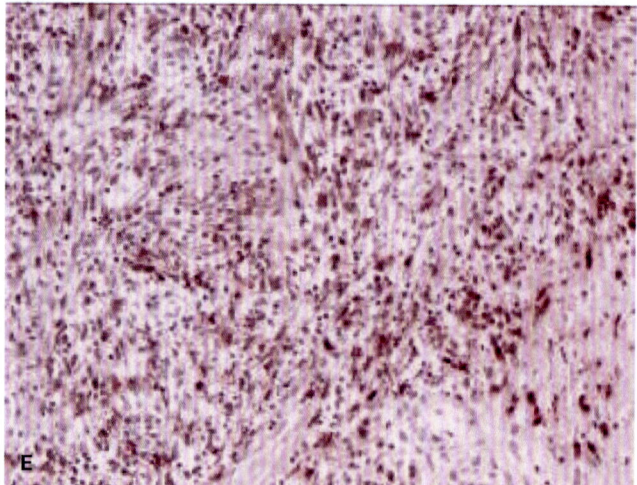 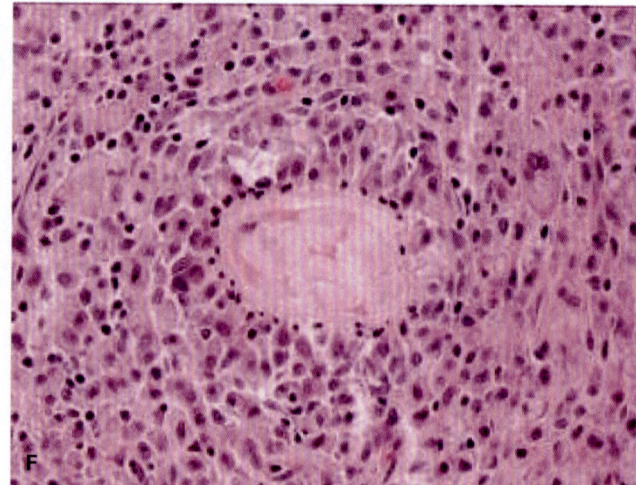

Figure 7-53. (*Continued*) **E:** CD68 immunohistochemistry confirms the histiocytic nature of the lesion. **F:** Occasional partially digested food particles were noted within the lesion.

Xanthogranulomatous Pseudotumor

Xanthogranulomatous inflammation rarely affects the GI tract, usually in areas of ulceration or perforation, sometimes producing mass lesions that mimic mesenchymal neoplasms.[355,356] Early lesions may be cellular with complex interlacing fascicles of spindled cells resembling a stromal tumor. Striking cytologic atypia and proliferative activity can be seen. Longer standing lesions show typical xanthogranulomatous changes including sheets or aggregates of lipid laden macrophages, admixed inflammatory cells, multinucleated giant cell, and occasionally foreign material[355] (Fig. 7-53).

Mycobacterial Spindle Cell Pseudotumor

This rare pseudotumor is associated with mycobacterial infection in immunocompromised patients and mostly affects lymph nodes but has been described in the appendix.[357] Histologically, they are composed of sheets of spindle-shaped histiocytes packed with acid-fast bacilli. A Ziehl–Neelsen stain should be performed on all spindle cell lesions in immunocompromised patients.

References

1. Miettinen M, Majidi M, Lasota J. Pathology and diagnostic criteria of gastrointestinal stromal tumors (GISTs): a review. *Eur J Cancer*. 2002;38(suppl 5):S39–S51.
2. Miettinen M, Makhlouf H, Sobin LH, Lasota J. Gastrointestinal stromal tumors of the jejunum and ileum: a clinicopathologic, immunohistochemical, and molecular genetic study of 906 cases before imatinib with long-term follow-up. *Am J Surg Pathol*. 2006;30(4):477–489.
3. Miettinen M, Sobin LH, Lasota J. Gastrointestinal stromal tumors of the stomach: a clinicopathologic, immunohistochemical, and molecular genetic study of 1765 cases with long-term follow-up. *Am J Surg Pathol*. 2005;29(1):52–68.
4. Rubin BP. Gastrointestinal stromal tumours: an update. *Histopathology*. 2006;48(1):83–96.
5. Mazur MT, Clark HB. Gastric stromal tumors. Reappraisal of histogenesis. *Am J Surg Pathol*. 1983;7(6):507–519.
6. Hirota S, Isozaki K, Moriyama Y, et al. Gain-of-function mutations of c-kit in human gastrointestinal stromal tumors. *Science*. 1998;279(5350):577–580.
7. Kindblom LG, Remotti HE, Aldenborg F, Meis-Kindblom JM. Gastrointestinal pacemaker cell tumor (GIPACT): gastrointestinal stromal tumors show phenotypic characteristics of the interstitial cells of Cajal. *Am J Pathol*. 1998;152(5):1259–1269.
8. Sarlomo-Rikala M, Kovatich AJ, Barusevicius A, Miettinen M. CD117: a sensitive marker for gastrointestinal stromal tumors that is more specific than CD34. *Mod Pathol*. 1998;11(8):728–734.
9. Goettsch WG, Bos SD, Breekveldt-Postma N, et al. Incidence of gastrointestinal stromal tumours is underestimated: results of a nation-wide study. *Eur J Cancer*. 2005;41(18):2868–2872.
10. Nilsson B, Bumming P, Meis-Kindblom JM, et al. Gastrointestinal stromal tumors: the incidence, prevalence, clinical course, and prognostication in the preimatinib mesylate era—a population-based study in western Sweden. *Cancer*. 2005;103(4):821–829.
11. Rubio J, Marcos-Gragera R, Ortiz MR, et al. Population-based incidence and survival of gastrointestinal stromal tumours (GIST) in Girona, Spain. *Eur J Cancer*. 2007;43(1):144–148.
12. Tran T, Davila JA, El-Serag HB. The epidemiology of malignant gastrointestinal stromal tumors: an analysis of 1,458 cases from 1992 to 2000. *Am J Gastroenterol*. 2005;100(1):162–168.
13. Tryggvason G, Gislason HG, Magnusson MK, Jonasson JG. Gastrointestinal stromal tumors in Iceland, 1990–2003: the icelandic GIST study, a population-based incidence and pathologic risk stratification study. *Int J Cancer*. 2005;117(2):289–293.
14. Bussolati G. Of GISTs and EGISTs, ICCs and ICs. *Virchows Arch*. 2005;447(6):907–908.
15. Miettinen M, Lasota J. Gastrointestinal stromal tumors: review on morphology, molecular pathology, prognosis, and differential diagnosis. *Arch Pathol Lab Med*. 2006;130(10):1466–1478.
16. De Chiara A, De Rosa V, Lastoria S, et al. Primary gastrointestinal stromal tumor of the liver with lung metastases successfully treated with STI-571 (imatinib mesylate). *Front Biosci*. 2006;11:498–501.

17. Furihata M, Fujimori T, Imura J, et al. Malignant stromal tumor, so called "gastrointestinal stromal tumor", with rhabdomyomatous differentiation occurring in the gallbladder. *Pathol Res Pract*. 2005;201(8–9):609–613.
18. Lasota J, Carlson JA, Miettinen M. Spindle cell tumor of urinary bladder serosa with phenotypic and genotypic features of gastrointestinal stromal tumor. *Arch Pathol Lab Med*. 2000;124(6):894–897.
19. Uchida H, Sasaki A, Iwaki K, et al. An extramural gastrointestinal stromal tumor of the duodenum mimicking a pancreatic head tumor. *J Hepatobiliary Pancreat Surg*. 2005;12(4):324–327.
20. Demetri GD, Benjamin RS, Blanke CD, et al. NCCN Task Force report: management of patients with gastrointestinal stromal tumor (GIST)—update of the NCCN clinical practice guidelines. *J Natl Compr Canc Netw*. 2007;5(suppl 2):S1–S29; quiz S30.
21. Gupta P, Tewari M, Shukla HS. Gastrointestinal stromal tumor. *Surg Oncol*. 2008;17(2):129–138.
22. Nishida T, Hirota S, Yanagisawa A, et al. Clinical practice guidelines for gastrointestinal stromal tumor (GIST) in Japan: English version. *Int J Clin Oncol*. 2008;13(5):416–430.
23. Riddell RH, Petras RE, Williams GT, et al. Mesenchymal tumors. In: *Atlas of Tumor Pathology: Tumors of the Intestines*. Washington, DC: Armed Forces Institute of Pathology; 2003(Third series):325–394.
24. Chak A, Canto MI, Rosch T, et al. Endosonographic differentiation of benign and malignant stromal cell tumors. *Gastrointest Endosc*. 1997;45(6):468–473.
24a. Tuveson DA, Willis NA, Jacks T, et al. STI571 inactivation of the gastrointestinal stromal tumor c-KIT oncoprotein: biological and clinical implications. *Oncogene*. 2001;20(36):5054–5058.
24b. von Mehren M, Benjamin RS, Bui MM, Casper ES, et al. Soft tissue sarcoma, version 2.2012: featured updates to the NCCN guidelines. *J Natl Compr Canc Netw*. 2012;10(8):951–960.
24c. Demetri GD, Reichardt P, Kang YK, et al. Efficacy and safety of regorafenib for advanced gastrointestinal stromal tumours after failure of imatinib and sunitinib (GRID): an international, multicentre, randomised, placebo-controlled, phase 3 trial. *Lancet*. 2013;381(9863):295–302.
24d. Patil DT, Rubin BP. Gastrointestinal stromal tumor: advances in diagnosis and management. *Arch Pathol Lab Med*. 2011;135(10):1298–1310.
25. Miettinen M, Kopczynski J, Makhlouf HR, et al. Gastrointestinal stromal tumors, intramural leiomyomas, and leiomyosarcomas in the duodenum: a clinicopathologic, immunohistochemical, and molecular genetic study of 167 cases. *Am J Surg Pathol*. 2003;27(5):625–641.
26. Miettinen M, Sarlomo-Rikala M, Sobin LH, Lasota J. Esophageal stromal tumors: a clinicopathologic, immunohistochemical, and molecular genetic study of 17 cases and comparison with esophageal leiomyomas and leiomyosarcomas. *Am J Surg Pathol*. 2000;24(2):211–222.
27. Miettinen M, Sarlomo-Rikala M, Sobin LH, Lasota J. Gastrointestinal stromal tumors and leiomyosarcomas in the colon: a clinicopathologic, immunohistochemical, and molecular genetic study of 44 cases. *Am J Surg Pathol*. 2000;24(10):1339–1352.
28. Zamecnik M, Sosna B, Chlumska A. Gastrointestinal stromal tumor (GIST) with glandular component. A report of an unusual tumor resembling adenosarcoma. *Cesk Patol*. 2005;41(4):150–156.
29. Suster S, Fisher C, Moran CA. Expression of bcl-2 oncoprotein in benign and malignant spindle cell tumors of soft tissue, skin, serosal surfaces, and gastrointestinal tract. *Am J Surg Pathol*. 1998;22(7):863–872.
30. Richmond JA, Mount SL, Schwarz JE. Gastrointestinal stromal tumor of the stomach with rhabdoid phenotype: immunohistochemical, ultrastructural, and immunoelectron microscopic evaluation. *Ultrastruct Pathol*. 2004;28(3):165–170.
31. Insabato L, Di Vizio D, Ciancia G, et al. Malignant gastrointestinal leiomyosarcoma and gastrointestinal stromal tumor with prominent osteoclast-like giant cells. *Arch Pathol Lab Med*. 2004;128(4):440–443.
32. Wong NA. Gastrointestinal stromal tumours—an update for histopathologists. *Histopathology*. 2011;59(5):807–821.
33. Agaram NP, Besmer P, Wong GC, et al. Pathologic and molecular heterogeneity in imatinib-stable or imatinib-responsive gastrointestinal stromal tumors. *Clin Cancer Res*. 2007;13(1):170–181.
34. Goh BK, Chow PK, Chuah KL, et al. Pathologic, radiologic and PET scan response of gastrointestinal stromal tumors after neoadjuvant treatment with imatinib mesylate. *Eur J Surg Oncol*. 2006;32(9):961–963.
35. Pauwels P, Debiec-Rychter M, Stul M, et al. Changing phenotype of gastrointestinal stromal tumours under imatinib mesylate treatment: a potential diagnostic pitfall. *Histopathology*. 2005;47(1):41–47.
36. Antonescu CR, Besmer P, Guo T, et al. Acquired resistance to imatinib in gastrointestinal stromal tumor occurs through secondary gene mutation. *Clin Cancer Res*. 2005;11(11):4182–4190.
37. Espinosa I, Lee CH, Kim MK, et al. A novel monoclonal antibody against DOG1 is a sensitive and specific marker for gastrointestinal stromal tumors. *Am J Surg Pathol*. 2008;32(2):210–218.
38. Miettinen M, Wang ZF, Lasota J. DOG1 antibody in the differential diagnosis of gastrointestinal stromal tumors: a study of 1840 cases. *Am J Surg Pathol*. 2009;33(9):1401–1408.
39. Miselli F, Millefanti C, Conca E, et al. PDGFRA immunostaining can help in the diagnosis of gastrointestinal stromal tumors. *Am J Surg Pathol*. 2008;32(5):738–743.
40. Rossi G, Valli R, Bertolini F, et al. PDGFR expression in differential diagnosis between KIT-negative gastrointestinal stromal tumours and other primary soft-tissue tumours of the gastrointestinal tract. *Histopathology*. 2005;46(5):522–531.
41. Hornick JL, Fletcher CD. The role of KIT in the management of patients with gastrointestinal stromal tumors. *Hum Pathol*. 2007;38(5):679-87.
42. Corless CL, Fletcher JA, Heinrich MC. Biology of gastrointestinal stromal tumors. *J Clin Oncol*. 2004;22(18):3813–3825.
43. Miettinen M, Lasota J. Gastrointestinal stromal tumors (GISTs): definition, occurrence, pathology, differential diagnosis and molecular genetics. *Pol J Pathol*. 2003;54(1):3–24.
44. Orosz Z, Tornoczky T, Sapi Z. Gastrointestinal stromal tumors: a clinicopathologic and immunohistochemical study of 136 cases. *Pathol Oncol Res*. 2005;11(1):11–21.
45. Kaifi JT, Strelow A, Schurr PG, et al. L1 (CD171) is highly expressed in gastrointestinal stromal tumors. *Mod Pathol*. 2006;19(3):399–406.
46. Sarlomo-Rikala M, Tsujimura T, Lendahl U, Miettinen M. Patterns of nestin and other intermediate filament expression distinguish between gastrointestinal stromal tumors, leiomyomas and schwannomas. *Apmis*. 2002;110(6):499–507.
47. Miettinen M, Furlong M, Sarlomo-Rikala M, et al. Gastrointestinal stromal tumors, intramural leiomyomas, and leiomyosarcomas in the rectum and anus: a clinicopathologic, immunohistochemical, and molecular genetic study of 144 cases. *Am J Surg Pathol*. 2001;25(9):1121–1133.
48. Hasegawa T, Matsuno Y, Shimoda T, Hirohashi S. Gastrointestinal stromal tumor: consistent CD117 immunostaining for diagnosis, and prognostic classification based on tumor size and MIB-1 grade. *Hum Pathol*. 2002;33(6):669–676.

49. Montgomery E, Torbenson MS, Kaushal M, et al. Beta-catenin immunohistochemistry separates mesenteric fibromatosis from gastrointestinal stromal tumor and sclerosing mesenteritis. *Am J Surg Pathol.* 2002;26(10):1296–1301.
50. Hornick JL, Fletcher CD. Immunohistochemical staining for KIT (CD117) in soft tissue sarcomas is very limited in distribution. *Am J Clin Pathol.* 2002;117(2):188–193.
51. Hornick JL, Fletcher CD. Validating immunohistochemical staining for KIT (CD117). *Am J Clin Pathol.* 2003;119(3):325–327.
52. Miettinen M, Lasota J. KIT (CD117): a review on expression in normal and neoplastic tissues, and mutations and their clinicopathologic correlation. *Appl Immunohistochem Mol Morphol.* 2005;13(3):205–220.
53. Lucas DR, Al-Abbadi M, Tabaczka P, et al. c-Kit expression in desmoid fibromatosis. Comparative immunohistochemical evaluation of two commercial antibodies. *Am J Clin Pathol.* 2003;119(3):339–345.
54. Blay JY, Bonvalot S, Casali P, et al. Consensus meeting for the management of gastrointestinal stromal tumors. Report of the GIST Consensus Conference of 20–21 March 2004, under the auspices of ESMO. *Ann Oncol.* 2005;16(4):566–578.
55. Loughrey MB, Trivett M, Beshay V, et al. KIT immunohistochemistry and mutation status in gastrointestinal stromal tumours (GISTs) evaluated for treatment with imatinib. *Histopathology.* 2006;49(1):52–65.
56. Badalamenti G, Rodolico V, Fulfaro F, et al. Gastrointestinal stromal tumors (GISTs): focus on histopathological diagnosis and biomolecular features. *Ann Oncol.* 2007(suppl 6):vi136–140.
57. Lopes LF, West RB, Bacchi LM, et al. DOG1 for the diagnosis of gastrointestinal stromal tumor (GIST): comparison between 2 different antibodies. *Appl Immunohistochem Mol Morphol.* 2010;18(4):333–337.
58. Novelli M, Rossi S, Rodriguez-Justo M, et al. DOG1 and CD117 are the antibodies of choice in the diagnosis of gastrointestinal stromal tumours. *Histopathology.* 2010;57(2):259–270.
59. Heinrich MC, Corless CL, Duensing A, et al. PDGFRA activating mutations in gastrointestinal stromal tumors. *Science.* 2003;299(5607):708–710.
60. Hirota S, Ohashi A, Nishida T, et al. Gain-of-function mutations of platelet-derived growth factor receptor alpha gene in gastrointestinal stromal tumors. *Gastroenterology.* 2003;125(3):660–667.
61. Medeiros F, Corless CL, Duensing A, et al. KIT-negative gastrointestinal stromal tumors: proof of concept and therapeutic implications. *Am J Surg Pathol.* 2004;28(7):889–894.
62. Chute DJ, Cousar JB, Mills SE. Anorectal malignant melanoma: morphologic and immunohistochemical features. *Am J Clin Pathol.* 2006;126(1):1–8.
63. Miettinen M, Sarlomo-Rikala M, Lasota J. KIT expression in angiosarcomas and fetal endothelial cells: lack of mutations of exon 11 and exon 17 of C-kit. *Mod Pathol.* 2000;13(5):536–541.
64. Geller MA, Argenta P, Bradley W, et al. Treatment and recurrence patterns in endometrial stromal sarcomas and the relation to c-kit expression. *Gynecol Oncol.* 2004;95(3):632–636.
65. Evert M, Wardelmann E, Nestler G, et al. Abdominopelvic perivascular epithelioid cell sarcoma (malignant PEComa) mimicking gastrointestinal stromal tumour of the rectum. *Histopathology.* 2005;46(1):115–117.
66. Bellone G, Smirne C, Carbone A, et al. KIT/stem cell factor expression in premalignant and malignant lesions of the colon mucosa in relationship to disease progression and outcomes. *Int J Oncol.* 2006;29(4):851–859.
67. Reed J, Ouban A, Schickor FK, et al. Immunohistochemical staining for c-Kit (CD117) is a rare event in human colorectal carcinoma. *Clin Colorectal Cancer.* 2002;2(2):119–122.
68. Yorke R, Chirala M, Younes M. c-kit proto-oncogene product is rarely detected in colorectal adenocarcinoma. *J Clin Oncol.* 2003 15;21(20):3885–3886; discussion 6–7.
69. Butnor KJ, Burchette JL, Sporn TA, et al. The spectrum of Kit (CD117) immunoreactivity in lung and pleural tumors: a study of 96 cases using a single-source antibody with a review of the literature. *Arch Pathol Lab Med.* 2004;128(5):538–543.
70. Parfitt JR, Streutker CJ, Riddell RH, Driman DK. Gastrointestinal stromal tumors: a contemporary review. *Pathol Res Pract.* 2006;202(12):837–847.
71. Rutkowski P, Debiec-Rychter M, Ruka W. Gastrointestinal stromal tumors: key to diagnosis and choice of therapy. *Mol Diagn Ther.* 2008;12(3):131–143.
72. Hirota S, Isozaki K. Pathology of gastrointestinal stromal tumors. *Pathol Int.* 2006;56(1):1–9.
73. Patil DT, Rubin BP. Gastrointestinal stromal tumor: advances in diagnosis and management. *Arch Pathol Lab Med.* 2011;135(10):1298–1310.
74. Huss S, Kunstlinger H, Wardelmann E, et al. A subset of gastrointestinal stromal tumors previously regarded as wild-type tumors carries somatic activating mutations in KIT exon 8 (p.D419del). *Mod Pathol.* 2013;26(7):1004–1012.
75. Corless CL, Schroeder A, Griffith D, et al. PDGFRA mutations in gastrointestinal stromal tumors: frequency, spectrum and in vitro sensitivity to imatinib. *J Clin Oncol.* 2005;23(23):5357–5364.
76. Lasota J, Stachura J, Miettinen M. GISTs with PDGFRA exon 14 mutations represent subset of clinically favorable gastric tumors with epithelioid morphology. *Lab Invest.* 2006;86(1):94–100.
77. Postow MA, Carvajal RD. Therapeutic implications of KIT in melanoma. *Cancer J.* 2012;18(2):137–141.
78. Debiec-Rychter M, Sciot R, Le Cesne A, et al. KIT mutations and dose selection for imatinib in patients with advanced gastrointestinal stromal tumours. *Eur J Cancer.* 2006;42(8):1093–1103.
79. Hostein I, Faur N, Primois C, et al. BRAF mutation status in gastrointestinal stromal tumors. *Am J Clin Pathol.* 2010;133(1):141–148.
80. Agaimy A, Terracciano LM, Dirnhofer S, et al. V600E BRAF mutations are alternative early molecular events in a subset of KIT/PDGFRA wild-type gastrointestinal stromal tumours. *J Clin Pathol.* 2009;62(7):613–616.
81. Miettinen M, Wang ZF, Sarlomo-Rikala M, et al. Succinate dehydrogenase-deficient GISTs: a clinicopathologic, immunohistochemical, and molecular genetic study of 66 gastric GISTs with predilection to young age. *Am J Surg Pathol.* 2011;35(11):1712–1721.
82. Gill AJ, Chou A, Vilain R, et al. Immunohistochemistry for SDHB divides gastrointestinal stromal tumors (GISTs) into 2 distinct types. *Am J Surg Pathol.* 2010;34(5):636–644.
83. Wagner AJ, Remillard SP, Zhang YX, et al. Loss of expression of SDHA predicts SDHA mutations in gastrointestinal stromal tumors. *Mod Pathol.* 2013;26(2):289–294.
84. Chou A, Chen J, Clarkson A, Samra JS, et al. Succinate dehydrogenase-deficient GISTs are characterized by IGF1R overexpression. *Mod Pathol.* 2012;25(9):1307–1313.
85. El-Rifai W, Sarlomo-Rikala M, Andersson LC, et al. DNA sequence copy number changes in gastrointestinal stromal tumors: tumor progression and prognostic significance. *Cancer Res.* 2000;60(14):3899–3903.
86. Takahashi T, Nakajima K, Nishitani A, et al. An enhanced risk-group stratification system for more practical prognostication of clinically malignant gastrointestinal stromal tumors. *Int J Clin Oncol.* 2007;12(5):369–374.
87. Joensuu H. Risk stratification of patients diagnosed with gastrointestinal stromal tumor. *Hum Pathol.* 2008;39(10):1411–1419.

88. Fletcher CD, Berman JJ, Corless C, et al. Diagnosis of gastrointestinal stromal tumors: a consensus approach. *Hum Pathol.* 2002;33(5):459–465.
89. Appelman H, Helwig EB. Cellular leiomyomas of the stomach in 40 patients. *Arch Pathol Lab Med.* 1977;101(7):373–377.
90. Emory TS, Sobin LH, Lukes L, et al. Prognosis of gastrointestinal smooth-muscle (stromal) tumors: dependence on anatomic site. *Am J Surg Pathol.* 1999;23(1):82–87.
91. Ueyama T, Guo KJ, Hashimoto H, et al. A clinicopathologic and immunohistochemical study of gastrointestinal stromal tumors. *Cancer.* 1992;69(4):947–955.
92. Lagarde P, Perot G, Kauffmann A, et al. Mitotic checkpoints and chromosome instability are strong predictors of clinical outcome in gastrointestinal stromal tumors. *Clin Cancer Res.* 2012;18(3):826–838.
93. Bertucci F, Finetti P, Ostrowski J, et al. Genomic Grade Index predicts postoperative clinical outcome of GIST. *Br J Cancer.* 2012;107(8):1433–1441.
94. Beghini A, Tibiletti MG, Roversi G, et al. Germline mutation in the juxtamembrane domain of the kit gene in a family with gastrointestinal stromal tumors and urticaria pigmentosa. *Cancer.* 2001;92(3):657–662.
95. Hirota S, Nishida T, Isozaki K, et al. Familial gastrointestinal stromal tumors associated with dysphagia and novel type germline mutation of KIT gene. *Gastroenterology.* 2002;122(5):1493–1499.
96. Isozaki K, Terris B, Belghiti J, et al. Germline-activating mutation in the kinase domain of KIT gene in familial gastrointestinal stromal tumors. *Am J Pathol.* 2000;157(5):1581–1585.
97. Li FP, Fletcher JA, Heinrich MC, et al. Familial gastrointestinal stromal tumor syndrome: phenotypic and molecular features in a kindred. *J Clin Oncol.* 2005;23(12):2735–2743.
98. Maeyama H, Hidaka E, Ota H, et al. Familial gastrointestinal stromal tumor with hyperpigmentation: association with a germline mutation of the c-kit gene. *Gastroenterology.* 2001;120(1):210–215.
99. Nishida T, Hirota S, Taniguchi M, et al. Familial gastrointestinal stromal tumours with germline mutation of the KIT gene. *Nat Genet.* 1998;19(4):323–324.
100. Thalheimer A, Schlemmer M, Bueter M, et al. Familial gastrointestinal stromal tumors caused by the novel KIT exon 17 germline mutation N822Y. *Am J Surg Pathol.* 2008;32(10):1560–1565.
101. Chompret A, Kannengiesser C, Barrois M, et al. PDGFRA germline mutation in a family with multiple cases of gastrointestinal stromal tumor. *Gastroenterology.* 2004;126(1):318–321.
102. Wozniak A, Rutkowski P, Sciot R, et al. Rectal gastrointestinal stromal tumors associated with a novel germline KIT mutation. *Int J Cancer.* 2008;122(9):2160–2164.
103. Neuhann TM, Mansmann V, Merkelbach Bruse S, et al. A novel germline KIT mutation (p.L576P) in a family presenting with juvenile onset of multiple gastrointestinal stromal tumors, skin hyperpigmentations, and esophageal stenosis. *Am J Surg Pathol.* 2013;37(6):898–905.
104. Zoller ME, Rembeck B, Oden A, et al. Malignant and benign tumors in patients with neurofibromatosis type 1 in a defined Swedish population. *Cancer.* 1997;79(11):2125–2131.
105. Andersson J, Sihto H, Meis-Kindblom JM, et al. NF1-associated gastrointestinal stromal tumors have unique clinical, phenotypic, and genotypic characteristics. *Am J Surg Pathol.* 2005;29(9):1170–1176.
106. Miettinen M, Fetsch JF, Sobin LH, Lasota J. Gastrointestinal stromal tumors in patients with neurofibromatosis 1: a clinicopathologic and molecular genetic study of 45 cases. *Am J Surg Pathol.* 2006;30(1):90–96.
107. Kinoshita K, Hirota S, Isozaki K, et al. Absence of c-kit gene mutations in gastrointestinal stromal tumours from neurofibromatosis type 1 patients. *J Pathol.* 2004;202(1):80–85.
108. Yantiss RK, Rosenberg AE, Sarran L, et al. Multiple gastrointestinal stromal tumors in type I neurofibromatosis: a pathologic and molecular study. *Mod Pathol.* 2005;18(4):475–484.
109. Takazawa Y, Sakurai S, Sakuma Y, et al. Gastrointestinal stromal tumors of neurofibromatosis type I (von Recklinghausen's disease). *Am J Surg Pathol.* 2005;29(6):755–763.
110. Boldorini R, Tosoni A, Leutner M, et al. Multiple small intestinal stromal tumours in a patient with previously unrecognised neurofibromatosis type 1: immunohistochemical and ultrastructural evaluation. *Pathology.* 2001;33(3):390–395.
111. Carney JA. Gastric stromal sarcoma, pulmonary chondroma, and extra-adrenal paraganglioma (Carney Triad): natural history, adrenocortical component, and possible familial occurrence. *Mayo Clin Proc.* 1999;74(6):543–552.
112. Carney JA, Sheps SG, Go VL, Gordon H. The triad of gastric leiomyosarcoma, functioning extra-adrenal paraganglioma and pulmonary chondroma. *N Engl J Med.* 1977;296(26):1517–1518.
113. Agaimy A, Pelz AF, Corless CL, et al. Epithelioid gastric stromal tumours of the antrum in young females with the Carney triad: a report of three new cases with mutational analysis and comparative genomic hybridization. *Oncol Rep.* 2007;18(1):9–15.
114. Diment J, Tamborini E, Casali P, et al. Carney triad: case report and molecular analysis of gastric tumor. *Hum Pathol.* 2005;36(1):112–116.
115. Carney JA, Stratakis CA. Familial paraganglioma and gastric stromal sarcoma: a new syndrome distinct from the Carney triad. *Am J Med Genet.* 2002;108(2):132–139.
116. Pasini B, McWhinney SR, Bei T, et al. Clinical and molecular genetics of patients with the Carney–Stratakis syndrome and germline mutations of the genes coding for the succinate dehydrogenase subunits SDHB, SDHC, and SDHD. *Eur J Hum Genet.* 2008;16(1):79–88.
117. Agaimy A, Dirnhofer S, Wunsch PH, et al. Multiple sporadic gastrointestinal stromal tumors (GISTs) of the proximal stomach are caused by different somatic KIT mutations suggesting a field effect. *Am J Surg Pathol.* 2008;32(10):1553–1559.
118. Gasparotto D, Rossi S, Bearzi I, et al. Multiple primary sporadic gastrointestinal stromal tumors in the adult: an underestimated entity. *Clin Cancer Res.* 2008;14(18):5715–5721.
119. Haller F, Schulten HJ, Armbrust T, et al. Multicentric sporadic gastrointestinal stromal tumors (GISTs) of the stomach with distinct clonal origin: differential diagnosis to familial and syndromal GIST variants and peritoneal metastasis. *Am J Surg Pathol.* 2007;31(6):933–937.
120. Kang DY, Park CK, Choi JS, et al. Multiple gastrointestinal stromal tumors: clinicopathologic and genetic analysis of 12 patients. *Am J Surg Pathol.* 2007;31(2):224–232.
121. Kerr JZ, Hicks MJ, Nuchtern JG, et al. Gastrointestinal autonomic nerve tumors in the pediatric population: a report of four cases and a review of the literature. *Cancer.* 1999;85(1):220–230.
122. Miettinen M, Lasota J, Sobin LH. Gastrointestinal stromal tumors of the stomach in children and young adults: a clinicopathologic, immunohistochemical, and molecular genetic study of 44 cases with long-term follow-up and review of the literature. *Am J Surg Pathol.* 2005;29(10):1373–1381.
123. Prakash S, Sarran L, Socci N, et al. Gastrointestinal stromal tumors in children and young adults: a clinicopathologic,

molecular, and genomic study of 15 cases and review of the literature. *J Pediatr Hematol Oncol.* 2005;27(4):179–187.
124. Price VE, Zielenska M, Chilton-MacNeill S, et al. Clinical and molecular characteristics of pediatric gastrointestinal stromal tumors (GISTs). *Pediatr Blood Cancer.* 2005;45(1):20–24.
125. Chetty R. Small and microscopically detected gastrointestinal stromal tumours: an overview. *Pathology.* 2008;40(1): 9–12.
126. Agaimy A, Wunsch PH, Hofstaedter F, et al. Minute gastric sclerosing stromal tumors (GIST tumorlets) are common in adults and frequently show c-KIT mutations. *Am J Surg Pathol.* 2007;31(1):113–120.
127. Kawanowa K, Sakuma Y, Sakurai S, et al. High incidence of microscopic gastrointestinal stromal tumors in the stomach. *Hum Pathol.* 2006;37(12):1527–1535.
128. Abraham SC, Krasinskas AM, Hofstetter WL, et al. "Seedling" mesenchymal tumors (gastrointestinal stromal tumors and leiomyomas) are common incidental tumors of the esophagogastric junction. *Am J Surg Pathol.* 2007;31(11): 1629–1635.
129. Agaimy A, Wunsch PH. Sporadic Cajal cell hyperplasia is common in resection specimens for distal oesophageal carcinoma. A retrospective review of 77 consecutive surgical resection specimens. *Virchows Arch.* 2006;448(3):288–294.
130. Corless CL, McGreevey L, Haley A, et al. KIT mutations are common in incidental gastrointestinal stromal tumors one centimeter or less in size. *Am J Pathol.* 2002;160(5):1567–1572.
131. Abraham SC. Distinguishing gastrointestinal stromal tumors from their mimics: an update. *Adv Anat Pathol.* 2007; 14(3):178–188.
132. Kirsch R, Gao ZH, Riddell R. Gastrointestinal stromal tumors: diagnostic challenges and practical approach to differential diagnosis. *Adv Anat Pathol.* 2007;14(4):261–285.
133. Higa S, Matsumoto M, Tamai O, et al. Plexiform leiomyoma of the esophagus: a peculiar gross variant simulating plexiform neurofibroma. *J Gastroenterol.* 1996;31(1):100–104.
134. Mutrie CJ, Donahue DM, Wain JC, et al. Esophageal leiomyoma: a 40-year experience. *Ann Thorac Surg.* 2005;79(4): 1122–1125.
135. Miettinen M, Sarlomo-Rikala M, Sobin LH. Mesenchymal tumors of muscularis mucosae of colon and rectum are benign leiomyomas that should be separated from gastrointestinal stromal tumors—a clinicopathologic and immunohistochemical study of eighty-eight cases. *Mod Pathol.* 2001;14(10):950–966.
136. Matsukuma S, Takeo H, Ohara I, Sakai Y. Endoscopically resected colorectal leiomyomas often containing eosinophilic globules. *Histopathology.* 2004;45(3):302–303.
137. Deyrup AT, Lee VK, Hill CE, et al. Epstein-Barr virus-associated smooth muscle tumors are distinctive mesenchymal tumors reflecting multiple infection events: a clinicopathologic and molecular analysis of 29 tumors from 19 patients. *Am J Surg Pathol.* 2006;30(1):75–82.
138. Ho-Yen C, Chang F, van der Walt J, Lucas S. Gastrointestinal malignancies in HIV-infected or immunosuppressed patients: pathologic features and review of the literature. *Adv Anat Pathol.* 2007;14(6):431–443.
139. Calabrese C, Fabbri A, Fusaroli P, et al. Diffuse esophageal leiomyomatosis: case report and review. *Gastrointest Endosc.* 2002;55(4):590–593.
140. McKeeby JL, Li X, Zhuang Z, et al. Multiple leiomyomas of the esophagus, lung, and uterus in multiple endocrine neoplasia type 1. *Am J Pathol.* 2001;159(3):1121–1127.
141. Siegler RW, Rothstein RI, Beecham JB, Dunn JL. Gastroesophageal-vulvar leiomyomatosis presenting over the course of 20 years. *Arch Pathol Lab Med.* 1996;120(12):1141–1144.
142. Vallaeys JH, Cuvelier CA, Bekaert L, Roels H. Combined leiomyomatosis of the small intestine and colon. *Arch Pathol Lab Med.* 1992;116(3):281–283.
143. Goh SG, Ho JM, Chuah KL, et al. Leiomyomatosis-like lymphangioleiomyomatosis of the colon in a female with tuberous sclerosis. *Mod Pathol.* 2001;14(11):1141–1146.
144. Hizawa K, Iida M, Matsumoto T, et al. Gastrointestinal involvement in tuberous sclerosis. Two case reports. *J Clin Gastroenterol.* 1994;19(1):46–49.
145. Hardman WJ, III, Majmudar B. Leiomyomatosis peritonealis disseminata: clinicopathologic analysis of five cases. *South Med J.* 1996;89(3):291–294.
146. Papadatos D, Taourel P, Bret PM. CT of leiomyomatosis peritonealis disseminata mimicking peritoneal carcinomatosis. *AJR Am J Roentgenol.* 1996;167(2):475–476.
147. Randrianjafisamindrakotroka NS, Baldauf JJ, Philippe E, et al. Leiomyomatosis peritonealis disseminata. Report on two cases and differential diagnosis with peritoneal metastases of a low-grade stromal sarcoma of the ovary. *Pathol Res Pract.* 1995;191(12):1252–1257; discussion 8.
148. Fulcher AS, Szucs RA. Leiomyomatosis peritonealis disseminata complicated by sarcomatous transformation and ovarian torsion: presentation of two cases and review of the literature. *Abdom Imag.* 1998;23(6):640–644.
149. Valente PT, Fine BA, Parra C, Schroeder B. Gastric stromal tumor with peritoneal nodules in pregnancy: tumor spread or rare variant of diffuse leiomyomatosis. *Gynecol Oncol.* 1996;63(3):392–397.
150. Yasuda K, Adachi Y, Kitano S, et al. Gastrointestinal stromal tumor with diffuse mesenteric metastases. *Int Surg.* 2005;90(4):215–218.
151. Saglam EA, Usubutun A, Kart C, et al. Reactive nodular fibrous pseudotumor involving the pelvic and abdominal cavity: a case report and review of literature. *Virchows Arch.* 2005;447(5):879–882.
152. Appelman HD, Helwig EB. Glomus tumors of the stomach. *Cancer.* 1969;23(1):203–213.
153. Miettinen M, Paal E, Lasota J, Sobin LH. Gastrointestinal glomus tumors: a clinicopathologic, immunohistochemical, and molecular genetic study of 32 cases. *Am J Surg Pathol.* 2002;26(3):301–311.
154. Barua R. Glomus tumor of the colon. First reported case. *Dis Colon Rectum.* 1988;31(2):138–140.
155. Geraghty JM, Everitt NJ, Blundell JW. Glomus tumour of the small bowel. *Histopathology.* 1991;19(3):287–289.
156. Folpe AL, Fanburg-Smith JC, Miettinen M, Weiss SW. Atypical and malignant glomus tumors: analysis of 52 cases, with a proposal for the reclassification of glomus tumors. *Am J Surg Pathol.* 2001;25(1):1–12.
157. Kapur U, Hobbs CM, McDermott E, Mooney EE. Gastric glomus tumor. *Ann Diagn Pathol.* 2004;8(1):32–35.
158. Aggarwal G, Sharma S, Zheng M, et al. Primary leiomyosarcomas of the gastrointestinal tract in the post-gastrointestinal stromal tumor era. *Ann Diagn Pathol.* 2012;16(6):532–540.
159. Kwon MS, Lee SS, Ahn GH. Schwannomas of the gastrointestinal tract: clinicopathological features of 12 cases including a case of esophageal tumor compared with those of gastrointestinal stromal tumors and leiomyomas of the gastrointestinal tract. *Pathol Res Pract.* 2002;198(9):605–613.
160. Lasota J, Wasag B, Dansonka-Mieszkowska A, et al. Evaluation of NF2 and NF1 tumor suppressor genes in distinctive gastrointestinal nerve sheath tumors traditionally diagnosed as benign schwannomas: s study of 20 cases. *Lab Invest.* 2003;83(9):1361–1371.
161. Miettinen M, Shekitka KM, Sobin LH. Schwannomas in the colon and rectum: a clinicopathologic and

immunohistochemical study of 20 cases. *Am J Surg Pathol.* 2001;25(7):846-855.
162. Hou YY, Tan YS, Xu JF, et al. Schwannoma of the gastrointestinal tract: a clinicopathological, immunohistochemical and ultrastructural study of 33 cases. *Histopathology.* 2006;48(5):536-545.
163. Voltaggio L, Murray R, Lasota J, et al. Gastric schwannoma: a clinicopathologic study of 51 cases and critical review of the literature. *Hum Pathol.* 2012;43(5):650-659.
164. Iida A, Imamura Y, Katayama K, et al. Plexiform schwannoma of the small intestine: report of a case. *Surg Today.* 2003;33(12):940-943.
165. Brown RM, Darnton SJ, Papadaki L, et al. A primary tumour of the oesophagus with both melanocytic and schwannian differentiation. Melanocytic schwannoma or malignant melanoma? *J Clin Pathol.* 2002;55(4):318-320.
166. Chetty R, Vajpeyi R, Penwick JL. Psammomatous melanotic schwannoma presenting as colonic polyps. *Virchows Arch.* 2007;451(3):717-720.
167. Lewin MR, Dilworth HP, Abu Alfa AK, et al. Mucosal benign epithelioid nerve sheath tumors. *Am J Surg Pathol.* 2005;29(10):1310-1315.
168. Petersen JM, Ferguson DR. Gastrointestinal neurofibromatosis. *J Clin Gastroenterol.* 1984;6(6):529-534.
169. Bakker JR, Haber MM, Garcia FU. Gastrointestinal neurofibromatosis: an unusual cause of gastric outlet obstruction. *Am Surg.* 2005;71(2):100-105.
170. Fuller CE, Williams GT. Gastrointestinal manifestations of type 1 neurofibromatosis (von Recklinghausen's disease). *Histopathology.* 1991;19(1):1-11.
171. Liu T, Willmore-Payne C, Layfield LJ, et al. A gastrointestinal stromal tumor of the stomach morphologically resembling a neurofibroma: demonstration of a novel platelet-derived growth factor receptor alpha exon 18 mutation. *Hum Pathol.* 2008;39(12):1849-1853.
172. Chan OT, Haghighi P. Hamartomatous polyps of the colon: ganglioneuromatous, stromal, and lipomatous. *Arch Pathol Lab Med.* 2006;130(10):1561-1566.
173. Shekitka KM, Sobin LH. Ganglioneuromas of the gastrointestinal tract. Relation to Von Recklinghausen disease and other multiple tumor syndromes. *Am J Surg Pathol.* 1994;18(3):250-257.
174. d'Amore ES, Manivel JC, Pettinato G, et al. Intestinal ganglioneuromatosis: mucosal and transmural types. A clinicopathologic and immunohistochemical study of six cases. *Hum Pathol.* 1991;22(3):276-286.
175. Gibson JA, Hornick JL. Mucosal Schwann Cell "Hamartoma": clinicopathologic study of 26 neural colorectal polyps distinct from neurofibromas and mucosal neuromas. *Am J Surg Pathol.* 2009;33(5):781-787.
176. Carr NJ, Sobin LH. Unusual tumors of the appendix and pseudomyxoma peritonei. *Semin Diagn Pathol.* 1996;13(4):314-325.
177. Agaimy A, Wuensch PH. Perineurioma of the stomach. A rare spindle cell neoplasm that should be distinguished from gastrointestinal stromal tumor. *Pathol Res Pract.* 2005;201(6):463-467.
178. Hornick JL, Fletcher CD. Intestinal perineuriomas: clinicopathologic definition of a new anatomic subset in a series of 10 cases. *Am J Surg Pathol.* 2005;29(7):859-865.
179. Eslami-Varzaneh F, Washington K, Robert ME, et al. Benign fibroblastic polyps of the colon: a histologic, immunohistochemical, and ultrastructural study. *Am J Surg Pathol.* 2004;28(3):374-378.
180. Agaimy A, Stoehr R, Vieth M, et al. Benign serrated colorectal fibroblastic polyps/intramucosal perineuriomas are true mixed epithelial-stromal polyps (hybrid hyperplastic polyp/mucosal perineurioma) with frequent BRAF mutations. *Am J Surg Pathol.* 2010;34(11):1663-1671.
181. Pai RK, Mojtahed A, Rouse RV, et al. Histologic and molecular analyses of colonic perineurial-like proliferations in serrated polyps: perineurial-like stromal proliferations are seen in sessile serrated adenomas. *Am J Surg Pathol.* 2011;35(9):1373-1380.
182. Groisman GM, Polak-Charcon S. Fibroblastic polyp of the colon and colonic perineurioma: 2 names for a single entity? *Am J Surg Pathol.* 2008;32(7):1088-1094.
183. Zamecnik M, Chlumska A. Perineurioma versus fibroblastic polyp of the colon. *Am J Surg Pathol.* 2006;30(10):1337-1339.
184. Rittershaus AC, Appelman HD. Benign gastrointestinal mesenchymal BUMPS: a brief review of some spindle cell polyps with published names. *Arch Pathol Lab Med.* 2011;135(10):1311-1319.
185. Bucher P, Mathe Z, Buhler L, et al. Paraganglioma of the ampulla of Vater: a potentially malignant neoplasm. *Scand J Gastroenterol.* 2004;39(3):291-295.
186. Burke AP, Helwig EB. Gangliocytic paraganglioma. *Am J Clin Pathol.* 1989;92(1):1-9.
187. Scheithauer BW, Nora FE, LeChago J, et al. Duodenal gangliocytic paraganglioma. Clinicopathologic and immunocytochemical study of 11 cases. *Am J Clin Pathol.* 1986;86(5):559-565.
188. Narra SL, Tombazzi C, Datta V, Ismail MK. Granular cell tumor of the esophagus: report of five cases and review of the literature. *Am J Med Sci.* 2008;335(5):338-341.
189. Johnston J, Helwig EB. Granular cell tumors of the gastrointestinal tract and perianal region: a study of 74 cases. *Dig Dis Sci.* 1981;26(9):807-816.
190. Gertsch P, Mosimann R. A rare tumor of the esophagus: the granular cell myoblastoma. Report of a case and review of the literature. *Endoscopy.* 1980;12(5):245-249.
191. Fanburg-Smith JC, Meis-Kindblom JM, Fante R, Kindblom LG. Malignant granular cell tumor of soft tissue: diagnostic criteria and clinicopathologic correlation. *Am J Surg Pathol.* 1998;22(7):779-794.
192. Al-Nafussi A, Wong NA. Intra-abdominal spindle cell lesions: a review and practical aids to diagnosis. *Histopathology.* 2001;38(5):387-402.
193. Lee YJ, Moon H, Park ST, et al. Malignant peripheral nerve sheath tumor arising from the colon in a newborn: report of a case and review of the literatures. *J Pediatr Surg.* 2006;41(2):e19-e22.
194. Murase K, Hino A, Ozeki Y, et al. Malignant schwannoma of the esophagus with lymph node metastasis: literature review of schwannoma of the esophagus. *J Gastroenterol.* 2001;36(11):772-777.
195. Chambonniere ML, Mosnier-Damet M, Cavillon C, Mosnier JF. Mixed neuronal-glial tumor of the digestive tract: distinctive entity from gastrointestinal stromal tumor? *Pathol Int.* 2002;52(2):153-157.
196. Burke AP, Sobin LH, Shekitka KM, et al. Intra-abdominal fibromatosis. A pathologic analysis of 130 tumors with comparison of clinical subgroups. *Am J Surg Pathol.* 1990;14(4):335-341.
197. Dong-Heup K, Kim DH, Goldsmith HS, et al. Intra-abdominal desmoid tumor. *Cancer.* 1971;27(5):1041-1045.
198. Rodriguez JA, Guarda LA, Rosai J. Mesenteric fibromatosis with involvement of the gastrointestinal tract. A GIST simulator: a study of 25 cases. *Am J Clin Pathol.* 2004;121(1):93-98.
199. Yantiss RK, Spiro IJ, Compton CC, Rosenberg AE. Gastrointestinal stromal tumor versus intra-abdominal fibromatosis of the bowel wall: a clinically important differential diagnosis. *Am J Surg Pathol.* 2000;24(7):947-957.

200. Miettinen M. Are desmoid tumors kit positive? *Am J Surg Pathol.* 2001;25(4):549-550.
201. Daum O, Hes O, Vanecek T, et al. Vanek's tumor (inflammatory fibroid polyp). Report of 18 cases and comparison with three cases of original Vanek's series. *Ann Diagn Pathol.* 2003;7(6):337-347.
202. Schildhaus HU, Cavlar T, Binot E, et al. Inflammatory fibroid polyps harbour mutations in the platelet-derived growth factor receptor alpha (PDGFRA) gene. *J Pathol.* 2008;216(2):176-182.
203. Gonul II, Erdem O, Ataoglu O. Inflammatory fibroid polyp of the ileum causing intussusception: a case report. *Turk J Gastroenterol.* 2004;15(1):59-62.
204. Nkanza NK, King M, Hutt MS. Intussusception due to inflammatory fibroid polyps of the ileum: a report of 12 cases from Africa. *Br J Surg.* 1980;67(4):271-274.
205. Vanek. Gastric submucosal granuloma with eosinophilic infiltration. *Am J Pathol.* 1949;25:397-412.
206. Pantanowitz L, Antonioli DA, Pinkus GS, et al. Inflammatory fibroid polyps of the gastrointestinal tract: evidence for a dendritic cell origin. *Am J Surg Pathol.* 2004;28(1):107-114.
207. Huss S, Wardelmann E, Goltz D, et al. Activating PDGFRA mutations in inflammatory fibroid polyps occur in exons 12, 14 and 18 and are associated with tumour localization. *Histopathology.* 2012;61(1):59-68.
208. Lasota J, Wang ZF, Sobin LH, et al. Gain-of-function PDGFRA mutations, earlier reported in gastrointestinal stromal tumors, are common in small intestinal inflammatory fibroid polyps. A study of 60 cases. *Mod Pathol.* 2009;22(8):1049-1056.
209. Allibone RO, Nanson JK, Anthony PP. Multiple and recurrent inflammatory fibroid polyps in a Devon family ('Devon polyposis syndrome'): an update. *Gut.* 1992;33(7):1004-1005.
210. Abu-Abed S KR, Chen CH, Riddell RH, et al. Multiple, recurrent inflammatory fibroid polyps associated with an exon 18 PDGFRA germline mutation. *Gastroenterology.* 2013;144:S-523.
211. Carney JA, Stratakis CA. Stromal, fibrous, and fatty gastrointestinal tumors in a patient with a PDGFRA gene mutation. *Am J Surg Pathol.* 2008;32(9):1412-1420.
212. Makhlouf HR, Sobin LH. Inflammatory myofibroblastic tumors (inflammatory pseudotumors) of the gastrointestinal tract: how closely are they related to inflammatory fibroid polyps? *Hum Pathol.* 2002;33(3):307-315.
213. Miettinen M, Makhlouf HR, Sobin LH, Lasota J. Plexiform fibromyxoma: a distinctive benign gastric antral neoplasm not to be confused with a myxoid GIST. *Am J Surg Pathol.* 2009;33(11):1624-1632.
214. Tripathi M LCH, Divaris D, Pace R, et al. Plexiform fibromyxoma of the gastric antrum: clinicopathologic and molecular characterization of 5 cases. *Lab Invest.* 2013;93(183A).
215. Coffin CM, Watterson J, Priest JR, Dehner LP. Extrapulmonary inflammatory myofibroblastic tumor (inflammatory pseudotumor). A clinicopathologic and immunohistochemical study of 84 cases. *Am J Surg Pathol.* 1995;19(8):859-872.
216. Cook JR, Dehner LP, Collins MH, Ma Z, et al. Anaplastic lymphoma kinase (ALK) expression in the inflammatory myofibroblastic tumor: a comparative immunohistochemical study. *Am J Surg Pathol.* 2001;25(11):1364-1371.
217. Coffin CM, Humphrey PA, Dehner LP. Extrapulmonary inflammatory myofibroblastic tumor: a clinical and pathological survey. *Semin Diagn Pathol.* 1998;15(2):85-101.
218. Sanders BM, West KW, Gingalewski C, et al. Inflammatory pseudotumor of the alimentary tract: clinical and surgical experience. *J Pediatr Surg.* 2001;36(1):169-173.
219. Coffin CM, Patel A, Perkins S, et al. ALK1 and p80 expression and chromosomal rearrangements involving 2p23 in inflammatory myofibroblastic tumor. *Mod Pathol.* 2001;14(6):569-576.
220. Mariño-Enríquez A, Wang WL, Roy A, et al. Epithelioid inflammatory myofibroblastic sarcoma: an aggressive intra-abdominal variant of inflammatory myofibroblastic tumor with nuclear membrane or perinuclear ALK. *Am J Surg Pathol.* 2011;35(1):135-144.
221. Donner LR, Trompler RA, White RRt. Progression of inflammatory myofibroblastic tumor (inflammatory pseudotumor) of soft tissue into sarcoma after several recurrences. *Hum Pathol.* 1996;27(10):1095-1098.
222. Hussong JW, Brown M, Perkins SL, et al. Comparison of DNA ploidy, histologic, and immunohistochemical findings with clinical outcome in inflammatory myofibroblastic tumors. *Mod Pathol.* 1999;12(3):279-286.
223. Moran CA, Suster S, Koss MN. The spectrum of histologic growth patterns in benign and malignant fibrous tumors of the pleura. *Semin Diagn Pathol.* 1992;9(2):169-180.
224. Hasegawa T, Matsuno Y, Shimoda T, et al. Extrathoracic solitary fibrous tumors: their histological variability and potentially aggressive behavior. *Hum Pathol.* 1999;30(12):1464-1473.
225. Doucet J, Dardick I, Srigley JR, et al. Localized fibrous tumour of serosal surfaces. Immunohistochemical and ultrastructural evidence for a type of mesothelioma. *Virchows Arch A Pathol Anat Histopathol.* 1986;409(3):349-363.
226. Lee WA, Lee MK, Jeen YM, et al. Solitary fibrous tumor arising in gastric serosa. *Pathol Int.* 2004;54(6):436-439.
227. Young RH, Clement PB, McCaughey WT. Solitary fibrous tumors ('fibrous mesotheliomas') of the peritoneum. A report of three cases and a review of the literature. *Arch Pathol Lab Med.* 1990;114(5):493-495.
228. Goodlad JR, Fletcher CD. Solitary fibrous tumour arising at unusual sites: analysis of a series. *Histopathology.* 1991;19(6):515-522.
229. Brunnemann RB, Ro JY, Ordonez NG, et al. Extrapleural solitary fibrous tumor: a clinicopathologic study of 24 cases. *Mod Pathol.* 1999;12(11):1034-1042.
230. Gengler C, Guillou L. Solitary fibrous tumour and haemangiopericytoma: evolution of a concept. *Histopathology.* 2006;48(1):63-74.
231. Binder SC, Wolfe HJ, Deterling RA Jr. Intra-abdominal hemangiopericytoma. Report of four cases and review of the literature. *Arch Surg.* 1973;107(4):536-543.
232. McMaster MJ, Soule EH, Ivins JC. Hemangiopericytoma. A clinicopathologic study and long-term followup of 60 patients. *Cancer.* 1975;36(6):2232-2244.
233. Attila T, Chen D, Gardiner GW, et al. Gastric calcifying fibrous tumor. *Can J Gastroenterol.* 2006;20(7):487-489.
234. Chen KT. Familial peritoneal multifocal calcifying fibrous tumor. *Am J Clin Pathol.* 2003;119(6):811-815.
235. Delbecque K, Legrand M, Boniver J, et al. Calcifying fibrous tumour of the gastric wall. *Histopathology.* 2004;44(4):399-400.
236. Elpek GO, Kupesiz GY, Ogus M. Incidental calcifying fibrous tumor of the stomach presenting as a polyp. *Pathol Int.* 2006;56(4):227-31.
237. Kocova L, Michal M, Sulc M, Zamecnik M. Calcifying fibrous pseudotumour of visceral peritoneum. *Histopathology.* 1997;31(2):182-184.
238. Nascimento AF, Ruiz R, Hornick JL, Fletcher CD. Calcifying fibrous 'pseudotumor': clinicopathologic study of 15 cases and analysis of its relationship to inflammatory myofibroblastic tumor. *Int J Surg Pathol.* 2002;10(3):189-196.

239. Puccio F, Solazzo M, Marciano P, Benzi F. Laparoscopic resection of calcifying fibrous pseudotumor of the gastric wall. A unique case report. *Surg Endosc.* 2001;15(10):1227.
240. Emanuel P, Qin L, Harpaz N. Calcifying fibrous tumor of small intestine. *Ann Diagn Pathol.* 2008;12(2):138–141.
241. Van Dorpe J, Ectors N, Geboes K, et al. Is calcifying fibrous pseudotumor a late sclerosing stage of inflammatory myofibroblastic tumor? *Am J Surg Pathol.* 1999;23(3):329–335.
242. Enjoji M, Sumiyoshi K, Sueyoshi K. Elastofibromatous lesion of the stomach in a patient with elastofibroma dorsi. *Am J Surg Pathol.* 1985;9(3):233–237.
243. Saint-Paul MC, Musso S, Cardot-Leccia N, et al. Elastofibroma of the stomach. *Pathol Res Pract.* 2003;199(9):637–639.
244. Sakatani T, Shomori K, Adachi H, et al. Elastofibroma of the sigmoid colon. *Pathol Res Pract.* 2000;196(3):205–207.
245. Vesoulis Z, Ravichandran P, Agamanolis D, Roe D. Elastofibromatous polyp of the sigmoid colon—a case report and review of gastrointestinal elastofibromas. *Can J Gastroenterol.* 2003;17(4):275–277.
246. Goldblum JR, Beals T, Weiss SW. Elastofibromatous change of the rectum. A lesion mimicking amyloidosis. *Am J Surg Pathol.* 1992;16(8):793–795.
247. Markl B, Kerwel TG, Langer E, et al. Elastosis of the colon and the ileum as polyp causing lesions: a study of six cases and review of the literature. *Pathol Res Pract.* 2008;204(6):395–399.
248. Tawfik OW, McGregor DH. Lipohyperplasia of the ileocecal valve. *Am J Gastroenterol.* 1992;87(1):82–87.
249. Geboes K, De Wolf-Peeters C, Rutgeerts P, et al. Submucosal tumors of the colon: experience with twenty-five cases. *Dis Colon Rectum.* 1978;21(6):420–425.
250. Imamura K, Fuchigami T, Iida M, et al. Duodenal lipoma—a report of three cases. *Gastrointest Endosc.* 1983;29(3):223–224.
251. Chiang JM, Lin YS. Tumor spectrum of adult intussusception. *J Surg Oncol.* 2008;98(6):444–447.
252. Martin P, Sklow B, Adler DG. Large colonic lipoma mimicking colon cancer and causing colonic intussusception. *Dig Dis Sci.* 2008;53(10):2826–2827.
253. Snover DC. Atypical lipomas of the colon. Report of two cases with pseudomalignant features. *Dis Colon Rectum.* 1984;27(7):485–488.
254. Kato K, Matsuda M, Onodera K, et al. Angiolipoma of the colon with right lower quadrant abdominal pain. *Dig Surg.* 1999;16(5):441–444.
255. McGregor DH, Kerley SW, McGregor MS. Case report: gastric angiolipoma with chronic hemorrhage and severe anemia. *Am J Med Sci.* 1993;305(4):229–235.
256. Mohl W, Fischinger J, Moser C, et al. Duodenal angiolipoma—endoscopic diagnosis and therapy. *Z Gastroenterol.* 2004;42(12):1381–1383.
257. Ling CS, Leagus C, Stahlgren LH. Intestinal lipomatosis. *Surgery.* 1959;46:1054–1059.
258. Climie AR, Wylin RF. Small-intestinal lipomatosis. *Arch Pathol Lab Med.* 1981;105(1):40–42.
259. Margolin FR, Lagios MD. Polypoid lipomatosis of the small bowel. *Gastrointest Radiol.* 1980;5(1):59–60.
260. O'Connell DJ, Shaw DG, Swain VA. Epiploic lipomatosis and lipomatous polyposis of the colon. *Br J Radiol.* 1976;49(587):969–971.
261. Amato G, Martella A, Ferraraccio F, et al. Well differentiated "lipoma-like" liposarcoma of the sigmoid mesocolon and multiple lipomatosis of the rectosigmoid colon. Report of a case. *Hepatogastroenterology.* 1998;45(24):2151–2156.
262. Ranchod M, French TJ, Novis BH, et al. Diffuse nodular lipomatosis and diverticulosis of the small intestine. *Gastroenterology.* 1972;63(4):667–671.
263. Young TH, Ho P, Lee HS, et al. A rare case of multiple intussusceptions: intense segmentary lipomatosis of the ileum. *Am J Gastroenterol.* 1996;91(1):162–163.
264. Tayal S, Classen E, Bemis L, et al. C-kit expression in dedifferentiated and well-differentiated liposarcomas; immunohistochemistry and genetic analysis. *Anticancer Res.* 2005;25(3B):2215–2220.
265. Wallander ML, Layfield LJ, Tripp SR, et al. Gastrointestinal stromal tumors: clinical significance of p53 expression, MDM2 amplification, and KIT mutation status. *Appl Immunohistochem Mol Morphol.* 2013;21(4):308–312.
266. Tornillo L, Duchini G, Carafa V, et al. Patterns of gene amplification in gastrointestinal stromal tumors (GIST). *Lab Invest.* 2005;85(7):921–931.
267. Kang JY, Chan-Wilde C, Wee A, et al. Role of computed tomography and endoscopy in the management of alimentary tract lipomas. *Gut.* 1990;31(5):550–553.
268. Weiss SW, Goldblum JR. Benign tumors and tumor-like lesions of blood vessels. In: *Enzinger and Weiss's Soft Tissue Tumors.* Philadelphia, PA: Elsevier; 2008:Chapter 22.
269. Sylla P, Deutsch G, Luo J, et al. Cavernous, arteriovenous, and mixed hemangioma-lymphangioma of the rectosigmoid: rare causes of rectal bleeding—case series and review of the literature. *Int J Colorectal Dis.* 2008;23(7):653–658.
270. Allred HW Jr. Hemangiomas of the colon, rectum, and anus. *Mayo Clin Proc.* 1974;49(10):739–741.
271. Coppa GF, Eng K, Localio SA. Surgical management of diffuse cavernous hemangioma of the colon, rectum and anus. *Surg Gynecol Obstet.* 1984;159(1):17–22.
272. Stening SG, Heptinstall DP. Diffuse cavernous haemangioma of the rectum and sigmoid colon. *Br J Surg.* 1970;57(3):186–189.
273. Camilleri M, Chadwick VS, Hodgson HJ. Vascular anomalies of the gastrointestinal tract. *Hepatogastroenterology.* 1984;31(3):149–153.
274. Allison KH, Yoder BJ, Bronner MP, et al. Angiosarcoma involving the gastrointestinal tract: a series of primary and metastatic cases. *Am J Surg Pathol.* 2004;28(3):298–307.
275. Bavikatty NR, Goldblum JR, Abdul-Karim FW, et al. Florid vascular proliferation of the colon related to intussusception and mucosal prolapse: potential diagnostic confusion with angiosarcoma. *Mod Pathol.* 2001;14(11):1114–1118.
276. Aase S, Gundersen R. Submucous lymphatic cysts of the small intestine. An autopsy study. *Acta Pathol Microbiol Immunol Scand A.* 1983;91(3):191–194.
277. Axiotis CA, Zeman RK, Chuong JJ, Barwick KW. Intra-abdominal lymphangiectatic cysts: an uncommon abdominal lesion in children and young adults. *J Clin Gastroenterol.* 1983;5(6):541–548.
278. Loludice T, West D, Rosenblum S, et al. Chylous cyst of the transverse colon. *J Clin Gastroenterol.* 1986;8(5):580–581.
279. Lapner PC, Chou S, Jimenez C. Perianal fetal rhabdomyoma: case report. *Pediatr Surg Int.* 1997;12(7):544–547.
280. Roberts F, Kirk AJ, More IA, et al. Oesophageal rhabdomyoma. *J Clin Pathol.* 2000;53(7):554–557.
281. Tuazon R. Rhabdomyoma of the stomach. Report of a case. *Am J Clin Pathol.* 1969;52(1):37–41.
282. Okamura K, Yamamoto H, Ishimaru Y, et al. Clinical characteristics and surgical treatment of perianal and perineal rhabdomyosarcoma: analysis of Japanese patients and comparison with IRSG reports. *Pediatr Surg Int.* 2006;22(2):129–134.
283. Caty MG, Oldham KT, Prochownik EV. Embryonal rhabdomyosarcoma of the ampulla of Vater with long-term survival following pancreaticoduodenectomy. *J Pediatr Surg.* 1990;25(12):1256–1258.

284. Fox KR, Moussa SM, Mitre RJ, et al. Clinical and pathologic features of primary gastric rhabdomyosarcoma. *Cancer.* 1990;66(4):772–778.
285. Moses I, Coodley EL. Rhabdomyosarcoma of duodenum. *Am J Gastroenterol.* 1969;51(1):48–54.
286. Willen R, Lillo-Gil R, Willen H, et al. Embryonal rhabdomyosarcoma of the oesophagus. Case report. *Acta Chir Scand.* 1989;155(1):59–64.
287. Deenik W, Mooi WJ, Rutgers EJ, et al. Clear cell sarcoma (malignant melanoma) of soft parts: a clinicopathologic study of 30 cases. *Cancer.* 1999;86(6):969–975.
288. Enzinger FM. Clear-cell sarcoma of tendons and aponeuroses. An Analysis of 21 cases. *Cancer.* 1965;18:1163–1174.
289. Covinsky M, Gong S, Rajaram V, et al. EWS-ATF1 fusion transcripts in gastrointestinal tumors previously diagnosed as malignant melanoma. *Hum Pathol.* 2005;36(1):74–81.
290. Friedrichs N, Testi MA, Moiraghi L, et al. Clear cell sarcoma-like tumor with osteoclast-like giant cells in the small bowel: further evidence for a new tumor entity. *Int J Surg Pathol.* 2005;13(4):313–318.
291. Huang W, Zhang X, Li D, et al. Osteoclast-rich tumor of the gastrointestinal tract with features resembling those of clear cell sarcoma of soft parts. *Virchows Arch.* 2006;448(2):200–203.
292. Taminelli L, Zaman K, Gengler C, et al. Primary clear cell sarcoma of the ileum: an uncommon and misleading site. *Virchows Arch.* 2005;447(4):772–777.
293. Venkataraman G, Quinn AM, Williams J, Hammadeh R. Clear cell sarcoma of the small bowel: a potential pitfall. Case report. *Apmis.* 2005;113(10):716–719.
294. Zambrano E, Reyes-Mugica M, Franchi A, Rosai J. An osteoclast-rich tumor of the gastrointestinal tract with features resembling clear cell sarcoma of soft parts: reports of 6 cases of a GIST simulator. *Int J Surg Pathol.* 2003;11(2):75–81.
295. Abdulkader I, Cameselle-Teijeiro J, de Alava E, Ruiz-Ponte C, et al. Intestinal clear cell sarcoma with melanocytic differentiation and EWS [corrected] rearrangement: report of a case. *Int J Surg Pathol.* 2008;16(2):189–193.
296. Rosai J. Editorial: clear cell sarcoma and osteoclast-rich clear cell sarcoma-like tumor of the gastrointestinal tract: one tumor type or two? Melanoma or sarcoma? *Int J Surg Pathol.* 2005;13(4):309–311.
297. Lyle PL, Amato CM, Fitzpatrick JE, Robinson WA. Gastrointestinal melanoma or clear cell sarcoma? Molecular evaluation of 7 cases previously diagnosed as malignant melanoma. *Am J Surg Pathol.* 2008;32(6):858–866.
298. Stockman DL, Miettinen M, Suster S, et al. Malignant gastrointestinal neuroectodermal tumor: clinicopathologic, immunohistochemical, ultrastructural, and molecular analysis of 16 cases with a reappraisal of clear cell sarcoma-like tumors of the gastrointestinal tract. *Am J Surg Pathol.* 2012;36(6):857–868.
299. Asada Y, Isomoto H, Akama F, et al. Metastatic low-grade endometrial stromal sarcoma of the sigmoid colon three years after hysterectomy. *World J Gastroenterol.* 2005;11(15):2367–2369.
300. Kethu SR, Zheng S, Eid R. Metastatic low-grade endometrial stromal sarcoma presented as a subepithelial mass in the stomach was diagnosed by EUS-guided FNA. *Gastrointest Endosc.* 2005;62(5):814–816.
301. Kovac D, Gasparovic I, Jasic M, et al. Endometrial stromal sarcoma arising in extrauterine endometriosis: a case report. *Eur J Gynaecol Oncol.* 2005;26(1):113–6.
302. Yantiss RK, Clement PB, Young RH. Neoplastic and preneoplastic changes in gastrointestinal endometriosis: a study of 17 cases. *Am J Surg Pathol.* 2000;24(4):513–524.
303. Mourra N, Tiret E, Parc Y, et al. Endometrial stromal sarcoma of the rectosigmoid colon arising in extragonadal endometriosis and revealed by portal vein thrombosis. *Arch Pathol Lab Med.* 2001;125(8):1088–1090.
304. Cho HY, Kim MK, Cho SJ, et al. Endometrial stromal sarcoma of the sigmoid colon arising in endometriosis: a case report with a review of literatures. *J Korean Med Sci.* 2002;17(3):412–414.
305. Kusaka M, Mikuni M, Nishiya M. A case of high-grade endometrial stromal sarcoma arising from endometriosis in the cul-de-sac. *Int J Gynecol Cancer.* 2006;16(2):895–899.
306. Agaimy A, Gaumann A, Schroeder J, et al. Primary and metastatic high-grade pleomorphic sarcoma/malignant fibrous histiocytoma of the gastrointestinal tract: an approach to the differential diagnosis in a series of five cases with emphasis on myofibroblastic differentiation. *Virchows Arch.* 2007;451(5):949–957.
307. Coindre JM, Mariani O, Chibon F, et al. Most malignant fibrous histiocytomas developed in the retroperitoneum are dedifferentiated liposarcomas: a review of 25 cases initially diagnosed as malignant fibrous histiocytoma. *Mod Pathol.* 2003;16(3):256–262.
308. Genevay M, Mc Kee T, Zimmer G, et al. Digestive PEComas: a solution when the diagnosis fails to "fit". *Ann Diagn Pathol.* 2004;8(6):367–372.
309. Hornick JL, Fletcher CD. PEComa: what do we know so far? *Histopathology.* 2006;48(1):75–82.
310. Ryan P, Nguyen VH, Gholoum S, et al. Polypoid PEComa in the rectum of a 15-year-old girl: case report and review of PEComa in the gastrointestinal tract. *Am J Surg Pathol.* 2009;33(3):475–482.
311. Shi HY, Wei LX, Sun L, et al. Clinicopathologic analysis of 4 perivascular epithelioid cell tumors (PEComas) of the gastrointestinal tract. *Int J Surg Pathol.* 2010;18(4):243–247.
312. Park SH, Ro JY, Kim HS, Lee ES. Perivascular epithelioid cell tumor of the uterus: immunohistochemical, ultrastructural and molecular study. *Pathol Int.* 2003;53(11):800–805.
313. Folpe AL, Mentzel T, Lehr HA, et al. Perivascular epithelioid cell neoplasms of soft tissue and gynecologic origin: a clinicopathologic study of 26 cases and review of the literature. *Am J Surg Pathol.* 2005;29(12):1558–1575.
314. De Padua M, Gupta N, Broor SL, Govil D. Duodenal angiomyolipoma: a case report. *Ind J Pathol Microbiol.* 2007;50(3):568–569.
315. Lin CY, Chen HY, Jwo SC, Chan SC. Ileal angiomyolipoma as an unusual cause of small-intestinal intussusception. *J Gastroenterol.* 2005;40(2):200–203.
316. Billings SD, Meisner LF, Cummings OW, Tejada E. Synovial sarcoma of the upper digestive tract: a report of two cases with demonstration of the X;18 translocation by fluorescence in situ hybridization. *Mod Pathol.* 2000;13(1):68–76.
317. Butori C, Hofman V, Attias R, et al. Diagnosis of primary esophageal synovial sarcoma by demonstration of t(X;18) translocation: a case report. *Virchows Arch.* 2006;449(2):262–267.
318. Makhlouf HR, Ahrens W, Agarwal B, et al. Synovial sarcoma of the stomach: a clinicopathologic, immunohistochemical, and molecular genetic study of 10 cases. *Am J Surg Pathol.* 2008;32(2):275–281.
319. Parfitt JR, Xu J, Kontozoglou T, et al. Primary monophasic synovial sarcoma of the colon. *Histopathology.* 2007;50(4):521–523.
320. Schreiber-Facklam H, Bode-Lesniewska B, Frigerio S, Flury R. Primary monophasic synovial sarcoma of the duodenum with SYT/SSX2 type of translocation. *Hum Pathol.* 2007;38(6):946–949.

321. Gal AA, Martin SE, Kernen JA, Patterson MJ. Esophageal carcinoma with prominent spindle cells. *Cancer.* 1987;60(9):2244-2250.
322. Iezzoni JC, Mills SE. Sarcomatoid carcinomas (carcinosarcomas) of the gastrointestinal tract: a review. *Semin Diagn Pathol.* 1993;10(2):176-187.
323. Kayaselcuk F, Tuncer I, Toyganozu Y, et al. Carcinosarcoma of the stomach. *Pathol Oncol Res.* 2002;8(4):275-277.
324. Tsukadaira A, Koizumi T, Okubo Y, et al. Small-intestinal sarcomatoid carcinoma with superior vena cava syndrome. *J Gastroenterol.* 2002;37(6):471-475.
325. Ishida H, Ohsawa T, Nakada H, et al. Carcinosarcoma of the rectosigmoid colon: report of a case. *Surg Today.* 2003;33(7):545-549.
326. Kalogeropoulos NK, Antonakopoulos GN, Agapitos MB, Papacharalampous NX. Spindle cell carcinoma (pseudosarcoma) of the anus: a light, electron microscopic and immunocytochemical study of a case. *Histopathology.* 1985;9(9):987-994.
327. Lewin KJ, Appelman HA. Squamous carcinoma. In: *Atlas of Tumor Pathology: Tumors of the Esophagus and Stomach.* Fascicle 18. Washington, DC: Armed Forces Institute of Pathology; 1996:43-97.
328. Miettinen M, Dow N, Lasota J, Sobin LH. A distinctive novel epitheliomesenchymal biphasic tumor of the stomach in young adults ("gastroblastoma"): a series of 3 cases. *Am J Surg Pathol.* 2009;33(9):1370-137.
329. Wey EA, Britton AJ, Sferra JJ, et al. Gastroblastoma in a 28-year-old man with nodal metastasis: proof of the malignant potential. *Arch Pathol Lab Med.* 2012;136(8):961-964.
330. Dasgupta TK, Brasfield RD. Metastatic melanoma of the gastrointestinal tract. *Arch Surg.* 1964;88:969-973.
331. Klaase JM, Kroon BB. Surgery for melanoma metastatic to the gastrointestinal tract. *Br J Surg.* 1990;77(1):60-61.
332. Cooper PH, Mills SE, Allen MS, Jr. Malignant melanoma of the anus: report of 12 patients and analysis of 255 additional cases. *Dis Colon Rectum.* 1982;25(7):693-703.
333. DiCostanzo DP, Urmacher C. Primary malignant melanoma of the esophagus. *Am J Surg Pathol.* 1987;11(1):46-52.
334. Riddell R, Petras RE, Williams GT, et al. Malignant melanomas. In: *Atlas of Tumor Pathology: Tumors of the Intestines.* Washington, DC: Armed Forces Institute of Pathology; 2003; Third Series: 266-267.
335. Lewin KJ, Appelman HA. Unusual malignant neoplasms of the esophagus. In: *Atlas of Tumor Pathology: Tumors of the Esophagus and Stomach.* Washington, DC: Armed Forces Institute of Pathology; 1996;Third Series:163-173.
336. Chang KC, Jin YT, Chen FF, Su IJ. Follicular dendritic cell sarcoma of the colon mimicking stromal tumour. *Histopathology.* 2001;38(1):25-29.
337. Pileri SA, Grogan TM, Harris NL, et al. Tumours of histiocytes and accessory dendritic cells: an immunohistochemical approach to classification from the International Lymphoma Study Group based on 61 cases. *Histopathology.* 2002;41(1):1-29.
338. Geerts A, Lagae E, Dhaene K, et al. Metastatic follicular dendritic cell sarcoma of the stomach: a case report and review of the literature. *Acta Gastroenterol Belg.* 2004;67(2):223-227.
339. Chan JK, Fletcher CD, Nayler SJ, Cooper K. Follicular dendritic cell sarcoma. Clinicopathologic analysis of 17 cases suggesting a malignant potential higher than currently recognized. *Cancer.* 1997;79(2):294-313.
340. Perez-Ordonez B, Rosai J. Follicular dendritic cell tumor: review of the entity. *Semin Diagn Pathol.* 1998;15(2):144-154.
341. Shah VI, Freites ON, Maxwell P, McCluggage WG. Inhibin is more specific than calretinin as an immunohistochemical marker for differentiating sarcomatoid granulosa cell tumour of the ovary from other spindle cell neoplasms. *J Clin Pathol.* 2003;56(3):221-224.
342. Flemming P, Wellmann A, Maschek H, et al. Monoclonal antibodies against inhibin represent key markers of adult granulosa cell tumors of the ovary even in their metastases. A report of three cases with late metastasis, being previously misinterpreted as hemangiopericytoma. *Am J Surg Pathol.* 1995;19(8):927-933.
343. Chen TS, Montgomery EA. Are tumefactive lesions classified as sclerosing mesenteritis a subset of IgG4-related sclerosing disorders? *J Clin Pathol.* 2008;61(10):1093-1097.
344. Bala A, Coderre SP, Johnson DR, Nayak V. Treatment of sclerosing mesenteritis with corticosteroids and azathioprine. *Can J Gastroenterol.* 2001;15(8):533-535.
345. Genereau T, Bellin MF, Wechsler B, et al. Demonstration of efficacy of combining corticosteroids and colchicine in two patients with idiopathic sclerosing mesenteritis. *Dig Dis Sci.* 1996;41(4):684-688.
346. Mazure R, Fernandez Marty P, Niveloni S, et al. Successful treatment of retractile mesenteritis with oral progesterone. *Gastroenterology.* 1998;114(6):1313-1317.
347. Levy AD, Rimola J, Mehrotra AK, Sobin LH. From the archives of the AFIP: benign fibrous tumors and tumor-like lesions of the mesentery: radiologic-pathologic correlation. *Radiographics.* 2006;26(1):245-264.
348. Vaglio A, Salvarani C, Buzio C. Retroperitoneal fibrosis. *Lancet.* 2006;367(9506):241-251.
349. Yantiss RK, Nielsen GP, Lauwers GY, Rosenberg AE. Reactive nodular fibrous pseudotumor of the gastrointestinal tract and mesentery: a clinicopathologic study of five cases. *Am J Surg Pathol.* 2003;27(4):532-540.
350. Chatelain D, Manaouil D, Levy P, et al. Reactive nodular fibrous pseudotumor of the gastrointestinal tract and mesentery. *Am J Surg Pathol.* 2004;28(3):416; author reply 7.
351. Daum O, Vanecek T, Sima R, et al. Reactive nodular fibrous pseudotumors of the gastrointestinal tract: report of 8 cases. *Int J Surg Pathol.* 2004;12(4):365-374.
352. Zardawi IM, Catterall N, Cox SA. Reactive nodular fibrous pseudotumor of the gastrointestinal tract and mesentery. *Am J Surg Pathol.* 2004;28(2):276-277.
353. Nash S. Benign lesions of the gastrointestinal tract that may be misdiagnosed as malignant tumors. *Semin Diagn Pathol.* 1990;7(2):102-114.
354. Patel RM, Weiss SW, Folpe AL. Heterotopic mesenteric ossification: a distinctive pseudosarcoma commonly associated with intestinal obstruction. *Am J Surg Pathol.* 2006;30(1):119-122.
355. Kubosawa H, Yano K, Oda K, et al. Xanthogranulomatous gastritis with pseudosarcomatous changes. *Pathol Int.* 2007;57(5):291-295.
356. Lai HY, Chen JH, Chen CK, et al. Xanthogranulomatous pseudotumor of stomach induced by perforated peptic ulcer mimicking a stromal tumor. *Eur Radiol.* 2006;16(10):2371-2372.
357. Basilio-de-Oliveira C, Eyer-Silva WA, Valle HA, et al. Mycobacterial spindle cell pseudotumor of the appendix vermiformis in a patient with aids. *Braz J Infect Dis.* 2001;5(2):98-100.

8. Gastrointestinal Manifestations of Extraintestinal Disorders and Systemic Disease

Chapter Outline

INTRODUCTION
CONNECTIVE TISSUE DISORDERS (COLLAGEN VASCULAR DISEASES)
SCLERODERMA (PROGRESSIVE SYSTEMIC SCLEROSIS)
  Pathogenesis and Clinical Features
  Gross Pathology and Histology
  Clinical Implications
  Dermatomyositis and Polymyositis
  Systemic Lupus Erythematosus
  Mixed Connective Tissue Diseases and the Overlap Syndrome
  Rheumatoid Arthritis
  Miscellaneous Disorders
GASTROINTESTINAL MANIFESTATIONS IN ENDOCRINE DISORDERS
  Thyroid Gland
    Hyperthyroidism
  Hypothyroidism
  Autoimmune Thyroid Disease
  Thyroid Neoplasms
  Parathyroid Gland
    Hyperparathyroidism
  Hypoparathyroidism
  Endocrine Pancreas
    Diabetes
  Hyperfunction of Islets of Langerhans
  Gastrinoma
  VIPoma Syndrome (Verner–Morrisons Syndrome)
  Somatostatinoma
  Other Islet Cell Tumors
  Adrenal Gland
  Gonads
    Pregnancy
  Hypothalamus and Pituitary
  Hypopituitarism
  Pituitary Adenoma
  Autoimmune Polyendocrinopathy Syndrome Type 1
    The IPEX syndrome

GASTROINTESTINAL MANIFESTATIONS IN RENAL DISEASE
  Acute Renal Failure
  Chronic Renal Failure
  Endoscopic and Histologic Appearances
  Other Findings
  Renal Transplantation
  Role of the Pathologist and Clinical Implications
GASTROINTESTINAL MANIFESTATIONS OF HEPATIC DISORDERS
  Portal Hypertension
  Primary Sclerosing Cholangitis and Autoimmune Hepatitis
  Liver Transplantation
GASTROINTESTINAL MANIFESTATIONS OF SKIN DISORDERS
  Bullous Disorders
    Epidermolysis bullosa
  Epidermolysis Bullosa Acquisita
  Pemphigus Vulgaris
  Cicatricial Pemphigoid (Benign Mucous Membrane Pemphigoid)
  Stevens–Johnson Syndrome
  Herpes Simplex Virus Infection
  Hyperkeratotic Disorders
    Lichen planus
  Tylosis
  Miscellaneous Disorders
    Acrodermatitis enteropathica
  Darier's Disease
  Dermatogenic Enteropathy
  Malignant Disease of the Gastrointestinal Tract and Skin Disease
  Acanthosis Nigricans
  Cowden's Disease
  Dermatomyositis
  Miscellaneous

GASTROINTESTINAL MANIFESTATIONS OF CARDIAC DISEASE
  Congestive Cardiac Failure
  Infective Endocarditis
  Open Heart Surgery, Extracorporeal Circulation, and Cardiac Transplantation
HEMATOLOGIC DISORDERS
  Dysproteinemias
  Hemolytic Uremic Syndrome
  Coagulation Disorders
    Hemophilia
  Other Coagulation Disorders
  Mastocytosis
  Rosai–Dorfman Disease (Sinus Histiocytosis with Massive Lymphadenopathy)
  Miscellaneous Disorders
GASTROINTESTINAL AMYLOID DEPOSITION
  General Properties and Classification
  Clinical Features
  Histologic Features
  Diagnosis and Clinical Implications
DISORDERS OF LIPID METABOLISM
  Fabry's Disease
  Tangier Disease
  Wolman's Disease
  Abetalipoproteinemia
GRANULOMATOUS DISORDERS
  Sarcoidosis
  Chronic Granulomatous Disease
MISCELLANEOUS DISORDERS
  Endometriosis
  Pellagra
  Familial Mediterranean Fever (Familial Paroxysmal Polyserositis)
NEOPLASTIC DISEASE

Chapter 8 Gastrointestinal Manifestations of Extraintestinal Disorders and Systemic Disease

INTRODUCTION

Gastrointestinal symptoms are common in primary extraintestinal diseases as well as in systemic disorders. Such manifestations may occur in a variety of scenarios including

1. Conditions with pathologic changes common to intestinal and extraintestinal organs, for example, connective tissue disorders
2. Functional abnormalities in the absence of morphologic changes, reflecting altered hormonal or electrolyte changes or neurologic abnormalities, for example, hyperthyroidism or hypothyroidism
3. Mechanical factors, for example, congestive gastropathy or colopathy in portal hypertension or congestive cardiac failure
4. Complications such as infections and neoplasms, in immunocompromised patients
5. Medications frequently administered in certain extraintestinal diseases, for example, nonsteroidal anti-inflammatory drugs (NSAIDs) in rheumatoid arthritis
6. Metastases from extraintestinal neoplasms

The purpose of this chapter is to describe the well-documented morphologic changes that occur in the gastrointestinal tract in extraintestinal disease and systemic disorders and to mention briefly the important functional abnormalities. It should also be noted that there are numerous reports, especially from the older literature, of gastrointestinal abnormalities in extraintestinal disorders whose morphology is poorly documented. We have chosen not to refer to these reports unless they have been confirmed by carefully controlled studies. Finally, some disorders, such as the neuromuscular disorders, are covered in other sections (see Chapter 6), and to avoid duplication, discussion of these conditions is referred to other chapters.

CONNECTIVE TISSUE DISORDERS (COLLAGEN VASCULAR DISEASES)

Gastrointestinal manifestations are common in some of the connective tissue disorders. There are three predominant pathologic changes: (a) deposition of collagen with submucosal fibrosis and muscle atrophy, resulting in motility disorders; (b) arteritis or vasculitis, leading to mucosal erosions, ulceration, or infarction depending on the size of vessel involved; and (c) complications associated with therapy such as NSAIDs and corticosteroids.[1,2]

The collagen abnormalities are seen mainly in scleroderma and dermatomyositis, while the arteritic lesions occur predominantly in systemic lupus erythematosus (SLE), rheumatoid arthritis, and polyarteritis nodosa. However, not infrequently, there is some overlap between these disorders. Sometimes it is impossible to know if a given lesion is due to the disorder itself or to its therapy or complications. Examples include

1. Patients with rheumatoid arthritis who are on NSAIDs and have gastric ulcers or erosions. Here the drugs rather than the underlying disease are the most likely culprit.
2. Patients with SLE who have renal failure and are on high-dose corticosteroids. In this setting, ulcerative lesions may be due to stress lesions that occur in any seriously ill patient or to opportunistic infections, especially *Candida* or cytomegalovirus (CMV).

Also see Chapter 2 for a more detailed description of the vascular changes in the connective tissue disorders.

SCLERODERMA (PROGRESSIVE SYSTEMIC SCLEROSIS)

Pathogenesis and Clinical Features

Scleroderma is a systemic disease of unknown etiology, characterized by chronic inflammation, collagen deposition, smooth muscle atrophy and telangiectasia and less commonly, by a vasculitis or immune-mediated enteric autonomic neuron dysfunction. Over 80% of patients have alterations in gastrointestinal function,[3] about 50% have serious gastrointestinal involvement, and 5% to 10% die from a gastrointestinal-related cause.[4] Gastrointestinal involvement is characterized primarily by motility disorders, including gastroesophageal reflux disease, pseudo-obstruction, and bacterial overgrowth, and gastrointestinal hemorrhage.[5-7] Gastrointestinal hemorrhage is particularly prominent in patients with CREST (calcinosis, Raynaud's disease, esophageal dysmotility, sclerodactyly, and gastrointestinal telangiectasia) and is secondary to telangiectasia.[8,9] The "watermelon stomach" or gastric antral vascular ectasia (GAVE) is being increasingly recognized as being associated with scleroderma and responsible for upper gastrointestinal hemorrhage in some of these patients.[3,10,11]

The esophagus is the most commonly involved gastrointestinal site in scleroderma.[3,12] As the muscularis externa of the proximal esophagus is composed of striated muscle, involvement is typically confined to the distal two thirds.[13] Lower esophageal sphincter pressure is reduced, and compounding this is ineffective peristalsis with delayed esophageal clearance.[3] Delayed gastric emptying (see below) contributes to reflux by increasing the volume of reflux, which is poorly cleared as a result of the esophageal motor disorder.[14,15] Thus erosive esophagitis may be severe and associated with stricture formation.[12,16] In the end stages, the esophagus may appear dilated, with a stricture at the lower esophageal sphincter region and little or no peristalsis in the body of the esophagus. Patients are additionally predisposed to candidal esophagitis due to a combination of poor esophageal emptying, frequent use of immunosuppressive agents, and acid suppression. Dysmotility also predisposes to "pill esophagitis" due to increased mucosal contact with the pill. Bisphosphonates, NSAIDs, quinidine, and potassium chloride have been implicated in these patients. Appropriate counseling is important to prevent this unpleasant complication.[3,12] Any putative increased incidence of squamous carcinoma or adenocarcinoma of the esophagus in scleroderma is probably due to the associated gastroesophageal reflux disease rather than due to any intrinsic risk conferred by the connective tissue disease itself.[3,17]

In the stomach, significantly delayed gastric emptying occurs in approximately 50% of patients.[3] This results in early satiety, worsening of reflux, and accompanying vomiting.

Small intestinal involvement has been reported in 15% to 57% of patients depending on the method of detection and primarily relates to dysmotility.[10] The initial manifestation is that of a dilated bowel, sometimes associated with scattered wide-mouthed diverticula[18] (Fig. 8-1). This may be followed by intestinal pseudo-obstruction (see Chapter 7) of which scleroderma is the most common cause. Stasis predisposes to small intestinal overgrowth, which occurs in 33% to 40% of patients with scleroderma[10] and may result in malabsorption and diarrhea.[10,19] The frequent use of strong acid-suppressing medications may contribute to bacterial overgrowth by removing the acid barrier to colonization by oropharyngeal bacteria.[20] Bacterial overgrowth may be associated with malabsorption and diarrhea. Other causes of diarrhea and malabsorption in these patients include pancreatic and vascular insufficiency.[10] Malabsorption is often a late event in the disease probably because of the large reserve function of the small intestine. In disorders such as scleroderma and diabetes where malabsorption may be a complication, one must always be open to the possibility that a second disorder (e.g., celiac disease) may be responsible for, or contributing to, the malabsorption.[19,21]

In the colon a similar process may also result in pseudo-obstruction or symptoms of severe constipation, with the risk of stool impaction and stercoral ulceration, or sometimes diarrhea.[3,22] Impaired function of the internal anal sphincter may lead to fecal incontinence.[3,10,22,23] Vascular ectasia may involve the small and large bowel.[5] Rarely, pneumatosis intestinalis, intussusception, and volvulus of the small intestine may complicate scleroderma.[23-27] A few patients with scleroderma present with vasculitis, leading to ischemic lesions resulting in gastrointestinal hemorrhage, ulcers, or intestinal infarction, depending on the size of vessels involved[28] (see Chapter 2).

Gross Pathology and Histology

The major abnormality consists of smooth muscle atrophy and fibrosis[10,27,29-32] (Figs. 8-2 and 8-3). Most

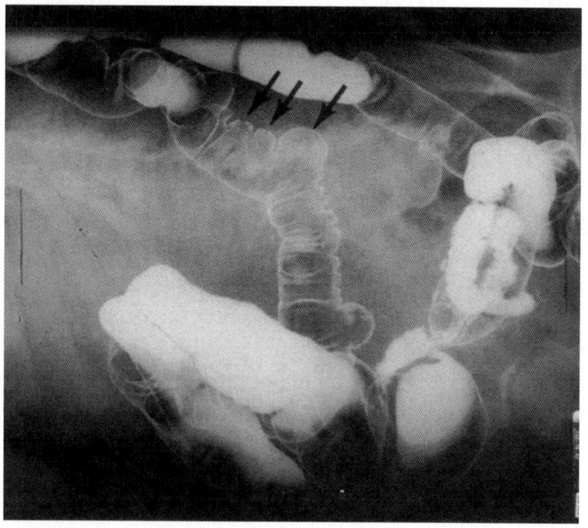

Figure 8-1. Scleroderma of the gastrointestinal tract. Barium enema examination to show wide-mouthed diverticula (*arrows*). (Courtesy of Dr M Weiner UCLA.)

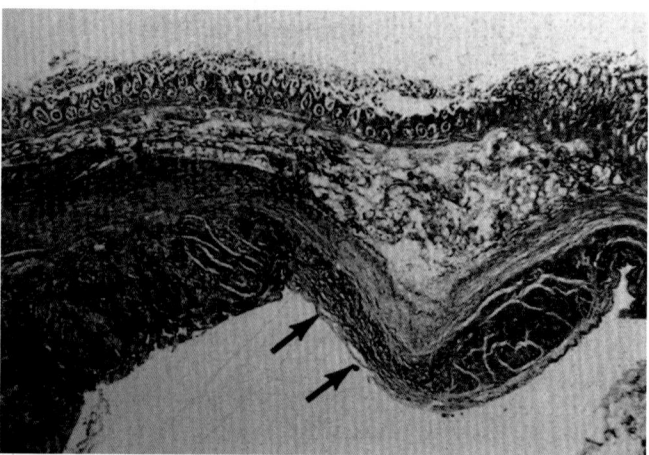

Figure 8-2. Scleroderma of the gastrointestinal tract. Scanning-power view of the colon showing atrophy and fibrous replacement of the muscularis propria. Note that one segment of the muscularis propria (*arrows*) is completely replaced by fibrous tissue (trichrome stain).

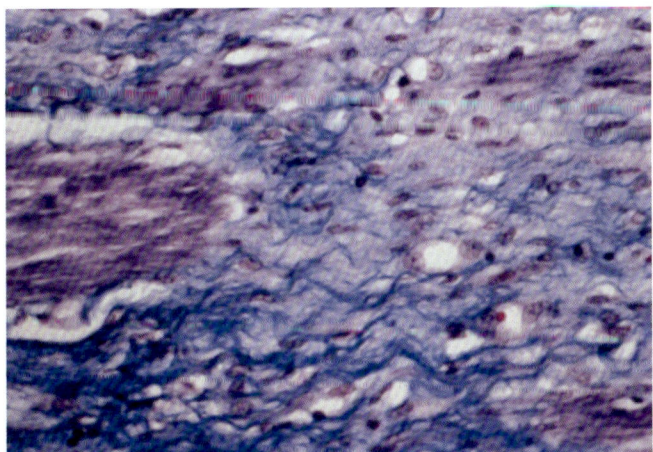

Figure 8-3. Detail of Figure 8-2 to show atrophy of muscularis propria. Note the replacement of muscle fibers (stained purple) by collagenous fibrous tissue (trichrome stain).

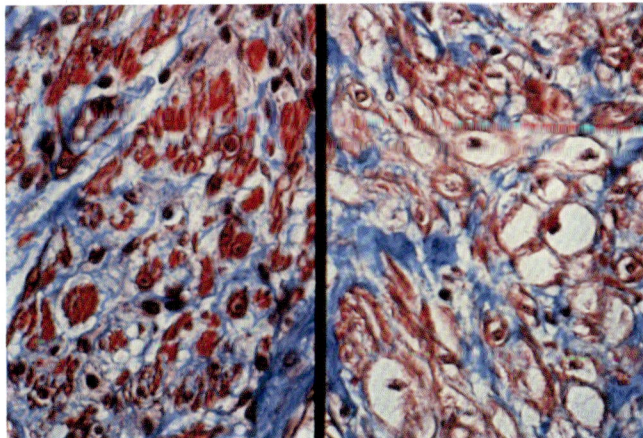

Figure 8-4. Composite photomicrograph comparing intestinal scleroderma (**left**) with idiopathic visceral myopathy (**right**). In scleroderma there is atrophy of the smooth muscle fibers and replacement by collagen (*stained blue*). In contrast, in idiopathic visceral myopathy, there is vacuolar degeneration of muscle fibers encircled by collagen, often resulting in clear spaces surrounded by acellular collagen. (Courtesy of Schuffler, M. M.D., Seattle.)

commonly, the former affects the circular muscle coat. Fibrosis accompanies the muscle atrophy but appears to be the replacement of the atrophied muscle rather than active fibroblastic proliferation. Collagen deposition in the submucosa and subserosa is very variable. Muscle atrophy results in atony and dilatation and may produce flaccid, wide-mouthed diverticula (Fig. 8-1), and, less commonly, megaduodenum or megacolon.[33] Diverticula are better appreciated radiologically when distended with barium than when collapsed at autopsy or in resection specimens. They are not generally complicated by diverticulitis because their wide necks are less prone to obstruction.[10] The muscle changes of scleroderma most closely resemble those of idiopathic familial and sporadic visceral myopathy. The major difference between the two entities consists of muscle atrophy with fibrous replacement in scleroderma compared to vacuolar degeneration resulting in clear spaces surrounded by collagen in visceral myopathy (Fig. 8-4) (see Chapter 7 for further details). Mucosal changes in scleroderma are secondary to motor dysfunction. In the esophagus, severe erosive esophagitis and superinfection with *Candida* may be seen.[34] Associated stricture formation is common in scleroderma, and it may be made more intractable by submucosal collagen formation. In the stomach, submucosal and mural fibrosis may result in a lack of distensibility with consequent early satiety. Occasionally, severe atrophy of the gastric wall musculature may result in a small, shrunken stomach (Fig. 8-5). Collagen encapsulation of Brunner's glands has been reported in duodenal biopsies,[35-37] but this is not a consistent finding[38,39] and is often present in duodenal biopsies in general.

Vascular lesions vary in their endoscopic appearances depending on their type and size. Appearances may range from those of telangiectasia to the broad red antral stripes of the watermelon stomach.

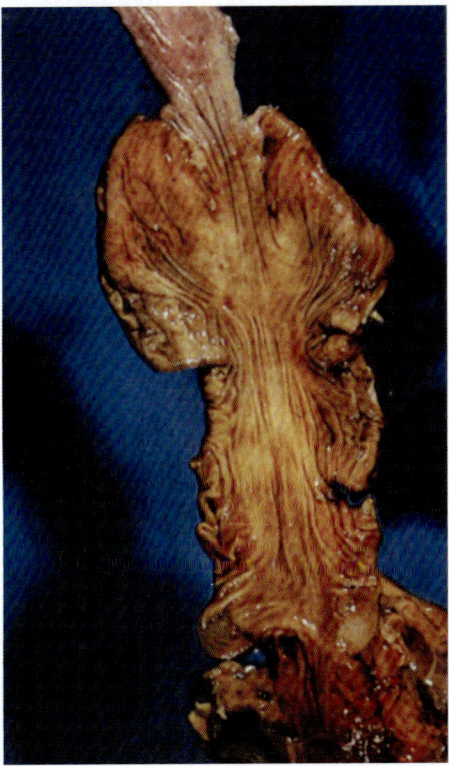

Figure 8-5. Scleroderma of the gastrointestinal tract. Autopsy specimen showing terminal portion of esophagus and a small, shrunken stomach.

Sometimes the associated vascular abnormality may be masked at endoscopy by an area of subepithelial hemorrhage. If vasculitic lesions have progressed, then the changes may be those of erosions or ulcerations. Lesions vary from small, ischemic ulcers to transmural infarction and perforation, depending on the size and number of vessels involved.[28] Patients are also prone to pneumatosis intestinalis. Histologically, the small vessels of the bowel frequently show a proliferative endarteritis with endothelial swelling, intimal proliferation,[10] and a peculiar mucinous change of the media [40] (Fig. 8-6). In addition, there may be a vasculitis, which can affect the mesenteric arteries at any level.

Clinical Implications

The pathologist most commonly receives tissue in scleroderma from esophageal erosions or ulcers. Here the differential diagnosis includes *Candida*-associated esophagitis, "pill" esophagitis, reflux esophagitis, Barrett's esophagus, and carcinoma. Less commonly, small bowel biopsies may be received from patients with malabsorption. The mucosa may exhibit a mild abnormality in the villous architecture and epithelial lymphocytosis compatible with small intestinal bacterial overgrowth (SIBO). Vasculitis, when encountered, is usually an incidental finding. Biopsies of suspected vascular lesions such as in "watermelon stomach" (see Chapter 2) may be disappointing because the mucosal vessels may collapse with the major abnormality being in the submucosa. This difficulty in verifying vascular lesions by endoscopic mucosal biopsy is not unique in scleroderma or to any particular region of the gastrointestinal tract (see Chapter 1).

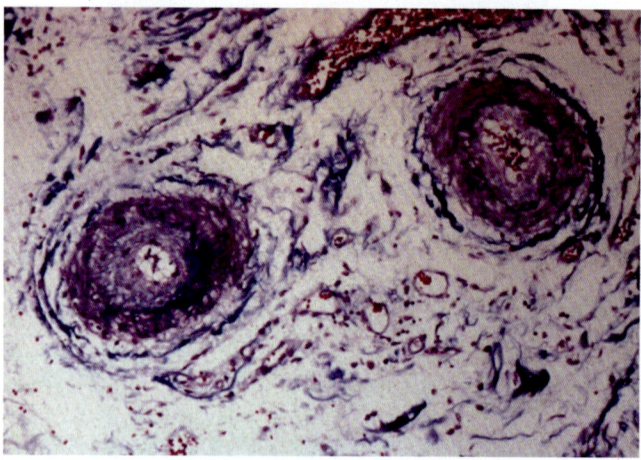

Figure 8-6. Intestinal scleroderma. Overview demonstrating proliferative endarteritis in two small submucosal vessels characterized by a subintimal mucinous deposition.

Dermatomyositis and Polymyositis

Dermatomyositis and polymyositis are rare connective tissue disorders characterized by symmetric proximal muscle weakness, elevated serum levels of muscle enzymes, and an inflammatory myopathy on muscle biopsy. Skin involvement occurs in dermatomyositis, but not in polymyositis.[41] Gastrointestinal symptoms are not that uncommon, but major complications are rare.[42–45] The striated muscle of the hypopharynx and cervical esophagus is most frequently affected and, as with the changes in muscle and skin, is manifested by chronic inflammation, edema, muscle atrophy, and on rare occasions spontaneous esophageal rupture.[43,46] Impaired swallowing, tracheal aspiration, and aspiration pneumonia are common complications. In addition, occasionally, as in scleroderma, smooth muscle atrophy and fibrosis may occur, resulting in dysfunction of the lower esophageal sphincter. Dysmotility in other parts of the gastrointestinal tract may result in delayed gastric emptying, colonic dilatation, constipation, and pseudodiverticula.[41,47] A small minority of adult patients have been reported to experience more acute and severe gastrointestinal symptoms including abdominal pain, diarrhea, and gastrointestinal bleeding. In such cases gastrointestinal involvement may be diffuse.[45] Histologic findings included ulcers and erosions, severe acute and chronic inflammation, and prominent mucosal and submucosal telangiectasia, but not vasculitis. By contrast, severe gastrointestinal involvement due to vasculitis of the bowel wall is a well-recognized complication of juvenile dermatomyositis.[45]

A variety of malignancies have been reported in dermatomyositis including colorectal and gastric adenocarcinomas.[41] Many or most of the malignancies in this disease are found at presentation or shortly thereafter. In these cases, it is likely that dermatomyositis is of paraneoplastic etiology.[48] The prevalence of associated cancers is that which is unique to a locale or population group.[49] For example, in Singapore and Tunisia nasopharyngeal cancer predominates,[48,50] whereas in elderly Danish patients it is colon cancer.[51] Once these initial or early cases are detected, there does not appear to be any increased risk with time beyond 1 year.[52] Gastroenterologists are frequently asked to perform endoscopic examinations of the upper and lower gastrointestinal tract to look for cancer. There is however no generally accepted standard for cancer screening in these patients. The starting point is to carefully evaluate for clinical and laboratory clues that might point to a cancer at the time of presentation and in the early follow-up period after diagnosis. The risk of neoplasia in polymyositis is much lower.

Systemic Lupus Erythematosus

SLE is a multisystem disease characterized by immunologic abnormalities, with numerous autoantibodies to a host of nuclear and cytoplasmic antigens (e.g., antinuclear, anti–double-stranded DNA, and anticardiolipin antibodies) and associated with tissue damage. Gastrointestinal manifestations occur in about 25% to 40% of cases and are primarily related to vasculitis or to complications of therapy.[41] Vasculitis is the most important intrinsic feature of this disorder, and ischemia is responsible for many of the gastrointestinal manifestations. Small vessels of the submucosa and muscularis propria are typically involved rather than the medium-sized mesenteric vessels.[53,54] Fibrinoid necrosis is characteristic. Vasculitis may affect the small and large bowel (especially terminal ileum and cecum) and less commonly the esophagus[41,55] (see Chapter 2). Lupus anticoagulants and anticardiolipin antibodies may contribute to ischemia from vasculitis.[56] The most dramatic gastrointestinal manifestations of SLE include abdominal pain with peritoneal signs,[57] penetrating ulcers, and outright transmural infarction.[58-60] Fortunately these occur uncommonly.[61] Strictures may develop in cases where the ischemia progresses slowly or resolves after a major insult.[62] Whenever diffuse or focal mucosal lesions such as ulcers or erosions are found, the challenge is to try to determine whether these are due to vasculitis or represent infectious complications of the immunosuppressive therapy that these patients receive. Such infections range from common types such as *Candida*, CMV, and herpes simplex to more exotic types.[41,63-65] The challenge is compounded by the fact that endoscopic mucosal biopsies usually do not contain the vasculitic lesions.[53]

Other complications of connective tissue disorders in general have been reported in SLE including amyloidosis[66] and pneumatosis cystoides intestinalis.[67] Reports of functional disorders such as malabsorption or protein-losing enteropathy are presumed to be due to ischemia or perhaps other mechanisms, for example, autoantibodies and bacterial overgrowth, but without proof.[41,68,69] When malabsorption is found in a patient with SLE, other known causes of malabsorption, such as celiac disease, should be excluded.[70] Intestinal pseudo-obstruction occurs uncommonly.[71] Esophageal dysmotility can often be demonstrated by manometry but does not correlate well with esophageal symptoms.[41,55] Peptic ulcer disease is common in patients treated with NSAIDs and corticosteroids. In diseases such as SLE with diverse manifestations, it is not surprising that associated disorders will be reported, such as hypereosinophilia without knowing whether it is coincidence or somehow unmasked by the presence of SLE.[72] Patients treated with steroids may also develop lesions secondary to the steroids such as perforating diseases (stomach, diverticular disease, appendix) that may escape detection until advanced with widespread peritonitis.

Mixed Connective Tissue Diseases and the Overlap Syndrome

Mixed connective tissue disease is characterized by features of scleroderma, SLE, and polymyositis. When some of these features are missing, the disorder is referred to as the overlap syndrome. Gastrointestinal manifestations are common and most frequently resemble those seen in scleroderma.[15,73,74]

Rheumatoid Arthritis

Many patients with rheumatoid arthritis have gastrointestinal symptoms, mostly due to drug therapy, especially NSAIDs[41,75] (see Chapters 14 and 18). The poor correlation between symptoms and the presence of gastroduodenal erosions or ulcers is well recognized. Fifty percent or more of patients on these drugs have gastroduodenal lesions.[76,77] Gold therapy for rheumatoid arthritis may also cause a colitis or enteritis.[78,79]

Vasculitis was documented even with blind suction biopsy in rheumatoid arthritis, illustrating that at times the gut may be a mirror or a source of diagnosis for vasculitis in connective tissue disorders.[80] The complications listed previously for SLE may occur in rheumatoid arthritis, albeit with a lesser frequency.[62,81] Involvement of smaller vessels results in multiple ischemic ulcers (Fig. 8-7), which may perforate.[41,82] Nondescript mucosal lesions such as those described in seronegative spondyloarthropathy have been reported also in rheumatoid arthritis but with a lesser prevalence[83] (see Chapter 18). Lymphonodular hyperplasia and increased intraepithelial lymphocytes have been reported in patients with juvenile idiopathic arthritis who experience gastrointestinal symptoms. It is uncertain whether these findings are related to the underlying disease or treatment.[84]

Miscellaneous Disorders

Intestinal complications may occasionally develop in persons with other connective tissue disorders such as Sjögren's syndrome, Reiter's syndrome, Behçet's disease, and the hereditary connective tissue disorders.

Patients with Sjögren's syndrome frequently experience dysphagia, which has been variously ascribed

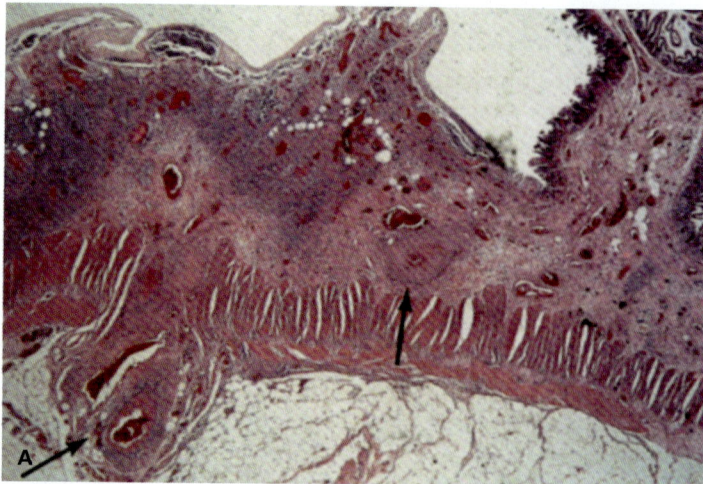
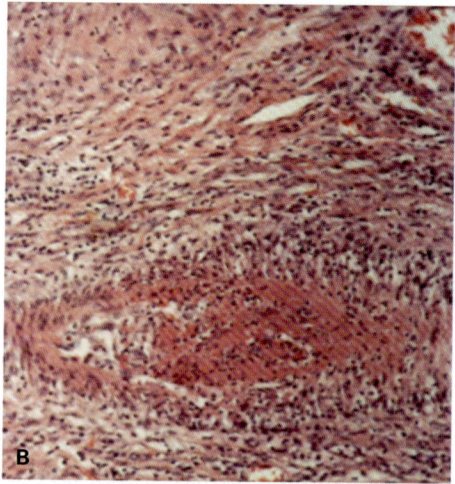

Figure 8-7. Rheumatoid arthritis with intestinal vasculitis and ischemic necrosis. **A:** Low-power view of a segment of small intestine showing ischemic ulceration involving the mucosa and submucosa. Note the vasculitic involvement of submucosal and subserosal vessels (*arrows*). **B:** High-power view of one of the vessels showing inflammation of the adventitia and media. (Courtesy of Mitros, F M.D., Iowa City.)

to decreased production of saliva, upper esophageal webs, parasympathetic dysfunction, and esophageal dysmotility,[41,85-87] although the role of the latter has been questioned.[85,86] Atrophic gastritis and duodenal ulcers have been described,[41,87] but whether this is a true association and not ulcers secondary to medications and long-standing *Helicobacter* is unclear. Patients with Sjögren's may also be at increased risk for the development of lymphomas including MALT lymphomas of the stomach,[87-89] and this should be borne in mind when evaluating endoscopic biopsies from such patients.

Reiter's syndrome is characterized by arthritis, urethritis, conjunctivitis, and mucocutaneous lesions and usually follows an attack of infectious diarrhea or urethritis.[90] It appears that some patients have a subclinical colitis characterized by normal endoscopy and microscopic colitis.[91]

In Behçet's disease there is gastrointestinal involvement in up to 50% of patients. In addition to the typical aphthous ulceration of the mouth, patients may have ulcerative lesions throughout the gastrointestinal tract, in particular the ileocecal region, which can mimic Crohn's disease. The underlying abnormality is a vasculitis of small veins and venules, but sometimes affecting larger vessels.[41,92] Behçet's disease is more fully described in Chapter 23.

The hereditary connective tissue disorders, such as Ehlers–Danlos syndrome and pseudoxanthoma elasticum, are due to structural derangements of elastic tissue and fragility of blood vessels. This results in a variety of gastrointestinal disorders, such as gastrointestinal hemorrhage, ulceration, secondary diverticula, bowel rupture, and rectal prolapse.[93-95] For a more detailed description, see Chapter 2.

GASTROINTESTINAL MANIFESTATIONS IN ENDOCRINE DISORDERS

Altered hormonal homeostasis due to endocrine-related disorders and functioning tumors can produce disordered function often in the absence of recognized structural change in the gastrointestinal tract. Symptoms may be due to altered motility, altered absorption and secretion, or both. Symptoms of altered motility and mucosal function may include vomiting, diarrhea, or constipation.[96-99] There is also an association between endocrine disorders and certain gastrointestinal diseases, for example, autoimmune gastritis and thyroiditis. These will be discussed in the chapters dealing with these conditions. In this chapter, we shall concentrate our discussion primarily on the morphologic abnormalities accompanying diseases of the endocrine system.

Thyroid Gland

Hyperthyroidism. The main gastrointestinal manifestation of hyperthyroidism is diarrhea, but some patients have constipation. Accelerated intestinal transit has been a long-standing explanation for the diarrhea,[100,101] but absorptive or secretory abnormalities might be contributing. Steatorrhea is usually mild.[100] Patients frequently have chronic dyspeptic symptoms including epigastric pain, fullness, and nausea and vomiting.[101] Altered gastroenteric myoelectrical activity has been documented by electrogastrography but does not appear to correlate with gastric emptying or dyspepsia.[102,103] There is no convincing evidence that intrinsic gut lesions occur in this disorder. Putative associations with gastritis were claimed on the basis of studies with blind suction biopsies,[104] and claims of mild small bowel lesions need confirmation because the illustrations in one published report are not convincing.[105] A small study in autoimmune thyroid disease suggested that there were more lymphoid follicles present in Helicobacter pylori–positive patients than in controls with H. pylori infection. The significance of this is unclear.[106] An ileus-like picture with vomiting has been reported in a case of "thyroid storm."[107] Uncommonly dysphagia occurs in thyrotoxicosis and may be secondary to direct compression from a goiter, neurohumoral dysregulation, or a generalized myopathy including striated muscles of the pharynx and smooth muscle of the esophagus.[101,108,109] Histologic changes in the esophagus have not been reported.

Hypothyroidism

A variety of gastrointestinal hypomotility disorders have been described in hypothyroidism, such as disturbance of esophageal sphincter function and atony and dilatation of the esophagus, stomach, small intestine, and colon, with consequent reflux esophagitis, bezoar formation, abdominal distention, ileus, and megacolon.[101,104,110-112] The pathophysiologic abnormalities producing these motility changes are not clearly understood, although they appear to be reversible after treatment of hypothyroidism.[110,113] SIBO was reported in up to 54% (27/50) patients in one study compared to only 2% of matched controls. In these patients, abdominal symptoms were significantly improved following decontamination therapy.[114]

The pathologic changes in the gut consist of marked dilatation and thickening of the bowel wall and microscopic accumulation of mucopolysaccharide substances within the submucosa, muscularis propria, and subserosa. An accompanying increase in the number of mast cells has also been described. These histologic changes have been likened to those found in the subcutaneous tissue of myxedematous patients.[115,116] Most of the reported pathologic studies were done some time ago on autopsy material, without control groups for comparison, and are poorly illustrated. Thus, the precise histologic changes remain to be confirmed.

Autoimmune Thyroid Disease

The association of autoimmune thyroid disease and autoimmune diseases of the gastrointestinal tract, namely, atrophic gastritis, celiac disease, and microscopic colitis, is well recognized. These conditions may all display the HLA-DR3-DQ2 haplotype common to many autoimmune diseases.[101,117] These associations are discussed further in the chapters dealing with these conditions.

Thyroid Neoplasms

Medullary thyroid carcinoma (MTC) is a tumor of the calcitonin-producing endocrine C cells of the thyroid. It is often familial and associated with the multiple endocrine neoplasia (MEN) syndromes, primarily types IIa and IIb. About one-third of the patients have a secretory (i.e., resistant to fasting) diarrhea.[118,119] The latter has been attributed to the excessive production of certain peptides including calcitonin, serotonin, and vasoactive intestinal polypeptide.[118] The histology of the intestinal mucosa is normal.

A number of other thyroid neoplasms may sometimes occur concurrently with gastrointestinal tumors. Thus, patients with primary lymphoma of the thyroid are reported to have an increased incidence of lymphomatous involvement of the gastrointestinal tract,[120] and papillary carcinoma of the thyroid is sometimes associated with Gardner's syndrome, in particular the cribriform (morular) variant.[121]

Parathyroid Gland

Hyperparathyroidism. The classical presentation of hyperparathyroidism as "stones, bones and abdominal groans" as described by St. Goar[122] is now a rarity in most Western countries although still seen in some parts of the world. With routine measurement of blood calcium, most patients now present with asymptomatic hypercalcemia. Even those left untreated rarely develop the "classical" picture.[123] Gastrointestinal symptoms, including abdominal pain and distention, vomiting, and constipation, described in up to 50% of patients in the earlier literature were ascribed to the effects of hypercalcemia, possibly via altered neuronal transmission and neuromuscular excitability.[124-126] Despite the historical association with peptic ulcer disease, the prevalence of peptic ulcers in sporadic hyperparathyroidism is probably similar to that of the general population.[123] However, in the setting of MEN1, hyperparathyroidism and peptic ulcer disease frequently coexist due to the presence of gastrinomas in 40% of these patients.

Hypoparathyroidism

Hypoparathyroidism is associated with diarrhea and sometimes steatorrhea and malabsorption.[127-129] These changes are related to hypocalcemia and are not associated with any apparent morphologic abnormalities.[128,129] The precise mechanisms for the diarrhea remain to be elucidated but impaired enteropancreatic peptide secretion following caloric stimulus and increased epithelial permeability due to cytoskeletal alterations have been suggested to play a role.[129]

Endocrine Pancreas

Diabetes

Pathogenesis and Clinical Manifestations Several population-based studies suggest an increased prevalence of upper and lower gastrointestinal symptoms among patients with diabetes, although epidemiologic data are inconsistent.[130-133] Gastrointestinal symptoms in diabetics may be due to gastroparesis, altered intestinal motility/function, loss of sphincteric control, infection, or associated autoimmune disorders such as celiac disease and atrophic gastritis.[130,131,134]

Gastroparesis occurs in both type 1 and 2 diabetics but seems to be particularly prevalent in patients with long-standing type 1 diabetes.[131,135] Symptoms of gastroparesis include nausea, vomiting, epigastric fullness, bloating, and abdominal discomfort. Bezoar formation may sometimes ensue, exacerbating the symptoms of gastroparesis or producing a palpable mass, ulceration, perforation, or small bowel obstruction[131,135] (Fig. 8-8). The cause of gastric dysmotility appears to be multifactorial with postulated mechanisms including autonomic dysfunction, impaired glycemic control (hyperglycemia disrupts antral motor complexes, delaying gastric emptying), hormonal imbalances (elevations in postprandial glucagon delays gastric emptying), loss of interstitial cells of Cajal, microangiopathy, and psychological distress.[130,131,134,135]

Diarrhea affects 4% to 22% of diabetics with up to 75% also having steatorrhea.[131,134] Occasionally this is severe and intractable.[136,137] Segments of bowel may undergo dilatation with secondary bacterial overgrowth, which may cause or exacerbate diarrhea.[138] Bacterial overgrowth is present in up to 43% of diabetics with chronic diarrhea.[139] As with gastroparesis the etiology of diabetic diarrhea appears to be multifactorial. A role of visceral autonomic neuropathy is supported by morphologic changes in both the parasympathetic and sympathetic nervous systems in diabetics (see below) and by the occurrence of diarrhea in other conditions affecting the autonomic nervous system including vagotomy.[131,140-142] Other postulated mechanisms include pancreatic insufficiency, small bowel bacterial overgrowth, infections, drugs (e.g., metformin) or associated celiac disease or hyperthyroidism,[131,134,139,143] and a decrease in interstitial cells of Cajal.

In the colon, dysmotility may result in severe constipation and even stercoral ulceration.[144,145] Autonomic neuropathy is likely a major factor, but a deficiency of ICC[146] and decreased production of substance P (a stimulant of colonic motility and fluid secretion)[147] may also contribute. Sometimes, patients develop dysfunction of anal sphincters, resulting in fecal incontinence, often in association with diarrhea.[131] They may also develop severe, unexplained abdominal pain (diabetic radiculopathy).[131,140-142]

Although esophageal abnormalities are commonly demonstrated with manometry, esophageal symptoms are uncommon. Diabetics are known to be

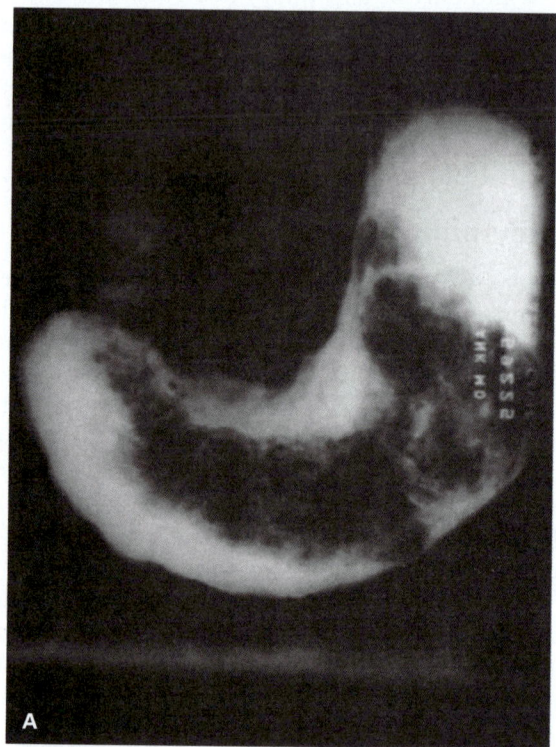

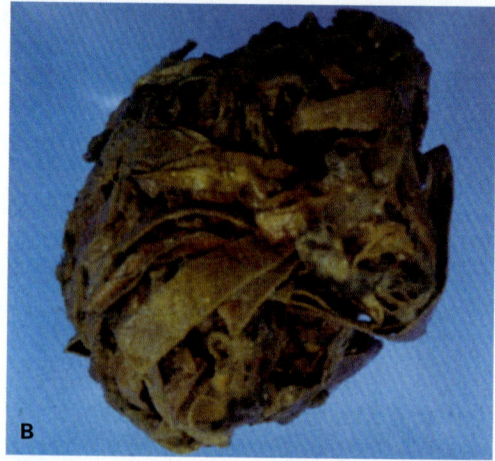

Figure 8-8. Gastric bezoar. **A:** Barium study of the stomach from a diabetic patient with gastroparesis diabeticorum showing extensive radiolucency due to the presence of a large bezoar. **B:** Gross appearance of bezoar, which is composed of retained, partially digested food.

susceptible to infections in the gut, especially esophageal candidiasis,[148] and in ketoacidosis there may be severe upper gastrointestinal bleeding from gastric erosions, presumably of the stress type. There is an increased incidence of atrophic gastritis with pernicious anemia and celiac sprue among type 1 diabetics. These cases are associated with significant titers of circulating parietal cell antibodies and often thyroid antibodies.[149-152] The prevalence of autoimmune gastritis in type 1 diabetics is three- to fivefold higher than that of the general population. Celiac disease is reported in up to 5% to 10% of patients with type 1 diabetes[152-154] compared to 0.55% to 1% in the general population in Europe and North America. In most cases the diagnosis of diabetes precedes that of celiac disease. One study found the prevalence of symptomatic celiac disease at diagnosis to be 0.7%, but this increased to 10% after 5 years of annual screening.[154] Many centers advocate routine annual screening for celiac disease in type 1 diabetics with a minimum of 2 years suggested.[154] (Celiac disease is further discussed in Chapter 20.)

Most studies support an association between diabetes and colorectal carcinoma. A meta-analysis of 15 studies including over 2,500,000 patients confirmed this association, demonstrating a relative risk of 1.3 (95% CI = 1.2–1.4) in diabetic patients compared to nondiabetics. This relative risk was maintained when analysis was restricted to the seven studies, which controlled for body mass index and physical inactivity.[155]

Pathology Surgical pathologists encountering material from the gastrointestinal tract of diabetics are most likely to see esophageal candidiasis, the mucosal lesion of celiac disease, or autoimmune gastritis (see Chapters 14 and 20). Other findings include erosive gastritis in diabetic ketoacidosis, SIBO, and stercoral ulceration. Resection specimens may show features of autonomic neuropathy, which are frequently patchy and may involve both the vagal and the sympathetic nervous systems. Such changes include a marked decrease in the density of unmyelinated axons, axonal degeneration, thickening of the basement membrane of Schwann cells, decreased caliber of vagal nerves, and decreased fiber density of sympathetic nerves.[131,156] Myenteric ganglia may also show degenerative changes characterized by distended neurons; enlarged, club-shaped neuronal processes; and accompanying chronic inflammation. Secondary degenerative changes in the muscularis propria may be found.[157] A marked decrease in interstitial cells of Cajal has been reported both in the stomach and the colon of diabetics[146,158,159] as well as animal models of diabetic gastroparesis[143] and may be related to lack of Heme oxygenase 1.[159a] Patients with diabetes are also at increased risk of atherosclerosis and its complications, such as acute mesenteric arterial ischemia. Microangiopathy is frequently mentioned in the literature, but it has not been conclusively demonstrated in the gut.[160,161]

Hyperfunction of Islets of Langerhans

The hormones produced by the pancreas play an important role in intestinal function. Consequently, alteration of hormonal homeostasis may have profound effects on normal digestion and motility. Islet cell hyperfunction can result from diffuse hyperplasia (nesidioblastosis) or neoplasia,[162,163] with the production of a variety of hormones, although in most instances one hormone predominates.[164] The hormones produced are those normally found in the cells of the islets of Langerhans such as insulin, glucagon, somatostatin, and pancreatic polypeptide. Sometimes, however, ectopic hormones, such as gastrin, ACTH, calcitonin, parathormone, and serotonin, are the major secretion products. In almost all instances, the gastrointestinal manifestations are a reflection of altered digestive function and motility and are unaccompanied by morphologic changes in the gastrointestinal mucosa. The major islet cell proliferations and their gastrointestinal manifestations are as follows.

Gastrinoma

This lesion results in the Zollinger–Ellison syndrome characterized by aggressive peptic ulcer disease, severe diarrhea, or both (see "Gastrointestinal Endocrine Disorders," Chapter 6). In addition to peptic ulceration, gastrin induces prominent trophic changes in the oxyntic mucosa including increased mucosal thickness, increased parietal cell mass, lingulate parietal cytoplasmic projections into the gland lumen, hyperplasia of mucin neck cells, mucin hypersecretion, and ECL cell hyperplasia and microcarcinoids. The antral mucosa is diminished in size to accommodate the expanded oxyntic zone, and there is a decrease in the density of antral G cells.[165]

VIPoma Syndrome (Verner–Morrisons Syndrome)

VIPomas constitute about 5% of pancreatic endocrine tumors of which the vast majority are malignant based on the presence of lymph node, hepatic, or distant metastases.[166] The VIPoma syndrome may also result from diffuse hyperplasia of the islets[162] and occasionally from ganglioneuromas or ganglioneuroblastomas, which secrete vasoactive intestinal peptide (VIP).[167,168] The syndrome is characterized by profuse watery secretory diarrhea (i.e., resistant to fasting), with hypersecretion of water and electrolytes, resulting in severe dehydration, hypokalemia, and metabolic acidosis. VIPomas may secrete other products such as gastrin, serotonin, gastrin inhibitory polypeptide, and somatostatin, which may contribute to the diarrhea.[166] No morphologic abnormalities have been described in the gastrointestinal tract.

Somatostatinoma

Somatostatin-producing tumors including somatostatinoma (and less commonly gangliocytic paraganglioma and poorly differentiated neuroendocrine carcinoma) may occasionally produce the clinical triad of diabetes mellitus, gallstones, and diarrhea ("somatostatinoma syndrome").[169] The vast majority of somatostatin-producing tumors are nonfunctional (probably due to the very short half-life of somatostatin), and full-blown somatostatinoma syndrome appears to be uncommon.[170] Diarrhea results from the physiological actions of somatostatin, namely, diminished pancreatic enzyme secretion and delayed intestinal absorption of nutrients. Somatostatinomas are frequently periampullary in location, and psammoma bodies are a typical feature (see Chapter 6).

Other Islet Cell Tumors

The other islet cell tumors, such as insulinomas and glucagonomas, may be accompanied by severe angular stomatitis and glossitis. Giant intestinal villi have been described with glucagonomas.[171-173] Such enterotrophic effects have been reproduced in animals administered glucagon-like peptide 2.[174]

Adrenal Gland

Gastrointestinal symptoms are common in Addison's disease with anorexia, nausea, and vomiting occurring in almost all advanced cases. Other symptoms include abdominal pain and diarrhea, sometimes with steatorrhea.[175,176] The diagnosis is frequently overlooked due to the nonspecific nature of the complaints, particularly when skin pigmentation is absent (5%–8% of cases).[176] Celiac disease is common in patients with autoimmune Addison's disease, with a prevalence of 8% to 12% reported in several European studies.[177-179] There have been isolated reports of atrophic gastritis with pernicious anemia in Addison's disease,[175,180] but its overall prevalence is uncertain. Peptic ulceration occurs uncommonly.[176]

Cushing's disease is frequently accompanied by gastrointestinal symptoms including anorexia, nausea, and vomiting.

Adrenal tumors may form part of syndromes affecting the gastrointestinal tract for example, adrenal cortical adenoma in Gardner's syndrome[181,182] and pheochromocytomas in MEN IIa and IIb and von Recklinghausen's disease (sometimes with somatostatin-rich duodenal carcinoids).[183,184]

Adrenal pheochromocytoma may have a number of gastrointestinal manifestations including nausea and vomiting, abdominal pain, and constipation. In addition, intestinal pseudo-obstruction and megacolon may occur due to the inhibition of gastrointestinal smooth muscle activity due to very high circulating catecholamine levels.[185-188] Rarely, patients may present with ischemic colitis due to catecholamine-mediated vasospasm.[189] Occasionally tumors may produce VIP and present with watery diarrhea, hypokalemia, and achlorhydria syndrome.[190,191] No recognized histologic changes have been demonstrated in these patients, and symptoms are often reversible with intravenous phentolamine or after surgical excision of the tumor. Rarely gastrointestinal hemorrhage may occur secondary to multiple varices associated with the tumor mass.[192]

Gonads

Pregnancy. Gastrointestinal symptoms are extremely common in pregnancy and include nausea (80%–90%), vomiting (50%), heartburn (40%–80%), bloating, and constipation (25%–40%). Altered levels of female sex hormones are considered to play a major role in these symptoms by lowering esophageal sphincter pressure, delaying gastric emptying, and decreasing intestinal motility. Other factors, especially mechanical, may contribute but are considered of lesser importance.[193-195] Severe, intractable vomiting (hyperemesis gravidarum) affects 0.3% to 2% of pregnancies and is strongly associated with elevated levels of human chorionic gonadotrophin (HCG) and estrogen.[196] HCG is thought to act via a stimulatory effect on secretory processes in the upper gastrointestinal tract (and possibly through binding to TSH receptor) while estrogen delays gastric emptying and motility. Patients with hyperemesis gravidarum have an increased prevalence of *H. pylori* infection compared to controls.[196]

Hypothalamus and Pituitary

The hypothalamus and pituitary normally function as an integrated unit, and disorders of either may involve gastrointestinal function.

Hypopituitarism

This affects gastrointestinal motility in much the same way as hypothyroidism. For example, a patient may develop nausea and vomiting secondary to gastroparesis on account of L-thyroxine deficiency. Replacement of the latter will relieve these symptoms.[197]

Pituitary Adenoma

Acromegaly, a disorder associated with excess growth hormone production, is characterized by overgrowth of the musculoskeletal system and all organs, including the gastrointestinal tract. Acromegalics are at increased risk of developing a variety of neoplasms including those arising in the gastrointestinal tract.[96,198–200] They have a three- to eightfold risk of developing colorectal carcinoma or premalignant polyps compared to the general population.[96] Risk factors for colorectal cancer in acromegalics include male gender, age >50 years, disease duration >5 years, three or more skin tags (to which these patients are prone), a family history of colorectal carcinoma, and a prior history of adenomatous polyps.[96,199] One study found elevated levels of insulin-like growth factor 1 (IGF-1) to be associated with an especially high risk of colorectal carcinoma in acromegalics,[201] but others have not.[199] More recently, it has been shown that the risk of colorectal neoplasms is markedly increased in patients with elevated fasting insulin levels.[199] Screening colonoscopy is recommended in all patients with acromegaly, with more frequent surveillance in those with additional risk factors for colorectal neoplasia.[96,200]

Autoimmune Polyendocrinopathy Syndrome Type 1

This rare monogenic autoimmune syndrome, caused by a defect in the *AIRE* gene on chromosome 21, is characterized by polyendocrinopathy and chronic *Candida* infection.[202,203] The condition usually manifests in childhood or early teenage years with chronic candidiasis (affecting tongue, esophagus, and nails) followed by autoimmune hypoparathyroidism and Addison's disease. At least two of the three aforementioned conditions are required for diagnosis. Other autoimmune disorders such as type 1 diabetes, autoimmune thyroid disease, autoimmune gastritis with pernicious anemia, celiac disease, and hypogonadism may be present. Patients may also have alopecia, vitiligo, urticaria-like erythema, ectodermal dystrophies affecting nails and enamel, and keratoconjunctivitis. Affected patients may present with chronic unexplained diarrhea and have decreased enteroendocrine cells relative to controls.[202] Thus, examination of mucosal biopsies for enteroendocrine cells in patients with unexplained diarrhea may alert the pathologist to the possibility of autoimmune polyglandular syndrome. Chronic diarrhea accompanied by loss of enteroendocrine cells may also be seen in enteroendocrine cell dysgenesis.[202] The precise cause of candidiasis is unclear but is thought to result from defective T-cell responses or immunological dysregulation. Patients are treated with hormone replacement therapy and systemic antifungal agents against *Candida* infection.[204]

The IPEX syndrome. The IPEX syndrome (immune dysregulation, polyendocrinopathy, enteropathy, and X-linkage syndrome) is due to a germline mutation in the forkhead box protein 3 (*FOXP3*) gene on the X chromosome, which in young males results in defective development of CD4+CD25+ T-regulatory cells. This leads to a variety of autoimmune phenomena including autoimmune enteropathy, gastritis, colitis, dermatitis, thyroiditis, and type 1 diabetes and frequently results in death within the first 2 years of life. Some patients have antigoblet cell antibodies, while others may have antiparietal cell and antiislet cell antibodies as well. It is discussed in more detail in Chapter 3.

Multiple Endocrine Neoplasia The MEN syndromes consist of a group of autosomal-dominant inherited disorders, characterized by hyperplastic or neoplastic involvement of a variety of endocrine glands.[205,205a,206] The major manifestations are listed in Table 8-1. The main variants of this syndrome are: MEN I, MEN IIa, MEN IIb, together with FMTC (familial medullary thyroid cancer) that does not have GI involvement. Their gastrointestinal symptoms result mainly from the products of endocrine proliferations, which stimulate or inhibit one or more functions of the gastrointestinal tract.[101,207,208] MEN IIb most commonly has major intestinal manifestations.[209,210] Patients have a characteristic marfanoid habitus and facies, along with nodular thickening of the lips and anterior tongue. They frequently have chronic constipation, dating from birth, associated with megacolon and narrowing of the lower sigmoid or upper rectum, which mimics Hirschsprung's disease. This disease is often associated with ganglioneuromatosis, which is thought to be responsible for the constipation, although the pathogenetic mechanism is unclear. A possible association with adenomatous polyposis throughout the gastrointestinal tract and with mucosal ganglioneuromatosis has also been noted.[211–213] MTC is the main morbidity in patients with MEN II, and early prophylactic thyroidectomy is indicated in these patients.[214] The gastrointestinal manifestations of MEN I and MEN IIa are due to hormone hypersecretion resulting from the endocrine cell proliferations, for example, peptic ulceration in patients with gastrinomas

Table 8-1 Gastrointestinal Manifestations of Multiple Endocrine Neoplasia (MEN) Syndromes

	COMPONENT	PENETRANCE (%)	GASTROINTESTINAL MANIFESTATIONS

MEN I (MEN1 gene mutations, rarely CDKN1B gene mutations encoding p27, sometimes referred to as MEN4)	Primary hyperparathyroidism
	Enteropancreatic neuroendocrine tumors
	  Gastrinoma
	  Insulinoma
	Pituitary adenomas
	Adrenocortical neoplasms
	Foregut neuroendocrine tumors (gastric, thymic, bronchial)
	Multiple facial angiofibroma
	Collagenoma
	Multiple lipomas
		90–100
		60
		
		40
		10
		30
		20–30
		10–15
		
		85
		70
		30
			Peptic ulceration associated with gastrinoma. Diarrhea associated with carcinoid syndrome or VIPoma.

MEN IIa (RET gene mutations—classically codon 634)	Medullary thyroid carcinoma Pheochromocytoma Primary hyperparathyroidism Hirschsprung's disease	95–100 50 20–30 Uncommon	Watery (secretory) diarrhea associated with medullary carcinoma (?) due to calcitonin overproduction
MEN IIb (RET gene mutations—classically codon 918)	Mucosal ganglioneuromatosis Medullary thyroid carcinoma Pheochromocytoma	100 95–100 50	Nodularities of lips and anterior tongue, gastric and intestinal dilatation, megacolon mimicking Hirschsprung's disease, constipation or diarrhea, hematochezia.

Modified from Giusti F, Marini F, Brandi ML. Multiple endocrine neoplasia type 1. In: Pagon RA, Adam MP, Bird TD, et al., eds. *Gene Reviews.* Available at: http://www.ncbi.nlm.nih.gov/books/NBK1538/. September 2012; Moline J, Eng C. Multiple endocrine neoplasia type 2. In: Pagon RA, Adam MP, Bird TD, et al., eds. *Gene Reviews.* Available at: http://www.ncbi.nlm.nih.gov/books/NBK1257/. January 2013.

(50% of patients with Zollinger–Ellison have MEN I),[206] or diarrhea due to the carcinoid syndrome, VIPoma, or medullary carcinoma of the thyroid. Hirschsprung's disease is occasionally seen in patients with MEN IIa.[208]

GASTROINTESTINAL MANIFESTATIONS IN RENAL DISEASE

A large number of gastrointestinal complications of renal failure have been reported and are listed in Table 8-2. The major problems, however, are upper gastrointestinal bleeding from erosions, ulcers, or gastric vascular ectasia; infarcts due to nonocclusive intestinal ischemia; and perforated diverticula. Most of these complications seem to be associated with renal dialysis and renal transplantation for reasons that are not always clear.

The pathogenesis of gastrointestinal manifestations of uremia is likely multifactorial and often difficult to dissect. However, gastric hypomotility with delayed gastric emptying,[215-217] capillary fragility and disordered hemostasis of uremia,[218-221] effects of unfiltered humoral factors or toxins,[222] comorbidities (including other organ failures or underlying causes, e.g., diabetes or amyloid), and medications (e.g., NSAIDs) may all play a role.

Acute Renal Failure

These patients, most of whom are postsurgical or trauma patients, frequently develop multiple gastric and duodenal erosions with gastrointestinal hemorrhage and occasionally perforation. Although high serum gastrin levels are found in some patients, it is probable that the gastrointestinal complications are the result of the physiologic stress with multiple organ failure (see Chapter 14) rather than acute renal failure.[223,224]

Chronic Renal Failure

Seventy five percent of patients with end-stage renal disease have gastrointestinal symptoms. Nausea, vomiting, and anorexia are most prevalent, with each affecting over 60% of patients. Other common complaints include bloating, heartburn, abdominal pain, and constipation.[222] Major but less common complications include bleeding from GAVE, erosions or ulcers, and infarcts due to nonocclusive intestinal ischemia. Gastrointestinal hemorrhage is particularly important, occurring in up to 15% of patients with chronic renal failure[225] and accounting for up to 15% to 20%

Table 8-2 Interrelationship of Gastrointestinal and Renal Diseases

GASTROINTESTINAL MANIFESTATIONS OF RENAL DISEASE

Acute renal failure
- Gastric and duodenal erosions
- Gastric perforation

Chronic renal failure
- Erosive esophagitis
- Erosive and hemorrhagic gastritis
- (Nodular) duodenitis
- ? Peptic ulcer disease
- ? Angiodysplasia
- Intussusception secondary to mucosal hemorrhage
- Diverticula in adult polycystic kidney disease (APCKD)
- Salmonella enteritis
- Calcific uremic arteriolopathy

Complications of therapy
- Kayexalate sorbitol associated GI mucosal injury
- Anticoagulant and antiplatelet therapy associated GI bleeding
- Mycophenylate mofetil associated GI mucosal injury (transplants)

Complications of dialysis
- Acute fluid loss resulting in nonocclusive intestinal ischemia
- Peritonitis (bacterial or chemical) in peritoneal dialysis
- Hernia (+/− obstruction or incarceration) in peritoneal dialysis
- Sclerosing peritonitis in long-term peritoneal dialysis

Renal transplantation
- Gastric and duodenal erosions and ulcers
- Esophagitis (often candida)
- Mycophenylate mofetil associated GI mucosal injury
- Perforation of colonic diverticula (especially APCKD)
- Cecal ulceration
- Pseudomembranous colitis (50% of patients receiving antibiotics)
- Nonocclusive vascular insufficiency
- Infections due to chronic immunosupression, especially cytomegalovirus infection and intestinal strongyloidiasis
- Posttransplant GI lymphoproliferative disorders

DISEASES AFFECTING BOTH GASTROINTESTINAL AND RENAL SYSTEMS
- Collagen vascular diseases
  - Scleroderma
  - Vasculitides
- Diabetes mellitus
- Hyperparathyroidism
- Amyloidosis
- Myeloma
- Henoch–Schonlein purpura
- Hemolytic uremic syndrome

RENAL MANIFESTATIONS OF GASTROINTESTINAL DISEASE

Crohn's disease
- Calcium oxalate stones
- Ureteral obstruction
- Entero or colovesical fistula
- Perinephric abscess

---

of deaths in patients on maintenance dialysis.[220,225] Cardiovascular complications of chronic renal failure, such as hypertension and arteriosclerosis, may predispose to intestinal ischemia.

Gastritis and duodenitis have long been recognized in patients with uremia. An autopsy series from 1934, which included 136 consecutive patients with untreated uremia, found diffuse hemorrhagic gastritis to be present in 42% of patients and diffuse hemorrhagic duodenitis in 24%.[226] Pseudomembranous colitis was also a frequent feature. A subsequent review of 265 untreated uremic patients reported similar findings.[227] Studies in uremic patients on maintenance hemodialysis have produced varied and often conflicting data.[222,228] Several have reported an increased prevalence of gastroduodenal lesions including gastritis, duodenitis, and peptic ulcers in uremic patients,[229-235] while others have found their prevalence to be similar to general population.[225,236-242] Such variations may reflect differences in patient populations, comorbidities, sample sizes, investigative techniques used, prevalence of *H. pylori* infection, use of NSAID agents, and others. The prevalence of gastrointestinal lesions in patients with chronic renal failure does not appear to correlate with the severity of renal dysfunction or duration of hemodialysis.[236,238,242] The reported prevalence of *H. pylori* infection in patients with uremia varies from 21% to 73%[242,243] and overall does not appear to exceed that of the general population.[222]

Gastrointestinal bleeding (mostly occult) is common in patients with uremia, particularly those on hemodialysis. Gastritis, duodenitis, peptic ulcers, and telangiectasias are more prone to bleed in uremic patients than in the general population. This is due to the disordered hemostasis of uremia resulting from platelet and endothelial dysfunction, associated anemia, and antiplatelet and anticoagulant therapies frequently taken by these patients.[221] Patients with chronic renal failure may lose 3 to 4 mL of blood via the gastrointestinal tract per day (compared to around 1 mL/d in the general population), increasing to 6 mL in patients on hemodialysis.[221] Overt gastrointestinal hemorrhage is a serious complication in uremic patients and is associated with a higher rate of blood transfusion, emergency surgery, and mortality than in the general population.[228] Angiodysplasia (or vascular ectasia) is well described in chronic uremia and may be a cause of severe upper gastrointestinal bleeding. However, it remains unclear whether it has a higher prevalence in uremics than in the general population.[222]

Finally, uremic patients who receive kayexalate sorbitol for the treatment of hyperkalemia may develop mucosal injury and often necrosis, in the lower and upper gastrointestinal tract.[244-246] In H&E sections kayexalate crystals appear as basophilic polygonal crystals with a characteristic striped or mosaic pattern.

Patients undergoing dialysis are prone to additional complications including

1. Acute fluid loss during dialysis, producing hypotension, which may result in nonocclusive vascular ischemia[247]
2. Peritonitis, the most common complication of peritoneal dialysis, which can be bacterial (most commonly due to staphylococcal or streptococcal species) or chemical[222]
3. Hernias, a common complication of peritoneal dialysis, posing a risk of acute bowel obstruction or incarceration[248,249]
4. Sclerosing peritonitis, which is a rare complication of long-term peritoneal dialysis[222]

Endoscopic and Histologic Appearances

The gross and histologic features of erosive esophagitis, gastritis, and duodenitis are discussed in their respective chapters.

Other Findings

A number of other abnormalities have been described in association with chronic renal failure, namely, massive small bowel infarction secondary to nonocclusive vascular insufficiency, colonic intussusception secondary to intramural hemorrhage, duodenal pseudomelanosis, and susceptibility to *Salmonella* enteritis in hemodialysis patients.[218,250-253] Diverticulosis is common in patients with autosomal dominant polycystic kidney disease and is particularly prone to complications in the posttransplant period (see below)[254,255] A peculiar form of "nodular duodenitis" associated with Brunner's gland hyperplasia has been described in renal failure[256] (see Chapter 14). Calcific uremic arteriolopathy is a rare complication of end-stage renal disease, which may present with intestinal ischemia or infarction.[257] Uremic colitis per se probably does not exist as a distinct entity but is due to other causes such as infection and ischemic colitis.

There are a number of diseases, which affect both the renal system and the gut, for example, the collagen vascular diseases, hyperparathyroidism, amyloidosis, and myeloma. These are described separately in other parts of this chapter. In addition, the kidney can be secondarily involved in primary intestinal disease, for example, oxalate stones in Crohn's disease. These conditions are listed in Table 8-2 and will not be further discussed.

Renal Transplantation

Gastrointestinal complications are an important cause of morbidity following renal transplantation, with an incidence of around 20%[258] (Table 8-2). Many complications are related to immunosuppressive therapy (especially mycophenolate mofetil [MMF] and corticosteroids), preexisting gastrointestinal pathology, antibiotic therapy, and infections.[258,259] The most common gastrointestinal complications include nausea, vomiting, and abdominal discomfort (frequent in patients receiving MMF, corticosteroids, or both), candidal and less commonly CMV- or herpes-related esophagitis, peptic ulcer disease, diarrhea, and colonic hemorrhage or perforation. The complications common to organ transplant–related immunosuppression are discussed in detail in Chapter 4 and are mentioned only briefly here.

Until fairly recently, peptic ulcer disease was a frequent cause of morbidity and mortality in renal transplant recipients, accounting for around 4% of deaths in these patients. This picture has changed dramatically with active screening and treatment of patients for *Helicobacter* and ulcerogenic medications prior to transplantation and with the routine use of prophylactic H2 receptor antagonists, proton pump inhibitors, or sucralfate in the postoperative period by many transplant groups.[258,260] This practice has reduced the mortality from gastroduodenal perforation or hemorrhage to near zero.

Diarrhea is frequent in renal transplant recipients and is mostly related to infections, drugs, or antibiotics. Self-limited and short-lived viral gastroenteritis is the most frequent cause of diarrhea. Certain immunosuppressives, especially MMF, are associated with diarrhea. Pseudomembranous colitis occurs in about 50% of transplant recipients receiving antibiotics. Other infective agents responsible for diarrhea include bacteria (*Shigella*, *Salmonella*, and *Campylobacter*, etc.), viruses (CMV, herpes simplex virus), and parasites (*Cryptosporidium*, *Giardia*, and *Strongyloides*).[258]

Renal transplant recipients are at increased risk for a variety of colonic complications, which seem to be more common in the elderly and in patients with polycystic kidney disease. These include ruptured colonic diverticula, bleeding from cecal ulceration, and nonocclusive vascular insufficiency.[258,261,262] The latter may be patchy and mimic inflammatory bowel disease (IBD).[261] The cause of ruptured diverticula and its relationship to steroids and immunosuppressive therapy are not understood, but its high incidence in renal transplant patients at one stage prompted some to advocate prophylactic sigmoid colectomies in patients with symptomatic disease.[263-266] Although more common in the elderly, young patients may also be affected.

Chronically immunosuppressed patients are prone to unusual infections. Thus, renal transplant recipients, especially following treatment for rejection, are prone to CMV infection, which in some instances results in colonic perforation[267,268]; parasitic infections such as cryptosporidiosis, giardia, and blastocystosis[269]; and hyperinfection with *Strongyloides stercoralis*. The latter may, on rare occasions, result in severe colitis and perforation.[270,271] Finally, the gastrointestinal tract is a common site for posttransplant-associated lymphoproliferative disorders (see Chapter 5).

Role of the Pathologist and Clinical Implications

In examining biopsy and resection specimens from patients with renal failure, renal transplants, or both, the pathologist should always be on the lookout for potentially treatable conditions. This refers mainly to infections such as candidiasis, herpes virus, CMV, and strongyloides. Pathologists should be aware that the commonly used immunosuppressive drug MMF may cause toxic injury throughout the gastrointestinal tract including ulcerative esophagitis, reactive gastropathy, graft versus host disease (GVHD)-like features (i.e., dilated damaged intestinal crypts with increased epithelial apoptosis), crypt architectural distortion, and increased lamina propria inflammation. Caution is thus required when considering a diagnosis of IBD or GVHD in such patients.[272] Finally, if the cause of a patient's renal failure is undetermined, gut specimens from the patient should be examined carefully for the presence of amyloid.

GASTROINTESTINAL MANIFESTATIONS OF HEPATIC DISORDERS

The major gastrointestinal disorders associated with liver disease are related to portal hypertension and liver transplantation.

Portal Hypertension

Portal hypertension is most commonly associated with cirrhosis but can also result from noncirrhotic portal fibrosis, extrahepatic portal vein obstruction, hepatocellular carcinoma, and other hepatic lesions such as polycystic liver disease.[273] Portal hypertension commonly results in esophageal and gastric varices and portal congestive gastropathy, often causing severe upper gastrointestinal hemorrhage. Endoscopic treatment of varices appears to predispose to the development of congestive gastropathy due to the redistribution of blood flow.[274] It has now been shown that similar congestive colonic lesions and rectal varices (portal colopathy) are not uncommon and can also result in frequent hemorrhage.[274-278] A study, using capsule endoscopy, found small intestinal varices in 3 of 19 patients (16%) who had previously undergone eradication of esophageal varices.[279] Morphologically, the gastrointestinal mucosal changes in portal hypertension involve primarily the mucosal vessels, resulting in an increased number of mucosal capillaries and venules in all portions of the mucosa, with prominent branching and marked dilatation. The best recognized of these is portal hypertensive gastropathy in which dilated mucosal capillaries are present, which by definition have a greater diameter than the gastric pits. Unlike GAVE, they are usually not thrombosed. In addition, some of the venules are tortuous and show thick-walled arterialization. In addition to the varices, other vascular changes are sometimes found in hepatic cirrhosis such as vascular ectasia, erythematous mucosal patches, red macules, and telangiectasia, all of which may also give rise to gastrointestinal hemorrhage. However, some of these lesions, such as vascular ectasia, may be unrelated to portal hypertension and due to other causes such as liver dysfunction.[280]

Up to 60% of cirrhotic patients have evidence of SIBO, thought to result from small intestinal dysmotility and impaired antimicrobial defenses. SIBO is considered a predictor of spontaneous bacterial peritonitis.[274] Patients with alcoholic liver disease may display many of the small intestinal mucosal abnormalities seen in SIBO, including partial villous atrophy, increased lamina propria cellularity, increased intraepithelial lymphocytes, and brush border abnormalities.[281]

Primary Sclerosing Cholangitis and Autoimmune Hepatitis

Fifty five to seventy percent of patients with primary sclerosing cholangitis (PSC) and four to thirteen percent of patients with autoimmune hepatitis have IBD, mainly ulcerative colitis.[282] The finding of PSC therefore demands colonoscopy, and if colitis is present, this counts as the first surveillance colonoscopy, as it is unclear how long the colitis has been present. Patients with PSC are at increased risk for the development of IBD-associated colorectal carcinoma[283] as well as the development of pouchitis following ileoanal pouch anastomosis.[284] One of the problems of PSC is that if the patient is close to a liver transplantation, dysplasia or even carcinoma may be present in the large bowel, raising the question of which needs to be carried out first.

Liver Transplantation

Liver transplantation can give rise to the usual posttransplant complications involving the gastrointestinal tract such as infections, lymphoproliferative disorders, etc. Other complications described include intestinal perforation due to operative injury or infection[285] and eosinophilic gastroenteropathy with intense eosinophilic mucosal infiltration. The latter may be due to immunomodulatory medications such as corticosteroids as suggested by disappearance of the infiltrate after discontinuation of therapy.[286] IBD may develop de novo following liver transplantation,[282,287] mostly in patients with autoimmune hepatitis or PSC. Continuous immunosuppressive therapy in transplant patients does not prevent flares or de novo occurrence of IBD. In fact the disease may follow a more aggressive course than that prior to liver transplantation; this may be related to immunosuppressive regimens used.[288] Interestingly, in one study of patients transplanted for PSC or autoimmune cirrhosis, de novo IBD was strongly associated with postoperative CMV infection.[287] A causative role of CMV infection in this setting remains to be determined.

GASTROINTESTINAL MANIFESTATIONS OF SKIN DISORDERS

Skin and gastrointestinal tract disorders may occur simultaneously in a number of settings:

1. The skin disorder may be secondary to a primary disease of the gut, for example, ulcerative colitis with erythema nodosum and pyoderma gangrenosum.
2. The gut lesion is in contiguity with the skin disorder, for example, pemphigus and blistering lesions in the esophagus, or is associated with a primary dermatologic disorder, such as dermatitis herpetiformis and celiac sprue.
3. The skin and gut disorders are both manifestations of generalized disease or a genetic disorder, for example, skin and gut disorders in scleroderma, colonic polyps and dermal tumors in Gardner's syndrome, eczema and eosinophilic esophagitis in atopic patients, and vascular malformations of the skin and mucous membranes in Rendu–Osler–Weber syndrome.

Table 8-3 lists the major disorders in which skin and gastrointestinal manifestations are found. This section will focus on gastrointestinal lesions with documented pathology occurring in the setting of primary skin disorders or generalized disorders in which skin manifestations are the major abnormalities.

The esophagus is the most frequently affected extracutaneous site. Although esophageal involvement is rare in common diseases such as dermatitis and psoriasis, it may be a major manifestation of a number of uncommon skin disorders. Such disorders can be broadly divided into bullous, hyperkeratotic, malignant, and group of miscellaneous disorders.

Bullous Disorders

Epidermolysis bullosa. This heterogeneous group of inherited blistering diseases can involve all organs lined by squamous epithelium, with the esophagus one of the most common extracutaneous sites involved.[289] Gastrointestinal symptoms are reported in up to 58% of patients.[290] The hallmark of epidermolysis bullosa is the development of bullae due to the separation of the dermis and epidermis following minimal trauma. This is seen histologically as subepidermal bullae. The bullae become tense and rupture, producing erosions or ulcers, which often heal poorly with scarring.[289,291] In the esophagus the scars vary from minor webs in the postcricoid region to long strictures of the esophagus. Because the blisters are so fragile and rupture easily, endoscopy is often avoided[292-294] (see Chapter 11). The anorectal region may also be involved giving rise to pain on defecation and constipation. Pyloric stenosis or atresia and duodenal obstruction have been described in some patients.[290,295-297]

There are 20 different phenotypes associated with mutations in 10 different genes, but they can be broadly classified into four groups based on the plane of cleavage of the basement membrane zone and pattern of inheritance. These include (a) epidermolysis bullosa simplex, (b) junctional epidermolysis bullosa, (c) dominant dystrophic epidermolysis bullosa, and (d) recessive dystrophic epidermolysis bullosa. Esophageal manifestations are very common in dystrophic epidermolysis bullosa, particularly the recessive form.[289-291] Dysphagia (70%–94%) and esophageal strictures (65%–80%) are frequent findings in patients with recessive dystrophic epidermolysis bullosa.[289,290] Some patients may have diarrhea associated with endoscopic and histologic features of colitis, including increased lamina propria cellularity and neutrophil infiltrates. Gastroesophageal reflux and constipation are frequent in both simplex and dystrophic forms (with painful perianal disease likely contributing to the latter), whereas failure to thrive is frequent in patients with junctional and recessive dystrophic forms of the disease.[290] A subgroup of junctional epidermolysis bullosa is associated with pyloric and rarely duodenal atresia (pyloric atresia–junctional epidermolysis bullosa syndrome).[290,296] Patients with esophageal disease require nutritional support in the

Table 8-3 Primary Skin Disorders Associated with Gastrointestinal Disease

SKIN DISORDER	GASTROINTESTINAL PATHOLOGY	COMMENT
SKIN DISORDERS WITH GASTROINTESTINAL MANIFESTATIONS		
Dermatogenic Enteropathy		
Severe eczema	Malabsorption; pathogenesis unclear.	
Psoriasis		
Bullous Eruptions		
Epidermolysis bullosa dystrophica	Dysphagia, constipation, pain on defecation, esophageal bullae, rupture of bullae, esophageal webs, fibrosis and stricture, pyloric stenosis.	See esophageal disease, Chapter 11.
Epidermolysis bullosa acquisita	Bullae, proximal esophageal webs and strictures, association with Crohn's disease.	
Pemphigus vulgaris	Dysphagia, esophageal bullae, erosions, stricture.	
Bullous pemphigoid	Dysphagia, esophageal bullae, erosions and stricture on rare occasions.	
Stevens–Johnson syndrome	Dysphagia, occasionally severe hemorrhage.	
Dermatitis herpetiformis	Celiac sprue, rarely esophageal bullae, erosions and stricture.	See small bowel mucosal disease, Chapter 20. See inflammatory disorders of the esophagus, Chapter 11.
Herpes simplex virus	Yellow-white plaque with surrounding erythematous base throughout gastrointestinal tract, especially esophagus; vesicles and small, punched-out erosions. Later, diffuse, intensely erythematous mucosa. Intranuclear inclusions in epithelial cells around vesicles or at ulcer margin.	
Hyperkeratotic Disorders		
Lichen planus	Dysphagia, strictures (usually proximal).	
Tylosis	Esophagitis, esophageal webs, stricture, squamous carcinoma of esophagus.	
Miscellaneous		
Darier's disease	Esophageal keratotic papules.	
Acrodermatitis enteropathica	Patchy, variable villous lesion. Abnormal inclusions in Paneth cells. May follow Crohn's disease.	See small bowel mucosal disease, Chapter 2.
SKIN DISORDERS ASSOCIATED WITH GASTROINTESTINAL MALIGNANCY		
Tylosis	Squamous carcinoma of esophagus.	
Acanthosis nigricans	Adenocarcinoma of stomach and colon.	
Dermatomyositis	Adenocarcinoma of stomach and colon.	
Multiple seborrheic keratosis (Leser–Trelat sign)	Gastrointestinal carcinoma.	
Erythema multiforme	Adenocarcinoma of colon.	See connective tissue disorders, Chapter 5.
Ataxia telagiectasia	Adenocarcinoma of stomach, nodular lymphoid hyperplasia.	See immune deficiency disorders, Chapter 4.
SYSTEMIC DISORDERS INVOLVING THE SKIN AND GUT		
Connective Tissue Disorders		
Scleroderma	Motility disorder resulting in esophagitis and pseudo-obstruction. Atrophy of circular muscle and replacement fibrosis, esophagitis and esophageal stricture. Intestinal atony and pseudodiverticula.	See connective tissue disorders, Chapter 3.

(Continued)

Table 8-3 Primary Skin Disorders Associated with Gastrointestinal Disease (Continued)

SKIN DISORDER	GASTROINTESTINAL PATHOLOGY	COMMENT
Dermatomyositis	Arteritis, ischemia, infarctions and perforations. Cervical esophagus—inflammation, edema and muscle atrophy. Lower esophagus—inflammation, muscle atrophy and stricture.	
Systemic lupus erythematosus	Arteritis, ischemic ulcers, segmental bowel infarction, gastrointestinal hemorrhage and perforation, depending on the size of the vessel involved.	See vascular disorders, Chapter 2.
Vascular Disorders and Malformations		
Malignant atrophic papulosis (Degos' disease)	Progressive occlusive vascular disease of small and medium-sized vessels resulting in patchy necrosis, infarction and peritonitis.	
Ehlers–Danlos syndrome	Structural derangement of elastic tissue with fragility of blood vessels, rupture and ischemic necrosis, diverticula.	
Pseudoxanthoma elasticum	Gastrointestinal hemorrhage, yellow mucosal nodules, proliferation of elastic fibers, which may be calcified.	
Rendu–Osler–Weber syndrome	Mucosal telangiectasia, gastrointestinal bleeding.	
Blue rubber bleb nevus syndrome	Mucosal cavernous hemangiomas.	
Henoch–Schonlein purpura	Mucosal hemorrhage, abdominal pain.	See vascular disorders, Chapter 2.
Cutaneous visceral hemangiomatosis	Mucosal cavernous hemangiomata.	
Kaposi sarcoma	Mucosal and submucosal hemorrhagic nodules.	
Miscellaneous Diseases		
Behçet's disease	Crohn's-like colitis.	See colitis, Chapter 23.
Fabry's disease	Angiokeratomas on scrotum, extremities, lips and mouth, crampy abdominal pain, nausea, diarrhea, impaired intestinal motility.	See disorders of lipid metabolism, Chapter 9.
SKIN LESION ASSOCIATED WITH MAJOR GASTROINTESINAL DISEASES		
Erythema nodosa, pyoderma gangrenosum	Inflammatory bowel disease.	
Dermatitis herpetiformis	Celiac sprue.	
Sebaceous cysts, lipomas	Polyposis syndromes *Gardner syndrome*.	See polyposis syndromes, Chapter 26.
Pigmented macules on lips, mouth and feet	*Peutz–Jegher syndrome*.	
Alopecia, nail dystrophy, skin pigmentation	*Cronkhite–Canada syndrome*.	
Carcinoid syndrome—flushing, telangiectasia on face and neck.	Carcinoid tumor.	
Flushing, telangiectasia, pigmented macules and papules	Systemic mastocytosis.	

form of liquid/pureed diets, gastrostomy feeding, or sometimes total parenteral nutrition. Esophageal dilatation may be beneficial in some patients who fail to respond to conservative measures, but requires caution since new bullae may be induced, leading to further structuring.[291]

Epidermolysis Bullosa Acquisita

As with genetic epidermolysis bullosa above, epidermolysis bullosa acquisita (EBA) is characterized by bullae following minor trauma. It differs from the former in its adult onset, lack of family history, milder skin disease, and rarity of esophageal involvement. Affected patients may present with dysphagia. Endoscopic findings include bullae, proximal esophageal webs, and strictures.[291,298] Bullae may be induced by endoscopy. EBA is associated with circulating autoantibodies against collagen VII.[299] As in skin biopsies, endoscopic biopsies may show subepidermal bullae with linear deposition of IgG along the basement membrane. EBA may occur in association with Crohn's disease[300,301] (see also Chapter 11).

Pemphigus Vulgaris

This rare autoimmune blistering disease is associated with autoantibodies to the cell adhesion molecule desmoglein 3.[291] This results in loss of cohesion between epithelial cells of the suprabasal stratum spinosum, with characteristic acantholytic, suprabasal blister formation. Eighty to ninety percent of patients have both skin and mucous membrane involvement, with 70% presenting initially with oral lesions.[291] Esophageal involvement is fairly common if looked for, being reported in 42% to 88% of patients in several small series.[302–306] Dysphagia and odynophagia are the most common symptoms associated with esophageal lesions. Endoscopy is considered safe in skilled hands,[305] provided care is taken not to damage fragile mucosa or induce new lesions.[291] Biopsies should be taken from the junction between the floor and the roof of the blister and the adjacent mucosa (not the blister itself) to best evaluate suprabasal clefting and acantholysis.[305] Both formalin-fixed and fresh tissue should be submitted for routine histologic assessment and immunofluorescence studies, respectively. Diagnosis is based on demonstration of characteristic acantholytic lesions on routine stains, intercellular "lace-like" deposition of IgG and C3 by direct immunofluorescence, and binding of circulating antibodies to squamous epithelium by indirect immunofluorescence (a marker of active disease). Esophageal lesions are treated as for other mucocutaneous lesions, that is, with combinations of steroids and other immunomodulatory agents and sometimes plasmapheresis.[291] Rare examples of esophageal involvement by pemphigus vegetans are reported.[307]

Cicatricial Pemphigoid (Benign Mucous Membrane Pemphigoid)

This rare autoimmune disease occurs in middle age and predominantly affects women.[291,308] Patients have circulating antibodies to bullous pemphigoid antigen 2. The ocular and oral mucosa is most frequently involved, but the upper aerodigestive tract, esophagus, and anogenital regions can also be involved. Skin involvement is present in a minority of patients (25%).[291] Esophageal involvement is reported in 2% to 13% of cases. Symptoms include dysphagia, odynophagia, heartburn, or chronic cough due to aspiration.[308] Endoscopic findings include bullae, ulcers, webs, and strictures in the upper esophagus. As with other blistering conditions, bullae can be a direct consequence of endoscopy.[291,308,309] Characteristic histologic findings include subepidermal bullae with abundant eosinophils, mononuclear cells, and some neutrophils. Direct immunofluorescence shows linear deposition of IgG and C3 at the dermal–epidermal junction.[309] Biopsies taken from the edge of the blister and containing underlying stroma have the best diagnostic yield. Treatment is with oral corticosteroids and other immunomodulatory agents or endoscopic esophageal dilation. The latter may provide rapid symptomatic improvement and avoid the need for prolonged therapy, but reports of mucosal injury, bulla formation, and even perforation are on record. Colonic interposition may sometimes be required for refractory dysphagia.[308]

Stevens–Johnson Syndrome

This rare, life-threatening mucocutaneous disorder is characterized by widespread epidermal necrosis secondary to keratinocyte apoptosis. It is most frequently associated with adverse drug-induced reactions and infections such as *Mycoplasma pneumoniae*. It presents with fever and acute bullous skin eruptions, which involve the mucous membranes in over 90% of cases.[291,310] The lips, oral cavity, conjunctiva, urethral meatus, vagina, and anus are most frequently involved.[291] Gastrointestinal involvement is rare and primarily affects the esophagus.[310,311] Patients present with dysphagia or occasionally severe hemorrhage. The endoscopic appearance ranges from solitary or multiple erosions to large erythematous areas of denuded mucosa with overlying white plaques. The histology ranges from an erythema multiforme-like picture to overt necrosis.[291] Late sequelae may include esophageal webs or strictures.[291,310,311] Gastric and intestinal involvement in Stevens–Johnson syndrome is extremely rare.[310,312]

Herpes Simplex Virus Infection

Herpes simplex may involve the mouth and pharynx and, not uncommonly, extend to the esophagus, especially in the immunosuppressed patient. In disseminated herpes simplex virus infection, the esophagus is the most common organ involved. The typical endoscopic appearance is that of multiple oval ulcers in the distal esophagus without overlying pseudomembranes.[291] Herpes simplex virus proctitis is not uncommon and occurs in homosexual males.[313]

Hyperkeratotic Disorders

Lichen planus. This idiopathic inflammatory disorder of skin, nails, and mucous membranes is characterized by eruptions of violaceous, polygonal pruritic plaques, predominantly on flexor skin surfaces. Clinically significant esophageal involvement occurs in about 1% of cases and tends to occur proximally.[291,314,315] Patients usually present with dysphagia and sometimes odynophagia. Endoscopic findings are usually nonspecific. Histology shows a band-like lichenoid infiltrate involving the superficial lamina propria and basal epithelium with basal keratinocyte degeneration, Civatte bodies, and overlying parakeratosis. Sawtooth acanthosis and hypergranulosis, typical of skin lesions, do not feature in esophageal lesions (the esophageal epithelium lacks a granular layer).[314] Strictures complicate symptomatic esophageal involvement in about 80% of cases.[314] Most patients respond to corticosteroids but tend to relapse when the dose is reduced or treatment discontinued. Multiple esophageal dilatations are often required for relief of recurring strictures but may exacerbate the condition as patients are prone to developing new lesions in traumatized areas of uninvolved mucosa.[314,315] Esophageal squamous carcinoma has been reported in a patient with long-standing lichen planus.[316]

Tylosis

This rare autosomal dominant condition, also known as hyperkeratosis plantaris et palmaris, is characterized by hyperkeratotic thickening of the palms and soles.[291,317,318] Two major subtypes have been described. Type A is later onset (5–15 years) and is associated with a high risk of esophageal squamous cell carcinoma. Type B is earlier onset (first year) and does not carry an increased cancer risk.[291,317] Type A tylosis is associated with a genetic abnormality, the *tylosis with esophageal cancer* (TOC) locus on chromosome 17q25. Importantly, this locus has also been implicated in sporadic esophageal squamous cell carcinomas.[319] Patients with tylosis patients are prone to reflux esophagitis and develop minor esophageal webs or strictures. Esophageal papillomatosis is a typical finding.[291] There is a 40% to 95% lifetime risk of esophageal squamous carcinoma, complicating tylosis depending on the pedigree,[318] although it can take up to 30 years to develop.[320] Gastric cancer has also rarely been reported. It has been recommended that patients undergo at least annual screening endoscopy with multiple biopsies, but there is no guarantee that this will impact mortality.[318]

Miscellaneous Disorders

Acrodermatitis enteropathica. This rare autosomal recessive disorder is thought to be due to an inability to absorb sufficient intestinal zinc. The gene responsible for acrodermatitis enteropathica has been mapped to chromosome 8q24.3 and shown to be a member of the solute carrier 39A superfamily, historically known as the Zrt–Irt-like protein family, which function as zinc transporters.[321] Acrodermatitis enteropathica presents, usually at the time of weaning, with eczematous pink scaly plaques on the hands and feet and around the mouth and anus, in addition to paronychia and nail dystrophy. The plaques can become bullous, pustular, or desquamative.[322] It is reversed by giving zinc orally. Gastrointestinal symptoms are often intermittent and consist of diarrhea and malabsorption.[323] The small bowel shows a patchy villous lesion of variable severity. Abnormal inclusions are found in the Paneth cells (see Chapter 20). Acrodermatitis enteropathica may also result from zinc deficiency secondary to Crohn's disease and malnutrition.[324,325]

Darier's Disease

This uncommon inherited disorder, characterized by abnormal keratinization of the skin, nails, and mucous membranes, may rarely involve the esophagus.[291,326,327] Endoscopy may show keratotic papules,[291] while histology shows acantholysis, suprabasal clefts, and submucosal villi projecting into lacunae as seen in Darier's skin lesions. Esophageal squamous carcinoma has been reported in a patient with long-standing Darier's disease.[326]

Dermatogenic Enteropathy

Patients with extensive skin disease such as eczema and psoriasis may develop steatorrhea; this condition has been named "dermatogenic enteropathy."[328–330] The malabsorption is proportional to the extent of the rash and improves as the rash subsides. The cause for the malabsorption is not known, and initial claims that it might be due to a small bowel lesion have never been verified.

Malignant Disease of the Gastrointestinal Tract and Skin Disease

Some skin disorders are specific for particular tumors, for example, carcinoma of the esophagus, while others indicate malignant disease in general, for example, generalized skin pigmentation and dermatomyositis. In a third group, skin manifestations are those of wasting disease associated with malignancy.

Acanthosis Nigricans

This rare mucocutaneous disorder is characterized by brown or black warty, velvety plaques in the axillae and groins. The oral mucosa is affected in 40% to 50% of patients, and the esophagus is rarely involved. The esophageal lesions appear as multiple squamous papillomatous lesions, which may enlarge and obstruct the lumen.[291] Acanthosis nigricans is commonly associated with insulin resistance, type II diabetes, and obesity (i.e., metabolic syndrome) but may also be seen with polycystic ovary syndrome, certain congenital disorders, acromegaly, certain drugs, and a number of rarer conditions reviewed elsewhere.[331] In the absence of an underlying condition, there is a high association with malignancy, often carcinoma of the stomach and colon.[332] The skin changes may appear before, after, or simultaneously with the tumor and may regress after extirpation of the tumor. However, by the time acanthosis develops, the associated tumors are usually advanced and often metastatic and inoperable.[330,333] The pathogenesis of acanthosis nigricans appears multifactorial with a likely role for IGF-1 receptors on keratinocytes and fibroblasts, which are activated by elevated insulin levels. Other growth factor receptors such as EGFR and FGFR may also play a role.[331]

Cowden's Disease

This rare autosomal dominant condition is characterized by multiple hamartomas in tissues from all embryonic germ cell layers; mucocutaneous lesions (e.g., facial trichilemmomas, mucocutaneous papillomatous papules, acral keratoses, esophageal glycogen acanthosis); and an increased risk of breast, thyroid, and endometrial cancers.[334] The hamartomatous polyps in the gastrointestinal tract may be indistinguishable from juvenile polyps, but also include inflammatory, lipomatous, and ganglioneuromatous polyps.[335] Cowden's syndrome is associated with a germline mutation in the PTEN tumor suppressor gene as are Bannayan–Riley–Ruvalcaba and Proteus syndromes; together these are classified under the broad term "PTEN hamartoma tumor syndromes."[336] (see Chapter 26). A subset of individuals with CS and CS-like symptoms not having germline PTEN mutations have germline variants of dehydrogenase complex subunits B or dehydrogenase complex subunits D.

Dermatomyositis

Dermatomyosis has a strong association with malignancy in general, including gastric and colonic carcinomas (see "Connective Tissue Disorders")

Miscellaneous

Other nonspecific skin disorders associated with neoplasms, including gastrointestinal carcinomas, are generalized dermal pigmentation, postulated to be due to tumor production of melanocyte-stimulating hormone; migratory thrombophlebitis; and multiple seborrheic keratoses (the Leser–Trélat sign).[337,338] Familial gastrointestinal stromal tumors due to germline mutations in *KIT* may be associated with a variety of cutaneous lesions (including hyperpigmentation of perioral, axillary, perineal regions and hands, lentigines, café au lait macules, benign nevi, urticaria pigmentosa, and melanoma) depending on the mutation involved (see Chapter 7).

GASTROINTESTINAL MANIFESTATIONS OF CARDIAC DISEASE

Congestive Cardiac Failure

Patients with congestive cardiac failure frequently show alterations in gastrointestinal morphology, permeability, and absorption, due to a combination of ischemia and congestion. Nonocclusive mesenteric ischemia can result from both low cardiac output and splanchnic vasoconstriction. Diversion of blood away from the splanchnic system is a well-recognized adaptive mechanism to counteract low cardiac output in congestive cardiac failure.[339] Elevated venous pressure in right heart failure results in splanchnic congestion and mucosal edema, further impairing the mucosal microcirculation.[340]

An upper gastrointestinal endoscopic study of 57 patients with congestive cardiac failure and upper gastrointestinal symptoms found gastric and duodenal mucosal alterations in 88% and 54% of patients, respectively. These changes, termed "congestive gastropathy/duodenopathy," correlated with the severity of symptoms and inferior vena cava and hepatic vein diameters. The most frequent endoscopic findings were a mosaic-like pattern and punctate speckling, whereas less common findings included thickened folds, watermelon stomach, and telangiectasias.[341] Patients with congestive cardiac failure have been shown to develop increased intramucosal carbon dioxide pressure (pCO_2) at low levels of exercise, likely reflecting splanchnic hypoperfusion.[342] Cardiogenic shock is associated with early elevations in intragastric pCO_2, whereas persistent elevations (>24 hours) indicate prolonged gastrointestinal mucosal ischemia.[343,344]

Morphologic and functional changes in the small and large intestine have been described in patients with congestive cardiac failure. Increased ileal and colonic permeability and wall thickening (likely edema) have been reported in patients with a left ventricular ejection fraction of <40%,[345] whereas decreased protein and fat absorption has been demonstrated in advanced stages of the disease.[346-348] Morphometric studies have revealed a striking increase in lamina propria collagen in small intestinal biopsies from patients with severe cardiac failure, which is most marked in cachectic patients.[348] At the extreme end of the spectrum, low perfusion states may be associated with nonocclusive intestinal ischemia or infarction (see Chapter 2). Drugs used in the treatment of cardiac failure, such as the cardiac glycosides, often produce anorexia, nausea, vomiting, abdominal pain, and distention.

Infective Endocarditis

Infective endocarditis due to *Streptococcus bovis* has been associated with a high rate of neoplasms (adenomas and carcinomas) in the colon and less frequently upper gastrointestinal tract. Upper and lower gastrointestinal endoscopy has been recommended in patients with *S. bovis* endocarditis, for which no other cause is found.[349-351] There are also isolated reports of colorectal neoplasia in association with *Gemella morbillorum*[352] and *Streptococcus gallolyticus* endocarditis.[353]

Open Heart Surgery, Extracorporeal Circulation, and Cardiac Transplantation

Gastrointestinal complications following open heart surgery are rare, occurring in 0.3% to 2% of cases, and are usually associated with cardiopulmonary bypass and extracorporeal circulation.[354,355] The major clinical features consist of upper gastrointestinal hemorrhage secondary to stress ulcers or duodenal ulcers, massive bowel necrosis due to intestinal ischemia from low cardiac output, and acute diverticulitis. Symptoms commonly occur within 7 days of surgery, and the mortality rate is high (about 30%).[354,356,357] In contrast to open-heart surgery, gastrointestinal complications are common following cardiac surgery with extracorporeal circulation, including cardiac transplantation, occurring in 25% to 40% of patients.[358-360] The most frequent include diarrhea, heartburn, abdominal pain, nausea, and vomiting. Less common but serious complications include gastrointestinal hemorrhage (associated with esophagitis, erosive gastritis, or gastric ulceration), intestinal ischemia, perforated colonic diverticula, and pancreatitis.[354,358,360] Since patients are on maintenance immunosuppressive therapy, they are also prone to all the complications of immunosuppression, such as bacterial, fungal, and viral infections and gastrointestinal neoplasms.[359,361-363] Similar gastrointestinal complications may also occur after lung transplantation.[364]

HEMATOLOGIC DISORDERS

Gastrointestinal manifestations of leukemia and lymphoma are described with the lymphoproliferative disorders in Chapter 5 and bone marrow transplantation with the immunodeficiency disorders in Chapter 4.

Dysproteinemias

Multiple myeloma may affect the gastrointestinal tract in the form of tumor masses (plasmacytomas) or amyloidosis. Plasmacytomas are described with the lymphoproliferative disorders (Chapter 5) and amyloid, separately in this chapter. The dysproteinemias associated with alpha-heavy chain and gamma-heavy chain disease are described with the lymphoproliferative disorders. In Waldenstrom's macroglobulinemia there is extracellular deposition of IgM in the lamina propria of the small bowel, resulting in malabsorption. This is described further in Chapter 20.

Hemolytic Uremic Syndrome

This syndrome is characterized by a microangiopathic hemolytic anemia, thrombocytopenia, and acute renal failure.[365,366] It is a frequent cause of acute renal failure in childhood[367] but can occur in adults.[368] About 90% of childhood cases in developed countries are caused by enterohemorrhagic *Escherichia coli* O157:H7, which produce a Shiga-like toxin (verotoxin). This toxin is similar to the cytotoxin produced by *Shigella dysenteriae* type 1 (another cause of HUS).[366] This cytotoxin causes damage to the vascular endothelium, thrombosis, and hemorrhage. Acute transient gastrointestinal symptoms occur frequently, producing hemorrhagic enterocolitis with bloody diarrhea. Other complications include transmural necrosis, perforation, and colonic stricture.[367,369]

Coagulation Disorders

Hemophilia. About 10% to 25% of patients with hemophilia suffer from gastrointestinal hemorrhage.[370,371] The hemorrhage originates most often from the upper gastrointestinal tract and is usually spontaneous but may be secondary to peptic ulceration. Gastrointestinal hemorrhage may also result from esophagitis, Mallory-Weiss tears, and erosive gastritis, but the incidence of these conditions in hemophilia seems to parallel that of the general population.[370,371] Clinically significant upper gastrointestinal bleeding (esophageal varices excluded) has been reported in about 1% of patients per year. The risk was significantly increased in patients taking NSAIDs.[371] Endoscopy is helpful in these patients to determine the cause of hemorrhage.[372] Patients occasionally present with signs and symptoms of an acute abdomen, sometimes in association with a tender abdominal mass due to intramural hematoma.[370,373-376] The latter produces a fairly characteristic x-ray appearance consisting of a segment of bowel with uniform thickened, rigid mucosal folds and a sharply delineated margin.[373,377] Intussusception is a rare complication of submucosal hemorrhage.[370] Histologically, there is intramural hemorrhage, which can involve all layers but is usually most prominent in the submucosa. Hemorrhage may also involve the mesentery and retroperitoneal tissues. Surgical intervention is rarely necessary for gastrointestinal hemorrhage as replacement of the clotting factors usually leads to rapid recovery.[373]

Other Coagulation Disorders

Von Willebrand's disease, heparin or warfarin overdose, vitamin K deficiencies, and platelet deficiency disorders resulting from bone marrow replacement by tumor or the myeloproliferative disorders can all produce gastrointestinal manifestations similar to hemophilia.[378] Thrombocytosis, resulting from conditions such as thrombotic thrombocytopenic purpura and polycythemia rubra vera, can also produce gastrointestinal bleeding. Clinically, they may resemble hemolytic uremic syndrome, described previously.[379,380]

Mastocytosis

This uncommon condition is characterized by an abnormal proliferation of mast cells in one or more organs. Most cases are confined to the skin (urticaria pigmentosa), but approximately 10% involve extracutaneous sites, most commonly bone, liver, spleen, gastrointestinal tract, and lymph nodes. Gastrointestinal symptoms are second only to pruritis as a cause of morbidity in these patients. Seventy to eighty percent of patients report gastrointestinal symptoms when a careful history is taken.[381] These include abdominal pain (dyspeptic and nondyspeptic), nausea, vomiting, diarrhea, malabsorption, weight loss, and occasionally gastrointestinal hemorrhage secondary to ulcers or erosions.[381-386] Increased systemic levels of mast cell mediators (e.g., histamine, leukotrienes, heparin, and proteases) are likely to play an important role in gastrointestinal symptoms, since the latter are not always associated with mucosal mast cell infiltrates.[387] The pathogenesis of the malabsorption is unclear.[381,388]

Endoscopically, the gastrointestinal mucosa may show a variety of changes including mucosal nodularity, urticaria-like mucosal lesions, mucosal thickening, friability, and gastric erosions. Peptic ulceration is found primarily in the duodenum. Mucosal nodularity is a frequent and distinctive finding in these patients, both endoscopically and radiologically[381,385,386,388-395] (Fig. 8-9). Sometimes colonoscopic findings may closely resemble IBD.

Histologically, mucosal and submucosal mast cell infiltrates vary from heavy to absent.[381,386,387,396] Mast cells are arranged in sheets, aggregates, or concentric pericryptal whorls and may expand the lamina propria[386,396] (Fig. 8-10A,B). They may resemble normal mast cells or can be spindled, fusiform, or histiocytoid (Fig. 8-10C-E). The latter appearances may lead to confusion with a histiocytic infiltrate, compounded by the fact that mast cells are immunoreactive for

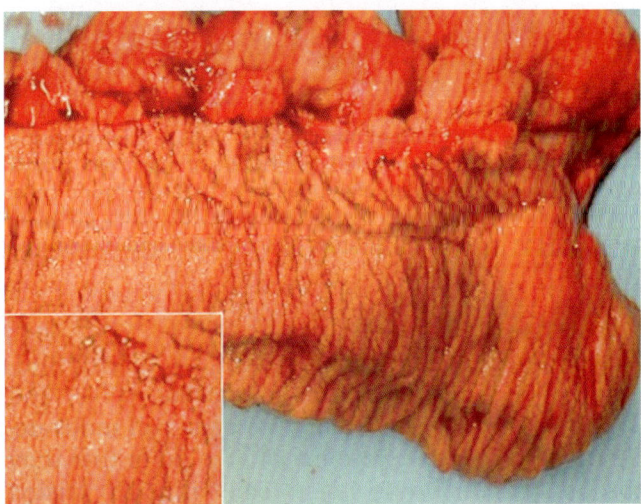

Figure 8-9. Mastocytosis of the right colon. Mucosal nodularity is a frequent feature observed grossly or at endoscopy (**inset**).

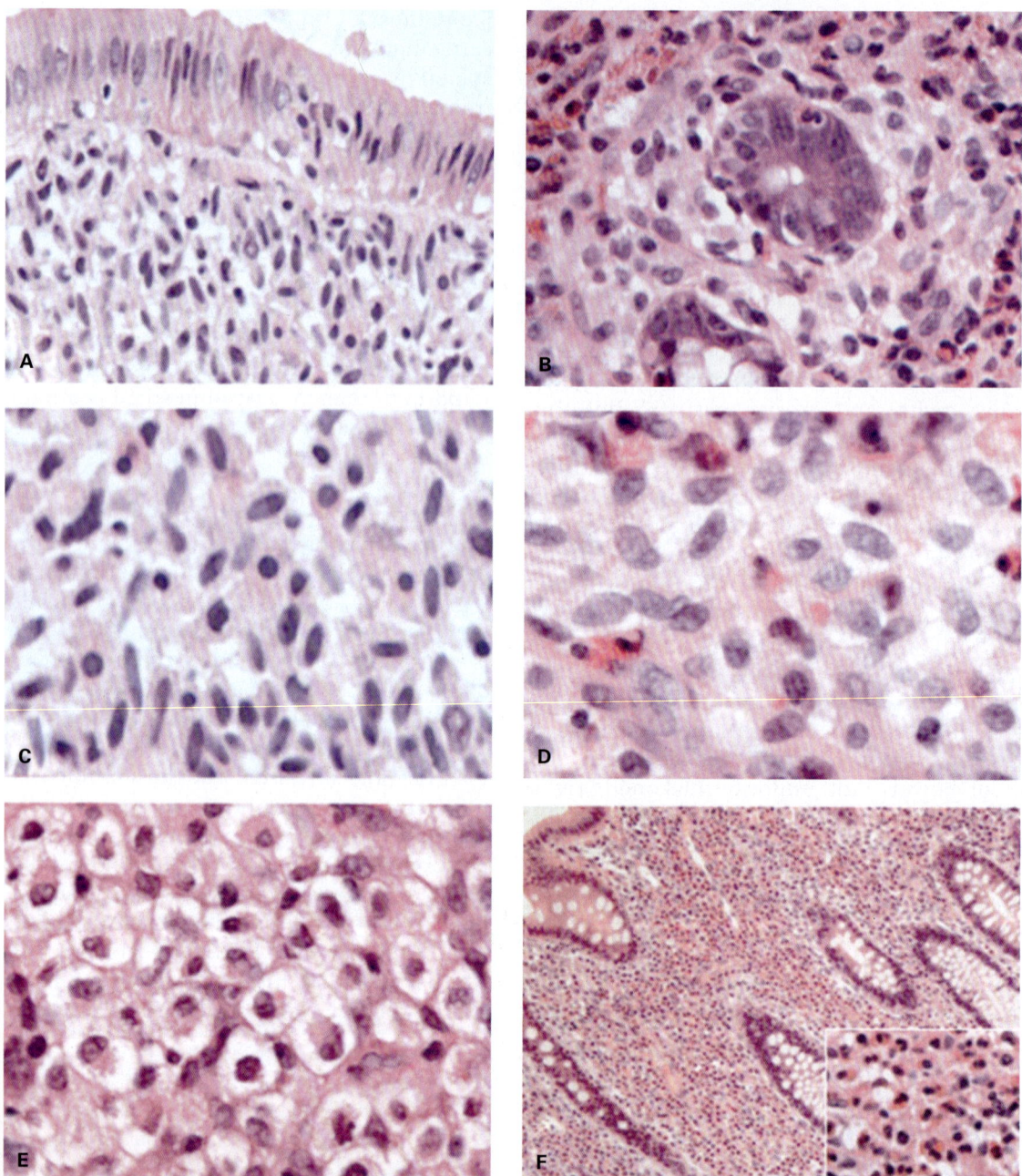

Figure 8-10. Spectrum of histologic findings in gastrointestinal mastocytosis. **A:** Expansion of the lamina propria by the mast cell infiltrate. **B:** Pericryptal whorled distribution of mast cells, which is a frequent feature. **C–E:** Range of appearances of mast cells including elongated or spindled, plump fusiform or large, round cells with abundant pale to clear cytoplasm; the latter is a result of retraction artifact. The latter two appearances may be easily confused with histiocyte infiltrates. **F:** Heavy eosinophil infiltrate, which may dominate the picture and at times obscured the underlying mast cell infiltrate (**inset:** eosinophils at higher magnification).

CD68. Mucosal edema and a patchy mixed infiltrate (including lymphocytes, plasma cells, and eosinophils) may accompany the mast cell infiltrate. Eosinophils may be prominent to the point that they obscure the underlying mast cell infiltrate, raising the possibility of an eosinophilic gastroenteritis[386] (Fig. 8-10F). Mucosal architectural distortion is not uncommon[383,389–391,396–399] and may lead to confusion with IBD, particularly when the colonoscopic findings are suggestive.[386,390] Changes secondary to the release of histamine and other vasoactive substances include erosive gastritis, mucosal congestion, and hemorrhage.

The mast cell infiltrate can be confirmed with histochemical stains that highlight mast cell granules (e.g., Giemsa, Leder) as well as immunohistochemical markers including CD117, mast cell tryptase, and CD25.[386,390,396] The latter marks neoplastic but not reactive mast cell infiltrates.[396] More than 90% of patients with systemic exhibit the characteristic D816V exon 17 *KIT* mutation in lesional tissue,[100] and this holds true for cases with gastrointestinal involvement.[386]

Rosai–Dorfman Disease (Sinus Histiocytosis with Massive Lymphadenopathy)

Rosai–Dorfman disease is a rare disease of unknown etiopathogenesis, generally presenting with nodal enlargement usually in the young, who are usually amazingly well considering their huge adenopathy. It is characterized by polyclonal proliferation of histiocytes that show many engulfed lymphocytes and plasma cells in their cytoplasm. The engulfed cells show intact cytologic and nuclear details, and this phenomenon is thought to represent emperipolesis rather than true phagocytosis by the histiocytes. It is believed to be a reactive process due to an abnormal immune response, leading to hyperactivation of the macrophages. Although an underlying infection is suspected, no consistent association with an infection has been shown so far. Few studies showing association with HHV-6 and HIV have been reported; however, several others have failed to confirm these findings. The disease can involve virtually any extranodal site. Gastrointestinal tract is the least common organ system involved, and to date only about nine patients (jejunum *n* = 1, appendix *n* = 2, colorectum *n* = 6) have been reported, many of whom were incidentally detected at resection or autopsy and in some it was the only site of involvement.[401–403] The gastrointestinal manifestations are generally nonspecific; however, rarely it may present with gastrointestinal bleeding or intestinal obstruction.[401,402]

The lesions are poorly circumscribed and largely centered in the submucosa. The overlying mucosa often appears smooth and not involved, and hence mucosal biopsies are likely to be negative. Histology is similar to nodal disease with the presence of abundant large histiocytes admixed with various other inflammatory cells, mostly lymphocytes and plasma cells. The histiocytes show pale foamy or lightly eosinophilic granular cytoplasm. They characteristically show prominent emperipolesis with lymphoplasmacytic cells. Such histiocytes may also be seen in dilated lymphatics, and the regional lymph nodes may also be involved. The differential diagnosis includes langerhans histiocytosis and familial hemophagocytosis syndrome. The langerhans cells are easily distinguished by their grooved nuclei and positivity for CD1a, and the background frequently contains a prominent eosinophilic infiltrate. In hemophagocytosis the histiocytes show prominent phagocytosis of red cells, rather than emperipolesis of lymphoplasmacytic cells. The treatment of Rosai–Dorfman disease includes surgical debulking, steroids, and radiotherapy.[401,402] With multisystemic involvement the prognosis appears to be protracted, and patients reported to date with more than 1 year of follow-up were either alive with disease or died of disease.[401]

Miscellaneous Disorders

A number of other hematologic disorders are associated with gastrointestinal manifestations and morphologic abnormalities. In the *Plummer–Vinson syndrome*, there is an association between iron deficiency anemia and postcricoid esophageal webs, atrophic gastritis, and achlorhydria. Granulomatous colitis has been reported in chronic granulomatous disease (see "Granulomatous Disorders" below). Patients with thrombocytosis due to myeloproliferative disorders may develop thrombotic or hemorrhagic complications involving gastrointestinal tract. Aspirin or corticosteroids predispose to the latter complication.[404,405]

GASTROINTESTINAL AMYLOID DEPOSITION

General Properties and Classification

Amyloidosis is the final common pathway of a number of unrelated disorders, which have in common the abnormal production and extracellular deposition of proteins with a common tertiary molecular structure. This structure includes antiparallel twisted β-pleated sheet fibrils that have a number of distinct morphologic properties including[406–408]

1. A glassy, homogenous red appearance by hematoxylin and eosin and Congo red stains (Figs. 8-11–8-14)
2. A red/green birefringence under polarized light after Congo red staining (Fig. 8-13)
3. A characteristic fibrillary, nonbranched structure by electron microscopy

The most widely accepted classifications of amyloid are based on the biochemical composition of the amyloid fibrils. The current nomenclature assigns the letter A (for amyloid) followed by a description of the precursor protein. The most common form is AL (light chain) or primary amyloidosis, derived from portions of immunoglobulin light chains produced in plasma cell

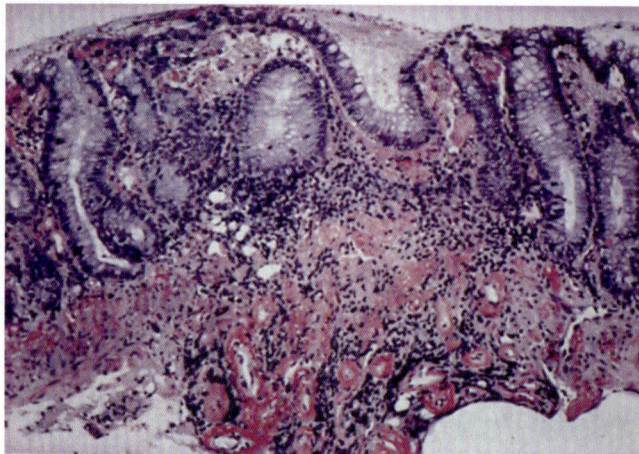

Figure 8-11. Amyloid deposition in the colon. Colonic biopsy specimen stained by hematoxylin and eosin showing homogenous, glassy, red amyloid deposition within arterioles of the superficial submucosa.

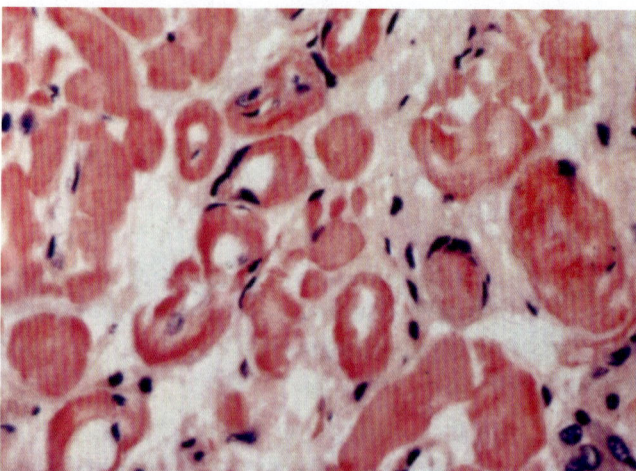

Figure 8-12. Rectal biopsy specimen from a patient with FMF and advanced amyloidosis. Congo red stain showing extensive amyloid deposition within arterioles.

dyscrasias. Most patients have a monoclonal protein that is demonstrable by immunoelectrophoresis of the serum or urine, even in the absence of multiple myeloma. The next most prevalent is AA (or secondary) amyloidosis associated with overproduction of the acute phase reactant serum amyloid A protein (A) in various inflammatory, infective, or neoplastic disorders. Up to 48% of such patients have rheumatoid arthritis.[407,408] Some of the other more common forms of amyloid include dialysis-related amyloid (Aβ2MG, β_2-microglobulin), senile amyloid (AβPP, amyloid beta precursor protein), and familial amyloidotic polyneuropathy (transthyretin—ATTR). A number of rarer forms exist.[408] Amyloid per se is quite inert and does not cause tissue injury. However, with progressive accumulation in tissues, it encroaches on adjacent cells to produce pressure atrophy in the muscularis externa, diffusion problems in the mucosa, and ischemia with vascular obliteration.

Clinical Features

Gastrointestinal involvement is common—as reflected by the 85% diagnostic yield for rectal biopsies—but does not necessarily produce symptoms. All levels of the gut may be affected.[406,409,410] Infiltration of the mucosa, muscularis externa, and blood vessels may result in a variety of symptoms, such as dysphagia, ulcer symptoms, diarrhea, steatorrhea, malabsorption, intestinal pseudo-obstruction, and hemorrhage.[407,408] The latter occurs in up to 57% of patients with amyloidosis[408] and may be massive. Motility disorders are

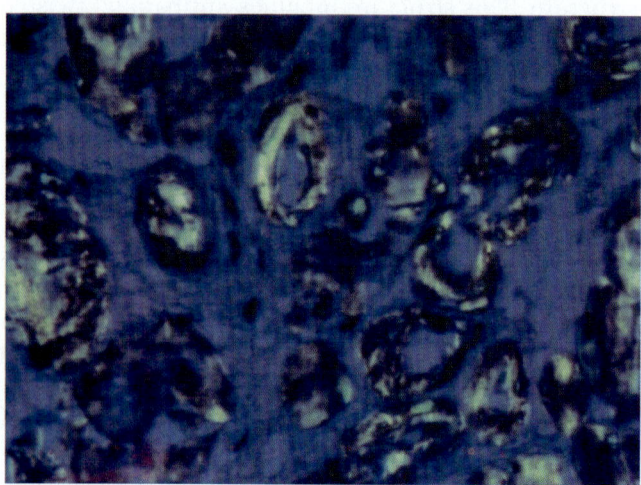

Figure 8-13. Same specimen as Figure 8-10 viewed under polarized light to show green birefringence.

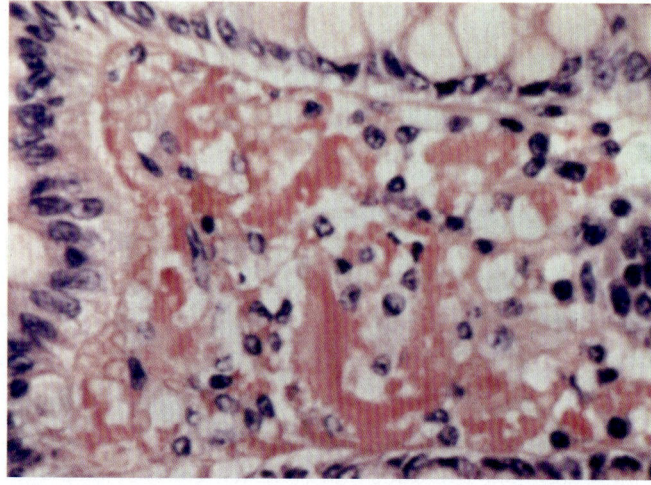

Figure 8-14. Rectal biopsy from a patient with FMF showing extensive amyloid deposition within the lamina propria.

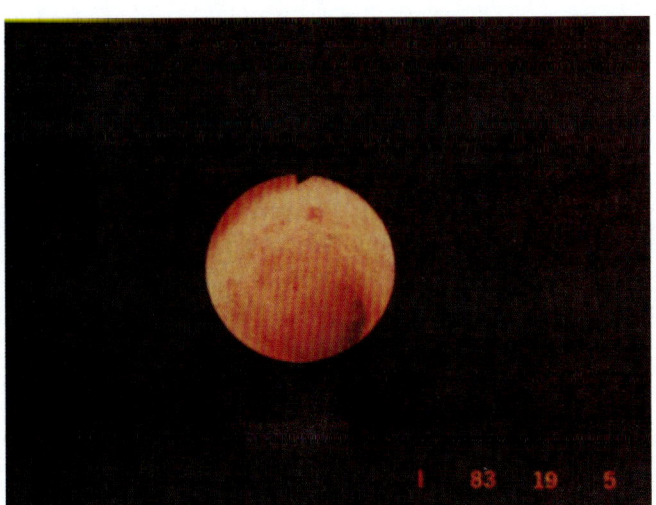

Figure 8-15. Petechial hemorrhages in the sigmoid colon in a patient with amyloidosis.

caused by amyloid infiltration of the enteric muscles or nerves or both.[407,408,411] Malabsorption results from a number of different mechanisms such as stasis with bacterial overgrowth due to dysmotility, diffusion problems from amyloid infiltration of the mucosa, and vascular infiltration. Vascular involvement by amyloid can also produce petechial hemorrhages of the mucosa (Fig 8-15), ischemic lesions with hemorrhage, mucosal ulceration, occasionally diverticular disease, and lesions that may mimic IBD.[412-414] Amyloidosis can sometimes produce solitary masses in the stomach or intestine. These can be confused clinically and radiologically with carcinoma and other intestinal polyps.[415-417]

Histologic Features

Amyloid is found throughout the length of the gut and is distributed primarily within submucosal arterioles; the muscularis propria and mucosae, around the myenteric nerves; and in advanced cases within the lamina propria (Fig. 8-14). On rare occasions a lamina propria amyloid infiltrate may mimic collagenous colitis.[418] With progressive accumulation, amyloid causes narrowing of vessels, with consequent ischemic ulcers; hemorrhage; and pressure atrophy of adjacent tissues such as the muscularis externa. With routine hematoxylin and eosin stains, amyloid appears as extracellular amorphous, glassy pink deposits (Figs. 8-11 and 8-12), often with a prominent cracking artifact. Amyloid stains pink-red with the Congo red stain and under polarized light exhibits apple-green birefringence (Fig. 8-13). With thioflavin T, amyloid fluoresces when viewed under ultraviolet light. By electron microscopy, amyloid appears as an interlocking meshwork of nonbranching fibrils measuring 7.5 to 10 nm in diameter but of variable length. Immunohistochemistry is the routine method for determining amyloid type but has limitations. AA amyloid stains consistently with the appropriate antibody, whereas AL deposits fail to stain in a significant proportion of cases. In such cases, AL becomes a diagnosis of exclusion supported somewhat by the demonstration of monoclonal gammopathy (although subtle plasma cell dyscrasias are not uncommon in elderly patients without amyloidosis).[407] Other techniques available for amyloid typing include amino acid analysis and proteomics on microdissected tissue.[419] The latter is emerging as a highly sensitive and specific technique for the typing of amyloid deposits but is only available at a few specialized centers.

Diagnosis and Clinical Implications

Rectal biopsy is a widely used procedure for the diagnosis of amyloidosis, with a diagnostic yield of around 85%.[408] However, several reports indicate that amyloid deposition is more marked in the small bowel and stomach,[420,421] and the latter are preferred over rectal biopsies in cases of suspected AL amyloid.[408,421] Although AL amyloid tends to form polypoid lesions and AA amyloid has a more finely granular appearance,[407] a characteristic or even visible endoscopic lesion may be lacking. This is another reason why we believe in biopsying all endoscopically normal patients to exclude such lesions as amyloid. Furthermore, it is important to remember that in biopsy material, amyloid is most likely to be found in submucosal arterioles; therefore, the biopsies must be sufficiently deep to include the superficial submucosa.

DISORDERS OF LIPID METABOLISM

Fabry's Disease

Fabry's disease is an X-linked disorder of glycolipid metabolism due to deficiency or absence of the lysosomal enzyme alpha-galactosidase A. This results in the cellular deposition of glycosphingolipids in most tissues.[422,423] Clinically, there may be dysfunction of the renal, pulmonary, cardiovascular, gastrointestinal, muscular, and nervous systems. Gastrointestinal symptoms consist of impaired motility with crampy postprandial abdominal pain, nausea, and diarrhea. Secondary bacterial overgrowth may also occur.[422,424,425] Gastrointestinal symptoms may improve with replacement therapy.[426,427] Histologically, lipid inclusions are found in the dorsal root ganglia and peripheral autonomic ganglia, including ganglia in the myenteric and submucosal nerve plexuses. Glycolipid deposition may also occur in the small vessels of the bowel with secondary thrombosis, resulting in ischemic bowel lesions and perforation.[425,428]

Tangier Disease

This is an autosomal recessive disorder characterized by accumulation of cholesterol esters in macrophages of reticuloendothelial tissues including tonsils, thymus, lymph nodes, bone marrow, liver, spleen, and gut, and a demyelinating neuropathy[429,430] Mutations in the adenosine triphosphate–binding cassette A1 gene that encodes a cellular phospholipid and cholesterol transporter essential for high-density lipoprotein (HDL) biogenesis underlie this condition. Patients have low levels of low-density lipoprotein cholesterol and HDL and high blood levels of triglycerides.[429,430] Clinically, patients have enlarged, yellow-orange streaked tonsils; hepatosplenomegaly; and peripheral neuropathy.[429,431] They may also have diarrhea for reasons that are unclear. Histologically, there is diffuse accumulation of cholesterol esters in foamy histiocytes. Ultrastructurally, the lipid deposition occurs within vacuoles not bounded by a membrane.[432] Foamy macrophages are also found in the mucosa throughout the gastrointestinal tract and appear as orange-brown spots in the rectum on colonoscopy.[431,433] Histologically, they consist of clusters of foamy histiocytes in the subcryptal space. Lipid accumulation may also occur in Schwann cells of the myenteric plexus.

Wolman's Disease

This rare autosomal recessive disorder results from mutations in the gene encoding lysosomal acid lipase, an enzyme essential for intracellular hydrolysis of cholesterol esters and triglycerides. It is characterized by massive accumulation of cholesterol ester and triglycerides in several tissues. Wolman's disease presents early in infancy with vomiting, diarrhea, hepatosplenomegaly, malabsorption, abdominal distention, failure to thrive, and ultimately cirrhosis. It is almost uniformly fatal in the first year of life. Adrenal gland enlargement with conspicuous calcific deposits is a characteristic finding. Intestinal biopsy may be undertaken to exclude a malabsorption syndrome and can show features of a lipid storage disorder, that is, numerous vacuolated lipid-laden macrophages in the lamina propria and submucosa sometimes with crystalline inclusions. Diagnosis is based on reduced acid lipase activity in cultured skin fibroblasts or peripheral blood lymphocytes.[434]

Abetalipoproteinemia

This is an autosomal recessive disorder characterized by acanthocytic erythrocytes, serum lipid abnormalities, ataxia, and steatorrhea. It is due to complete absence of all lipoproteins containing apolipoprotein B. Histologically, the small intestine is characterized by accumulation of fine lipid droplets within mucosal epithelial cells. For further details, see Chapter 20.

GRANULOMATOUS DISORDERS

Sarcoidosis

Sarcoidosis is a multisystem, granulomatous disease of unknown etiology. The most frequently involved organs are the lungs and mediastinal and hilar lymph nodes, but the liver, eyes, skin, spleen, and central nervous system are also commonly involved.[435] Reports of gastrointestinal sarcoidosis are rare.[435-437] A number of autopsy series reported no gastrointestinal involvement in sarcoidosis,[438-441] but others report gastrointestinal involvement in 5% to 10% of cases.[442-444] The vast majority of these cases are subclinical. Symptomatic gastrointestinal sarcoidosis occurs in <1% of patients with systemic sarcoidosis.[435,436]

The stomach, particularly the antrum, is the most frequently involved site, usually with subclinical granulomas.[435,445] Endoscopy may be normal or show a range of features including mucosal hyperemia, thickening of gastric folds, ulcers, nodular polypoid lesions, or narrowing. The latter may be due to mural infiltration or secondary to diffuse ulceration with fibrosis.[435,446,447] Infiltrative gastric sarcoidosis may be localized to the distal stomach, with cone-shaped narrowing, or diffuse resembling *linitis plastica*. Superficial biopsies may not sample these lesions so that the diagnosis may only be made after resection for suspected gastric carcinoma or gastric outlet obstruction.[435] When symptomatic, gastric sarcoidosis most commonly presents with epigastric pain but may also result in nausea, vomiting, early satiety, bloating, or bleeding.

The esophagus, small intestine, and colon are rarely involved. Depending on the site, patients may present with dysphagia, diarrhea, malabsorption, protein-losing enteropathy, abdominal pain, tenesmus, or hematochezia.[435,437,448-450]

Histologically, sarcoidosis of the gastrointestinal tract is characterized by noncaseating granulomatous inflammation. In the stomach this may be associated with ulceration or fibrosis, which may be diffuse.[447,451] In the differential diagnosis, it is necessary to exclude other causes of granulomatous inflammation such as tuberculosis, fungal infections, foreign body reactions, drug reactions, syphilis, neoplasia, parasitic disease, vasculitis, Whipple's disease, and Crohn's disease.[435,437,452] The latter can be difficult, since Crohn's disease may also have extraintestinal manifestations, although not normally pulmonary fibrosis or mediastinal lymphadenopathy. Conversely, gastrointestinal sarcoidosis does not produce active mucosal inflammation or perianal fistulae. Schaumann bodies (intracellular concentric calcifications) favor sarcoid, but are not specific. Serum angiotensin converting enzyme (SACE) is elevated in 60% of patients with sarcoid but not in Crohn's. SACE may, however, be elevated in other granulomatous conditions.[437] In cases of uncertain etiology, a symptomatic response to steroids would favor sarcoidosis. In some cases an unequivocal diagnosis of sarcoid may not be possible. In such patients, careful follow-up with frequent re-evaluation is prudent.

Chronic Granulomatous Disease

Chronic granulomatous disease is an inherited disorder of phagocyte function in which defective reactive oxygen species production results in deficient microbicidal activity.[453] Clinically, these patients suffer from recurrent life-threatening infections, and nearly half of them develop a number of gastrointestinal complications such as granulomatous colitis, gastric outlet obstruction, or perirectal abscess and may respond to granulocyte-stimulating factor.[454,455] Intestinal manifestations of chronic granulomatous disease show striking overlap with Crohn's disease including discontinuous inflammation, perianal involvement, and frequent presence of epithelioid granulomata on histology.[456] One of the characteristic features of this disorder is the presence of large pigmented macrophages distributed in the basal mucosa and superficial submucosa.

MISCELLANEOUS DISORDERS

Endometriosis

Endometriosis is characterized by the presence of endometrial glands, or stroma in abnormal sites, or both. It occurs most frequently in the pelvis, involving the ovaries, uterine ligaments, rectovaginal septum, and less commonly laparotomy scars, vagina, and vulva. Fifteen to thirty-seven percent of patients with pelvic endometriosis have intestinal involvement,[457] but only a minority has clinically significant disease. The lesion most commonly involves the rectosigmoid region, but other sites, such as the terminal ileum, cecum, colon and only occasionally the appendix, may be involved.[450-461] Clinically, gastrointestinal symptoms are frequently pelvic, abdominal, and rectal pain, most commonly related to intestinal obstruction. This usually results from marked angulation or kinking of the bowel. Less commonly, obstruction results from luminal narrowing, volvulus, intussusception,[458-464] or intramural hemorrhage.[465] Occasionally, patients present with rectal bleeding.[457,466] Rarely, patients present with perforation, usually in pregnancy or postpartum, and associated with decidual necrosis and contraction.[459] In some cases a temporal relationship between symptoms and menses may provide a diagnostic clue. However, in most cases the diagnosis is very difficult and often delayed due to the lack of pathognomonic symptoms.[457,463,467] Endometriosis may masquerade as a variety of conditions, including irritable bowel syndrome, Crohn's disease, acute self-limited colitis, ischemic colitis or enteritis, diverticular disease, or neoplasia.[457,458,467] To add to the challenge, endoscopic biopsy has a low yield due to the propensity for endometriosis to involve the deeper layers.[457,458,463] Mucosal biopsies may show a range of nonspecific features, which range from mild to severe and include architectural changes and a lymphoplasmacytic infiltrate mimicking IBD, ischemic type changes, villous blunting, and features of mucosal prolapse. Rarely pyloric metaplasia may be seen.[457] A preoperative diagnosis is often difficult to establish.[467] Intestinal resection can be performed safely in most women with severe endometriosis and bowel involvement, although symptoms may recur due to the recurrence of endometriosis in other sites.[464] Rectovaginal fistula is an uncommon complication that occurs in up to 3% of patients undergoing surgery for endometriosis.[468]

Grossly, lesions may be solitary (commonly the rectal lesions) but are usually multifocal. They are frequently confined to the serosa but may involve the muscularis propria. Occasionally they appear as ulcers with rolled margins or polyps that mimic neoplasms (Fig. 8-16). On cut section they appear as firm fibrotic masses, with mural thickening and stenosis.[457] Hemorrhagic punctate areas may be seen. Serosal adhesions may be prominent. Microscopically, endometriotic foci are seen in the subserosal tissue often extending through the bowel wall to the mucosa.[469] Histologically, the foci are characterized by endometrial glands and stroma, are surrounded by fibrosis and smooth muscle proliferation, and often show fresh hemorrhage and hemosiderin-laden macrophages (Fig. 8-17).

Rarely, neoplasms may arise in endometriotic foci, notably endometrioid and clear cell sarcoma but also endometrioid stromal sarcoma.[457,470,471] The underlying endometriotic focus is often overrun by the tumor, presenting a diagnostic challenge when tumors arise in the gastrointestinal tract.

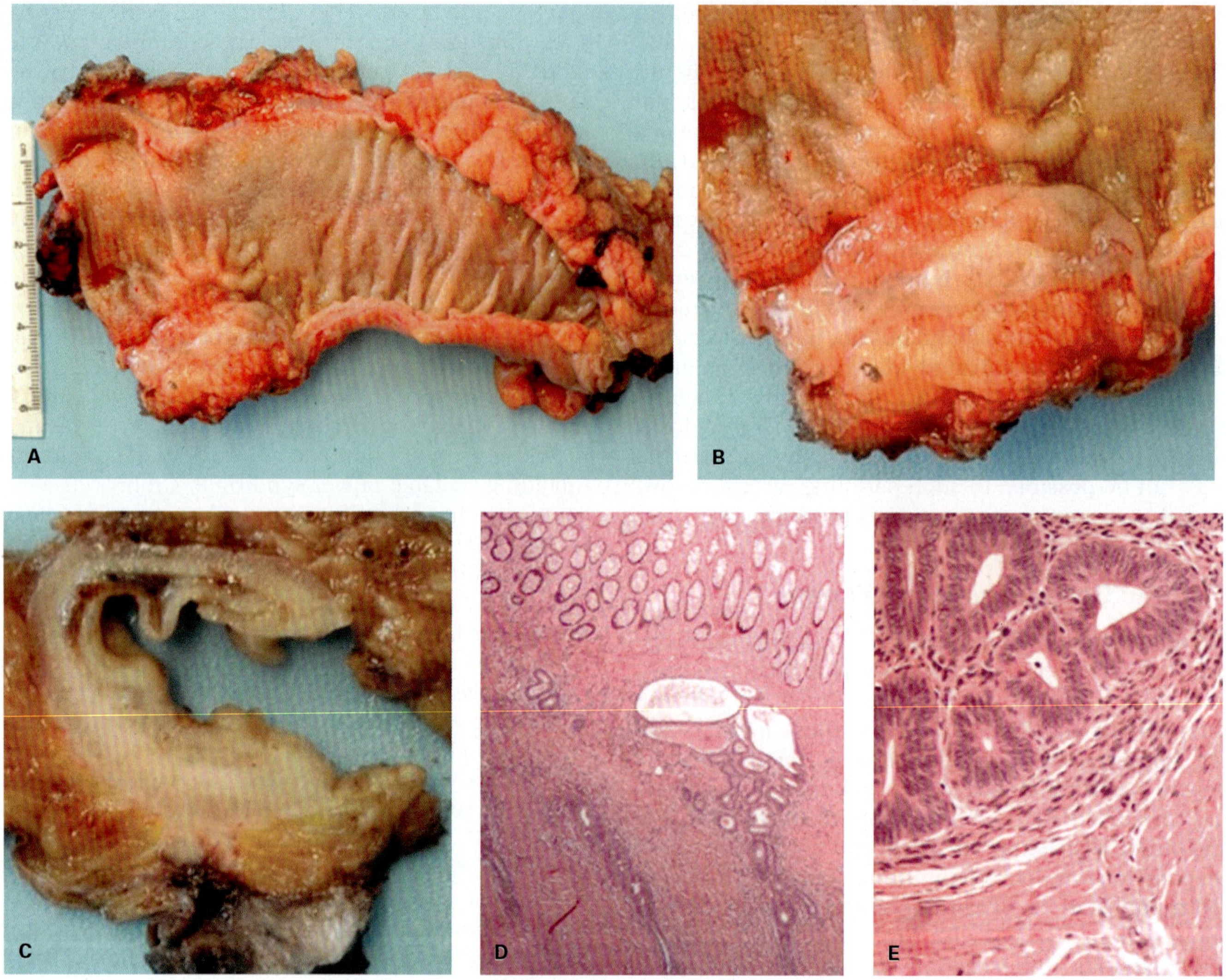

Figure 8-16. Endometriosis of the rectum. **A,B:** Gross specimen showing an ulcerated lesion with rolled margins that was initially thought to be a carcinoma clinically. **C:** Cut section shows an irregular fibrotic mass. **D:** Histology showing endometrial glands and stroma throughout the muscularis propria of the rectum. **E:** Higher magnification showing endometrial glands surrounded by a cuff of stroma.

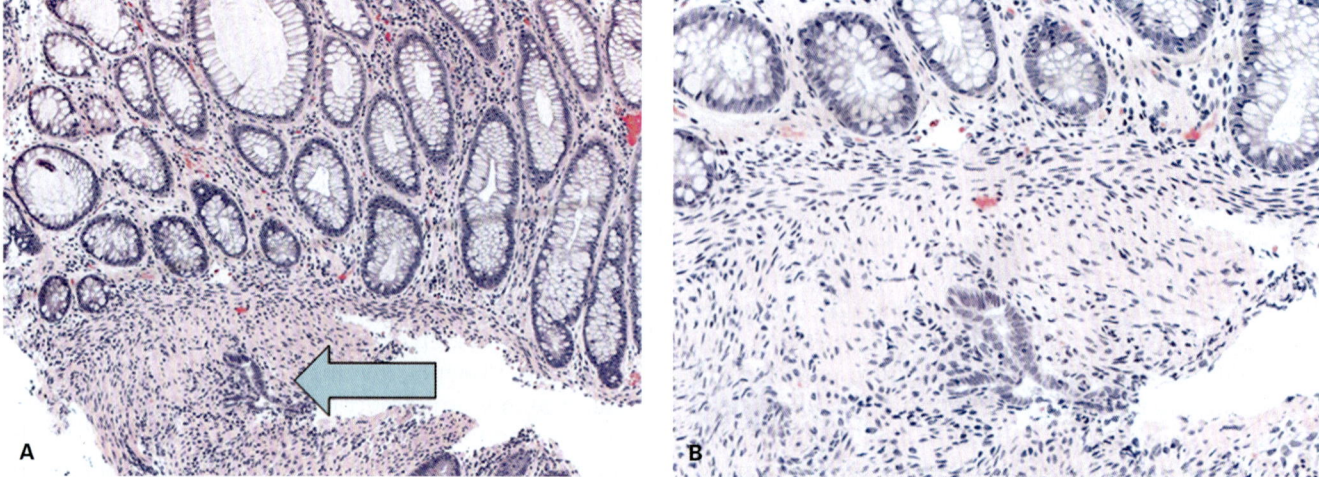

Figure 8-17. Endometriosis in a large bowel biopsy. **A:** Biopsy with a small isolated gland within the muscularis mucosae (*arrow*). **B:** Detail of **(A)**.

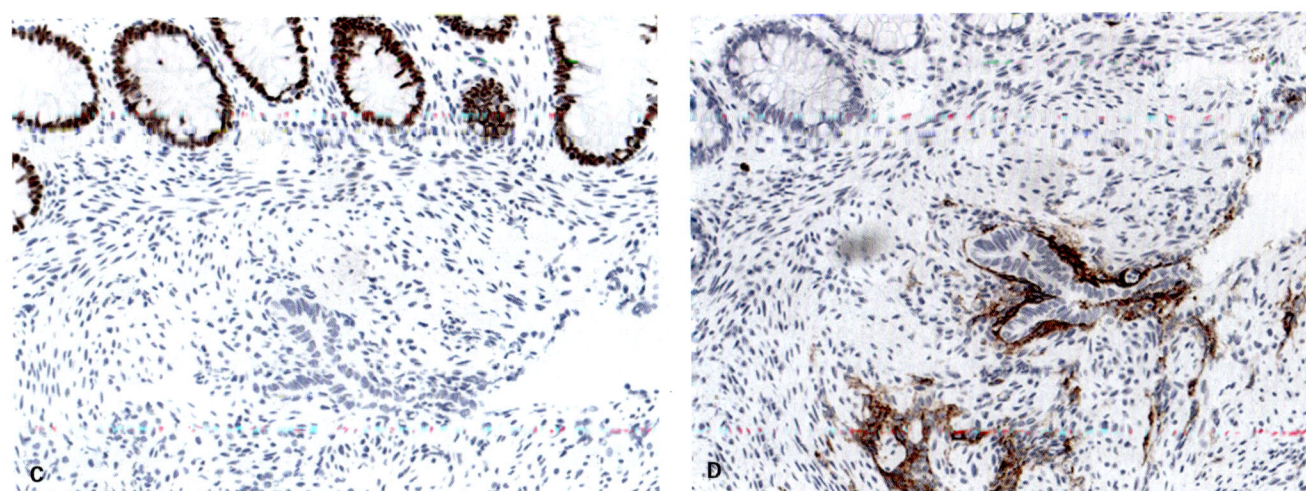

Figure 8-17. (*Continued*) **C:** CDX2 stain that stains nuclei of the normal large bowel but not the endometriosis tissue. **D:** CD10 decorating the endometriotic stroma. (Courtesy of Dr A Medline, Toronto.)

Pellagra

Pellagra is a vitamin deficiency syndrome caused by dietary deficiency or impaired absorption of niacin. Frequently, there is concomitant protein malnutrition and other deficiencies, such as those involving riboflavin, thiamin, and tryptophan. In many parts of Africa and some parts of Asia where maize or certain cereals are the staple foods, niacin is present in the bound form and is not nutritionally available. Thus, unless alternate foods containing niacin are available or added as supplements, pellagra may ensue. Pellagra may also have a number of secondary causes including chronic alcoholism, anorexia nervosa, IBD, carcinoid tumor, and certain drugs (e.g., isoniazid).[472–474]

Clinically, pellagra is characterized by the three Ds—diarrhea, dermatitis, and dementia. Patients commonly suffer from glossitis and stomatitis. Gastrointestinal manifestations consist predominantly of diarrhea, abdominal pain, and sometimes steatorrhea.[472,475] On sigmoidoscopy, inflammation is seen in over one-half of all patients. However, histologically, colitis is present in all patients.[474] In the majority of cases, the inflammation is mild or moderate, often with features of colitis cystica superficialis, characterized by cystic dilatation of the crypts and crypt abscesses. Occasionally, inflammation may be severe and necrotizing. The small intestine is usually normal unless there are concomitant multiple nutritional deficiencies.[476]

Familial Mediterranean Fever (Familial Paroxysmal Polyserositis)

Familial mediterranean fever (FMF) is a hereditary disorder transmitted as an autosomal recessive trait. The gene responsible, *MEFV* (on the short arm of chromosome 16), encodes the inflammatory mediator pyrin, expressed only in myeloid cells. FMF occurs almost exclusively in Sephardic Jews, Arabs, and Turks.[477,478] Clinically, it is characterized by brief but disabling, self-limited, febrile attacks of peritonitis, synovitis, pleuritis, or an erysipelas-like erythema affecting the legs or feet. It usually starts in childhood or adolescence and recurs at irregular intervals throughout life. Systemic amyloidosis develops frequently in untreated patients, leading to death from renal failure.[477–483]

Gastrointestinal involvement is characterized by acute inflammation limited to the serosal surfaces of the bowel. Usually, this resolves spontaneously within a few days, but occasionally it may give rise to peritoneal adhesions. Patients who develop

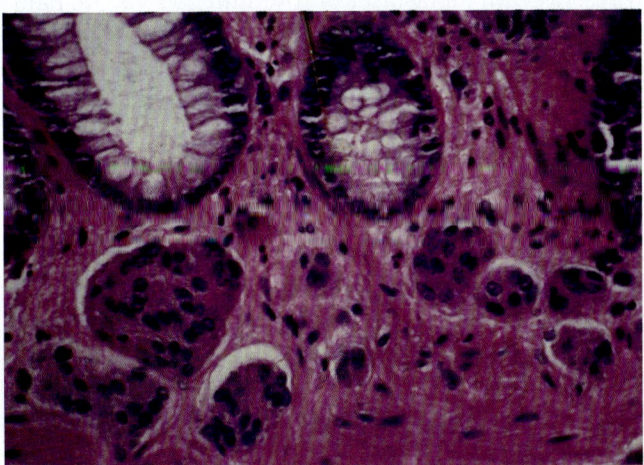

Figure 8-18. Carcinoma of the prostate metastatic to the rectum. Rectal biopsy specimen showing poorly differentiated epithelial cell nests lying in the subcryptal space beneath normal-appearing rectal glands.

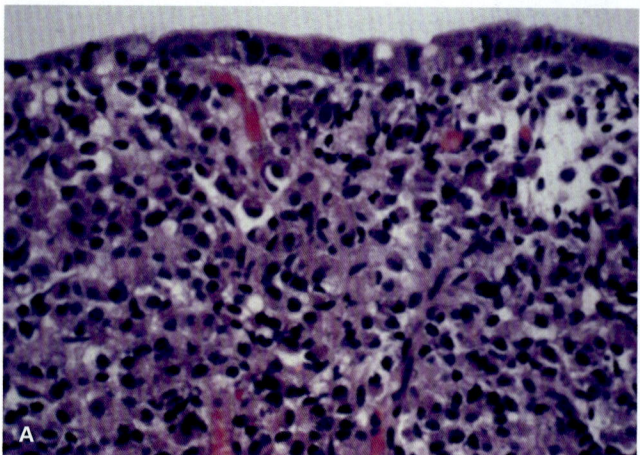 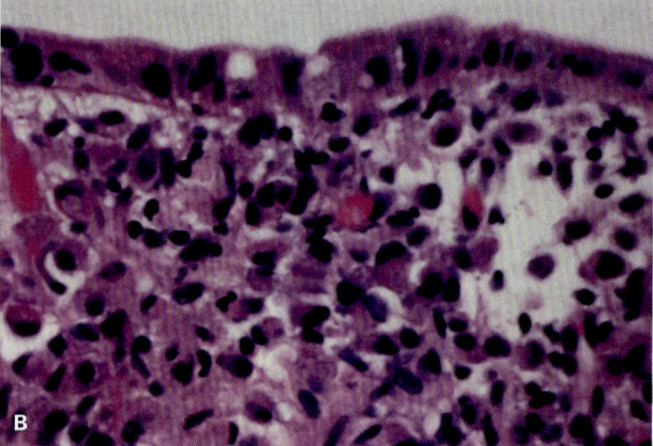

Figure 8-19. Carcinoma of the breast metastatic to the colon. **A:** There is diffuse infiltration of the lamina propria by signet ring cells. **B:** Higher-power magnification showing the neoplastic signet ring cells and attenuated but nondysplastic surface epithelium.

systemic amyloidosis usually die of renal complications.[480] They may have gastrointestinal deposition of amyloid within the lamina propria and submucosal vessels, although this is usually unassociated with any symptoms.[481,482] The disease and its complications can be controlled with colchicine treatment although increased intestinal permeability and mild intestinal mucosal injury often occurs.[483–485] Also, studies have documented a potential role for interferon-alpha in aborting or preventing attacks,[485a] and multiple immunosuppressive agents have been used in colchicine-resistant FMF patients.

NEOPLASTIC DISEASE

Extraintestinal tumors can involve the bowel in two ways: (a) with metastases or (b) indirectly via the paraneoplastic syndromes. The paraneoplastic syndromes present either as intestinal pseudo-obstruction, often in association with oat cell carcinoma of the lung, or as an isolated acute colonic dilatation (Ogilvie's syndrome). These are further described in Chapter 7.

Up to 20% of extraintestinal tumors metastasize or invade the bowel.[486] Frequently, this occurs by direct invasion from adjacent organs, such as prostate (Fig. 8-18); gynecologic and bladder cancers; or peritoneal seeding, primarily from ovarian tumors. In peritoneal seeding the tumor is usually confined to the subserosal tissues; rarely does it penetrate the muscularis propria and into the submucosa and mucosa. Hematogenous and lymphatic spread occurs less frequently, mainly in tumors from the breast, lung, and malignant melanomas.[487–489] Some metastatic lesions are fairly characteristic, such as the radiologic "bull's eye" lesions in malignant melanoma.[490] Others may resemble primary tumors. A lack of epithelial dysplasia adjacent to the tumorous infiltration, sparing of the overlying mucosa, prominent lymphatic infiltration, and multiplicity of tumors often allows for differentiation of primary from metastatic lesions. However, in a few instances, distinction may be difficult based on morphology alone. For example, metastatic breast carcinoma to the stomach produces a pattern that may closely mimic those of signet ring cell carcinoma and linitis plastica[491] (Fig 8-19).

References

1. Morris AJ. Nonsteroidal anti-inflammatory drug enteropathy. *Gastrointest Endosc Clin N Am*. 1999;9(1):125–133.
2. Wolfe MM, Lichtenstein DR, Singh G. Gastrointestinal toxicity of nonsteroidal antiinflammatory drugs.[see comment] [erratum appears in N Engl J Med. 1999;341(7):548]. *N Engl J Med*. 1999;340(24):1888–1899.
3. Domsic R, et al. Gastrointestinal manifestations of systemic sclerosis. *Digest Dis Sci*. 2008;53(5):1163–1174.
4. Steen VD, Medsger TA Jr. Severe organ involvement in systemic sclerosis with diffuse scleroderma. *Arthritis Rheum*. 2000;43(11):2437–2444.
5. Khanlou H, et al. Jejunal telangiectasias as a cause of massive bleeding in a patient with scleroderma. *Revue du Rhumatisme (English Edition)*. 1999;66(2):119–121.
6. Lock G, et al. Association of autonomic nervous dysfunction and esophageal dysmotility in systemic sclerosis. *J Rheumatol*. 1998;25(7):1330–1335.
7. Reynolds JC, Immune-mediated enteric neuron dysfunction in scleroderma [comment]. *J Lab Clin Med*. 1999;133(6):523–524.
8. Cohen S. The gastrointestinal manifestations of scleroderma: pathogenesis and management. *Gastroenterology*. 1980;79(1):155–166.
9. Duchini A, Sessoms SL. Gastrointestinal hemorrhage in patients with systemic sclerosis and CREST syndrome. *Am J Gastroenterol*. 1998;93(9):1453–1456.
10. Ebert EC, Ebert EC. Gastric and enteric involvement in progressive systemic sclerosis. *J Clin Gastroenterol*. 2008;42(1):5–12.

11. Watson M, et al. Gastric antral vascular ectasia (watermelon stomach) in patients with systemic sclerosis. *Arthritis Rheum.* 1996;39(2):341–346.
12. Ebert EC, Ebert EC. Esophageal disease in scleroderma. *J Clin Gastroenterol.* 2006;40(0):769–775.
13. Roberts CG, et al. A case-control study of the pathology of oesophageal disease in systemic sclerosis (scleroderma). *Gut.* 2006;55(12):1697–1703.
14. Sridhar KR, et al. Prevalence of impaired gastric emptying of solids in systemic sclerosis: diagnostic and therapeutic implications. *J Lab Clin Med.* 1998;132(6):541–546.
15. Weston S, et al. Clinical and upper gastrointestinal motility features in systemic sclerosis and related disorders. *Am J Gastroenterol.* 1998;93(7):1085–1089.
16. Zamost BJ, et al. Esophagitis in scleroderma. Prevalence and risk factors. *Gastroenterology.* 1987;92(2):421–428.
17. Segel MC, et al. Systemic sclerosis (scleroderma) and esophageal adenocarcinoma: Is increased patient screening necessary? *Gastroenterology.* 1985;89(3):485–488.
18. Meszaros WT. The colon in systemic sclerosis (scleroderma). *Am J Roentgenol, Radium Ther Nucl Med.* 1959;82:100–102.
19. Marguerie C, et al. Malabsorption caused by coeliac disease in patients who have scleroderma [see comment]. *Br J Rheumatol.* 1995;34(9):858–861.
20. Shindo K, et al. Deconjugation ability of bacteria isolated from the jejunal fluid of patients with progressive systemic sclerosis and its gastric pH. *Hepatogastroenterology.* 1998;45(23):1643–1650.
21. Sheehan NJ, Stanton-King K. Co-existent coeliac disease and scleroderma.[comment]. *Br J Rheumatol.* 1996;35(8):807.
22. Rose S, Young MA, Reynolds JC. Gastrointestinal manifestations of scleroderma. *Gastroenterol Clin North Am.* 1998;27(3):563–594.
23. Lock G, et al. Gastrointestinal manifestations of progressive systemic sclerosis. *Am J Gastroenterol.* 1997;92(5):763–771.
24. Fraback RC, et al. Sigmoid volvulus in two patients with progressive systemic sclerosis. *J Rheumatol.* 1978;5(2):195–198.
25. Hendy MS, Torrance HB, Warnes TW. Small-bowel volvulus in association with progressive systemic sclerosis. *Br Med J.* 1979;1(6170):1051–1052.
26. Netscher DT, Richardson JD. Complications requiring operative intervention in scleroderma. *Surg Gynecol Obstet.* 1984;158(5):507–512.
27. Rohrmann CA Jr, et al. Radiologic and histologic differentiation of neuromuscular disorders of the gastrointestinal tract: visceral myopathies, visceral neuropathies, and progressive systemic sclerosis. *Am J Roentgenol.* 1984;143(5):933–941.
28. Ebert EC, Ruggiero FM, Seibold JR. Intestinal perforation. A common complication of scleroderma. *Digest Dis Sci.* 1997;42(3):549–553.
29. Cerinic MM, et al. The nervous system in systemic sclerosis (scleroderma). Clinical features and pathogenetic mechanisms. *Rheum Dis Clin North Am.* 1996;22(4):879–892.
30. D'Angelo WA, et al. Pathologic observations in systemic sclerosis (scleroderma). A study of fifty-eight autopsy cases and fifty-eight matched controls. *Am J Med.* 1969;46(3):428–440.
31. Meyers AR. Progressive systemic sclerosis: gastrointestinal involvement. *Clin Rheum Dis.* 1979(5):115–129.
32. Peachey, RD, Creamer B, Pierce JW. Sclerodermatous involvement of the stomach and the small and large bowel. *Gut.* 1969;10(4):285–292.
33. Shamberger RC, Crawford JL, Kirkham SE. Progressive systemic sclerosis resulting in megacolon. A case report. *JAMA.* 1983;250(8):1063–1065.
34. Hendel L, et al. Esophageal candidosis in progressive systemic sclerosis: occurrence, significance, and treatment with fluconazole. *Scand J Gastroenterol.* 1988;23(10):1182–1186.
35. Hoskins LC, et al. Functional and morphologic alterations of the gastrointestinal tract in progressive systemic sclerosis (scleroderma). *Am J Med.* 1962;33:459–470.
36. McBrien DJ, Mummery HEL. Steatorrhea in progressive systemic sclerosis (scleroderma). *Br Med J.* 1962,2. 1653–1656.
37. Rosson RS. Yesner R. Peroral duodenal biopsy in progressive systemic sclerosis. *N Engl J Med.* 1965;272:391–394.
38. Bluestone R, Macmahon M, Dawson JM. Systemic sclerosis and small bowel involvement. *Gut.* 1969;10(3):185–193.
39. Cobden I, et al. Small intestinal structure and passive permeability in systemic sclerosis. *Gut.* 1980;21(4):293–298.
40. Regan PT Weiland LH, Geall MG. Scleroderma and intestinal perforation. *Am J Gastroenterol.* 1977;68(6):566–571.
41. Schneider A, Merikhi A, Frank BB. Autoimmune disorders: gastrointestinal manifestations and endoscopic findings. *Gastrointest Endosc Clin N Am.* 2006;16(1):133–151.
42. Eshraghi N, et al. Adult-onset dermatomyositis with severe gastrointestinal manifestations: case report and review of the literature. *Surgery.* 1998;123(3):356–358.
43. Kleckner FS. Dermatomyositis and its manifestations in the gastrointestinal tract. *Am J Gastroenterol.* 1970;53(2): 141–146.
44. Shehata R, et al. Juvenile dermatomyositis: clinical profile and disease course in 25 patients. *Clin Exp Rheumatol.* 1999; 17(1):115–118.
45. Tweezer-Zaks N, et al. Severe gastrointestinal inflammation in adult dermatomyositis: characterization of a novel clinical association. *Am J Med Sci.* 2006;332(6):308–313.
46. Dougenis D, et al. Spontaneous esophageal rupture in adult dermatomyositis. *Eur J Cardiothorac Surg.* 1996;10(11): 1021–1023.
47. de Merieux P, et al. Esophageal abnormalities and dysphagia in polymyositis and dermatomyositis. *Arthritis Rheum.* 1983; 26(8):961–968.
48. Mebazaa A, et al. Dermatomyositis and malignancy in Tunisia: a multicenter national retrospective study of 20 cases. *J Am Acad Dermatol.* 2003;48(4):530–534.
49. Bernard P, Bonnetblanc JM. Dermatomyositis and malignancy. *J Invest Dermatol.* 1993;100(1):128S–132S.
50. Leow YH, Goh CL. Malignancy in adult dermatomyositis. *Int J Dermatol.* 1997;36(12):904–907.
51. Marie I, et al. Influence of age on characteristics of polymyositis and dermatomyositis in adults. *Medicine.* 1999;78(3):139–147.
52. Chow WH, et al. Cancer risk following polymyositis and dermatomyositis: a nationwide cohort study in Denmark. *Cancer Causes Control.* 1995;6(1):9–13.
53. Miyahara S, et al. Two cases of systemic lupus erythematosus complicated with colonic ulcers [see comment]. *Intern Med.* 2005;44(12):1298–1306.
54. Lee J, et al. Mechanisms of carvacrol-induced expression of type 1 collagen gene. *J Dermatol Sci.* 2008;52(3):160–169.
55. Sultan SM, Ioannou Y, Isenberg DA. A review of gastrointestinal manifestations of systemic lupus erythematosus. *Rheumatology.* 1999;38(10):917–932.
56. Triplett DA. Many faces of lupus anticoagulants. *Lupus.* 1998;7(suppl 2):S18–S22.
57. Andoh A, et al. Acute lupus peritonitis successfully treated with steroid pulse therapy. *J Gastroenterol.* 1997;32(5): 654–657.
58. Papa MZ Shiloni E, McDonald HD. Total colonic necrosis. A catastrophic complication of systemic lupus erythematosus. *Dis Colon Rectum.* 1986;29(9):576–578.
59. Reissman P, et al. Gangrenous ischemic colitis of the rectum: a rare complication of systemic lupus erythematosus. *Am J Gastroenterol.* 1994;89(12):2234–2236.

60. Teramoto J, et al. Systemic lupus erythematosus with a giant rectal ulcer and perforation. *Intern Med.* 1999;38(8):643–649.
61. Lee JR, et al. Ischemic colitis associated with intestinal vasculitis: histological proof in systemic lupus erythematosus. *World J Gastroenterol.* 2008;14(22):3591–3593.
62. Keating JP, et al. Vasculitis-induced colonic strictures: report of two cases. *Dis Colon Rectum.* 1998;41(10):1316–1321.
63. Hayden GM, Atlas SA. Strongyloidiasis masquerading as inflammatory bowel disease in a patient with lupus erythematosus: a case report. *Conn Med.* 1995;59(11):649–650.
64. Hosseini M, Lee J. Gastrointestinal mucormycosis mimicking ischemic colitis in a patient with systemic lupus erythematosus. *Am J Gastroenterol.* 1998;93(8):1360–1362.
65. Ramos-Casals M, et al. Acute viral infections in patients with systemic lupus erythematosus: description of 23 cases and review of the literature. *Medicine.* 2008;87(6):311–318.
66. Al-Hoqail I, et al. Systemic lupus erythematosus and amyloidosis. *Clin Rheumatol.* 1997;16(4):422–424.
67. Cabrera GE, et al. Pneumatosis cystoides intestinalis in systemic lupus erythematosus with intestinal vasculitis: treatment with high dose prednisone. *Clin Rheumatol.* 1994;13(2):312–316.
68. Kashihara T, et al. Protein-losing enteropathy and pancreatic involvement in a case of connective tissue disease. *Gastroenterol Jpn.* 1992;27(2):246–251.
69. Mader R, Adawi M, Schonfeld S. Malabsorption in systemic lupus erythematosus. *Clin Exp Rheumatol.* 1997;15(6):659–661.
70. Komatireddy GR, et al. Association of systemic lupus erythematosus and gluten enteropathy. *South Med J.* 1995;88(6):673–676.
71. Perlemuter G, et al. Chronic intestinal pseudo-obstruction in systemic lupus erythematosus. *Gut.* 1998;43(1):117–122.
72. Markusse HM, Schravenhoff R, Beerman H. Hypereosinophilic syndrome presenting with diarrhoea and anaemia in a patient with systemic lupus erythematosus. *Neth J Med.* 1998;52(2):79–81.
73. Marshall JB, et al. Gastrointestinal manifestations of mixed connective tissue disease. *Gastroenterology.* 1990;98(5 pt 1):1232–1238.
74. Smolen JS, Steiner G. Mixed connective tissue disease: to be or not to be? [see comment]. *Arthritis Rheum.* 1998;41(5):768–777.
75. Raskin JB. Gastrointestinal effects of nonsteroidal anti-inflammatory therapy. *Am J Med.* 1999;106(5B):3S–12S.
76. Voutilainen M, et al. Nonsteroidal anti-inflammatory drug-associated upper gastrointestinal lesions in rheumatoid arthritis patients. Relationships to gastric histology, *Helicobacter pylori* infection, and other risk factors for peptic ulcer. *Scand J Gastroenterol.* 1998;33(8):811–816.
77. Cheatum DE, et al. An endoscopic study of gastroduodenal lesions induced by nonsteroidal anti-inflammatory drugs. *Clin Therap.* 1999;21(6):992–1003.
78. Teodorescu V, et al. Gold-induced colitis: a case report and review of the literature. *Mt Sinai J Med.* 1993;60(3):238–241.
79. Evron E, et al. Correlation between gold-induced enterocolitis and the presence of the HLA-DRB1*0404 allele. *Arthritis Rheum.* 1995;38(6):755–759.
80. Schneider RE, Dobbins WO III. Suction biopsy of the rectal mucosa for diagnosis of arteritis in rheumatoid arthritis and related diseases. *Ann Intern Med.* 1968;68(3):561–568.
81. Babian M, Nasef S, Soloway G. Gastrointestinal infarction as a manifestation of rheumatoid vasculitis. *Am J Gastroenterol.* 1998;93(1):119–120.
82. Parker B, Chattopadhyay C. A case of rheumatoid vasculitis involving the gastrointestinal tract in early disease. *Rheumatology.* 2007;46(11):1737–1738.
83. Porzio V, et al. Intestinal histological and ultrastructural inflammatory changes in spondyloarthropathy and rheumatoid arthritis. *Scand J Rheumatol.* 1997;26(2):92–98.
84. Kokkonen J, et al. Intestinal immune activation in juvenile idiopathic arthritis and connective tissue disease. *Scand J Rheumatol.* 2007;36(5):386–389.
85. Volter F, et al. Esophageal function and Sjogren's syndrome. *Digest Dis Sci.* 2004;49(2):248–253.
86. Mandl T, et al. Dysphagia and dysmotility of the pharynx and oesophagus in patients with primary Sjogren's syndrome. *Scand J Rheumatol.* 2007;36(5):394–401.
87. Tzioufas AG, et al. Update on Sjogren's syndrome autoimmune epithelitis: from classification to increased neoplasias. *Best Pract Res Clin Rheumatol.* 2007;21(6):989–1010.
88. De Vita S, et al. Widespread clonal B-cell disorder in Sjogren's syndrome predisposing to *Helicobacter pylori*-related gastric lymphoma. *Gastroenterology.* 1996;110(6):1969–1974.
89. Queneau PE, et al. Diagnosis of a gastric mucosa-associated lymphoid tissue lymphoma by endoscopic ultrasonography-guided biopsies in a patient with a parotid gland localization. *Scand J Gastroenterol.* 2002;37(4):493–496.
90. Wu IB, et al. Reiter's syndrome: the classic triad and more. *J Am Acad Dermatol.* 2008;59(1):113–121.
91. Mielants H, et al. HLA-B27 related arthritis and bowel inflammation. Part 2. Ileocolonoscopy and bowel histology in patients with HLA-B27 related arthritis. *J Rheumatol.* 1985;12(2):294–298.
92. Ebert EC. Gastrointestinal manifestations of Behcet's disease. *Digest Dis Sci.* 2009(54):201–207.
93. Collins MH, et al. Multiple vascular and bowel ruptures in an adolescent male with sporadic Ehlers-Danlos syndrome type IV. *Pediatr Dev Pathol.* 1999;2(1):86–93.
94. Blaker H, et al. Pathology of the large intestine in patients with vascular type Ehlers-Danlos syndrome. *Virchows Arch.* 2007;450(6):713–717.
95. Sur MD, et al. Pseudoxanthoma elasticum: a case of total gastrectomy for gastric hemorrhage. *Am Surg.* 2008;74(4):361–362.
96. Sharma S, et al. Colorectal manifestations of endocrine disease. *Dis Colon Rectum.* 1995;38(3):318–323.
97. Deen KI, Seneviratne SL, de Silva HJ. Anorectal physiology and transit in patients with disorders of thyroid metabolism. *J Gastroenterol Hepatol.* 1999;14(4):384–387.
98. Lew EA, et al. Adenocarcinoma of the colon with neuroendocrine features and secretory diarrhea. *Am J Gastroenterol.* 1999;94(6):1692–1694.
99. Matosin-Matekalo M, et al. Glucose and thyroid hormone co-regulate the expression of the intestinal fructose transporter GLUT5. *Biochem J.* 1999;339(pt 2):233–239.
100. Papa A, et al. Effects of propylthiouracil on intestinal transit time and symptoms in hyperthyroid patients. *Hepatogastroenterology.* 1997;44(14):426–429.
101. Maser C, et al. Gastrointestinal manifestations of endocrine disease. *World J Gastroenterol.* 2006;12(20):3174–3179.
102. Pfaffenbach B, et al. Effect of hyperthyroidism on antral myoelectrical activity, gastric emptying and dyspepsia in man. *Hepatogastroenterology.* 1997;44(17):1500–1508.
103. Gunsar F, et al. Effect of hypo- and hyperthyroidism on gastric myoelectrical activity. *Digest Dis Sci.* 2003;48(4):706–712.

104. Miller LJ, Corman CA, Go VL. Gut-thyroid interrelationships. *Gastroenterology*. 1978;75(5):901–911.
105. Hellesen C, et al. Small intestinal histology, radiology and absorption in hyperthyroidism. *Scand J Gastroenterol*. 1969;4(2):169–175.
106. Cammarota G, et al. Gastric mucosa-associated lymphoid tissue in autoimmune thyroid diseases. *Scand J Gastroenterol*. 1997;32(9):869–872.
107. Cansler CL, et al. Duodenal obstruction in thyroid storm. *South Med J*. 1997;90(11):1143–1146.
108. Marks P, Anderson J. Vincent R. Thyrotoxic myopathy presenting as dysphagia. *Postgrad Med J*. 1980;56(659):669–670.
109. Buchholz DW. Neurogenic dysphagia: what is the cause when the cause is not obvious? *Dysphagia*. 1994;9(4):245–255.
110. Eastwood GL, et al. Reversal of lower esophageal sphincter hypotension and esophageal aperistalsis after treatment for hypothyroidism. *J Clin Gastroenterol*. 1982;4(4):307–310.
111. Borrie MJ, et al. Myxedema megacolon after external neck irradiation. *J Am Geriatr Soc*. 1983;31(4):228–230.
112. Patel R, Hughes RW Jr. An unusual case of myxedema megacolon with features of ischemic and pseudomembranous colitis. *Mayo Clin Proc*. 1992;67(4):369–372.
113. Abbasi AA, et al. Myxedema ileus. A form of intestinal pseudo-obstruction. *JAMA*. 1975;234(2):181–183.
114. Lauritano EC, et al. Association between hypothyroidism and small intestinal bacterial overgrowth. *J Clin Endocrinol Metab*. 2007;92(11):4180–4184.
115. Bastenie PA. Paralytic ileus in severe hypothyroidism. *Lancet*. 1946;1:413–416.
116. Douglass RC, Jacobson SD. Pathologic changes in adult myxedema: survey of 10 necropsies. *J Clin Endocrinol Metab*. 1957;17(11):1354–1364.
117. Tysk C, et al. Diagnosis and management of microscopic colitis. *World J Gastroenterol*. 2008;14(28):7280–7288.
118. Hanna FW, et al. Regulatory peptides and other neuroendocrine markers in medullary carcinoma of the thyroid. *J Endocrinol*. 1997;152(2):275–281.
119. Guyetant S, et al. Medullary thyroid microcarcinoma: a clinicopathologic retrospective study of 38 patients with no prior familial disease. *Hum Pathol*. 1999;30(8):957–963.
120. Stone CW, et al. Thyroid lymphoma with gastrointestinal involvement: report of three cases. *Am J Hematol*. 1986;21(4):357–365.
121. Groen EJ, et al. Extra-intestinal manifestations of familial adenomatous polyposis. *Ann Surg Oncol*. 2008;15(9):2439–2450.
122. St. Goar WT. Gastrointestinal symptoms as a clue to the diagnosis of primary hyperparathyrodism: a review of 45 cases. *Ann Intern Med*. 1957;46:102–118.
123. Silverberg SJ, et al. The diagnosis and management of asymptomatic primary hyperparathyroidism. *Nat Clin Pract Endocrinol Metab*. 2006;2(9):494–503.
124. Eversman JJ, Farmer RG, Brown CH. Gastrointestinal manifestations of hyperparathyroidism. *Arch Intern Med*. 1967;119(6):605–609.
125. Gardner EC, Hersh T. Primary hyperparathyroidism and the gastrointestinal tract. *South Med J*. 1981;74:197–199.
126. Palmer FJ. The clinical manifestations of primary hyperparathyroidism. *Compr Ther*. 1983;9(2):56–64.
127. Clarkson B, et al. Clinical and metabolic study of a patient with malabsorption and hypoparathyroidism. *Metabolism*. 1960(9):1093–1106.
128. Peracchi M, Bardella MT, Conte D. Late-onset idiopathic hypoparathyroidism as a cause of diarrhoea. *Eur J Gastroenterol Hepatol*. 1998;10(2):163–165.
129. Landauer N, et al. A rare but endocrine cause of chronic diarrhea. *Am J Gastroenterol*. 2003;98(1):227–228.
130. Bytzer P, et al. Prevalence of gastrointestinal symptoms associated with diabetes mellitus: a population-based survey of 15,000 adults [see comment]. *Arch Intern Med*. 2001;161(16):1989–1996.
131. Ebert EC, Ebert EC. Gastrointestinal complications of diabetes mellitus. *Dis Mon*. 2005;51(12):620–663.
132. Koch CA, et al. Are gastrointestinal symptoms related to diabetes mellitus and glycemic control? [comment]. *Eur J Gastroenterol Hepatol*. 2008;20(9):822–825.
133. Quan C, et al. Gastrointestinal symptoms and glycemic control in diabetes mellitus: a longitudinal population study.[see comment]. *Eur J Gastroenterol Hepatol*. 2008;20(9):888–897.
134. Shakil A, et al. Gastrointestinal complications of diabetes [summary for patients in Am Fam Physician. 2008 Jun 15;77(12):1703–1704; PMID: 18619080]. *Am Fam Physician*. 2008;77(12):1697–1702.
135. Hasler WL. Type 1 diabetes and gastroparesis: diagnosis and treatment. *Curr Gastroenterol Rep*. 2007;9(4):261–269.
136. Malins JM, Mayne N. Diabetic diarrhea. A study of thirteen patients with jejunal biopsy. *Diabetes*. 1969;18(12):858–866.
137. Feldman M, Schiller LR. Disorders of gastrointestinal motility associated with diabetes mellitus. *Ann Intern Med*. 1983;98(3):378–384.
138. Glouberman S. Diabetes mellitus and the gastrointestinal tract. Part II: Small and large intestine and gallbladder. *Ariz Med*. 1977;34(3):174–175.
139. Virally-Monod M, et al. Chronic diarrhoea and diabetes mellitus: prevalence of small intestinal bacterial overgrowth. *Diabetes Metab*. 1998;24(6):530–536.
140. Hosking DJ, et al. Vagal impairment of gastric secretion in diabetic autonomic neuropathy. *Br Med J*. 1975;2(5971):588–590.
141. Stewart IM, et al. Oesophageal motor changes in diabetes mellitus. *Thorax*. 1976;31(3):278–283.
142. Yang R, Arem R, Chan L. Gastrointestinal tract complications of diabetes mellitus. Pathophysiology and management. *Arch Intern Med*. 1984;144(6):1251–1256.
143. Ordog T, et al. Remodeling of networks of interstitial cells of Cajal in a murine model of diabetic gastroparesis. *Diabetes*. 2000;49(10):1731–1739.
144. Katz LA, Spiro HM. Gastrointestinal manifestations of diabetes. *N Engl J Med*. 1966;275(24):1350–1361.
145. Paley RG, Mitchell W, Watkinson G. Terminal colonic dilatation following intractable diarrhea in a diabetic. *Gastroenterology*. 1961;41:401–407.
146. Nakahara M, et al. Deficiency of KIT-positive cells in the colon of patients with diabetes mellitus. *J Gastroenterol Hepatol*. 2002;17(6):666–670.
147. Lysy J, et al. Decreased substance P content in the rectal mucosa of diabetics with diarrhea and constipation. *Metabolism*. 1997;46(7):730–734.
148. Kodsi BE, et al. *Candida* esophagitis: a prospective study of 27 cases. *Gastroenterology*. 1976;71(5):715–719.
149. Arapakis G, et al. Diabetes mellitus and pernicious anaemia. *Br Med J*. 1963;1(5324):159–161.
150. Irvine WJ, et al. Thyroid and gastric autoimmunity in patients with diabetes mellitus. *Lancet*. 1970;2(7665):163–168.
151. Walsh CH, et al. Diabetes mellitus and coeliac disease: a clinical study. *Q J Med*. 1978;47(185):89–100.
152. De Block CE, et al. Autoimmune gastritis in type 1 diabetes: a clinically oriented review. *J Clin Endocrinol Metab*. 2008;93(2):363–371.

153. Barker JM, et al. Celiac disease: pathophysiology, clinical manifestations, and associated autoimmune conditions. *Adv Pediatr*. 2008;55:349-365.
154. Larsson K, et al. Annual screening detects celiac disease in children with type 1 diabetes. *Pediatr Diabetes*. 2008;9(4 pt 2): 354-359.
155. Larsson SC, et al. Diabetes mellitus and risk of colorectal cancer: a meta-analysis. *J Natl Canc Inst*. 2005;97(22): 1679-1687.
156. Schmidt H, et al. Ultrastructure of diabetic autonomic neuropathy of the gastrointestinal tract. *Klin Wochenschr*. 1984;62(9):399-405.
157. Duchen LW, et al. Pathology of autonomic neuropathy in diabetes mellitus. *Ann Intern Med*. 1980;92(2 pt 2):301-303.
158. He CL, et al. Loss of interstitial cells of cajal and inhibitory innervation in insulin-dependent diabetes. *Gastroenterology*. 2001;121(2):427-434.
159. Forster J, et al. Absence of the interstitial cells of Cajal in patients with gastroparesis and correlation with clinical findings. *J Gastrointest Surg*. 2005;9(1):102-108.
159a. Choi KM, et al. Heme oxygenase-1 protects interstitial cells of Cajal from oxidative stress and reverses diabetic gastroparesis. *Gastroenterology*. 2008;135(6):2055-2064.
160. Bojsen-Moller F, Gronbaek P, Rostgaard J. Light microscopic study of gastrointestinal and skin capillaries in diabetes mellitus. *Diabetes*. 1963;12:429-432.
161. Goyal RK, Spiro HM. Gastrointestinal manifestations of diabetes mellitus. *Med Clin North Am*. 1971;55(4):1031-1044.
162. Verner JV, Morrison AB. Endocrine pancreatic islet disease with diarrhea. Report of a case due to diffuse hyperplasia of nonbeta islet tissue with a review of 54 additional cases. *Arch Intern Med*. 1974;133(3):492-499.
163. Tomita T, et al. Pancreatic polypeptide cell hyperplasia with and without watery diarrhea syndrome. *J Surg Oncol*. 1980;14(1):11-20.
164. Rigaud D, Rene E, Mignon M. Pancreatic endocrine tumors with digestive effects. Physiopathological and clinical aspects. *Ann Med Intern*. 1984;135(5):396-399.
165. Lehy T, Roucayrol AM, Mignon M. Histomorphological characteristics of gastric mucosa in patients with Zollinger-Ellison syndrome or autoimmune gastric atrophy: role of gastrin and atrophying gastritis. *Microsc Res Tech*. 2000;48(6):327-338.
166. Ghaferi AA, et al. Pancreatic VIPomas: subject review and one institutional experience. *J Gastrointest Surg*. 2008; 12(2):382-393.
167. Long RG, et al. Clinicopathological study of pancreatic and neural VIPomas. *Gut*. 1979;20:A934.
168. Shulman DI, et al. Ganglioneuromatosis involving the small intestine and pancreas of a child and causing hypersecretion of vasoactive intestinal polypeptide. *J Pediatr Gastroenterol Nutr*. 1996;22(2):212-218.
169. Krejs GJ, et al. Somatostatinoma syndrome. Biochemical, morphologic and clinical features. *N Engl J Med*. 1979; 301(6):285-292.
170. Garbrecht N, et al. Somatostatin-producing neuroendocrine tumors of the duodenum and pancreas: incidence, types, biological behavior, association with inherited syndromes, and functional activity. *Endocr Relat Cancer*. 2008;15(1): 229-241.
171. Mallinson CN, et al. A glucagonoma syndrome. *Lancet*. 1974;2(7871):1-5.
172. Jones B, et al. Villous hypertrophy of the small bowel in a patient with glucagonoma. *J Comput Assist Tomogr*. 1983;7(2):334-337.
173. Stevens FM, et al. Glucagonoma syndrome demonstrating giant duodenal villi. *Gut*. 1984;25(7):784-791.
174. Litvak DA, et al. Enterotrophic effects of glucagon-like peptide 2 are enhanced by neurotensin. *J Gastrointest Surg*. 1999;3(4):432-439; discussion 439-440.
175. McBrien DJ, Jones RV, Creamer B. Steatorrhea in Addison's disease. *Lancet*. 1963(1):25-26.
176. Tobin MV, et al. Gastrointestinal manifestations of Addison's disease. *Am J Gastroenterol*. 1989;84(10):1302-1305.
177. O'Leary C, et al. Coeliac disease and autoimmune Addison's disease: a clinical pitfall. *Q J Med*. 2002;95(2):79-82.
178. Betterle C, et al. Celiac disease in North Italian patients with autoimmune Addison's disease. *Eur J Endocrinol*. 2006; 154(2):275-279.
179. Myhre AG, et al. High frequency of coeliac disease among patients with autoimmune adrenocortical failure. *Scand J Gastroenterol*. 2003;38(5):511-515.
180. Bergwitz C, et al. A patient with autoimmune hepatitis type I, Addison's disease, atrophic thyroiditis, atrophic gastritis, exocrine pancreatic insufficiency, and heterozygous alpha1-antitrypsin deficiency. *Am J Gastroenterol*. 2002;97(4):1050-1052.
181. Naylor EW, Gardner EJ. Adrenal adenomas in a patient with Gardner's syndrome. *Clin Genet*. 1981;20(1):67-73.
182. Beuschlein F, et al. Cortisol producing adrenal adenoma— a new manifestation of Gardner's syndrome. *Endocr Res*. 2000;26(4):783-790.
183. Dayal Y, et al. Duodenal carcinoids in patients with and without neurofibromatosis. A comparative study. *Am J Surg Pathol*. 1986;10(5):348-357.
184. Wheeler MH, Curley IR, Williams ED. The association of neurofibromatosis, pheochromocytoma, and somatostatin-rich duodenal carcinoid tumor. *Surgery*. 1986;100(6):1163-1169.
185. Mullen JP, et al. Pathogenesis and pharmacologic management of pseudo-obstruction of the bowel in pheochromocytoma. *Am J Med Sci*. 1985;290(4):155-158.
186. Khafagi FA, Lloyd HM, Gough IR. Intestinal pseudo-obstruction in pheochromocytoma. *Aust N Z J Med*. 1987; 17(2):246-248.
187. Nigawara K, et al. A case of recurrent malignant pheochromocytoma complicated by watery diarrhea, hypokalemia, achlorhydria syndrome. *J Clin Endocrinol Metab*. 1987; 65(5):1053-1056.
188. Wu HW, et al. Pheochromocytoma presented as intestinal pseudo-obstruction and hyperamylasemia. *Am J Emerg Med*. 2008;26(8):971 e1-e4.
189. Szmulowicz UM, et al. Ischemic colitis: an uncommon manifestation of pheochromocytoma. *Am Surg*. 2007;73(4): 400-403.
190. Smith SL, et al. Pheochromocytoma producing vasoactive intestinal peptide. *Mayo Clin Proc*. 2002;77(1):97-100.
191. Ikuta S, et al. Watery diarrhea, hypokalemia and achlorhydria syndrome due to an adrenal pheochromocytoma. *World J Gastroenterol*. 2007;13(34):4649-4652.
192. Vazquez-Quintana E, et al. Pheocromocytoma and gastrointestinal bleeding. *Am Surg*. 1995;61(11):937-939.
193. Ali RA, et al. Gastroesophageal reflux disease in pregnancy. *Best Pract Res Clin Gastroenterol*. 2007;21(5):793-806.
194. Cullen G, et al. Constipation and pregnancy. *Best Pract Res Clin Gastroenterol*. 2007;21(5):807-818.
195. Keller J, et al. The spectrum and treatment of gastrointestinal disorders during pregnancy. *Nat Clin Pract Gastroenterol Hepatol*. 2008;5(8):430-443.
196. Ismail SK, et al. Review on hyperemesis gravidarum. *Best Pract Res Clin Gastroenterol*. 2007;21(5):755-769.
197. Krishna AY, Blevins LS Jr. Case report: reversible gastroparesis in patients with hypopituitary disease. *Am J Med Sci*. 1996;312(1):43-45.

198. Popovic V, et al. Increased incidence of neoplasia in patients with pituitary adenomas. *Clin Endocrinol (Oxf)*. 1998;49(4):441–445.
199. Colao A, et al. The association of fasting insulin concentrations and colonic neoplasms in acromegaly, a colonoscopy-based study in 210 patients. *J Clin Endocrinol Metab*. 2007;92(10):3854–3860.
200. Resmini E, et al. Computed Tomography Colonography in Acromegaly. *J Clin Endocrinol Metab*. 2009;94(1):218–222.
201. Jenkins PJ, et al. Insulin-like growth factor I and the development of colorectal neoplasia in acromegaly. *J Clin Endocrinol Metab*. 2000;85(9):3218–3221.
202. Ohsie S, et al. A paucity of colonic enteroendocrine and/or enterochromaffin cells characterizes a subset of patients with chronic unexplained diarrhea/malabsorption. *Hum Pathol*. 2009.
203. Cortina G, et al. Enteroendocrine cell dysgenesis and malabsorption, a histopathologic and immunohistochemical characterization. *Hum Pathol*. 2007;38(4):570–580.
204. Peterson P, Peltonen L. Autoimmune polyendocrinopathy syndrome type 1 (APS1) and AIRE gene: new views on molecular basis of autoimmunity. *J Autoimmun*. 2005;25(suppl):49–55.
205. Giusti F, Marini F, Brandi ML. Multiple endocrine neoplasia type 1. In: Pagon RA, Adam MP, Bird TD, et al., eds. *Gene Reviews*. Available at: http://www.ncbi.nlm.nih.gov/books/NBK1538/. September 2012.
205a. Moline J, Eng C. Multiple endocrine neoplasia type 2. In: Pagon RA, Adam MP, Bird TD, et al., eds. *Gene Reviews*. Available at: http://www.ncbi.nlm.nih.gov/books/NBK1257/. January 2013.
206. DeLellis RA, et al. Multiple endocrine neoplasia (MEN) syndromes: cellular origins and interrelationships. *Int Rev Exp Pathol*. 1986;28:163–215.
207. Grobmyer SR, et al. Colonic manifestations of multiple endocrine neoplasia type 2B: report of four cases. *Dis Colon Rectum*. 1999;42(9):1216–1219.
208. Cohen MS, et al. Gastrointestinal manifestations of multiple endocrine neoplasia type 2. *Ann Surg*. 2002;235(5):648–654; discussion 654–655.
209. Carney AJ, Hayles AB. Alimentary tract manifestations of multiple endocrine neoplasia, type 2b. *Mayo Clin Proc*. 1977(52):543–548.
210. Cope R. Schleinitz PF. Multiple endocrine neoplasia, type 2b, as a cause of megacolon. *Am J Gastroenterol*. 1983;78(12):802–805.
211. Snover DC, Weigent CE, Sumner HW. Diffuse mucosal ganglioneuromatosis of the colon associated with adenocarcinoma. *Am J Clin Pathol*. 1981;75(2):225–229.
212. Weidner N, Flanders DJ, Mitros FA. Mucosal ganglioneuromatosis associated with multiple colonic polyps. *Am J Surg Pathol*. 1984;8(10):779–786.
213. Perkins JT, Blackstone MO, Riddell RH. Adenomatous polyposis coli and multiple endocrine neoplasia type 2b. A pathogenetic relationship. *Cancer*. 1985;55(2):375–381.
214. Lewis CE, et al. Inherited endocrinopathies: an update. *Mol Genet Metab*. 2008;94(3):271–282.
215. Van Vlem B, et al. Dyspepsia and gastric emptying in chronic renal failure patients. *Clin Nephrol*. 2001;56(4):302–307.
216. Schoonjans R, et al. Dyspepsia and gastroparesis in chronic renal failure: the role of *Helicobacter pylori*. *Clin Nephrol*. 2002;57(3):201–207.
217. Hirako M, et al. Impaired gastric motility and its relationship to gastrointestinal symptoms in patients with chronic renal failure. *J Gastroenterol*. 2005;40(12):1116–122.
218. Boyle JM, Johnston D. Acute upper gastrointestinal hemorrhage in patients with chronic renal disease. *Am J Med*. 1983;75(3):409–412.
219. Mitchell CJ, et al. Gastric function and histology in chronic renal failure. *J Clin Pathol*. 1979;32(3):209–213.
220. Zuckerman GR, et al. Upper gastrointestinal bleeding in patients with chronic renal failure. *Annals of Intern Med*. 1985;102(5):588–592.
221. Sohal AS, et al. Uremic bleeding: pathophysiology and clinical risk factors. *Thromb Res*. 2006;118(3):417–422.
222. Etemad B. Gastrointestinal complications of renal failure. *Gastroenterol Clin North Am*. 1998;27(4):875–892.
223. Bumaschny, E., et al. Postoperative acute gastrointestinal tract hemorrhage and multiple-organ failure. *Arch Surg*. 1988;123(6):722–726.
224. Wesdorp RI, et al. Gastrin and gastric acid secretion in renal failure. *Am J Surg*. 1981;141(3):334–338.
225. Tani N, et al. Lesions of the upper gastrointestinal tract in patients with chronic renal failure. *Gastroenterol Jpn*. 1980;15(5):480–484.
226. Jaffe RH, Laing DR. Changes of the digestive tract in uremia; pathologic anatomy study. *Arch Intern Med*. 1934;53:851–864.
227. Mason EE. Gastrointestinal lesions occurring in uremia. *Ann Intern Med*. 1952;37(1):96–105.
228. Kang JY. The gastrointestinal tract in uremia. *Digest Dis Sci*. 1993;38(2):257–268.
229. Goldstein H, et al. Gastric acid secretion in patients undergoing chronic dialysis. *Arch Intern Med*. 1967;120(6):645–653.
230. Doherty CC, McGeown MG. Peptic ulceration, gastric secretion, and renal transplantation. *Br Med J*. 1977;2(6080):188.
231. Milito, G., et al. The gastrointestinal tract in uremic patients on long-term hemodialysis. *Kidney Int Suppl*. 1985;17:S157–S160.
232. Kang JY, et al. Erosive prepyloric changes in patients with end-stage renal failure undergoing maintenance dialysis treatment. *Scand J Gastroenterol*. 1990;25(7):746–750.
233. Shousha S, et al. Antral *Helicobacter pylori* in patients with chronic renal failure. *J Clin Pathol*. 1990;43(5):397–399.
234. Var C, et al. The effects of hemodialysis on duodenal and gastric mucosal changes in uremic patients. *Clin Nephrol*. 1996;45(5):310–314.
235. Khedmat H, et al. Gastro-duodenal lesions and *Helicobacter pylori* infection in uremic patients and renal transplant recipients. *Transplant Proc*. 2007;39(4):1003–1007.
236. Margolis DM, et al. Upper gastrointestinal disease in chronic renal failure. A prospective evaluation. *Arch Intern Med*. 1978;138(8):1214–1217.
237. Musola R, et al. Prevalence of gastroduodenal lesions in uremic patients undergoing dialysis and after renal transplantation. *Gastrointest Endosc*. 1984;30(6):343–346.
238. Andriulli A, et al. Patients with chronic renal failure are not at a risk of developing chronic peptic ulcers. *Clin Nephrol*. 1985;23(5):245–248.
239. Kang JY, et al. Prevalence of peptic ulcer in patients undergoing maintenance hemodialysis. *Digest Dis Sci*. 1988;33(7):774–778.
240. Kang JY, et al. Peptic ulcer and gastritis in uraemia, with particular reference to the effect of *Helicobacter pylori* infection. *J Gastroenterol Hepatol*. 1999;14(8):771–778.
241. Boudville N. The predictable effect that renal failure has on H2 receptor antagonists–increasing the half-life along with increasing prescribing errors. *Nephrol Dial Transplant*. 2005;20(11):2315–2317.
242. Stolic RV, et al. Influence of the level of renal insufficiency on endoscopic changes in the upper gastrointestinal tract. *Am J Med Sci*. 2008;336(1):39–43.

243. Cocchiara G, et al. Advantage of eradication therapy for *Helicobacter pylori* before kidney transplantation in uremic patients. *Transplant Proc.* 2007;39(10):3041–3043.
244. Rashid A, Hamilton SR. Necrosis of the gastrointestinal tract in uremic patients as a result of sodium polystyrene sulfonate (Kayexalate) in sorbitol: an underrecognized condition. *Am J Surg Pathol.* 1997;21(1):60–69.
245. Abraham SC, et al. Upper gastrointestinal tract injury in patients receiving kayexalate (sodium polystyrene sulfonate) in sorbitol: clinical, endoscopic, and histopathologic findings. *Am J Surg Pathol.* 2001;25(5):637–644.
246. Chatelain D, et al. Rectal stenosis caused by foreign body reaction to sodium polystyrene sulfonate crystals (Kayexalate). *Ann Diagn Pathol.* 2007;11(3):217–219.
247. Diamond SM, Emmett M, Henrich WL. Bowel infarction as a cause of death in dialysis patients. *JAMA.* 1986;256(18):2545–2547.
248. Madden, MA, et al. Acute bowel obstruction: an unusual complication of chronic peritoneal dialysis. *Am J Kidney Dis.* 1982;1(4):219–221.
249. Bargman JM. Hernias in peritoneal dialysis patients: limiting occurrence and recurrence. *Perit Dial Int.* 2008;28(4):349–351.
250. Herbstman D, Kraft SC. Extraintestinal manifestations of gastrointestinal disease and gastrointestinal manifestations of extraintestinal disease. In: Gitnik GL, ed. *Current Gastroenterology.* 6th ed. Chicago, IL: Year Book Medical Publichers; 1986.
251. Kraft SC, Wang NS. Extraintestinal manifestations of gastrointestinal disease and gastrointestinal manifestations of extraintestinal disease. In: Gitnik GL, ed. *Current Gastroenterology.* Boston, MA: Houghton Mifflin; 1985:299–351.
252. Lockyer WA, et al. An outbreak of *Salmonella* enteritis and septicemia in a population of uremic patients. A review of four cases, including infection of an arteriovenous fistula. *Arch Intern Med.* 1980;140(7):943–945.
253. Young R, Bryk D. Colonic intussusception in uremia. *Am J Gastroenterol.* 1979;71(2):229–232.
254. Pourfarziani V, et al. The outcome of diverticulosis in kidney recipients with polycystic kidney disease. *Transplant Proc.* 2007;39(4):1054–1056.
255. Lederman ED, et al. Diverticulitis and polycystic kidney disease. *Am Surg.* 2000;66(2):200–203.
256. Paimela H, et al. Relation between serum group II pepsinogen concentration and the degree of Brunner's gland hyperplasia in patients with chronic renal failure. *Gut.* 1985;26(2):198–202.
257. Tuthill MH, Stratton J, Warrens AN. Calcific uremic arteriolopathy presenting with small and large bowel involvement. *J Nephrol.* 2006;19(1):115–118.
258. Ponticelli C, Passerini P. Gastrointestinal complications in renal transplant recipients. *Transpl Int.* 2005;18(6):643–650.
259. Davies NM, et al. Gastrointestinal side effects of mycophenolic acid in renal transplant patients: a reappraisal. *Nephrol Dial Transplant.* 2007;22(9):2440–2448.
260. Walter S, et al. Effect of cimetidine on upper gastrointestinal bleeding after renal transplantation: a prospective study. *Br Med J Clin Res Ed.* 1984;289(6453):1175–1176.
261. Komorowski RA, et al. Gastrointestinal complications in renal transplant recipients. *Am J Clin Pathol.* 1986;86(2):161–167.
262. Dominguez Fernandez E, et al. Prevalence of diverticulosis and incidence of bowel perforation after kidney transplantation in patients with polycystic kidney disease. *Transpl Int.* 1998;11(1):28–31.
263. Carson SD, et al. Colon perforation after kidney transplantation. *Ann Surg.* 1978;188(1):109–113.
264. Sawyerr OI, et al. Colorectal complications of renal allograft transplantation. *Arch Surg.* 1978;113(1):84–86.
265. Meyers WC, et al. Alimentary tract complications after renal transplantation. *Ann Surg.* 1979;190(4):535–542.
266. Scheff RT, et al. Diverticular disease in patients with chronic renal failure due to polycystic kidney disease. *Ann Intern Med.* 1980;92(2 pt 1):202–204.
267. Toogood GJ, et al. Cytomegalovirus infection and colonic perforation in renal transplant patients. *Transplant Int.* 1996;9(3):248–251.
268. Kashyap R, et al. The clinical significance of cytomegaloviral inclusions in the allograft kidney. *Transplantation.* 1999;67(1):98–103.
269. Ok UZ, et al. Cryptosporidiosis and blastocystosis in renal transplant recipients. *Nephron.* 1997;75(2):171–174.
270. Schumaker JD, et al. Thiabendazole treatment of severe strongyloidiasis in a hemodialyzed patient. *Ann Intern Med.* 1978;89(5 pt 1):644–645.
271. Leapman SB, et al. Strongyloides stercoralis in chronic renal failure: safe therapy with thiabendazole. *South Med J.* 1980;73(10):1400–1402.
272. Parfitt JR, Jayakumar S, Driman DK. Mycophenolate mofetil-related gastrointestinal mucosal injury: variable injury patterns, including graft-versus-host disease-like changes. *Am J Surg Pathol.* 2008;32(9):1367–1372.
273. Srinivasan R, Polycystic liver disease: an unusual cause of bleeding varices. *Digest Dis Sci.* 1999;44(2):389–392.
274. Norman K, Pirlich M. Gastrointestinal tract in liver disease: which organ is sick? *Curr Opin Clin Nutr Metab Care.* 2008;11(5):613–619.
275. Ganguly S, et al. The prevalence and spectrum of colonic lesions in patients with cirrhotic and noncirrhotic portal hypertension. *Hepatology.* 1995;21(5):1226–1231.
276. Lamps LW, et al. Alterations in colonic mucosal vessels in patients with cirrhosis and noncirrhotic portal hypertension. *Hum Pathol.* 1998;29(5):527–535.
277. Ohtani T, et al. Ileal varices associated with recurrent bleeding in a patient with liver cirrhosis. *J Gastroenterol.* 1999;34(2):264–268.
278. Zaman A, et al. Prevalence of upper and lower gastrointestinal tract findings in liver transplant candidates undergoing screening endoscopic evaluation [see comment]. *Am J Gastroenterol.* 1999;94(4):895–899.
279. Canlas KR, et al. Using capsule endoscopy to identify GI tract lesions in cirrhotic patients with portal hypertension and chronic anemia. *J Clin Gastroenterol.* 2008;42(7):844–848.
280. Spahr L, et al. Gastric antral vascular ectasia in cirrhotic patients: absence of relation with portal hypertension [see comment]. *Gut.* 1999;44(5):739–742.
281. Bhonchal S, et al. Functional and morphological alterations in small intestine mucosa of chronic alcoholics. *J Gastroenterol Hepatol.* 2008;23(7 pt 2):e43–e48.
282. Worns MA, et al. Five cases of de novo inflammatory bowel disease after orthotopic liver transplantation. *Am J Gastroenterol.* 2006;101(8):1931–1937.
283. Lakatos PL, Lakatos L. Risk for colorectal cancer in ulcerative colitis: changes, causes and management strategies. *World J Gastroenterol.* 2008;14(25):3937–3947.
284. Abdelrazeq AS, et al. Predictors for acute and chronic pouchitis following restorative proctocolectomy for ulcerative colitis. *Colorectal Dis.* 2008;10(8):805–813.
285. Beierle EA, et al. Gastrointestinal perforation after pediatric orthotopic liver transplantation. *J Pediatr Surg.* 1998;33(2):240–242.
286. Dhawan A, et al. Posttransplant eosinophilic gastroenteritis in children. *Liver Transplant Surg.* 1997;3(6):591–593.

287. Verdonk RC, et al. Inflammatory bowel disease after liver transplantation: a role for cytomegalovirus infection. *Scand J Gastroenterol.* 2006;41(2):205–211.
288. Dvorchik I, et al. Effect of liver transplantation on inflammatory bowel disease in patients with primary sclerosing cholangitis. *Hepatology.* 2002;35(2):380–384.
289. Fine JD, et al. Gastrointestinal complications of inherited epidermolysis bullosa: cumulative experience of the National Epidermolysis Bullosa Registry. *J Pediatr Gastroenterol Nutr.* 2008;46(2):147–158.
290. Freeman EB, et al. Gastrointestinal complications of epidermolysis bullosa in children. *Br J Dermatol.* 2008;158(6):1308–1314.
291. Wise JL, Murray JA. Esophageal manifestations of dermatologic disease. *Curr Gastroenterol Rep.* 2002;4(3):205–212.
292. Marsden RA, et al. Epidermolysis bullosa of the oesophagus with oesophageal web formation. *Thorax.* 1974;29(3):287–295.
293. Orlando RC, et al. Epidermolysis bullosa: gastrointestinal manifestations. *Ann Intern Med.* 1974;81(2):203–206.
294. Harmel RP Jr. Esophageal replacement in two siblings with epidermolysis bullosa. *J Pediatr Surg.* 1986;21(2):175–176.
295. Berger TG, Detlefs RL, Donatucci CF. Junctional epidermolysis bullosa, pyloric atresia, and genitourinary disease. *Pediatr Dermatol.* 1986;3(2):130–134.
296. Shaw DW, et al. Gastric outlet obstruction and epidermolysis bullosa. *J Am Acad Dermatol.* 1997;36(2 pt 2):304–310.
297. Mellerio JE, et al. Pyloric atresia-junctional epidermolysis bullosa syndrome: mutations in the integrin beta4 gene (ITGB4) in two unrelated patients with mild disease. *Br J Dermatol.* 1998;139(5):862–871.
298. Taniuchi K, et al. Nonscarring inflammatory epidermolysis bullosa acquisita with esophageal involvement and linear IgG deposits. *J Am Acad Dermatol.* 1997;36(2 pt 2):320–322.
299. Remington J, et al. Autoimmunity to type VII collagen: epidermolysis bullosa acquisita. *Curr Dir Autoimmun.* 2008;10:195–205.
300. Cheesbrough MJ, Epidermolysis bullosa acquisita and Crohn's disease. *Br J Dermatol.* 1978;99(suppl 16):53–54.
301. Hallel-Halevy D, et al. Epidermolysis bullosa acquisita: update and review. *Clin Dermatol.* 2001;19(6):712–718.
302. Trattner A, et al. Esophageal involvement in pemphigus vulgaris: a clinical, histologic, and immunopathologic study. *J Am Acad Dermatol.* 1991;24(2 pt 1):223–226.
303. Mignogna MD, et al. Oral pemphigus: clinical significance of esophageal involvement: report of eight cases. *Oral Surg Oral Med Oral Pathol Oral Radiol Endod.* 1997;84(2):179–184.
304. Gomi H, et al. Oesophageal involvement in pemphigus vulgaris [see comment]. *Lancet.* 1999;354(9192):1794.
305. Galloro G, et al. The role of upper endoscopy in identifying oesophageal involvement in patients with oral pemphigus vulgaris. *Digest Liver Dis.* 2005;37(3):195–199.
306. Calka O, et al. Oesophageal involvement during attacks in pemphigus vulgaris patients. *Clin Exp Dermatol.* 2006;31(4):515–519.
307. Ichimiya M, Nakano J, Muto M. Pemphigus vegetans involving the esophagus. *J Dermatol.* 1998;25(3):195–198.
308. Syn WK, Ahmed MM. Esophageal involvement in cicatricial pemphigoid: a rare cause of dysphagia. *Dis Esophagus.* 2004;17(2):180–182.
309. Stallmach A, et al. Esophageal involvement in cicatricial pemphigoid. *Endoscopy.* 1998;30(7):657–661.
310. Hazin R, et al. Stevens-Johnson syndrome: pathogenesis, diagnosis, and management. *Ann Med.* 2008;40(2):129–138.
311. Misra SP, Dwivedi M, Misra V. Esophageal stricture as a late sequel of Stevens-Johnson syndrome in adults: incidental detection because of foreign body impaction. *Gastrointest Endosc.* 2004;59(3):437–440.
312. Zweiban B, Cohen H, Chandrasoma P. Gastrointestinal involvement complicating Stevens-Johnson syndrome. *Gastroenterology.* 1986;91(2):469–474.
313. Lavery EA, Coyle WJ. Herpes simplex virus and the alimentary tract. *Curr Gastroenterol Rep.* 2008;10(4):417–423.
314. Chandan VS, Murray JA, Abraham SC. Esophageal lichen planus. *Arch Pathol Lab Med.* 2008;132(6):1026–1029.
315. Westbrook R, Riley S. Esophageal lichen planus: case report and literature review. *Dysphagia.* 2008;23(3):331–334.
316. Calabrese C, et al. Squamous cell carcinoma arising in esophageal lichen planus. *Gastrointest Endosc.* 2003;57(4):596–569.
317. McRonald FE, et al. Down-regulation of the cytoglobin gene, located on 17q25, in tylosis with oesophageal cancer (TOC): evidence for trans-allele repression. *Hum Mol Genet.* 2006;15(8):1271–1277.
318. Robertson EV, Jankowski JA. Genetics of gastroesophageal cancer: paradigms, paradoxes, and prognostic utility. *Am J Gastroenterol.* 2008;103(2):443–449.
319. von Brevern M, et al. Loss of heterozygosity in sporadic oesophageal tumors in the tylosis oesophageal cancer (TOC) gene region of chromosome 17q. *Oncogene.* 1998;17(16):2101–2105.
320. Howel-Evans W, et al. Carcinoma of the oesophagus with keratosis palmaris et plantaris (tylosis): a study of two families. *Q J Med.* 1958;27(107):413–429.
321. Andrews GK. Regulation and function of Zip4, the acrodermatitis enteropathica gene. *Biochem Soc Trans.* 2008;36(pt 6):1242–1246.
322. Maverakis E, et al. Acrodermatitis enteropathica and an overview of zinc metabolism. *J Am Acad Dermatol.* 2007;56(1):116–124.
323. Granel F, et al. Acrodermatitis enteropathica-like rash and enterocolitis. *Eur J Dermatol.* 1998;8(6):445–446.
324. Ecker RI, Schroeter AL. Acrodermatitis and acquired zinc deficiency. *Arch Dermatol.* 1978;114(6):937–939.
325. McClain C, Soutor C, Zieve L. Zinc deficiency: a complication of Crohn's disease. *Gastroenterology.* 1980;78(2):272–279.
326. Shimizu H, Tan Kinoshita MT, Suzuki H. Darier's disease with esophageal carcinoma. *Eur J Dermatol.* 2000;10(6):470–472.
327. Vieites B, et al. Darier's disease with esophageal involvement. *Scand J Gastroenterol.* 2008;43(8):1020–1021.
328. Shuster S, Marks J. Dermatogenic enteropathy: a new cause for steatorrhea. *Lancet.* 1965;1:1367–1368.
329. Shuster S. Systemic effects of skin disease. *Lancet.* 1967;1(7496):907–912.
330. Marks J. The relationship of gastrointestinal disease and the skin. *Clin Gastroenterol.* 1983;12(3):693–712.
331. Higgins SP, Freemark M, Prose NS. Acanthosis nigricans: a practical approach to evaluation and management. *Dermatol Online J.* 2008;14(9):2.
332. Lenzner U, et al. Acanthosis nigricans maligna. Case report and review of the literature. *Hautarzt.* 1998;49(1):41–47.
333. Curth HO, Aschner BM. Genetic studies on acanthosis nigricans. *AMA Arch Dermatol.* 1959;79(1):55–66.
334. Lopiccolo J, Ballas MS, Dennis PA. PTEN hamartomatous tumor syndromes (PHTS): rare syndromes with great relevance to common cancers and targeted drug development. *Crit Rev Oncol Hematol.* 2007;63(3):203–214.

335. Schreibman IR, et al. The hamartomatous polyposis syndromes: a clinical and molecular review. *Am J Gastroenterol.* 2005;100(2):476-490.
336. Zbuk KM, Eng C. Hamartomatous polyposis syndromes. *Nat Clin Pract Gastroenterol Hepatol.* 2007;4(9):492-502.
337. Liddell K, White JE, Caldwell IW. Seborrhoeic keratoses and carcinoma of the large bowel. Three cases exhibiting the sign of Lester-trelat. *Br J Dermatol.* 1975;92(4):449-452.
338. Wagner RF, Wagner KD. Malignant neoplasms and the Leser-Trelat sign. *Arch Dermatol.* 1981;117(9):598-599.
339. Parks DA, Jacobson ED. Physiology of the splanchnic circulation. *Arch Intern Med.* 1985;145(7):1278-1281.
340. Sandek A, et al. The emerging role of the gut in chronic heart failure. *Curr Opin Clin Nutr Metab Care.* 2008;11(5):632-639.
341. Raja K, et al. An endoscopic study of upper-GI mucosal changes in patients with congestive heart failure. *Gastrointest Endosc.* 2004;60(6):887-893.
342. Krack A, et al. Studies on intragastric PCO2 at rest and during exercise as a marker of intestinal perfusion in patients with chronic heart failure. *Eur J Heart Fail.* 2004;6(4):403-407.
343. Boyd O, et al. Comparison of clinical information gained from routine blood-gas analysis and from gastric tonometry for intramural pH. *Lancet.* 1993;341(8838):142-146.
344. Janssens U, et al. Gastric tonometry in patients with cardiogenic shock and intra-aortic balloon counterpulsation. *Crit Care Med.* 2000;28(10):3449-3455.
345. Sandek A, et al. Altered intestinal function in patients with chronic heart failure. *J Am Coll Cardiol.* 2007;50(16):1561-1569.
346. Sondheimer JM, Hamilton JR. Intestinal function in infants with severe congenital heart disease. *J Pediatr.* 1978;92(4):572-578.
347. King D, et al. Fat malabsorption in elderly patients with cardiac cachexia. *Age Ageing.* 1996;25(2):144-149.
348. Arutyunov GP, et al. Collagen accumulation and dysfunctional mucosal barrier of the small intestine in patients with chronic heart failure. *Int J Cardiol.* 2008;125(2):240-245.
349. Kupferwasser I, et al. Clinical and morphological characteristics in *Streptococcus bovis* endocarditis: a comparison with other causative microorganisms in 177 cases. *Heart.* 1998;80(3):276-280.
350. Gonzalez-Juanatey C, et al. Infective endocarditis due to *Streptococcus bovis* in a series of nonaddict patients: clinical and morphological characteristics of 20 cases and review of the literature. *Can J Cardiol.* 2003;19(10):1139-1145.
351. Ferrari A, et al. Colonoscopy is mandatory after *Streptococcus bovis* endocarditis: a lesson still not learned. Case report. *World J Surg Oncol.* 2008;6:49.
352. FitzGerald SF, et al. Gemella endocarditis: consider the colon. *J Heart Valve Dis.* 2006;15(6):833-835.
353. Kok H, et al. Colon cancer presenting as *Streptococcus gallolyticus* infective endocarditis. *Singapore Med J.* 2007;48(2):e43-e45.
354. Aouifi A, et al. Severe digestive complications after heart surgery using extracorporeal circulation. *Can J Anaesth.* 1999;46(2):114-121.
355. Ohri SK, Velissaris T. Gastrointestinal dysfunction following cardiac surgery. *Perfusion.* 2006;21(4):215-223.
356. Aranha GV, et al. The reasons for gastrointestinal consultation after cardiac surgery. *Am Surg.* 1984;50(6):301-304.
357. Lebovics E, et al. Endoscopy for gastrointestinal complications of open heart surgery: predominant findings of aggressive duodenal ulcer disease. *Gastroenterology.* 1989;96A.
358. Steed DL, et al. General surgical complications in heart and heart-lung transplantation. *Surgery.* 1985;98(4):739-745.
359. Johnson R, et al. Upper gastrointestinal endoscopy after cardiac transplantation. *Surgery.* 1988;103(3):300-304.
360. Diaz B, et al. Gastrointestinal complications in heart transplant patients: MITOS study. *Transplant Proc.* 2007;39(7):2397-2400.
361. Sinnott JT, Cullison JP, Rogers K. Treatment of cytomegalovirus gastrointestinal ulceration in a heart transplant patient. *J Heart Transplant.* 1987;6(3):186-188.
362. Huwez FU, et al. Infective dyspepsia in a heart transplant recipient. *J Gastroenterol.* 1996;31(6):848-850.
363. Knoop C, et al. Gastric perforation due to mucormycosis after heart-lung and heart transplantation. *Transplantation.* 1998;66(7):932-935.
364. Lubetkin EI, et al. GI complications after orthotopic lung transplantation. *Am J Gastroenterol.* 1996;91(11):2382-2390.
365. Franchini M. Thrombotic microangiopathies: an update. *Hematology.* 2006;11(3):139-146.
366. Johnson S, Taylor CM. What's new in haemolytic uraemic syndrome? *Eur J Pediatr.* 2008;167(9):965-971.
367. Scheiring J, Andreoli SP, Zimmerhackl LB. Treatment and outcome of Shiga-toxin-associated hemolytic uremic syndrome (HUS). *Pediatr Nephrol.* 2008;23(10):1749-1760.
368. Morel-Maroger L. Adult hemolytic-uremic syndrome. *Kidney Int.* 1980;18(1):125-134.
369. Razzaq S. Hemolytic uremic syndrome: an emerging health risk. *Am Fam Physician.* 2006;74(6):991-996.
370. Pauly MP, Watson-Williams E, Trudeau WL. Intussusception presenting with lower gastrointestinal hemorrhage in a hemophiliac. *Gastrointest Endosc.* 1987;33(2):115-118.
371. Eyster ME, et al. Upper gastrointestinal bleeding in haemophiliacs: incidence and relation to use of non-steroidal anti-inflammatory drugs. *Haemophilia.* 2007;13(3):279-286.
372. Mittal R, et al. Patterns of gastrointestinal hemorrhage in hemophilia. *Gastroenterology.* 1985;88(2):515-522.
373. Griffin PH, et al. Intramural gastrointestinal hemorrhage. *J Clin Gastroenterol.* 1986;8(3 pt 2):389-394.
374. Santoro R, Iannaccaro P. Spontaneous intramural intestinal haemorrhage in a haemophiliac patient. *Br J Haematol.* 2004;125(4):419.
375. Ramadan KM, et al. Acute intestinal obstruction due to intramural haemorrhage in small intestine in a patient with severe haemophilia A and inhibitor. *Eur J Haematol.* 2005;75(2):164-166.
376. Jarry J, et al. Spontaneous intramural haematoma of the sigmoid colon causing acute intestinal obstruction in a haemophiliac: report of a case. *Haemophilia.* 2008;14(2):383-384.
377. Dodds WJ, Spitzer RM, Friedland GW. Gastrointestinal roentgenographic manifestations of hemophilia. *Am J Roentgenol Radium Ther Nucl Med.* 1970;110(2):413-416.
378. Prentice CR. Acquired coagulation disorders. *Clin Haematol.* 1985;14(2):413-442.
379. Myers TJ, Steinberg WM, Rickles FR. Polycythemia vera and mesenteric arterial thrombosis. A disease association resulting from decreased platelet sensitivity to aspirin. *Arch Intern Med.* 1979;139(6):695-698.
380. Lichtin AE, Silberstein LE, Schreiber AD. Thrombotic thrombocytopenic purpura with colitis in an elderly woman. *JAMA.* 1986;255(11):1435-1436.
381. Jensen RT. Gastrointestinal abnormalities and involvement in systemic mastocytosis. *Hematol Oncol Clin North Am.* 2000;14(3):579-623.
382. Soter NA, Austen KF, Wasserman SI. Oral disodium cromoglycate in the treatment of systemic mastocytosis. *N Engl J Med.* 1979;301(9):465-469.

383. Bredfeldt JE, et al. Malabsorption and gastric hyperacidity in systemic mastocytosis. Results of cimetidine therapy. *Am J Gastroenterol.* 1980;74(2):133–137.
384. Cherner JA, et al. Gastrointestinal dysfunction in systemic mastocytosis. A prospective study. *Gastroenterology.* 1988;95(3):657–667.
385. Johnson AC, et al. Systemic mastocytosis and mastocytosis-like syndrome: radiologic features of gastrointestinal manifestations. *South Med J.* 1988;81(6):729–733, 750.
386. Kirsch R, et al. Systemic mastocytosis involving the gastrointestinal tract: clinicopathologic and molecular study of five cases. *Mod Pathol.* 2008;21(12):1508–1516.
387. Siegert SI, et al. Are gastrointestinal mucosal mast cells increased in patients with systemic mastocytosis? *Am J Clin Pathol.* 2004;122(4):560–565.
388. Reisberg IR, Oyakawa S. Mastocytosis with malabsorption, myelofibrosis, and massive ascites. *Am J Gastroenterol.* 1987;82(1):54–60.
389. Ammann RW, et al. Gastrointestinal involvement in systemic mastocytosis. *Gut.* 1976;17(2):107–112.
390. Bedeir A, et al. Systemic mastocytosis mimicking inflammatory bowel disease: a case report and discussion of gastrointestinal pathology in systemic mastocytosis. *Am J Surg Pathol.* 2006;30(11):1478–1482.
391. Braverman DZ, Dollberg L, Shiner M. Clinical, histological, and electron microscopic study of mast cell disease of the small bowel. *Am J Gastroenterol.* 1985;80(1):30–37.
392. Huang TY, Yam LT, Li CY. Radiological features of systemic mast-cell disease. *Br J Radiol.* 1987;60(716):765–770.
393. Mahood JM, et al. Forty years of diarrhoea in a patient with urticaria pigmentosa. *Acta Derm Venereol.* 1982;62(3):264–265.
394. Mutter RD, Tannenbaum M, Ultmann JE. Systemic Mast Cell Disease. *Ann Intern Med.* 1963;59:887–906.
395. Quinn SF, et al. Bull's-eye lesions: a new gastrointestinal presentation of mastocytosis. *Gastrointest Radiol.* 1984;9(1):13–15.
396. Hahn HP, Hornick JL. Immunoreactivity for CD25 in gastrointestinal mucosal mast cells is specific for systemic mastocytosis. *Am J Surg Pathol.* 2007;31(11):1669–1676.
397. Dantzig PI. Tetany, malabsorption, and mastocytosis. *Arch Intern Med.* 1975;135(11):1514–1518.
398. Debray C, et al. Gastrointestinal mastocytosis. Report of a case and review of the literature. *Arch Fr Mal App Dig.* 1973;62(5):411–417.
399. Bank S, Marks IN. Malabsorption in Systemic Mast Cell Disease. *Gastroenterology.* 1963;45:535–549.
400. Garcia-Montero AC, et al. KIT mutation in mast cells and other bone marrow hematopoietic cell lineages in systemic mast cell disorders: a prospective study of the Spanish Network on Mastocytosis (REMA) in a series of 113 patients. *Blood.* 2006;108(7):2366–2372.
401. Long E, et al. Intestinal occlusion caused by Rosai-Dorfman disease mimicking colonic diverticulitis. *Pathol Res Pract.* 2007;203(4):233–237.
402. Lauwers GY, et al. The digestive system manifestations of Rosai-Dorfman disease (sinus histiocytosis with massive lymphadenopathy): review of 11 cases. *Hum Pathol.* 2000;31(3):380–385.
403. Alatassi H, et al. Rosai-Dorfman disease of the gastrointestinal tract: report of a case and review of the literature. *Int J Surg Pathol.* 2006;14(1):95–99.
404. Buss DH, Stuart JJ, Lipscomb GE. The incidence of thrombotic and hemorrhagic disorders in association with extreme thrombocytosis: an analysis of 129 cases. *Am J Hematol.* 1985;20(4):365–372.
405. Davis RB. Acute thrombotic complications of myeloproliferative disorders in young adults. *Am J Clin Pathol.* 1985;84(2):180–185.
406. Glenner GG. Amyloid deposits and amyloidosis: the beta-fibrilloses (second of two parts). *N Engl J Med.* 1980;302(24):1333–1343.
407. Ebert EC, Nagar M. Gastrointestinal manifestations of amyloidosis. *Am J Gastroenterol.* 2008;103(3):776–787.
408. Petre S, Shah IA, Gilani N. Review article: gastrointestinal amyloidosis—clinical features, diagnosis and therapy. *Aliment Pharmacol Therap.* 2008;27(11):1006–1016.
409. Friedman S, Janowitz HD. Systemic amyloidosis and the gastrointestinal tract. *Gastroenterol Clin North Am.* 27(3):595–614.
410. Kisslevsky R. Amyloidosis: a familiar problem in the light of current pathogenic developments. *Lab Invest.* 1983;(49):381–390.
411. Yoshimatsu S, et al. Endoscopic and pathological manifestations of the gastrointestinal tract in familial amyloidotic polyneuropathy type I (Met30). *J Intern Med.* 1998;243(1):65–72.
412. Vernon SE. Amyloid colitis. *Dis Colon Rectum.* 1982;25(7):728–730.
413. Kaiserling E, Krober S. Massive intestinal hemorrhage associated with intestinal amyloidosis. An investigation of underlying pathologic processes. *Gen Diagn Pathol.* 1995;141(2):147–154.
414. Diaz Candamio MJ, Pombo F, Yebra MT. Amyloidosis presenting as a perforated giant colonic diverticulum. *Eur Radiol.* 1999;9(4):715–718.
415. Kumar SS, et al. Amyloidosis of the colon. Report of a case and review of the literature. *Dis Colon Rectum.* 1983;26(8):541–544.
416. Shimizu S, et al. A case of primary amyloidosis confined to the small intestine. *Gastroenterol Jpn.* 1986;21(5):513–517.
417. Bjornsson S, Johannsson JH, Sigurjonsson F. Localized primary amyloidosis of the stomach presenting with gastric hemorrhage. *Acta Med Scand.* 1987;221(1):115–119.
418. Garcia-Gonzalez R, et al. Amyloidosis of the rectum mimicking collagenous colitis. *Pathol Res Pract.* 1998;194(10):731–735.
419. Pettersson T, Konttinen YT. Amyloidosis-recent developments. *Semin Arthritis Rheum.* 2010;39(5):356–368.
420. Kyle RA, Greipp PR. Amyloidosis (AL). Clinical and laboratory features in 229 cases. *Mayo Clin Proc.* 1983;58(10):665–683.
421. Yamada M, Hatakeyama S, Tsukagoshi H. Gastrointestinal amyloid deposition in AL (primary or myeloma-associated) and AA (secondary) amyloidosis: diagnostic value of gastric biopsy. *Hum Pathol.* 1985;16(12):1206–1211.
422. Zarate YA, Hopkin RJ. Fabry's disease. *Lancet.* 2008;372(9647):1427–1435.
423. Peters FP, et al. Fabry's disease: a multidisciplinary disorder. *Postgrad Med J.* 1997;73(865):710–712.
424. Bryan A, Knauft RF, Burns WA. Small bowel perforation in Fabry's disease. *Ann Intern Med.* 1977;86(3):315–316.
425. O'Brien BD, et al. Pathophysiologic and ultrastructural basis for intestinal symptoms in Fabry's disease. *Gastroenterology.* 1982;82(5 pt 1):957–962.
426. Hoffmann B, Keshav S. Gastrointestinal symptoms in Fabry disease: everything is possible, including treatment. *Acta Paediatr Suppl.* 2007;96(455):84–86.
427. Banikazemi M, Ullman T, Desnick RJ. Gastrointestinal manifestations of Fabry disease: clinical response to enzyme replacement therapy. *Mol Genet Metab.* 2005;85(4):255–259.
428. Kaye EM, et al. Nervous system involvement in Fabry's disease: clinicopathological and biochemical correlation. *Ann Neurol.* 1988;23(5):505–509.
429. Malloy MJ, Kane JP. Hypolipidemia. *Med Clin North Am.* 1982;66(2):469–484.

430. Iatan I, et al. Effect of ABCA1 mutations on risk for myocardial infarction. *Curr Atheroscler Rep.* 2008;10(5):413–426.
431. Tarao K, et al. Japanese adult siblings with Tangier disease and statistical analysis of reported cases. *Tokai J Exp Clin Med.* 1984;9(5–6):379–387.
432. Dechelotte P, et al. Tangier disease. A histological and ultrastructural study. *Pathol Res Pract.* 1985;180(4):424–430.
433. Bektas M, et al. An unusual presentation of Tangier disease with gallbladder involvement. *Acta Gastroenterol Belg.* 2008;71(4):397–400.
434. Boldrini R, et al. Wolman disease and cholesteryl ester storage disease diagnosed by histological and ultrastructural examination of intestinal and liver biopsy. *Pathol Res Pract.* 2004;200(3):231–240.
435. Vahid B, et al. Sarcoidosis of gastrointestinal tract: a rare disease. *Dig Dis Sci.* 2007;52(12):3316–3320.
436. Friedman M, Ali MA, Borum ML. Gastric sarcoidosis: a case report and review of the literature. *South Med J.* 2007;100(3):301–303.
437. Ebert EC, Kierson M, Hagspiel KD. Gastrointestinal and hepatic manifestations of sarcoidosis. *Am J Gastroenterol.* 2008;103(12):3184–3192; quiz 3193.
438. Ricker W, Clark M. Sarcoidosis; a clinicopathologic review of 300 cases, including 22 autopsies. *Am J Clin Pathol.* 1949;19(8):725–749.
439. Longcope WT, Freiman DG. A study of sarcoidosis; based on a combined investigation of 160 cases including 30 autopsies from The Johns Hopkins Hospital and Massachusetts General Hospital. *Medicine (Baltimore).* 1952;31(1):1–132.
440. Engle RL Jr. Sarcoid and sarcoid-like granulomas; a study of twenty-seven post-mortem examinations. *Am J Pathol.* 1953;29(1):53–69.
441. Mayock RL, et al. Manifestations of sarcoidosis. analysis of 145 patients, with a review of nine series selected from the literature. *Am J Med.* 1963;35:67–89.
442. Branson JH, Park JH. Sarcoidosishepatic involvement: presentation of a case with fatal liver involvement; including autopsy findings and review of the evidence for sarcoid involvement of the liver as found in the literature. *Ann Intern Med.* 1954;40(1):111–145.
443. Palmer ED, Note on silent sarcoidosis of the gastric mucosa. *J Lab Clin Med.* 1958;52(2):231–234.
444. Iwai K, et al. Sarcoidosis autopsies in Japan. Frequency and trend in the last 28 years. *Sarcoidosis.* 1988;5(1):60–65.
445. Ebert EC, et al. Gastrointestinal and hepatic manifestations of sarcoidosis. *Am J Gastroenterol.* 2008;103(12):3184–3192; quiz 3193.
446. Ona FV. Gastric sarcoid: unusual cause of upper gastrointestinal hemorrhage. *Am J Gastroenterol.* 1981;75(4):286–288.
447. Chinitz MA, et al. Symptomatic sarcoidosis of the stomach. *Digest Dis Sci.* 1985;30(7):682–688.
448. Popovic OS, et al. Sarcoidosis and protein losing enteropathy. *Gastroenterology.* 1980;78(1):119–125.
449. Sprague R, et al. Disseminated gastrointestinal sarcoidosis. Case report and review of the literature. *Gastroenterology.* 1984;87(2):421–425.
450. Rauf A, Davis P, Levendoglu H. Sarcoidosis of the small intestine [see comment]. *Am J Gastroenterol.* 1988;83(2):187–189.
451. Bellan L, Semelka R, Warren CP. Sarcoidosis as a cause of linitis plastica. *Can Assoc Radiol J.* 1988;39(1):72–74.
452. Tukiainen H, et al. Granulomatous gastritis as a diagnostic problem between sarcoidosis and other granulomatous disorders. *Sarcoidosis.* 1988;5(1):66–67.
453. Newburger PE. Disorders of neutrophil number and function. *Hematology Am Soc Hematol Educ Prog.* 2006; 104–110.
454. Werlin SL, et al. Colitis in chronic granulomatous disease. *Gastroenterology.* 1982;82(2):328–331.
455. Foster CB, et al. Host defense molecule polymorphisms influence the risk for immune-mediated complications in chronic granulomatous disease. *J Clin Invest.* 1998; 102(12):2146–2155.
456. Marks DJ, et al. Inflammatory bowel disease in CGD reproduces the clinicopathological features of Crohn's disease. *Am J Gastroenterol.* 2009;104(1):117–124.
457. Yantiss RK, Clement PB, Young RH. Endometriosis of the intestinal tract: a study of 44 cases of a disease that may cause diverse challenges in clinical and pathologic evaluation. *Am J Surg Pathol.* 2001;25(4):445–454.
458. De Ceglie A, et al. Acute small bowel obstruction caused by endometriosis: a case report and review of the literature. *World J Gastroenterol.* 2008;14(21):3430–3434.
459. Garg NK, et al. Intestinal endometriosis—A rare cause of colonic perforation. *World J Gastroenterol.* 2009;15(5): 612–614.
460. Ijaz S, et al. Intussusception of the appendix secondary to endometriosis: a case report. *J Med Case Rep.* 2008;2:12.
461. Mann WJ, et al. Endometriosis associated with appendiceal intussusception. A report of two cases. *J Reprod Med.* 1984;29(8):625–629.
462. Midorikawa Y, et al. Endometriosis of the rectum causing bowel obstruction: a case report. *Hepatogastroenterology.* 1997;44(15):706–709.
463. Shaw A, et al. Large bowel obstruction and perforation secondary to endometriosis complicated by a ventriculoperitoneal shunt. *Colorectal Dis.* 2008;10(5):520–521.
464. Urbach DR, et al. Bowel resection for intestinal endometriosis. *Dis Colon Rectum.* 1998;41(9):1158–1164.
465. Wynn TE. Endometriosis of the sigmoid colon. Massive intramural hematoma. *Arch Pathol Lab Med.* 1971;92(1): 24–27.
466. Azzena A, et al. Rectosigmoid endometriosis: diagnosis and surgical management. *Clin Exp Obstetr Gynecol.* 1998; 25(3):94–96.
467. Cameron IC, et al. Intestinal endometriosis: presentation, investigation, and surgical management. *Int J Colorectal Dis.* 1995;10(2):83–86.
468. Slack A, et al. Urological and colorectal complications following surgery for rectovaginal endometriosis. *BJOG.* 2007;114(10):1278–1282.
469. Insabato L, Pettinato G. Endometriosis of the bowel with lymph node involvement. A report of three cases and review of the literature. *Pathol Res Pract.* 1996;192(9): 957–961; discussion 962.
470. Leiserowitz GS, et al. Endometriosis-related malignancies. *Int J Gynecol Cancer.* 2003;13(4):466–471.
471. Mourra N, et al. Endometrial stromal sarcoma of the rectosigmoid colon arising in extragonadal endometriosis and revealed by portal vein thrombosis. *Arch Pathol Lab Med.* 2001;125(8):1088–1090.
472. Hegyi J, Schwartz RA, Hegyi V. Pellagra: dermatitis, dementia, and diarrhea. *Int J Dermatol.* 2004;43(1):1–5.
473. Karthikeyan K, Thappa DM. Pellagra and skin. *Int J Dermatol.* 2002;41(8):476–481.
474. Segal I, et al. Rectal manifestations of pellagra. *Int J Colorectal Dis.* 1986;1(4):238–243.
475. Spivak JL, Jackson DL. Pellagra: an analysis of 18 patients and a review of the literature. *Johns Hopkins Med J.* 1977; 140(6):295–309.

476. Cook GC. D-xylose absorption and jejunal morphology in African patients with pellagra (niacin tryptophan deficiency). *Trans R Soc Trop Med Hyg.* 1976;70(4):349–351.
477. El-Shanti H, Majeed HA, El-Khateeb M. Familial mediterranean fever in Arabs. *Lancet.* 2006;367(9515):1016–1024.
478. Samuels J, Ozen S. Familial Mediterranean fever and the other autoinflammatory syndromes: evaluation of the patient with recurrent fever. *Curr Opin Rheumatol.* 2006;18(1):108–117.
479. Ciftci AO, et al. Adhesive small bowel obstruction caused by familial Mediterranean fever: the incidence and outcome. *J Pediatr Surg.* 1995;30(4):577–579.
480. Kavukcu S, et al. Renal, gastric and thyroidal amyloidosis due to familial Mediterranean fever. *Pediatr Nephrol.* 1997;11(2):210–212.
481. Meyerhoff J, Familial Mediterranean fever: report of a large family, review of the literature, and discussion of the frequency of amyloidosis. *Medicine.* 1980;59(1):66–77.
482. Sohar E, et al. Familial Mediterranean fever. A survey of 470 cases and review of the literature. *Am J Med.* 1967;43(2):227–253.
483. Zemer D, et al. Colchicine in the prevention and treatment of the amyloidosis of familial Mediterranean fever. *N Engl J Med.* 1986;314(16):1001–1005.
484. Fradkin A, et al. Colchicine enhances intestinal permeability in patients with familial Mediterranean fever. *Eur J Clin Pharmacol.* 1996;51(3–4):241–245.
485. Hart J, et al. Effect of long-term colchicine therapy on jejunal mucosa. *Digest Dis Sci.* 1993;38(11):2017–2021.
485a. Tunca M, et al. The efficacy of interferon alpha on colchicine-resistant familial Mediterranean fever attacks: a pilot study. *Br J Rheumatol.* 1997;36(9):1005–1008.
486. Abrams HL, Spiro R, Goldstein N. Metastases in carcinoma; analysis of 1000 autopsied cases. *Cancer.* 1950;3(1):74–85.
487. Ricaniadis N, et al. Gastrointestinal metastases from malignant melanoma. *Surg Oncol.* 1995;4(2):105–110.
488. Garwood RA, et al. A case and review of bowel perforation secondary to metastatic lung cancer. *Am Surg.* 2005;71(2):110–116.
489. Idelevich E, et al. Small bowel obstruction caused by secondary tumors. *Surg Oncol.* 2006;15(1):29–32.
490. Goldstein HM, Beydoun MT, Dodd GD. Radiologic spectrum of melanoma metastatic to the gastrointestinal tract. *Am J Roentgenol.* 1977;129(4):605–612.
491. Washington K, McDonagh D. Secondary tumors of the gastrointestinal tract: surgical pathologic findings and comparison with autopsy survey. *Mod Pathol.* 1995;8(4):427–433.

9. Esophagus: Normal Structures, Developmental Abnormalities, and Miscellaneous Disorders

Chapter Outline

STRUCTURE OF THE ESOPHAGUS
  Anatomy
  Histology
    Mucosa
    Submucosa and muscularis propria
ESOPHAGEAL FUNCTION
  Age-Dependent Changes
EMBRYOLOGY AND DEVELOPMENT OF THE ESOPHAGUS
DEVELOPMENTAL AND CONGENITAL ANOMALIES
  Esophageal Atresia and Tracheoesophageal Fistulas
  Bronchoesophageal Fistula
  Developmental and Congenital Cysts
    Duplication and congenital cysts
    Neurenteric cysts/remnants
    Bronchogenic cysts
    Other cysts
  Heterotopias
    Gastric heterotopia in the esophagus
    Other heterotopias

  Other Developmental Anomalies
    Congenital esophageal stenosis or stricture
    Short esophagus
    Pulmonary sequestrations
ESOPHAGEAL PERFORATION
  Spontaneous Rupture (Boerhaave's Syndrome)
    Pathogenesis and clinical features
    Pathology
  Nonspontaneous Rupture and Penetration
    Pathogenesis and clinical features
    Pathology
ESOPHAGEAL HEMORRHAGE
  Esophageal Tears (Mallory–Weiss Syndrome)
    Pathogenesis and clinical features
    Pathology
  Esophageal Varices
    Pathogenesis and clinical features
    Pathology

ESOPHAGEAL FISTULA
  Acquired Esophageal Stenosis or Stricture
    Esophageal webs and rings
DIVERTICULA AND PSEUDODIVERTICULA
  Upper Esophageal Diverticula (Zenker's)
    Pathogenesis and clinical features
    Pathology
  Mid- and Lower Esophageal Diverticula
    Pathogenesis and clinical features
    Pathology
  Atypical Esophageal Diverticula in Scleroderma
  Esophageal Intramural Pseudodiverticulosis/Retention Cysts
    Pathogenesis and clinical features
    Pathology
OTHER MISCELLANEOUS CONDITIONS
  Mucosal Bridge
  Glycogenic Acanthosis
  Esophageal Xanthelasma

STRUCTURE OF THE ESOPHAGUS

Anatomy

The esophagus is a muscular tube that is lined with stratified squamous epithelium. Its average length is about 11 cm in newborn and about 25 cm in adults. The upper boundary of the esophagus consists of cricopharyngeal muscle that forms the upper esophageal sphincter at the level of the sixth cervical vertebra. The esophagus enters the stomach at an oblique angle (angle of His) several centimeters below the diaphragm.

Endoscopists measure esophageal landmarks as the number of centimeters from the incisors. The upper esophageal sphincter is located 15 to 18 cm from the incisors. The gastroesophageal junction is classically described as being approximately 40 cm (range 37–42 cm) from the incisors, but this location varies considerably according to the individual's height and whether a hiatal hernia is present (Fig. 9-1). In the latter instance, the gastroesophageal junction is located, on average, 36 cm from the incisors; however, in a short person with a hiatal hernia, it may be located as little as 30 cm from the incisors.

The endoscopic determination of the location of the gastroesophageal junction is based on visualizing the zigzag ora serrata, known more popularly as the *Z-line*; this is the interface between the pearly, gray-white squamous epithelium of the esophagus and the pink-orange columnar epithelium of the stomach (Fig. 9-2). It straddles the region of the lower esophageal sphincter (LES), which appears endoscopically as an indented or contracted part of the distal esophagus. There may not be a strict correlation between the location of the LES zone and the histologic esophagogastric (squamocolumnar) mucosal

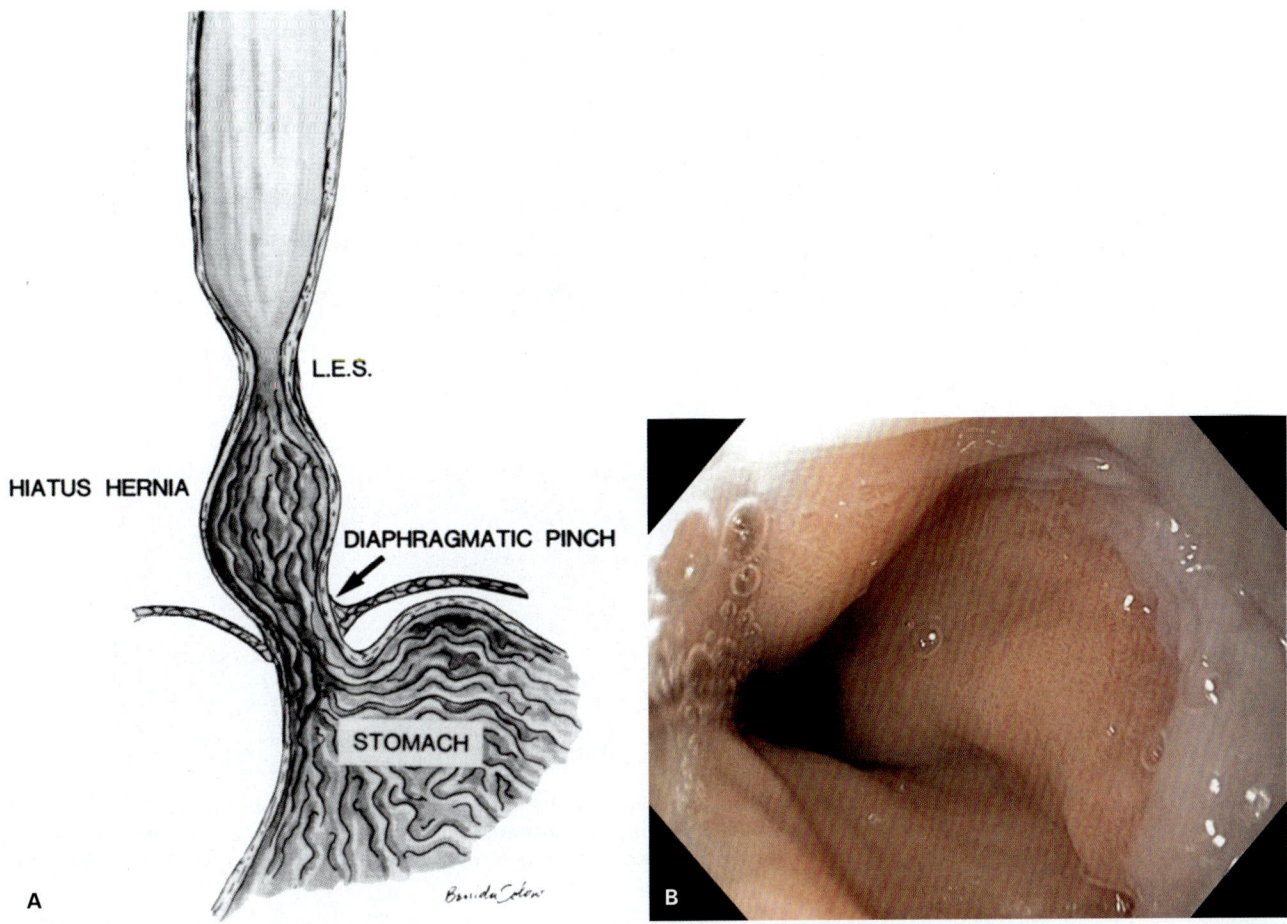

Figure 9-1. A: Sketch of the LES region and the proximal stomach. A hiatus hernia is present above the diaphragmatic pinch. **B:** Endoscopic view (prograde) of the squamocolumnar junction (Z-line). The distal end of the esophagus is defined as the proximal end of the gastric folds. The Z-line is almost straight with very few small indentations. (Courtesy of Steffen Muehldorfer, M.D.)

junction. This is reflected in the endoscopic appearance of the Z-line. Gastric mucosa may thus normally extend into the esophagus in this irregular (Z-line) fashion. Endoscopically the junction of tubular esophagus with the saccular stomach is defined by the upper border of convergence of the gastric folds, as neither the squamocolumnar junction nor the lower sphincter defined by manometry is considered reliable or accurate.

The blood supply to the esophagus is from the inferior thyroid artery in the upper segment; bronchial arteries, direct aortic branches, accessory branch of subclavian artery, and sometimes branches from the intercostal arteries in the midsegment; and the left gastric artery and the left phrenic artery in the distal segment. The venous drainage arises from intercommunicating plexuses that are both superficial and deep to the muscle coats. The upper third of the esophagus drains through the inferior thyroid veins into the superior vena cava. The middle third of the esophagus drains into the azygous system, and the lower third into gastric veins and ultimately into the portal vein.

The innervation of the esophagus is from both the vagus nerve and the sympathetic nervous system. Most of the esophageal musculature is supplied from the vagus nerve. Its fibers anastomose with short postganglionic fibers in the myenteric (Auerbach's) plexuses. The sympathetic fibers to the esophagus are derived from cervical and thoracic sympathetic ganglia. As is true throughout the gastrointestinal (GI) tract, regulatory peptides interact with neural and muscle elements in the control of normal function.[1]

The mucosal and submucosal lymphatics communicate with longitudinal lymphatic channels in the muscle coats. The upper third of the esophagus drains into the cervical nodes, the middle third into the paraesophageal and paratracheal nodes of the mediastinum, and the lower third into the para-aortic nodes, nodes in the celiac axis, or both.

Histology

Mucosa. The mucosal lining consists of stratified squamous epithelium of the nonkeratinized type (Fig. 9-3). Occasionally, keratohyalin particles are present, although a well-developed granular cell layer is absent, which differentiates it from the squamous

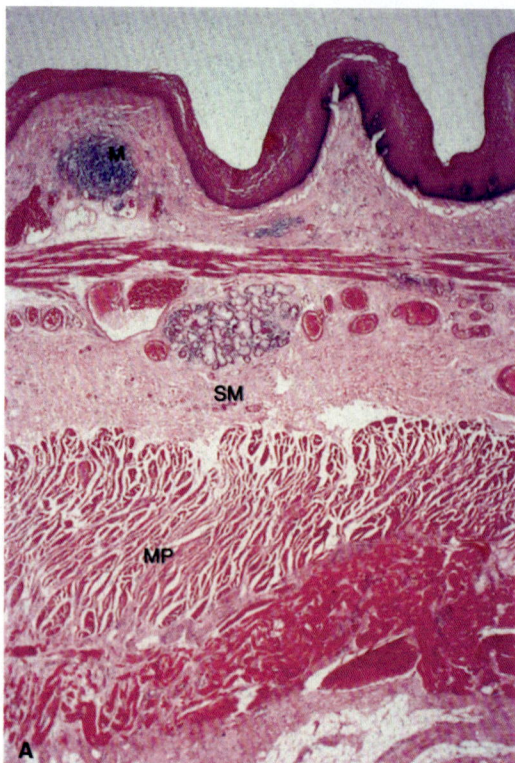 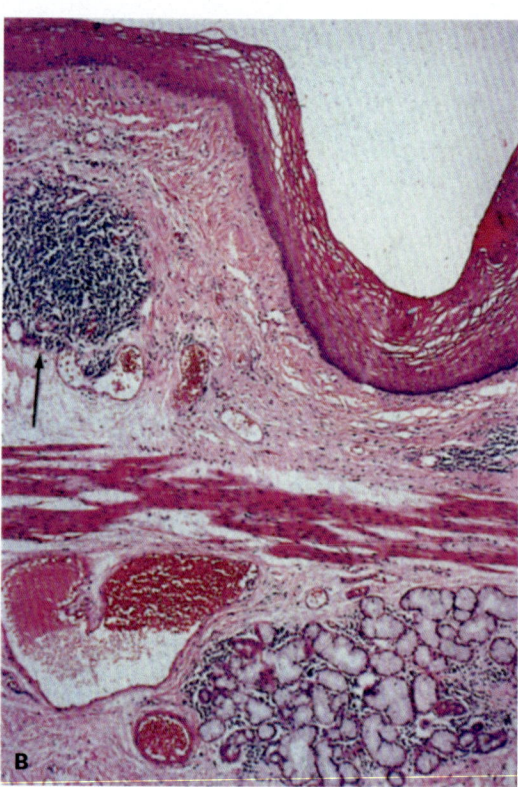

Figure 9-2. Normal histology of the esophagus. **A:** Low-power view showing the mucosa (M), the submucosa (SM), and the two layers of the muscularis propria (MP). **B:** High-power view showing that scattered lymphoid aggregates are normally found in the lamina propria (*arrow*) and that mucous glands are located in the submucosa (proper esophageal glands) (G), here just below the muscularis mucosae.

epithelium of skin. With electron microscopy the cell layers have been characterized as basal, prickle, and functional, the last referring to the flattened surface cells.[2] The epithelium is generally 15 cell layer thick (350–450 μm). In clinical practice, one need to only distinguish between the basal and overlying nonbasal cells. The basal cell zone is one to four cells thick and does not exceed 15% of the thickness of the squamous layer except in the most distal centimeters of the esophagus.[3,4] The cells above the basal zone contain flattened nuclei and a glycogen-rich cytoplasm. The cells at the surface are elongated, with a very narrow margin of cytoplasm surrounding pyknotic-appearing nuclei. Basal cells are distinguished from nonbasal cells by the fact that the former do not contain glycogen. In clinical practice, using conventionally stained sections, basal cells appear juxtaposed. One rule of thumb used to define the upper margin of the basal layer is to determine where nuclei are separated by a distance of at least one nuclear diameter.[5] Sometimes the tongues of columnar mucosa of the gastric type normally extend several centimeters on either side of the apparent LES zone. In addition, glands similar to those of the gastric cardia, with mucous glands and scattered fundic gland elements, commonly extend up into the lamina propria of the esophagus for a short distance.

Mitoses can be observed in the parabasal cell layer and are associated with increased proliferative activity. No mitoses are detected in the basal cell layer, and presumably the cells move higher up once they enter mitotic cycle. The exact time for cells to move from basal zone to surface for shedding is believed to be <10 days, while in mice and rats this is between 4 and 7 days.

Melanocytes have also been described in some esophagi.[6] Melanocytes are believed to occur in between 4% and 8% of esophagi. The latter are likely relevant to the rare primary malignant melanomas of the esophagus (see Chapter 12), in which *melanosis* may surround the neoplasms.[7] The number of melanocytes seems to be increased in many esophageal resections (27%–34%) performed for squamous cell carcinoma for yet unclear reasons. *Pseudomelanosis* of the esophagus has been reported, but the cause is still unknown.[8]

Endocrine cells can be observed in the esophageal epithelium as well. The incidence is reported to be about 28%. Mostly these cells are found in the basal cell layer of squamous epithelium. There is an ongoing discussion whether these cells contribute to the regulation of esophageal sphincters. Langerhans cells are also present in the esophageal squamous epithelium that can be highlighted with S100 and CD1a immunostains. Their function is likely to be antigen presentation similar to their role in skin, and their

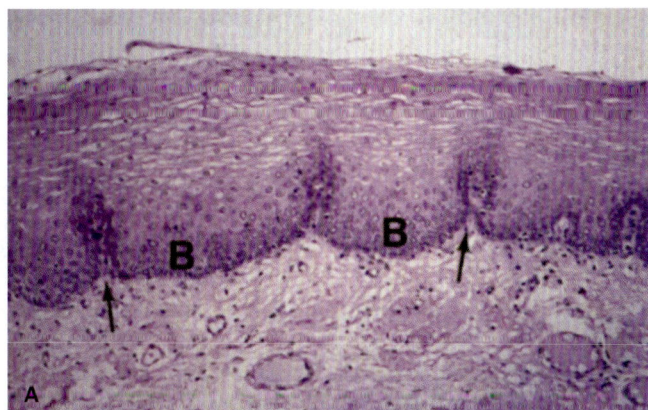
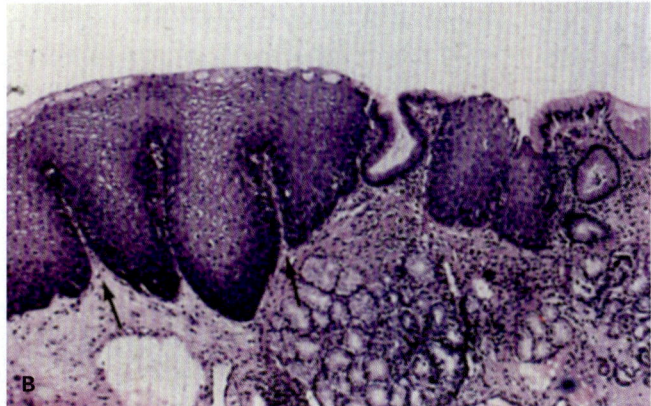
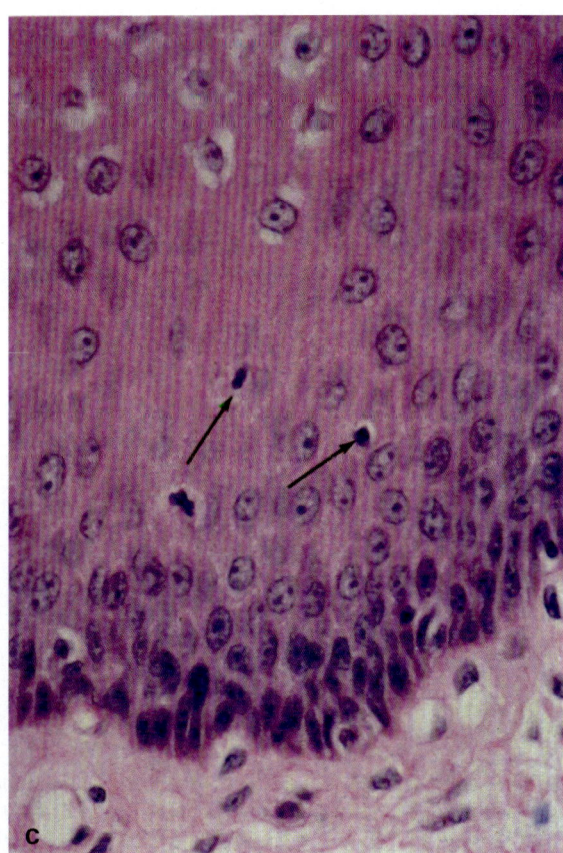

Figure 9-3. **A:** Normal squamous epithelium with a thin basal cell zone (B) and epithelial papillae (*arrows*) that extend upwards. **B:** Biopsy specimen from the gastroesophageal junction. Epithelial papillae close to the Z-line are believed to be more elongated physiologically compared to the upper esophagus. The squamocolumnar junction is rarely abrupt, as illustrated by the alternating columnar and squamous epithelium in the right half of the photograph. The mucous glands (G) in the lamina propria are believed to represent a sign that the biopsy was taken from the esophagus but are almost indistinguishable from cardiac glands. **C:** Detail of the basal cell zone; the *arrows* point to mononuclear cells. Sometimes fragments of these cells (squiggle cells) give a false impression of neutrophils.

number seems to increase in esophagitis. Merkel cells are also found in the esophageal mucosa.[9] Compared to fetuses their numbers are slightly increased in adults (1.2/cm vs. 2.2/cm). The numbers of Merkel cells vary markedly among individuals (Fig. 9-4). Immunohistochemically Merkel cells are positive for CK20. Merkel cells with their long dendritic processes can be identified from the 13th week of gestation onward. They are associated with light touch and in the skin can discriminate shape and textures, but it is unclear if they can do this in the esophagus.

Lymphocytes may be scattered throughout the squamous cell layer, interspersed between epithelial cells. Their nuclei may be compressed (squiggle cells) or lobulated and thus may be mistaken for neutrophils (Fig. 9-5A). Some tiny cell fragments in the epithelium may defy identification of their origin. Immunocytochemical studies show that these are mostly T lymphocytes[10] and are CD8 immunoreactive. Intraepithelial mast cells and B cells can also be found.[11]

The basal cell zone is invaginated by extensions of the lamina propria termed *dermal papillae* (see Fig. 9-3B). They generally do not extend more than two-thirds of the thickness of the epithelium, except in the distal 2 to 3 cm of the esophagus.[3,4] These papillae contain narrow capillaries; sometimes they are engorged with erythrocytes.

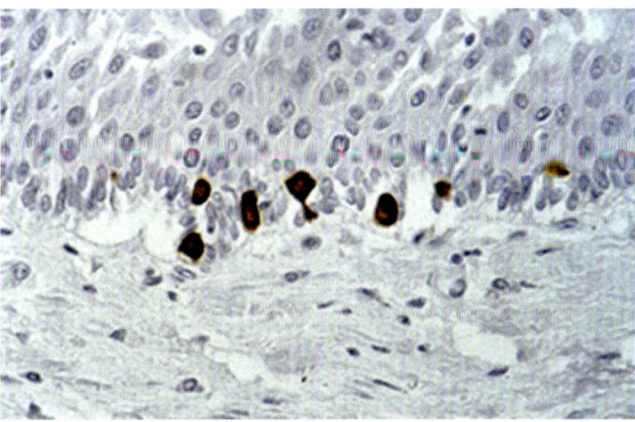

Figure 9-4. Esophageal Merkel cells in the basal layer demonstrated with a CK20 immunostain. (Courtesy of Tilman Schulz, M.D.). These cells likely develop in *situ* in mammals and do not migrate in, but their precise function in the esophagus remains unclear.

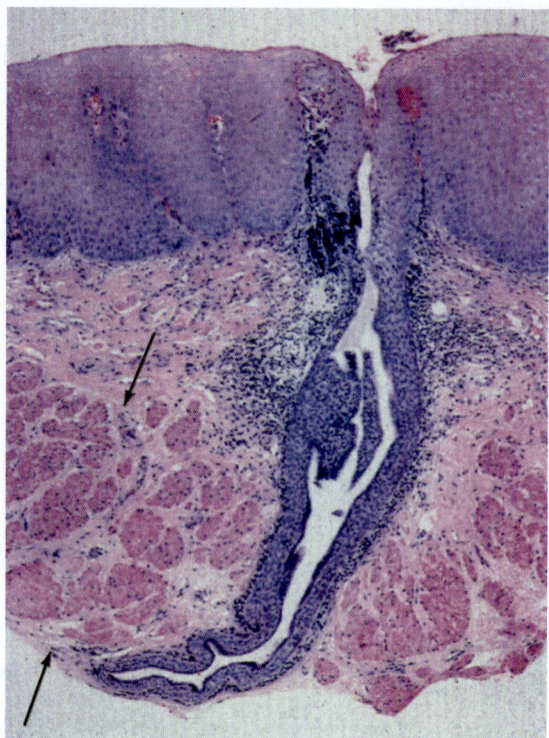

Figure 9-5. Mucosal biopsy specimen of the esophagus illustrating that the muscularis mucosae (*arrows*) may normally be thickened to the point where the unwary may mistakenly interpret this as muscularis propria. Also seen is a squamous duct from a submucosal gland penetrating the muscularis mucosae and opening onto the luminal surface of the esophagus. These ducts are commonly cuffed by mononuclear cells.

The lamina propria consists of connective tissue, which contains scattered plasma cells and occasional lymphoid nodules (see Fig. 9-3B). Sparsely distributed mucous glands are present in the lamina propria of the distal esophagus. These have been termed *esophageal cardiac glands*. Near the gastroesophageal junction, these glands may contain oxyntic mucosa glands, such as parietal cells.[12]

The muscularis mucosae become progressively thicker in the distal part of the esophagus. In biopsy specimens, the unwary morphologist may make the frightening mistake of confusing the thick muscularis mucosae for the muscularis propria (Fig. 9-5). The muscularis mucosa is particularly thick in cases of Barrett's associated distal esophageal or GE junction cancers and can form multiple layers (duplication of muscularis mucosa).[13,14]

Submucosa and muscularis propria. The submucosa consists of loose connective tissue containing blood vessels, nerve fibers, scattered lymphocytes, and small lymphoid follicles. Ganglion cells of Meissner's submucosal plexus are very sparse in the esophagus. Submucosal esophageal mucous glands are distributed throughout the esophagus (Fig. 9-3B). Ducts from these glands penetrate the muscularis mucosae and end in the epithelium. The ducts are covered with a cuboidal epithelium and then by a stratified epithelium in their terminal parts (Fig. 9-5).[15] Focal cystic dilatation of these ducts and glands and surrounding lymphoid collections may be seen in some autopsy specimens of "normal" esophagi.[16]

The muscle coats that lie outside the submucosa consist of striated muscle in the upper one-quarter to one-third of the esophagus and of smooth muscle in the lower two-thirds of the esophagus. Much of the striated muscle portion (except for the upper esophageal sphincter) is actually a blend of striated and smooth muscles.[17] Individual muscle fibers are arranged in a spiral fashion, with inner horizontally curved bands and outer bands with a more longitudinal orientation.[15,17] The ganglion cells of the myenteric plexus (Auerbach's) are more dense in the distal esophagus. The number of cells of Cajal is related to the plexus density. In achalasia cells of Cajal are more sparse.[18] Thus, it is proposed in the esophagus also that cells of Cajal are necessary for a neural-controlled motor function.[19,20]

The LES consists of a thickened zone of inner circular fibers in a spiral or oval arrangement. Some of these fibers blend with inner oblique muscle fibers of the stomach.[21,22] The esophagus lacks a serosa, except in the distal few centimeters.

ESOPHAGEAL FUNCTION

Food is transported through the esophagus into the stomach at a speed of about 2 to 4 cm/s by peristalsis. The gastroesophageal sphincter relaxes for few seconds before and after the passage of food. Repeated swallowing results in the relaxation of the sphincter for a longer period. During vomiting the LES relaxes and the gastric content is transported upward due to contractions of abdominal musculature and stomach. Numerous transmitters (prostaglandins, VIP, 5HT3, nitrogen oxide, dopaminergic and H2 receptors, gastrin, motilin, cholecystokinin, etc.) are responsible for the physiological motility of the esophagus and the sphincter activity.

Age-Dependent Changes

The data on age-dependent esophageal changes are very limited. It is known that the smooth musculature does not change with age, but in the elderly the number of ganglia in the Auerbach's plexus is reduced.[23] With age the esophageal lumen is believed to become wider, and the wall consistency and sensitivity to stretching are said to decrease.[24]

EMBRYOLOGY AND DEVELOPMENT OF THE ESOPHAGUS

Prenatal life is divided into embryonic (until 9 weeks) and fetal (9 weeks to birth) periods. Around 14th day the embryo develops into a bilaminar disk of ectoderm and endoderm (Fig. 9-6A). The endoderm forms the lining of the yolk sac and is the scaffold for the future GI tract. The mesoderm appears as the third layer around 15th day and gives rise to the connective tissue, vessels, smooth muscle, and serosal layers of the GI tract. Proliferation and segmentation of the mesoderm into somites that takes place between the endoderm and ectoderm induces numerous transformations in the endoderm. During this time the embryo continues to elongate craniocaudally and folds laterally. The embryo thus becomes a cylindrical tube lined with endoderm, which divides the yolk sac into intraembryonic and extraembryonic parts (Fig. 9-6). The intraembryonic part forms the GI tract and its accessory glands (pancreas, gall bladder, and liver). The extraembryonic part regresses and disappears around 12th week. At this point, based on the arterial supply the primitive digestive tube can be divided into foregut, midgut, and hindgut supplied by celiac, superior mesenteric, and inferior mesenteric arteries, respectively.

Development of the GI tract takes place in four axes: Anterior–posterior, dorsal–ventral, left–right, and craniocaudal. Development along each axis is based on the epithelial–mesenchymal interactions mediated by specific molecular pathways and growth factors such as Wnt5a (expressed by mesoderm), endodermal proteins Six2/Sox2, as well as Hoxa-2, Hoxa-3, and Hoxb-4, which control esophageal development in the anterior–posterior axis. These factors affect both the esophageal environment and the migration of the neural crest cells.

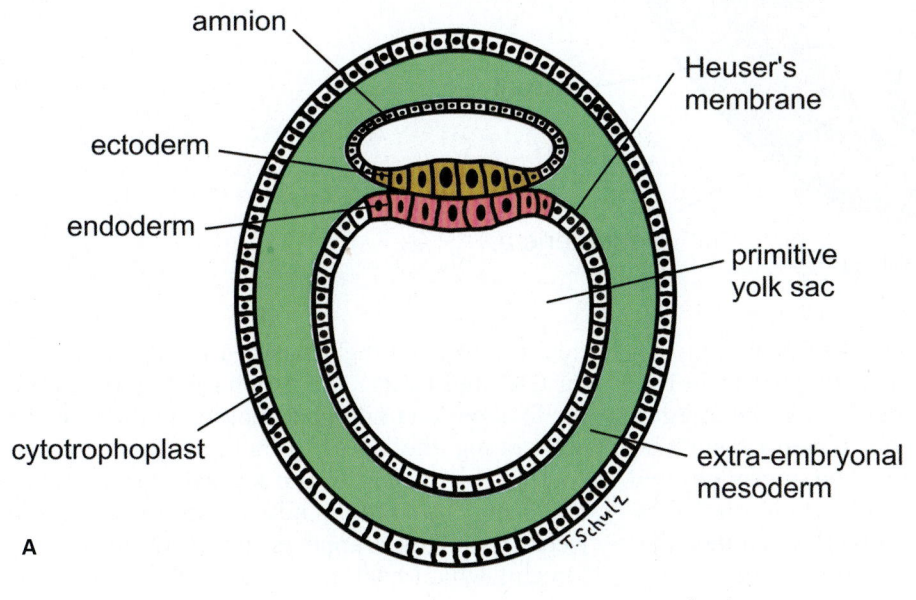
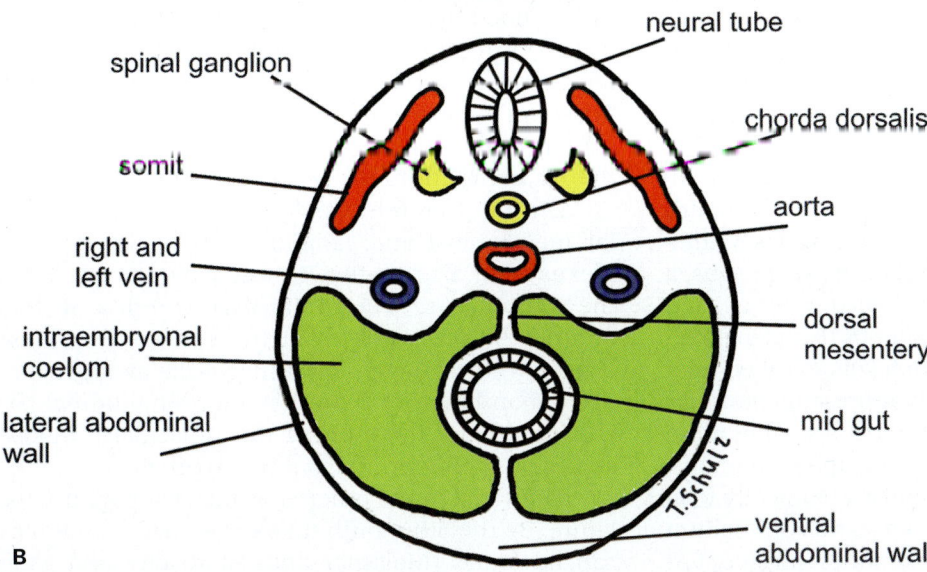

Figure 9-6. Schematic representation of the development of foregut, midgut, and hindgut in the embryo. A: Second week of gestation with development of ecto- and endoderm. B: Transversal cut of the embryo at 4th week of gestation displaying early embryological parenchyma development.

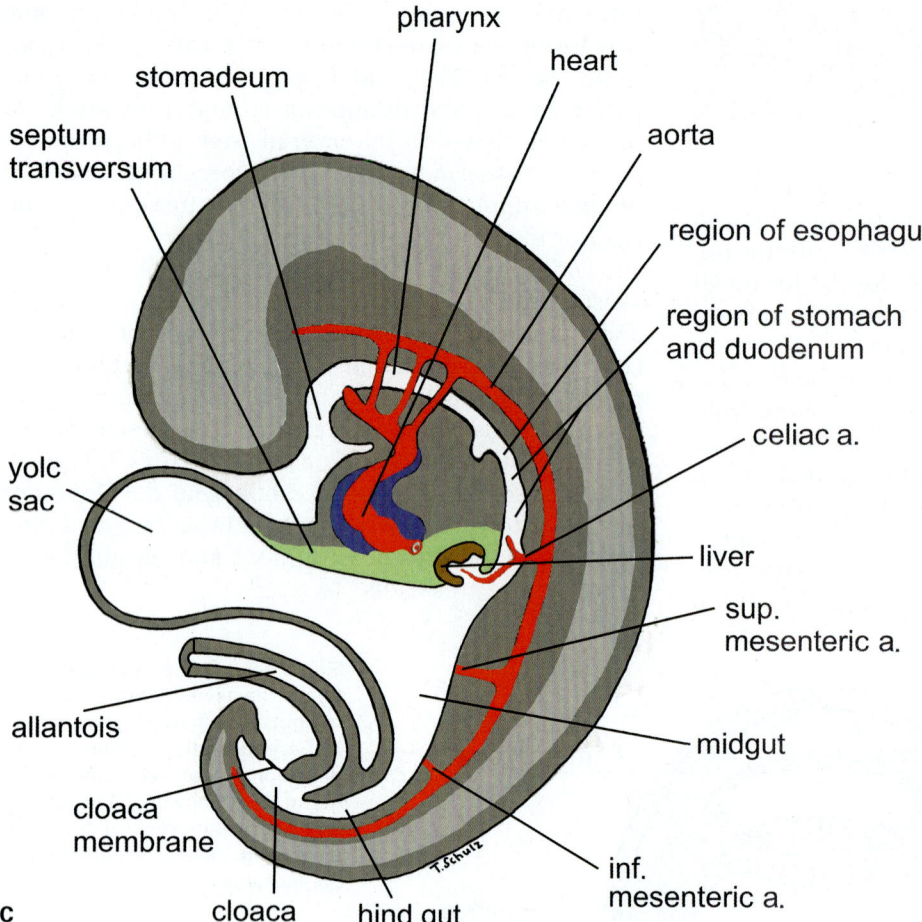

Figure 9-6. *(Continued)* **C:** Saggital cut of the embryo at 5th week of gestation showing various developing vascular structures and their relationship to the gut.

Between the 3rd and 4th weeks of gestation the esophagus becomes recognizable as distinct from the stomach and the pharynx. During week 4, the foregut develops a small diverticulum on its ventral surface adjacent to the pharyngeal gut. The mesenchyme between the esophagus and this diverticulum forms the esophagotracheal septum, which separates the esophagus from trachea during subsequent development. This tracheobronchial diverticulum subsequently elongates caudally and forms the primitive respiratory tract, including the lungs around 26th day.

The remaining part of the foregut rapidly elongates along with the craniocaudal growth of the embryo. Initially the esophagus is lined by ciliated columnar epithelium (Fig. 9-7), and during the 14th week to 4th month it starts getting replaced by stratified squamous epithelium starting from the middle third of the esophagus, a process that continues until birth.[25] Portions of ciliated columnar epithelium can persist after birth and even till adulthood.[26-28] In the proximal esophagus so-called inlet patches (gastric heterotopia) likely represent columnar mucosa that develops into gastric mucosa seen in more than 10% of all individuals undergoing upper GI endoscopy.[29] Histologically and immunohistochemically fetal esophageal epithelium differs from cardia-epithelium and gastric heterotopia in the proximal esophagus.[30] At this time it is strongly positive for CK19 and negative for CK7 and CK20. The esophageal epithelium during the fetal period undergoes marked proliferation, nearly obliterating the entire lumen. Unlike other species, complete occlusion of the foregut by this process has not been observed in human embryos. By the 10th week, vacuolation appears in the luminal cells of the foregut, which coalesce to form a central esophageal lumen lined by a superficial layer of ciliated epithelial cells. During the 4th month the longitudinal mucosal folds develop.[31] The primitive foregut endoderm is the origin for both the future esophageal epithelium and submucosal glands. Esophageal glands develop during the 7th month from the esophageal epithelium.

During the 6th week of gestation, the circular muscle coat and ganglion cells of the myenteric plexus form. During the 7th week, blood vessels enter the submucosa. The muscularis propria develops around the 6th week from the surrounding mesenchyme. Interestingly, the inner circular layer develops a month earlier than the outer longitudinal layer. During 4th to 7th months the muscularis mucosae start developing from distal to proximal.

The vagal nerve innervates the esophageal musculature. By the 5th month fully developed neural plexus can be found (Meissner and Auerbach), and ganglia

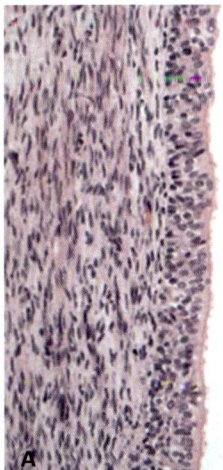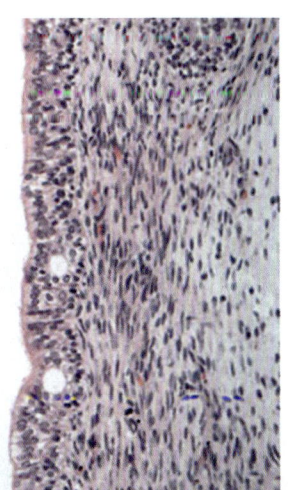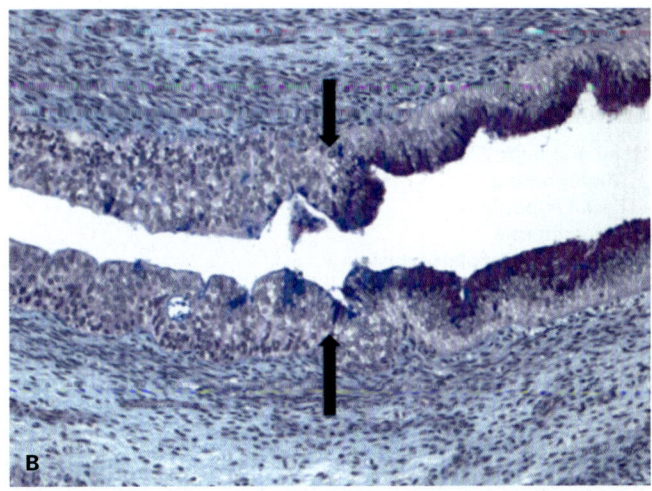

Figure 9-7. **A:** Histology of the early stages of esophageal development when it is lined by columnar epithelium. **B:** Embryonic gastroesophageal junction (PAS–AB stain). The *arrows* mark the junction between ciliated columnar epithelium-lined esophagus and mucus-secreting cells of the stomach. Few scattered mucin-secreting cells seem to be extending into the esophagus as well.

can also be identified by the 7th week.[25] From animal experiments it is known that interstitial cells of Cajal in the neural plexus and the circular muscle build networks for neural motor function. At time of birth it is concluded that neural networks are more mature in esophagus and stomach. Esophageal development of nerve and Cajal cell activity precede that in the remaining gut but have not achieved adult organization at time of birth. The timepoint of migration of Cajal cells into esophageal tissue is not yet known in detail. These findings explain that gut motility at birth does not show an adult pattern.[32] The smooth muscle of the lower esophagus and the LES is derived from the mesenchyme of the somites surrounding the foregut. The striated muscle in the muscularis propria of the upper part of the esophagus and the upper esophageal sphincter is derived from mesenchyme of the fourth, fifth, and sixth branchial arches. This explains the innervation of the upper esophageal sphincter by the vagal nerve (the nerve of fifth branchial arch) and by the recurrent laryngeal nerve (a branch of the vagus nerve and the nerve of sixth branchial arch). The embryologic origin of the gastroesophageal junction is still controversial, but gastric rotation, together with augmentation of the fundus of the stomach, is believed to determine its formation.

DEVELOPMENTAL AND CONGENITAL ANOMALIES

Esophageal Atresia and Tracheoesophageal Fistulas

Esophageal atresia along with tracheoesophageal fistula is the most frequent esophageal anomaly (1:3,000–5,000 births), although isolated esophageal atresia is quite rare.[33] It is unclear whether this results from lack of proper separation of foregut into respiratory and intestinal tracts by the growth of tracheoesophageal septum or improper recanalization of the esophagus following esophageal epithelial proliferation.[25] The use of teratogenic substances during pregnancy has been implicated in the development of esophageal atresia. Frequently additional anomalies involving other organ systems are also present (Table 9-1; Fig. 9-8).

Esophageal atresia occurs in five different forms (Table 9-2).[34,35] Unfortunately, the terminology in the literature is not consistent and many different classification schemes are in use resulting in some confusion (A–E, Type I–V, Type 1–5, Type I–IIIc). The most common variant is type C (Table 9-2) with a proximal blind esophageal pouch and a fistula between the trachea and the distal esophagus. The fistula often enters the trachea close to the carina. The second most common anomaly is type A—pure esophageal atresia without tracheoesophageal fistula.

The clinical presentation depends on the type of atresia and the presence of a tracheoesophageal fistula. Lack of swallowing and absorption of the amniotic fluid due to esophageal atresia result in polyhydramnios during pregnancy, which may be the first sign of the problem. When the proximal esophagus ends as a blind loop, drooling of saliva or recurrent vomiting in the neonatal period is the most common presentation. In the presence of a tracheoesophageal fistula the child is at risk of aspiration pneumonia and repeated respiratory infections. In addition, entry of air through tracheoesophageal fistula into the GI tract distal to the atretic segment results in overinflation seen on imaging. In contrast, cases that have no connection with the respiratory tract show absence of gas shadow on imaging. The diagnosis of so-called H-fistula can be very difficult, and some cases are

Table 9-1	Concomitant Anomalies in Individuals with Esophageal Atresia

Head and neck (5%)
  Micrognathia
  Facial hypoplasia
  Macrostomia
  Cheilognathopalatoschisis
  Microencephalopathy
  Midcerebellum agenesis
  Olfactory nerve agenesis
Upper airways and thorax (15%)
  Choanal stenosis
  Pharyngeal clefts
  Subglottic stenosis
  Bronchial stenosis
  Pulmonary agenesis
  Diaphragmatic hernia
Cardiovascular system (30%)
  Atrial and ventricular wall defects
  Coarctation of aorta, open
  Ductus of Botalli (patent ductus arteriosus)
  Peripheral pulmonary artery stenosis
  Patent foramen ovale
  Truncus arteriosus communis
  Transposition of great vessels
  Tetralogy of Fallot
  Ventricular hypoplasia
  Dextrocardia
Gastrointestinal tract (30%)
  Small bowel atresia
  Meckel's diverticulum
  Pancreas annulare
  Malrotation
  Bile duct atresia
  Anorectal atresia
Genitourinary tract (15%)
  Agenesia of kidney (single sided)
  Horse shoe kidney
  Multicystic kidneys
  Hydronephrosis
  Ureter duplex
  Urethra duplex
  Posterior urethral valves
  Epispadias and hypospadias
Skeleton and musculature (5%)
  Spine and rip anomalies
  Anomalies of extremities

Source: References[162–166].

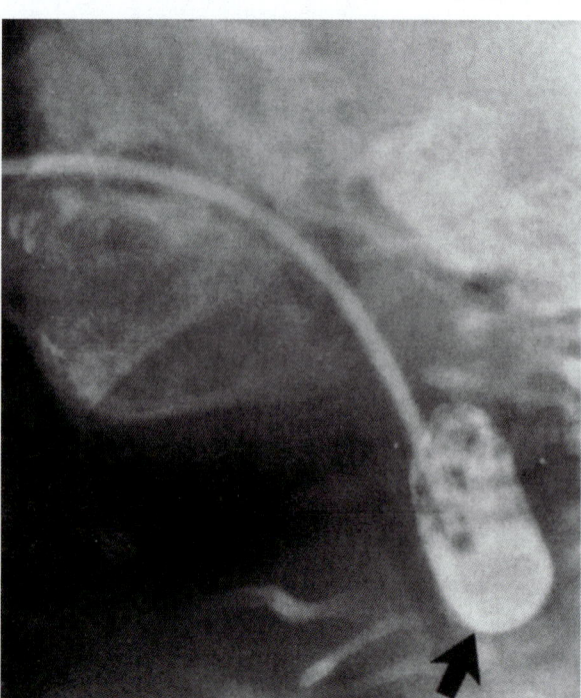

Figure 9-8. Esophageal atresia. Contrast placed via a tube fills the blind upper end of the esophagus. In this patient there was a distal tracheoesophageal fistula; see Figure 9-7, panel 1. (Courtesy of Marvin Weiner, M.D.)

birth weight, and wide distance between the atretic segments are believed to represent unfavorable factors. Sequelae following surgical correction include, for example, secondary stenosis, secondary fistula, dehiscence of sutures, stridor, and hiatal hernia.

Bronchoesophageal Fistula

Congenital bronchoesophageal fistulas are rare (<10%), and most lesions encountered in practice are acquired.[37] Esophageal atresia as discussed above is associated in some cases. Often the fistula is recognized for the first time during adulthood due to recurrent respiratory infections.[36]

The diagnosis is established using imaging studies with contrast (Fig. 9-9), although the exact type of fistula may not be established till the surgical correction is undertaken. The overall mortality of these patients has improved over the years, and the prognosis is largely dependent on the presence of other associated anomalies that occurs in up to 50% of affected individuals (see Table 9-1). Tracheomalacia with attendant tracheal collapse and respiratory complications is an additional source of morbidity. Early delivery, low

Table 9-2	The Different Types of Esophageal Atresia	
TYPE	ANOMALY	PERCENTAGE (%)
Type A	Isolated esophageal atresia	7.6
Type B	Esophageal atresia with proximal tracheoesophageal fistula	0.8
Type C	Esophageal atresia with distal tracheoesophageal fistula	86.5
Type D	Esophageal atresia with proximal and distal tracheoesophageal fistula	0.7
Type E	H-type tracheoesophageal fistula without esophageal atresia	4.4

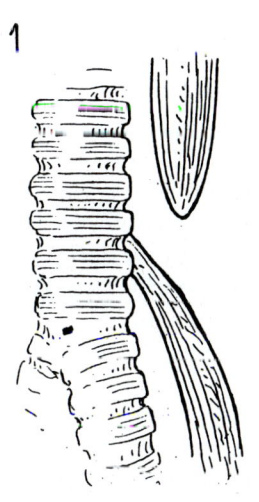
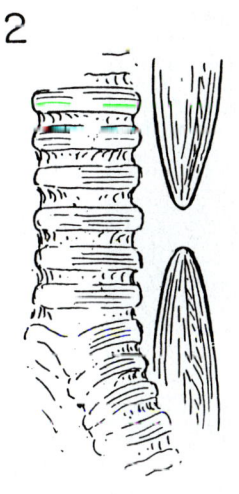
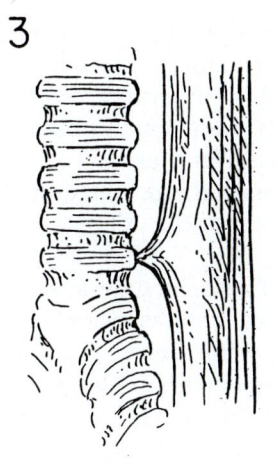
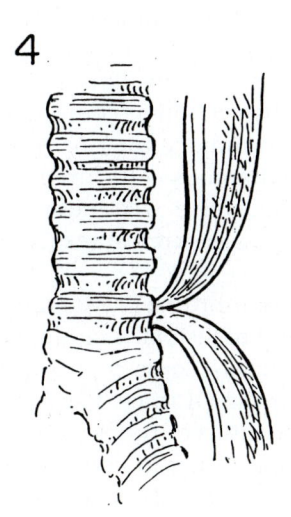
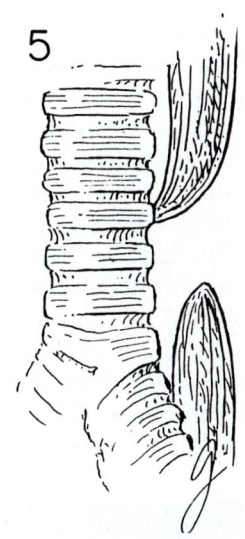

Figure 9-9. Various types of congenital tracheoesophageal fistulas and atresias. Approximately 85% are of the type illustrated in panel 1. Those represented in panels 4 and 5 are rare.

connected to the right main bronchus.[38] The fistulous tract may be lined by a squamous, respiratory, or a transitional-type epithelium.[39] Grossly several types of bronchoesophageal fistulas can be identified:

1. Short-segment fistulas between esophagus and a lobar or segmental bronchus
2. Fistula that is connected to a lung cyst
3. Fistula with a sequestration of lung that has aortic blood supply
4. Esophageal diverticulum with penetration into lung (acquired)

In adults it could be difficult to differentiate congenital from an acquired fistula. Congenital fistulas are believed to be identified on the basis of the following criteria: (a) lack of inflammatory reaction in the surrounding connective tissue at the point of resection, (b) lack of adhesion between fistula and adjacent lymph nodes, (c) lack of esophageal mucosa containing muscularis mucosae, and (d) lack of focal vascular inflammatory changes.

Acquired benign broncho- or tracheoesophageal fistulas are mostly secondary to either inflammatory causes, for example, tuberculosis, or are posttraumatic.[40] Acquired fistulas may also form secondary to infiltration by esophageal squamous cell carcinomas. Sometimes the etiology of the fistula remains unclear.

Developmental and Congenital Cysts

Duplication and congenital cysts. These represent a variety of confusing lesions, for which a wide variety of names have been used in the past, some of which include dorsal enteric cysts, enterogenous cysts, neurenteric cysts, giant diverticula, and persistent neurenteric canal. A simple classification would be to divide them into duplications, congenital enteric/esophageal cysts, and neurenteric cysts/remnants.

Duplications of the GI tract conceptually represent an extra copy or a replica of a GI segment that is often imperfect. General duplications have an organization similar to the gut with muscular wall, neural plexus, and a lining epithelium (either embryonic

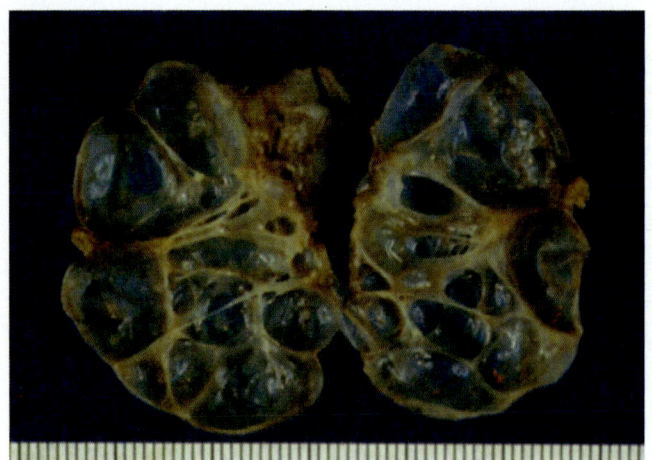

Figure 9-10. Gross appearance of reduplication of the esophagus.

or mature type typical for that site). These need not communicate with the lumen. The esophageal duplications can become cystic, and it then becomes difficult to differentiate them from other congenital cysts (see later), and currently there are no reliable criteria to differentiate between these. Most would agree that an esophageal duplication should be contiguous with esophagus and have smooth muscle layers (Figs. 9-10 and 9-11). Most often these cysts are not connected to the esophageal lumen and are partially intramural or attached to the wall. Those that are connected to the esophageal lumen could be considered as esophageal diverticula.[41-43] The lesions may become cystic or remain tubular. Histologically duplications show all the layers of the esophageal wall that include mucosa, muscularis mucosae, submucosa, and muscularis propria.[44] The lining epithelium could be nonkeratinizing squamous epithelium, pseudostratified ciliated respiratory epithelium, or simple flat cuboidal to columnar epithelium. Rarely gastric fundic-type mucosa may be present, and some cases fail to show any lining epithelium at all. Many of the cysts defy classification and show a variety of lining epithelium and a fibrous wall. Depending on the appearance and the lining epithelium, a variety of names are in use. Some that are lined by gastric[45] or small bowel-type epithelium[46] have also been described that are referred to as gastroenteric cysts, while others are simply referred to as congenital esophageal cysts. The congenital cysts have a predilection for the lower third of the esophagus and rarely involve the upper esophagus.[47]

These duplications and other cysts are usually asymptomatic and detected incidentally. However, they may result in a mass effect causing symptoms of obstruction or compression of adjacent structures like respiratory tract or heart. Rarely adenocarcinoma or squamous cell carcinoma can arise in these cysts.[48,49] Definitive treatment of duplications and congenital cysts is surgical resection.

Neurenteric cysts/remnants. These include a variety of lesions including diverticula, fistulas, cysts, and fibrous cords that originate from the dorsal midline of the GI tract. They are often associated with abnormalities of the vertebral column, spinal cord, or both. Many of the abnormalities are not compatible with life and only detected at autopsy. They can occur at any level but are most common at the cervicothoracic and lumbosacral areas. The walls of these structures are composed of the normal layers of the GI tract, and neuroglial tissues or less likely leptomeningeal tissues may be found in and around the lesions that are close to or involve the vertebra and spinal cord. The lining epithelium is variable and may be similar to the gut at that site or could be a mixture of different types.

Bronchogenic cysts. Bronchogenic cysts are often seen anteriorly and are often attached to a bronchus rather than esophagus. The lining epithelium is most often pseudostratified ciliated columnar and less commonly squamous, gastric, or intestinal type. The wall contains bronchial-type mucus glands and cartilage and lacks esophagus-like muscularis mucosae and muscularis propria.[44] Despite these differences differentiation from an esophageal duplication can be sometimes very difficult.

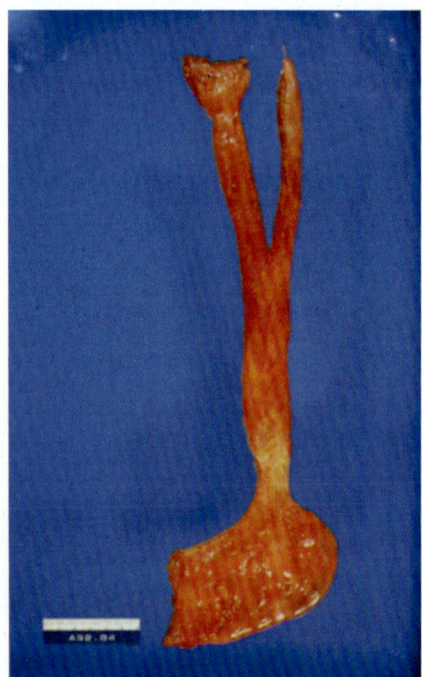

Figure 9-11. Gross appearance of a Y-shaped communicating duplication of the esophagus. A portion of the stomach is shown at the bottom of the picture.

Other cysts. These are the cysts that cannot be assigned to other specific categories.[44] The lining epithelium is variable, and the wall does not contain the GI wall structures or cartilage.

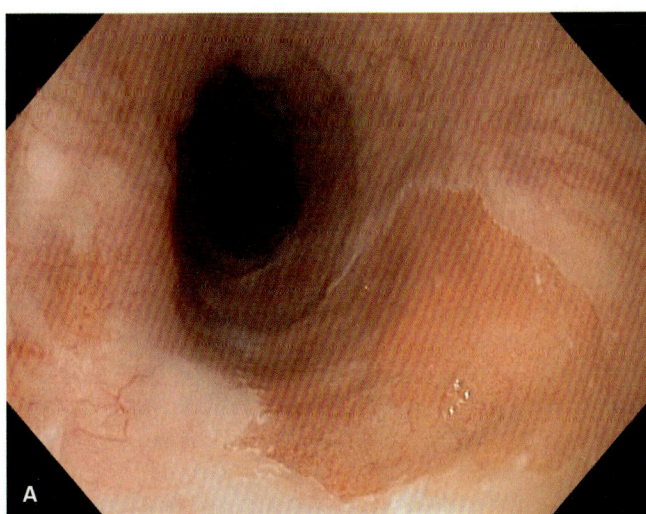
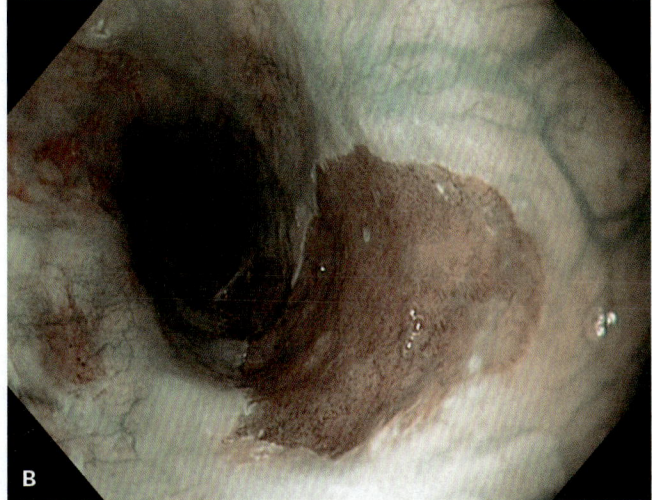
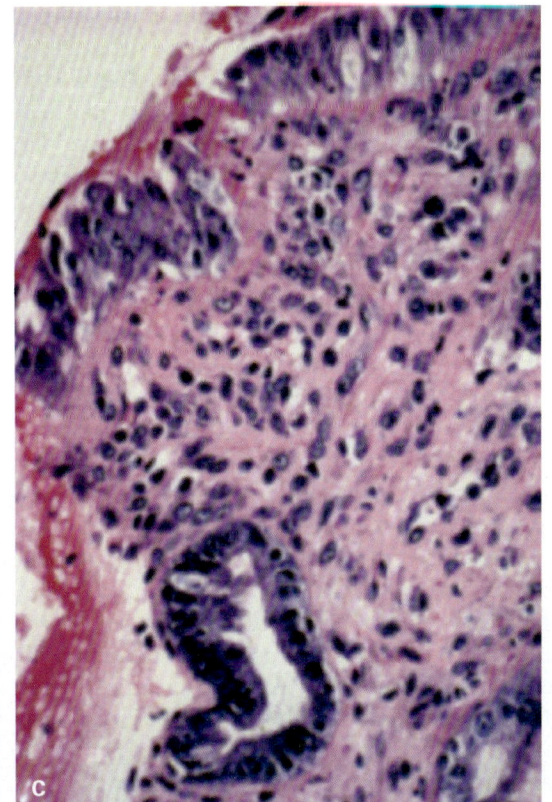
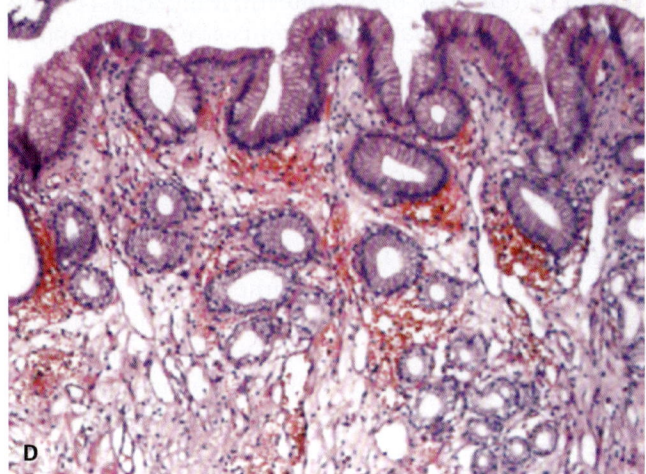

Figure 9-12. Gastric heterotopia. **A:** Endoscopic view of a pink patch of gastric mucosa just below the upper esophageal sphincter—an *inlet patch*. **B:** Same example as seen by narrow band imaging. **C:** Biopsy specimen from an inlet patch. The basophilic surface epithelium appears to be very reactive, with an underlying inflammatory reaction and a suggestion of fibrosis. **D:** Biopsy of an inlet patch from a different patient. Such type of (cardia or antrum-like) mucosa is mainly found at the transition to the adjacent squamous epithelium. The center often shows corpus-like mucosa (not shown here).

Heterotopias

Gastric heterotopia in the esophagus

Pathogenesis and Clinical Features For decades it has been known that heterotopic gastric tissue can occur anywhere between the mouth and the anus.[50] Interest in this condition has been rejuvenated because endoscopists have rediscovered it.[50-52] These tissue nests are easily missed at endoscopy because they are usually located in the proximal esophagus, within or just below the upper esophageal sphincter (Fig. 9-12), hence the colloquial term *inlet patch*.[52] So-called inlet patches can be observed in more than 10% of all upper GI endoscopies. The prevalence at endoscopy of about 4% may be an underestimate because of difficulty in endoscopically visualizing the mucosa within or just below the upper esophageal sphincter.[51] By contrast, the prevalence of 21% in an autopsy study of children is likely an overestimate because some of the subjects had other congenital anomalies, and there was an inverse relation with age up to 14 years. Perhaps some of these congenital nests are overgrown by squamous epithelium later in life.[53]

It should be stressed that despite a flurry of reports detailing complications of these nests, they are overwhelmingly incidental and do not require surveillance of any kind. Because they are capable of secreting acid, it is not surprising that they are rarely associated with burning sensations in the neck or with ulceration or cause strictures with resultant dysphagia.[54-57] Adenocarcinoma may arise in these ectopic patches but is rare.[58] Some carcinomas have been described as arising from heterotopic gastric patches further downstream in the esophagus.[58,59] When inlet patches are encountered, there is no indication for biopsy. However, it is difficult for many endoscopists to resist the urge to biopsy the first few they encounter.

Pathology The typical endoscopic appearance is that of a circular area of orange-pink mucosa standing out in stark contrast to the whitish squamous mucosa (Fig. 9-12A). Sometimes the patches are larger, exceeding the usual size of 1 to 2 cm. Circumferential involvement is very uncommon. The surface epithelium is of the gastric foveolar type, and the underlying glands are usually of the cardiofundic type, with variable amount of mucous glands (Fig. 9-12B) intermixed with fundic gland elements. In this regard, it is not uncommon to see parietal cells without distinct chief cells. In a minority of cases, there are only mucous glands, without any fundic gland elements. Some patients have variable amounts of mucosal inflammation, with a reactive surface epithelium (Fig. 9-12C). *Helicobacter pylori* infection may occur. Intestinal metaplasia may be seen and presumably represents a reaction to peptic or some other type of injury, as elsewhere in the stomach.[58] Gastrin and a few other peptides have been identified with immunohistochemical staining.[55] Intestinal metaplasia in a zone of gastric heterotopia should not be regarded as Barrett's esophagus.

Other heterotopias. The esophagus begins to change from ciliated to columnar epithelium in the 14th week.[60] Ciliated epithelium has been described in the esophagus of premature infants but not in those who live beyond 3 days.[61] The tracheobronchial remnants described in the next section on congenital stenosis may represent a variant of tracheoesophageal fistula.

Rarely heterotopic sebaceous glands, liver, pancreas, or thyroid tissue can be found in the esophagus.[62,63] Often with sebaceous gland heterotopia the duct of the glands is lined by squamous epithelium. Endoscopically this appears like a yellowish nodule. Rarely hair follicles may also be present (hairy esophagus). More often this condition is a sequela of pharyngoesophageal procedures.[64] The histology of the various heterotopic tissues is fairly typical, and the lesions seldom cause diagnostic difficulties.

Other Developmental Anomalies

Congenital esophageal stenosis or stricture. Congenital esophageal strictures are rare (1 in 25,000 births). The stenotic segment can be up to 1.5 cm in length. The stenosis may result from membranous diaphragm or web, postulated to be due to improper recanalization of the esophagus during the fetal period. This is most frequently seen in the middle third of the esophagus. Other congenital anomalies including tracheoesophageal fistula and atresias of the other segments of the GI tract are frequently seen. Other causes of esophageal stenosis include mural lesions that can compromise the lumen and include various types of heterotopic tissues, cartilaginous nodules suggestive of tracheobronchial remnants, or benign mesenchymal tumors (Table 9-3). Esophageal strictures due to tracheobronchial remnants tend to occur in the lower third of the esophagus. Rarely strictures can be caused by vascular anomalies. In children the tracheal system and in adults the esophagus tend to be more often affected.[65]

Short esophagus. This is also a very rare congenital anomaly of the esophagus that largely remains asymptomatic. The stomach pulled up in the thorax similar to a sliding-type of hiatal hernia. This part of the stomach is supplied by arterial branches from the descending aorta rather than the gastric artery, a feature that helps in differentiating this from a true sliding-type of hiatal hernia.[66]

Pulmonary sequestrations. In these anomalies, collections of lung tissue communicate with the lower end of the esophagus.[67,68] Pulmonary sequestrations

Table 9-3 Esophageal Stenosis

Congenital:
  Membrane or web
    Vessel anomalies (e.g., dysphagia lusoria caused by compression of the esophagus by the right subclavian artery arising abnormally from the descending aorta and passing behind the esophagus)
    Other esophageal anomalies (atresia, duplication, cysts, diverticula)
Acquired:
  Achalasia
  Inflammation (GERD, Crohn's disease)
  Infections (mycotic infections)
  Tumors (benign and malignant)
  Iatrogenic
    - After probe insertion
    - Postoperative
    - After endoscopic therapy (mucosal ablation, endoscopic resection, APC, photodynamic therapy)
  Posttraumatic
    - Acidic or alkali injury
    - Scarring
  Others
    Collagen vascular disease (e.g., scleroderma)
    - Rheumatic diseases
    - Retroperitoneal fibrosis
    - Pneumatosis cystoides

may be located within or outside the lung and have a separate systemic blood supply. Patients present with pulmonary infections or a chest mass.

ESOPHAGEAL PERFORATION

Spontaneous Rupture (Boerhaave's Syndrome)

Pathogenesis and clinical features. A spontaneous rupture is one in which there is no apparent cause such as an ingested foreign body or instrumentation.[69-72] Strictly speaking, the rupture is usually not spontaneous. There is often a history of vomiting or straining for various reasons. There is often a preceding history of voluminous meals, with or without alcohol. Some patients have predisposing conditions such as erosive esophagitis, tumors, hiatal hernia, strictures, or rings, but the majority do not.[73] The pathogenesis is related to a rapid rise in intraluminal pressure in the esophagus, and at least about 140 mm Hg of pressure is needed for perforation to occur. Elderly males are more frequently affected as the tensile strength and elasticity of the esophagus is believed to decrease with age. Patients present with any combination of mediastinitis, pneumothorax, and peritonitis, depending on the location and the extent of the perforation. The diagnosis is best established by contrast x-ray. These patients require immediate surgery to repair the perforation and provide drainage. A fortunate few, who present late, survive with nonoperative management.[74] The mortality ranges from 10% to 30% (Table 9-4).[71,75]

Pathology. Most of the perforations occur in the left rear wall of distal esophagus, few centimeters above the diaphragm. The average length of the tears is 2 to 3 cm, but they can be more extensive (6–12 cm). The mucosal part of the tear is usually longer than the muscular part.[71] The degree of surrounding mediastinitis, pleuritis, and peritonitis depends upon the delay in operative intervention and upon the nature of the spilled gastroesophageal contents. Abscesses may have formed by the time this condition is recognized. *Intramural hematoma* is an occasional accompaniment, although it is rarely the sole manifestation of spontaneous trauma when there is an underlying coagulation defect.[76,77]

Nonspontaneous Rupture and Penetration

Pathogenesis and clinical features. Esophageal (Mallory–Weiss) tears are considered separately in the next section. Iatrogenic causes of nonspontaneous rupture and penetration account for more than 50% of cases.[69] In this group are endoscopic diagnostic procedures and therapeutic interventions such as endoscopic stent placement for obstructing carcinomas, dilatation of esophageal strictures, and pneumatic dilatation for achalasia.[78] Ingested *foreign bodies* and trauma (e.g., penetrating chest injuries or sword swallowing) each account for 10% to 14%.[69,79,80] The miscellaneous group consists of any esophageal disorder that may be characterized by deep ulceration. Such lesions may perforate or, more commonly, penetrate the wall more slowly, sometimes producing a fistula.

Perforations during endoscopy are rare (<1%) but account for 75% of all esophageal perforations. The other common type of iatrogenic injury is induced by prolonged nasogastric intubation (which predisposes to gastroesophageal reflux), trauma from difficult or forceful endoscopic intubation, and large-bore-tube intubation for gastric lavage to treat poisoning or to clear blood prior to endoscopy. Perforation during therapeutic procedures like Bougie dilations are rare and account for <5% of all cases. Intramural hematomas can lead to perforation later. Aortoesophageal fistulas after long time nasogastric intubation or malfunction of metal stents are also very rare.

Esophageal perforations can follow soon after radiation and surgery. Scarring with strictures and motility disorders associated with late phases of radiation or postsurgical trauma may also result in perforation. Postoperative suture dehiscence is a life-threatening complication that can lead to mediastinitis, sepsis, and fatal outcome.

Complication of sclerotherapy for esophageal varices with injection of alcohol or oily liquids also includes esophageal perforation, besides esophageal ulceration, hemorrhage, mediastinitis, and sepsis. Patients with liver cirrhosis have a higher risk of complications. About one-third of patients after emergency

Table 9-4	Causes of Esophageal Perforation

Iatrogenic:
  Endoscopy
  Bougie dilation
  Probe insertion
  Intubation
  Radiation
  Drug induced
  Periesophageal and esophageal surgery
  Endoscopic therapy (resection, ablation, APC, PDT)
  Graft versus host disease
Acid and alkali ingestion
Foreign bodies (e.g., forks, razor blades, sword swallowing) (Fig. 9-13)
Trauma
Spontaneous esophageal rupture (Boerhaave's syndrome)

sclerotherapy develop a septic complication. Bronchoesophageal fistulas do occur rarely as a late complication.

Drugs that cause perforations due to deep ulcerations are most commonly NSAIDs, but also include tetracycline, potassium chloride tablets (if not properly dissolved in water), iron sulfate/succinate, vitamin C, and bisphosphonates, and others for treating of osteoporosis can cause perforations. The duration of contact with the pills seems to play a role in the perforation, even if drug acts systemically. That is why it is always recommended to swallow the pills with enough water. Drug-induced lesions are often found in the mid and lower esophagus (Fig. 9-13).

Graft versus host disease can also rarely lead to severe desquamation of the esophageal epithelium and perforation. Prior radiation and concomitant esophagitis might play a role in this setting. Perforation during endoscopic resections or other mucosal ablative therapy (cryoablation or laser phototherapy) is rare and directly related to the experience of the endoscopist.

Acidic or alkaline injuries and other toxic chemicals (e.g., heavy metals) have harmful effects on the epithelium. The nature of the injury depends on the type, concentration, and quantity of the chemical swallowed and its duration of contact. Late complications include strictures and squamous cell carcinomas. Therefore patients with alkali-induced esophageal injury need regular endoscopic follow-up.

Perforation can occur secondary to impacted foreign bodies in the esophagus, especially in early childhood. Sharp-tipped foreign bodies like fish bones or bone splinters are more likely to lead to perforation. Foreign bodies often get stuck at one of the three physiological areas of esophageal narrowing. Sometimes the perforation occurs during the process of removal of the foreign body.

Trauma caused by blunt injuries such as car accidents, exposure to high-pressure air inflation into the GI tract, and penetrating injuries can all lead to perforations of the esophageal wall as well.

The clinical presentation varies according to the underlying disease and the site of perforation. Localized symptoms and signs (abscess) occur in upper (cervical) esophageal perforations in both neonates and adults.[81] In lower esophageal perforations, which constitute the majority, signs and symptoms are the same as those for spontaneous rupture. However, if the leak is small, there may be less severe chest pain, fever, and leukocytosis. With prompt detection and institution of antibiotic therapy and nasogastric drainage, increasing numbers of these patients are being managed conservatively.[69,78,81] The presenting features of fistulas (discussed later in this chapter) depend on where the communication leads.

Pathology. The pathology of penetrating or perforating injury depends upon the underlying cause and the timing of institution of therapy. The findings are similar

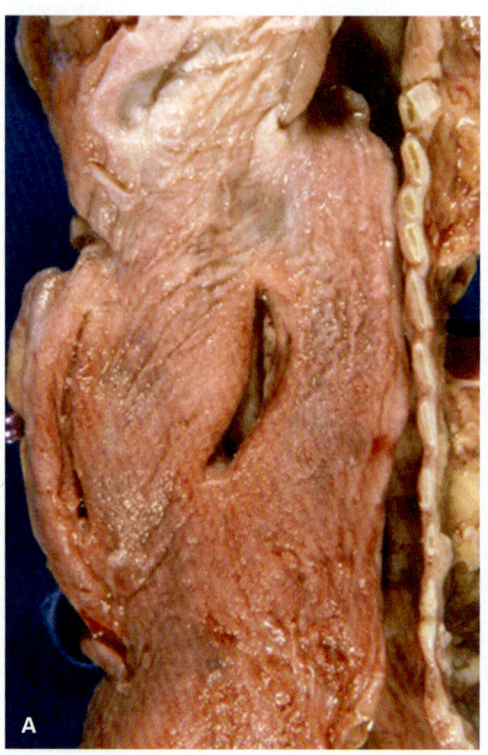
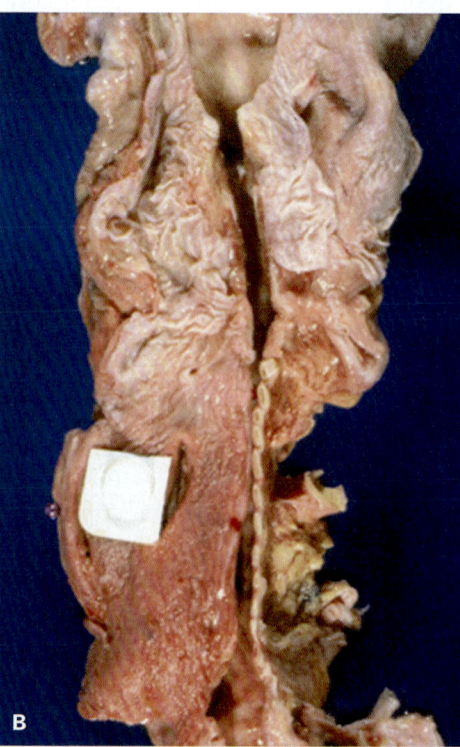

Figure 9-13. Autopsy case of an esophageal perforation **(A)** by a tablet still in the ulcer **(B)**. The patient died from septic shock from refractory mediastinitis.

to those described in the previous section on spontaneous perforation. The appearance of the esophagus ranges from subepithelial hemorrhages and erosions to penetrations or perforations, as described subsequently. Microscopically pill-induced mucosal injury tends to show homogenous eosinophilic coagulative necrosis on the mucosal surface similar to that seen in the stomach or colon. Penetration along the wall with the formation of a double-barreled esophagus has been reported.[82] In perforation after foreign body ingestion and after instrumentation, it is essential to determine whether underlying esophageal disease (e.g., ulcerative esophagitis, strictures, rings) is present.

ESOPHAGEAL HEMORRHAGE

Bleeding from esophagus can result from mucosal injury, varices, or hemorrhagic diathesis. Various forms of esophageal trauma (e.g., foreign body, iatrogenic traumas, etc.) can cause bleeding also. A rare form of acute esophageal necrosis resulting in GI hemorrhage is the so-called black esophagus.[83]

Esophageal Tears (Mallory–Weiss Syndrome)

Pathogenesis and clinical features. There is a moderately voluminous literature on this popular topic since the initial description by Mallory and Weiss in 1929.[84-88] The syndrome refers to a linear tear of the lower esophagus, usually just below the gastroesophageal sphincter region, accompanied by upper GI bleeding.[86]

Spontaneous rupture (Boerhaave's syndrome) may rarely occur. It has been reported to account for approximately 10% to 15% of the cases of upper GI bleeding.[85,86] The prevalence varies according to the type of patient population.

Previously, it was thought that these tears were induced by repeated retching from any cause, especially in actively drinking alcoholics. However, increased recognition of this lesion at endoscopy in patients with upper GI bleeding has revealed some tears that are unexplained by retching, alcoholism, or even some other logical causes, such as nonsteroidal anti-inflammatory drugs or other types of pill-induced esophagitis. The other risk factors include hiatal hernia, pregnancy, cough, external heart massage, and disseminated intravascular coagulation with impaired mucosal blood supply. When this diagnosis is made, especially in the absence of risk factors, the lesion may be a solitary erosion or ulcer at the gastroesophageal junction, with a tear representing only an educated guess. Bleeding stops spontaneously in the majority of patients. Endoscopic hemostasis techniques with injection or coagulation are employed when bleeding does not cease; surgery to oversee the defect is rarely required. Relapses are rare.

Pathology. Information is limited largely to gross descriptions because the condition is self-limited or easily controlled at endoscopy. The tears predominate on the cardia side of the gastroesophageal junction.[87] When early endoscopy is done, the lesions look like simple linear, longitudinal tears (Fig. 9-14A). When there is a delay in the endoscopic examination, there is more of an ulcer-like appearance, with an apparent

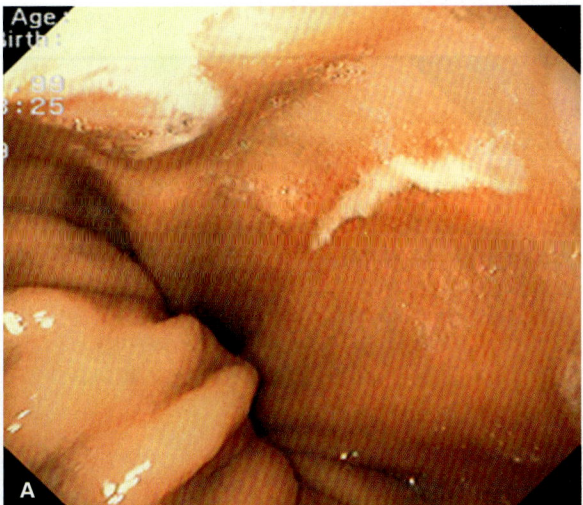
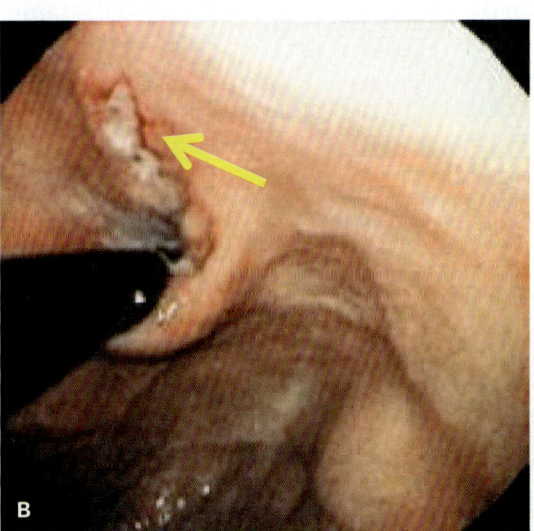

Figure 9-14. Endoscopic appearance of Mallory–Weiss tears. **A:** Early endoscopic appearance. The linear bloody tear straddles the gastroesophageal junction, with whitish squamous-type mucosa on the left and pink gastric-type mucosa on the right. (Courtesy of Steffen Mühldorfer, M.D.) **B:** Endoscopic appearance of a healing Mallory–Weiss tear with a whitish exudate at the base and no signs of active bleeding.

exudate at the base (Fig. 9-14B). Many lesions are extremely evanescent, capable of vanishing within 72 hours. It is presumed that the tears do not extend deeper than the submucosa; intramural dissection and hematoma are extremely rare.[88]

Esophageal Varices

Pathogenesis and clinical features.
Esophageal varices are due to portal hypertension; however, in very few cases no liver cirrhosis can be found.[89] When the portal hypertension is due to active cirrhosis, as in an actively drinking alcoholic, the prognosis is poor. In primary extrahepatic portal vein obstruction, the prognosis is excellent. *Downhill varices* are varices that arise when there is superior vena caval obstruction. These rarely bleed.

The esophageal venous system is an integral part of the portacaval collateral flow pathway. It receives blood from the left gastric vein and drains mainly through the azygous system into the superior vena cava. This plexus quickly fills in response to increases in portal venous pressure. Most bleeding from esophageal varices occurs in the distal 5 cm of the esophagus, even though large varices may be present throughout its length.

A better understanding of the structure and location of varices has come from studies utilizing special techniques that include Doppler ultrasound and resin casting.[90–92] In earlier studies, the normal venous anatomy was defined as consisting of an intrinsic plexus, which was subdivided into a subepithelial plexus in the lamina propria, and a submucosal plexus and veins, which perforated the muscularis propria.[93] In the distal 5 cm of the esophagus, a greater proportion (both the number and size of veins) of the lamina propria is occupied by veins than that in the more proximal esophagus. With resin casting, four layers of veins have been identified[94]: intraepithelial channels that drain into a superficial venous plexus, which connect to larger deep intrinsic veins, and perforating veins connected the deeper veins with veins in the adventitia outside the esophageal wall. The deep intrinsic veins appear to communicate with gastric veins. It has been proposed that minor bleeding from esophageal varices may be due to rupture of the superficial intraepithelial channels, whereas major bleeding is due to rupture of one of the larger deep venous trunks.[90]

Esophageal varices are detected most reliably at endoscopy (Fig. 9-15A) in the setting of GI bleeding or incidentally in nonbleeding patients with portal hypertension. When they bleed, one can see oozing from these, but a rent or defect is not seen (Fig. 9-15B).

Endoscopic Sclerotherapy
Endoscopic variceal ligation (EVL) is used to obliterate varices in patients who are actively bleeding or who have bled from previously. This is a very effective procedure in controlling bleeding and obliterates varices by causing thrombosis and inducing vessel fibrosis. In the past decade, EVL has replaced sclerotherapy as the preferred endoscopic therapy for variceal hemorrhage management because it is safer, more effective, and associated with lower rebleeding rates, resulting in a reduced morbidity.[95] In addition, nonselective β-blockers have been recommended for the prophylaxis of varceal hemorrhage.[96] In patients awaiting liver transplant, control of bleeding saves life by "buying time" until a transplant can be done. Pathologists today are less involved with the detection of varices at autopsy and more involved with

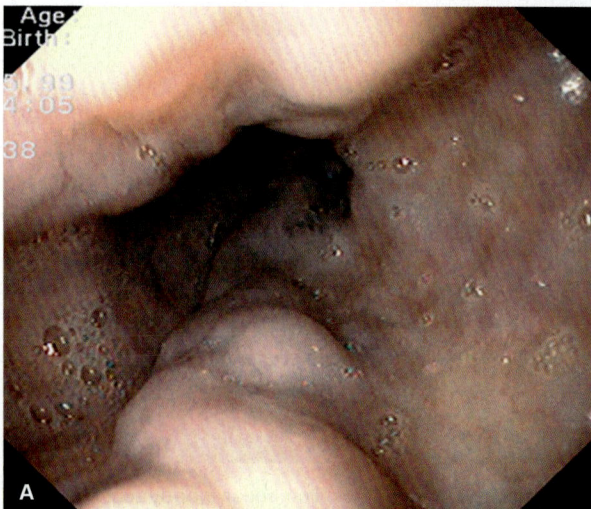 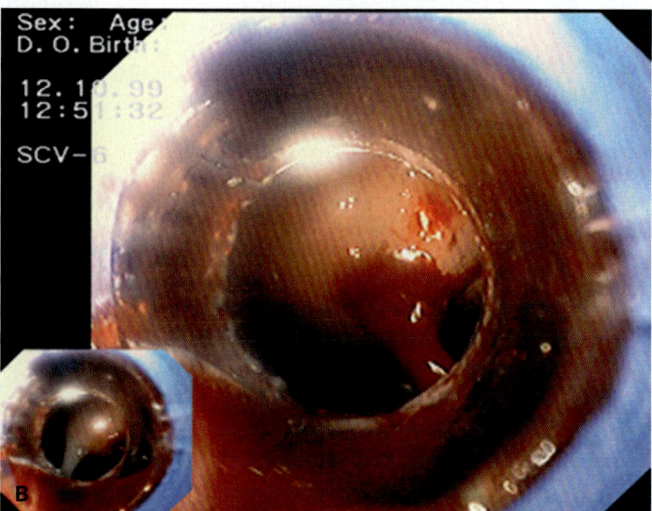

Figure 9-15. **A:** Endoscopic appearance of esophageal varices with striking tortuosity and mild blue color. (Courtesy of Steffen Mühldorfer, M.D.) **B:** Bleeding varices in the distal esophagus during endoscopic ligation. (Courtesy of Steffen Mühldorfer, M.D.)

the observation at autopsy of the consequences and complications of endoscopic sclerotherapy of varices (see Chapter 11).

An alternative technique, *endoscopic banding*, may be equally effective in controlling bleeding.

Pathology. Varices are best appreciated at endoscopy (Fig. 9-15): longitudinal, tortuous (snaky), bluish bulges into the esophageal lumen; when large, they obliterate the lumen as viewed from above. The size of varices, red spots on their surfaces, and red wale markings (longitudinal dilated venules resembling whip marks) tend to be associated with a greater risk of bleeding from varices at a population level but may not be highly specific at the individual patient level.[97-101] Adherent blood clots may identify varices as the site of upper GI bleeding at endoscopy. The finding of erosions or ulcers on variceal surfaces is uncommon. At autopsy, the bluish appearance of varices may not be evident. The varices may be demonstrated by inversion of the transected esophagus and massaging down of the blood.

Accurate histologic documentation of esophageal varices at autopsy requires casting techniques, as described in the section on pathogenesis. Dilated vascular channels may be observed, but vessel collapse may make some varices inapparent. Some vessels demonstrate thrombosis, organization, and recanalization. As already indicated, if the patient had received endoscopic sclerotherapy, a host of new lesions may be seen, as discussed in Chapter 10.

Acute Esophageal Necrosis (Black Esophagus) Acute esophageal necrosis is a rare disorder that is poorly described in the medical literature.[102-105] Risk factors include age, male sex, cardiovascular disease, hemodynamic compromise, gastric outlet obstruction, alcohol use, malnutrition, diabetes, renal insufficiency, hypoxemia, hypercoagulable state, and trauma. Patients generally present with GI bleeding (hematemesis, melena, or both) and cardiovascular shock. Upper endoscopy showed black, diffusely necrotic esophageal mucosa predominantly affecting the distal third of the organ. Histologically entire mucosa is necrotic. Mechanism of damage is usually multifactorial secondary to ischemic compromise, acute gastric outlet obstruction, and malnutrition. Complications include strictures or stenoses, mediastinitis/abscesses, and perforations. The mortality in these patients is about 31%. Overall, it is a poor prognostic factor, associated with high mortality from the underlying clinical disease.

ESOPHAGEAL FISTULA

Adults may present with esophageal fistulas (Fig. 9-16) from congenital causes such as ulceration in gastric heterotopia and from H-type congenital tracheoesophageal fistulas, described previously in this chapter. Acquired causes include Barrett's associated ulcers, necrotic tumors of the esophageal wall, foreign bodies, and some exotic infections of the esophagus.[56,106-108] The presentation may be dramatic when the fistula communicates with the heart or aorta.[109]

Acquired Esophageal Stenosis or Stricture

Acquired causes of esophageal stenosis are many (Table 9-3), of which inflammatory disorders leading to scarring are the most frequent followed by tumors.

Esophageal webs and rings. The distinction between a ring and a web is unclear.[110] A web is considered to be a thin, partially or completely circumferential

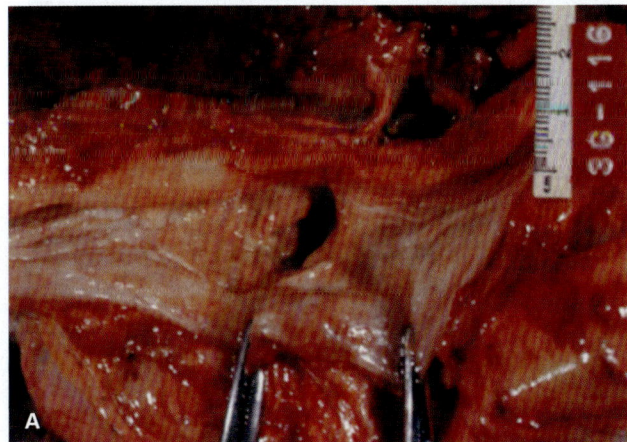
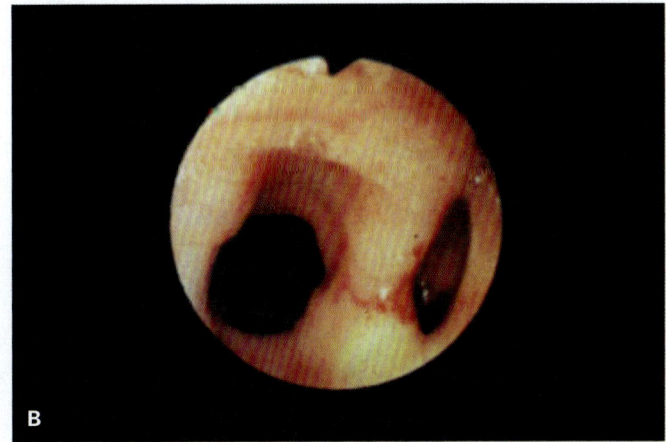

Figure 9-16. Esophageal fistula. **A:** Gross pathology at autopsy. **B:** Endoscopic view. The fistula's opening is on the right. (American Society for Gastrointestinal Endoscopy; courtesy of Worth Boyce, M.D.)

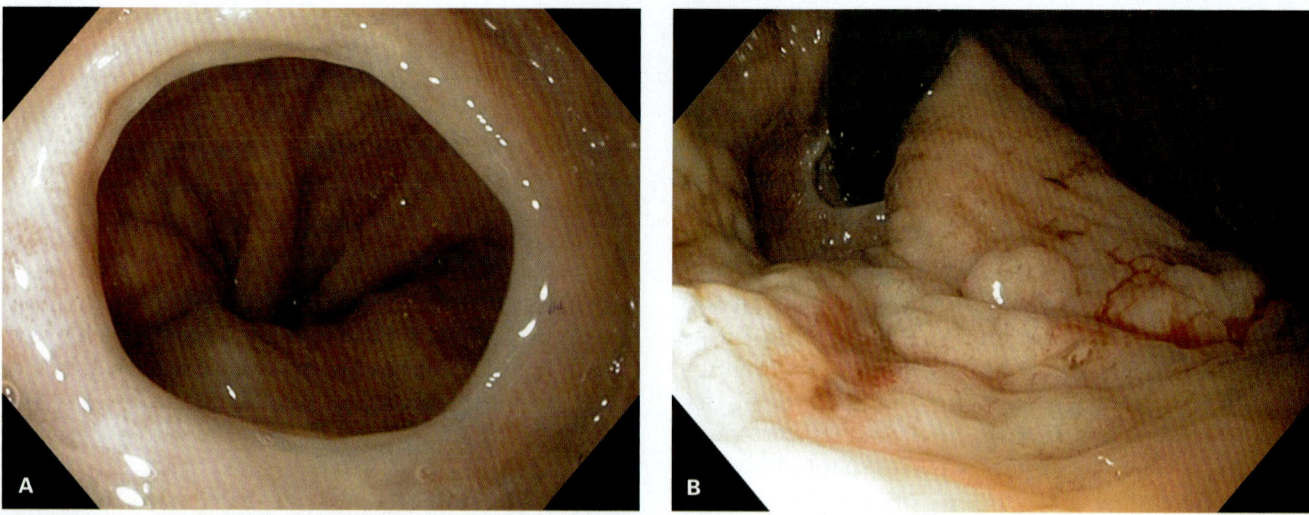

Figure 9-17. **A:** Endoscopic view of a single esophageal ring, prograde view. **B:** Endoscopic view of an esophageal ring, retroflexed view. (Courtesy of Steffen Mühldorfer, M.D.)

structure that intuitively is presumed to be entirely mucosal or, at most, to contain mucosa and submucosa.[110] A ring implies a thicker structure, generally circumferential, and presumed to contain muscularis propria. The reader who is interested in these curious lesions should be aware that what is a web for one author is a ring for another. Further confusion results when the term *web* or *ring* (Fig. 9-17) is used to describe a lesion that is clearly an inflammatory stricture on clinical grounds (e.g., caustic, reflux) but is sharply demarcated. In this instance, the stricture is better described as a "web-like stricture," describing its appearance rather than including it in the group discussed subsequently.

The pathologist generally becomes involved with webs and rings when presented with endoscopic biopsy specimens from these lesions, with the endoscopist standing by, hoping that some new insight will be gained. Unfortunately, most of the time, all one can say is that the biopsy specimen consists of squamous epithelium. There might be variable amount of inflammatory or reactive epithelial changes, and the main role of the biopsy is to exclude dysplasia and malignancy.

We will consider these conditions by site of origin and match that with the pathogenesis or associations whenever possible.[110] We have seen rare instances of multiple webs and rings (Fig. 9-18) that defy classification, and we wonder whether they represent some form of inappropriate muscular (muscularis mucosae or muscularis propria) contracture.

Upper Esophageal Webs and Rings

These webs and rings are located in the upper third of the esophagus. The best way to visualize them (without inadvertently rupturing them at endoscopy) is with a barium x-ray (Fig. 9-19). The popular syndrome of webs causing dysphagia and associated with iron deficiency anemia (Plummer–Vinson or Paterson–Kelly syndrome) may be extinct.[111] The webs disappear after anemia recovers. An increased risk of postcricoid carcinoma has been reported in this syndrome.[111,112] Biopsy specimens from these webs are normal or reveal changes of regenerative hyperplasia (elongated dermal papillae and basal cell hyperplasia) and mononuclear cell infiltrates.[113,114]

Other associations with upper esophageal webs include chronic graft versus host disease and gastric

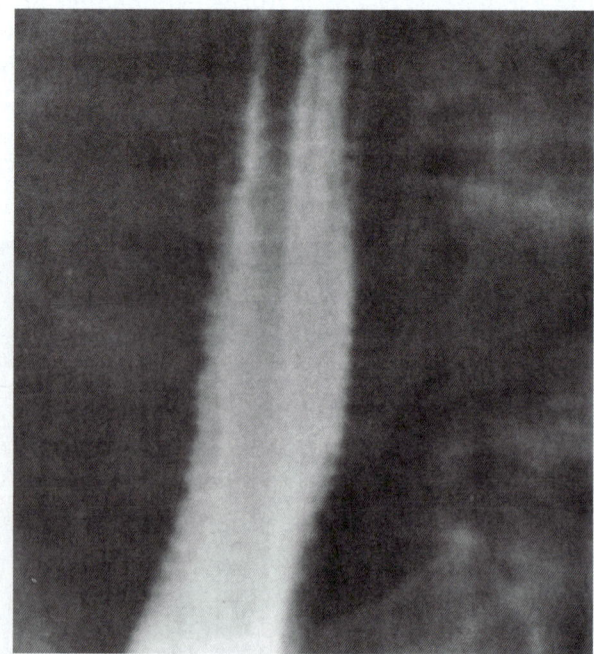

Figure 9-18. Multiple esophageal rings. The walls of the esophagus have a corrugated appearance. (Courtesy of Marvin Weiner, M.D.)

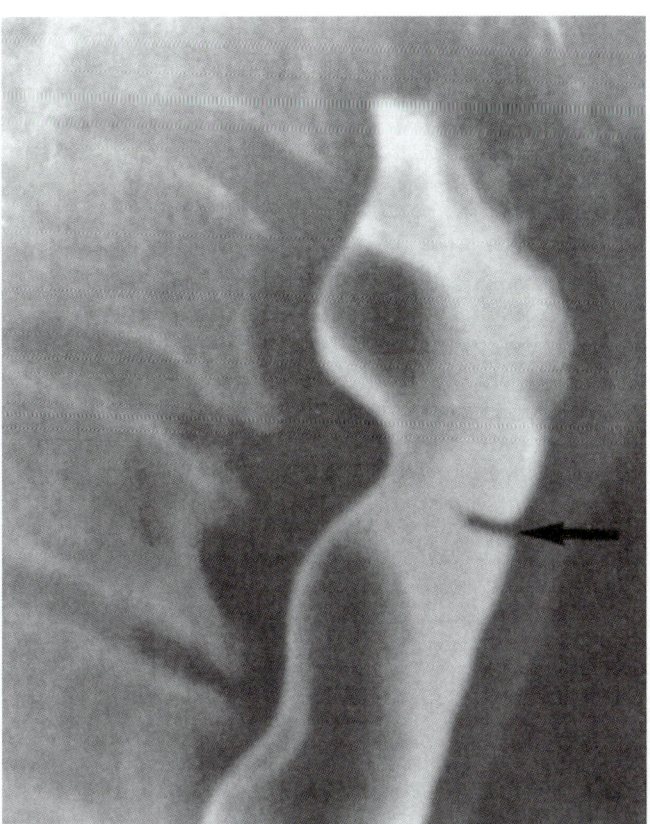

Figure 9-19. Upper esophageal web, seen as an indentation (*arrow*) in the barium-filled esophagus. (Courtesy of Marvin Weiner, M.D.)

heterotopias.[115,116] Not infrequently, the astute radiologist (Fig. 9-19) points out (as an incidental finding) asymmetric indentations in the upper esophagus that are thought to represent webs. Multiple webs or rings throughout the esophagus have been illustrated and found to be associated histologically with regenerative hyperplastic changes.[114]

Midesophageal Webs and Rings

Webs or rings are rare in the midesophageal region.[117,118] Here the concern is to differentiate a benign from a malignant stricture.

Lower Esophageal Webs and Rings

PATHOGENESIS AND CLINICAL FEATURES. The lower esophageal (Schatzki) ring is a circumferential indentation of the distal esophagus (Fig. 9-20) that consists of squamous mucosa (sometimes squamocolumnar) and submucosa.[119] It is believed to correspond to the gastroesophageal junction, although this issue is not completely settled.[119-121] Just above this mucosal ring an apparent muscular ring may exist, although some believe it to be an artifact.[119]

The pathogenesis of the lower esophageal ring is unknown. Gastroesophageal reflux may be a contributing factor, causing progressive luminal narrowing sufficient to produce dysphagia.[122]

These rings may be discovered incidentally or in the course of an evaluation for dysphagia. With minimal encroachment of the lumen, they can be easily overlooked. In this setting, expert radiologic examination may be superior to endoscopic examination.[123]

The backbone of treatment is dilatation. Some physicians perform it under direct vision after taking biopsy specimens at several quadrants to help loosen the ring. In those with very tight rings, a more

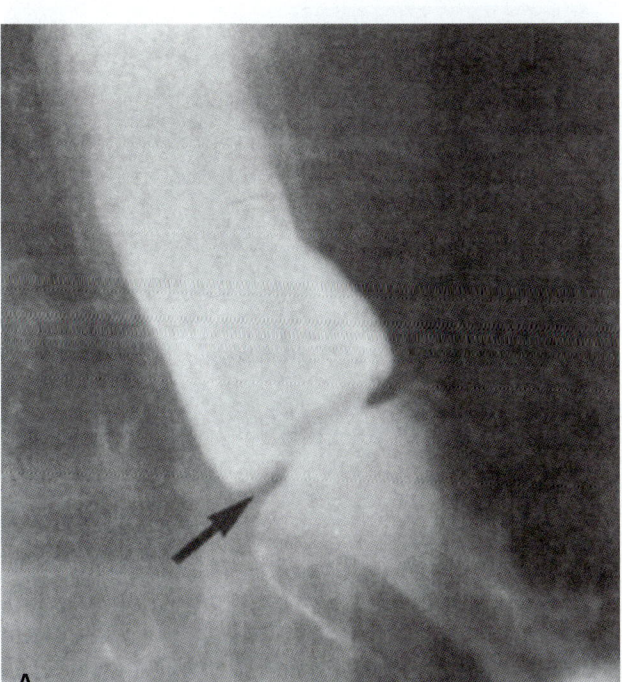
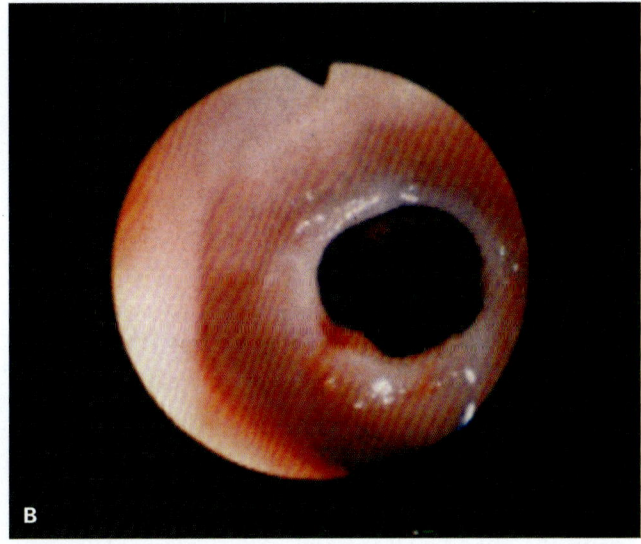

Figure 9-20. Schatzki ring. **A:** Barium x-ray. The *arrow* points to the ring. (Courtesy of Marvin Weiner, M.D.). **B:** Endoscopic appearance.

high-technology solution is to perform electrosurgical incision of the ring.[124]

PATHOLOGY. There are only a very few histologic descriptions on esophageal webs available. The endoscopic appearance is that of a narrow indentation, which often appears paler and more glistening than the rest of the squamous epithelium (Fig. 9-20B). Usually the webs are not thicker than 2 mm and are completely covered by squamous epithelium. Erosion and ulceration are usually absent, except when there has been food or foreign body impaction. The mucosal histology is either normal or shows signs of regenerative hyperplasia (elongation of papillae, thickened basal cell layer, etc.). The latter cannot be taken as evidence of gastroesophageal reflux as the cause of the ring because similar histologic changes are seen in the distal 2 to 3 cm of the esophagus in normal individuals.[3] Webs are believed not to have muscularis mucosae and are built only from lamina mucosa and epithelium. The main consideration in the differential diagnosis is a sharply delimited peptic stricture, but this is usually not a difficult problem.

DIVERTICULA AND PSEUDODIVERTICULA

Table 9-2 outlines the major categories of diverticula and pseudodiverticula. The current semantic convention is that diverticula represent an outpouching of one or more layers of the esophageal wall. Pseudodiverticula or intramural pseudodiverticulosis is characterized by dilated ducts of submucosal glands. Squamous carcinomas have been reported with both Zenker's (upper) and lower esophageal diverticula, perhaps reflecting chronic stasis in the sacs.[125,126]

The pathogenic descriptor terms *pulsion* and *traction diverticula* are now less fashionable. The former refers to presumed intraluminal pressure increases or defects in the wall, and the latter refers to the rare cases in which mediastinal inflammation pulls on the esophagus to create diverticula.

Upper Esophageal Diverticula (Zenker's)

Pathogenesis and clinical features. These are not infrequent and reported to occur in 0.11% of the population. Other than Zenker's, unilateral or Killian–Jamieson (bilateral) diverticula are rarely noted in the cervical esophagus. This type of diverticulum is an outpouching from the lateral wall of cervical esophagus.[127] These were once thought to arise from motor incoordination of the cricopharyngeal musculature.[128] Possibility of a congenital weakness of the dorsal pharyngeal wall (Kilian's triangle) just above the proximal esophageal opening with an increased intraluminal pressure (pulsion diverticulum) has been also suggested. Considerable doubt has now been cast on that notion.[129,130] It is believed that gastroesophageal reflux leads to cricopharyngeal spasm, which may lead to formation of the diverticulum. Also in countries where gastroesophageal reflux disease is uncommon, Zenker's diverticulum is rare too. Currently, the most widely accepted theory is that upper esophageal sphincter relaxation is inadequate, resulting in the incomplete opening and high intraluminal pressure.[131] Classic symptoms include gurgling, a mass in the neck, and regurgitation into the mouth or lungs. Therapy is surgical, consisting of cricopharyngeal myotomy, with or without resection of the diverticulum, depending on its size. For high-risk individuals, flexible endoscopic-based needle-knife technique for cricopharyngeal myotomy has been quite promising.[132]

Pathology. The gross appearance is distinctive with barium x-ray (Fig. 9-21). All layers of the wall are represented in the diverticulum, which generally faces posteriorly, just above the upper esophageal sphincter. Histologically, stasis and distention may be indicated by erosions or inflammatory infiltrates.

Mid- and Lower Esophageal Diverticula

Pathogenesis and clinical features. Midesophageal diverticula are usually single (Fig. 9-22) and, by themselves, do not cause symptoms. They were once attributed to mediastinal inflammations such as tuberculosis, with traction being considered responsible for

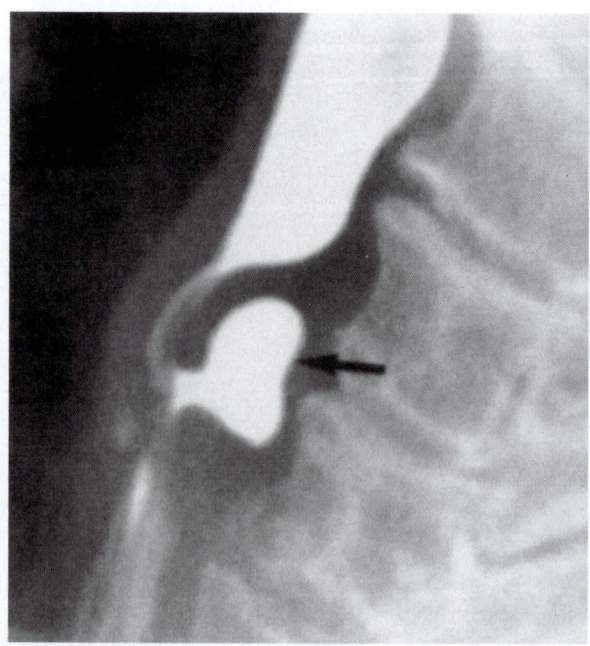

Figure 9-21. Small Zenker's diverticulum (*arrow*) on barium x-ray. (Courtesy of Marvin Weiner, M.D.)

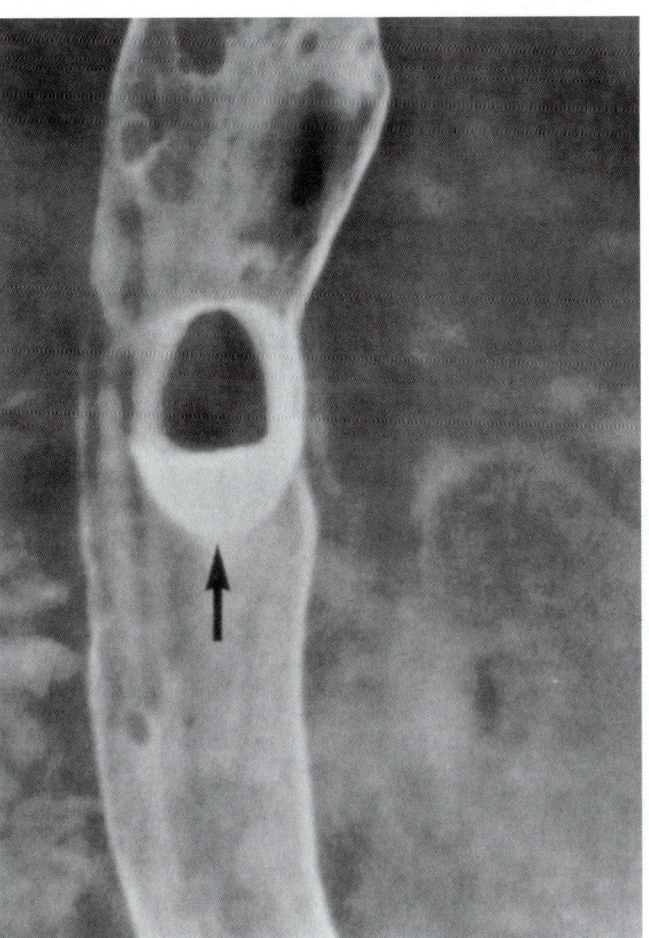

Figure 9-22. Midesophageal diverticulum with a barium–air interface within the diverticulum. (Courtesy of Marvin Weiner, M.D.)

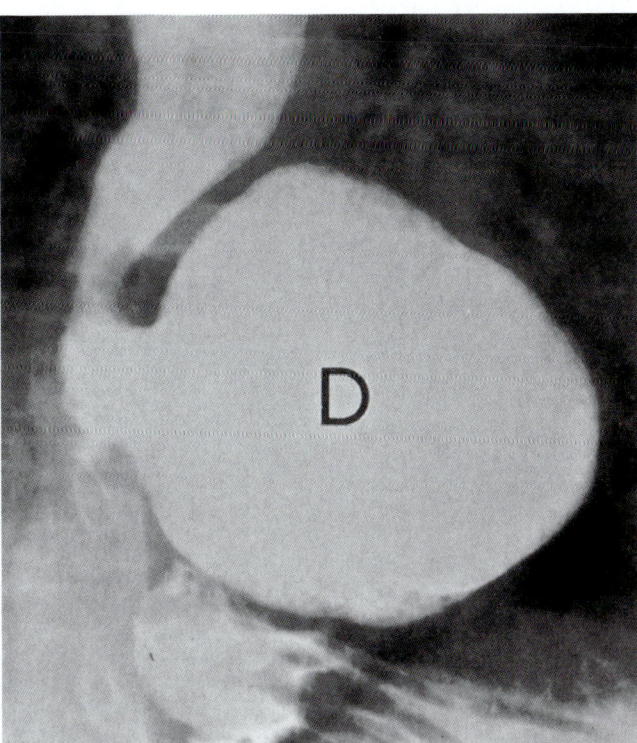

Figure 9-23. Huge epiphrenic diverticulum (D). An esophageal stricture is present just above the entrance to the diverticulum. (Courtesy of Marvin Weiner, M.D.)

the diverticulum. Now it appears that some of them may be a reflection of motor disorders of the esophagus.[129]

Lower esophageal or epiphrenic diverticula commonly reflect more severe motor disorders of the esophagus, such as achalasia and diffuse esophageal spasm[133,134] (see Chapter 7). They may grow very large (Fig. 9-23) and sometimes are multiple. Association with esophageal leiomyoma has been described in the literature, but is probably a chance phenomenon.[135–139] Subphrenic diverticula are found very rarely, and in the literature there are only a few case reports available.[138,140]

The main symptom is dysphagia, due mainly to the motor disorder of the esophagus. When surgery is required, it is primarily a procedure for the motor disorder (esophagomyotomy); diverticulectomy is performed if the sacs are large.[133]

Pathology. The size of these diverticula is best appreciated radiologically. Large diverticula may have a stretched muscularis propria, and, depending upon the amount of debris in the lumen, there may be mucosal ulceration. Leiomyomas have been found in the wall in a few cases.[133]

Atypical Esophageal Diverticula in Scleroderma

Elongated sacculations similar to those seen in the colon in scleroderma are found less commonly in the esophagus at any level.[141]

Esophageal Intramural Pseudodiverticulosis/Retention Cysts

Pathogenesis and clinical features. This entity was first described from Germany and Italy in 1899 as "cystic esophagitis." Around 100 cases have been reported to date.[142,143] This uncommon disease manifests as dysphagia, usually in adults, but may also occur in childhood. The peak incidence is around seventh to eighth decade. Men are slightly more often affected. It is characterized by multiple epithelium-lined cysts within the esophageal wall. These cysts are due to dilated ducts from submucosal glands. On barium swallow x-rays, they appear as tiny flask-shaped (collar button) outpouchings (Fig. 9-24) because the cysts communicate with the esophageal lumen via narrow openings.

The genesis of this peculiar disorder may be due in part to underlying motor abnormalities of the esophagus; on the other hand, so few cases have been subjected to manometric studies that it is possible that any observed motility disturbances may be

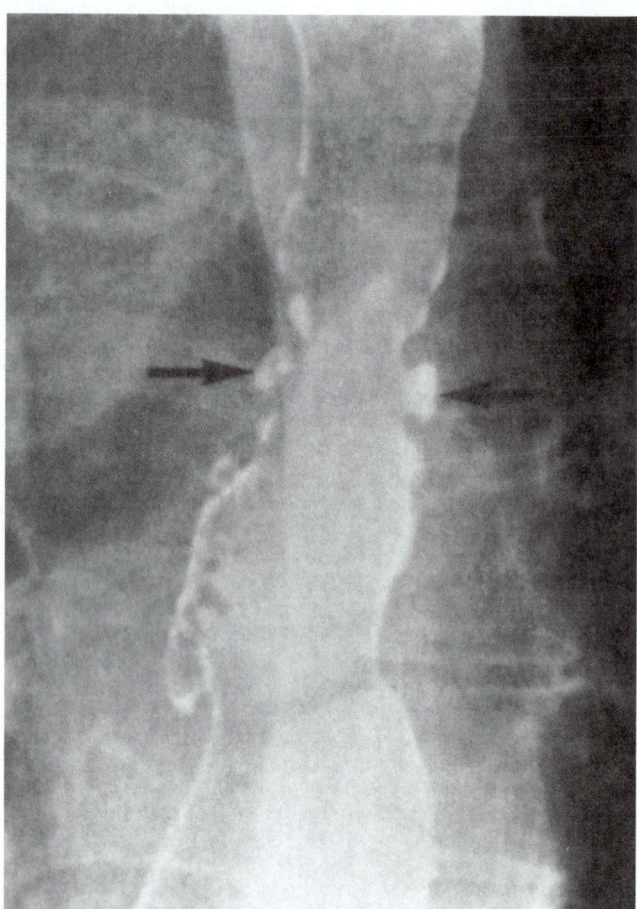

Figure 9-24. Diffuse intramural pseudodiverticulosis of barium x-ray. *Arrows* point to the outpouchings. (Courtesy of Marvin Weiner, M.D.)

secondary to the intramural changes.[144] It is suggested that esophageal inflammation (e.g., reflux esophagitis, sialadenitis of esophageal glands, candidiasis) precedes development of these cysts. It is also possible that scarring and duct obstruction leads to retention of secretion of the esophageal glands, resulting in cyst formation.[16] Esophageal strictures, candidiasis, or both may contribute to the patients' dysphagia.[145–147]

The diagnosis is established with barium x-ray. Endoscopically smooth mucosal elevations can be seen. Strictures and candidiasis are evaluated by endoscopy, biopsy, and smears. Therapy is directed to the candidiasis and to dilatation of esophageal strictures.

Pathology. The typical barium x-ray appearance (Fig. 9-24) parallels the findings seen in autopsy specimens.[16,148] Numerous submucosal-appearing nodules are present, resulting in marked thickening of the submucosa. Numerous duct openings (ostia) are visible. The cysts may be filled with a white viscous material.[16]

Mononuclear cell aggregates commonly surround the dilated submucosal ducts. The pseudodiverticula are lined with squamous epithelium and their ducts with an attenuated low cuboidal epithelium.[148] The pseudodiverticula may contain inflammatory cells, desquamated squames, and necrotic debris. The squamous mucosa between the pseudodiverticula may be inflamed, with or without evidence of accompanying candidiasis. Squamous metaplasia can be sometimes seen. In practice, esophageal inflammation that does not respond to medical therapy should raise the question of pseudodiverticulosis. In a comparative autopsy study, 15% of apparently, it was found that "normal" esophagi had microscopic cyst formation. An associated mononuclear cell infiltrate and duct dilatation was present in approximately half of the cases.[16] There may be an increased number of submucosal glands with advancing age.[16] Thus, in a sense, diffuse intramural pseudodiverticula may represent an exaggeration of a normal phenomenon.

OTHER MISCELLANEOUS CONDITIONS

Mucosal Bridge

This is a rare condition, and only about 80 cases have been reported in the literature to date. More than 80% of these cases have been reported from Japan. Mucosal bridges can be vertical or horizontal and be found anywhere within the esophagus. Mucosal bridges are rarely congenital when they are associated with other anomalies or can be acquired. In acquired cases prior variceal sclerotherapy, Barrett's esophagus, GERD,[149] acidic injury, drug-induced injury, radiation, collagenosis,[150] Mallory–Weiss tears, and candidiasis may have played a role.[151] In one Japanese series 20% of all cases occurred after prior variceal sclerotherapy, 12% were associated with GERD, 9% with Mallory–Weiss, and 5% were associated with other diseases such as candidiasis. In 29% of the patients the etiology remained unclear.[152] There are specific clinical symptoms, other than those that led to the development of mucosal bridges. The epithelium shows regenerative changes for the most part. A rare case with squamous cell carcinoma has been described, but whether it is merely a chance association is not yet clear.[152]

Glycogenic Acanthosis

Glycogenic acanthosis is not a disease; in fact, it may represent a variant of normal. It is characterized by tiny gray-white nodules or plaques, which are due to enlarged cells of the prickle cell layer above the basal zone (Fig. 9-25).[153–157] Occasionally, the nodularity is prominent or is confluent on x-ray or at endoscopy. In the clinical differential diagnosis, the concern is to rule out candidiasis or squamous carcinoma.

No symptoms or disease associations are associated with this very common finding. Endoscopists are generally aware of this entity and do not biopsy these tiny bumps with their former regularity.

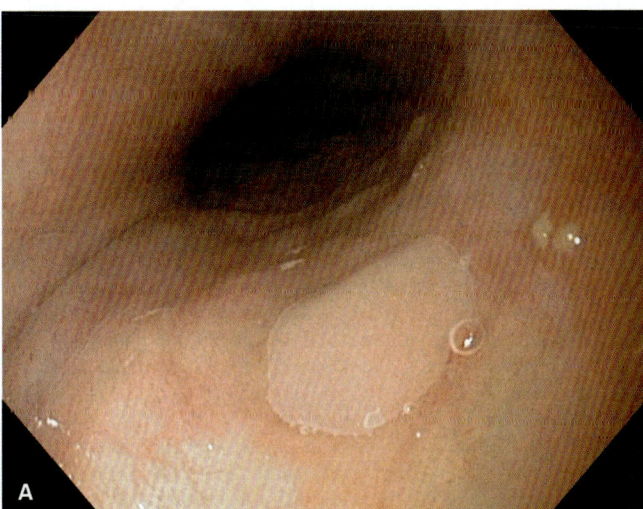
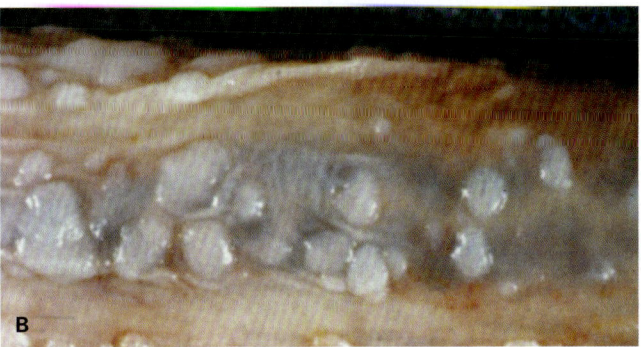
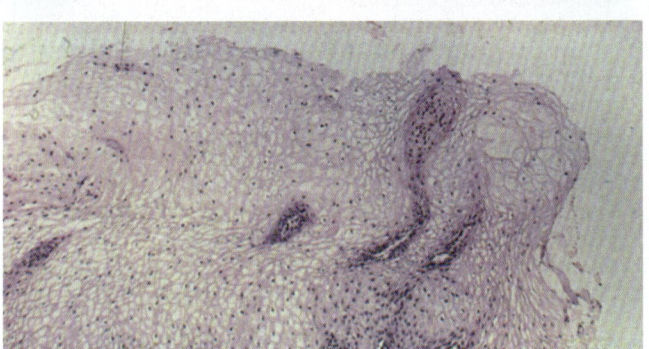
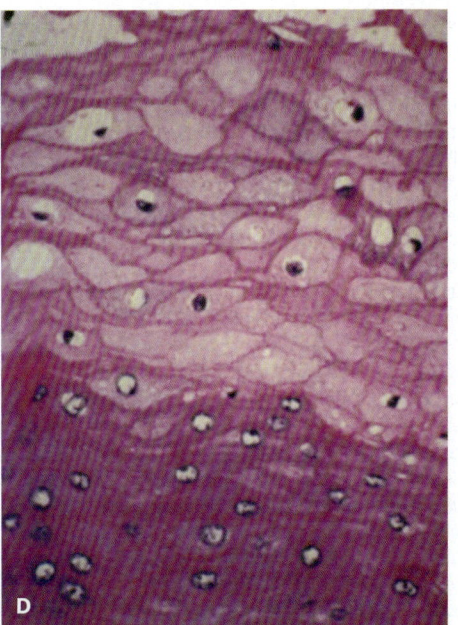
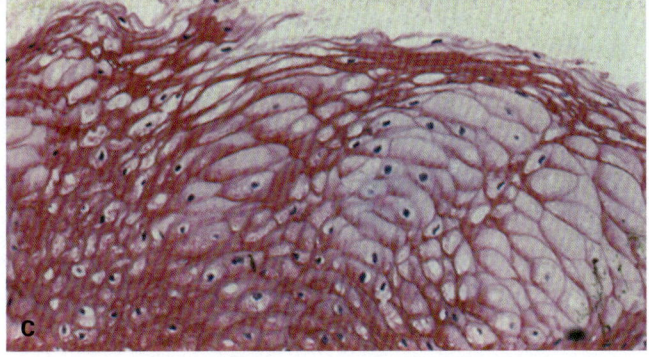

Figure 9-25. Glycogenic acanthosis. **A:** Endoscopic appearance of a white plaque (9 o'clock position), which proved to be glycogenic acanthosis on biopsy. **B:** Autopsy appearance of multiple large whitish nodules of glycogenic acanthosis—an incidental and unusual (for nodules this large) finding. **C: Top:** Hematoxylin and eosin stain of a glycogenic acanthosis nodule. **Bottom:** High-power view of the luminal surface (PAS stain). **D:** A 1-pm epon-embedded section demonstrates the bloated cells even more dramatically (Huber stain).

The enlarged cells in the expanded zone above the basal cell layer can be enhanced for aesthetic reasons with the periodic acid-Schiff (PAS) stain (Fig. 9-25C). Not all of the cellular enlargement is due to glycogen accumulation. The PAS stain can also be used if either the pathologist or the endoscopist has an interest in differentiating glycogenic acanthosis from ballooned cells containing plasma proteins, discussed subsequently. In biopsy specimens we have the impression that mechanical dislodgement of superficial layers of cells may occur. This may result in under-representation of the actual thickness of the squamous cell layer in biopsy specimens from distinct nodules of apparent classic glycogenic acanthosis.

Sometimes ballooned cells have been described to contain albumin and immunoglobulin.[158] The appearance in hematoxylin- and eosin-stained sections may be identical to that of glycogenic acanthosis; however, the ballooned cells stained relatively negatively with PAS. The retrospective nature of this report made it impossible to know if grossly visible nodules can be attributed to these cell collections; also, it is not known whether these ballooned cells represent a marker of mucosal injury.

Esophageal Xanthelasma

The lesion consists of accumulation of foamy histiocytes in the lamina propria. In contrast to gastric xanthelasma, esophageal xanthelasma are rather rare, and very few cases have been reported in the literature.[159–161]

References

1. Aggestrup S, Uddman R, Jensen SL, et al. Regulatory peptides in lower esophageal sphincter of pig and man. *Dig Dis Sci*. 1986;31(12):1370–1375.
2. Hopwood D, Logan KR, Bouchier IA. The electron microscopy of normal human oesophageal epithelium. *Virchows Arch B Cell Pathol*. 1978;26(4):345–358.
3. Weinstein WM, Bogoch ER, Bowes KL. The normal human esophageal mucosa: a histological reappraisal. *Gastroenterology*. 1975;68(1):40–44.
4. Ismail-Beigi F, Horton PF, Pope CE II. Histological consequences of gastroesophageal reflux in man. *Gastroenterology*. 1970;58(2):163–174.
5. Johnson LF, Demeester TR, Haggitt RC. Esophageal epithelial response to gastroesophageal reflux. A quantitative study. *Am J Dig Dis*. 1978;23(6):498–509.
6. Tateishi R, Taniguchi H, Wada A, et al. Argyrophil cells and melanocytes in esophageal mucosa. *Arch Pathol*. 1974;98(2):87–89.
7. DiCostanzo DP, Urmacher C. Primary malignant melanoma of the esophagus. *Am J Surg Pathol*. 1987;11(1):46–52.
8. Kimball MW. Pseudomelanosis of the esophagus. *Gastrointest Endosc*. 1978;24(3):121–122.
9. Harmse JL, Carey FA, Baird AR, et al. Merkel cells in the human oesophagus. *J Pathol*. 1999;189(2):176–179.
10. Geboes K, De Wolf-Peeters C, Rutgeerts P, et al. Lymphocytes and Langerhans cells in the human oesophageal epithelium. *Virchows Arch A Pathol Anat Histopathol*. 1983;401(1):45–55.
11. Vicario M, Blanchard C, Stringer KF, et al. Local B cells and IgE production in the oesophageal mucosa in eosinophilic oesophagitis. *Gut*. 2010;59(1):12–20.
12. Cestari R, Villanacci V, Bassotti G, et al. The pathology of gastric cardia: a prospective, endoscopic, and morphologic study. *Am J Surg Pathol*. 2007;31(5):706–710.
13. Lewis JT, Wang KK, Abraham SC. Muscularis mucosae duplication and the musculo-fibrous anomaly in endoscopic mucosal resections for barrett esophagus: implications for staging of adenocarcinoma. *Am J Surg Pathol*. 2008;32(4):566–571.
14. Abraham SC, Krasinskas AM, Correa AM, et al. Duplication of the muscularis mucosae in Barrett esophagus: an underrecognized feature and its implication for staging of adenocarcinoma. *Am J Surg Pathol*. 2007;31(11):1719–1725.
15. Geboes K, Desmet V. Histology of the esophagus. *Front Gastrointest Res*. 1978;3:1–17.
16. Medeiros LJ, Doos WG, Balogh K. Esophageal intramural pseudodiverticulosis: a report of two cases with analysis of similar, less extensive changes in "normal" autopsy esophagi. *Hum Pathol*. 1988;19(8):928–931.
17. Meyer GW, Austin RM, Brady CE III, Castell DO. Muscle anatomy of the human esophagus. *J Clin Gastroenterol*. 1986;8(2):131–134.
18. Gockel I, Bohl JR, Eckardt VF, Junginger T. Reduction of interstitial cells of Cajal (ICC) associated with neuronal nitric oxide synthase (n-NOS) in patients with achalasia. *Am J Gastroenterol*. 2008;103(4):856–864.
19. Negreanu LM, Assor P, Mateescu B, Cirstoiu C. Interstitial cells of Cajal in the gut–a gastroenterologist's point of view. *World J Gastroenterol*. 2008;14(41):6285–6288.
20. Berezin I, Daniel EE, Huizinga JD. Ultrastructure of interstitial cells of Cajal in the canine distal esophagus. *Can J Physiol Pharmacol*. 1994;72(9):1049–1059.
21. Liebermann-Meffert D, Allgower M, Schmid P, Blum AL. Muscular equivalent of the lower esophageal sphincter. *Gastroenterology*. 1979;76(1):31–38.
22. Jackson AJ. The spiral constrictor of the gastroesophageal junction. *Am J Anat*. 1978;151(2):265–275.
23. Eckardt VF, LeCompte PM. Esophageal ganglia and smooth muscle in the elderly. *Am J Dig Dis*. 1978;23(5):443–448.
24. Rao SS, Mudipalli RS, Mujica VR, et al. Effects of gender and age on esophageal biomechanical properties and sensation. *Am J Gastroenterol*. 2003;98(8):1688–1695.
25. Moore KL. *Embryologie: Lehrbuch und Atlas der Entwicklungsgeschichte des Menschen*. 3rd ed. Stuttgart, Germany: Schattauer; 1990.
26. Elster K, Schlegl A. Untersuchungen von Kinder-und Säuglingsmägen unter besonderer Berücksichtigung des Vorkommens von Becherzellen und saumetragenden Zylinderepithelien. *Z Gastroenterol*. 1965;3:131–137.
27. Neumann E. Flimmerepithel im Ösophagus menschlicher Embryonen. *Arch Microskop Anat*. 1876;12:570–574.
28. Takubo K, Vieth M, Honma N, et al. Ciliated surface in the esophagogastric junction zone: a precursor of Barrett's mucosa or ciliated pseudostratified metaplasia? *Am J Surg Pathol*. 2005;29(2):211–217.
29. Borhan-Manesh F, Farnum JB. Incidence of heterotopic gastric mucosa in the upper oesophagus. *Gut*. 1991;32(9):968–972.
30. Bechman S, Vieth M, Stolte M, Moll R. Cytokeratins and cell-cell adhesion molecules in Barrett's esophagus: implications for its histogenesis. *Pathol Res Pract*. 2003;199:268–269.
31. Boening H. *Leitfaden der Entwicklungsgeschichte des Menschen*. Leipzig, Germany: Edition Leipzig; 1965.
32. Daniel EE, Wang YF. Control systems of gastrointestinal motility are immature at birth in dogs. *Neurogastroenterol Motil*. 1999;11(5):375–392.
33. Konkin DE, O'Hali WA, Webber EM, Blair GK. Outcomes in esophageal atresia and tracheoesophageal fistula. *J Pediatr Surg*. 2003;38(12):1726–1729.
34. Holder TM, Ashcraft KW. Esophageal atresia and tracheoesophageal fistula. *Ann Thorac Surg*. 1970;9(5):445–467.
35. Spitz L, Kiely E, Brereton RJ. Esophageal atresia: five year experience with 148 cases. *J Pediatr Surg*. 1987;22(2):103–108.
36. Kirk JM, Dicks-Mireaux C. Difficulties in diagnosis of congenital H-type tracheo-oesophageal fistulae. *Clin Radiol*. 1989;40(2):150–153.
37. Blackburn WR, Amoury RA. Congenital esophagopulmonary fistulas without esophageal atresia: an analysis of 260 fistulas in infants, children and adults. *Rev Surg*. 1966;23(3):153–175.
38. Moreno Azcoita M, Ruiz de Adana JC, Sanchez Urdazpal L, et al. Congenital oesophagobronchial fistula in an adult involving left main bronchus. *Thorax*. 1994;49(8):835–836.
39. Nakamura Y, Yamazumi T, Hatama T. Congenital bronchoesophageal fistula in adult. *Surg Diagn Treat (Geka Shinryo)*. 1972;14:1067–1072.
40. Wesselhoeft CW Jr, Keshishian JM. Acquired nonmalignant esophagotracheal and esophagobronchial fistulas. *Ann Thorac Surg*. 1968;6(2):187–195.
41. Iseki K, Ito O, Kusakari K. Tubular-type duplication of the esophagus, report of a case. *I to Cho (Stomach and Intestine)*. 1985;20:555–559.
42. Ratan ML, Anand R, Mittal SK, Taneja S. Communicating oesophageal duplication: a report of two cases. *Gut*. 1988;29(2):254–256.
43. Robison RJ, Pavlina PM, Scherer LR, Grosfeld JL. Multiple esophageal duplication cysts. *J Thorac Cardiovasc Surg*. 1987;94(1):144–147.
44. Arbona JL, Fazzi JG, Mayoral J. Congenital esophageal cysts: case report and review of literature. *Am J Gastroenterol*. 1984;79(3):177–182.

45. Kaneko E, Kohda A, Honda N, Kino I. Incomplete tubular duplication of esophagus with heterotopic gastric mucosa. *Dig Dis Sci.* 1989;34(6):948–951.
46. Salyer DC, Salyer WR, Eggleston JC. Benign developmental cysts of the mediastinum. *Arch Pathol Lab Med.* 1977;101(3):136–139.
47. Gatzinsky P, Fasth S, Hansson G. Intramural oesophageal cyst with massive mediastinal bleeding. A case report. *Scand J Thorac Cardiovasc Surg.* 1978;12(2):143–145.
48. Singh S, Lal P, Sikora SS, Datta NR. Squamous cell carcinoma arising from a congenital duplication cyst of the esophagus in a young adult. *Dis Esophagus.* 2001;14(3–4):258–261.
49. Tapia RH, White VA. Squamous cell carcinoma arising in a duplication cyst of the esophagus. *Am J Gastroenterol.* 1985;80(5):325–329.
50. Taylor AL. The epithelial heterotopias of the alimentary tract. *J Pathol Bacteriol.* 1927;30:415–449.
51. Truong LD, Stroehlein JR, McKechnie JC. Gastric heterotopia of the proximal esophagus: a report of four cases detected by endoscopy and review of literature. *Am J Gastroenterol.* 1986;81(12):1162–1166.
52. Jabbari M, Goresky CA, Lough J, et al. The inlet patch: heterotopic gastric mucosa in the upper esophagus. *Gastroenterology.* 1985;89(2):352–356.
53. Variend S, Howat AJ. Upper oesophageal gastric heterotopia: a prospective necropsy study in children. *J Clin Pathol.* 1988;41(7):742–745.
54. Steadman C, Kerlin P, Teague C, Stephenson P. High esophageal stricture: a complication of "inlet patch" mucosa. *Gastroenterology.* 1988;94(2):521–524.
55. Shah KK, DeRidder PH. Ectopic gastric mucosa in proximal esophagus. Its clinical significance and hormonal profile. *J Clin Gastroenterol.* 1986;8(5):509–513.
56. Kohler B, Kohler G, Riemann JF. Spontaneous esophagotracheal fistula resulting from ulcer in heterotopic gastric mucosa. *Gastroenterology.* 1988;95(3):828–830.
57. Hamilton JW, Thune RG, Morrissey JF. Symptomatic ectopic gastric epithelium of the cervical esophagus. Demonstration of acid production with Congo red. *Dig Dis Sci.* 1986;31(4):337–342.
58. Christensen WN, Sternberg SS. Adenocarcinoma of the upper esophagus arising in ectopic gastric mucosa. Two case reports and review of the literature. *Am J Surg Pathol.* 1987;11(5):397–402.
59. Pech O, May A, Gossner L, et al. Early stage adenocarcinoma of the esophagus arising in circular heterotopic gastric mucosa treated by endoscopic mucosal resection. *Gastrointest Endosc.* 2001;54(5):656–658.
60. Schaller G. Luminal surface of human esophagus during ontogeny. *Z Mikrosk Anat Forsch.* 1978;92(4):675–699.
61. Rector L, Connerley ML. Aberrant mucosa in the oesophagus in infants and in children. *Arch Pathol.* 1941;31:285–294.
62. Merino MJ, Brand M, LiVolsi VA, McCallum RW. Sebaceous glands in the esophagus diagnosed in a clinical setting. *Arch Pathol Lab Med.* 1982;106(1):47–48.
63. De La Pava S, Pickren JW. Ectopic sebaceous glands in the esophagus. *Arch Pathol.* 1962;73:397–399.
64. McLean G, Laufer I. Hairy esophagus: a complication of pharyngoesophageal reconstructive surgery in two cases. *Am J Roentgenol.* 1979;132(2):269–270.
65. Takubo K. *Pathology of the Esophagus.* 2nd ed. Tokyo, Japan: Springer; 2007.
66. Leung AW, Lam HS, Chu WC, et al. Congenital intrathoracic stomach: short esophagus or hiatal hernia? *Neonatology.* 2008;93(3):178–181.
67. Gerle RD, Jaretzki A III, Ashley CA, Berne AS. Congenital bronchopulmonary-foregut malformation. Pulmonary sequestration communicating with the gastrointestinal tract. *N Engl J Med.* 1968;278(26):1413–1419.
68. Heithoff KB, Sane SM, Williams HJ, et al. Bronchopulmonary foregut malformations. A unifying etiological concept. *Am J Roentgenol.* 1976;126(1):46–55.
69. Bladergroen MR, Lowe JE, Postlethwait RW. Diagnosis and recommended management of esophageal perforation and rupture. *Ann Thorac Surg.* 1986;42(3):235–239.
70. Michel L. Post-emetic laceration and rupture of the gastroesophageal junction. *Acta Chir Belg.* 1982;82(1):13–24.
71. Curci JJ, Horman MJ. Boerhaave's syndrome: the importance of early diagnosis and treatment. *Ann Surg.* 1976;183(4):401–408.
72. Case records of the Massachusetts General Hospital. Weekly Clinicopathological exercises. Case 4–1989. Sudden onset of abdominal pain and hematemesis in a 56-year-old woman. *N Engl J Med.* 1989;320(4):235–244.
73. Miller S, Hines C Jr, Ochsner JL. Spontaneous perforation of the esophagus associated with a lower esophageal ring. *Am J Gastroenterol.* 1988;83(12):1405–1408.
74. Ivey TD, Simonowitz DA, Dillard DH, Miller DW Jr. Boerhaave syndrome. Successful conservative management in three patients with late presentation. *Am J Surg.* 1981;141(5):531–533.
75. Wilde PH, Mullany CJ. Oesophageal perforation—a review of 37 cases. *Aust N Z J Surg.* 1987;57(10):743–747.
76. Ashman FC, Hill MC, Saba GP, Diaconis JN. Esophageal hematoma associated with thrombocytopenia. *Gastrointest Radiol.* 1978;3(2):115–118.
77. Shay SS, Berendson RA, Johnson LF. Esophageal hematoma. Four new cases, a review, and proposed etiology. *Dig Dis Sci.* 1981;26(11):1019–1024.
78. van den Brandt-Gradel V, den Hartog Jager FC, Tytgat GN. Palliative intubation of malignant esophagogastric obstruction. *J Clin Gastroenterol.* 1987;9(3):290–297.
79. Webb WA. Management of foreign bodies of the upper gastrointestinal tract. *Gastroenterology.* 1988;94(1):204–216.
80. Witcombe B, Meyer D. Sword swallowing and its side effects. *Br Med J.* 2006;333(7582):1285–1287.
81. Krasna IH, Rosenfeld D, Benjamin BG. Esophageal perforation in the neonate: an emerging problem in the newborn nursery. *J Pediatr Surg.* 1987;22(8):784–790.
82. Pellicano A, Watier A, Gentile J. Spontaneous double-barrelled esophagus. Report of two cases and review of the literature. *J Clin Gastroenterol.* 1987;9(2):149–154.
83. Le K, Ahmed A. Acute necrotizing esophagitis: case report and review of the literature. *J La State Med Soc.* 2007;159(6):330, 3–8.
84. Mallory GK, Weiss S. Hemorrhages from lacerations of the cardiac orifice due to vomiting. *Am J Med Sci.* 1929;170:506–511.
85. Sugawa C, Benishek D, Walt AJ. Mallory-Weiss syndrome. A study of 224 patients. *Am J Surg.* 1983;145(1):30–33.
86. Graham DY, Schwartz JT. The spectrum of the Mallory-Weiss tear. *Medicine (Baltimore).* 1978;57(4):307–318.
87. Knauer CM. Mallory-Weiss syndrome. Characterization of 75 Mallory-Weiss lacerations in 528 patients with upper gastrointestinal hemorrhage. *Gastroenterology.* 1976;71(1):5–8.
88. Thompson NW, Ernst CB, Fry WJ. The spectrum of emetogenic injury to the esophagus and stomach. *Am J Surg.* 1967;113(1):13–26.
89. Lytkin MI, Zubarev PN, Kalashnikov SA. Idiopathic portal hypertension. *Vestn Khir Im I I Grek.* 2001;160(1):101–105.
90. Hashizume M, Kitano S, Sugimachi K, Sueishi K. Three-dimensional view of the vascular structure of the lower

esophagus in clinical portal hypertension. *Hepatology.* 1988;8(6):1482–1487.
91. Spence RA, Terblanche J. Venous anatomy of the lower oesophagus: a new perspective on varices. *Br J Surg.* 1987;74(8):659–660.
92. McCormack TT, Rose JD, Smith PM, Johnson AG. Perforating veins and blood flow in oesophageal varices. *Lancet.* 1983;2(8365-66):1442–1444.
93. Butler H. The veins of the oesophagus. *Thorax.* 1951;6(3):276–296.
94. Kitano S, Terblanche J, Kahn D, Bornman PC. Venous anatomy of the lower oesophagus in portal hypertension: practical implications. *Br J Surg.* 1986;73(7):525–531.
95. Laine L, Cook D. Endoscopic ligation compared with sclerotherapy for treatment of esophageal variceal bleeding. A meta-analysis. *Ann Intern Med.* 1995;123(4):280–287.
96. Garcia-Tsao G, Sanyal AJ, Grace ND, Carey W. Prevention and management of gastroesophageal varices and variceal hemorrhage in cirrhosis. *Hepatology.* 2007;46(3):922–938.
97. Prediction of the first variceal hemorrhage in patients with cirrhosis of the liver and esophageal varices. A prospective multicenter study. *N Engl J Med.* 1988;319(15):983–989.
98. Paquet KJ. Prophylactic endoscopic sclerosing treatment of the esophageal wall in varices—a prospective controlled randomized trial. *Endoscopy.* 1982;14(1):4–5.
99. Beppu K, Inokuchi K, Koyanagi N, et al. Prediction of variceal hemorrhage by esophageal endoscopy. *Gastrointest Endosc.* 1981;27(4):213–218.
100. Terblanche J, Burroughs AK, Hobbs KE. Controversies in the management of bleeding esophageal varices (2). *N Engl J Med.* 1989;320(22):1469–1475.
101. Terblanche J, Burroughs AK, Hobbs KE. Controversies in the management of bleeding esophageal varices (1). *N Engl J Med.* 1989;320(21):1393–1398.
102. Gurvits GE, Shapsis A, Lau N, et al. Acute esophageal necrosis: a rare syndrome. *J Gastroenterol.* 2007;42(1):29–38.
103. Nagri S, Hwang R, Anand S, Kurz J. Herpes simplex esophagitis presenting as acute necrotizing esophagitis ("black esophagus") in an immunocompetent patient. *Endoscopy.* 2007;39(suppl 1):E169.
104. Akkinepally S, Poreddy V, Moreno A. Black esophagus. *Cleve Clin J Med.* 2009;76(7):400.
105. Grudell AB, Mueller PS, Viggiano TR. Black esophagus: report of six cases and review of the literature, 1963-2003. *Dis Esophagus.* 2006;19(2):105–110.
106. Catinella FP, Kittle CF. Tuberculous esophagitis with aortic aneurysm fistula. *Ann Thorac Surg.* 1988;45(1):87–88.
107. Coss KC, Wheat LJ, Conces DJ Jr, et al. Esophageal fistula complicating mediastinal histoplasmosis. Response to amphotericin B. *Am J Med.* 1987;83(2):343–346.
108. West AB, Nolan N, O'Briain DS. Benign peptic ulcers penetrating pericardium and heart: clinicopathological features and factors favoring survival. *Gastroenterology.* 1988;94(6):1478–1487.
109. Grey TC, Mittleman RE, Wetli CV, Horowitz S. Aortoesophageal fistula and sudden death. A report of two cases and review of the literature. *Am J Forensic Med Pathol.* 1988;9(1):19–22.
110. Pope CE II. Rings and webs. In: Sleisenger MH, Fordtran JE, eds. *Gastrointestinal Disease.* Philadelphia, PA: W.B. Saunders Co.; 1989.
111. Chisholm M, Ardran GM, Callender ST, Wright R. Iron deficiency and autoimmunity in post-cricoid webs. *Q J Med.* 1971;40(159):421–433.
112. Chisholm M, Ardran GM, Callender ST, Wright R. A follow-up study of patients with post-cricoid webs. *Q J Med.* 1971;40(159):409–420.
113. Okamura H, Tsutsumi S, Inaki S, Mori T. Esophageal web in Plummer-Vinson syndrome. *Laryngoscope.* 1988;98(9):994–998.
114. Janisch HD, Eckardt VF. Histological abnormalities in patients with multiple esophageal webs. *Dig Dis Sci.* 1982;27(6):503–506.
115. McDonald GB, Sullivan KM, Schuffler MD, et al. Esophageal abnormalities in chronic graft-versus-host disease in humans. *Gastroenterology.* 1981;80(5 pt 1):914–921.
116. Weaver GA. Upper esophageal web due to a ring formed by a squamocolumnar junction with ectopic gastric mucosa (another explanation of the Paterson-Kelly, Plummer-Vinson syndrome). *Dig Dis Sci.* 1979;24(12):959–963.
117. Longstreth GF, Wolochow DA, Tu RT. Double congenital midesophageal webs in adults. *Dig Dis Sci.* 1979;24(2):162–165.
118. Ikard RW, Rosen HE. Midesophageal web in adults. *Ann Thorac Surg.* 1977;24(4):355–358.
119. Goyal RK, Bauer JL, Spiro HM. The nature and location of lower esophageal ring. *N Engl J Med.* 1971;284(21):1175–1180.
120. Eckardt VF, Adami B, Hucker H, Leeder H. The esophagogastric junction in patients with asymptomatic lower esophageal mucosal rings. *Gastroenterology.* 1980;79(3):426–430.
121. Hendrix TR. Schatzki ring, epithelial junction, and hiatal hernia—an unresolved controversy. *Gastroenterology.* 1980;79(3):584–585.
122. Chen YM, Gelfand DW, Ott DJ, Munitz HA. Natural progression of the lower esophageal mucosal ring. *Gastrointest Radiol.* 1987;12(2):93–98.
123. Ott DJ, Chen YM, Wu WC, et al. Radiographic and endoscopic sensitivity in detecting lower esophageal mucosal ring. *Am J Roentgenol.* 1986;147(2):261–265.
124. Guelrud M, Villasmil L, Mendez R. Late results in patients with Schatzki ring treated by endoscopic electrosurgical incision of the ring. *Gastrointest Endosc.* 1987;33(2):96–98.
125. Saldana JA, Cone RO, Hopens TA, Bannayan GA. Carcinoma arising in an epiphrenic esophageal diverticulum. *Gastrointest Radiol.* 1982;7(1):15–18.
126. Huang BS, Unni KK, Payne WS. Long-term survival following diverticulectomy for cancer in pharyngoesophageal (Zenker's) diverticulum. *Ann Thorac Surg.* 1984;38(3):207–210.
127. Boisvert RD, Bethune DC, Acton D, Klassen DR. Bilateral Killian-Jamieson diverticula: a case report and literature review. *Can J Gastroenterol.* 2010;24(3):173–174.
128. Catalano PJ. Zenker's diverticulum: case report and review. *Mt Sinai J Med.* 1987;54(6):535–540.
129. Pope CE II. Diverticula. In: Sleisenger M, Fordtran JS, eds. *Gastrointestinal Disease.* Philadelphia, PA: W.B. Saunders Co.; 1989.
130. Knuff TE, Benjamin SB, Castell DO. Pharyngoesophageal (Zenker's) diverticulum: a reappraisal. *Gastroenterology.* 1982;82(4):734–736.
131. Cook IJ, Gabb M, Panagopoulos V, et al. Pharyngeal (Zenker's) diverticulum is a disorder of upper esophageal sphincter opening. *Gastroenterology.* 1992;103(4):1229–1235.
132. Ferreira LE, Simmons DT, Baron TH. Zenker's diverticula: pathophysiology, clinical presentation, and flexible endoscopic management. *Dis Esophagus.* 2008;21(1):1–8.
133. Mulder DG, Rosenkranz E, DenBesten L. Management of huge epiphrenic esophageal diverticula. *Am J Surg.* 1989;157(3):303–307.

134. Debas HT, Payne WS, Cameron AJ, Carlson HC. Physiopathology of lower esophageal diverticulum and its implications for treatment. *Surg Gynecol Obstet.* 1980;151(5):593-600.
135. Wallner B, Friedrich JM, Kunz R. Leiomyoma of the esophagus in a subphrenic diverticulum. *Rofo.* 1988;148(6):717-718.
136. Gothlin J, Bloch R, Sundgren R. Intraphrenic esophageal leiomyoma associated with diverticula preoperatively diagnosed by angiography. *Acta Radiol Diagn (Stockh).* 1975;16(6):673-678.
137. Bozorgi S, Migliorelli FA, Cook WA. Leiomyoma of the esophagus presenting as a bleeding epiphrenic diverticulum. *Chest.* 1973;63(2):281-284.
138. Coburn WM Jr, Dana ER, Gayler BW. Subphrenic esophageal diverticulum: a case studied by cine-manometry. *Johns Hopkins Med J* 1971;128(1):41-44.
139. Hodge GB. Esophageal leiomyoma associated with an epiphrenic diverticulum and hiatus hernia. *Am Surg.* 1970;36(9):538-543.
140. Wenzel KP. Subphrenic esophageal diverticula following Starck's cardia dilatation. *Zentralbl Chir.* 1970;95(29):849-851.
141. Clements JL Jr, Abernathy J, Weens HS. Atypical esophageal diverticula associated with progressive systemic sclerosis. *Gastrointest Radiol.* 1978;3(4):383-386.
142. Sabanathan S, Salama FD, Morgan WE. Oesophageal intramural pseudodiverticulosis. *Thorax.* 1985;40(11):849-857.
143. Koyama S, Watanabe M, Iijima T. Esophageal intramural pseudodiverticulosis (diffuse type). *J Gastroenterol.* 2002;37(8):644-648.
144. Murney RG Jr, Linne JH, Curtis J. High-amplitude peristaltic contractions in a patient with esophageal intramural pseudodiverticulosis. *Dig Dis Sci.* 1983;28(9):843-847.
145. Levine MS, Moolten DN, Herlinger H, Laufer I. Esophageal intramural pseudodiverticulosis: a reevaluation. *Am J Roentgenol.* 1986;147(6):1165-1170.
146. Fromkes J, Thomas FB, Mekhjian H, et al. Esophageal intramural pseudodiverticulosis. *Am J Dig Dis.* 1977;22(8):690-700.
147. Castillo S, Aburashed A, Kimmelman J, Alexander LC. Diffuse intramural esophageal pseudodiverticulosis. New cases and review. *Gastroenterology.* 1977;72(3):541-545.
148. Umlas J, Sakhuja R. The pathology of esophageal intramural pseudodiverticulosis. *Am J Clin Pathol.* 1976;65(3):314-320.
149. Papazian A, Capron JP, Sevenet F. Mucosal bridges of the distal esophagus related to reflux esophagitis. *Gastrointest Endosc.* 1984;30(3):217-218.
150. Sood A, Midha V, Sood N, Kaushal V. Multiple mucosal bridges in the oesophagus after sclerotherapy for varices. *Trop Gastroenterol.* 2001;22(2):94-95.
151. Simson JN, Kinder RB, Isaacs PE, Jourdan MH. Mucosal bridges of the oesophagus in Candida oesophagitis. *Br J Surg.* 1985;72(3):209-210.
152. Hanai H, Honda S, Sugimoto K, et al. Endoscopic therapy for multiple mucosal bridges in the esophagus of a patient with Crohn's disease. *Gastrointest Endosc.* 1999;50(5):715-717.
153. Ghahremani GG, Rushovich AM. Glycogenic acanthosis of the esophagus: radiographic and pathologic features. *Gastrointest Radiol.* 1984;9(2):93-98.
154. Glick SN, Teplick SK, Goldstein J, et al. Glycogenic acanthosis of the esophagus. *AJR Am J Roentgenol.* 1982;139(4):683-688.
155. Stern Z, Sharon P, Ligumsky M, et al. Glycogenic acanthosis of the esophagus. A benign but confusing endoscopic lesion. *Am J Gastroenterol.* 1980;74(3):261-263.
156. Bender MD, Allison J, Cuartas F, Montgomery C. Glycogenic acanthosis of the esophagus: a form of benign epithelial hyperplasia. *Gastroenterology.* 1973;65(3):373-380.
157. Rywlin AM, Ortega R. Glycogenic acanthosis of the esophagus. *Arch Pathol.* 1970;90(5):439-443.
158. Jessurun J, Yardley JH, Giardiello FM, Hamilton SR. Intracytoplasmic plasma proteins in distended esophageal squamous cells (balloon cells). *Mod Pathol.* 1988;1(3):175-181.
159. Remmele W, Engelsing B. Lipid island of the esophagus. Case report. *Endoscopy.* 1984;16(6):240-241.
160. Stolte M, Seifert E. Lipid islands in the esophagus. *Leber Magen Darm.* 1985;15(4):137-139.
161. Vimala R, Ananthalakshmi V, Murthy M, et al. Xanthelasma of esophagus and stomach. *Indian J Gastroenterol.* 2000;19(3):135.
162. Brereton RJ. Skeletal anomalies in oesophageal atresia. *Z Kinderchir.* 1979;26:258-270.
163. German JC, Mahour GH, Woolley MM. Esophageal atresia and associated anomalies. *J Pediatr Surg.* 1976;11(3):299-306.
164. Greenwood RD, Rosenthal A. Cardiovascular malformations associated with tracheoesophageal fistula and esophageal atresia. *Pediatrics.* 1976;57(1):87-91.
165. Töndury G. Zur Pathogenese der Ösophagusatresie. *Z Kinderchir.* 1975;16:118-133.
166. Weigel W, Kaufmann HJ. The frequency and types of other congenital anomalies in association with tracheoesophageal malformations. Radiologic studies of 83 such infants. *Clin Pediatr (Phila).* 1976;15(9):819-820, 27-29, 32-34.

10 Inflammatory Disorders of the Esophagus: Reflux and Nonreflux Types

Chapter Outline

GASTROESOPHAGEAL REFLUX DISEASE (REFLUX ESOPHAGITIS–GERD/GORD)
Definition of GERD
Symptoms of GERD
  Correlation between GERD, symptoms, and endoscopy
  Therapy
  Long-term therapy for GERD and prognosis
The Gastroesophageal Junction and Z-Line
Etiology and Pathogenesis of GERD
Endoscopic Grading of Reflux Disease in Squamous Mucosa
Los Angeles Grading System for Reflux Disease in Squamous Mucosa
Nonerosive Reflux Disease and Its Pathology
Gross/Endoscopic Appearances of GERD
Where to Biopsy for GERD and Criteria Used
  Erosions
  Traditional biopsy sites
  Cardia biopsies
Histologic Diagnosis and Criteria for GERD in Biopsies
  Evaluating reactive changes
  Grading reactive epithelial changes
INFLAMMATORY CELLS
Intraepithelial Mononuclear Cells
  Minor changes
Inflammatory Polyps
  Reactive changes versus neoplasia following erosions and ulcers
Atypical Cells in Squamous Mucosa
Carditis as a Manifestation of GERD
  Progression of GERD
Complications of GERD
  GERD-related strictures
Cameron's Ulcer
BARRETT'S ESOPHAGUS (BE)
Definition
Practical Aspects of Making the Diagnosis of BE
  Irregular Z-line versus "ultrashort" BE

  Definitions of BE: short- versus long-segment BE
When BE Does Not Have Goblet Cells, Does It Matter?
  When are goblet cells not present?
  Risk of carcinoma in patients with non–goblet cell BE
  Conclusions regarding the definition and cancer risk in Barrett's (columnar-lined) esophagus
Epidemiology and Pathophysiology of Barrett's Esophagus
Morphologic Development of Barrett's Esophagus
Endoscopic Grading of Barrett's Mucosa
Histology
  Double muscularis mucosae
  Palisaded vessels
Handling of Patients and Biopsies Postablation or Postendoscopic Resection
Differential Diagnosis of BE and Other Mucosal Types Encountered
Barrett-associated Neoplasia
Diagnosing and Grading Dysplasia
Indefinite for Dysplasia
Low-grade Dysplasia (Low-grade Intraepithelial Neoplasia—LGNIN)
High-grade Dysplasia (High-grade Intraepithelial Neoplasia—HGIEN)
  Implication
Intramucosal Carcinoma
Invasive Carcinoma (Submucosal invasion)
Interobserver Variability and Need for a Second Opinion for Dysplasia
Ancillary Techniques
  Surveillance biopsies
NONREFLUX ESOPHAGITIS
INFECTIONS
Viral Infections
  Herpes virus infection
  Cytomegalovirus esophagitis
  Human papillomavirus

  Acute HIV infection
  Other viral infections
Fungal Infections
  Clinic symptoms and prognosis
  Other fungal infections
Bacterial Esophagitis
  Luetic infection
  Other bacteria
DESCRIPTIVE ESOPHAGITIDES
Lymphocytic Esophagitis
Exfoliative (Sloughing) Esophagitis (Esophagitis Dissecans Superficialis)
Acute Necrotizing Esophagitis (Black Esophagus)
Eosinophilic Esophagitis
  Pathogenesis
  Symptoms
  Clinical
  Biopsy sites
  Pathology
  Differential diagnosis
Corrosive Esophagitis
Drug-induced Esophagitis (Pill Esophagitis)
SYSTEMIC DISEASES INVOLVING THE ESOPHAGUS
Skin Diseases and Esophageal Inflammation
  Glycogenic acanthosis
Skin Diseases and Esophageal Inflammation
Pseudoepitheliomatous Hyperplasia
Leukoplakia
Graft versus Host Disease
Behçet's Disease
Crohn's Disease
  Lymphocytic esophagitis in Crohn's disease
Granulomatous Esophagitis and Sarcoid
Ulcerative Colitis
Brown Bowel Syndrome (Ceroid Lipofuscinosis)
Diabetes Mellitus
Parkinson's Disease

GASTROESOPHAGEAL REFLUX DISEASE (REFLUX ESOPHAGITIS—GERD/GORD)

Definition of GERD

Gastroesophageal reflux disease (GERD) is defined as at least weekly heartburn, acid regurgitation, or both, or extraesophageal symptoms with impairment of quality of life.[1] GERD is quite common and affects around 20% to 30% of the population in industrialized countries. In the United States, 21% to 44% are said to suffer from regular heartburn, while GERD is actually diagnosed in 10% to 20%, with mucosal breaks (endoscopic erosions) being present in 2% to 5% of all refluxers. Around one-third of the affected individuals seek professional help. It is now clear that lifestyle factors, in particular obesity and smoking, are associated with increased reflux symptoms.[2] In overweight individuals, the presence of a hiatal hernia increases the risk of reflux disease about ninefold compared to individuals without hiatal hernia.[3]

GERD is readily diagnosed in most patients from the characteristic history, and is treated by medications that decrease the amount of gastric acid. These range from over-the-counter antacids to medications reducing gastric acid secretion, of which there are two major classes. H2 receptor antagonists (H2RA) block the secretion of acid by blocking the histamine 2 receptors (hence H2) that mediate acid secretion in response to gastrin (released from the gastric antrum and duodenum) or acetylcholine. They usually have the suffix -tidine (cimetidine, ranitidine, etc.). Proton pump inhibitors (PPIs), as their name implies, inhibit secretion of hydrogen ions (protons) from parietal cells, and tend to be more potent although a little slower to act. They usually have the suffix -prazole (omeprazole, esomeprazole, lanzoprazole, etc.). Response to therapy is usually almost immediate, and further serves as a confirmation of the diagnosis.

Some patients have periodic symptoms and can take medications as the need arises, but for many it is chronic, so medications may be lifelong. Some patients become aware of the increased quality of life with PPIs when they undergo Helicobacter pylori eradication therapy, of which a PPI is a key ingredient. When the course of therapy ceases, their symptoms quickly recur so they become "hooked" on PPIs. While these are a remarkably safe group of drugs, they do increase the risk of gastrointestinal (GI) infections, and in the long term, gastric fundic gland polyps, which fortunately appear quite harmless. PPIs may increase the risk of osteopenia and fractures. In patients on long-term high-dose PPIs, the risk of vitamin B_{12} deficiency is increased, as both acid and B_{12} are required for its absorption, and the secretion of both from parietal cells is diminished by PPIs. Endoscopy, potentially with biopsies, is therefore reserved for patients who are not responding to therapy or have atypical symptoms such as chest pain in which it is unclear whether this is of cardiac, esophageal, or some other cause. While endoscopic erythema, erosions (mucosal breaks), and ulcers can all be seen, patients may have GERD without these changes (nonerosive reflux disease [NERD]), although on biopsy a variety of abnormalities can be found in these patients. Some of these patients appear to simply have exquisite esophageal sensitivity to acid.

There are numerous other causes of esophageal ulceration, especially medication, which may become stuck in the esophagus (pill-induced esophagitis), so that a history of medications used is also key (discussed subsequently). Infections (herpes, cytomegalovirus [CMV]) can also be painful and cause ulcers while there are numerous other less common causes (Table 10-1) that can affect the esophagus. Further, GERD has numerous complications but especially Barrett's esophagus (BE), which increases the risk of esophageal adenocarcinoma, usually in association

Table 10-1 Classification of Esophagitis by Etiology

1. Reflux—acid or alkaline reflux
2. Infectious
   Fungal (e.g., moniliasis, Mucor)
   Bacterial (e.g., mycobacteria)
   Viral (e.g., herpes, CMV, HPV, HIV, varicella zoster)
3. Ingested substances
   Medications
      NSAID/ASA
      Tetracyclines
      Bisphosphonates (antiosteoporosis drugs)
      Chemotherapy
      Iron and Plummer–Vinson syndrome (ulcer due to iron–sulfur preparations for anemia)
   Chemicals (acute)
      Ingested acid or alkali
      Silicates/metals/porcelain dust
      Extremely hot or cold drinks
4. Trauma
   Iatrogenic tubes (naso-gastric, pH-metry)
   Bolus—injury due to foreign bodies
   Radiotherapy
   Ulceration of anastomosis (ischemic or insufficiency)
5. Systemic diseases
   Collagenous diseases
   Crohn's disease
   Sarcoidosis
   Eosinophilic esophagitis
6. Tumors and their complications
   Luminal obstruction
   External compression
   Necrosis
   Neoangiogenesis
7. Miscellaneous
   Exfoliative (sloughing) esophagitis

with hiatal hernia, which tends to promote free gastroesophageal reflux, as the additional safety valve of the diaphragmatic pinch is less effective. Other patients have motility problems that allow reflux of gastric contents into the esophagus or have a degree of peristaltic failure.

Symptoms of GERD

The leading symptom of GERD is heartburn, which needs to be differentiated from other causes of retrosternal pain, such as dysphagia, odynophagia, and cardiac pain. Further, GERD can lead to extraesophageal symptoms such as hoarseness, laryngitis, dyspnoea, cough, bronchitis and reflux-induced asthmatic disease, dental erosions, and retrosternal pain that need to be differentiated from ischemic heart disease.[1] The frequency of these extraesophageal symptoms is probably underestimated in the population, but on the other hand laryngitis as a sequel of GERD is probably overestimated.[4]

Correlation between GERD, symptoms, and endoscopy. An ill-defined proportion of patients clearly have reflux-induced esophageal lesions endoscopically, but are asymptomatic, while another group have symptoms but little to see endoscopically (nonerosive [endoscopy-negative] reflux disease—NERD/ENRD).[5,6] A more troublesome group of patients appear to have persistent symptoms despite being on high-dose PPIs but have nothing evident endoscopically. These patients may have "visceral hypersensitivity" to esophageal acid, possibly mediated through dilated intercellular spaces (DISs) allowing acid (and other molecules) to pass through the pericellular space into the lamina propria and the nerves there.[7] DISs are readily visible on biopsies, but it is unclear where physiology stops and pathology starts.

Therapy. In classical reflux disease, symptoms are treated with antisecretory therapy, usually PPIs. A 1-week course of PPI that proves to be therapeutic can serve as a diagnostic test, and endoscopy is limited to those that do not respond, or have atypical symptoms, so that biopsies are not usually necessary.

Long-term therapy for GERD and prognosis. If long-term (usually lifetime) treatment with PPIs[8] is refused, there are intraluminal endoscopic procedures available besides open or endoscopic fundoplication. What all of these procedures have in common is that they narrow the distal esophagus to imitate the distal esophageal sphincter to avoid regurgitation of gastric contents into the esophagus. Many of these endoscopic procedures have fallen out of favor because of either failure or complications. The surgical equivalent of these techniques has a small but definite mortality, related to some extent on the experience of the surgeon. However, patients who benefit most from a fundoplication are also those who show the best response to medical treatment. Also, fundoplication does not last forever (they become lax over time) and ultimately about 60% of operated patients need PPIs to manage symptoms. Approximately 20% of individuals who undergo surgical fundoplication may suffer from a gas-bloat syndrome where there is difficulty with eructation and air feels trapped and some develop dysphagia secondary to the fundoplication wrap being too tight, and dilation is required. General health (losing weight, sleeping with bed head raised) recommendations do not have long-lasting benefits in reflux disease. Nevertheless, there are always patients who report symptom relief after losing weight or after changes in lifestyle.

The Gastroesophageal Junction and Z-Line

One major problem is the difficulty in the definition of the gastroesophageal junction (GEJ), which differs worldwide. Practically by far, the most important definition is that used endoscopically in which the GEJ is now defined as the upper limit of the proximal gastric folds. Endoscopically, the Z-line is defined as the transition of columnar epithelium into stratified squamous epithelium. The Z-line is usually irregular (hence Z-line) and should be within the lower esophageal sphincter (LES), which itself extends for several centimeters (see Chapter 9). Histologically, squamous mucosa may be in direct continuity with:

1. Gastric cardiac, cardio-oxyntic, or less frequently oxyntic (acid-producing) mucosa
2. Undermining cardiac glands below the squamous epithelium (that can also be seen in treated GERD)
3. The presence of multilayered (hybrid) epithelium
4. Pancreatic metaplasia

The last three are usually not recognizable endoscopically.

In Japan, the GEJ is defined by the distal end of esophageal palisade vessels. However, this is an approximation, as the end of these vessels can be present above, at, and even below the Z-line in normal individuals.

Etiology and Pathogenesis of GERD

Temporary mild reflux of gastric contents into the distal esophagus is thought to be physiologic. Pathologic reflux is diagnosed clinically whenever, in the supine position, a prolonged contact of gastric refluxate is present combined with a pH < 4 for more than 4% of 24 hours (at least 1 hour a day). It is believed that low basal lower esophageal sphincter (LES) pressure along with increased transient LES relaxations (tLESR) cause reflux disease. Besides increased relaxation, or insufficiency of the distal esophageal sphincter, there are other factors that can either cause or unmask prior existing reflux disease. These include the presence of a hiatal hernia (Fig. 10-1), the increased acid secretion that often follows *H. pylori* eradication therapy (or rarely Zollinger–Ellison syndrome), obesity, medications that decrease the LES pressure,[9] possibly excess alcohol, impairments of esophageal emptying (motility disorders), impaired salivary and esophageal gland secretions, duodenogastric reflux, delayed gastric emptying (mostly in diabetic patients with autonomic neuropathy), stenosis or strictures, impaired esophageal resistance to acid, and failure of clearance. Numerous changes occur in the esophageal nerves (described under morphologic changes in nerves).

Gastric heterotopia (inlet patch) in the proximal esophagus can contribute to acid secretion, depending on its size and the presence of oxyntic mucosa.

For NERD, dilated intercellular spaces (DISs—see subsequent discussion) and visceral hypersensitivity are postulated mechanisms. The DIS experimentally can be induced by acid plus sodium nitrite,[10] which is present in saliva.[11,12] In addition, the presence of duodenal contents containing bile and activated pancreatic juice, both known to be considered as etiologic factors in generating BE, might also be involved in the etiology of reflux disease. In large-scale studies, alcohol and smoking appeared not to be risk factors for reflux disease or its complications. General recommendations such as reducing weight may not impact reflux disease but in some contribute to reduced symptoms and of course make sense for general health.

The role of hormonal effects is controversial: Gastrin and cholinomimetics increase the lower sphincter pressure, whereas secretin, glucagon, cholecystokinin, and prostaglandins inhibit the effect of gastrin.[13]

Endoscopic Grading of Reflux Disease in Squamous Mucosa

If endoscopy is carried out, there are numerous schemes available, but the Los Angeles classification (Fig. 10-2)[14] is the best-validated classification scheme and is the most frequently used classification. It grades the extent of erosions and ulcers, which are together called "mucosal breaks." A mucosal break is defined as a lesion covered by slough and is sharply delineated from the adjacent epithelium, often showing increased vascularity at the margin.

Grading is undertaken with letters A to D to avoid confusion with other classifications. Two additional grades were also proposed that would incorporate changes found in nonerosive reflux disease (NERD—discussed subsequently) with minimal changes (M) and without visible minimal changes (N)[15] but these are not widely accepted or used outside of Japan. However, in common with the other classification systems, the Los Angeles system does not recommend taking biopsies.

Los Angeles Grading System for Reflux Disease in Squamous Mucosa

The Los Angeles classification (Fig. 10-2A–D) grades changes in squamous mucosa as follows:

Grade A—One or more mucosal breaks (= erosions) no longer than 5 mm, none of which extends between the tops of the mucosal folds

Grade B—One or more mucosal breaks more than 5 mm long, none of which extends between the tops of two mucosal folds

Grade C—Mucosal breaks that extend between the tops of two or more mucosal folds, but which involve <75% of the esophageal circumference

Grade D—Mucosal breaks that involve at least 75% of the esophageal circumference

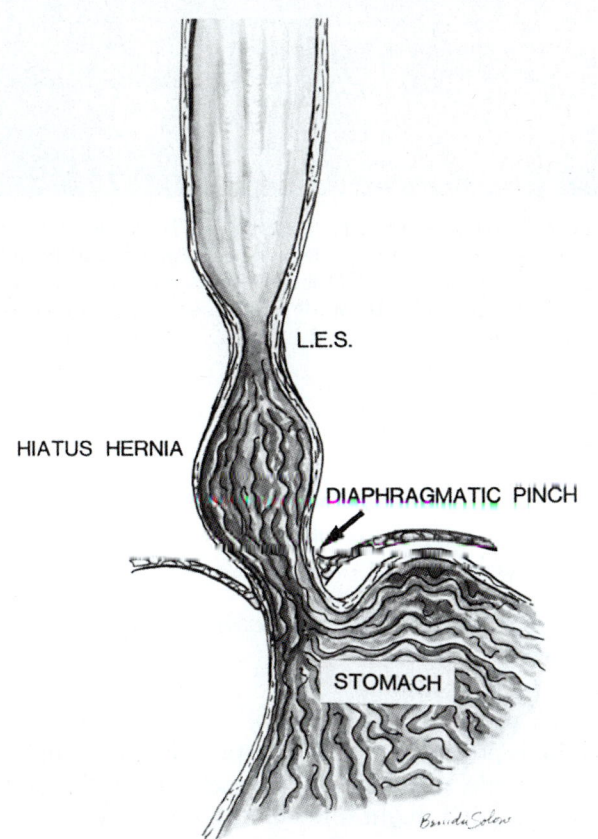

Figure 10-1. Sketch of a sliding hiatus hernia. The LES is located in the chest above the diaphragm. (Courtesy of E. Hassall, MD.)

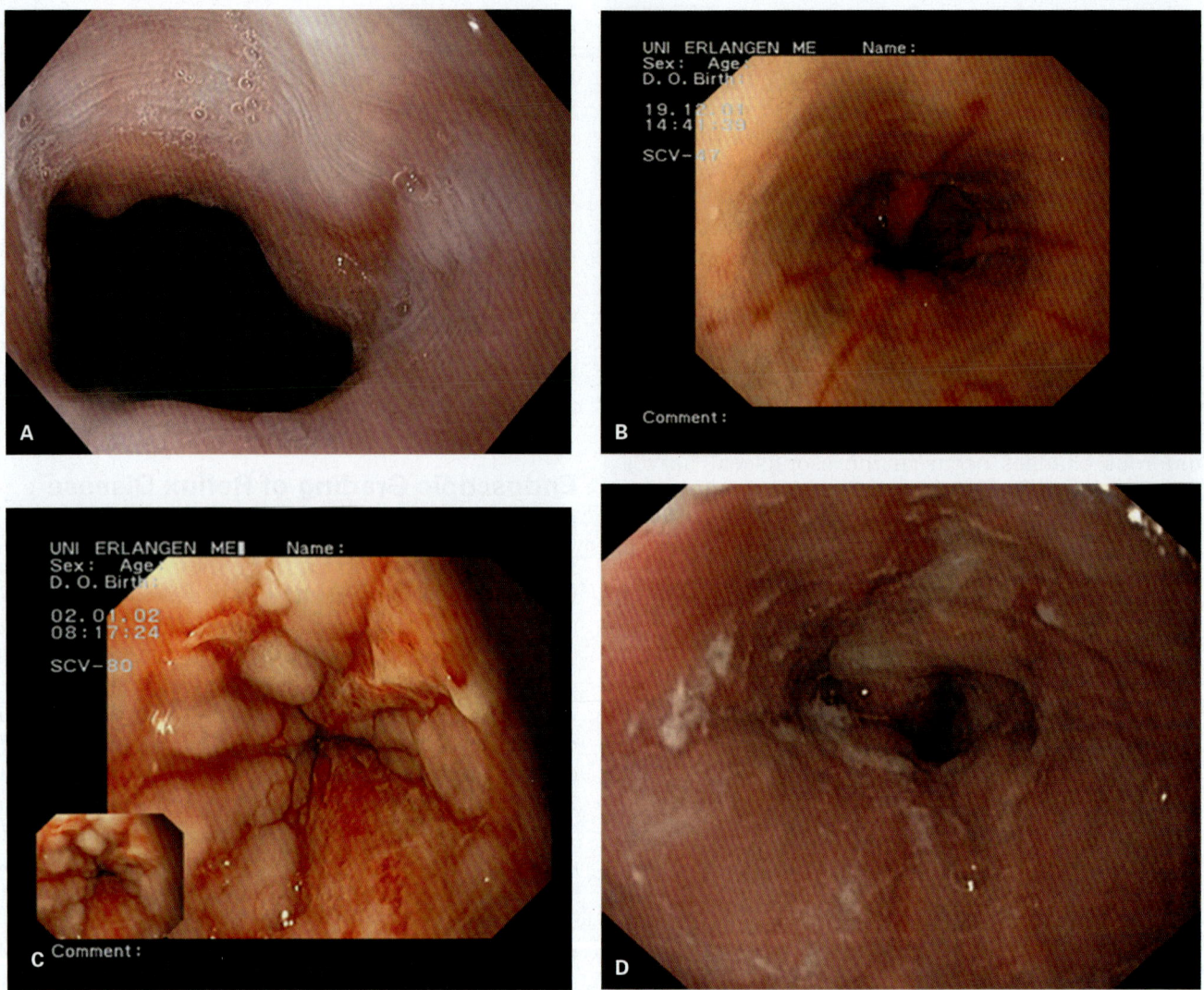

Figure 10-2. Reflux esophagitis: Endoscopic appearance of Los Angeles A–D reflux esophagitis. (Courtesy of Steffen Muehldorfer, MD.) **A**: Grade A: A mucosal break <5 mm long between the tops of the mucosal folds at the right side of the esophageal wall. **B**: Grade B: Six mucosal breaks more than 5 mm long between the tops of the mucosal folds. **C**: Grade C: Mucosal breaks that extend between the tops of two or more mucosal folds, but involve <75% of the esophageal circumference. **D**: Grade D: Mucosal breaks that involve more than 75% of the esophageal circumference.

Proposed additions that would precede grades A to D[15] are also occasionally used:

Grade N—Reflux disease with normal endoscopic appearance and absence of minimal signs and mucosal breaks

Grade M—Minimal changes other than mucosal breaks

In Europe, the *Savary-Miller* classification is often used.[16] However, there have been several modifications, and interobserver variation is considered poor. *The MUSE classification* (*M*etaplasia, *U*lcer, *S*tricture, *E*rosion)[17] is very logical but not used.

For routine clinical practice, in endoscopic examination, the esophagus in patients with GERD, only five things are relevant:

1. Are erosions (called mucosal breaks in the LA system) present?
2. Is stenosis present?
3. Is BE present?
4. If BE is present, the detection of dysplasia/neoplasia.
5. Are subtle/minimal features present (redness, red streaks) that might reflect NERD?

Endoscopic grading is of less interest in a clinical routine setting, but erosions (mucosal breaks) may be relevant, while stenosis may need to be dilated and BE might need PPIs (even if asymptomatic) and follow-up surveillance.

Nonerosive Reflux Disease and Its Pathology

It is now accepted that the vast majority of patients with reflux disease do not present with esophageal lesions (mucosal breaks/erosions) but do suffer from reflux symptoms.[1] These patients are believed to belong to a group of patients with nonerosive (endoscopy-negative or with minimal changes) reflux disease.[6] However, using magnifying zoom endoscopy (magnification between 110 and 150 times), it has been shown that minimal lesions that do not fulfill the criteria of a mucosal break that occur in this group of patients are for the most part dilated intraepithelial capillary loops in the lower esophagus.[18] Further, some patients may just be hypersensitive to esophageal acid.

This group can further be subdivided into true normals and those with minimal lesions such as vascular ectasia, an increase in DISs, and an increase in basal cell height or papillary height that is not in the pathologic range yet decreases considerably on PPIs. This suggests that NERD may consist of both patients with minimal lesions that can be demonstrated with appropriate endoscopes and a further subgroup of patients who may be very sensitive to acid (visceral hypersensitivity) but who are completely normal endoscopically.[19] In both groups of patients, PPIs cause all of these changes to disappear, and the normal palisaded vessels at the Z-line become visible again, while many of the hypersensitive groups also become symptom free. The diagnosis of endoscopic-negative reflux disease is still somewhat difficult. pH-metry is considered to be the "gold standard" but is uncommonly carried out, although it can be done with a portable device at home.

Histology can help in this respect, depending mostly on the site of the biopsy. Biopsies close to the GEJ often show typical features of GERD but in biopsies close to the Z-line these probably have to be interpreted as normal, even though in some it represents genuine reflux disease as there may well be some differences between normal and abnormal (see previous discussion[18,40,41]).

The other features that can be found in patients with NERD are DISs (spongiosis) of the epithelium. This accentuates the intercellular prickles ("ladders") between two adjacent cells, but at the intersection between three cells these form intercellular canals that appear rounded (bubbles) (Fig. 10-3). This intercellular edema is a good marker of epithelial damage, so it is not specific and is also common in eosinophilic esophagitis (EoE). In addition, small amounts of intercellular edema are common and probably normal, so when normal becomes pathologic is unclear. Care must be taken to not misinterpret cytoplasmic vacuolation as DIS.

Gross/Endoscopic Appearances of GERD

Endoscopically, early signs of reflux disease are for the most part found in the distal 2 cm of the esophagus (see Fig. 10-2), likely being most marked between the right and posterior wall of the esophagus.[20] Within the valleys of the mucosal folds, esophageal gland ducts open and secrete bicarbonate and acid-neutralizing mucous. The top of the mucosal folds are therefore likely to be damaged mechanically during esophageal contractions with higher mechanical pressure, as well as by acid. If severe enough erosions form, in the Los Angeles system these are called "mucosal breaks." Minimal changes that are not covered by this definition are not further defined in classifications on reflux esophagitis and are considered to represent their own group, rather than classified as true endoscopic-negative reflux disease.[21] One example

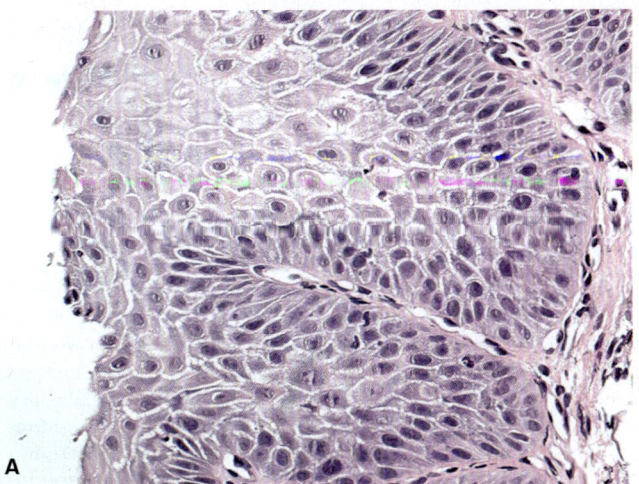
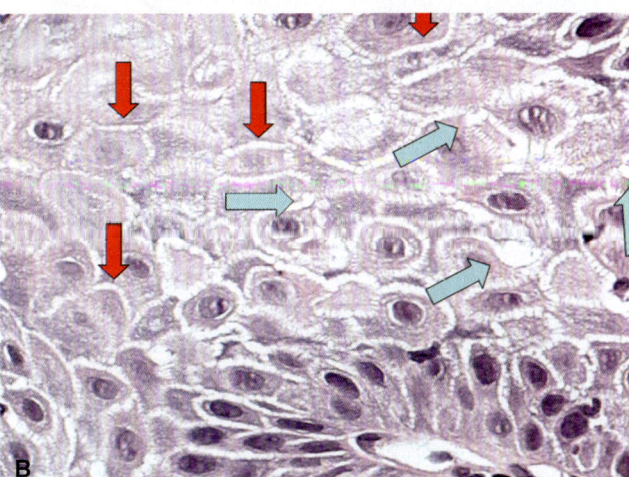

Figure 10-3. Dilated intercellular spaces. **A:** Overview of an esophageal biopsy with overt basal cell hyperplasia. DIS tends to be maximal around the papillae. **B:** Detail showing DIS that can take the form of exaggerated intercellular prickles (ladders) between any two cells (*red arrows*), or "bubbles" at the junctions of three cells (*blue arrows*).

is that of *red streaks* of the distal esophagus. These are covered by a thin layer of newly re-epithelialized squamous epithelium with underlying capillary-rich granulation tissue.[21] Frequently, such lesions can be seen after healing of erosions (mucosal breaks).

Biopsies (see subsequent section) can be useful whenever atypical symptoms or questionable lesions are present endoscopically to exclude neoplasia. Changes may also be present in endoscopically normal mucosa that can support the clinical diagnosis of reflux disease.[8]

Where to Biopsy for GERD and Criteria Used

Erosions. Although erosions are not often biopsied to confirm their presence if they are multiple or atypical, consideration may be given to exclude other treatable causes such as *Candida* or herpes. Biopsies from erosions are easy to interpret when at the edge of a biopsy, as they consist of granulation tissue, sometimes with atypical stromal cells. However, small fragments may show only basal cells and underlying capillaries representing granulation tissue that is being re-epithelialized, some of which correspond to the red streaks seen endoscopically (Fig. 10-4A). Marked reactive changes may also be problematic as they may be confused with invasive squamous carcinoma. Initially they are part of re-epithelialization (Fig. 10-4B–E). The regularity of these "prongs" is the key to their reactive nature. More usually there are typical reactive changes with overt basal cell hyperplasia and papillary elongation (Fig. 10-4).

If no erosions are seen, biopsies from just above the Z-line can show evidence of healing erosion (Fig. 10-4),

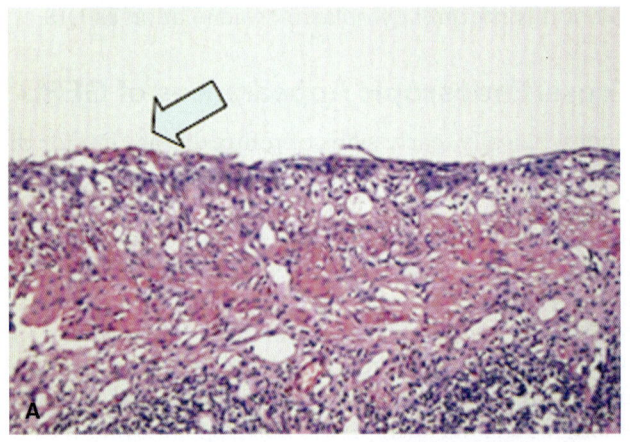
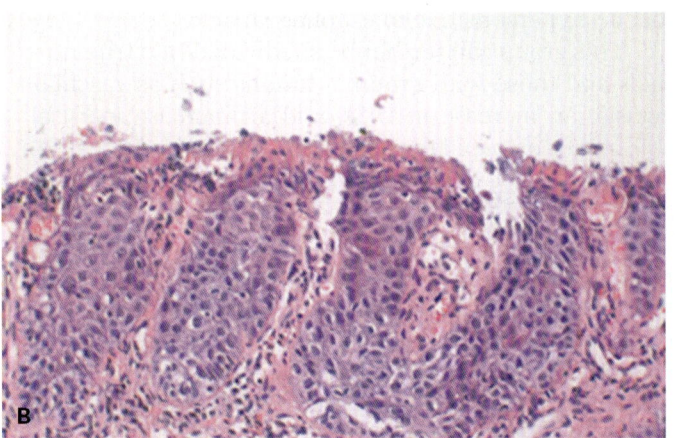
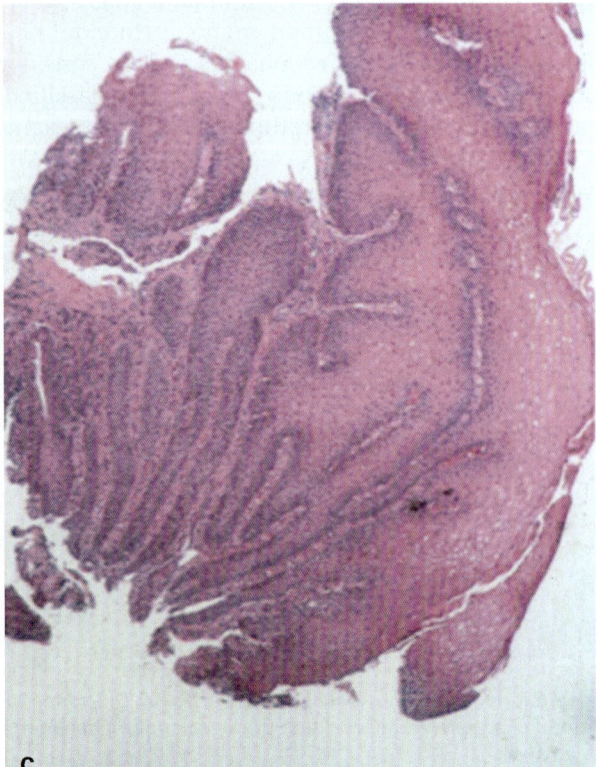
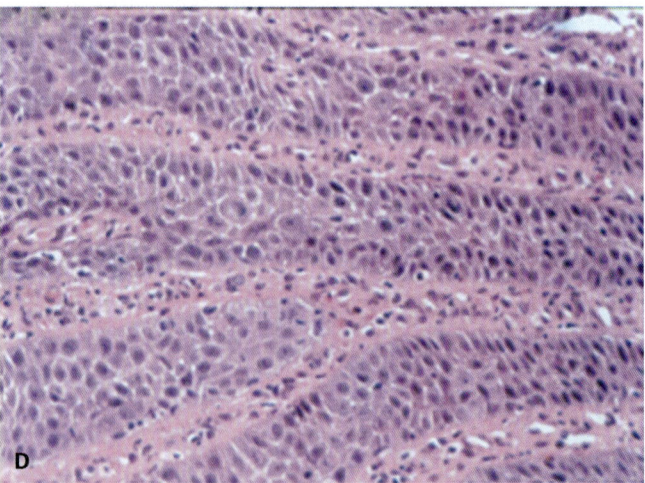

Figure 10-4. Erosions and sequela. **A:** Erosion with a wisp of superficial restituting epithelium (*left arrow*). Lesions such as these can be seen when *red streaks* seen endoscopically are biopsied. **B:** Erosion undergoing re-epithelialization. The epithelium consists entirely of basal cells dipping into the underlying granulation tissue. **C–E:** Healing erosion with marked pseudo-epitheliomatous hyperplasia. The distinction from neoplasia at low power is the regularity of the "prongs."

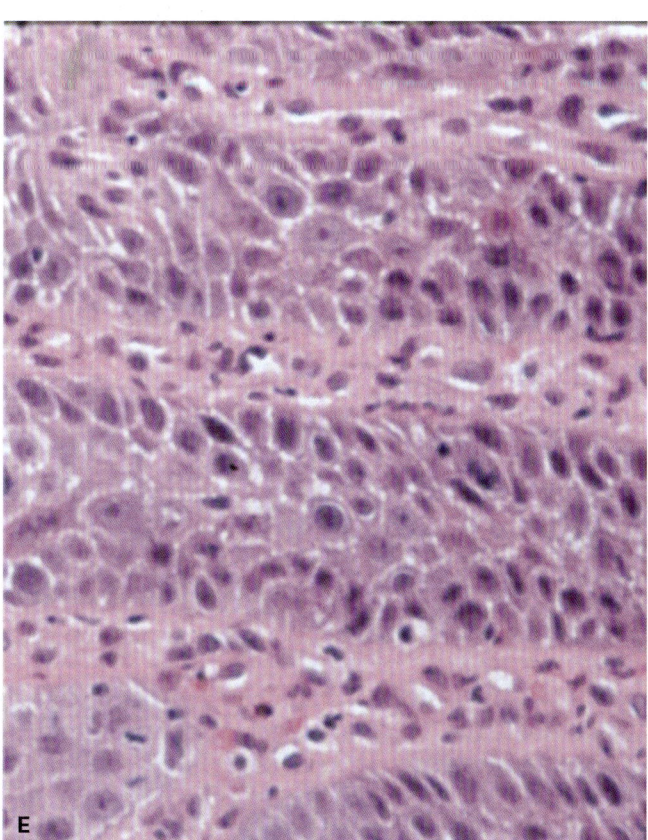
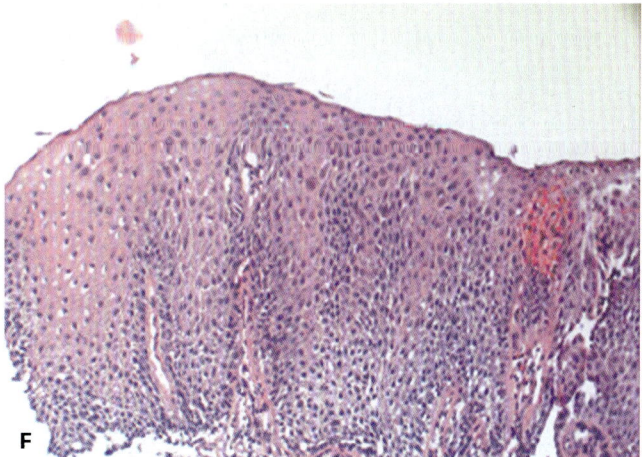

Figure 10-4. *(Continued)* **F:** More typical reactive changes in which the acanthotic epithelium has basal cell hyperplasia and papillae extend about 80% of the way to the surface. To the right there is a hemorrhagic papilla and the remnants of granulation tissue.

neutrophils that are initially superficial (Fig. 10-5), and a sprinkling of *eosinophils* (Fig. 10-5) that are less than those seen in EoE (<25 in 1 high-power field [HPF] or 15 in each of 2 in the same biopsy, and usually far fewer than this) but are usually sufficiently uncommon that one usually has to search for them. There is an overlap with EoE (see that section); patients with typical clinical, endoscopic, and histologic features of EoE are usually treated as such but where these are not all present (and in some patients with typical features of EoE), they are often treated for GERD, at least initially. A rare eosinophil is thought to be acceptable in adults, although they remain uncommon, but in children eosinophils are always regarded as abnormal. An excess of *intraepithelial lymphocytes* (IELs) (lymphocytic esophagitis) is seen in GERD but appears

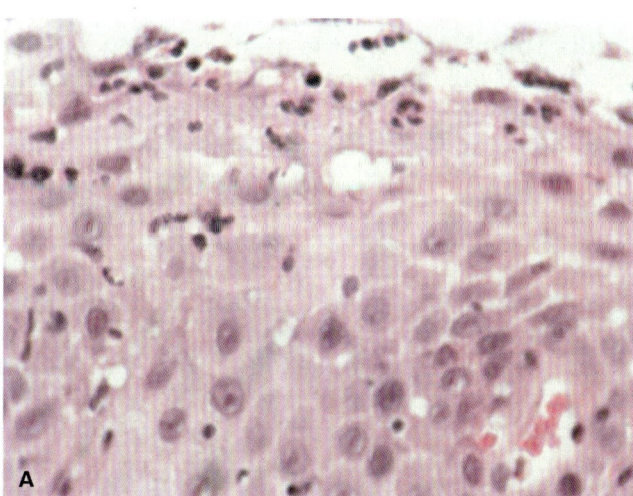
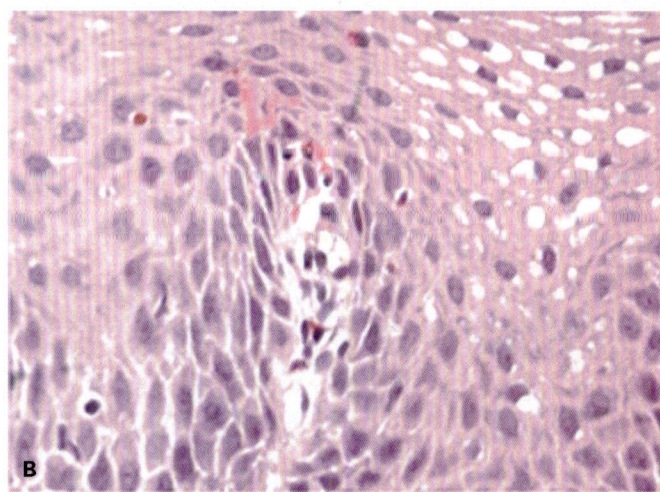

Figure 10-5. GERD. **A:** (detail **C**) Esophageal mucosa with superficial neutrophils. While this can be seen in GERD, it can also be part of drug-induced injury and infections such as *Candida*.

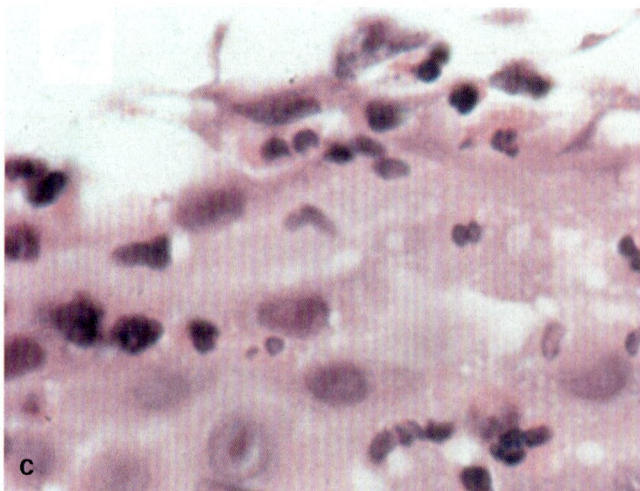
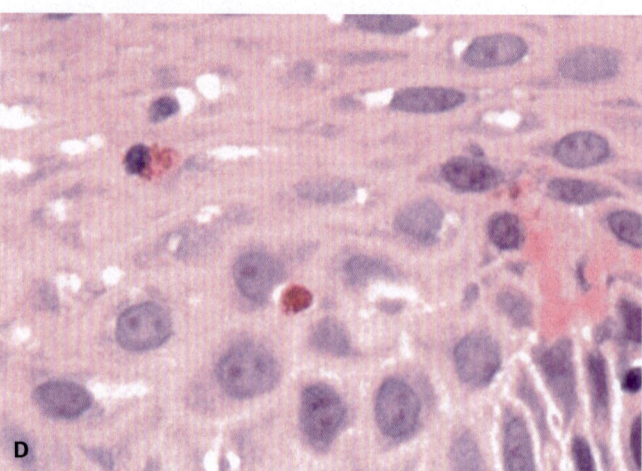

Figure 10-5. *(Continued)* **B:** (detail **D**) Epithelium with scattered eosinophils indicative of GERD.

to be neither sensitive nor specific; nor has the cut-off for normals been well defined. As such, this cannot reasonably be used to make a diagnosis of GERD.

Biopsies 3 cm above the Z-line may show reactive epithelial changes (basal cell hyperplasia, elongation of papillary length) (Fig. 10-6). Biopsies also exclude imitations of reflux disease (Table 10-2) even if there are minor changes such as red streaks or areas of redness,[22] and to recognize BE with or without dysplasia or carcinoma. Theoretically, a periodic acid–Schiff (PAS) stain can also be used to delineate the basal layer as these cells are glycogen deficient (Fig. 10-7), but this is rarely used as the hyperplasia is obvious on H&E sections (see Figs. 10-4F and 10-8). Another feature of basal cells is that they have a high proliferative index (see Fig. 10-6). In comparison, not only does normal mucosa have a much lower proliferative index, but in a Ki-67 immunostain the basal layer is unstained, but this disappears as soon as proliferation increases, suggesting that these may be part of the stem cell population of the esophagus.

Traditional biopsy sites. Distal esophageal biopsies are usually taken at the Z-line or 3, or 5, or 7 cm above the Z-line (depending on the author), but are said to play a minor role in diagnosis because in early papers basal cell hyperplasia and papillary elongation may be seen physiologically in the distal 3 cm.[23] The closer these are taken to the Z-line the more likely these reactive changes are assumed to be present. It is likely that most of the regenerative changes are found between the right esophageal and the rear esophageal wall[20] due to the asymmetrical structure of the LES. This seems to be the region where the valve-like mechanism of the LES opens first.[24] However, this does not take into account that the other changes associated with GERD are all *maximal close to the Z-line*, so this is where biopsies should be taken to detect erosions or their healing phase (often red streaks), neutrophils, eosinophils, and markedly DIS even when the mucosa appears absolutely normal. Thus biopsies from this region should show more changes compared to other quadrants.

In the squamous mucosa, biopsies for features of GERD should therefore be taken

1. immediately above the Z-line for erosions, neutrophils, eosinophils, and DIS, preferably from the right esophageal wall (basal cell hyperplasia or papillary hyperplasia in this zone have to be interpreted as being within normal limits).
2. 3 cm above the Z-line for traditional reactive changes in the squamous mucosa.
3. from the mid or upper esophagus when EoE is in the diagnosis, hopefully to demonstrate their proximal persistence in that disease.

Cardia biopsies. A little-used criterion is the presence of inflammation limited to the cardia. The rationale for taking biopsies from the cardia is that there are only two major causes of cardiac inflammation: that associated with *H. pylori* and that associated with GERD. However to establish the latter, it is necessary to also take standard biopsies for *Helicobacter* from the gastric antrum and body—the latter are particularly important if patients are taking PPIs, and organisms may only be found in oxyntic mucosa. In the absence of inflammation in the remainder of the stomach, cardia inflammation is assumed to be secondary to GERD.[25] A similar theoretical argument can be made with the incidental finding of intestinal metaplasia in cardiac biopsies; this should either be associated with intestinal metaplasia in the distal stomach, and therefore part of more widespread

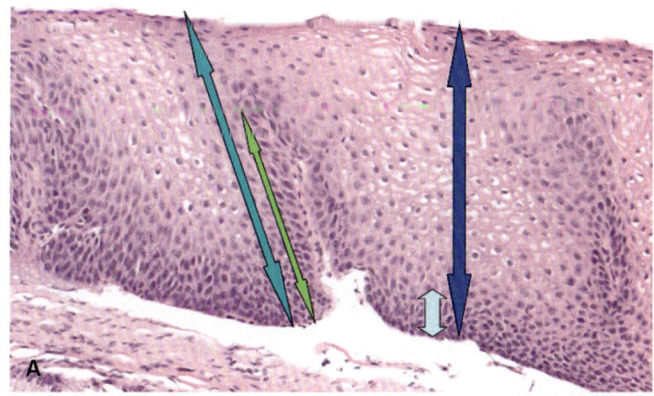
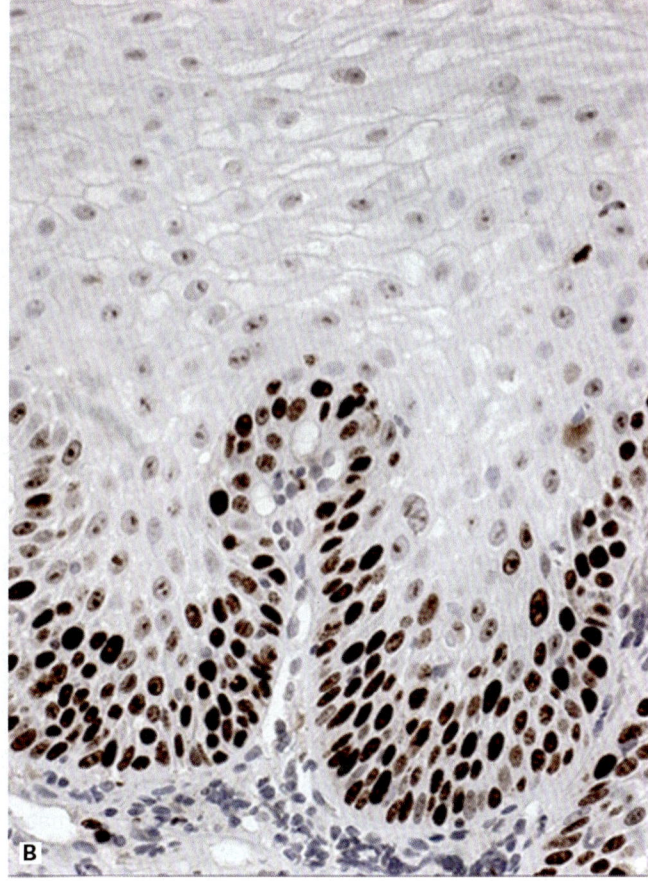
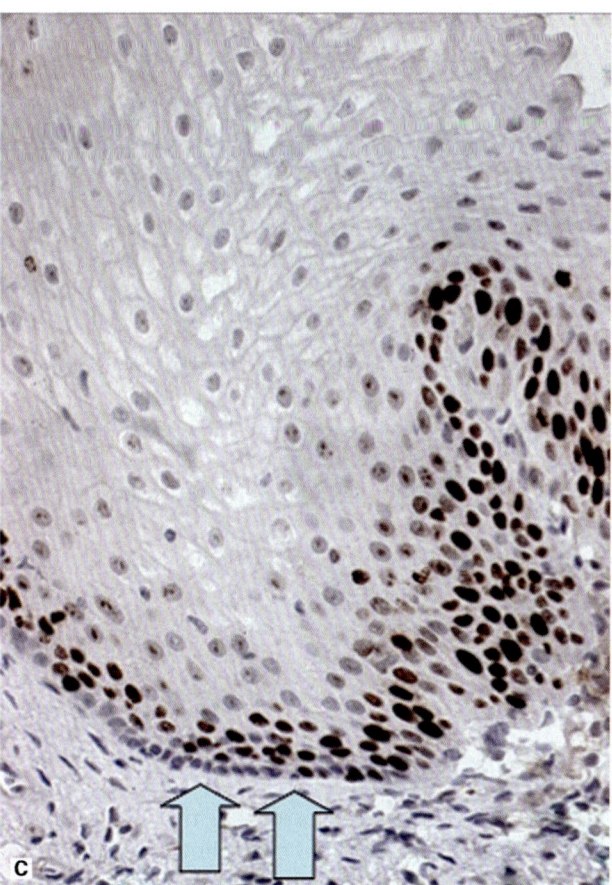

Figure 10-6. Reactive changes in squamous mucosa. **A:** Normal squamous epithelium with small layer of basal cells extending about one-sixth of the distance to the surface (*light blue* and *dark blue arrows right*). The epithelial papillae do not extend more than about two-thirds of the entire epithelial thickness. This can be gauged by dividing the epithelium into thirds (*light green* and *dark green arrows* left). The papillae should not extend into the upper one-third, while if the basal third is mentally divided into thirds, the basal layer should not occupy more the half of this. The basal layer stops where the distance between nuclei is greater than the nuclear diameter. **B,C:** Ki-67 immunostain in reactive hyperplasia (**B**) and normal mucosa (**C**). In normal mucosa (**right**) the proliferative zone is above the most basal layer (*arrows*) suggesting that the nonproliferating cells are "stem cells." In reactive changes (**left**) they are all reincorporated into the proliferative zone.

gastric intestinal metaplasia, or limited to the cardia, and be GERD related.

Histologic Diagnosis and Criteria for GERD in Biopsies

The following criteria are used in the morphologic diagnosis of reflux disease; however, as with inflammatory diseases elsewhere, no criteria are specific for reflux disease, and can be seen in other diseases also, causing erosions and ulcers such as infections (e.g., *Candida*, herpes simplex virus [HSV], cytomegalovirus [CMV]), medications causing ulceration (NSAIDs, bisphosphonates, etc.) that tends to be higher in the esophagus, although not often enough to be relied on, and rarely other causes (e.g., Crohn's disease). (See subsequent discussion.):

1. Erosions or ulcers, usually close to the Z-line (other causes: infections, medication)
2. Re-epithelializing erosions (regenerative papillae elongation with attenuated overlying epithelium, and then with marked hyperplasia of the basal layer) (see Fig. 10-4)

Table 10-2.	Reflux-independent Esophageal Lesions	
	NONNEOPLASTIC LESIONS WITHOUT REFLUX DISEASE	**NEOPLASTIC LESIONS WITHOUT REFLUX DISEASE**
Erosion	Drug-induced, mechanical (probes), ischemia, moniliasis, bacterial and viral infections, eosinophilic esophagitis	Early carcinoma
	Systematic diseases with esophageal involvement	Dysplasia

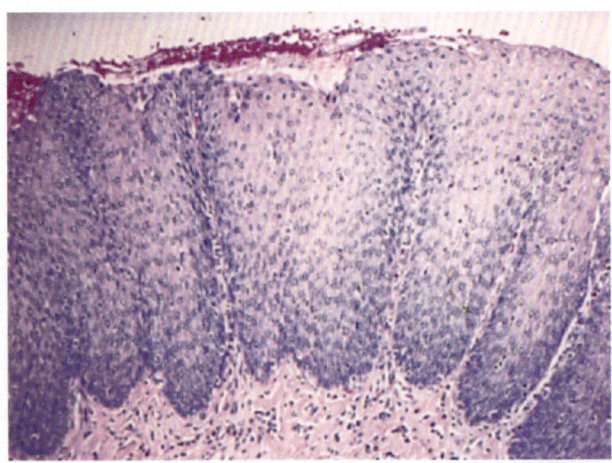

Figure 10-8. The dermal papillae are elongated, and the basal cell zone is expanded to more than 15% of the squamous layer's thickness. If these changes were found in a biopsy that included the Z-line, or were stated as being within 3 cm of the Z-line, it is appropriate to say that "reactive changes are present but in this location they may be physiologic."

3. Neutrophils (same differential diagnosis as 1) (see Fig. 10-5)
4. Eosinophils (differential is primarily EoE if numerous) (see Fig. 10-5)
5. Reactive epithelial changes—basal cell layer >15% to the surface or papillary height >two-thirds of the way to the surface (3 cm or more above the Z-line only)

Evaluating reactive changes. In practice, no one measures reactive changes other than in research protocols, but the "rule of thirds" works well. The mucosa is divided mentally into thirds. Papillae extending into the upper one-third are abnormal. The basal one-third is mentally halved. Basal cells extending into the upper third of these are abnormal (in practice, 16.7% of the epithelial thickness, but close enough). The upper end of the basal cell layer is where the distance between the nuclei exceeds their diameter that is, where it becomes possible to fit in a nucleus between nuclei (see Fig. 10-5). This can also be demonstrated using the presence of glycogen (PAS stain) (see Fig. 10-7) that accumulates in cells above the basal layer, but this is rarely used. In a well-orientated biopsy, both basal cell hyperplasia and papillary elongation can be evaluated with relative ease (see Fig. 10-8).

Less Reliable Criteria
1. Increased peripapillary hemorrhage (increased fragility of capillaries) (Fig. 10-9)
2. Presence of so-called balloon cells (acid-damaged squamous cells)
3. Eosinophilic "densification" of superficial squamous epithelium
4. DISs (likely a sensitive marker of any sort of epithelial damage but no good data on how much is normal)
5. Increase in IELs

Standardized criteria have been difficult to achieve as few of the criteria are specific for reflux disease, although very sensitive markers of esophageal damage.[23]

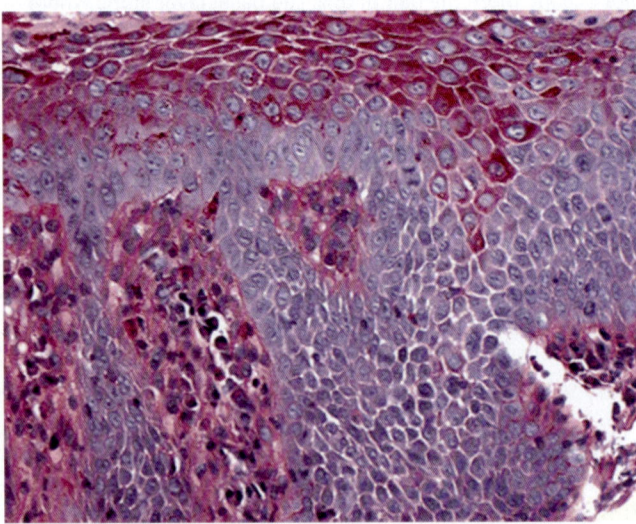

Figure 10-7. PAS stain showing PAS-positive glycogen-containing cells that are not present in the basal cells and are limited to the nonbasal superficial cells.

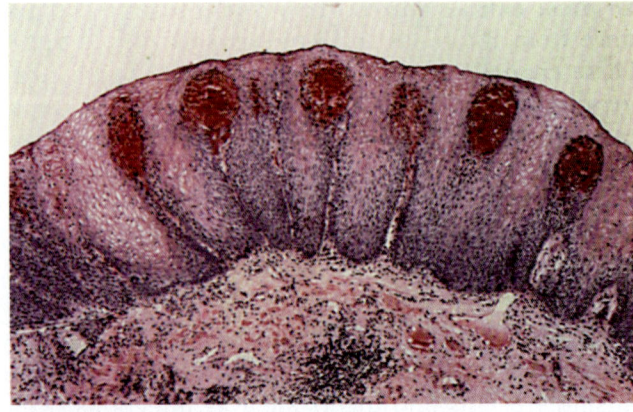

Figure 10-9. Dilated vessels in papillae (vascular "lakes").

In practice, the most relevant (specific) criteria are thickness of the basal cell layer (>15%) and proportional length of papillae (>2/3),[26-28] the latter invariably coming out as the best criteria in clinical studies. This may be useful as it suggests that the presence of an erosion or ulcer without immediately adjacent reactive changes in the squamous mucosa may be an indicator of acute damage (pills) rather than more chronic intermittent disease (reflux).

Dilated Intercellular Spaces It is clear that DIS (spongiosis) are a very sensitive marker of esophageal damage, and are seen especially in GERD, EoE, and "pill"-associated damage. However, the literature is relatively vague on criteria for their use. It has been suggested that although this initially referred to dilatation of the round spaces where pericellular spaces between more than two cells join ("bubbles"), this can also be applied to the spongiotic zone between two cells ("ladders").[29] Further, a degree of DIS can always be seen in the basal and prickle layers, so a small amount of this is always normal.

The question then is when can this be regarded as pathologic. In one study using oil immersion and electron microscopy, mean diameters were 0.58 ± 0.16 μm for controls, 1.07 ± 0.30 mm for NERD, and 1.29 ± 0.20 μm for erosive disease. The optimal cut-off value from receiver operator characteristic analysis was 0.85 μm.[30-32] There are also data showing that DIS get smaller following antisecretory (proton pump) therapy, but this happens to some extent in controls as well as in patients, suggesting that DIS are largely acid reflux related.[30] Anecdotally, we have found that numerous markers of intercellular junctions can facilitate demonstration of DIS including desmocollins, desmogleins, cadherins, catenins, occludins, and claudins. However β-catenin, which is available in many laboratories, works well and reliably until one can routinely identify these changes at routine H&E light microscopy.

Grading reactive epithelial changes. The original criteria for reactive esophageal squamous changes (basal cell hyperplasia, papillary elongation)[26] were subsequently graded by Elster,[33] which is difficult if biopsies are not well orientated, but grading has proven useful in routine practice. The system was
- Grade I: The thickness of the basal cell layer reaches up to 10% of total epithelial thickness, papillae reach up to 40% of total epithelial thickness (i.e., normal).
- Grade II: The basal cell layer reaches up to 30% (abnormal) and papillae reach up to 60% of total epithelial thickness (still just normal).
- Grade III: The basal cell thickness is more than 50% and papillae reach up to 90% of total epithelial thickness.

In virtually all studies where both of these criteria have been measured, papillary elongation (height) is the most reliable criterion. A potential weakness of this system is that using papillary height, the abnormal range is in grade III, whereas using basal cell hyperplasia it is in grade II.

Signing Out Reactive Changes in Biopsies In routine practice, no criteria really need to be graded, although frequently that is the case, as it is almost second nature for pathologists to add "mild, moderate or marked/severe" as a prefix to anything that is a variable criterion. At the mild end, the pathologist may be trying to be helpful in providing a diagnosis. However, if the squamocolumnar junction is included in the biopsies then unless there is evidence of an erosion, all changes based entirely on the morphology of the squamous mucosa may be physiologic. While it is usually easy to say that basal cell hyperplasia or papillary elongation or marked dilatation of intercellular spaces (together often called "reactive changes") are present, the issue is in their interpretation. It is not incorrect to say that they are "consistent with reflux disease," as this may be true. However, this can be frankly misleading as they are also quite consistent with being within normal limits. One approach is simply to state that "reactive changes are present but these are normal in this location." Of course, the additional presence of occasional neutrophils or eosinophils changes this immediately, but any change is based entirely on the presence of these cells, the changes in the squamous mucosa being irrelevant. Conversely, if it is clear that the biopsies come from 3 cm or more above the squamocolumnar changes, then they are pathologic, although a degree of caution is required because reactive changes can have numerous causes other than GERD, especially medications, as well as infection. Caution should therefore be exercised before mindlessly stating that reactive changes are "consistent with GERD" as it may be overtly misleading.

EROSIVE ESOPHAGITIS. In erosive esophagitis, the mucosa is reddened, the lesions are covered by debris, and whitish slough is found. Histologically, the margin of esophageal lesions shows the most marked regenerative changes reaching into hemorrhagic or necrosis with marked active inflammation including neutrophils, eosinophils, and less frequently lymphocytes and plasma cells. By definition, erosions do not extend into the submucosa while ulcers do. However, as the lamina propria underlies the epithelium, it is possible to completely lose the epithelium without satisfying the pathologic definition of an ulcer. This is usually impossible to assess in biopsies that may show only hyalinized lamina propria or granulation tissue

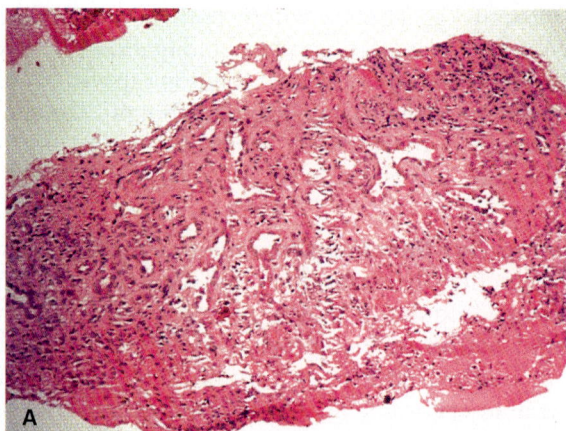
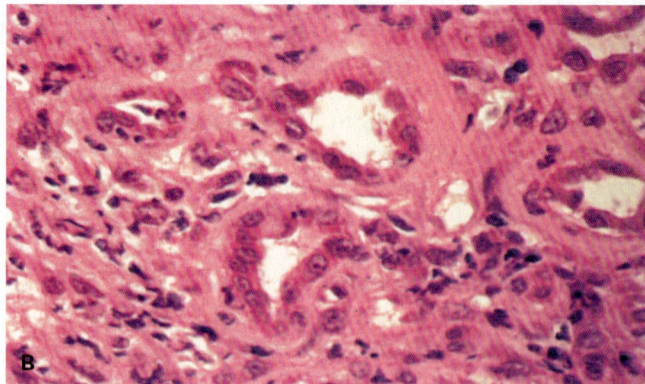

Figure 10-10. Exuberant granulation tissue in ulcerative esophagitis can mimic adenocarcinoma. **A:** Low-power view of a biopsy specimen from an esophageal ulcer. **B:** High-power view shows the microvessels of the granulation tissue.

(Fig. 10-10), so it is usually assessed more precisely endoscopically.

Interestingly, although it would be reasonable to think that GERD-associated ulcers occur in association with reactive changes in the adjacent squamous mucosa, as opposed to no reactive changes, our own experience is that this is not the case, and that in biopsies from clinical studies from patients with erosive esophagitis who have a well-controlled drug history, that GERD-associated ulcers are frequently accompanied by a virtually normal adjacent mucosa. Further, biopsies from "mucosal" breaks may show a variety of changes from genuine erosions and ulcers through reactive changes to inflamed and normal mucosa. Whether the latter represents inadequate sectioning through the block or an endoscopic "miss" is unclear; the esophagus is constantly moving with respiration and heartbeat so is not the easiest organ to biopsy accurately. Therapy with PPIs is the therapy of choice.

INFLAMMATORY CELLS

Neutrophils are usually only found close to lesions, but can be helpful in biopsies from the Z-line when reflux disease is by far the most common cause. Neutrophils are usually found in the apical layer of squamous epithelium (see Fig. 10-5A–C), although when they start forming clusters it is wise to carry out special stains to exclude moniliasis, which can be easily missed on an H&E section.

However, asthmatics can also have reflux disease.[34]

Intraepithelial Mononuclear Cells

These are primarily lymphocytes (CD3+, usually CD8+) with a varying portion of S-100–positive antigen-presenting cells, but mast cells can also be present. Intraepithelial mononuclear cells (IEMs) are *eosinophils* that can be observed at the margin of esophageal lesions (especially pill-associated ulcers with homogenous eosinophilic necrosis) but, apart from a rare cell, are not found in normal squamous epithelium. Scattered eosinophils (see Fig. 10-5B–D) imply GERD until proven otherwise. In children, they are always assumed to be abnormal. In this respect, EoE should always be excluded. Asthmatics can have an increased number of intraepithelial eosinophils, possibly related to the asthma therapy increased in reflux disease (Fig. 10-11), but there are no controlled studies available that help in grading this finding.[35] Although there is an association with GERD and numerous other disorders including inflammatory bowel disease, it is wise to be cautious about interpreting an esophageal lymphocytosis (vide infra section on lymphocytic esophagitis).

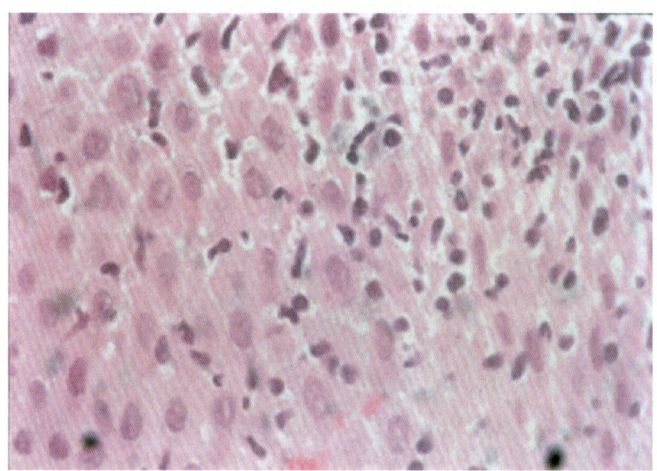

Figure 10-11. Esophageal mucosa with myriad IEMs, most of which are lymphocytes, but antigen-presenting cells and sometimes mast cells may all be present.

Minor changes

Nerves Numerous neuropeptides and changes in them are reported in reflux disease (such as CGRP, neuropeptide Y, Substance P, and VIP). Generic neural markers (such as PGP 9.5) have been evaluated in the esophageal epithelium. For VIP and PGP 9.5 a relation to inflammation and thus symptoms in reflux disease has been shown.[36] The relevance of these findings is not yet known. Increased capsaicin receptor TRPV1 (transient receptor potential cation channel, subfamily V, member 1) nerve fibers have been found in the inflamed human esophagus, but the potential diagnostic utility of this finding is unclear.[37] In the mouse esophagus, capsaicin inhibits the vagally mediated striated muscle contractions mainly through its action on mucosal primary afferents, which in turn activate the presumed inhibitory local reflex arc.[38] Inhibition of contractions would promote reflux. Cholinergic and nonadrenergic noncholinergic inhibitory nerves that are nitric oxide mediated play important roles in regulating contraction and relaxation of the human LES. A decrease of the action of cholinergic nerves and an increase of the action of nonadrenergic noncholinergic inhibitory nerves by nitric oxide may be largely related to the low LES pressure observed in patients with reflux esophagitis,[39] while increased serum levels of both nitrous oxide and VIP that mediate esophageal inhibitory neurons are elevated resulting in relaxation.[40] Nitrous oxide is also implicated in the DISs associated with GERD.[12] It may cause relaxation of the LES and, in the presence of acid, result in DIS that are also the direct result of reflux.[10,12,41] Further, DIS may also be potentiated by direct central vagal stimulation.[42]

Inflammatory Polyps

These are by far the most common polyps in the vicinity of the Z-line, and follow erosions and ulcers irrespective of the etiology. Most begin as granulation tissue but are then re-epithelialized by mucosa that may come from squamous mucosa, or are the glandular mucosal types found at the Z-line. However, squamous mucosa is by far the most common. There are several potential diagnostic pitfalls with these polyps:

1. Pseudoepitheliomatous hyperplasia.
2. The cuboidal-like endothelium can appear almost epithelial, so that their random nature may be mistaken for invasive carcinoma. This is particularly likely if frozen sections are carried out (see Fig. 10-10).
3. Atypical reactive stromal cells (pseudosarcomatous changes in the stroma) (Fig. 10-12). These have a range of appearances but can look overtly malignant, but are always single, stain only with vimentin, sometimes CG10, while Ki-67 can vary from entirely negative to most cells staining, although when the latter occurs, mitotic figures, which can be atypical, are invariably present. Because these cells are seen in inflammatory polyps, invariably adjacent to erosions or ulcers in a variety of locations, they are sometimes colloquially referred to as "ulcerocytes," which at least gives them the harmless name they deserve. The trap is to regard these as spindle cell carcinomas, or "sarcoma" in an inflammatory polyp.

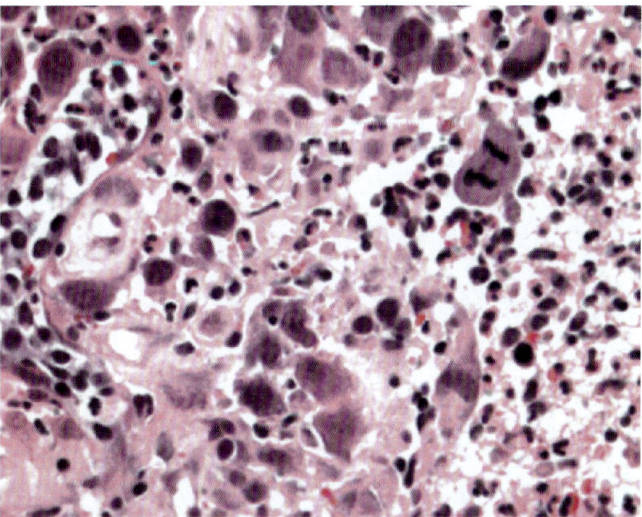

Figure 10-12. Reactive (pseudosarcomatous) changes in the stroma. Note the lack of cohesion, large nuclei but with indistinct chromatin, and, in this example, mitotic figures. These cells are immunoreactive to vimentin, sometimes CD10, and occasionally Ki-67.

Reactive changes versus neoplasia following erosions and ulcers. There are two main circumstances where this is a problem:

A. Distinguishing basal cell hyperplasia from squamous dysplasia
B. Distinguishing the marked hyperplasia of rete pegs from invasive squamous carcinoma

Basal Cell Hyperplasia versus Squamous Dysplasia
A side-by-side comparison with low-grade dysplasia is shown in Figure 10-13, with low grade dysplasia. Typically, squamous dysplasia ranges from mild to in situ carcinoma (low- to high-grade dysplasia [HGD]/intraepithelial neoplasia [IEN]). The nuclei are usually open, vesicular, contain more chromatin, are punctate, and small nucleoli may be present. It is usually fairly regular throughout the biopsy although in resections junctions and different grades may be present. There is invariably loss of polarity in the basal layer so the nuclear features of one nucleus cannot be readily predicted from its neighbor. Whenever this issue arises, it is always worth ensuring that there is no another cause for the epithelial hyperplasia, especially a granular cell tumor or fungal infection, so both are worth a search.

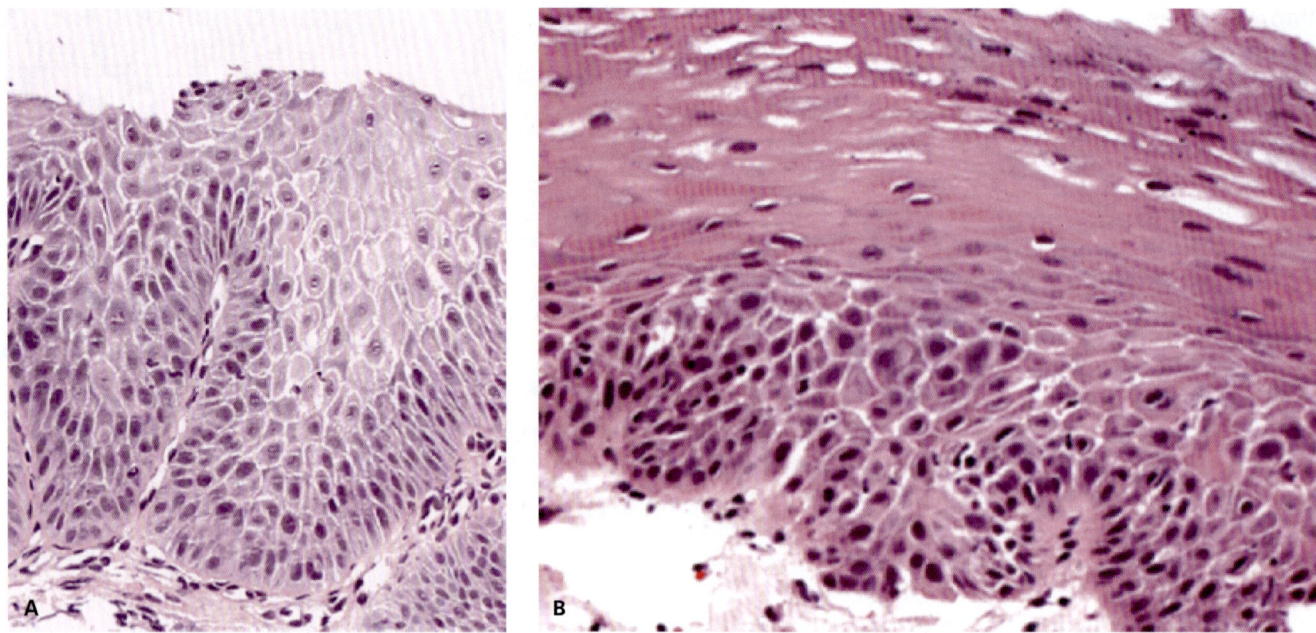

Figure 10-13. Reactive hyperplasia (A) versus low-grade squamous dysplasia (B). Note the orderly maturation in the squamous mucosa but disorderly maturation, sometimes with almost an abrupt transition from immature to mature epithelium as shown here. A helpful clue is that other features of reactive changes (papillary hyperplasia, extensive dilatation of intercellular spaces) are present on the left, but rarely present in squamous mucosa. Although dilated intercellular spaces are present in the dysplastic mucosa on the right, they stop abruptly where the squamous dysplasia stops.

Marked Hyperplasia of Rete Pegs versus Invasive Squamous Carcinoma In this the regularity of the rete pegs which is orderly is contrasted with the disorder and randomness of the neoplastic pegs that is the key to this diagnosis. This is also best illustrated (Fig. 10-14).

Perhaps the most difficult of these is when verrucous carcinoma is in the differential diagnosis. These are also discussed in Chapter 11, but dysplasia/atypia in the basal layer may be the only feature that allows this distinction morphologically short of invasion, which can be quite subtle. It also differs from reactive changes in that the architecture is also not predictable. Rete pegs in carcinomas are irregular, cannot be predicted, can have little or no orientation to the point that one assumes the biopsy is very poorly oriented, and when well oriented, the pegs vary in size and shape with some often being club shaped amidst others that are tapering or anastomsing. The second feature is that the nuclei are different in that they are more open, vesicular, may have small nucleoli, and, at least in the basal layer, there is a lack of predictability with loss of polarity. However, the latter may be limited only to the basal layer, and even within it may be focal, although readily identified. Although usually HPV related, HPV effects may be present but may also be focal; similarly in situ hybridization for HPV may also be focal. If p16 is strong and diffuse that should help, but it is usually weak or absent, even in those associated with HPV, usually subtypes 6 or 11. Sometimes one gets the impression that reactive changes are admixed with verrucous changes. The saving grace in this situation is that the biopsy invariably comes not from a possible ulcer or erosion but from an endoscopic lesion. The presence of an endoscopic tumor should also raise the possibility that one is dealing with an inflammatory polyp, especially close to the GEJ. These are relatively common. Verrucous carcinomas are also discussed in the following chapter.

Atypical Cells in Squamous Mucosa

A degree of individual nuclear changes can be seen in changes that are not overtly reactive or dysplastic, but these are better demonstrated than described (Fig. 10-15).

Carditis as a Manifestation of GERD

Several studies suggest changes even distal to the Z-line can be part of reflux disease. Apart from *H. pylori*, there does appear to be an association between GERD and inflammation limited to the gastric cardia.[25,43] In these studies, active and chronic inflammation was only found in patients with reflux disease (neutrophils, lymphocytes, and plasma cells). Unfortunately, these findings could not be reproduced in larger studies.[44,25] It is not clear yet whether cardia mucosa is a metaplastic mucosa per se.[45] Conversely, fetuses and children do have cardia mucosa.[46,47]

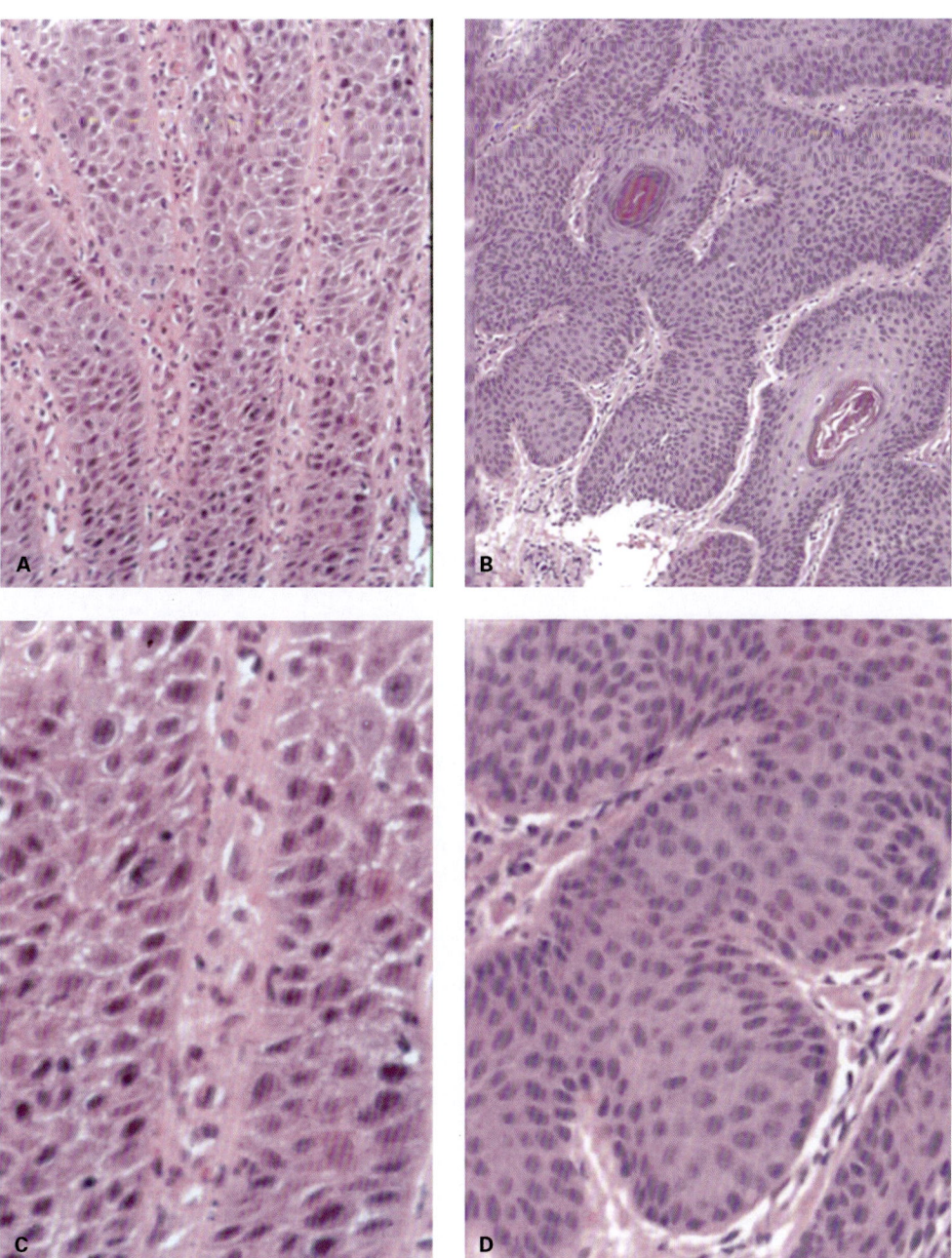

Figure 10-14. Reactive versus neoplasia. The panels on the left **(A,C)** show orderly reactive hyperplasia where the squamous rete pegs (prongs) are orderly and predictable in their regularity. In comparison, in this example of one of the best-differentiated squamous carcinomas we could find **(B,D)**, the major difference is at low power (A,B) where the tumor grows in a disorderly and unpredictable manner. The details (C,D) show dysplastic mucosa to primarily have greater cellularity. Loss of polarity, especially in the basal layer, together with lack of reproducibility between adjacent cells, and greater hyperchromatism in dysplastic mucosa tend to be the best features.

For routine diagnosis, the presence or absence of carditis seems not to be in standard use, possibly because it is necessary to not only take biopsies of the cardia, but also do the usual two antral and two oxyntic mucosa biopsies to exclude *Helicobacter* as a cause, for if these are present, the presence of carditis cannot be used to confirm the diagnosis of reflux disease, as the carditis is presumably *Helicobacter* related. Is it possible to have carditis in the absence of both GERD and *Helicobacter*? To date only one study that we are aware of has suggested that this might occur.[44] The combination of normal (*Helicobacter*-negative) biopsies from the gastric antrum and corpus, along with chronic or chronic active cardia inflammation, needs an explanation. In the absence of other explanations, it seems very likely that these are GERD related (Fig. 10-16).

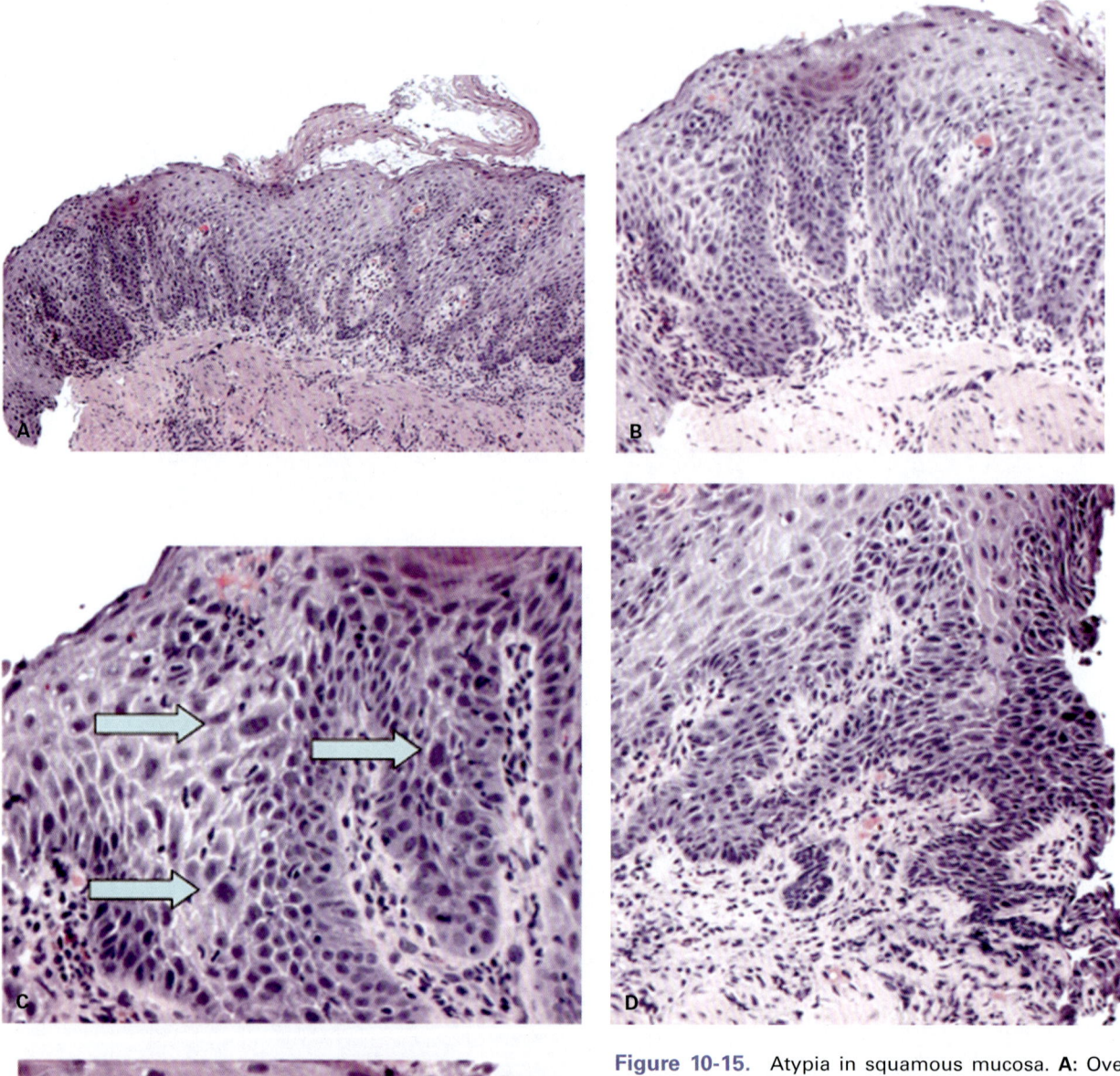

Figure 10-15. Atypia in squamous mucosa. A: Overview of lower esophageal biopsy showing marked nuclear changes, especially in the papillae that extend very close to the surface. Note that the epithelium rests almost on top of the muscularis mucosae with virtually no lamina propria, suggesting that this is a re-epithelialized erosion. B,C: Details of the left end of (A), with enlarged atypical nuclei (*arrows*). D,E: Adjacent field from (A) showing the restituting edge of an erosion lower right (E), immediately adjacent mucosa to (D), with further individual atypical cells, the largest **(right)** in E being binucleate (*arrows*). Situations such as these are best handled by treating with PPIs and repeating the biopsies within a month or two. Endoscopy should be carried out with high a resolution endoscope, biopsies being directed at atypical areas.

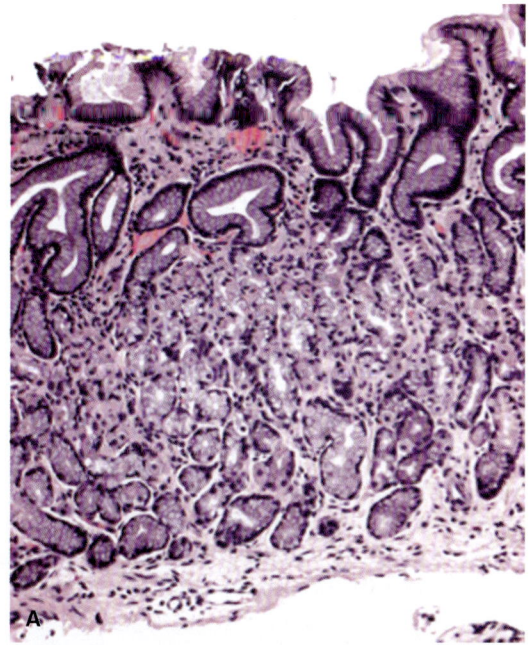
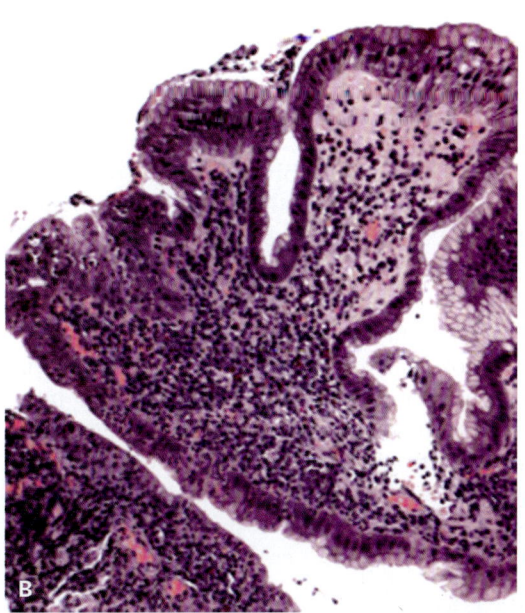
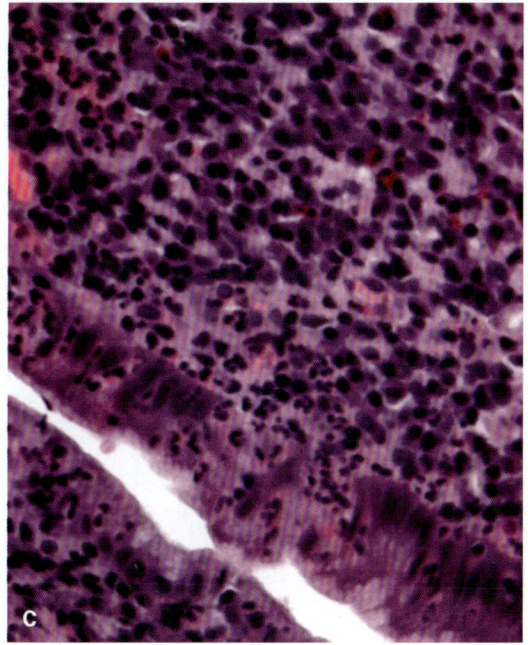

Figure 10-16. Chronic active carditis. **A:** Antral biopsy with no hint of *Helicobacter* gastritis (key in determining that this is the case, as antral and cardiac mucosa tend to resemble each other in *Helicobacter* infection). **B:** Biopsy from cardia—same patient and same magnification as "A" showing marked inflammation. **C:** Detail of (B) showing the chronic active inflammation. In the differential diagnosis, the severe chronic inflammation makes medication use unlikely and Crohn's disease is unlikely as a presenting manifestation. This essentially leaves GERD or an "idiopathic" etiology. The former seems the most likely choice. Diagnosis was "chronic active carditis that, in the absence of *Helicobacter*, is most likely GERD-related."

Progression of GERD. In adults, there appears to be almost no progression of reflux disease with time, although in children the situation is unclear. Over time, repeated healing and damage of the epithelium can be noted but progression from endoscopically negative to erosive and to BE seems not to occur—or if it does it is appears to be uncommon.[48] The more accepted model of reflux disease is therefore a steady-state model. Furthermore, it is unknown why there is much variation between patients, with some patients showing alterations of the very few distal centimeters and others showing lesions 15 cm and more above the GEJ.

Complications of GERD

These include ulcers that can penetrate but do not perforate the esophageal wall. Fistulas can occur between esophagus, bronchus, pericardium, or aorta but are extremely rare, although they do occur in squamous cell carcinoma. Strictures are for the most part a sequel of long-standing ulcerative reflux disease, but are becoming rare as a result of sufficient acid suppression. Severe hemorrhage is also rare but bleeding can lead to chronic iron deficiency.

Reflux-induced neoplasms are always adenocarcinomas associated with BE. The risk for the development of carcinoma is 40- to 125-fold higher in BE compared to in the normal population (see following Section and Chapter).

GERD-related strictures. Strictures are usually managed by endoscopic dilatation, but occasionally need to be resected. They invariably occur immediately proximal to the Z-line and are 1 to 4 cm long. When resected, the stricture itself may be ulcerated, and the stricture is seen to be due to marked submucosal fibrosis and smooth muscle proliferation, the latter penetrating extensively into the muscularis propria. Immediately proximal to the stricture the muscle is markedly hypertrophied, and the epithelium may be thickened and hyperplastic. Reactive changes are present at the junction of ulcerated and nonulcerated mucosa; residual esophageal glands are often visible in the submucosa, and sometimes in the lamina propria.

Cameron's Ulcer

This is an ulcer, usually longitudinal, but can involve much of the circumference of the mucosa, that occurs in a hiatal hernia as it goes through the diaphragm, and so is found at that constriction. These ulcers can bleed, and be associated with hematemesis or anemia. The etiology of these ulcers is not known, but the few that we have seen have been surprisingly severe, sometimes almost purulent but without identifiable organisms, and sometimes with an overt ischemic component (Fig. 10-17).

There are many postulated mechanisms, but if these ulcers by definition occur at the diaphragmatic hiatus, this is likely involved in its pathogenesis. If there is an ischemic element, then some form of pressure-induced ischemia seems most likely. In patients taking appropriate medications, pill damage needs to be considered, as these can cause ischemic-type damage and injury might be caused if they are held up at the diaphragmatic pinch. Other factors that have been implicated inevitably include gastric acid exposure, although this is likely to potentiate or prevent healing in established ulcers rather than being the primary cause. PPIs therefore tend to be used in their therapy and appear effective, presumably confirming a role for acid, unless this is a placebo effect. Gastric stasis and lymphatic obstruction have also been implicated.

A potential clue to the diagnosis in biopsies is that because these are in a hiatal hernia, accompanying squamous mucosa is absent in the ulcerated fragments, the background mucosa being cardiac or oxyntic. However, it needs either knowledge of the clinical location or recognition of a potential ischemic component in the biopsy, or both.

BARRETT'S ESOPHAGUS (BE)

Definition

BE is defined in the United States as "the condition in which any extent of metaplastic columnar epithelium that predisposes to cancer development replaces the stratified squamous epithelium that normally lines the distal esophagus."[49,50] This "political" definition still begs the question of which types of metaplasia are actually being referred to, but does appear to parallel the definition in the United Kingdom,[51] that just uses any columnar metaplasia, but on the grounds

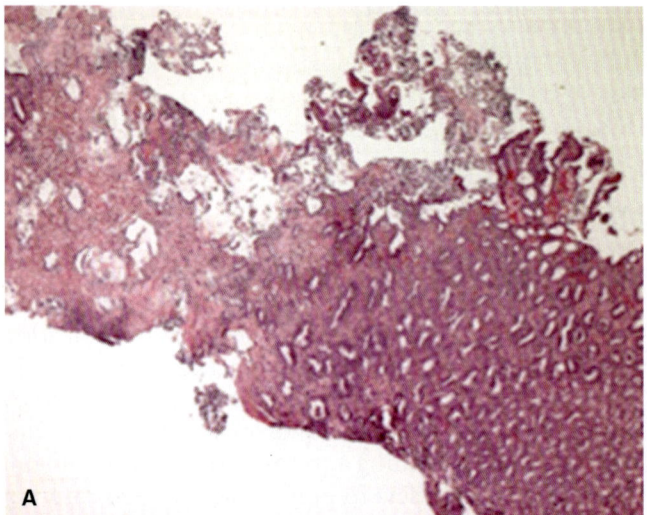
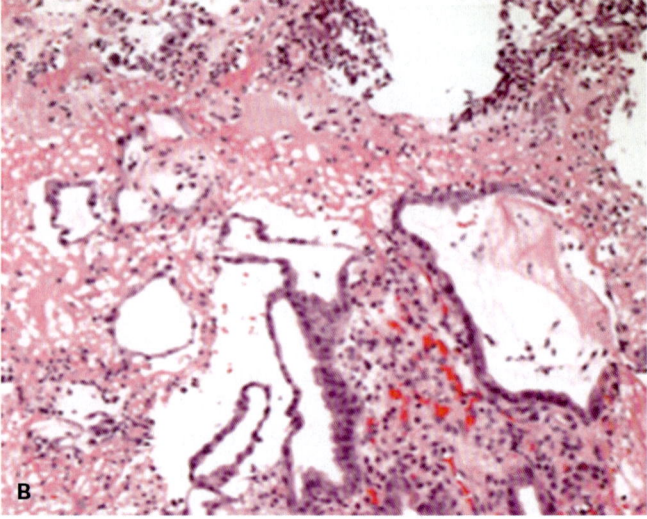

Figure 10-17. Cameron's ulcer in a hiatal hernia. **A:** Oxyntic mucosa **(right)** with an exudate on the surface **(left)**. **B:** Detail of part of the pseudomembrane showing pits with attenuated restituting epithelium in a fibrin neutrophil exudate and bearing considerable resemblance to pseudomembranous colitis. Although no fibrin thrombi are present in this biopsy, its apparent acute ischemic nature is apparent.

that goblet cells are lurking in there somewhere and just need to be found.

Both definitions therefore *initially* seem to

1. remove the need for goblet cells to be present to diagnose BE
2. remove the need to state whether goblet cells are present or not
3. remove the need to state whether it is called BE or columnar-lined-esopahgus (CLE).

However, in the more recent guidelines,[50] the American Gastroenterological Association (AGA) position becomes more ambiguous, specifically stating that goblet cells *are* required for the diagnosis of BE, and also stating that "the inclusion of patients with cardia-type epithelium under the rubric of 'Barrett's esophagus' in what is otherwise typical Barrett's esophagus would substantially increase the number of patients with that disorder, which would substantially increase treatment costs" possibly implying that the definition has been swayed by costs of long-term surveillance if implemented. The logic is that if it is fiscally difficult to justify surveillance in BE with goblet cells where there are reasonable data, it is even harder if goblet cells are not present and there are even fewer data. This is far from the spirit of the UK definition in which such patients would have BE.

According to the AGA, the term "Barrett's esophagus" presently should therefore be used only for patients who have intestinal metaplasia (goblet cells) in the esophagus, while in the United Kingdom and Japan they are not required. In other countries, local guidelines need to be followed. For now, only patients with intestinal-type columnar metaplasia in the esophagus are known to have an increased cancer risk, and in North America only those patients meet our criteria for the diagnosis of BE.

In the AGA position paper with regard to the issue of what to call endoscopic BE when goblet cells are not identified in the biopsies, further confusion arises with the statements "Whether patients who have only cardia-type epithelium lining the distal esophagus have Barrett's esophagus is primarily a semantic issue." Life insurance companies would disagree. It goes on to give no recommendation on what to call patients who clearly have BE endoscopically whether circumferential or overt tongues or both, if they have no goblet cells. This does not help the practicing endoscopist or pathologist know what to call patients with BE endoscopically, and whether to follow them for neoplastic sequela if they do not have goblet cells, when in practice there are data to suggest that they are also at substantial risk from carcinoma, although it may be less than in the case of those with overt goblet cells.[52] We would therefore suggest that for pathologists, the following definitions be used for practical reasons.

Columnar-lined esophagus is used for all mucosa with overt extensions of glandular mucosa into the lower esophagus, and that is then subdivided into those without goblet cells that are simply called CLE, while those with goblet cells are called *Barrett's esophagus*. An lesion that is clearly BE endoscopically, whether circumferential or a tongue, but in which multiple biopsies fail to reveal goblet cells, is called "columnar-lined esophagus but without identifiable goblet cells." Should the endoscopist then ask "well does the patient have BE or not?," one would have to defer to local guidelines (and whether they are believed if the answer is "no").

It seems likely that endoscopists will use an endoscopic appearance of BE to call it BE irrespective of whether goblet cells are present or not, although they may be completely lost as to whether these patients need surveillance or not. If these patients are rescoped and biopsied at least once more, a good proportion will have goblet cells at the second endoscopy, thereby resolving the issue. It is not unreasonable that surveillance interval can be gradually lengthened if there is no dysplasia or goblet cells. In the future, hopefully further data will clarify the risk of dysplasia and carcinoma in patients with CLE, but not BE as defined above. The important implication of this definition is that patients with apparent non–goblet cell BE are also at increased risk of adenocarcinoma so should not be lost to surveillance or follow-up, and the first (diagnostic) endoscopy is in practice the first surveillance endoscopy,[50] so appropriate biopsies are required.

Practical Aspects of Making the Diagnosis of BE

In many countries, including much of North America and Europe, clinicians and pathologists are much more confident in making the diagnosis of BE if goblet cells are present. The presence or absence of goblet cells in biopsies should therefore be stated, if only for traditional reasons.

Nevertheless, the definition of BE still requires two components,

1. demonstration of a proximal shift in the Z-line endoscopically, and
2. histologic demonstration that the mucosa that has shifted proximal is columnar (with or without goblet cells depending on the country).

Usually the presence of a proximal shift in the Z-line is apparent endoscopically as tongues, circumferential spread, and occasionally squamous islands as judged by proximal extension from the endoscopic landmarks (proximal limit of the gastric folds, although recognition of the diaphragmatic pinch can also be useful, especially in establishing the presence of a hiatal hernia that invariably accompanies BE (Fig. 10-18), but when the squamous mucosa is inflamed it becomes red, so the proximal limit of the Z-line may not be apparent, and it is here that biopsies may be required to confirm that the proximal mucosa is indeed columnar and not squamous. The top of the gastric folds marks the proximal limit of the stomach (Fig. 10-19), although this is not as easy as it seems, as it depends in part on the degree of insufflation.

The exception to this two-part practical definition is Japan, where the CLE is defined on endoscopy alone, by the distal limit of the lower esophageal palisade vessels[53] (Fig. 10-20). However, use of these anatomic landmarks to define the length of BE results in a large number of patients with this condition, hence all patients with BE < 5 mm in length, without any other factors associated with typical BE, are excluded.[54,55] It is unclear how this correlates with BE as defined above, and what proportion of these patients have intestinalization in this mucosa, and if so how much of this is otherwise typical cardia-type mucosa.

In much of Europe, intestinal metaplasia (i.e., goblet cells) is required on biopsy from the suspected segment of endoscopic BE to establish the diagnosis[56] (Fig. 10-21A,B). In the United Kingdom, the presence of columnar metaplasia alone with or without goblet cells (Fig. 10-21C,D) in the distal esophagus defines BE, the assumption being that every columnar mucosa has goblet cells somewhere.[51] The diagnosis of BE is therefore primarily endoscopic, biopsy being used to confirm the diagnosis and to ensure that, as this is also the first surveillance endoscopy, as far as possible dysplasia or carcinoma is not already present.

Irregular Z-line versus "ultrashort" BE. Apart from in Japan, the top of the gastric folds marks the beginning of the cardia, from which the Z-line has to be shifted proximally to make a diagnosis of BE. The most difficult endoscopic decision is where an irregular Z-line becomes a tongue of BE. In an interobserver endoscopic study of "experts," there was no agreement until the tongue was 1 cm or more in length,[54] reflecting the difficulties in reliably measuring columnar tongues < 1 cm. The implication of

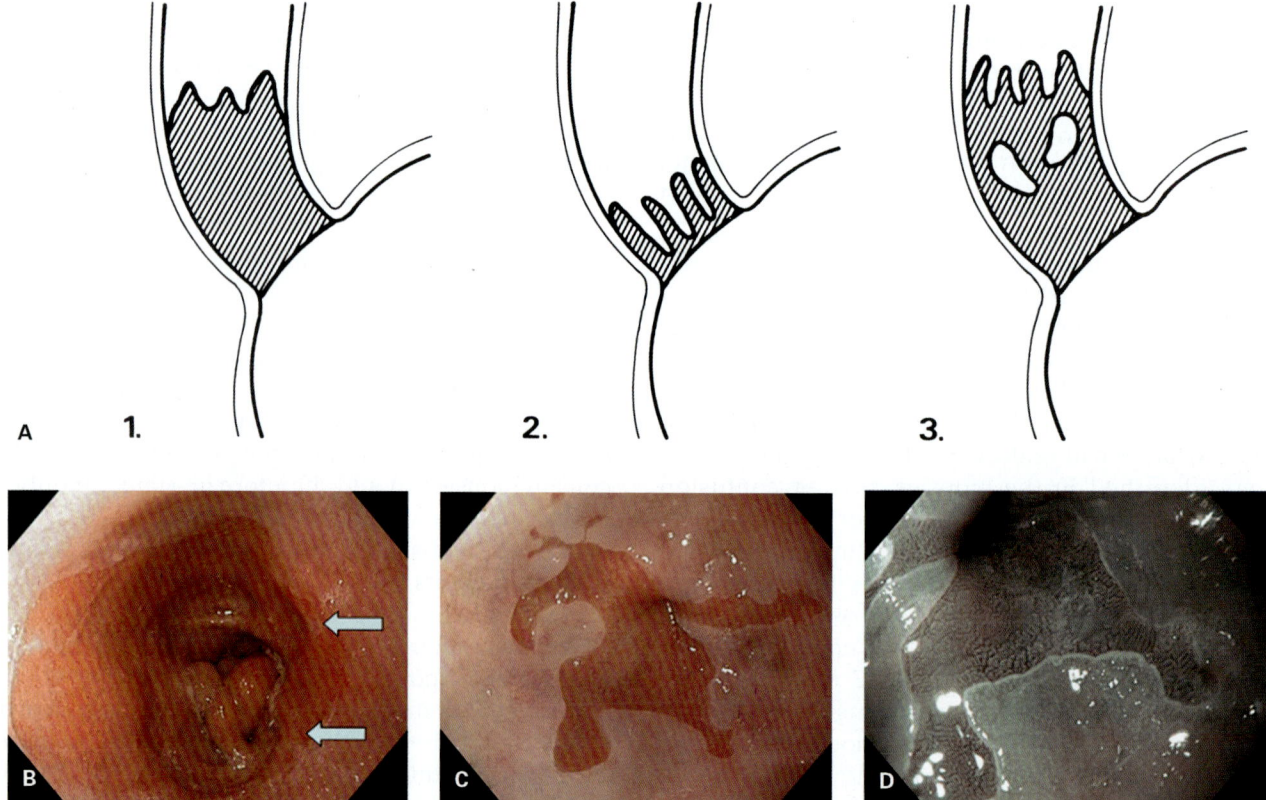

Figure 10-18. Endoscopic appearances of BE. **A:** Sketch illustrating the patterns. A common pattern is shown in *panel 1.* The interface between the Barrett's (hatched) and squamous mucosa is often wavy, as shown, similar to the Z-line at the GEJ. *Panel 2*: Short segment with tongues only, that is, no circumferential involvement. *Panel 3*: Residual whitish squamous islands are commonly present, especially near the upper end of Barrett's mucosa. **B:** Endoscopic view of long-segment Barrett's with circular columnar metaplasia and small islands of squamous epithelium (*arrows*). **C:** Tongues of columnar metaplasia in the distal esophagus (BE) in white light. **D:** NBI technique with regular gyriform surface epithelium pattern. (Images courtesy of Steffen Muehldorfer, MD.)

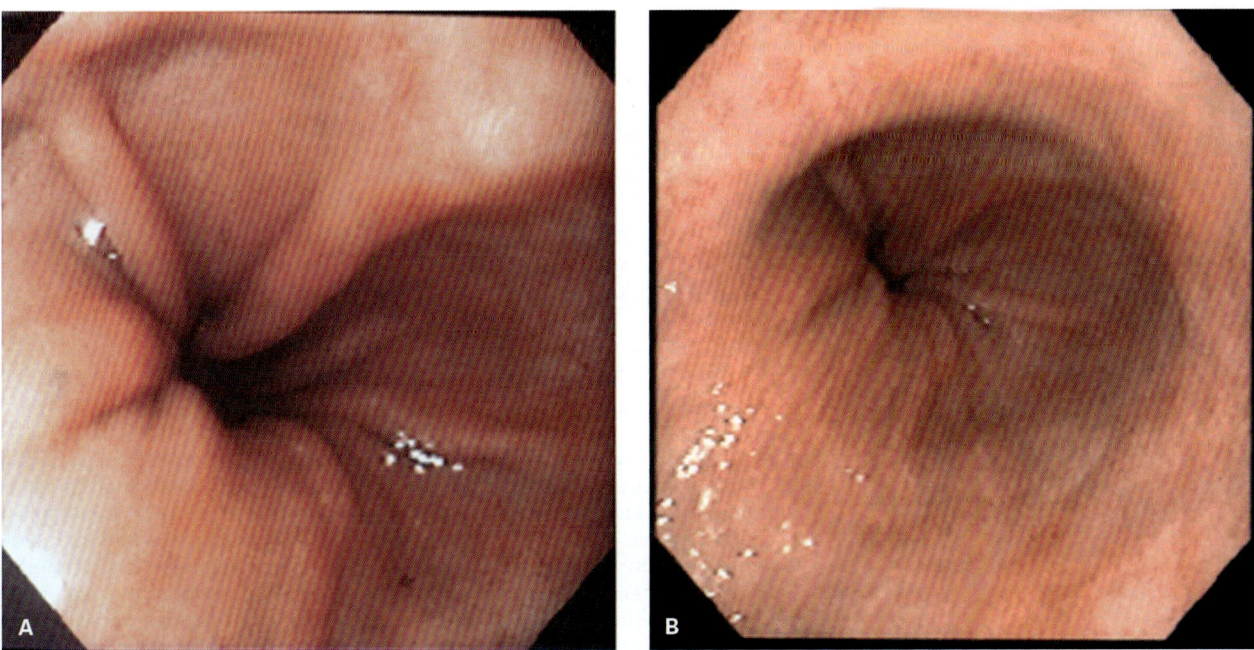

Figure 10-19. Endoscopic Landmarks: Recognizing the GEJ. **A:** Top of the gastric folds. **B:** LES pinch that is frequently lax in patients with GERD-associated disorders. Here it is at the top of the gastric folds.

this is that it is impossible to make a confident diagnosis of BE until the proximal extension of columnar mucosa, whether a tongue or circumferential extension, is at least 1 cm in length. Less than this it is simply an irregular Z-line by definition. The corollary of this is that it is impossible to separate "ultra-short" BE (<1 cm of BE) from intestinal metaplasia in native cardiac mucosa. Although ultrashort BE presumably must exist, at the time of writing there is no good way to make that diagnosis by biopsy of this region

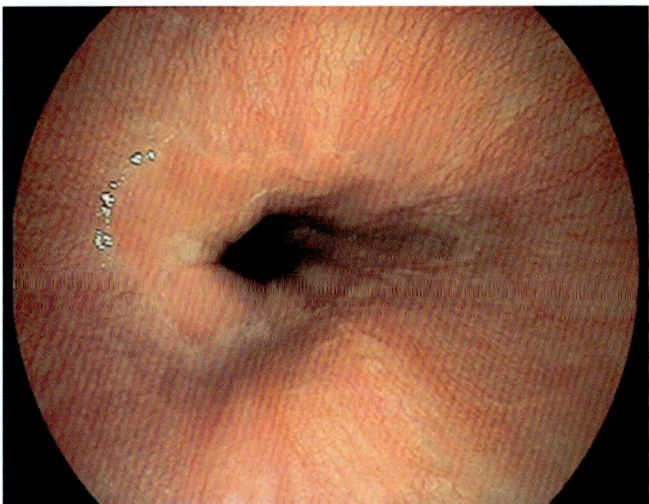

Figure 10-20. Endoscopic landmarks of the distal end of the esophagus (in Japan) showing the limits of the palisaded vessels. In this example, they focally descend beyond the upper limit of the gastric folds.

alone. If intestinal metaplasia is isolated to the cardia region without the rest of the stomach being involved, this implies that it may well be GERD related and therefore Barrett's related, but this remains implied and not definitive. The latter requires biopsies of that area most likely to have intestinal metaplasia, namely, the antrum and incisura region of the stomach, the most likely cause of which is Helicobacter, and which is mirrored at the cardia. If biopsies are carried out to ascertain this, those from the cardia must necessarily be placed into a separate container to allow identification of cardiac and antral pathology separately.

With this proviso, intestinal metaplasia limited to the cardia (no metaplasia in the antrum or rest of the stomach) is likely to be reflux related.

Definitions of BE: short- versus long-segment BE. Endoscopically, BE has been divided into short segment (<3 cm) or long segment (3 cm+). This is a historical feature that is slowly losing favor due to lack of relevance. It was developed because it was known that the Z-line should be somewhere within the LES, which is about 3 cm long. Anything more than 3 cm was therefore "unequivocal" BE, whereas anything less than this was open to question. However, it was clear that some of the excluded patients also had to have BE, so the issue became how best to make that diagnosis, particularly when biopsies of that region showed that some of these patients also had intestinal metaplasia, the presumed precursor of esophageal carcinoma.

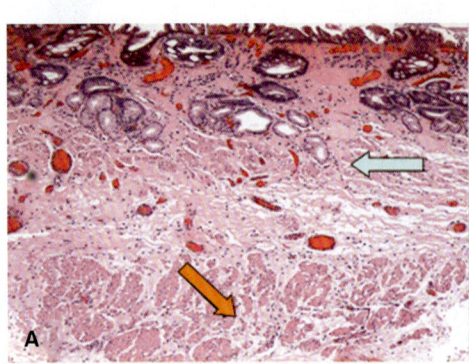
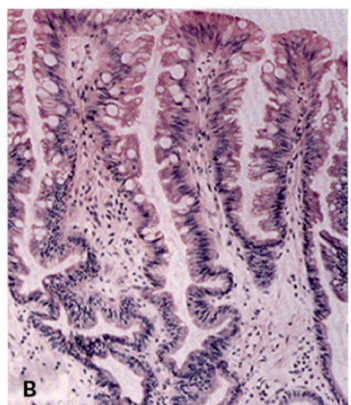
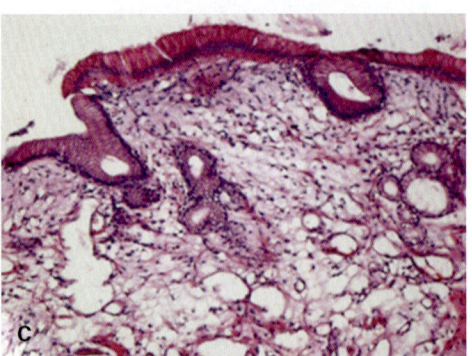
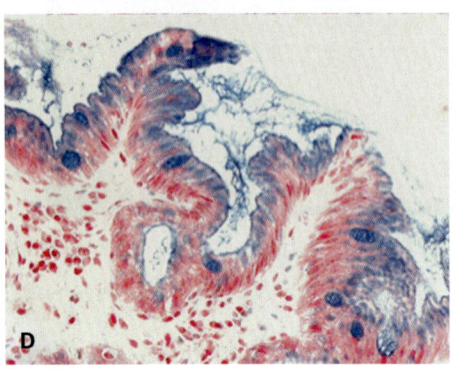

Figure 10-21. **A:** Histology of columnar metaplasia with goblet cells/specialized intestinal metaplasia and double muscularis mucosae. The marked and diffuse intestinalization in the lower esophagus is virtually diagnostic of BE as such metaplasia is only seen in gastric mucosa with diffuse intestinal metaplasia. In addition, the duplicated muscularis mucosa is clearly visible with a superficial (neo) layer immediately beneath the epithelium (*blue arrow*) and the original muscularis mucosae beneath (*orange arrow*). Courtesy of Dr. C Streutker. **B:** Typical biopsy appearances of BE with incomplete intestinal metaplasia and branching pits. **C:** Histology of columnar metaplasia without goblet cells. This patient had a 3.5-cm circular segment of columnar metaplasia in the distal esophagus with no significant hiatal hernia. Repeated endoscopy and multiple biopsies still did not show goblet cells. **D:** Alcian blue stain at pH 2.5. While the goblet cells stain, many of the intervening columnar cells also stain. Not only can interpretation be difficult but it can sometimes be positively misleading. We rarely carry out this stain for diagnostic purposes.

When BE Does Not Have Goblet Cells, Does It Matter?

The requirement of goblet cells for the diagnosis of BE is based on the notion that carcinoma only develops if intestinal metaplasia is present. Yet there are abundant data to suggest that the non–goblet cell population in BE already have most of the abnormalities found in goblet cells, including many of the characteristics of an intestinal phenotype,[52,57] and the necessity of having goblet cell required for the diagnosis of BE has been questioned.[54]

When are goblet cells not present? There are numerous circumstances when BE is present endoscopically but goblet cells are not found. These include the following:

1. Children with BE do not usually develop goblet cells until into the second decade of life.
2. Some patients with tongues of columnar mucosa do not have goblet cells when first biopsied. While some have them on repeat biopsy (presumably sampling problems first time), some never seem to develop them; do these patients have "a tongue of BE," and if not, what does one call this appearance if not a tongue of BE? Perhaps just "a tongue of columnar-lined esophagus."
3. Several large studies appear to show that some patients with unequivocal BE endoscopically never seem to develop intestinal metaplasia. From our own unpublished data about 80% of segments <1 cm do not have goblet cells. With increasing length the probability of detecting goblet cells increases but never reaches 100% even in very long segments. It is not clear how much this reflects reality and what proportion is due to sampling error.

The first paper to suggest this was by Kim et al.,[58] in a Veterans Administration study that included only patients with long-segment BE (>3 cm). They found that 20% of patients with BE did not exhibit intestinal metaplasia in biopsies from two endoscopies, a figure similar to that obtained by Harrison et al.[59] over a decade later. Also, in the latter study, of 125 patients with BE, only 35% of patients would have been diagnosed with BE if only one to four biopsies were obtained; 68% if five to eight biopsies were obtained; and 74% if more than eight biopsies were obtained.

In another multicenter study looking at 3,568 nondysplastic biopsies from 1,751 patients, intestinal metaplasia was detected more commonly in males (odds ratio 1.24) and in patients with a longer columnar segment length.[60] In that study, the chance of detecting goblet cells was also proportional to the number of biopsies obtained. About 55% of patients without intestinal metaplasia at index endoscopy showed intestinal metaplasia after 5 years, while at 10 years the figure reached 91%. Thus, 9% of patients in these cohorts never had goblet cells detected over that time period.

Another quirk is that goblet cells may be easier to find in short- rather than long-segment BE as goblet cells are preferentially found proximally in columnar-lined mucosa. In one study, 70% of patients with 1 to 2 cm and 90% of patients with 3 to 4 cm of columnar metaplasia had goblet cells—more than that seen in many patients with long-segment BE. In this study, 94% of proximal biopsies had goblet cells compared with only 39% of biopsies from the distal esophagus.[45] Obtaining biopsies from the distal esophagus only could have resulted in BE being missed in more than 50% of patients. There are therefore many reasons why goblet cells may not be detected: They may be present but not detected; they may not be present; they may come and go.

Risk of carcinoma in patients with non–goblet cell BE. It is difficult to decide what type of follow-up the individuals without goblet cells within columnar metaplasia should receive, but this should likely be the same as for those with goblet cells. The important thing is that if goblet cells are not found, that the patient is not lost to follow-up assuming they still have a risk of cancer. But do they?

Several studies have shown a similar risk of neoplastic progression in patients with BE, irrespective of the presence of goblet cells. Gatenby et al.[60] looked at 322 patients with and 612 patients without intestinal metaplasia, and found that 19.8% of the former and 15.2% of the latter developed LGD or HGD or adenocarcinoma on follow-up (no significant difference). Similarly, in another follow-up study by Kelty et al.,[61] the rate of development of adenocarcinoma was 4.5% in those with intestinal metaplasia and 3.6% in those without. Putting both studies together, perhaps there is a slight additional risk if goblet cells are present, but it is also clear that the dictum "no goblet cells, no cancer risk" is incorrect.[52,62]

However, possibly the proof is suggested in a detailed morphologic study of 141 small (minute) esophageal adenocarcinomas and areas of dysplasia removed by endoscopic mucosal resection (EMR), by Takubo et al.,[63] in which the mucosa on each side of the tumors was examined for the type of epithelium. More than 70% of adenocarcinomas were located adjacent to the cardiac/fundic-type rather than the intestinal-type mucosa. Even more surprisingly, intestinal metaplasia was not observed in any other areas of the EMR specimens in over half (56.6%) of the cases. These data challenge directly the long-held belief that BE-associated adenocarcinoma is always accompanied and is preceded by intestinal-type epithelium. It remains to be seen whether other studies support these data.

Conclusions regarding the definition and cancer risk in Barrett's (columnar-lined) esophagus

1. The dictum, "no goblet cells, no cancer risk," appears to be wrong, although the size of the risk in patients without goblet cells remains to be fully determined.
2. Patients with endoscopic CLE should almost certainly have some type of surveillance for potential cancer risk, if clinically appropriate, irrespective of the presence of goblet cells. The interval is unclear, but like other BE patients, after the first few endoscopies without dysplasia, the interval can likely be lengthened.
3. When endoscopic BE is seen, then this is also the first surveillance endoscopy for this patient. The purpose of taking biopsies is therefore to establish that the epithelium is indeed columnar and that no dysplasia is present. Indeed, dysplasia, and carcinoma, is much more likely to be found at the first endoscopy at which BE is found than in subsequent surveillance endoscopy. However, dysplasia in nonmetaplastic mucosa (foveolar dysplasia) can be much more subtle than that in metaplastic mucosa.[64] This is discussed subsequently.

Epidemiology and Pathophysiology of Barrett's Esophagus

BE is clearly acquired as a result of both acid and alkaline reflux (presumably duodenogastroesophageal) and is not a congenital condition, so terms like endobrachyesophagus and related terms implying a congenital origin for BE[65] are obsolete, despite the fact that Barrett himself thought this to be the case.

Men are affected twice as often as women. Children can also be affected. Surprisingly, the length of columnar metaplasia seems not to change with patients' age. The yearly incidence of Barrett's adenocarcinoma is between 0.12% and 1%. Less than 5% of patients with BE are believed to develop Barrett's adenocarcinoma. The mean average age of patients with BE is about 55 years whereas patients with Barrett's adenocarcinoma are about 10 years older.[66,67] Patients with BE tend to have higher body mass index, more obesity, and virtually all have a hiatal hernia.[68] Patients with BE are more likely to die of ischemic heart death and bronchopneumonia rather than esophageal adenocarcinoma.[69]

Often patients with BE report severe reflux disease in the past with change into milder symptoms years prior to the first diagnosis. It is believed that this might represent the time of development of columnar metaplasia since this epithelium is more resistant to acid than squamous epithelium and probably innervation has been somehow modified at this point. However, if true, it suggests that patients can develop or extend the length of their BE segment over time, which is not what is seen endoscopically, although the possibility that this develops quickly following an episode of ulceration cannot be excluded. Given that most patients with BE are receiving PPIs, they are therefore selected clinically as having a very low-risk group for ulceration.

Morphologic Development of Barrett's Esophagus

Columnar metaplasia in the esophagus can show a mosaic distribution of different types of epithelium, and there are several hypotheses regarding how BE might develop. Whether any or all of these develop by gradual "creeping" metaplasia, or in one or two major episodes, for example, immediately following ulceration, and whether they are different if they occur from any or many of the following is unclear.

Multilayered (transitional) epithelium (Fig. 10-22) is one potential candidate and consists of a stratified squamous mucosa basally but with a superficial layer of columnar cells, occasionally with cilia. Occasionally the nuclear stratification is mistaken for dysplastic epithelium, primarily by those not familiar with this type of epithelium. Other candidates in the genesis of BE include the following:

1. Metaplasia of gastric epithelium[70,71]
2. Metaplasia of cardia epithelium[72,73]
3. An origin from (stem) cells in the ducts of esophageal glands[74-77]
4. Re-epithelialization (regeneration) directly from the upper (squamous) mucosa. While this almost certainly occurs following esophageal ulceration, it necessarily results in squamous mucosa, so it is not a contender for the genesis of columnar epithelium, unless this includes metaplasia of esophageal stem cells (whatever these are),[78-80] or gut regenerative cell lineage[81]

Endoscopic Grading of Barrett's Mucosa

The Prague criteria[54] include a grading system for BE. The Prague criteria for BE recommend measuring the length of the circumferential (C) segment of BE and also the maximum (M) extent of columnar mucosa in the distal esophagus and coding it as C,M[54]; for example, a segment of BE 4 cm in circumference and of 6 cm maximum length (= C4, M6 Barrett's).

Histology

Because BE is a mosaic of tissue types, a variety of epithelial types can be found in the CLE.

These can be

1. intestinalized (complete or incomplete)
2. nonintestinalized (Fig. 10-23)
   - oxyntic (rare), cardio-oxyntic, and cardiac (common)
   - pancreatic metaplasia, multilayered epithelium (relatively frequent)
3. squamous islands (native or regenerative—the latter being derived from esophageal gland ducts)
4. esophageal gland ducts (useful for confirming that one is unequivocally in the esophagus and that any glandular mucosa present must be part of "columnar lined esophagus")
5. subsquamous glandular/intestinalized mucosa in which usually the squamous mucosa extends distally to cover the previous glandular mucosa. This is primarily a repair phenomenon, so is only seen when reflux is diminished or prevented (PPIs, fundoplication, proximal to tumors, postablation, possibly spontaneously). However, this change can occur in intestinalized cardia mucosa where its significance is less clear.

The most characteristic type of BE has incomplete intestinal metaplasia (see Fig. 10-21). Complete intestinal metaplasia can also be found in which the gastric foveolar mucin-producing cells found in "classical" BE are replaced by a full intestinal phenotype with absorptive cells, often Paneth cells and intestinal-type endocrine cells. After total gastrectomy, metaplasia to small bowel type can be found in the esophagus,[82] suggesting a role for duodenogastroesophageal reflux of bile and activated pancreatic juice.[45]

The mucosa in BE often has an atrophic appearance, analogous to the architectural distortion seen in ulcerative colitis, likely by an identical mechanism. This can be very useful as it is rarely seen in intestinal

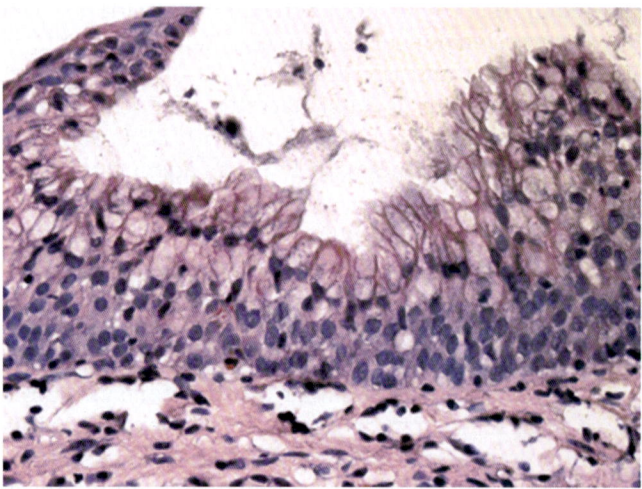

Figure 10-22. Multilayered/transitional mucosa consisting of pseudostratified squamous epithelium that bears characteristics of columnar and squamous epithelium and probably represents a kind of transitional epithelium that can span a fraction of a millimeter and up to several millimeters in length. For the unsuspecting, the stratified nuclei can raise the question of dysplasia.

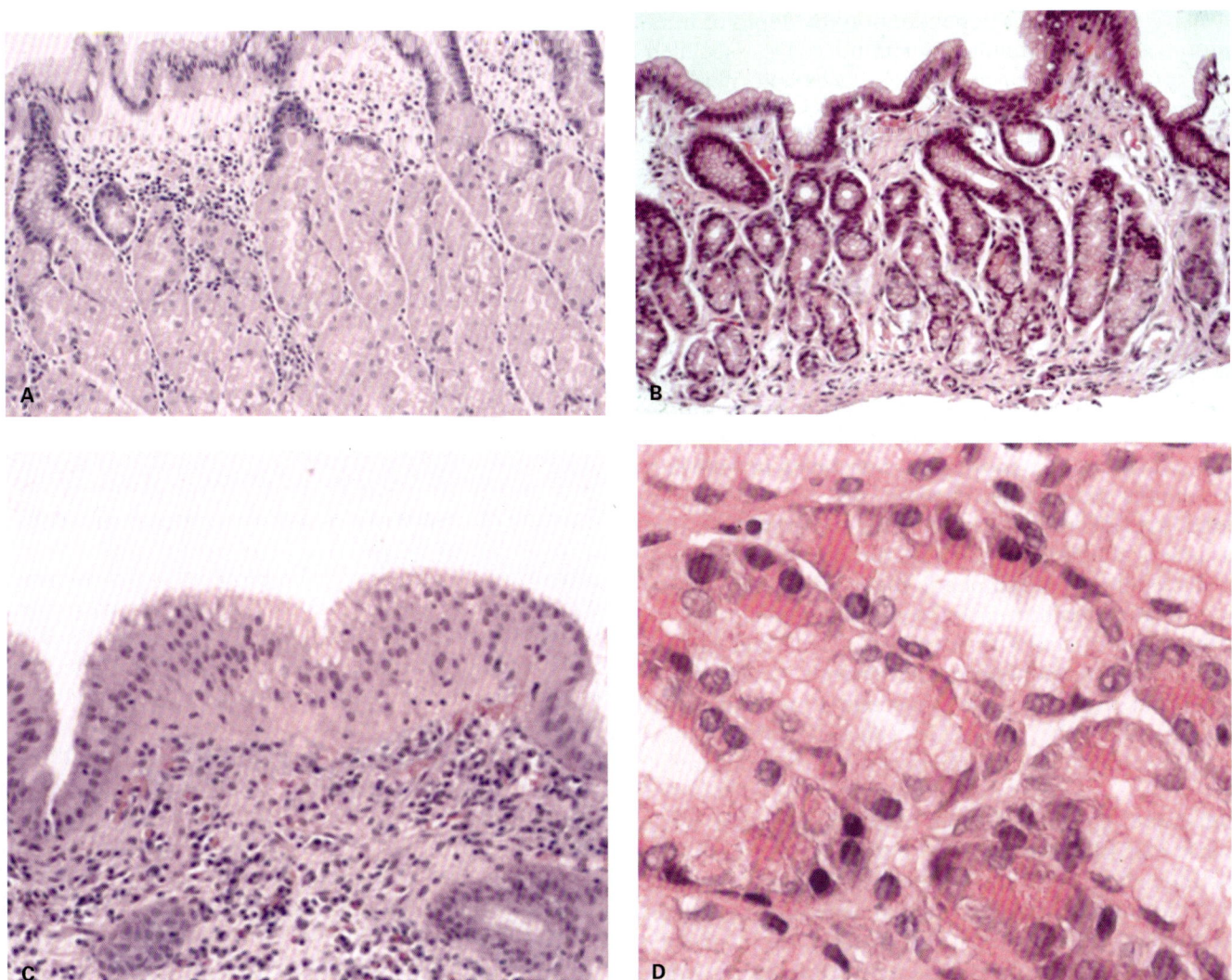

Figure 10-23. Other types of mucosa that can be seen in BE. **A:** Full oxyntic mucosa is rarely seen although aggregates of parietal cells are common distally. Mucosa of this type usually comes from within a hiatal hernia. **B:** Cardia type mucosa. Unless overtly atrophic it may be impossible to know if this originated from within native cardia or BE. **C:** Multilayered epithelium. **D:** Pancreatic metaplasia.

metaplasia in the cardia, so is virtually diagnostic of BE, and is not seen in normal cardiac mucosa (see Fig. 10-21A). Sometimes esophageal glands and their ducts are found in biopsies that allow an unequivocal diagnosis of CLE or BE. On top of these ducts, small squamous islands can sometimes be detected, which give rise to the squamous mucosa from which re-epithelialization of the esophagus with squamous mucosa can occur following therapy.[83]

The surface epithelium of intestinalized mucosa has a brush border, goblet cells, mucus-producing cells that are virtually pregoblet cells, occasional neuroendocrine cells (serotonin, somatostatin, secretin, gastrin, and pancreatic polypeptides), mucous neck cells, Paneth cells, and sometimes chief and parietal cells, especially in the more distal parts of the columnar segment. This indicates the mosaic of cell types and distribution of different types of epithelium within columnar metaplasia.

Double muscularis mucosae. A common feature of BE is the presence of a double (duplicated) muscularis mucosae.[84] As in inflammatory bowel disease, this is likely the result of mucosal erosion with preservation of the native muscularis mucosae. However, when the epithelium regenerates there is also formation of a neo-muscularis mucosae, which inevitably is superficial to the original one, so that the real submucosa is deep to the second layer of muscularis mucosae. This fact is only of importance in the presence of neoplasia, where the question has arisen as to whether the space between both layers of muscularis mucosae behaves as lamina propria, as it should, or as neo-submucosa with an increased risk of nodal metastases. The prognosis of invasive carcinoma is dependent on the depth of infiltration, as infiltration into the submucosa is associated with a greater risk of nodal metastases and therefore a worse prognosis. With a double layer of muscularis mucosae, the submucosa is not reached until the second layer is breached. The double muscularis mucosae are present in all resection specimens but are not necessarily identified in every section as neoplasia may have destroyed the upper layer. A subdivision of the layers analogous to those used in esophageal squamous cell carcinoma has been proposed: In squamous cell carcinoma, there are three layers (m1 to m3), but in BE, due to the double-layer adenocarcinomas, there are four layers (m1: neoplasia limited to upper mucosal layer, m2: infiltration of upper layer of the muscularis mucosae, m3: infiltration into layer in between the double muscularis mucosae, m4: infiltration into deep layer of muscularis mucosae). Fortunately, this is largely theoretical, as most tumors limited to m1 to m4 rarely show lymphatic metastasis.[8] Smoothelin is a novel smooth muscle protein expressed only by fully differentiated smooth muscle cells and not by proliferative or noncontractile smooth muscle cells, and stains the deep (true) muscularis mucosae more strongly than the superficial (neo) layer,[85] but any muscle stain can show if there is more than one layer.

Palisaded vessels. Although these are used as a marker of BE, especially in Japan, where their size distinguished them from the mucosa above the LES and the stomach distally, their morphologic counterpart is not well studied. These vessels are invariably >85 µm, while the use of the figure 100 µm provides even greater separation from proximal or distal vessels.[86] However, endoscopically these vessels do sometimes get down to the level of the upper end of the gastric folds, the traditional upper end of the stomach. Nevertheless, in endoscopic resections, mucosal vessels >100 µm or submucosal vessels >260 µm (veins proximal or distal) are smaller than this.[86]

Handling of Patients and Biopsies Postablation or Postendoscopic Resection

Perhaps the most important thing is that after successful ablation or endoscopic resection of Barrett's neoplasia, the patient needs continued follow-up, since there is at least a 25% rate of metachronous neoplasia,[87] especially where Barrett's epithelium is left after endoscopic resection. With ablation techniques a second problem lies in potential remnants of BE or Barrett's neoplasia below the neosquamous epithelium. Several studies after ablation have shown that there may be remnants of Barrett's epithelium in the surface mucosa, or they may be detected below the squamous epithelium (subsquamous Barrett's) in a small proportion of patients.[88] The problem is that biopsies are often very flat and rarely contain lamina propria below the squamous epithelium in routine settings.[89,90] This means that the biopsies may well be inadequate to answer the question of whether persistent subsquamous Barrett's mucosa is present, which might be dysplastic or even carcinomatous (Fig. 10-24). The presence of squamous papillae should not be taken as evidence of lamina propria and therefore of adequacy of the biopsy to make this determination. Lamina propria in papillae is very superficial so does not exclude deeper lamina propria invasion; indeed lamina propria invasion only occasionally extends up into the papillae. Lamina propria beneath the squamous mucosa is required. Subsquamous columnar epithelium may be visible endoscopically as flat elevations of the mucosa. Long-term follow-up for more than 5 years has shown that ablation is a safe technique.[91] Our own observations suggest that subsquamous columnar epithelium is much more likely to consist of complete intestinalized mucosa rather than the incomplete type with foveolar mucous-producing cells. As this mucosa is likely shielded from mucosal duodenogastroesophageal reflux, our suspicion is that subsquamous mucosa may be less susceptible to neoplastic transformation than surface Barrett's mucosa, except when it has already undergone some form of neoplastic transformation. Subsquamous intestinal metaplasia is therefore highly suggestive of BE. Cytokeratin staining seems not to help in this respect.[92]

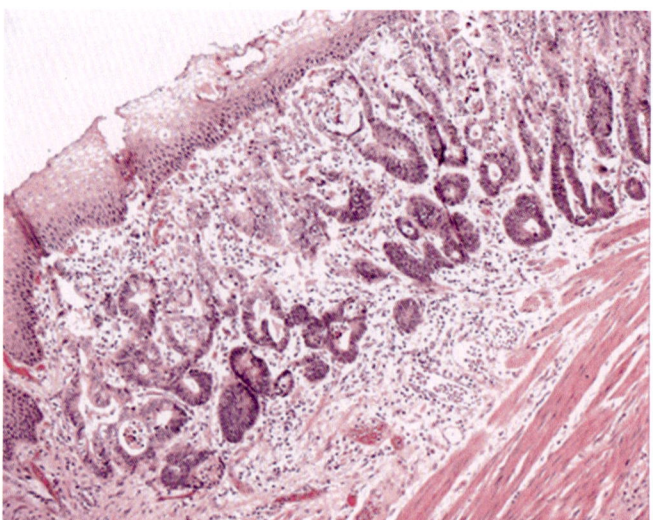

Figure 10-24. Subsquamous carcinoma postendoscopic ablation.

Differential Diagnosis of BE and Other Mucosal Types Encountered

The most complicated differential diagnosis is intestinal metaplasia of the cardia or the proximal stomach. In practice, this is becoming less of an issue, as

It is clear that endoscopists appear not to be able to distinguish an irregular Z line from BE if the latter is <1 cm, so on simple endoscopic grounds the two appear to be inseparable. The new question becomes whether it is possible histologically to separate what is truly ultrashort-segment BE (<1 cm of BE) from intestinal metaplasia at the cardia. Some criteria can help, but likely not sufficiently to confidently distinguish between the two all the time. Cardia mucosa is a nonatrophic mucosa with a proliferation zone within the upper body of the glands. Deep glands are composed of mucous glands that show larger diameter compared to esophageal mucous-producing glands.

Pancreatic acinar metaplasia can also be identified in the cardia, and in some individuals in the so-called hybrid epithelium.

Multilayered epithelium (pseudostratified squamous metaplasia) can be seen. One group[92] interprets such a lesion as a precursor lesion for BE while others have arguments against it.[22] It is commonly seen in BE. Because of the nuclear stratification present, that may reach close to the surface, this occasionally is misinterpreted as low-grade dysplasia (LGD).

Pseudogoblet cells do not react strongly by Alcian blue staining, although it may be part of weak diffuse staining as shown in Figure 10-21D, in which real goblet cells are also apparent. Because the notion of BE without goblet cells is sometimes seen, routine Alcian blue staining is not required and also has its own pitfalls in staining mucous cells strongly when they are not goblet cells (columnar blues). The proliferative zone is situated in the middle or bottom part of the mucosa when completely intestinalized. Intestinal metaplasia of the incomplete type is found at the surface with goblet cells and foveolar cells in between.

The subtype of intestinal metaplasia (complete vs. incomplete) also helps little. Certainly BE is usually incomplete, unless subsquamous, when it is usually complete.[93]

If the answer is really required as to whether IM at the cardia is really part of BE or part of more diffuse intestinal metaplasia in the stomach, that is part of atrophic gastritis, the latter should be accompanied by identical changes in the distal stomach. Taking multiple biopsies from the antrum, especially from the angulus distally as part of routine, *Helicobacter* sampling should resolve the issue, as metaplasia should be present in these biopsies also. Normal distal biopsies indicate that the cardia biopsies are not part of diffuse atrophic gastritis, and are therefore very likely isolated to the cardia.

Barrett-associated Neoplasia

Patients with specialized intestinal metaplasia have up to 125-fold risk for Barrett's adenocarcinoma compared to a normal population, which in practice translates to about 0.12% per annum and is almost certainly lower in patients without intestinal metaplasia. Risk factors for carcinoma are long standing reflux disease, white males, and the presence of dysplasia/IEN. Dysplasia/IEN is subdivided into low-grade dysplasia (LGD or LGIEN) (Figs. 10-25 and 10-26) and high-grade dysplasia (HGD or high-grade intraepithelial neoplasia [HGIEN]) (Figs. 10-27 and 10-28). The latter includes carcinoma in situ (Fig. 10-29).

The use of a three-grade system (*mild, moderate, and severe*) for dysplasia is obsolete as there are no guidelines for their management. Similarly, the term "atypia" is not encouraged in view of its ambiguity and should never be used as a synonym for dysplasia, although it can be used if preceded by "regenerative," although even here "regenerative changes" are preferred.

There is recognized interobserver variability, especially between LGD and indefinite for dysplasia (IFD). One reason for this is the issue of whether surface maturation precludes a diagnosis of LGD. In practice it does *not*, as basal crypt dysplasia occurs at all sites within the GI tract and is the hallmark of most serrated neoplasia, but it is necessary to be absolutely certain that basal dysplasia is present. If *not* certain, *and* there is surface maturation, then the diagnosis reverts to IFD. In practice it may make a difference, for while both demand further biopsies, ideally after an increase in therapy, there is much less reluctance to refer patients for endoscopic ablation if a diagnosis of dysplasia is made. An example of maturing LGD is shown in Figure 10-30. As the subsequent follow-up is usually similar (repeat to ensure that unequivocal dysplasia or worse is not present), it should matter little. However, with endoscopic ablation techniques becoming so readily available, there is a distinct "left shift" so that lower grades of dysplasia

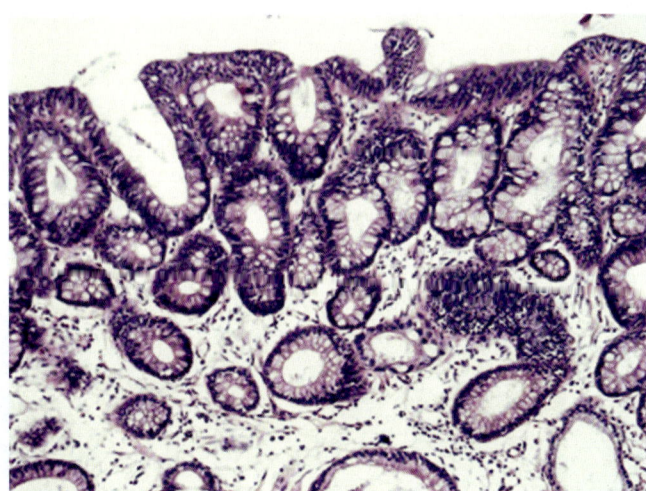

Figure 10-25. Low-grade dysplasia. The tip-off is that the changes are increasing as the surface is reached, where the mucosa looks very similar to adenomas seen in other parts of the GI tract.

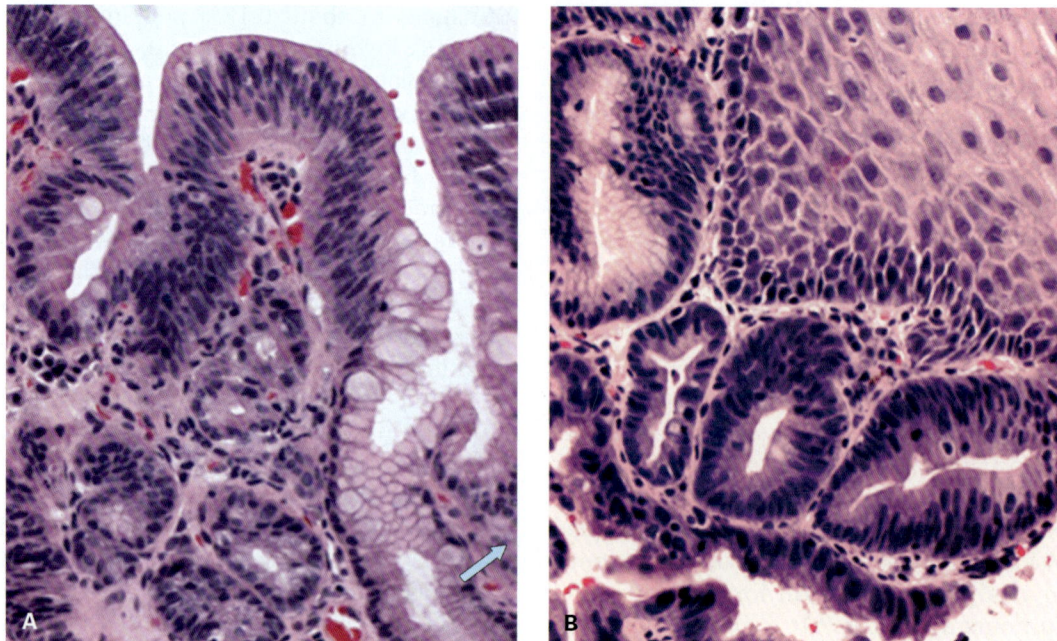

Figure 10-26. **A,B:** Overt ("rock solid") low-grade dysplasia. In fields like this, there should be virtually no interobserver variability. The abrupt junction with nondysplastic Barrett's mucosa (*arrow*) is a very useful indicator of neoplastic epithelium. Similar changes in a subsquamous location.

(sometimes none) are treated with these techniques. A more typical IFD is shown in Figure 10-31.

An emerging problem is reactive changes in inflamed multilayered epithelium. These cause problems because when inflamed, the superficial mucous vacuole is lost so the appearances are those of stratified nuclei reaching the surface. When a degree of nuclear atypia is added, the problem is compounded, and the question of LGD is raised (Fig. 10-31C–F). The clue is in recognizing that the epithelium is multilayered, either because the nuclei look relatively bland, much less cellular than seen in typical LGD, or because it is inflamed. Being familiar with the appearance of multi-layered epithelium clearly helps.

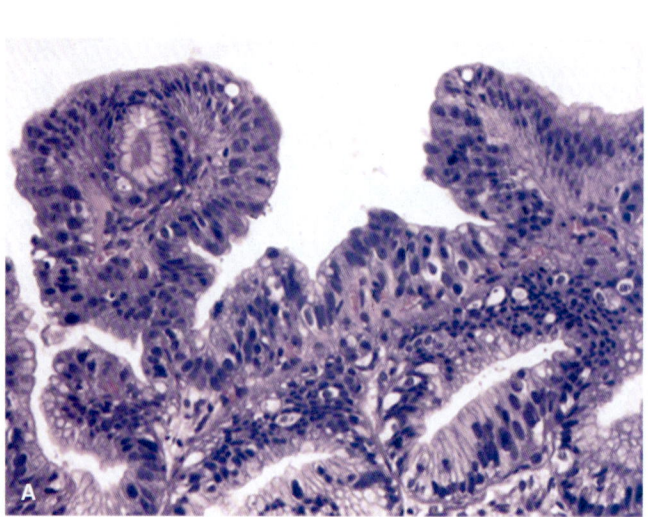
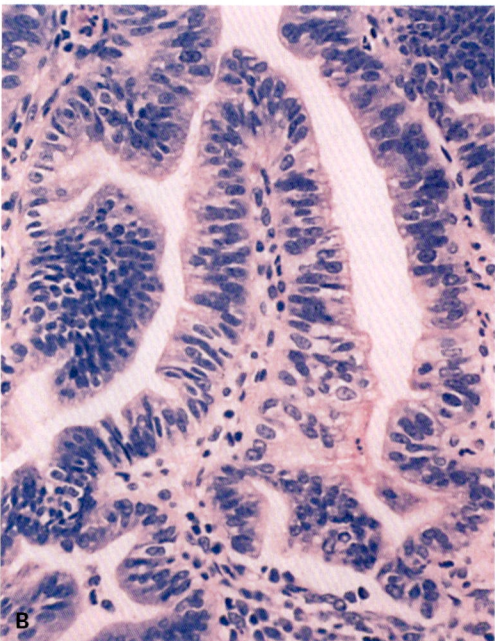

Figure 10-27. High-grade dysplasia. **A:** There is stratification to the surface and also a degree of loss of polarity. **B:** HGD with marked pseudostratification.

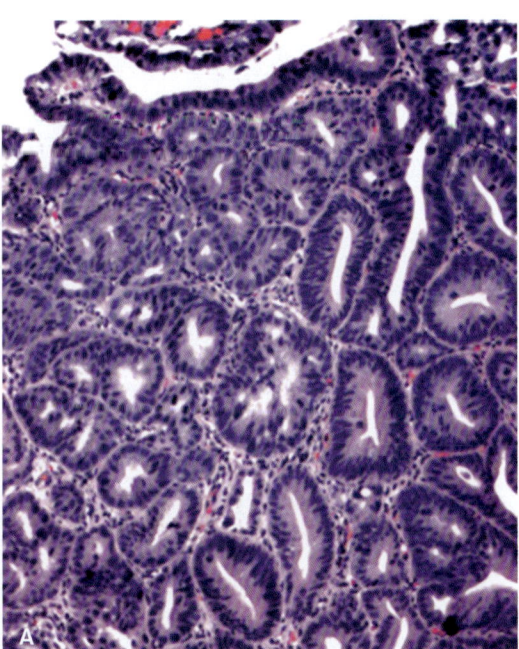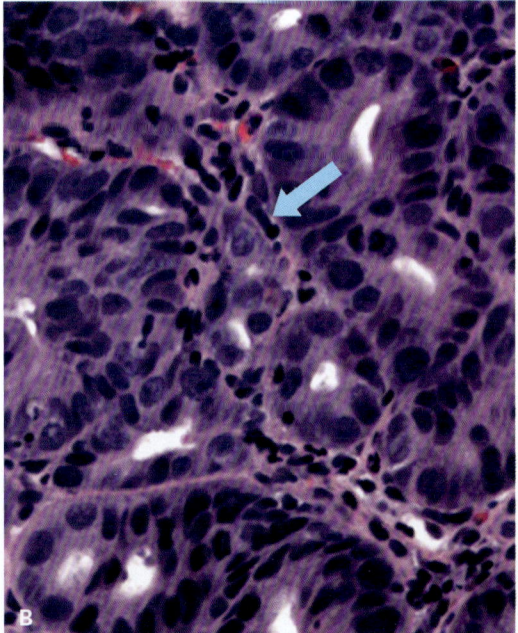

Figure 10-28. Variable dysplasia. **A:** Lower right there is LGD, but upper left there is architectural complexity far greater than seen in usual Barrett's. **B:** Detail with single and small groups of cells (*arrow*) infiltrating the lamina propria indicative of intramucosal carcinoma.

The risk of having or developing a carcinoma increases with the grade of dysplasia, and is also increased in IFD, which seems to better resemble LGD than negative for dysplasia in its neoplastic potential. The frequency of LGD in a consecutive series is believed to be around 1%.[94]

Diagnosing and Grading Dysplasia

It is easy to be simplistic and not appreciate that while there is a spectrum of change from negative through HGD, that there is more than one morphological, and therefore molecular, pathway, (complete and incomplete intestinal metaplasia, foveolar dysplasia), all of which can be complicated by reactive/regenerative changes. These pathways are virtually identical to those seen in the stomach, which are also described and illustrated in detail in Chapter 14. Further, all have their own spectra of changes, so that all cut-offs are to some degree arbitrary, subjective, and therefore subject to inter- (and also intra)observer variation. The spectrum of changes seen in BE are as follows:

- Negative for dysplasia/intraepithelial neoplasia
- Indefinite for dysplasia/intraepithelial neoplasia
- Low-grade dysplasia
- HGD, which includes "carcinoma in situ"—a term that we tend not to use except as an alarm term when suspicious that underlying invasion is likely present. It corresponds to "suspicious for invasive carcinoma" of the Vienna classification:
  - Intramucosal carcinoma (invasion into the lamina propria)
  - Invasive carcinoma (invasion into the submucosa or beyond)

Indefinite for Dysplasia

The distinction of normal or reactive changes from IFD affects the interval to the next endoscopy, and so should not be taken lightly. Conversely, the distinction between IFD and LGD usually does not result in a change in surveillance, although increasingly patients may undergo some form of endoscopic ablation to remove the entire Barrett's segment. A comment along the lines of "please

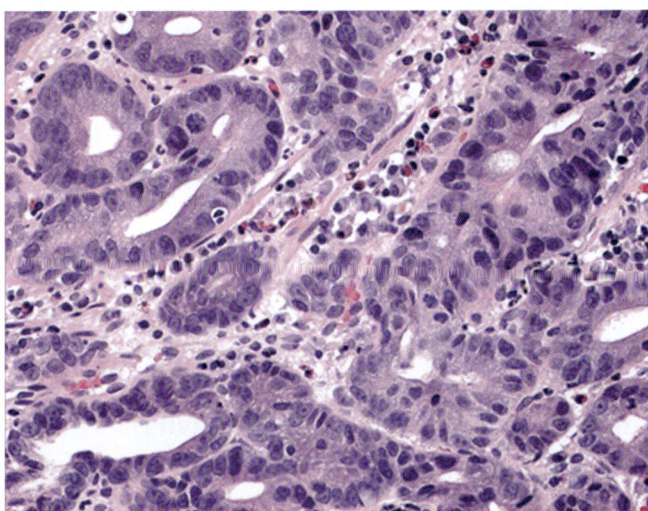

Figure 10-29. Intramucosal carcinoma, probably in foveolar mucosa. In the top left, apart from the lack of polarity, the nuclei are basal. Elsewhere, the crypts are totally random as seen in carcinoma. No muscularis mucosae is present to assess deeper invasion.

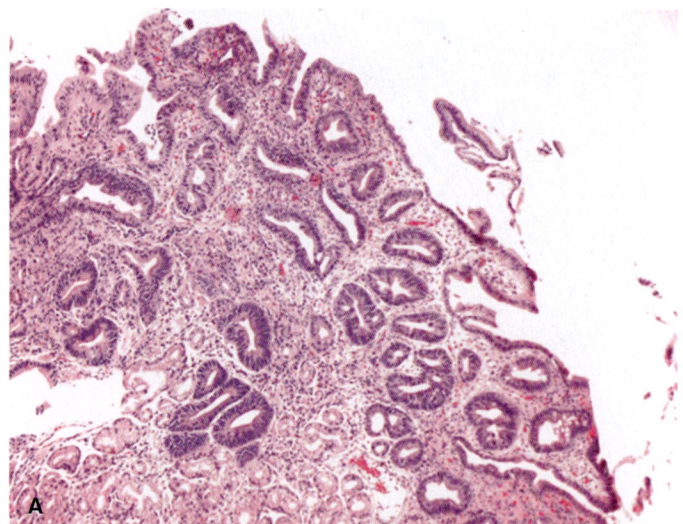
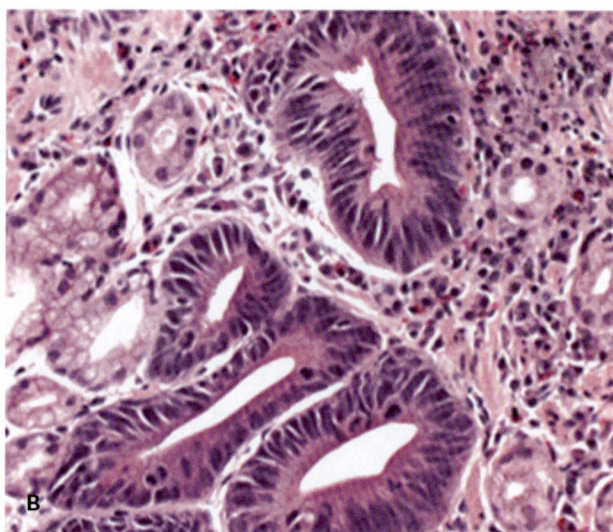
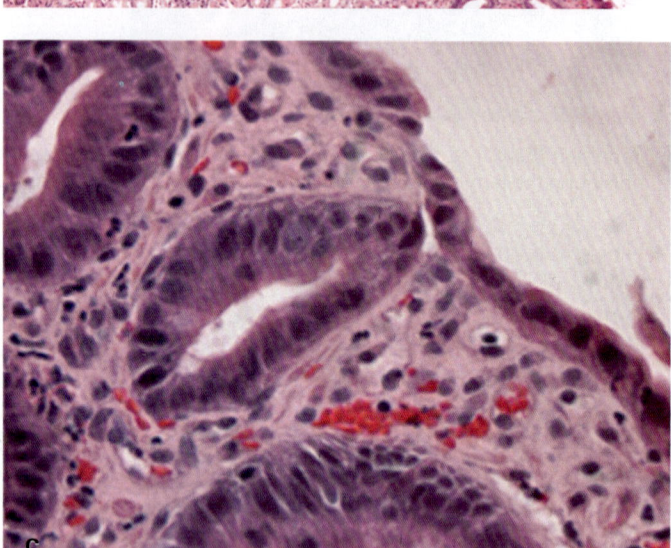

Figure 10-30. **A:** Low-grade dysplasia with maturation or indefinite for dysplasia? The dysplastic crypts are readily visible at low power. **B:** Detail of crypt base. Showing features that are quite acceptable for LGD (compare with Fig. 10-26). **C:** The problem is the attenuated restituting surface mucosa. Those demanding surface involvement for a diagnosis of LGE would have to call this IFD, while others might be persuaded by the crypt changes. Biopsies such as this result in the interobserver disagreement between these categories. Either diagnosis demands rescoping and rebiopsy to ensure that HGD or worse are not present.

ensure that these changes are not part of unequivocal dysplasia, or worse, at the patient's next endoscopy" certainly underscores the potential risk for the endoscopist.

Histologically, the likelihood is that one is dealing with IFD whenever there is restituting epithelium (cuboidal to low columnar epithelium with widely separated nuclei that are re-epithelializing erosions) and that the crypts from which they arise, and the immediately adjacent crypts, can show changes that mimic dysplasia but are usually limited to the crypt bases. So whenever attenuated mucosa is present in the upper parts of the crypts or on the surface, any grade of possible dysplasia should be regarded with suspicion and only diagnosed with the greatest confidence (see Figs. 10-30 and 10-31). While a small proportion of dysplasias are genuinely maximal in the crypt bases ("bottom-up dysplasia"), this is sufficiently uncommon that in the presence of surface maturation a diagnosis of dysplasia again needs to be made with caution. Downgrading to "indefinite for dysplasia" is appropriate in this situation, with subsequent rebiopsy to ensure that unequivocal dysplasia (or worse) is not present. Theoretically, an easy way of arriving at this diagnosis is to ask oneself two questions:

1. Are these changes unequivocally dysplastic/neoplastic/those of intraepithelial neoplasia?
2. Are these changes unequivocally negative for dysplasia or overtly reparative?

If the answer to both questions is "no," then by definition one is dealing with changes IFD (see Fig. 10-31).

Low-grade Dysplasia (Low-grade Intraepithelial Neoplasia—LGNIN)

In LGD/IEN, the glands are usually somewhat parallel and regular. The diagnosis is usually made on nuclear and not architectural changes (see Figs. 10-25 and 10-26). However, one of the problems with BE is that the architecture can be markedly distorted in nonneoplastic mucosa, even to the point of having a

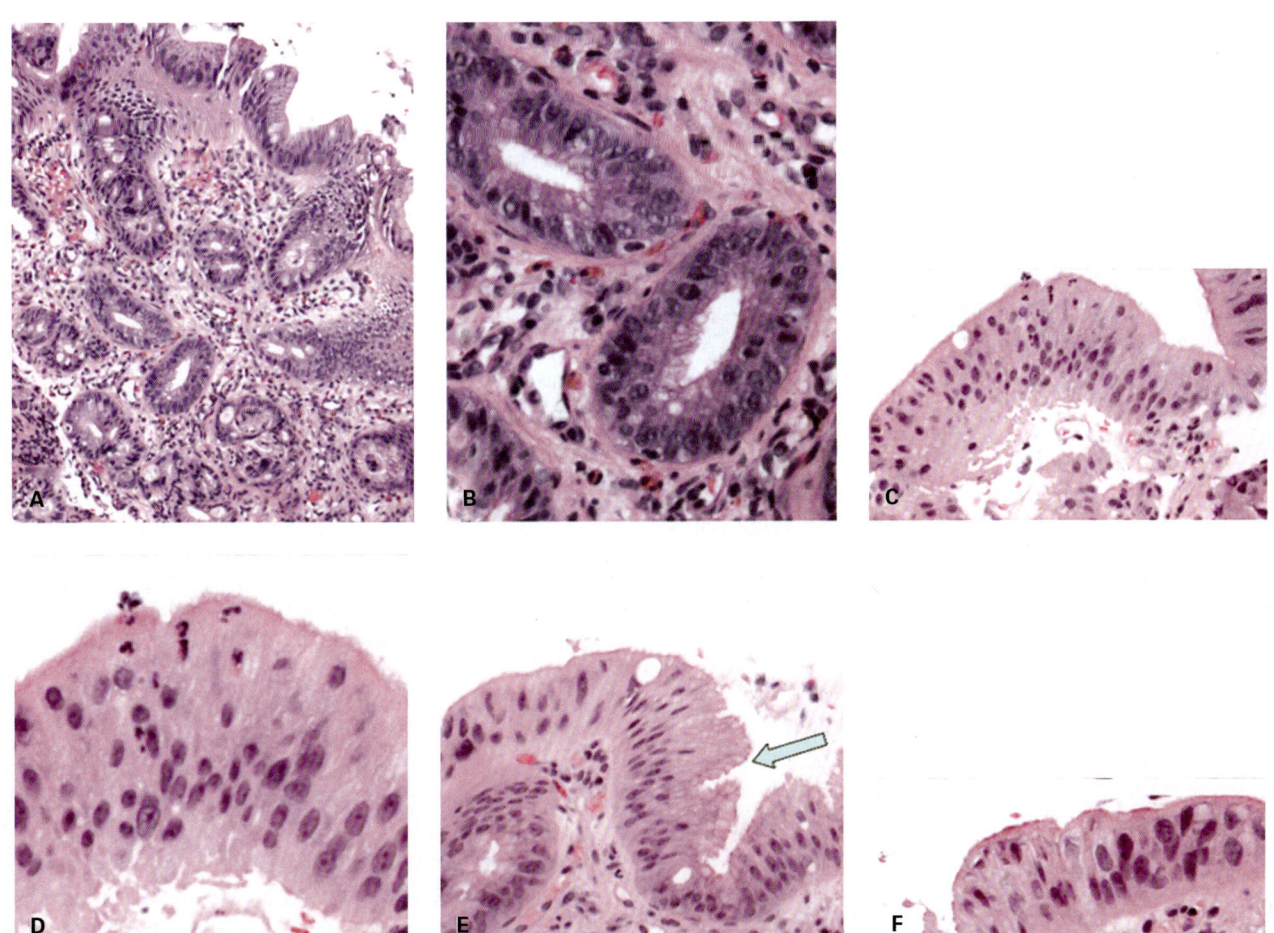

Figure 10-31. Indefinite for dysplasia. **A, B:** More typical IFD with nuclei that are neither clearly dysplastic or negative for dysplasia. Our suspicion is that these are likely reactive (likely = IFD as we are not sure). However, notice the extensive architectural back to back/gland within gland appearance, the addition to which of LGD would likely result in interpretation as HGD. **C–F:** Inflamed multilayered epithelium with reactive changes that can be mistaken for LGD in view of the nuclear stratification and nuclear atypicality. **C:** Multilayered epithelium with depleted mucous cells secondary to acute inflammation and repair. **D:** Detail of C showing neutrophils in the epithelium. **E:** Similar biopsy but mucous vacuoles can just be identified in the epithelium (*arrow*). **F:** Detail of mucosa immediately adjacent to E demonstrating the reactive atypia present. In practice all of these changes in multilayered epithelium are almost certainly reactive in nature.

back-to-back (gland within gland) appearance, so that the addition of any amount of nuclear atypia immediately causes concern that HGD may be present (Fig. 10-31A). In LGD, the crypt bases often consist of preexisting nonneoplastic glands, often resembling pyloric glands. Sudden transitions to normal epithelium are always a pointer of neoplasia, since junctions between two types of nonneoplastic mucosa is quite uncommon. Such abrupt transitions are even regarded as "proof" of neoplasia, as regenerative changes should be in direct continuity with the crypt giving rise to it, and should therefore be without an abrupt transition.

In the usual complete intestinal type of dysplasia, the changes essentially resemble a large bowel adenoma, sometimes so closely that it is called an adenoma, and may even form a localized polyp (Figs. 10-26, 10-28, and 10-29). Further, there is rarely doubt about whether one is dealing with dysplasia as the changes are so obvious and unambiguously dysplastic. Nuclei are typically elongated, hyperchromatic, and can leave their basal location. In low-grade IEN not more than two to three rows of nuclei are to be expected. The epithelium usually shows little evidence of differentiation toward the lumen or the base. In most cases, the numbers of goblet cells are reduced but can be present even in clear carcinomas.

Foveolar dysplasias can be more difficult as there are several variants, and comparison with gastric foveolar dysplasia is often worthwhile (Figs. 10-29 and 10-32). However, foveolar dysplasia does occasionally mature superficially as its most marked changes tend to be in the mucous neck region, so care has to be taken in this respect. Unless there is overt loss of polarity, the distinction between LGD and HGD can be notoriously difficult (see top left of Fig. 10-29). More often the problem is whether the lesion is high grade or intramucosal carcinoma. The spectrum of reactive changes are also discussed and illustrated in Chapters 13 and 14.

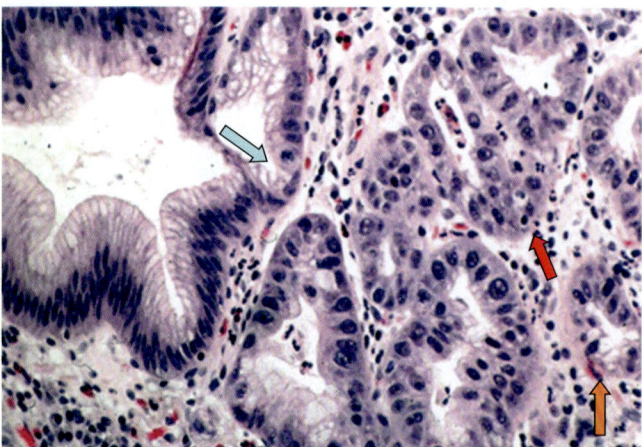

Figure 10-32. Spectrum of foveolar dysplasia. **Top left** is low-grade foveolar dysplasia with stratified nuclei but every cell is mucous producing as seen in normal superficial gastric mucosa. However, there is also a junction—usually a marker between dysplastic and nondysplastic epithelium—that here shows the cells of HGD taking over the LGD (*blue arrow*). On the extreme right the nuclei are fairly bland and the epithelium attenuated so regeneration might be considered (*orange arrow*). However, the glands in the center that have overt loss of polarity could have architectural distortion, and in one area the question is whether the glands might be trying to infiltrate the lamina propria between the position in which regular crypts are expected (*red arrow*), which would indicate intramucosal carcinoma—for which this is "suspicious."

High-grade Dysplasia (High-grade Intraepithelial Neoplasia—HGIEN)

In the classical (intestinal) pathway, biopsies with HGD (IEN), including "carcinoma in situ" (see Fig. 10-27 and 10-28), are defined using the above-mentioned criteria, but are present "to a greater degree." And herein lies the problem, as the dividing line between LGD and HGD is entirely subjective, and therefore inevitably subject to inter- (and intra) observer variability. Nuclei should reach the lumen of the pits unless overt loss of polarity is present.

Implication. This distinction between LGD and HGD seems to be gradually becoming less important. The diagnosis of HGD is still an "action" diagnosis, meaning that it is not usually left untreated. However, with newer modes of endoscopic therapy able to remove or destroy large or small areas of BE with little morbidity and no mortality, there is also a trend to treat overt LGD (Fig. 10-26) endoscopically as well as HGD.

In HGD/HGIEN, three to five nuclei can be found, with nuclei reaching the luminal surface. The number of goblet cells is further reduced but can be absent in both LGD and HGD. Further, if mucous is present it is often present in every cell, resembling the large bowel. Nuclei are not only enlarged, but they are more open with prominent single nucleoli, and may lose their polarity. At the crypt bases, preexisting glands may still be identified. Architectural changes may be present with budding of glands. If the latter is used as a criterion to separate HGD from intramucosal carcinoma, then, care has to be taken if based on one area, because nondysplastic mucosa can have occasional crypts with a back-to-back configuration. Adding even LGD to this can result in an interpretation of HGD—again a subjective interpretation.[94]

The glands may also be connected by lateral anastomoses (lateral expansion). Loss of nuclear polarity can be seen also.

Not surprisingly, patients with extensive HGD are more likely to have or develop invasive carcinoma in the following year than those with focal HGD.[95] Features in HGD that suggest there is likely an invasive component include

1. Architectural complexity
2. Necrotic debris in tubules
3. Neutrophils in dysplastic epithelium
4. Ulcers
5. Pagetoid spread into squamous epithelium

The likelihood of finding invasive carcinoma on resection was 79% overall but increased with the number of these features found such that when one factor was present on biopsy specimens, cancer was found in 39% of resections, whereas when all factors were identified, 88% of the resections showed invasion.[96] Conversely, when these features were not present (otherwise "unremarkable" HGD), none of the patients proved to have invasive carcinoma. This is potentially useful therapeutically, especially if the decision is a borderline one between endoscopic therapy. Unless an overtly infiltrating lesion is present, EMR (or submucosal dissection) is often a good start as the presence of invasion can be determined, and often the margins of resection on which further management can be based.

Intramucosal Carcinoma

This implies the presence of lamina propria invasion (see Figs. 10-28 and 10-29). Unfortunately, the myth that invasion occurs when tumor cells "break through the basement membrane" is good in theory, but practically tumor cells form their own basal membrane,[97] even if partial, around themselves both in the lamina propria and in metastases. Further, areas of mucosa without basement membrane can sometimes be seen in carcinoma in situ, especially in squamous mucosa. If this concept was credible, we would have been carrying out basement membranes stains long ago. However, the need for an equivalent in the GI tract to actin immunohistochemistry in the breast or high molecular weight cytokeratins in the prostate to indicate invasion would be useful. Unfortunately, there is no equivalent in the

GI tract (at least yet). Terms such as "confined to the basement membrane" to indicate that we are still dealing with dysplasia sound better in print than they do in practice. So under what criteria can the term intramucosal carcinoma be used, if one is not using a Japanese nomenclature where "carcinoma" is diagnosed on purely cytologic grounds, and therefore includes many things called dysplasia, both low and high, in the West?

There are two main features, both of which are thought to indicate lamina propria invasion by tumor cells. Both depend on the fact that neoplastic glands are present between what are thought to be preexisting glands, and therefore within the lamina propria.

1. Single tumor cells or small groups of them can sometimes be seen in the lamina propria apparently between glands—this is the best indication for a diagnosis of intramucosal carcinoma.
2. A mucosa with very tightly packed glands, often of smaller caliber than those usually seen. The implication here is that the normal lamina propria is no longer present and therefore must have been invaded (see Figs. 1-28, 19-29, and 10-32).

Using the latter definition, there are no criteria for where the line between HGD and intramucosal carcinoma is drawn, and is a diagnosis about which there is varying inter agreement,[98] so is not reproducible. This does not mean that many do not use it as it seems to have a frequent association with underlying invasion.

Is this distinction worth making? In practice, anything that is HGD or worse needs serious consideration for some sort of therapeutic intervention. Increasingly, this is endoscopic resection that if demonstrably complete is sufficient treatment, but it also allows evaluation of the presence of invasion into the submucosa, at which point the risk of metastases increases so that serious consideration of risks and benefits of esophagectomy need to be considered. It must always be remembered that the ultimate outcome is to preserve the life of the patient for as long as possible.

Invasive Carcinoma (Submucosal invasion)

The presence of a desmoplastic stromal reaction is indicative of invasion. These signs of invasive growth are found in deep invading tumors but not in early carcinomas since these tumors can build their own basal membrane.[97] Invasion and penetration of muscularis mucosae is not necessary for the diagnosis of Barrett's carcinoma since mucosal carcinoma has well been recognized in BE.

A desmoplastic stromal reaction is not usually present until submucosal invasion is present. If desmoplasia is not present, the diagnosis of invasion of the submucosa needs to be made carefully, with full awareness that there may be a double layer of muscularis mucosae (see Histology of BE section above). In an endoscopic resection an awareness that this double muscularis is usually present is required so that submucosal invasion is not diagnosed when the tumor is still intramucosal, but through the neo-muscularis mucosae. Usually the most difficult issue is that during the repair process nondysplastic glands can be found within the neomuscularis mucosae. When dysplasia is present in these glands it is easy to overcall them as overt invasive carcinoma. Conversely it is also impossible to exclude this so a comment that "underlying invasion cannot be excluded" is often made. As the dysplasia in the biopsies is necessarily deep in the biopsy this can be justified.

Interobserver Variability and Need for a Second Opinion for Dysplasia

Due to the inter- and (intra)observer variability, it is recommended that dysplasia be confirmed by "an experienced GI pathologist" (someone who (a) sees a lot of Barrett's biopsies or (b) is known to have a reliable opinion regarding the diagnosis of dysplasia, and ideally both). This was formerly more important as HGD was an indication for esophagectomy, with its attendant morbidity and mortality. Increasingly, patients with dysplasia are treated by EMR or endoscopic submucosal dissection (carried out with precision in one piece), which has minimal morbidity and virtually no mortality. However, ESD is much more time-consuming that EMR so is not often carried out outside of Japan. It can be argued that the distinction of HGD from LGD matters less if EMR is carried out, provided the epithelium in question really is dysplastic.

Both ends of the spectrum (negative for dysplasia and HGD/intramucosal carcinoma) have much higher interobserver agreement than IFD and LGD, so the latter tend to be combined for diagnostic and management purposes.[99] While this implies that the latter cannot be distinguished, there are biopsies, especially in the intestinal pathway that are clearly LGD (Fig. 10-26), and others that are overtly IFD, but there are inevitably biopsies that remain problematic.

Biopsies IFD are probably those with greatest interobserver variation, as criteria for its diagnosis are effectively the result of getting a negative reply to the following two questions:

1. Is the biopsy unequivocally negative for dysplasia?
2. Is the biopsy unequivocally dysplastic?

LGD is probably the lesion most commonly misdiagnosed, usually because the implications of the inflammatory, regenerative, and restituting changes are not appreciated. In one study, in which all biopsies from six non-University hospitals diagnosed over a 6-year period were reviewed, only 15% were confirmed as LGD after "expert" review, the remainder being downgraded to either negative or IFD. For patients with a consensus diagnosis of LGD, the cumulative risk of progressing to HGD or carcinoma was 85.0% in 109 months compared with 4.6% in 107 months for patients that were downgraded. The incidence rate of HGD or Ca was 13.4% per patient per year for patients in whom the diagnosis of LGD was confirmed, but only 0.49% for patients downgraded.[100] Fortunately, the management of both IFD and LGD is usually to repeat the endoscopy, after further treatment if necessary, and take multiple biopsies to ensure as far as possible that unequivocal dysplasia, or worse, is not present. A second opinion is also recommended in cases where HGD/HGIEN and early carcinoma cannot be made readily, and in patients in whom the diagnosis will result in esophagectomy in centers/areas where endoscopic ablation techniques/EMR are not available.[101]

Ancillary Techniques

Additional methods (proliferation index, p53, racemase) can support but not exclude the diagnosis of neoplasia.[102] Some recommend a second opinion instead of generating costly immunohistochemical or molecular evaluations,[103] but second opinions are seldom free. While dysplasia may be intensely immunoreactive for p53 and proliferation markers, they are unreliable, insensitive, and lack specificity. In our hands, racemase (AMACR) is also of little value for similar reasons. While we have found that it is often positive with unequivocal dysplasia, especially intestinal (non-foveolar), usually these do not need ancillary techniques to help with the diagnosis, and we have occasionally seen immunoreactivity in overtly normal epithelium albeit in high-risk patients, where its utility has not (yet) been evaluated. The diagnosis of dysplasia, as well as its grade, therefore relies solely on H&E, and while it is comforting to see strong immunoreactivity for these markers, it does not change the diagnosis. Similarly, p53 may show clear intense foci of clonal proliferation, invariably in mucosa that is dysplastic. In mucosa IFD it may show strong basal immunoreactivity with surface maturation. The significance is also unclear but may well portend an increased risk of subsequent dysplasia/IEN. Mib-1 often reflects p53 immunoreactivity when the latter is enhanced. While the finding of aneuploidy is likely the best indicator of dysplasia or an increased risk of carcinoma, it is rarely practical to do it, and again does not change the morphological diagnosis.

Surveillance biopsies. To enhance endoscopic sensitivity four-quadrant biopsies each 1 or 2 cm are recommended. In practice, this protocol is often not followed because of the resulting bleeding and the "blind" nature of the following biopsies. However, any sort of endoscopically visible abnormality, nodule, plaque should be biopsied—(i.e., targeted biopsies), which are aided by high-magnification endoscopes with and without chromoendoscopy, and especially by narrow-band imaging (NBI) where vascular anomalies acting as a marker for neoplastic lesions may be better detected. These can reduce the number but enhance the sensitivity of individual biopsies.

Neoplasia within Barrett's epithelium can be multifocal. This may go part of the way to explain the high rate (25%+) of metachronous carcinomas after prior endoscopic resection of neoplasia.[87] Therefore the remaining Barrett's mucosa should always be ablated, coagulated, or otherwise removed. Ablation by argon plasma ablation can lead to almost 90% complete ablation after 5 years,[104] while the figures may be even higher for radio-frequency ablation. Radio-frequency ablation has become the standard approach, including over photodynamic therapy, mostly because of increased efficacy but also reduced side effects.

Atypical localization, shape, or morphology should raise the suspicion of possible esophageal adenocarcinomas. If there is doubt between neoplasia and regenerative changes, high-dose PPI therapy should be recommended to exclude regenerative changes before performing the control biopsy, but does assume the same site can be identified and biopsied.

NONREFLUX ESOPHAGITIS

These include infections, inflammatory, especially from other diseases that can affect any part of the GI tract, and medications ("pill esophagitis").

INFECTIONS

Candida infection (Monilia) is the most common infection of the esophagus. Herpes esophagitis is possibly the most common viral infection, with CMV the next most common.[105]

Viral Infections

Herpes virus infection. HSV Type I is said to be the most frequent cause of viral infection of the esophagus,[106,107] although we suspect that this "prize" likely belongs to HPV infection (see below), as it is largely asymptomatic and undetectable unless specifically looked for. Esophageal HSV is also associated with

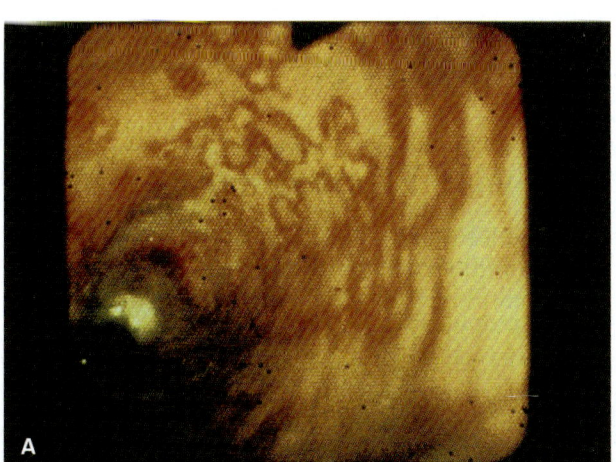
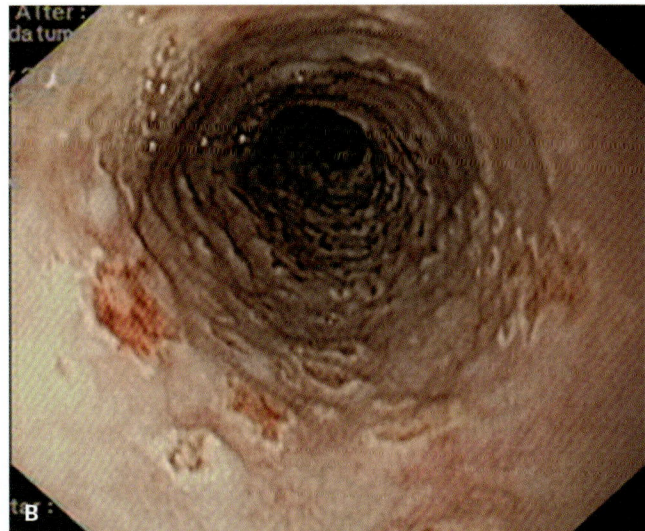

Figure 10-33. Herpes esophagitis. A,B: Endoscopic view of herpes esophagitis with numerous small sharply demarcated erosions and whitish slough at the edges of the lesions.

most infections of visceral organs. Autopsy series, which are inevitably biased, show an incidence of HSV between 1.4% and 6%, often in combination with malignant lymphomas, leukemias, or other causes of immunosuppression. Complications include dysphagia/odynophagia, and sometimes bleedings, perforation, and fistula. Common risk factors for all viral infections[108] are an impaired immune system, malignant diseases, immunosuppression of all kinds, and radio- or chemotherapy. In patients on combinations of steroids and cyclosporin A after organ transplantation, viral infection should always be considered when esophageal lesions are found. Also, other severe diseases like toxoplasmosis, tuberculosis, aspergillosis, and moniliasis are risk factors. HSV infections can also be found in immunocompetent individuals. Injuries and mucosal "damage" may also predispose to infections.

The typical endoscopic appearance includes multiple 2- to 3-mm sized mucosal breaks with elevated margins that tend to become confluent (Fig. 10-33A–B). Typical blisters, similar to those seen in the skin, are not seen, since the keratin layer is missing in esophageal squamous epithelium.

Histologically, the superficial part or whole epithelial layer is infiltrated with lymphocytes and plasma cells. Viral inclusions in epithelial cells are found within the areas of necrosis and can affect nuclei eccentrically or replace the entire nucleus (Fig. 10-34). This is the reason why biopsies should not be shaken when putting them in formalin. These fragile, largely necrotic, specimens can fall apart, making diagnosis very difficult or impossible. In H&E stains, the eosinophilic inclusion bodies tend to appear larger than the nucleoli (Cowdry Type A). Sometimes multinucleated giant cells with loose chromatin and ground-glass nuclei can be found (Fig. 10-34). Immunohistochemical detection readily confirms the diagnosis. Rarely, submucosal esophageal glands and their ducts are affected. Cytologically, the diagnosis becomes easy when multinucleated giant cells with loose chromatin in a "dirty" background are found. This finding is identical with vaginal/cervical herpes infections.

Varicella zoster infection is a rare finding that can be diagnosed by specific immunohistochemical antibodies. In varicella zoster infection, it is believed that inclusion bodies are found within the epithelium and in the stromal tissue of the lamina propria. Patients may have clinical evidence of this infection elsewhere but are usually immunosuppressed.[109] Rare

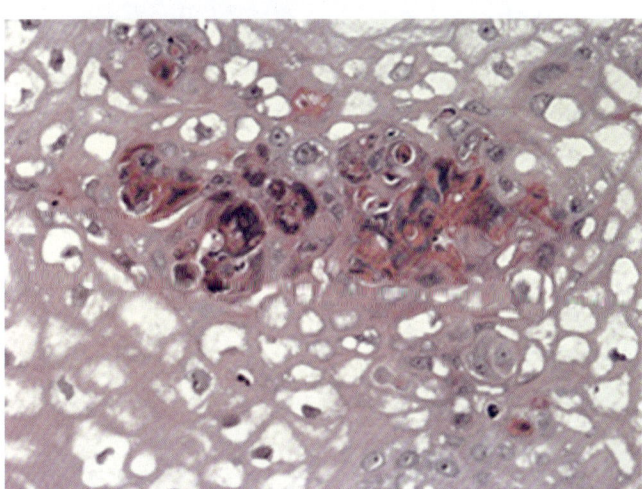

Figure 10-34. Intraepithelial varicella esophagitis indicated by the presence of bizarre large virus inclusion bodies within the squamous epithelium with only a little surrounding inflammatory reaction.

examples of congenital varicella affecting the esophagus are described.[110]

Cytomegalovirus esophagitis. Most frequently, esophageal CMV infection is found in patients with leukemia, and is much less common than large bowel disease.[111] Infants can also be affected.[112] In immunosuppressed patients with pulmonary CMV infection, the esophagus is very often affected as well. In CMV infection, the esophageal mucosa is reddened and shows mucosal breaks. These mucosal breaks can sometimes become confluent to very large lesions. In immunosuppressed patients, there may be diffuse esophageal necrosis ("black esophagus").[113] Cases with nodular and polypoid lesions are also described. Viral inclusion bodies are found exclusively within stromal fibroblasts and endothelial cells (Fig. 10-35) but not in squamous epithelial cells. Biopsies from the base of an ulcer show inclusion bodies with the typical halo within fibroblasts, endothelial cells, and capillary-rich granulation tissue. Immunohistochemistry helps confirm the diagnosis. CMV infections are increasing in prevalence due to increased use of immunosuppressive therapy. Spontaneous healing of ulcerations and disappearance of viral inclusion bodies have been described.

Human papillomavirus. Human papillomavirus (HPV) infection may well be the most frequent esophageal viral infection on a worldwide basis. Infections with HPV[114] can be found in normal squamous epithelium, esophageal papillomas, and papillomatosis, and in squamous cell carcinoma (Fig. 10-36). HPV is believed to play a role in the development of esophageal squamous cell carcinoma. Especially HPV types 16 and 18 can be detected with in situ hybridization in almost 25% of carcinomas. It is possible to detect HPV-DNA in 15% of normal squamous epithelium. These results have mainly been reported from the United States. Rare instances of ulcers apparently caused by HPV have been reported.[115]

Acute HIV infection. Patients with HIV infection can have odynophagia and dysphagia. In general, these symptoms are caused by secondary opportunistic infections. It is unclear whether HIV-1 can

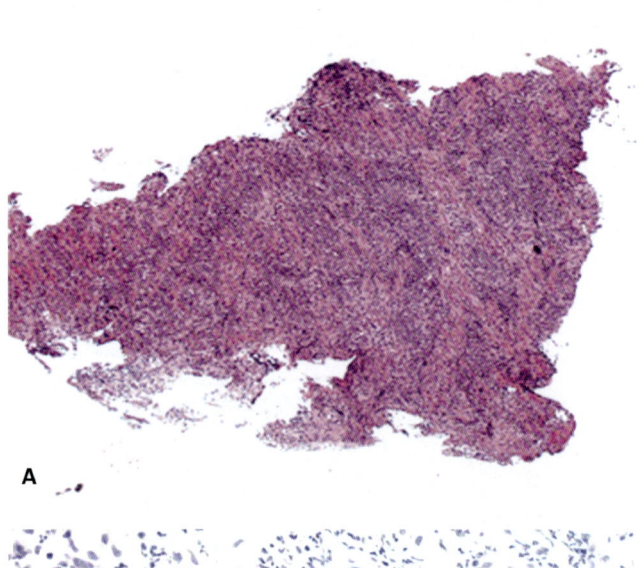

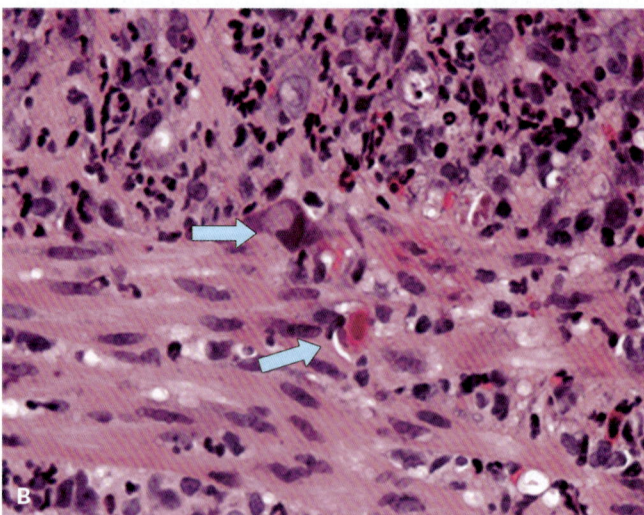

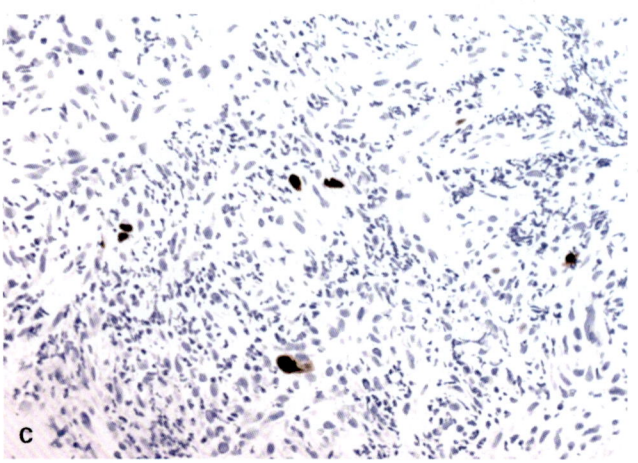

Figure 10-35. CMV esophagitis. Inclusions are found in ulcer bases and may be in either muscle or endothelial cells. **A:** Ulcer base extending into the muscle. **B:** Smooth muscle with a necrotic cell (*lower arrow*) and inclusion (*upper arrow*). **C:** The diagnosis is readily confirmed immunohistochemically in which inclusions are readily demonstrated.

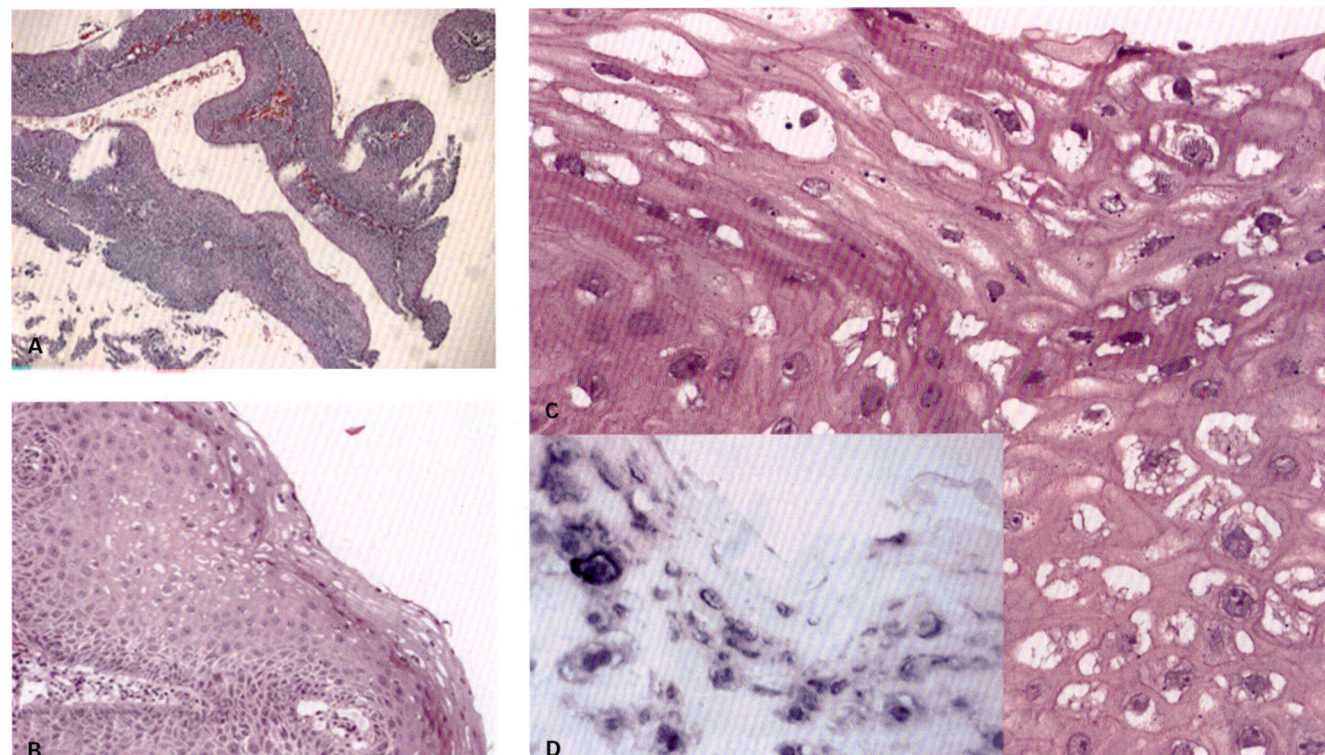

Figure 10-36. HPV-associated esophageal papillomatosis **(A)** with **(B)** the superficial pale zone that is often the mark of HPV infection. **C:** Koilocytes with wrinkled nuclei, occasionally binucleate with surrounding retraction artifact so that the cells appear to be in vacuoles. **D:** Detection of HPV 6 by in situ hybridization (positive signal is *black*).

cause small erosions itself,[116] but endoscopically these small erosions are believed to have an appearance like herpes infections. Histologically, necrosis with abundant neutrophils as seen in any other erosion can be seen. Giant cells or viral inclusion bodies have not yet been described. Electron microscopically, intracellular viral inclusion could be detected within the lesions (lymphocytes/Langerhans cells).[117] Confluent ulcerations and fibroid inflammatory polyps have been described in HIV-positive individuals.[118,119]

Other viral infections. Rarely, esophageal lesions are caused by rubella,[120] variola (smallpox), Epstein–Barr,[121] and Papovavirus infections. Despite animal experiments, these seem to be of no clinical significance.

Fungal Infections

After reflux disease, and almost certainly "pill" esophagitis, esophageal fungal infections are the next most common cause for esophagitis, primarily *Candida*.

Candida albicans is a saprophyte of human skin and mucosa, and in about 50% of healthy individuals *Candida* is present in the oral cavity and in 30% in the GI tract. Risk factors for *Candida* primarily include immunosuppression, whether congenital, iatrogenic, or acquired.[122] A gender predisposition has not been detected. In autopsy series, in patients dying of carcinoma, fungal infections can be found in about 5%, which increases to 15% in patients with leukemia. It is believed that colonization is pathologic in the first 12 months of life and in the elderly.[123] Food bolus predispose to fungal infections in a variety of conditions including achalasia, stenosing tumors, diverticula, fistulas, stenosis, stricture, and so on, and postoperatively.

Diabetes mellitus is a predisposing disease, as are a variety of diseases associated with increased risk of infection. These include malignant neoplasms in general, hematologic diseases, immunodeficiency syndromes whether congenital or acquired including HIV, systemic lupus erythematosus, cachexia/malnutrition, and alcoholism. Spontaneous infection does occur in otherwise healthy individuals but, like HPV infection elsewhere, is at lest initially, asymptomatic.

Endoscopically, typical slightly elevated whitish membranes with hyperemic margins can be seen (Fig. 10-37A). If the membranes are removed, bleeding occurs easily. Partially nodular elevations can be

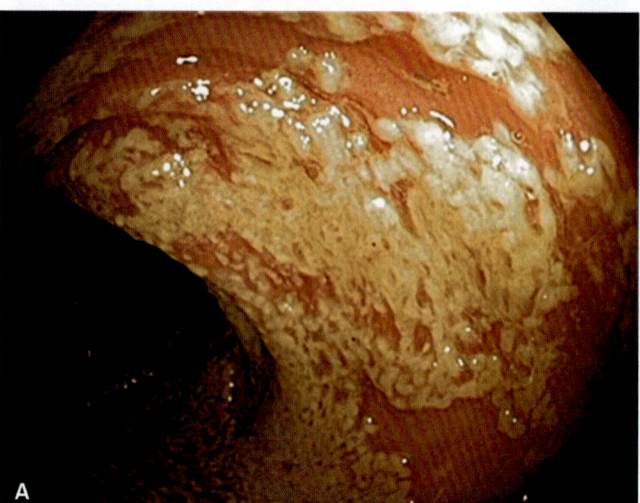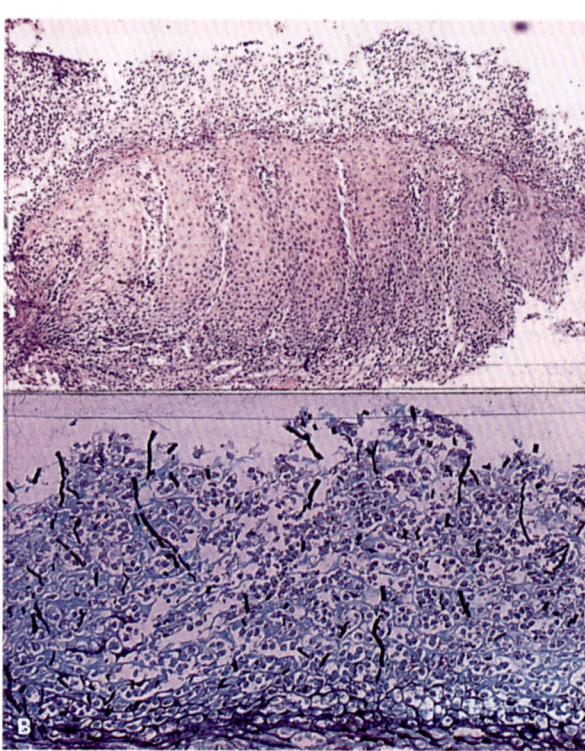

Figure 10-37. Esophageal moniliasis. **A:** Endoscopic view of esophageal moniliasis with yellow plaques and slough. (Courtesy of Steffen Muehldorfer, MD.) **B: Top panel:** Overview of esophageal biopsy with an overlying plaque. **Bottom panel:** Gomori methenamine silver stain with budding spores. Numerous other coccoid bacteria are also present.

observed. These lesions can be confluent and affect the whole esophagus. Histologically, the diagnosis can usually be made in H&E sections (Fig. 10-37B). Infiltration of neutrophils within the superficial layers of the squamous epithelium is indicative of fungal infections.[124] In reflux disease, there is more diffuse epithelial infiltration by neutrophils close to mucosal breaks but this is not reliable. Neutrophilic infiltrates are so typical that the diagnosis of moniliasis can be strongly suspected on the basis of this observation. Grocott or PAS stain enhance the structures of hyphae, and should be considered whenever neutrophils are seen as they can be quite subtle (Fig. 10-37).

In *Mucor* infection (Fig. 10-38), invariably occurring following chemotherapy, and while invariably identifiable on an H&E stain, Grocott or Warthin–Starry silver stain should be used for confirmation since these angioinvasive fungi are negative for the PAS reaction. The adjacent epithelium can show regenerative acanthosis and pseudoepitheliomatous hyperplasia that must not be misinterpreted as neoplasia. Lesions may be localized to the middle or proximal esophagus, compared to reflux, which is almost exclusively distal. Cytologically, in fungal infections a strong inflammatory background with regenerating epithelium can be found. In a Papanicolaou stain, the mycelia appears brown. If there are fungal structures (often in combination with coccoid bacteria), they are invariably in acanthotic squamous epithelium.

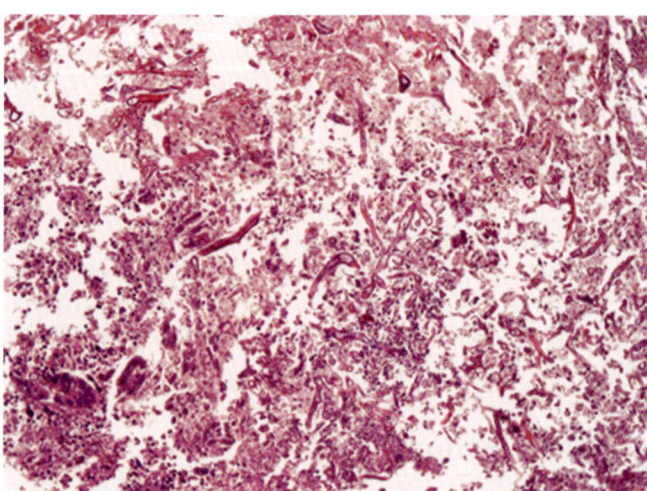

Figure 10-38. *Mucor* infection of esophagus and stomach during chemotherapy course in a patient with colorectal carcinoma. The patient succumbed shortly after initial diagnosis from respiratory insufficiency due to *Mucor* infection of the lung and concomitant *Mucor* sepsis. Note the large hyphae with a folded irregular shape within the necrosis.

Clinic symptoms and prognosis. The clinical symptoms in fungal infections are dominated by dysphagia and much less so odynophagia. Retrosternal sensations, heartburn, foreign body sensation, vomiting, regurgitation, epigastric pain, and cachexia can be observed, but do not need to correlate with the severity of the findings. Complications include bleeding, stenosis, fistula, aspiration pneumonia, and perforation. In immunodeficient individuals, the fungal infection can involve the entire GI tract.

Other fungal infections. Especially in eastern United States, histoplasmosis is an important differential diagnosis and derives from an infection of mediastinal lymph node with compression and infiltration of the esophagus.[125,126] Histoplasma capsulatum can be visualized by silver stains. Cultures are possible.

Besides *C. albicans*, other *Candida* (krusei, tropicalis, *Torulopsis glabrata*)[127] or *Aspergillus* species[128] have been described. Rarely, infections are caused by Phycomycetes,[129] *Sporotrichum* species, Paracoccidioides, and *Mucor*.[130,131]

Bacterial Esophagitis

Bacterial infections of the esophagus are rare. The most frequent bacterial infection is tuberculosis,[132] but it is rare and only about 200 cases are described.[133] The exact pathogenesis of esophageal infections is still somewhat unclear and most probably occurs due to secondary involvement. Direct involvement from mediastinal lymph nodes seems likely, but direct infection of ingested organisms or ingestion of infected material in open lung tuberculosis, as discussed, has been suggested. Hematogenous spread, descending pharyngitis, tuberculosis, or retrograde lymphatic spread in the case of paratracheal and peribronchial lymph nodes are rare.[134–137]

Due to the increased mobility of the population, the number of infections because of tuberculosis is increasing again and cases with severe infections can also be seen again.

Morphologically, in advanced stages, three types of esophageal involvement can be distinguished:

1. A hypertrophic or stenosing form with luminal obstruction and tumorous aspect
2. Ulcerative form with solitary or multiple ulcerations
3. Granular tuberculosis with numerous mucosal granulomas

Histologically, the typical central necroses need not be present; in many cases only epithelioid giant cells are found. Specific PCR with detection of bacterial DNA can be helpful.

Late complications include traction diverticula (due to scarring and traction due to involved mediastinal and paratracheal lymph nodes, perforations, esophageal strictures, recurrence paresis, fistulas between esophagus and bronchial system/pleura, pericardium and erosion of an aortic aneurysm). In secondary stages, meningeal involvement is life threatening. In HIV-infected patients, esophageal infections through atypical mycobacteria have been described.

Luetic infection. Syphilitic involvement of the esophagus is extremely rare. The number of published case reports is < 100[138] with very few recent descriptions, possibly because it is not considered, but it is likely genuinely rare. It causes granulomata and ulcerations, so odynophagia and dysphagia tend to occur, especially for food rich in fiber. Strictures can occur.[139] Histologically, numerous plasma cells and perivascular lymphocytic infiltrations can be seen. Periarteritis and endarteritis can also be seen depending on the nature of the specimen. Rarely, esophago-tracheal fistulas are diagnosed. Late complications include esophageal stenosis due to scarring. Warthin–Starry stain–specific immunohistochemistry or PCR can be used to detect the presence of organisms.

Other bacteria. Only very rarely are opportunistic infections of Corynebacteria, Actinomycetes,[140] and Lactobacillus acidophilus[141] found. In immunodeficient patients, bacteremia can lead to systemic infection. Chagas infection can lead to achalasia.[142,143] In an HIV-infected patient, an infection by Leishmania was observed.[144,145] In exfoliative (sloughing) esophagitis, bacterial superinfections are the underlying cause for infiltrations by neutrophils that cannot be seen in ordinary exfoliative esophagitis.

DESCRIPTIVE ESOPHAGITIDES

These are a series of descriptive diagnoses, terms that represent a reaction, usually to a variety of underlying insults. It is important to recognize that some have relatively few causes and others many, and that therapy is directed at the underlying cause, which must therefore be sought.

Lymphocytic Esophagitis

Lymphocytic esophagitis is an ill-defined entity[146] with an excess of IELs, (formerly called "squiggle cells" due to their ability to squeeze through intraepithelial spaces so that their nuclei became "squiggly")

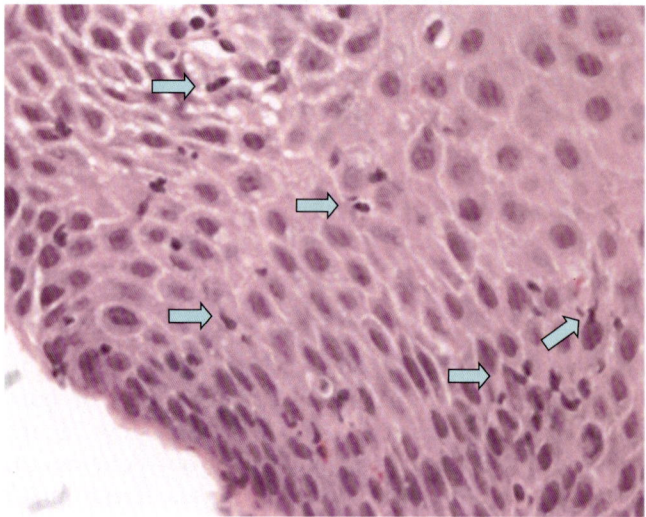

Figure 10-39. Intraepithelial mononuclear (squiggle) cells (*arrows*).

(Fig. 10-39). It appears to have numerous causes. The major problems are as follows:

1. The lack of a definition of where normal starts and pathology starts so unless there are numerous cells present (Fig. 10-40), it is difficult (or impossible) to make the diagnosis.
2. The term is a misnomer, as the exact nature of the cells present is still an issue, there being several different cell types of IEMs including lymphocytes that are invariably T-suppressor cells (CD3+, CD4−, CD8+), antigen-presenting cells (S100+), and mast cells (CD117 or mast cell tryptase+). It is therefore really an increase in IEMs or a mononuclear lymphocytosis (although we suspect that "mononuclear esophagitis" is not going to catch on).

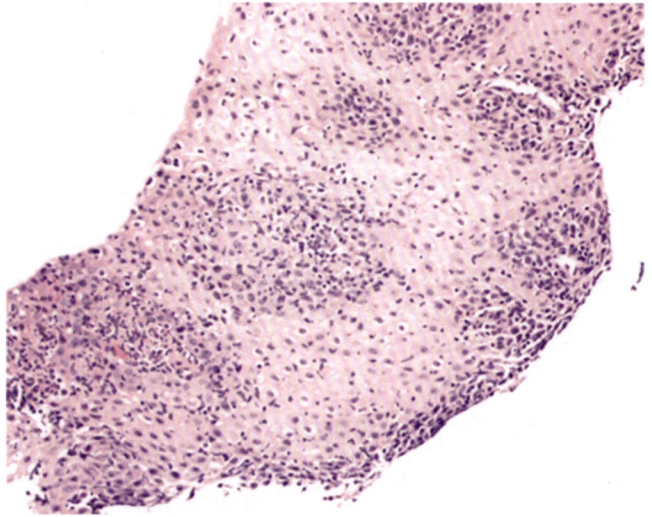

Figure 10-40. "Lymphocytic" esophagitis with myriad mononuclear cells primarily around the papillae.

The most common cause is likely reflux disease, and is limited to the lower esophagus. Relation to an esophageal contact dermatitis-like reaction has been postulated,[147] although anecdotally we know that infiltrate of lymphocytes can be seen in cases with motility disorders (prolonged contact of food), Crohn's disease,[148] and other esophageal diseases. No gender or age prevalence has been identified so far. Typically, peripapillary and parabasal intraepithelial infiltrates of CD3+ lymphocytes are seen. A diffuse dilation of intercellular spaces is observed in almost all cases. The number of lymphocytes range from a very few up to more than 100 per HPF. The normal mid and upper esophagus rarely shows more than an occasional lymphocyte per HPF. Thus, all intraepithelial infiltrates by lymphocytes in the upper and likely mid esophagus can be regarded as "lymphocytic esophagitis." An effort to identify the underlying disease should always be made, and specific therapy is directed at the underlying disease, if treatment is required at all.

Exfoliative (Sloughing) Esophagitis (Esophagitis Dissecans Superficialis)

Exfoliative esophagitis was first described in 1890[149] by Reichmann, but is frequently unrecognized or misinterpreted.[150] In this condition the superficial esophageal mucosa separates from the underlying squamous mucosa. The desquamated epithelium can be expectorated. Patients often complain of severe pain, are often elderly, have other debilitating illnesses, and are taking multiple medications.[151] Malignant transformation has not been described, and the esophagus seems to heal without complications.

The desquamated epithelium has a surprisingly normal appearance, so the diagnosis is easily missed unless the split is seen, or recognized if it has become separated. It depends on identifying[152]:

1. The split in the superficial part of the epithelium; this can usually only be appreciated if the junction where the separation is occurring is included (Fig. 10-41).
2. The split can be bullous in the midpart of the epithelium and even form multiple adjacent bullous spaces.
3. There is often a tinctorial change in the H&E section with an eosinophilic band where the separation occurs.
4. The separated epithelium does not have papillae, so can look like a superficial fragment of stripped epithelium. (Conversely, whenever a superficial strip of esophageal mucosa is seen, the possibility of this condition needs to be considered.)
5. Typically, basal fibrinoid membranes can be seen close to the desquamated basal cell layer.
6. Neutrophils can be seen in biopsies with bacterial or fungal superinfections.

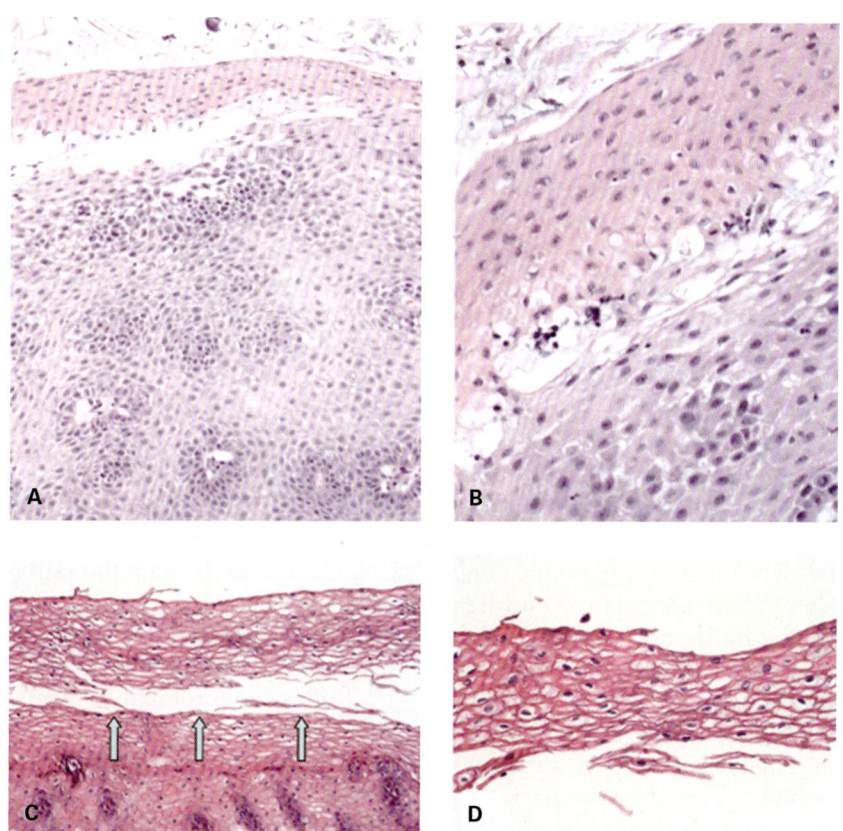

Figure 10-41. Exfoliative/sloughing esophagitis. **A:** Early lesion showing partial detachment of the superficial and basal halves of the epithelium that is typical of this condition. **B:** Junction of the separation zone showing apoptotic cells and edema. A few apoptotic bodies can also be seen in the epithelium that is more luminal. **C:** Edge of esophageal segment with a reactive desquamation of superficial half of the epithelial layer with clear intraepithelial gap (*arrows*). If this is not identified, the diagnosis will not be made. **D:** Occasionally only the slough is present in biopsies, and may be interpreted as a very superficial biopsy. However, under these circumstances, it is always worth finding out whether the endoscopic appearances were normal or not. Rarely, fibrinoid necrosis can be seen at the basal part of the desquamated necrobiotic squamous epithelium.

Medications are always suspect, and patients with this disease were found to be taking multiple medications and have more debilitating illnesses than the control population.

Acute Necrotizing Esophagitis (Black Esophagus)

In the English literature, this disease has been described as "black esophagus" and is caused by prior severe ischemia, which is very difficult to document unless there is an overt cause or previous antibiotic treatment. Histologically, necrosis with numerous neutrophils can be seen. Epithelium most often is not detected. Endoscopically, the involved esophageal segments appear black and this led to the name "black esophagus."[153-155] Given the potential for numerous medications to cause severe esophageal damage, it is perhaps surprising that this has not been indicted. In immunosuppressed patients there may be diffuse esophageal necrosis ("black esophagus").[113]

Eosinophilic Esophagitis

EoE is a disease characterized by an excess of eosinophils that are usually present throughout the entire esophagus that is being recognized with increasing frequency, and appears to be the most common cause of dysphagia and bolus obstruction. It predominates in younger males; individuals often have other atopic or allergic features and appear to respond well to swallowed oral fluticasone spray. Interestingly, it may well be part of Kaijser's eosinophilic gastroenteritis, first reported in 1937.[156] Often this disease is limited to the esophagus.

More than 60% of the affected individuals have a positive clinical or familiar history for allergic/atopic diseases. The prevalence of EoE has been shown to be 0.1% in a Northern Swedish normal population.[157] From this population-based study, it is apparent that there are individuals with an eosinophilic esophageal infiltrate but no (or unrecognized) clinical symptoms, although there can be a long lead time before the diagnosis is made.

Pathogenesis. The etiology and long-term clinical prognosis of these cases are unclear, but presumably is a response to something swallowed in food, or refluxed, or inhaled antigens that are then swallowed. Normally there are no, or only rare, eosinophils within the esophageal squamous epithelium and the blood supply is limited to capillaries within the epithelial papillae. Several studies suggest an allergic-type pathway.[158] Specifically, there has been evidence of increased T-cells, mast cells, IL-5, and tumor necrosis factor-α, which may stimulate eotaxin, all of which can be central to an allergic (Th-2 helper–induced) reaction, and were detected in biopsy studies in EoE. Furthermore, T-cell subsets were characterized as CD3, CD8, and CD1a antigen-presenting cells, also fitting in with an allergic type of reaction. It seems that esophageal eosinophils depend on greater levels of activating cytokines such as CD25, IL-3, IL-4, IL-5, and IL-13 in comparison with healthy individuals and other sites of the GI tract. Cytokines seem to be elevated even preceding eosinophilic infiltration of the esophagus.[159,160] These findings favor a systemic predisposition for EoE. It is not clear at the moment why the esophagus is often the sole site to be involved in eosinophilic infiltration within gut epithelial tissue.[161] A particular subpopulation of eosinophils (bone marrow derived?) that homes the esophagus more selectively is discussed. Recent theories discuss early antigen priming as a prerequisite for later EoE. Anti-interleukin treatment such as with anti-interleukin-5[162] seems to have a similar therapeutic effect compared to treatment based on topical steroids such as fluticasone, which are sprayed into the mouth and then swallowed rather than inhaled.[163,164]

Symptoms. Patients classically have dysphagia, odynophagia, and bolus obstructions, especially with food rich in fibers.[165,166] EoE and Schatzki rings are likely the most common causes of dysphagia, and this symptom, or that of food impaction, should immediately lead to the suspicion of EoE, and biopsies should be taken from at least the lower and mid esophagus to confirm the diagnosis.

Clinical. There is a male predominance and younger patients predominate. A family history is also common if asked, and there are often seasonal peaks (spring). Endoscopically, the esophagus can appear almost normal to having a multiringed esophagus (aka trachealization because of its resemblance to trachea) or feline esophagus (Fig. 10-42A, as cats' esophagi appear similar, often with longitudinal furrows, with whitish elevations that represent eosinophilic abscesses). The mucosa is fragile and often has erosions. It is common for endoscopists to notice "tearing" of the mucosa as the scope is passed through the esophagus. There is considerable fibrosis of the submucosa, and perforation can occur if strictures are dilated. Stenoses may be present and they may be associated with food impaction.

Endosonographically, the esophageal wall is thickened due to edema, and lamina propria and submucosal fibrosis, although infiltration of deeper layers by eosinophilic granulocytes is also likely. In extreme cases, the esophageal wall can be 2 cm thick, pointing to an involvement of submucosa and muscularis propria.[167] Esophageal eosinophils can be detected in patients with asthmatic disease as well; the number is related to the sufficiency of asthmatic therapy.[168]

Biopsy sites. Changes are marked immediately above the Z-line, but, unlike reflux disease, frequently involve the whole esophagus. Sometimes this is at the same level of eosinophilic infiltration, and sometimes

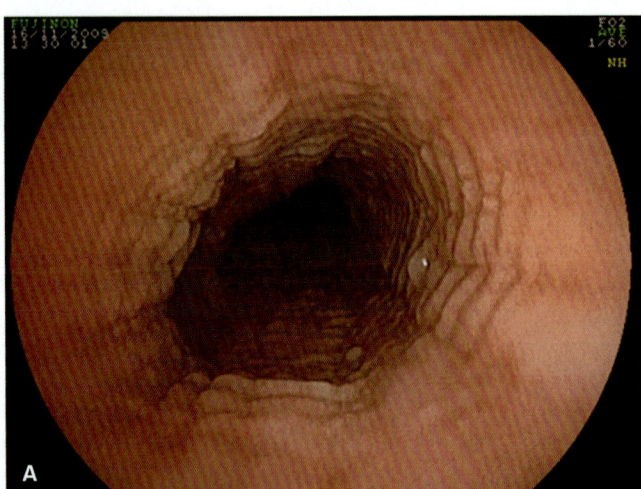
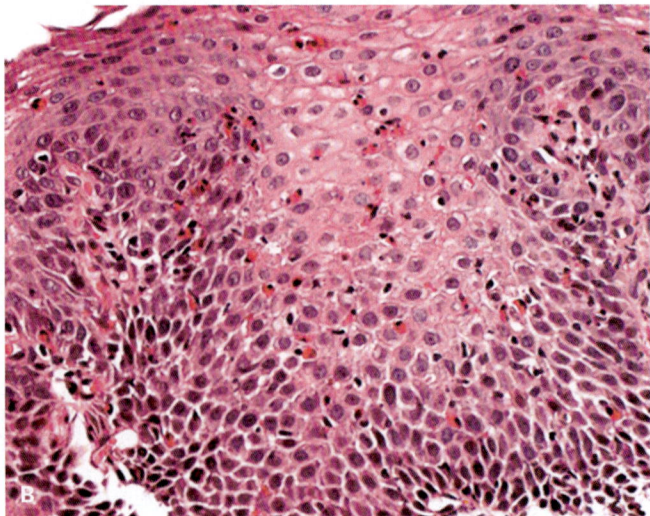

Figure 10-42. Eosinophilic esophagitis. **A:** Endoscopic view of EoE with typically multiringed esophagus with furrows and with whitish elevations that are the counterpart of eosinophilic abscesses, so should be targeted for biopsy. (Courtesy of Hartmut Bordel, MD.) **B:** Biopsy specimen of a patient with EoE with numerous intraepithelial eosinophils, marked dilation of intercellular spaces, and marked regeneration (increased length of papillae, increased thickness of basal cell layer). These changes were present in biopsies from both lower and mid esophagus.

it drops off proximally. In some patients, it only affects the lower esophagus, but it is unclear if this is a genuine change or reflects sampling. Even more interesting is that some patients with "classical" symptoms have absolutely normal biopsies, and (anecdotally) some appear to have a modest lymphocytic esophagitis. Biopsies (preferably two from each location) should be taken from at least (a) the region of the Z-line and (b) a proximal site—ideally around 5 to 10 cm proximally to determine proximal involvement. Most pathologists would probably like two from the Z-line, and two each from the mid (5 to 10 cm) and also upper esophagus. Biopsies from whitish elevations are most likely to show eosinophilic abscesses. Biopsies of other structural abnormalities present ensure that if a mosaic of different densities of eosinophils is present, these are sampled.[169] Each needs to be in separate containers so that the sites of origin are clear.

Pathology. Biopsies show marked reactive changes with elongation of dermal papillae and thickened basal cell layer and very DISs.[170] Typically, numerous eosinophils are found that are often grouped together to form intraepithelial eosinophilic microabscesses (Fig. 10-42B). The mean number of intraepithelial eosinophils varies by author and *there is no good number that absolutely establishes the diagnosis*. The usual figures quoted are >20 (or 25) per ×40 HPF, or 2 × 40 HPF with 15 or more eosinophils.[171] An eosinophilic infiltrate should be present at all sites in EoE but only in the distal esophageal biopsies in GERD (Fig. 10-43).

Differential diagnosis. Both GERD and EoE are distinct entities, but there are occasions when the criteria can overlap, and almost certainly some patients either have both or EoE is potentiated by coexistent GERD. It is perhaps not surprising that if the allergen for EoE is in food, that reflux will exacerbate any allergic reactions to food, and that any reaction will predominate in the lower esophagus. Conversely, if it is primarily a systemic disease then this will have less impact.

It can be difficult to distinguish eosinophils as a sequel of reflux disease from EoE in biopsies limited to the distal esophagus, especially when few eosinophils are present, and under these circumstances it increasingly becomes a clinicopathologic diagnosis requiring the appropriate clinical scenario and biopsy appearances for a confident diagnosis. Patients with EoE may get some benefit from PPIs, although there are exceptions, but most get almost immediate relief from swallowed topical steroids such as fluticasone. In a subgroup of patients, PPIs can resolve clinical symptoms and lead to a lesser extent to histologic improvement concerning the number of eosinophils.[172–174]

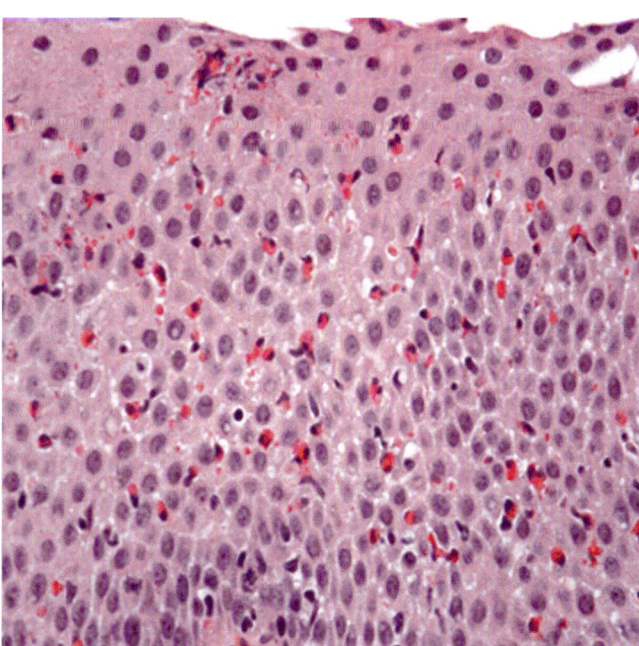

Figure 10-43. Morphologic comparison between EoE and GERD. This biopsy is from patient with GERD but numerous eosinophils in the biopsies from the lower esophagus only. The overlap with the biopsy from a patient with EoE shown in Fig. 10-42B is apparent.

Therapeutic approaches include PPIs swallowed topical steroids,[163] and less commonly systemic steroids as well as mast cell stabilizers.[175] It can sometimes be helpful to search for food allergies.[176] Eosinophils are rare in the normal esophageal epithelium, considered to always be abnormal in children, and are less frequently seen in reflux disease than previously anticipated.

There can also be issues because some patients that clinically have typical symptoms of EoE have no eosinophils in their biopsies, or have them only at one site. It is unclear if the eosinophilia is present but missed because of sampling problems, or whether these patients have completely separate, even new, disorders.

Corrosive Esophagitis

Ingestion of corrosive substances such as acids and alkalis can induce extensive necrosis in the upper GI tract. Corrosion with alkaline substances is more pronounced in the esophagus than in the stomach since alkaline chemicals are neutralized in the gastric acid environment. Household cleaners containing lye are particularly likely to be ingested by children in view of their widespread use and ready availability, often being stored within the reach of children. Most corrosive ingestion is accidental although a proportion is clearly premeditated.

Corrosive esophagitis can be confused with drug-induced esophagitis, although they potentially have features in common. However, maintaining the difference makes sense and the term "corrosive esophagitis" should be reserved to cases of alkaline, acid, or even ingestions of liquid glue or other corrosive chemicals,[177] whereas terms like "drug-induced esophagitis or pill esophagitis" should be reserved to cases connected to medications.

Corrosive esophagitis can be classified into three grades[178,179]:

Grade I: hyperaemia and desquamation of the apical mucosal layer
Grade II: injury of the full thickness of the esophageal wall
Grade III: involvement of other organs adjacent to the esophagus

As a consequence, stenoses develop in most of Grade II and regularly in all of Grade III cases.

Corrosive esophagitis can also be subdivided chronologically according to the course the damage took into the following stages:[149]

A. Acute necrotizing stage
B. Ulcerative and granulation stage
C. Scarring stenotic stage

In some ways, these are equivalent for I and A, and II and B, while III presumably preceded C.

Complications of corrosive injury also include squamous cell carcinoma, which is believed to increase the risk 1,000- to 3,000-fold after ingestion in survivors, and develop more than a decade, and usually two decades, after ingestion. Such carcinomas are believed to develop more often just above the stenotic segment. This should lead to a careful endoscopic inspection above the stenosis during follow-up. Rarely, adenocarcinomas, adenosquamous, and spindle cell carcinomas are reported after corrosive esophagitis.[180] One possibility is that these neoplasms occur due to the food retention proximal to the stenosis, possibly akin to those seen in achalasia.

The type of damage depends on the causative agent and may imply different clinical decisions.

Drug-induced Esophagitis (Pill Esophagitis)

Drug-induced esophagitis continues to be a problem both clinically and histologically. It has been known for a long time that KCL tablets, NSAIDs, and ASA that are available over the counter likely represent the most common cause of esophageal injury. In addition, antibiotics (in particular doxycycline), iron tablets, and anticancer agents, kayexalate, among others, can cause erosions and ulcers in the esophagus, while bisphosphonates, used for osteopenia, also cause esophagogastroduodenal injury.[181-185] Indeed, most of the drugs that injure the stomach and duodenum can injure the esophagus, the possible exception being occasional reports of PPIs, which are described in the esophagus but not the stomach or duodenum where they are protective. Typically, there is a history of patients swallowing pills dry, without liquid. In most cases, the histologic picture with capillary-rich granulation tissue is completely nonspecific but the type of the necrosis is often homogenous eosinophilic compared to infections showing a granulocyte-rich type of necrosis (see gastritis chapter were a similar situation applies between NSAIDs and *Helicobacter* ulcers). Iron tablets produce a typical band of chemical in the ulcer bed (always a good place to look in any ulcer for evidence of medication), which stains positive with stains for ferric and ferrous iron.[186]

Characteristically, one would expect the adjacent squamous epithelium not to show changes suggestive of reflux disease with enhanced regeneration, but anecdotally GERD-associated ulcers seem sometimes to have the same lack of adjacent changes, possibly as it is also a chemical injury, albeit usually more chronic. So, unless the patient is also using medications surreptitiously, it seems not to be useful in separating the two. Endoscopically, there are usually focal erosions or ulcerations but cases with semi- and circumferential lesions can be observed. Sometimes pills or their remnants are visible in the ulcer base, where they are presumed to be the primary cause. However, sometimes they become stuck in diverticula. What they all have in common is that abrupt changes to the adjacent normal epithelium can be noted.

Risk factors include taking medication with an insufficient volume of fluid ("on the fly") or taking tablets shortly before going to bed. Patients should be advised to take medication in an upright position, and with adequate fluid. Strictures, whether physiologic (aortic arch, right main stem bronchus, right atrium) or pathologic, and motility disorders may also increase the probability of lesions. The mid esophagus (aortic arch) is a common site, which is far proximal to the usual GERD injury, which is in the distal esophagus. Most individuals get self-limited pain, but esophageal hemorrhage, stricture, and perforation may occur, and rarely the outcome may be fatal.

SYSTEMIC DISEASES INVOLVING THE ESOPHAGUS

Skin Diseases and Esophageal Inflammation

These are described in Chapter 8, but the following are also included here.

Glycogenic acanthosis. Esophageal glycogenic acanthosis is harmless but has been associated with Cowden's syndrome, part of the PTEN hamartoma family.[187–190] In autopsy series, glycogenic acanthosis is found in up to 23% of all autopsies. A male predominance has been described. A relationship with reflux disease has been questioned but not verified, although more than two-thirds of all affected individuals have GERD.[191] Alcohol and tobacco are not considered risk factors. Changes do affect the whole esophagus, with changes usually maximal in the distal esophagus. Endoscopically, multiple whitish elevations can be seen that measure a few millimeter in size with most located on the tips of the longitudinal folds.[192] Lugol's solution readily visualizes these lesions. Histologically, a focal acanthosis with an extended zone of cells with clear cytoplasm (Fig. 10-44) due to cells rich in glycogen (PAS-positive) can be observed.[193]

Skin Diseases and Esophageal Inflammation

Esophageal involvement in lichen planus[194,195] is well known though rarely biopsied (Fig. 10-45), and may also be affected by Darier's disease,[196] acanthosis nigricans,[197] and also in bullous diseases such as pemphigus vulgaris (Fig. 10-46) and pemphigoid. The histologic findings in oral, pharyngeal, and esophageal epithelium are comparable with the outer skin manifestations. Mucosal epithelium and epidermis can be affected together or isolated from each other. Clinically, hoarseness, bolus feelings, or even asymptomatic cases have been described. Biopsies might reveal acute fibrinoid necrosis. The basal layer often shows a bullous degeneration. The basal cell layer is infiltrated by diffuse accumulations of lymphocytes that extend to the submucosa.

In bullous diseases, the epithelial layer can be detached within the epithelium, above or below the basal cell layer. These patients suffer from marked dysphagia. In pemphigus vulgaris, the vulnerable, often bleeding, epithelium is detached and shows acantholysis with suprabasal bullae.[198,199] With immunofluorescence typical IgG deposits can be visualized along the basal membrane. The blisters contain aggregates of eosinophils. Esophageal stenoses and obstructions have been described but the exact etiology in pemphigoid disease is not clear yet.

About 25% of patients with bullous pemphigoid show mucosal involvement, especially stomatitis with

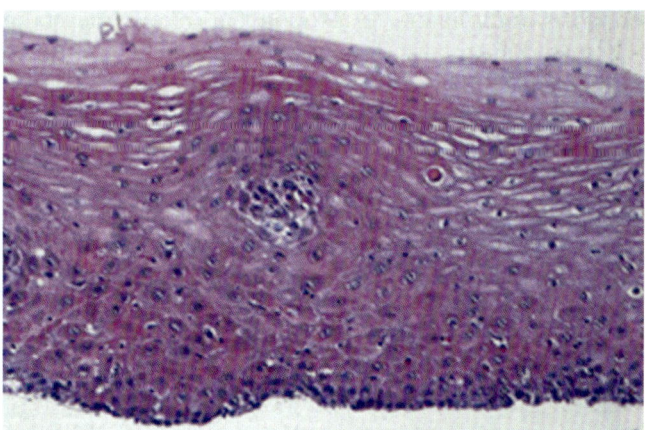

Figure 10-45. Lichen planus. Biopsy from a patient with esophageal involvement of lichen planus with basal accentuation of sparse IELs, eosinophilic granulocytes, Langerhans cells, and apoptotic squamous cells. Basal dilatation of intercellular spaces. It is apparent that changes can be minimal.

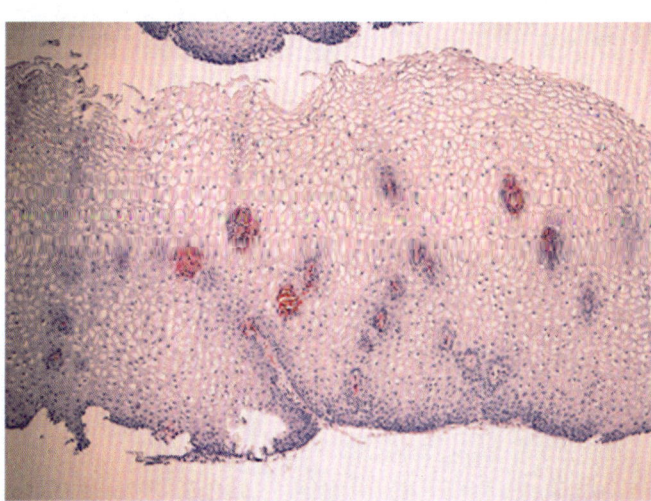

Figure 10-44. Glycogenic acanthosis of squamous epithelium with optically empty squamous cells in the upper half of the epithelium. The epithelium is thicker than usual.

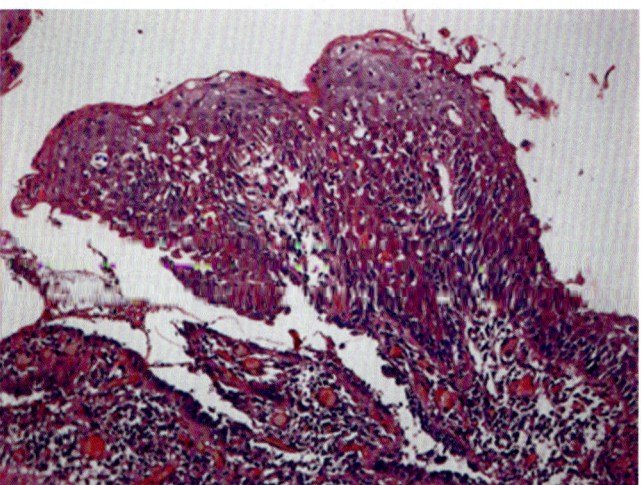

Figure 10-46. Pemphigus vulgaris. Histologic view of marked esophageal pemphigus vulgaris with suprabasal blister, marked proliferation of squamous epithelium, dilation of intercellular spaces, desquamation of suprabasal epithelial layer, and sparse eosinophilic granulocytes

erosions and blisters. In esophageal involvement the whole esophagus is affected with diffuse erosions and hemorrhage. The blisters are found subepithelial. Blisters contain eosinophils, neutrophils, and fibrin.

Acanthosis nigricans is often observed as a paraneoplastic complication of gastric carcinomas and affects the epidermis but also esophageal mucosa.[197,200,201] Histologically, there can be finely granular elevations with epithelial hyperplasia and papillomatosis.[202] Pigmentation is not always observed. Histologic data need to be interpreted with caution since descriptions are often vague. Etiologically, involvement of transforming growth factor-alpha secretion from the tumor has been proposed.[203] Complete regression after gastrectomy has been described.[204]

Pseudoepitheliomatous Hyperplasia

Pseudoepitheliomatous hyperplasia shows a pseudo-invasive growth pattern of epithelial nests with an intact basal cell layer. The basal layer in the "infiltrating" component can be quite atypical as it is restituting type epithelium, but the overlying epithelium from which it is arising is usually much less atypical and the "infiltrating" component lacks any sort of desmoplastic reaction (Fig. 10-47). These changes must not be mistaken as neoplasia, although the distinction can be problematic if only the pattern is taken into account.[205] Mitoses can be seen, but without any further meaning being regenerative. Epithelial stratification with regenerative changes (elongation of papillae, thickened basal cell layer) is preserved. While pseudoepitheliomatous hyperplasia is classically seen above esophageal granular cell tumors,[206] they are much more frequent close to ulcerative esophagitis and healing erosions.[207] Often such changes can also be seen at the margin of a Barrett's adenocarcinoma. The diagnosis and differential diagnosis is discussed previously with GERD.

Leukoplakia

The definition of leukoplakia is not precise. In the literature "whitish lesions" are often interpreted as the histologic diagnosis of keratosis. There is no consensus whether leukoplakias of the esophagus really exist. If so, they must be very rare. In the literature, esophageal leukoplakias are most often misinterpreted as glycogenic acanthosis.[208] Therefore, an exact prognostic relevance cannot be drawn from the data so far available. In the oral mucosa, leukoplakias are regarded as facultative precancerous lesions that need treatment (removal). In the esophagus data are too sparse to give a clear recommendation.

Graft versus Host Disease

Only sparse information is available concerning acute esophageal graft versus host disease (GVHD). Patients can have dysphagia and motility disorders, but it is often an incidental histologic finding in patients undergoing endoscopy and biopsy for suspected GVHD. Histologically, necrosis with apoptosis and regenerative changes of the epithelium with IELs and sometimes neutrophils or eosinophils can be seen,[209] affecting the whole esophagus. Chronic GVHD show fibrosis of the muscularis mucosae and submucosa but not of the muscularis propria.[210] GVHD is discussed in detail in Chapter 8.

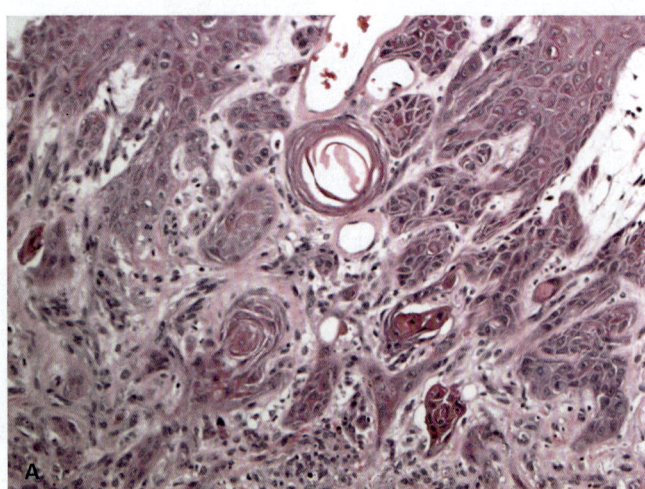 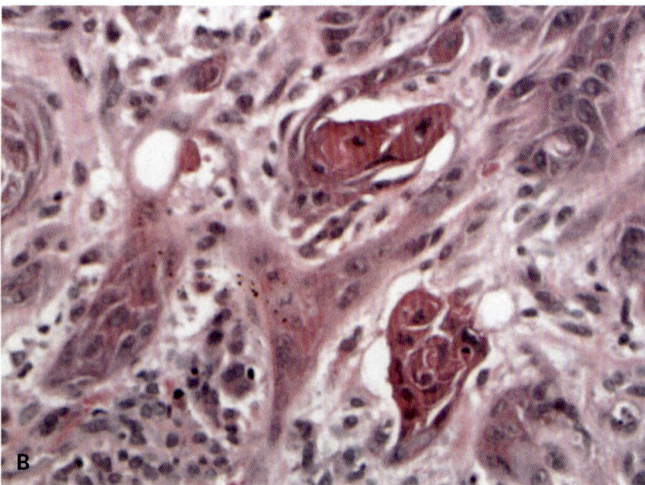

Figure 10-47. Pseudoepitheliomatous hyperplasia. **A:** Overview showing the infiltrating pattern, but note the regularity if the nuclei in the base of the epithelium from which it is arising (**top right**). **B:** Detail showing the quite marked nuclear variability but without the typical nuclear features usually associated with squamous carcinoma and with no hint of desmoplasia.

Behçet's Disease

Less than 50 cases of esophageal involvement of Behçet's disease have been reported, but lesions can be found throughout the GI tract.[211] The GI tract can be affected in up to 60%, and can present with mesenteric arteritis or spontaneous perforations.[212] Esophageal involvement is uncommon. Dysphagia is most frequently reported, followed by chest pain. Most cases have been described in Japan. Patients' age in the Japanese series are between 12 and 71 years. There is a slight male predominance (1.5:1).[213] The diagnosis is mainly based on the clinical symptoms. As an initial event, bacterial infections (streptococcus) or viral infections (herpes) in conjunction with the genetic background have been proposed. It is considered to represent an inflammatory disease that starts with oral ulcerations and has a poor prognosis if systemic with a certain genetic background.[214] It is seen endemically in Eastern Asia, China, Japan, Korea, Iran, and Turkey.[215]

The histologic picture is that of ischemic necrosis due to involvement of small vessel vasculitis. Lesions are found in the mid and sometimes the upper esophagus and are irregular in shape[216] with development of esophageal erosions and ulcerations, sometimes progressing to stricture formation.[217,218] In chronic lesions the ischemic and vasculitic lesions may no longer be present. In these cases the diagnoses have to be made in conjunction with the clinical history. A primary diagnosis of Behçet's esophagitis in the absence of other features of the disease is untenable, so that besides esophageal and other GI lesions, a combination of any of aphthous stomatitis, episcleritis, uveitis, conjunctivitis, and hypopyon iritis can be found. The triad is completed by genitourinary ulceration. Rarely, pulmonary involvement is present. Histologically, the ulceration has no specific features, and the underlying angiitis can be difficult to prove.[219] In the remaining GI tract, in Japan the lesions tend to be large ileal or cecal lesions that can perforate, but in the West the features are indistinguishable from Crohn's disease. The main problem is that both esophageal and ileocecal disease, including perforation, are also seen with NSAIDs. It seems to be difficult to exclude this. Treatment includes immunosuppression by steroids and monoclonal antibodies.

Crohn's Disease

Esophageal involvement disease affects around 1.8% to 2.4% of patients with Crohn's disease.[220] Lesions are usually found in patients with established Crohn's disease,[221] but rarely is the presenting feature.[148] Histologically, the features are usually those of capillary-rich granulation tissue with erosions and esophageal ulcerations in which the inflammatory infiltrate is often deep and severe (Fig. 10-48).[222] Typical granulomas are rare.[223] When they are the presenting lesion the differential diagnosis is that of all other causes of esophageal granulomas.

If the lesion is ulcerative and biopsies show only inflammation, a primary diagnosis is often impossible. In particular, an infectious etiology, possibly HIV related, may be considered, although organisms are not found unless superficial secondary invaders. *Candida*, other fungi, syphilis, and other rare infections may all be considered. A neoplastic etiology always enters the diagnosis but workup is negative. The possibility of medications or recreational drugs may be considered. Crohn's disease may be thought of, and some form of small bowel and large bowel imaging or endoscopy should always be considered. However, if it is the presenting manifestation, these may be normal also. A hint may come from the response to steroids, which may be given more out of desperation to relieve symptoms, but Crohn's disease is not unique in this respect. From our routine biopsy cases with Crohn's involvement we have the impression that broad parts of the lamina propria are attached to the epithelium (Fig. 10-47A). Anecdotally, this may be a clue for Crohn's disease and seems to be rare in biopsies from individuals without Crohn's disease. Within the lamina propria prominent lymphoid tissue and occasionally follicles can be identified. Immunohistochemically, the normal-appearing squamous epithelium in Crohn's patients is said to show a transepithelial expression of HLA-DR in one-third of patients but is said to be rare in controls. This has been observed only in Crohn's disease so far.[224]

Lymphocytic esophagitis in Crohn's disease. An increase in IEMs ("lymphocytic esophagitis") may also be present (see section on lymphocytic esophagitis). However, it is common in numerous other disorders, especially reflux disease, and sometimes appears to be idiopathic. It should not be construed as esophageal involvement by Crohn's disease, and may reflect an upregulation of the immune system, similar to that which can be seen in other parts of the GI tract.

Granulomatous Esophagitis and Sarcoid

Very few symptomatic cases with esophageal granulomatous disease are described, and sarcoid seems the most prevalent. Dysphagia is most often reported, and may cause esophageal stenosis.[225] Histologic changes with typical epithelioid granulomas are similar to those changes found elsewhere in the sarcoid. The differential diagnosis includes other granulomatous diseases such as Crohn's disease or tuberculosis that do not need to show central necrosis or caseation. The

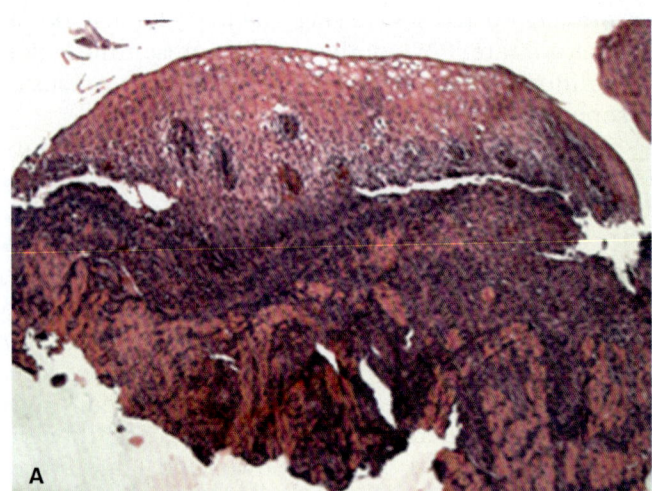
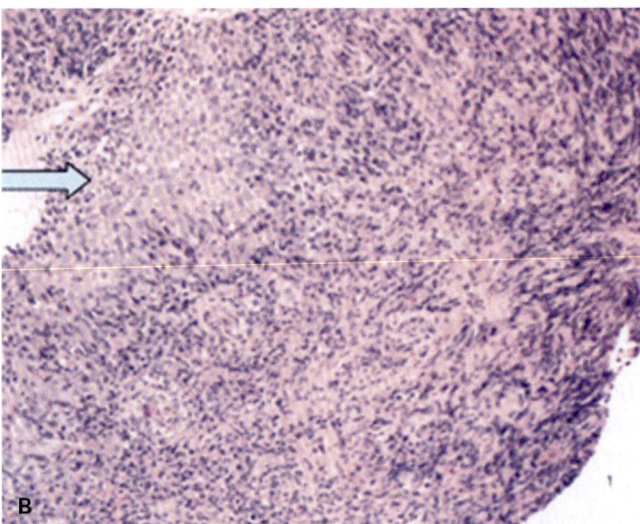
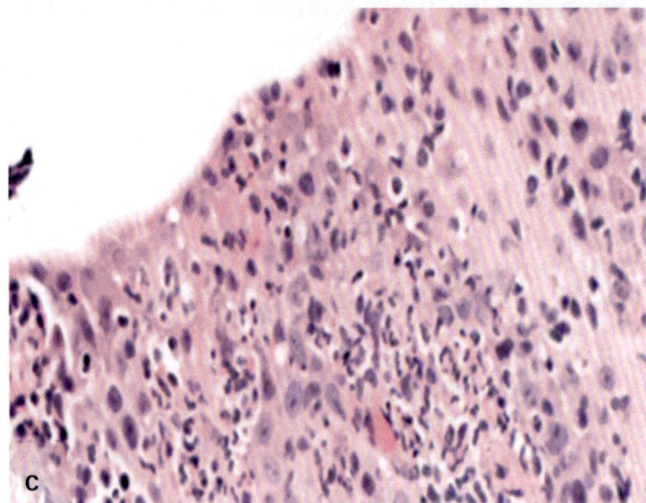

Figure 10-48. Crohn's disease involving the esophagus. **A:** There is focal marked subepithelial inflammation. Large part of esophageal tunica propria attached to the epithelium in this biopsy as an indirect marker of Crohn's esophageal involvement. **B,C:** Squamous mucosa (*arrow*) with a marked inflammatory infiltrate. **C:** Detail of (B) showing the chronic inflammatory infiltrate.

endoscopic findings can be variable.[226] In tuberculosis, following therapy, granulomas can persist for a long time without any activity.

Ulcerative Colitis

Esophagitis in patients with ulcerative colitis has been described with erosions and ulcerations.[227,228] The etiology is completely unclear. One might assume a concomitant reflux disease, an infectious esophagitis, or an underlying Crohn's disease rather than ulcerative colitis. Or like its gastroduodenal counterpart, assuming that it really exists, it may be a sympathetic reaction to large bowel active disease and regress during remissions.

Brown Bowel Syndrome (Ceroid Lipofuscinosis)

Ceroid deposits in brown bowel syndrome due to vitamin E deficiency have been reported in the esophageal smooth muscles as well[229] but are characteristically found in the smooth muscle fibers of the colon.[230] Often these deposits are found systemically.[231,232] Brown granules are readily identified in routine H&E sections. PAS, Giemsa, methenamine silver, oil-red O stains enhance the contrast to identify these brown granules.

Diabetes Mellitus

Patients with diabetes mellitus can have dysphagia with prolonged bolus passage due to the microangiopathy and neuropathy that might impair peristalsis and delayed relaxation of the LES.[233,234] There may therefore be an association with GERD, BE, and neoplasia.[235] Descriptions of typical histologic findings are not available.[236] Sometimes patients with poorly controlled diabetes present with esophageal ulcers that do not heal with PPI therapy, but respond to control of the diabetes.

Parkinson's Disease

About half of patients with Parkinson's disease report a degree of dysphagia.[237,239] Lewy corpuscles can also be seen in ganglia of the Auerbach's plexus but less often in Meissner's plexus Lewy bodies are intracytoplasmic or intraneural. Often the lower esophagus is affected.[240] Immunohistochemically, Lewy bodies are immunoreactive for anti-ubiquitin and anti–alpha-Synuclein antibodies. The differential diagnosis includes other diseases with presence of Lewy bodies, such as diffuse Lewy body disease.

References

1. Dent J, El-Serag HB, Wallander MA, et al. Epidemiology of gastro-oesophageal reflux disease: a systematic review. *Gut.* 2005;54(5):710–717.
2. Nocon M, Labenz J, Willich SN. Lifestyle factors and symptoms of gastro-oesophageal reflux—a population-based study. *Aliment Pharmacol Ther.* 2006;23(1):169–174.
3. Vieth M, Gossner L, Stolte M. Volkskrankheit Refluxkrankheit. *Leber Magen Darm.* 1999(suppl 2):3–28.
4. Jaspersen D, Labenz J, Willich SN, et al. Long-term clinical course of extra-oesophageal manifestations in patients with gastro-oesophageal reflux disease. A prospective follow-up analysis based on the ProGERD study. *Dig Liver Dis.* 2006;38(4):233–238.
5. Vakil N, van Zanten SV, Kahrilas P, et al. The Montreal definition and classification of gastroesophageal reflux disease: a global evidence-based consensus. *Am J Gastroenterol.* 2006;101(8):1900–1920;quiz 43.
6. Hershcovici T, Fass R. Nonerosive reflux disease (NERD)—an update. *J Neurogastroenterol Motil.* 2010;16(1):8–21.
7. Dellon ES, Shaheen NJ. Persistent reflux symptoms in the proton pump inhibitor era: the changing face of gastroesophageal reflux disease. *Gastroenterology.* 2010;139(1):7–13.e3.
8. Vieth M, Kulig M, Leodolter A, et al. Histological effects of esomeprazole therapy on the squamous epithelium of the distal oesophagus. *Aliment Pharmacol Ther.* 2006;23(2):313–319.
9. Sifrim D, Silny J, Holloway RH, et al. Patterns of gas and liquid reflux during transient lower oesophageal sphincter relaxation: a study using intraluminal electrical impedance. *Gut.* 1999;44(1):47–54.
10. Ito H, Iijima K, Ara N, et al. Reactive nitrogen oxide species induce dilatation of the intercellular space of rat esophagus. *Scand J Gastroenterol.* 2010;45(3):282–291.
11. Manning JJ, Wirz AA, McColl KE. Nitrogenous chemicals generated from acidification of saliva influence transient lower oesophageal sphincter relaxations. *Scand J Gastroenterol.* 2007;42(12):1413–1421.
12. Winter JW, Paterson S, Scobie G, et al. N-nitrosamine generation from ingested nitrate via nitric oxide in subjects with and without gastroesophageal reflux. *Gastroenterology.* 2007;133(1):164–174.
13. Piche T, Galmiche JP. Pharmacological targets in gastro-oesophageal reflux disease. *Basic Clin Pharmacol Toxicol.* 2005;97(6):333–341.
14. Lundell LR, Dent J, Bennett JR, et al. Endoscopic assessment of oesophagitis: clinical and functional correlates and further validation of the Los Angeles classification. *Gut.* 1999;45(2):172–180.
15. Hoshihara Y, Hashimoto M. Endoscopic classification of reflux esophagitis. *Nippon Rinsho.* 2000;58(9):1808–1812.
16. Savary M. The problem of gastro-esophageal reflux from the endoscopic viewpoint. *Pract Otorhinolaryngol (Basel).* 1965;27:20–29.
17. Armstrong D, Emde C, Inauen W, et al. Diagnostic assessment of gastroesophageal reflux disease: what is possible vs. what is practical? *Hepatogastroenterology.* 1992;39(suppl 1):3–13.
18. Kiesslich R, Kanzler S, Vieth M, et al. Minimal change esophagitis: prospective comparison of endoscopic and histological markers between patients with non-erosive reflux disease and normal controls using magnifying endoscopy. *Dig Dis.* 2004;22(2):221–227.
19. Chua YC, Aziz Q. Perception of gastro-oesophageal reflux. *Best Pract Res Clin Gastroenterol.* 2010;24(6):883–891.
20. Edebo A, Vieth M, Tam W, et al. Circumferential and axial distribution of esophageal mucosal damage in reflux disease. *Dis Esophagus.* 2007;20(3):232–238.
21. Vieth M, Haringsma J, Delarive J, et al. Red streaks in the oesophagus in patients with reflux disease: is there a histomorphological correlate? *Scand J Gastroenterol.* 2001;36(11):1123–1127.
22. Takubo K, Vieth M, Honma N, et al. Ciliated surface in the esophagogastric junction zone: a precursor of Barrett's mucosa or ciliated pseudostratified metaplasia? *Am J Surg Pathol.* 2005;29(2):211–217.
23. Weinstein WM, Bogoch ER, Bowes KL. The normal human esophageal mucosa: a histological reappraisal. *Gastroenterology.* 1975;68(1):40–44.
24. Pandolfino JE, Zhang Q, Ghosh SK, et al. Acidity surrounding the squamocolumnar junction in GERD patients: "acid pocket" versus "acid film." *Am J Gastroenterol.* 2007;102(12):2633–2641.
25. Der R, Tsao-Wei DD, Demeester T, et al. Carditis: a manifestation of gastroesophageal reflux disease. *Am J Surg Pathol.* 2001;25(2):245–252.
26. Ismail-Beigi F, Horton PF, Pope CE II. Histological consequences of gastroesophageal reflux in man. *Gastroenterology.* 1970;58(2):163–174.
27. Ismail-Beigi F, Pope CE II. Distribution of the histological changes of gastroesophageal reflux in the distal esophagus of man. *Gastroenterology.* 1974;66(6):1109–1113.
28. Leape LL, Bhan I, Ramenofsky ML. Esophageal biopsy in the diagnosis of reflux esophagitis. *J Pediatr Surg.* 1981;16(3):379–384.
29. Fiocca R, Mastracci L, Riddell R, et al. Development of consensus guidelines for the histologic recognition of microscopic esophagitis in patients with gastroesophageal reflux disease: the Esohisto project. *Hum Pathol.* 2010;41(2):223–231.
30. Xue Y, Zhou LY, Lin SR. Dilated intercellular spaces in gastroesophageal reflux disease patients and the changes of intercellular spaces after omeprazole treatment. *Chin Med J (Engl).* 2008;121(14):1297–1301.
31. Cui R, Zhou L, Lin S, et al. The feasibility of light microscopic measurements of intercellular spaces in squamous epithelium in the lower oesophagus of GERD patients. *Dis Esophagus.* 2011;24(1):1–5.
32. Neumann H, Monkemuller K, Fry LC, et al. Intercellular space volume is mainly increased in the basal layer of esophageal squamous epithelium in patients with GERD. *Dig Dis Sci.* 2011;56(5):1404–1411.
33. Elster K. Morphology of esophagitis. *Leber Magen Darm.* 1972;2(2):44–47.
34. Thakkar K, Boatright RO, Gilger MA, et al. Gastroesophageal reflux and asthma in children: a systematic review. *Pediatrics.* 2010;125(4):e925–e930.
35. Ireland-Jenkin K, Wu X, Heine RG, et al. Oesophagitis in children: reflux or allergy? *Pathology.* 2008;40(2):188–195.

36. Newton M, Kamm MA, Soediono PO, et al. Oesophageal epithelial innervation in health and reflux oesophagitis. *Gut.* 1999;44(3):317–322.
37. Matthews PJ, Aziz Q, Facer P, et al. Increased capsaicin receptor TRPV1 nerve fibres in the inflamed human oesophagus. *Eur J Gastroenterol Hepatol.* 2004;16(9):897–902.
38. Boudaka A, Worl J, Shiina T, et al. Key role of mucosal primary afferents in mediating the inhibitory influence of capsaicin on vagally mediated contractions in the mouse esophagus. *J Vet Med Sci.* 2007;69(4):365–372.
39. Tomita R, Tanjoh K, Fujisaki S, et al. Physiological studies on nitric oxide in the lower esophageal sphincter of patients with reflux esophagitis. *Hepatogastroenterology.* 2003;50(49):110–114.
40. Kassim SK, El Touny M, El Guinaidy M, et al. Serum nitrates and vasoactive intestinal peptide in patients with gastroesophageal reflux disease. *Clin Biochem.* 2002;35(8):641–646.
41. Caviglia R, Ribolsi M, Maggiano N, et al. Dilated intercellular spaces of esophageal epithelium in nonerosive reflux disease patients with physiological esophageal acid exposure. *Am J Gastroenterol.* 2005;100(3):543–548.
42. Abrahams TP, Partosoedarso ER, Hornby PJ. Lower oesophageal sphincter relaxation evoked by stimulation of the dorsal motor nucleus of the vagus in ferrets. *Neurogastroenterol Motil.* 2002;14(3):295–304.
43. Cestari R, Villanacci V, Bassotti G, et al. The pathology of gastric cardia: a prospective, endoscopic, and morphologic study. *Am J Surg Pathol.* 2007;31(5):706–710.
44. El-Serag HB, Graham DY, Rabeneck L, et al. Prevalence and determinants of histological abnormalities of the gastric cardia in volunteers. *Scand J Gastroenterol.* 2007;42(10):1158–1166.
45. Chandrasoma PT, Der R, Ma Y, et al. Histologic classification of patients based on mapping biopsies of the gastroesophageal junction. *Am J Surg Pathol.* 2003;27(7):929–936.
46. De Hertogh G, Van Eyken P, Ectors N, et al. On the existence and location of cardiac mucosa: an autopsy study in embryos, fetuses, and infants. *Gut.* 2003;52(6):791–796.
47. El-Serag HB, Pilgrim P, Tatevian N, et al. Prevalence and histological features of the gastric cardia-type mucosa in children. *Dig Dis Sci.* 2008;53(7):1792–1796.
48. Labenz J, Nocon M, Lind T, et al. Prospective follow-up data from the ProGERD study suggest that GERD is not a categorial disease. *Am J Gastroenterol.* 2006;101(11):2457–2462.
49. Spechler SJ, Fitzgerald RC, Prasad GA, et al. History, molecular mechanisms, and endoscopic treatment of Barrett's esophagus. *Gastroenterology.* 2010;138(3):854–869.
50. Spechler SJ, Sharma P, Souza RF, et al. American Gastroenterological Association technical review on the management of Barrett's esophagus. *Gastroenterology.* 2011;140(3):e18–e52;quiz e13.
51. Playford RJ. New British Society of Gastroenterology (BSG) guidelines for the diagnosis and management of Barrett's oesophagus. *Gut.* 2006;55(4):442.
52. Riddell RH, Odze RD. Definition of Barrett's esophagus: time for a rethink—is intestinal metaplasia dead? *Am J Gastroenterol.* 2009;104(10):2588–2594.
53. Ogiya K, Kawano T, Ito E, et al. Lower esophageal palisade vessels and the definition of Barrett's esophagus. *Dis Esophagus.* 2008;21(7):645–649.
54. Sharma P, Dent J, Armstrong D, et al. The development and validation of an endoscopic grading system for Barrett's esophagus: the Prague C & M criteria. *Gastroenterology.* 2006;131(5):1392–1399.
55. Takubo K, Vieth M, Aida J, et al. Differences in the definitions used for esophageal and gastric diseases in different countries: endoscopic definition of the esophagogastric junction, the precursor of Barrett's adenocarcinoma, the definition of Barrett's esophagus, and histologic criteria for mucosal adenocarcinoma or high-grade dysplasia. *Digestion.* 2009;80(4):248–257.
56. Wang KK, Sampliner RE. Updated guidelines 2008 for the diagnosis, surveillance and therapy of Barrett's esophagus. *Am J Gastroenterol.* 2008;103(3):788–797.
57. Liu W, Hahn H, Odze RD, et al. Metaplastic esophageal columnar epithelium without goblet cells shows DNA content abnormalities similar to goblet cell-containing epithelium. *Am J Gastroenterol.* 2009;104(4):816–824.
58. Kim SL, Waring JP, Spechler SJ, et al. Diagnostic inconsistencies in Barrett's esophagus. Department of Veterans Affairs Gastroesophageal Reflux Study Group. *Gastroenterology.* 1994;107(4):945–949.
59. Harrison R, Perry I, Haddadin W, et al. Detection of intestinal metaplasia in Barrett's esophagus: an observational comparator study suggests the need for a minimum of eight biopsies. *Am J Gastroenterol.* 2007;102(6):1154–1161.
60. Gatenby PA, Ramus JR, Caygill CP, et al. Relevance of the detection of intestinal metaplasia in non-dysplastic columnar-lined oesophagus. *Scand J Gastroenterol.* 2008;43(5):524–530.
61. Kelty CJ, Gough MD, Van Wyk Q, et al. Barrett's oesophagus: intestinal metaplasia is not essential for cancer risk. *Scand J Gastroenterol.* 2007;42(11):1271–1274.
62. Vieth M, Barr H. Editorial: defining a bad Barrett's segment: is it dependent on goblet cells? *Am J Gastroenterol.* 2009;104(4):825–827.
63. Takubo K, Aida J, Naomoto Y, et al. Cardiac rather than intestinal-type background in endoscopic resection specimens of minute Barrett adenocarcinoma. *Hum Pathol.* 2009;40(1):65–74.
64. Mahajan D, Bennett AE, Liu X, et al. Grading of gastric foveolar-type dysplasia in Barrett's esophagus. *Mod Pathol.* 2010;23(1):1–11.
65. Barrett NR. Chronic peptic ulcer of the oesophagus and "oesophagitis." *Br J Surg.* 1950;38(150):175–182.
66. Vieth M, Schubert B, Lang-Schwarz K, et al. Frequency of Barrett's neoplasia after initial negative endoscopy with biopsy: a long-term histopathological follow-up study. *Endoscopy.* 2006;38(12):1201–1205.
67. Grunewald M, Vieth M, Kreibich H, et al. The status of diagnosis of Barrett esophagus. An analysis of 1,000 histologically diagnosed cases. *Dtsch Med Wochenschr.* 1997;122(14):427–431.
68. Westhoff B, Brotze S, Weston A, et al. The frequency of Barrett's esophagus in high-risk patients with chronic GERD. *Gastrointest Endosc.* 2005;61(2):226–231.
69. Pavlov K, Maley CC. New models of neoplastic progression in Barrett's oesophagus. *Biochem Soc Trans.* 2010;38(2):331–336.
70. Barrett NR. The lower esophagus lined by columnar epithelium. *Surgery.* 1957;41(6):881–894.
71. Levine DS, Rubin CE, Reid BJ, et al. Specialized metaplastic columnar epithelium in Barrett's esophagus. A comparative transmission electron microscopic study. *Lab Invest.* 1989;60(3):418–432.
72. Bremner CG, Lynch VP, Ellis FH Jr. Barrett's esophagus: congenital or acquired? An experimental study of esophageal mucosal regeneration in the dog. *Surgery.* 1970;68(1):209–216.
73. Hage E, Pedersen SA. Morphological characteristics of the columnar epithelium lining the lower oesophagus in patients with Barrett's syndrome. *Virchows Arch A Pathol Pathol Anat.* 1972;357(3):219–229.
74. Gillen P, Keeling P, Byrne PJ, et al. Experimental columnar metaplasia in the canine oesophagus. *Br J Surg.* 1988;75(2):113–115.

75. Li H, Walsh TN, O'Dowd G, et al. Mechanisms of columnar metaplasia and squamous regeneration in experimental Barrett's esophagus. *Surgery*. 1994;115(2):176–181.
76. Glickman JN, Chen YY, Wang HH, et al. Phenotypic characteristics of a distinctive multilayered epithelium suggests that it is a precursor in the development of Barrett's esophagus. *Am J Surg Pathol*. 2001;25(5):569–578.
77. Nicholson AM, Graham TA, Simpson A, et al. Barrett's metaplasia glands are clonal, contain multiple stem cells and share a common squamous progenitor. *Gut*. 2012;61(10):1380–1389.
78. Shields HM, Zwas F, Antonioli DA, et al. Detection by scanning electron microscopy of a distinctive esophageal surface cell at the junction of squamous and Barrett's epithelium. *Dig Dis Sci*. 1993;38(1):97–108.
79. Boch JA, Shields HM, Antonioli DA, et al. Distribution of cytokeratin markers in Barrett's specialized columnar epithelium. *Gastroenterology*. 1997;112(3):760–765.
80. Salo JA, Kivilaakso EO, Kiviluoto TA, et al. Cytokeratin profile suggests metaplastic epithelial transformation in Barrett's oesophagus. *Ann Med*. 1996;28(4):305–309.
81. Kumagai H, Mukaisho K, Sugihara H, et al. Cell kinetic study on histogenesis of Barrett's esophagus using rat reflux model. *Scand J Gastroenterol*. 2003;38(7):687–692.
82. Peitz U, Vieth M, Ebert M, et al. Small-bowel metaplasia arising in the remnant esophagus after esophagojejunostomy—a [corrected] prospective study in patients with a history of total gastrectomy. *Am J Gastroenterol*. 2005;100(9):2062–2070.
83. Coad RA, Woodman AC, Warner PJ, et al. On the histogenesis of Barrett's oesophagus and its associated squamous islands: a three-dimensional study of their morphological relationship with native oesophageal gland ducts. *J Pathol*. 2005;206(4):388–394.
84. Abraham SC, Krasinskas AM, Correa AM, et al. Duplication of the muscularis mucosae in Barrett esophagus: an under-recognized feature and its implication for staging of adenocarcinoma. *Am J Surg Pathol*. 2007;31(11):1719–1725.
85. Faragalla HF, Marcon NE, Yousef GM, et al. Immunohistochemical staining for smoothelin in the duplicated versus the true muscularis mucosae of Barrett esophagus. *Am J Surg Pathol*. 2011;35(1):55–59.
86. Aida J, Vieth M, Ell C, et al. Palisade vessels as a new histologic marker of esophageal origin in endoscopically resected specimens from columnar-lined esophagus. *Am J Surg Pathol*. 2011;35(8):1140–1145.
87. Pech O, Behrens A, May A, et al. Long-term results and risk factor analysis for recurrence after curative endoscopic therapy in 349 patients with high-grade intraepithelial neoplasia and mucosal adenocarcinoma in Barrett's oesophagus. *Gut*. 2008;57(9):1200–1206.
88. Pouw RE, Gondrie JJ, Rygiel AM, et al. Properties of the neosquamous epithelium after radiofrequency ablation of Barrett's esophagus containing neoplasia. *Am J Gastroenterol*. 2009;104(6):1366–1373.
89. Overholt BF, Dean PJ, Galanko JA, et al. Does ablative therapy for Barrett esophagus affect the depth of subsequent esophageal biopsy as compared with controls? *J Clin Gastroenterol*. 2010;44(10):676–681.
90. Shaheen NJ, Peery AF, Overholt BF, et al. Biopsy depth after radiofrequency ablation of dysplastic Barrett's esophagus. *Gastrointest Endosc*. 2010;72(3):490–496.e1.
91. Fleischer DE, Overholt BF, Sharma VK, et al. Endoscopic radiofrequency ablation for Barrett's esophagus: 5-year outcomes from a prospective multicenter trial. *Endoscopy*. 2010;42(10):781–789.
92. Chen X, Qin R, Liu B, et al. Multilayered epithelium in a rat model and human Barrett's esophagus: similar expression patterns of transcription factors and differentiation markers. *BMC Gastroenterol*. 2008;8:1.
93. Mohammed IA, Streutker CJ, Riddell RH. Utilization of cytokeratins 7 and 20 does not differentiate between Barrett's esophagus and gastric cardiac intestinal metaplasia. *Mod Pathol*. 2002;15(6):611–616.
94. Vieth M, Stolte M. Barrett's esophagus and neoplasia: data from the Bayreuth Barrett's archive. *Gastroenterology*. 2002;122(2):590–591.
95. Buttar NS, Wang KK, Sebo TJ, et al. Extent of high-grade dysplasia in Barrett's esophagus correlates with risk of adenocarcinoma. *Gastroenterology*. 2001;120(7):1630–1639.
96. Zhu W, Appelman HD, Greenson JK, et al. A histologically defined subset of high-grade dysplasia in Barrett mucosa is predictive of associated carcinoma. *Am J Clin Pathol*. 2009;132(1):94–100.
97. Borchard F. Forms and nomenclature of gastrointestinal epithelial expansion: what is invasion? *Verh Dtsch Ges Pathol*. 2000;84:50–61.
98. Downs-Kelly E, Mendelin JE, Bennett AE, et al. Poor interobserver agreement in the distinction of high-grade dysplasia and adenocarcinoma in pretreatment Barrett's esophagus biopsies. *Am J Gastroenterol*. 2008;103(9):2333–2340;quiz 41.
99. Montgomery E, Bronner MP, Goldblum JR, et al. Reproducibility of the diagnosis of dysplasia in Barrett esophagus: a reaffirmation. *Hum Pathol*. 2001;32(4):368–378.
100. Curvers WL, ten Kate FJ, Krishnadath KK, et al. Low-grade dysplasia in Barrett's esophagus: overdiagnosed and underestimated. *Am J Gastroenterol*. 2010;105(7):1523–1530.
101. Faller G, Borchard F, Ell C, et al. Histopathological diagnosis of Barrett's mucosa and associated neoplasias: results of a consensus conference of the Working Group for Gastroenterological Pathology of the German Society for Pathology on 22 September 2001 in Erlangen. *Virchows Arch*. 2003;443(5):597–601.
102. Vieth M, Seitz G. 50 years of Barrett esophagus. Current diagnostic possibilities in pathology. *Pathologe*. 2001;22(1):62–71.
103. Faller G, Berndt R, Borchard F, et al. Histopathological diagnosis of Barrett's mucosa and associated neoplasias. Results of a consensus conference of the Working Group for "Gastroenterological Pathology of the German Society for Pathology" on 22 September 2001. *Pathologe*. 2003;24(1):9–14.
104. Madisch A, Miehlke S, Bayerdorffer E, et al. Long-term follow-up after complete ablation of Barrett's esophagus with argon plasma coagulation. *World J Gastroenterol*. 2005;11(8):1182–1186.
105. Laguna F, Garcia-Samaniego J, Alonso MJ, et al. Pseudotumoral appearance of cytomegalovirus esophagitis and gastritis in AIDS patients. *Am J Gastroenterol*. 1993;88(7):1108–1111.
106. McDonald GB, Sharma P, Hackman RC, et al. Esophageal infections in immunosuppressed patients after marrow transplantation. *Gastroenterology*. 1985;88(5 pt 1):1111–1117.
107. Nash G, Ross JS. Herpetic esophagitis. A common cause of esophageal ulceration. *Hum Pathol*. 1974;5(3):339–345.
108. Hamilton S. Esophagitis due to infectious agents. In: Ming SC, Goldman H, eds. *Pathology of the gastrointestinal tract*. Philadelphia, PA: WB Saunders; 1992:386–401.
109. Takatoku M, Muroi K, Kawano-Yamamoto C, et al. Involvement of the esophagus and stomach as a first manifestation of varicella zoster virus infection after allogeneic bone marrow transplantation. *Intern Med*. 2004;43(9):861–864.
110. Ussery XT, Annunziato P, Gershon AA, et al. Congenital varicella-zoster virus infection and Barrett's esophagus. *J Infect Dis*. 1998;178(2):539–543.

111. Villar LA, Massanari RM, Mitros FA. Cytomegalovirus infection with acute erosive esophagitis. *Am J Med.* 1984;76(5):924–928.
112. Weinstein M, Ford-Jones E, Cutz E. Esophagatis and perinatal cytomegalovirus infection. *Pediatr Infect Dis J.* 2001;20(5):545–546.
113. Trappe R, Pohl H, Forberger A, et al. Acute esophageal necrosis (black esophagus) in the renal transplant recipient: manifestation of primary cytomegalovirus infection. *Transpl Infect Dis.* 2007;9(1):42–45.
114. Odze R, Antonioli D, Shocket D, et al. Esophageal squamous papillomas. A clinicopathologic study of 38 lesions and analysis for human papillomavirus by the polymerase chain reaction. *Am J Surg Pathol.* 1993;17(8):803–812.
115. Quarto G, Sivero L, Somma P, et al. A case of infectious esophagitis caused by human papilloma virus. *Minerva Gastroenterol Dietol.* 2008;54(3):317–321.
116. Bach MC, Valenti AJ, Howell DA, et al. Odynophagia from aphthous ulcers of the pharynx and esophagus in the acquired immunodeficiency syndrome (AIDS). *Ann Intern Med.* 1988;109(4):338–339.
117. Rabeneck L, Boyko WJ, McLean DM, et al. Unusual esophageal ulcers containing enveloped viruslike particles in homosexual men. *Gastroenterology.* 1986;90(6):1882–1889.
118. Rabeneck L, Popovic M, Gartner S, et al. Acute HIV infection presenting with painful swallowing and esophageal ulcers. *JAMA.* 1990;263(17):2318–2322.
119. Levine MS, Loercher G, Katzka DA, et al. Giant, human immunodeficiency virus-related ulcers in the esophagus. *Radiology.* 1991;180(2):323–326.
120. Chatty EM, Tomeh MO, Mercer RD, et al. Congenital rubella syndrome with viral esophagitis. An electron microscopic study. *Cleve Clin Q.* 1971;38(2):73–78.
121. Kitchen VS, Helbert M, Francis ND, et al. Epstein–Barr virus associated oesophageal ulcers in AIDS. *Gut.* 1990;31(11):1223–1225.
122. Jensen KB, Stenderup A, Thomsen JB, et al. Oesophageal moniliasis in malignant neoplastic disease. *Acta Med Scand.* 1964;175:455–459.
123. Parker JC Jr, McCloskey JJ, Knauer KA. Pathobiologic features of human candidiasis. A common deep mycosis of the brain, heart and kidney in the altered host. *Am J Clin Pathol.* 1976;65(6):991–1000.
124. Scherwitz C. Candidiases of the skin and mucous membrane. *Med Klin.* 1976;71:1172–1182.
125. Khandekar A, Moser D, Fidler WJ. Blastomycosis of the esophagus. *Ann Thorac Surg.* 1980;30(1):76–79.
126. Ziliotto Junior A, Kunzle JE, Takeda Fde A. Paracoccidioidomycosis of the esophagus. Report of a case. *Rev Inst Med Trop Sao Paulo.* 1980;22(5):261–264.
127. Bentlif PS, Wiedermann B. Esophagitis caused by *Torulopsis glabrata*. Case report. *Am J Gastroenterol.* 1979;71(4):395–397.
128. Young RC, Bennett JE, Vogel CL, et al. Aspergillosis. The spectrum of the disease in 98 patients. *Medicine (Baltimore).* 1970;49(2):147–173.
129. Lyon DT, Schubert TT, Mantia AG, et al. Phycomycosis of the gastrointestinal tract. *Am J Gastroenterol.* 1979;72(4):379–394.
130. McBride R, Corson J, Dammin G. Mucormycosis. Two cases of disseminated disease with cultural identification of Rhizopus. Review of the literature. *Am J Med.* 1960;28:832–846.
131. Whiteway DE, Virata RL. Mucormycosis. *Arch Intern Med.* 1979;139(8):944.
132. Catinella FP, Kittle CF. Tuberculous esophagitis with aortic aneurysm fistula. *Ann Thorac Surg.* 1988;45(1):87–88.
133. Ito Y, Kobayashi S, Kasugai T. Tuberculosis of the esophagus. *Am J Gastroenterol.* 1976;65(5):454–456.
134. Hadlich E, Galperim B, Rizzon CF. Esophageal ulcers caused by reactivation of ganglionary tuberculosis: a case report. *Braz J Infect Dis.* 2007;11(2):293–296.
135. Vahid B, Huda N, Esmaili A. An unusual case of dysphagia and chest pain in a non-HIV patient: esophageal tuberculosis. *Am J Med.* 2007;120(4):e1–e2.
136. Gordon AH, Marshall JB. Esophageal tuberculosis: definitive diagnosis by endoscopy. *Am J Gastroenterol.* 1990;85(2):174–177.
137. Rovekamp BT, van der Linde K, Dees J, et al. A solitary tuberculous ulcer in the oesophagus. *Eur J Gastroenterol Hepatol.* 2005;17(4):435–439.
138. Hudson TR, Head JR. Syphilis of the esophagus. *J Thorac Surg.* 1950;20(2):216–221.
139. Ibbotson W. Syphilitic stricture of oesophagus. *Proc R Soc Med.* 1931;25(2):232.
140. Abdalla J, Myers J, Moorman J. Actinomycotic infection of the oesophagus. *J Infect.* 2005;51(2):E39–E43.
141. McManus JP, Webb JN. A yeast-like infection of the esophagus caused by *Lactobacillus acidophilus*. *Gastroenterology.* 1975;68(3):583–586.
142. Zucoloto S, de Rezende JM. Mucosal alterations in human chronic chagasic esophagopathy. *Digestion* 1990;47(3):138–142.
143. Pimenta APA, Carneiro FMH, Capela JA. Esophageal schistosomiasis and achalasia. Cause or consequence? Report of a case. *Dis Esophagus.* 1996;9:63–66.
144. Villanueva JL, Torre-Cisneros J, Jurado R, et al. Leishmania esophagitis in an AIDS patient: an unusual form of visceral leishmaniasis. *Am J Gastroenterol.* 1994;89(2):273–275.
145. Gutierrez-Macias A, Alonso-Alonso JJ, Aguirre-Errasti C. Esophageal leishmaniasis in a patient infected with the human immunodeficiency virus. *Clin Infect Dis.* 1995;21(1):229–230.
146. Rubio CA, Sjodahl K, Lagergren J. Lymphocytic esophagitis: a histologic subset of chronic esophagitis. *Am J Clin Pathol.* 2006;125(3):432–437.
147. Purdy JK, Appelman HD, Golembeski CP, et al. Lymphocytic esophagitis: a chronic or recurring pattern of esophagitis resembling allergic contact dermatitis. *Am J Clin Pathol.* 2008;130(4):508–513.
148. Oberhuber G. Histology of Crohn disease type lesions in the upper gastrointestinal tract. *Pathologe.* 2001;22(2):91–96.
149. Takubo K. *Pathology of the Esophagus*. 2nd ed. Tokyo, Japan: Springer; 2007.
150. Patterson T. A simple superficial oesophageal cast. (oesophagitis exfoliativa: oesophagitis dissecans superficialis). *J Path Bact.* 1935;40:559–569.
151. Purdy JK, Appelman HD, McKenna BJ. Sloughing esophagitis is associated with chronic debilitation and medications that injury the esophageal mucosa. *Mod Pathol.* 2012;25(5):767–775.
152. Carmack SW, Vemulapalli R, Spechler SJ, et al. Esophagitis dissecans superficialis ("sloughing esophagitis"): a clinicopathologic study of 12 cases. *Am J Surg Pathol.* 2009;33(12):1789–1794.
153. Obermeyer R, Kasirajan K, Erzurum V, et al. Necrotizing esophagitis presenting as a black esophagus. *Surg Endosc.* 1998;12(12):1430–1433.
154. Goldenberg SP, Wain SL, Marignani P. Acute necrotizing esophagitis. *Gastroenterology.* 1990;98(2):493–496.
155. Augusto F, Fernandes V, Cremers MI, et al. Acute necrotizing esophagitis: a large retrospective case series. *Endoscopy.* 2004;36(5):411–415.

156. Vieth M, Stolte M. Eosinophilic esophagitis: a largely unknown entity? *Z Gastroenterol*. 2000;38(5):447–448.
157. Ronkainen J, Talley NJ, Aro P, et al. Prevalence of oesophageal eosinophils and eosinophilic oesophagitis in adults: the population-based Kalixanda study. *Gut*. 2007;56(5):615–620.
158. Moawad FJ, Veerappan GR, Lake JM, et al. Correlation between eosinophilic oesophagitis and aeroallergens. *Aliment Pharmacol Ther*. 2010;31(4):509–515.
159. Atkins D, Furuta GT. Mucosal immunology, eosinophilic esophagitis, and other intestinal inflammatory diseases. *J Allergy Clin Immunol*. 2010;125(2 suppl 2):S255–S261.
160. Rothenberg ME. Biology and treatment of eosinophilic esophagitis. *Gastroenterology*. 2009;137(4):1238–1249.
161. Moawad FJ, Veerappan GR, Wong RK. Eosinophilic esophagitis. *Dig Dis Sci*. 2009;54(9):1818–1828.
162. Straumann A, Conus S, Grzonka P, et al. Anti-interleukin-5 antibody treatment (mepolizumab) in active eosinophilic oesophagitis: a randomised, placebo-controlled, double-blind trial. *Gut*. 2010;59(1):21–30.
163. Straumann A, Conus S, Degen L, et al. Budesonide is effective in adolescent and adult patients with active eosinophilic esophagitis. *Gastroenterology*. 2010;139(5):1526–1537, 37e1.
164. Dohil R, Newbury R, Fox L, et al. Oral viscous budesonide is effective in children with eosinophilic esophagitis in a randomized, placebo-controlled trial. *Gastroenterology*. 2010;139(2):418–429.
165. Straumann A, Spichtin HP, Grize L, et al. Natural history of primary eosinophilic esophagitis: a follow-up of 30 adult patients for up to 11.5 years. *Gastroenterology*. 2003;125(6):1660–1669.
166. Straumann A. Eosinophilic esophagitis: a novel entity? *Praxis (Bern 1994)*. 2006;95(6):191–195.
167. Fox VL, Nurko S, Furuta GT. Eosinophilic esophagitis: it's not just kid's stuff. *Gastrointest Endosc*. 2002;56(2):260–270.
168. Thompson DM, Arora AS, Romero Y, et al. Eosinophilic esophagitis: its role in aerodigestive tract disorders. *Otolaryngol Clin North Am*. 2006;39(1):205–221.
169. Shah A, Kagalwalla AF, Gonsalves N, et al. Histopathologic variability in children with eosinophilic esophagitis. *Am J Gastroenterol*. 2009;104(3):716–721.
170. Noel RJ, Tipnis NA. Eosinophilic esophagitis—a mimic of GERD. *Int J Pediatr Otorhinolaryngol*. 2006;70(7):1147–1153.
171. Genevay M, Rubbia-Brandt L, Rougemont AL. Do eosinophil numbers differentiate eosinophilic esophagitis from gastroesophageal reflux disease? *Arch Pathol Lab Med*. 2010;134(6):815–825.
172. Molina-Infante J, Ferrando-Lamana L, Mateos-Rodriguez JM, et al. Overlap of reflux and eosinophilic esophagitis in two patients requiring different therapies: a review of the literature. *World J Gastroenterol*. 2008;14(9):1463–1466.
173. Sayej WN, Patel R, Baker RD, et al. Treatment with high-dose proton pump inhibitors helps distinguish eosinophilic esophagitis from noneosinophilic esophagitis. *J Pediatr Gastroenterol Nutr*. 2009;49(4):393–399.
174. Ngo P, Furuta GT, Antonioli DA, et al. Eosinophils in the esophagus—peptic or allergic eosinophilic esophagitis? Case series of three patients with esophageal eosinophilia. *Am J Gastroenterol*. 2006;101(7):1666–1670.
175. Remedios M, Campbell C, Jones DM, et al. Eosinophilic esophagitis in adults: clinical, endoscopic, histologic findings, and response to treatment with fluticasone propionate. *Gastrointest Endosc*. 2006;63(1):3–12.
176. Liacouras CA, Spergel JM, Ruchelli E, et al. Eosinophilic esophagitis: a 10-year experience in 381 children. *Clin Gastroenterol Hepatol*. 2005;3(12):1198–1206.
177. Pace F, Greco S, Pallotta S, et al. An uncommon cause of corrosive esophageal injury. *World J Gastroenterol*. 2008;14(4):636–637.
178. Gumaste VV, Dave PB. Ingestion of corrosive substances by adults. *Am J Gastroenterol*. 1992;87(1):1–5.
179. Ramasamy K, Gumaste VV. Corrosive ingestion in adults. *J Clin Gastroenterol*. 2003;37(2):119–124.
180. Oak JH, Chung WC, Jung JH, et al. A case of carcinosarcoma in a patient with corrosive esophagitis. *Korean J Gastroenterol*. 2008;52(1):42–47.
181. Abraham SC, Cruz-Correa M, Lee LA, et al. Alendronate-associated esophageal injury: pathologic and endoscopic features. *Mod Pathol*. 1999;12(12):1152–1157.
182. Winstead NS, Bulat R. Pill Esophagitis. *Curr Treat Options Gastroenterol*. 2004;7(1):71–76.
183. Abid S, Mumtaz K, Jafri W, et al. Pill-induced esophageal injury: endoscopic features and clinical outcomes. *Endoscopy*. 2005;37(8):740–744.
184. Leong RW, Chan FK. Drug-induced side effects affecting the gastrointestinal tract. *Expert Opin Drug Saf*. 2006;5(4):585–592.
185. Singh NP, Rizk JG. Oesophageal perforation following ingestion of over-the-counter ibuprofen capsules. *J Laryngol Otol*. 2008;122(8):864–866.
186. Parfitt JR, Driman DK. Pathological effects of drugs on the gastrointestinal tract: a review. *Hum Pathol*. 2007;38(4):527–536.
187. Nishizawa A, Satoh T, Watanabe R, et al. Cowden syndrome: a novel mutation and overlooked glycogenic acanthosis in gingiva. *Br J Dermatol*. 2009;160(5):1116–1118.
188. Umemura K, Takagi S, Ishigaki Y, et al. Gastrointestinal polyposis with esophageal polyposis is useful for early diagnosis of Cowden's disease. *World J Gastroenterol*. 2008;14(37):5755–5759.
189. Kay PS, Soetikno RM, Mindelzun R, et al. Diffuse esophageal glycogenic acanthosis: an endoscopic marker of Cowden's disease. *Am J Gastroenterol*. 1997;92(6):1038–1040.
190. Vadva MD, Triadafilopoulos G. Glycogenic acanthosis of the esophagus and gastroesophageal reflux. *J Clin Gastroenterol*. 1993;17(1):79–83.
191. Glick SN, Teplick SK, Goldstein J, et al. Glycogenic acanthosis of the esophagus. *AJR Am J Roentgenol*. 1982;139(4):683–688.
192. Ghahremani GG, Rushovich AM. Glycogenic acanthosis of the esophagus: radiographic and pathologic features. *Gastrointest Radiol*. 1984;9(2):93–98.
193. Bender MD, Allison J, Cuartas F, et al. Glycogenic acanthosis of the esophagus: a form of benign epithelial hyperplasia. *Gastroenterology*. 1973;65(3):373–380.
194. Al-Shihabi BM, Jackson JM. Dysphagia due to pharyngeal and oesophageal lichen planus. *J Laryngol Otol*. 1982;96(6):567–571.
195. Lefer LG. Lichen planus of the esophagus. *Am J Dermatopathol*. 1982;4(3):267–269.
196. Shimizu H, Tan Kinoshita MT, Suzuki H. Darier's disease with esophageal carcinoma. *Eur J Dermatol*. 2000;10(6):470–472.
197. Krebs A. Acanthosis nigricans with involvement of the esophagus and vitamin A deficiency. *Schweiz Med Wochenschr*. 1962;92:545–552.
198. Raque CJ, Stein KM, Samitz MH. Pemphigus vulagis involving the esophagus. *Arch Dermatol*. 1970;102(4):371–373.
199. Sami N, Bhol KC, Beutner EH, et al. Diagnostic features of pemphigus vulgaris in patients with bullous pemphigoid. Molecular analysis of autoantibody profile. *Dermatology*. 2002;204(2):108–117.
200. Sher AM. Cutaneous signs of gastrointestinal disease. *Compr Ther*. 1986;12(5):50–57.

201. Itai Y, Kogure T, Okuyama Y, et al. Radiological manifestations of oesophageal involvement in acanthosis nigricans. *Br J Radiol.* 1976;49(583):592–593.
202. Itai Y, Kogure T, Okuyama Y, et al. Diffuse finely nodular lesions of the esophagus. *AJR Am J Roentgenol.* 1977;128(4):563–566.
203. Wilgenbus K, Lentner A, Kuckelkorn R, et al. Further evidence that acanthosis nigricans maligna is linked to enhanced secretion by the tumour of transforming growth factor alpha. *Arch Dermatol Res.* 1992;284(5):266–270.
204. Umeda T, Kito T, Yamamura Y, et al. A case of long surviving gastric cancer with an malignant acanthosis nigricans. *Gan No Rinsho.* 1990;36(9):1042–1046.
205. Haim N, Krugliak P, Cohen Y, et al. Esophageal metastasis from breast carcinoma associated with pseudoepitheliomatous hyperplasia: an unusual endoscopic diagnosis. *J Surg Oncol.* 1989;41(4):278–281.
206. Schlick T, Junginger T. Abrikossoff granular cell tumor: a rare tumor of the esophagus. *Chirurg.* 1997;68(9):932–935.
207. Lack EE, Worsham GF, Callihan MD, et al. Granular cell tumor: a clinicopathologic study of 110 patients. *J Surg Oncol.* 1980;13(4):301–316.
208. Ishii Y, Sayama K, Ohtsuka H, et al. Oral florid papillomatosis and leukoplakia of the esophagus associated with keratoderma and showing transepidermal elimination. *J Dermatol.* 1994;21(12):974–978.
209. Nakshabendi IM, Maldonado ME, Coppola D, et al. Esophageal cast: a manifestation of graft-versus-host disease. *Dig Dis.* 2000;18(2):103–105.
210. McDonald GB, Sullivan KM, Schuffler MD, et al. Esophageal abnormalities in chronic graft-versus-host disease in humans. *Gastroenterology.* 1981;80(5, pt 1):914–921.
211. Donghi D, Mainetti C. Infliximab for the treatment of refractory Adamantiades-Behcet disease with articular, intestinal, cerebral and ocular involvement. *Dermatology.* 2010;220(3):282–286.
212. Glosemeyer R, Deppe H, Dormann AJ, et al. Ulcerative esophagitis and colitis as rare manifestations of Adamantiades-Behcet disease. *Z Gastroenterol.* 2001;39(2):167–171.
213. Yashiro K, Nagasako K, Hasegawa K, et al. Esophageal lesions in intestinal Behcet's disease. *Endoscopy.* 1986;18(2):57–60.
214. Durrani K, Papaliodis GN. The genetics of Adamantiades-Behcet's disease. *Semin Ophthalmol.* 2008;23(1):73–79.
215. Zouboulis CC, Kotter I, Djawari D, et al. Epidemiological features of Adamantiades-Behcet's disease in Germany and in Europe. *Yonsei Med J.* 1997;38(6):411–422.
216. Mori S, Yoshihira A, Kawamura H, et al. Esophageal involvement in Behcet's disease. *Am J Gastroenterol.* 1983;78(9):548–553.
217. Bektas M, Altan M, Alkan M, et al. Manometric evaluation of the esophagus in patients with Behcet's disease. *Digestion.* 2007;76(3–4):192–195.
218. Bottomley WW, Dakkak M, Walton S, et al. Esophageal involvement in Behcet's disease. Is endoscopy necessary? *Dig Dis Sci.* 1992;37(4):594–597.
219. Anti M, Marra G, Rapaccini GL, et al. Esophageal involvement in Behcet's syndrome. *J Clin Gastroenterol.* 1986;8(5):514–519.
220. Ramaswamy K, Jacobson K, Jevon G, et al. Esophageal Crohn disease in children: a clinical spectrum. *J Pediatr Gastroenterol Nutr.* 2003;36(4):454–458.
221. Bona D, Incarbone R, Chella B, et al. Heartburn and multiple-site foregut perforations as primary manifestation of Crohn's disease. *Dis Esophagus.* 2005;18(3):199–201.
222. Weigand K, Wagner-Thiessen E, Stolte M. Esophagitis in an adolescent patient with Crohn's disease after changing treatment from prednisolone to budesonide. *Z Gastroenterol.* 2004;42(10):1179–1181.
223. Decker GA, Loftus EV Jr, Pasha TM, et al. Crohn's disease of the esophagus: clinical features and outcomes. *Inflamm Bowel Dis.* 2001;7(2):113–119.
224. Oberhuber G, Puspok A, Peck-Radosavlevic M, et al. Aberrant esophageal HLA-DR expression in a high percentage of patients with Crohn's disease. *Am J Surg Pathol.* 1999;23(8):970–976.
225. Wiesner PJ, Kleinman MS, Condemi JJ, et al. Sarcoidosis of the esophagus. *Am J Dig Dis.* 1971;16(10):943–951.
226. Murdock A, Jacob G. Sarcoidosis of the esophagus presenting macroscopically as Barrett's esophagitis. *Am J Gastroenterol.* 2003;98(7):1661–1662.
227. Asakawa A, Kojima Y, Fujii E, et al. Case of ulcerative colitis associated with oesophageal ulcer. *J Int Med Res.* 2000;28(4):191–196.
228. Rosendorff C, Grieve NW. Ulcerative oesophagitis in association with ulcerative colitis. *Gut.* 1967;8(4):344–347.
229. Stamp GW, Evans DJ. Accumulation of ceroid in smooth muscle indicates severe malabsorption and vitamin E deficiency. *J Clin Pathol.* 1987;40(7):798–802.
230. Vieth M, Kansy A, Bethke B, et al. Brown-bowel-syndrome association with ascending colon adenocarcinoma. *Leber Magen Darm.* 1999;29:104–107.
231. Pappenheimer AM, Victor J. "Ceroid" pigment in human tissues. *Am J Pathol.* 1946;22(2):395–413.
232. Takahashi K, Oka K, Hakozaki H, et al. Ceroid-like histiocytic granuloma of gall-bladder—a previously undescribed lesion. *Acta Pathol Jpn.* 1976;26(1):25–46.
233. Feldman M, Schiller LR. Disorders of gastrointestinal motility associated with diabetes mellitus. *Ann Intern Med.* 1983;98(3):378–384.
234. Nguyen NQ, Holloway RH. Recent developments in esophageal motor disorders. *Curr Opin Gastroenterol.* 2005;21(4):478–484.
235. Rubenstein JH, Davis J, Marrero JA, et al. Relationship between diabetes mellitus and adenocarcinoma of the oesophagus and gastric cardia. *Aliment Pharmacol Ther.* 2005;22(3):267–271.
236. Goyal RK, Spiro HM. Gastrointestinal manifestations of diabetes mellitus. *Med Clin North Am.* 1971;55(4):1031–1044.
237. Castell JA, Johnston BT, Colcher A, et al. Manometric abnormalities of the oesophagus in patients with Parkinson's disease. *Neurogastroenterol Motil.* 2001;13(4):361–364.
238. Pfeiffer RF. Gastrointestinal dysfunction in Parkinson's disease. *Lancet Neurol.* 2003;2(2):107–116.
239. Lieberman AN, Horowitz L, Redmond P, et al. Dysphagia in Parkinson's disease. *Am J Gastroenterol.* 1980;74(2):157–160.
240. Wakabayashi K, Takahashi H, Ohama E. *Lewy bodies in the visceral autonomic nervous system in Parkinson's disease.* Amsterdam, The Netherlands: Elsevier; 1991.

Polyps and Tumors of the Esophagus

Chapter Outline

ROLE OF THE PATHOLOGIST
SQUAMOUS CELL CARCINOMA
  Pathogenesis and Clinical Features
  Risk Factors
    Geographic distribution: association with smoking and alcohol
    Diet
    Genetic factors
    Human papillomavirus infection
    Other risk or protective factors
  Predisposing Conditions
    Celiac sprue
    Tylosis palmaris et plantaris
    Other carcinomas
    Prior irradiation
  Premalignant Lesions: Dysplasia and Intraepithelial Neoplasia
  Gross and Endoscopic Appearances
  Microscopic Appearances
  Spread of Tumor, Staging, and Prognosis
    TNM classification
    Local spread and prognostic factors
    Effect of chemotherapy and irradiation
    DNA ploidy
    Molecular factors as prognosticator
    Failure and causes of death

UNUSUAL VARIANTS OF SQUAMOUS CELL CARCINOMA
  Superficial Esophageal Carcinoma
    Endoscopic mucosal resection
    Superficial spreading carcinoma
  Verrucous Carcinoma
  Spindle Cell Carcinoma
    Gross appearances
    Microscopic appearances
    Histogenesis
    Biopsy diagnosis
  Small Cell Carcinoma
  Basaloid Squamous Cell Carcinoma
ADENOCARCINOMA
  Adenocarcinoma in the Columnar-lined Esophagus (Barrett's Esophagus)
    Risk and pathogenesis
  Clinical Features
  Gross and Endoscopic Appearances
    Microscopic appearances
  Endoscopic Ablation Techniques
    Endoscopic mucosal resection
  Prognosis
UNUSUAL VARIANTS OF ADENOCARCINOMA
  Adenoid Cystic Carcinoma
  Mucoepidermoid Carcinoma

  Adenocarcinoma in Heterotopic Gastric Mucosa
  Adenocarcinoma in Submucosal Glands
  Adenosquamous Carcinoma and Adenoacanthoma
  Choriocarcinoma and Hepatoid Adenocarcinoma
BIOPSY DIAGNOSIS OF SQUAMOUS AND ADENOCARCINOMA AND ASSOCIATED PROBLEMS
  Regenerative changes
  Granulation tissue
  Barrett's esophagus
  Other Polyps and Tumors
  Squamous papilloma and papillomatosis
  Inflammatory Polyps
  Pseudosarcomatous changes in inflammatory polyps
  Mucosal Tags
  Fibrovascular Polyps
  Hamartomas, Choristomas, Thyroid Rests, Parathyroid Rests
  Malignant Melanoma
  Secondary Tumors
  Mesenchymal Tumors

Most tumors of the esophagus that cause symptoms are malignant. Of these, over 95% are either squamous cell carcinoma or adenocarcinoma. Squamous cell carcinoma has been the most common esophageal malignancy worldwide in the past and continues to be so in Eastern countries and in many developing countries. However, the incidence of adenocarcinoma has increased dramatically in the Western world with approximately a sixfold increase from 1975 to 2001 in the United States where currently adenocarcinomas constitute 50% to 80% of esophageal cancers diagnosed and have replaced squamous cell carcinoma as the predominant type of esophageal cancer.[1,2] The majority of these cancers arise on the background of the columnar-lined (Barrett's) esophagus, or intestinal metaplasia in native cardiac mucosa, which may be related, at least in some instances. A classification of esophageal tumors is presented in Table 11-1.

Table 11-1 Classification of Esophageal Tumors

Malignant Tumors
- Epithelial tumors
  - Squamous cell carcinoma
    - Typical (including carcinoma in situ)
    - Superficial spreading carcinoma
    - Verrucous carcinoma
    - Spindle cell variant
    - Basaloid cell variant
  - Adenocarcinoma
    - Arising in Barrett's mucosa
    - Arising in heterotopic gastric mucosa
    - Arising in submucosal glands
  - Other rare tumors
    - Adenoid cystic carcinoma
    - Mucoepidermoid carcinoma
    - Adenosquamous carcinoma
    - Small cell carcinoma
    - Undifferentiated carcinoma
    - Others
- Mesenchymal tumors
  - Leiomyosarcoma GISTs
  - Rhabdomyosarcoma
  - Other rare sarcomas
- Other tumors
  - Malignant melanoma
  - Malignant lymphoma
  - Choriocarcinoma
  - Secondary tumors

Potentially Malignant Tumors
- Gastrointestinal stromal tumor
- Carcinoid tumor

Benign Tumors
- Squamous cell papilloma
- Leiomyoma
- Granular cell tumor
- Inflammatory polyp
- Fibrovascular polyp
- Others

ROLE OF THE PATHOLOGIST

In the biopsy diagnosis of tumors, the major challenge for the pathologist is in being aware of diagnostic pitfalls, particularly at the edge of an ulcer, where, in squamous mucosa, severe basal cell hyperplasia can be mistaken for carcinoma in situ or even early invasion; on frozen sections, endothelial channels in granulation tissue can be mistaken for adenocarcinoma; and in any form of erosion, bizarre stromal cells can be mistaken for an undifferentiated neoplasm.

In resections of all esophageal carcinoma, if there is any possibility of extending the proximal resected margin, frozen section of the proximal margin should be considered so that if tumor extends close to it, an additional margin can be resected. The presumption is that this provides at least the possibility for the resection to be curative and is less likely to result in anastomotic recurrences. A practical problem is whether the frozen section should be taken transversely or longitudinally, and arguments for and against both ways can be made. A transverse section may need to be partially or completely circumferential in several frozen sections. Longitudinal sections immediately proximal to the epicenter of the tumor have the advantages that the submucosa is more readily visualized and the resected margin is clear, but several frozen sections may be required to increase the chance of detecting focal lymphatic involvement. Some surgeons begin a thoracoabdominal approach by requesting a frozen section of a celiac lymph node, knowing that if it is positive, a curative resection will not be carried out.

Many unusual tumors of the esophagus are polypoid. For this reason, when polypoid lesions are encountered, the index of suspicion that an unusual tumor such as spindle cell carcinoma and melanoma may be present should be high. It is therefore wise to anticipate that these tumors may well require electron microscopy and immunohistochemistry for diagnosis.

The pathologist has come to have an increasing role in the diagnosis of dysplasia and microinvasive carcinoma in both squamous and Barrett's esophagus. In addition, the apparent increase in the prevalence of adenocarcinoma of the lower esophagus requires accurate documentation in distinguishing tumors that are primarily in the lower esophagus, from those in the gastric cardiac, or from those in the stomach. Although this distinction may seem academic, it may be of much greater significance epidemiologically; it is best accomplished at the time of resection. The epicenter of the tumor in relationship to the upper end of the gastric folds internally as this provides the best landmarks. This is discussed with adenocarcinoma

SQUAMOUS CELL CARCINOMA

Squamous cell carcinoma is a malignant epithelial tumor with squamous differentiation, which is microscopically characterized by keratinocyte-like cells with or without intercellular bridges, keratinization, or both. This type of esophageal cancer is declining in Western countries but is still most common in the Eastern countries. Most carcinomas of the esophagus still present at an advanced stage, frequently with transmural spread, lymph node metastasis, or both; either of these features portends a very poor prognosis. The approximate percentage of each tumor stage is stage I in 8%, stage II in 42%, stage III in 33%, and stage IV in 13%.[3] In parts of the world where this tumor is very common, attempts at early detection have yielded tumors of earlier pathologic stages. The incidence of stage IV tumors has also been declining in the United States and survival has been steadily improving, independent of all other risk factors. Part of this may be due to finding early tumors endoscopically, especially with more early lesions being found and resected endoscopically. In advanced tumors, neoadjuvant chemoradiotherapy mostly with cisplatin and 5-fluorouracil improves local tumor control leading to more R0 curative resections with clear margins. However, this may not significantly improve overall survival.[2,4–7]

Pathogenesis and Clinical Features

In general, half of squamous cell carcinomas occur in the middle third of the esophagus, a third in the lower third, and the rest in the upper third. Tumors arising at the gastroesophageal junction are called exactly that and are judged by their center and relation to the esophagi gastric junction externally and from the upper end of the gastric folds and relationship to the squamoesophageal junction internally.

The median age for esophageal carcinoma is around 65 in both males and females, and males are affected far more frequently than females.[8] In the United States, squamous cell carcinoma is two to three times more frequent among African Americans than among Whites, Asians, or Native Americans.[9]

The most common clinical symptom is dysphagia, which is usually progressive and frequently accompanied by anorexia and weight loss. While carcinomas limited to the mucosa or submucosa are frequently asymptomatic, dysplasia sometimes produces odynophagia, possibly because of failure of keratinization. Retrosternal pain, food sticking, dry throat, and back soreness may occur. These symptoms suggesting an esophageal tumor are usually investigated initially with barium swallow or endoscopy. However, if barium testing is used initially, ultimately an upper endoscopy will be required to facilitate biopsy. In screening programs in high-risk populations, esophageal balloon cytology, endoscopy, iodine stain, and multipoint biopsy may be the best approach for early detection of carcinoma.[10] Balloon cytology is reported to have a sensitivity of 89% and a specificity of 91%.[11]

Risk Factors

Geographic distribution: association with smoking and alcohol. There are several high-incidence regions throughout the world; however, the likely major predisposing cause varies markedly from one to the other. These areas include northwestern France, northern Italy, parts of southern and eastern Africa, and southern Brazil as well as the Asian belt stretching from Iran through Afghanistan to central China. The incidence varies from about 30 to 200/100,000 with a strong male predominance of up to 6:1.[12,13] In these regions, esophageal cancer is usually the most prevalent cancer and results in 30% of all cancer-related deaths. The comparable figure for North America and remaining Europe does not exceed 8/100,000.[11]

Smoking and alcohol drinking appear to be the major risk factors with dose-response.[15,16,253] Several studies have suggested that smoking increases the likelihood of developing squamous cell carcinoma of the esophagus two to six times.[14,17,18] Chewing tobacco may well be as harmful as smoking it, and in India it seems to be associated with about a threefold increase in the disease. In Africa, North America, and the rest of Europe, it is quite unusual to encounter squamous cell carcinoma in patients who are not heavy drinkers.[17] This association is independent of tobacco use; in France, alcohol alone seems to be the major predisposing factor.

Although much work has been done on dietary factors, the major etiologic links seem to be with opium in Iran and possibly in the Transkei region of Africa. In Iran, households with a patient having esophageal cancer have much higher levels of urinary opiate metabolites than control households from the same village.[19]

Diet. A variety of dietary deficiencies resulting from malnutrition have been postulated as predisposing to esophageal cancer, including deficiencies in vitamins A, C, E, and riboflavin, as well as in trace elements such as zinc and molybdenum; indeed these have been postulated for the weak association with celiac disease. A low-protein or low-calorie diet is a possible risk factor. Indeed, increased consumption of meat, eggs, and increased BMI have been reported to be protective factors for squamous cell carcinoma.[20] In high-risk areas of China, drinking shallow ground water and frequent intake of pickled vegetables and fermented fish sauce are associated with the development of esophageal cancer.[16,21] Consumption of fresh fruits and fresh vegetables may decrease the risk.[16,20,21] Although drinking of very hot beverages, which causes thermal injury leading to chronic esophagitis, has also been proposed, these beverages are not associated with risk of esophageal squamous cell carcinoma or adenocarcinoma in a Western population.[22]

Genetic factors. Family history of esophageal squamous cell carcinoma is a risk factor for this disease.[23,24] A meta-analysis using data from three case-control studies conducted in Italy and Switzerland shows that the alcohol- and tobacco-adjusted odds ratio for a family history of esophageal cancer was 3.2 in first-degree relatives; an odds ratio is more than 100 for subjects who currently intake both tobacco and alcohol and also have the family history.[24] The risk of esophageal squamous cell carcinoma is increased in subjects with a family history of cancer of the oral cavity/pharynx and stomach, but not of other cancers.[24]

Human papillomavirus infection. Although human papillomavirus (HPV) is well known to be strongly associated with dysplasia and squamous cell carcinoma of the uterine cervix, its role in esophageal cancer is controversial. In high-risk areas of China, the incidence rate for HPV in squamous cell carcinoma tissue is 17% by in situ hybridization and 65% by polymerase chain reaction.[25,26] Further analysis in the latter study shows that the high-risk HPV type 16 and 18 are found in the cancer cells (43%), whereas the low-risk HPV type 6 and 11 are seen mainly in the normal mucosa (52%).[25] HPV and p16 silencing may have an etiologic role in esophageal carcinogenesis at least in the high-incidence areas such as China, Korea, Iran, and Greek.[25-29] The silencing of p16 was reported also from the United States.[30] However, conflicting results with the incidence rates of 0 to 5% have been reported mainly from Western countries.[31,32]

Other risk or protective factors. Free silica dust is suggested to be a possible etiologic factor of esophageal cancer. Among caisson workers who had a higher exposure to silica dust, the relative risk of esophageal cancer has been reported to be more than four and significantly high even after adjusting for the effects of smoking and alcohol drinking.[33] In contrast, chronic intake of rofecoxib and celecoxib (selective cyclooxygenase 2 [COX-2] inhibitors) and nonselective nonsteroidal anti-inflammatory drugs (NSAIDs) appears to be associated with a decreased incidence of esophageal cancer.[34] A randomized control trial suggested that selenomethionine, a synthetic form of organic selenium, might have a protective effect.[35] Infection with *Helicobacter* pylori may reduce the risk of esophageal adenocarcinoma, but gastric atrophy and infection with CagA-positive strains may increase the risk for esophageal squamous cell carcinoma.[36]

Predisposing Conditions

Celiac sprue. This may be associated with squamous carcinoma of the esophagus,[37] possibly because of deficient absorption of vitamins and trace metals[38]; however, excessive permeability of jejunal epithelium to carcinogens may be an additional factor.

Tylosis palmaris et plantaris. This very rare autosomal dominant condition is characterized by hyperkeratosis of palms and soles, and is associated with a very high frequency of esophageal carcinoma in those who inherit the defect.[39]

Other carcinomas. Esophageal squamous carcinoma may also be associated with other smoking-related carcinomas, such as those of laryngeal, oral, or bronchogenic origin. Synchronous tumors have been reported in up to 10% to 15% of patients,[40,41] while metachronous tumors in survivors are typical smoking-related tumors in 60%.[41] A similar argument can be made for the presence of alcoholic cirrhosis, in view of the propensity of alcohol to predispose to both cirrhosis and esophageal carcinoma.

In up to 15% of patients, a second esophageal carcinoma may be present that may represent either a second primary tumor or a submucosal deposit, invariably proximal to the main tumor. The distinction can be made only by the presence of overlying dysplasia (intraepithelial neoplasia) from which tumor arises in further primary tumors, and its absence or dissociation in metastases that are presumed to have spread through submucosal lymphatics.[40]

Prior irradiation. There are numerous case reports of patients who developed squamous esophageal carcinoma following irradiation to the thyroid or to the cervical spine. The doses of radiation received were often low and the interval to develop carcinoma was long, sometimes up to 50 years.[42] Thus the magnitude of increased risk, if any, is probably low.

Premalignant Lesions: Dysplasia and Intraepithelial Neoplasia

In three major high-risk populations, those of Iran, China, and South Africa, the sequence of events seems to consist of basal cell hyperplasia, dysplasia, and carcinoma. Further change includes esophagitis, which tends to affect the middle and lower esophagus while sparing the gastroesophageal junction, suggesting that it may not be reflux associated, as the latter is usually in continuity with the gastroesophageal junction. Endoscopic esophagitis is seen in about 85% of all high-risk populations and is already present in some persons in their teens. However, in over half of the patients, the esophagitis is endoscopically mild, and severe changes are seen in only a small percentage. A recent study adjusting for potential confounding factors reported that esophagitis was not a risk factor for squamous cell carcinoma.[43] In this study, relative risks for the incidence of squamous cell carcinoma, by initial histological diagnosis, were normal 1.0, esophagitis 0.8, basal cell hyperplasia 1.9 (95% CI 0.8–4.5), mild dysplasia 2.9 (1.6–5.2), moderate dysplasia 9.8 (5.3–18.3), severe dysplasia 28.3 (15.3–52.3), and carcinoma in situ 34.4 (16.6–71.4), during the follow-up period of 13.5 years after endoscopy. Some patients have lesser degrees of dysplasia and sometimes no evidence of dysplasia on follow-up; in these patients, it is unclear whether this represents regression or sampling problems. Dysplasia in other sites such as uterine cervix is known to regress, and the esophagus may be no exception. Mild dysplasia appears more likely to regress than severe dysplasia, but all degrees of dysplasia may remain stable over considerable periods of time.[44]

It has long been recognized that the mucosa immediately adjacent to squamous cell carcinoma may show dysplasia or in situ carcinoma.[45,46] The expression of p53 protein gradually increases from 12% in normal mucosa to 36% in low-grade dysplasia, and 100% in high-grade dysplasia and squamous cell carcinoma.[47] These observations strongly suggest that dysplasia and carcinoma in situ are precursor lesions. Caspase-3, TRAIL, Fas-L, Fas, Smad 4, VHL, E-cadherin, and EGFR may be involved in the progression from dysplasia to invasive esophageal squamous cell carcinoma.[48] Dysplasia is more frequently found in the mucosa adjacent to early mucosal cancer than with advanced cancer invading into the adjacent structures. This suggests that it is destroyed by the invasive component as the tumor grows. The relatively widespread nature of the dysplasia in some patients was reflected by the fact that when the tumor was limited to the muscularis propria, both proximal and distal margins were involved in 71%.[45]

Dysplasia is defined morphologically by the presence of atypical cells that always include the basal layer and extend throughout varying portions of the thickness of the mucosa. The atypical cells are invariably hyperchromatic with an increase in nuclear/cytoplasmic ratio, but the chromatin may be chunky and distributed irregularly throughout the nucleus. One or more nucleoli are often visible. The common form of dysplasia is composed of atypical basal-type cells that are often monomorphic and is most easily recognized in practice. Pleomorphism, loss of polarity, and sometimes atypical mitotic figures are the major features by which this type of dysplasia is distinguished from simple basal cell hyperplasia associated with reflux or other injuries. An endoscopic "front," meaning the border between atypical and normal epithelium, is a useful endoscopic sign of dysplasia rather than reactive change. Histologically, in some biopsies, the dysplastic epithelium shows variable extent of maturation and can resemble normal squamous epithelium, except for the dysplasia in the basal layer that can be quite subtle and extremely difficult to recognize. The nuclear atypia, loss of polarity, and dyskeratosis are often subtle, but present. The presence of normal epithelium, if any, in the same slide for comparison is of great help.

Dysplasia or intraepithelial neoplasia had been graded into mild, moderate, and severe dysplasia and carcinoma in situ. In this system, dysplasia affecting only the lower third of the epithelium is called *mild*; dysplasia extending up to two-thirds of the epithelium is called *moderate*; dysplasia reaching into the upper third of the epithelium is called *severe*, or *carcinoma in situ* (Fig. 11-1). It is interesting that in glandular mucosa the dysplasia is usually at the surface initially in most examples, with only a small proportion being "bottom up," while in squamous mucosa the dysplasia always begins in the basal epithelium. In the esophageal squamous mucosa, some prefer not to use the term *carcinoma in situ* when surface maturation is present. However, severe dysplasia and carcinoma in situ have equivalent relative risks for incidence of squamous cell carcinoma, and thus they may have the same clinical implications.[43,49] To improve the comparability of research data, it has been recommended to use the terms *low-* and *high-grade dysplasia* (intraepithelial neoplasia),[49,50] and this system has been employed in the WHO classification from 2000,[51] as well as in the 2010 version. The abnormal cells in low-grade dysplasia are usually confined to the lower half of the epithelium, whereas those in high-grade dysplasia occur in the upper half of the epithelium and exhibit a greater degree of atypia. The distinction from reactive changes is discussed subsequently.

In Japan, carcinoma in situ has morphologically also been divided into two types as total-layer type or basal-layer type.[52,53]

In the total-layer type, the full thickness of the epithelium is involved by atypical cells and would be called carcinoma in situ in all other classification schemes. The basal-layer type comprises atypical cells that are present only in the lower half of the epithelium, which would be classified as low-grade dysplasia by Western criteria. However, it appears that the basal-type more often shows signs of early stromal invasion and progression to invasive carcinoma compared to total-layer type.[52]

Gross and Endoscopic Appearances

Esophageal carcinomas are typically advanced when diagnosed. Advanced cancers are macroscopically classified into three major types: fungating, ulcerative, and infiltrating. Fungating tumors are well-demarcated lesions with primarily exophytic growth and are less likely to be deeply infiltrating, at least in early stages (Fig. 11-2). Ulcerative tumors are predominantly intramural, with a central ulceration and elevated ulcer edges. These two types are the most common, forming 60% of tumors in some series.[54] Infiltrating tumors are the least common (15%), but there is tremendous overlap between these groups of tumors. Most tumors infiltrate through the muscularis propria into the adventitia and frequently into adjacent organs, especially in the infiltrating gross variant.[54] Barium swallow may roughly predict the depth of tumor invasion. In one

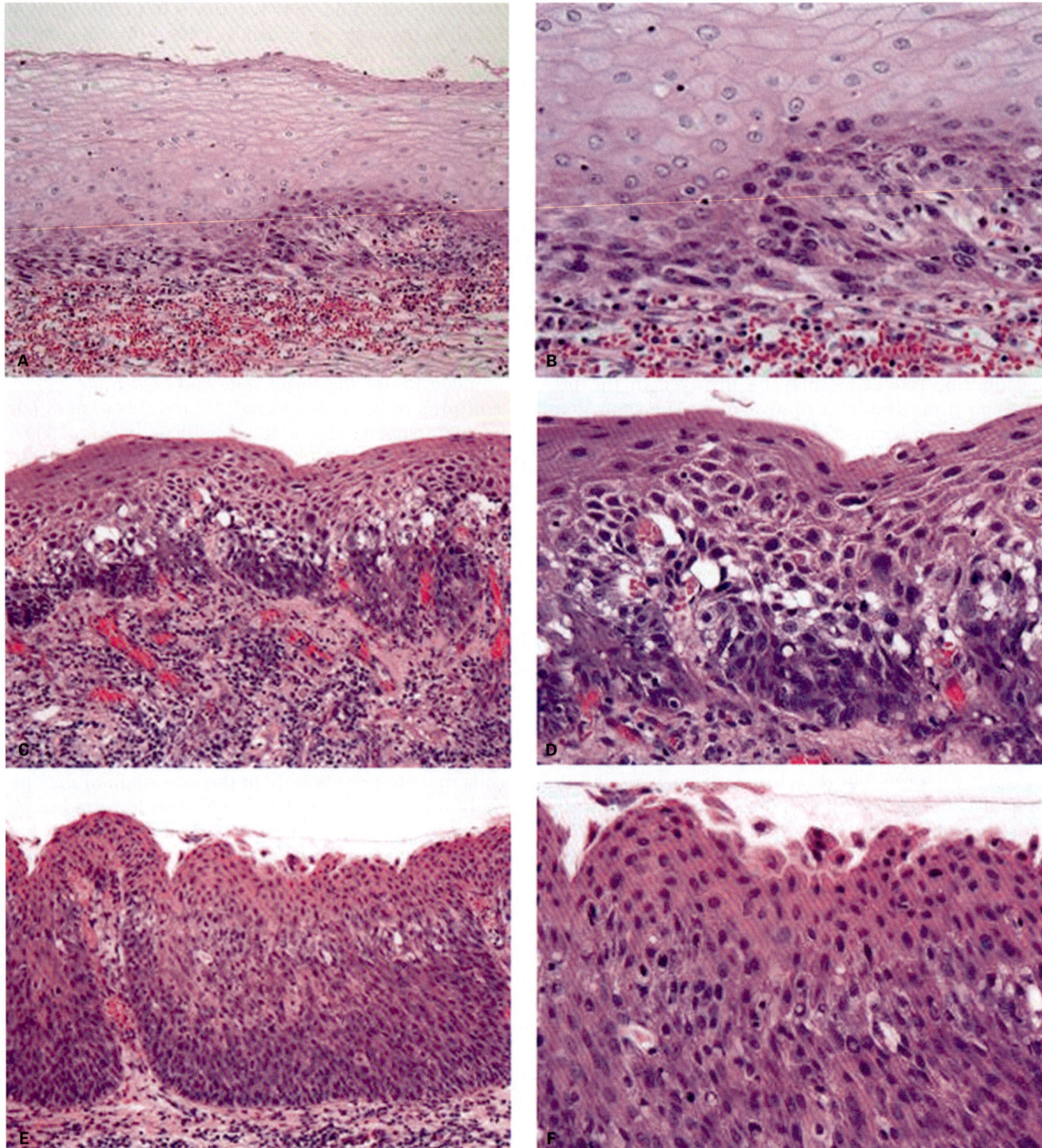

Figure 11-1. Degrees of esophageal dysplasia. **A,B:** Dysplastic cells confined to the basal third of the mucosa (low-grade dysplasia). **C,D:** Dysplastic cells reaching into the upper third of the mucosa but not reaching the surface (high-grade dysplasia). **E,F:** Dysplastic cells reaching the surface (high-grade dysplasia/carcinoma in situ). Note the relative lack of inflammation in the lamina propria, which can be a useful aid in the distinction form reactive changes.

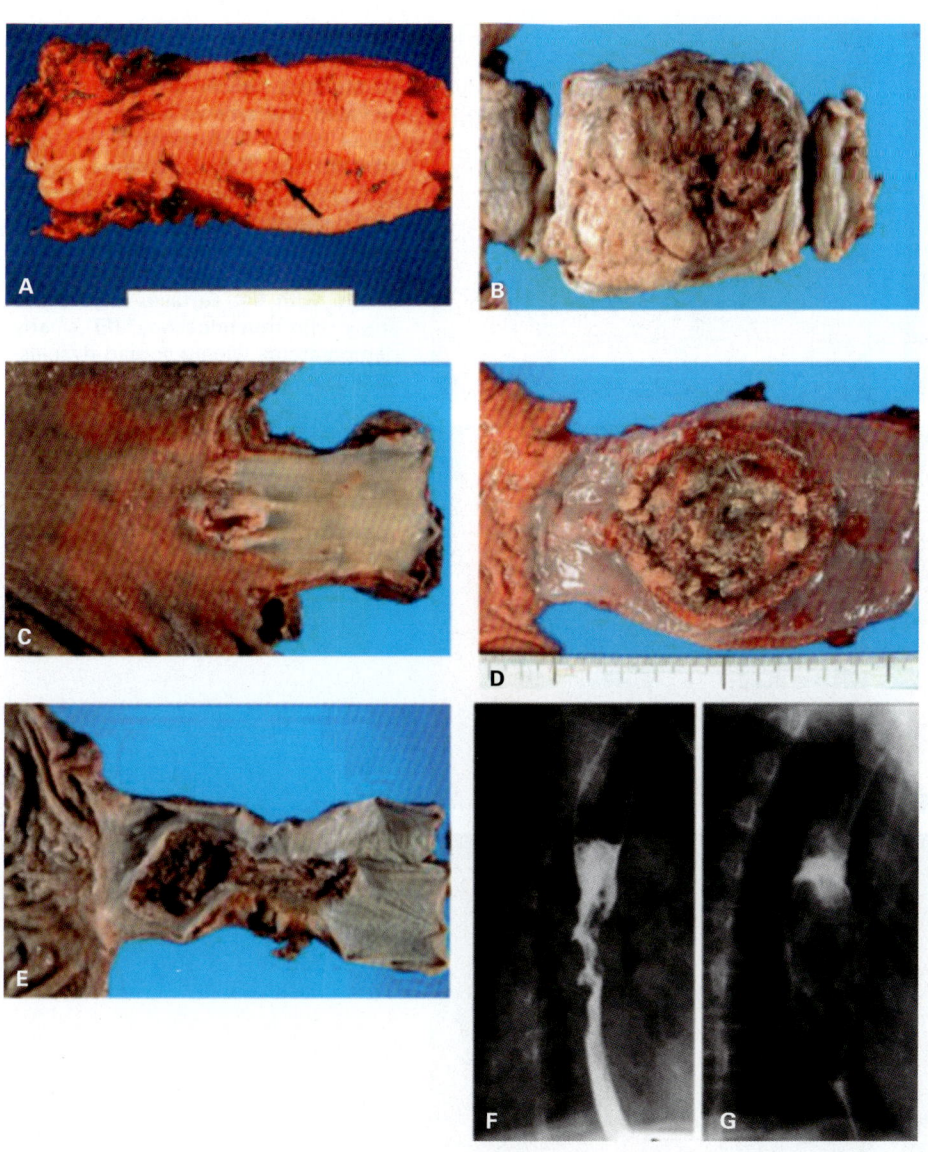

Figure 11-2. Gross appearances of squamous cell carcinoma. A: Small elevated tumor in which invasion is confined to the submucosa. B: Large exophytic and ulcerative mass occupying most of the circumference. C: Small ulcerative tumor with elevated ulcer edge. D: Large ulcerative tumor in which the elevated rim has partially collapsed. E: Ulcerative tumor infiltrating proximally. F: Radiograph of an esophageal stricture resulting from advanced carcinoma. G: Radiograph of an exophytic carcinoma dilating the esophagus.

series, rates of complete resection were 90% in tumors with no deviation of the axis on the barium swallow, 74% in those with deviation of the axis and with partial or complete response to chemoradiotherapy, and 51% in those with deviation of the axis and with no response to chemoradiotherapy, respectively.[33]

Invasive tumors limited to the mucosa or submucosa and with or without lymph node involvement were originally called superficial carcinomas by the Japanese authors,[56] and this concept is now generally accepted.[57] The definition of early esophageal carcinoma is different from that of early gastric carcinoma in Japan. The former is confined to mucosal carcinoma without lymph node metastasis, while the latter includes also submucosal carcinoma; this difference in the definition reflects a considerable prognostic difference in submucosal carcinoma.

Superficial carcinomas may appear papillary, protruding, plaque-like, erosive, or ulcerated, and sometimes may be invisible (flat), grossly or endoscopically, or may appear as a mucosal granularity, with or without erosions grossly (Fig. 11-3).[56] The detection of these lesions, as well as of carcinoma in situ, is enhanced by the use of Lugol's dye spray chromoendoscopy; both fail to stain, in contrast to the normal mucosa, which stains strongly because of its high glycogen content.[37] In one series, standard endoscopy and chromoendoscopy detected 55% and 100% of high-grade intraepithelial neoplasia, respectively.[58] Confocal endomicroscopy and narrow-band imaging has also been used to facilitate the detection of early lesions.[59,60] However, endoscopic diagnosis of submucosal invasion is not easy even if using high-resolution endosonography (EUS); sensitivity for submucosal tumors is around 50%.[61]

Submucosal extension of tumor may be marked in all forms of esophageal carcinoma and occurs

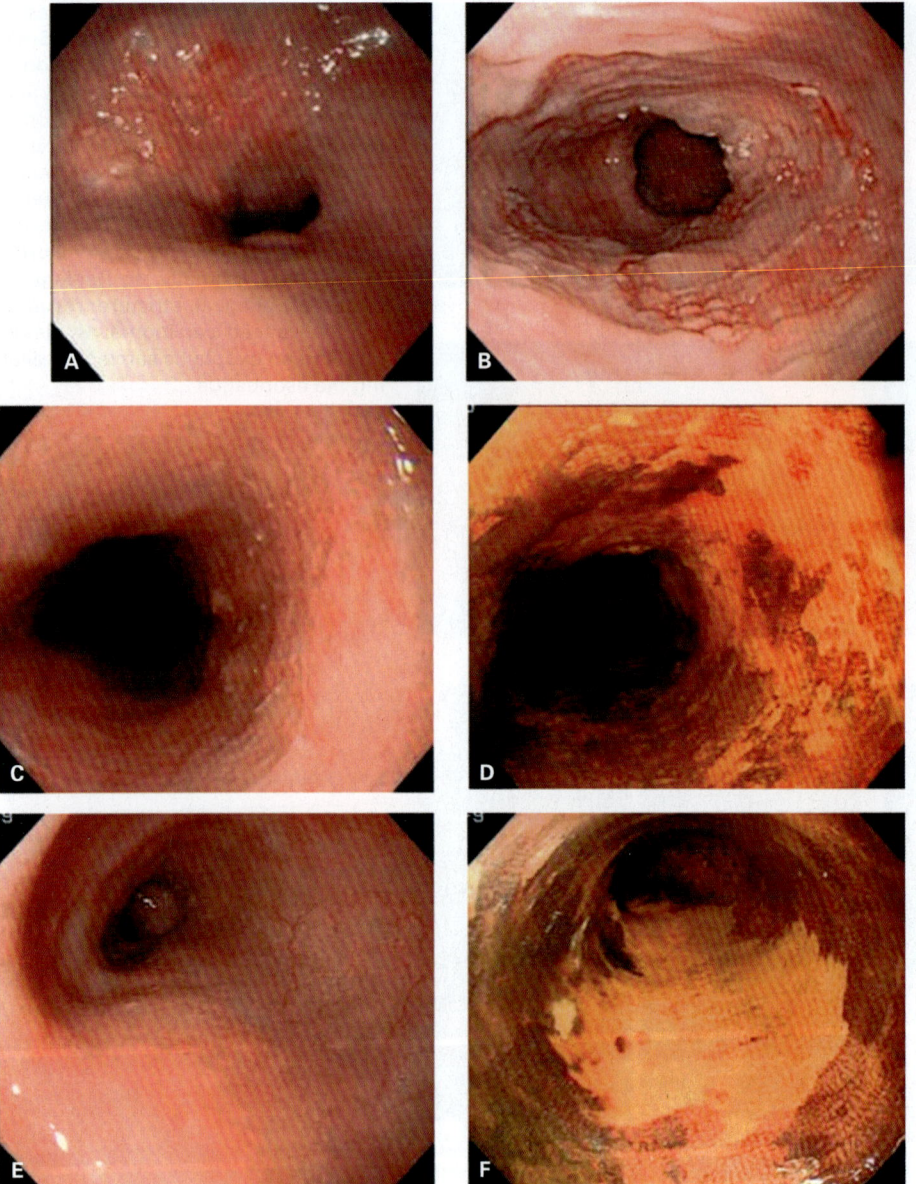

Figure 11-3. Endoscopic features of mucosal cancer and carcinoma in situ. **A:** Mucosal cancer showing slightly elevated and erosive lesion. **B:** Carcinoma in situ with granular and erosive surface. **C,D:** Carcinoma in situ with irregular surface. Lugol's dye spray chromoendoscopy **(D)** reveals widely spread lesions, most of which are severe dysplasia. **E,F:** Carcinoma in situ with flat surface. Lugol's dye spray chromoendoscopy **(F)** clearly demonstrates widely spread dysplastic areas.

primarily proximal to the tumor, particularly in the submucosal esophageal lymphatics. This has particular relevance at resection because it may be detected only microscopically. Frozen section of the proximal margin is advocated in all patients in whom, should unexpected submucosal tumor spread be found, the resection can be extended proximally. If submucosal tumor extension is marked, it may fill out the submucosal lymphatics to such a degree that they may resemble varices radiologically. This appearance has been termed varicoid carcinoma.[62] Endoscopically, there is little room for confusion because the bluish hue and softness of varices are not apparent.

Multiple tumors are encountered in about 15% of patients.[40,57] They may reflect either proximal submucosal tumor metastasis with ulceration of the overlying epithelium or truly multiple primaries. It can be argued that such metastases should lack dysplasia or carcinoma in situ in the immediately adjacent mucosa, but coincidental dysplasia or even intramucosal spread of carcinoma can never be entirely excluded, although the latter is quite rare. If small submucosal metastases are examined following radiotherapy, ulceration of the overlying epithelium may be seen. Such ulcers heal following the full course of radiotherapy, causing regression of the underlying tumor. This has been called the Ebb effect.[63]

When an esophageal cancer is diagnosed endoscopically unless there are known metastases and particularly if surgery is being contemplated, then the patient should undergo an EUS to stage the extent of local invasion.

Microscopic Appearances

The whole range of morphologic appearances can be found, from well-differentiated tumors to nests of poorly cohesive cells, or sometimes single cells, often in a desmoplastic stroma (Fig. 11-4). Well-differentiated tumors are characterized by squamous pearl formation, individual cell keratinization, and intercellular prickles; the keratinization has been interpreted as a sign of differentiation. The tumors, in which none of these features are found, may be diagnosed as poorly differentiated if the pattern of infiltration is similar to that found in other squamous cell carcinomas; we prefer to call them undifferentiated and add that they are most likely of squamous origin. Use of immunohistochemical markers (CK5/6 and P63) may help (see later). We are reluctant to call tumors squamous on the basis of intercellular bridges (prickles) alone unless such bridges are very well formed, as formalin fixation sometimes causes cytoplasmic retraction between cells, forming structures resembling prickles. Some tumors can only be inferred to be squamous because of the presence of dysplasia or carcinoma in situ in the overlying epithelium. Other variants include a pseudoglandular variant and a centrally necrotic variant (Fig. 11-5).

Grading tumors is very subjective and, unless reproducible, probably of little value. Some grade the best-differentiated areas, others the worst, and some use Broder's grading and try to assess the proportion of differentiating cells, with grade I having more than 75% keratinized cells, in 25% increments to grade IV, which has <25% of keratinized cells. Some grade IV tumors merge imperceptibly with anaplastic variants, some of which have the characteristics of small cell undifferentiated tumors. Grading is probably of little prognostic significance, this being largely related to tumor stage, although one study[64] suggests that in superficial carcinoma, lymph node metastasis is liable to occur in the tumors with high nuclear atypia and infiltrative growth pattern. Apart from the cellular atypia, the presence of lymphocyte infiltration around cancerous lesions results in favorable prognosis;

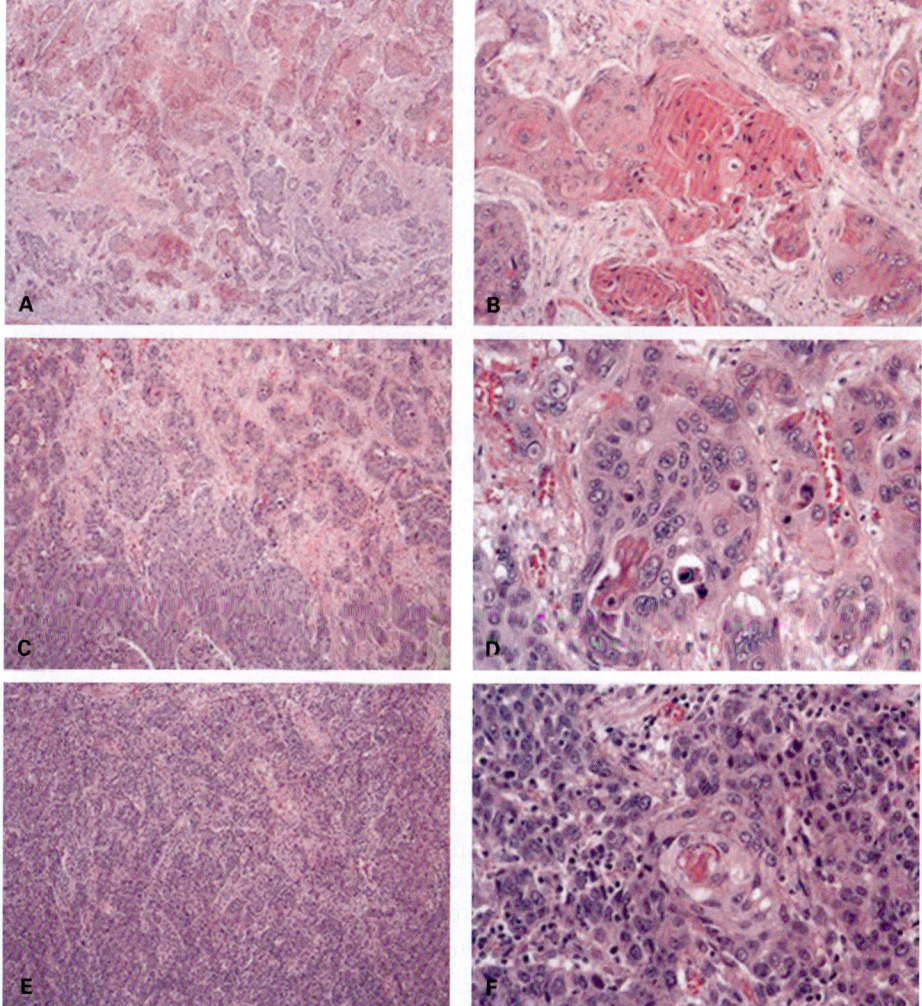

Figure 11-4. The degrees of differentiation in squamous cell carcinoma. The keratinization has been interpreted as a sign of differentiation. **A,B:** Well-differentiated squamous cell carcinoma characterized by numerous squamous pearls. **C,D:** In moderately differentiated squamous cell carcinoma, squamous pearl formation and individual cell keratinization are not numerous but can be found easily. **E,F:** Nests of poorly differentiated squamous cell carcinoma show minimal keratinization. Carcinomas without keratinization or well-formed intercellular bridges are diagnosed as undifferentiated rather than squamous.

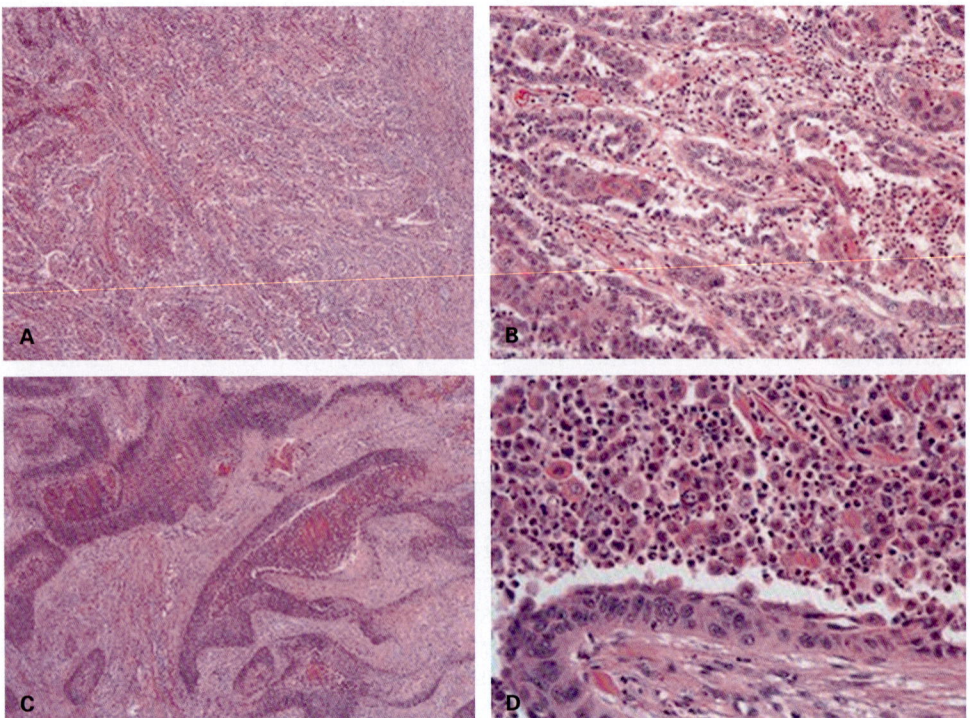

Figure 11-5. Variants of squamous cell carcinoma. **A,B:** Pseudoglandular variant resembles adenocarcinoma, but keratinization can be seen and mucin stains are negative. **C,D:** Centrally necrosing variant giving a comedocarcinoma-like appearance. The similarity to the pseudoglandular variant can be appreciated, but numerous necrotic tumor cells are present in the lumen.

the 5-year survival rates of patients with marked and minimal lymphocyte infiltration were reported to be 75.5% and 27.8%, respectively.[65]

Spread of Tumor, Staging, and Prognosis

Esophageal carcinoma presenting with symptoms has a very poor prognosis, because its clinicopathological characteristics include the frequent presence of intraepithelial spread, blood vessel and lymphatic permeation, and consequently intramural and lymph node metastasis. Widespread lymphatic dissemination can be present at the time of exploratory thoracoceliotomy even in individuals who do not appear to have metastatic disease clinically. In one series, all of the patients with carcinoma of the lower third of the esophagus and approximately 45% of those with carcinoma of the middle third had celiac node involvement.[66] A major factor in the high mortality of this disease is that 30% to 40% of patients have evidence of advanced local or metastatic disease at presentation; in one series the mean time from first symptoms to autopsy was 10.6 months,[67] although there are increasing data that chemoradiotherapy, particularly that includes cisplatin, can cause considerable shrinkage of tumor, and sometimes prolonged remission even in advanced tumors. The introduction of preoperative chemoradiotherapy resulted in more curative (R0—no residual disease) resections, increasing from 63% to 78% to 79% to 94% of patients.[2,4,7] However, a meta-analysis across six studies showed that neoadjuvant chemoradiotherapy followed by surgery had only a small, nonstatistically significant trend toward improved survival.[6] Even after R0 resection, overall 1-, 3-, and 5-year survival rates are 91%, 54%, and 41%, respectively; the pattern of recurrence is local in 12%, regional in 21%, and distant in 20%.[68] The perioperative mortality for esophageal resection was on the order of $10 \pm 5\%$ in the past but is now 1.2% to 6% in many recent reports, although this does depend on patient selection.[2,4,7,10,69–73]

TNM classification. Posttherapy pathologic stage was the best available predictor of outcome for patients with esophageal carcinoma.[74] The depth of invasion and the presence of nodal or distant metastases are independent predictors of survival, and these are reflected in the recent TNM classification, being the most widely used staging system. The classification is summarized as follows:

T0 is high-grade dysplasia (see previous discussion—includes the former carcinoma in situ)

T1 invades the lamina propria or muscularis mucosae (T1a) or submucosa (T1b)

T2 invades the muscularis propria

T3 invades the adventitia

T4 invades adjacent structures (Pleura, pericardium or diaphragm—T4a), or other adjacent structures (e.g., aorta, vertebral bodies, trachea, etc., T4b)

Lymph nodes and distant metastases are classified as negative (0), positive (1), or inaccessible (x), for example, N0 (no regional metastases), N1 (1–2 positive nodes), N2 (3–6 positive nodes), N3 (7 or more positive nodes), M0 (no distant metastases), M1 (distant metastases, or unknown NX, MX).[75]

Local spread and prognostic factors

T Stage The most important factor for prognosis is the histopathological extent of tumor spread. Advanced T stage is a factor predictive of recurrent disease and an independent prognostic indicator.[8,68,76,77] After R0 resection with histologically node-negative (pN0), the survival for patients with T2 or T3 tumors is significantly worse than for those with Tis or T1 tumors.[8] T1 tumors with and without lymph node involvement have a 5-year survival in excess of 60% and 75%, respectively.[78–80] Intraluminal polypoid or pedunculated tumors and verrucous carcinomas are particularly likely to be in this group.[81] Lymph node metastasis is rarely found in tumors limited to the lamina propria or muscularis mucosae, but occurs in about 40% of tumors invading the submucosa.[64,80,82] (See also subsequent section on superficial esophageal carcinoma.) In T2 and T3 tumors, the 5-year survival rate drops to 30% and 10%, respectively[83]; however, these rates are more than 50% and 30% in patients successfully undergoing R0 esophagectomy with 3-field lymphadenectomy.[69] The tumor size is an additional independent predictor of mortality when controlling for depth of invasion in patients with localized disease.[3,84] In one series, cause-specific 5-year survival is 51% for tumors ≤3 cm in diameter, 32% for 3.1 to 4 cm, and 16% for 4.1 to 5 cm; no patient with a tumor ≥6 cm survived.[85]

Lymphovascular invasion allows nodal metastasis and hematogenous dissemination and thus results in a frequent tumor relapse and a poor prognosis.[77] Vascular endothelial growth factor (VEGF)-C may play a role in tumor progression via lymphangiogenesis and angiogenesis.[86] Lymphatic invasion is an independent prognostic factor; in one series the 5-year survival rate in patients with lymphatic invasion is 11.1%, compared with 46.6% in those without the invasion.[87]

Intramural metastases, probably via a lymphatic duct, are associated with an advanced stage of disease and with a shorter survival.

Radial margin There is some evidence that the presence of tumor within 1 mm of the circumferential margin following potentially curative resection is an important prognostic factor[88] and that a wide proximal margin of excision of at least 10 cm and extensive radical lymphadenectomy may improve survival.[89]

Lymph node metastasis indicates a poor prognosis; 5-year survival is 80% and 25% for node-negative and positive patients, respectively.[69] Recent studies have also demonstrated that both the number of positive lymph nodes and the ratio of positive to negative lymph nodes have a prognostic significance.[76,84,90] The 2009 CAP guidelines divide these into

_____ pN1: Regional lymph node metastasis involving 1 to 2 nodes
_____ pN2: 3 to 6 nodes involved
_____ pN3: 7 or more nodes involved

In patients with T3 tumor, 5-year survival rates for those without, those with pN1 or pN2 or higher stage are approximately 50%, 30%, and 10%, respectively.[90] Because there is no significant correlation between lymph node size and the frequency of nodal metastases, evaluation of the nodal status is entirely based on histologic analysis.[91] For accurately defining pN category, it is recommended that more than 12 nodes should be examined histologically.[92] Another study from the United States suggested a minimum number of 18 lymph nodes to be examined in such cases.[93]

Immunohistochemical detection of lymph node micrometastasis may be an indicator of lymphatic dissemination of tumor cells, but is not associated with recurrence-free survival rate.[8,77]

Effect of chemotherapy and irradiation. There is an increasing trend toward preoperative chemoradiotherapy, particularly with regimens employing cisplatin and 5-fluorouracil, since patients with squamous cell carcinoma tend to have better progression-free survival with this therapy than those with nonsquamous tumors.[94] A meta-analysis of randomized controlled trials showed that preoperative chemoradiotherapy is associated with a lower rate of esophageal resection but a higher rate of complete resection, and that this therapy does not increase treatment-related mortality.[5] However, chemoradiotherapy followed by surgery does not significantly improve overall survival for patients with advanced esophageal cancer compared with surgery alone,[3,5,6,73,94] although patients downstaged to pathologic stage 0 or I have a longer survival than those patients who were not downstaged.[73] Note that esophageal biopsy after chemoradiation therapy is not a sensitive (sensitivity 23%) predictor of residual cancer following esophagectomy.[95] The prolonged survival in responders is evident also in chemotherapy plus surgery; 5-year survivals for complete responders, nonresponders, and patients with surgery alone are 60%, 12%, and 26%, respectively.[4] Radiation therapy is very effective for tumors limited to the mucosa and considered to be an alternative modality when endoscopic mucosal resection (EMR) or surgical treatment cannot be available.[96] However, chemoradiotherapy should be considered for patients with tumor invading into the submucosa, since recurrences are noted in 30% of these patients treated by irradiation alone.[96]

2009 CAP guidelines suggest the following for assessment of treatment effects (http://www.cap.org/apps/docs/committees/cancer/cancer_protocols/2009/Esophagus_09protocol.pdf):

No viable cancer cells	0 (Complete response)
Single cells or small groups of cancer cells	1 (Moderate response)
Residual cancer outgrown by fibrosis	2 (Minimal response)
Minimal or no tumor kill; extensive residual cancer	3 (Poor response)

DNA ploidy. The nuclear DNA ploidy is determined by flow cytometry or image analysis. In patients with esophageal squamous cell carcinoma, diploid DNA histogram patterns are usually observed not only in cancer cells but also in nonpathologic tissues, either distant or proximal to the lesion.[97] Aneuploidy of cancer cells is identified in 55% to 95%, but not statistically associated with the differentiation of the tumor.[97,98] It has been suggested that early malignant changes in the esophagus are already associated with alteration in DNA content, and that aneuploidy tends to correlate with progression to invasive cancer; in one series, aneuploidy was observed in 63% of early carcinomas and 91% of advanced carcinomas.[97] However, it is unclear whether ploidy status represents an independent variable for prognosis. A prognostic impact independent of tumor stage has been shown only in a few studies,[99,100] whereas the majority of studies have not verified this finding.[98] One study suggested that aneuploid tumors may be more sensitive to chemoradiotherapy with hyperthermia.[101]

Molecular factors as prognosticator. There is growing evidence that preoperative genetic assessment of biopsy specimens provides useful information concerning selection of treatment modalities. Preoperative chemoradiotherapy is a recent trend and pathologic complete responders have a significant better 5-year survival rate compared with nonresponders. The good response to this therapy has been suggested in tumors with strong expression of 14-3-3 sigma (one of the p53 family proteins) or CDC25B, while expressions of p53, metallothionein, and COX-2 are associated with the poor response.[102] The combined evaluation of these biomarkers may therefore help to identify patients who will benefit from chemoradiotherapy.[103-105]

Matrix metalloproteinases (MMPs) such as MMP-2, MMP-7, MMP-9, stomelysin-3 (MMP-11), and MMP-13 have been thought to function in an early stage of squamous cell carcinoma.[106,107] The expression of MMP-9 is mainly found in cancer cells at the invasive front and is positively correlated with existence of vessel permeation and lymph node metastasis.[107,108] Regarding the prognostic impact, the coexpression of MMP-7, MMP-9, and MMP-13, and the combined phenotype of positive stomelysin-3 and negative tissue inhibitors of MMP-2 may be adverse prognosticators for relatively early stage tumors.[106-108] The diminished expression of E-cadherin correlates to poor prognosis,[109] but a Cox multivariate analysis revealed that the expression of dysadherin, which downregulates E-cadherin expression and promotes metastasis, is an independent prognostic factor.[110] Other potential indicators of poor survival include p53 null mutation, endothelin (vasoactive peptide), VEGF, fascin (actine bundling protein), PGP9.5 methylation, Mina53 (a novel Myc target gene), valosin-containing protein (VCP), survivin, and EphA2 (a receptor tyrosine kinases).[86,111-118] The reduced expressions of transforming growth factor-beta (TGF-β) receptors, gamma-catenin, mismatch repair gene MLH1, and bcl-2 are also candidates predicting poor survival.[48,109,119,120] However, the majority of these genetic factors are closely associated with pathologic stage. It is unclear, therefore, whether these factors represent independent indicators for prognosis.

Failure and causes of death. These can be divided into perioperative death within 30 days of resection and death related to the tumor growth such as local recurrence and distant metastasis. An increased risk of the perioperative death includes increasing age at diagnosis, increasing tumor size and depth of invasion, and impaired preoperative respiratory function.[72,84] Apart from progression of the tumor, pulmonary complications and anastomotic failure are the leading causes of perioperative death; these account for about 50% and 10% of deaths, respectively.[3,121] The pulmonary complications, which are also the most common causes of morbidity, consist of pneumonia, atelectasis, adult respiratory distress syndrome, pleural effusion, tracheal fistula, and chylothorax.[3] The perioperative mortality has decreased dramatically; it was on the order of 10% ± 5% in the past but is now 1.2% to 6% in many recent reports.[2,4,7,10,69-73,121] This improvement might be due to exclusion of high-risk patients from surgical resection,[70] induction of preoperative chemoradiotherapy, or both.[2] The latter reason may be controversial as there are conflicting results suggesting that hospital mortality is higher in patients with chemoradiotherapy and surgery than in those undergoing surgery alone.[122] On the other hand, a meta-analysis of randomized controlled trials showed that preoperative chemoradiotherapy does not increase treatment-related mortality.[5]

Metastases to other organs, particularly liver, lung, and bone occur in 25% to 30% of patients within the first 3 years, and 40% to 45% of patients develop nodal metastases in the superior mediastinum, supraclavicular fossa, or cervical lymph nodes within 5 years. Between 5 and 10 years, 30% of all deaths are due to late recurrence of tumor. At autopsy, local recurrence is prominent in 50% to 75% of patients, with direct invasion into every conceivable adjacent structure, particularly the trachea and bronchus in about 40%, tracheoesophageal fistula being the cause of death in 10% to 15%. Nodal deposits are common; the mediastinal and cervical nodes are positive in about half and the intra-abdominal nodes in a quarter of the patients. Haematogenous dissemination is also common and is present in about half of the patients, affecting the lung in 25% to 30%, the liver in 20%, the bone in 10% to 15%, and the adrenal, thyroid, and other organs in 10% or less.[67,123] Bronchopneumonia is the most common immediate cause of death and is associated with tracheoesophageal or bronchoesophageal fistulae in a high proportion of cases.[67] In rare cases aortoesophageal fistula may form leading to torrential upper GI hemorrhage and death from exsanguination.

UNUSUAL VARIANTS OF SQUAMOUS CELL CARCINOMA

Superficial Esophageal Carcinoma

Superficial esophageal carcinoma is an early form of invasive carcinoma, with involvement limited to the mucosa or submucosa, and represents the esophageal counterpart of early gastric cancer[56,57]; in Japan, the term "early esophageal carcinoma" is used only for a mucosal carcinoma with or without nodal metastasis, since the implication of early cancer is that of a good prognosis. According to the 2010 WHO classification, this term is defined irrespective of the presence or absence of lymph node involvement. The lesions vary from <1 cm to 5 cm in size, may involve varying proportion of the wall, sometimes even being circumferential, and present grossly as mucosal irregularity that may be coarse at one extreme and flat at the other, only being identifiable using Lugol's iodine.[57] Protruded and plaque-like lesions are more frequent among submucosal cancers, whereas most flat lesions are mucosal cancers.[124] Superficial carcinomas carry a much better prognosis than conventional squamous cell carcinomas; the tumors with and without lymph node involvement have a 5-year survival in excess of 60% and 75%, respectively.[78-80]

Endoscopic mucosal resection. Superficial carcinomas have lymph node metastasis in 20% to 40% of patients,[80,82,125] and the highest figures are obtained in those with an ulceroinfiltrative gross appearance.[57] Two major histologic factors associated with nodal metastasis are tumor depth and lymphatic invasion.[64,82,125] In a large series of superficial squamous carcinomas,[125] nodal metastasis was noted in

0% of m1 (intraepithelial) tumors, (dysplasia)

5.6% of m2 tumors limited to the lamina propria but not reaching the muscularis mucosae

18.0% of m3 tumors, defined as both invading the muscularis mucosae but also in contact with or invading the muscularis mucosa. (Recall that in the esophagus, the lamina propria is also beneath the epithelium with a gap between the base of the squamous or glandular mucosa and the muscularis mucosae, although it can be lost in Barrett's esophagus. Also, the distinction between m2 and m3 can be difficult or impossible in biopsies, as the orientation may be suboptimal, while if there are no muscularis mucosae, as is often the case, it is impossible to determine whether it has been reached.)

53.1% of sm1 tumors invading the shallowest 1/3 of the submucosa

53.9% of sm2/sm3 tumors invading deeper than the sm1 level (Fig. 11-6). So effectively once in the submucosa about a half of all carcinomas have nodal metastses (Note: For surgically resected specimens, the submucosal layer is evenly divided into three (sm1, sm2, and sm3), as the entire submucosa can be seen. However, in endoscopically resected specimens, sm1 is defined as <200 microns, sm2 ≥200 microns, and sm3 can not be defined.)

The majority of other studies also support that carcinomas invading beyond the lamina propria run the risk of nodal metastasis and recurrence, and stress that only patients with m1/m2 lesions (see subsequent discussion) are good candidates for EMR and endoscopic submucosal dissection (ESD), the latter of which enables en bloc resection for large lesions (Fig. 11-7).[64,126,127] However, note that multiple Lugol-voiding lesions are an independent risk factor for local recurrence after EMR, with the cumulative local recurrence rates of 39% and 14% in patients with and without these multiple lesions, respectively.[128] Before considering EMR or ESD an EUS must be performed.

The ducts of esophageal glands may be involved by superficial carcinomas. In one series, 43 (21.3%) of 201 superficial carcinomas had ductal involvement, which always remained in situ; lymph node metastasis was rarely found and the 5-year survival rate was 100% in the patients having mucosal cancer even with ductal involvement extending to the submucosal layer.[129] The ductal involvement itself is of little significance in squamous cell carcinoma, and therefore the in situ extending to the submucosa should not be classified as submucosal carcinoma.

Superficial spreading carcinoma. Superficial spreading carcinoma is defined as superficial carcinoma measuring >5 cm and consisting mainly of intraepithelial carcinoma.[130,131] These lesions make up about 20% of superficial carcinomas. Between superficial spreading and nonspreading carcinomas, there is no significant difference in lymphatic invasion, venous invasion, intramural metastasis, or lymph node metastasis.[131] However, patients with spreading type

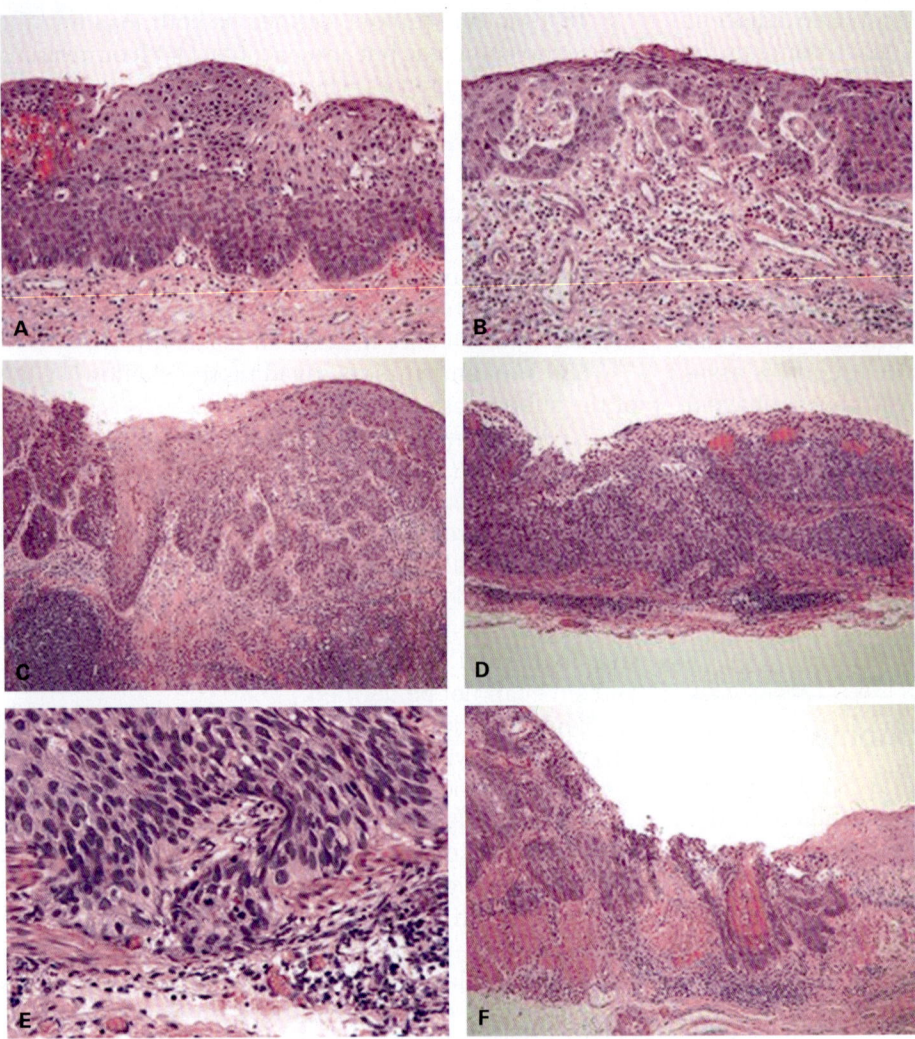

Figure 11-6. Superficial squamous cell carcinoma. (Depth determines the likelihood of nodal metastases being present.) **A:** M1 tumor synonymous with dysplasia, or, as seen here, carcinoma in situ. **B,C:** The m2 tumors invade into the lamina propria but do not reach the muscularis mucosae. **D,E:** The m3 tumors are in contact with or invading the muscularis mucosae. **F:** This sm1 tumor invades just though the muscularis mucosae and so has just reached the superficial one-third of the submucosa.

carcinoma have a higher prevalence of associated multiple cancerous lesions.[130] Preoperative examination to detect the resection margin should include Lugol's dye spray chromoendoscopy.

Verrucous Carcinoma

Verrucous carcinoma is a rare and relatively indolent variant of squamous cell carcinoma. Its appearance is similar to that of verrucous carcinoma occurring in other organs such as the mouth, larynx, and anus. It is an exophytic papillary tumor that grows slowly and has virtually no metastasizing potential. Invasion is often relatively limited locally, but the tumor may infiltrate through the wall of the esophagus, involve pericardium or pleura, and even line subsequent fistula tracts. The importance of these lesions is that their prognosis seems to be considerably better than that of the usual squamous cell carcinoma, but they can be very difficult to diagnose in biopsies (Fig. 11-8).

Cytological atypia in verrucous carcinoma tends to be minimal and located primarily in the basal layer. Single cell keratinization may also be present. The tumor is characterized by papillary fronds with a delicate fibrovascular stalk, by marked acanthosis and parakeratosis with broad pegs, sometimes central areas of degenerated keratin within these pegs, and some degree of vacuolation superficially; the last is, of course, entirely nonspecific and thus is of little help. On biopsy, unless the papillary architecture and basal dysplasia can be identified, it may be almost impossible to distinguish this lesion from squamous papilloma. Because the tumor surface consists of well-differentiated squamous epithelium, superficial biopsies may be reported as benign. Even deep biopsies may be inadequate to make the diagnosis, which may depend on knowledge both of the lesion's existence and of the problems of biopsy interpretation of these tumors (Fig. 11-8) so that the possibility of this being the underlying lesion can be raised.[132]

Small foci of minimal invasion may be present, which helps make the diagnosis of carcinoma (Fig. 11-8). Some prefer to call this very well differentiated squamous carcinoma, but they still have no

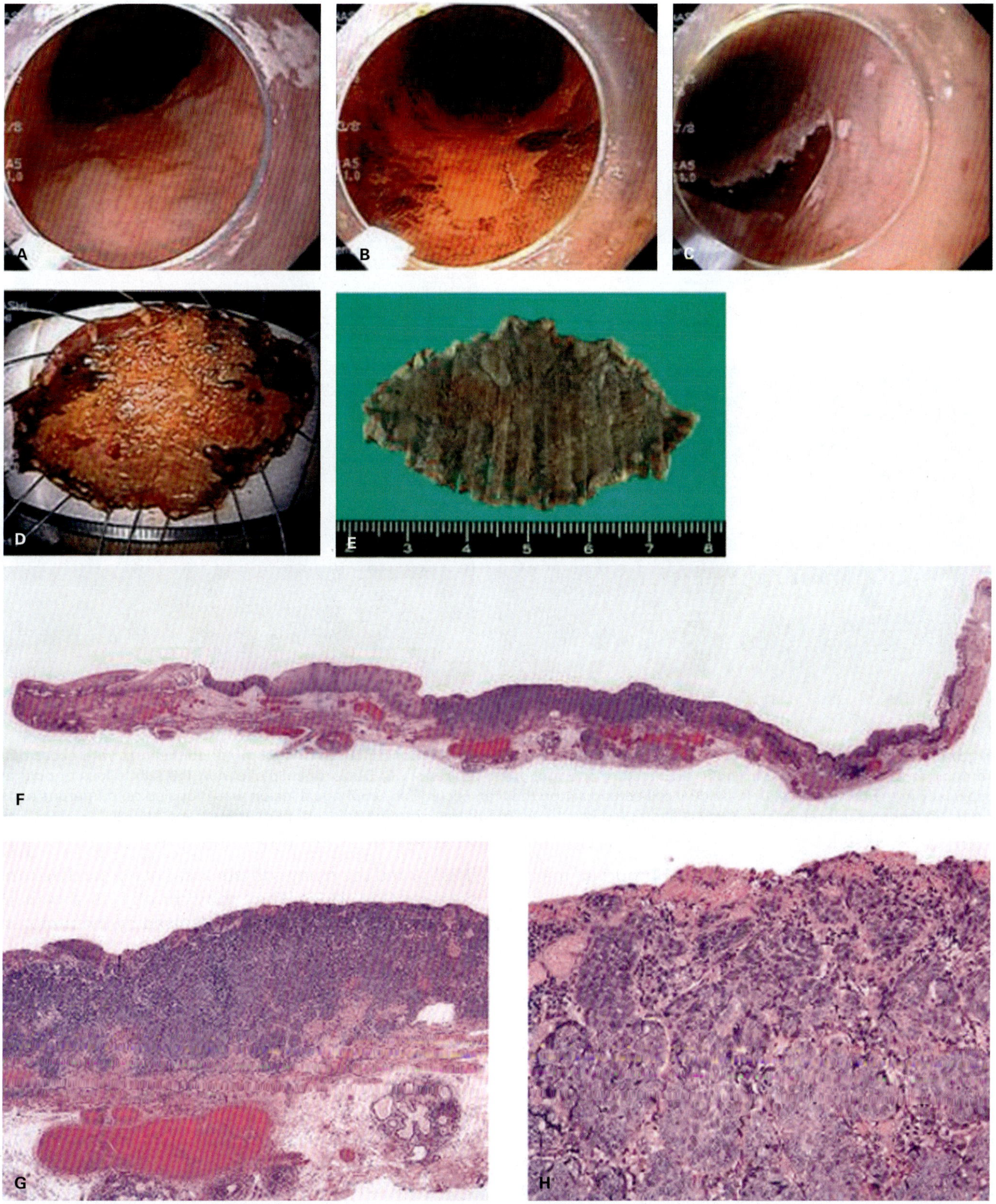

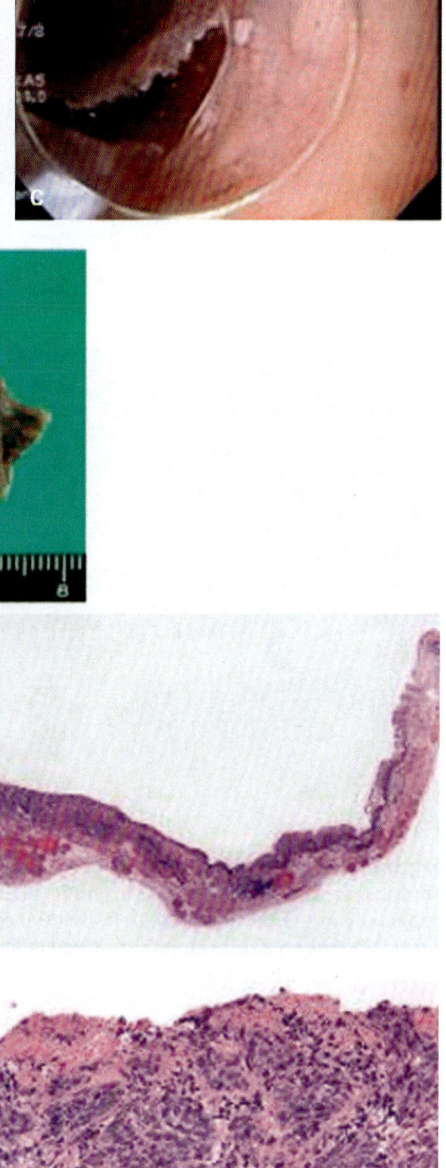

Figure 11-7. ESD for superficial squamous cell carcinoma. **A,B:** Superficial carcinoma is often poorly circumscribed but Lugol's dye spray chromoendoscopy can clearly detect the whole area of the dysplastic lesion. **C,D:** ESD enables en bloc resection for superficial carcinoma. **E:** The resected specimen is serially cut to examine depth of invasion and condition of all margins. **F–H:** This m3 tumor reaching to or into, but not through, the muscularis mucosae was completely resected with free margins. (Courtesy of Dr. Y. Sasaki M.D.)

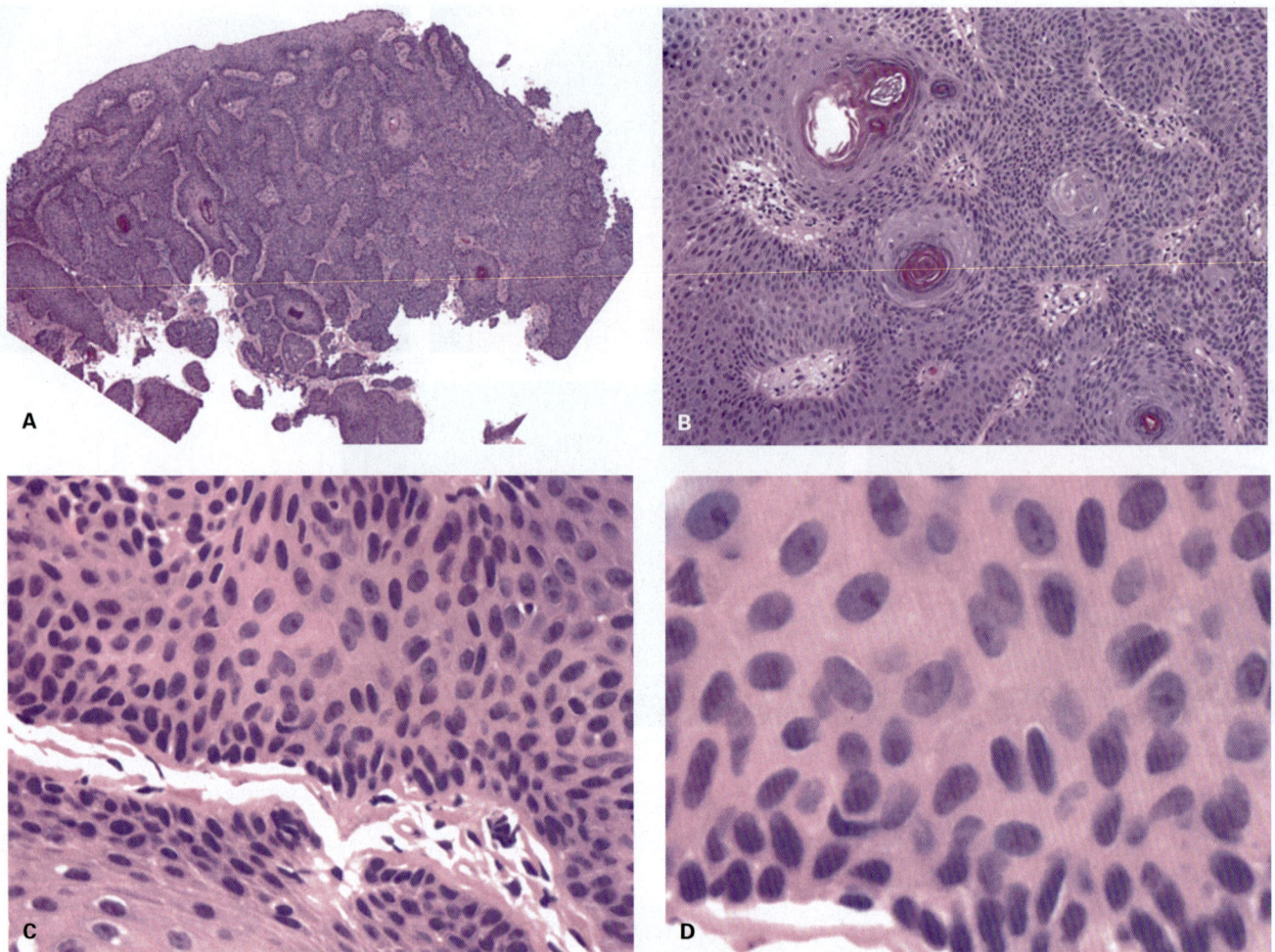

Figure 11-8. Esophageal verrucous carcinoma. **A:** Overview with anastomosing cords of squamous epithelium, with occasional keratin pearls. **B:** Detail of the irregular architecture and foci of keratinization. **C:** Detail of cells showing the subtle loss of polarity especially in the basal layers. **D:** Individual cell keratinization that can occur. This esophageal lesion was biopsied on numerous occasions, and when exploratory surgery was attempted was found to infiltrate into the adjacent pericardium and pleura.

metastasizing potential, so it is still appropriate to call this verrucous carcinoma.

Spindle Cell Carcinoma

This unusual variant of squamous cell carcinoma is also known by a variety of other terms such as carcinosarcoma, pseudosarcomatous squamous cell carcinoma, polypoid carcinoma, and squamous cell carcinoma with a spindle cell component. It occurs predominantly in the middle and lower esophagus, and often presents as a polypoid lesion containing an exuberant spindle cell component.[133–136] Survival figures suggest an overall 5-year mortality rate of 50% to 60%, with a better prognosis because of a relatively small number of patients with infiltration through the muscularis propria.[133,137]

Gross appearances. These tumors may reach a considerable size; tumors up to 15 cm in diameter have been reported.[138] Their surface is often ulcerated superficially, and they may contain areas of hemorrhage and necrosis (Fig. 11-9). They are typically on a pedicle, but the pedicle may become involved by the tumor, so that its polypoid nature is less apparent.[134,135,139]

Microscopic appearances. The histologic hallmark of these tumors is the presence of malignant epithelial and spindle cell elements, sometimes with evidence of mesenchymal differentiation. The epithelial component is almost invariably squamous, although adenocarcinoma and undifferentiated carcinoma have been reported.[132,138] The squamous component is variable, ranging from an obvious infiltrating squamous cell carcinoma to only dysplastic epithelium or carcinoma in situ in the mucosa immediately overlying or adjacent to the tumor (Fig. 11-9). The spindle cell component is also variable. At one end of the spectrum, these cells are rather innocuous with virtually no pleomorphism and few or no mitotic figures. In these cases, murine double minute-2 (MDM2) and

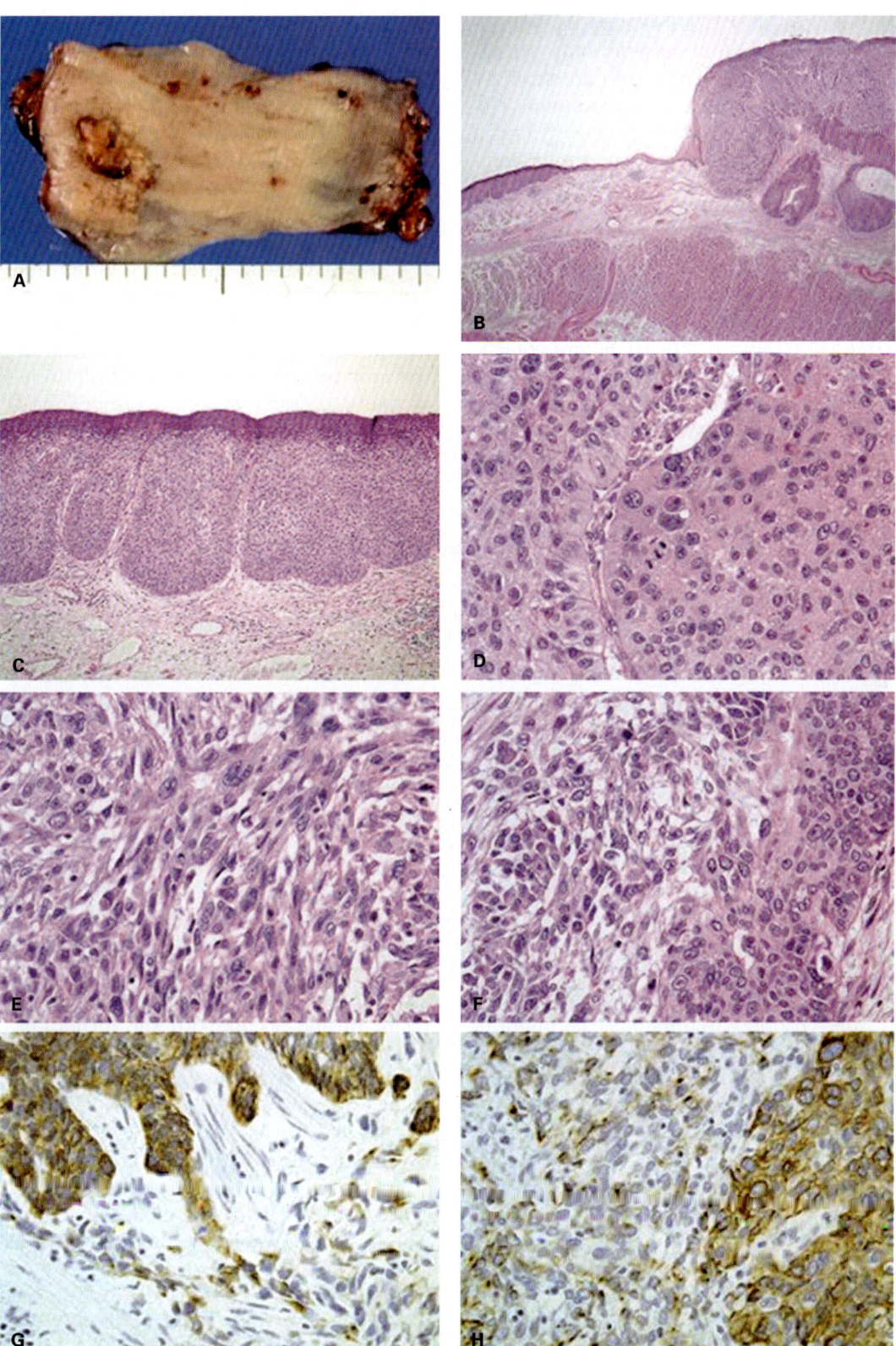

Figure 11-9. Spindle cell carcinoma. **A,B:** Gross appearance and scanning view of spindle cell carcinomas, which characteristically have a polypoid component. **C:** Detail of the adjacent flat mucosa showing carcinoma in situ; the serial sections demonstrated that the lesion was continuous with the polypoid tumor. **D:** Detail of the polypoid tumor showing conventional poorly differentiated squamous cell carcinoma with individual cell keratinization. **E:** Spindle cell component with nuclear pleomorphism and mitotic figures. **F:** The transitional part between squamous and spindle components. **G,H:** Keratin immunoreactivity in some of the spindle cells as well as squamous cells. (Courtesy of Dr. H. Kawasaki M.D.)

cycline-dependent kinase 4 (CDK4) may be helpful to distinguish spindle cell element from only prominent stromal reaction; MDM2 and CDK4 are strongly positive in both carcinomatous and sarcomatous elements, but not in the reactive stromal cells.[140] At the other extreme, the spindle cell component is composed of more pleomorphic cells, occasionally with bizarre giant cells and numerous mitoses. The entire spectrum may exist within the same tumor and even in the same histologic section. Larger cells may bear a striking resemblance to rhabdomyoblasts, and cross-striations can sometimes be seen within the cytoplasm, confirming that they are true rhabdomyoblasts. Other mesenchymal components that may be found within these tumors include smooth muscle, cartilage, osteoid, bone, and myxoid or fibrohistiocytic tissue. In some tumors, one component may completely dominate the morphology, which may explain the description of rhabdomyosarcomas and osteogenic sarcomas in the esophagus. The significance for the pathologist is that even armed with this knowledge, it may be impossible to find a focus of dysplasia or invasive squamous carcinoma to confirm the histogenesis of these purely spindle cell or apparent mesenchymal tumors. One case seen by us was ultimately reported as a leiomyosarcoma, evidence of its origin being apparent only in a subsequent cerebral metastasis.

Histogenesis. The confusion has arisen because different proportions of any one or several elements have resulted in a variety of interpretations of their histogenesis and their relationship to each other. In 1957, two publications[135,141] described a subgroup of these tumors having either dysplasia or small foci of infiltrating squamous cell carcinoma in the overlying squamous mucosa, accompanied by an exuberant spindle cell component that was often bizarre. It was thought that this "pseudosarcomatous" component was benign and never metastasized, although rare instances of metastases occurred from the associated well-differentiated infiltrating squamous cell carcinoma. The authors proposed the term pseudosarcoma for these tumors in order to emphasize the benign nature of the spindle cell component and to separate them from genuine carcinosarcomas in which either or both of these elements were noted to be capable of metastasis. However, evidence accumulated that cast doubt on the benignity of the pseudosarcomatous element of these tumors. Both local recurrence and lymph node metastases of pseudosarcoma were documented.[133,137] These findings and critical reviews[54,134,139] suggested that the spindle cell element occurring in pseudosarcomas was neoplastic, albeit with a relatively low metastasizing potential.

Electron microscopy and immunocytochemistry of the spindle cell component showed a range of features that added to the confusion in terminology regarding these tumors. Some reports suggested that these spindle cells show only mesenchymal characteristics.[133,142] In contrast, the majority of other reports showed the spindle cell component to contain tonofilaments and desmosomes, as seen in squamous cell carcinomas, thereby suggesting that this element was derived from squamous epithelium and is in fact a spindle cell variant of squamous cell carcinoma.[137,139,140,142] Immunocytochemically, the spindle cell component is invariably vimentin positive and frequently keratin positive; vimentin positivity may also be present in the carcinomatous component.[136,137] In our experience, p63 is also frequently positive in the spindle cell component. In addition, p53 protein is overexpressed in most tumors, and the similar expression pattern in the two components suggests their common origin.[136]

Squamous cell carcinoma therefore develop a spindle cell component, which may retain epithelial features, as reflected by electron microscopy or immunohistochemistry, and that this component may undergo further transformation or metaplasia to one that, while retaining a spindle cell appearance, is essentially mesenchymal. This transition was noted by electron microscopy and it was pointed out that although the cytoplasmic features of some of the spindle cells were mesenchymal, they retained the nuclear characteristics in the component showing evidence of squamous differentiation.[142] Handra-Luca et al.[136] found that E-cadherin was expressed in the carcinomatous component of most tumors but absent in the spindle cell component. Loss of E-cadherin expression therefore appears to be associated with the acquisition of spindle cell morphology. Further, it is apparent that once mesenchymal transformation has occurred within this population of cells, they may continue to differentiate along a variety of mesenchymal pathways. This may result in and account for the formation of the other mesenchymal elements such as fibroblasts, myofibroblasts, cartilage, osteoid, bone, myxoid tissue, and both smooth and striated muscle cells.

Biopsy diagnosis. Interpretation of multiple biopsies from these tumors may cause diagnostic problems due to the presence of elements mentioned above. The unwary pathologist may therefore interpret such a specimen as indicating a benign mesenchymal tumor (e.g., leiomyoma), resulting in inadequate surgical treatment. The biopsy of any polypoid tumor of the esophagus should lead to consideration that this may be the underlying lesion, with recognition of its potential malignancy.

Small Cell Carcinoma

Small cell carcinomas of the esophagus are indistinguishable from their pulmonary counterparts (see also

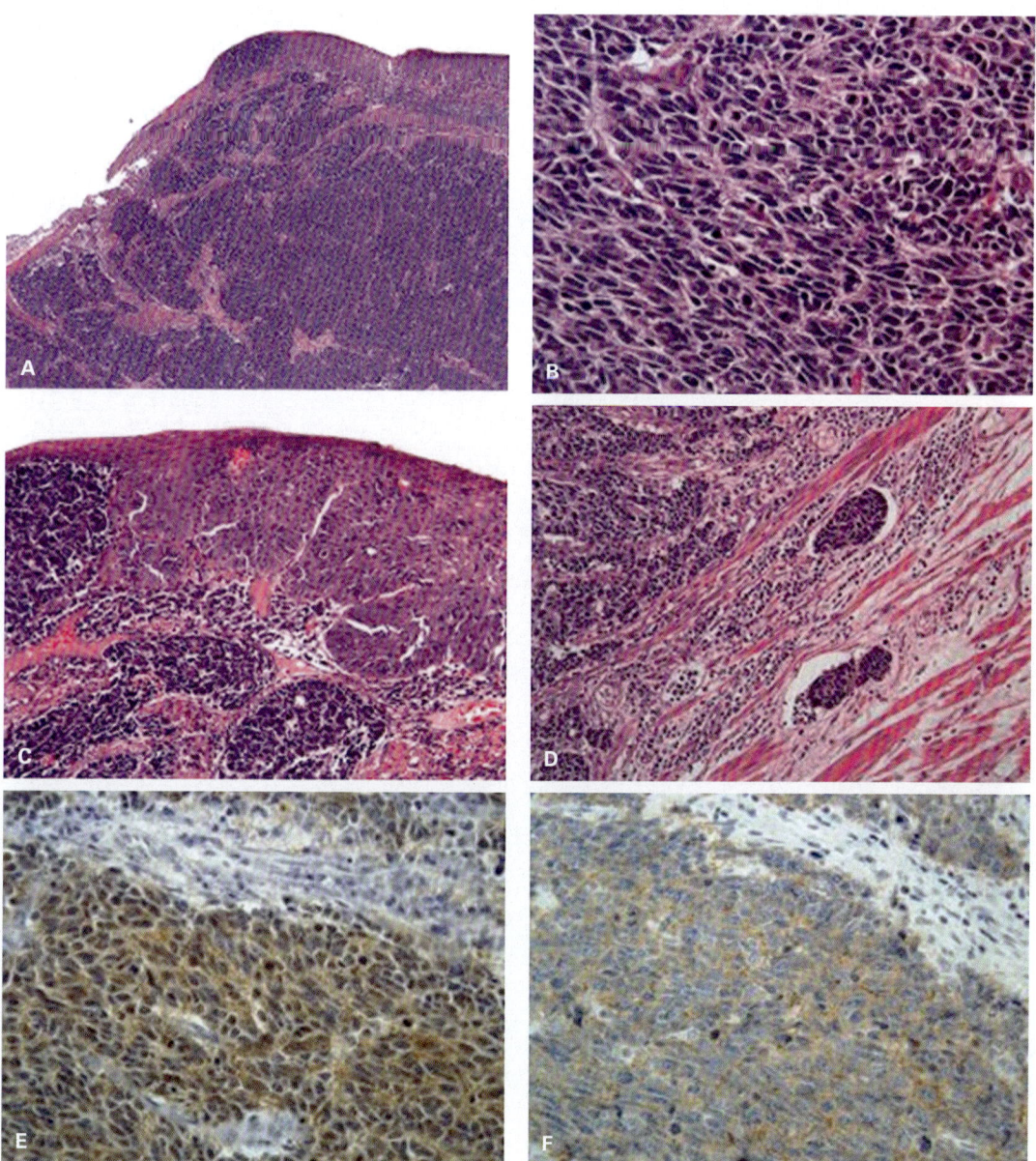

Figure 11-10. Small cell carcinoma. **A,B:** The tumor is composed of undifferentiated small cells with scant cytoplasm, and strongly resembles pulmonary counterpart. **C:** They may have components of in situ or invasive squamous cell carcinoma. **D:** Aggressive lymphatic invasion may be present. **E,F:** Positive immunohistochemical reactions for neuron-specific enolase and synaptophysin in this tumor.

Chapter 5). The incidence is about 2% of all esophageal malignancies.[143,144] Adults between the fifth and seventh decades are primarily affected[145] and patients may present with dysphagia, weight loss, and chest pain.[146] Almost all of the tumors occur in the middle or distal third of the esophagus, with the average length of 5 cm.[146] The tumors show more ulcerative and infiltrative growth than ordinary squamous cell carcinoma.[143]

Microscopically, small cell carcinomas are seen to grow in sheets, cords, and trabecular- or alveolar-like patterns, and occasionally exhibit glands, rosettes, and hyalinization (Fig. 11-10). They are composed of undifferentiated small cells with scant cytoplasm and exhibiting nuclear molding. Some subdivide them into oat and intermediate subtypes,[147] but there is no evidence that this is of prognostic value. The pathogenesis of these tumors is not known. About one-third of these have heterogeneous components of in situ or invasive squamous cell carcinoma with squamous pearls,[146,148] and the evidence raises the possibility that this tumor represents a small cell variant of squamous cell carcinoma. However, there may be foci of adenocarcinoma and mucoepidermoid carcinoma. Endocrine differentiation is usually demonstrated by the presence of positive immunohistochemical reactions for, synaptophysin, chromogranin A, CD56 or CD57 (Leu7).[146,148] They can often also be seen as argyrophylic granules on Grimelius stain, numerous dense core granules on electron microscopy, or both. Some are associated with the production of ectopic hormones such as

ACTH and calcitonin.[147] These features may support the possibility that small cell carcinomas arise from pluripotent cells present in the squamous epithelium, including those giving rise to Merkel cells, raising the possibility that at least some small cell carcinomas may reflect Merkel cell differentiation, or ducts of the submucosal glands. Interestingly, the tumors with squamous cell carcinoma components were positive

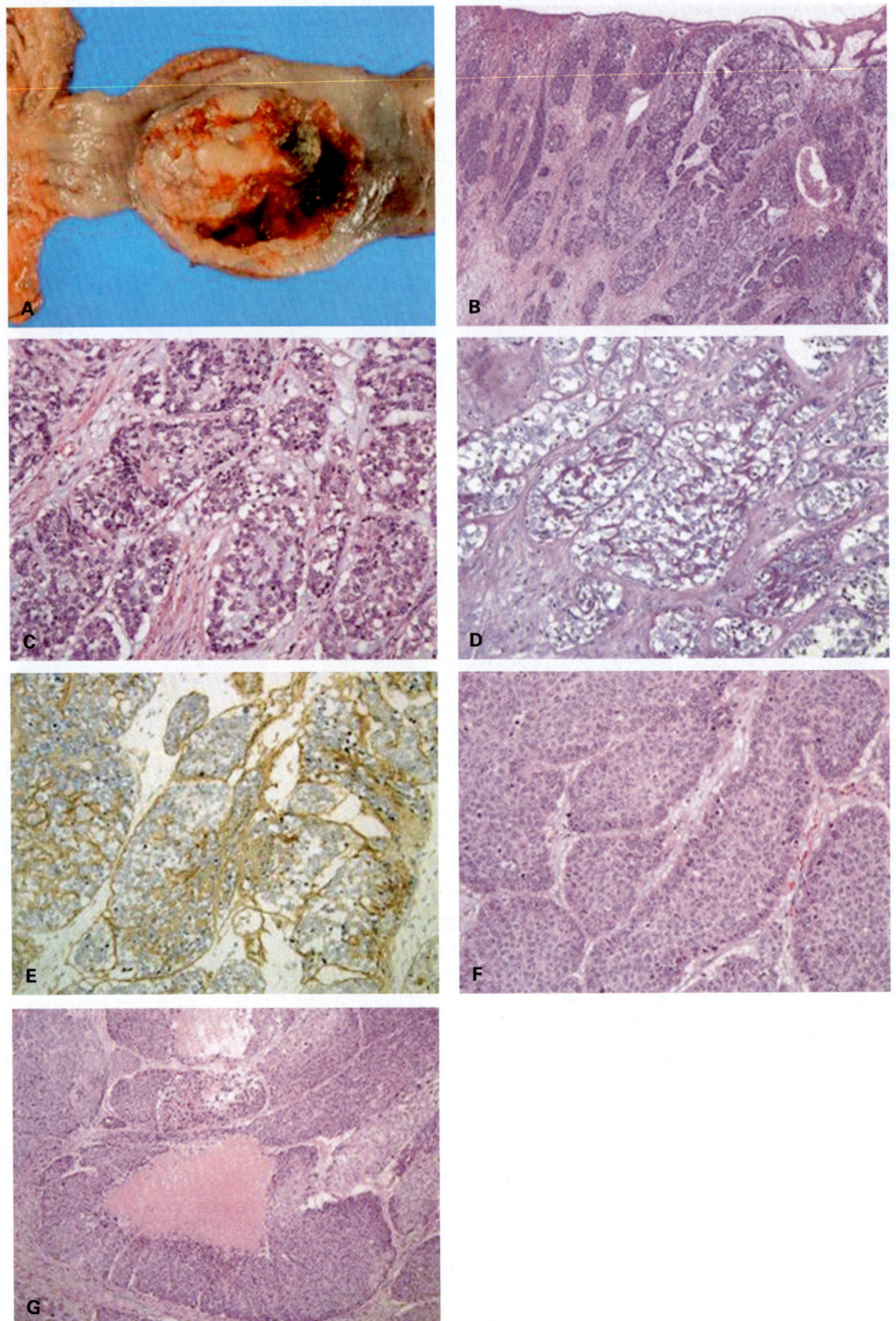

Figure 11-11. Basaloid squamous cell carcinoma. **A:** Gross appearance with polypoid growth and ulceration. **B:** The tumor is composed of nests with pseudoglandular luminal formation and solid lobules. **C:** The pseudoglandular nests have abundant hyaline material deposition. **D,E:** The hyaline material is positive for PAS and also immunohistochemically positive for laminin. **F:** Solid lobules with peripheral palisading of basaloid cells. **G:** Another part of the tumor with foci of comedo-type necrosis. (Courtesy of Dr. H. Kawasaki M.D.)

for CEA and E-cadherin, whereas others were negative.[148] Small cell carcinomas have a high incidence of metastatic disease at presentation; the commonly affected distant organs are liver, followed by lung, bone, and brain.[145,146] They show more aggressive lymphatic spread than squamous cell carcinoma, with metastases into the thoracic lymph nodes in almost all patients and the abdominal nodes in two-thirds of patients.[143,146] The prognosis is poor; many die within the first year, and nearly all die within 2 or 3 years of diagnosis.[144,146] Although patients treated with surgery and adjuvant chemotherapy are reported to have a better survival, the overall median survival is still only 6 to 15 months.[143-145]

Basaloid Squamous Cell Carcinoma

Basaloid squamous cell carcinoma is a rare malignant tumor, accounting for 2% to 5% of all primary esophageal malignancies.[149-151] The tumor has a strong male predominance,[149,150] and occurs primarily in the middle third of the esophagus.[150] These tumors usually have an intraepithelial or invasive squamous cell carcinoma component and are thought to be a variant of squamous cell carcinoma similar to their anal counterpart.[152,153] It is composed of solid lobules or nests of basaloid cells with foci of comedo-type necrosis and well-demarcated outlines surrounded by a fibrous stroma (Fig. 11-11).[151] Basaloid squamous cell carcinomas are often misdiagnosed as adenoid cystic carcinoma due to areas of cribriforming and pseudoglandular lumina formation. The most important features differentiating basaloid squamous cell carcinoma from adenoid cystic carcinoma are peripheral palisading and abundant hyaline material deposition. Immunohistochemically, AE1/3 and CAM5.2 are positive in tumor cells, and laminin is positive in the periphery of the nests.[154] A predominant expression of keratins 14 and 19 at the periphery of the basaloid nest is also helpful.[155] Ultrastructurally, the tumor cells exhibit relatively undifferentiated phenotype with undeveloped cell organelles.[151] These immunohistochemical and ultrastructural features are important because genuine adenoid cystic carcinoma is much less aggressive than basaloid squamous cell carcinoma. The long-term prognosis of patients with basaloid squamous cell carcinoma is reported no worse than that of squamous cell carcinoma.[150,156]

ADENOCARCINOMA

Primary adenocarcinoma of the esophagus was a relatively uncommon tumor, but its incidence has dramatically increased in the Western countries over the past 20 years.[157] In the United States, the incidence of these cancers has risen approximately sixfold and the mortality has increased more than sevenfold from 1975 to 2001.[1] Adenocarcinoma has replaced squamous cell carcinoma as the predominant histology.[7] Although adenocarcinoma is still rare in Japan, the annual death rate has doubled during the recent 35 years.[158] Adenocarcinoma of the esophagus merges imperceptibly with that of the cardia. The definition of "cardia" stops when the epicenter of the cancer is thought to be no more than 1 cm above the upper end of the gastric folds (Siewert-Stein classification—see Chapter 14). Above this, it is considered to be an esophageal primary.

The current evidence suggests that significant risk factors of adenocarcinoma include male sex, Caucasian race, and the presence of gastroesophageal reflux disease (GERD).[157-159] The CCND1 A/A genotype is associated with increased risk for GERD, columnar-lined (Barrett's) esophagus, and adenocarcinoma.[160] It is universally accepted that Barrett's esophagus is an acquired condition resulting from GERD. The majority of adenocarcinomas arise in the lower third of the esophagus within a segment of Barrett's esophagus. In one study,[161] as the incidence of Barrett's esophagus increased from 14.3 in 1997 to 23.1/100,000 person years in 2002, the incidence of adenocarcinoma also increased from 1.7 to 6.0/100,000 person years during the same period. A recent meta-analysis estimated the incidence of adenocarcinoma was 6.3/1,000 person years of follow-up.[162] This increase in incidence of distal esophageal adenocarcinoma, gastroesophageal junction (GEJ), and proximal stomach is intriguing as the diagnosis of Barrett's esophagus has been aggressively pursued in patients in the last 2 decades, stronger acid suppressant therapies have evolved and widely used, better control of *H. Pylori* infection has been achieved and surveillance of patients at high risk has increased. Indeed the risk of Barrett's adenocarcinoma is reduced markedly in patients treated with PPIs (El-Serag 04).

Adenocarcinoma can also arise from the submucosal glands and their mucosal and submucosal ducts of the middle and lower thirds and from the heterotopic gastric mucosa in the upper end of the esophagus as well as from the Barrett's esophagus.

Adenocarcinomas arising in Barrett's esophagus or in heterotopic gastric mucosa show a microscopic spectrum similar to that seen in gastric carcinomas, particularly those of the intestinal type.

Adenocarcinoma in the Columnar-lined Esophagus (Barrett's Esophagus)

Risk and pathogenesis. Columnar-lined (Barrett's) esophagus increases the risk of esophageal adenocarcinoma approximately 30 times compared with the general population without the condition.[163] However, the overall mortality rate in patients with Barrett's esophagus is closely similar to that of the general population, and esophageal cancer is an uncommon cause of death in these patients.[164]

Patients with Barrett's esophagus of length ≥3 cm have a significantly greater prevalence of dysplasia compared to length <3 cm (23% vs. 9%).[165] The annual risk of developing high-grade dysplasia or adenocarcinoma is estimated to be 0.8% in those with long-segment Barrett's esophagus.[166] Severe esophagitis, nodularity, Barrett's ulcer and stricture are macroscopic markers associated with this risk; patients with one of these factors are approximately 7 times more likely to develop high-grade dysplasia or adenocarcinoma, and those with two or more factors have 14 times the risk.[167] Adequate sampling and possibly rebiopsy of ulcerated areas should be considered. In one study, 15 of 21 (71%) patients with ulcers contained cancers.[168] Dysplasia development is significantly less common after antireflux surgery compared with conventional medical therapy.[169]

Absence of H. pylori infection and long duration of reflux symptoms are significantly associated with an increased risk of development of high-grade dysplasia and adenocarcinoma.[169-171] Conversely, H. pylori infection is associated with a reduced risk for esophageal adenocarcinoma,[36] although it is debatable whether it is due to reduced acidity from atrophy of the gastric mucosa. The other risk factors for development of adenocarcinoma include BMI >25, hiatal hernia, and cigarette smoking,[170-174] but drinking very hot beverages is not associated with the risk.[22] Interestingly, daily use of nonaspirin, NSAIDs is a protective factor against adenocarcinoma.[175] Although genetic susceptibility has been suggested by its predominance in white males and the early age of onset of Barrett's esophagus in some families,[172,173] few candidates including glutathione S-transferase P1 gene and its variants have not clinically been available yet.[176]

Dysplasia, Aneuploidy, and Other Markers of Increased Risk Dysplasia is the most reliable marker for developing adenocarcinoma at the present time (See Chapter 10). Invasive carcinoma is present in 30% to 60% of patients with high-grade dysplasia within a Barrett's area.[168,177-179] Long-term cancer-related survivals are almost 100% in patients treated promptly, but only about 50% in patients with expectant management; almost all of the former patients have stage I disease. Prompt decision regarding an esophageal resection as soon as high-grade dysplasia is found is much safer than an expectant management.

Low-grade dysplasia and indefinite for dysplasia are also to be associated with an increased risk of developing high-grade dysplasia or adenocarcinoma.[168,169] In one series, carcinomas were detected in 4 of 22 (18%) cases submitted as indefinite for dysplasia, in 4 of 25 (15%) cases of low-grade dysplasia, and in 20 of 33 (61%) cases of high-grade dysplasia.[168] Initial grading appears to well correlate with progression to invasive carcinoma. Not enrolling a patient with low-grade dysplasia and possibly with indefinite for dysplasia in an endoscopic surveillance program can lead to the development of extramural invasive cancer with poor outcomes. A large multicenter cohort study stressed that the majority (66%) of patients with low-grade dysplasia regressed and had a cancer incidence similar to all Barrett's patients, raising the question of whether there may have been a degree of over-interpretation of reactive changes.[180] However, there was no pathologist on the authorship, no illustrations, and the reference given for "established criteria for low-grade and high-grade dysplasia" was the original 1983 paper for inflammatory bowel disease. This casts considerable doubt on the validity of these changes, despite all of the pathologists reading the slides being "specialized" pathologists, and still does not exclude a systematic error. In another large study with similar results,[181] the illustration of low-grade dysplasia would be indefinite or reactive for many pathologists. Further, there are data suggesting that the risk of carcinoma is related to the length of low-grade dysplasia present, suggesting a definite relationship between low-grade dysplasia and carcinoma.[182]

The current perioperative mortality of esophagectomy is 1.2% to 6%,[2,4,7,10,69-73,121] which is high for a prophylactic procedure. Alternative therapies have emerged for high-grade dysplasia and early stage cancer. Photodynamic therapy (PDT) using photosensitizer drugs activated by laser light for mucosal ablation has been used. Porfimer sodium PDT has been used extensively with suggested long-term efficacy and durability for the ablation of Barrett's esophagus and high-grade dysplasia and early esophageal adenocarcinoma. However, continued use is hampered by an associated stricture risk and prolonged photosensitivity (4–6 weeks). An endoscopic ablative therapy has emerged called radiofrequency endoluminal ablation (the BARRX device). In a multicenter, randomized sham-controlled trial of 127 patients with dysplastic Barrett's esophagus, complete eradication of low-grade dysplasia occurred in 90.5% of those in the radiofrequency ablation group, as compared with 22.7% of those in the sham group ($p < 0.001$). Among patients with high-grade dysplasia, complete eradication occurred in 81.0% of those in the radiofrequency ablation group, as compared with 19.0% of those in the sham group ($p < 0.001$). Overall, 77.4% of patients in the radiofrequency ablation group had complete eradication of intestinal metaplasia, as compared with 2.3% of those in the sham group ($p < 0.001$). Patients in the radiofrequency ablation group also had less disease progression (3.6% vs. 16.3%, $p = 0.03$) and fewer cancers (1.2% vs. 9.3%, $p = 0.045$). A meta-analysis of ablative therapies in Barrett's esophagus showed that patients with nondysplastic Barrett's esophagus, low-grade dysplasia, or high-grade dysplasia followed for at least 6 months showed a cancer incidence of 6/1,000 patient-years in nondysplastic Barrett's; 17/1,000 patient-years in low-grade dysplasia; and 66/1,000 patient-years in high-grade dysplasia patients. The incidence rate for cancer was 1.63/1,000 patient-years for nondysplastic Barrett's, 1.58/1,000 patient-years for low grade dysplasia; and 16.76/1,000 patient-years for high-grade dysplasia patients. The greatest benefit of ablation seemed to be observed in Barrett's esophagus with high-grade dysplasia.

There have been few direct comparisons of ablation therapy with esophagectomy. In a retrospective study, endotherapy (with any of PDT, argon plasma coagulation or EMR) and esophagectomy effectively treated high-grade dysplasia and intramucosal carcinoma associated with Barrett's esophagus. However, endotherapy was also associated with a higher risk of tumor progression, although this is uncommon (occurred in 6%). Esophagectomy incurred higher initial costs and resulted in more frequent minor complications but was usually curative. Hence, age might be an important factor to consider when deciding upon esophagectomy versus endoscopic therapy. For instance, older patients at greater risk for surgery could do better with endoscopic therapy, whereas younger patients who might be facing years of frequent endoscopic treatments might do better with surgery.

There are problems with surveillance in Barrett's esophagus. One of the major problems in diagnosing dysplasia for the pathologist is the significant interobserver variation. For the endoscopist, there is difficulty in its endoscopic recognition, because dysplasia in Barrett's esophagus may have no distinctive gross features. Dysplasia may be focal and multiple, so that there may be considerable sampling problems in its detection. While much dysplasia is an unexpected finding in incidental biopsies, systematic sampling in a protocol of a single biopsy every 2-cm was reported to miss 50% of cancers that were detected by a four-quadrant 1-cm protocol.[183] Chromoendoscopy with the spraying of a dye is said to accentuate dysplastic lesions when present. Methylene blue as chromogen is taken up by actively absorbing intestinal-type epithelial cells and dysplastic cells but not by squamous or gastric mucosa. A lighter intensity of staining would highlight an area of dysplasia. However, a meta-analysis of nine studies comparing methylene blue chromoendoscopy with routine white light endoscopy plus biopsy revealed no incremental benefit of methylene blue chromoendoscopy over white light endoscopy.[184]

An alternative to the time-consuming and often messy spraying of dye solutions is narrow band imaging (NBI). NBI involves light of a short wavelength (blue light in the visible spectrum) penetrating superficially into the mucosa allowing for improved surface detail. As blue light is highly absorbed by hemoglobin, the vascular pattern is especially accentuated. The major advantages of NBI are that it involves merely the switch of a button on the head of the endoscope and hence requires little time and is also less messy. Further, it is uniformly applied, whereas dye spraying can be non-uniform. Autofluorescence imaging uses blue light for excitation of endogenous tissue fluorophores, which emit fluorescent green light of longer wavelength. It can also highlight neoplastic tissue without the need for exogenous fluorophores. These latter two modalities have the potential advantage of not just identifying neoplasia when present that might be missed by white light endoscopy but also by highlighting the superficial pit patterns of the lesion in question.

In a prospective study of 65 patients with Barrett's esophagus, NBI identified more subjects with higher grades of dysplasia than white light endoscopy (18% vs. 0%), while standard endoscopy was associated with more biopsies (8.5 vs. 4.7, $p < 0.001$).[185] While NBI is easy to use, a study of eight endoscopists scoring 1,600 NBI images of Barrett's esophagus found moderate interobserver agreement at best, including for high-grade dysplasia. This suggests that NBI could not replace histologic evaluation for neoplasia in Barrett's esophagus.[186] In another study that assessed NBI chromoendoscopy, the chromoendoscopy techniques added nothing to the interobserver agreement achieved on white light endoscopy.[187]

Fluorescence-aided confocal laser endomicroscopy may also be a promising tool. This predicted Barrett's esophagus and associated neoplasias with a sensitivity of 98.1% and 92.9% and a specificity of 94.1% and 98.4%, respectively.[188] These types of data need to be reproduced by other studies; however, confocal laser endomicroscopy requires considerable expertise and is sufficiently expensive to render this technique impractical for commonplace use in the near future.

The benefit of surveillance is controversial. There are data that pathologic stage of carcinomas is 0 or 1 in 75% of patients in the surveillance group compared to 10% to 20% of those without surveillance and that median survival is 107 months for the former group but 12 months for the latter group.[189,190] However, endoscopic surveillance has limited value in patients with Barrett's esophagus, because surveillance failures are common due to inconsistent endoscopic findings and sampling errors. It may be appropriate to restrict surveillance to patients with additional risk factors such as stricture, ulcer, long segment (>8 cm) Barrett's esophagus, or previous diagnosis of low-grade dysplasia.

DNA aneuploidy has been suggested to be a useful marker for predicting carcinoma. Among patients with negative, indefinite, or low-grade dysplasia, those with neither aneuploidy nor increased 4N fractions had a 0% 5-year cumulative cancer incidence compared with 28% for those with either aneuploidy or increased 4N. Patients with baseline-increased 4N, aneuploidy, and high-grade dysplasia had 5-year cancer incidences of 56%, 43%, and 59%, respectively.[191] The utility of finding aneuploidy is still unclear but surveillance endoscopy with a longer interval could potentially be allowed in patients without aneuploidy.

An increased Ki-67 proliferation fraction and a decreased E-cadherin expression have been reported not only in adenocarcinoma but even in dysplasia, and may represent an early phenomenon in the malignant progression of Barrett's esophagus.[192] The p53 expression is an additional marker of risk for malignancy in Barrett's esophagus,[193,194] being positive in 15% of patients without dysplasia, 37% with dysplasia, and 44% with adenocarcinoma in one series.[195]

Carcinoma in Short Segment Barrett's Esophagus

Short segment Barrett's esophagus is diagnosed by the presence of <3 cm of columnar epithelium in the lower esophagus. However, it has been shown that endoscopists cannot reproducibly separate a tongue of <1 cm from an irregular Z-line,[196] so that short segment Barrett's esophagus is defined as being 1 to 3 cm above the top of the gastric folds, and "ultra-short Barrett's esophagus," although it has to exist, cannot be diagnosed with any confidence. Any tongue of metaplastic mucosa longer than 3 cm satisfies conventional definitions of long segment Barrett's esophagus. A longer length of Barrett's esophagus is associated with an increased risk of dysplasia and adenocarcinoma,[165] and thus the risk of adenocarcinoma developing in short segment Barrett's esophagus is expected to be small. However, there is a conflicting report that the risk is not substantially lower than that in long segment Barrett's esophagus.[197] Adenocarcinomas in short and long segment Barrett's esophagus are suggested to occur through similar genetic alterations by one study on allelic loss of 3p, 5q, 9p, and 17p.[198] The true risk for carcinoma in patients with short segment Barrett's esophagus cannot be estimated until more data are available.

Adenocarcinomas of the proximal stomach and those in short segment Barrett's esophagus are often confused with each other particularly in patients with hiatal hernia. The former and latter can be diagnosed when the tumor located entirely below and entirely above the esophagogastric junction, respectively; the term "adenocarcinoma of the esophagogastric junction" is applied to the rest of tumors that cross this junction. In normal individuals without Barrett's esophagus, an endoscopic landmark of the esophagogastric junction is the squamocolumnar junction (Z-line), which is irregular but clearly recognizable, while this landmark is often useless for patients with Barrett's esophagus. Alternatively, the Siewert-Stein classification can be used (see Chapter 14). The anatomic esophagogastric junction can be determined from either the proximal ends of the gastric rugae, or by paying attention to the trabecular capillaries, which run longitudinally parallel and are located only in the lower esophagus within 2 cm from the proximal margin of the stomach (see Chapter 12 and Fig. 11-12).[199] The columnar epithelium showing through the trabecular capillaries is highly suggestive of Barrett's esophagus. These capillaries may be unclear in the mucosa with ulceration or deep inflammation, but Barrett's esophagus is probable in the mucosa without gastric folds and adjacent to the squamous epithelium without the trabecular capillaries.

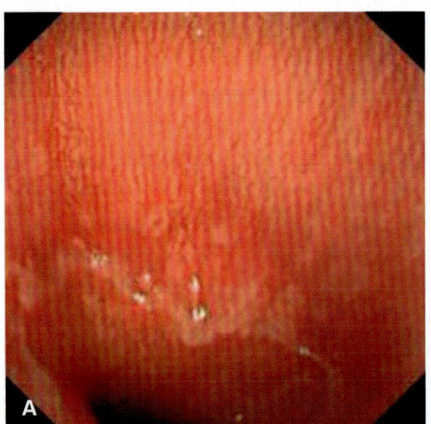 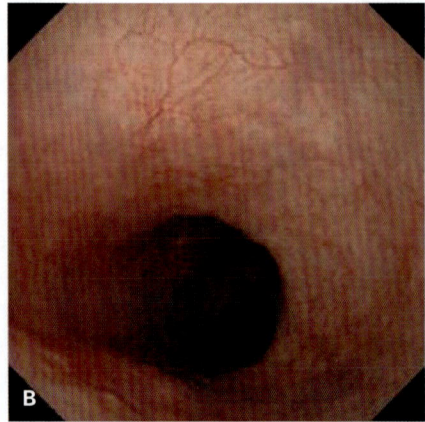 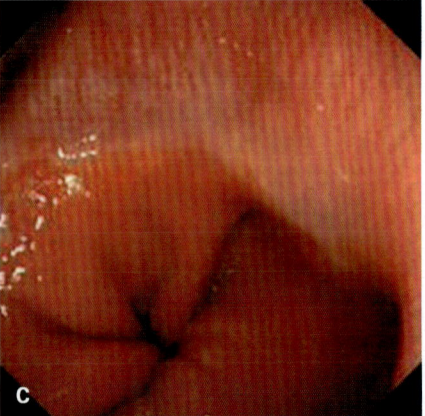

Figure 11-12. A: Endoscopic appearance of the normal lower esophagus within 2 cm from the proximal margin of the stomach (Z-line). The trabecular capillaries run longitudinally parallel. **B:** Reticular capillaries are distributed throughout the rest of esophagus. **C:** Endoscopic picture not showing Barrett's esophagus, but a sliding hernia of the stomach, in which the true Z-line can be recognized if paying attention to the trabecular capillaries, and the location of the upper end of the gastric rugae.

Clinical Features

Most studies have found a heavy predominance of white males, in marked contrast to squamous cell carcinoma, which has a high prevalence in African Americans.[9,157] The age range is wide with a mean of about 60; the median age is about 5 years higher in patients who had Barrett's esophagus with carcinoma compared to those without carcinoma.[200] The majority of adenocarcinomas arise in the lower third of the esophagus, while half of squamous cell carcinomas occur in the middle third of the esophagus. The rare adenocarcinomas arising from ectopic gastric glands and esophageal glands are also found in the upper and middle third of the esophagus. A change in symptoms such as progressive dysphagia is likely to portend advanced disease.

Gross and Endoscopic Appearances

These appearances are similar to those of squamous cell carcinomas and have a similar range, varying from slight mucosal irregularities or plaques that may be virtually invisible endoscopically and in resected esophagi to obvious exophytic, fungating, or deeply ulcerated masses, which may occlude varying proportions of the lumen (Fig. 11-13). In

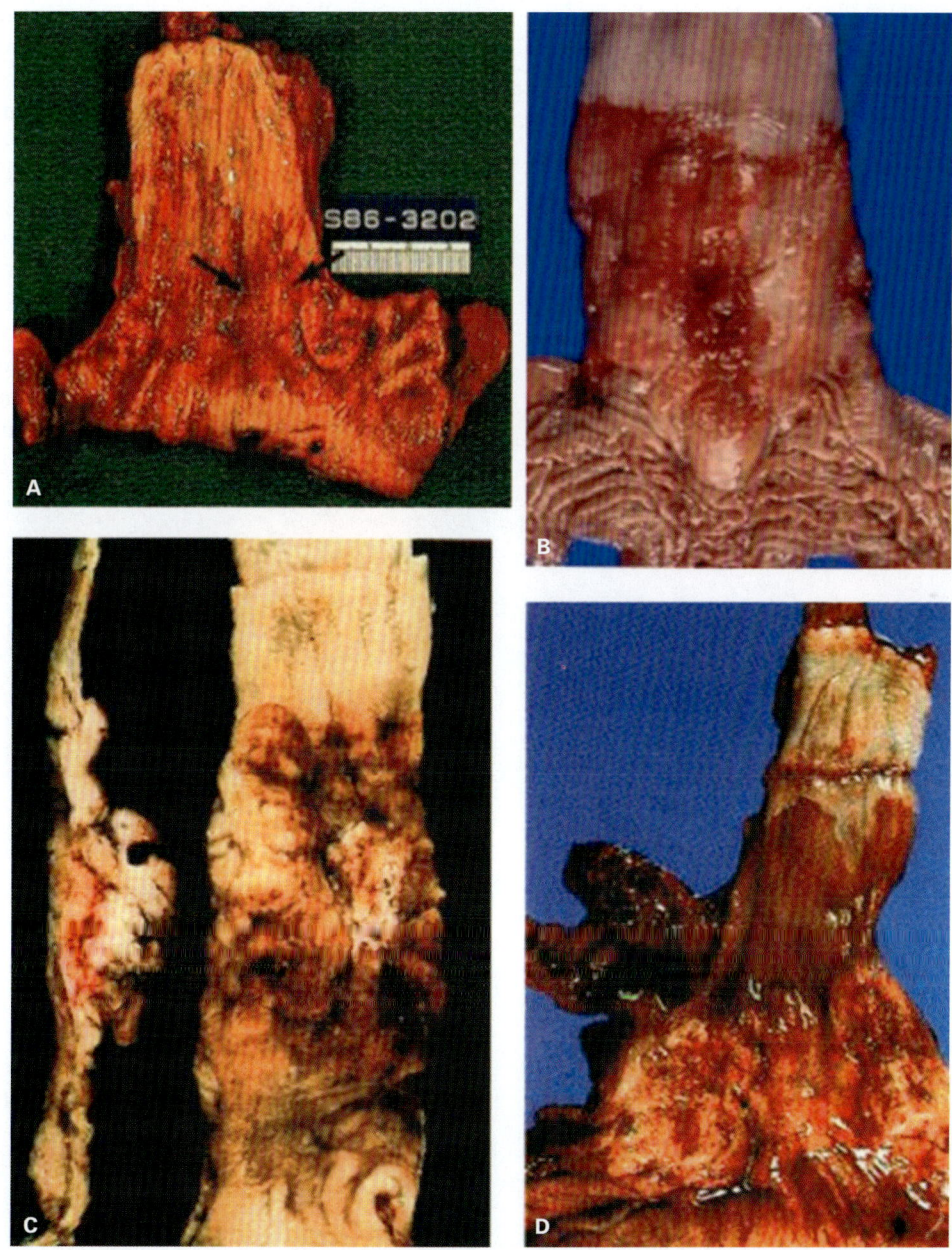

Figure 11-13. Gross appearance of carcinomas in Barrett's esophagus. In all, the squamocolumnar junction extends for varying distances proximal to its usual location in the distal 2 cm of the tubular esophagus. **A:** Carcinoma biopsied incidentally at endoscopy (poorly circumscribed area at *arrow*). **B:** Plateau-like raised tumor with the irregular surface (Courtesy of Dr. H. Kawasaki M.D.). **C,D:** Carcinomas presenting symptomatically. One of them is markedly exophytic but is not deeply infiltrating; the second is deeply infiltrating.

patients with Barrett's esophagus, the presence of an ulcer with high-grade dysplasia increases the likelihood of adenocarcinoma in the resection specimen, as 80% of high-grade dysplasia patients with ulcers have carcinoma compared to 50% of those without ulcers.[201]

Because adenocarcinomas tend to spread proximally in the submucosal lymphatics, it is always wise to obtain frozen sections from the proximal resected margin in order to detect tumor in the margin in patients in whom further proximal resection can be carried out. Although adenocarcinoma of the lower third of the esophagus is particularly likely to be accompanied by abdominal nodal metastasis, submucosal extension to the distal resected margin appears to be uncommon.

Microscopic appearances. Adenocarcinomas of the esophagus show a virtually identical histologic spectrum to gastric carcinomas (see Chapter 14). Adenocarcinomas arising in Barrett's esophagus are predominantly tubular, papillary, or combinations of them.[202] A few tumors are of the diffuse type, and signet-ring cell or mucinous carcinomas also occur (Fig. 11-14). Differentiation may include endocrine, Paneth cell, or ciliated cells, together with varying degrees of dysplasia. Some carcinomas are of the so-called pylorocardiac type. The latter, as well as other well-differentiated tumors, may pose a problem on biopsy because the infiltrating component may be difficult to recognize and therefore reported as high-grade dysplasia or carcinoma in situ. A proportion is adenosquamous,[203,204] and the squamous component may predominate.

Endoscopic Ablation Techniques

A variety of ablation techniques are now available in Barrett's esophagus, including endoscopic mucosal resection (EMR), endoscopic submucosal dissection (ESD), and a variety of endoscopic ablation techniques, primarily radiofrequency ablation (RFA). These are rapidly becoming the treatment of choice for all dysplasias, intramucosal carcinomas, and superficial submucosal carcinomas as EMR (or ESD) allows staging regarding depth of invasion, and therefore an indication of the risk of nodal metastases, which in turn dictates consideration of surgical resection including lymph nodes. A combination of these may be used. The huge advantage of these techniques is that they have minimal morbidity and virtually no mortality, which contrasts with their surgical counterparts. Further, a combination of these may be used, so EMR may be used to resect an area of known dysplasia to assess for possible invasive carcinoma, while RFA may be used to destroy the reminder of the Barrett's segment. All of these techniques are

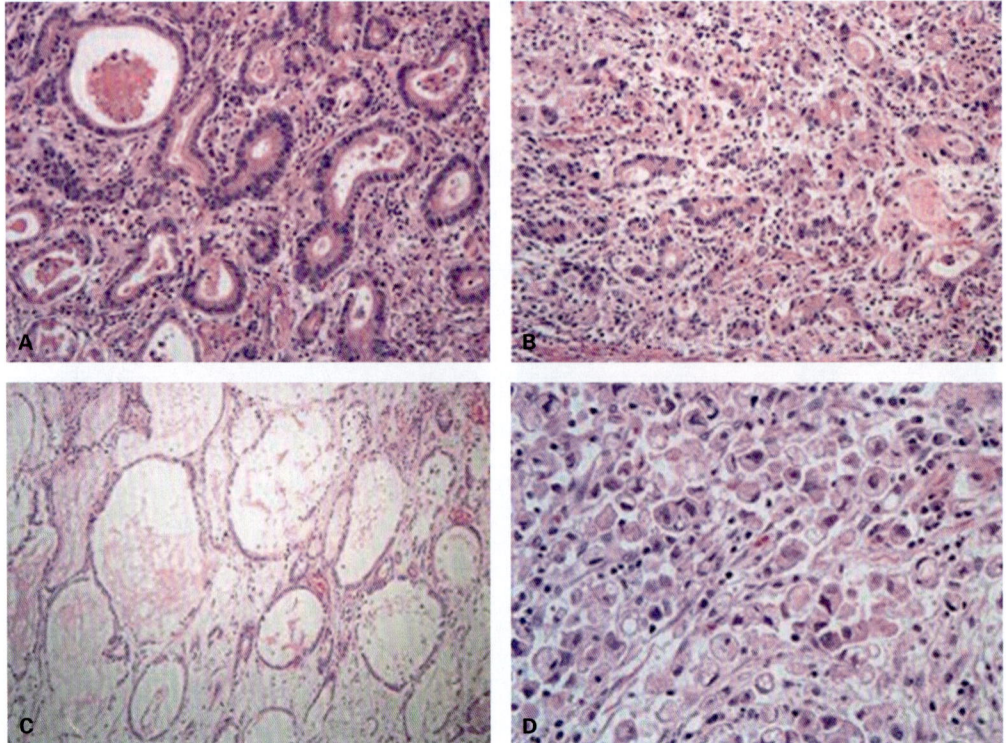

Figure 11-14. Examples of the spectrum of infiltrating carcinomas that are associated with Barrett's esophagus. **A:** Well-differentiated tubular adenocarcinoma. **B:** Moderately differentiated tubular adenocarcinoma. **C:** Tubular adenocarcinoma with attenuated epithelium that tend to be aggressive. **D:** Signet-ring cell carcinoma.

followed (often preceded) by high dose PPIs to allow regeneration of the destroyed mucosa by squamous mucosa from the peripheral squamous mucosa and, mostly, from the esophageal gland ducts. RFA can be local or circumferential. The problems with handling post-ablative/EMR therapy are those of residual Barrett's epithelium, dysplasia, and the potential for residual dysplastic glands to become invasive, although the question of whether the invasion was already present at the time of ablation/EMR is often unanswerable.

Endoscopic mucosal resection. EMR (Fig. 11-15) and ESD (Fig. 11-7) are promising therapies for mucosal neoplasia in Barrett's esophagus. Under the condition of small neoplastic lesions <2 cm in diameter and no sign of submucosal infiltration, positive lymph nodes, or distant metastasis, EMR is successfully performed in more than 90% of patients[205,206]; 20% may have a recurrence of high-grade dysplasia but all are successfully re-treated with EMR.[206] However, mucosal neoplasias in Barrett's esophagus are often distributed diffusely with unclear margin, and thus the complete ablation should be confirmed by the subsequent biopsy. Theoretically, frozen section analysis of EMR specimens could allow endoscopists to make decisions regarding further therapy if margins are involved[207]; however usually EMR results in multiple fragments, so this can be difficult or impossible to carry out. Further presence of cautery artifacts on the edges of the fragments can make interpretation of dysplasia difficult even on permanent sections. Papillary architecture on pre-EMR biopsy is one of the features predicting failure in EMR.[202] Stricture requiring dilation occurred in 20% of patients is the most common serious complication of EMR.[208]

Endoscopic delineation of the entire lesion prior to endoscopic resection appears the most promising means of ensuring complete excision.

Prognosis

The important prognostic factors are similar to those affecting squamous cell carcinoma, and include completeness of tumor resection, depth and size of tumors, lymphovascular invasion, and lymph node status.[209–211] The perioperative mortality for esophageal resection is currently reported to be 1.2% to 6%[2,4,7,10,69–73,121]; the mortality is predominantly affected by pulmonary complications.[212] The overall 5-year survival after esophageal resection is <30% in most series. R0 resections improve the rates to 50%,[211,213] and the subsequent neoadjuvant chemotherapy (paclitaxel and cisplatin) may further improve survival.[214]

The 5-year recurrence-free survival is significantly better in patients with tumors confined to mucosa (97%–100%) than with those invasive into submucosa (around 60%); the data for tumors limited to superficial one-third of the submucosa (sm1) are almost equal to those confined to mucosa.[209,215] Since pathologic stage is the most important factor affecting R0 resection, endoscopic surveillance of Barrett's patients results in better prognosis. However, to assess the depth of submucosal invasion by these criteria, the entire submucosa needs to be present.

Lymph node metastasis is significantly associated with tumor recurrence but may not directly with overall survival.[209] Factors that predict the presence of lymph node metastasis are multiple, including tumor diameter >3 cm, infiltration beyond sm1, and lymphatic invasion.[216] Among these factors, the depth of tumor invasion is the most important. Nodal metastases are extremely rare in adenocarcinomas limited to lamina propria but occur in 35% to 50% of those invading deep submucosa. The reported percentages vary from 0% to 10% in those invading into muscularis mucosae or superficial submucosa.[209,215–217]

Lymphatic spread is initially limited to the regional lymph nodes. Skipping of regional lymph node with distant metastases to the upper mediastinum or the

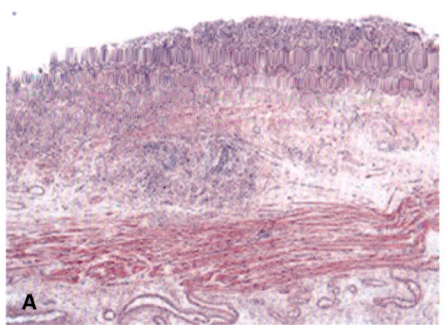
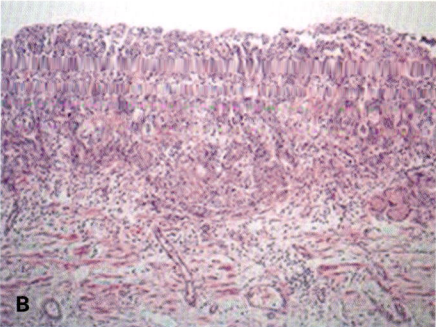
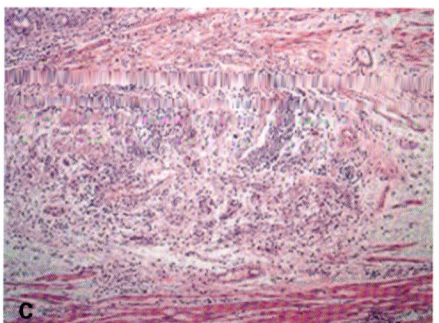

Figure 11-15. **A:** Mucosal cancer (m2 tumor) associated with Barrett's esophagus, in which the muscularis mucosae is often duplicated, the original being the lower that is hypertrophied and the upper that was formed with the neomucosa following ulceration. **B,C:** Details of adenocarcinoma. The carcinoma has infiltrated to the upper surface of the original muscularis mucosae so is still intramucosal.

celiac lymph nodes occurs in <5% of the patients.[218] EUS correctly predicts the absence of nodal metastasis in 93% of node-negative patients.[216]

Sentinel lymph nodes can be detected by endoscopic peritumoral injection of radiolabelled nanocolloid, and the overall accuracy of biopsy from these nodes is 96% in all of node-positive patients.[219] For patients with positive sentinel lymph node, the best chance for cure comes from esophagectomy with two-field lymphadenectomy compared to less extensive operation; 50% versus 23% survival at 5 years.[213]

Although immunohistochemical expressions of COX-2 protein and tissue inhibitor of metalloproteinase-3 protein correlate with patient survival, they are not carried out routinely. COX is the best-known target of NSAIDs, which are associated with a reduced risk of cancer in the digestive tract.

UNUSUAL VARIANTS OF ADENOCARCINOMA

Adenoid Cystic Carcinoma

Adenoid cystic carcinoma tends to occur distally and do not appear to have a major gender predominance.[220] However, given the male predilection in virtually all other esophageal carcinomas, this may reflect an increased tendency toward adenoid cystic differentiation in women; this is of interest in that the salivary gland counterpart of this tumor also has a strong female predominance. It is characterized by islands of neoplastic epithelium forming well-defined regular glands (a cribriform pattern) containing mucin. It has been considered to arise from submucosal ducts or glands,[221,222] but doubt has been cast on this notion because many cases are associated with, or in direct continuity with, overlying squamous mucosa with dysplasia or carcinoma in situ, suggesting that at least some of these tumors originate from squamous epithelium and therefore represent variants of, or metaplasia in, squamous carcinoma. However, some early adenocarcinomas thought to be of submucosal gland origin may be accompanied by in situ squamous carcinoma,[223] so that this whole issue is rather controversial. The prognosis of adenoid cystic carcinoma may not be worse than that of ordinary or basaloid squamous cell carcinoma.[151]

Mucoepidermoid Carcinoma

Mucoepidermoid carcinoma, which has been believed to arise from esophageal glands, is often confused and used interchangeably, perhaps not unreasonably, with adenosquamous carcinoma.[204] Mucoepidermoid carcinoma typically has islands of tumor, some of which are distinctly squamous but containing a glandular component. The glandular component sometimes consists of well-formed glands but also of groups of cells in which intracellular mucin can be demonstrated with periodic acid-Schiff (PAS) and Alcian blue at pH 2.5, or mucicarmine stains. The tumor shows an intimate mixture of squamous cells and mucus secreting cells, but, in contrast, both elements are not intimately admixed in adenosquamous carcinoma. The glandular component is often low-grade and there are intermediate cells similar to their salivary gland counterparts. Although, in eight patients with mucoepidermoid carcinoma, it was reported that neither chemotherapy and radiotherapy were effective and overall median survival period was shorter than that in those with squamous carcinoma (11 vs. 32 months),[224] there are too few cases in the literature to allow us to judge whether they really behave more aggressively than other squamous carcinomas.

Adenocarcinoma in Heterotopic Gastric Mucosa

Heterotopic (ectopic) gastric mucosa is relatively common at autopsy or endoscopy. Most patients are asymptomatic but some patients complain of dysphagia, odynophagia, and extraesophageal manifestations such as hoarseness and coughing.[225] Rarely, this mucosa may undergo ulceration, stricture, or esophagotracheal fistula formation,. The ulcers are likely peptic in origin, being at the distal end of the ectopic mucosa.

Adenocarcinoma arising from heterotopic gastric mucosa is considered a source of adenocarcinoma in the upper esophagus (Fig. 11-16). This malignant transformation via intestinal metaplasia and dysplasia may occur particularly in larger areas of heterotopia but is exceedingly rare with only 25 reported cases.[225-227] In a reported case of adenocarcinoma, intestinal metaplasia was immunoreactive for both CK7 and CK20, which is a common pattern in Barrett's mucosa.[226]

Adenocarcinoma in Submucosal Glands

These are the extremely rare salivary gland-type tumors that are occasionally found in the esophagus and classically include adenoid cystic and mucoepidermoid tumors.[228-230] Unlike their salivary gland counterparts, these tumors are as aggressive as other variants of esophageal carcinoma and are rapidly lethal. They are supposed to arise from the esophageal submucosal glands mainly based on their submucosal position or overlying intact squamous epithelium. However, involvement of these structures is not uncommon in other adenocarcinomas such as those associated with Barrett's esophagus.[223] Except the cases of in situ adenocarcinoma arising in submucosal mucous glands,[231]

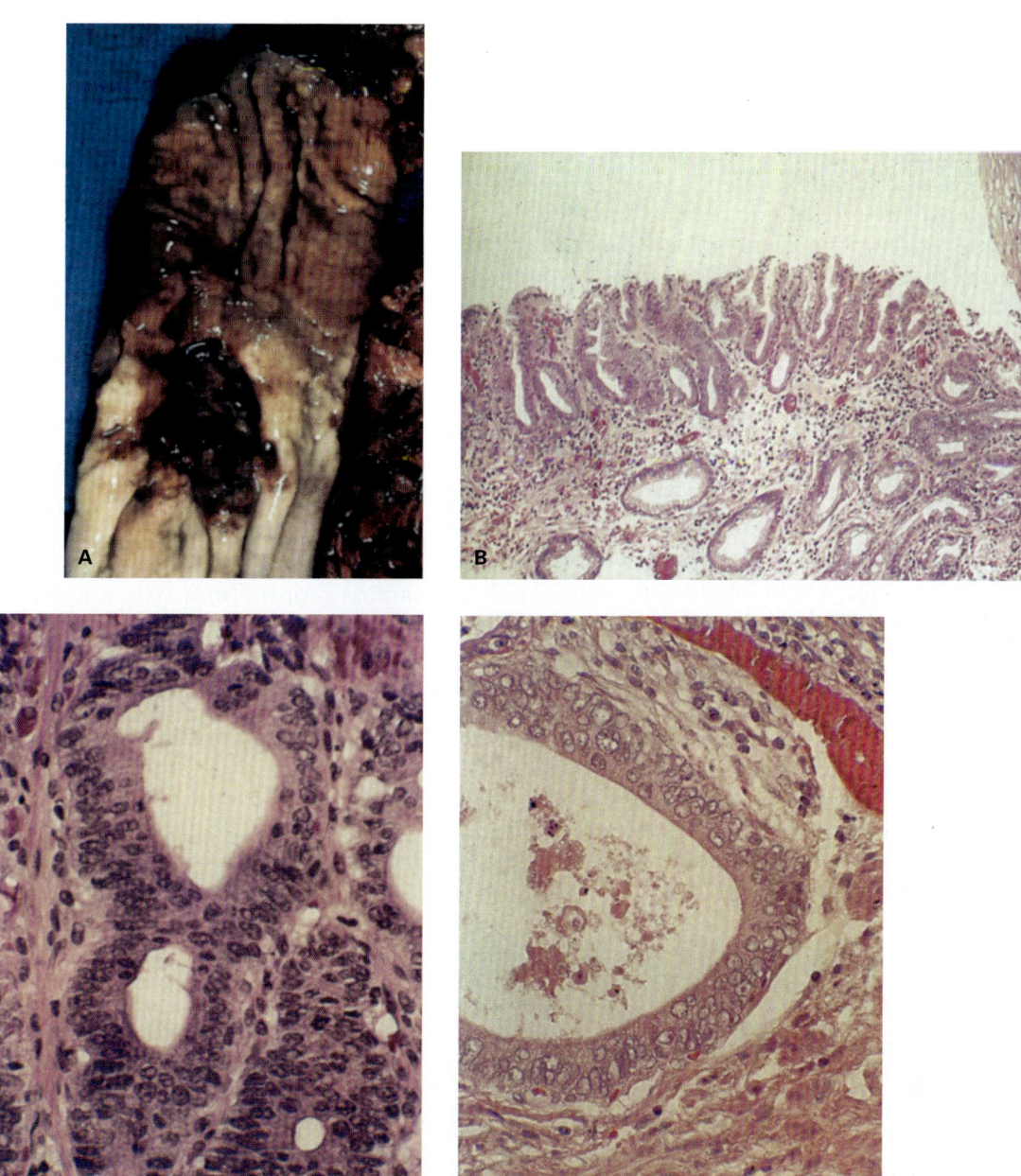

Figure 11-16. Adenocarcinoma arising in heterotopic gastric mucosa in the cervical esophagus. **A:** Cervical esophagus with circumferential heterotopic gastric mucosa extending to the upper margin. At the lower margin there is a deep peptic ulcer, at the distal edge of which was a focus of intestinal metaplasia, dysplasia, and infiltrating, well-differentiated adenocarcinoma. **B:** Heterotopic gastric mucosa with dysplasia. **C:** Detail of low grade dysplasia. **D:** Part of the invasive carcinoma.

many of reported cases do not stand critical review and we therefore suspect that they are extremely rare.

Adenosquamous Carcinoma and Adenoacanthoma

Adenosquamous carcinomas are tumors containing coexisting infiltrating adenocarcinoma and squamous cell carcinoma; they tend to occur primarily in association with Barrett's esophagus.[203,204] Some of these tumors may represent or be confused with high-grade mucoepidermoid carcinoma. These can be distinguished from each other because, in mucoepidermoid carcinomas, mucus-secreting cells occur within islands of squamous carcinoma with intermediate cells, whereas in true adenosquamous carcinomas both elements coexist, but without intimate admixture in this manner.

The histogenesis of adenosquamous carcinomas is controversial. Only if adjacent mucosal dysplasia is identified in both squamous and glandular epithelium can tumors be considered to be arising from both types of epithelium simultaneously. More likely these tumors may be primarily adenocarcinomas with areas of squamous metaplasia or possibly squamous carcinomas with glandular metaplasia.[223] Apparently mature but phenotypically malignant squamous epithelium is very rarely present in adenocarcinomas, in which case some prefer to call these tumors adenoacanthomas.[220]

Choriocarcinoma and Hepatoid Adenocarcinoma

Primary choriocarcinoma of the esophagus is an extremely rare tumor and represents an unusual pattern of differentiation of adenocarcinoma rather than a true germ cell tumor. Such lesions are well documented in the lung, where the bizarre, atypical giant cells have been found to contain human chorionic gonadotropin. While it appears that such tumors have trophoblastic differentiation, their origin from typical adenocarcinoma can often be demonstrated.[232,233] Hepatoid carcinomas resemble their counterparts elsewhere. Unlike most hepatomas, they are invariably α-fetoprotein immunoreactive, and also can be strongly immunoreactive for cdx2, features which are both useful in the distinction from primary or metastatic hepatocellular carcinoma.

BIOPSY DIAGNOSIS OF SQUAMOUS AND ADENOCARCINOMA AND ASSOCIATED PROBLEMS

In most instances, this diagnosis presents little problem, and biopsy is both accurate and sensitive. In one series, it has been estimated that one biopsy specimen will provide the correct diagnosis in 93% of tumors, while up to seven specimens are necessary for a diagnosis in all cases.[234] A small proportion of tumors may be more resistant to diagnosis, especially those associated with strictures and widespread inflammation. Strictures located proximal to the gastroesophageal junction are very likely to be malignant unless they are associated with Barrett's esophagus. The most difficult is often in deciding whether a lesion is simply dysplastic (m1) or whether there is invasion into the lamina propria (m2). When glands seem to bud into the lamina and are tightly packed, this appearance is frequently interpreted as intramucosal carcinoma, correctly or incorrectly (see Chapter 10).

When tight strictures are present, vigorous brushing and cytology may allow the diagnosis to be made where biopsies fail. An unequivocally positive cytologic smear in the presence of an endoscopic tumor usually provides adequate evidence for the diagnosis. Some tumors are so poorly differentiated that it may be difficult to be certain whether they are of

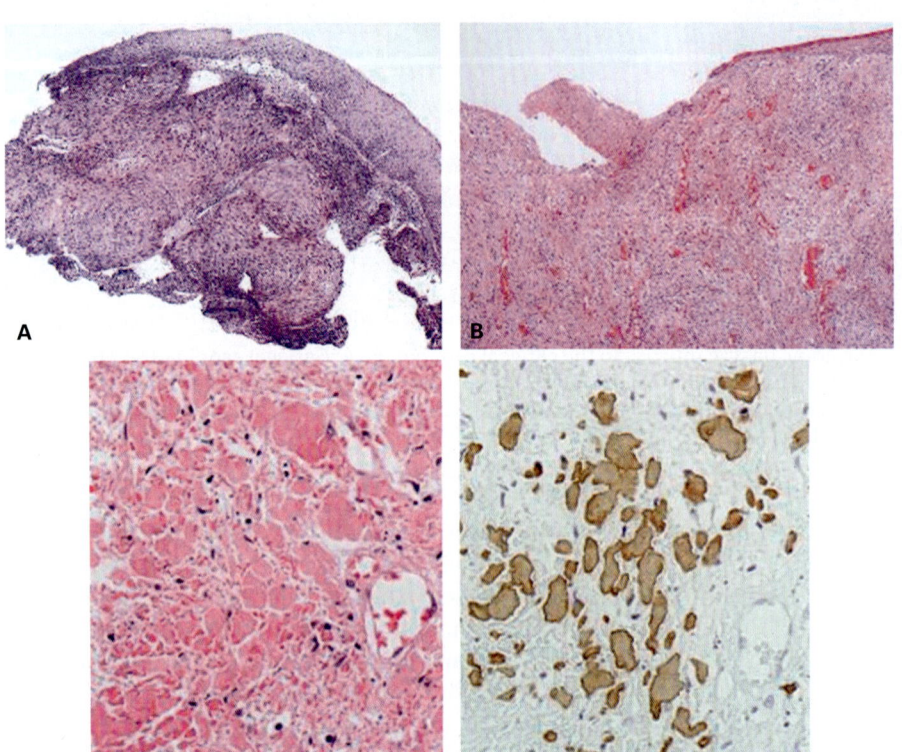

Figure 11-17. **A:** Biopsy of an esophageal tumor shows squamous cell carcinoma. **B,C:** Resection following chemoradiotherapy showed there is no residual tumor. **D:** Immunohistochemistry using AE1/AE3 demonstrated cytokeratin, indicative of residual squamous cell carcinoma.

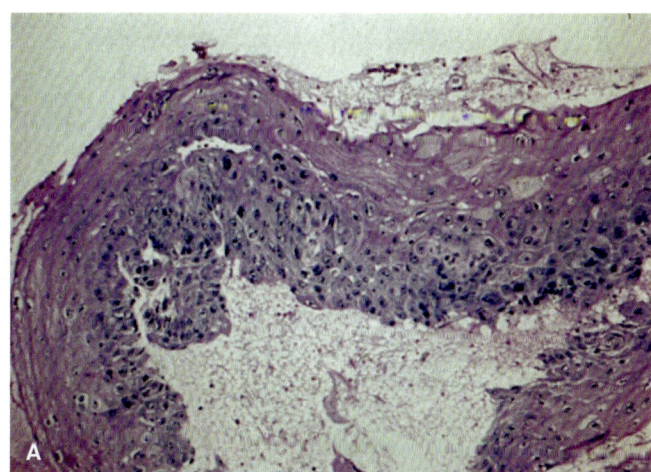
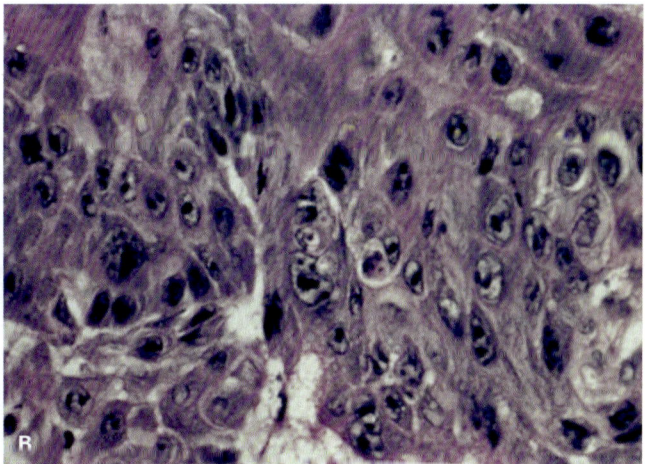

Figure 11-18. A,B: Biopsy specimen following radiation therapy for invasive squamous carcinoma showing residual dysplasia. The biopsy is too superficial to assess invasion.

the squamous or glandular origin. Carcinomas of the lower esophagus, including those arising in Barrett's epithelium, are sometimes adenosquamous. Squamous cell carcinomas can be a problem if resection is contemplated following neoadjuvant chemotherapy or chemoradiotherapy as the entire tumor may disappear (Fig. 11-17). Residual dysplasia is difficult to interpret as it may also be therapy related (Fig. 11-18). However, subsequent therapy is based on the presence of residual invasive carcinoma and not dysplasia, unless a decision to resect following therapy is made initially.

The decision to undertake esophagectomy for squamous carcinoma in situ alone can be difficult, particularly given the relatively high mortality of this procedure. As with analogous problems in other sites, the risks and benefits of the operation must be weighed and each patient must be treated individually, and increasingly endoscopic ablation, primarily endoscopic mucosal resection is being used for these lesions where possible.

Most other difficulties are caused when an unusual type of tumor is biopsied, such as a verrucous carcinoma that can be mistaken for hyperplastic mucosa or the spindle cell variant of squamous carcinoma that can be mistaken for a sarcoma.

Regenerative changes. A false-positive diagnosis of squamous cell carcinoma may sometimes be made when either marked basal cell hyperplasia is present or pseudoepitheliomatous hyperplasia is present. Severe basal hyperplasia without maturation can be misinterpreted as carcinoma in situ, but in the latter, severe dysplasia, usually including loss of polarity, must also be present. In the presence of a stricture secondary to reflux, the lack of dysplasia may be all that prevents this combination from being interpreted as a squamous carcinoma (Fig. 11-19). Rebiopsy to search for invasion is frequently required.

The problem in pseudoepitheliomatous hyperplasia is primarily with the pattern of long thin prongs of squamous mucosa apparently infiltrating into underlying fibrous or granulation tissue (Fig. 11-20). On closer inspection there is little evidence of dysplasia, and sometimes actively regenerating mucosa is clearly associated. Once this appearance is appreciated it does not cause difficulty. This problem may be compounded if actively regenerating epithelium is biopsied because, as in other sites, regeneration is accompanied by prominent eosinophilic nucleoli, which can be interpreted as evidence of either malignancy or viral inclusions (Fig. 11-21).

Granulation tissue. This is a problem primarily of frozen section diagnosis, where the presence of

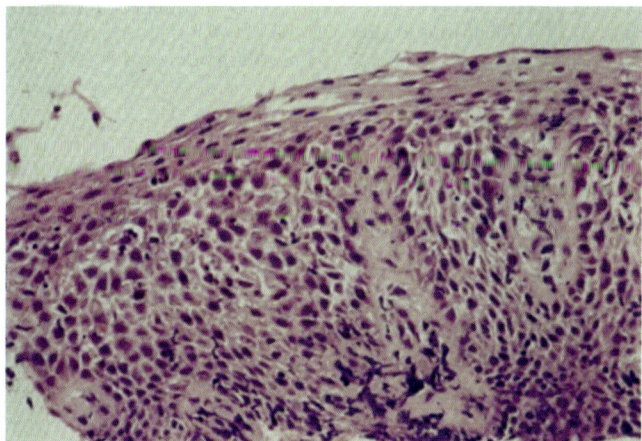

Figure 11-19. Severe basal cell hyperplasia extending close to the surface. However, additional dysplasia is required for a diagnosis of high-grade dysplasia/carcinoma in situ.

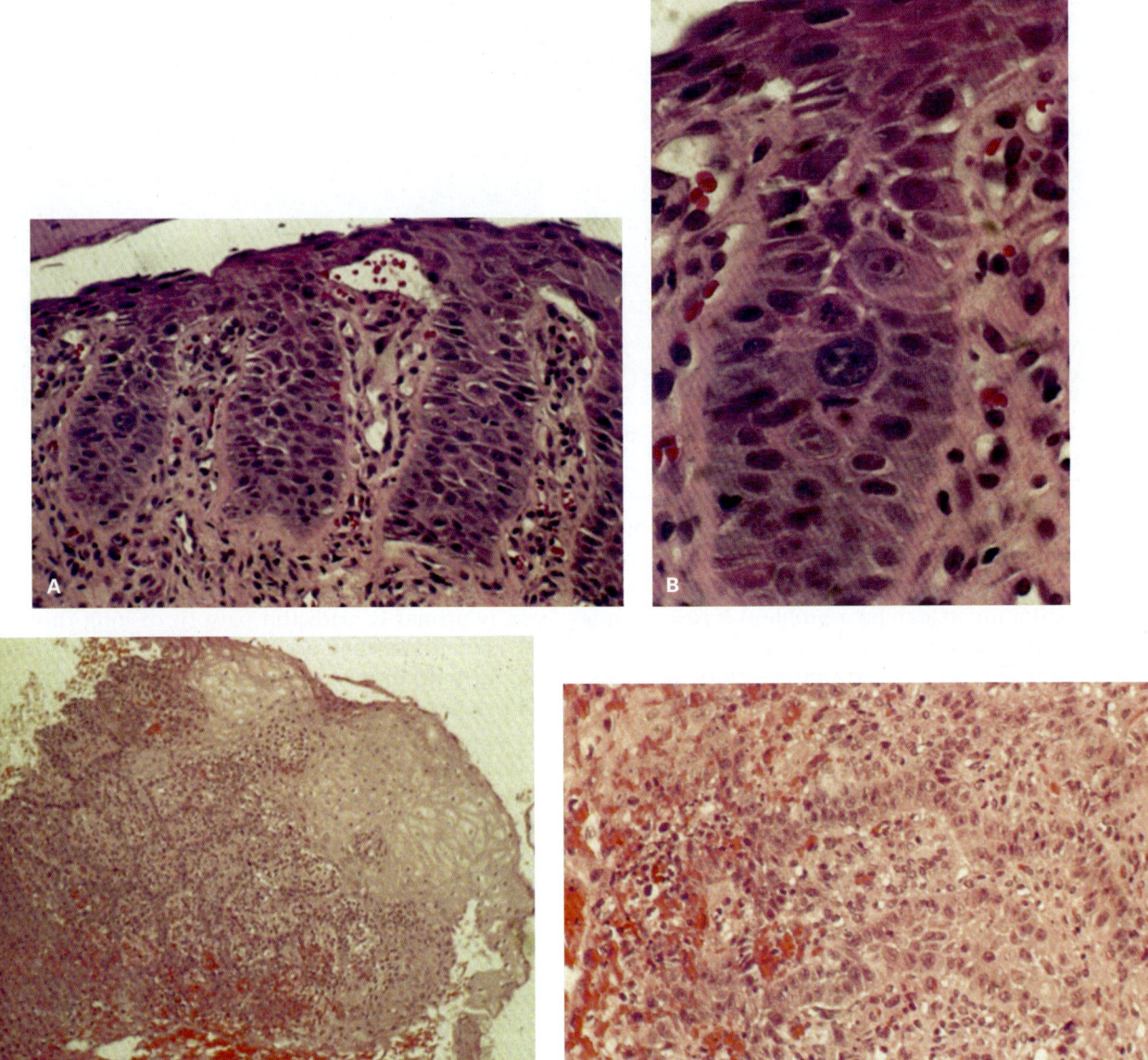

Figure 11-20. A,B: Reactive hyperplasia of squamous mucosa with papillomatosis. Note the occasional atypical nucleus but regular pattern of surface maturation. **C,D:** Tangential cutting adds to the problem by increasing the apparent length of the epithelial prongs mimicking invasion. However, the regularity of all of these "invasive" cords of cells provides the clue that this is organized and therefore reparative.

plump, gland-like endothelial lined vessels may be misinterpreted as adenocarcinoma or possibly a capillary hemangioma if its endothelial nature is recognized (Fig. 11-22). The presence of other inflammatory cells commonly associated with granulation tissue is of help in the differential diagnosis.

Barrett's esophagus. In Barrett's esophagus, regenerated glands can occasionally form a gland-within-gland (back-to-back) appearance (Fig. 11-23). The presence of minimal additional nuclear atypia can readily lead to overdiagnosis of high-grade dysplasia/carcinoma in situ. Under these circumstances, nuclear rather than architectural changes are the most reliable.

In glandular dysplasia, the biggest problems are whether one is dealing with dysplasia or intramucosal carcinoma, and especially whether underlying invasion might be present. The presence of trapped dysplastic glands in the thickened re-duplicated muscularis mucosae can mimic dysplasia and interpretation may be impossible. Features suggesting underlying invasion include a cribriform/solid growth, dilated tubules with necrotic debris, ulcerated high-grade dysplasia and a polymorphonuclear neutrophils in dysplasia (See Chapter 10).

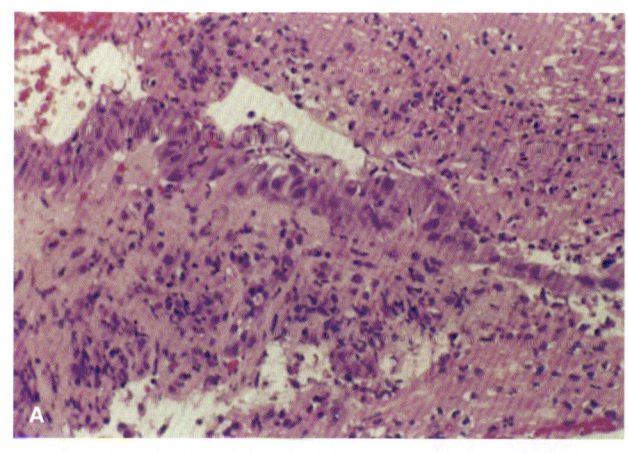
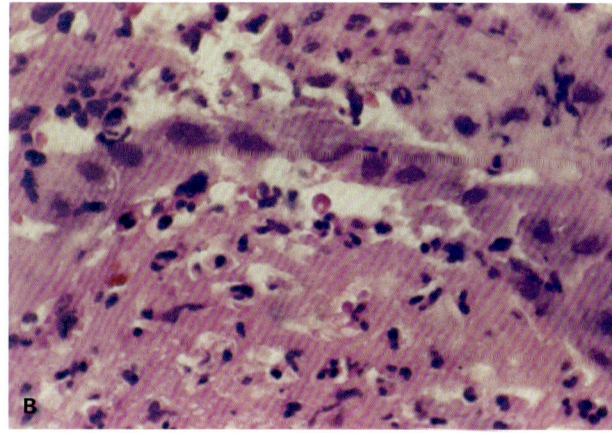

Figure 11-21. A–C: Reparative changes in epithelium actively regenerating over an ulcerated surface.

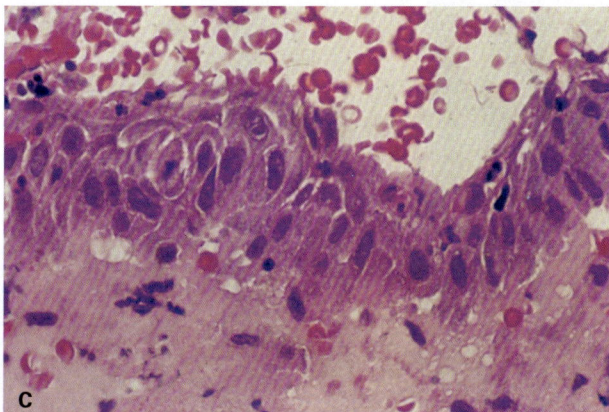

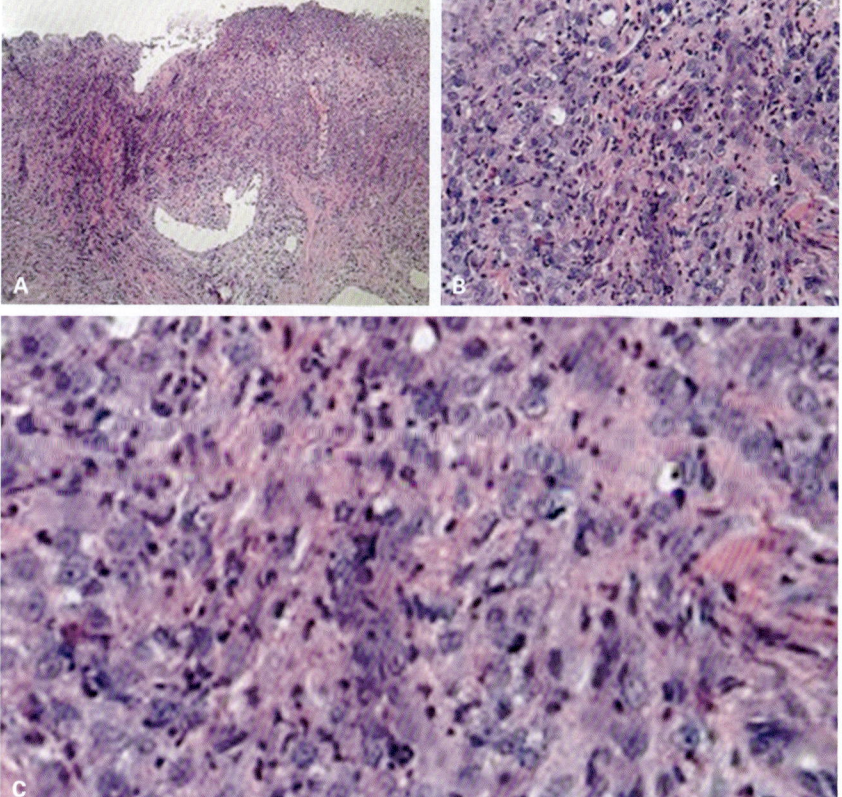

Figure 11-22. A,B: Granulation tissue with inflammatory cell infiltration. Note the numerous endothelial channels with prominent nucleoli (C), which can be misinterpreted as gland, and therefore as adenocarcinoma. The residual inflammatory tissue indicates the diagnosis.

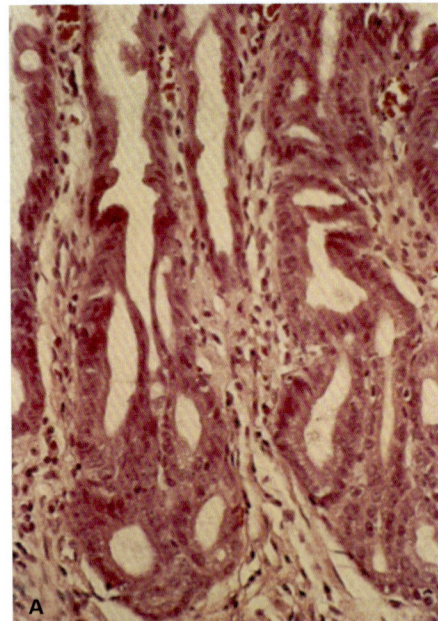

Figure 11-23. **A,B:** Regenerative changes in Barrett's esophagus. Note the back-to-back appearance that can result in over-interpretation as carcinoma in situ. Other evidence of regeneration or lack of dysplasia is necessary to arrive at the correct interpretation.

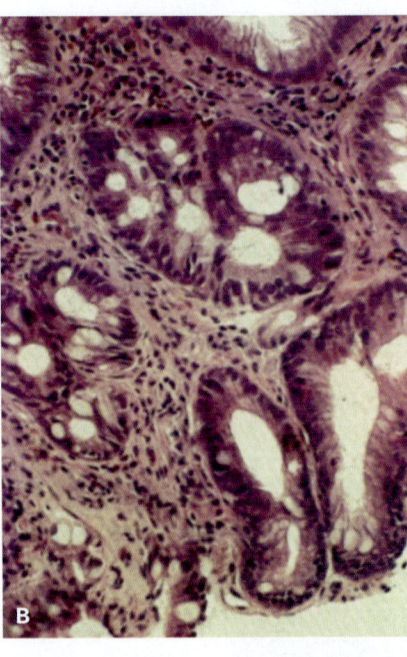

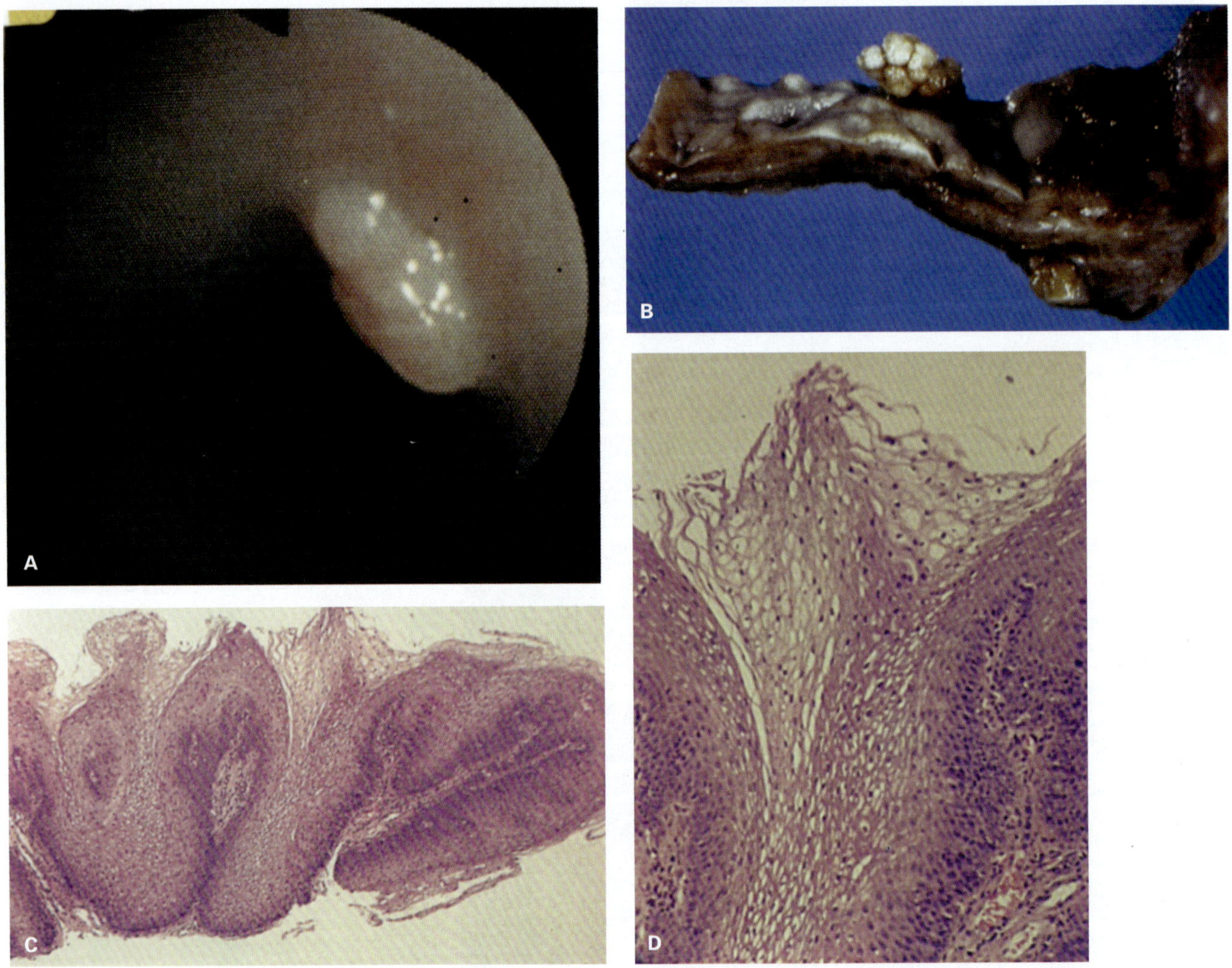

Figure 11-24. Squamous papilloma. **A:** Endoscopic image of papilloma. **B:** Resection showing numerous pearly-white nodules of esophageal papillomatosis. **C, D:** Detail showing acanthosis, mild papillomatosis, and clearing of the cytoplasm superficially.

Other Polyps and Tumors

Squamous papilloma and papillomatosis. Squamous papillomas are rare with the prevalence varying from 0.01% to 0.43%.[235] They are typically located in the mid-esophagus and macroscopically vary from small protrusions to sessile tumors (Fig. 11-24). The diameter is usually 5 mm or less but rarely up to 5 cm.[236] They may rarely cause dysphagia, but usually they are incidentally found in patients without specific symptoms. Squamous papillomatosis is seen primarily in infants and may involve the entire esophageal mucosa. These lesions seem ultimately to disappear, sometimes spontaneously.[237,238]

Histologically, they consist of papillary projections with a central core of connective tissue and well-organized, nondysplastic overlying epithelium. The possibility that larger tumors represent fibrovascular polyps should be considered, although the distinction may be arbitrary in the presence of normal epithelium. Although some lesions display koilocytosis suggesting HPV infection, the etiological role of this virus is controversial in several studies using immunohistochemical method, in situ hybridization, and polymerase chain reaction.[239] Nevertheless, it can occasionally be demonstrated (Fig. 11-25). Malignant progression to squamous cell carcinoma is extremely rare.[235]

Inflammatory Polyps

These are probably the most common esophageal polyps. They occur primarily in males and in the lower esophagus or at the esophagogastric junction, and are usually associated with gastroesophageal reflux.[240] Polyps may consist entirely of vascular granulation tissue and may bleed on contact, sometimes severely. Occasionally, the granulation tissue may be so exuberant that it occludes the esophageal lumen, primarily at anastomosis or radiation sites,[241] and may be misinterpreted as a hemangioma. Identical polyps may sometimes be found undergoing active reepithelialization. Care must be taken not to overinterpret squamous epithelium growing into this granulation tissue as invasive squamous carcinoma.

Pseudosarcomatous changes in inflammatory polyps. Inflammatory polyps can generate very bizarre stromal cells with nuclei that can be pleomorphic, have giant nuclei, numerous mitotic figures, and vary from round to spindled (Fig. 11-26). The surface of the polyp is invariably ulcerated. The concern for the pathologist is whether a neoplasm, especially a carcinoma of some sort, is present. However, cytokeratins stains, endothelial markers, and lymphatic markers are always negative, and the only immunoreactivity demonstrable is with vimentin, and often CD10.

Mucosal Tags

Sometimes small fronds of epithelium are found incidentally, which consist of normal squamous epithelium thrown into a small polyp. Although we call them mucosal tags or fibroepithelial polyps, some may also represent the remnants of inflammatory polyp, which has become reepithelialized and the granulation tissue resolved. Histologically, they are usually indistinguishable from normal mucosa, and it

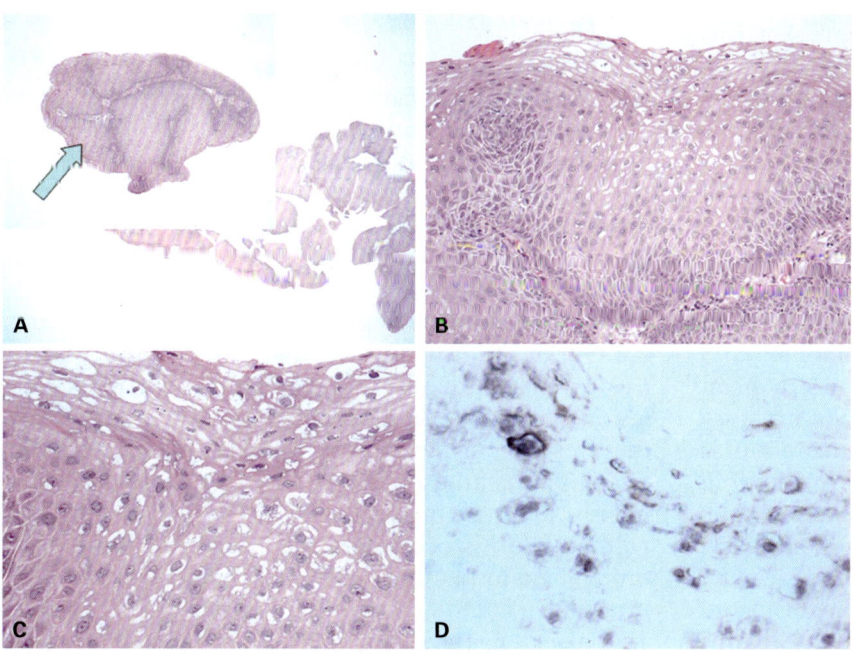

Figure 11-25. Squamous papilloma. **A:** Fragments of squamous mucosa that are overtly acanthotic in part (*arrow*). **B** and **C:** Acanthotic epithelium with superficial cytoplasmic clearing and raisinoid nuclei is seen in HPV infection. **D:** In situ hybridization for HPV 16, 18, and 33.

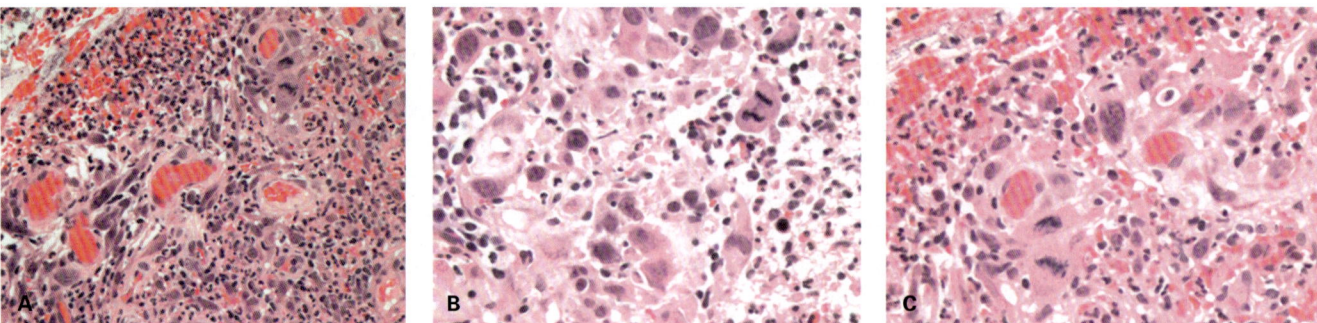

Figure 11-26. Inflammatory polyps with pseudosarcomatous stroma (A–C). The surface is ulcerated, but beneath it (B,C) numerous large bizarre pleomorphic cells "ulcerocytes" (term courtesy of Dr. Henry Appelman) with prominent mitotic figures are present in the stroma. Cytokeratin stains are always negative (unless it really is carcinoma), but these cells are immunoreactive for vimentin, and sometimes CD10.

is only the clinical "polyp" that prompts a second look to ensure that nothing more sinister is being missed, and levels just to ensure that this is the case.

Fibrovascular Polyps

They are benign polypoid or pedunculated tumors that tend to occur in males and usually arise from the proximal third of the esophagus, often in the vicinity of the cricoid (Fig. 11-27). After smooth muscle tumors, most of which occur in the lower third of the esophagus, fibrovascular polyps are probably the most frequent nonepithelial tumors of the esophagus. They often reach a considerable size.[242–244] Larger tumors tend to be sausage-shaped, presumably conforming to the shape of the esophagus and may be multilobular; they may have a pedicle long enough for the patient to regurgitate the tumor into the mouth,[245] although patients more frequently present with dysphagia or awareness of a lump in the throat. They are a potential threat to life as they occasionally occlude the larynx. For this reason they are best removed. They are primarily submucosal tumors covered by normal squamous epithelium, which may be focally ulcerated. Rapid growth has been reported but is likely a complication following torsion or hemorrhage into the tumor.

Histologically, fibrovascular polyps consist of spindle cells occasionally arranged in whorls and loose edematous vascular connective tissue, sometimes with islands of lipocytes. They have variously been reported as lipomas, fibromas, fibrolipomas, and fibromyxomas. Similar lesions in colon have been called mucosal submucosal polyps. Inflammatory cells are mononuclear unless surface ulceration is present, which tends to occur distally. The eosinophil-mast cell-plasma cell combination so characteristic of inflammatory fibroid polyps is not seen, although eosinophils are sometimes numerous. They lack the cellularity of smooth muscle tumors. The histogenesis of these tumors is unclear; however, mechanisms similar to mucosal prolapse combined with weakness in the wall has been postulated. The differential diagnosis is with other mesenchymal tumors, hamartomas, and inflammatory fibroid polyps that are excessively rare in the esophagus.

Hamartomas, Choristomas, Thyroid Rests, Parathyroid Rests

Occasional examples of mature tissues occurring in the esophageal wall have been described. These include sebaceous glands, gastric, and respiratory epithelium. Nodules of cartilage may be a variant of the abnormalities associated with tracheobronchial fistula or possibly part of a duplication (see Chapter 9).[246,247] Nodules of ectopic thyroid tissue and parathyroid tissue, sometimes in the form of a functioning adenoma, have also been described.[248]

Malignant Melanoma

Primary melanoma is a rare tumor accounting for 0.1% to 0.2% of malignancies of the esophagus.[249] The majority of melanomas occur in the sixth to eighth decades of life with a male predominance, and are located in the mid to distal esophagus. The mean tumor size at the time of diagnosis is around 6 cm.[250] Melanomas present as a polypoid intraluminal tumor and a half of the tumors are amelanotic.[250] Junctional activity (melanocytic proliferation in the basal layer of the squamous epithelium) is required to demonstrate its primary nature or to exclude the possibility of a metastatic lesion (Fig. 11-28). In the absence of junctional activity, the presence of melanocytes in the adjacent mucosa also supports an esophageal origin, as these are found in only about 4% of esophagi examined.[251] Macroscopic pigmentation is occasionally apparent in the mucosa uninvolved by the tumor.[252,253] It is important to recognize that melanoma exhibits extensive lateral growth, and the extension of the tumor is often underestimated when a resection is contemplated.[252,254] Melanoma is typically aggressive and disseminates early via the bloodstream and lymphatics. Most patients have metastatic disease at the time of presentation. The prognosis is extremely poor, with 5% surviving for 5 years, even when resected at an early stage.[255]

The histologic spectrum is wide, including appearances mimicking lymphoma, poorly differentiated adenocarcinoma or sarcoma. The diagnosis can be confirmed either by finding premelanosomes electron microscopically or by immunohistochemical staining with a variety of melanoma markers such as HMB-45, Melan-A, tyrosinase, and S-100.

Malignant melanomas arising in the skin have a distinct tendency to metastasize to the submucosa of the entire intestinal tract, including the esophagus, where they may also form polypoid tumors.[251] In patients with disseminated melanoma of an unknown primary site, care should be taken not to interpret the polypoid esophageal tumor as being the primary unless other evidence, such as the presence of junctional activity, is found. If this is absent, the esophagus may still be the only reasonable primary site, but in this situation the interpretation of the esophageal tumor is clearly speculative in the absence of any other primary tumor.

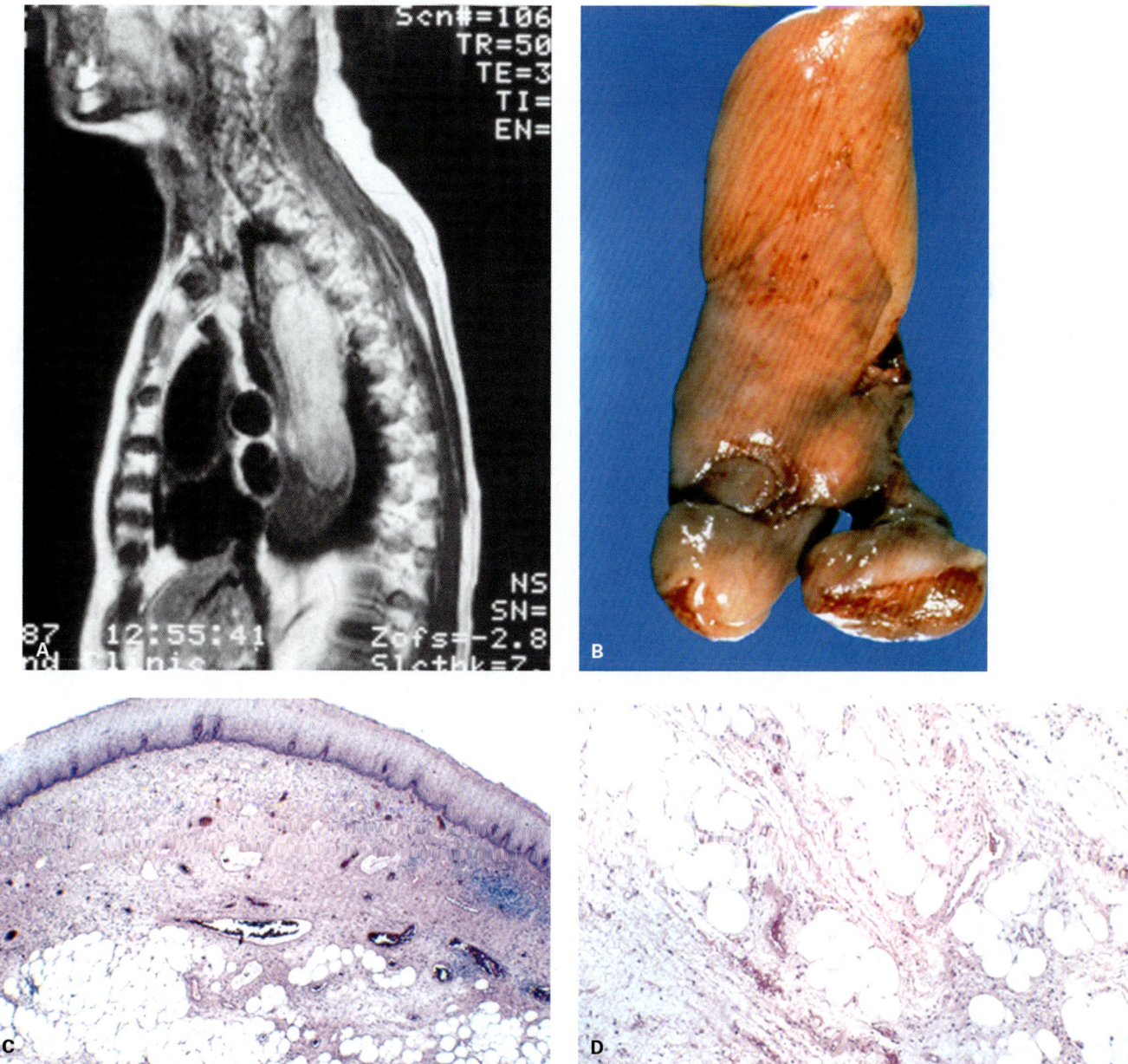

Figure 11-27. Giant fibrovascular polyp of the esophagus. **A:** Gross appearance showing the long sausage shape because of molding within the esophagus. This example is multilobated. **B–D:** Histologic appearance showing the epithelial covered surface but underlying mesenchymal tissue which is loose, modestly vascular, and myxoid, with a scattering of inflammatory cells. (Courtesy of Dr. R. E. Petras.)

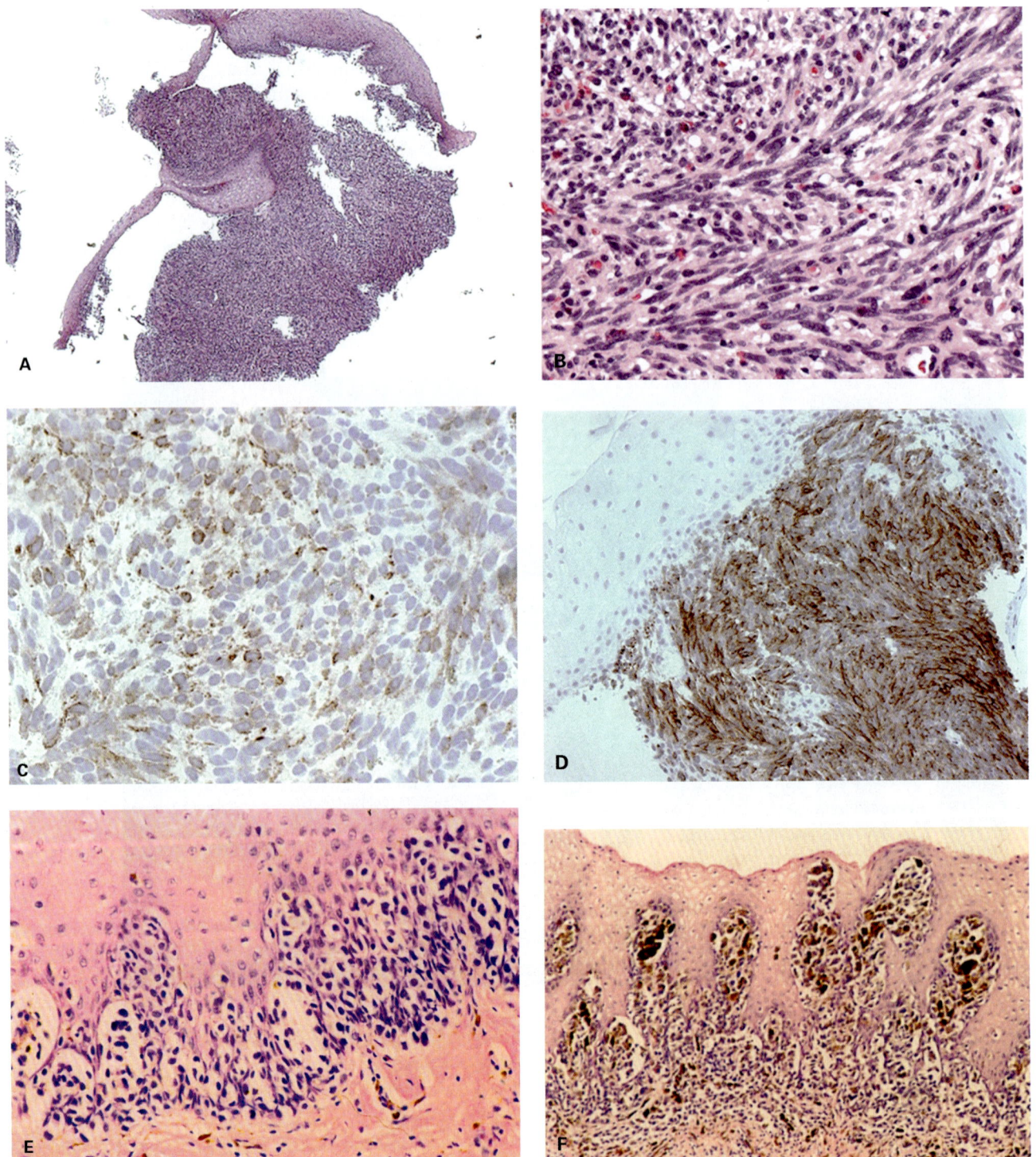

Figure 11-28. A,B: Mucosa adjacent to the esophageal tumor showing a proliferation of melanocytes in the basal layer. **C–F:** In some areas, these replace the papillae and extend close to the surface.

Secondary Tumors

Metastatic involvement of the esophagus from distant primary tumors is rare. Most commonly, secondary involvement occurs by direct spread from tumors from adjacent sites, such as those of the hypopharynx, larynx, trachea, thyroid, bronchus, and stomach (Fig. 11-29).[135] Secondary involvement can also occur from metastases to periesophageal lymph nodes and is most commonly seen in patients with lung and breast primaries.

Patients with squamous carcinoma of the head and neck have a high incidence of concomitant carcinoma of the esophagus because of exposure to similar etiologic agents, particularly tobacco. On rare occasions, differentiation between secondary esophageal

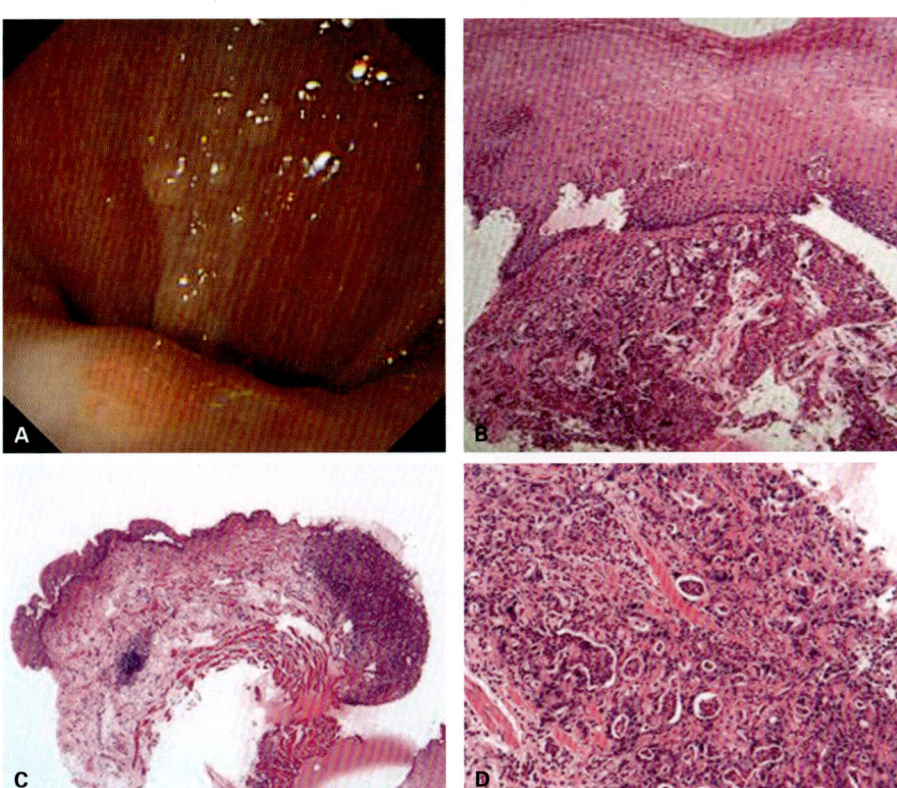

Figure 11-29. Metastatic involvement of the esophagus from a gastric cancer. **A:** Endoscopic appearance of multiple metastases. **B:** Adenocarcinoma covered by normal squamous epithelium. **C,D.** Carcinoma subsequently destroys the overlying epithelium.

involvement and a second primary may present difficulties or may be impossible.

Esophageal involvement in leukemia is not infrequent and is manifested by hemorrhagic lesions in the mucosa or submucosa. Leukemic infiltrates may range from microscopic to grossly nodular lesions. Mucosal erosions or ulcerations may become infected by fungi, especially *Candida*, or bacteria, with the formation of a pseudomembrane containing necrotic debris and fibrin.

Mesenchymal Tumors

Specific entities are discussed in more details in Chapter 7 and esophagus specific issues are dealt here. The most common benign mesenchymal tumors of the esophagus are of smooth muscle origin. Leiomyomas occur primarily in the third decade of life with a male predominance.[256,257] They are located in the middle or lower esophagus.[258] Almost all of the tumors show intramural growth,[259] and esophagography showed them as smoothly elevated defects. The larger tumors may extend to mediastinum forming mediastinal masses. Enhanced CT scan reveals a smooth or lobulated tumor margin, and attenuation is homogeneously low or iso.[258] Esophageal leiomyomas are usually very slow growing and often asymptomatic. Symptomatic tumors are usually >5 cm in diameter,[260] and dysphagia and chest or epigastric pain were the most common presenting symptoms. Endoscopic tissue sampling is usually difficult and the assessment of malignancy is not very reliable. Histologically, leiomyoma is composed of spindle cells, which are typically positive for desmin and α-smooth muscle actin but are negative for CD34 or CD117 (c-kit) (see also Chapter 7).[257]

Leiomyomatosis is a rare lesion and can be associated with Alport's syndrome in familial cases. It can involve the upper part of the stomach and is frequently associated with genital or tracheobronchial localizations. Characteristically there is diffuse proliferation of smooth muscle cells in the esophageal wall forming a worm-like intramural structure or a localized circumferential thickening (Fig. 11-30).[260] A curious feature of these tumors is that they are invariably admixed with interstitial cells of Cajal, which are visible on the CD117 or DOG-1 immunostains used to exclude gastrointestinal stromal tumors (GISTs). However, neural processes, which are invariably very prominent in normal smooth muscle of the GI tract, are very hard to locate (Fig. 11-30). Esophageal resection is the only suitable treatment in symptomatic cases.

Leiomyosarcomas of the esophagus are rare malignant smooth muscle tumors and occur primarily in males between the sixth and the eighth decades. Dysphagia is one of the most common presenting symptoms, which are indistinguishable from other esophageal

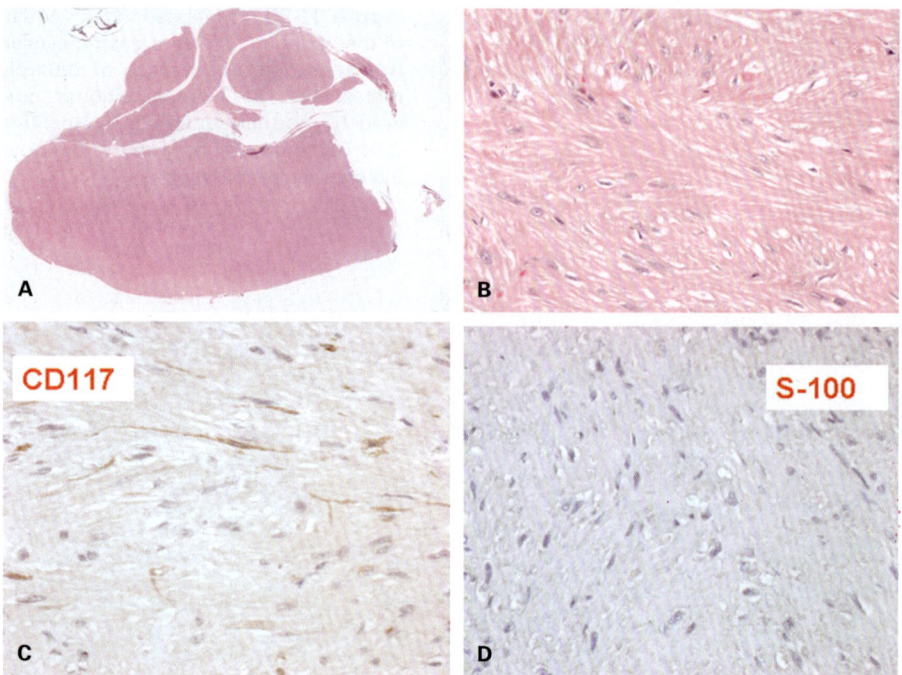

Figure 11-30. Leiomyoma (leiomyomatosis) of the lower esophagus. **A:** Scanning shows a multilobated polypoid mass, which is very characteristic of these lesions **B:** Typical paucicellular densely eosinophilic cytoplasm of a smooth muscle tumor **C:** CD117 showing abundant interstitial cells of Cajal. **D:** S-100 immunostain with no identifiable neural pricesses.

neoplasms, though the history may be longer due to the slow growth of these tumors. Barium studies may show large intramural masses with ulceration or tracking, expansile intraluminal masses or areas of luminal narrowing. Endoscopic biopsies may give a high false negative rate especially in cases where the mucosa is intact. The commonly used criteria for malignancy are nuclear pleomorphism and over 10 mitoses per 10 HPF (see also Chapter 7). Prognosis is poor but better than in patients with squamous cell carcinoma.[261]

GISTs rarely occur primarily in the lowest third of the esophagus; of all GISTs, only 1% to 2% are found in the esophagus (Fig. 11-31).[262] The predisposing age and sex are similar to those of leiomyosarcoma, from which they need to be differentiated because of different prognosis and management issues (see Chapter 7).

Granular cell tumors are endoscopically detected usually as yellow nodules or small sessile polyps. The majority of the tumors are solitary (95%), <10 mm in diameter (75%), and localized in the distal esophagus (75%).[263] Histologically, they are similar to granular cell tumors elsewhere (see Chapter 7). and consist of spindle or polyhedral cells with small central nucleus, and the cytoplasm contains eosinophilic granules, which reflect extensive accumulation of lysosomes. They are typically PAS and S-100 protein positive. They are generally believed to be of neurogenic origin but are benign; interestingly, endoscopic follow-up (1–60 months) in 16 out of 17 patients left untreated showed either a stable tumor size or regression of the tumor. In one case with multiple GCTs, a slight tumor growth was seen after a follow-up period of 48 months.[263]

Synovial sarcomas, which are histologically indistinguishable from their peripheral counterparts, rarely occur in the upper esophagus of children and older adults (see also Chapter 7). They usually present as polypoid masses and are not associated with dysplasia of the overlying epithelium. It therefore appears to be a distinct entity and unlike the peripheral one seems not to metastasize so that local removal may well be curative.[264–266]

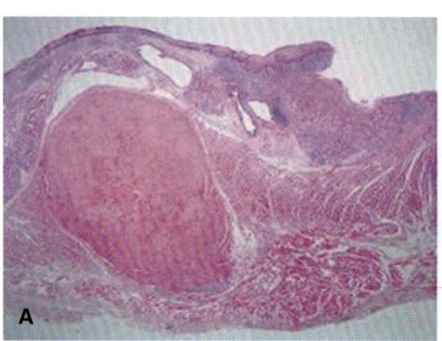
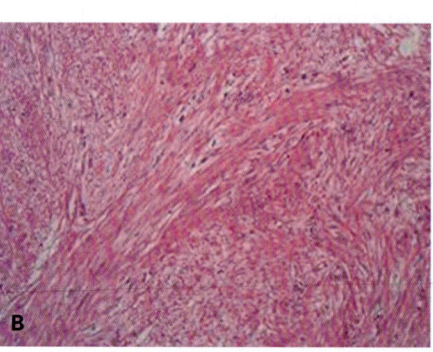

Figure 11-31. **A,B:** GIST arising in the muscularis propria of the esophagus. The diagnosis of spindle cell tumors requires immunohistochemical studies (CD117 was diffusely immunoreactive).

References

1. Pohl H, Welch HG. The role of overdiagnosis and reclassification in the marked increase of esophageal adenocarcinoma incidence. *J Natl Cancer Inst.* 2005;97(2):142–146.
2. Hofstetter W, Swisher SG, Correa AM, et al. Treatment outcomes of resected esophageal cancer. *Ann Surg.* 2002;236(3):376–384; discussion 84–85.
3. Wang HW, Kuo KT, Wu YC, et al. Surgical results of upper thoracic esophageal carcinoma. *J Chin Med Assoc.* 2004;67(9):447–457.
4. Ancona E, Ruol A, Santi S, et al. Only pathologic complete response to neoadjuvant chemotherapy improves significantly the long term survival of patients with resectable esophageal squamous cell carcinoma: final report of a randomized, controlled trial of preoperative chemotherapy versus surgery alone. *Cancer.* 2001;91(11):2165–2174.
5. Urschel JD, Vasan H, Blewett CJ. A meta-analysis of randomized controlled trials that compared neoadjuvant chemotherapy and surgery to surgery alone for resectable esophageal cancer. *Am J Surg.* 2002;183(3):274–279.
6. Greer SE, Goodney PP, Sutton JE, Birkmeyer JD. Neoadjuvant chemoradiotherapy for esophageal carcinoma: a meta-analysis. *Surgery.* 2005;137(2):172–177.
7. Law S, Kwong DL, Kwok KF, et al. Improvement in treatment results and long-term survival of patients with esophageal cancer: impact of chemoradiation and change in treatment strategy. *Ann Surg.* 2003;238(3):339–347; discussion 47–48.
8. Tabira Y, Yasunaga M, Sakaguchi T, et al. Outcome of histologically node-negative esophageal squamous cell carcinoma. *World J Surg.* 2002;26(12):1446–1451.
9. El-Serag HB, Sonnenberg A. Ethnic variations in the occurrence of gastroesophageal cancers. *J Clin Gastroenterol.* 1999;28(2):135–139.
10. Wang GQ, Jiao GG, Chang FB, et al. Long-term results of operation for 420 patients with early squamous cell esophageal carcinoma discovered by screening. *Ann Thorac Surg.* 2004;77(5):1740–1744.
11. Leoni-Parvex S, Mihaescu A, Pellanda A, et al. Esophageal cytology in the follow-up of patients with treated upper aerodigestive tract malignancies. *Cancer.* 2000;90(1):10–16.
12. Negri E, La Vecchia C, Levi F, et al. Comparative descriptive epidemiology of oral and oesophageal cancers in Europe. *Eur J Cancer Prev.* 1996;5(4):267–279.
13. Launoy G, Milan CH, Faivre J, et al. Alcohol, tobacco and oesophageal cancer: effects of the duration of consumption, mean intake and current and former consumption. *Br J Cancer.* 1997;75(9):1389–1396.
14. Wynder EL, Mabuchi K. Cancer of the gastrointestinal tract. Etiological and environmental factors. *JAMA.* 1973;226(13):1546–158.
15. Boffeta P, Hashibe M. Alcohol and cancer. *Lancet Oncol.* 2006;7:149–156.
16. Yang CX, Wang HY, Wang ZM, et al. Risk factors for esophageal cancer: a case-control study in South-western China. *Asian Pac J Cancer Prev.* 2005;6(1):48–53.
17. La Rosa F, Cresci A, Orpianesi C, et al. Esophageal cancer mortality: relationship with alcohol intake and cigarette smoking in Italy. *Eur J Epidemiol.* 1988;4(1):93–98.
18. Yun YH, Jung KW, Bae JM, et al. Cigarette smoking and cancer incidence risk in adult men: National Health Insurance Corporation Study. *Cancer Detect Prev.* 2005;29(1):15–24.
19. Ghadirian P, Stein GF, Gorodetzky C, et al. Oesophageal cancer studies in the Caspian littoral of Iran: some residual results, including opium use as a risk factor. *Int J Cancer.* 1985;35(5):593–597.
20. Tran GD, Sun XD, Abnet CC, et al. Prospective study of risk factors for esophageal and gastric cancers in the Linxian general population trial cohort in China. *Int J Cancer.* 2005;113(3):456–463.
21. Li K, Yu P. Food groups and risk of esophageal cancer in Chaoshan region of China: a high-risk area of esophageal cancer. *Cancer Invest.* 2003;21(2):237–240.
22. Terry P, Lagergren J, Wolk A, Nyren O. Drinking hot beverages is not associated with risk of oesophageal cancers in a Western population. *Br J Cancer.* 2001;84(1):120–121.
23. Wei WQ, Abnet CC, Lu N, et al. Risk factors for oesophageal squamous dysplasia in adult inhabitants of a high risk region of China. *Gut.* 2005;54(6):759–763.
24. Garavello W, Negri E, Talamini R, et al. Family history of cancer, its combination with smoking and drinking, and risk of squamous cell carcinoma of the esophagus. *Cancer Epidemiol Biomarkers Prev.* 2005;14(6):1390–1393.
25. Shen ZY, Hu SP, Lu LC, et al. Detection of human papillomavirus in esophageal carcinoma. *J Med Virol.* 2002;68(3):412–416.
26. Chang F, Syrjanen S, Shen Q, et al. Human papillomavirus involvement in esophageal carcinogenesis in the high-incidence area of China. A study of 700 cases by screening and type-specific in situ hybridization. *Scand J Gastroenterol.* 2000;35(2):123–130.
27. Kim SG, Hong SJ, Kwon KW, et al. The expression of p53, p16, cyclin D1 in esophageal squamous cell carcinoma and esophageal dysplasia]. *Korean J Gastroenterol.* 2006;48(4):269–276.
28. Lyronis ID, Baritaki S, Bizakis I, Tsardi M, Spandidos DA. Evaluation of the prevalence of human papillomavirus and Epstein-Barr virus in esophageal squamous cell carcinomas. *Int J Biol Markers.* 2005;20(1):5–10.
29. Farhadi M, Tahmasebi Z, Merat S, Kamangar F, Nasrollahzadeh D, Malekzadeh R. Human papillomavirus in squamous cell carcinoma of esophagus in a high-risk population. *World J Gastroenterol.* 2005;11(8):1200–1203.
30. Guo M, Ren J, House MG, Qi Y, Brock MV, Herman JG. Accumulation of promoter methylation suggests epigenetic progression in squamous cell carcinoma of the esophagus. *Clin Cancer Res.* 2006;12(15):4515–4522.
31. Lambot MA, Haot J, Peny MO, Fayt I, Noel JC. Evaluation of the role of human papillomavirus in oesophageal squamous cell carcinoma in Belgium. *Acta Gastroenterol Belg.* 2000;63(2):154–156.
32. White RE, Mungatana C, Mutuma G, et al. Absence of human papillomavirus in esophageal carcinomas from southwestern Kenya. *Dis Esophagus.* 2005;18(1):28–30.
33. Yu IT, Tse LA, Wong TW, Leung CC, Tam CM, Chan AC. Further evidence for a link between silica dust and esophageal cancer. *Int J Cancer.* 2005;114(3):479–483.
34. Bardou M, Barkun AN, Ghosn J, Hudson M, Rahme E. Effect of chronic intake of NSAIDs and cyclooxygenase 2-selective inhibitors on esophageal cancer incidence. *Clin Gastroenterol Hepatol.* 2004;2(10):880–887.
35. Limburg PJ, Wei W, Ahnen DJ, et al. Randomized, placebo-controlled, esophageal squamous cell cancer chemoprevention trial of selenomethionine and celecoxib. *Gastroenterology.* 2005;129(3):863–873.
36. Ye W, Held M, Lagergren J, et al. Helicobacter pylori infection and gastric atrophy: risk of adenocarcinoma and squamous-cell carcinoma of the esophagus and adenocarcinoma of the gastric cardia. *J Natl Cancer Inst.* 2004;96(5):388–396.
37. Swinson CM, Slavin G, Coles EC, Booth CC. Coeliac disease and malignancy. *Lancet.* 1983;1(8316):111–115.
38. Cooper BT, Holmes GK, Ferguson R, Cooke WT. Celiac disease and malignancy. *Medicine (Baltimore).* 1980;59(4):249–261.
39. Harper PS, Harper RM, Howel-Evans AW. Carcinoma of the oesophagus with tylosis. *Q J Med.* 1970;39(155):317–333.

40. Kuwano H, Ohno S, Matsuda H, Mori M, Sugimachi K. Serial histologic evaluation of multiple primary squamous cell carcinomas of the esophagus. *Cancer.* 1988;61(8):1635-1638.
41. Norton GA, Postlethwait RW, Thompson WM. Esophageal carcinoma: a survey of populations at risk. *South Med J.* 1980;73(1):25-27.
42. Charles J, Fiasse R, Pringot J, Heller F. [Radiation induced cancer of pharynx and esophagus. Report of three cases (author's transl)]. *Acta Gastroenterol Belg.* 1979;42(1-2):7-29.
43. Wang GQ, Abnet CC, Shen Q, et al. Histological precursors of oesophageal squamous cell carcinoma: results from a 13 year prospective follow up study in a high risk population. *Gut.* 2005;54(2):187-192.
44. Yanjin M, Guangyi L, Xianzhi G, Wenheng C. Detection and natural progression of early oesophageal carcinoma: preliminary communication. *J R Soc Med.* 1981;74(12):884-886.
45. Kuwano H, Matsuda H, Matsuoka H, Kai H, Okudaira Y, Sugimachi K. Intra-epithelial carcinoma concomitant with esophageal squamous cell carcinoma. *Cancer.* 1987;59(4):783-787.
46. Mandard AM, Marnay J, Herlin P, Elie H, Tuyns AJ, Le Talaer JY. [Cancer of the esophagus induced in the Wistar rat by ethyl-N-butyl-nitrosamine]. *Bull Cancer.* 1984;71(5):419-424.
47. Fagundes RB, Mello CR, Tollens P, et al. p53 protein in esophageal mucosa of individuals at high risk of squamous cell carcinoma of the esophagus. *Dis Esophagus.* 2001;14(3-4):185-190.
48. Chang MS, Lee HS, Lee BL, Kim YT, Lee JS, Kim WH. Differential protein expression between esophageal squamous cell carcinoma and dysplasia, and prognostic significance of protein markers. *Pathol Res Pract.* 2005;201(6):417-425.
49. Rubio CA, Liu FS, Zhao HZ. Histological classification of intraepithelial neoplasias and microinvasive squamous carcinoma of the esophagus. *Am J Surg Pathol.* 1989;13(8):685-690.
50. Schlemper RJ, Dawsey SM, Itabashi M, et al. Differences in diagnostic criteria for esophageal squamous cell carcinoma between Japanese and Western pathologists. *Cancer.* 2000;88(5):996-1006.
51. Gabbert H, Shimoda T, Hainaut P, Nakamura Y, Field J, Inoue H. Squamous cell carcinoma of the esophagus. In: Hamilton S, Aaltonen, LA, eds. World Health Organization Classification of Tumour Pathology and Genetics of Tumours of the Digestive System. Lyon: IARC Press; 2000:11-19.
52. Takubo K, Aida J, Sawabe M, et al. Early squamous cell carcinoma of the oesophagus: the Japanese viewpoint. *Histopathology.* 2007;51(6):733-742.
53. Shimizu M, Ban S, Odze RD. Squamous dysplasia and other precursor lesions related to esophageal squamous cell carcinoma. *Gastroenterol Clin North Am.* 2007;36(4):797-811, v-vi.
54. Ming S. Tumors of the esophagus and stomach. In: *Atlas of Tumor Pathology, Series 2, Fascicle 7.* Washington, DC: Armed Forces Institute of Pathology; 1973.
55. Mariette C, Finzi L, Fabre S, Balon JM, Van Seuningen I, Triboulet JP. Factors predictive of complete resection of operable esophageal cancer: a prospective study. *Ann Thorac Surg.* 2003;75(6):1720-1726.
56. Ide H, Endo M, Kinoshita Y, et al. Clinicopathological aspect of superficial esophageal cancer (22 cases of our experience). *Chir Gastroenterol.* 1976;10:9-16.
57. Bogomoletz WV, Molas G, Gayet B, Potet F. Superficial squamous cell carcinoma of the esophagus. A report of 76 cases and review of the literature. *Am J Surg Pathol.* 1989;13(7):535-546.
58. Hashimoto CL, Iriya K, Baba ER, et al. Lugol's dye spray chromoendoscopy establishes early diagnosis of esophageal cancer in patients with primary head and neck cancer. *Am J Gastroenterol.* 2005;100(2):275-282.
59. Kuraoka K, Hoshino E, Tsuchida T, Fujisaki J, Takahashi H, Fujita R. Early esophageal cancer can be detected by screening endoscopy assisted with narrow-band imaging (NBI). *Hepatogastroenterology.* 2009;56(89):63-66.
60. Pech O, Rabenstein T, Manner H, et al. Confocal laser endomicroscopy for in vivo diagnosis of early squamous cell carcinoma in the esophagus. *Clin Gastroenterol Hepatol.* 2008;6(1):89-94.
61. May A, Gunter E, Roth F, et al. Accuracy of staging in early oesophageal cancer using high resolution endoscopy and high resolution endosonography: a comparative, prospective, and blinded trial. *Gut.* 2004;53(5):634-640.
62. Brombard M. *Clinical Radiology of the Esophagus.* Baltimore, MD: Williams & Wilkins; 1961.
63. Kumagai Y, Makuuchi H, Fujita H, Miyoshi H, Suguro Y. "Ebb phenomenon"—diagnosis of submucosal diffuse invasion of esophageal cancer. *Endoscopy.* 1982;14(1):6-8.
64. Tajima Y, Nakanishi Y, Ochiai A, et al. Histopathologic findings predicting lymph node metastasis and prognosis of patients with superficial esophageal carcinoma: analysis of 240 surgically resected tumors. *Cancer.* 2000;88(6):1285-1293.
65. Morita M, Kuwano H, Araki K, et al. Prognostic significance of lymphocyte infiltration following preoperative chemoradiotherapy and hyperthermia for esophageal cancer. *Int J Radiat Oncol Biol Phys.* 2001;49(5):1259-1266.
66. Guernsey JM, Knudsen DF, Mark JB. Abdominal exploration in the evaluation of patients with carcinoma of the thoracic esophagus. *J Thorac Cardiovasc Surg.* 1970;59(1):62-66.
67. Mandard AM, Chasle J, Marnay J, et al. Autopsy findings in 111 cases of esophageal cancer. *Cancer* 1981;48(2):329-335.
68. Mariette C, Balon JM, Piessen G, et al. Pattern of recurrence following complete resection of esophageal carcinoma and factors predictive of recurrent disease. *Cancer* 2003;97(7):1616-1623.
69. Lerut T, Nafteux P, Moons J, et al. Three-field lymphadenectomy for carcinoma of the esophagus and gastroesophageal junction in 174 R0 resections: impact on staging, disease-free survival, and outcome: a plea for adaptation of TNM classification in upper-half esophageal carcinoma. *Ann Surg.* 2004;240(6):962-972; discussion 72-74.
70. Siewert JR, Stein HJ, Feith M, Bruecher BL, Bartels H, Fink U. Histologic tumor type is an independent prognostic parameter in esophageal cancer: lessons from more than 1,000 consecutive resections at a single center in the Western world. *Ann Surg.* 2001;234(3):360-367; discussion 8-9.
71. Mariette C, Piessen G, Balon JM, Van Seuningen I, Triboulet JP. Surgery alone in the curative treatment of localised oesophageal carcinoma. *Eur J Surg Oncol.* 2004;30(8):869-876.
72. Abunasra H, Lewis S, Beggs L, Duffy J, Beggs D, Morgan E. Predictors of operative death after oesophagectomy for carcinoma. *Br J Surg.* 2005;92(8):1029-1033.
73. Berger AC, Farma J, Scott WJ, et al. Complete response to neoadjuvant chemoradiotherapy in esophageal carcinoma is associated with significantly improved survival. *J Clin Oncol.* 2005;23(19):4330-4337.
74. Chirieac LR, Swisher SG, Ajani JA, et al. Posttherapy pathologic stage predicts survival in patients with esophageal carcinoma receiving preoperative chemoradiation. *Cancer.* 2005;103(7):1347-1355.
75. Edge SB, Compton CC. The American Joint Committee on Cancer: the 7th edition of the AJCC cancer staging manual and the future of TNM. *Ann Surg Oncol.* 2010;17(6):1471-1474.

76. Igaki H, Kato H, Tachimori Y, Nakanishi Y. Prognostic evaluation of patients with clinical T1 and T2 squamous cell carcinomas of the thoracic esophagus after 3-field lymph node dissection. *Surgery.* 2003;133(4):368–374.
77. Vazquez-Sequeiros E, Wang L, Burgart L, et al. Occult lymph node metastases as a predictor of tumor relapse in patients with node-negative esophageal carcinoma. *Gastroenterology.* 2002;122(7):1815–1821.
78. Shimizu Y, Tsukagoshi H, Fujita M, Hosokawa M, Kato M, Asaka M. Long-term outcome after endoscopic mucosal resection in patients with esophageal squamous cell carcinoma invading the muscularis mucosae or deeper. *Gastrointest Endosc.* 2002;56(3):387–390.
79. Igaki H, Kato H, Tachimori Y, et al. Clinicopathologic characteristics and survival of patients with clinical Stage I squamous cell carcinomas of the thoracic esophagus treated with three-field lymph node dissection. *Eur J Cardiothorac Surg.* 2001;20(6):1089–1094.
80. Gotohda N, Nishimura M, Yoshida J, Nagai K, Tanaka N. The pattern of lymphatic metastases in superficial squamous cell carcinoma of the esophagus. *Hepatogastroenterology.* 2005;52(61):105–107.
81. Sasajima K, Takai A, Taniguchi Y, et al. Polypoid squamous cell carcinoma of the esophagus. *Cancer.* 1989;64(1):94–97.
82. Nakajima Y, Nagai K, Miyake S, Ohashi K, Kawano T, Iwai T. Evaluation of an indicator for lymph node metastasis of esophageal squamous cell carcinoma invading the submucosal layer. *Jpn J Cancer Res.* 2002;93(3):305–312.
83. Iizuka T, Hirata K, Watanabe H, Senba T. Factors controlling five-year survival in patients with esophageal carcinoma. *Jpn J Clin Oncol.* 1979;9:41–48.
84. Eloubeidi MA, Desmond R, Arguedas MR, Reed CE, Wilcox CM. Prognostic factors for the survival of patients with esophageal carcinoma in the U.S.: the importance of tumor length and lymph node status. *Cancer.* 2002;95(7):1434–1443.
85. Yeh AM, Mendenhall WM, Morris CG, et al. Factors predictive of survival for esophageal carcinoma treated with preoperative radiotherapy with or without chemotherapy followed by surgery. *J Surg Oncol.* 2003;83(1):14–23.
86. Kimura Y, Watanabe M, Ohga T, et al. Vascular endothelial growth factor C expression correlates with lymphatic involvement and poor prognosis in patients with esophageal squamous cell carcinoma. *Oncol Rep.* 2003;10(6):1747–1751.
87. Brucher BL, Stein HJ, Werner M, Siewert JR. Lymphatic vessel invasion is an independent prognostic factor in patients with a primary resected tumor with esophageal squamous cell carcinoma. *Cancer.* 2001;92(8):2228–2233.
88. Dexter SP, Sue-Ling H, McMahon MJ, Quirke P, Mapstone N, Martin IG. Circumferential resection margin involvement: an independent predictor of survival following surgery for oesophageal cancer. *Gut.* 2001;48(5):667–670.
89. Khoury GA. Oesophageal surgery under Akiyama. *Lancet.* 1989;1(8620):101–02.
90. Xiao ZF, Yang ZY, Miao YJ, et al. Influence of number of metastatic lymph nodes on survival of curative resected thoracic esophageal cancer patients and value of radiotherapy: report of 549 cases. *Int J Radiat Oncol Biol Phys.* 2005;62(1):82–90.
91. Schroder W, Baldus SE, Monig SP, Beckurts TK, Dienes HP, Holscher AH. Lymph node staging of esophageal squamous cell carcinoma in patients with and without neoadjuvant radiochemotherapy: histomorphologic analysis. *World J Surg.* 2002;26(5):584–587.
92. Dutkowski P, Hommel G, Bottger T, Schlick T, Junginger T. How many lymph nodes are needed for an accurate pN classification in esophageal cancer? Evidence for a new threshold value. *Hepatogastroenterology.* 2002;49(43):176–180.
93. Rizk NP, Seshan VE, Bains MS, et al. Prognostic factors after combined modality treatment of squamous cell carcinoma of the esophagus. *J Thorac Oncol.* 2007;2(12):1117–1123.
94. Burmeister BH, Smithers BM, Gebski V, et al. Surgery alone versus chemoradiotherapy followed by surgery for resectable cancer of the oesophagus: a randomised controlled phase III trial. *Lancet Oncol.* 2005;6(9):659–668.
95. Yang Q, Cleary KR, Yao JC, et al. Significance of post-chemoradiation biopsy in predicting residual esophageal carcinoma in the surgical specimen. *Dis Esophagus.* 2004;17(1):38–43.
96. Ishikawa H, Sakurai H, Yamakawa M, et al. Clinical outcomes and prognostic factors for patients with early esophageal squamous cell carcinoma treated with definitive radiation therapy alone. *J Clin Gastroenterol.* 2005;39(6):495–500.
97. Blant SA, Ballini JP, Caron CT, Fontolliet C, Monnier P, Laurini NR. Evolution of DNA ploidy during squamous cell carcinogenesis in the esophagus. *Dis Esophagus.* 2001;14(3–4):178–184.
98. Klimstra DS. Pathologic prognostic factors in esophageal carcinoma. *Semin Oncol.* 1994;21(4):425–430.
99. Doki Y, Shiozaki H, Tahara H, et al. Prognostic value of DNA ploidy in squamous cell carcinoma of esophagus. Analyzed with improved flow cytometric measurement. *Cancer.* 1993;72(6):1813–1818.
100. Matsuura H, Sugimachi K, Ueo H, et al. Malignant potentiality of squamous cell carcinoma of the esophagus predictable by DNA analysis. *Cancer.* 1986;57(9):1810–1814.
101. Ohno S, Korenaga D, Kuwano H, et al. DNA aneuploidy assessment of the effectiveness of hyperthermo-chemo-radiotherapy for esophageal carcinoma. *Cancer.* 1989;63(10):1951–1955.
102. Okumura H, Natsugoe S, Matsumoto M, et al. Predictive value of p53 and 14-3-3sigma for the effect of chemoradiation therapy on esophageal squamous cell carcinoma. *J Surg Oncol.* 2005;91(1):84–89.
103. Uemura N, Nakanishi Y, Kato H, et al. Transglutaminase 3 as a prognostic biomarker in esophageal cancer revealed by proteomics. *Int J Cancer.* 2009;124(9):2106–2115.
104. Ishikawa N, Takano A, Yasui W, et al. Cancer-testis antigen lymphocyte antigen 6 complex locus K is a serologic biomarker and a therapeutic target for lung and esophageal carcinomas. *Cancer Res.* 2007;67(24):11601–11611.
105. Yamabuki T, Takano A, Hayama S, et al. Dikkopf-1 as a novel serologic and prognostic biomarker for lung and esophageal carcinomas. *Cancer Res.* 2007;67(6):2517–2525.
106. Sharma R, Chattopadhyay TK, Mathur M, Ralhan R. Prognostic significance of stromelysin-3 and tissue inhibitor of matrix metalloproteinase-2 in esophageal cancer. *Oncology.* 2004;67(3–4):300–309.
107. Gu ZD, Li JY, Li M, et al. Matrix metalloproteinases expression correlates with survival in patients with esophageal squamous cell carcinoma. *Am J Gastroenterol.* 2005;100(8):1835–1843.
108. Tanioka Y, Yoshida T, Yagawa T, et al. Matrix metalloproteinase-7 and matrix metalloproteinase-9 are associated with unfavourable prognosis in superficial oesophageal cancer. *Br J Cancer.* 2003;89(11):2116–2121.
109. Lin Y, Wu M, Li D, et al. Prognostic and clinicopathological features of E-cadherin, beta-catenin, gamma-catenin, and cyclin D1 expression in human esophageal squamous cell carcinoma. *World J Gastroenterol.* 2004;10:3235–3239.
110. Shimada Y, Hashimoto Y, Kan T, et al. Prognostic significance of dysadherin expression in esophageal squamous cell carcinoma. *Oncology.* 2004;67(1):73–80.

111. Osugi H, Morimura K, Okuda E, et al. p53 null mutations detected by a p53 yeast functional assay predict a poor outcome in young esophageal carcinoma patients. *Int J Oncol.* 2002;21(3):637–641.
112. Miyazaki T, Kato H, Fukuchi M, et al. EphA2 overexpression correlates with poor prognosis in esophageal squamous cell carcinoma. *Int J Cancer.* 2003;103(5):657–663.
113. Grabowski P, Kuhnel T, Muhr-Wilkenshoff F, et al. Prognostic value of nuclear survivin expression in oesophageal squamous cell carcinoma. *Br J Cancer.* 2003;88(1):115–119.
114. Yamamoto S, Tomita Y, Hoshida Y, et al. Expression level of valosin-containing protein (p97) is associated with prognosis of esophageal carcinoma. *Clin Cancer Res.* 2004;10(16):5558–5565.
115. Tsuneoka M, Fujita H, Arima N et al. Mina53 as a potential prognostic factor for esophageal squamous cell carcinoma. *Clin Cancer Res.* 2004;10(21):7347–7356.
116. Mandelker DL, Yamashita K, Tokumaru Y, et al. PGP9.5 promoter methylation is an independent prognostic factor for esophageal squamous cell carcinoma. *Cancer Res.* 2005;65(11):4963–4968.
117. Hashimoto Y, Ito T, Inoue H, et al. Prognostic significance of fascin overexpression in human esophageal squamous cell carcinoma. *Clin Cancer Res.* 2005;11(7):2597–2605.
118. Ishibashi Y, Hanyu N, Nakada K, et al. Endothelin protein expression as a significant prognostic factor in oesophageal squamous cell carcinoma. *Eur J Cancer.* 2003;39(10):1409–1415.
119. Kishi K, Doki Y, Yano M, et al. Reduced MLH1 expression after chemotherapy is an indicator for poor prognosis in esophageal cancers. *Clin Cancer Res.* 2003;9(12):4368–4375.
120. Fukai Y, Fukuchi M, Masuda N, et al. Reduced expression of transforming growth factor-beta receptors is an unfavorable prognostic factor in human esophageal squamous cell carcinoma. *Int J Cancer.* 2003;104(2):161–166.
121. Whooley BP, Law S, Murthy SC, et al. Analysis of reduced death and complication rates after esophageal resection. *Ann Surg.* 2001;233(3):338–344.
122. Makary MA, Kiernan PD, Sheridan MJ, et al. Multimodality treatment for esophageal cancer: the role of surgery and neoadjuvant therapy. *Am Surg.* 2003;69(8):693–700; discussion -2.
123. Takita H, Vincent RG, Caicedo V, Gutierrez AC. Squamous cell carcinoma of the esophagus: a study of 153 cases. *J Surg Oncol.* 1977;9(6):547–554.
124. Lee SS, Ha HK, Byun JH, et al. Superficial esophageal cancer: esophagographic findings correlated with histopathologic findings. *Radiology.* 2005;236(2):535–544.
125. Eguchi T, Nakanishi Y, Shimoda T, et al. Histopathological criteria for additional treatment after endoscopic mucosal resection for esophageal cancer: analysis of 464 surgically resected cases. *Mod Pathol.* 2006;19(3):475–480.
126. Araki K, Ohno S, Egashira A, et al. Pathologic features of superficial esophageal squamous cell carcinoma with lymph node and distal metastasis. *Cancer.* 2002;94(2):570–575.
127. Fujishiro M, Yahagi N, Kakushima N, et al. Endoscopic submucosal dissection of esophageal squamous cell neoplasms. *Clin Gastroenterol Hepatol.* 2006;4(6):688–694.
128. Katada C, Muto M, Manabe T, et al. Local recurrence of squamous-cell carcinoma of the esophagus after EMR. *Gastrointest Endosc.* 2005;61(2):219–225.
129. Tajima Y, Nakanishi Y, Tachimori Y, et al. Significance of involvement by squamous cell carcinoma of the ducts of esophageal submucosal glands. Analysis of 201 surgically resected superficial squamous cell carcinomas. *Cancer.* 2000;89(2):248–254.
130. Yuasa N, Miyachi M, Yasui A, et al. Clinicopathological features of superficial spreading and nonspreading squamous cell carcinoma of the esophagus. *Am J Gastroenterol.* 2001;96(2):315–321.
131. Nozoe T, Saeki H, Ohga T, Sugimachi K. Clinicopathologic characteristics of superficial spreading type squamous cell carcinoma of the esophagus. *Oncol Rep.* 2002;9(2):313–316.
132. Mayerowitz B, Shea L. The natural history of squamous verrucous carcinoma of the esophagus. *J Thorac Cardiovasc Surg.* 1972;61:646–649.
133. Martin MR, Kahn LB. So-called pseudosarcoma of the esophagus: nodal metastases of the spindle cell element. *Arch Pathol Lab Med.* 1977;101(11):604–609.
134. Matsusaka T, Watanabe H, Enjoji M. Anaplastic carcinoma of the esophagus. Report of three cases and their histogenetic consideration. *Cancer.* 1976;37(3):1352–1358.
135. Stout A, Lattes R. Tumors of the esophagus.In: *Atlas of Tumor Pathology, Series 1, Section 5, Fascicle 20.* Washington, DC: Armed Forces Institute of Pathology; 1957:78–95.
136. Handra-Luca A, Terris B, Couvelard A, et al. Spindle cell squamous carcinoma of the oesophagus: an analysis of 17 cases, with new immunohistochemical evidence for a clonal origin. *Histopathology.* 2001;39(2):125–132.
137. Osamura RY, Shimamura K, Hata J, et al. Polypoid carcinoma of the esophagus. A unifying term for "carcinosarcoma" and "pseudosarcoma". *Am J Surg Pathol.* 1978;2(2):201–208.
138. Moore T, Battersby J, Vellios F, Loehr W. Carcinosarcoma of eso;hagus. *J Thorac Cardiovasc Surg.* 1983;45:281–288.
139. Du Boulay CE, Isaacson P. Carcinoma of the oesophagus with spindle cell features. *Histopathology.* 1981;5(4):403–414.
140. Nikitakis NG, Drachenberg CB, Papadimitriou JC. MDM2 and CDK4 expression in carcinosarcoma of the esophagus: comparison with squamous cell carcinoma and review of the literature. *Exp Mol Pathol.* 2002;73(3):198–208.
141. Lane N. Pseudosarcoma (polypoid sarcoma-like masses) associated with squamous-cell carcinoma of the mouth, fauces, and larynx; report of ten cases. *Cancer.* 1957;10(1):19–41.
142. Battifora H. Spindle cell carcinoma: ultrastructural evidence of squamous origin and collagen production by the tumor cells. *Cancer.* 1976;37(5):2275–2282.
143. Osugi H, Takemura M, Morimura K, et al. Clinicopathologic and immunohistochemical features of surgically resected small cell carcinoma of the esophagus. *Oncol Rep.* 2002;9(6):1245–1249.
144. Bennouna J, Bardet E, Deguiral P, Douillard JY. Small cell carcinoma of the esophagus: analysis of 10 cases and review of the published data. *Am J Clin Oncol.* 2000;23(5):455–459.
145. Pantvaidya GH, Pramesh CS, Deshpande MS, et al. Small cell carcinoma of the esophagus: the Tata Memorial Hospital experience. *Ann Thorac Surg.* 2002;74(6):1924–1927.
146. Wu Z, Ma JY, Yang JJ, et al. Primary small cell carcinoma of esophagus: report of 9 cases and review of literature. *World J Gastroenterol.* 2004;10(24):3680–3682.
147. Mori M, Matsukuma A, Adachi Y, et al. Small cell carcinoma of the esophagus. *Cancer.* 1989;63(3):564–573.
148. Yamamoto J, Ohshima K, Ikeda S, et al. Primary esophageal small cell carcinoma with concomitant invasive squamous cell carcinoma or carcinoma in situ. *Hum Pathol.* 2003;34(11):1108–1115.
149. Cho KJ, Jang JJ, Lee SS, Zo JI. Basaloid squamous carcinoma of the oesophagus: a distinct neoplasm with multipotential differentiation. *Histopathology.* 2000;36(4):331–340.
150. Lam KY, Law S, Luk JM, Wong J. Oesophageal basaloid squamous cell carcinoma: a unique clinicopathological entity with telomerase activity as a prognostic indicator. *J Pathol.* 2001;195(4):435–442.

151. Li TJ, Zhang YX, Wen J, et al. Basaloid squamous cell carcinoma of the esophagus with or without adenoid cystic features. *Arch Pathol Lab Med.* 2004;128(10):1124-1230.
152. Wain SL, Kier R, Vollmer RT, Bossen EH. Basaloid-squamous carcinoma of the tongue, hypopharynx, and larynx: report of 10 cases. *Hum Pathol.* 1986;17(11):1158-1166.
153. Tsang WY, Chan JK, Lee KC, et al. Basaloid-squamous carcinoma of the upper aerodigestive tract and so-called adenoid cystic carcinoma of the oesophagus: the same tumour type? *Histopathology.* 1991;19(1):35-46.
154. Nishimura W, Naomoto Y, Hamaya K, et al. Basaloid-squamous cell carcinoma of the esophagus: diagnosis based on immunohistochemical analysis. *J Gastroenterol Hepatol.* 2001;16(5):586-590.
155. Abe K, Sasano H, Itakura Y, et al. Basaloid-squamous carcinoma of the esophagus. A clinicopathologic, DNA ploidy, and immunohistochemical study of seven cases. *Am J Surg Pathol.* 1996;20(4):453-461.
156. Sarbia M, Verreet P, Bittinger F, et al. Basaloid squamous cell carcinoma of the esophagus: diagnosis and prognosis. *Cancer.* 1997;79(10):1871-1878.
157. Wong A, Fitzgerald RC. Epidemiologic risk factors for Barrett's esophagus and associated adenocarcinoma. *Clin Gastroenterol Hepatol.* 2005;3(1):1-10.
158. Hongo M. Barrett's oesophagus and carcinoma in Japan. *Aliment Pharmacol Ther.* 2004;20(suppl 8):50-54.
159. Falk GW, Thota PN, Richter JE, et al. Barrett's esophagus in women: demographic features and progression to high-grade dysplasia and cancer. *Clin Gastroenterol Hepatol.* 2005;3(11):1089-1094.
160. Casson AG, Zheng Z, Evans SC, et al. Cyclin D1 polymorphism (G870A) and risk for esophageal adenocarcinoma. *Cancer.* 2005;104(4):730-739.
161. van Soest EM, Dieleman JP, Siersema PD, et al. Increasing incidence of Barrett's oesophagus in the general population. *Gut.* 2005;54(8):1062-1066.
162. Sikkema M, de Jonge PJ, Steyerberg EW, Kuipers EJ. Risk of esophageal adenocarcinoma and mortality in patients with Barrett's esophagus: a systematic review and meta-analysis. *Clin Gastroenterol Hepatol.* 2010;8(3):235-244; quiz e32.
163. Solaymani-Dodaran M, Logan RF, West J, et al. Risk of oesophageal cancer in Barrett's oesophagus and gastro-oesophageal reflux. *Gut.* 2004;53(8):1070-1074.
164. Anderson LA, Murray LJ, Murphy SJ, et al. Mortality in Barrett's oesophagus: results from a population based study. *Gut.* 2003;52(8):1081-1084.
165. Gopal DV, Lieberman DA, Magaret N, et al. Risk factors for dysplasia in patients with Barrett's esophagus (BE): results from a multicenter consortium. *Dig Dis Sci.* 2003;48(8):1537-1541.
166. Hage M, Siersema PD, van Dekken H, et al. Oesophageal cancer incidence and mortality in patients with long-segment Barrett's oesophagus after a mean follow-up of 12.7 years. *Scand J Gastroenterol.* 2004;39(12):1175-1179.
167. Hillman LC, Chiragakis L, Clarke AC, et al. Barrett's esophagus: Macroscopic markers and the prediction of dysplasia and adenocarcinoma. *J Gastroenterol Hepatol.* 2003;18(5):526-533.
168. Montgomery E, Goldblum JR, Greenson JK, et al. Dysplasia as a predictive marker for invasive carcinoma in Barrett esophagus: a follow-up study based on 138 cases from a diagnostic variability study. *Hum Pathol.* 2001;32(4):379-388.
169. Oberg S, Wenner J, Johansson J, et al. Barrett esophagus: risk factors for progression to dysplasia and adenocarcinoma. *Ann Surg.* 2005;242(1):49-54.
170. de Martel C, Llosa AE, Farr SM, et al. Helicobacter pylori infection and the risk of development of esophageal adenocarcinoma. *J Infect Dis.* 2005;191(5):761-767.
171. Weston AP, Sharma P, Mathur S, et al. Risk stratification of Barrett's esophagus: updated prospective multivariate analysis. *Am J Gastroenterol.* 2004;99(9):1657-1666.
172. Chak A, Lee T, Kinnard MF, et al. Familial aggregation of Barrett's oesophagus, oesophageal adenocarcinoma, and oesophagogastric junctional adenocarcinoma in Caucasian adults. *Gut.* 2002;51(3):323-328.
173. Ji J, Hemminki K. Familial risk for esophageal cancer: an updated epidemiologic study from Sweden. *Clin Gastroenterol Hepatol.* 2006;4(7):840-845.
174. Sasco AJ, Secretan MB, Straif K. Tobacco smoking and cancer: a brief review of recent epidemiological evidence. *Lung Cancer.* 2004;45(suppl 2):S3-S9.
175. Tsibouris P, Hendrickse MT, Isaacs PE. Daily use of non-steroidal anti-inflammatory drugs is less frequent in patients with Barrett's oesophagus who develop an oesophageal adenocarcinoma. *Aliment Pharmacol Ther.* 2004;20(6):645-655.
176. Casson AG, Zheng Z, Porter GA, Guernsey DL. Genetic polymorphisms of microsomal epoxide hydroxylase and glutathione S-transferases M1, T1 and P1, interactions with smoking, and risk for esophageal (Barrett) adenocarcinoma. *Cancer Detect Prev.* 2006;30(5):423-431.
177. Zaninotto G, Parenti AR, Ruol A, et al. Oesophageal resection for high-grade dysplasia in Barrett's oesophagus. *Br J Surg.* 2000;87(8):1102-1105.
178. Romagnoli R, Collard JM, Gutschow C, et al. Outcomes of dysplasia arising in Barrett's esophagus: a dynamic view. *J Am Coll Surg.* 2003;197(3):365-371.
179. Tseng EE, Wu TT, Yeo CJ, Heitmiller RF. Barrett's esophagus with high grade dysplasia: surgical results and long-term outcome—an update. *J Gastrointest Surg.* 2003;7(2):164-170; discussion 70-71.
180. Sharma P, Falk GW, Weston AP, et al. Dysplasia and cancer in a large multicenter cohort of patients with Barrett's esophagus. *Clin Gastroenterol Hepatol.* 2006;4(5):566-572.
181. Schnell TG, Sontag SJ, Chejfec G, et al. Long-term nonsurgical management of Barrett's esophagus with high-grade dysplasia. *Gastroenterology.* 2001;120(7):1607-1619.
182. Srivastava A, Hornick JL, Li X, et al. Extent of low-grade dysplasia is a risk factor for the development of esophageal adenocarcinoma in Barrett's esophagus. *Am J Gastroenterol.* 2007;102(3):483-493; quiz 694.
183. Reid BJ, Blount PL, Feng Z, Levine DS. Optimizing endoscopic biopsy detection of early cancers in Barrett's high-grade dysplasia. *Am J Gastroenterol.* 2000;95(11):3089-3096.
184. Ngamruengphong S, Sharma VK, Das A. Diagnostic yield of methylene blue chromoendoscopy for detecting specialized intestinal metaplasia and dysplasia in Barrett's esophagus: a meta-analysis. *Gastrointest Endosc.* 2009;69(6):1021-1028.
185. Wolfsen HC, Crook JE, Krishna M, et al. Prospective, controlled tandem endoscopy study of narrow band imaging for dysplasia detection in Barrett's Esophagus. *Gastroenterology.* 2008;135(1):24-31.
186. Herrero LA, Curvers WL, Bansal A, et al. Zooming in on Barrett oesophagus using narrow-band imaging: an international observer agreement study. *Eur J Gastroenterol Hepatol* 2009;21(9):1068-1075.
187. Curvers W, Baak L, Kiesslich R, et al. Chromoendoscopy and narrow-band imaging compared with high-resolution magnification endoscopy in Barrett's esophagus. *Gastroenterology.* 2008;134(3):670-679.
188. Kiesslich R, Gossner L, Goetz M, et al. In vivo histology of Barrett's esophagus and associated neoplasia by confocal laser endomicroscopy. *Clin Gastroenterol Hepatol.* 2006;4(8):979-987.
189. Incarbone R, Bonavina L, Saino G, Bona D, Peracchia A. Outcome of esophageal adenocarcinoma detected during

189. endoscopic biopsy surveillance for Barrett's esophagus. *Surg Endosc.* 2002;16(2):263–266.
190. Ferguson MK, Durkin A. Long-term survival after esophagectomy for Barrett's adenocarcinoma in endoscopically surveyed and nonsurveyed patients. *J Gastrointest Surg.* 2002;6(1):29–35; discussion 6.
191. Reid BJ, Levine DS, Longton G, et al. Predictors of progression to cancer in Barrett's esophagus: baseline histology and flow cytometry identify low- and high-risk patient subsets. *Am J Gastroenterol.* 2000;95(7):1669–1676.
192. Feith M, Stein HJ, Mueller J, Siewert JR. Malignant degeneration of Barrett's esophagus: the role of the Ki-67 proliferation fraction, expression of E-cadherin and p53. *Dis Esophagus.* 2004;17(4):322–327.
193. Murray L, Sedo A, Scott M, et al. TP53 and progression from Barrett's metaplasia to oesophageal adenocarcinoma in a UK population cohort. *Gut.* 2006;55(10):1390–1397.
194. Skacel M, Petras RE, Rybicki LA, et al. p53 expression in low grade dysplasia in Barrett's esophagus: correlation with interobserver agreement and disease progression. *Am J Gastroenterol.* 2002;97(10):2508–2513.
195. Illueca C, Llombart-Bosch A, Ferrando Cucarella J. Prognostic factors in Barrett's esophagus: an immunohistochemical and morphometric study of 120 cases. *Rev Esp Enferm Dig.* 2000;92:726–737.
196. Sharma P, Dent J, Armstrong D, et al. The development and validation of an endoscopic grading system for Barrett's esophagus: the Prague C & M criteria. *Gastroenterology.* 2006;131(5):1392–1399.
197. Rudolph RE, Vaughan TL, Storer BE, et al. Effect of segment length on risk for neoplastic progression in patients with Barrett esophagus. *Ann Intern Med.* 2000;132(8):612–620.
198. Nobukawa B, Abraham SC, Gill J, et al. Clinicopathologic and molecular analysis of high-grade dysplasia and early adenocarcinoma in short- versus long-segment Barrett esophagus. *Hum Pathol.* 2001;32(4):447–454.
199. De Carvalho C. Sur l'architectgureveineuse de la zone de transition oesophagogastrique et soninterpretation functionnele. *Acta Anat.* 1966;64:125–162.
200. Skinner DB, Walther BC, Riddell RH, et al. Barrett's esophagus. Comparison of benign and malignant cases. *Ann Surg.* 1983;198(4):554–565.
201. Montgomery E, Bronner MP, Greenson JK, et al. Are ulcers a marker for invasive carcinoma in Barrett's esophagus? Data from a diagnostic variability study with clinical follow-up. *Am J Gastroenterol.* 2002;97(1):27–31.
202. Ban S, Mino M, Nishioka NS, et al. Histopathologic aspects of photodynamic therapy for dysplasia and early adenocarcinoma arising in Barrett's esophagus. *Am J Surg Pathol.* 2004;28(11):1466–1473.
203. Banner BF, Memoli VA, Warren WH, Gould VE. Carcinoma with multidirectional differentiation arising in Barrett's esophagus. *Ultrastruct Pathol.* 1983;4(2–3):205–217.
204. Pascal RR, Clearfield HR. Mucoepidermoid (adenosquamous) carcinoma arising in Barrett's esophagus. *Dig Dis Sci.* 1987;32(4):428–432.
205. Chennat J, Konda VJ, Ross AS, et al. Complete Barrett's eradication endoscopic mucosal resection: an effective treatment modality for high-grade dysplasia and intramucosal carcinoma—an American single-center experience. *Am J Gastroenterol.* 2009;104(11):2684–2692.
206. Peters FP, Kara MA, Rosmolen WD, et al. Endoscopic treatment of high-grade dysplasia and early stage cancer in Barrett's esophagus. *Gastrointest Endosc.* 2005;61(4):506–514.
207. Prasad GA, Wang KK, Lutzke LS, et al. Frozen section analysis of esophageal endoscopic mucosal resection specimens in the real-time management of Barrett's esophagus. *Clin Gastroenterol Hepatol.* 2006;4(2):173–178.
208. Wolfsen HC, Hemminger LL, Wallace MB, Devault KR. Clinical experience of patients undergoing photodynamic therapy for Barrett's dysplasia or cancer. *Aliment Pharmacol Ther.* 2004;20(10):1125–1131.
209. Liu L, Hofstetter WL, Rashid A, et al. Significance of the depth of tumor invasion and lymph node metastasis in superficially invasive (T1) esophageal adenocarcinoma. *Am J Surg Pathol.* 2005;29(8):1079–1085.
210. Sabel MS, Pastore K, Toon H, Smith JL. Adenocarcinoma of the esophagus with and without Barrett mucosa. *Arch Surg.* 2000;135(7):831–835; discussion 6.
211. Bonavina L, Via A, Incarbone R, et al. Results of surgical therapy in patients with Barrett's adenocarcinoma. *World J Surg.* 2003;27(9):1062–1066.
212. Meyer W, Popp M, Klinger L, et al. Results of surgical therapy of adenocarcinomas of the esophagogastric junction according to a standardized surgical resection technique. *Dig Surg.* 2002;19(4):269–274; discussion 75.
213. Sihvo EI, Luostarinen ME, Salo JA. Fate of patients with adenocarcinoma of the esophagus and the esophagogastric junction: a population-based analysis. *Am J Gastroenterol.* 2004;99(3):419–424.
214. Armanios M, Xu R, Forastiere AA, et al. Adjuvant chemotherapy for resected adenocarcinoma of the esophagus, gastro-esophageal junction, and cardia: phase II trial (E8296) of the Eastern Cooperative Oncology Group. *J Clin Oncol.* 2004;22(22):4495–4499.
215. Westerterp M, Koppert LB, Buskens CJ, et al. Outcome of surgical treatment for early adenocarcinoma of the esophagus or gastro-esophageal junction. *Virchows Arch.* 2005;446(5):497–504.
216. Buskens CJ, Westerterp M, Lagarde SM, et al. Prediction of appropriateness of local endoscopic treatment for high-grade dysplasia and early adenocarcinoma by EUS and histopathologic features. *Gastrointest Endosc.* 2004;60(5):703–710.
217. Mandal RV, Forcione DG, Brugge WR, et al. Effect of tumor characteristics and duplication of the muscularis mucosae on the endoscopic staging of superficial Barrett esophagus-related neoplasia. *Am J Surg Pathol.* 2009;33(4):620–625.
218. Feith M, Stein HJ, Siewert JR. Pattern of lymphatic spread of Barrett's cancer. *World J Surg.* 2003;27(9):1052–1057.
219. Lamb PJ, Griffin SM, Burt AD, et al. Sentinel node biopsy to evaluate the metastatic dissemination of oesophageal adenocarcinoma. *Br J Surg.* 2005;92(1):60–67.
220. Bell-Thomson J, Haggitt RC, Ellis FH, Jr. Mucoepidermoid and adenoid cystic carcinomas of the esophagus. *J Thorac Cardiovasc Surg.* 1980;79(3):438–446.
221. Watanabe H, Jass J, Sobin L. *WHO: Hisgtological Typing of Oesophagel and Gastric Tumours.* Berlin, Germany: Springer-Verlag; 1977.
222. Cerar A, Jutersek A, Vidmar S. Adenoid cystic carcinoma of the esophagus. A clinicopathologic study of three cases. *Cancer.* 1991;67(8):2159–2164.
223. Kuwano H, Nagamatsu M, Ohno S, et al. Coexistence of intraepithelial carcinoma and glandular differentiation in esophageal squamous cell carcinoma. *Cancer.* 1988;62(8):1568–1572.
224. Hagiwara N, Tajiri T, Miyashita M, et al. Biological behavior of mucoepidermoid carcinoma of the esophagus. *J Nippon Med Sch.* 2003;70(5):401–407.
225. von Rahden BH, Stein HJ, Becker K, et al. Heterotopic gastric mucosa of the esophagus: literature-review and proposal of a clinicopathologic classification. *Am J Gastroenterol.* 2004;99(3):543–551.
226. Chatelain D, de Lajarte-Thirouard AS, Tiret E, Flejou JF. Adenocarcinoma of the upper esophagus arising in heterotopic gastric mucosa: common pathogenesis with

Barrett's adenocarcinoma? *Virchows Arch.* 2002;441(4): 406–411.
227. Abe T, Hosokawa M, Kusumi T, et al. Adenocarcinoma arising from ectopic gastric mucosa in the cervical esophagus. *Am J Clin Oncol.* 2004;27(6):644–645.
228. Woodward B, Shelburne J, Vollmer R, Postlethwait R. Mucoepidermoid carcinoma of the esophagus: a case report. *Hum Pathol.* 1978;9:352–354.
229. Yoshida M, Ide H, Yamada A, Endo M. Early detection of adenocarcinoma of the esophagus. *Endoscopy.* 1986;18(suppl 3):44–48.
230. Azzopardi J, Menzies T. Primary oesophageal adenocarcinoma: confirmation of its existence by the finding of mucous gland tumors. *Br J Surg.* 1961;49:497–506.
231. Fabre A, Tansey DK, Dave U, et al. Adenocarcinoma in situ arising from the submucosal oesophageal mucous glands. *Eur J Gastroenterol Hepatol.* 2003;15(9):1047–1049.
232. McKechnie JC, Fechner RE. Choriocarcinoma and adenocarcinoma of the esophagus with gonadotropin secretion. *Cancer.* 1971;27(3):694–702.
233. Trilo A, Accettullo L, Yeiter T. Choriocarcinoma of the esohagus: histologic and cytologic findings. A case report. *Acta Cytol.* 1978;23:69–74.
234. Graham DY, Schwartz JT, Cain GD, Gyorkey F. Prospective evaluation of biopsy number in the diagnosis of esophageal and gastric carcinoma. *Gastroenterology.* 1982;82(2):228–231.
235. Mosca S, Manes G, Monaco R, et al. Squamous papilloma of the esophagus: long-term follow up. *J Gastroenterol Hepatol.* 2001;16(8):857–861.
236. Walker JH. Giant papilloma of the thoracic esophagus. *Am J Roentgenol.* 1978;131(3):519–520.
237. Nuwayhid NS, Ballard ET, Cotton R. Esophageal papillomatosis: case report. *Ann Otol Rhinol Laryngol.* 1977;86(5 pt 1):623–625.
238. Frootko NJ, Rogers JH. Oesophageal papillomata in the child. *J Laryngol Otol.* 1978;92(9):823–827.
239. Carr NJ, Bratthauer GL, Lichy JH, et al. Squamous cell papillomas of the esophagus: a study of 23 lesions for human papillomavirus by in situ hybridization and the polymerase chain reaction. *Hum Pathol.* 1994;25(5):536–540.
240. Rabin MS, Bremner CG, Botha JR. The reflux gastroesophageal polyp. *Am J Gastroenterol.* 1980;73(5):451–452.
241. Philp T, Gunning AJ, Bennett MK. Inflammatory obstruction of oesophageal tubes. *Gut.* 1983;24(10):960–963.
242. Schuhmacher C, Becker K, Dittler HJ, et al. Fibrovascular esophageal polyp as a diagnostic challenge. *Dis Esophagus.* 2000;13(4):324–327.
243. Fries MR, Galindo RL, Flint PW, Abraham SC. Giant fibrovascular polyp of the esophagus. A lesion causing upper airway obstruction and syncope. *Arch Pathol Lab Med.* 2003;127(4):485–487.
244. Ogunseyinde AO, Mamman M, Edino ST, Kazuere I. Giant fibrolipomatous polyp of the oesophagus: a case report. *Niger Postgrad Med J.* 2004;11(4):298–300.
245. Jang GC, Clouse ME, Fleischner FG. Fibrovascular polyp– a benign intraluminal tumor of the esophagus. *Radiology.* 1969;92(6):1196–1200.
246. Anderson LS, Shackelford GD, Mancilla-Jimenez R, McAlister WH. Cartilaginous esophageal ring: a cause of esophageal stenosis in infants and children. *Radiology.* 1973;108(3):665–666.
247. Shah B, Unger L, Heimlich HJ. Hamartomatous polyp of the esophagus. *Arch Surg.* 1975;110(3):326–328.
248. Postlethwait RW, Detmer DE. Ectopic thyroid nodule in the esophagus. *Ann Thorac Surg.* 1975;19(1):98–100.
249. Archer HA, Owen WJ. Primary malignant melanoma of the esophagus. *Dis Esophagus.* 2000;13(4):320–323.
250. Lohmann CM, Hwu WJ, Iversen K, et al. Primary malignant melanoma of the oesophagus: a clinical and pathological study with emphasis on the immunophenotype of the tumours for melanocyte differentiation markers and cancer/testis antigens. *Melanoma Res.* 2003;13(6): 595–601.
251. Kreuser ED. Primary malignant melanoma of the esophagus. *Virchows Arch A Pathol Anat Histol.* 1979;385(1): 49–59.
252. Ludwig ME, Shaw R, de Suto-Nagy G. Primary malignant melanoma of the esophagus. *Cancer.* 1981;48(11): 2528–2534.
253. Piccone VA, Klopstock R, LeVeen HH, Sika J. Primary malignant melanoma of the esophagus associated with melanosis of the entire esophagus. First case report. *J Thorac Cardiovasc Surg.* 1970;59(6):864–870.
254. DiCostanzo DP, Urmacher C. Primary malignant melanoma of the esophagus. *Am J Surg Pathol.* 1987;11(1):46–52.
255. Boni L, Benevento A, Dionigi G, Dionigi R. Primary malignant melanoma of the esophagus: a case report. *Surg Endosc.* 2002;16(2):359–360.
256. Seremetis MG, Lyons WS, deGuzman VC, Peabody JW Jr. Leiomyomata of the esophagus. An analysis of 838 cases. *Cancer.* 1976;38(5):2166–2177.
257. Miettinen M, Sarlomo-Rikala M, Sobin LH, Lasota J. Esophageal stromal tumors: a clinicopathologic, immunohistochemical, and molecular genetic study of 17 cases and comparison with esophageal leiomyomas and leiomyosarcomas. *Am J Surg Pathol.* 2000;24(2):211–222.
258. Yang PS, Lee KS, Lee SJ, et al. Esophageal leiomyoma: radiologic findings in 12 patients. *Korean J Radiol.* 2001;2(3):132–137.
259. Wang Y, Zhang R, Ouyang Z, et al. Diagnosis and surgical treatment of esophageal leiomyoma. *Zhonghua Zhong Liu Za Zhi.* 2002;24(4):394–396.
260. Misra M, Maziak DE, Shamji FM, Michaud C, Perkins DG, Matzinger F. Esophageal leiomyomatosis. *Med Sci Monit.* 2003;9(11):CS98–CS101.
261. Pramesh CS, Pantvaidya GH, Moonim MT, et al. Leiomyosarcoma of the esophagus. *Dis Esophagus.* 2003;16(2): 142–144.
262. Hasegawa T, Matsuno Y, Shimoda T, Hirohashi S. Gastrointestinal stromal tumor: consistent CD117 immunostaining for diagnosis, and prognostic classification based on tumor size and MIB-1 grade. *Hum Pathol.* 2002;33(6):669–676.
263. Voskuil JH, van Dijk MM, Wagenaar SS, et al. Occurrence of esophageal granular cell tumors in The Netherlands between 1988 and 1994. *Dig Dis Sci.* 2001;46(8):1610–1614.
264. Bloch MJ, Iozzo RV, Edmunds LH Jr, Brooks JJ. Polypoid synovial sarcoma of the esophagus. *Gastroenterology.* 1987;92(1):229–233.
265. Amr SS, Shihabi NK, Al Hajj H. Synovial sarcoma of the esophagus. *Am J Otolaryngol.* 1984;5(4):266–269.
266. Palmer BV, Levene A, Shaw HJ. Synovial sarcoma of the pharynx and oesophagus. *J Laryngol Otol.* 1983;97(12): 1173–1176.

12 Stomach: Normal Structures and Developmental Abnormalities

Chapter Outline

EMBRYOLOGY
  Stomach
  Cardia
  Duodenum
NORMAL STRUCTURE OF THE STOMACH
  Anatomy

Gastric surfaces (relations of the stomach)
Anatomic regions
Blood vessels and lymphatics
Nerve supply
Histology

Mucosa
Submucosa
Muscularis propria, ICCs, and serosa
DEVELOPMENTAL ABNORMALITIES OF THE STOMACH
  Pathogenesis and Clinical Features

EMBRYOLOGY

Stomach

The stomach appears at 14 weeks as a fusiform dilation of the caudal part of the foregut. The dorsal border grows faster than the ventral border, establishing the greater curvature of the stomach. As the stomach acquires its adult shape, it rotates 90 degrees in a clockwise direction on its longitudinal axis. The adult orientation of the stomach is established as the ventral border (lesser curvature) moves to the right, the dorsal border (greater curvature) moves to the left, the original left side becomes the ventral surface, and the original right side becomes the dorsal surface. These changes explain why the left vagus nerve supplies the anterior (ventral) wall of the adult stomach and the right vagus innervates the posterior (dorsal) wall (Fig. 12-1).[1]

The epithelial lining and gastric glands develop from foregut endoderm. Splanchnic mesoderm produces gastric smooth muscle, the lesser omentum, and the dorsal mesentery (dorsal mesogaster and greater omentum). Gastric epithelial cells express a range of peptide hormones known to regulate gastric functions including digestive enzymes, mucus, and hormones that regulate gastric motility. At 8 weeks, the developing human stomach has gastrin-containing cells in the antrum, and somatostatin cells in both the antrum and the fundus. At 10 weeks, glucagon-containing cells are seen the gastric fundus; these are preceded by glicentin (enteroglucagon—the precursor of glucagon) but have disappeared postnatally, although occasional glicentin or glucagon-containing cells can be found in various poly and cancers.[2] Serotonin-containing cells are seen in the antrum and fundus by 11 weeks.[3–6]

Cardia

There has been considerable controversy regarding whether the cardia is normal or is acquired in response to reflux.[7,8] In embryos, there can be either a direct transition from oxyntic to esophageal squamous mucosa or a transition from oxyntic to cardiac to esophageal[7,9] suggesting that cardia is physiological and may even develop in response to gastroesophageal reflux in utero. The issue assumes potential importance in adults, where a direct oxynto-squamous transition is rare, so that an argument can be made for the cardia being acquired in at least some adults. While this should be analogous to how much gastric metaplasia is present in the first part of the duodenum, which likely also develops in response to acid reaching that part of the duodenum, it assumes potential importance in the esophagus if it is acquired in response to gastroesophageal reflux disease. This could potentially be interpreted as acquired and therefore to have potential for neoplastic transformation—with or without goblet cells. It can therefore be argued that, unless this starts acquiring intestinal mucosa features, it likely has little risk.[10] However, this is a moving target, as in some studies intestinal metaplasia can be present in over a third of the population if looked for.[11] We therefore suspect that normal cardia has no increased risk of neoplasia.

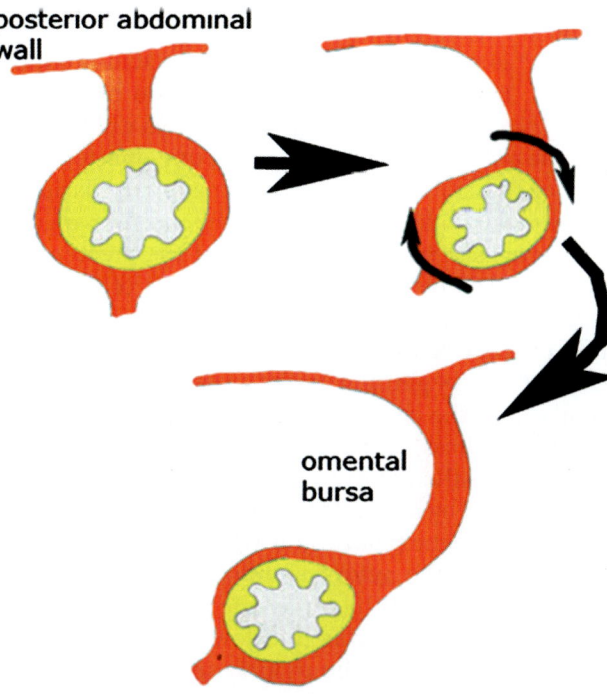

Figure 12-1. The adult orientation of the stomach is established as the ventral border (lesser curvature) moves to the right, the dorsal border (greater curvature) moves to the left, the original left side becomes the ventral surface, and the original right side becomes the dorsal surface.

Duodenum

The duodenum develops from the most caudal part of the foregut and the most cranial part of the midgut. These parts grow rapidly and form a C-shaped loop that projects ventrally. The junction of the foregut and the midgut is at the apex of this embryonic duodenal loop usually immediately below the ampulla of Vater. Because of its derivation from both the foregut and the midgut, the duodenum is supplied by branches of the celiac and superior mesenteric arteries. During the 5th and 6th weeks, the duodenal lumen is reduced and may be obliterated by epithelial cells, but it recanalizes by the end of the embryonic period (8th week).[1] Most of the duodenal ventral mesentery disappears, but the free border remains and forms the ventral border of the epiploic foramen.

NORMAL STRUCTURE OF THE STOMACH

Anatomy

The stomach is J-shaped, although there is considerable variation, depending on the degree of distention and the body habitus. Between its two areas of fixation at each end, the stomach is quite mobile. It is fixed above at the esophagogastric junction and below at the gastroduodenal junction. The two curvatures of the stomach are designated the *lesser* and *greater curvatures* (Fig. 12-2). Externally, the stomach is covered completely by peritoneum, except where the blood vessels run along its curvatures (Fig. 12-2), and a small bare area posterior to the cardiac orifice. The peritoneum is reflected at the lesser curvature forming the lesser omentum that extends to the liver. Likewise, the peritoneum is reflected at the greater curvature to become the greater omentum (a double layer of fatty peritoneum suspended from the greater

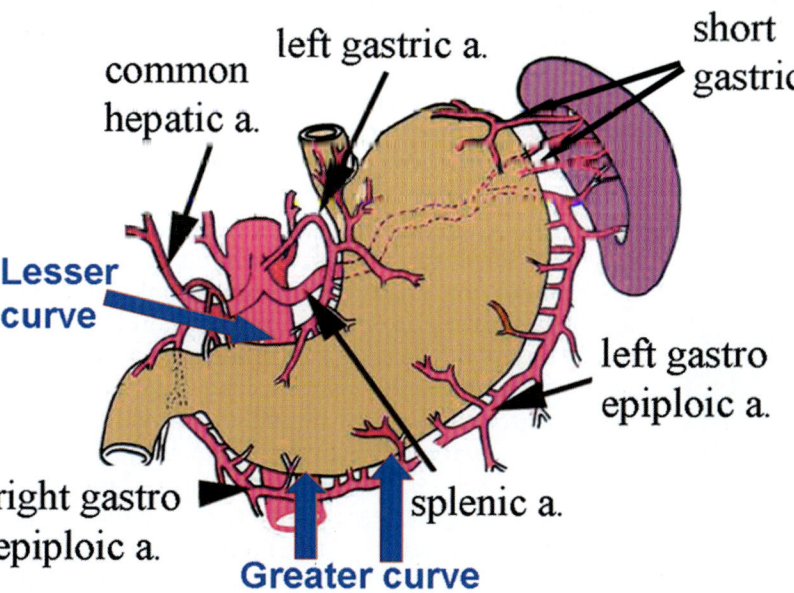

Figure 12-2. Outline of the stomach with its rich blood supply from all three branches of the celiac trunk, namely the left gastric, splenic, and common hepatic arteries (a. = artery).

curvature). The greater omentum is an apron-like structure hanging off the stomach that has a remarkable ability to stick to damaged or perforated parts of the gastrointestinal tract, sealing off leaks and giving some protection against peritonitis. Excess fat may be stored on the greater omentum, especially in men (hence beer belly).[12]

Gastric surfaces (relations of the stomach). The antero-superior surface of the stomach is in contact with the diaphragm (fundal region), gastric surface of the spleen, left and quadrate lobes of the liver, the anterior abdominal wall, and the transverse colon—when the stomach is empty. The postero-inferior surface (stomach bed) is formed by the posterior wall of the omental bursa and retroperitoneal structures between it and the posterior abdominal wall. Superiorly, the stomach bed includes part of the diaphragm (left crus), the spleen, the left suprarenal gland, and upper pole of the left kidney. Inferiorly, the stomach bed includes the body and tail of pancreas, transverse mesocolon, left colic flexure, the splenic artery, and, in some people, the transverse colon.

Anatomic regions. Anatomically, the stomach is subdivided arbitrarily into four regions: the fundus, body (corpus), cardia, and antrum (Fig. 12-3). It connects with the esophagus and duodenum through the cardia and pyloric canal, respectively. The *fundus* (superior part of the stomach) is a dome-shaped area that lies above an imaginary horizontal plane passing through the cardiac orifice. The *fundus* extends to the left and superiorly from the cardia region. The body lies between the fundus and the antrum. It is the largest part of the stomach and extends to the level of the incisura angularis on the lesser curve. Confusion can arise when *fundus* is used as a gross anatomic term including both the body and the fundus, and this use of the term should be avoided.[13] The term "oxyntic mucosa" is a useful term to describe acid-producing mucosa. It is useful histologically when biopsies are clearly "oxyntic" but their precise site is unknown.

The *antrum* occupies the lower one-quarter to one-third of the stomach. Its approximate boundaries can be defined by a line drawn from the incisura angularis to the opposite wall; its junction on the greater curve is determined by the approximate ends of the gastric rugae (Fig. 12-3). When the stomach is distended with air at endoscopy to permit visualization, the antrum is designated as beginning on the greater curvature at the point where the gastric body folds end and where the smooth, "foldless" antrum begins. The opening into the duodenum is the pyloric orifice, and its position is usually indicated by a circular groove on the surface of the organ, termed the pyloric constriction, which indicates the position of the pyloric sphincter.

The pyloric sphincter is the most distal part of the antrum and controls the flow of gastric contents into the duodenum. The pyloric sphincter, similar to the lower esophageal sphincter, is several centimeters long (Fig. 12-3). Its narrow lumen, which passes between the antrum and the duodenum, is referred to as the *pyloric canal*. In endoscopic parlance, the term *pylorus* is commonly used interchangeably with *pyloric canal* and *pyloric sphincter region*. Some use the term *pyloric antrum* to designate the gastric antrum and *pyloric canal* to indicate the pyloric sphincter region. We prefer to avoid the prefix term *pyloric* in order to avoid confusion and to use the simpler terms *antrum* and *pylorus*.

The *cardia region* refers to a short zone measuring from a few millimeters to several centimeters where the stomach immediately adjoins the esophagus. It is so named because of the mucus-secreting glands (cardiac glands) it contains. When the term *cardia region* is used in clinical or macroscopic terms, it usually denotes the most proximal (juxtaesophageal) stomach. The gastric cardia starts at the gastroesophageal junction where the squamous mucosa terminates (in patients in whom Barrett's esophagus is not a consideration). There is no consensus on the endoscopic landmarks for the gastric cardia. Western gastroenterologists arbitrarily define the distal extent of the cardia as the level of the most proximal gastric folds (Fig. 12-4).[14] Japanese gastroenterologists define the proximal extent of the EGJ as the distal end of the lower esophageal palisade vessels.[15,16] These palisades are the termination of esophageal vessels that run longitudinally in the submucosal layer of the body of the esophagus, where their structure is truncal and consists of a few

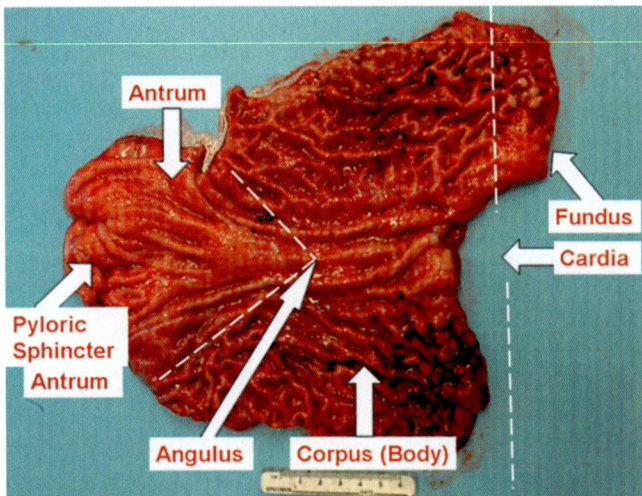

Figure 12-3. Areas of the stomach shown in this total gastrectomy specimen in a patient with an E-cadherin germline mutation but no gross abnormality. The pyloric sphincter is clearly identified on the left as a circular constriction.

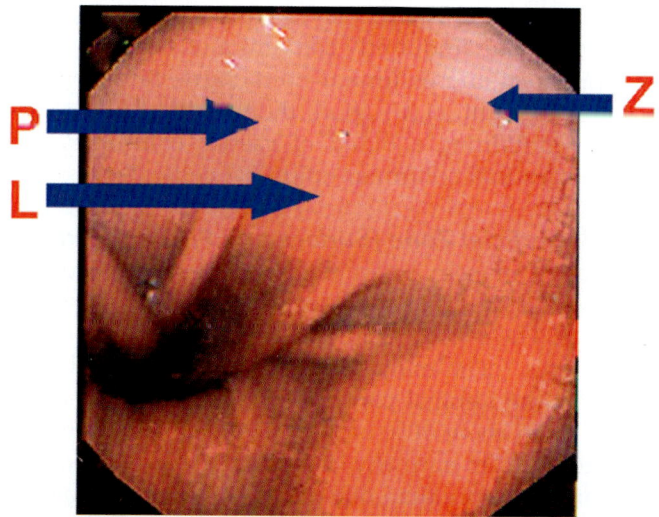

Figure 12-4. Endoscopic image of the cardia region. In Western countries, the cardia begins distally at the proximal end of the gastric longitudinal folds in the partially deflated stomach (P). In Japan, the lower end of the cardia is determined by the lower limit of palisade vessels (L). While both of these definitions are almost the same, as can be seen here, the palisade vessels actually extend a little distal to the upper end of the gastric folds. The upper end of the cardia is the squamocolumnar junction or Z-line (Z). (Image courtesy of Dr. Worth Boyce.)

large columns.[16] At the cardia, the veins penetrate the muscularis mucosae and become superficial, forming the palisade vessels in the lamina propria beneath the epithelium. At the distal end of the palisade vessels, these veins merge with the submucosal venous network of the stomach. These two landmarks are similar but not always identical (Fig. 12-4).

The *squamocolumnar junction* between the esophagus and the stomach is not an abrupt horizontal transition. Rather, there are grossly visible interdigitating tongues referred to as the *ora serrata* or, more commonly in endoscopic circles, as the *Z-line* (Fig. 12-4).

As indicated subsequently in the section on histology, the histologic zones of the stomach do not correspond precisely to the gross anatomic regions. The mucosa in the body of the stomach, especially on the greater curvature, is thrown into numerous thick folds, or rugae, which run in a longitudinal direction. In the fundus, the lesser curvature of the body and, in the antrum, the mucosal folds commonly flatten when the stomach is distended with air or barium. With isotopically labeled meals, a midgastric *transverse band* can be identified in the food-filled stomach. There is no known anatomic correlate to explain its appearance.[17] When the gastric body mucosa is viewed with a hand lens or close up at endoscopy, shallow slits or furrows, the *areae gastricae,* are seen. These represent the furrows between undulations of the mucosa that range up to 5 mm in diameter.

Blood vessels and lymphatics

Arterial Supply The stomach has a rich blood supply from all three branches of the celiac axis (left gastric, splenic, and common hepatic arteries. The lesser curvature receives blood from two sources. The lesser curvature of the stomach is supplied by the right gastric artery (that arises from the hepatic branch of the celiac near the pylorus) inferiorly and the left gastric artery (that arises directly from the celiac artery) superiorly, which also supplies the cardiac region. The greater curvature receives blood from two sources. The greater curvature is supplied by the right gastroepiploic artery (that originates from the gastroduodenal branch of the hepatic artery) inferiorly and the left gastroepiploic artery (which arises from the splenic artery) superiorly. The fundus of the stomach is supplied by short gastric branches from the splenic artery.

Venous Drainage The lesser curvature is drained by the right and left gastric veins, which run next to the arteries and drain into the portal vein. The fundus is supplied by short gastric veins that ultimately join the splenic vein, again finishing in the portal vein. Branches of the short gastric veins and the left coronary gastric vein at the cardia drain the lower esophagus. Blood from the lower portion of the greater curvature is drained by the right gastroepiploic vein, which enters the superior mesenteric vein and thence the portal vein.

Lymphatics The lymphatic drainage from the stomach generally follows the main arteries and is named accordingly. Beginning in the gastric mucosa, the lymphatics pass through the gastric wall and go toward one or the other of the curvatures, draining to four main areas, along the routes of the arteries and veins. The largest is for most of the lesser curvature and the lower end of the esophagus, along the left gastric artery to the *left gastric nodes*. The distal portion of the lesser curvature in the region of the pylorus drains to the *right gastric nodes* that drain to the *hepatic nodes*. The proximal part of the greater curvature drains along the gastroepiploic and splenic vessels, terminating in *splenic nodes* in the hilum of the spleen. The distal portion of the greater curvature drains to the *right gastroepiploic* nodes in the greater omentum and to *pyloric nodes* at the head of the pancreas. Ultimately, the branches from all of these groups drain into the *celiac nodes* located around the celiac trunk as it arises from the abdominal aorta. From the celiac nodes, lymph drains directly into the *thoracic duct*. It is important to understand gastric lymphatic drainage as veins provide routes for spread of gastric cancer, when present, directly to the liver, while from the celiac nodes, the thoracic duct provides direct access to the systemic circulation.

Nerve supply. The parasympathetic nerve supply is from the vagus nerve and its branches. The right vagus nerve enters the abdomen as one or two trunks on the posterior side of the esophagogastric junction. It supplies branches to both surfaces of the stomach. The left vagus nerve also has one or two trunks, and it enters the abdomen on the anterior surface of the stomach, where it is present because of the rotation of the stomach early in its development (see "Embryology" section above). Shortly after entering the abdomen, the anterior vagal nerve gives off a hepatic branch and the posterior trunk gives off a celiac branch. Thus, transection of these trunks below these branches only results in gastric denervation. Even more selective denervation of the fundic gland mucosa (highly selective vagotomy) can be achieved by preserving the terminal portions of the vagal nerves that supply the gastric antrum. Vagal nerve fibers connect with ganglion cells located between the circular and longitudinal fibers of the muscularis propria (Auerbach's plexus) and with submucosal ganglion cells (Meissner's plexus). From these plexi, postganglionic fibers innervate both glands and muscle.

The sympathetic nerve supply to the stomach is from the celiac plexus via branches that follow the gastric and gastroepiploic arteries. There are also sympathetic branches from the right and left phrenic nerves. These nerves contain afferent pain fibers as well as motor fibers to the pyloric sphincter region. Vagal stimulation from ghrelin mediated pituitary stimulation produces release of ghrelin and orexin that stimulates gastric secretion prior to food ingestion, the former resulting in increased gastric acid secretion via acetyl choline, and the latter that also stimulates a craving for food.

Histology

This section focuses on the light microscopic appearance of the stomach. Comprehensive reviews of the electron microscopic appearance are available.[18-20] All parts of the stomach have the same basic structural layers (mucosa, submucosa, muscularis propria, subserosa, and serosa).

Mucosa. Traditionally, but for no good reason that we are aware of, the term crypt (crypts of Lieberkuhn) is applied to the small and large intestine, but in the stomach, they are pits. We are willing to accept either terminology but will use "pit" as terms such as "pit pattern" are now generally accepted. Gastric pits are divided into three histologic zones: superficial zone (surface and pit epithelium); neck zone, which is the regenerative region of the stomach; and deep or glandular zone. While the surface and neck zone cells are uniform throughout the stomach, the underlying glands differ in structure and function by region, and the histologic zones of the stomach are classified according to these types of glands: cardiac, oxyntic, antral.

At the microscopic level, this esophagogastric transition zone frequently contains alternating islands of squamous and columnar epithelium. Similarly, in the pyloric sphincter region, there may be short segments containing a blend of gastric columnar and small intestinal columnar epithelial cells.

The Superficial Zone (Surface and Pit Epithelium)

The gastric mucosa is covered by tall (20–40 μm) columnar mucous cells that are invaginated to form the pits or foveolae. The surface epithelial cells are replaced every 4 to 6 days.[21] The mucus in the surface epithelial cells occupies the luminal part of the cells (Fig. 12-5), occupying up to about 80% of the cell. Nuclei are regularly oriented and are normally located in the basal part of the cell, and no more than one-fifth of the distance toward the lumen; when reactive changes are present, the

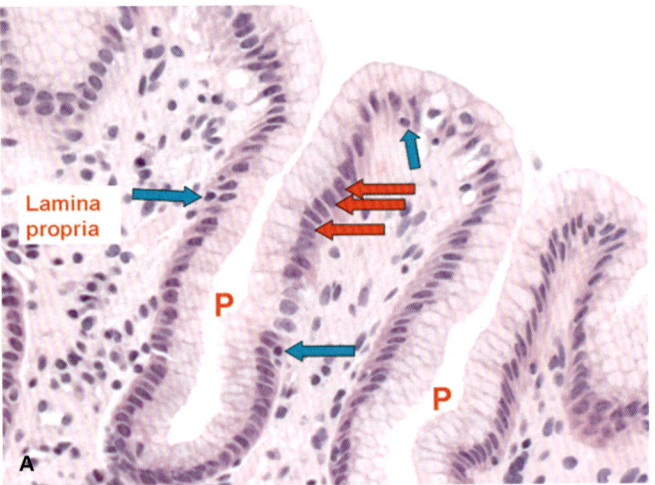

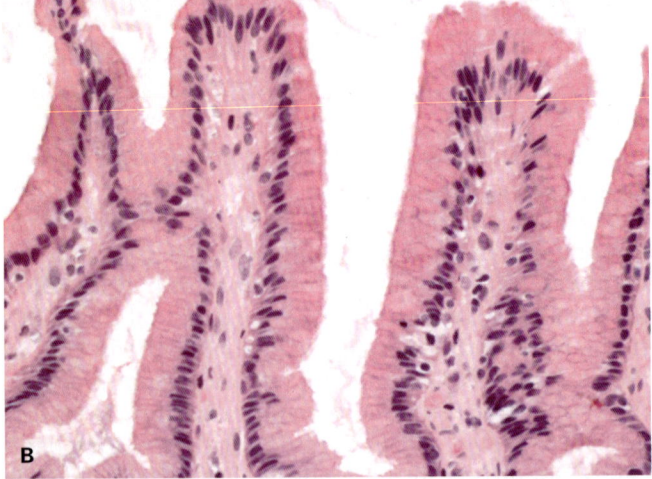

Figure 12-5. A: In the gastric pits (P), superficial cells in the stomach are mucin-producing throughout the entire stomach. Each nucleus has an apical mucin vacuole that usually occupies well over 50% of the cell (*red arrows*). Occasional intraepithelial lymphocytes are also visible (*blue arrows*). Depending on the staining technique employed, the mucous cells maybe almost clear as in (**A**), or eosinophilic as in (**B**).

Table 12-1 Endocrine Cells of the Stomach

CELL TYPE	CORPUS	ANTRUM	HORMONE AMINE	HORMONE PEPTIDE	MARKER (ANTIBODY)	SILVER STAIN MASSON–FONTANA	SILVER STAIN OTHERS
ECL	30%	0	Histamine	Unknown	Synaptophysin, Chromogranin A, VMAT2, Histamine	Negative	Positive
EC	7%	10%	Serotonin (5HT)	Unknown	Synaptophysin, Chromogranin A serotonin	Positive	Positive
D	22%	20%		Somatostatin	Synaptophysin, Chromogranin A somatostatin MAb	Negative	Positive
G	0	60%		Gastrin	Synaptophysin, Chromogranin A Gastrin	Negative	Positive
D1, A/X	20%	Unknown		Ghrelin	Chromogranin, Ghrelin	Negative	Positive

Modified from Sachs G, Zeng N, Prinz C. Physiology of isolated gastric endocrine cells. *Annu Rev Physiol.* 1997;59:243–256; and Rindi G, Leiter AB, Kopin AS, et al. The "normal" endocrine cell of the gut: changing concepts and new evidences. *Ann N Y Acad Sci.* 2004;1014:1–12.

mucin is reduced and the nuclei occupy correspondingly more of the cell (see Chapter 13). Mucous cells lining the gastric lumen secrete mucus as well as bicarbonate ions. The bases of these pits are in direct continuity with the underlying glands. The surface epithelial cells appear similar to each other in all gland zones except those in the cardia region, where they may be taller and narrower. Occasional intraepithelial lymphocytes are normally present. Sometimes, the surface configuration of the mucosa of the antral and cardiac gland mucosa has a villous configuration. This appearance is a normal variant and should not be confused with intestinal metaplasia of the stomach, because the epithelial cells are normal, not metaplastic. The entire superficial zone of the stomach including the superficial part of the mucous secreting glands are immunoreactive to MUC5, and the deeper parts with MUC6, a staining pattern also seen in antral mucosa, Table 12-1, and illustrated in Chapter 14. These cells are strongly diastase PAS positive but do not stain with Alcian blue except in the cardia.

The Neck Zone (Middle Zone)
The neck zone (middle zone) has mucous cells as well as immature stem cells. This is the generative zone for the stomach, and all cells above and below are derived from this region. Mitotic figures are surprisingly sparse, although stains for Ki-67 show virtually all of the cells to be in the proliferative phase (Fig. 12-6). The immature stem cells migrate upward to renew the surface epithelium or downward to form the differentiated cells of the glands. These cells are also PAS positive.

The Deep (Glandular) Zone
Glands are found in the deep zone. In contrast to surface mucous cell that is continuous over the entire stomach surface, regional differences are mainly in the composition of gastric tubular glands within each compartment.

Cardiac Gland Mucosa
The gastric cardia has branched tubular glands that are primarily mucous-type glands, oxyntic-type glands, or both.[22,23] Those that are mucous but clearly have residual specialized elements are called cardio-oxyntic. Unlike the antrum, in which the deep glands are diffuse, in the cardia, they often are compartmentalized, akin to lobules, which in normal stomachs allow ease of identification at low power. Mucus-secreting glands are similar in appearance on conventional stains to those of the gastric antrum and Brunner's glands, except for the compartmentalization and lack of overt endocrine cells so readily seen in the gastric antrum (Fig. 12-7). In contrast to antral glands, portions of the cardiac glands may contain sialomucins that stain with Alcian blue at pH 2.5. Parietal cells are commonly scattered within the cardiac glands, although endocrine and chief cells are rare. Mucous cell–lined cysts are a frequent finding

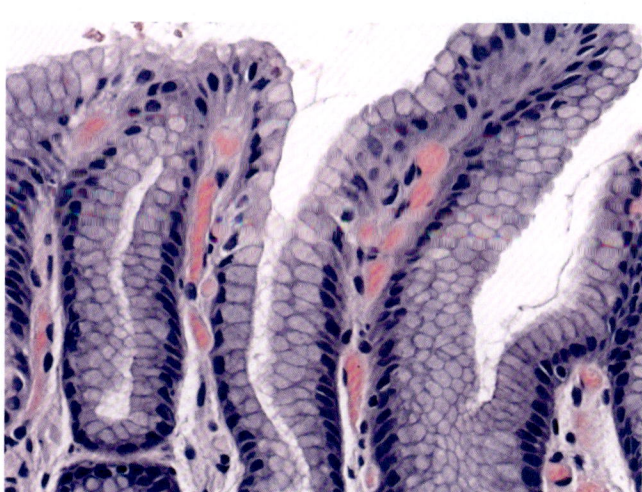

Figure 12-6. Mucous neck region stained with Mib-1 to show the marked proliferation of this region. The paradox is how inconspicuous mitotic figures are in this region.

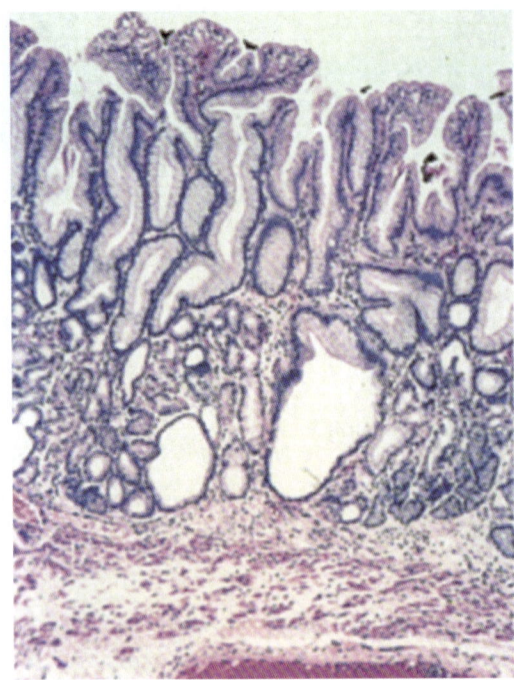

Figure 12-7. Cardiac gland mucosa. The glands in the bottom half of the section are a mix of mucous glands (cardiac glands) and fundic gland elements. Mucosal cysts, as seen here, are a common finding in cardiac gland mucosa. Note the vague lobularity that is very characteristic of cardia. Occasionally, pancreatic-type cells can be seen in these glands but appear to be without significance.

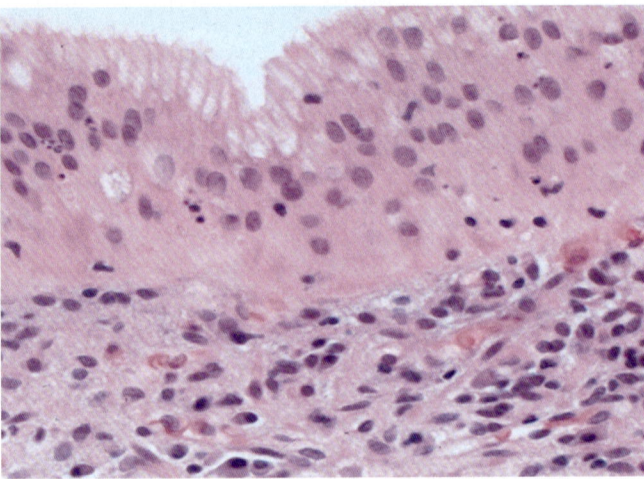

Figure 12-9. Transitional mucosa (mutilayered epithelium) that is sometimes seen in the cardiac region. The most superficial cells are mucous secreting, but beneath that, the cells and their nuclei are stratified as seen in squamous mucosa of the esophagus. These are discussed further in Chapter 10.

(Fig. 12-7). The pits in the cardiac region are very shallow, occupying less than one-quarter of the overall mucosal thickness (Fig. 12-8)—ranging from 0.5 to 1.5 mm—and are immunoreactive with MUC6. There are at best rare endocrine cells in the gastric cardia—there are no data to suggest that they have physiologic or pathologic significance.

Occasionally, pancreatic-type glands can be seen in the cardia in the form of exocrine cells that are immunoreactive with lipase or trypsin. They can be admixed with simple mucous-producing cells or oxyntocardiac mucosa with parietal and mucous-producing glands. Chief cells appear to be rare in the cardia. Endocrine components admixed with heterotopic pancreas are vanishingly rare, and endocrine neoplasms even more so. Also, at the squamocolumnar junction, the so-called multilayered epithelium can be seen (Fig. 12-9), which seems to be associated with the development of Barrett's esophagus. They are sometimes ciliated. They are discussed in more detail in Chapter 10.

Oxyntic Mucosa (Fundic and Corpus Gland Mucosa)

Oxyntic gland literally means acid producing so is a good name for normal corpus and fundic gland mucosa. Surprisingly, the thickness of the oxyntic mucosa varies. It is thickest in the greater curve, gradually thins as the antrum is approached, and is thinnest on the lesser curve (Fig. 12-10).

In the oxyntic gastric corpus, pits have four major cell types (Fig. 12-11): chief cells responsible for pepsinogen production, which can be demonstrated using pepsinogen 1 (Fig. 12-11A), parietal (oxyntic) cells that secrete acid and the intrinsic factor necessary for vitamin B_{12} absorption and apart from antibodies to H^+K^+ ATPase can be demonstrated with PDGFRα (Fig. 12-11B), mucous neck cells, and a variety of endocrine cells (Fig. 12-11C,D). At the interface between the pits and the parietal cell zone, and scattered throughout it, are tiny (~7 μm-wide) mucin-containing neck cells. They are not easily seen with conventionally stained sections, but they can be visualized with the use of the PAS (neutral mucin) stains and sometimes with Alcian blue pH 2.5. In addition, there are a scattering of mucous-producing cells seen throughout

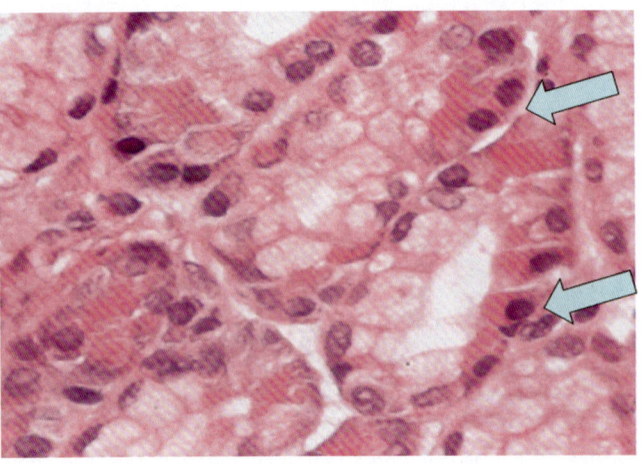

Figure 12-8. Cardiac glands with pancreatic-type *cells (arrows)*.

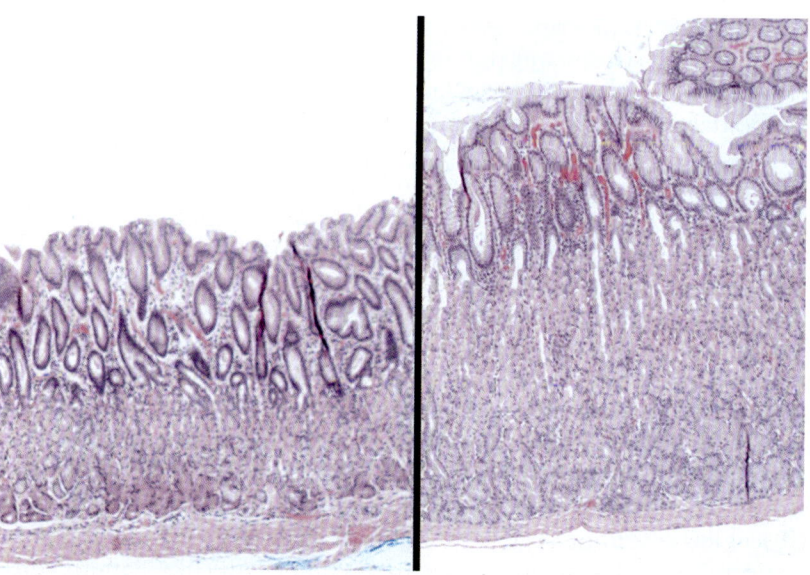

Figure 12-10. Oxyntic mucosa varies in thickness depending on its location.

the specialized mucosa in a small proportion of patients, and they appear to be present and increase toward the distal end of the oxyntic mucosa.

In the oxyntic mucosa, parietal cells predominate in the upper half of the glands, and chief cells dominate in the lower half Figure 12-12. The parietal cells have a round or pyramidal shape, an eosinophilic cytoplasm, and a centrally placed nucleus. The cytoplasm appears vacuolated or finely reticular, especially in the perinuclear area, because of the extensive secretory canaliculae. These can be demonstrated with electron microscopy,[24] or as shown in Figure 12-12B. Parietal cells produce hydrogen ions as hydrochloric acid which facilitates the digestion of protein and absorption of vitamin B_{12}, iron, and calcium. It also prevents bacterial overgrowth and reduces the chances of enteric infection. However, parietal cells also secrete intrinsic factor, transforming growth factor-alpha, amphiregulin, heparin-binding epidermal growth factor–like growth factor, and sonic hedgehog.[25] The major stimulants of acid secretion are gastrin, histamine, and acetylcholine, along with ghrelin (centrally but also produced in the stomach) and orexin (produced centrally and stimulating a craving for food). Indeed, the weight loss following gastrectomy, especially proximal, is due to the loss of this stimulus to eat. The main inhibitor of acid secretion is somatostatin, along with nitric oxide and dopamine.

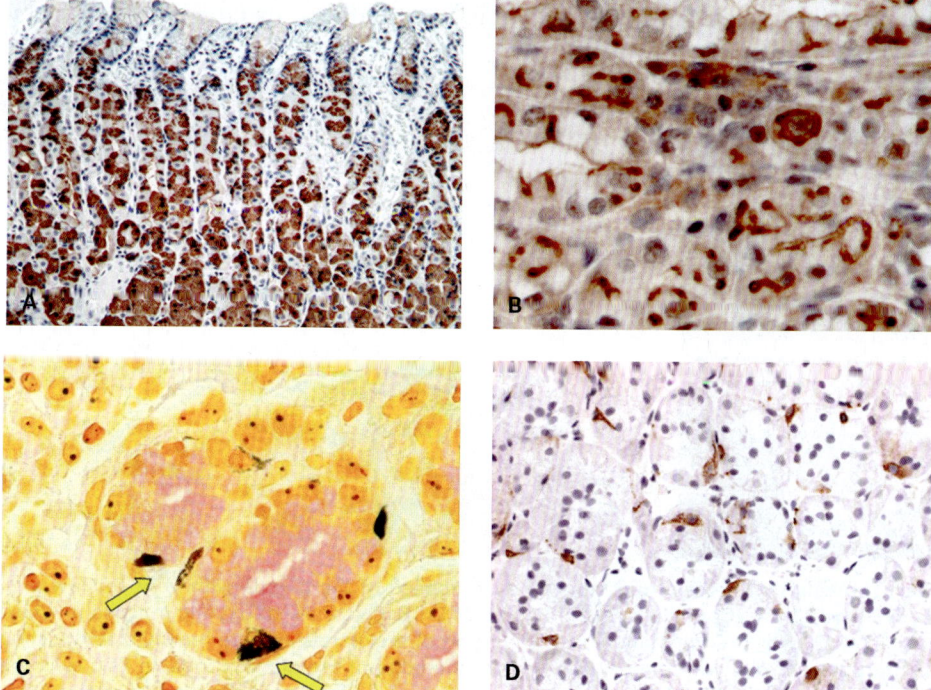

Figure 12-11. Specialized cells of the oxyntic mucosa can be appreciated with (A) immunostains for pepsinogen 1, which stains chief cells and (B) platelet-derived growth factor receptor alpha (PDGFRα) that appears to outline the secretory apparatus (canliculi) of the parietal cells. In addition, (C) endocrine cells of the gastric body can be demonstrated with either argyrophylic stains, here surrounding chief cells at the base of the glands, or (D) division of the numerous diffusely immunoreactive endocrine cells in the oxyntic mucosa, here stained with chromogranin A, which contrasts markedly with the band-like distribution consisting mainly of G cells, seen in the antrum.

The chief cells contain zymogen granules that are basophilic, but the degree of basophilia can vary and can be quite faint, especially in transition zones. Chief cells have a large basal nucleus and a more cuboidal shape. They secrete pepsinogens I and II, and these products can be demonstrated immunocytochemically (Fig. 12-11A).[26,27] However, in addition, chief cells also release pepsinogen, gastric lipase, and the protease chymosin (formerly known as rennin—to be distinguished from renin), which commercially is used to produce cheese from milk. Chief cells release the zymogen pepsinogen when stimulated by a variety of factors including cholinergic activity from the vagus nerve and acidic condition in the stomach. Gastrin and secretin may also act as secretagogues. These cells have the same gastrin and CCK2 receptors found on parietal cells, enterochromaffin-like (ECL) cells, and D (somatostatin) cells suggesting similar control.

The parietal and chief cell turnover rates have not been clearly defined because they are much slower. In rodents, the turnover for parietal cells has been estimated to be about 164 days.[28] The key feature is that the specialized compartment in the stomach is renewed, but the turnover time is in months. Under stress, both parietal and chief cells appear to be able to undergo cell division, parietal cells with hypergastrinemia from, for example, PPIs, while chief cells may also be able to replicate.

The endocrine cells of the fundic gland mucosa are distributed fairly diffusely throughout the oxyntic mucosa. The presence of endocrine cells is sometimes suggested by a degree of perinuclear clearing (halo), although far less than that seen in G-cells in the antrum, while the nuclei are far less hyperchromatic than the intraepithelial lymphocytes that may be present. Endocrine cells can sometimes be identified on H&E sections in the oxyntic mucosa as nuclei immediately above the basal lamina of the gland that are not in the middle of parietal cells and not clearly associated with chief cell granules (Fig. 12-6B). However, the nuclei need to be observed carefully, for, if very densely hyperchromatic, they could represent intraepithelial lymphocytes (demonstrable on CD3 immunostains).

Antral Mucosa The antral glands are coiled branched tubular glands that appear diffusely located with no, or at best minimal, hint of the lobular compartmentalization seen in the cardia (Fig. 12-13B), unless atrophy is present. Glands are predominantly mucous, and while most are clear, in some patients, the mucous cells have distinctly eosinophilic granules that can be either very fine or almost as large as Paneth cell granules, which they can resemble. All (like Paneth cells) secrete lysozyme. Gastric cells can also upregulate specific defensins in response to *Helicobacter* infection, but it is so far unclear if these are produced by lysozyme-producing cells.[29]

Numerous endocrine cells are also present and are primarily gastrin-producing cells (G cells), sertonin-producing (EC) cells, and somatostatin-producing cells (D cells) (Fig. 12-14). Endocrine cells appear more frequent in the antrum than in the corpus[22] but are concentrated in a band (Fig. 12-12) rather than being diffusely dispersed (see Fig. 12-11D) and with a little practice are readily visible at scanning power on H&E sections (Fig. 12-13). They are easily seen at high power with virtually any stain (Fig. 12-14). Specific immunostaining for gastrin shows that the vast majority of these are G cells (Figs. 12-13 and 12-15). If there is any doubt about whether a specific biopsy is antral

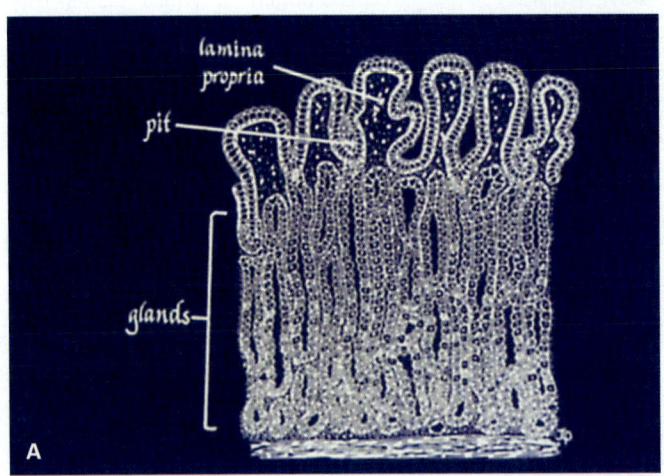 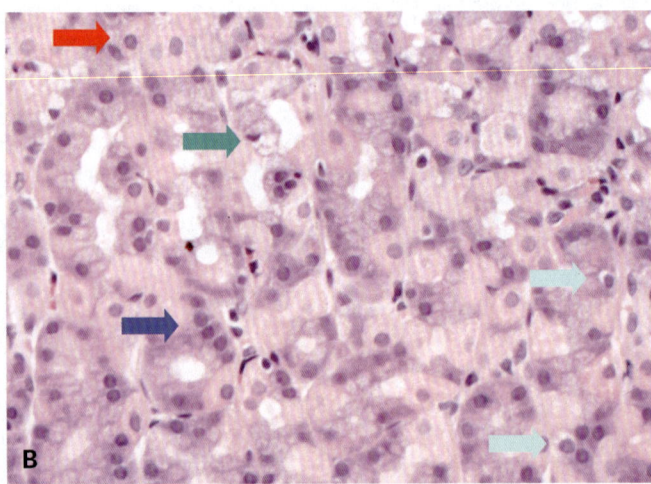

Figure 12-12. Oxyntic mucosa. **A:** Sketch showing that most of the mucosa is composed of the glands with very shallow pits. Contrast this with the antral gland sketch in Figure 13-6A. (Courtesy of John Petrini, M.D.) **B:** Overview of oxyntic mucosa in which the pink parietal cells with their central nuclei (*red arrow*) predominate in the upper part of the glands and are readily distinguished from the more purple staining chief cells (*dark blue arrow*) with their nuclei against the edge of the gland. Probable ECL cells are insignificant but have a central nucleus and pale cytoplasm (*light blue arrows*) and occasional mucous-producing cells are also present (*green arrow*).

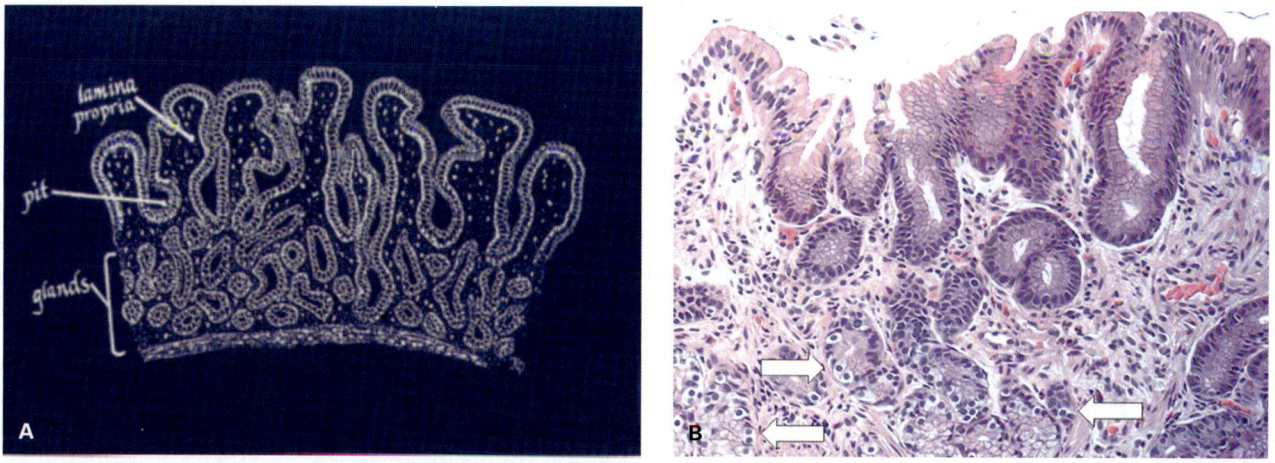

Figure 12-13. Antral gland mucosa. **A:** Sketch showing that the thickness of the mucosa is usually less than that of the fundic gland mucosa. The gastric pits occupy one-half or more of the mucosal thickness. (Courtesy of John Petrini, M.D.) **B:** Low-power histologic section in which the "fried egg" or "halo" (originally "waterclear" cells) are readily seen (*arrowed*).

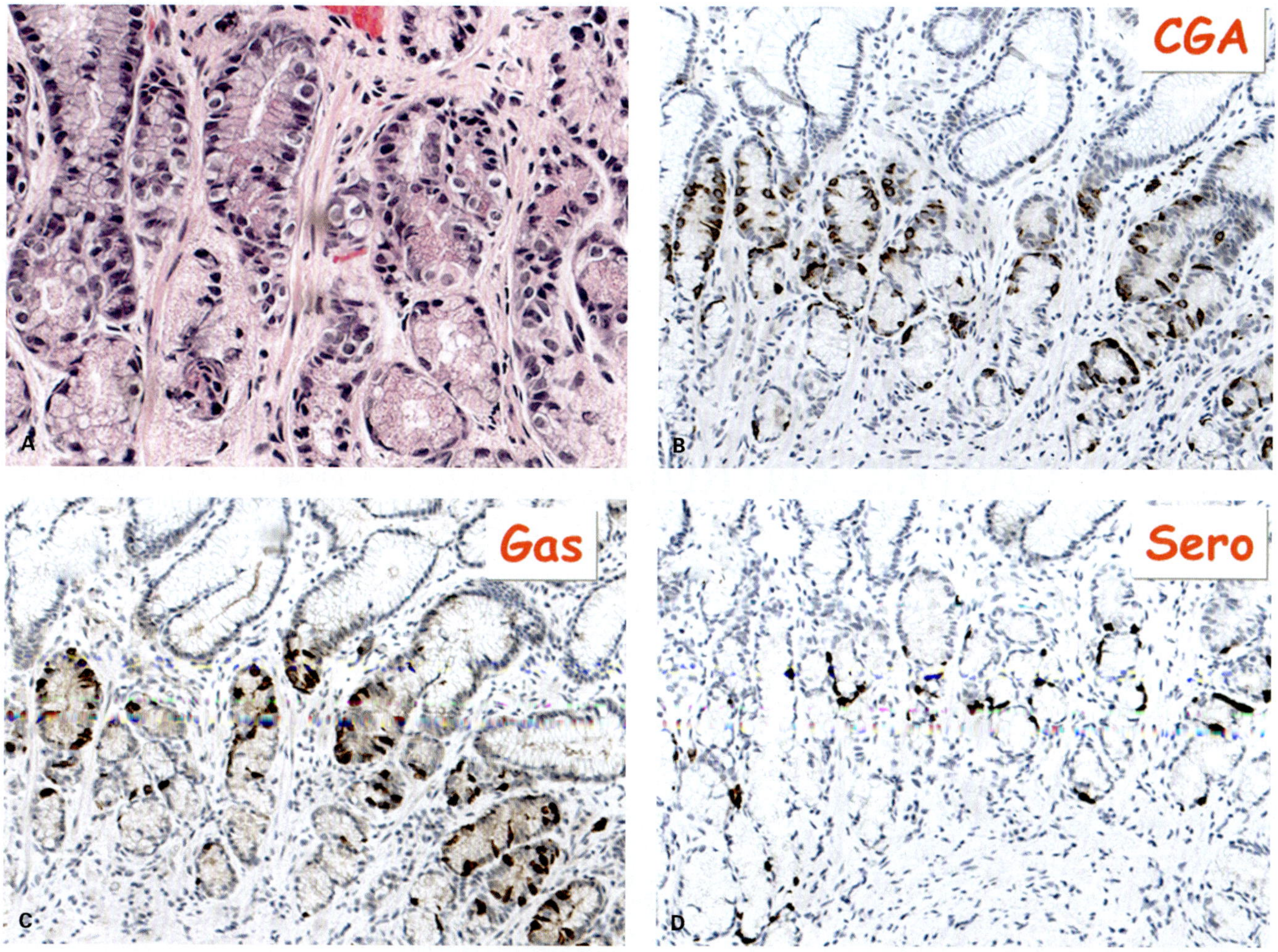

Figure 12-14. **A:** Antral mucosa with occasional endocrine "halo" cells scattered regularly down the sides of the midportion of each crypt. **B–D:** Immunostains for chromogranin A, which immunostains virtually all of the endocrine cells, and specific stains for gastrin **(C)** and serotonin **(D)**, which make up about 2/3 and 1/3 of the cells, while somatostatin are about 5%.

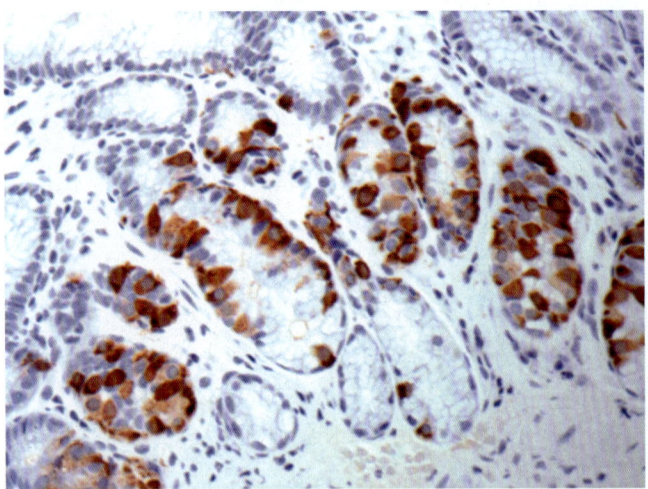

Figure 12-15. Immunohistochemical stain for gastrin showing the band of G cells in the antrum, here accentuated as there is hyperplasia from long term PPIs.

so absolute distinction can be difficult. It also needs to be appreciated that the G-cell containing portion of the antrum is relatively distal in the "anatomical" antrum, the more proximal mucosa being more transitional as it acquires oxyntic characteristics. This becomes important as biopsies from histological antrum need to be taken quite distally—ideally from the prepyloric region, to guarantee getting the endocrine portion of the antrum. Whether this matters in looking at biopsies for *Helicobacter* has not been determined. Gastric endocrine cells are also discussed subsequently.

Parietal cells can be quite conspicuous in the antrum and should not be taken as an indication that one is not in the antrum (Fig. 12-18); indeed, they often appear to increase in density toward the pylorus, rather than petering out as might be expected, but detection of the G-cells, even on H&E stains, is usually easy and confirms the location as being antrum. The density of parietal cells in the antrum decreases in the face of moderate to severe antral gland gastritis.[30]

or not, additional immunostaining for pepsinogen 1, if available, help, as they stain oxyntic glands but are immunonegative in antral mucosa (Fig. 12-16). However, there is a transition zone between antrum and oxyntic mucosa; in this location, practically, the presence of gastrin cells puts the biopsy in the antrum. In chromogranin A stains staining (for some reason, this seems to detect G cells much more readily than synaptophysin, but this may vary from lab to lab), the band of G cells can be detected. Differences between these two endocrine cell stains are shown in Figure 12-17. However, in the transition zones, these become more diffuse and intermixed with oxyntic endocrine cells,

Mucosal Transition Zones As indicated previously, all of the cardiac gland mucosa may contain scattered fundic gland elements, especially parietal cells. This mixed-gland phenomenon may be equally prominent in antral–fundic gland transition zones. The transition zone between fundic gland and antral gland mucosa does not usually follow the gross anatomic boundaries. It is not uncommon to find a mixed-gland mucosa extending 5 cm or more, especially along the lesser curvature. At endoscopy, biopsy specimens taken from what is considered to be the proximal third of the antrum may consist entirely of fundic gland mucosa,

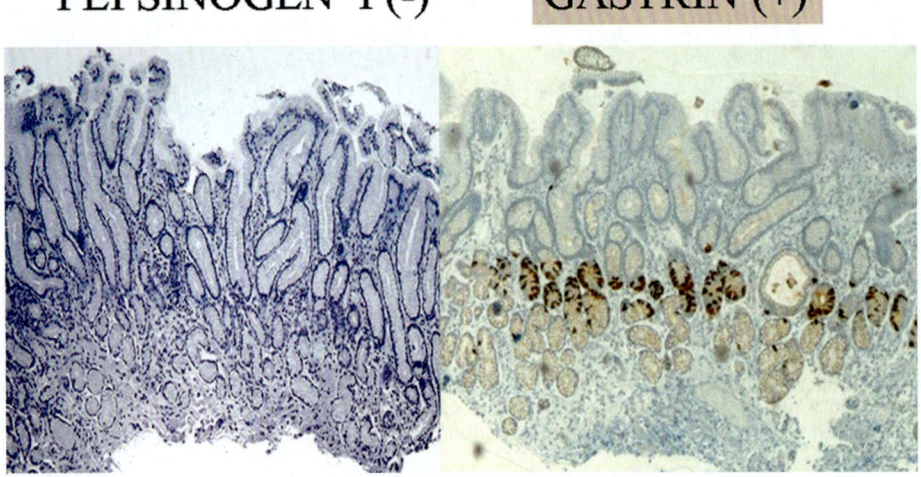

Figure 12-16. Typical immunophenotype of gastric antrum with no pepsinogen 1 immunoreactivity and strong gastrin immunoreactivity.

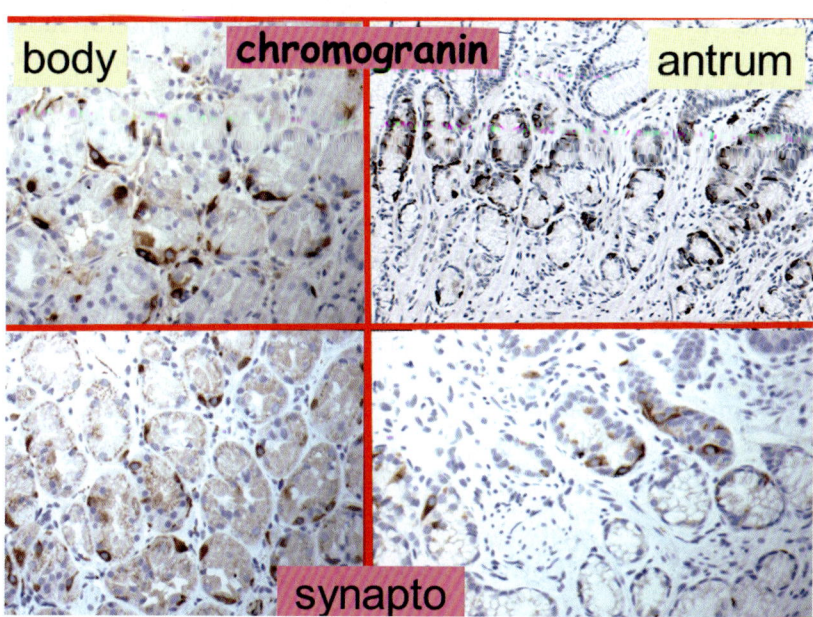

Figure 12-17. Comparative immunoreactivity of chromogranin A and synaptophysin in normal antrum and body. Synaptophysin seems to stain G cells preferentially, while in the oxyntic mucosa, they are much more similar, with perhaps chromogranin A getting the edge in numbers of endocrine cells stained.

which likely does matter if looking for *Helicobacter* in what is thought to be antral mucosa; these need to be taken more distally (we advise from the distal or prepyloric antrum). Furthermore, parietal cells are commonly found scattered throughout the antral gland mucosa down to the pylorus (Fig. 12-18).[30] The presence of parietal cells in a biopsy does not therefore preclude an antral origin. Although chief cells may be found in the immediate transition zone between fundic gland and antral gland mucosae, they are usually absent in the more distal antrum.

Gastric Mucins The gastric mucosa is covered by mucin-producing cells that play important roles in protecting gastrointestinal mucosa from a variety of physical, chemical, and microbial damage.[31–33] Mucins are highly glycosylated glycoproteins and their core proteins (mucin core proteins: MUC).[34] The expression of these mucins and intestinal enzyme are cell-type specific; hence, they are useful phenotypic indicators of cell differentiation in normal, metaplastic, or neoplastic epithelial cells in the gastrointestinal tract.[35–37] MUC5AC (sometimes just abbreviated to MUC5) is expressed in gastric surface mucous cells, MUC6 is expressed in gastric gland mucous cells (cardiac gland cells, mucous neck cells, and pyloric gland cells), and MUC2 is expressed in intestinal goblet cells,[38–40] The histochemistry and immunohistochemistry of gastrointestinal mucins are discussed in Chapter 14.

Histochemically, mucins of the surface and pit epithelium are predominantly of the neutral polysaccharide type and thus stain positively with the periodic acid–Schiff (PAS) stain.[41] Much fainter staining with PAS is seen in parietal cells and in the mucous glands of the antral and cardiac gland regions. Acid, nonsulfated mucins (sialomucins) are absent from the

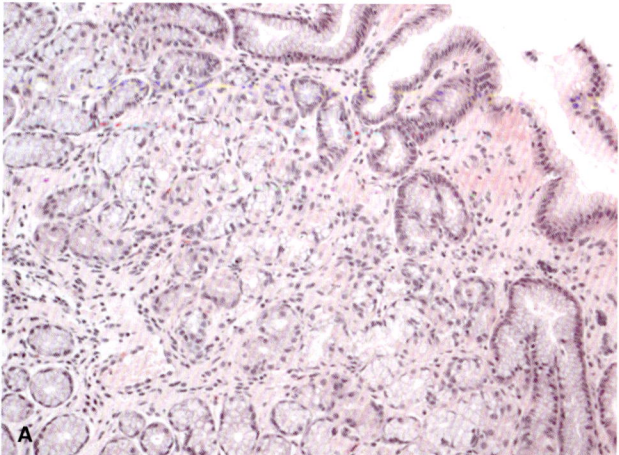
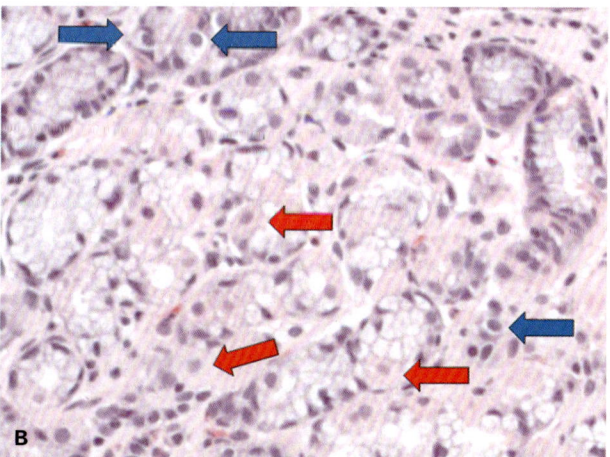

Figure 12-18. Parietal cells in the antrum. **A:** At scanning power, numerous parietal cells are visible. **B:** Detail shows the parietal cells (*red arrows*) and endocrine cells (*blue arrows*), the latter confirming that this is antral mucosa.

surface epithelium but are present in small amounts in the deep pit regions and mucous neck cells. These can be highlighted by staining with Alcian blue at pH 2.5.[41]

Gastric Endocrine Cells Enteroendocrine cells (also defined as the diffuse endocrine system) are specialized endocrine cells of the gastrointestinal tract that produce hormones such as gastrin, histamine, ghrelin, serotonin, and somatostatin.[42,43] The enteroendocrine cells are derived from the same stem cells as the rest of the epithelium and are not derived from the migratory neural crest source that provides the enteric nervous system.[44] The enteroendocrine system of the gut is heterogeneous and is composed of as many as 14 highly specialized cells, some with unknown function.[42,43] Table 12-2 lists gastric endocrine cells with known function.

Most endocrine cells historically can be identified immunohistochemically or with silver stains, which were among the first methods to assess gastric endocrine cells. Endocrine cells in the antrum can be identified without special stains. The staining properties of endocrine cells displaying intrinsic silver reducing power either with or without ammonium ions being provided. Interaction of some of these cells with chromium salts (hence enterochromaffin [EC] cells) proved to be the same cells that could precipitate silver salts in the absence of ammonium ions (e.g., Masson–Fontana stain—argentaffin cells), while all other cells required the addition of ammonium ions for the silver to precipitate (e.g., Grimelius, or Sevier–Munger stains—argyrophil cells). (It will not have escaped some that the terms argyrophil and argentaffin have identical meanings, except that the first is of Greek derivation and the second of Latin.) The staining of endocrine cells requiring the presence of added reducing agents (argyrophilia) resulted in the term enterochromaffin-like cells (ECL cells).[43] Because silver stains tend to be capricious, numerous arghyrophil stains exist, and some were found to be more specific for certain cell types (e.g., Sevier–Munger for G cells). Silver impregnation techniques, although effective and reproducible, have now been largely replaced with immunohistochemistry (Table 12-1).

In the antral mucosa, most endocrine cells are G cells, producing gastrin, while most of the remainder are D (somatostatin-producing) cells (see Table 12-1). In the oxyntic mucosa, ECL cells secrete histamine and directly stimulate acid secretion; they can specifically be demonstrated with antibodies to Human Vesicular Monoamine Transporter 2 (VMAT2). Ghrelin is a peptide hormone that has been localized to the oxyntic mucosa X/A-like (Gr) cells.[45,46] X/A-like cells that resemble pancreatic A cell (glucagon-producing cells—hence the A part of the name) are the most abundant endocrine cells in the stomach after the histamine-producing cells.[46,47] Though ghrelin most widely known function is growth hormone release from the pituitary gland; it also plays a role in mediating immune and inflammatory processes.[48] Ghrelin plays an important role in regulating appetite, feeding, and energy metabolism[49] in addition to stimulating gastric motility.[50] D cells are also the "turn-off" cell in the oxyntic mucosa.

Acid Secretion Gastric acid secretion is regulated by a complex set of mechanisms acting at the central, peripheral, and cellular level. A detailed description of neural regulation (both central and peripheral) is beyond the scope of this chapter (interested readers should refer to 22,25). This section is a simplified view of acid secretion in the normal physiologic state, but is required to understand gastric pathophysiology.

Though the capacity of the stomach to secrete acid is almost linearly related to parietal cell mass, the major endocrine cells known to play an important role in acid secretion are the ECL cell of the fundus, the gastrin (G) cell of the antrum, and the somatostatin (D) cells of the fundus and antrum. Physiologically, the thought of food enhances release of ghrelin that initiates acid secretion prior to food ingestion and orexin that stimulates a craving for food. Gastric distension and the presence of food in the stomach stimulate the release of gastrin from antral G cells. Gastrin diffuses into the circulation via an autocrine process to stimulate the parietal cell to produce gastric acid, both directly acting on parietal cells and indirectly by stimulating ECL cells to secrete histamine[51] via the CCK2 receptors[25] that are found on D cell, ECL cells, and parietal cells. Parietal cells specifically have the H2-histaimine receptor, which is why suppression of acid secretion with H2-receptor antagonists was key in acid suppressive therapy, especially prior to the PPI era.

Histamine (and possibly gastrin directly) activates the parietal cell to secrete acid. Thus, in a normal physiologic state, acid secretion is directly related to histamine receptor stimulation by ECL cells. Histamine release from ECL cells is continuous in the presence of gastrin. As the acidity of the stomach and duodenum increases, further acid secretion is inhibited through the release of somatostatin by D cells.[52-54] Somatostatin inhibits the secretion of gastrin and histamine and appears to have a direct inhibitory effect on the parietal cell.[22] Figure 12-19 is a simplified diagram of mechanisms involved in gastric acid secretion.

Lamina Propria The lamina propria is located between the pits and contains smooth muscle cells that have very eosinophilic, and sometimes wavy, cytoplasm and are

Table 12-2 Developmental Abnormalities of the Stomach

DISORDER (REF.)	PATHOGENESIS	PREVALENCE	CLINICAL FEATURES	GROSS APPEARANCES	HISTOLOGY	COMMENT
Pyloric stenosis Infantile[62-66]	May be familial	0.3% of live births, mainly firstborn and male; rare in blacks	Projectile vomiting in 3rd wk of life; visible gastric peristalsis; palpable pylorus	A 2- to 3-cm ovoid mass in pylorus; knob-like projection into duodenum	Hypertrophy and hyperplasia of circular muscle; normal autonomic ganglia	
Adult[67]	Persistence of mild infantile form	Very rare	Nausea, vomiting	Pyloric channel elongated and narrowed	Hypertrophy and hyperplasia of circular muscle	Exclude peptic ulcer and malignancy
Pancreatic Heterotopias[68,69]	Cephalad displacement of pancreatic bud during embryonic life	2% of population at autopsy	Often asymptomatic; epigastric pain or outlet obstruction; 1–3 cm in diameter within 6 cm of pylorus	Gastric filling defect with central umbilication; may be cystic	Usually submucosal; pancreatic ducts or acini; islets less common	Pancreatitis, carcinoma (rare)
Aplasia[62,70]	Found in anencephalics	Rare				
Atresia[62,70-79]	Arrested phase of normal development; vascular factors; autosomal recessive	Very rare	Depends on severity of lesion and age; infants: outlet obstruction, vomiting, gastric distention; older children and adults: peptic ulcer symptoms	Complete segmental defect; stomach ends blindly Fibrous cord. Atretic strand of mucosa and seromuscular layer Webs: by endoscopy, portion distal to web can be mistaken for duodenal bulb	Gastric mucosa; rarely, squamous epithelium	
Microgastria[74,75]	Arrested development of foregut; familial; autosomal trait	Very rare	Feeding abnormalities	Small stomach Failure to rotate and differentiate into different parts		Other congenital malformations
Duplications[62,76-80]	Embryonic epithelial nodules that fail to regress	Very rare account for ~4% of gastrointestinal duplications; more common in females than in males	Young patients; symptoms depend on location and size; most gastric emptying problems; upper abdominal mass; perforation; peritonitis	Variably sized cyst; often greater curvature Usually no communication with gastric lumen	All layers of stomach; rarely lined by squamous epithelium	May also involve esophagus; one-third of patients have other anomalies
Diverticula[81,82]	As for duplications	Very rare	As for duplications	Posterior wall 2 cm below esophagogastric junction		As for duplications
Positional Defects[83]		Very rare		Right-sided stomach Inversion: pylorus more cephalad than esophagogastric junction		Situs inversus
Muscle defect[84,85]	Developmental defect in muscle	Very rare	Gastric perforation more common in premature babies	Mainly greater curvature rupture and perforation		
Volvulus[86,87]	Long gastric ligaments	Very rare	Vomiting	Antrum rotates up and to left or right		

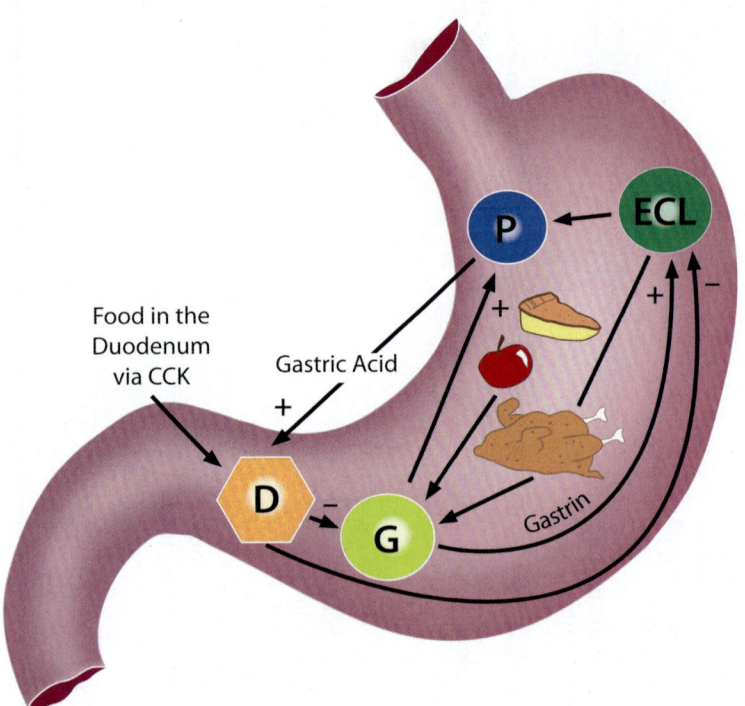

Figure 12-19. Diagram of known mechanisms involved in gastric acid secretion.

frequently confused with other cells, very few fibroblasts, macrophages, eosinophils, plasma cells, and lymphocytes. Mast cells are scattered in the interpit regions as well as between the fundic glands.[55] In the gastric corpus, glands are so tightly packed that it may be hard to see the lamina propria, except just beneath the surface mucous cells. Small lymphoid follicles may be seen just above the muscularis mucosae; these are normal and physiological[56]—we disagree with the notion that no lymphoid aggregates are present normally. They are usually small but present nonetheless. There is also a finely dispersed network of reticulin and collagen fibers. These, as well as fibers of smooth muscle, extend upward from the muscularis mucosae and may appear as fern-like streamers in the lamina propria, reaching the superficial portion of the mucosa. This is a more prominent finding in the antrum, especially near the pylorus.

Tiny vessels are seen in the lamina propria, but it may be impossible to differentiate lymph capillaries from blood capillaries without the use of immunohistochemistry. With electron microscopy, it has been demonstrated that, like the large bowel, lymph capillaries are primarily confined to the basal portion of the mucosa just above the muscularis mucosae. In contrast, blood capillaries are distributed throughout the mucosa.[57]

There is considerable normal variation in the density of the lamina propria cells located between the pits. This variability is more prominent in antral gland mucosa, where the pits are longer. However, while occasional lymphocytes, histiocytes, mast cells, and eosinophils are present, plasma cells are uncommon, and more that occasional cells reflect chronic inflammation. Neutrophils are normally absent.

Muscularis Mucosae As elsewhere throughout the intestinal tract, the muscularis mucosae has both a thin layer of internal, primarily circular, muscle and an outer longitudinal layer. In the cardiac and antral glands, mucosal strands of muscle fibers may radiate into the lamina propria from the muscularis mucosae. This may be very prominent in the distal antrum and, on first glance, may be misinterpreted as fibrosis. Sometimes, lymphoid follicles are located at the bases of the glands above the muscularis mucosae, or they may actually breach it and occupy part of the upper submucosa.

Submucosa. The submucosa consists of loose connective tissue, a rich plexus of blood vessels, sizable lymphatic vessels, the ganglion cells of Meissner's plexus, scattered mast cells, and mononuclear cells.

Muscularis propria, ICCs, and serosa. The muscularis propria consists of three layers: outer longitudinal, middle circular, and inner oblique. The outer longitudinal layer is most concentrated along both curvatures. The middle circular zone encircles the body of the stomach and is thickened distally to form the pyloric sphincter. The inner oblique fibers pass down from the fundus over both the anterior and posterior walls.

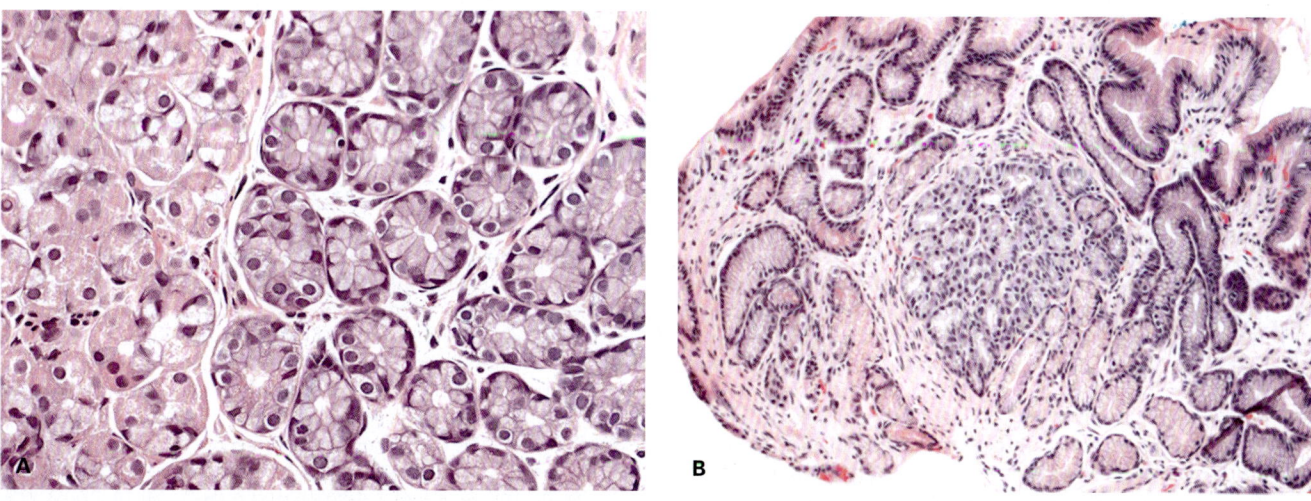

Figure 12-20. Heterotopic islands of endocrine mucosa (**A**) in the oxyntic mucosa (adjacent normal oxyntic mucosa is seen right) and (**B**) in the antrum. In both, the waterclear "halo" cells are present in abundance.

The muscularis propria is bounded on its outer surface by a serosa similar to that of the other regions of the gut. It consists of loose connective tissue and contains blood vessels, lymphatics, and nerve fibers. The muscularis propria is richly innervated with nerves, while interstitial cells of Cajal are present both in and immediately around the myenteric plexus, while intramuscular interstitial cells are also present in all layers of the muscle. If interstitial cells are being assessed, it is very wise to have normal controls, ideally from the same area of the stomach, with which they can be compared.[58]

DEVELOPMENTAL ABNORMALITIES OF THE STOMACH

With the exception of infantile pyloric stenosis and pancreatic heterotopia, most of the other developmental abnormalities of the stomach are rare. Some findings, such as goblet cells in the stomach of adults, are difficult to classify as a rare congenital cause,[59,60] because intestinal metaplasia is such a common accompaniment of noncrosive gastritis or focal injury.

Gastric heterotopias, in which gastric tissue is located outside of the stomach, are not discussed here. These are discussed in the chapters dealing with specific regions of the gastrointestinal tract as in gastric heterotopia in the upper esophagus and in Meckel's diverticulum. Gastric heteroptopia occurs in a variety of organs and is discussed there. Gastric hamartomas are discussed in Chapter 14. Within the stomach, occasionally, small islands of islet tissue can be found in both the antral or oxyntic mucosa in the absence of any other features (Fig. 12-20).

Pathogenesis and Clinical Features

The pathogenesis of developmental disorders is poorly understood.[61] Table 12-2 outlines and references the various disorders. With the exception of pancreatic heterotopia, most congenital anomalies present in the postnatal period or in childhood. Rarely, pyloric stenosis gastric duplications and gastric webs present in adulthood.

References

1. Moore KL, ed. *The Developing Human: Clinically Oriented Embryology*. 7th ed. Philadelphia, London, Toronto: W.B. Saunders Company; 2013.
2. Tsutsumi Y. Immunohistochemical studies on glucagon, glicentin and pancreatic polypeptide in human stomach: normal and pathological conditions. *Histochem J*. 1984;16(8):869–883.
3. Stein BA, Buchan AM, Morris J, et al. The ontogeny of regulatory peptide-containing cells in the human fetal stomach: an immunocytochemical study. *J Histochem Cytochem*. 1983;31(9):1117–1125.
4. Yasugi S. Regulation of pepsinogen gene expression in epithelial cells of vertebrate stomach during development. *Int J Dev Biol*. 1994;38(2):273–279.
5. Johnson LR. Functional development of the stomach. *Annu Rev Physiol*. 1985;47:199–215.
6. Deren JS. Development of structure and function in the fetal and newborn stomach. *Am J Clin Nutr*. 1971;24(1):144–159.
7. Park YS, Park HJ, Kang GH, et al. Histology of gastroesophageal junction in fetal and pediatric autopsy. *Arch Pathol Lab Med*. 2003;127(4):451–455.
8. Chandrasoma PT. Fetal "cardiac mucosa" is not adult cardiac mucosa. *Gut*. 2003;52(12):1798; author reply 9.
9. De Hertogh G, Van Eyken P, Ectors N, Geboes K. On the origin of cardiac mucosa: a histological and immunohistochemical study of cytokeratin expression patterns in the developing esophagogastric junction region and stomach. *World J Gastroenterol*. 2005;11(29):4490–4496.

10. Riddell RH, Odze RD. Definition of Barrett's esophagus: time for a rethink–is intestinal metaplasia dead? *Am J Gastroenterol.* 2009;104(10):2588-2594.
11. Ronkainen J, Aro P, Storskrubb T, et al. Prevalence of Barrett's esophagus in the general population: an endoscopic study. *Gastroenterology.* 2005;129(6):1825-1831.
12. Schutze M, Schulz M, Steffen A, et al. Beer consumption and the 'beer belly': scientific basis or common belief? *Eur J Clin Nutr.* 2009;63(9):1143-1149.
13. Owen DA. Normal histology of the stomach. *Am J Surg Pathol.* 1986;10(1):48-61.
14. Gottfried MR, McClave SA, Boyce HW. Incomplete intestinal metaplasia in the diagnosis of columnar lined esophagus (Barrett's esophagus). *Am J Clin Pathol.* 1989;92(6):741-746.
15. Ishimura N, Amano Y, Kinoshita Y. Endoscopic definition of esophagogastric junction for diagnosis of Barrett's esophagus: importance of systematic education and training. *Dig Endosc.* 2009;21(4):213-218.
16. Sato T, Kato Y, Matsuura M, et al. Significance of palisading longitudinal esophagus vessels: identification of the true esophagogastric junction has histopathological and oncological considerations. *Dig Dis Sci.* 2010;55(11):3095-3101.
17. Moore JG, Dubois A, Christian PE, et al. Evidence for a midgastric transverse band in humans. *Gastroenterology.* 1986;91(3):540-545.
18. Rubin W, Ross LL, Sleisenger MH, et al. The normal human gastric epithelia. A fine structural study. *Lab Invest.* 1968;19(6):598-626.
19. Helander HF. The cells of the gastric mucosa. *Int Rev Cytol.* 1981;70:217-289.
20. Day DW, Morson BC. Structure and infrastructure. *Front Gastrointest Res.* 1980;6:1-19.
21. Macdonald WC, Trier JS, Everett NB. Cell proliferation and migration in the stomach, duodenum, and rectum of man: radioautographic studies. *Gastroenterology.* 1964;46:405-417.
22. Hersey SJ, Sachs G. Gastric acid secretion. *Physiol Rev.* 1995;75(1):155-189.
23. el-Zimaity HM, Verghese VJ, Ramchatesingh J, et al. The gastric cardia in gastro-oesophageal disease. *J Clin Pathol.* 2000;53(8):619-625.
24. Helander HF, Leth R, Olbe L. Stereological investigations on human gastric mucosa: I. Normal oxyntic mucosa. *Anat Rec.* 1986;216(3):373-380.
25. Schubert ML. Gastric exocrine and endocrine secretion. *Curr Opin Gastroenterol.* 2009;25(6):529-536.
26. Samloff IM. Cellular localization of group I pepsinogens in human gastric mucosa by immunofluorescence. *Gastroenterology.* 1971;61(2):185-188.
27. Samloff IM, Liebman WM. Cellular localization of the group II pepsinogens in human stomach and duodenum by immunofluorescence. *Gastroenterology.* 1973;65(1):36-42.
28. Li H, Helander HF. Parietal cell kinetics after administration of omeprazole and ranitidine in the rat. *Scand J Gastroenterol.* 1995;30(3):205-209.
29. Otte JM, Neumann HM, Brand S, et al. Expression of beta-defensin 4 is increased in human gastritis. *Eur J Clin Invest.* 2009;39(2):126-138.
30. Tominaga K. Distribution of parietal cells in the antral mucosa of human stomachs. *Gastroenterology.* 1975;69(6):1201-1207.
31. Slomiany BL, Slomiany A. Role of mucus in gastric mucosal protection. *J Physiol Pharmacol.* 1991;42(2):147-161.
32. Ota H, Katsuyama T. Alternating laminated array of two types of mucin in the human gastric surface mucous layer. *Histochem J.* 1992;24(2):86-92.
33. Matsuo K, Ota H, Akamatsu T, et al. Histochemistry of the surface mucous gel layer of the human colon. *Gut.* 1997;40(6):782-789.
34. Moniaux N, Escande F, Porchet N, et al. Structural organization and classification of the human mucin genes. *Front Biosci.* 2001;6:D1192-D1206.
35. Akamatsu T, Katsuyama T. Histochemical demonstration of mucins in the intramucosal laminated structure of human gastric signet ring cell carcinoma and its relation to submucosal invasion. *Histochem J.* 1990;22(8):416-425.
36. Tatematsu M, Tsukamoto T, Inada K. Stem cells and gastric cancer: role of gastric and intestinal mixed intestinal metaplasia. *Cancer Sci.* 2003;94(2):135-141.
37. Ota H, Katsuyama T, Ishii K, et al. A dual staining method for identifying mucins of different gastric epithelial mucous cells. *Histochem J.* 1991;23(1):22-28.
38. Buisine MP, Devisme L, Maunoury V, et al. Developmental mucin gene expression in the gastroduodenal tract and accessory digestive glands. I. Stomach. A relationship to gastric carcinoma. *J Histochem Cytochem.* 2000;48(12):1657-1666.
39. Buisine MP, Devisme L, Degand P, et al. Developmental mucin gene expression in the gastroduodenal tract and accessory digestive glands. II. Duodenum and liver, gallbladder, and pancreas. *J Histochem Cytochem.* 2000;48(12):1667-1676.
40. Nakajima K, Ota H, Zhang MX, et al. Expression of gastric gland mucous cell-type mucin in normal and neoplastic human tissues. *J Histochem Cytochem.* 2003;51(12):1689-1698.
41. Filipe MI. Mucins in the human gastrointestinal epithelium: a review. *Invest Cell Pathol.* 1979;2(3):195-216.
42. Sachs G, Zeng N, Prinz C. Physiology of isolated gastric endocrine cells. *Annu Rev Physiol.* 1997;59:243-256.
43. Rindi G, Leiter AB, Kopin AS, et al. The "normal" endocrine cell of the gut: changing concepts and new evidences. *Ann N Y Acad Sci.* 2004;1014:1-12.
44. Thompson M, Fleming KA, Evans DJ, et al. Gastric endocrine cells share a clonal origin with other gut cell lineages. *Development.* 1990;110(2):477-481.
45. Kojima M, Hosoda H, Date Y, et al. Ghrelin is a growth-hormone-releasing acylated peptide from stomach. *Nature.* 1999;402(6762):656-660.
46. Date Y, Kojima M, Hosoda H, et al. Ghrelin, a novel growth hormone-releasing acylated peptide, is synthesized in a distinct endocrine cell type in the gastrointestinal tracts of rats and humans. *Endocrinology.* 2000;141(11):4255-4261.
47. Simonsson M, Eriksson S, Hakanson R, et al. Endocrine cells in the human oxyntic mucosa. A histochemical study. *Scand J Gastroenterol.* 1988;23(9):1089-1099.
48. Tesauro M, Schinzari F, Caramanti M, et al. Cardiovascular and metabolic effects of Ghrelin. *Curr Diabetes Rev.* 2010;6(4):228-235.
49. Suzuki K, Simpson KA, Minnion JS, et al. The role of gut hormones and the hypothalamus in appetite regulation. *Endocr J.* 201057(5):359-372.
50. Falken Y, Hellstrom PM, Sanger GJ, et al. Actions of prolonged ghrelin infusion on gastrointestinal transit and glucose homeostasis in humans. *Neurogastroenterol Motil.* 201022(6):e192-e200.
51. Prinz C, Zanner R, Gratzl M. Physiology of gastric enterochromaffin-like cells. *Annu Rev Physiol.* 2003;65:371-382.
52. Lloyd KC, Wang J, Aurang K, et al. Activation of somatostatin receptor subtype 2 inhibits acid secretion in rats. *Am J Physiol.* 1995;268(1 pt 1):G102-G106.
53. Martinez V, Curi AP, Torkian B, et al. High basal gastric acid secretion in somatostatin receptor subtype 2 knockout mice. *Gastroenterology.* 1998;114(6):1125-1132.

54. Schubert ML, Edwards NF, Makhlouf GM. Regulation of gastric somatostatin secretion in the mouse by luminal acidity: a local feedback mechanism. *Gastroenterology.* 1988;94(2):317–322.
55. Steer HW. Mast cells of the human stomach. *J Anat.* 1976;121(pt 2):385–397.
56. Graham DY, Opekun AR, Osato MS, et al. Challenge model for Helicobacter pylori infection in human volunteers. *Gut.* 2004;53(9):1235–1243.
57. Lehnert T, Erlandson RA, Decosse JJ. Lymph and blood capillaries of the human gastric mucosa. A morphologic basis for metastasis in early gastric carcinoma. *Gastroenterology.* 1985;89(5):939–950.
58. Harberson J, Thomas RM, Harbison SP, et al. Gastric neuromuscular pathology in gastroparesis: analysis of full-thickness antral biopsies. *Dig Dis Sci.* 2010;55(2):359–370.
59. Kimura K. Chronological transition of the fundic-pyloric border determined by stepwise biopsy of the lesser and greater curvatures of the stomach. *Gastroenterology.* 1972;63(4):584–592.
60. Salenius P. On the ontogenesis of the human gastric epithelial cells. A histologic and histochemical study. *Acta Anat Suppl (Basel).* 1962;50(46):1–76.
61. Berant M, Aviad I, Jacobs J. Heterotopic duodenal mucosa in the stomach. *Am J Dis Child.* 1965;110(5):566–569.
62. Simstein NL. Congenital gastric anomalies. *Am Surg.* 1986;52(5):264–268.
63. Shim WK, Campbell A, Wright SW. 276 cases of pyloric stenosis in Hawaii. II. Racial aspects. *Hawaii Med J.* 1970;29(4):292–295.
64. Friesen SR, Pearse AG. Pathogenesis of congenital pyloric stenosis: histochemical analyses of pyloric ganglion cells. *Surgery.* 1963;53:604–608.
65. Grant GA, McAleer JA. Increasing incidence of infantile hypertrophic pyloric stenosis, 1971–1983. *Ir Med J.* 1986;79(5):118–119.
66. Leahy PF, Farrell R, O'Donnell B. 300 infants with hypertrophic pyloric stenosis: presentation and outcome. *Ir Med J.* 1986;79(5):114–116.
67. Wellmann KF, Kagan A, Fang H. Hypertrophic Pyloric Stenosis in Adults. Survey of the Literature and Report of a Case of the Localized Form (Torus Hyperplasia). *Gastroenterology.* 1964;46:601–608.
68. Dolan RV, ReMine WH, Dockerty MB. The fate of heterotopic pancreatic tissue. A study of 212 cases. *Arch Surg.* 1974;109(6):762–765.
69. Rose C, Kessaram RA, Lind JF. Ectopic gastric pancreas: a review and report of 4 cases. *Diagn Imaging.* 1980;49(4):214–218.
70. Guttman FM, Braun P, Garance PH, et al. Multiple atresias and a new syndrome of hereditary multiple atresias involving the gastrointestinal tract from stomach to rectum. *J Pediatr Surg.* 1973;8(5):633–640.
71. Bar-Maor JA, Nissan S, Nevo S. Pyloric atresia. A hereditary congenital anomaly with autosomal recessive transmission. *J Med Genet.* 1972;9(1):70–72.
72. Clements JL Jr, Jinkins JR, Torres WE, et al. Antral mucosal diaphragms in adults. *Am J Roentgenol.* 1979;133(6):1105–1111.
73. Feliciano DV, van Heerden JA. Pyloric antral mucosal webs. *Mayo Clin Proc.* 1977;52(10):650–653.
74. Shackelford GD, McAlister WH, Brodeur AE, et al. Congenital microgastria. *Am J Roentgenol Radium Ther Nucl Med.* 1973;118(1):72–76.
75. Kessler H, Smulewicz JJ. Microgastria associated with agenesis of the spleen. *Radiology.* 1973;107(2):393–396.
76. Chen YM, Teague RS, Ott DJ, et al. Gastric duplication cyst simulating leiomyoma. *Gastrointest Endosc.* 1987;33(3):250–252.
77. Bidwell JK, Nelson A. Prenatal ultrasonic diagnosis of congenital duplication of the stomach. *J Ultrasound Med.* 1986;5(10):589–591.
78. Tihansky DP, Sukarochana K, Hanrahan JB. Pyloroduodenal duplication cyst. *Am J Gastroenterol.* 1986;81(3):189–191.
79. Abrami G, Dennison WM. Duplication of the stomach. *Surgery.* 1961;49:794–801.
80. Wieczorek RL, Seidman I, Ranson JH, et al. Congenital duplication of the stomach: case report and review of the English literature. *Am J Gastroenterol.* 1984;79(8):597–602.
81. Meeroff M, Gollan JR, Meeroff JC. Gastric diverticulum. *Am J Gastroenterol.* 1967;47(3):189–203.
82. Mc LN, Purves JK, Saunders RL. The genesis of gastric and certain intestinal diverticula and enterogenous cysts. *Surg Gynecol Obstet.* 1954;92(2):135–141.
83. Hewlett PM. Isolated dextrogastria. *Br J Radiol.* 1982;55(657):678–681.
84. Shaw A, Blanc WA, Santulli TV, et al. Spontaneous rupture of the stomach in the newborn: a clinical and experimental study. *Surgery.* 1965;58:561–571.
85. Bayatpour M, Bernard L, McCune F, et al. Spontaneous gastric rupture in the newborn. *Am J Surg.* 1979;137(2):267–269.
86. Patel NM. Chronic gastric volvulus: report of a case and review of literature. *Am J Gastroenterol.* 1985;80(3):170–173.
87. Idowu J, Aitken DR, Georgeson KE. Gastric volvulus in the newborn. *Arch Surg.* 1980;115(9):1046–1049.

# 13 Stomach and Proximal Duodenum: Inflammatory and Miscellaneous Disorders

Chapter Outline

CLASSIFICATION OF GASTRITIS AND GASTROPATHY
  Current Classification of Gastritis
GASTRITIS
  Distinctive (Specific) Types of Gastropathies
  Reactive (Predominant Epithelial) Changes
    Reactive gastropathy
    Toxic gastropathy
  Reactive Changes with Erosions in Helicobacter—One or Two Diseases?
  Distinction of Reactive Changes from Dysplasia
    Reactive changes in intestinal metaplasia
    Alcoholic gastropathy
    Caustic-induced injury
    Graft versus host disease
    Chemotherapy and radiation
    Ischemia
  Predominantly Vascular Changes
    Gastric antral vascular ectasia
    Portal hypertension (congestive gastropathy)
    Hemorrhagic gastropathy ("gastritis") and "Curling's ulcer"
  Distinctive (Specific) Types of Gastritis
    Infections
    A H. pylori infection
    Histology of H. pylori–associated gastritis
    H. pylori diagnosis
    Noninvasive methods
    Invasive methods
    Atrophic gastritis and gastric atrophy
    Staging gastric atrophy
    Disorders associated with H. pylori gastritis
    Gastroduodenal erosions and ulcers ("peptic ulcers")
    Pathogenetic factors
    Epidemiology
    Atypical clinical presentations
    Endoscopic appearance of peptic erosions and ulcers
"PEPTIC DISEASES" OF THE DUODENAL BULB AND THE PROXIMAL DUODENUM
  Pathogenesis and Clinical Features of Duodenitis
    Duodenal ulcer
    Clinical features
  Pathology of Duodenitis and Duodenal Erosions and Ulcer
    Gross pathology
    Histology
    Differential diagnosis of duodenitis
    Healing and healed ulcers
    Complications of gastroduodenal ulcers
  Treatment
    The role of the pathologist and clinical implications
  Autoimmune Gastritis
    Pathogenesis
    Subtypes of autoimmune gastritis (AIG) and their etiology
    Clinical features
    Pathology
LYMPHOCYTIC GASTRITIS
  Morphologic Separation of Etiologies
GRANULOMATOUS GASTRITIS
CARDITIS
NON–H. PYLORI BACTERIAL INFECTIONS
  Non–H. pylori Helicobacter Species (NHPH)/"Helicobacter heilmannii"
    Gastric disease associated with non–H. pylori Helicobacter species/"Helicobacter heilmannii"
    Diagnosis
  Tuberculosis
  Syphilis
  Enterococcal Gastritis
  Phlegmonous and Emphysematous Gastritis
VIRAL INFECTIONS
  Cytomegalovirus Infection (HHV-5)
  Herpes Viruses (HHV-1,2)
  Epstein–Barr Virus (EBV—HHV-4)
  Other HHV Viruses
  Other Viruses
FUNGAL INFECTIONS
  Candida albicans
  Histoplasmosis
  Mucormycosis (Zygomycosis)
  Aspergillosis
PARASITES AND NEMATODES
  Cryptosporidium
  Anisakiasis
  Other Parasites and Nematodes
OTHER GASTRITIDES
  Clinical features
  Endoscopic features
  Histologic features
  Eosinophilic Gastritis
    Eosinophilic gastritis as part of gastric involvement in eosinophilic gastroenteritis
    Differential diagnosis
  Collagenous Gastritis
    Diffuse collagenous gastroenterocolitis
  Gastric Malakoplakia
  Drug- and Chemotherapy-induced Gastritis
HYPERTROPHIC GASTROPATHIES AND MÉNÉTRIER'S DISEASE
  Primary/Idiopathic Ménétrier's Disease
  Clinical Presentation
  Pathology of Primary Ménétrier's Disease
  Carcinoma Complicating Ménétrier's Disease
  Secondary Ménétrier's Disease
HYPERTROPHIC GASTROPATHY-ASSOCIATED WITH PROTEIN LOSS
  Cytomegalovirus-associated Hypertrophic Gastropathy
  Hypertrophic Lymphocytic Gastritis
  Helicobacter pylori–associated Hypertrophic Gastritis
  HIV-associated Hypertrophic Gastritis
  Large Gastric Folds Associated with Other Conditions
  Other Types of Large Gastric Folds
DISTINCTIVE ENDOSCOPIC ENTITIES
MISCELLANEOUS DISORDERS OF THE STOMACH
  Gastric Calcinosis
  Gastric Glandular Siderosis
  Approach to the Interpretation of Gastric Biopsies
    Surface epithelium
HISTOLOGY

CLASSIFICATION OF GASTRITIS AND GASTROPATHY

Though no classification of gastritis satisfies everyone, the overall goal of any classification is to help clear thinking and be clinically useful. Inevitably much of the early thinking regarding gastritis was centered on "peptic ulcer disease" (PUD). Ignorance regarding the role of both *Helicobacter* and medications gave rise to theories that were to some extent flawed, yet they still dominate traditional teaching. Gastritis was considered physiologic and intestinal metaplasia an aging phenomenon. We also need to recall that

1. Gastritis originally meant "redness"—which now is usually associated with a gastropathy rather than gastritis; conversely, most histologic gastritis has a normal endoscopic appearance.
2. Many disorders that are characterized by abnormal endoscopy also have a typical biopsy appearance. From a classification viewpoint are these best considered from an endoscopic or histologic viewpoint? Most classifications can only be viewed from one vantage point.
3. From a clinical viewpoint, "ulcers" have played a major role in gastric disease because of the symptoms with which they or their complications are associated (pain, bleeding, perforation, and obstruction/stenosis). However, the term "peptic ulcer disease" has been in common parlance for decades, with the implication that this is associated with acid, the "proof" being that symptoms are markedly ameliorated with therapy, whether antacids, H2-receptor antagonists, or proton pump inhibitors (PPIs). In the early 1980s, it was ultimately shown that some ulcer disease, especially in the duodenum, was related to *Helicobacter pylori*, so that its eradication virtually guaranteed that duodenal ulcer, the archetypal peptic ulcer, would not recur. Thus PUD changed from being primarily acid related to primarily bacterial, or a combination of both.
4. Nonsteroidal anti-inflammatory drugs (NSAIDs), aspirin (acetylsalicylic acid—ASA), and other medications now play a huge role in gastric pathology. While the introduction of NSAIDs around 1970 was a major step forward therapeutically, it came at a price that included numerous gastrointestinal (GI) side effects. Prior to this time, ASA had been "the" analgesic and antipyretic of choice. Bayer introduced ASA in the market around 1900, and within a decade or two this "wonderdrug" was present in virtually every household in the more developed countries, and used widely for numerous ailments—colds, coughs, headaches, migraines, and all arthritides. Yet the erosive, ulcerative, and bleeding diathesis associated with this drug was not widely appreciated. In retrospect, from about 1900 on, many "peptic ulcers" may well have been as much ASA associated as *Helicobacter* associated, and this association even creeps, almost inadvertently, into case reports back in the 1950s.[1] So while we typically think of "peptic ulcer disease" historically as unrecognized *Helicobacter* infection, ASA was very likely a major contributor. This continued until acetaminophen/paracetamol/Tylenol came into the market in to the 1960s. Further, it is now well recognized that, especially in the very young[2,3] and elderly,[4] not only that NSAIDs are likely "the" culprit irrespective of the presence of *H. pylori*, but that the risk of complications such as bleeding (and therefore the erosions and ulcers that bleed) can be largely prevented using PPIs. Thus, historically, the disease we consider to be "peptic ulcer disease" may have been as much NSAID/ASA associated as *Helicobacter* associated, especially in the presence of abundant acid.
5. Historically, alcohol, which not only has a social role in many societies but is also an analgesic in large doses, has been around much longer than any other gastric damaging agent except for *Helicobacter*, and produces histologic changes similar to NSAIDs (i.e., a chemical/reactive gastropathy). From around 1900 on when aspirin became available, the big three, became *Helicobacter*, alcohol, and ASA, and from 1970 on, NSAIDs was added to these.
6. The notion of "peptic ulcer disease" and "no acid—no ulcer" is therefore likely true in that in the major causes of gastroduodenal erosions and ulcers, namely, *Helicobacter* and NSAIDs/ASA, and other medications or chemicals, especially alcohol, the presence of acid facilitated the development of injury caused by these agents. Although the nature of the interaction of these common causes of peptic ulcer is still unclear, it would make most sense if, when antral-predominant *H. pylori* is present, that the risk of NSAID/ASA and alcohol-induced damage was increased, but that when the organism spread proximally, resulting in a decrease in acid output, that there may well be a degree of protection from NSAID/ASA, and possibly alcohol associated damage (Table 13-1).

Current Classification of Gastritis

Until the early 1970s, chronic gastritis was classified into three main varieties (superficial, atrophic, and hypertrophic) as suggested by Schindler in 1939[5] (Table 13-2). Wood as well as Schindler later concluded that chronic hypertrophic gastritis is a variation of normal mucosal function.[6,7] Thus, chronic gastritis was classified as superficial or atrophic.

Whitehead's classification was the first to understand the importance of noting location, and grading

Table 13-1	ABC Classification of Gastritis
Autoimmune	Pernicious anemia
Bacterial	Bugs including post-Rx effects: *Helicobacter pylori*
	Enterococcus
	Syphilis
Chemical	Bile reflux
Drug-associated/ Iatrogenic	NSAIDs/ASA
	Anti-platelet medications
	Chemotherapy/GVHD
	Iron
	Alcohol
Eosinophilic	Eosinophilic gastritis/ gastroenteritis
	Food allergies, medications
Focal	Crohn's disease
Granulomatous	Tuberculosis
	Sarcoid
	Crohn's disease
	Foreign body
	Helicobacter pylori
Hypertrophic (big folds)	"Ménétrier's disease"
	Lymphocytic gastritis
	Eosinophilic gastritis
	Gastric varices
	Gastritis cystica profunda
	Lymphoma (MALT)
	Gastric adenocarcinoma
	Helicobacter pylori gastritis (lymphocytic), CMV
	Zollinger–Ellison syndrome
	Multiple polyps/polyposis
Idiopathic	
Juvenile (pediatric)	Follicular with *H. pylori*, CMV
Lymphocytic	*Helicobacter pylori*, celiac disease
	Chronic erosive (varioliform) gastritis
Multifocal intestinal metaplasia with/ without atrophic front	In atrophic gastritis, isolated

Modified from Wyatt JI, Dixon MF. Chronic gastritis—a pathogenetic approach. *J Pathol.* 1988;154(2):113–124.

With the rediscovery of *H. pylori* (originally *Campylobacter pylori*) by Warren and Marshall in the early 1980s,[9] it became clear that *H. pylori* is a principal component of most gastritides. In 1988, two classification systems emerged. That by Wyatt and Dixon incorporated reactive gastropathy (then called chemical gastritis/gastropathy) as the "C" of the ABC classification system, A being autoimmune and B being bacterial (=*Helicobacter* but, at that time, *C. pylori*).[10] The same year, Correa proposed classifying gastritis based on clinical and etiopathogenetic information. He classified chronic gastritis into superficial gastritis, diffuse antral gastritis (DAG), usually *Helicobacter* associated and related to duodenal ulcer disease, diffuse corporal atrophic gastritis (autoimmune), and multifocal atrophic gastritis (MAG—considered to be "environmental"). MAG was related to intestinal-type adenocarcinoma and gastric ulcer, and intestinal metaplasia in the antrum and body.[11] Diffuse corporal atrophic gastritis was often related to AIG and pernicious anemia, with inflammation and atrophy in the corpus and relative sparing of the antrum[11,12] (Fig. 13-1).

The *Sydney system is the basis of most contemporary classifications of gastritis.* Proposed by a group of European pathologists and clinicians (World Congress of Gastroenterology, Sydney, August 1990),[12] it recommended incorporating the topography of gastric mucosal changes with the immunology and microbiology of the disease. The classification depends on separate assessment of the antrum and corpus by taking a minimum of two biopsies from the *anterior* and *posterior* walls of the respective gastric compartments as well as any specific lesions identified. An important feature is a standard three-tier grade of mild, moderate, and severe applicable to a selected number of morphologic variables. As a broad guideline, each successive grade represents an increment in severity of about one-third. Graded variables included inflammation (acute and chronic), atrophy, metaplasia, and density of *H. pylori*. The Sydney system also expanded previous classifications by adding a variety of other "special forms" of gastritides (collagenous, eosinophilic, granulomatous, lymphocytic, etc.).

The *Sydney classification* was updated in 1994,[13] which expanded the section on specific entities (special forms) and includes a 4-point visual analog (equivalent to none, mild, moderate, and severe) to aid with morphologic grading of inflammation and atrophy.[13] Gastric atrophy is loss of normal glands, often with replacement by an epithelium that could be either native or metaplastic (Table 13-3). The score is an average from each region's biopsies. Antral atrophy was the average score for atrophy from all antral biopsies and corpus atrophy (the average score for atrophy from all corpus biopsies).[13] The updated Sydney classification depends on the separate assessment of the

the depth and degree of inflammation and the presence or absence of both intestinal and pseudopyloric metaplasia, separating them from atrophic changes[8] (Table 13-2). This really formed the basis of all subsequent morphologic classifications of gastritis. In 1973, Strickland and Mackay classified gastritis based on detecting parietal cell (PC) antibodies, clarifying the etiology of autoimmune gastritis (AIG) (type A) despite the fact that these can develop in *Helicobacter* infected patients. It is associated with atrophic changes in body and fundic (oxyntic) mucosa. Antral predominant gastritis was type B. Glass and Pitchumon added type AB into Strickland–Mackay classification to encompass cases that did not fit type A or type B, essentially pangastritis.

Table 13-2 Gastritis Classification "Historical Prospective"

YEAR, AUTHOR	CLASSIFICATION		
1942, Schindler		*Gastritis* Superficial Atrophic Hypertrophic (later dropped as Schindler and others concluded hypertrophy is normal function variation)	
1972, Whitehead et al.[8]	*Mucosa type* Pyloric Body Cardiac Transitional Indeterminate	*Gastritis grade* Superficial Quiescent Active Atrophic (used synonymous with deep inflammation). Mild (quiescent or active) Moderate (quiescent or active) Severe (quiescent or active)	*Metaplasia* Pseudopyloric Intestinal
1973, Strickland and Mackay[828]	Type A or autoimmune gastric atrophy of pernicious anemia Type B—nonautoimmune (pyloro-cardial extension type in connection with PUD (Kimura, 1972)[181]		
1976, Glass and Pitchumoni modification of Strickland and Mackay[829]	Type A (autoimmune) Type B (antrum) Type AB (cases that did not fit Type A or Type B)		

1988, Correa[11]	*Morphologic*
	Not atrophic
	  Superficial
	  Diffuse antral (DAG)
	
	Atrophic
	  Postgastrectomy
	  Diffuse corporal
	  Multifocal
		Mechanistic
		
		Initial stage of other types?
		Hypersecretory?
		Psychosomatic?
		Infectious? (*C. pylori*)
		
		Reflux
		Autoimmune
		Dietary?
			Synonyms
			
			Simple?
			Antral
			Type B
			
			Chemical
			Type A
			Environmental
			Type B
			Type AB
			Pangastritis

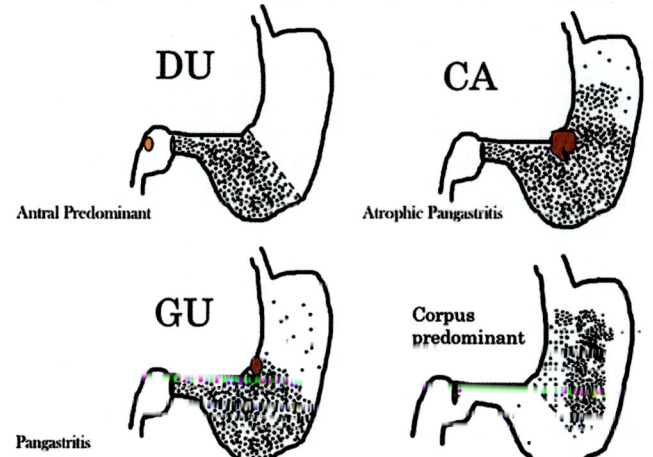

Figure 13-1. Prototypes of gastritis pattern predict disease outcome. In practice, all tend to have some degree of both antral and corpus inflammation. **Top left:** Duodenal ulcer (DU) patients have antral predominant inflammation with little corpus inflammation. **Bottom left:** Pangastritis is seen in gastric ulcer (GU) patients. Corpus mucosa is inflamed and often extends into the specialized mucosa but still tends to be antral predominant. **Top right:** Pangastritis with atrophy is seen in patients with the intestinal type of gastric adenocarcinoma (CA). **Bottom right:** Corpus-predominant gastritis is usually seen in AIG or end-stage *Helicobacter* infection.

antrum and corpus. It needs a minimum of two biopsies from the *lesser* and *greater* curvature of the respective gastric compartments as well as the incisura and any specific lesions identified (Fig. 13-2).[13] On all occasions accurate grading depends on correctly oriented full-thickness mucosal biopsies. In practice, other than for academic studies, grading is rarely required.

GASTRITIS

Gastritis (in its broadest sense) and its complications account for millions of doctors' office visits each year. Symptoms are often associated with acute changes or complications described as mild upper abdominal discomfort, indigestion, heartburn, coated tongue, foul breath, and bad taste to more ominous symptoms such as loss of appetite, nausea, vomiting blood or coffee-ground material, diarrhea, and dark stools. Most patients with chronic gastritis have no symptoms. Even so, these symptoms are not specific and include broad differentials such as *H. pylori* infection, other infections, bile reflux, inflammatory

Table 13-3 Gastritis Classification "Sydney System"

	GASTRITIS TYPE	ETIOLOGY	SYNONYMS
1996, Updated Sydney[13]	Non-atrophic	*Helicobacter pylori* ? Other factors	Superficial Diffuse antral, Chronic atrophic Interstitial—follicular Hypersecretory Type B
	Atrophic		
	Autoimmune	Autoimmunity	Type A Diffuse corporal Pernicious-anaemia associated
	Multifocal	*Helicobacter pylori* Dietary ? Environmental	Type B Type AB Environmental
	Special forms		Metaplastic

	Chemical	Chemical irritation:
		  Bile
		  NSAIDs/Antiplatelet
		  Other medications
			
			Reactive, Reflux
			NSAID
			Type C

	Radiation	Radiation injury	
	Lymphocytic	Idiopathic? Immune mechanism Gluten Drug (ticlopidine)	Varioliform (endoscopic) Celiac disease–associated
	Noninfectious granulomatous	? *H. pylori* Crohn's disease Sarcoidosis Wegener's granulomatosis and other vasculitides Idiopathic	Isolated granulomatous
	Eosinophilic	Food sensitivity, drugs, Churg-Straus	Allergic
	Other infectious gastritis	Bacteria (other than *H. pylori*) Viruses Fungi Parasites	Phlegmonous

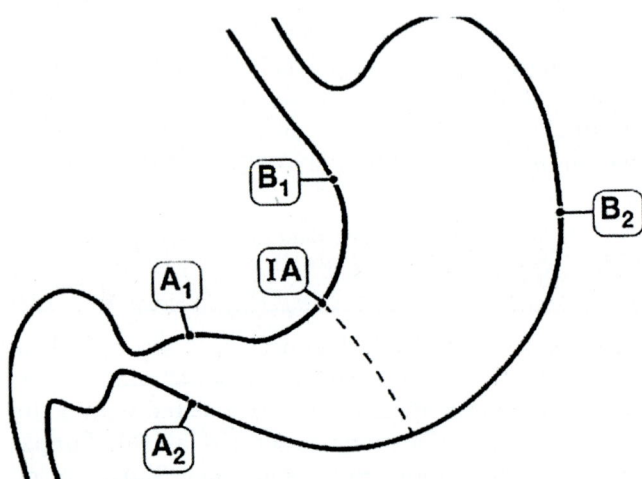

Figure 13-2. The updated Sydney biopsy protocol requires a minimum of two biopsies from the *lesser* and *greater* curvature of the respective gastric compartments as well as the incisura and any specific lesions identified. This identifies all of the patterns of gastritis illustrated in Figure 13-1, as well as estimating the extent of atrophy present, which often starts at the incisura/angulus (IA), affects the antrum (A_1, A_2), and then extends proximally to the oxyntic zone (B_1, B_2), so that, as antral inflammation extends proximally, biopsy site B_1 is first affected, and B_2 is the last site affected.

bowel disease (IBD), and side effects of medications (Table 13-4). As treatment depends on the cause, it is important to know the cause for appropriate management. Occasionally, it may be necessary to list possible etiologies for gastric inflammation, rather that reporting "nonspecific chronic inflammation"—which is an unnecessarily complex term as all inflammation is "nonspecific," so these words can always be omitted from reports without deleterious effect. If it is specific, the cause (e.g., *Helicobacter*) should be stated.

Distinctive (Specific) Types of Gastropathies

Gastropathies are biopsies in which epithelial (noninflammatory) changes predominate. The mucosa is often mucin depleted, causing it to appear red endoscopically (invariably interpreted by endoscopists as "gastritis" rather than areas of redness). They include biopsies with primary epithelial reactive changes (such as chemical/reflux (bile) gastropathy, chemotherapy effect) and a smaller subset of biopsies with predominant vascular pathology (such as gastric antral

Table 13-4 Classification by Predominant Histologic Change

CATEGORY	SUBCATEGORY	
Gastropathy (predominantly noninflammatory)	Predominant epithelial changes	(a) Medications/reflux (bile) gastropathy (b) Alcoholic gastropathy (c) Caustic-induced injury (d) GVHD (e) Radiation/chemotherapy (f) Ischemia
	Predominant vascular pathology	(a) GAVE (b) Portal hypertension (c) Hemorrhagic/shock gastropathy

Gastritis (predominant inflammatory)	Infectious	1. Bacterial
		  (a) *Helicobacter pylori* bacterial infection (autoimmune gastritis, lymphocytic gastritis, granulomatous gastritis, carditis)
		  (b) NHPH infections—"*H. heilmanii*"
		  Other bacteria—TB, syphilis, phlegmonous and emphysematous gastritis
		2. Viral (CMV, Herpes)
		3. Fungal (*Candida*, histoplasma, mucormycosis, Aspergillosis)
		4. Parasitic (*Cryptosporidium*, Anisadikosis, other parasites, and nematodes)

	Noninfectious	1. IBD (endoscopic, histologic features, clinical implication) 2. Eosinophilic gastroenteritis
	Part of systemic involvement	1. GVHD 2. Vasculitis (including Churg–Strauss)

Endoscopic gastropathies	Distinctive macroscopic (endoscopic) appearance with appropriate histology	1. Erosive and hemorrhagic
		  Varioliform gastritis
		  Watermelon stomach (GAVE)
		  Portal gastropathy
		  Hemorrhagic gastritis/gastropathy
		2. Nonerosive
		  Nodular gastritis, children
		  Atrophic front, adults
		3. Distinctive hypertrophic gastropathy

vascular ectasia [GAVE], portal hypertension gastropathy, Dieulafoy, and hemorrhagic/shock) (Table 13-4). Graft versus host disease (GVHD) is usually normal endoscopically.

Reactive (Predominant Epithelial) Changes

Reactive (chemical/reflux-associated) gastropathy is a reaction to noninfectious irritants. This can be due to protracted exposure to bile and pancreatic juice (especially postgastric surgery[14]). The most infamous of irritants are NSAIDs, which include over-the-counter drugs such as aspirin and ibuprofen, and many prescription medicines. Other medications—such as bisphosphonates used for osteopenia, iron pills and irritants in food such as capsaicin in peppers and chilies and alcohol—can all cause this lesion.[15] These irritants usually cause no clinical problems when taken for the short term, although endoscopic damage can be seen even with short-term use. However, regular (or excessive) use can lead to a more severe gastropathy as well as erosions and ulcers. With the increasing use of aspirin and other NSAIDs, and decreasing prevalence of *Helicobacter*, chemical/reactive gastropathy is increasingly seen in gastric biopsies, and may co-exist. Anti-platelet mediations also cause similar injury.

Pathogenesis: Aspirin is the best-studied NSAID, the mechanism of injury is inhibition of prostaglandin synthesis by inhibiting cyclooxygenase (COX) 1 and 2.[16] Aspirin also changes the ability of the mucosa to maintain a pH gradient causing gastric acid back-diffusion with resultant mucosal injury.[16] Further, its anticoagulant properties increase the risk of bleeding once erosions or ulcers are present. Conversely, some other NSAIDs have antiplatelet properties but do not possess this therapeutic anticoagulant effect. NSAIDs produce mucosal injury by both local and systemic effects.[16] Newer NSAIDs are predominantly COX-2 inhibitors, which make them less likely to cause gastric injury and the risk of gastric (or duodenal) injury is reduced, but not abolished. A variety of antiplatelet medications are increasingly being implicated causing similar injury.

Histology: The histology of reactive gastropathies has both an acute and a chronic phase, although in practice it is often reported without qualifying it as acute or chronic. In some patients both are present together.

Reactive gastropathy. The morphologic changes that accompany ingestion of medications such as NSAIDs have been known for decades,15 but they are now more commonly recognized.

In the acute phase, as in any reparative process, the main changes are

1. Mucin depletion—the amount of supranuclear mucin is markedly reduced or absent, so that at low power the cells appear more basophilic—often the most apparent low-power indication that this change is present
2. A reduction of the normal cell size so that the cells are frequently low columnar to cuboidal
3. A corresponding increase in nuclear size, and also an increase in hyperchromatism; nuclei that are normally compressed at the cell base markedly increase in size, and in conjunction with the smaller cell size cause a marked increase in nuclear–cytoplasmic ratio.
4. Because this appears to be a reparative, partly restitutional process, the number of cells and nuclei appears reduced; this results in nuclei being distinct and separated, one of the best indicators that this is not dysplasia. However, especially following erosions, the reactive changes can be more marked so that the nuclei become more open and vesicular with distinct nucleoli, and there may also be concomitant increase in nuclear hyperchromatism (Fig. 13-3).
5. Changes are usually most marked in the mucous neck region, and tend to decrease superficially. Interestingly, some of these changes appear on the surface, especially the mucin depletion, but most of the other changes are maximal in the mucous neck region suggesting that these are all a reaction to injury and not dysplasia. These changes can be easily missed in the fundic glands as the foveolae are shorter and changes can be mistaken for biopsy artifacts. Occasionally, the changes may extend deeper to involve the entire length of the oxyntic or antral glands (Fig. 13-3E).
6. Erosions or ulcers may be present. When this occurs, careful examination of the erosion or ulcer base should be carried out for the presence of crystals or foreign material representing medications. Iron encrustation can readily be confirmed using Perl's stain (Fig. 13-3). When erosions or ulcers occur, the immediately adjacent epithelium may be

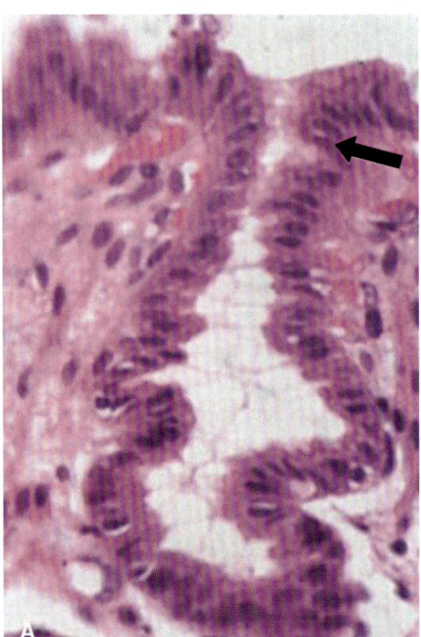
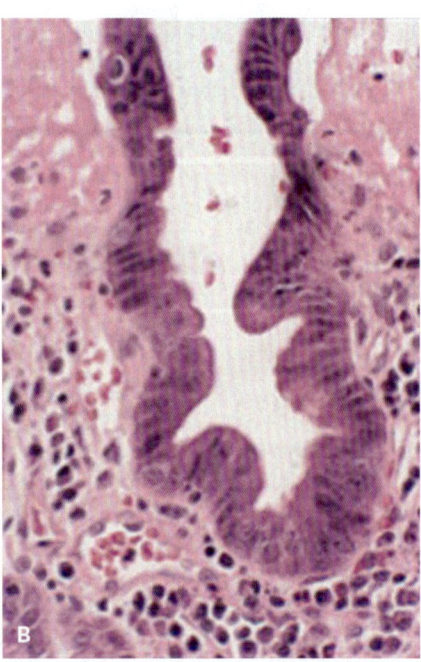
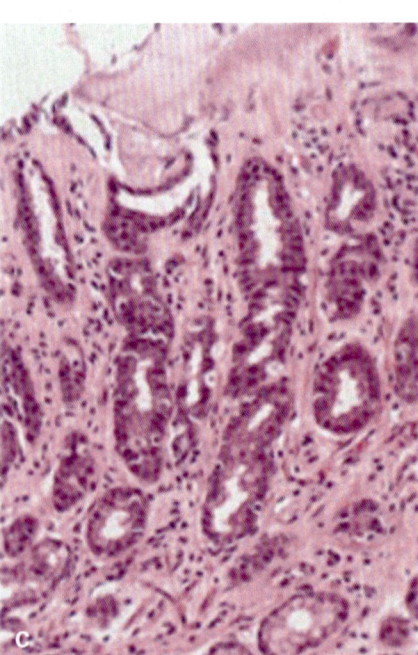

Figure 13-3. Reactive changes in gastric mucosa. **A:** Pit in which there is total mucin loss but nuclei are separated from each other. This is most marked superficially where the epithelial cells are more cuboidal and attenuated. Hints of mucin secretion are reappearing superficially (*arrow*) at the apex of the cell—an indication of maturation. Note the lack of any inflammation in the lamina propria in this biopsy. **B:** Similar features but there is more attenuation of epithelium superficially, and in the generative zone at the bottom nuclei are becoming stratified. The hyperchromatism associated with most dysplasias is absent. A modest chronic inflammatory infiltrate is present in the lamina propria but this disappears superficially. **C:** Chemical (NSAID) erosion. The attenuated epithelium is visible superficially with diffuse mucin depletion. Foveolar hyperplasia (corkscrewed pits) are visible, as is the normal architecture. At the surface the hyalinized zone is typical of NSAID damage. The lamina propria is largely empty indicating that this cannot be a *Helicobacter*-associated erosion.

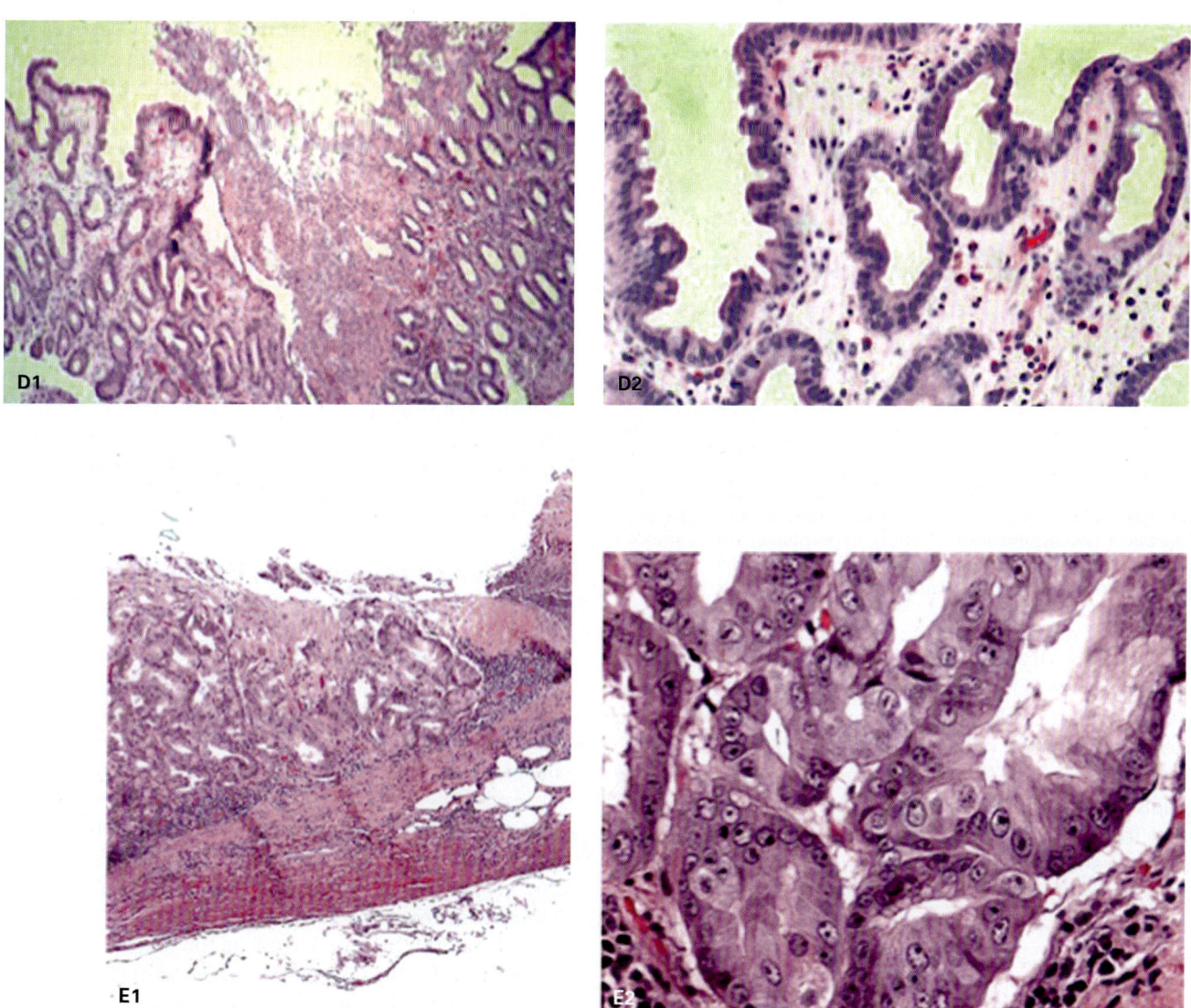

Figure 13-3. *(Continued)* **D: D1.** An erosion with almost a pseudomembranous appearance. **D2.** The adjacent mucosa has typical reactive changes and scattered eosinophils predominate. **E1:** Further NSAID erosion with the superficial hyalinized band that approaches the muscularis mucosae and **E2:** Very reactive nuclei, again most marked at the bases of the pits, nuclei remain separated but here have a prominent nucleolus. More superficially nuclei are even more widely separated indicating restitution. Note also that these nuclear changes do not correspond to intestinal, foveolar, or pyloric dysplasia.

restituting, and appears attenuated as seen in any restitutional processes.

7. Occasionally there is focal edema in the lamina propria, which may also be devoid of inflammatory cells or have a predominantly acute or eosinophilic (sometimes both) infiltrate. A sparse chronic inflammatory infiltrate can also be seen, but in most biopsies chronic inflammation is usually conspicuous by its absence or minimal presence (Fig. 13-3), indicating that *Helicobacter* infection is not the etiology of the changes present.

In the chronic phase, other changes become apparent. Sometimes the acute and chronic phases coexist, sometimes only the chronic changes persist, and it is presumed that they followed the acute changes (Fig. 13-4).

1. Foveolar hyperplasia can develop that results in tortuosity of pits in the mucous neck region.
2. Proliferation of smooth muscle in the lamina propria above that normally seen
3. A degree of vasodilatation of capillaries with congestion and edema.[17,18]
4. If erosions have occurred, a degree of lamina propria fibrosis ensues.

Iron toxicity, especially in children, may result in gastric mucosal necrosis, sometimes with extension into the submucosa.[19] The encrustation is often visible (Fig. 13-5).

Biopsies show reactive mucosal changes (mucin depletion, foveolar hyperplasia, and smooth muscle hyperplasia) without the severe inflammatory component seen in infectious gastritis (Fig. 13-5).

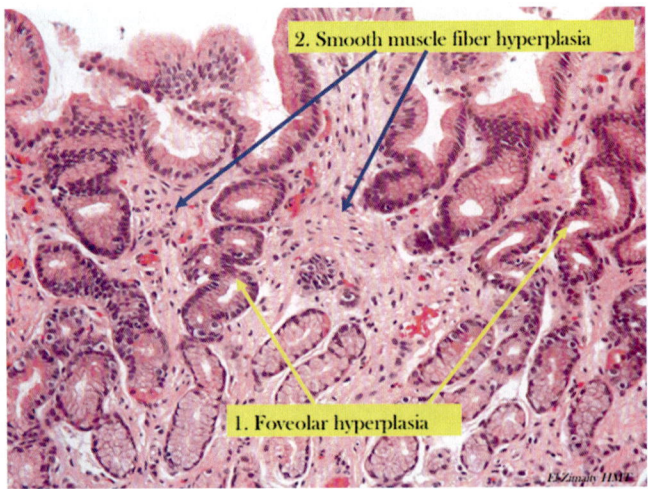

Figure 13-4. Chronic reactive gastropathy. The pits have foveolar hyperplasia, being elongated and have a corkscrew configuration (*yellow arrows*). There is hyperplasia of the smooth muscle fibers (*blue arrow*) that are normally found in the stomach. Note the lack of inflammation.

Foveolar hyperplasia appears to be a result of excessive cell exfoliation from the surface epithelium over a period of time and, accordingly, is likely to be seen in all types of active gastritis.[17] Further, if the insult is ongoing, superimposed changes of acute reactive gastropathy may also be present, and this may include erosions. These histopathologic changes are not seen in all patients and when present are usually patchy (postgastrectomy states usually being more diffuse and therefore the exception). Pathology is more likely to be seen in biopsies obtained from incisura angularis.[20] If biopsies are taken, then those from areas of endoscopic abnormality are preferred.

Gastric glands may be distorted and dilated, with an absence or paucity of plasma cells. In some areas there is no gland distortion, just simple thinning of the mucosa.[21] Other features include stomal erosions,[22] lipid islands, and intramucosal cysts[21] (Fig. 13-6). Sometimes the cysts become large enough to be visible grossly and extend into the submucosa. These cysts have been labeled with a variety of names, including *gastritis cystica polyposa* and *gastritis cystica* profunda.[23] Adenocarcinoma in the postoperative stomach has been reported in association with these cysts, but this association appears to be coincidental, especially because the cysts are so commonly found microscopically in the postoperative stomach.[21,24]

Toxic gastropathy. Changes can be seen characterized by vacuolated cells in the specialized mucosa. The cause is not always apparent but may be prominent in uremic patients, the vacuolation tending to occur in chief cells rather than PCs (Fig. 13-7).

Reactive Changes with Erosions in *Helicobacter*—One or Two Diseases?

It should be appreciated that while "reactive gastropathy" is usually applied to changes with minimal chronic inflammation, identical epithelial and lamina propria changes can be seen in other etiologies such as *Helicobacter* infections, especially if acute inflammation is present. However, in the presence of *Helicobacter* gastritis with relatively little acute inflammation, erosions are almost certainly not related to the underlying infection, and the possibility that the patient has medication-related erosions or ulcers superimposed on *Helicobacter* gastritis should be considered as the distinction can be made in many instances.[25] *Helicobacter*-type associated erosions invariably occur on a background of severe chronic active gastritis, so if this is not present they should always be viewed with suspicion, and a second etiology considered. Further, the nature of the erosion (see Fig. 13-3) can distinguish the two on biopsy, with a dense hyalinized band in the superficial mucosa being indicative of NSAID type-associated injury.[26] Indeed, in patients with both diseases it is likely that a medication caused the damage.[25,26]

Caveat: Severe (disproportionate) reactive changes resembling those seen in, for example, NSAID gastropathy in patients with only a modest chronic *Helicobacter* gastritis may well be related to medications rather than the concurrent *Helicobacter* infection. This is discussed subsequently.

Distinction of Reactive Changes from Dysplasia

It is imperative to distinguish reactive changes from dysplasia as they resolve when the acute insult is withdrawn. The most helpful feature is that at the surface there is invariably maturation in the form of

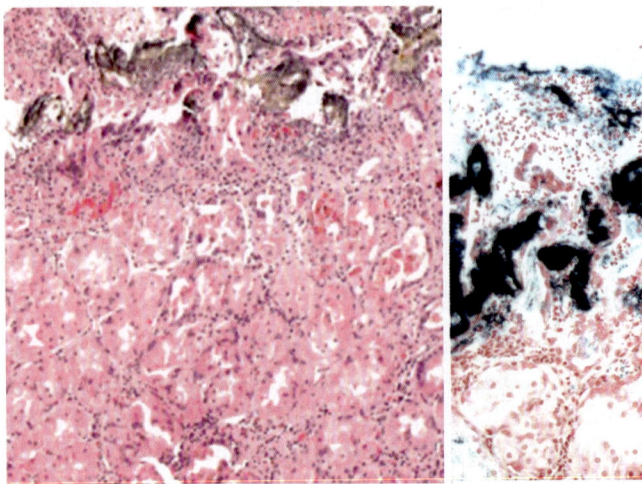

Figure 13-5. Reactive gastropathy. Iron medication may result in gastric mucosal necrosis (H&E stain) with iron encrustation (Perl's stain—**right**)

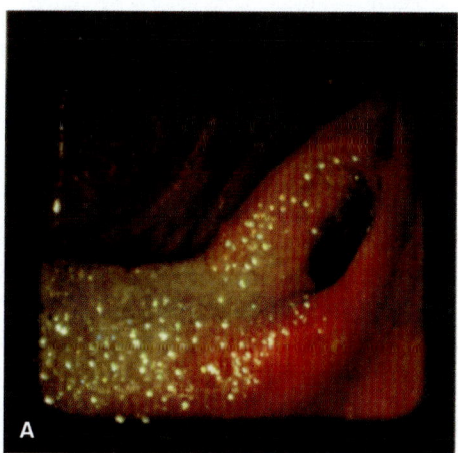
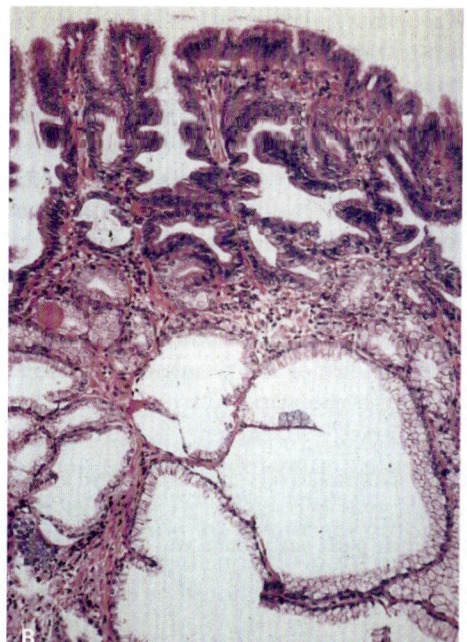
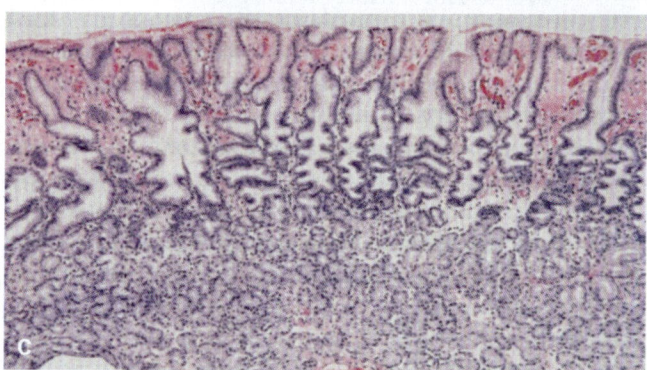
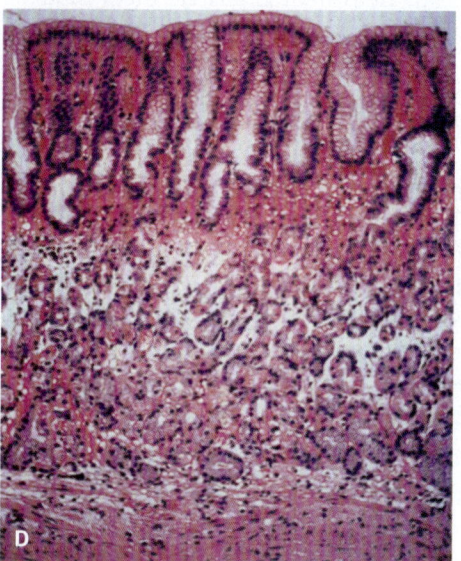

Figure 13-6. The postoperative stomach. **A:** Endoscopic view of a Billroth II stoma, which is typically red. Bile-stained fluid is refluxing into the gastric remnant. **B:** Biopsy specimen from the stoma of a Billroth II anastomosis. There is marked foveolar hyperplasia (corkscrew pattern), with minimal or no increase in the number of inflammatory cells. The epithelium in the surface and pits is dark and mucin depleted. Large intramucosal cysts are present. **C:** Fundic gland mucosa from the gastric body after Billroth II anastomosis. There is mild interfoveolar edema and marked foveolar hyperplasia with the corkscrew pattern, but an intact gland zone without increased numbers of inflammatory cells. **D:** Biopsy specimen from the greater curvature of the midbody region after Billroth II anastomosis. Many biopsy specimens in such patients simply show a thin fundic gland mucosa with a shallow epithelial gland zone, especially when the antrum has been removed as the gastrin drive for growth is lost. This specimen also shows subepithelial hemorrhage and edema in the interface between the pits and glands. It is not possible to exclude endoscope trauma as the cause of this finding.

small mucin droplets at the surface. While "bottom-up" dysplasia (dysplasia maximal in the pit bases) does occur, it is quite rare, so the diagnosis of dysplasia should only be made if the diagnosis is absolutely clear, and ideally conforms to one of the usual forms of foveolar dysplasia (see following chapter). The adage that dysplasia should never be diagnosed in the presence of overlying or adjacent ulcers, erosions, or restituting epithelium unless absolutely clear is a good one. Making a diagnosis of dysplasia under these circumstances is fraught with danger. Unless there is absolutely no diagnostic uncertainty, it is usually best to rebiopsy the area following antisecretory therapy (e.g., PPIs) to ensure that the changes persist when the erosions have healed. Fortunately, even if dysplasia is diagnosed and graded, most can be visualized and treated endoscopically (Fig. 13-8).

Reactive gastropathy may be confused with dysplasia and may be one reason why some have reported large numbers of cases of dysplasia in the postoperative stomach.[21] We suspect that the vast majority of these changes represent "regenerative atypia" rather than dysplasia. Highly reactive cytologic changes are seen in other conditions, such as in the mucosa

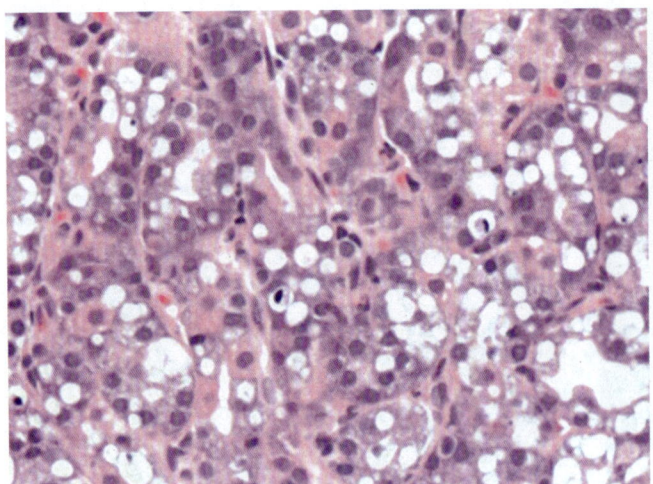

Figure 13-7. Vacuolated cells that are prominent in toxic states, in this patient the association was uremia.

adjacent to alcohol- and NSAID-induced erosions[27] in some patients without erosions on NSAIDs[17] and in the mucosa at or near-healed gastric ulcer sites. Though, at times, it can be challenging, atypical reparative changes can be distinguished from dysplasia (intraepithelial neoplasia or dysplasia) as discussed in the previous section.

Reactive changes in intestinal metaplasia. It should also be recognized that gastric intestinal metaplasia, whether incomplete (residual foveolar epithelium admixed with goblet cells) or complete (goblet and absorptive cells with or without Paneth cells), can be subject to surface injury and reactive changes. However, the same principles apply regarding using surface maturation as an indicator of reactive changes and not diagnosing it in the presence of ulcers, erosions, or restituting epithelium. These can also be recognized by the presence of metaplasia in the adjacent mucosa. However, complete intestinal metaplasia starts with intestinal nuclei that are already considerably larger than native gastric mucosa. Nuclei in incomplete intestinal metaplasia are more open and vesicular with distinct small nucleoli. Reactive changes enhance all of these features, so this needs to be taken into account. All forms of reactive mucosa have both mucin depletion and enlarged pleomorphic nuclei occupying most of the cell, and may be accompanied by erosions or ulcer. The tip-off is the presence of (a) restituting mucosa (low cuboidal or columnar) with nuclei that are usually more widely separated than in normal mucosa, especially superficially, and (b) usually a degree of maturation superficially, to the degree that a diagnosis of dysplasia should be made very cautiously in the presence of active restitution. It is worthwhile to remember that in the bases of these pits, nuclei can overlap and be stratified and hyperchromatic causing confusion with adenoma/dysplasia.

Reporting reactive gastropathy: Minor degrees of superficial mucin depletion are relatively common, and it is unclear how much surface mucin depletion is required to report the changes, or indeed whether they can be seen physiologically. As a guide we do not report reactive changes unless the mucin droplet in the superficial epithelial cells (usually about 75%–80% of the cell) is <50%, but there are no data to support this. However, when reported we usually indicate the most common causes.

Reporting chronic changes: Usually mild chronic reactive changes alone, such as isolated foveolar hyperplasia, are not reported unless marked, as they

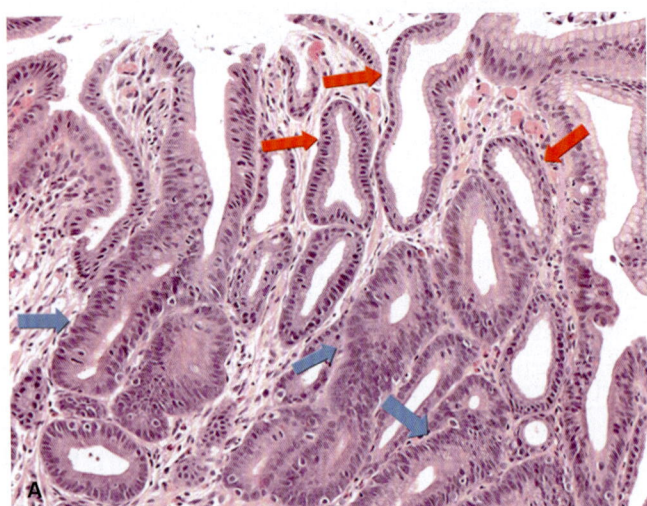 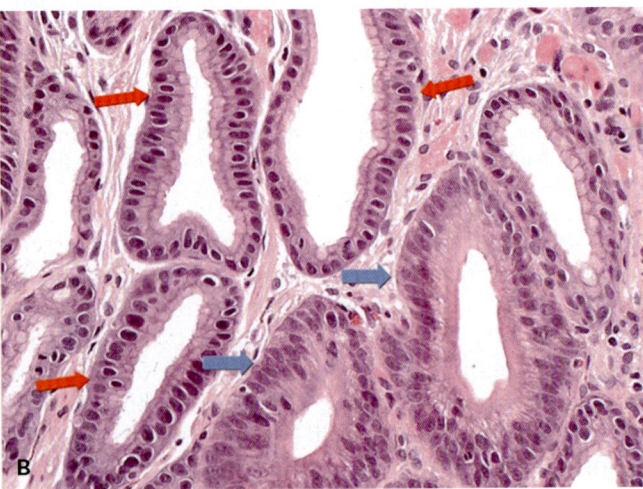

Figure 13-8. A: Reactive changes versus dysplasia. Typical reactive changes with mucin depletion, but widely spaced nuclei and superficially attenuated epithelium (*red arrows*). These contrast with the closely packed stratified nuclei in the dysplastic crypts (*blue arrows*). **B:** Detail of (A). Reactive changes (*red arrows*) versus low-grade dysplasia (*blue arrows*).

tend to refer to events that happened at some point in the past, and it is unclear how long these changes take to reverse. If accompanied by acute changes of damage, then "reactive changes" covers both acute and chronic changes without the need to specify.

Clinical Implications: Of the millions of patients who every day ingest NSAIDs/ASA, only about 2% per year develop a GI complication severe enough to require medical attention, usually a bleeding gastric ulcer. Yet even 2% of a million is 20,000 events. It is possible that these patients represent a subset of individuals with a predisposition (increased sensitivity) to greater loss of their physiologic mucosal defense mechanisms. The risk of GI bleeding with NSAID use increases with age, duration of use, comorbidities, anticoagulant use (including aspirin that may also cause the damage itself), and a history of bleeding ulcers. However, it also causes bleeding in infants.[28] A subset of patients (about one-third in one series[20]) may suffer a modest mucosal injury that results in one of the characteristic chronic changes of reactive gastropathy. However, in a series looking at the protective use of PPIs on naproxen 500 mg b.i.d.,[4] within a week 25% developed antral ulcers, 12.5% duodenal ulcers, and 9.4% ulcers in multiple locations (one developed ulcers in the antrum and body; two in the antrum and duodenum). Of those taking PPIs, only 11.8% developed ulcers, all of which were antral. Anecdotally we have seen inflammatory masses in the cardia and proximal duodenal that seem likely NSAID related. They may take weeks/months to resolve or persist for months.

The gastric mucosa of the majority of users may therefore never develop changes that can be detected by endoscopic or histopathologic examination. In practice, however, most NSAID users have been taking them for long periods of time, and it is less clear how well the stomach is able to adapt to chronic NSAID ingestion. Overall, only a small subset of chronic NSAID users have biopsies with all features we commonly associate with chemical gastropathy; most may only have foveolar hyperplasia.[20] In addition, such changes may occasionally occur in persons with no history of chemical injury. Concurrent *H. pylori* infection makes a firm diagnosis of chemical gastropathy extremely arduous.[20]

Alcoholic gastropathy. The term *alcoholic gastritis (or gastropathy)* is commonly used in a clinical or endoscopic context to explain abdominal pain or gastric lesions in alcoholic patients. Gastric hemorrhages, erosions, or both are found in 20% or less of actively drinking alcoholics with GI bleeding[27] (Fig. 13-9A). In humans, there are few data concerning the histologic basis of gastric erosions or subepithelial (lamina propria, rarely with submucosal) hemorrhages. However, in 1954 (pre-*Helicobacter* days), servicemen had their gastric mucosa examined after acute alcoholic ingestion.[29] In most, a variety of lesions were noted: patchy hyperemia, erosions, petechiae, and "exudate." Biopsy specimens showed mainly superficial gastritis with prominent neutrophils.[29] Some specimens exhibited edema of the foveolar region. More recently, actively drinking alcoholics had biopsy specimens taken from either subepithelial (lamina propria) hemorrhages or erosions, with specimens for comparison from adjacent sites.[27] The subepithelial hemorrhage specimens revealed foveolar region hemorrhage in target lesions and sometimes striking edema in the adjacent mucosa (Fig. 13-9B). The erosions were verified histologically in 70% and commonly exhibited a pseudomembranous appearance. In both the erosions and the hemorrhages, the associated inflammatory change

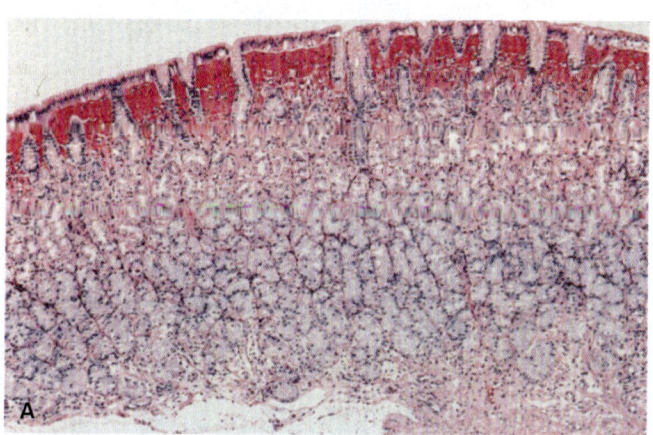 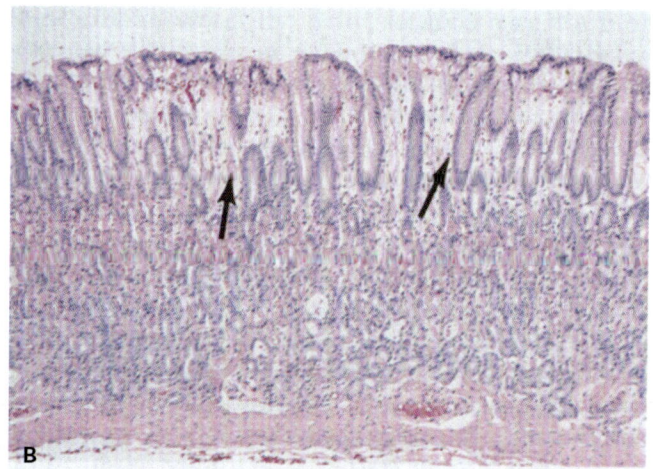

Figure 13-9. **A:** Biopsy specimen of a subepithelial hemorrhage in a patient with alcoholism. There is diffuse subepithelial hemorrhage across the full span of the fundic gland mucosa, but there is no inflammation present. **B:** Mucosal edema with an empty appearance of the interpit regions throughout the span of the biopsy (*arrows*). This is from a biopsy specimen adjacent to an area of subepithelial hemorrhage in a patient with alcoholism.

was mild and was similar in severity in the lesions and the adjacent mucosa. In actively drinking alcoholic patients, the gastric mucosa may, in addition, exhibit the features of *congestive gastropathy* if there is portal hypertension. This is discussed in the next section.

Caustic-induced injury. Accidental or suicidal ingestion of acids or alkalis (commonly in the form of household cleaners) may cause a wide range of oral, esophageal, and gastric lesions.[30,31] The gastric antrum is especially vulnerable, with lesions ranging from superficial erosions to gangrene. A late complication in some cases is the development of gastric antral strictures.[31]

Graft versus host disease. is discussed in detail in Chapter 3. GVHD is seen in severely immunosuppressed patients after allogeneic bone marrow transplant where the donor T cells attack host cells leading to cell necrosis. Upper endoscopic examination in the context of suspected or proven GVHD is done if upper GI symptoms are prominent. The severity of change in the upper gastrointestinal tract (UGT) frequently do not parallel the colonic changes (see Chapter 3). The endoscopic spectrum ranges from normal to subtle swelling to erosions, ulcers, and mucosal sloughing. In addition to mild reactive changes, variable degrees of epithelial injury are seen in a background of few inflammatory cells. In general, the histopathology is that of epithelial injury/death at variance with the amount of inflammation present. In the acute phase, epithelial injury can be seen as increased apoptosis (occasionally more numerous in the neck area), attenuated regenerative-appearing epithelial cells in less injured glands, granular eosinophilic debris intermixed occasionally with nuclear debris within dilated glands, sloughed mucosa, and total destruction of gastric glands in severely injured glands. The histopathology in chronic cases can include crypt loss, inflammatory polyps in severe disease, and architectural distortion with crypt branching and atrophy.[32-34] Telangiectatic vessels suggestive of gastric vascular ectasia have been identified.[34] Biopsy specimens are commonly taken to also rule out infections such as cytomegalovirus (CMV). Nonetheless, similar histopathology can be seen in CMV and human immunodeficiency virus (HIV) infection, transplant recipients, and in primary immunodeficiency.[34]

Chemotherapy and radiation. can cause both gastritis and stomach ulcers. The pathology is similar to that seen in chemical/reactive gastropathy with glandular atypia and increased apoptosis (apoptotic gastropathy), and there may be abnormal mitosis.[35] A typical feature, identifiable at low power, is that adjacent pits with relatively normal epithelium, and pits with attenuated mucosa, and all stages between, can be immediately adjacent to each other (Fig. 13-10). Gastric injury induced in short-term exposure is often temporary. The acute response to massive irradiation occurs largely in the antrum and the prepyloric region. Not uncommonly, gastric erosions or discrete ulcers are encountered in patients with malignancy who have received abdominal irradiation and are on chemotherapy. Biopsy specimens and cultures may be obtained to rule out recurrent or metastatic disease and opportunistic infection. With larger doses, the damage may be irreversible with destruction of acid-producing glands.

Ischemia. Ischemic disease of the stomach is extremely rare. See Chapter 2 for a more detailed discussion. Atheromatous embolization of cholesterol,[36] therapeutic

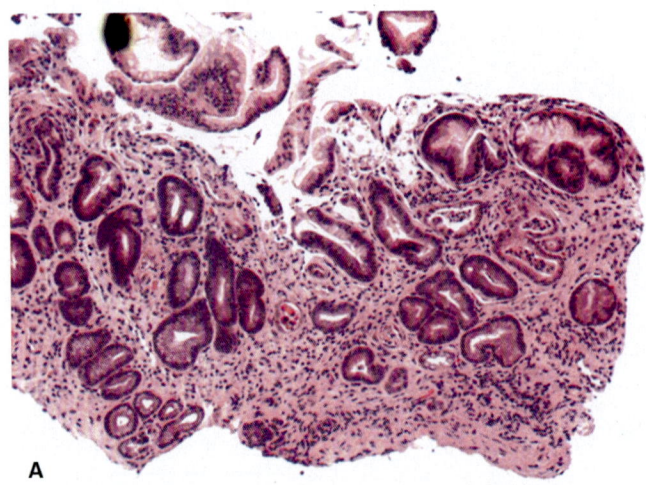
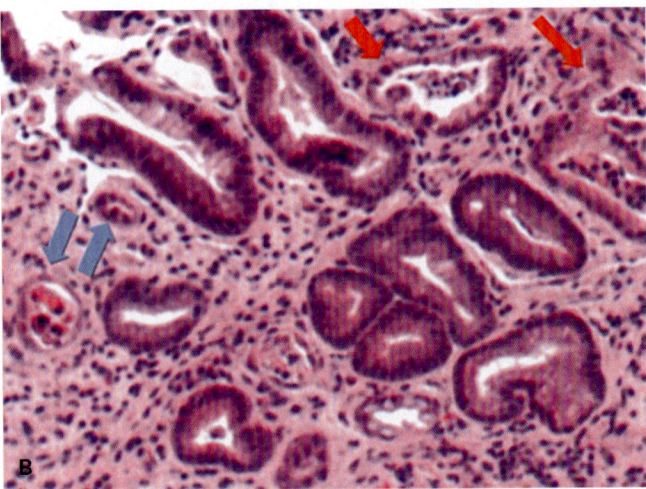

Figure 13-10. A: With chemotherapy, gastric injury is not uniform. There is architectural distortion and individual crypts are in various stages of repair. **B:** Individual crypts vary from some that are very attenuated and undergoing restitution (*blue arrow*) to others in which more typical regenerative changes can be found (*red arrows*). These are irregularly admixed with more normal-appearing pits.

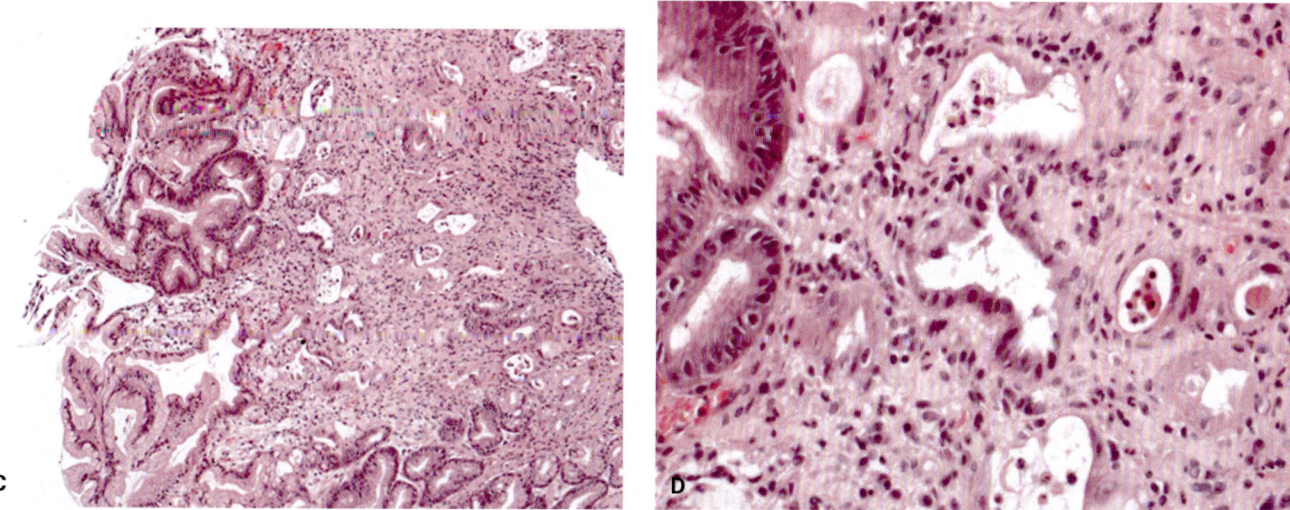

Figure 13-10. *(Continued)* **C:** Overview of second biopsy with more severe changes. The admixture of pits of different stages of degeneration and repair, some benign columnar and others lined by restituting epithelium. **D:** Severe chemotherapy changes with most glands being lined by restituting epithelium although focally they are more columnar.

embolization to help control bleeding, accidental entry of selective intra-arterial radiotherapy (SIRT) beads, and vasculitis[37,38] or hypovolemic states are reported causes of erosive gastritis and gastric ulcers. There have also been isolated reports of patients with chronic gastric ulcers and erosions that healed after intestinal revascularization.[39] The reported histology in these cases may lack the classic features of ischemia. In severe disease, epithelial and glandular cells are shed in the lumens of pits. Although this sounds innocuous, the mucous-producing cells can take on the appearances of signet ring cells, mimicking signet ring carcinoma (Fig. 13-11), analogous to similar lesions seen in pseudomembranous colitis. Another potential mimic of signet ring cells are the normal mucous-producing cells that appear in the oxyntic mucosa as it approaches the antrum. The polarity of these cells may appear abnormal, but these are terminally differentiated cells with no proliferative activity (Fig. 13-11E,F), while parietal cells can be shed into the lumen in oxyntic mucosa and raise the question of parietal cell carcinoma because of apparent disorderly sheets of cells (Fig. 13-12). The gastroduodenal subepithelial hemorrhages and erosions reported in some children with *Henoch–Schonlein* purpura might be due to vasculitis-induced mucosal ischemia.[40]

Predominantly Vascular Changes

Gastric antral vascular ectasia. is an uncommon cause of chronic GI bleeding with occult iron deficiency anemia. It is characterized by telangiectatic

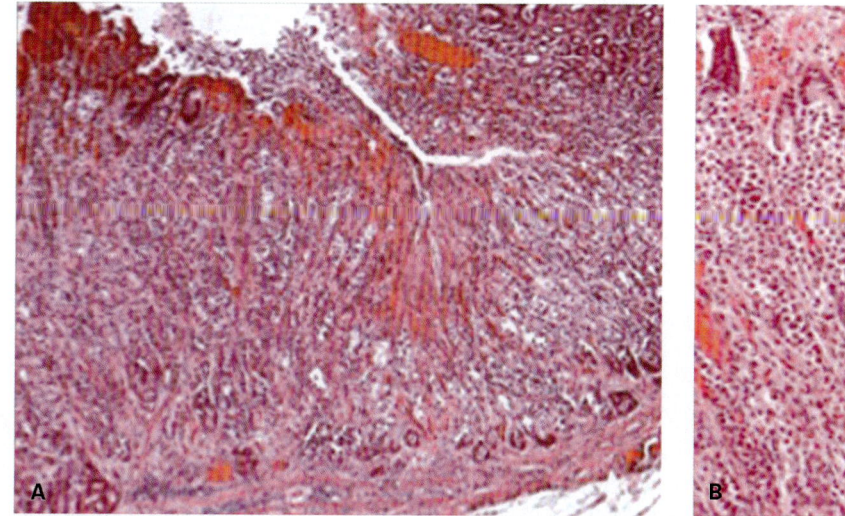
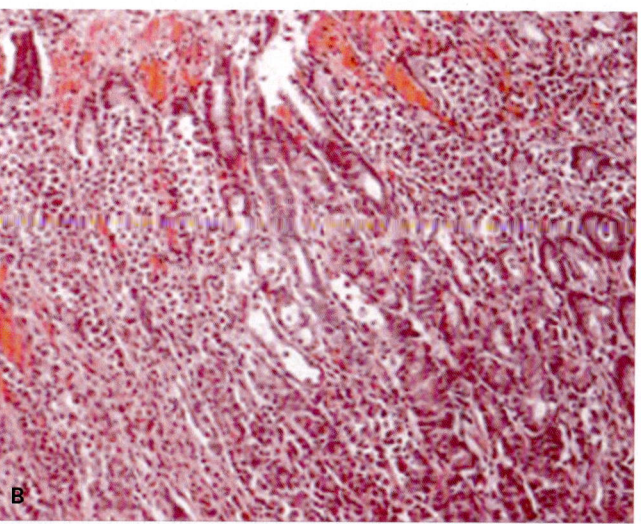

Figure 13-11. Ischemic change with signet ring cells. **A:** Active erosion with fibrinous exudes and hemorrhagic ischemic change. **B:** "Pseudomembranous gastritis"–like appearance with "signet ring" cells (SRCs) on the surface.

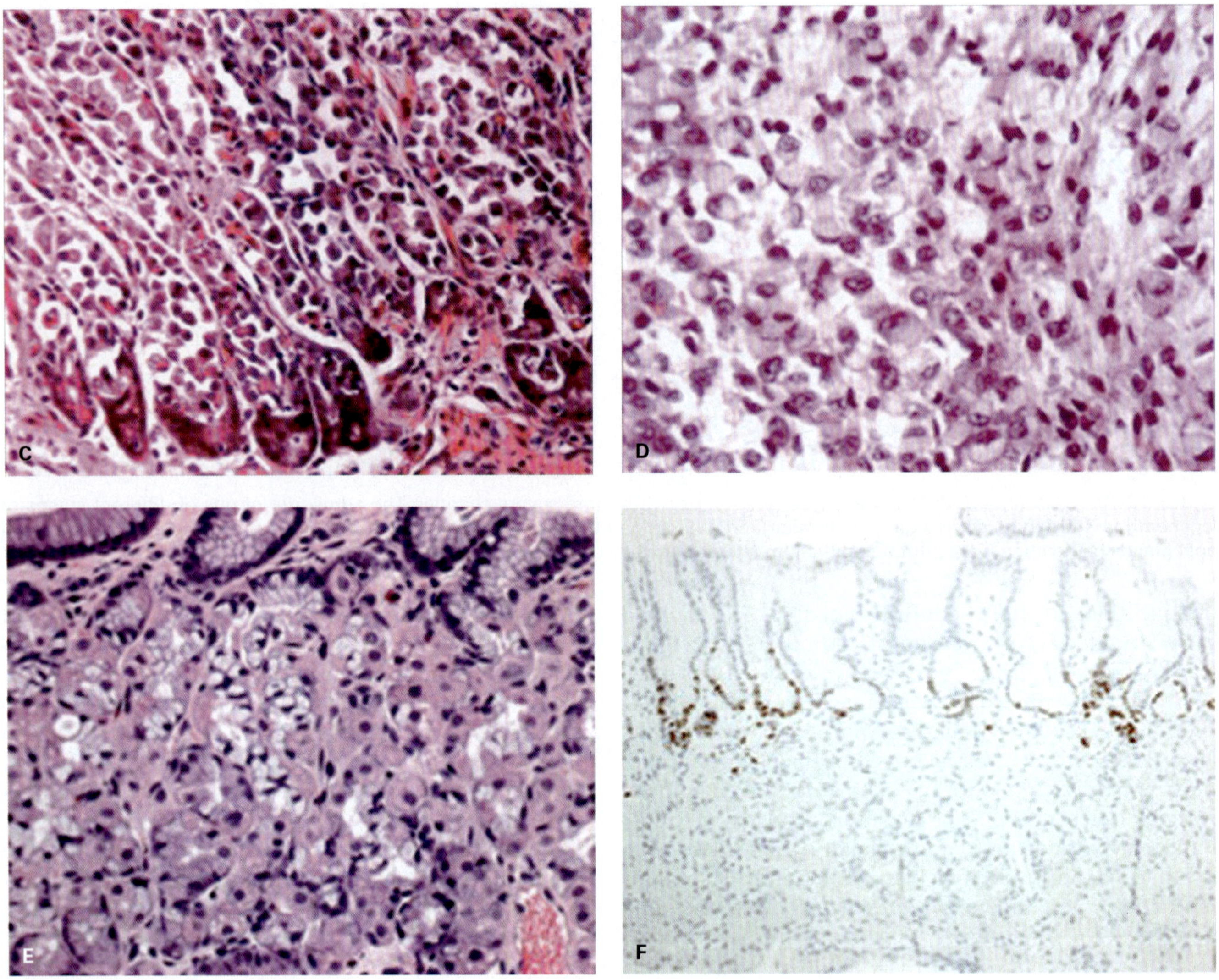

Figure 13-11. *(Continued)* **C:** Numerous SRCs observed in and out of degenerated glands on ischemic background. **D:** SRCs with abundant cytoplasm and compressed nuclei, mimicking infiltrative adenocarcinoma but almost too monomorphous for carcinoma. **E:** A further possible mimic of signet ring cells are the mucous cells normally found in the superficial midzone of the oxyntic mucosa toward the antrum. **F:** The mib-1 shows this zone to have no proliferative activity.

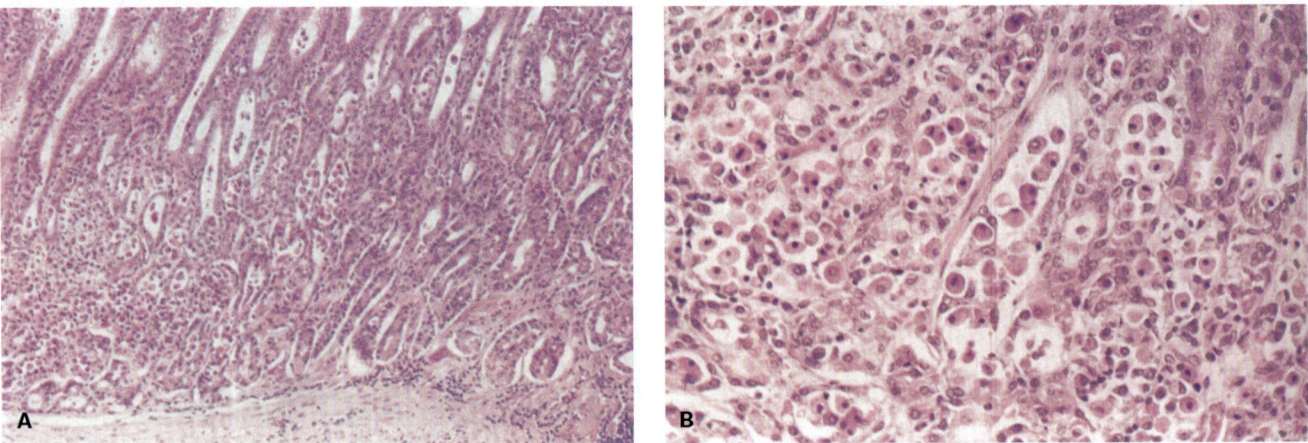

Figure 13-12. Gastric ischemia. **A:** The deep specialized compartment of the mucosa is ill-defined, lacking a crisp definition seen superficially. **B:** Detail reveals that the specialized glands have been shed into the lumen of the pits and that PCs are particularly conspicuous. The patient also had contiguous infarction of the small intestine. (Courtesy of Dr. R. Barr.)

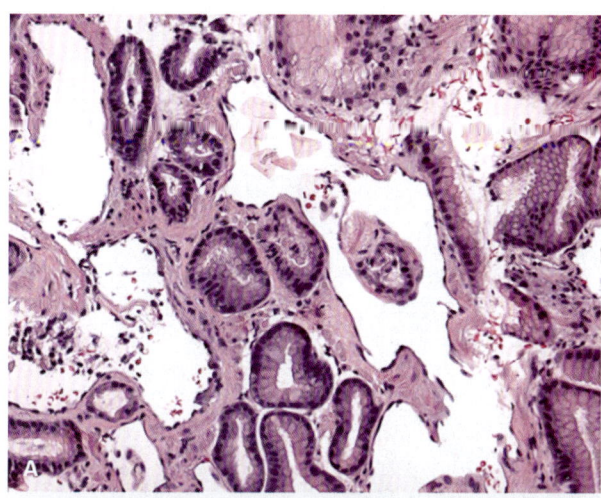
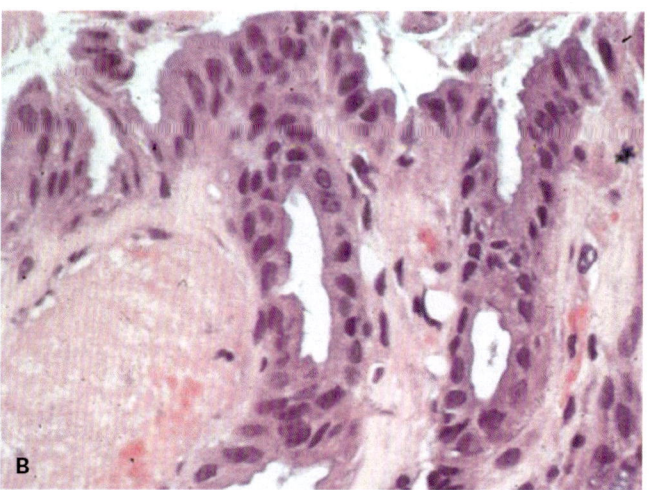
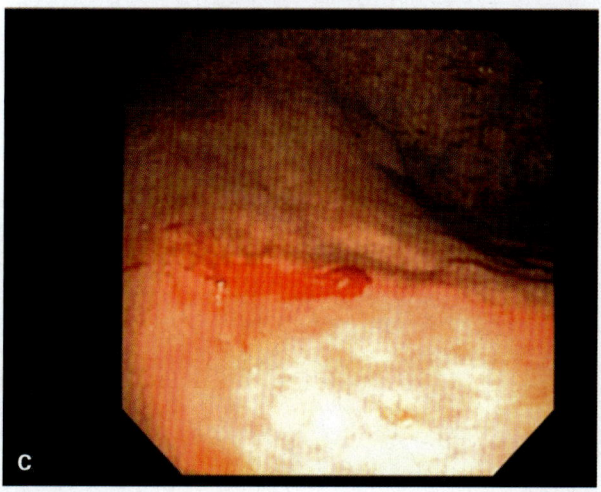

Figure 13-13. **A:** GAVE with numerous dilated capillaries and intervening muscle in the lamina propria, here quite marked, interweaving between the pits. **B:** GAVE with a thrombosed vessel in the lamina propria **(bottom left)** and marked reactive epithelium, which is seen frequently in this condition. **C:** Bleeding from GAVE.

capillaries with fibrin thrombi and marked fibromuscular hyperplasia of the lamina propria[41] (Fig. 13-13). Though it has been primarily described in the gastric antrum, proximal involvement has been reported.[42,43] Vascular ectasia can be seen in a number of other conditions, including portal hypertension,[44] end-stage renal disease,[45] and congestive heart failure.[46] Histology is rarely needed to confirm the diagnosis when the endoscopy has a characteristic watermelon appearance; however, sometimes differentiation from portal hypertensive gastropathy can be problematic (see Chapter 2).[47]

Portal hypertension (congestive gastropathy). In cirrhosis, especially when accompanied by portal hypertension, a number of endoscopic abnormalities have been described; they are thought to represent the consequences of portal hypertension and mucosal congestion.[48] These are considered here because sometimes they are associated with discrete subepithelial hemorrhages. In the fundus and proximal body there may be a mosaic pattern, sometimes described as a snakeskin appearance. These are red areas separated by fine white serpentine reticulations.[48] Another appearance is that of discrete red spots, especially in the antrum.[48] Biopsy specimens may reveal focal mucosal vascular ectasia[49] that can be mistaken for chronic inflammation to the unwary (Fig. 13-14), but the ectasia may be much more striking in the submucosa[50] deep to the zone usually sampled in endoscopic biopsies[50] (see Chapter 2).

Hemorrhagic gastropathy ("gastritis") and "Curling's ulcer". Stress/shock/burn-related ulcer is the most serious form of gastropathy that usually occurs in critically ill patients, including organ system failure, sepsis, burns, and intracranial disease.[51,52] The term "gastritis" may have a degree of truth historically in that many of these patients may well have had concomitant *Helicobacter* gastritis, but it is primarily a gastropathy.

This condition is usually a complication of severe trauma leading to profound physiologic stress with hypovolemia or hypoxia (as in shock), but can also be seen in binge drinking alcoholics. It used to be common post surgery, but with better intensive care and

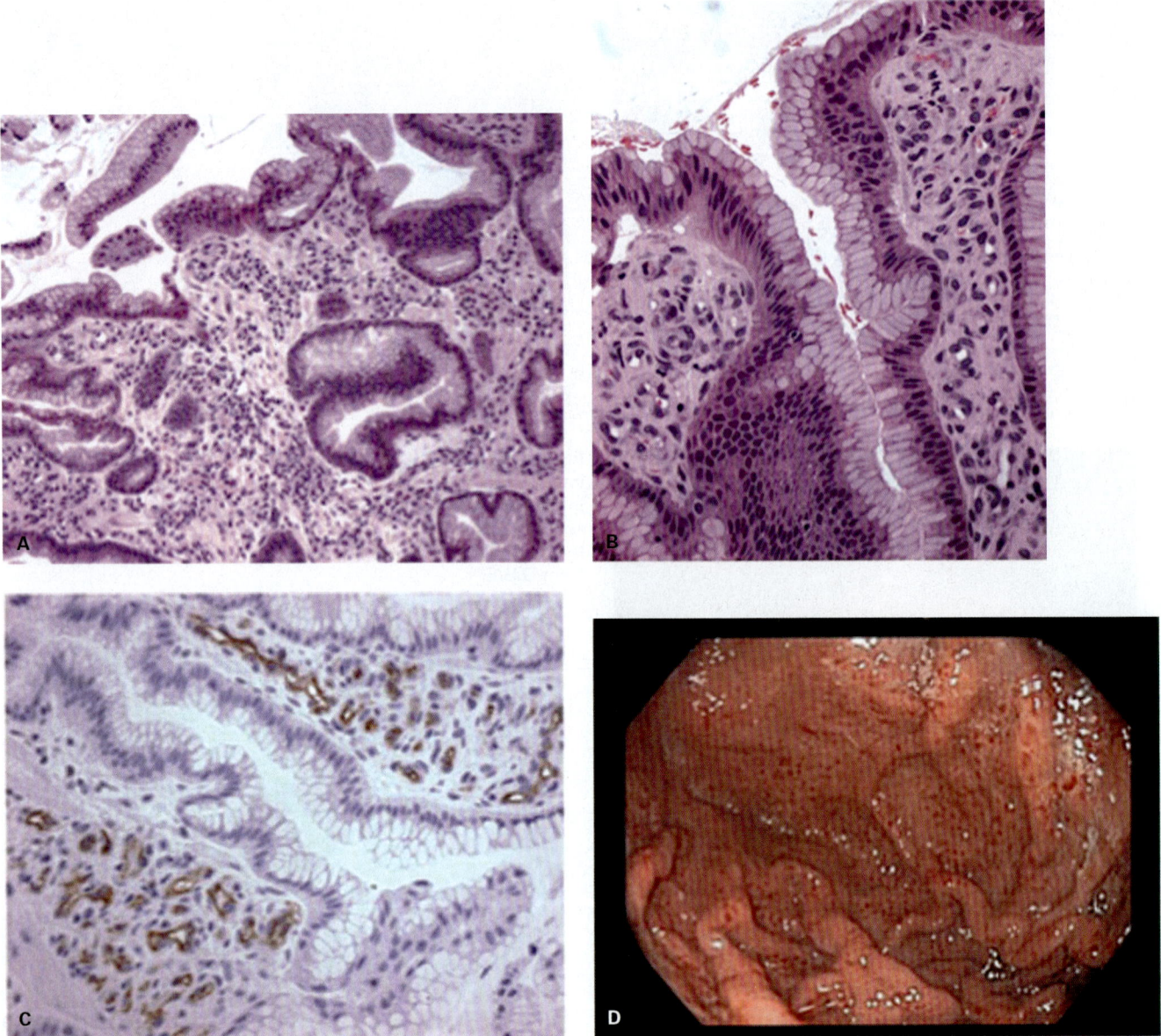

Figure 13-14. Portal hypertensive gastropathy. **A:** The overview suggest chronic gastritis. However, detail **(B)** suggests that these are all small endothelial-lined channels with small lumina. **C:** CD31 immunostain shows that these are endothelial. **D:** Endoscopic appearances of portal gastropathy. Note not only the varices but the numerous telangiectases in the background that are the endoscopic counterpart of the biopsy.

prophylactic antisecretory therapy, this is now rare. In shock and other low-flow conditions, mesenteric blood flow is shunted to the systemic circulation to maintain perfusion. Shunting mesenteric blood flow to the systemic circulation is often accomplished at the expense of adequate blood flow to the mucosa, with back perfusion of acid into the lamina propria and subsequent hemorrhage. Such shunting is a major contributing factor to stress-related mucosal disease and acute hemorrhagic gastritis.

The pathology is inconspicuous except for areas of mucosal hemorrhage that can precipitate significant acute blood loss. In pre-PPI days this condition was often fatal and involved the entire stomach. Early lesions seem to predominate in the fundus and more proximal body; later there is more distal spread to involve the antrum. It is very uncommon to have only antral involvement. Stress lesions are usually superficial. Areas of hemorrhage are seen at the tips of the mucosal folds down to the mucous neck region.[53-56] Hemorrhagic gastropathy, which frequently occurs in the early postburn period and is often manifested by coffee-ground emesis, damages the mucosa, rendering it more susceptible to ulceration "Curling's ulcer."[57] Bleeding from hemorrhagic gastropathy is commonly trivial and ceases with resumption of GI function. GI bleeding later in the postburn period should suggest the diagnosis of Curling's ulcer.

Curling's stress ulcers of the stomach or duodenum were once the most frequent life-threatening GI complications of burn patients. These are usually diagnosed at operation or at autopsy after the 3rd postburn day in patients with larger burns. These stress ulcers are usually preceded by hemorrhagic gastropathy ("gastritis"), and often result in hemorrhage and perforation more often than intestinal ulceration[58]—thus, they have correspondingly high mortality rates.[57] The limited literature on Curling's ulcers describe engorged submucosal capillaries, a paucity of inflammatory cells, and a sharp demarcation of necrotic mucosa showing cellular degeneration from viable apparently uninvolved mucosa.[57] The deeper lesions usually contain a base of necrotic debris without the scarring or well-formed granulation tissue seen in ordinary gastric ulcers.

The apparent decrease in major complications (bleeding and perforation) may be more due to improved cardiorespiratory and nutritional support[53] than to routine acid-neutralizing or acid-inhibiting prophylactic therapy.[59] Endoscopic studies have shown that the lesions develop within hours of the illness or trauma.[54–56,60] If the underlying disease is reversed, the lesions vanish in parallel. It is unlikely to receive a biopsy in this condition but it can be in the differential in a gastrectomy specimen of a patient with hypovolemia secondary to severe hemorrhage. Patients with stress/shock ulcer often are given continuous PPIs that are also given prophylactically to patients at risk before surgery.

Of interest, gastric mucosal damage seen in marathon runners can also be explained by shunting of mesenteric blood flow to the periphery.[61–64] Gastric erosions and ulcers in marathon runners are mainly localized in the corpus,[61–63] where stress or shock-associated gastritis is normally seen.[64] Mucosal erosions can also be seen in the antrum (sometimes primarily), suggesting altered gastric physiology and microcirculation induced by intense exercise.[65,66]

Distinctive (Specific) Types of Gastritis

The designation distinctive or specific refers to histologic features that markedly narrow the differential diagnosis or are occasionally pathognomonic. We subclassify these into infectious and noninfectious (Table 13-4).

Infections. The most common infection in immune competent patients is *H. pylori* infection. It has an acute phase as demonstrated by volunteers swallowing the organism, and then most pass on to a phase of chronic relatively asymptomatic infection. Although many organisms have urease and hence can potentially survive in the stomach for short periods, there are few data to suggest that other bacteria cause an acute infectious gastritis rather than what is euphemistically called infectious gastroenteritis; however, a patient with enterococcal gastritis has been described presenting with "dyspepsia"[67] (Fig. 13-15). These organisms are readily visible on an hematoxylin and eosin (H&E) stain but any bacterial stain can enhance their visibility. They are Gram positive. The challenge is not to interpret them as coccal forms of *Helicobacter*, which are not overtly adherent to the surface epithelium (they are dead), or as incidental organisms of oral or duodenal origin that can grow in the stomach in patients with marked hypo or achlorhydria, whether pathologic or iatrogenic (PPIs). They are negative with *Helicobacter* immunohistochemistry.

Amongst viral infections, CMV is the most common in the stomach and is found especially in children. How long the infection needs to be present before becoming symptomatic, and therefore whether it is really acute, is unclear. It is also the cause of childhood large gastric folds—pediatric "Ménétrier's disease." Apparent incidental inclusions are occasionally found, primarily in epithelial cells, and are thought to represent a carrier state. In immunodeficient patients, whether iatrogenic, acquired, or congenital, a variety of infections including CMV may be encountered (Fig. 13-16, Chapter 19, and subsequently in this chapter—Ménétrier's disease). General viremias may be associated with a variety of other viruses that may be found incidentally such as measles (Fig. 13-17), herpes, and Parvovirus infection.

A *H. pylori* **infection.** *Helicobacter pylori* is etiologically linked to histologic gastritis, PUD, marginal zone lymphoma, and gastric carcinoma in addition

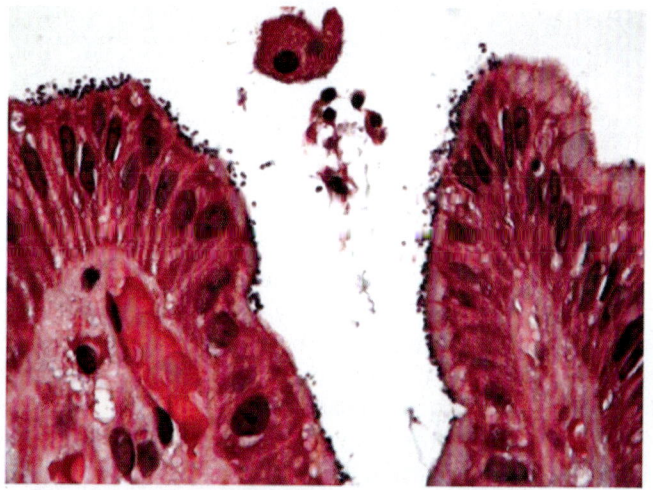

Figure 13-15. Enterococcal gastritis. It is important not to interpret these as coccal forms of *Helicobacter,* which never exist in the absence of typical forms of *Helicobacter* as they are not viable. (Triple stain with carbol fuchsin.)

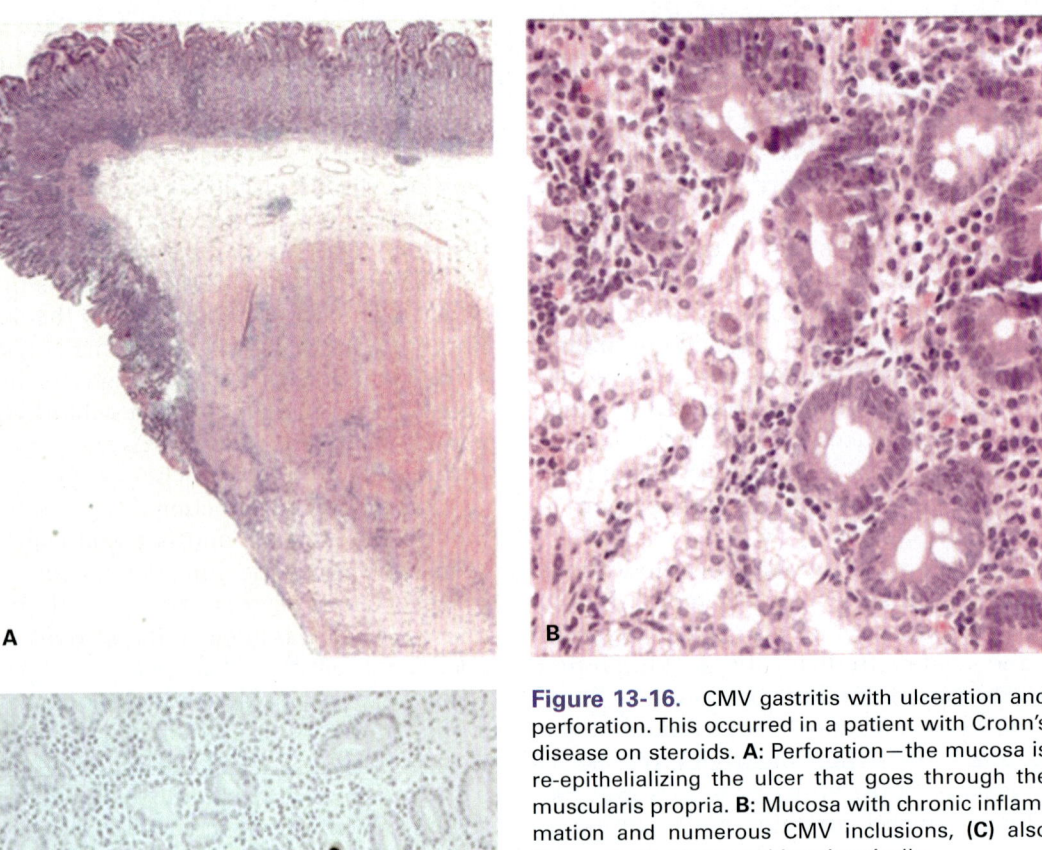

Figure 13-16. CMV gastritis with ulceration and perforation. This occurred in a patient with Crohn's disease on steroids. **A:** Perforation—the mucosa is re-epithelializing the ulcer that goes through the muscularis propria. **B:** Mucosa with chronic inflammation and numerous CMV inclusions, **(C)** also demonstrated immunohistochemically.

to other conditions (Table 13-5). The discovery of *Campylobacter pylori* by Warren and Marshall in 1982 and subsequently renamed *Helicobacter pylori*, was preceded by nearly 100 years of inconspicuous publications relating spiral bacteria to achlorhydria, gastritis, gastric urease, and antimicrobial therapy for ulcers.[68–71] Koch's postulates for *H. pylori* were fulfilled by volunteers who ingested the organism and produced gastritis, one self-limited[9] and the others more persistent.[72] In 1984, the bacterium was cultured from 88% of patients with gastritis and the bacteria was not cultured from any patient with histologically normal gastric mucosa.[73] Furthermore, the inflammation associated with *H. pylori* gastritis is reduced with antibiotics that suppress *H. pylori*.[74,75] This direct evidence of a causative role was complemented by indirect evidence that *H. pylori* may have been responsible for two miniepidemics of nonerosive, "nonspecific" gastritis.[76,77] These miniepidemics were reported in volunteers taking part in secretory studies. The individuals developed self-limited upper abdominal complaints, with hypochlorhydria that continued for months in some. In this "*epidemic gastritis*," the pattern of inflammation was a superficial gastritis, suggesting severe functional impairment of parietal cells rather than their obliteration. In 2005,

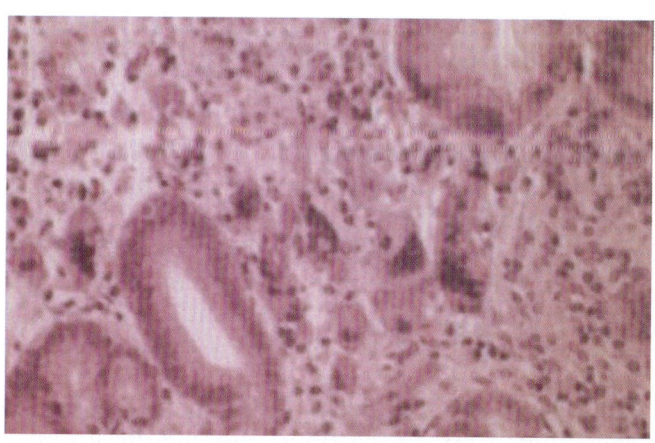 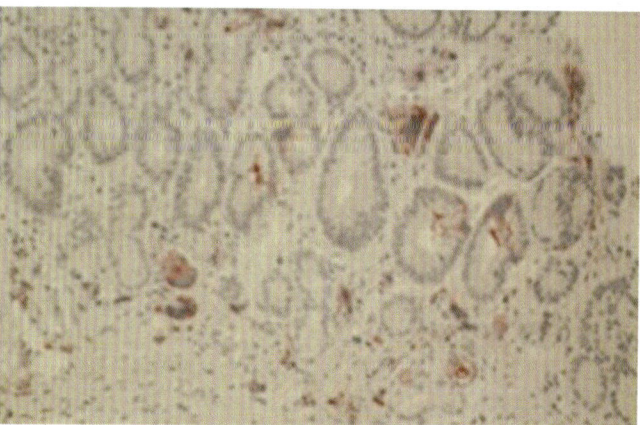

Figure 13-17. Measles in a gastric biopsy. Numerous Warthin–Finkeldey giant cells typical of measles can be seen. A specific anti-measles antibody was used to confirm the diagnosis immunohistochemically **(right)**. The patient was prodromal when the biopsies were taken and developed a typical rash soon after. (Courtesy of Dr. M Vieth, Bayreuth.)

Barry Marshall and Robin Warren jointly received the Nobel Prize in physiology and medicine for their "discovery of the bacterium *Helicobacter pylori* and its role in gastritis and peptic ulcer disease".

Epidemiology *Helicobacter pylori* infection almost certainly is the most common chronic bacterial infection in humans and is present in approximately 60% of the world population.[78] *Helicobacter pylori* gastritis is for the most part acquired before age 10.[79] The prevalence of *H. pylori* infection varies both between and within countries.[80] This relates to the known determinants of infection, particularly socioeconomic standards of living of the young.[81–85] Differences in prevalence among ethnic groups of similar socioeconomic status reflect differences in the environment and possible host genetics.[82,86] In countries where there has been rapid economic development with associated improvements in standards of living, there is some evidence that the prevalence of infection is declining.[87,88] In developed countries, it is currently uncommon to find infected children, but there is a cohort effect so that the percentage of infected people increases with age, being about 50% in those over the age of 60.[89–91] The higher prevalence among the elderly reflects higher infection rates when they were children rather than infection at later ages. Nonetheless, *H. pylori* infection remains common among the socially disadvantaged and in the large immigrant population in developed countries.[92,93]

Although the exact route of transmission is not known, person-to-person transmission, oral–oral or fecal–oral, as exemplified by data on intrafamilial clustering is most likely.[94,95] Possibilities include the common practice of (grand)parents masticating food before feeding to infants, bearing in mind that the act of burping showers the oral cavity with gastric organisms. The role of external reservoirs in *H. pylori* transmission has not been ruled out, particularly in rural and developing areas.[96] Nonetheless, studies on water, one of the most well-studied ecosystems, yielded inconsistent results.[97–99] The inconsistent results may reflect different water treatment modalities and/or variations in polymerase chain reaction (PCR) procedures. It is important to remember that mere presence of DNA in a potential environmental reservoir is not a clear evidence of the transmissibility of the organisms, as the organisms may or may not be viable. A culture of *H. pylori* organisms from these sources would provide stronger evidence—*H. pylori*

Table 13-5 A *Helicobacter*-associated Diseases

Gastric conditions associated with *H. pylori* infection
Gastritis
Duodenal ulcer
Gastric ulcer
Gastric carcinoma
Gastric lymphoma

Extragastric conditions possibly associated with *H. pylori* infection
Iron deficiency anemia[830,831]
Vitamin B_{12} deficiency
Pernicious anemia
Coronary artery disease
Cerebrovascular disease
Hypertension
Raynaud's phenomenon
Migraine headaches
Hyperemesis gravidarum[832]
Immune thrombocytopenic purpura
Hyperammonemia
Sudden infant death syndrome
Growth retardation "short stature"[833]
Anorexia of aging
Rosacea

has not been cultured to date from water reservoirs, but has been found in streams, possibly the result of fecal contamination.

Most interestingly, H. pylori strains from different geographical areas exhibit clear phylogeographic features that provide information about the migration of human populations.[100] Sequence differences in seven core housekeeping genes enabled grouping H. pylori into seven population types based on geographical associations (hpEurope, hpEastAsia, hpAfrica1, hpAfrica2, hpAsia2, hpNEAfrica, and hpSahul).[101-103] These studies suggest H. pylori has spread from East Africa over the same time period as modern humans, around 58,000 years ago.[104] Helicobacter pylori has remained intimately associated with the human host populations ever since.[102] Overall, H. pylori sequences can potentially provide details of human migrations that would otherwise be difficult.[104]

Some strains of Helicobacter are clearly associated with more inflammation, the ability to produce ulcers, atrophy, and carcinoma. The best known of these is the CagA gene that is present in 50% to 70% of H. pylori in Western societies. It resides in the CagA pathogenicity island (PAI), although a vacuolating toxin (VacA) can also be present. The CagAPAI contains about 30 genes, but is usually absent from H. pylori strains isolated from humans who are carriers of H. pylori but remain asymptomatic. The CagA gene codes for a relatively long (1,186 amino acid) protein. The CagAPAI also includes a gene coding for a complex type IV secretion system. About 50% to 70% of H. pylori strains in Western countries carry the cag PAI.[105] Western patients infected with strains carrying the cag PAI have a stronger inflammatory response in the stomach and are at a greater risk of developing peptic ulcers or stomach cancer than those infected with strains lacking the island.[106]

Following attachment of H. pylori to gastric epithelial cells, the type IV secretion system "injects" a pro-inflammatory peptidoglycan from the organisms' own cell wall into the epithelial cells. The injected peptidoglycan is recognized by NOD1, which is a cytoplasmic pattern recognition receptor (immune sensor), which then stimulates expression of pro-inflammatory cytokines.[107] The type IV secretion system also injects CagA into the epithelial cells, where it disrupts the cytoskeleton, adherence to adjacent cells, cell polarity, and intracellular signaling.[108] Once inside the cell, the CagA protein is phosphorylated on tyrosine residues by a host cell membrane tyrosine kinase. There may also be activation of the epidermal growth factor receptor (EGFR), a membrane protein that also has a tyrosine kinase domain, and this activation is associated with altered signal transduction and gene expression in host epithelial cells, all of which likely contribute to pathogenesis. A C-terminal region of the CagA protein can also regulate host cell gene transcription independent of protein tyrosine phosphorylation.[109]

H. Pylori–associated Gastritis

Helicobacter pylori gastritis is for the most part acquired before age 10.[79] Today, many believe the hypochlorhydria accompanying febrile childhood infections predisposes children to H. pylori infection, as hypo or achlorhydria often develops during and after acute infectious diseases such as influenza, tonsillitis, pneumonia, and bronchitis. In several cases, in spite of normal acid secretion before the disease, lowered secretion was documented for a long time after the disease. It is unclear if these changes are secondary to direct bacterial involvement or due to bacterial toxins as acute gastritis with complete achlorhydria can be produced following intravenous injection of dogs with diphtheria toxin. Also, a fall of secretion, amounting at times to achylia, is seen in toxemias of pregnancy, especially eclampsia.[110]

Disease outcome varies from no symptoms in many patients, to duodenal ulcers, gastric ulcers, gastric mucosa-associated lymphoid tissue (MALT) lymphoma (marginal zone lymphoma), and gastric carcinoma in others. While host and environmental factors play critical roles in disease outcome, it is well known that the development of a specific disease is associated with a specific gastritis pattern[111,112] (see Fig. 13-1). DU is typically associated with antral-predominant gastritis, little or no oxyntic gland (corpus and fundus) atrophy, and normal or increased acid secretion.[113-116] Gastric ulcer and the intestinal type of gastric cancer are typically associated with pangastritis, widespread oxyntic atrophy with varying degrees of intestinal metaplasia, and hypo- or achlorhydria,[113,117-119] (see Fig. 13-1).

The distribution and severity of H. pylori–related gastritis (and thus disease risk) is related to the distribution and density of H. pylori within the stomach.[120] The distribution of H. pylori within the stomach is influenced by a person's acid secretory status.[120-122] Helicobacter pylori are well adapted to the human stomach with its acidic environment that is hostile for most microorganisms by producing large amounts of the enzyme urease. Urease catalyzes hydrolysis of urea present in the stomach to yield ammonium ions (NH_4^-) and CO_2 in a thin neutral layer around the outer surface of the bacteria.[123] The ammonium ions markedly increase the pH in its surrounding environment to neutral (or above), which is necessary for its survival.[124] Helicobacter pylori further protects itself by swimming through the protective layer of gastric mucus away from the acidic contents of the lumen toward the more neutral pH environment of the epithelial cells beneath.[125] Nonetheless, H. pylori flourishes best at a pH range of 3.5 to 5[126] where in the presence of urea it can maintain a proton motive force across its periplasmic membrane, ensuring a continued supply of energy through ATP synthesis.[126] In a high acid output microenvironment, this protective mechanism cannot keep up with the high hydrogen ion influx and the bacterium dies.[126,127] This explains why early *H. pylori* gastritis is concentrated in the antrum, although the organism may also be able to produce a protein that reduces gastric acidity, facilitating colonization.

Similarly, when the microenvironment pH rises above about 5, the bacteria produces ammonia in excess of what is needed to neutralize the much-diminished influx of hydrogen ion. The microenvironment then becomes increasingly alkaline, which is also detrimental to the bacteria. If *Helicobacter pylori*'s continual production of ammonia raises the pH above 8, the bacteria cannot survive.[126-130] This explains why *H. pylori* may not be identified in achlorhydric states (gastric atrophy and with continued PPI use) when the inflammatory pattern is clearly that associated with low *H. pylori* density. Further, in patients on PPIs the organism may migrate to the oxyntic mucosa to find enough acid to survive, hence the frequently observed proximal migration of *Helicobacter* with both increasing atrophy and PPI use. Not only that, but the organisms seem to migrate deeper into the oxyntic glands as opposed to their usual superficial location, and can even be found within canaliculi of parietal cells.

Histology of *H. pylori*–associated gastritis. The histologic spectrum of *H. pylori*–associated gastritis ranges from minimal to severe inflammation. When present, neutrophils are concentrated in the pit regions; uncommonly, they infiltrate the surface in a dense fashion, often associated with erosions. The association with neutrophils has been stressed, in part because they are not normally present in the lamina propria. Thus, their presence indicates inflammation and active disease, whereas with mononuclear cells, an increase is much more difficult to appreciate unless quite marked. Occasional chronic inflammatory cells are acceptable as part of the normal.[131] In *H. pylori*–associated active gastritis, the number of mononuclear cells is also increased.[132] The inflammation is worse along the lesser curve than on the greater curve with the most severe inflammation at the antral-body transitional mucosa. Lymphoid hyperplasia (Fig. 13-18) with numerous lymphoid follicles is seen in some cases, especially in children.[133,134] Similar to mononuclear cells, unorganized lymphoid aggregate abutting the muscularis mucosae is normal.[131]

The epithelial mucin ranges from intact to markedly depleted (reactive changes), with mild depletion being the most common pattern. With progressive atrophic gastritis, especially when accompanied by intestinal metaplasia, there is a reduced frequency of association with *H. pylori*.[135] Indeed, it is rare to find *Helicobacter* when intestinal metaplasia is present.

Helicobacter pylori may be present in biopsy specimens that are histologically close to normal, especially in the gastric body[132,136,137] (Fig. 13-19), and in patients with much more active disease in the gastric antrum that may not have been well-sampled. In such examples, the mild inflammation is limited to the superficial lamina propria, especially in the oxyntic mucosa where it is easily overlooked on a cursory examination. This also tends to occur with *Helicobacter* species other than *H. pylori*. However, we have never seen an absolutely normal (noninflamed) mucosa in an infected patient if biopsies from both

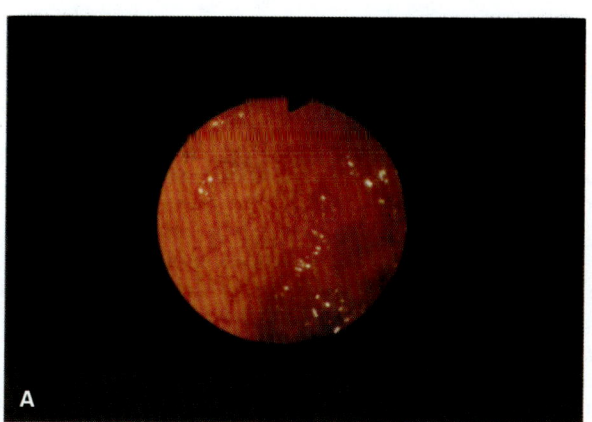
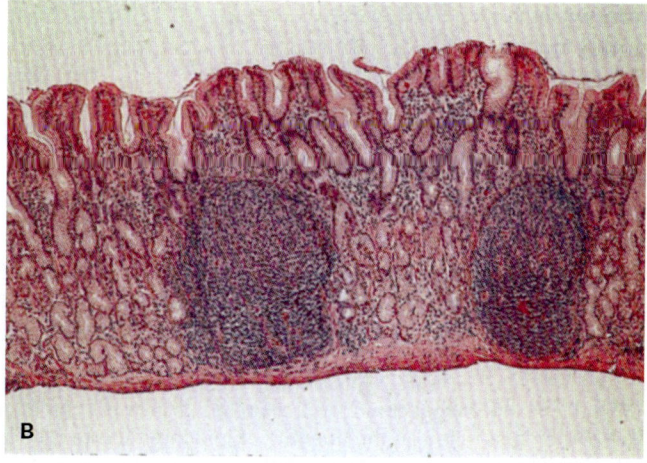

Figure 13-18. *Helicobacter pylori* in a child. **A:** Pronounced antral gland nodularity at endoscopy. **B:** Prominent lymphoid follicles and otherwise mild inflammation are revealed in this *H. pylori*–positive biopsy specimen. (Courtesy of Drs. E. Hassall and J. Dimmick.)

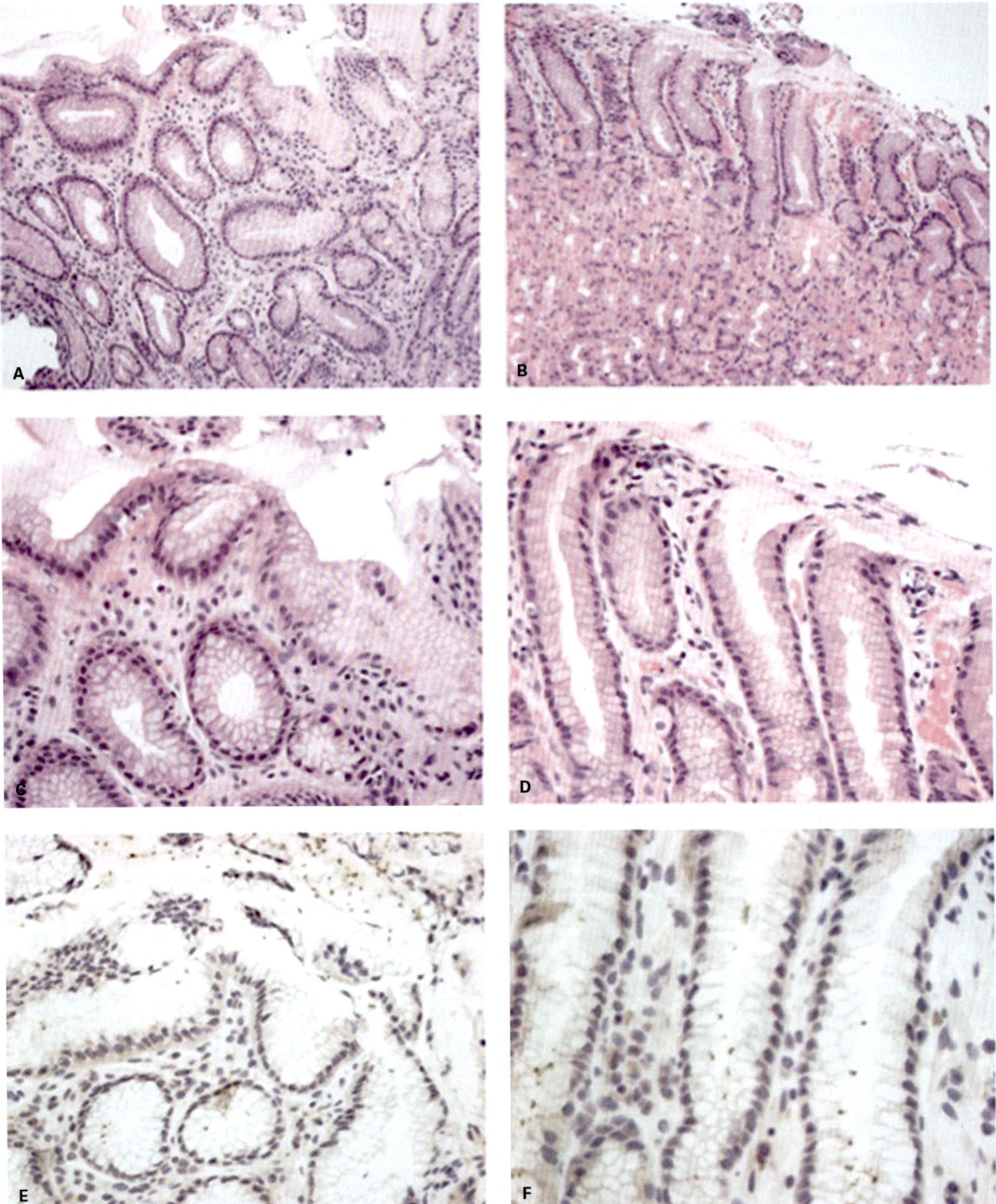

Figure 13-19. Our current minimal inflammation in a patient with *H. pylori* gastritis. Antral mucosa is in the **left three panels** and oxyntic mucosa in the **right three**. Appreciating this is important in laboratories in which some form of routine stain is not employed, and the pathologist relies on the quantity of inflammation to justify ordering a special stain or immunostain. The **lower two panels** are anti-*Helicobacter* immunostains at both sites. The numbers of organisms in both are readily appreciated.

antral and oxyntic mucosa have been taken. This becomes important practically.

1. When routine special stains for *Helicobacter* come with gastric biopsies, some meticulously examine them until they realize the time has been spent to no purpose, so they make a decision as to the minimal amount of inflammation required to seriously examine the special stain, and when they can rest assured that no organisms are present. In all likelihood absolutely normal (non-inflamed) biopsies need minimal examination of special stains provided. As shown in Figure 13-19 when *Helicobacter* are present in minimally inflamed biopsies organisms are invariably numerous so readily detected. They are also likely to be non-toxin producers and have virtually no pathogenic potential, as complications follow organisms producing considerable inflammation.
2. When no special stains are carried out routinely on all gastric biopsies, a decision has to be made on the minimal amount of inflammation to trigger this (Fig. 13-19).
3. If the special stain routinely carried out in a lab is a stain in which one cannot have real confidence (e.g., Giemsa stain), a backup is required (e.g., silver stain or an immunostain) in which one does have more confidence is required when inflammation equal to or more than that shown in Figure 13-29 is present, and organisms are not identified. Especially when one is convinced that the organism may be present.
4. When patients have recently undergone eradication therapy but still have chronic inflammation quantitatively compatible with *Helicobacter* being present, we usually revert to a silver or immunostain before declaring that "*Helicobacter* are not identified".

When organisms are present, especially if scant, although it seems mundane, it really is necessary to ensure that the organism is *H. pylori* or other *Helicobacter* species. Although therapy sounds easy, there is a risk of complications such as the NAP1 strain of *Clostridium difficile*, which can be potentially lethal. Our approach is that if organisms considered to be *Helicobacter* are identified, you should be able to photograph it and others will "buy it." We do not make the diagnosis on coccal forms unless accompanied by an immunostain with regular organisms as they are otherwise nonviable and easily mistaken for other cocci—discussed subsequently. Most biopsy specimens with diffuse chronic *active* gastritis are associated with *H. pylori*. Sampling error because of the patchy distribution of the organisms, and especially failure to biopsy both antral and oxyntic mucosa, may be one of the reasons that a minority of cases of diffuse chronic gastritis lack *H. pylori*.[136] However, recent use of antibiotics, PPIs, recent eradication therapy, atrophy and intestinal metaplasia, and other rare causes such as diffuse chronic gastritis are all reasons organisms may not be found.

ACUTE PHASE: The initial, acute phase of infection is subclinical in the great majority of subjects. As in any acute infection, there is lamina propria edema with neutrophilic infiltration of foveolar and surface epithelium—acute neutrophilic gastritis. Acute *H. pylori* infection can temporarily induce a period of hypochlorhydria, which probably facilitates widespread colonization and a pangastritis. In a small minority of people, and particularly in childhood, the organisms may be spontaneously cleared,[138] the polymorph infiltrate resolves, and appearances return to normal. Nonetheless, the acute phase is short-lived. Of those infected, the majority fail to eliminate the infection. Over a couple of weeks, there is a gradual accumulation of chronic inflammatory cells that come to dominate the histologic picture[131]—chronic active gastritis.[131,139] It may take weeks or months for acid output to return close to preinfection levels, and in a proportion of patients output remains low. In general, as the hypochlorhydria seen in the acute phase of infection is short-lived, early *H. pylori* gastritis is typically antrum-predominant.

EARLY H. PLYORI INFECTION: *H. pylori* colonization is usually accompanied by inflammation. This involves secretion of a protein that decreases acid secretion, allowing colonization, potent neutrophil chemokines, and mast cell degranulation that increases polymorph immigration.[140–142] *Helicobacter pylori* density, and the presence of a PAI (see previous discussion), influence the severity of inflammation and subsequent damage over the course of lifelong infection.

Early *H. pylori* gastritis is typically antral predominant where gastric acidity is reduced by antral mucin. The antrum shows diffuse superficial or full-thickness infiltration by lymphocytes, eosinophils and plasma cells, occasional lymphoid follicles, and variable infiltration with neutrophils within the lamina propria but more commonly infiltrating the foveolar and surface epithelium. In early *H. pylori* gastritis, inflammation in the gastric corpus is mild, superficial, or even absent[120,143] (Fig. 13-20A,B). Inflammatory sequelae, such as intestinal metaplasia, are for the most part (initially) confined to the antrum or angulus.

Early *H. pylori* gastritis is often characterized by an exaggerated gastrin response to meals and other stimuli,[144] which precipitates an increase in acid secretion enough to cause duodenal ulcer disease in some patients. A consistent histologic finding associated with marked duodenitis occurring in some patients with early *H. pylori* gastritis is surface

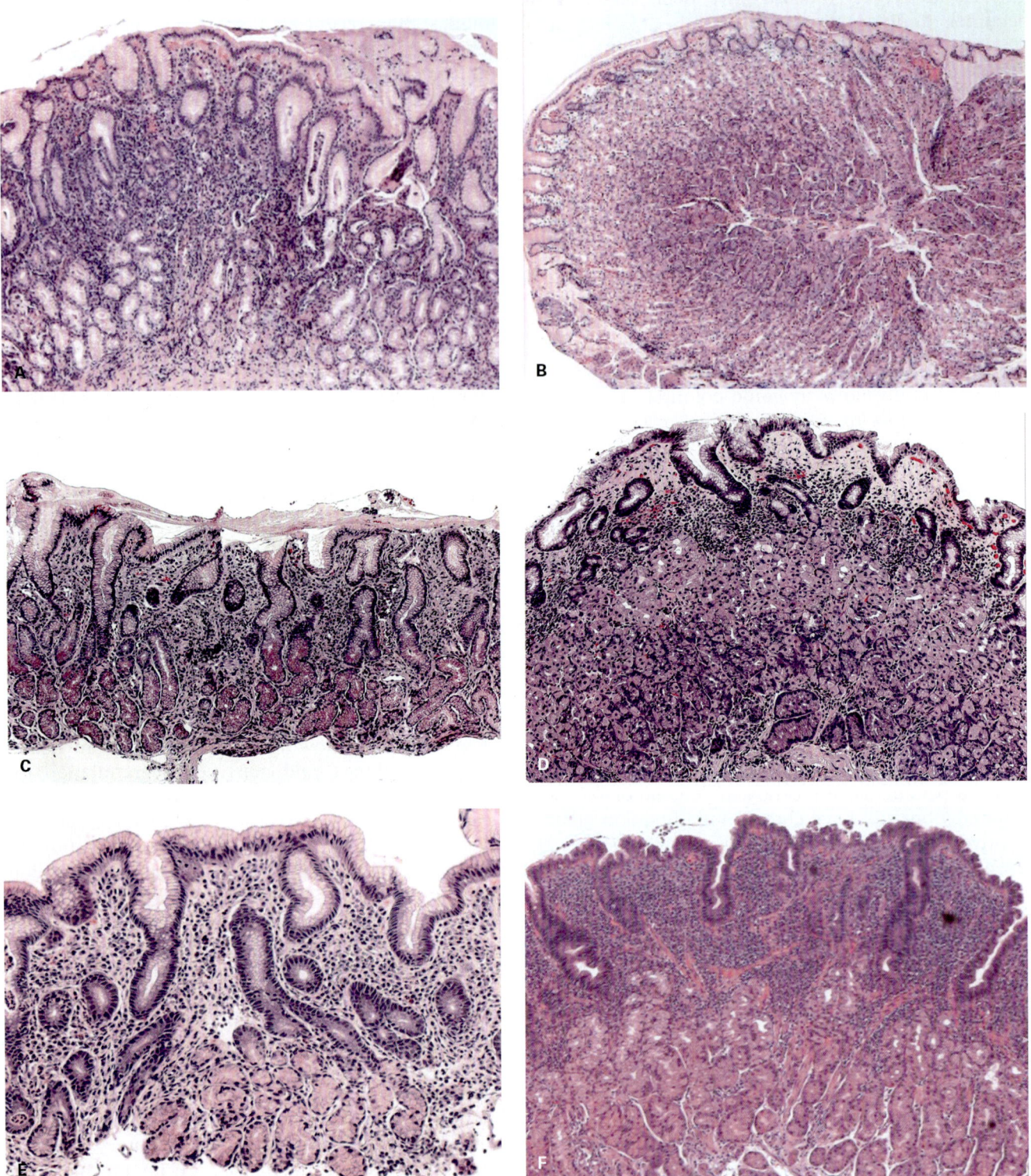

Figure 13-20. Stages in the natural history of *H. pylori*. Biopsies from the antrum are on the left and the oxyntic mucosa on the right. **A,B:** Initial infection affects the antrum with minimal involvement of the oxyntic mucosa. **C,D:** Over time this extends to the oxyntic mucosa so that there is superficial inflammation but no atrophy. **E,F:** Ultimately the chronic inflammation extends into the specialized mucosa with gland loss. (This can also be exaggerated or mimicked with long-term PPI use.)

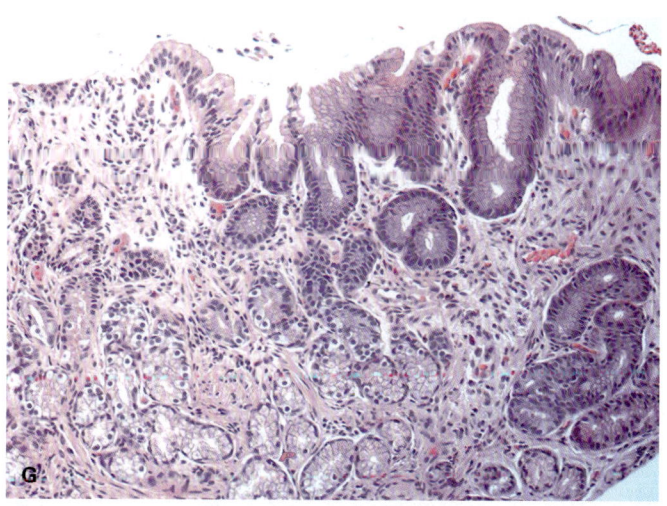
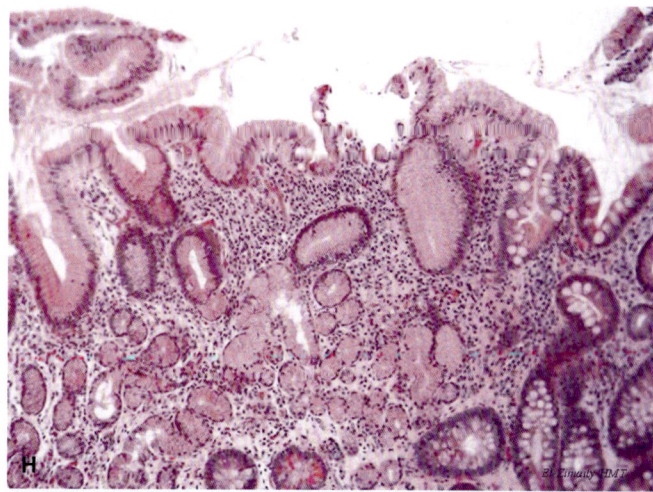

Figure 13-20. *(Continued)* **G,H:** Finally the oxyntic mucosa becomes lost completely and is replaced by pseudopyloric metaplasia, as shown here (invariably with endocrine cell hyperplasia), or with intestinal mucosa. The inflammation in the antral mucosa varies from virtually none when there is severe hypochlorhydria to modest if there is still sufficient acid secretion to support antral organisms (which require acid to prevent their urease causing too alkaline an environment).

gastric metaplasia—patches of gastric type mucous cells interspersed between the absorptive and goblet cells of the duodenal epithelium. *Helicobacter pylori*, when present in the duodenum, can only be identified in areas with gastric metaplasia. It is hypothesized that in the duodenum, similar to the gastric mucosa proper, *H. pylori* induces inflammation and erosions where it resides—gastric metaplasia (and heterotopia) patches,[145] although in our experience this has a low yield (see subsequent section on duodenal disease). As such, the prevalence of duodenal gastric metaplasia is much lower in "healthy" volunteers.[145]

ADVANCED H. PYLORI INFECTION: With sustained *H. pylori* infection, there is a gradual reduction of acid-producing mucosa because of gradual proximal spread of inflammation that facilitates *H. pylori*'s proximal migration. *Helicobacter pylori* colonization is accompanied by the inflammation. As there is a gradual reduction in the acid-producing mucosa,[146-148] the inflammatory front advances proximally with disease progression (Fig. 13-20B). The development of hypochlorhydria and even achlorhydria, including use of PPIs, facilitates proximal migration of the bacteria, which allows the development of corpus gastritis, and eventually corpus atrophy (Fig. 13-20C,D). This is the setting in which gastric ulcer and later gastric carcinoma develops (see Fig. 13-1).

The natural history of *H. pylori* gastritis is for the inflammation to progress diffusely from the antrum into the adjacent corpus resulting in an atrophic front of advancing corpus injury (that may be visible endoscopically to the trained eye—Fig. 13-21), leading to a reduction in acid secretion and eventually loss of parietal cells and development of corpus atrophy.[120,149,150] The front progresses uniformly and so appears to advance faster on the lesser curve (Fig. 13-22). This scenario is accelerated in clinical situations associated with low acid secretion such as chronic therapy with PPIs—widely used in gastroesophageal reflux disease (GERD)[151-153] (Fig. 13-23). Thus, antral-predominant gastritis may in some instances represent an earlier stage of atrophic pangastritis, these patterns representing two ends of the spectrum of "*H. pylori* infection" rather than mutually exclusive diseases.[14,120,154]

***H. pylori* diagnosis.** Depending on endoscopy need, diagnostic testing for *H. pylori* can be divided into invasive and noninvasive methods.[155] Noninvasive methods do not require endoscopy and include serology and urea breath test. Invasive tests require endoscopy; this group includes tests for urease, histology, and culture. The choice of test depends on the clinical situation (e.g., patient requires evaluation with upper endoscopy) and on other issues such as cost, availability, population prevalence of infection, pretest probability of infection, and factors such as the use of PPIs and antibiotics, which may influence certain test results.

Noninvasive methods

1. **Serology:** Antibodies to IgG and IgA have been used successfully to study the epidemiology of *H. pylori* in different populations in different parts of the world. However, serology remains positive long after successful treatment of the infection and cannot be used to assess treatment outcome.

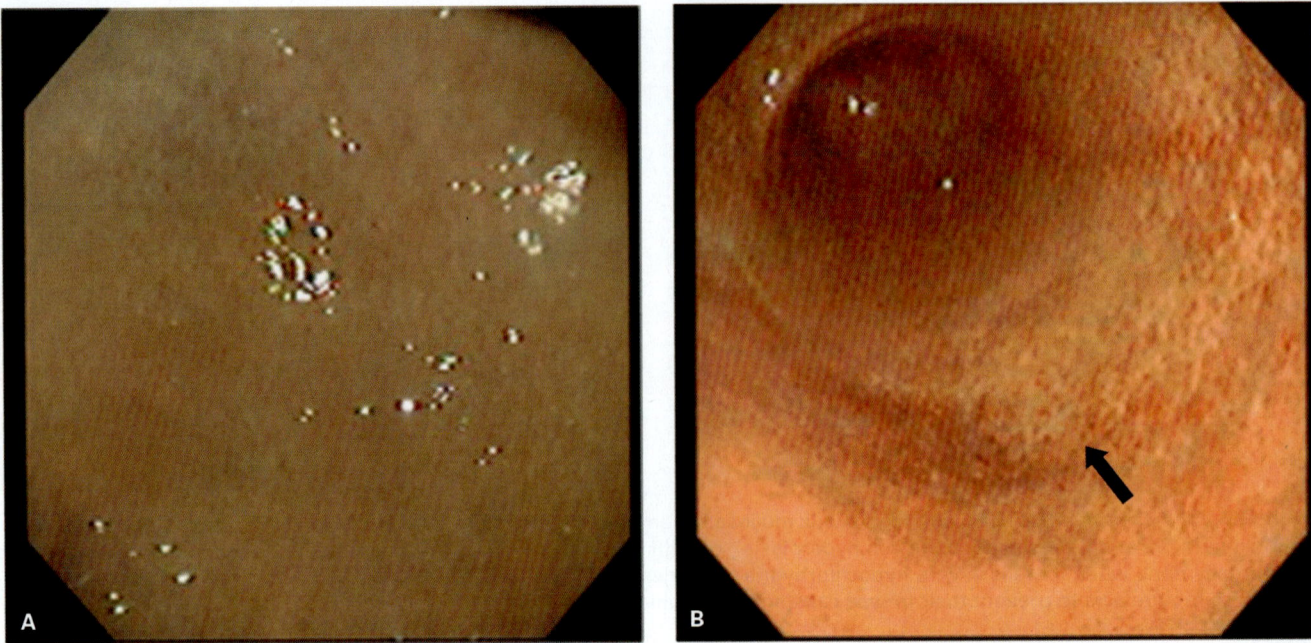

Figure 13-21. **Left panel** shows the natural and indistinct transition from antral oxyntic mucosa. That on the **right** shows the atrophic front (*arrow*). Prior to the rediscovery of *H. pylori*, this was thought to be an aging change. (Courtesy of Dr. Taiji Akamatsu.)

Serologic tests are often species specific (*H. pylori*) and can be negative with infection with other *Helicobacter* species, for example, *Helicobacter heilmannii*. In addition, inaccurate tests are also more common in the elderly and in patients with cirrhosis in whom specificity can be compromised. As a result, other techniques are preferred in these settings.[156–158]

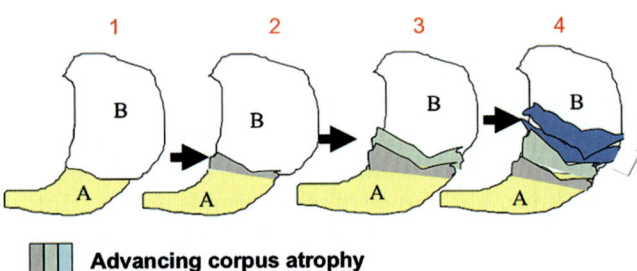

Figure 13-22. Advancing gastritis with time. "A" depicts *Helicobacter*-inflamed antrum and "B" *Helicobacter*-inflamed or possibly normal corpus/oxyntic mucosa. *1.* No atrophy. *2.* Atrophy is thought to begin at the junction of the antral–corpus junction and spreads proximally in a cone-like manner. Often this equates with the angulus but the histologic junction is variable. *3.* With time the cone extends proximally, but *4.* Because the lesser curve is much shorter than the greater curve, the lesser curve is completely atrophic long before the greater curve and fundus. It is therefore possible to have biopsies from the lesser curve with complete atrophy and metaplasia but relatively normal oxyntic mucosa on the greater curve.

2. **Urea breath tests**, with ^{13}C or more widely available ^{14}C, provide a powerful, noninvasive tool for research. The principle is that the carbon-labeled urea is hydrolyzed by the urease in the *H. pylori*, if present, resulting in the formation of ammonia and carbon dioxide. The amount of labeled carbon dioxide in the breath is then measured.[159] The urea breath test provides an accurate assessment of *H. pylori* status that rivals histology for being the gold standard,[159] but can be negative in cases with a very low level of infection.

3. **Stool antigen**: The presence of *H. pylori* in the stool of infected patients has led to the development of fecal assays.[160–162] The stool assay shares a limitation of tests that use urease as a marker for the organism.[163,164] Though this is a noninvasive method, any of us who has been asked for a stool specimen might sympathize with its difficulty.

Invasive methods

1. **Rapid urease test** is based on the organism's urease activity. It can be used at the "bedside" in the endoscopy unit. A gastric biopsy specimen is placed in contact with a pellet or solution that contains urea and a pH color indicator. The color changes when the pH rises above 6.0 as a result of hydrolysis of urea to ammonia.[165]

2. **Culture:** Although culture is the theoretical gold standard as there is an excellent correlation with histologic identification, in practice and in many research studies, histologic identification is used as the gold standard. One reason is that in many

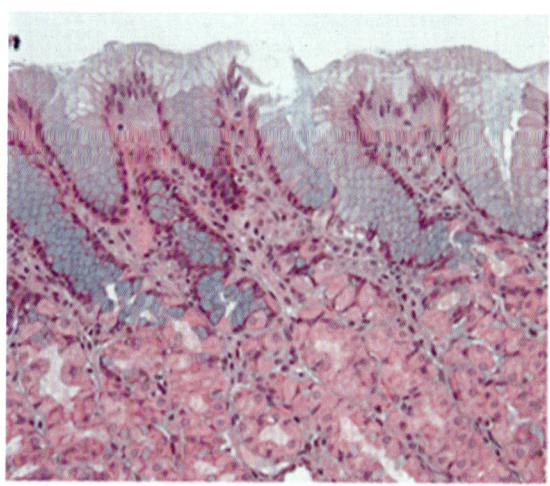 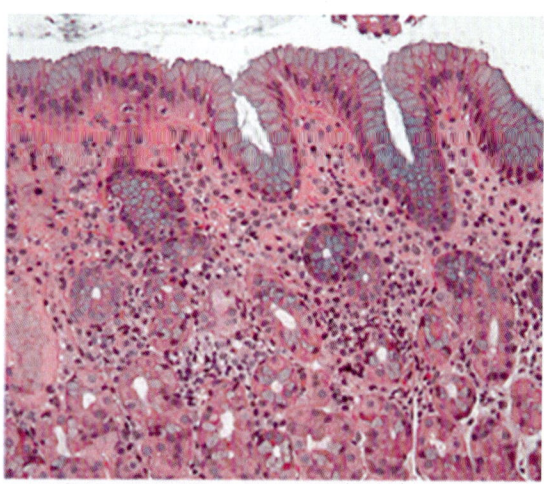

Figure 13-23. Oxyntic mucosa before and after a 2-week course of PPIs in a *Helicobacter*-positive patient. The increase in chronic inflammation over this time frame is readily apparent.

laboratories, cultures are less frequently positive than histology and serology. This may be due to the fact that small numbers of organisms cannot always be cultured or identified, and also because there is varying expertise in different laboratories for culturing these organisms. In general, *H. pylori* is a fastidious and slow-growing organism that is difficult to culture.[166]

3. **Histology** is currently considered the "gold standard" for detecting the infection for both untreated individuals and following therapy. The advantages of histology include the ability to document *H. pylori* infection, the degree of inflammation, and any associated pathology such as intestinal metaplasia, cancer, or lymphoma. The detection of organisms is enhanced by using special staining techniques discussed subsequently with their pros and cons in different clinical scenarios (see Table 13-9).

What are we looking for and where? *Helicobacter pylori* is a small (3 × 0.5 μm), gram-negative, wavy rod-shaped bacteria. The organisms can be visualized on the luminal side of gastric surface and pit mucous cells, in or near the adherent mucous. Often the organisms seem to cluster near more normal-appearing mucous cells (Fig. 13-24) rather than near those exhibiting severe mucous depletion. A similar situation applies when *H. pylori* is associated with erosive gastritis. That is, the organisms do not overlie the erosion or the very reactive mucosa immediately adjacent to it; rather, they are present in adjacent, less abnormal mucosa. Also, as discussed in the subsequent section on duodenitis, *H. pylori* can sometimes be seen in the duodenum only in association with gastric surface cell metaplasia. Although we look for its characteristic shape, only a small proportion of organisms are in the plane of section and so have the characteristic shape.

Hematoxylin and Eosin: Few studies report the accuracy of an H&E stain,[167,168] and it varies with the type of stain used. Experienced pathologists overall will have higher accuracy than junior pathologists in evaluating H&E-stained slides.[168] Even the staining intensity varies among biopsies within a given laboratory even in the same batch, and they are especially difficult to see if all are adherent to the epithelium. Nonetheless, within and between biopsy specimens there is often considerable variation in the numbers of organisms. H&E-stained slides have low sensitivity, in particular, in biopsies with low bacterial density.[168] This is particularly observed in patients using PPIs, in patients who recently received antibiotics, but also if biopsies are only taken from one part of the stomach instead of both antrum and oxyntic mucosa. Typically, there is chronic inflammation, but few or rare *H. pylori* organisms, and minimal or no active inflammation.

It is also important to remember that studies evaluating H&E stains are not evaluating the same stain. Though H&E stain is the most widely used stain in medical diagnosis, there are a large number of H&E protocols. Primary differences are dye composition, staining protocol, and intensity of the blue dye. Staining contrast (including *H. pylori*) differ depending upon the approach that is used. For example, there are actually two very closely related compounds commonly referred to as eosin. Eosin Y (also known as eosin Y ws or eosin yellowish) that is the most often used, and has a slightly yellowish cast. The other eosin compound is eosin B (eosin bluish or imperial

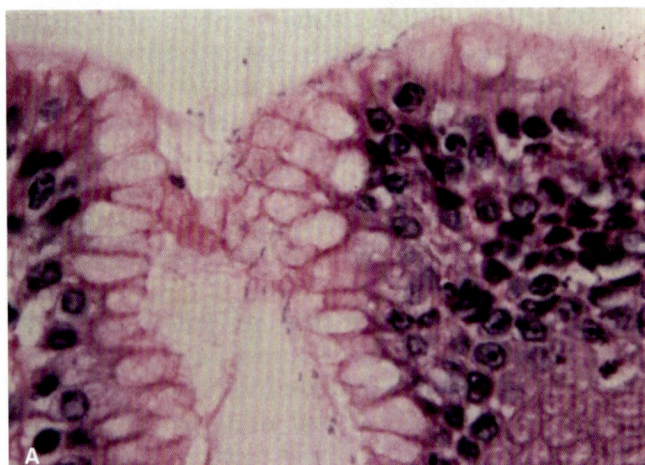
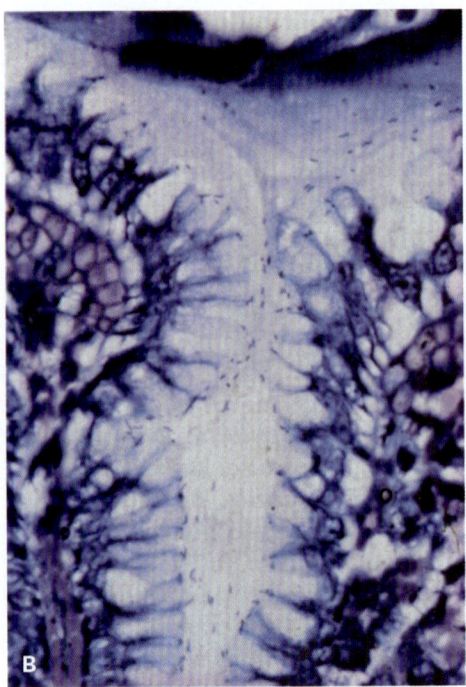

Figure 13-24. **A:** Detail (high dry) view of *H. pylori* organisms at the entrance of a gastric pit. With a little experience, they can be recognized (as gray-blue) in conventionally stained sections. **B:** Higher-power (×600) view showing the organisms more clearly with a modified Giemsa stain.

red) and has a faint bluish cast. The two dyes are interchangeable, and selection of a particular eosin (or H&E protocol) is more a matter of preference and tradition. Overall, evaluating sections stained only with H&E leads to inconsistent results and special stains have been recommended whenever inflammation is present and organisms are not readily identifiable on an H&E stain.[13]

However, if organisms are clearly identified on H&E stain in the presence of a compatible inflammatory infiltrate, this is usually adequate for diagnostic purposes. A useful rule of thumb is that, for any diagnosis of *H. pylori*, you have to be able to "photograph it and stand up in court and defend the diagnosis." If this cannot be done, then a special stain is needed. Deciding when to order a special stain is itself fraught with problems, and such a "pragmatic approach" leads to underdiagnosing *Helicobacter* infection about 10% of the time when a decision is made on whether "sufficient" inflammation is present to justify ordering the special stain. Overall, pathologists do not appreciate how little inflammation may be seen in some biopsies with *Helicobacter* (see Fig. 13-19). While one could argue that if there is little inflammation, then the chances of that organism producing complications are small. This may not hold true if, for example, only antral biopsies are obtained showing only scant inflammation and no *Helicobacter*, as these may be ravaging the oxyntic mucosa.

Policies for Detecting Helicobacter There is no "correct" protocol for histologic diagnosis of Helicobacter, and it depends on numerous factors that can be the driving force including the following:

1. The likelihood of organisms being present. In some populations, the positive rate is 10% to 20%, and in other >80%. In some commercial labs, it may even be supplier dependent; for an endoscopy group, serving a Western-white population may have an incidence that is <10%, whereas one serving, for example, a primary immigrant population from high *Helicobacter* prevalence areas, may have a rate in excess of 90%.
2. Commitment to turn-around time (TAT). Even though the vast majority of biopsies really are nonurgent, if a lab is committed to, for example, a 24-hour TAT, then this becomes the driving force. and an H&E and good special stain (silver or immunostain) may be done routinely. While in some biopsies the organisms may be easily visible at a first glance, opinions on how much time should one spend on one biopsy hunting for the organisms on H&E stain may vary when these are not that readily visible. This also gets into the issues of resource utilization and individual ego, where some take extra pride in their ability to find the organisms on H&E stain only and saving money (for the patient or institution). However, if the biopsies are normal, or the organisms are overtly detectable on the H&E stain, one can raise an ethical question of justification to bill for tests that were not really required. Unfortunately while opinions are many, evidence-based guidelines are lacking.

3. Economics—likely, the cheapest way to make the histologic diagnosis is to try and make the diagnosis on an H&E stain when there may be no inflammation or organisms and others with a typical *Helicobacter* pattern of inflammation and readily identifiable organisms. However, if inflammation is present but organisms are not identified, it is best to do a special stain. The choice of the stain is a matter of personal choice, available resources, and emphasis on TAT. One could start with a "quick and cheap" stain (e.g., Giemsa stain) that, if positive, solves the problem, but if it is negative or equivocal, one can order a more sensitive and specific stain (silver stain or immunostain) or alternatively do the more expensive but sensitive stains at the outset. Unfortunately, in this regard, any data on cost-efficiency are lacking.

4. Clinical factors—if the patient has a bleeding ulcer, this is far more critical than when biopsies are taken for long-standing symptoms, and the patient is returning in 2 weeks for the results.

Special stains for *H. pylori* identification—which is best? Most pathologists use H&E plus a second stain for *H. pylori* visualization. The appearance of the organism varies with the staining technique used. Commonly used special stains can be divided arbitrarily into (a) silver-based stains, (b) non–silver-based stains, and (c) immunohistochemistry. Silver stains are more expensive, but organisms appear larger and there is contrast with the background, so small numbers of organisms are easier to identify. With few exceptions, non–silver-based methods try to detect small blue organisms on a blue background, so unless organisms are numerous they can be difficult to detect. Immunohistochemistry is an alternative to silver stains, primarily because the organisms are readily identifiable. It has the potential advantage of not picking up other organisms that may be present in the stomach (enteric, oral), which can proliferate in patients with atrophy or who are taking PPIs. Some labs use an immunostain initially, while others use a silver stain. Pathologists are faced with several types of stains to choose from. No stain is perfect.

Pathology laboratories vary in their resources. Silver-based stains and immunohistochemistry stains can be ideal in some laboratories but a technician's (and a pathologist's) nightmare in others. The best stain is the one that works in your laboratory bearing in mind that an H&E stain interpreted by inexperienced pathology staff is the least sensitive and the least specific, although frequently possible, while absolutely normal biopsies can similarly be identified that do not require a special stain. Silver and immunostains done well are the most sensitive and specific. A special stain is recommended to facilitate *H. pylori* diagnosis (Table 13-6). However, the best stain in the world is of no value if the biopsies provided are insufficient or

Table 13-6 Stains for Detection of *Helicobacter pylori*

STAIN	SENSITIVE	TECHNICAL TIME	COST	COMMENTS
Cresyl violet/Diff-Quik and variants	Intermediate	10 min	Low	H&E necessary
El-Zimaity dual stain[169]	High	28 min (9 min with autostainer)	Intermediate	Good for duodenal gastric metaplasia and specimens with very few bacteria; epithelial and lymphoid nuclei can look atypical
El-Zimaity's modification of Genta[173]	High	28 min (9 min with autostainer)	Intermediate	Only stain needed; epithelial and lymphoid nuclei can look atypical
El-Zimaity triple stain[834,835]	High	5 min	Low	Only stain needed
Genta[170]	High	74 min (50 min with autostainer)	High	Only stain needed; epithelial and lymphoid nuclei can look atypical; some find it technically difficult[172]
Giemsa	Intermediate	11 min	Low	False positive[168]; H&E necessary
H&E	Low	17 min	Low	Another stain needed
Immunohistochemistry	High	As other immunostains	High	H&E also necessary
Leung[176]	High	10 min	Low	H&E also necessary
Steiner	High	28 min	High	Sometimes high background (deposits); epithelial and lymphoid nuclei can look atypical; H&E necessary
Warthin–Starry (or modified Steiner)	High	28 min	High	Sometimes high background (deposits)—autostainers tend to be much cleaner and reliable; epithelial and lymphoid nuclei can look atypical; H&E necessary

Stains are listed in alphabetic order. Other stains used for *H. pylori* identification but not included in this table include Half-Gram, Brown-Hopps, Toluidine Orange, Acridine Orange–ultraviolet fluorescence, and Butler Modified Wright stain.

inadequate to answer the question "Does the patient have *Helicobacter* gastritis?"

(a) **Silver-based stains** produce dense, black, fine deposit of silver and silver oxide where the silver ions have been reduced. Silver impregnation makes *H. pylori* appear larger, making detection easier (Fig. 13-25A–C). This is particularly useful in patients on PPI where bacteria present are fewer in number and generally smaller in size. The Warthin–Starry and the modified Steiner stains are commonly used. In addition, silver techniques are so sensitive that they can sometimes give nonspecific background deposits ("dirty preparations"). Background deposits are less frequently seen with El-Zimaity dual stain[169] and the Genta stain,[170] or on some automated staining machines. The El-Zimaity dual stain was introduced for the simultaneous visualization of the bacteria and gastric metaplasia in the duodenum. However, since gastric mucin is always positive for periodic acid-Schiff (PAS) (glycoprotein), this stain has proven

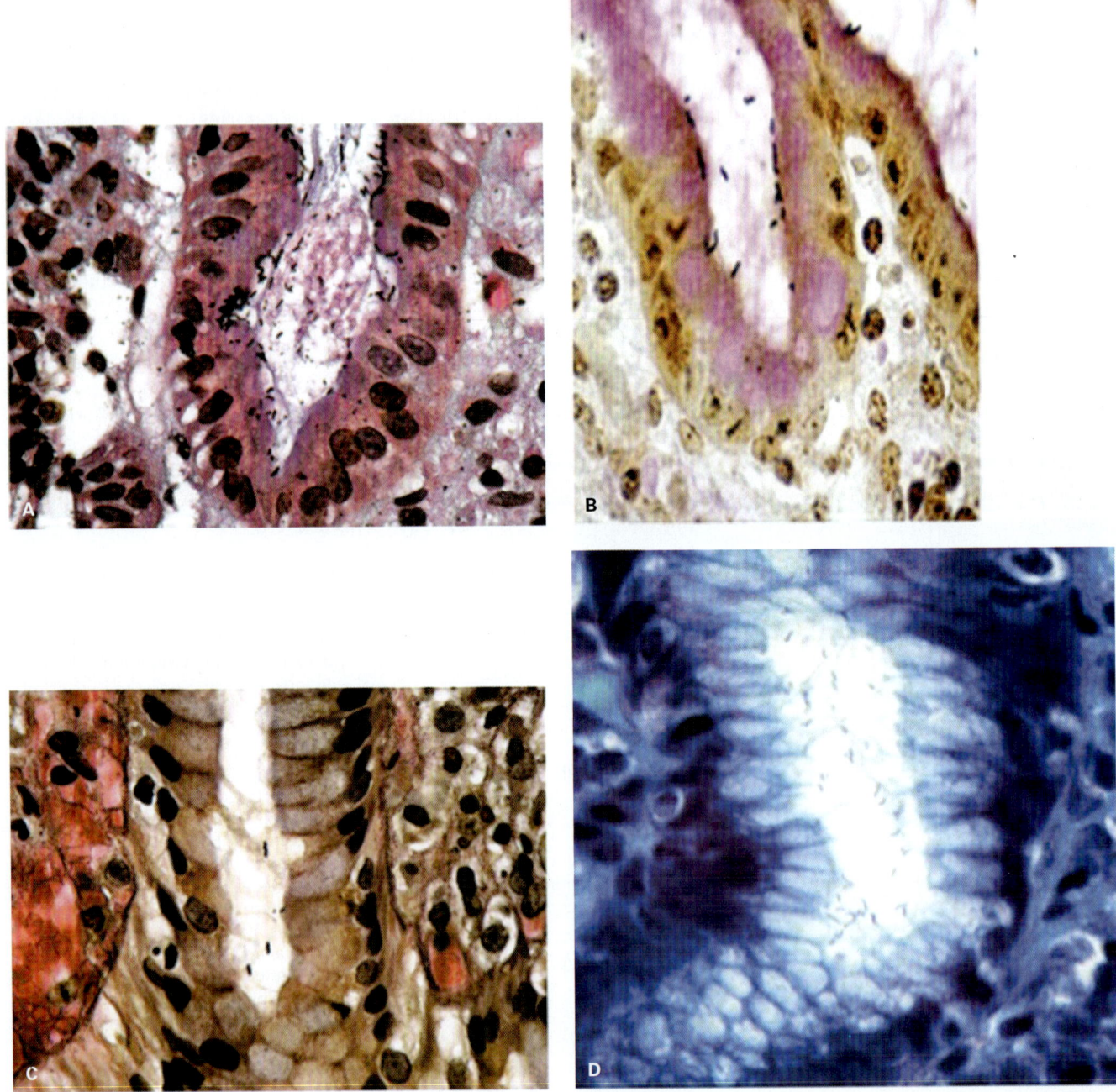

Figure 13-25. *Helicobacter pylori* as demonstrated by a variety of stains. The first three are silver stains—**A**: Genta. **B**: El-Zimaity Dual PAS Silver. **C**: Warthin–Starry. The second three are nonsilver stains—**D**: Diff-Quik.

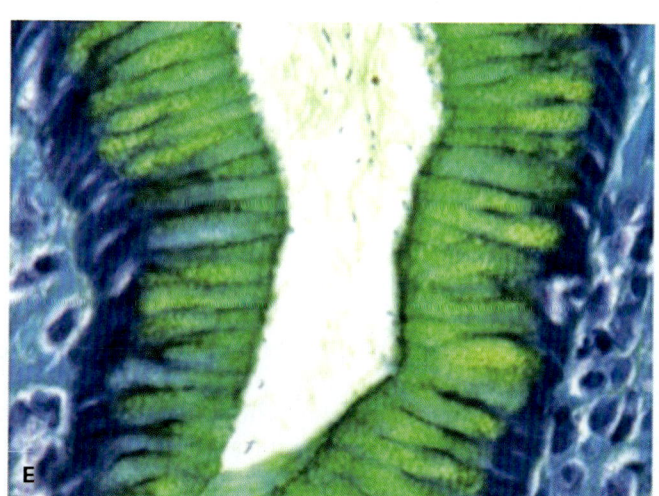
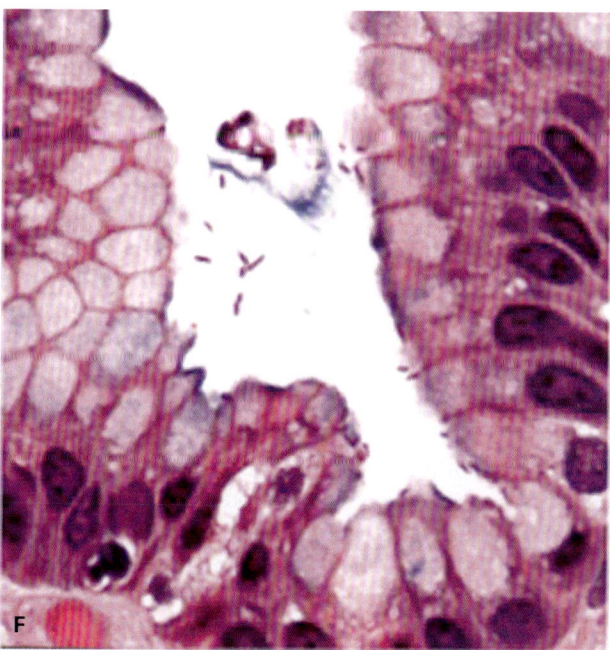

Figure 13-25. *(Continued)* **E:** Alcian yellow. **F:** Triple stain with carbol–fuchsin.

useful when only few bacteria are present.[171] The Genta stain is particularly useful in high-workload laboratories as only one slide is reviewed (instead of H&E and another stain); the stain can be technically challenging in some laboratories.[172] For laboratories that cannot use uranyl nitrate, the modified Genta stain[173] can be used instead; this uses lead nitrate as a substitute, together with Alcian blue and an H&E stain. In general, background deposits are less frequently seen with slides processed using the autostainer. Silver-based methods have the disadvantage of being relatively more expensive, cannot be discarded into the drains as it is a heavy metal poison, and the stain does not work in improperly fixed tissue (e.g., if the formalin used is too diluted).

(b) In **non–silver-based stains**, (Fig. 13-25D–F), the dye tints the bacteria with a color. For example, the bacteria are blue with Diff-Quik, crystal violet, and Giemsa stains.[168,174] In contrast to silver-based stains, visualizing the bacteria totally depends on the contrast between the bacteria and tissue sections. The Diff-Quik has the better sensitivity and specificity; the Giemsa stain has suboptimal accuracy (more false-positive results)[168,175] especially with less experienced pathologists. The lack of contrast between organism and background renders specimen evaluation for *H. pylori* infection rather arduous, which is reflected in the time required to examine slides, especially when multiple biopsies are present and several serial sections on the slide may need to be examined to be convinced that *H. pylori* is either present or absent.[168]

In this group, we prefer Leung's Alcian yellow stain;[176] it is easier to spot blue (but still small) bacteria against yellow gastric mucin, compared with blue organisms in paler blue mucin with other stains. These stains are relatively inexpensive and thus are commonly used. Though we prefer silver-based stains, tinctorial stains do not require optimum formalin fixation. This group of stains is particularly disadvantaged by mucus and debris that can mimic the presence of *H. pylori*. In equivocal situations (common with chronic PPI use), pathologists may err on the side of overcalling the presence of any bacteria present as *H. pylori*. This might seem unimportant. However, *H. pylori* infection is absent in up to 27% of patients with endoscopically proven duodenal ulcers.[177] Such patients appear to have a significantly worse outcome when treated empirically for the infection,[178] almost certainly because they were also ingesting NSAIDs.

(c) **Immunohistochemistry** is perceived as the gold standard by some investigators as in some settings immunohistochemistry reduces the false positive rate, providing greater accuracy over routine histochemistry.[179] Both polyclonal and monoclonal antibodies are commercially available. In addition, in some laboratories, immunohistochemical stains are performed using an autostainer, which translates into less technical time and less technical training. It is our experience that cases with few bacteria can also be missed with immunostains. We have also seen other *Helicobacter* species (*H. heilmannii*) stain positive with antibodies (especially polyclonal) for *H. pylori*, and morphologic differences in their spiral morphology are difficult to detect on immunostains. Importantly, anti–*H. pylori* antibodies also stain the coccoid forms of the bacteria. These forms may possibly be viable but are nonculturable, and one study suggests less virulent, and less likely to colonize and induce inflammation.[180] Coccoid forms have never (yet) been shown to be viable; further, coccoid organisms can come from the small bowel and oral cavity, so basing a diagnosis of *Helicobacter* gastritis only on coccoid forms of organisms should arguably never be made, or at least should be stated clearly in the pathology report. Similar to silver-based methods, optimal specimen processing (i.e., formalin fixative) is necessary for immunohistochemistry. Fluorescent antibodies are unpopular because in addition to requiring the use of fluorescent microscopes, they fade over time, and so do not provide a permanent record.

Role of Biopsy Site(s) in Determining H. pylori Infection

While histology may be considered a gold standard, the reliability of detecting *H. pylori* infection is actually dependent on the site, number, and size of gastric biopsies, as well as stain used and expertise in staining to visualize the bacteria. False-negative and -positive interpretations are all too easy. The standard of two biopsies from the antrum and two from the oxyntic mucosa covers most eventualities. Stripping of surface epithelium, that seems to occur readily in oxyntic mucosa, is a good reason to always take 2 oxyntic biopsies. Some use a combination of three biopsies (angulus, greater curvature of the corpus, and greater curvature of the antrum) (see Fig. 13-2), which seems to be the minimum for accurate diagnosis.[136] When biopsy specimens had few *H. pylori* per slide, the same patient had biopsies from other areas with more bacteria. This emphasizes the need to obtain multiple biopsies to exclude *H. pylori* infection.[136] In patients treated with PPIs, antibiotics or other antibacterials such as bismuth salts 2 to 4 weeks prior to biopsy, the bacteria may be restricted to the corpus or fundus, and as small numbers of organisms may be present, really need a silver or immunostain if not detected using other stains.

Failure to Biopsy Both Oxyntic and Antral Mucosa—Major Cause of Failure to Detect Helicobacter

When biopsies are taken for *Helicobacter* detection, it becomes important to ensure that both antral and oxyntic mucosa are biopsied, as when the organisms are present, biopsying only one site is a major reason for failure of detection. It will be recalled that *H. pylori* infection is initially primarily an antral disease, and oxyntic mucosa may show only minimal superficial inflammation, and organisms may be impossible to detect. Conversely with time, atrophy of oxyntic mucosa, or PPI therapy, may result in the organism moving proximally, at which point it may no longer be detectable in the antrum. When only antral or oxyntic mucosa is biopsied, the false-negative reading for *Helicobacter* is about 10% to 15% (El-Zimaity H e-pub Canadian J Gastroenterol).

Major reasons for failing to obtain both antral and oxyntic biopsies when the endoscopist believes both sites have been biopsied include the following:

1. The endoscopists believe that the antrum is the preferred site for *Helicobacter*, so never biopsy the oxyntic mucosa.
2. Many endoscopists do not appreciate that the histologic antrum is often quite distal in the anatomical antrum, so that the prepyloric region needs to be biopsied to guarantee getting antral mucosa, although this may also fail if the anrum has diffuse intestinal metaplasia. Some endoscopists always attempt to obtain biopsies from both antral and oxyntic mucosa, but others tend to obtain three oxyntic and one antral or all oxyntic mucosa, and are quite surprised when the "comment" states that all biopsies are from one site—invariably oxyntic when "random gastric biopsies" are taken.
3. If there is an atrophic front that passes unrecognized endoscopically (Fig. 13-21), and the mucosa is also not recognized as being atrophic, and it is as biopsied a presumed oxyntic mucosa, then the latter will not be obtained.

Differential diagnosis of the H. pylori organisms. Chains of cocci may be seen and only occasionally are confused with *H. pylori*. It is possible that in some instances these cocci represent degenerate forms of the organisms.[180] Confusion with enterococcal gastritis, which is rare, can occur, primarily if one is unaware of its existence, and when immunostains are not used[67] (see Fig. 13-15). Numerous organisms, often mixed cocci, rods, and even fungi can be seen on patients on long-term PPIs (Fig. 13-26). Determining whether *Helicobacter* are present amongst an admixture of organisms is one situation in which an immunostain is far superior to all other blanket bacterial stains including silver stains.

Another artifact is that the apices of mucous cells may be cut in a plane such that they may look like a curved organism, but always in the same direction, so that only one-half of the "wave" is present. *Helicobacter heilmannii* are larger (2.5–10 μm) than *H. pylori* and are much less frequently observed. These organisms contain four to nine even spirals along their length and are frequently arranged in stacks.

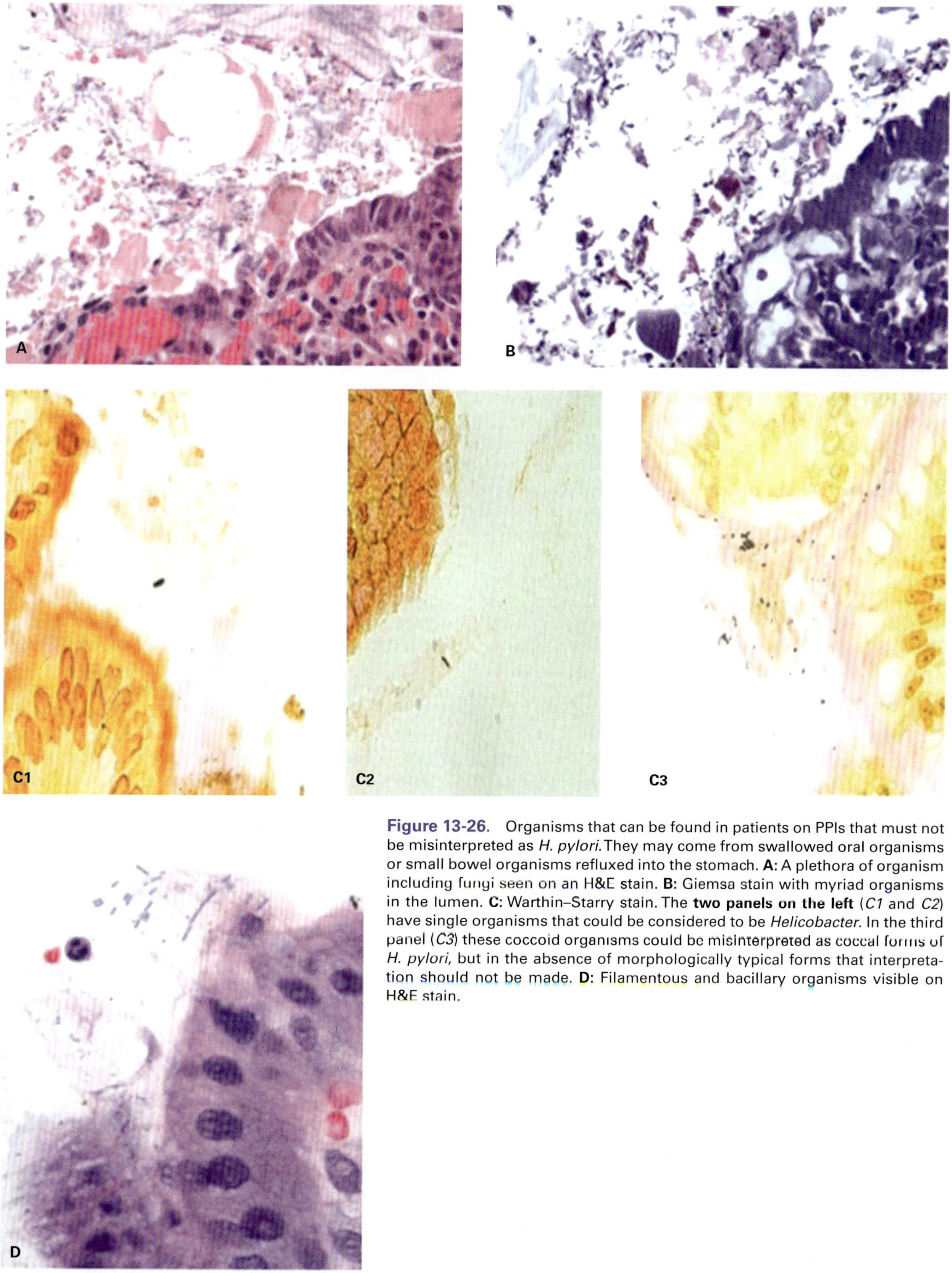

Chapter 13 Stomach and Proximal Duodenum: Inflammatory and Miscellaneous Disorders

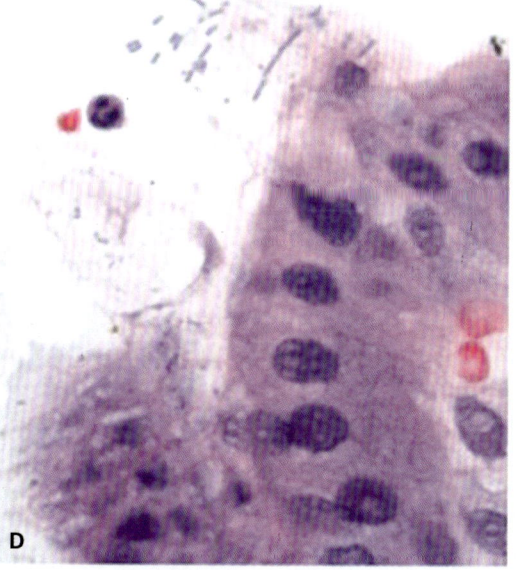

Figure 13-26. Organisms that can be found in patients on PPIs that must not be misinterpreted as *H. pylori*. They may come from swallowed oral organisms or small bowel organisms refluxed into the stomach. **A:** A plethora of organism including fungi seen on an H&E stain. **B:** Giemsa stain with myriad organisms in the lumen. **C:** Warthin–Starry stain. The **two panels on the left** (*C1* and *C2*) have single organisms that could be considered to be *Helicobacter*. In the third panel (*C3*) these coccoid organisms could be misinterpreted as coccal forms of *H. pylori*, but in the absence of morphologically typical forms that interpretation should not be made. **D:** Filamentous and bacillary organisms visible on H&E stain.

Algorithm for Failing to Detect Helicobacter When the Morphology Suggests That They Should Be Present It is not infrequent to have gastric biopsies with a clinical question to rule out *H. pylori* ("R/O Hp"), and be faced with a morphology that suggests that *Helicobacter* should be present, but special stains fail to detect the organism. It is useful to have an algorithm for dealing with such biopsies. All of these are discussed in various sections of this chapter, but have been compiled together here for convenience.

1. *Was an appropriate special stain ordered?* (just H&E is unreliable.)
2. *False-negative stain.* If a blue-on-blue stain (Cresyl violet, Giemsa, Diff-Quick, etc.) was carried out, do a silver, dual, or immunostain.
3. *PPI changes.* If oxyntic mucosa is present, are there changes of PPI ingestion? PPIs can reduce *Helicobacter* to undetectable levels. Sometimes they may only be present deep in the oxyntic mucosa, sometimes only within parietal cells, when either silver or immunostains are usually necessary to detect them (see Fig. 13-22). Recent administration of PPIs however rapidly reduces numbers of *Helicobacter*, but the morphologic changes are not detectable on histology as it takes weeks for these changes to develop, so requires clinical input. Because PPIs may result in numerous organisms being able to grow in the stomach—both oral and duodenal, a *Helicobacter* immunostain is the stain of choice for determining if *Helicobacter* are present in and admixture of bacteria.
4. *Lymphocytic gastritis.* In addition to the lamina propria infiltrate, and especially if this is active (neutrophilic), is there an intraepithelial lymphocytosis? If so, lymphocytic gastritis frequently has no *Helicobacter*, but serology is positive, and treatment with eradication therapy results in healing of the gastritis. This form of lymphocytic gastritis is usually easily distinguished from the mild intraepithelial lymphocytosis associated with celiac disease.
5. *Diffuse reactive gastropathy.* Organisms are rarely found in the absence of mucin, so when there is diffuse reactive (chemical) gastropathy, *Helicobacter* are rarely found. In some conditions such as post–gastric resection or gastroenterostomy, there is pathologic duodenogastric reflux with resulting diffuse gastropathy. Even if *Helicobacter* are present proximally, marked mucin depletion can prevent their identification in the part of the stomach affected by reflux.
6. *Sampling. Are both antral and oxyntic mucosa present?* If not, this could well be the reason as 10% to 15% of patients with *Helicobacter* have them in only one site (El-Zimaity, E-pub Canadian J Gastroenterology).
7. *Intestinal metaplasia. Helicobacter* will not grow in intestinal type mucosa whether native or metaplastic. So if, for example, two antral biopsies are taken and both are completely metaplastic, no organisms may be detected. Unless the proximal mucosa is also sampled, the organisms will not be found.
8. *Atrophy with pseudopyloric metaplasia imitating antral mucosa without (or with minimal) intestinal metaplasia. Helicobacter* are not found in either the residual antral or metaplastic mucosa. However, to recognize this requires the ability to distinguish antral mucosa from oxyntic mucosa that has undergone complete atrophy with pseudopyloric metaplasia. This is usually part of the creeping atrophy that takes place in *Helicobacter* gastritis with time, rather than autoimmune gastritis.

If all biopsies appear to be antral (nonoxyntic), a hint to help identify pseudopyloric metaplasia is that one needs to evaluate if all biopsies are similar regarding inflammation and architecture. If different (e.g., one/some are inflamed or architecturally different—especially holes between the glands [atrophy] and one/some are noninflamed or with regular architecture), the likelihood is that the inflamed biopsies, which invariably have a degree of gland loss, represent oxyntic mucosa with atrophy and pseudopyloric metaplasia. An immunostain for gastrin will show the antral biopsies by the presence of G cells, while their lack indicates atrophic oxyntic mucosa. If gastrin stain is not available, then chromogranin A stain can serve a similar function, but now the distribution of endocrine cells needs to be evaluated. G cells primarily form a band below the mucous neck, with few or no cells in the pyloric glands. Conversely oxyntic mucosa has regularly spaced endocrine cells if normal, but with long-standing hypergasrtinemia resulting in their hyperplasia, these form chains (linear hyperplasia) and small clusters of endocrine cells (microcarcinoids), and they also migrate to the base of the crypt close to the muscularis mucosae. In some patients, these changes are detectable on H&E stain as the crypt bases can develop a double layer of nuclei, the outer layer being the endocrine cells.

9. *Other causes of diffuse gastritis*
   (a) Infections—CMV, syphilis, and other bacteria (*Micrococcus*). Immunostains to CMV if not visible on the H&E sections and *Treponema pallidum* (together with good clinical suspicion) are required for these to be considered.
   (b) An up-regulated immune system—IBD, especially Crohn's disease, in which a modest diffuse chronic superficial inflammation is often present. Appropriate clinical input is required for this.

10. *Recent administration of antibiotics or* Helicobacter *eradication therapy.* (This clearly needs clinical input.) The chronic inflammation following *Helicobacter* eradication can take months and sometimes over a year to completely subside. It is likely that rare instances of spontaneous eradication occur, or that eradication occurs when patients are put on antibiotics or other reasons. Either way, the chronic inflammation persists for a time.

11. *Idiopathic gastritis.* If the above have been excluded, there remains a group of patients in whom there appears to be no known cause despite extensive investigation. Pathologists seeing gastric biopsies regularly are well aware of this subgroup as it is not small and may account for perhaps 15% to 25% of biopsies. It therefore has to be acknowledged that there are a group of patients with chronic (less commonly chronic active) gastritis with no known cause. Fortunately, most of the gastritis is relatively mild and is *Helicobacter* negative in multiple biopsies and serologically. These are signed out simply as "chronic gastritis; *Helicobacter* are not identified". However, this diagnosis should not be used casually and until all other identifiable causes of inflammation resembling *Helicobacter* have been excluded as outlined above.

Atrophic gastritis and gastric atrophy. *Atrophic gastritis* refers to the finding of variable gland loss resulting from mucosal inflammation, often associated with metaplasia to either pyloric or intestinal types of mucosa. Although this term is most frequently applied to oxyntic mucosa, it can be applied to oxyntic mucosa, antrum, or both. In the antrum, atrophy is often associated with intestinal metaplasia that occupies the full thickness of the mucosa in all or part of a biopsy (Fig. 13-27). Complete or almost complete replacement of the antrum with intestinal metaplasia is associated with a higher cancer risk, even in the absence of corpus atrophy.[150]

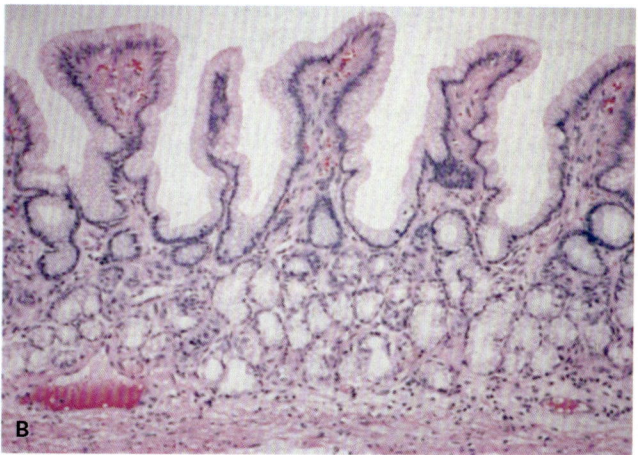

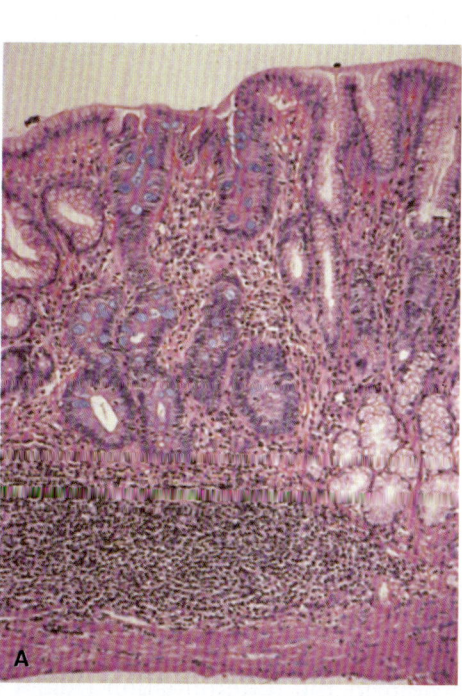

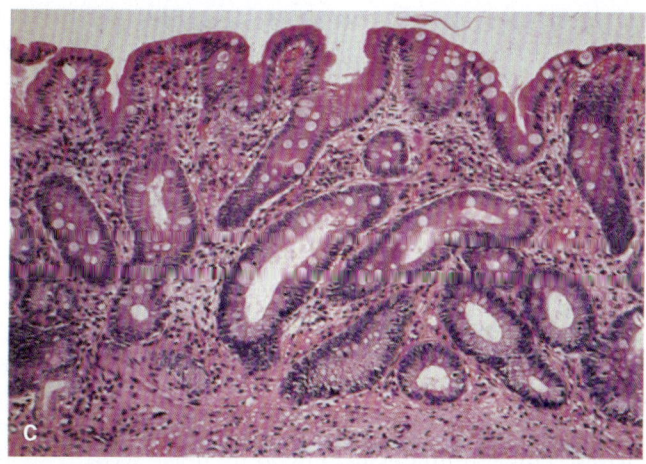

Figure 13-27. Atrophic antral gastritis. **A:** Atrophic antral gland gastritis. Much of the mucosa has been replaced (left two-thirds) by intestinal metaplasia and inflammatory cells in the lamina propria. Goblet cells stain blue in this H&E-Alcian blue, pH 2.5 stain. There are only a few residual antral mucous glands at the extreme right of the picture. **B:** Villiform normal antral gland mucosa (uncommon but not rare) should not be confused with intestinal metaplasia. The surface and pit epithelial cells are of the normal gastric mucous type. G-cells in the mucous neck region are not visible at this magnification. **C:** Complete atrophic gastritis of the antral gland mucosa with intestinal metaplasia occupying the full thickness of the mucosa.

Corpus atrophy begins at the junction between fundic and the antral mucosa.[85,181,182] This usually takes the form of loss of oxyntic glands with pseudopyloric, intestinal, and sometimes pancreatic metaplasia.[85,150,182] Corpus atrophy shifts proximally from the vicinity of the angulus circumferentially, such that the antrum appears to expand with advancing atrophic gastritis.[181,183] Corpus atrophy progresses at about the same rate in the contiguous greater curve, proximal half of the lesser curve, and neighboring anterior and posterior walls of the corpus.[150,181]

The rate of progression of *H. pylori* gastritis depends on the acid milieu. The natural history of *H. pylori* gastritis is to go through a cascade of events from nonatrophic gastritis, degrees of atrophic gastritis, and in some patients, dysplasia.[184-186] The atrophy involves loss of oxyntic glands with extension of mucous neck cells down into the pits (mucous cell hyperplasia—historically considered to be pseudopyloric metaplasia but the name persists). Intestinal metaplasia usually supervenes within this epithelium. However, on occasion isolated intestinal metaplasia may happen without adjacent pseudopyloric metaplasia. Presumably this is the result of focal injury, possibly related to NSAIDs or ASA, etc.

To increase our likelihood of identifying corpus atrophy—when present—it is important to remember five principles:

1. Corpus atrophy begins at the antrum–corpus junction. In the early stages of atrophic gastritis, for example, in children,[85] the location of early atrophy is only just proximal to the normal histologic antral–corpus border so that unless biopsies are taken from this region the atrophy will be missed (Fig. 13-22).[120]
2. Atrophy is gland loss with or without its replacement with fibrosis or metaplastic epithelium.[150,181,187]
3. The atrophic border extends proximally at a similar rate on both curvatures. However, because the lesser curve is much shorter than the greater curve, locations high on the greater curvature are among the last to undergo atrophy[150,181,187,188]; it is therefore also the best site to biopsy to find residual *Helicobacter* infection.
4. The presence of a dense mucosal mononuclear cells deep in the lamina propria is a predictor for the presence of gastric atrophy as the acid level will already be low.[189,190]
5. As the amount of atrophy increases, acid secretion diminishes. This stimulates G cells to increase gastrin secretion, G cells become hyperplastic, and there is hypertrophy of remaining parietal cells proximally, but a variable increase in the number of ECL cells in the body mucosa. This may be undetectable in residual oxyntic mucosa, but in the atrophic mucosa, there is ECL hyperplasia that varies from indiscernible to hyperplasia. It is basal and immediately above the muscularis mucosae, then linear hyperplasia; microcarcinoids may then form. However, while the tell-tale double row of nuclei may be visible above the muscularis mucosae, endocrine stains, especially chromogranin A (Fig. 13-28), and lack of gastrin staining, if that is available, help to make the diagnosis.

Recognizing Pseudopyloric Metaplasia (Mucous Cell Hyperplasia)

The normal oxyntic mucosa has straight glands composed of tightly packed chief and parietal cells, endocrine cells, and mucus cells. There is a higher ratio of glands to foveola (4–5:1) than the antrum (1–2:1). With continuous inflammation, there is a progressive loss of specialized cells. Eventually, the oxyntic glands are replaced by mucous cells extending down from the mucous neck regions, resembling antral/pyloric glands (pseudopyloric metaplasia), and failing to differentiate into parietal, chief, and endocrine cells (Fig. 13-28). The diagnosis of pseudopyloric metaplasia can be a diagnostic challenge as it is readily interpreted as antral mucosa. The diagnosis of pseudopyloric metaplasia, and its distinction from antral mucosa, can be facilitated by several methods (Fig. 13-28).

1. Because G cells are never seen in the body,[191] (other than rare cells in intestinal metaplasia), the absence of G cells is particularly useful in recognizing pseudopyloric metaplasia, or conversely the presence of G cells indicates that the mucosa is antral (Fig. 13-29). Gastrin immunostains are the easiest way of doing this.
2. Pepsinogen I (PGI), if available, is localized in chief cells, mucous-neck cells, and transitional mucous neck/chief cells of the human oxyntic mucosa[192]; it is not localized in antral gland cells (Fig. 13-29). Thus, it can also be used to differentiate antrum from oxyntic mucosa.[191]
3. Use both—ideal. Pseudopyloric metaplasia is identified by the presence of mucosa that superficially resembles antrum, stains positive for PGI, stains negative for G-cells, and is anatomically in a region where corpus would be expected[85,150] (Fig. 13-29).
4. The distribution of endocrine cells that can be highlighted with endocrine markers (chromogranin or synaptophysin—whichever works best) in the antrum and atrophic corpus mucosa can also help in the differentiation (Fig. 13-30). The normal endocrine cell staining in the antrum is intense, almost linear beneath the mucous neck region but above the bases of the crypts, while in oxyntic mucosa with pyloric metaplasia, it is initially represented by single cells diffusely

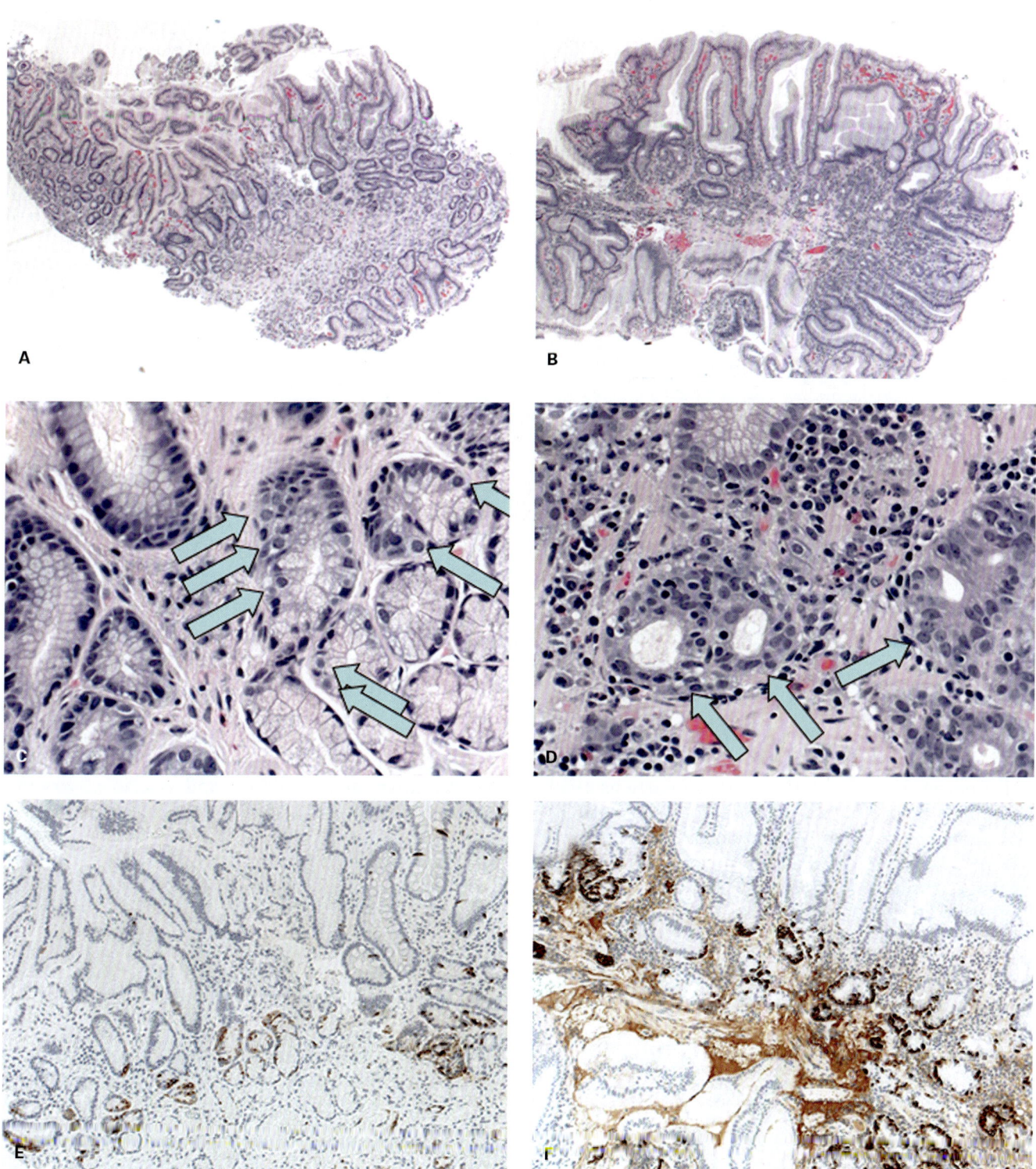

Figure 13-28. Two biopsies from the same patient to "rule out Hp." That on the left **(A)** is normal antral mucosa, and that on the right **(B)**, which is clearly not oxyntic, looks like inflamed antral mucosa. Note the architectural disarray in B at low power compared to A, as well as the additional inflammation. **C:** Numerous readily visible endocrine cells (mainly G cells—*arrows*) confirm that this is antrum. By contrast in **(D)**, the endocrine cells form a double layer (at least in this patient) indicative of ECL-cell hyperplasia at the bases of the crypts immediately above the muscularis mucosae. These appearances are confirmed in both biopsies using chromogranin. In (E), there is the usual band of endocrine cells seen in the antrum in the mid-third of the mucosa with rare deeper cells (a gastrin stain would have been even more specific for antral mucosa). In contrast in **(F)**, the endocrine cells are at the base of the mucosa, and here they form chains and completely encircle some pits, indicative of quite marked ECL hyperplasia. The gastrin stain was completely negative.

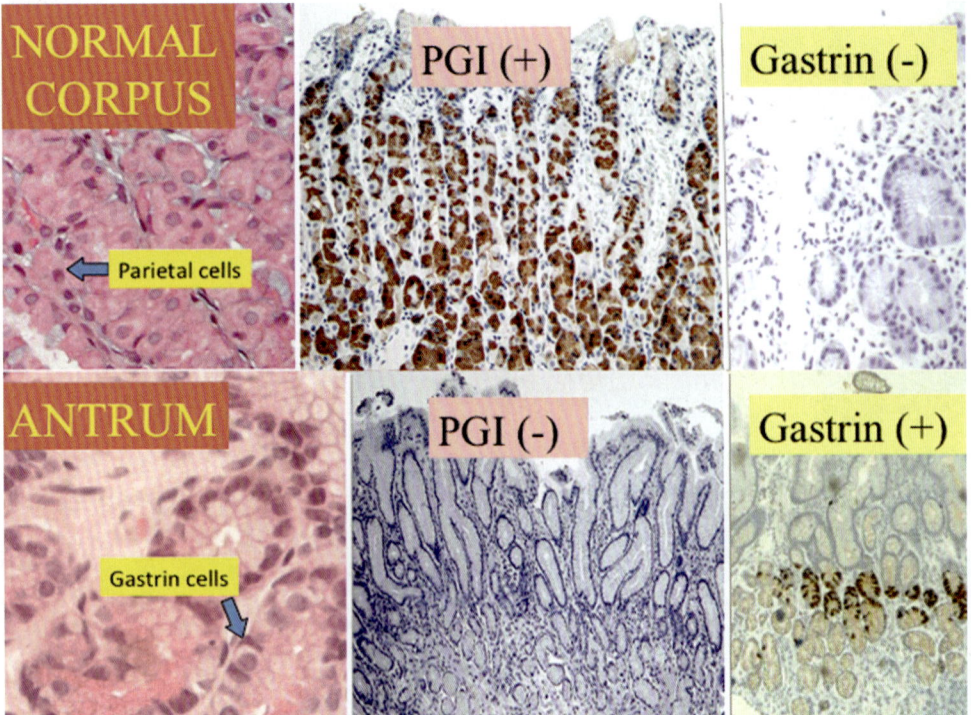

Figure 13-29. Normal corpus (oxyntic) mucosa in the **top three panels** and antral mucosa in the **lower three**. PGI is produced only in chief cells of the oxyntic mucosa and gastrin only in the G-cells of the antral mucosa. In practice G-cells can be recognized in H&E sections because of the perinuclear halos just below the mucous neck region.

scattered throughout the glands, but with progression there is increasing hyperplasia at the bases of the glands.

Pseudopyloric metaplasia (also called pyloric metaplasia or mucus metaplasia and ulcer-associated cell lineage[13,85,150,193] was described as early as 1959[188] in benign gastric ulcers proximal to the normal border zone (antrum–corpus junction). In fact, prior to the rediscovery of H. pylori, a proximally advancing atrophic front with pseudopyloric metaplasia was considered part of the normal gastric aging process.[181] Following the rediscovery of H. pylori, an association was demonstrated between the presence of mucous glands in corpus biopsies and the age of H. pylori–infected patients. Pseudopyloric metaplasia (downward extension of mucous neck cells) is considered regenerative in nature[194,195] and is also observed in gastric remnants following distal gastrectomy with gastroenteric anastomosis forming a "neo-antrum" although without new G-cells assuming that the antrum was completely removed.[196]

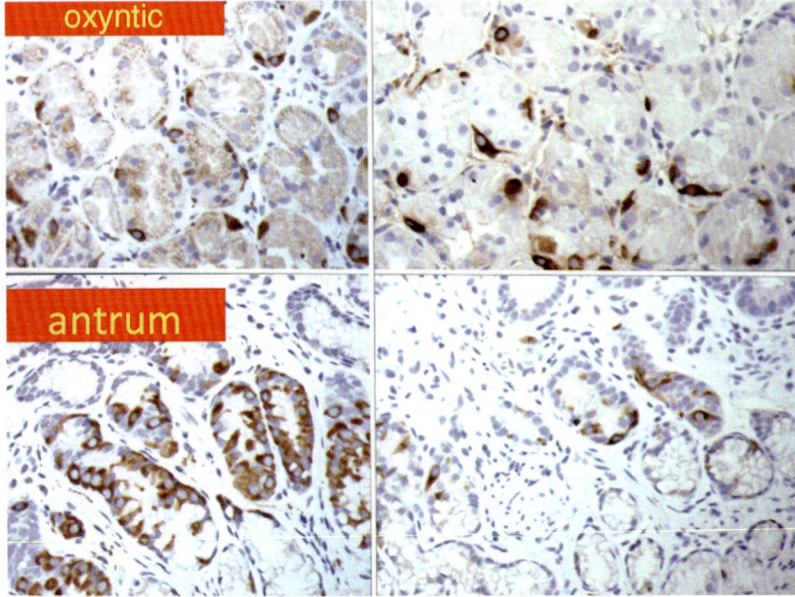

Figure 13-30. Use of standard endocrine stains to identify site by pattern of immunoreactivity. In normal oxyntic mucosa (**top 2 panels**) endocrine cells are distributed fairly regularly and singly. In antral mucosa G-cells form a zone in the midpart of the mucosa (**lower right**). Further, in atrophy with severe pseudopyloric metaplasia the atrophy results in hypergastrinemia and subsequent G-cell hyperplasia that affects the pits immediately beneath the mucous neck zone (**bottom left**).

In interpreting gastric biopsies, recognizing biopsy location and the location of the transitional zone is paramount. Although finding transitional mucosa (where antral mucosa becomes oxyntic which can be gradual or abrupt—also known as junctinal or intermediate mucosa) can help in determining the location of early atrophy, its recognition is not always obvious, especially on H&E sections. As discussed above, G cells are never seen in the body.[191] The complete disappearance of G cells is probably the most reliable method to define the proximal border of the antral body transitional zone. Other features including the change from single tubular glands in the body to branched glands in the antrum. The disappearance of parietal cells is not reliable as parietal cells can be normally present in the antrum and may extend to the duodenal junction.

Making the Diagnosis of Atrophy of Oxyntic Mucosa, Especially without Intestinal Metaplasia

The recognition of atrophic oxyntic mucosa with pseudopyloric metaplasia requires suspicion, experience, and the ability to confirm the diagnosis using immunohistochemistry.

Recognition. Recognizing pseudopyloric metaplasia should initially be endoscopic, for the atrophic front (see Figs. 13-21 and 13-22) should be recognized by this modality, so it may inadvertently be biopsied as oxyntic mucosa. Histologically it requires the ability to distinguish atrophic oxyntic mucosa from antral mucosa (Fig. 13-28). The three most useful features are the presence in atrophic oxyntic mucosa of (a) disordered pseudopyloric glands, (b) chronic inflammation, and (c) endocrine cell changes. The initial clue is to routinely look for G cells in H&E sections, where they are readily visible in antral mucosa beneath the mucous neck region (Figs. 13-28 and 13-29). With pseudopyloric metaplasia, G cells are absent. Endocrine cells in oxyntic mucosa are much more subtle to find on H&E sections. Native ECL cells are virtually invisible and initially retain the fairly diffuse and uniform pattern of endocrine cells seen in normal oxyntic mucosa on immunostaining. As expected, immunostains for gastrin are negative. With increasing serum gastrin levels, there is hyperplasia of endocrine cells that move to the pit base. This progresses to linear hyperplasia, and when this is marked, it can be recognized on the H&E stain by a double layer of nuclei, the outermost layer being pure endocrine cells, along with some of the inner layer (Fig. 13-28). Endocrine micronests often follow or are already present.

Conversely, antral mucosa is usually uniform in the distribution of antral glands; its G cells are readily recognized on H&E sections and are frequently hyperplastic, similar to the changes seen in patients on long-term PPIs as the mechanism (prolonged hypochlorhydria) is identical (Figs. 13-28 and 13-29). In the presence of atrophic oxyntic mucosa, there is usually little or no chronic inflammation in the antrum, and if present is usually considerably less than that in the atrophic oxyntic mucosa, as all of the *Helicobacter*-related inflammation has moved far proximally, and the pattern of endocrine cells is completely different. G cells can invariably be recognized and most of the time are overtly hyperplastic. This can be demonstrated by gastrin stains or the distribution of endocrine cells primarily in a band in or just above the mid-part of the mucosa. Thus, both types of mucosa can be recognized on H&E sections, although it takes most considerable time to understand this and remember to look for these changes in routine biopsies. When the antrum is not only atrophic but has diffuse intestinal metaplasia, defining antrum can be impossible unless residual clusters of G-cells can be identified.

When biopsies from both antral and corpus types of mucosa are present together, usually to "rule out H. pylori," the clue is that while initially all biopsies look like antral mucosa, it is usually apparent that there are two different biopsy types (Fig. 13-28). One has the features of uninflamed or minimally inflamed antral mucosa with appropriate G-cell populations, the other more inflamed with patchy pseudopyloric glands, no G-cell band, and possibly endocrine cell hyperplasia at the pit bases. There is virtually no recognized disorder that produces such variability in antral biopsies, so this combination of changes should immediately raise a red flag that at least one of the biopsies is not antral in origin.

Numerous variations in biopsy combinations can be found but the most common variants are the following: (a) the antral mucosa may be as inflamed as the atrophic mucosa, but all of the other features are present; (b) occasionally one of the oxyntic mucosal biopsies is proximal to the "atrophic front," so the biopsies consist of antral, atrophic oxyntic mucosa and either normal, but more commonly inflamed oxyntic mucosa, often with *Helicobacter* organisms; (c) occasionally the antral biopsies may not be present at all, so the biopsies are either all atrophic oxyntic alone or atrophic oxyntic and oxyntic. In our experience, this is uncommon.

Distinction from autoimmune gastritis. As discussed subsequently, the diagnosis of autoimmune gastritis (AIG) is often best made by a combination of the changes just described, together with serology, with antibodies to intrinsic factor and parietal cells, the latter also being present quite frequently in *Helicobacter* gastritis. However, it may also be appreciated because of the extent of disease (see subsequent section on autoimmune gastritis and Fig. 13-57). Although one might predict that AIG would occur diffusely throughout the oxyntic mucosa bearing the stomach, like other autoimmune conditions there is focality, at least until there is complete metaplasia. As it appears that AIG frequently results from *Helicobacter*, if *Helicobacter* have not been identified, serology for the organism is also appropriate as it is possible that its eradication may prevent further progression of the disease.

Intestinal Metaplasia Intestinal metaplasia comes in two major forms that often coexist, complete and incomplete (Fig. 13-31). The complete form essentially resembles the colon, with absorptive, goblet, Paneth, and endocrine cells, but when well developed may resemble small intestine with villi. Incomplete intestinal metaplasia consists of gastric mucous-producing cells with goblet cells interspersed amongst them. Intestinal metaplasia is a required precursor for intestinal-type carcinoma. The development of gastric carcinoma is a slow and unpredictable process, and intestinal metaplasia is an easily recognizable marker for atrophy.

Subtyping intestinal metaplasia using high iron diamine staining was thought to identify subgroups of patients with different risk potential (Fig. 13-31). Intestinal metaplasia subtype III (black-staining sulfomucin in goblet cells of incomplete intestinal metaplasia) is often considered the highest-risk precursor lesion for the intestinal form of gastric cancer,[197-200] but this is not uniformly accepted.

In addition, approximately equal number of studies have suggested that intestinal metaplasia regresses or does not regress after *H. pylori* treatment.[182,201-208] Sampling error is the likely factor responsible for this discrepancy. This question is a critical one, the corollary being whether eradication of *Helicobacter* prevents progression of intestinal metaplasia, but most importantly the associated cancer risk. Is there a point of no return? The assumption is that the greater the extent of metaplasia the greater the cancer risk, even though virtually all of the carcinomas arising from this etiologic pathway are in the antrum and lesser curve. If *Helicobacter* eradication prevents the risk, then all of the grading systems for atrophy are obsolete. However, currently this is still unclear, so a grading system for atrophy still has to be considered (see subsequent discussion).

Prior studies suggesting an association of type III intestinal metaplasia with the development of gastric cancer[197-200] did not take into account the higher prevalence of incomplete intestinal metaplasia (type III) in the gastric antrum.[23,150,197-200,209] In practice, areas of intestinal metaplasia (or a certain subtype) are generally small and can easily be missed at follow-up.[150,182]

A small percentage of cancer patients show complete replacement of the antral mucosa with intestinal metaplasia and have normal-appearing oxyntic mucosa.[150] It is unknown if these individuals lose their G-cells and have normal or reduced acid secretion. Continued inflammation with antral atrophy could possibly lead to sufficient destruction of G-cells,[210] which can result in a fall in acid secretion.[211,212] Alternatively, contiguous sheets of intestinal metaplasia may be an unstable epithelium especially upon exposure to persistent low-dose dietary or salivary carcinogens, and increase the risk of dysplasia and carcinoma.

Overall, it is apparent that it is not possible to make recommendations or prognoses-based comments on biopsies (single or multiple) showing sulfomucin expression in areas with intestinal metaplasia.[182,213-215] All data suggest that the extent of mucosal atrophy

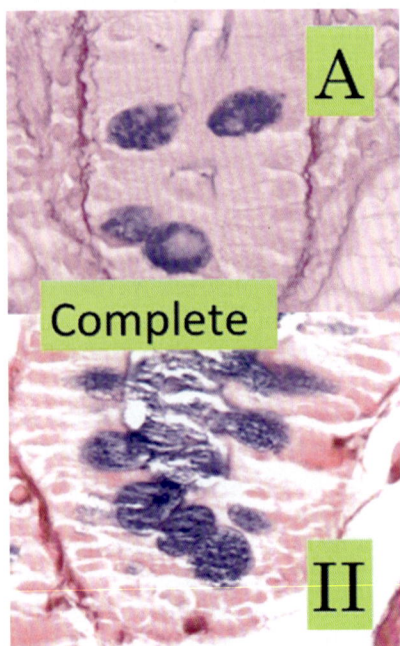
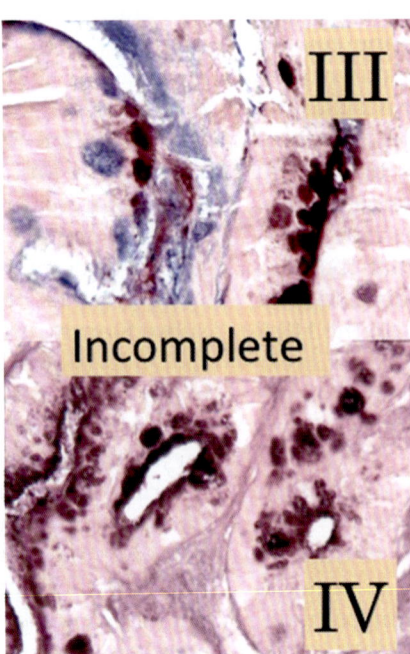

Figure 13-31. Types of intestinal metaplasia. Complete type refers to metaplastic glands composed of goblet cells, columnar cells with a distinctive brush border and in some cases Paneth cells. The type 1 goblet cell of the small intestine epithelium is the predominant element and is located chiefly in the villi **(A)**, while the type II goblet cell is preferentially located in the crypts. Using HID–AB stain, goblet cells are *blue* in type III whereas columnar cell mucus is blue. In type IV both the goblet cells and columnar cell mucus are sulphated (brown-stainnig).

within a region of the stomach is more important than the type of intestinal metaplasia in the development of intestinal type of gastric cancer.

While intestinal metaplasia is a form of atrophy that is easy for pathologists to recognize, it is also important to determine whether intestinal metaplasia is present as an isolated patch within nonatrophic mucosa or amidst an atrophic lawn.[120,150] Thus a patch of intestinal metaplasia in nonatrophic mucosa is a reparative phenomenon, and there are no data to suggest that it is associated with an increased risk of carcinoma.

Changes Associated with Long-term Proton Pump Inhibitors and Corpus Atrophy

PPIs are potent inhibitors of gastric acid secretion. They are widely used in the treatment of acid-peptic diseases and effectively alleviate acid-peptic symptoms and facilitate healing of inflamed or ulcerated mucosa. These drugs are increasingly used long term, frequently for a lifetime, in patients with typical or atypical symptoms of GERD, and in NSAID or aspirin users, such as patients with rheumatoid or osteoarthritis.[216] They give rise to the typically hypertrophied PCs that result from hypertrophy of endoplasmic reticulum (Fig. 13-32). This change is readily visible at scanning power because of the serrated, rather than round, shape of the pits lumen.

Although 20% to 50% of patients on long-term PPIs may still be infected with *H. pylori*, eradication of *Helicobacter* is not always carried out prior to starting PPIs. In these patients, *Helicobacter pylori* accelerates corpus gastritis with subsequent low acid secretion resulting from both the PPIs and the ensuing atrophy and resulting low acid secretion.[151–153,217–225] This in turn facilitates proximal migration and increased severity of *H. pylori* gastritis.[151,153,189,226] It also allows the development of a corpus-predominant gastritis rather than a pangastritis.[227] PPI therapy is associated with a reduction in bacterial load, both in the antrum and in the corpus, and a tendency for antral histology to improve and corpus gastritis to either not change or worsen. With PPI therapy, there is a significant progression of the inflammatory reaction deeper within the pit to involve the proliferative zone[189] (see Fig. 13-23) as seen in atrophic gastritis. This may be related to the migration of the bacteria deeper into the oxyntic glands secondary to PPI therapy.

Prolonged PPI use in *H. pylori*–negative patients showed no difference in gastric inflammation or atrophy over a 7-year period.[228] In contrast, *H. pylori*–positive patients followed over the same period showed increased inflammation and gastric atrophy.[228] Gastric atrophy with peripheral neuropathy and vitamin B_{12} deficiency has been described following 20-year treatment with PPI without *H. pylori* eradication.[229] These studies highlight the importance of considering *H. pylori* eradication in infected, long-term PPI users.

As PPI therapy reduces gastric acidity, it also reduces *H. pylori* density (average number of *H. pylori* per biopsy) in the stomach, *H. pylori* may not be identified in gastric biopsies.[219,230,231] One has to rely on the diffuse pattern of inflammation to diagnose the infection. Further, the *Helicobacter* seek out the acid to the point that they may invade the pits, and can even be found in the canaliculi of PCs (Fig. 13-33). Histopathologic features suggestive of long-term PPI use include not only PC hypertrophy but a degree of enterochromaffin-like (ECL) cell hyperplasia from long-standing hypergastrinemia, although this requires endocrine stains, and often counting to demonstrate the changes. These changes therefore resemble changes seen in the stomach in patients with Zollinger-Ellison syndrome, even to the point of small ECL-tumors.

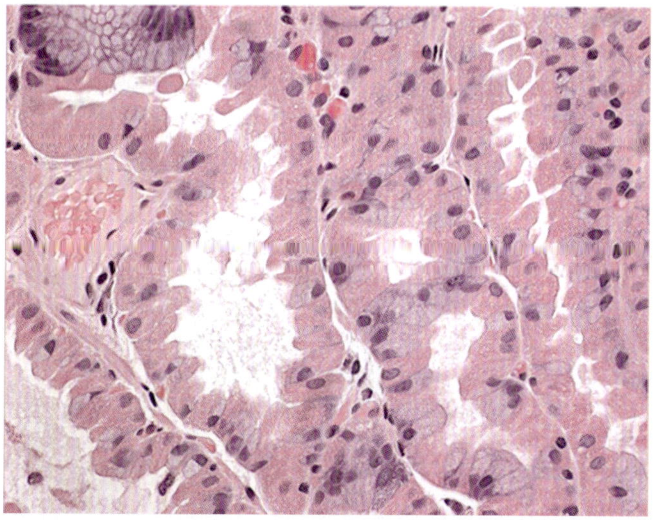

Figure 13-32. Hypertrophy of parietal cells as seen in long-standing hypergastrinemia. By far the most common cause of this is long-term ingestion of PPIs.

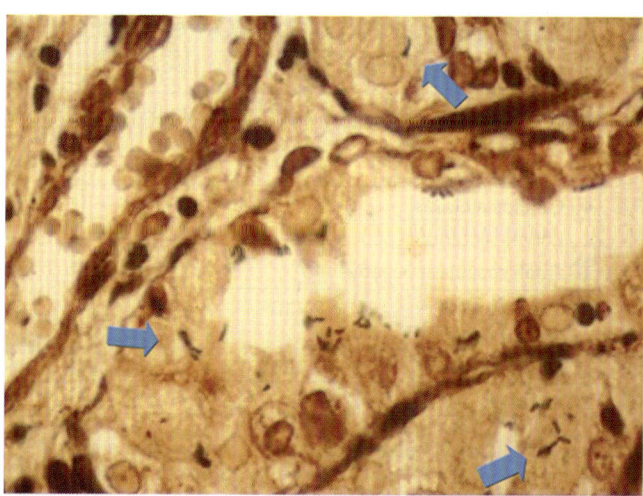

Figure 13-33. *Helicobacter* present deep in the pits and also in the canaliculi of PCs, some of which are *arrowed*. (Courtesy of Dr. M Vieth.)

PPI therapy, particularly with long-term or high-dose administration or both, is associated with several potential adverse effects, including vitamin B_{12} deficiency irrespective of *H. pylori* status,[229,232-234] enteric infections (e.g., *C. difficile*), community-acquired pneumonia, osteopenia and hip fractures, and small intestinal bacterial overgrowth. Proposed mechanisms are that reduced acidity impairs cobalamin release from dietary protein and bacterial overgrowth increases competitive consumption.[229,233,234]

Overgrowth of Other Organisms in the Hypo or Achlorhydric Stomach

It is not uncommon to see a variety of cocci and bacilli in gastric mucosa of patients on high-dose long-term PPIs (see Fig. 13-26) or with extensive atrophy from prolonged *H. pylori*. These organisms are either of oral or duodenal origin as PPIs can increase the median gastric pH from about 3.25 to 6.75 (Fig. 13-34). These should not be mistaken for *H. pylori* or its coccoid forms. While these colonies can be associated with inflammation, it is often difficult to be sure that the patient does not have *Helicobacter* that is being suppressed by the PPIs. *Helicobacter* immunohistochemistry is the obvious way of resolving this issue, but the typical morphology of *Helicobacter* needs to be present to make the diagnosis.

Staging gastric atrophy. Gastric atrophy and atrophic gastritis are often used synonymously in practice, although atrophic gastritis is the process resulting in atrophy. It also represents transmucosal inflammation (as opposed to superficial gastritis) that is likely to progress to glandular atrophy. Gastric atrophy simply refers to diffuse loss of gastric glands. As the presence of gastric atrophy, with or without intestinal metaplasia, is the critical determinant of a person's risk for gastric cancer,[120,235,236] recognizing its degree does have clinical implications. Most intestinal and some diffuse types of gastric carcinomas arise on a background of atrophic gastritis; an index of the extent of atrophy can be useful in predicting patients at greatest risk for carcinoma.[118,184,237] Screening protocols include endoscopic screening, serum biomarker tests, and histology.

Endoscopic Screening: Esophagogastroduodenoscopy has been used since the 1960s in Japan to detect the atrophic border,[181] and to simultaneously obtain biopsies for histologic exam.[238,239] For practical reasons, endoscopic mass screening can only be recommended in gastric cancer high-incidence areas such as Japan. In Western countries, limited experience with the endoscopic appearance of gastric atrophy (using conventional white-light endoscopy or newer endoscopic techniques) and conflicting data on endoscopic biopsy sites limit endoscopic screening of at-risk patients.

Serology: Noninvasive serum biomarker tests have been used since the 1990s to screen patients for gastric atrophy.[240-242] Determining serum pepsinogens, I and II (sPGI and sPGII), or sPGI:PGII ratio is an indirect measure of corpus function.[243-245] PGI is secreted only by oxyntic glands. PGII is produced by all gastric glands (oxyntic, cardiac, and pyloric) as well as duodenal (Brunner's) glands. With advancing corpus atrophy, secretion of PGI diminishes, so a low sPGI:PGII ratio is a serologic marker of corpus atrophy.[240,243-246] Screening using low sPGI:PII as an atrophy marker has made it possible to screen large populations[240-242] as it is convenient and economic.

Histopathology staging systems for gastric atrophy: Histology can also provide a direct measure of gastric function along with additional information about inflammation as well as the severity and topography of gastritis. A patient's risk for gastric cancer is determined by the degree and distribution of (a) atrophy, (b) intestinal metaplasia, and (c) inflammation. Several atrophy staging systems have been designed with varying degrees of success. As the predictive value of individual biopsy specimens for cancer risk is limited, this has led to the introduction of four histopathology indices (Gastritis Risk Index,[247] OLGA,[248,249] Baylor,[248,249] and Erasmus[250]) for gastric cancer relative risk. As each system uses different biopsy protocol systems and each has a different approach, a comparative study is of paramount importance but it is currently lacking. The various histopathology staging systems are as follows:

Gastritis Risk Index: This index uses the topographic grading of *H. pylori* gastritis in the antrum and corpus.[118] It uses the updated Sydney system biopsy site recommendations (2 antral, 2 corpus and angulus) and its 4-point scale (negative, mild, moderate, and

Microorganisms cultured in Omeprazole treated patients

N	Bacteria	CFU/ml in gastric juice
4	α-hemoloytic streptococci	$10^6 - 10^{10}$
4	Candida albicans	$8 \times 10^1 - 10^3$
2	Corynebacterium spp.	$10^9 - 10^{10}$
1	Staph coagulase negative	10^4
1	Streptococcus pneumoniae	8×10^2
1	Klebsiella pneumoniae	7×10^2
1	Klebsiella oxytoca	6.7×10^2

Figure 13-34. Principal organisms cultured from the stomach in patients taking omeprazole. Note the numbers of coccoid or cocco-bacillary organisms included. It is therefore important that these not be interpreted as coccoid forms or *Helicobacter*. (Adapted from Karmeli et al. *Dig Dis Sci* 1995;40:2070-2073.) (*N* is the number of patients.)

severe)[13] to grade active and chronic inflammation. Factored into the gastritis risk index are (1) infiltration with lymphocytes and plasma cells, that is, chronic inflammation, (2) neutrophil infiltration, that is, activity, and (3) intestinal metaplasia. If chronic inflammation in the corpus is greater than or equal to that in the antrum (antrum/corpus ratio), 1 point is scored. If active inflammation in the corpus is greater than or equal to that in the antrum (antrum/corpus ratio), 1 point is again scored. If intestinal metaplasia is found in the antrum or corpus (scored as absent or present), another point is scored. The maximum score is 3 points. Using the Gastritis Index in a German population, the positive predictive value for the presence of gastric carcinoma was 46% for score 1, 79% for score 2, and 94% for score 3 compared to 17% for score 0.[247] Except for intestinal metaplasia, Shimoyama et al.[251] did not find a similar predictive value. Nonetheless, the control group in Shimoyama's study included patients with atrophic gastritis.[251] It is difficult to assess the reproducibility of Gastritis Risk Index as studies in other populations (claiming to use the Gastritis Risk Index) dropped the predictive value of chronic inflammation.[252-254]

OLGA adopts the updated Sydney's biopsy protocol and its 4-point scale (negative, mild, moderate, and severe).[248] Atrophy is defined as the loss of normal glands with and without its replacement with fibrosis, intestinal metaplasia, and pseudopyloric metaplasia.[13,255] Following the updated Sydney recommendation the final atrophy score is calculated as the average score for each region (i.e., antral atrophy is the average score of all antral biopsies [n = 3] and corpus atrophy is the average score of the two corpus biopsies). OLGA combines antral and corpus atrophy scores for a final gastric atrophy stage that relates to cancer risk[248] (Table 13-7). It is noteworthy that if antral atrophy is moderate or severe (score 2 or 3) the presence of mild corpus atrophy does not increase OLGA's score further. Though gastric cancer risk is higher in patients with extensive intestinal metaplasia, OLGA's score equates all forms of atrophy. Elderly patients with antral fibrosis secondary to NSAID-induced ulcers will receive a high OLGA score irrespective of low cancer risk. Thus, OLGA does not take into account that gastric cancer risk increases with extensive intestinal metaplasia and with the advent of corpus atrophy.[110,120,181] In addition, in the original study, no new patients were included as being at risk of carcinoma as a result of the study, suggesting that in practice it was of little/no value. Other investigators have suggested replacing gastric atrophy by intestinal metaplasia "OLGAIM" to increase interobserver agreement and to increase the correlation with gastritis severity.[256]

Baylor. Sense can be made of the issues in OLGA by following a biopsy protocol similar to Sydney's biopsy protocol with two extra distal corpus biopsies (Fig. 13-35). Atrophy is defined as in the updated Sydney system.[13] Antral and corpus atrophy stage is recorded independent of each other. Intestinal metaplasia is recorded as an independent variable. The corpus atrophy stage (early, mid, and advanced corpus atrophy) is reported on the basis of the upward extension of atrophy along the lesser and greater curvature (Fig. 13-35). Antral atrophy is recorded on a 4-point scale (negative, mild, moderate, and severe) based on degree of replacement with intestinal metaplasia. Using low sPGI:PGII as a serologic marker of corpus atrophy, Baylor's stage showed a statistically significant inverse relationship with PGI:PGII serum levels ($p < 0.0001$).[249]

Erasmus Index uses a combination of clinical information, pepsinogen level serology, and histology to evaluate each patient's risk for gastric cancer.[250] Features factored into the Erasmus risk index are (1) family history of gastric cancer (2 points), (2) alcohol use >1 unit/d (1 point), (3) intestinal metaplasia grade (moderate 1 point, marked 3 points), and (4) pepsinogen I to II ratio <3 (3 points). Erasmus has a maximum score of 10; score ≥4 points was indicative of multifocal intestinal metaplasia in 96% and severe grades of intestinal metaplasia in 92%. The study examining the Erasmus Index used extensive intestinal metaplasia and not dysplasia or cancer (in follow-up biopsies) as a marker of gastric cancer risk. Dysplasia was identified

Table 13-7 OLGA

		CORPUS ATROPHY SCORE			
		No atrophy (score 0)	Mild atrophy (score 1)	Moderate atrophy (score 2)	Severe atrophy (score 3)
ANTRUM ATROPHY SCORE	No atrophy (score 0)	Stage 0	Stage I	Stage II	Stage II
	Mild atrophy (score 1)	Stage I	Stage I	Stage II	Stage III
	Moderate atrophy (score 2)	Stage II	Stage II	Stage III	Stage IV
	Severe atrophy (score 3)	Stage III	Stage III	Stage IV	Stage IV

All scores are between 0 and 3 for "mild, moderate, and severe" using a visual analogue scale.[248]

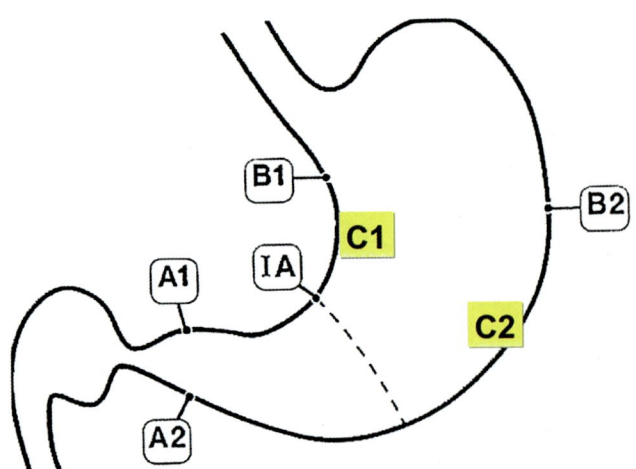

Figure 13-35. The updated Sydney biopsy protocol requires a minimum of five biopsies as shown in *white*. These can also identify the extent of atrophy present, albeit fairly crudely, as the first site involved is the angulus/incisura (IA), and should be followed by B1, and lastly B2. It is, however, essential that each biopsy site be submitted in its own container and the site labeled for identification. By adding biopsies C1 and C2, in which atrophic changes (especially intestinal metaplasia) appear to starts at the incisura/angulus (IA), affects the antrum (A1, A2), and then extends proximally to the oxyntic zone (C1, C2), so that after IA, C1, then C2, then B1 and lastly B2 are involved biopsy site B1 is first affected.

in follow-up biopsies of 7 out of 32 patients (22%); all had marked intestinal metaplasia.[250]

Disorders associated with *H. pylori* gastritis

Peptic Ulcer Disease An ulcer is a break in the mucosa involving both the epithelium and muscularis mucosae and therefore reaches the submucosa. It therefore differs from mucosal erosions, in which the epithelial break does not penetrate the muscularis mucosae to reach the submucosa. We tend not to use the term *acute ulcer*, which implies a temporal or recent lesion, when outside of clinical trials this knowledge is not available, while the depth of the lesion as an ulcer rather than an erosion is also subjective. The term *erosive gastritis or erosive gastropathy* is preferred, recognizing that some of these lesions may penetrate the muscularis mucosae, thus qualifying in the literal sense as ulcers, but that endoscopy does not distinguish between these perfectly. Similarly, the term *chronic ulcer* usually implies size or depth endoscopically, but long-standing changes, for example, (fibrosis) histologically.

Peptic ulcer disease is not a single entity but a heterogeneous group of disorders having in common mucosal erosion or ulceration. PUD results when aggressive factors (acid, pepsin, bile, activated pancreatic enzymes, medications, chemicals, ischemia, radiation, etc.) overwhelm intrinsic defense mechanisms and protective factors (mucin and bicarbonate secretion and numerous systems including the cyclo-oxygenase,

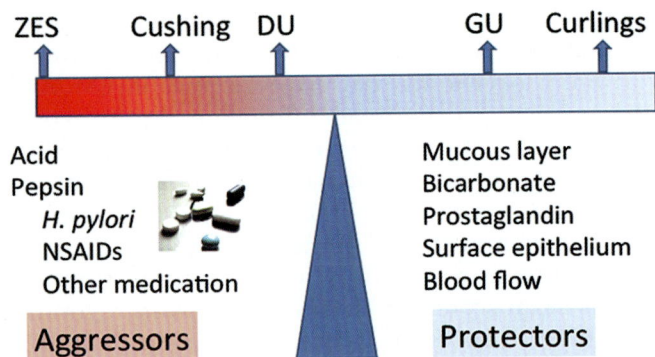

Figure 13-36. Imbalance between aggressive and protective factors in disease.

nitric oxide and transforming growth factor beta [TGF-β]–associated systems) (Fig. 13-36, Table 13-8). Ulcers occur primarily in the distal stomach and proximal duodenum but may occur anywhere acid and pepsin are found, for example, in the esophagus, in mucosa adjacent to surgically produced anastomoses on either side of the anastomotic line, and within ectopic gastric mucosa such as Meckel's diverticulum. This is perhaps best illustrated with medications (NSAIDs, aspirin, etc.) that specifically overwhelm the cyclo-oxygenase system, or situations where acid is deposited directly onto an epithelium not designed to withstand it (distal to gastroenterostomy lines, gastric heterotopia in the duodenum, or Meckel's diverticulum), and especially the Zollinger–Ellison syndrome (ZES) in which sheer volume of acid can overwhelm those parts of the intestinal tract not designed to deal with acid, and can result in other symptoms such as severe diarrhea and malabsorption.[257]

In practice, *H. pylori* infection and medication use such as NSAIDs are the most common etiologic factors for gastroduodenal ulcers.

The role of the pathologist is to exclude malignancy in the case of gastric ulcers, and to uncover causes of

Table 13-8	Factors That Damage or Protect the Gastric Mucosa
AGGRESSIVE FACTORS	**PROTECTIVE FACTORS**

Endogenous
  Hydrochloric acid
  Pepsin
  Bile
 	
Exogenous
  Nonsteroidal anti-inflammatory drugs
  Ethanol
  Other
	Gastric mucosal blood flow
	Mucus
	Bicarbonate secretion
	Prostaglandins
	Nitric oxide

gastroduodenal ulceration including unusual causes (e.g., those due to Crohn's disease [CD] or, opportunistic infection in the immunocompromised host), and to distinguish the main causes, namely, *Helicobacter* and medications, which is often fairly easy.

Gastroduodenal erosions and ulcers ("peptic ulcers"). In order to understand the development of ulcers, it is pertinent to discuss the mechanisms that help to maintain the integrity of the gastric mucosa. Mucosal integrity is maintained by numerous defense mechanisms, which include[258]

1. Pre-epithelial factors such as mucus–bicarbonate–phospholipid barrier
2. An epithelial barrier that includes surface epithelial cells connected by tight junctions and generating bicarbonate, mucus, phospholipids, trefoil peptides, prostaglandins, and heat shock proteins
3. Continuous cell renewal accomplished by proliferation of progenitor cells regulated by a variety of growth factors, for example, PGE2 and surviving TGF-β
4. An endothelial "barrier" that includes sensory innervation, generation of prostaglandins, and nitric oxide. Nitric oxide (NO) is protective and linked with NSAIDs (NO-NSAIDS), has the potential to form less injurious NSAIDs.
5. Continuous blood flow through mucosal microvessels.

Mucosal injury may occur either when noxious factors breach the intact mucosal defense system or when any of the components making up that mucosal defense is impaired. In mucosal erosions, when the surface epithelium is denuded, rapid cell restitution takes place to repair the break in the mucosa. For this to occur, intact mucosal blood flow is necessary, and prostaglandins and nitric oxide may mediate these changes. Thus an impairment of any of these factors may contribute to ulcer formation.

Patients hospitalized with severe burns have an enhanced risk of developing so-called Curling's ulcer. Despite the clear relationship between the severity of burns and the risk of PUD, these patients secrete less acid than control subjects. In fact, there is an inverse relationship between the extent of surface burns and the rate of acid secretion. Thus, while acid is necessary for the development of PUD in burn patients and can be prevented with medications that block acid secretion, mucosal damage is not due to increased acid secretion,[259] and is likely vagally mediated. In burn patients under stress, the primary factor causing ulcer disease appears to be impaired mucosal defense mechanisms against ulceration.[260] It is evident that although ulcers need a milieu of acid and pepsin for their development, factors affecting mucosal resistance to injury are critically important in the development of peptic ulcers.

1. **Gastric mucosal blood flow**: The high metabolic rate of the gastric and duodenal epithelium requires high blood flow to maintain mucosal integrity. Mucosal ischemia is believed to be important in the pathogenesis of "*stress*" lesions, but whether it contributes to chronic ulcers is unknown.[261-263] The role of acute ischemia in erosive gastritis is discussed subsequently.
2. **Mucus**: Surface columnar epithelium and mucus neck cells secrete a continuous layer of glycoprotein mucus gel (largely lost with conventional fixation and embedding[264]) that adheres to the mucosal surface.[265] Mucus protects the underlying epithelial cells in several ways: it acts as a lubricant protecting the mucosal surface from mechanical damage by food, as a neutralizer of gastric acid, and as a barrier to luminal pepsin, thereby protecting the underlying mucosa from proteolytic digestion.[266] The mucous layer has three trefoil peptides (TFFs) that have been shown to be key factors in stimulating cell migration and promoting epithelial repair after damage.[267-270] TFF1 is cosecreted with MUC5AC mucin in the superficial foveolar region of the stomach, TFF2 with MUC6 mucin in deep gastric and duodenal glands, and TFF3 with MUC2 mucin from goblet cells in the duodenum.[267-270]
3. **Bicarbonate secretion**: Surface epithelial cells secrete bicarbonate into the adherent layer of mucus gel creating a pH gradient with a near-neutral pH at the epithelial surfaces in the stomach and duodenum. Thus the mucosal surface is in contact with neutral fluid, regardless of the amount of acid in the lumen.[266] Bicarbonate secretion is depressed in the majority of peptic ulcer patients even after the ulcers have healed. Consequently, these patients have an impaired mucosal bicarbonate barrier against luminal acid and an increase in acidification at the mucosal surface.[271] Secreted acid appears to go through pores in this mucous gel to reach the lumen.
4. **Prostaglandins**: Prostaglandins are produced by GI tract cells as well as most other tissues. Prostaglandins of the E variety are major mucosal defense mediators. Animal experiments have shown that prostaglandins can protect the gastric mucosa from damage by several noxious agents, such as aspirin, bile salts, alcohol, and boiling water.[272,273] The mechanism by which this occurs is uncertain but probably includes stimulation of mucus and bicarbonate secretion in addition to enhancing blood flow to the gastric mucosa and augmenting cell proliferation.[274] Prostaglandins are responsible exclusively for maintaining mucosal integrity.[275]

Pathogenetic factors. Factors thought to be important in the pathogenesis of ulcer disease include genetic predisposition, increased acid and pepsin production, infections, and environmental factors, such as smoking and medications. Two important factors that disturb mucosal defense, and therefore may predispose to ulcer formation, are NSAIDS, including aspirin and *H. pylori* infection.[116] Today, with further decline in *H. pylori* prevalence, other etiologic factors primarily NSAIDs play a more important role even in less developed countries.[276] Indeed, we may never know the role aspirin played historically, as it was readily available prior to the rediscovery of *H. pylori* when it was "the" analgesic of choice until acetaminophen/paracetamol/Tylenol became available. Decreased mucosal resistance and rapid gastric emptying are also thought to play a role (see also discussion at the beginning of this chapter).

1. *Acid and pepsin.* It has long been known that peptic ulcers are dependent, at least in part, on an acid/peptic milieu, giving rise to the "no acid, no ulcer" dictum stated by Karl Schwartz in 1910.[277-279] Before *H. pylori* was rediscovered in 1984,[280] it was generally accepted that duodenal ulcer was due to high acid secretion. Effective measures to reduce acid output, surgical or medical, led to long-term healing.[281-284] The inhibition of acid secretion heals peptic ulcers that fail to respond to conventional ulcer therapy, although when therapy is stopped, there is often rapid recurrence of ulcers, unless the initiating agent, for example, *H. pylori* or NSAIDs/ASA, is removed. Ulcer healing correlates with the degree and duration of acid inhibition.[285] The validity of this generalization is supported by several observations. For example, peptic ulcers are exceedingly rare in atrophic gastritis associated with pernicious anemia.[278,279] Ulcers in patients with known achlorhydria strongly suggest the presence of a malignancy; patients with the most severe and intractable forms of PUD, such as the ZES/gastrinoma, have the highest rates of acid secretion.[286] However, it should be noted that 50% to 60% of ulcer patients secrete normal amounts of gastric acid.[287-293] While peptic damage is common, the fact that it does not occur with even greater frequency, despite the daily and nightly exposure of the stomach, distal esophagus, and duodenum to a very low pH, suggests that effective defensive factors are in place. Increased acid exposure alone is rarely sufficient to cause mucosal damage in the stomach or duodenum, although the squamous mucosa of the esophagus appears much more susceptible. The production of a gastric or duodenal ulcer at the individual level likely represents a consortium of events.

Fundic gland heterotopia, (Fig. 13-37) This refers to the presence of fundic-type glands with parietal and chief cells or commonly just parietal cells in the duodenum. This was reported to be more common (>50%) in resection specimens from duodenal ulcer patients than in nonulcer (20%) patients.[294,295] The gross findings may be those of nodules (commonly red-tipped) in the duodenal bulb. Sometimes these become very large, and ulcerate or obstruct the duodenal bulb or beyond, farther into the small bowel (see Chapter 20). Further these are known to actively secrete acid and almost certainly play a role in the genesis of duodenal ulcers. They are responsive to gastrin, and secrete acid directly into the adjacent duodenal mucosa, where the intestinal mucosa is susceptible to acid, and is frequently found at the edge of duodenal ulcers. While gastric *Helicobacter* clearly plays a role in duodenal ulcer disease (relative risk ×7) and especially when present in gastric surface metaplasia in the duodenum (relative risk ×51),[296] the role that it plays when heterotopic mucosa is infected is unknown.

Antral parietal cells: Although infrequently discussed, it is clear that there are huge variations in the numbers of parietal cells in the antrum. In some patients they cannot be found, while in others they are numerous. These are not accompanied by chief cells unlike normal corpus glands, so PGI staining is negative in the antrum. Whether these patients are resistant to *Helicobacter* because the gastric pH remains low in the antrum, or conversely, when infected they have a high prevalence of duodenal ulcer because of acid secretion almost directly into the pylorus, is unknown. However, they certainly increase the gastric parietal cell mass, and sometimes actually increase in the distal antrum. Further, most pathologists are very aware of the frequency with which biopsies designated as being "antral" by our clinical colleagues consist entirely of oxyntic mucosa. This is less likely to mean they have lost their way within the stomach than that the oxyntic mucosa extends well past the angulus on the lesser curve, and much closer to the pylorus than generally believed on the greater curve. Prepyloric biopsies are therefore ideally required to obtain antral mucosa.

Hypersecretory conditions associated with peptic ulcers. In these conditions there is excessive production of gastrin, resulting in continuous stimulation of acid secretion. This includes ZES, theoretically primary gastrin cell hyperplasia (if this exists—see Chapter 5), and the retained antrum syndrome.

Zollinger–Ellison syndrome is a rare disorder (see also Chapter 5) characterized by one or more gastrin-releasing tumors (gastrinomas) in the pancreas, duodenum, or both, often in association with syndromes such as multiple endocrine neoplasia type I (MEN I). Gastrinomas release abnormal amounts of gastrin that acts as a trophic or growth-promoting hormone that induces hyperplasia of parietal and ECL cells,[297,298] resulting in excess gastric acid in the stomach and duodenum. *Helicobacter pylori* infection

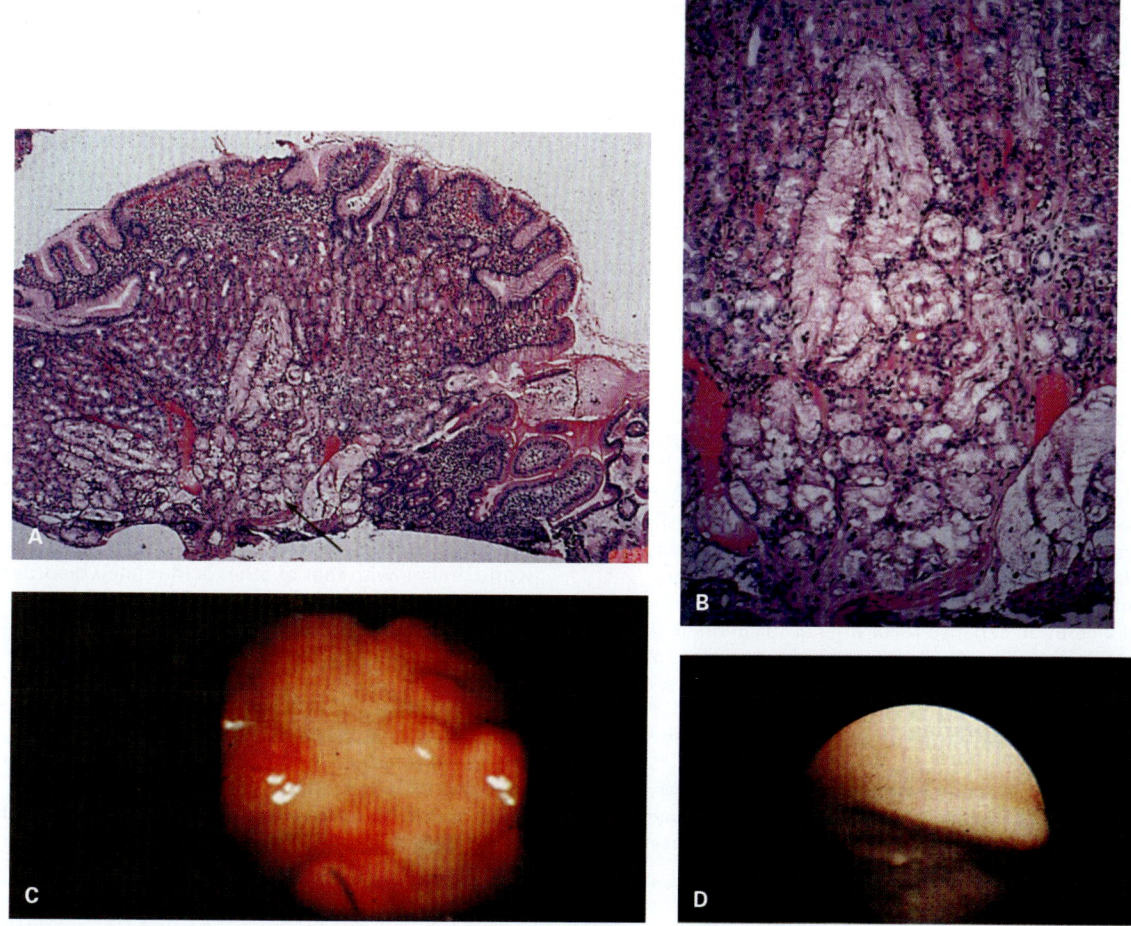

Figure 13-37. A,B: Fundic gland heterotopia in the duodenal bulb. **A:** Low-power view. Most of the lining epithelium is of the gastric type, with the only residual villi present at the **bottom right**. Brunner's glands are seen near the bottom of the section (*arrow*). **B:** High-power view showing the interface between Brunner's glands below and the fundic gland mucosa with parietal and chief cells above. **C,D:** These red bumps in the bulb represent nests of fundic gland heterotopia.

is not a major contributing factor in duodenal ulcer associated with ZES.[299] In fact, *H. pylori* infection, as well as transient acute inflammation of the gastric mucosa, is associated with decreased acid secretion in ZES (as it may in the rest of the population).[300,301] Only a very small number of patients with PUD have ZES. Its presence should be suspected in the absence of *H. pylori* infection or NSAIDs usage in patients with findings suggestive of acid hypersecretion (e.g., multiple refractory ulcers, severe peptic ulcers that bleed, perforation distal to the first portion of the duodenum), diarrhea, or a personal or family history of multiple endocrine neoplasia type 1.[302,303] Morphologically the combination of parietal cells hyperplasia and ECL hyperplasia at the base of the mucosa is virtually diagnostic of this syndrome. For further details, see hypertrophic gastropathies at the end of this chapter.

Retained antrum syndrome is an unusual complication of Billroth 2 surgery for gastric ulcer disease. In this procedure the antrum is resected, the duodenal stump is closed off, and a gastrojejunostomy is formed. If during surgery a portion of the antrum is inadvertently left behind within the duodenal stump the absence of acid in the antral remnant (and possibly duodenum where G-cells can also be found) will lead to continuous secretion of gastrin, resulting in a situation similar to gastrinoma or G-cell hyperplasia.

2. ***Helicobacter pylori.*** *Helicobacter pylori* infection of the stomach and duodenum is highly associated with the occurrence of peptic ulcers, especially with strains that produce the CagA.[116,304–309] Nonetheless, some doubt *H. pylori*'s role in ulcer genesis (reasons summarized in Table 13-9). In patients with duodenal ulcers, *H. pylori* infection induces antral gastritis, which leads to hypergastrinemia and acid hypersecretion. Excess acid enters the duodenal bulb causing or extending duodenal gastric metaplasia, allowing *H. pylori* colonization. This in turn induces an inflammatory response, and potentially focal erosions or ulceration. This is supported by Mongolian gerbil experiments; those infected

Table 13-9 Evidence Linking *H. pylori* to the Pathogenesis of Duodenal Ulcer[836–838]

EVIDENCE AGAINST	EVIDENCE FOR
Craters heal, even when bacteria persist	*Helicobacter pylori* prevalence in DU patients varies from 85% to 100%
Acid hypersecretion can lead to DU without bacterial infection	Antibiotics heal DU at the same rate as H2-receptor antagonists or PPIs
Most infected individuals never develop DU	DU recurrence is less after antimicrobial therapy than conventional treatment for DU
If *H. pylori* were the primary cause, we would not see regional variation in DU prevalence within areas of high *H. pylori* prevalence, particularly developing countries	DU recurrence is virtually always associated with failure to clear organisms or infection relapse
Helicobacter pylori infection has been present for many centuries, but duodenal ulcer emerged only around 1900—(around the time aspirin started becoming widely available!)	Koch's postulates have since been fulfilled for this histologic lesion
In developed countries, duodenal ulcers occur in people without *H. pylori* infection, raising the importance of factors such as aspirin and other NSAIDs and, much less commonly, CD	Mongolian gerbils injected with *H. pylori* develop duodenitis, gastric metaplasia, and duodenal ulcer
Ulcers are proportionately more common (up to 75% of all cases) in areas of low *H. pylori* prevalence. This may also reflect the emergence of medications as a major cause of gastroduodenal ulcers	If duodenal ulcer were predominantly (primarily) acid related, its incidence should be increasing in the Western world, in line with that of other acid-related disorders such as GERD.
Duodenal ulceration can also recur after eradication without reinfection	Successful eradication of the organism also leads to normalization of acid production by the stomach
Half of patients with acute perforations of a duodenal ulcer (i.e., with only a brief period of previous indigestion) are *H. pylori*–negative (medications again?)	
Working hypothesis: *Helicobacter pylori* infection is secondary, delaying healing and leading to chronicity. Aspirin and NSAIDs play a huge role in what we regard as "peptic ulcer disease"	**Working hypothesis:** Preexisting infection with *H. pylori* is significantly associated with subsequent development of duodenal ulcer

with *H. pylori* develop gastritis, gastric ulcer with gastritis cystica profunda, duodenitis, gastric metaplasia, and duodenal ulcer.[310] Today, the incidence of duodenal ulcers has decreased substantially in the Western world[311] mirroring the fall in *H. pylori* infection,[312] and possibly the replacement of aspirin by paracetamol/Tylenol as the analgesic of choice. In some Western countries, smoking, alcohol, and NSAIDs, but not *H. pylori* infection remain leading risk factors for duodenal or prepyloric ulcer.[313]

3. **Drugs**. Millions of people throughout the world are maintained on NSAID therapy, but with the use of over-the-counter NSAIDs, and aspirin, it is almost impossible to know how many are taken. The use of NSAIDs has increased dramatically since they came into the market in the early 1970s, and has been associated with increases in the relative risk of gastric ulcers and duodenal ulcer. During a course of NSAID therapy, approximately 15% of patients will develop gastric ulcers; 5% will develop duodenal ulcers.[314,315] Several studies have shown that chronic gastric ulcers occur more frequently in patients taking large doses of aspirin compared to control populations, and the risk of NSAID-associated ulcer bleeding is higher in elderly females, probably because of the increased consumption of NSAIDs by this group.[274,316–319] Interestingly, in the rare instances that gastric ulcers are resected in North America, we now find (personal experience) that chronic gastritis and *H. pylori* are rare, but the adjacent mucosa shows typical features of reactive gastropathy and particles of medication, presumably NSAIDs, can often be seen at the base of the ulcer (whether causative or therapeutic is a matter of debate). However, NSAID-associated upper GI bleeding does not originate from gastric ulcers alone. Duodenal ulcers may account for one-third or more of cases. Thus, although NSAIDs may only slightly increase the risk of duodenal ulcer, they appear to significantly increase the bleeding risk in those with a duodenal ulcer. Aspirin with its anticoagulant effect may potentiate this. The role that NSAIDs/ASA have played historically is outlined in the introduction to this chapter, including the association between ASA coming into the market around 1900 and the increasing numbers of patients with gastric and duodenal ulcers since that time.

The use of daily PPI therapy decreases symptoms and the development of NSAID-associated ulcers and recurrent NSAID-related ulcer complications. In patients using aspirin, the addition of a COX-2-specific inhibitor appears to significantly increase GI risk to the level of a nonselective NSAID; aspirin plus a nonselective NSAID appears to increase GI risk still higher. Patients taking low-dose aspirin who have risk factors for GI complications (including concomitant nonselective NSAID therapy) should receive medical cotherapy, such as a PPI.[320]

NSAID-associated ulcers are often clinically silent and probably account for about 30% of ulcer complications such as bleeding and perforation. Endoscopic erosions or ulcers are found in 15% to 30% of patients taking NSAIDS regularly, while the annual incidence of bleeding/perforation in these patients is 1% to 1.5%.[258] It has been estimated that NSAIDs account for about 3,000 deaths and 20,000 hospitalizations in the United States each year.[274,317,319,321-323] There were over 1,000 deaths annually in elderly patients in the United Kingdom in 2000,[324] so the figure in the United States may well be many times this.[325] Indeed, one estimate suggested 16,500 deaths from GI-related causes in 1997 from NSAIDs use in the United States.[326] However, the rates are likely lower now for various reasons including the concurrent use of PPI and also Coxibs.

The contribution of other drugs, such as corticosteroids, chemotherapeutic drugs, immunosuppressive agents (even embolization), and ischemia to the pathogenesis of erosions and ulcers, and their effects on healing of PUD, remain unclear.[327,328] Steroids reduce epithelial turnover so may potentiate other damaging factors.

4. **Duodenogastric reflux**. Duodenogastric reflux and gastroesophageal reflux represent physiologic phenomena occurring in the postprandial period and sporadically in the interdigestive state.[329-333] Duodenal contents contain not only bile but activated pancreatic enzymes, and so are potentially quite injurious. Episodes of "physiologic" reflux are typically postprandial, short-lived, asymptomatic, and are less common at night, although Barrett's esophagus is associated with nocturnal duodenal duodeno-gastroesophageal reflux. "Pathologic" reflux leads to histopathologic and clinical abnormalities. Bile reflux gastropathy is present in a significant proportion of patients with GERD, including Barrett's esophagus, and is associated with disease severity.[334] Duodenogastric reflux is greater in some gastric ulcer patients than in normal subjects.[335,336] However, its measurement and the data concerning what is normal are not yet definitive. Patients with gastroenterostomies are at particularly high risk and do develop gastric carcinomas close to the anastomotic line where they are accompanied by a severe reactive gastropathy.

The mechanism by which pathological amounts of duodenal reflux occur is unclear, although it may be due to motility abnormalities, such as incompetence of the pyloric sphincter, delayed clearance of refluxed contents, or increased gastric volume. However, reflux of duodenal contents per se may not be sufficient to cause ulceration and, at most, is just one potential risk factor.[336-339] A combination of bile salts and acid is more injurious to the stratified squamous mucosa than acid alone.[340-343] Though reflux gastropathy[47,344] is commonly seen after surgical procedures, such as distal gastrectomy, gastrojejunostomy, and pyloroplasty,[345,346] in a number of symptomatic patients who have not undergone previous gastric surgery a nonfunctioning gall bladder has been implicated in excessive abnormal duodenogastric reflux.[347-349]

5. **Environmental factors**. *Smoking* is a risk factor for PUD, the risk being directly proportional to the number of cigarettes smoked.[350-352] Cigarette smoking is an etiologic and is associated with the initiation, prolongation, and recurrence of gastric ulcer.[353,354] Although certain foods, beverages, and spices may cause dyspepsia, there are no convincing data to validate the previously held view that some foods, such as spicy meals, produce, perpetuate, or reactivate ulcers.[355]

Historically, *alcohol*, which not only has a social role in many societies, is also an analgesic in large doses, but can result in reactive and erosive gastropathy, has been around much longer than any other gastric damaging agent except for *Helicobacter*, and produces histologic changes similar to NSAIDs (i.e., a chemical/reactive gastropathy). From around 1900 on when aspirin became available, the big three became *Helicobacter*, alcohol, and ASA, and from 1970 on, NSAIDs were added to these. The use of analgesics to counteract alcohol-associated hangovers could well have been a lethal complication in some patients.

6. **Psychological stress.** Emotional factors or disturbances have long been suspected to play a role in the pathogenesis of PUD, for example, the type A "hard-driving executive" stereotype in duodenal ulcer disease. However, the role of psychological factors in the pathogenesis of ulcer disease is difficult to study because of methodologic problems in accurately quantifying stress.[356] Nevertheless, case-control studies have shown a strong association between psychological factors and ulcer disease.[357,358] Thus, although stressful life events occur with equal frequency in ulcer and control patients, the way these events are perceived and responded to differ between the two groups. Also, as a group, peptic ulcer patients have significantly more personality disturbances.[356] It should be recalled that the term *stress lesions* refers to erosions and ulcers in severely ill patients, and not to psychological stress.

7. **Heredity**. The observations of familial aggregation, blood groups, human leukocyte antigens (HLAs),

and secretory status in some cases of ulcer disease by earlier workers suggested that in some instances the tendency to develop a peptic ulcer is inherited. However, the patterns of inheritance are complex and were interpreted as polygenic, although the novel VEGF polymorphism −1780T/C could significantly predict the predisposition to gastroduodenal ulcer.[359] Also, the concept of genetic heterogeneity was proposed to explain the familial aggregation and the lack of a simple Mendelian pattern of inheritance.[360–362] Nonetheless, individuals who live in the same household carry the same *H. pylori* strains, independent of kinship.[363,364] Yet, in some cases, there is autosomal dominant hyperpepsinogenemia I.[365] Other rare genetic syndromes accompanied by ulcer disease include systemic mastocytosis, ulcer–tremor–nystagmus syndrome, type IV amyloidosis, and multiple lentigines–ulcer syndrome.[366–371]

8. **Associated diseases**. Several diseases appear to be associated with PUD, such as multiple endocrine neoplasia type I (MEN I with either gastrinoma or possibly hypercalcemia that may mediate a degree of acid secretion), chronic pulmonary disease, cirrhosis, systemic mastocytosis, and basophilic leukemia.[366,372–374] The pathogenetic mechanisms underlying ulcer formation in these disorders are not always clear. Because PUD is common, firm evidence of apparent associations of other disorders, such as heart disease, carcinoma of the lung, polycythemia, chronic pancreatitis, and chronic renal disease, including postrenal transplantation and renal dialysis, is lacking, and these diseases may be due to chance alone[375,376] (see also Chapter 8, Systemic Disease).

Epidemiology. The development and death of ulcer disease has been associated with the birth of urbanization in the last quarter of the 19th century.[377–379] At the turn of the century, annual hospital admissions for gastric ulcer exceeded those for duodenal ulcer[377,378] and the majority of gastric ulcers occurred among women; the majority of hospitalizations for duodenal ulcer occurred among men.[380,381] As discussed at the beginning of this chapter, it is easy to assume that these were all *H. pylori* related, although it should be noted that ASA came into the market around 1900, and, other than opiates, was the analgesic of choice until acetaminophen/paracetamol/Tylenol came into the market in the 1960s and regular NSAIDs around 1970. So many "peptic ulcers" from 1900 on may have been ASA rather than *H. pylori* related or a combination of both.

The age of presentation begins around 20 in duodenal ulcers and about 40 in gastric ulcers, though exceptions occur. In both conditions the incidence rises with age, peaking at around 40 for duodenal ulcers and in the late 50s and early 60s for gastric ulcers. It should be noted that no age group is exempt and that ulcer disease is well recognized in childhood. In children under 10 years of age, ulcers may occur in association with a severe underlying disease,[382] but increasingly appear to be NSAID related. There is an indication of regional differences, with higher incidence rates in urban compared to rural areas.[380] Although the incidence of peptic ulcers varies among different groups in the same country, and also among countries, such as the United States and Scandinavia, these differences are most likely due to environmental and not racial factors.

For the past 100 years, duodenal ulcer disease has been more common than gastric ulcer disease in Western countries.[383,384] From 1980 onward, there has been a decreasing incidence of both gastric and duodenal ulcers, with only a slight decline for gastric ulcer incidence.[385] The overall decline is likely to be due to a combination of factors including the introduction of acid-suppressive medication, a decreasing prevalence of *H. pylori* in subsequent birth cohorts, and the development of eradication treatment for *H. pylori*–positive ulcer patients, which prevents chronic relapsing ulcer disease.[386] However, there has been a concomitant increase in NSAIDs use, although more recently the use of PPIs, NO-NSAIDs, and Coxibs all helped to reduce the occurrences of erosions and ulcers.

Despite substantial advances, PUD remains an important clinical problem. The decreased incidence of ulcers was associated with a rise in the proportion of complicated ulcers. This rise was shown to be correlated with oral anticoagulants, NSAIDs, and oral corticosteroid intake.[386–388] NSAIDs and low-dose aspirin are an increasingly important cause of ulcers and their complications, especially in *H. pylori*–negative patients.[389–391] Other rare causes of ulcer disease in the absence of *H. pylori*, NSAIDs, and aspirin also exist, although some of these patients are found to have high serum salicylate levels despite repeatedly denying ASA use (that some cynically refer to as "essential hypersalicemia").

There seems to be no association between *H. pylori* eradication and the development of new cases of nonerosive GERD in dyspeptic patients, but in cohort studies, there seems to be a twofold higher risk of development of erosive GERD in subgroup of patients with PUD.[392] With a further decline in the prevalence of *H. pylori* and increasing use of NSAIDs, it has been speculated that the incidence of gastric ulcers is likely to exceed the incidence of duodenal ulcers in the very near future, revisiting a similar situation that was present at the beginning of the previous century.[386]

Clinical Features Symptoms of peptic ulceration are exceedingly variable, and a significant number of ulcers, especially in the elderly, are silent. The most common finding is epigastric pain, which is improved initially by eating (buffering action of food) but worsened hours later (further acid secretion). The abdominal pain is typically described as burning or gnawing, which may radiate to the back but can also consist of heartburn, abdominal cramping, or vague abdominal discomfort ("dyspepsia"). The pain is episodic in nature, both in a single day and over the span of weeks or months. Clearly, the symptoms of peptic ulceration are not specific and may be mimicked by numerous other disorders, such as cholelithiasis and gastric carcinoma. The other symptoms found in peptic ulcer patients are related to complications, such as bleeding with overt hemorrhage or occult bleeding resulting in anemia, perforation and peritonitis, obstruction, and penetration of the ulcer into adjacent organs such as the pancreas.

Helicobacter pylori infection is found most frequently in association with duodenal ulcers and is characterized by active antral gastritis and duodenitis in areas of gastric surface metaplasia. The persistence of *Helicobacter* infection appears to be important in ulcer recurrence. For instance, studies in which *H. pylori* infections were reliably eradicated showed a dramatic reduction in ulcer recurrence, whereas ulcers that did recur were invariably associated with an active infection or reinfection[116,393] or have other etiologies (NSAIDs, ASA, etc.).

Atypical clinical presentations. *Silent ulcers.* True incidence figures of silent ulcers are by definition difficult to elicit but have been reported to be as high as 70% in patients dying from complications of undiagnosed peptic ulcer and 71% in ulcer patients on treatment who are asymptomatic.[394] The recognition that ulcers are commonly silent has come from autopsy studies of patients dying from peptic ulcer and from endoscopic relapse studies after healing.[274,316] Silent ulcers occur in two important patient groups, namely, (1) elderly patients and (2) patients with arthritis on NSAIDs. These patients are especially prone to hemorrhage, perforation, and death. In fact, the majority of patients dying from peptic ulceration are elderly, frequently on NSAIDs, and asymptomatic until the presentation of their final illness.[274,316,395,396] This dissociation of pain and ulcer may be due to the analgesic effects of NSAIDs and to the fact that these patients may be conditioned to pain.[316] Unfortunately, the corollary of this is that one cannot rely on symptoms to reveal the presence of an ulcer in these patients, and there are no reliable tests currently available, other than an awareness of this complication, to detect these lesions before serious complications become manifest.

Pyloric channel ulcers. Patients with these ulcers differ from typical gastric ulcer patients in that they develop epigastric pain and vomiting shortly after eating and obtain little relief from antacids. Because of their strategic location, gastric outlet obstruction is more common than peptic ulcers elsewhere.[397,398]

Giant ulcers. These are defined as chronic peptic ulcers larger than 2 cm in diameter, and can be found in both the stomach and the duodenum. Because these ulcers may be intractable to medical therapy and have a high incidence of recurrence and complications, early surgery has been advocated for their management.[399-401] However, several reports have documented a successful response to medical therapy.[402,403] Some that we have seen are clearly NSAID related.

Postbulbar ulcers. Ulcers of the duodenum generally occur within 3 cm of the pyloric sphincter. Those found in the postbulbar region are almost always associated with hypersecretory states including ZES. The symptoms are generally indistinguishable from those of ordinary duodenal ulcers, although complications are often more severe, with intractable bleeding and obstruction.[404]

The diagnosis of PUD is largely made with endoscopy. However, the ability of the endoscopist to distinguish between an erosion and an ulcer may be arbitrary in some patients.

Endoscopic appearance of peptic erosions and ulcers. *Gastric erosions and ulcers.* Most ulcers are round, but oval or linear configurations are sometimes seen. The ulcer base is depressed beneath the level of the mucosa and is white, sometimes with a yellowish or green (bile-stained) tinge. Ulcers that have bled may contain clots, visible vessels, or have black staining of part of the ulcer base (Fig. 13-38). Erosions are more superficial and do not penetrate the submucosa, although the distinction is not always easy.

The edges are smooth and usually more erythematous than the surrounding mucosa. Ulcer edges that are markedly raised and nodular should raise a suspicion of malignancy. In clinical practice, most endoscopists make estimates concerning ulcer size without any formal measurements. Morphometrically oriented endoscopists or those engaged in ulcer healing studies commonly pass a biopsy forceps, open it, and relate the ulcer size to the known length of the opened forceps.

Duodenal ulcers. The appearances of these ulcers are similar to those of gastric ulcers, except that the surrounding mucosal folds are sometimes so swollen and deformed that it may be difficult to visualize the ulcer. Again, erosions are more superficial (Fig. 13-38C).

Gross Pathology The basic pathology of all ulcers is similar, irrespective of the site. The vast majority of ulcers are antroduodenal, and related to *Helicobacter* or NSAIDs/ASA. Ulcers occur much less frequently in the more proximal stomach, or atypical locations such as the esophagus, jejunum, and Meckel's diverticula containing functional gastric fundic mucosa. In the jejunum, they occur either adjacent to gastroenterostomy stomas (Fig. 13-39) or as part of the ZES, in which they may be multiple.[405] However, NSAIDs ulcers, as well as ulcers of other cause, occur throughout the small bowel.

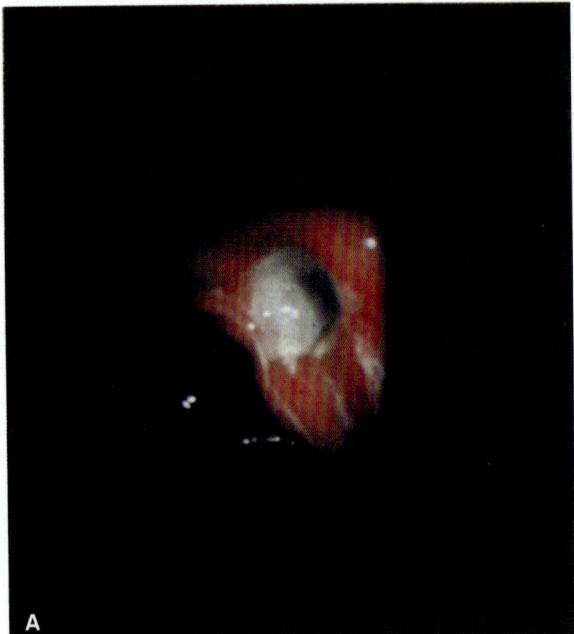
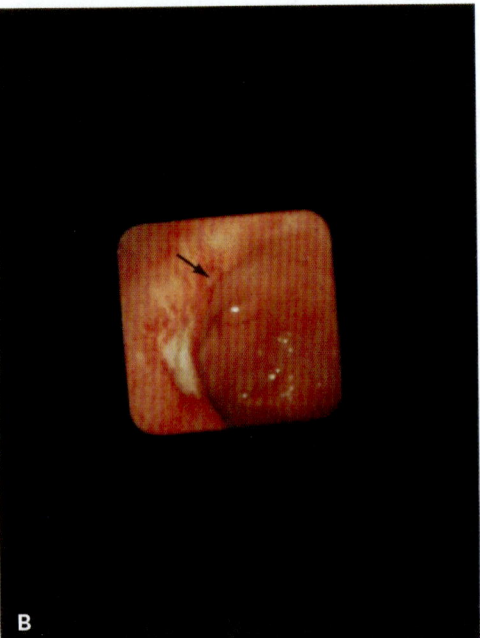
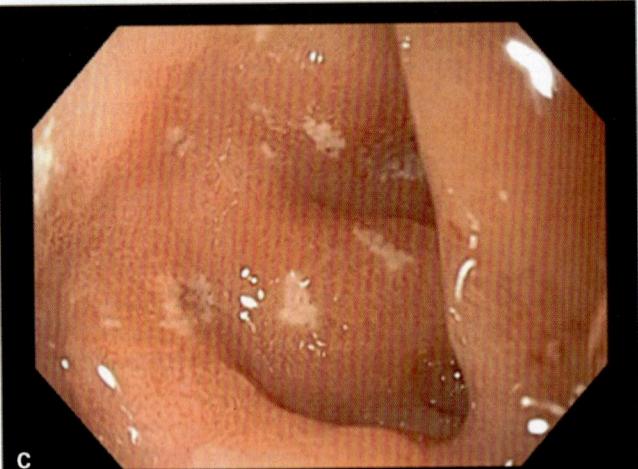

Figure 13-38. **A:** Chronic gastric ulcer. Endoscopic appearance demonstrating a punched-out ulcer covered by a greenish layer of pus. **B:** Endoscopic appearance of a small lesser curvature ulcer showing a depressed, ulcerated lesion lined by a yellowish-white exudate. A gastric erosion is present adjacent to the ulcer (*arrow*). **C:** Duodenal erosions.

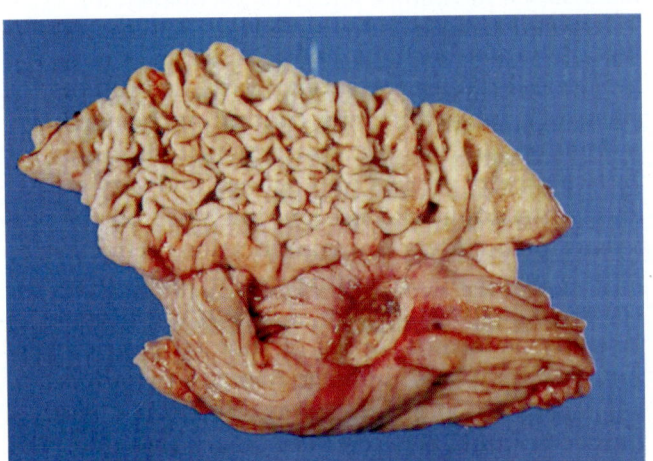

Figure 13-39. Large jejunal peptic ulcer adjacent to a gastrojejunostomy stoma. This patient had previously undergone a partial gastrectomy (Billroth 2) for PUD.

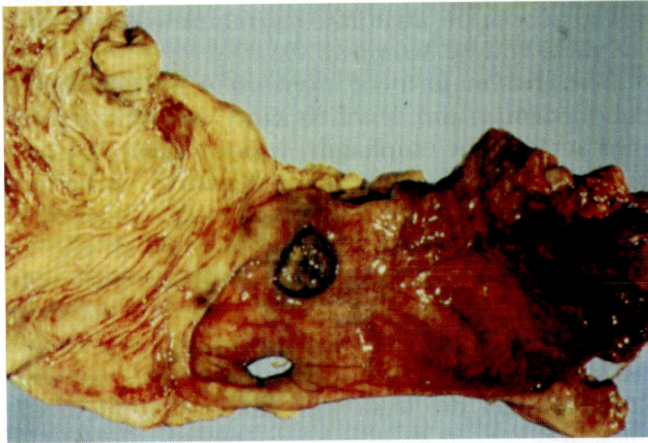

Figure 13-40. Two duodenal ulcers, so-called kissing ulcers, in the first part of the duodenum. The ulcers are about equal in size, located on opposite sides of the duodenum. One of them is covered by fibrinopurulent exudate, and the other is perforated. Note the severe mucosal erythema due to an accompanying duodenitis.

In the stomach the vast majority of peptic ulcers occur in the antrum, adjacent to the antral–fundic gland junction.[188] They are usually found on the lesser curvature, adjacent to the angularis, and only occasionally on the greater curvature. Occasionally they can be found in other parts of the stomach, such as the fundus. This supports the concept that the propensity of the mucous membrane for ulcer formation proceeds with age from the duodenum in the oral direction.[188,406] Up to one-third of patients with gastric ulcers also have duodenal ulcers,[407,408] which may also be NSAID related. In the duodenum, peptic ulcers most commonly occur in the first part, either on the anterior or on the posterior walls. Sometimes they occur at both sites simultaneously, so-called kissing ulcers (Fig. 13-40). Rarely they occur at the Z-line in hiatal hernias—so-called Camerons ulcers (see Chapter 10).

Chronic peptic ulcers are typically solitary, punched-out, oval, or elliptical lesions, occasionally with overhanging margins (Fig. 13-41). They are usually relatively small in size, measuring 0.5 to 2.0 cm in diameter, but occasionally may be very large (Fig. 13-42). Those measuring more than 2 (sometimes 3) cm in diameter have been defined as giant ulcers,[399,402] and are significant in that they may be misdiagnosed clinically as malignant (Fig. 13-43). The ulcer margins are typically level with the surrounding mucosa, in contrast to the heaped-up or beaded rim characteristic of most carcinomas (Fig. 13-43). In long-standing chronic ulcers, there are frequently folds of mucosa that radiate from the ulcer, probably because of the underlying scarring (see Figs. 13-40 and 13-43). The ulcer base is characteristically covered by an adherent, granular, grayish-white exudate (see Figs. 13-38A, 13-39, and 13-42). When the ulcer heals, the "healed" mucosa is often histologically abnormal[409] with lamina propria fibrosis, distortion of pits/crypts, and metaplasia.

The depth of penetration of ulcers varies. They may be confined to the submucosa but often reach into the muscularis propria and occasionally penetrate adjacent structures, most commonly the pancreas, or to the serosal surface, where they elicit a dense fibrosis and sometimes perforate (Fig. 13-44).

Histology of Gastroduodenal Ulcers
By definition, ulcers have extended beyond the muscularis mucosae, into the submucosa, and often into the muscularis propria and often beyond (Fig. 13-44), in contrast to erosions, which are limited to the mucosa. Those in the duodenum are the same as those seen in the stomach, and are characteristically composed of four layers.

The inflammation associated with duodenal ulcer is often localized to the immediate vicinity of the ulcer.[409–411] The uppermost portion of active ulcers consists of neutrophils and fibrin. Below this is a zone of necrosis made up of necrotic epithelial debris, inflammatory cells, and blood, all enmeshed in a fibrinous

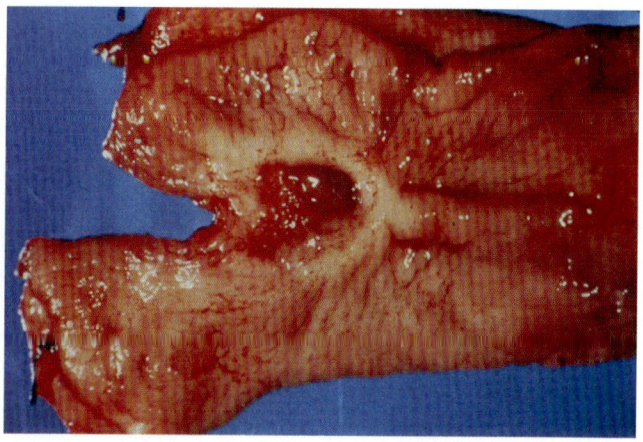

Figure 13-42. Chronic gastric ulcer with fibrosis resulting in thickened mucosal folds around the ulcer and radiating from the ulcer.

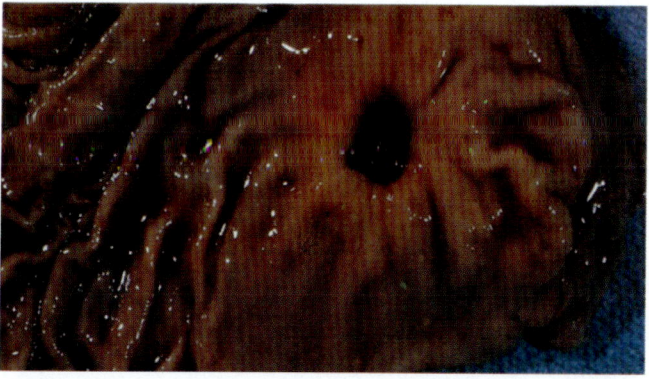

Figure 13-41. Gastrectomy specimen with a typical chronic gastric ulcer. Note the well-circumscribed, punched-out ulcer with smooth, edematous ulcer margins. Mucosal folds can be seen to be radiating from the ulcer margins.

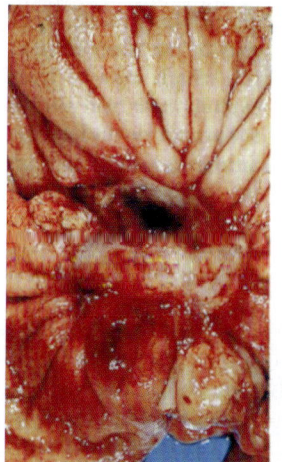 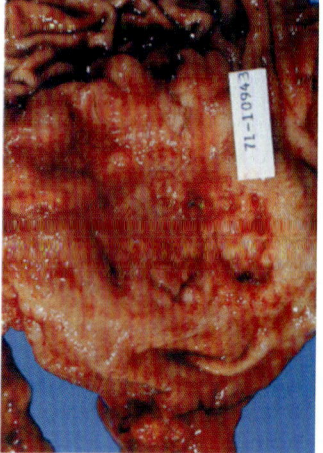

Figure 13-43. Giant ulcer (**left**) and gastric adenocarcinoma (**right**) for comparison. The ulcer margins are typically level with the surrounding mucosa, in contrast to the heaped-up or beaded rim that is characteristic of carcinoma. The gastric ulcer shows evidence of recent hemorrhage.

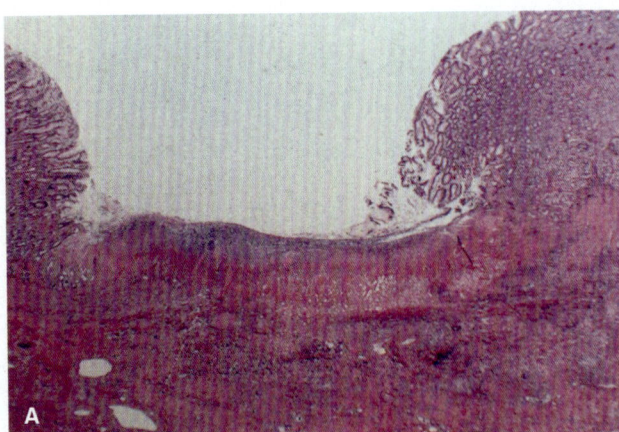
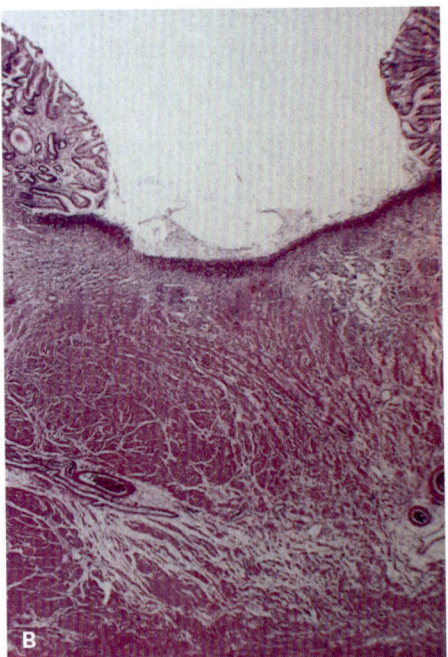
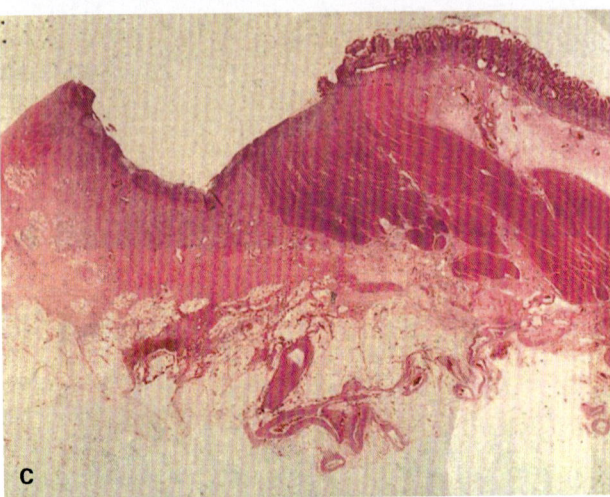

Figure 13-44. Chronic peptic ulcer. Scanning power view showing the histologic spectrum of appearances. **A:** Ulcer involving only the mucosa and submucosa. **B:** Ulcer extending to but not through the muscularis propria. **C:** Ulcer penetrating to the serosa and eliciting a marked fibrosis in the ulcer bed. Examination of the mucosa at the edge of the ulcer in all three specimens is surprisingly uninflamed, even at this power. This suggests an acute episode rather than *Helicobacter*, and therefore that these are medication (NSAID/ASA) related.

exudate (Fig. 13-45). Beneath the necrotic layer is a zone of granulation tissue (Fig. 13-45). The fourth layer consists of the ulcer base and is composed of fibrous tissue that may be hyalinized. This layer commonly extends into and through the muscularis propria to the serosa or underlying tissues such as the pancreas. In chronic ulcers, the muscularis mucosae and propria may be fused with dense submucosal fibrosis. A major key is the status of the adjacent mucosa, and especially if it is inflamed and *Helicobacter* related, or has severe reactive changes but relatively little inflammation (much more likely to be medication related). Sometimes there is a severe accompanying lymphoid infiltrate (see Fig. 13-18), (gastric lymphoid hyperplasia), which may mimic malignant lymphoma. Vessels in the ulcer bed commonly show marked endarteritic changes (see Fig. 13-45). They may be eroded and are the site of hemorrhage. Hypertrophy of nerve bundles is a common finding (Fig. 13-46). At the ulcer margin, the muscularis mucosae is usually thickened and often fused with the muscularis propria (Fig. 13-46B), and may also be accompanied by intestinal metaplasia that may be extensive (Fig. 13-46C).

At the edge of the ulcer mucosal regeneration occurs, and in the presence of inflammation the regenerative epithelium may sometimes be confused with dysplasia. The major histologic differences are described in detail in the discussion of gastric dysplasia (see Chapter 17). However, in regeneration there is usually evidence of surface maturation, mitotic activity is confined to the deeper foveolar regions, and cytologically the nuclei are blander and more uniform in appearance. In contrast, in dysplasia the appearances are essentially similar to those of adenoma, with marked cytologic atypia, loss of surface maturation, and cytoplasmic basophilia due to mucin depletion. However, these distinguishing features are sometimes not clear-cut, and it may not be possible to make a definitive diagnosis. In these cases, a repeat biopsy may be necessary.

In the proximal stomach ulceration in hiatal hernias (Cameron's ulcers) are associated with a pseudomembranous, almost ischemic appearance, which is rare at other sites. This may also cause necrosis of pit epithelium to form signet ring-like cells or sheets of parietal cells, both of which can be mistaken for carcinomas.

Chapter 13 Stomach and Proximal Duodenum: Inflammatory and Miscellaneous Disorders

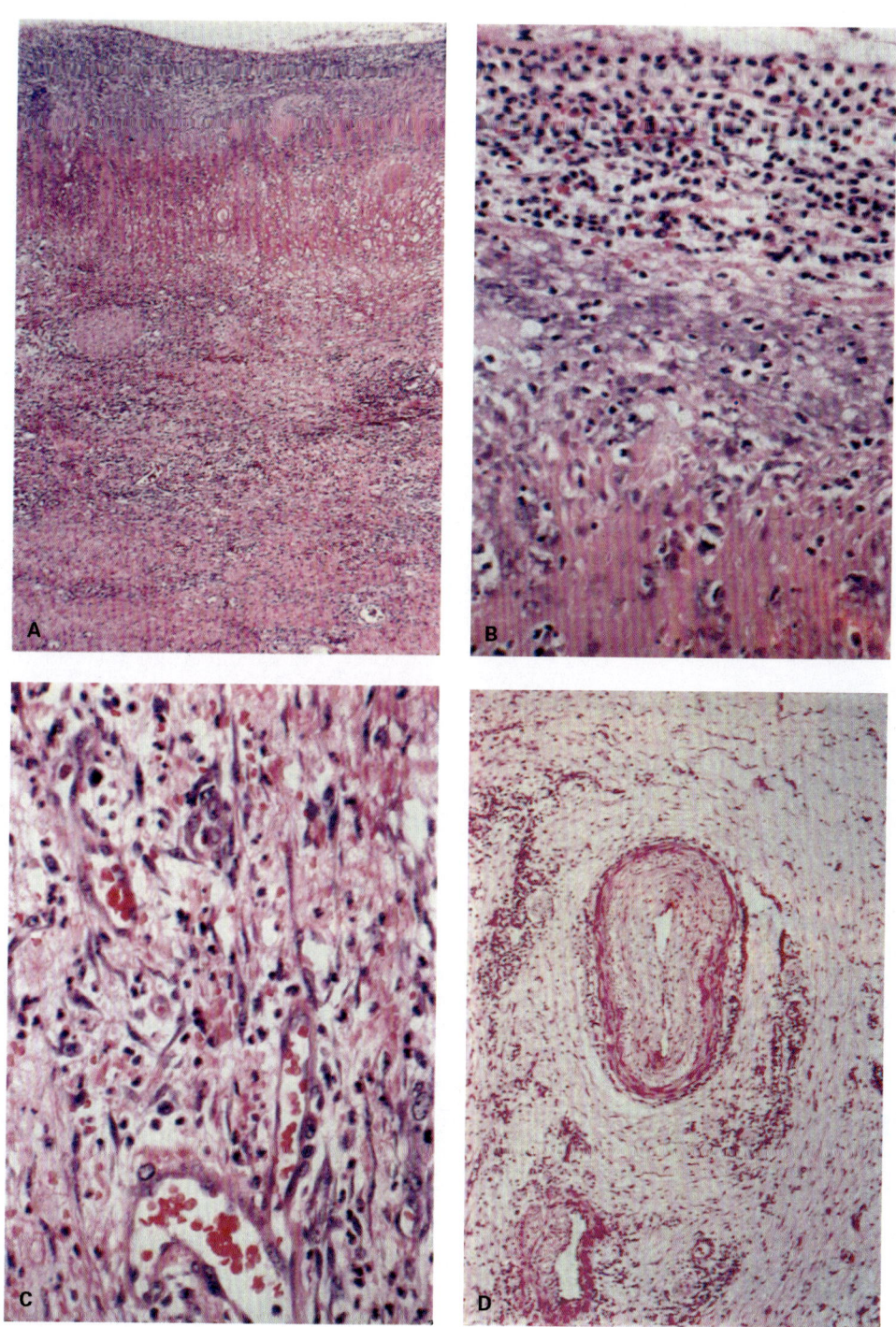

Figure 13-45. Sections of peptic ulcer bed showing the three layers. **A:** Low-power view demonstrating the superficial necrotic layer, middle layer of granulation tissue, and the deepest layer of fibrous tissue. **B:** Detail of the superficial necrotic zone. Note the superficial neutrophilic exudate and the underlying fibrinous exudate. **C:** Detail of the middle layer showing granulation tissue. **D:** Detail of the deepest layer showing fibrosis and endarteritis obliterans.

Differential diagnosis and etiology. The mucosa adjacent to gastric ulcers may show gastritis and the presence of *H. pylori* either in the adjacent gastric surface cell metaplasia or in the gastric antrum. Duodenitis surrounds duodenal ulcers that are associated with *H. pylori* and may be fairly diffuse.

In contrast, ulcers associated with medications (NSAIDs, etc.) may have virtually normal surrounding mucosa other than a few neutrophils or eosinophils—an etiologic clue, especially if (a) there are no gastric *Helicobacter* and (b) severe reactive gastropathy is seen (Fig. 13-47).

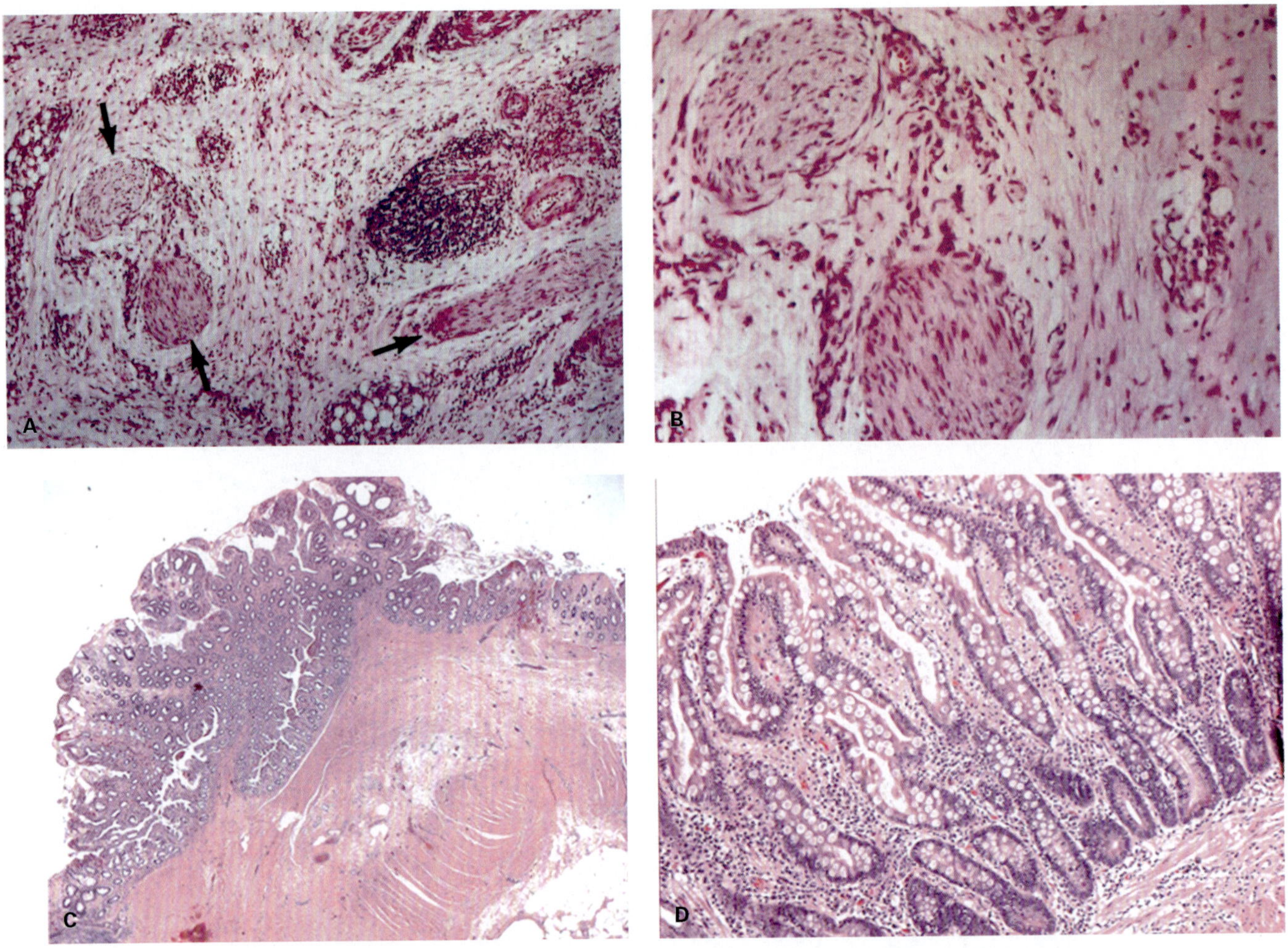

Figure 13-46. Ulcer bed from a chronic peptic ulcer with neural hyperplasia. **A:** Overview showing fibrosis, chronic inflammation, and several hypertrophied nerve bundles (*arrow*). **B:** Detail of hypertrophied nerves. **C:** Fusion of the muscularis mucosae and muscularis propria as they flow toward the bottom left of the illustration at site of healed GU. **D:** Extensive intestinal metaplasia in the gastric antrum; the villi having numerous goblet cells and therefore more reminiscent of ileal than duodenal villi.

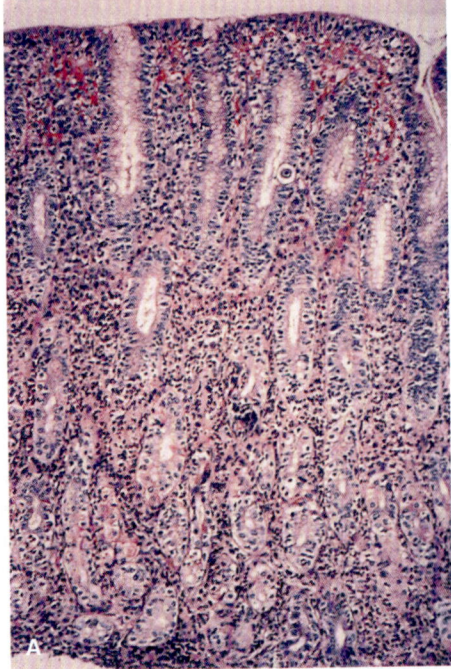

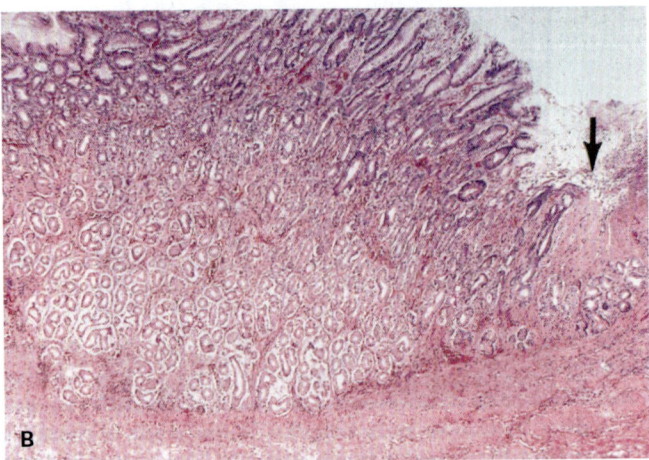

Figure 13-47. Overview of mucosa at the margins of two peptic ulcers. **A:** Severe gastritis compatible with *H. pylori* infection. **B:** Normal mucosa from the pyloric sphincter region with a small focus of coagulative necrosis (*arrow*). The coagulative necrosis and absence of inflammation should alert the clinician to the possibility of NSAID-associated peptic ulceration.

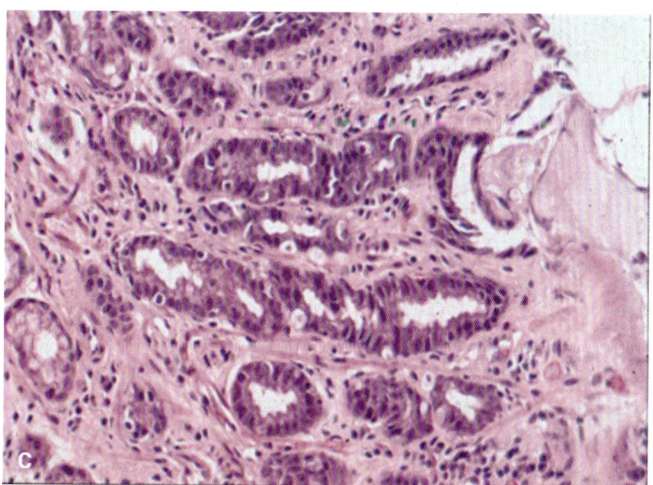
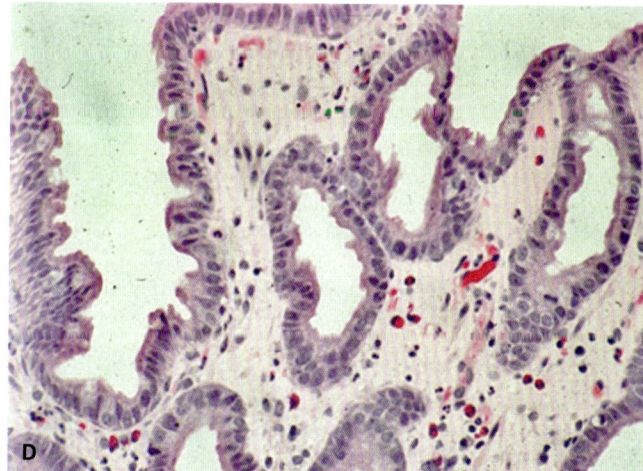
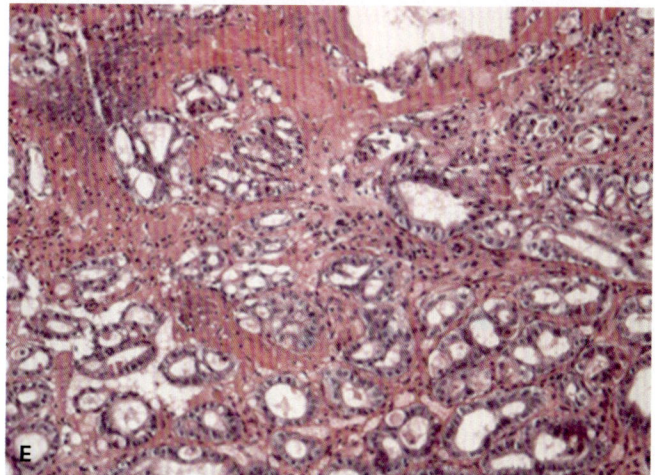

Figure 13-47. *(Continued)* **C:** Edge of an NSAID erosion. Note the total lack of chronic inflammation in the adjacent lamina propria that would be present in a *Helicobacter*-associated erosion and the uniform homogeneous eosinophilic erosion superficially. This is a typical NSAID erosion. **D:** Edge of an NSAID erosion. Note the reactive changes with eosinophils being the only recognizable cell in the lamina propria, and therefore not *Helicobacter*. In both (C) and (D) the lack of differentiation makes it difficult to know whether these are gastric or duodenal. **E:** NSAID erosion in the gastric body. Note the complex regenerative architecture that in the absence of the overt parietal cell differentiation could be mistaken for early carcinoma. (Fundic gland carcinomas have a completely different morphology—see Chapter 14.)

If the inflammation is focal with severe chronic active inflammation the possibility of Crohn's disease needs to be considered.

Healing. As the ulcer heals, the ulcer bed is gradually replaced by granulation tissue and fibrosis, and epithelial regeneration occurs, sometimes with intestinal metaplasia. In healed peptic ulcers the mucosa is often atrophic, frequently consisting of a thin, attenuated epithelium devoid of glands overlying dense fibrosis. The submucosa is usually gone, and the muscularis propria shows either irregular or complete replacement of muscle bundles by fibrous tissue. It should be remembered, however, that peptic ulceration is a dynamic process in which mucosal injury may persist or recur. Therefore, active superficial inflammation may persist in an apparently healed ulcer.

"PEPTIC DISEASES" OF THE DUODENAL BULB AND THE PROXIMAL DUODENUM

Duodenitis generally refers to inflammation confined to the duodenal bulb. Table 13-5 gives the associations with duodenitis. Erosive and nonerosive duodenitis are discussed together in this section because they coexist so commonly in the duodenal ulcer patient, especially in the course of ulcer healing. Most acute duodenitides are seen in patients with active erosions or ulcers, with recently healed ulcers, and in some with a more remote history of ulcer.[296,410,412–414] Also included in Table 13-10 is a reminder that the duodenal bulb is commonly involved in continuity with mucosal diseases of the small bowel, as discussed in Chapter 17. Strictly speaking, many of those disorders also represent duodenitis, but most use the term *duodenitis* in reference to inflammation primarily confined to the duodenal bulb.

Pathogenesis and Clinical Features of Duodenitis

Pathogenesis. The pathogenesis of duodenitis, when associated with duodenal ulcer, is also that of duodenal ulcer itself except for the superimposed features of ulceration discussed in the preceding section. Practically there are three major causes of duodenal erosions or ulcers. The "big 3" are *H. pylori*, medications/iatrogenic, and less commonly Crohn's disease. Some of the conditions associated with gastric hemorrhages and erosions (see Table 13-1) may be associated with erosive

Table 13-10	Associations of Erosive and Nonerosive Duodenitis

I. Duodenitis confined to the duodenal bulb
Duodenal ulcer spectrum,[a] active and after healing
In renal failure (nodular duodenitis)
Association with gastric erosions/subepithelial
   hemorrhages, especially:
     Medications: NSAIDs, ASA, bisophonates, other
     anti-platelet medications
No stress ulcers
No obvious association[a]

II. Nonspecific and specific duodenitis in continuity with disorders involving the rest of the small bowel[b]
Most commonly encountered are:
   Celiac sprue
   Postinfectious
   AIDS-associated
   More distinctive lesions
     Crohn's disease (if granulomatous)
     Giardia lamblia (intraepithelial lymphocytes)
     Cytomegalovirus

[a]*Helicobacter pylori* may be present and thus may also be associated with chronic active gastritis.
[b]All the potential contiguous small bowel mucosal diseases, as discussed in Chapter 20.

duodenitis or ulcers. This is especially true of patients on NSAIDs and also of some patients with stress lesions. Some of these may represent flare-ups of previous duodenal ulcers. This "spillover" from the stomach also applies to some rare cases of gastric ischemia.[39]

Duodenitis is encountered sporadically in dyspeptic and nondyspeptic patients with no history of duodenal ulcer disease. It is not known if these patients have a duodenal ulcer diathesis (however defined) or if their mucosal injury has some other basis. A clear implication of this is that if the duodenum has erosions or ulcers then it is also necessary to biopsy the stomach for *Helicobacter*, even if there is nothing obvious endoscopically as all of the major causes of duodenal erosions and ulcers (*H. pylori*, medications [NSAIDs/ASA], CD) may also have gastric lesions; clearly, duodenal *Helicobacter* cannot exist in the absence of gastric infection.

Duodenal ulcer. *Helicobacter*: CagA-producing strains are particularly associated with ulcer disease (see prior discussion for mechanisms[415,416]). This early stage of *H. pylori* gastritis is antral predominant with mild, superficial, or even absent inflammation in the gastric corpus.[120,143] This stage is often characterized by an exaggerated gastrin response to meals,[144] which precipitates an increase in acid secretion enough to cause duodenal ulcer disease in some patients. Gastric *Helicobacter* is commonly present in duodenitis, and in these instances the organisms are always present in the gastric antrum. Areas of gastric surface cell metaplasia (Fig. 13-48) are commonly present in duodenitis. When antral *H. pylori* is present, the relative risk of duodenal ulcers increases by a factor of 7, and when the organisms are present in the areas of the metaplasia,[296,417–420] the risk increases, possibly by a factor of 50.[421] It should be stressed, however, that small foci of gastric surface cell metaplasia (without accompanying inflammation) are physiological and have been documented in up to two-thirds of normal individuals and also in renal failure.[145,422] Yet the prevalence of *H. pylori* in these settings is uncommon.

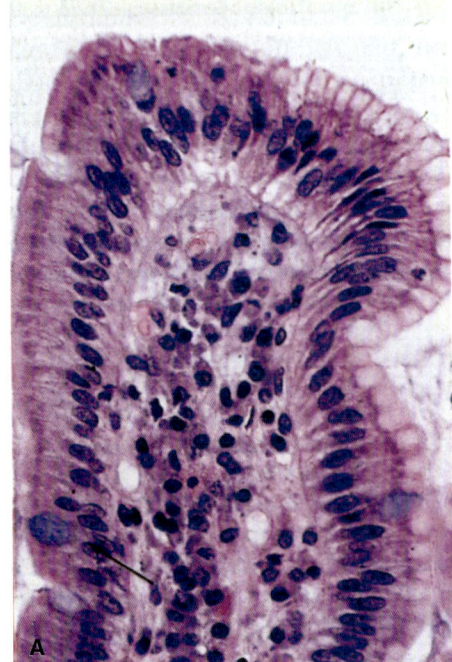

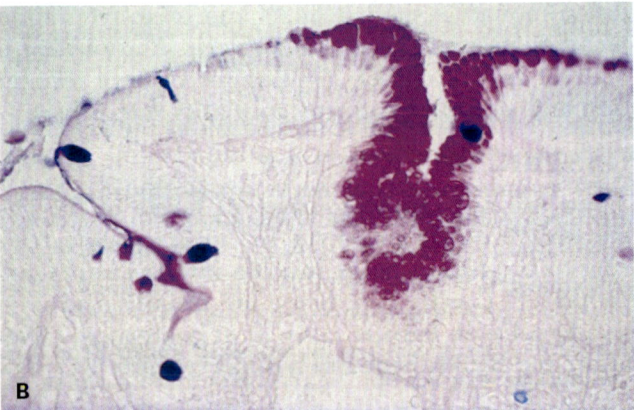

Figure 13-48. Gastric surface cell metaplasia. **A:** High-power view of a duodenal villus in which the right half is lined by typical gastric surface cells with their luminally displaced mucus. An intestinal-type blue goblet cell (*arrow*) is seen on the left, Alcian blue, pH 2.5. **B:** PAS highlights (red-staining) the gastric surface cell metaplasia.

Nonsteroidal Anti-inflammatory Drugs and Synergy with H. pylori: *H. pylori*– associated antral gastritis accompanies more than 90% of all duodenal ulcers, but as the prevalence of *H. pylori* decreases medications (NSAIDs/ASA) play a greater role in duodenal ulcers seen now. Given that NSAIDs (including aspirin) are gastric irritants, it could be predicted that such drugs would act synergistically with *H. pylori* gastritis to exacerbate mucosal damage. However, a role for *H. pylori* in increasing the risk of acute gastroduodenal injury has been difficult to establish or refute,[26,423] and *H. pylori* can be difficult to find in patients taking NSAIDs. Whether their anti-inflammatory effect includes decreasing the inflammation associated with *H. pylori,* and possibly the ability of *H. pylori* to grow in the stomach, is unknown.

Shiotani et al.[423] examined the relationship between the severity of endoscopic score for NSAID-induced gastric injury and gastric pathology including polymorphonuclear (PMN) leukocyte infiltration, *H. pylori* density, mucosal interleukin-8, and nitrite levels. Patients were assessed after receiving placebo and again after receiving 1,000 mg of naproxen daily for 3 days. All had normal-appearing gastric mucosa after placebo. Postnaproxen gastric damage included three with none, one with mild, three with moderate, two with severe, and three with very severe mucosal injury (including one with an 5 mm ulcer). There was an inverse correlation between endoscopic score and the pH of the gastric juice posttherapy. There was no significant change in histologic or biochemical parameters from pretreatment levels. In this study, none of the parameters (e.g., PMN density) predicted endoscopic outcome[423]—ischemic necrosis was not examined in the study.

Vieth et al.[26] studied the question whether NSAID/ASA-induced ulcerations can be identified in human gastric biopsy material on the basis of ischemic necrosis. NSAID/ASA ulcers were diagnosed when a homogeneous eosinophilic ischemic necrosis was found. *Helicobacter pylori*–induced ulcers were diagnosed when nonhomogeneous fibrinoid necrotic material containing granulocytes and cell debris was noted. The histologic diagnosis was compared with the data on medication use, endoscopy, and clinical history. Histology correctly identified all patients taking NSAIDS/ASA with no histologic evidence of *H. pylori* (100%). Histology correctly identified 66% of patients taking NSAID/ASA with histologic evidence of *H. pylori*. In infected patients with no such medication, histology correctly identified the pathogen in 76%. The sensitivity of the histologic diagnosis of NSAID/ASA-induced ulceration based on ischemic necrosis was 85%, and its specificity 53%.[26]

Overall, such drugs do act synergistically with *H. pylori* gastritis to exacerbate mucosal damage with an inverse correlation between the endoscopic score and the pH of the gastric juice posttherapy.[423] Though there is no relation between mucosal neutrophil density and endoscopic mucosal injury,[423] ischemic necrosis can be used as a good correlate of NSAID/ASA-induced ulcers in a high percentage of patients.[26]

Duodenal gastric oxyntic heterotopia: Islands of heterotopic oxyntic mucosa are quite common in the duodenum and are frequently biopsied. Yet the role of these in the genesis of duodenal ulcers has been largely ignored. In a fascinating study by Carrick et al.,[296] islands of oxyntic mucosa were demonstrated by giving subjects intravenous pentagastrin, then carrying out endoscopy and demonstrating acid production in the duodenum using Congo red spray, which is an indicator that becomes black at a pH of < 4. Congo red staining of the duodenal bulb showed that functioning endogenous acid-producing tissue could be found most often at the edges of duodenal ulcers, but also in nonulcer subjects. In those with active duodenal ulceration 20/23 patients had acid-producing mucosa at the edge of the ulcer, while 6/13 of those with healed ulcers had the same change. Interestingly, heterotopic gastric mucosa in the duodenum frequently has a chronically inflamed lamina propria as seen in normal duodenum, this is often a surprise when the gastric mucosa is completely uninflamed, as one expects it to have *Helicobacter*. Intrinsic duodenal acid secretion and *Helicobacter*, especially if duodenal, is therefore a potent association with duodenal ulceration.

Gastric ulcer: It is interesting that some patients develop both gastric and duodenal ulcers. In some the common predisposing cause is NSAIDs, but why this should happen in *Helicobacter*-related disease is less clear unless patients are taking NSAID-like medications in addition. Approximately 60% to 70% of patients with gastric ulcer have *H. pylori*–associated gastritis.[424,425] This is invariably associated with a pangastritis (inflammation of both the antrum and the body).[188,426-428] Inflammation is more severe in gastric than in duodenal ulcer.[426,427] The fundic gland zone is often inflamed as well, but initially less severely than the antrum. Like duodenal ulcers, NSAIDs play a significant role in *H. pylori*–negative gastric ulcers. As only one-half of NSAID users have the organism,[304,429] approximately one-half of the patients do not have antral gastritis.[304,429] The inflammation associated with duodenal ulcer is often localized to the immediate vicinity of the ulcer.[409-411] When the ulcer heals, the "healed" mucosa often remains histologically abnormal.[409]

Clinical features. Unlike nonerosive gastritis, duodenitis is not common in the population at large.[145,422] Attributing symptoms of dyspepsia to duodenitis is as difficult as it is with gastritis. The main reason is that duodenitis is extremely common in asymptomatic individuals, as exemplified by the healed or healing duodenal ulcer patient. Bleeding from erosive duodenitis is rare. Most of the symptoms come from complications (bleeding, penetration, perforation, stenosis, and obstruction).

Role of biopsy in duodenitis: The main indications for biopsy of the duodenum or the duodenal bulb are to rule out celiac disease, rule out infection in the immunocompromised, or when there is some reason to suspect that Crohn's disease or even rarer entities may be present. However, the golden rule of duodenal biopsy is that because duodenal disease is so closely related to gastric disease, that whenever the duodenum is biopsied, the usual five biopsies (incisura, two antral, and two oxyntic) need to be carried out to allow for evaluation of associated or concomitant gastric disease. Whenever duodenal injury is identified, the first question is inevitably that of what is going on in the stomach, whether it is *Helicobacter*- or NSAID-related change. When *H. pylori* is absent, a number of issues arise: sampling error because of focal distribution of the organisms; the potential role of NSAIDs, as in gastric ulcer (discussed previously; or a pathogenetically different type of mucosal injury, such as Crohn's disease or the other less common causes of duodenal ulceration.

Pathology of Duodenitis and Duodenal Erosions and Ulcer

Gross pathology. When erosions are present, they appear similar to those in the stomach (Fig. 13-49). Subepithelial hemorrhages are not as frequently encountered as in the stomach.

Unlike nonerosive gastritis, there appears to be a fairly good correlation between gross abnormalities at endoscopy and the finding of mucosal inflammation on biopsy.[145,430] In an endoscopically normal-appearing duodenal bulb, one is unlikely to find major inflammation on biopsy specimens. Intense focal erythema and mucosal swelling are very common when there is histologic duodenitis. Another finding is a diffuse pinpoint erythema, termed a *salt and pepper appearance*. Sometimes patches of erythema (Fig. 13-49C) appear to correspond to gastric surface cell metaplasia without much inflammation.

The gross changes around duodenal ulcers are confined generally to within 0.5 to 1.0 cm of the ulcer. A minority of patients have more diffuse change, suggesting that their duodenal bulb has been the battleground of numerous ulcer recurrences. If the gross changes spill into the descending duodenum, one should suspect other primary conditions, such as gastrinoma or Crohn's disease.[431]

Fundic gland heterotopia (see Fig. 13-37) has been previously discussed and is etiologically related to DU. It is reported to be more common (>50%) in resection specimens from duodenal ulcer patients than in nonulcer (20%) patients,[294,295] so is expected. When it is extensive, the gross findings may be those of nodules (commonly red-tipped) in the duodenal

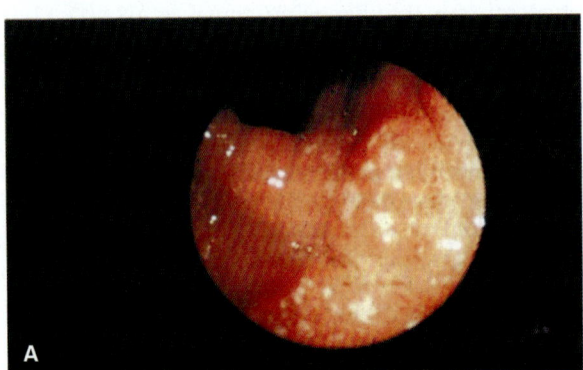
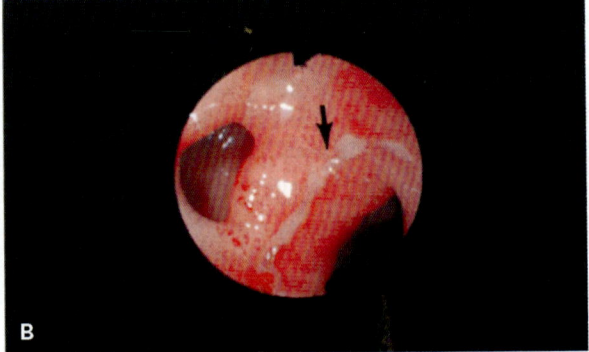
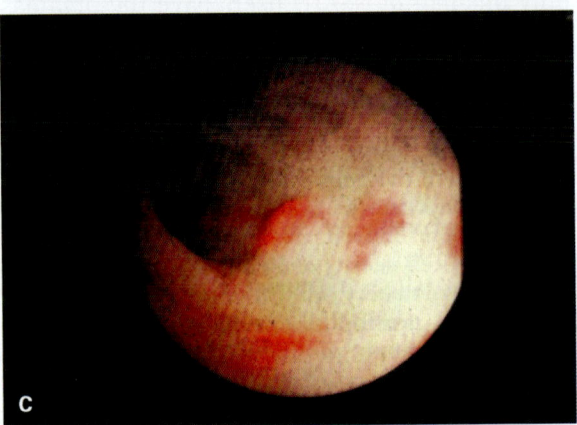

Figure 13-49. Endoscopically abnormal duodenal bulb. **A:** Erosive duodenitis with numerous white pus spots. **B:** Linear white erosion (*arrow*) in a patient endoscoped in the course of a healing study for the duodenal ulcer. The orifice of a pseudodiverticulum is at the left. **C:** Red patches. These commonly represent nonerosive duodenitis or just extensive areas of gastric surface cell metaplasia.

Histology. Villi are normally smaller ("blunter") in the proximal duodenum, and can even appear flat (Fig. 13-50). It is important to interpret these as normal, and particularly not to attach adjectives such as "atrophy" or "blunting" that are readily misinterpreted as suggesting celiac disease. Villous height is therefore not as important a criterion in grading mucosal abnormalities in the proximal duodenum as it is farther downstream in the duodenum. Instead, the focus is more on an intraepithelial lymphocytosis than the inflammatory cell density in the lamina propria and epithelial changes.

While duodenitis can be subjectively graded, (e.g., as mild, moderate, or severe—Fig. 13-51), whether it is worth stating anything other than inflammation is normal or abnormal is debatable, as there is normally chronic inflammation in the duodenum. Where a "mild increase" begins is therefore also debatable. It is certainly age-related and duodenal biopsies in children and infants have little cellularity normally, so degrees of inflammation may need to be tempered with the age of the patient, and what is normal in older patients may be pathological in children. The chronic inflammatory cell infiltrate normally consist of mononuclear cells, primarily plasma cells, lymphocytes with occasional histiocytes, and mast cells. Neutrophils are rare but occasional eosinophils may be present, and more marked in association with medications. Neutrophils are commonly present in the cap when *Helicobacter* are present in the antrum (Fig. 13-51B). When inflammatory cell density is overtly increased separation of crypts occurs (Fig. 13-51). This, rather than villous blunting, is a more reliable marker of severe change. Duodenal villi also (like the lamina propria of stomach) have considerable numbers of smooth muscle cells with small

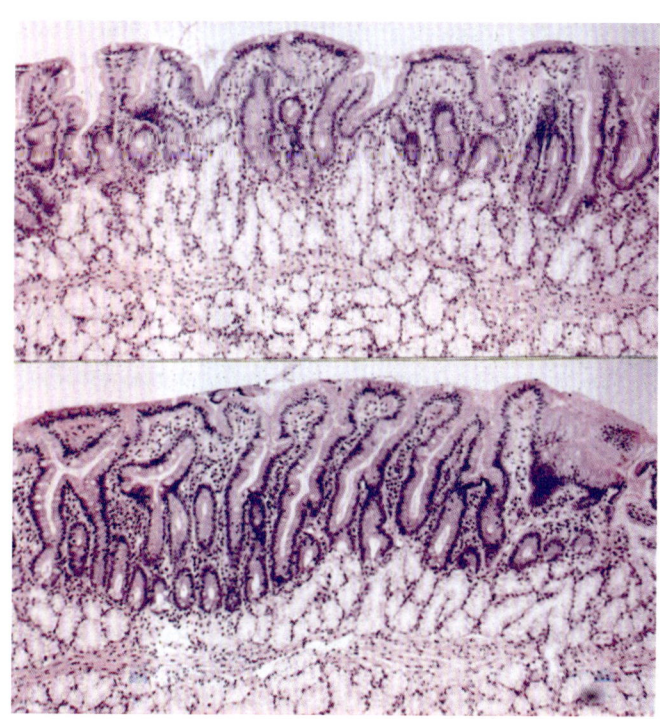

Figure 13-50. Variation in villous architecture in the duodenal bulb. The **top panel** shows an illusion of villous flattening, but without increased inflammation. The **bottom panel** shows more normal-appearing villi. The photographs are sections from different parts of the same duodenal biopsy specimen.

bulb (see Fig. 13-37). Sometimes these become very large and ulcerate or obstruct the duodenal bulb or beyond, farther into the small bowel (see Chapter 25).

Prominent nodularity of the duodenal bulb has numerous causes but the most common include nodular Brunner's glands, lymphoid nodules, or heterotopic oxyntic mucosa.

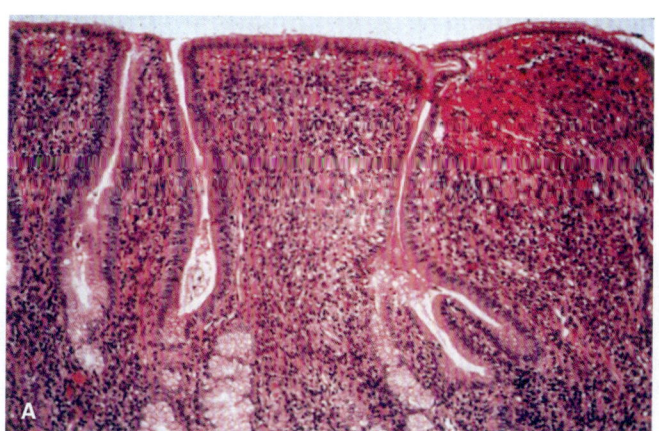 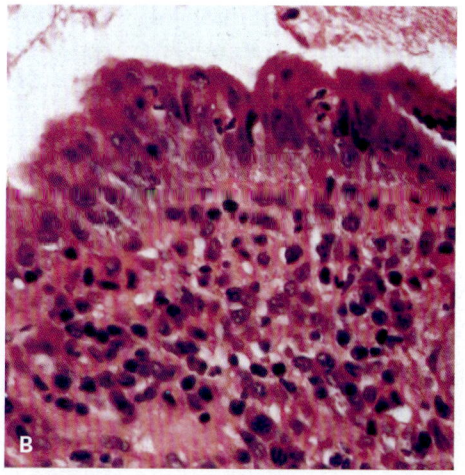

Figure 13-51. **A:** Severe nonerosive duodenitis with flattening of villi and marked expansion of the lamina propria by inflammatory cells. **B:** High-power view of the surface epithelium showing nuclear disarray, basophilia, and scattered neutrophils within the epithelium.

amounts of eosinophilic cytoplasm, which are easily mistaken for macrophage or mast cells by the unwary (see Chapter 16).

The three "major" causes of duodenal erosions are *Helicobacter*, medications, and Crohn's disease so this needs always to be borne in mind. *Helicobacter*-associated disease must by definition have contiguous gastric disease, and have a background of severe duodenitis, so that gastric biopsies for *Helicobacter* are mandatory whenever the cause of duodenal erosions or ulcers is being sought or they are being biopsied. Medication associated injury such as that seen with NSAIDs erosion give a characteristic acellular eosinophilic band (see subsequent section) but little or no chronic inflammation, while Crohn's disease, in the absence of granulomas, usually results in a quite marked focal chronic active inflammation but resultant erosions lack the eosinophilic acellular band associated with medications. It is rare for other causes of neutrophils (infections and bacterial overgrowth) to cause erosions or ulcers.

The reactive epithelial change in duodenitis (Fig. 13-52) may resemble the surface change of nonerosive gastritis that is common at gastroenterostomy stomas and adjacent to erosions. There may also be a comparable paucity of inflammatory cells accompanying the epithelial changes. Thus, in parallel with the disease of the stomach, the term *reactive duodenopathy (duodenitis)* has some appeal from a descriptive point of view. Interestingly, when these are marked, it may be impossible to ascertain with certainty whether the affected mucosa is duodenal or gastric type in the duodenum in view of the lack of recognizable gastric or duodenal differentiation.

Gastric surface cell metaplasia is a common if not invariable accompaniment of nonerosive duodenitis; its extent correlates, in general, with the severity of the inflammatory change.[145,296,418-420] This metaplasia is highlighted with a PAS stain (see Fig. 13-48) but is quite easily recognized in conventionally stained sections. It needs to be emphasized that small nests of surface gastric-type cells are seen in normal individuals without inflammatory change or *H. pylori*.

The morphology of *H. pylori* and its differential diagnosis are discussed in the previous section on nonerosive gastritis.

Differential diagnosis of duodenitis. When mucosal bumps are seen endoscopically in the duodenal bulb, the main possibilities include oxyntic (fundic) gland heterotopia, lymphoid follicles (rare), and Brunner's gland nodules (Fig. 13-53A,B), which were described by the anatomist Brunner in 1688 and are submucosal mucin-secreting glands.[432]

The principles of examining a biopsy specimen from the duodenal bulb are identical to those outlined for small bowel biopsy specimens in Chapter 17. In the bulb, biopsies should be compared with gastric biopsies because of the shared etiologies of many of the diseases found there, as described previously. For example, *H. pylori* gastritis is frequently accompanied by mild duodenitis and even an intraepithelial lymphocytosis (Marsh 1 lesions).[433] Architectural distortion secondary to NSAIDs use is frequently accompanied by reactive gastropathy. The presence of gastric surface cell metaplasia, *H. pylori*, and fundic gland heterotopia is noted, and CD, parasitic infestation (*Giardia, Cryptosporidium*), and celiac disease kept in mind. However, it is rare to uncover these entities when the clinical and endoscopic impressions are simply duodenitis (redness). In the immunocompromised patient, CMV is the main consideration in duodenitis. The cytomegalic cells seem to have a special affinity for Brunner's glands, where they are usually easy to recognize.

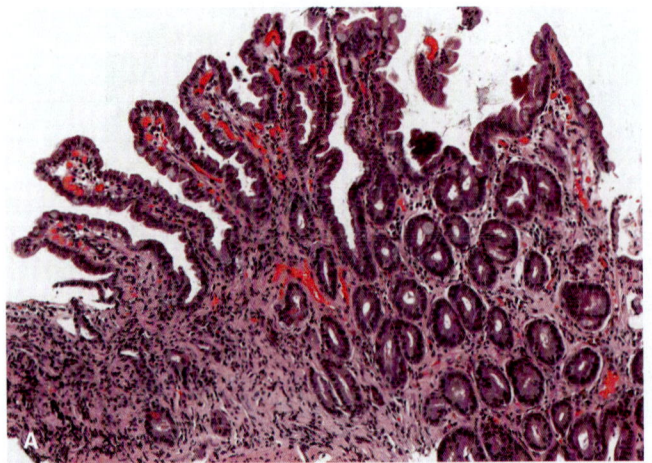
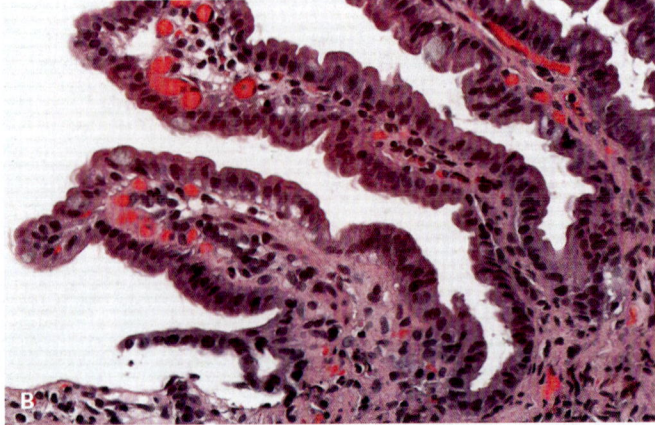

Figure 13-52. Reactive duodenitis. **A:** Very abnormal surface and crypt epithelium without an increase in inflammatory cells. **B:** High-power view of the crypt epithelium showing the reactive-appearing nuclei with large nucleoli and prominent mitotic figures.

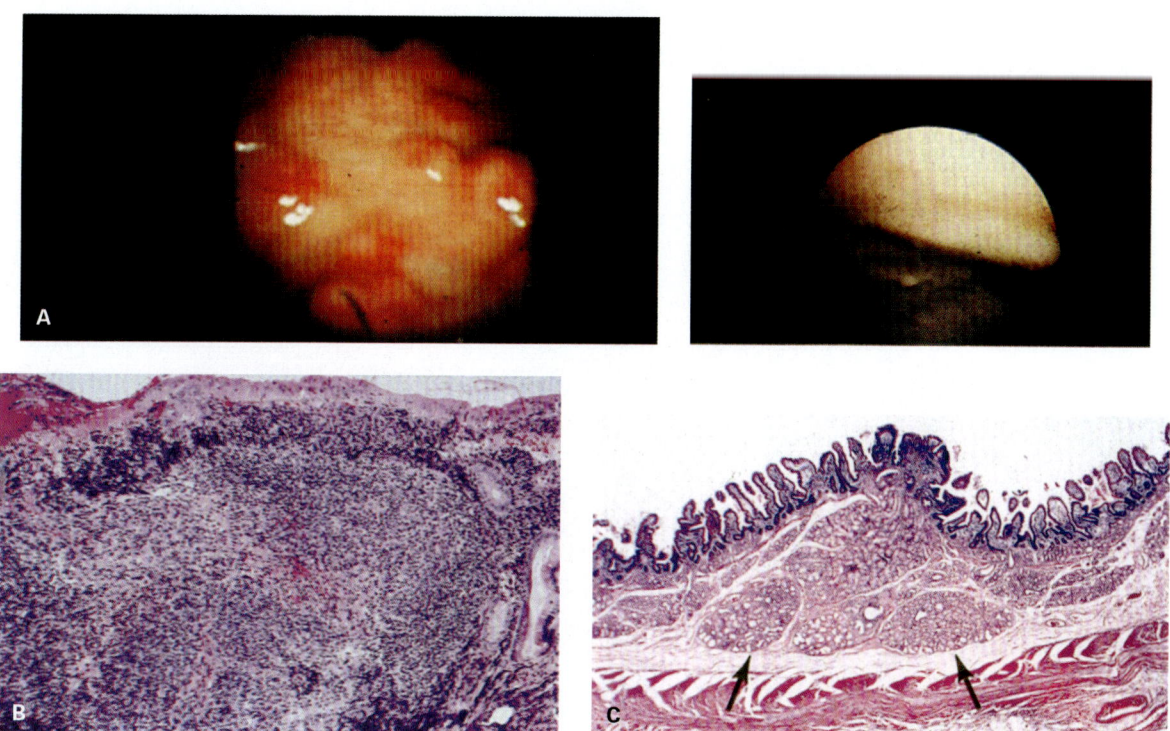

Figure 13-53. A: These red bumps in the bulb represent nests of fundic gland heterotopia. **B:** The tiny white bump in the duodenal bulb **(top panel)** is a histologically huge lymphoid aggregate **(bottom panel)**. Nodules due to large lymphoid follicles such as this are unusual in the duodenal bulb. **C:** Brunner's gland nodule. Overview of a surgical resection specimen with a Brunner's gland nodule (*arrows*). Endoscopic biopsy specimens cannot make the diagnosis because they cannot sample deeply enough.

Severe duodenitis in the absence of histopathologic features of celiac disease (e.g., secondary to bacterial over growth) can be associated with a flat or nearly flat mucosal lesions. This differs from celiac disease in several respects. In celiac disease prominent clusters of neutrophils are not common; neither is the reactive epithelium of duodenitis, which is more akin to that seen in gastritis. Nevertheless, if it is suspected on the basis of some of the histologic features, similar biopsy specimens beyond the duodenal bulb may help to confirm or to exclude celiac sprue, as this disease has lifelong therapeutic implications. If the edges of erosions are biopsied, it can be very difficult to know if one is really in gastric surface cell metaplasia or duodenal mucosa if there is no surface differentiation. Sometimes the differentiations (goblet cells or especially the small diffuse supranuclear vacuoles characteristic of gastric mucosa) are only seen in a small part of the biopsy.

Healing and healed ulcers. In the course of healing, the ulcers may assume an oval or linear shape. The ulcer base may no longer be depressed below the surface, thus resembling an erosion. As healing progresses with reepithelialization, bridges of mucosa between the residual ulcer base may create the appearance of localized multiple erosions.

Recent healed ulcers may exhibit a linear, whitish-appearing scar with variable or no surrounding puckering of the mucosa. In other instances there may only be residual erythema, and in later stages the mucosa may appear completely normal. Permanently deformed mucosal folds are more common after healing of duodenal than gastric ulcers.

Complications of gastroduodenal ulcers. Do any ulcer characteristics, such as the depth, size, and duration of the lesion, predict the likelihood of complications? The behavior of many ulcers is unpredictable, and their dimension is probably the best indicator of its behavior, lesions larger than 5 mm in diameter and deep lesions being more likely to produce significant complications. These lesions also heal more slowly and are more likely to recur.[274] However, what is probably more important than the morphologic characteristics is the question of associated *H. pylori* infection and NSAID medication.

Five major complications occur with peptic ulceration.

Bleeding. This results from erosions of arteries in the ulcer bed (Fig. 13-54), the severity of the hemorrhage depending on the size of the vessel involved. Consumption of NSAIDs accounts for about 30% of severe bleeding episodes, especially in the elderly,[316,386] and is enhanced by the anticoagulant effects of ASA and other platelet inhibitors.

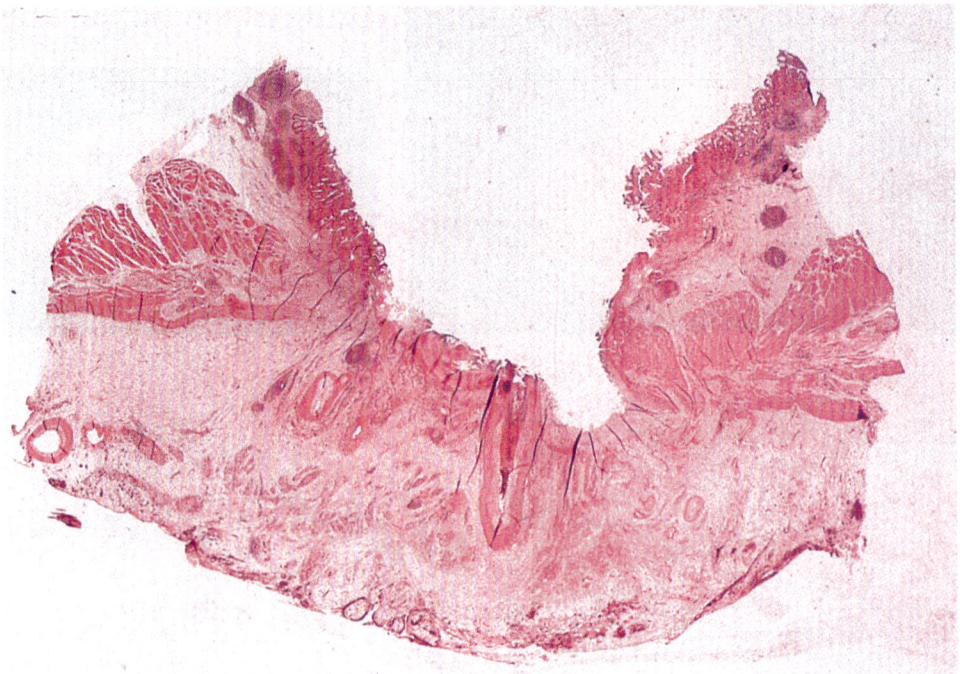

Figure 13-54. Ulcer extending to the serosa, with marked fibrosis in the ulcer bed. Note the erosion of a medium-sized artery in the ulcer bed that resulted in severe upper GI bleeding, necessitating surgery.

Penetration. An ulcer may extend beyond the bowel wall into an adjacent adherent organ, which functions as a seal and the ulcer is said to have penetrated the organ. This occurs most commonly with a posterior duodenal ulcer entering the pancreas, but other structures such as the colon, liver, or common bile duct may all occasionally be involved.

Perforation. When an ulcer extends through the intestinal wall with associated failure to be sealed by an adjacent organ, perforation occurs, with leakage of bacterially contaminated food and acid into the peritoneal cavity resulting in peritonitis (see Figs. 13-40 and 13-55). Interestingly, although *Helicobacter* must accompany the enteric organisms in the peritoneal cavity, it has never (to our knowledge) been cultured. This may be because other organisms overgrow it, it takes a long time to grow—beyond usual culture times, and it is also very sensitive to antibiotic therapy—enough for resolution to occur.

Obstruction. Ulcers may cause edema, spasm, or fibrosis, which may narrow the gastric outlet, often producing an hourglass deformity and impeding the emptying of the stomach.

Carcinoma. In the older literature, carcinoma of the stomach is frequently listed as a complication of gastric ulcer disease, occurring in as many as 5% of ulcer cases. Gastric carcinoma, in particular distal cancer, has decreased significantly with the decreasing prevalence of *H. pylori* infection and as a consequence of *H. pylori* eradication programs (see Chapter 14).

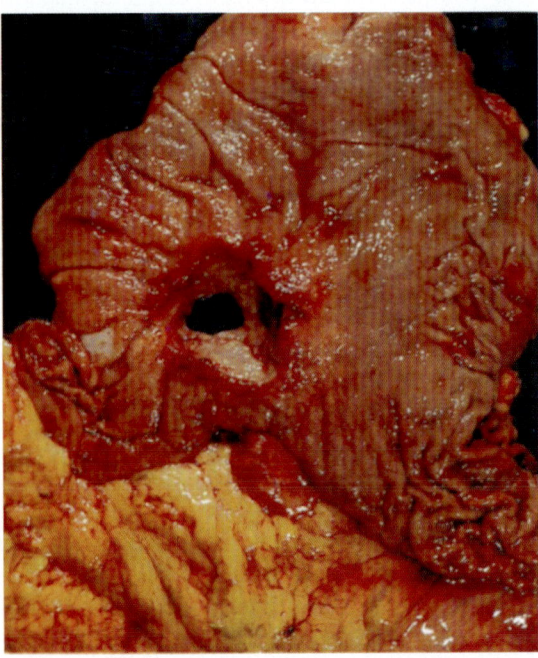

Figure 13-55. Perforated gastric ulcer. Note the typical punched-out ulceration with little mucosal abnormality around the margins of the ulcer. The wall of the stomach around the ulcer bed appears thickened.

Treatment

PUD was once considered a surgical disease, as it presented primarily with surgical complications. Our understanding of PUD has evolved from an acid-driven disease to one that requires acid but has become largely an infectious disease, a medication-associated disease, or both. Medical therapy has now become the mainstay of the treatment, which consists of agents that neutralize acid (antacids), inhibit acid secretion, as with the H2 receptor antagonists or PPIs, and eradicate *H. pylori* (e.g., antibiotics), or if possible remove injurious medication.

Indications for emergency surgery include continuing hemorrhage, perforation, and pyloric obstruction, and vary greatly among physicians.[434] Decisions are based on the persistence or occurrence of complications refractory to therapy or on the unwillingness or inability of the patient to continue therapy. The surgical procedures generally performed consist of subtotal gastric resection, vagotomy and drainage (usually pyloroplasty), and vagotomy and antrectomy. Following gastrectomy, continuity between the stomach and the small bowel is reestablished via either a gastroduodenostomy (Billroth 1) or a gastrojejunostomy (Billroth 2). However, these are vanishing procedures. Despite increased patient age and comorbidities, there has been a significant decrease in PUD mortality, a significant increase in the use of therapeutic endoscopy for bleeding ulcer, and a significant decrease in the use of definitive surgery (vagotomy or resection) for ulcer complications.[435]

The role of the pathologist and clinical implications. The role of the pathologist is threefold:

1. *To exclude malignancy* in gastric ulcers. Although cancer-complicating ulcer disease is rare, it is important for the endoscopist to be aware that early gastric cancer may resemble a peptic ulcer. In fact, because upper endoscopy is now so frequently performed, incidental early gastric cancers are being encountered more frequently. For the diagnosis of early gastric cancer to be excluded, adequate histologic examination is imperative. In general, it is recommended that four to six biopsy specimens be taken, most from the margins of the ulcer and at least one from the ulcer base. A potential difficulty arises in differentiating reactive hyperplasia in regenerating mucosa at the periphery of an ulcer from dysplasia and early gastric cancer. It should be stressed that if the histologic sections are small, crushed, or suboptimally fixed, this differentiation may be difficult. The pathologist should have no hesitation in requesting repeat biopsy specimens because of the serious implications of a diagnosis of cancer.

2. *Diagnosis of NSAID-induced gastric ulceration.* Clinically unsuspected NSAID ingestion in gastric ulceration can be suspected in gastric biopsy specimens because of the typical reactive changes described previously in the absence of *Helicobacter*. Histologically, these are commonly characterized not by mucosal erosion, but by foci of regenerative foveolar hyperplasia with minimal inflammation.

3. *To exclude other causes of gastroduodenal ulceration.* For example, sometimes "typical" gastric ulcers in immunocompromised patients result from opportunistic infections, such as *Candida* and CMV. Other less common causes of peptic ulceration also need to be considered and excluded, such as hyperchlorhydria due to hypergastrinemia.

Autoimmune Gastritis

Classical AIG results from immune-mediated progressive destruction of parietal cells leading to reduced acid production, and reduced or absent intrinsic factor (IF) necessary for vitamin B_{12} absorption.[436] Much of the autoimmunity may be related to a $CD4^+$ T-cell response to gastric H^+/K^+-ATPase in the canaliculi of parietal cells. Interestingly, although chief cells are the forgotten cell in this disease, they decrease at the same rate as parietal cells,[437] but this part of the immune response is not well-studied, and does not seem to be related to chief cell antibodies. In later stages of the disease vitamin B_{12} deficiency may result in severe anemia referred to as pernicious anemia. The name was originally chosen to reflect fatality in early sufferers who were anemic while the pathogenesis of the disease was unknown at that time.[438,439] The other scourge was subacute combined degeneration of the spinal cord, which was a major problem, although now virtually never seen in Westernized societies. George Whipple of "Whipple disease" fame won a Noble Prize in 1934 for his discovery that raw liver cured many anemias (including iron deficiency), and led to first cure for pernicious anemia, signifying the serious nature of this illness at that time. Full-blown pernicious anemia is now rare, and it is better referred to as AIG.

Pathogenesis. *Serology*: Approximately 90% of patients with AIG have antibodies to PCs, and 50% to 70% have antibodies to IF, and proton pump H^+, K^+-ATPase.[440-442] IF autoantibodies are considered by many as diagnostic of pernicious anemia.[440] The specificity of the autoantibody test is high as false positives in healthy controls have not yet been reported although antibodies to parietal cells are found in patients with *Helicobacter* gastritis and their incidence increases with age, and therefore (presumably) the duration which the organism has been present.[443-445]

In vitamin B_{12} deficiencies not due to AIG autoantibodies are rare and their prevalence may be 1%.[443–445] Cross-reacting autoantibodies initiated by *Helicobacter* may act against parietal cells resulting in AIG and hence *Helicobacter* is very much implicated in the genesis of AIG.[446,447] A major issue is that most of the definitive studies on AIG were carried out long before *Helicobacter* was rediscovered in 1983, and have not been repeated. Inevitably, studies dating back almost 100 years demonstrated the autoantibodies, but the fact that these represented immune mimicry to *Helicobacter* antigens could not have been appreciated.

Parietal cells loss can be widespread in *H. pylori*–induced gastritis atrophy and in some patients it is associated with a significant increase in antigastric autoantibodies.[448,449] The prevalence of antibodies to the canaliculi of the PCs increases significantly with the duration of *H. pylori* gastritis, in particular, with the development of atrophy of the corpus mucosa and subsequent hypergastrinemia.[450] In addition, a decrease of gastric autoantibodies after eradication of *H. pylori* infection has been reported by some.[451] Nonetheless, pernicious anemia following *H. pylori* infection is still rare and typically occurs in an elderly patient. For example, Chourasia et al.[229] reported gastric atrophy with peripheral neuropathy and vitamin B_{12} deficiency in a 74-year-old Indian patient following 20-year treatment with PPIs without *H. pylori* eradication.

For practical reasons, there are not many longitudinal autoantibody studies in patients with AIG, or in patients with *H. pylori*–induced gastric atrophy.[440] The only large longitudinal study in Caucasian patients with pernicious anemia ($n = 113$)[440] showed a trend for parietal cell autoantibodies to disappear gradually while IF autoantibodies became more prevalent. Unfortunately, this study relied on an insensitive and obsolete test for the detection of AIG. It may be preferable if AIG is restricted to patients showing typical corpus-predominant gastritis with positive serology for at least one of the gastric autoantibodies.[452] Thus while it is clear that *Helicobacter* is a major factor in the genesis of AIG, it is also clear that there is a subgroup in which *Helicobacter* play no role, these tending to occur in younger patients in whom there is an inherited predisposition. The inevitable possibility is that both are involved in some patients.

Subtypes of autoimmune gastritis (AIG) and their etiology. AIG is a corpus-predominant gastritis leading to severe atrophy of the oxyntic mucosa. The problem is that there are likely four variants of AIG:

1. Those related to *Helicobacter*-related that likely includes the well known predisposition typified by a Scandinavian ancestry.
2. Patients with other (auto)immune diseases, especially polyglandular syndromes and rarely IPEX syndrome, and therefore seen in both adults and children and occur in the absence of *Helicobacter*, although it is always possible they are potentiated by *Helicobacter*.
3. *Helicobacter*-related AIG. The most common cause of AIG is almost certainly *Helicobacter* related, with anti-*Helicobacter* antibodies cross-reacting with epitopes on or in parietal cells. The underlying disease is therefore *Helicobacter* gastritis that progresses proximally as described previously in atrophic gastritis, and increasingly involves oxyntic mucosa likely as an advancing front as seen in typical atrophic gastritis. AIG appears to be a late complication, as is any endocrine cell hyperplasia. Whether these patients have an inherited predisposition to AIG is unclear. Interestingly, when the advancing atrophic front with *Helicobacter* gastritis involves most, but not all of the oxyntic mucosa, a scenario can arise where the gastrin levels become high enough to begin driving ECL cell hyperplasia. One can therefore have the apparent paradox of ECL hyperplasia in the mid and distal corpus, but modest *Helicobacter* inflammation in the oxyntic mucosa, especially proximally on the greater curve.

This also casts an element of doubt on the role of antibodies, and why they should not affect the entire oxyntic mucosa. Nevertheless, virtually all autoimmune diseases have a degree of focality until completely endstage.

The form of AIG and PA that predominates in peoples of Scandinavian descent, but is almost certainly much more widespread but has been less studied in other races. It is oxyntic predominant, but its etiology is unclear. Assuming it conforms to other forms of AIG and PA, *Helicobacter* are likely required to precipitate it, potentiate it, but whether it can develop in the absence of *Helicobacter*, or be part of polyglandular syndrome (see next section) remains unclear. Both may well be involved. This is despite the fact that an autosomal recessive trait has been suggested.[436,469] Little is known of the pathology in these patients because initial studies were carried out in the pre-*Helicobacter* era. Now patients with anemia tend to go directly to hematologists for treatment of anemia who make the diagnosis on clinical and serologic grounds without gastric biopsies. Endocrine cell hyperplasia tends to develop early in this disease, most likely being in the same way as those with *Helicobacter*. However, when this occurs in patients in the first few decades of life, it is difficult to believe that an inherited trait is not present, either potentiated by *Helicobacter* or with a form of underlying polyglandular syndrome or other underlying inherited trait. These patients also invariably have antral G-cell hyperplasia, secondary to the profound hypo- or achlorhydria resulting in secondary hypergastrinemia.[244,453-456] While virtually all patients have or develop endocrine cell hyperplasia in the corpus, and some develop low grade endocrine tumors, which are largely harmless (see Chapter 5). Patients with corpus-predominant AIG who develop pernicious anemia have at least a three- to fivefold increased risk for gastric cancer and it may be as high as seven folds.[457,458] Pathologists can play a role by recognizing the ECL proliferation, although it can be subtle at times. Atrophic oxyntic mucosa with ECL hyperplasia can be misinterpreted as normal antral mucosa, so needs either expertise or a high index of suspicion or both.

4. AIG unrelated, or incidentally related to *Helicobacter*. *Helicobacter pylori* infection alone cannot explain AIG (latent or active) in the pediatric population,[459-461] nor the familial aggregation in the absence of *H. pylori* infection.[462] AIG associated with other autoimmune disorders has been described in teenagers.[459-461]

Polyglandular autoimmune syndromes: these include three major types, and pernicious anemia is seen mainly in types I and III. Type I is primarily seen in the pediatric age group, and types II and III in adults. Clinical features are described subsequently but organs involved include the thyroid, pancreas (type 1 diabetes mellitus), adrenal cortex, parathyroid (hypoparathyroidism), skin (candidiasis, alopecia, vitiligo). At least in the infantile form, the gastritis seems quite capable of developing in the absence of *Helicobacter*, but with formation of antiparietal cell antibodies. The prevalence of AIG and pernicious anemia is three- to fivefold higher in patients with type 1 diabetes mellitus, with respective frequencies of 5–10% and 2–4% compared to 2% and 0.5–1% in the general population.[463,464] Adults with autoimmune diseases (thyroiditis, rheumatoid arthritis etc) have an increased prevalence of parietal cell antibodies, but there are no correlative studies with gastric pathology, so it is unclear which proportion of these is associated with current *Helicobacter* infection, nor the severity or degree of inflammation and atrophy that might be present. There is no well-recognized association of other autoimmune disorders with *H. pylori* infection, although few investigators have examined this association.

The IPEX syndrome (immunodysregulation polyendocrinopathy enteropathy X-linked syndrome) can be accompanied by AIG and an autoimmune-type enteropathy, and is related to a mutation in the Fox P3 gene, whose function includes control of T-cell regulation. While the *Helicobacter* status in these children is unknown, given their very young age they are very likely to be negative.

It therefore seems likely that the pediatric forms of AIG are largely unrelated to *Helicobacter*, while the adult forms, are largely related to *Helicobacter*, some to type III polyglandular syndrome and other coexisting immune diseases. In the latter group, the role of coexisting *Helicobacter* infection is unknown.

Antral involvement in AIG: While most believe the antrum is uninvolved, this is often not the case.[465] It may represent either preexisting *Helicobacter* disease or an immune response aimed at parietal cells located within the antrum or a reactive gastropathy-type appearance.

Oxyntic mucosa involvement in AIG: The histopathologic diagnosis of AIG in its early stages can be challenging as biopsies only reveal chronic inflammation primarily in the oxyntic mucosa with minimal atrophy, and no metaplasia or endocrine cell hyperplasia. At its peak there is a severe chronic gastritis affecting the entire thickness of the oxyntic mucosa, usually with some residual *Helicobacter* inflammation in the antrum. In advanced disease, the degree of inflammation may decrease with loss of virtually all specialized glands of the upper stomach along with pseudopyloric, intestinal, and pancreatic metaplasia in both antral and corpus mucosa, occasionally with pyloric gland adenomas.[150,453,466]

Clinical features. AIG is far more common in Caucasians,[467,468] especially those of Scandinavian decent where an autosomal recessive trait has been suggested but it also occurs in other races but is just less well studied. As most result from longstanding *Helicobacter* infection this is not surprising.[436,469] Patients also tend to have other autoimmune diseases such as psoriasis, rosacea, autoimmune thyroid disorders, type I diabetes, Sjögren's syndrome, and celiac disease.[439,470-474] The association with other autoimmune diseases occurs in younger subjects as isolated AIG is rare before age 30 unless any congenital predisposing cause is present.[439,470-474]

Clinical symptoms in the early stages are no different from other forms of chronic gastritis, so are usually vague at best. If anemia develops, symptoms resemble those seen in other anemias (fatigue, pallor, and shortness of breath). Late complications of B_{12} deficiency include neurologic abnormalities such as peripheral neuropathy and subacute combined degeneration of the spinal cord.[475,476] Therapy for pernicious anemia centers on replacing vitamin B_{12} for life. In the presence of hypo- or achlorhydria, the absorption of nonheme iron is also decreased, leading to iron deficiency anemia.

As AIG is seen with *H. pylori*–induced gastric atrophy, vitamin B_{12} deficiency, common in Latin Americans and African Americans,[477] as well as severe vitamin B_{12} deficiency in the elderly,[478,479] has also

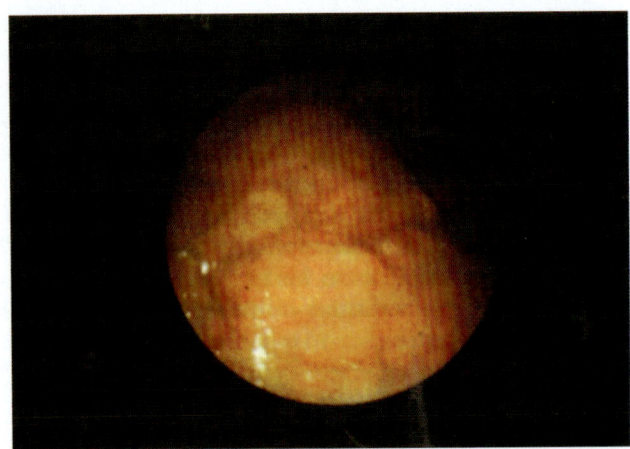

Figure 13-56. Thin gastric mucosa: endoscopic appearance. Folds in the body of the stomach are absent, and the blood vessels are easily visible.

been explained by a higher prevalence of *H. pylori* infection.[480,481] Further, severe vitamin B_{12} deficiency seen in *H. pylori* infection[477] has been reversed in some patients with antibiotics treatment.[232]

Endoscopy and biopsy—diagnosis and follow-up: Severe gastric atrophy may be evident as thinning (Fig. 13-56) of the mucosa, with a paucity of the gastric folds at the greater curvature and prominent vessels.[482] If there is extensive intestinal metaplasia, the mucosa may acquire whitish patches or a silvery sheen. The addition of other polyp other than fundic gland polyps (rarely seen in atrophic mucosa) which include numerous endocrine nodules causing polyposis in atrophic corpus mucosa. Also in the corpus mucosa hyperplastic or inflammatory polyps are found in 10% to 40% of patients on a background of an atrophic mucosa. Sometimes the polyps can be so numerous that it mimics a polyposis. Other polyps include intestinal type adenomas and carcinomas at any stage. All of these polyps may be clues for the alert. All require biopsy confirmation, and whether there are polyps or not, biopsying the background oxyntic and antral mucosa is key to making the diagnosis, especially the midbody region on the greater curve. The mucosa of the lesser curve and in transition zones (antral body, cardiac body) is commonly thinner than on the greater curve and could be erroneously interpreted as atrophic.

The question of endoscopic screening for neoplasms in patients with AIG is frequently raised. We agree with the recommendation that all patients with AIG should undergo endoscopy with biopsy at least once, either at or after the initial diagnosis.[483] We recommend taking four biopsies from the antrum and at least six from the body and fundus; these should be spaced equidistantly along the lesser and greater curvatures with additional biopsies from any nodules or polyps. If no carcinoids, adenomatous neoplasms, or high-grade dysplasia are discovered, the utility of screening at periodic intervals is likely not required.[484] Neuroendocrine tumors rarely increase in size, have no metastasizing potential until >1 cm and even if they do metastasize are rarely lethal and hence a case be made for no surveillance (see Chapter 5). However the risk of gastric carcinoma is significantly increased and the relative risk is about 7. Screening for dysplasia and early carcinomas every 3 years or so is therefore judicious, especially in those with widespread intestinal metaplasia. One additional concern is in patients with a history of gastric cancer in a first-degree relative; where again repeat examinations about every 3 years is appropriate. In the rare event that a patient is found to have high-grade dysplasia, more biopsy specimens should be taken immediately to rule out any coexisting carcinoma, and ideally treated with endoscopic mucosal resection or a similar ablative technique.[485]

Pathology. AIG is characterized by

1. ***Corpus (oxyntic) predominant gastritis***, that is moderate to marked but with little or no acute inflammation. It extends into the specialized mucosa where it is still present (Fig. 13-57).
2. ***Loss of specialized parietal and chief cells*** resulting in atrophy of oxyntic mucosa.
3. ***Pseudopyloric mucous gland (Fig. 13-28), endocrine cell (ECL) hyperplasia (ECL in corpus) (Fig. 13-58), and G-cell hyperplasia in the antrum, intestinal or pancreatic metaplasia or both.***
4. ***Numerous different polyps—hyperplastic, ECL (micro)carcinoids (Fig. 13-60), pyloric gland adenomas (see Chapters 5 and 14).***

In the areas of pseudopyloric metaplasia, there is invariably a degree of endocrine cell hyperplasia, and microcarcinoids may be present. However, these may be very difficult to identify in an H&E stain, but are brought out well with endocrine cell histochemistry or immunohistochemistry. If the patient has severe diffuse oxyntic atrophy and *no* ECL hyperplasia, the patient likely has had an antrectomy so that there are no G-cells to stimulate the ECL cells. The impressive endocrine cell hyperplasia in the fundic gland mucosa[486–490] is roughly correlated with the magnitude of serum gastrin elevation.[486] Table 13-11 summarizes the differential of corpus predominant gastritis.

Polyps: Apart from the mild nodularity often associated with endocrine cell hyperplasia or carcinoids, in the areas of intestinal metaplasia there may be dysplasia that can be flat or polypoid and rarely carcinoma. Rarely both endocrine and nonendocrine tumors are present. The much-discussed increased risk of gastric adenocarcinoma in pernicious anemia[484]

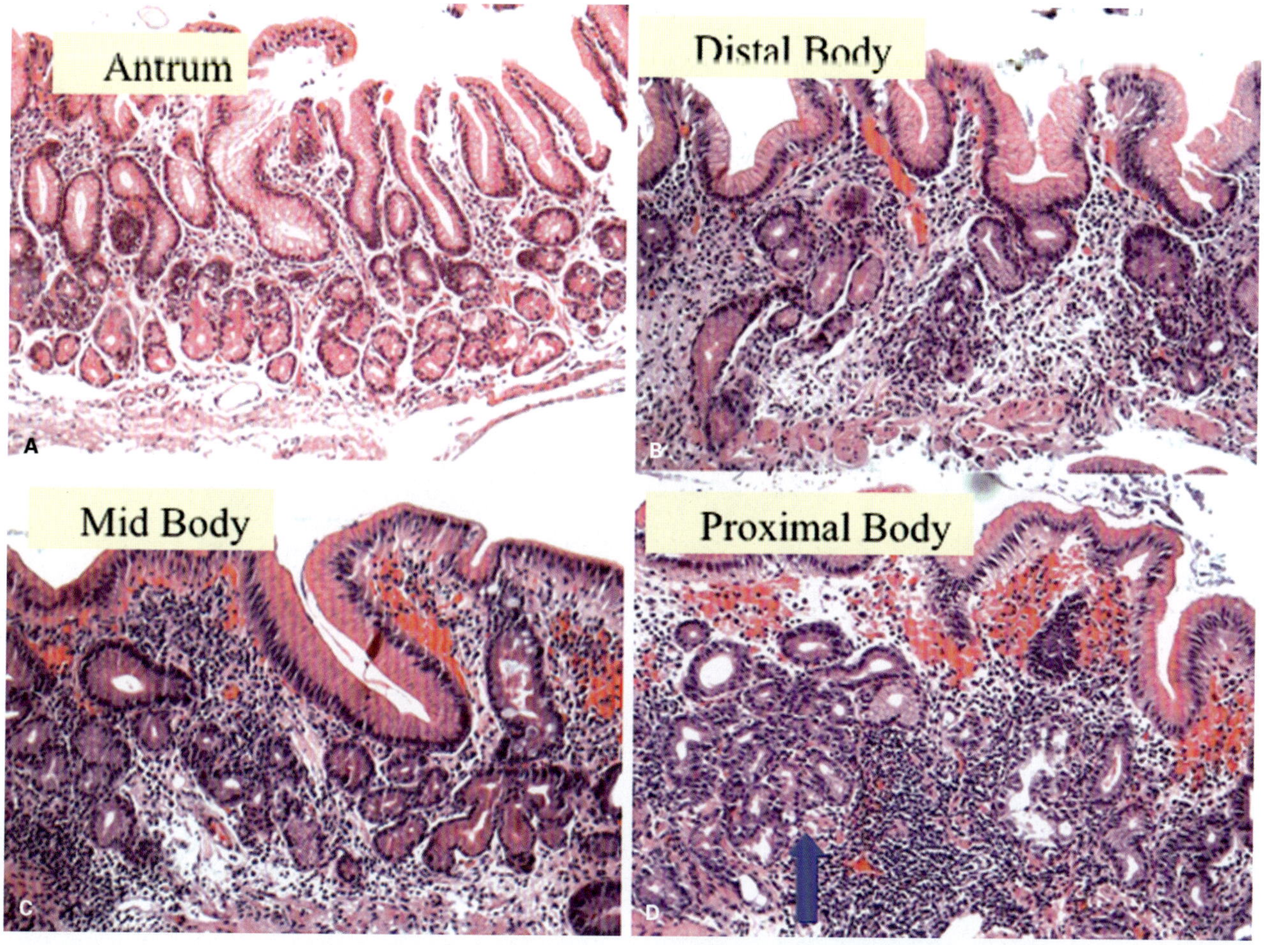

Figure 13-57. AIG with corpus/oxyntic-predominant gastritis. **A:** Antral mucosa that has at best minimal chronic inflammation. **B–D:** Distal, mid, and proximal body mucosa, showing complete loss of specialized mucosa, while all are chronically inflamed. There is pseudopyloric metaplasia and a focus of pancreatic metaplasia in **(D)** (*arrow*).

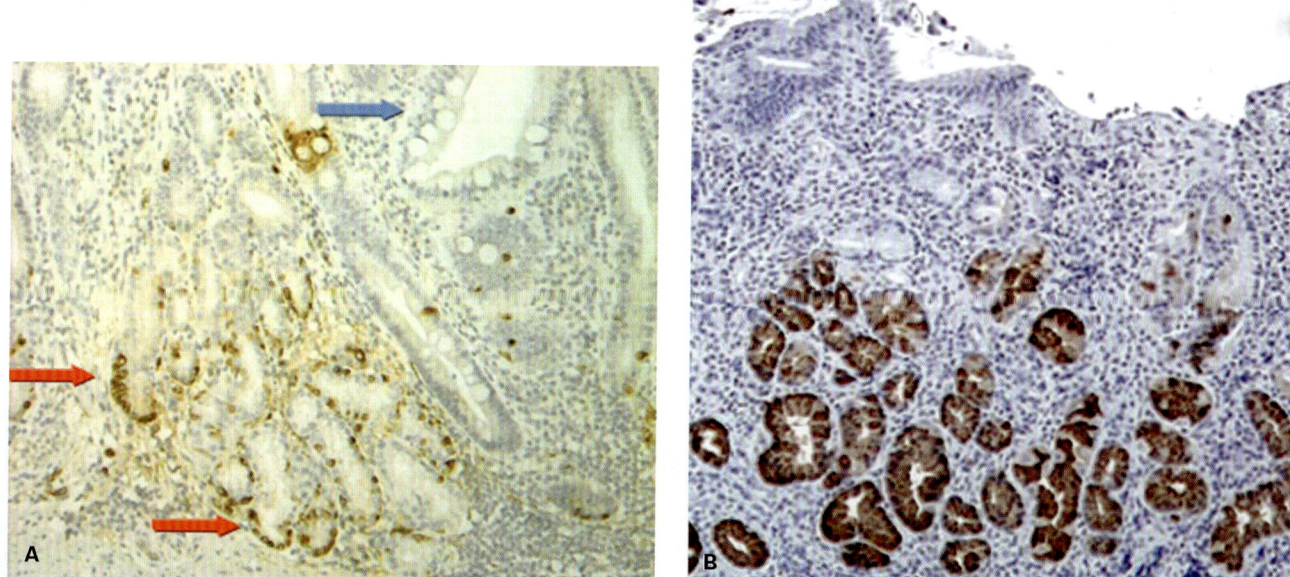

Figure 13-58. **A:** Anatomic corpus with pseudopyloric metaplasia **(left)** and intestinal metaplasia with goblet cell (*blue arrow*). Highlighted by the brown reactivity to synaptophysin are numerous brown-staining ECL cells that are increased in number (hyperplasia) and also forming chains (linear hyperplasia—*red arrows*). **B:** PGI immunostaining specifically stains corpus and not antral-type mucosa confirming that this is corpus mucosa.

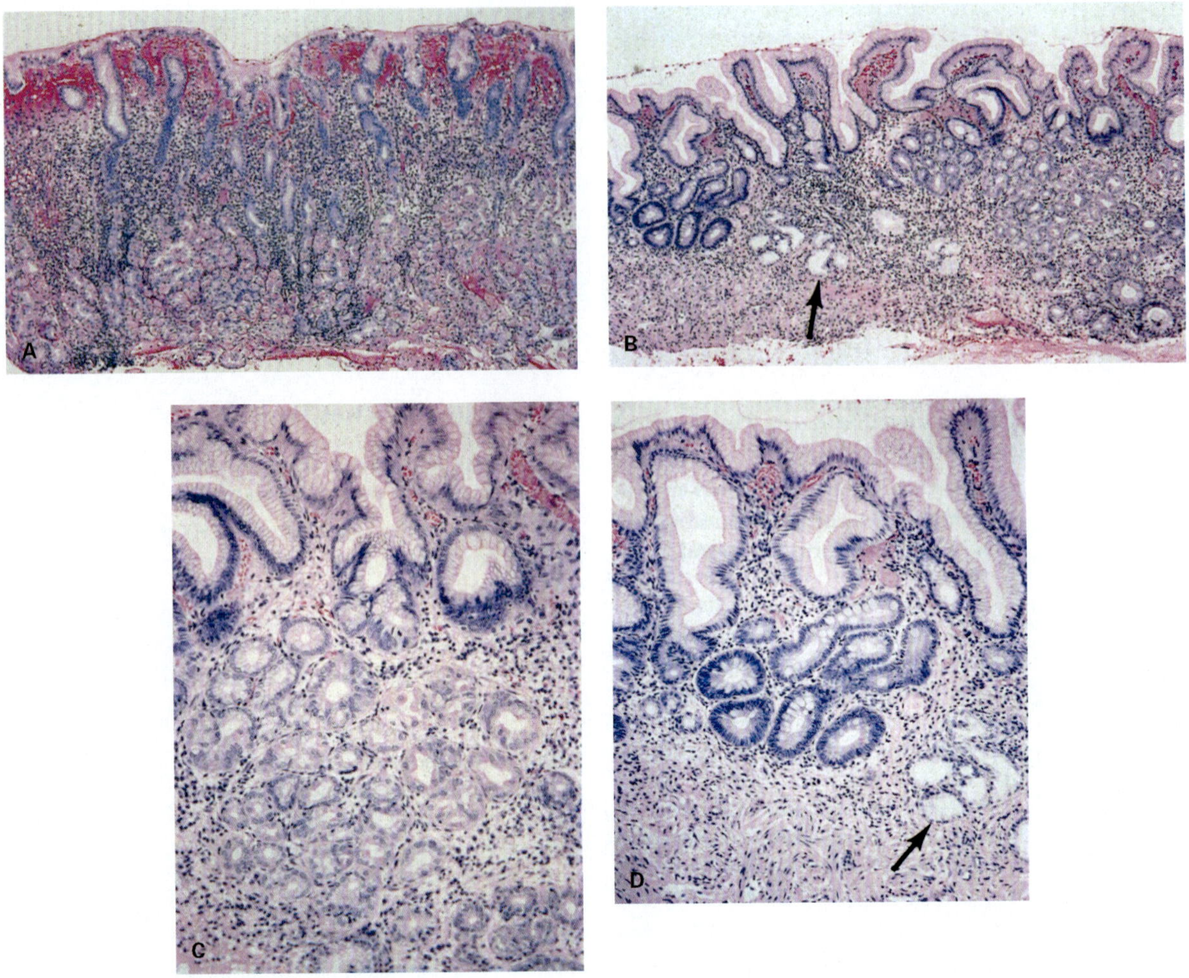

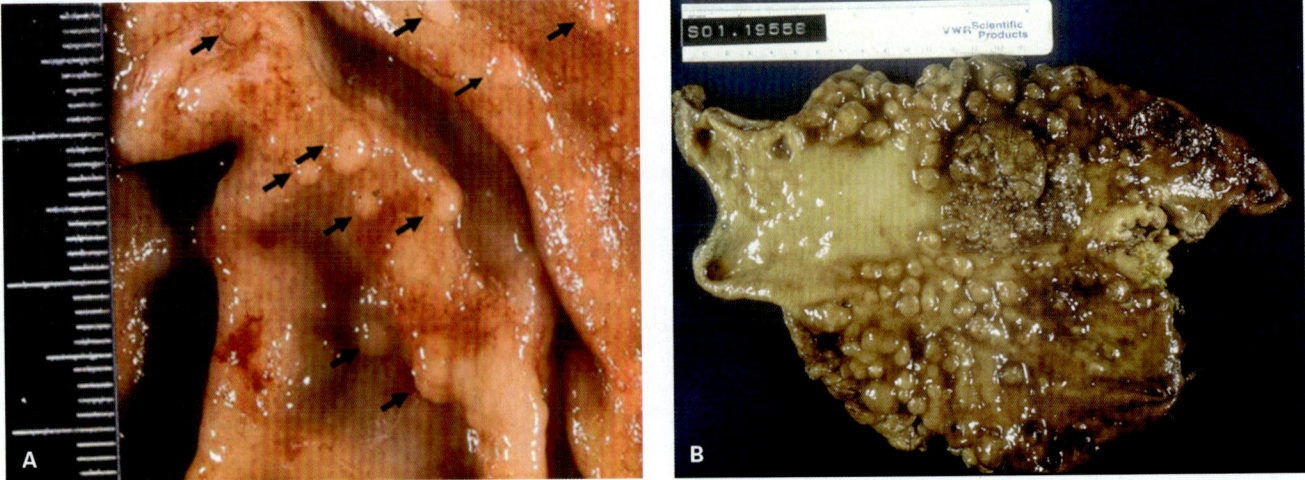

Figure 13-59. Atrophic fundic gland gastritis. **A:** Moderate atrophic fundic gland gastritis, with replacement of the top one-half to two-thirds of the glands by inflammatory cells. **B:** Severe atrophic gastritis overview. This biopsy is from the greater curvature of the midbody region. Surface epithelial cells contain abundant mucus. There are residual parietal and chief cells at the right, mucous gland metaplasia (pseudopyloric metaplasia) in the center (*arrow*), and a cluster of cross-sectioned intestinal-type crypts at the extreme left. **C:** Detail showing the residual parietal and chief cells from the right-hand portion of (B). **D:** Detail of (B) showing the cross-sectioned intestinal-type mucosa with goblet cells beneath the surface and pit epithelium. Also shown (*arrow*) is the small group of clear-staining mucous glands (pseudopyloric metaplasia). Only endocrine cell stains can determine if ECL hyperplasia is present, when as subtle as this.

Figure 13-60. **A:** Microcarcinoids/NETs in an atrophic stomach. **B:** Resection in atrophic gastritis with numerous hyperplastic polyps and also a carcinoma (**top center**).

has not been borne out in countries that have lower incidence rates in general for gastric cancer,[483,491] but may apply to populations with higher risks of gastric cancer, including Western and Asia populations.[492]

The most common lesions encountered in gastroscopic biopsy screening programs in AIG are hyperplastic or inflammatory polyps, found in 10% to 40% of patients (Fig. 13-60B). These innocuous, hyperplastic polyps tend to occur in the body in the background of an atrophic mucosa. Sometimes the polyps can be so numerous that it mimics a polyposis of some type, and can confuse the endoscopist or the gross pathologist in focusing their attention toward the polyps rather than the background atrophy (Fig. 13-61).[483,484,492] Less commonly, pyloric gland adenomas are found (see Chapter 14).

The antrum often has a mild degree of chronic inflammation (see Fig. 13-57), although whether this is the remnant of *Helicobacter* infection, or an autoimmune reaction to parietal cells that are often present in the antrum is unclear. On other occasions the antral changes may resemble a mild reactive gastropathy. In antral mucosa the presence of increased numbers of G cells is usually obvious on H&E stains but can be demonstrated with immunohistochemical techniques.[493] This increase in gastrin cell number is part of the reason for the elevated serum gastrin level that occurs in AIG.[486]

The distinction of atrophic oxyntic mucosa from antrum can usually be made because antral mucosa has regular glands and G-cells visible on a H&E stain as more open nuclei with cytoplasmic halos in the

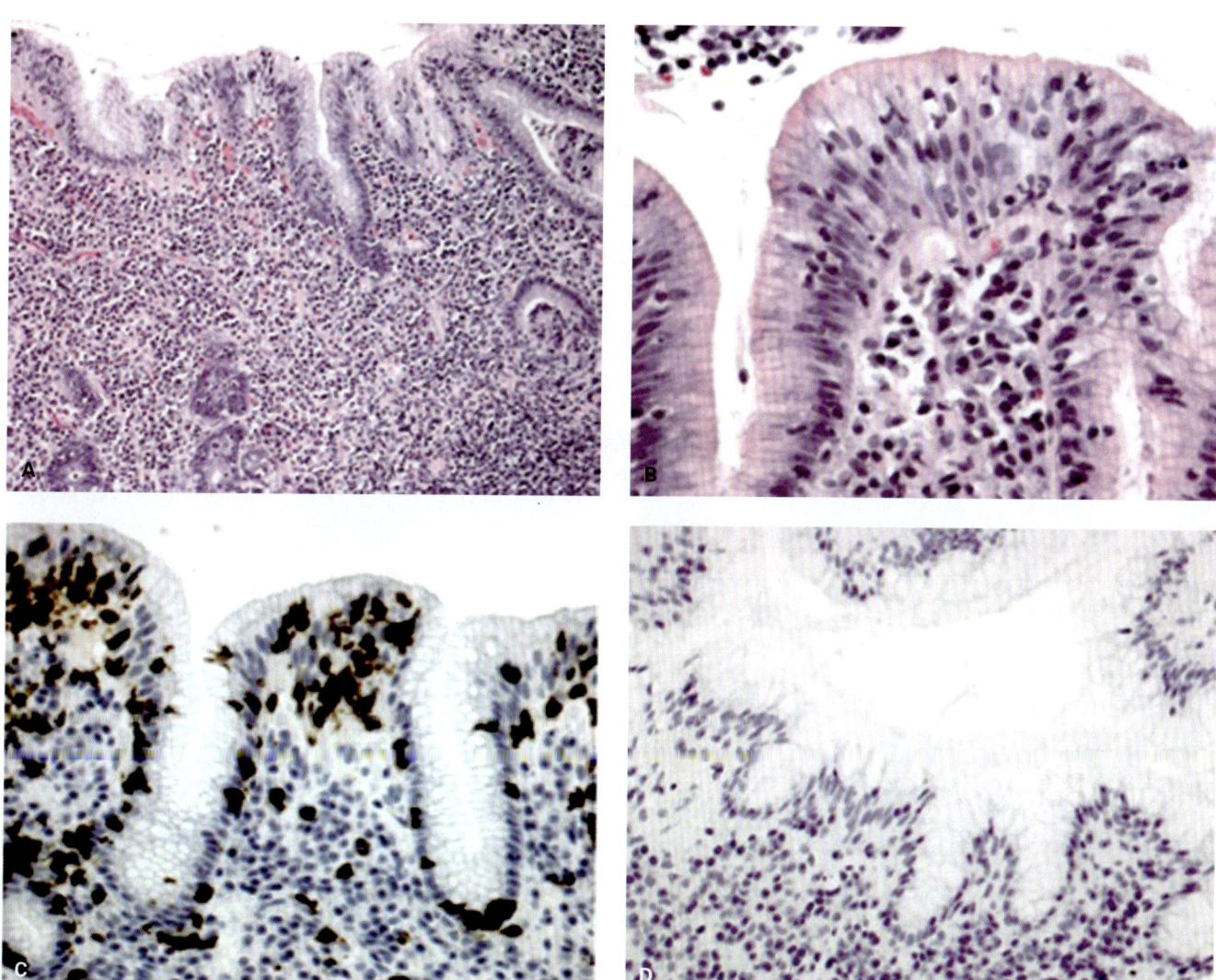

Figure 13-61. Lymphocytic gastritis (LG). **A:** Typical appearance of corpus-predominant *Helicobacter*-associated LG with a heavy chronic inflammatory infiltrate in a patient presenting with anemia. **B:** Detail of surface epithelium showing marked intraepithelial lymphocytosis. **C:** CD8 immunostain demonstrating the numerous intraepithelial suppressor cells. **D:** Immunostain for *Helicobacter* is frequently negative, but serology invariably positive.

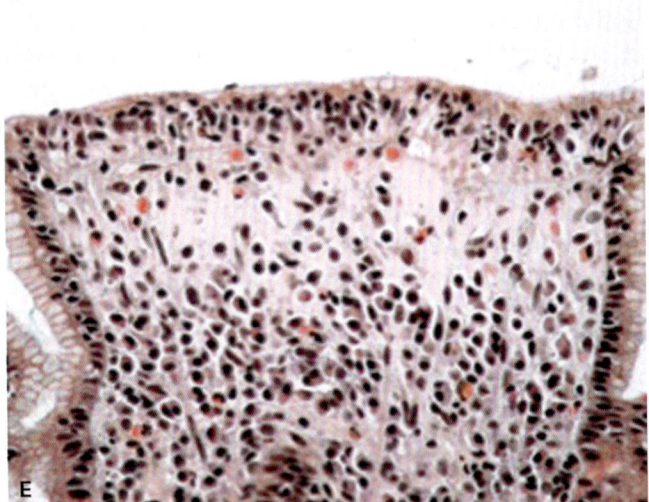
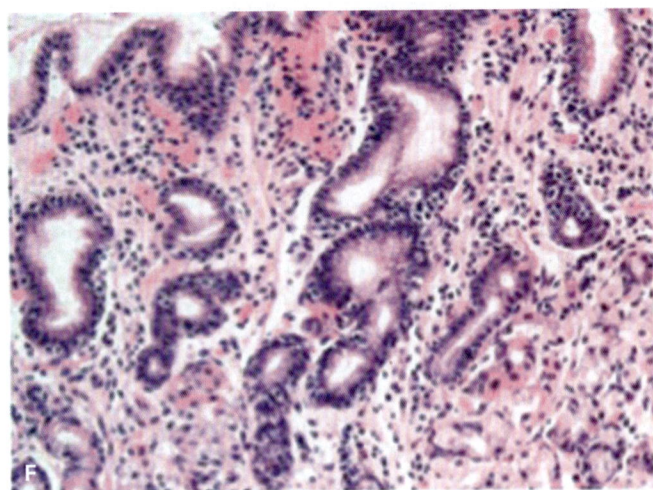

Figure 13-61. *(Continued)* **E:** In some patients rare *Helicobacter* are demonstrated (Genta stain). **F:** Sometimes the intraepithelial lymphocytosis in the pit epithelium is most apparent.

basal half of the mucosa. Whenever the proximal antrum is biopsied, or there is antral atrophy, it may require gastrin stains to identify the location of the biopsy. Sometimes just the pattern of endocrine cells (basal in oxyntic mucosa because of the ECL hyperplasia and mid to lower half of the mucosa in antrum) allows the distinction to be made on synaptophysin or chromogranin A immunostaining, or silver stains (see Fig. 13-58).

The antral surface epithelium is often remarkably well preserved. If there is accompanying inflammation it is usually much less severe than that of the fundic gland zones (see Fig. 13-57), but it can be quite severe and diffuse.[494] The possibility that this represents immune-mediated pangastritis also needs to be considered (next section).

Immune-mediated pangastritis: In some cases of *H. pylori*–negative gastritis the entire gastric mucosa is involved resulting in pangastritis that involves both antrum and body/fundus, unlike classic AIG.[495,496] This is usually seen in the setting of autoimmune enteropathy, other autoimmune disorders,

Table 13-11	Oxyntic (Corpus and Fundus) Predominant Gastritis			
	AUTOIMMUNE GASTRITIS	***HELICOBACTER PYLORI* GASTRITIS**	**PPI USERS (POSITIVE FOR *H. PYLORI*)**	**PPI USERS (NEGATIVE FOR *H. PYLORI*)**
Antral inflammation	Mild (?)	Present	Absent or mild	Absent
Antral atrophy	+/− (mild)	++/− (degree depends on stage)	+/− (mild when present)	Absent
ECL hyperplasia	Present, overt	Absent unless severe atrophy	Present, subtle	Present, subtle
Corpus inflammation	Present	Present (as disease progresses)	Present	Absent or mild
Corpus atrophy	Present earlier (?)	Present (late stage)	May be present	Absent
Autoantibodies:				
Parietal cell	Positive in 90% of cases[440]	Often	Often	No
Intrinsic factor	Positive in 88% of cases[452,839]	?Yes[840]	No	No
Gastrin	Abnormally high in 90%–100% of cases[456]	High in 31% of cases with severe vitamin B_{12} deficiency[477]	High	Higher
Vitamin B_{12} deficiency	Yes (late)	Sometimes (late)	Yes	Yes
Vitamin B_{12} deficiency treatment	Life-term vitamin B_{12} replacement	Antibiotics and vitamin B_{12} replacement (duration depends on corpus atrophy stage)	Antibiotics and vitamin B_{12} replacement (duration depends on corpus atrophy stage)	Short-term vitamin B_{12} replacement

or some immunodeficiency disorder (congenital or acquired). The underlying mechanisms are not fully understood. Anti-PC antibodies, anti-IF antibodies, or both have been detected in some patients while others have different autoantibodies such as antienterocyte antibodies or ANA. The infiltrate is mixed, composed of polyclonal plasma cells and numerous CD3+ T lymphocytes, with variable numbers of CD4- and CD8-positive T cells. Notably, secondary endocrine cell hyperplasia is absent, suggesting that all types of gastric cells are equally damaged, or there is no hypoacidity and secondary hypergastrinemia. While ECL hyperplasia and carcinoids are not seen in this setting, development of dysplasia has been rarely seen, suggesting a possible risk of adenocarcinoma.

LYMPHOCYTIC GASTRITIS

Lymphocytic gastritis is a description of a morphologic pattern, and not really an etiologic-specific diagnosis, although sometimes it gets treated that way. It is an uncommon type of gastritis characterized by an excess of intraepithelial lymphocytes (IELs), which is defined as more than 25 IEL/100 epithelial cells (1 in 4), this being considered the upper limit of normal. This is not usually counted but "eye-balled" because the number is usually far greater than this, although where close to physiologic a mental note of whether there are 3 or more IELs in 10 epithelial nuclei is easy to assess, when present. Even when focal (acceptable for the diagnosis), there are usually areas where there are almost as many IELs as epithelial cells. Typically, infiltrating lymphocytes are normal-appearing and seen involving both the surface and foveolar epithelium, but are usually maximal at the surface. In most cases of lymphocytic gastritis, there is an IEL for every two to three surface and glandular epithelial cells,[497] but this does depend to some extent on the underlying cause.

Lymphocytic gastritis is seen in about 1% of patients undergoing endoscopy for dyspepsia and 15% to 45% among patients with celiac disease.[498] Its pathogenesis is unknown, but it has been associated with several diseases (Table 13-12). Nonetheless, the most common associations include H. pylori infection and celiac disease,[499] and, in patients with IBD centers, CD. However, here the similarity between the two major forms stops.

Morphologic Separation of Etiologies

Lymphocytic gastritis secondary to *Helicobacter* and celiac disease are usually readily separated morphologically, but other etiologies, especially multiple polyps and Ménétrier's disease frequently have an intraepithelial lymphocytosis (Figs. 13-61 and 13-62). More commonly a focal intraepithelial lymphocytosis can be seen in patients with Crohn's disease, without necessarily meaning that the stomach is involved.

(a) ***Helicobacter***. *Helicobacter Pylori*–associated lymphocytic gastritis (Fig. 13-61) has overt chronic, and often acute, inflammation in the lamina propria. It usually, but not always, involves oxyntic mucosa, antral predominance only being seen in about 20% of patients.[500] There is a heavy lamina propria lymphoplasmacytosis, and there may be neutrophils and erosions, to the point that patients may present with anemia and a protein-losing state. The erosions may have a volcano-like appearance, which is called chronic erosive or "varioliform" gastritis (for the historically inclined because it resembles the rash of smallpox or variola, which itself was called "small" to distinguish it from "great pox," or syphilis, which can also affect the stomach—see later in this chapter).

Interestingly, in some patients *Helicobacter* are easily found, in which case the presence of the intraepithelial lymphocytosis may be overlooked as by itself it has very little significance. However, in most patients *Helicobacter* tend to be few or cannot be found (Fig. 13-61D,E), even with numerous antral and oxyntic mucosa biopsies. In varioliform gastritis *Helicobacter* may therefore not be found, and serology or other tests may be necessary to make the diagnosis.

It is estimated that one-third of patients with lymphocytic gastritis have *H. pylori* infection; approximately 4% of *H. pylori*–infected patients have lymphocytic gastritis.[500] Given that an unknown proportion of these may be false negatives, the true incidence is likely considerably more. The role of *H. pylori*

Table 13-12 Lymphocytic Gastritis Associations

Infections
   Helicobacter pylori
   HIV infection
Immune-mediated disorders
   Celiac disease
   Lymphocytic (gastro) enterocolitis
   Crohn's disease
   Common variable immunodeficiency
Endoscopic abnormalities
   Chronic erosive (varioliform) gastritis
   Large gastric folds
   Normal
Neoplasia
   Lymphoma
   Carcinoma
Medications
   E.g., ticlopidine, olmesartan

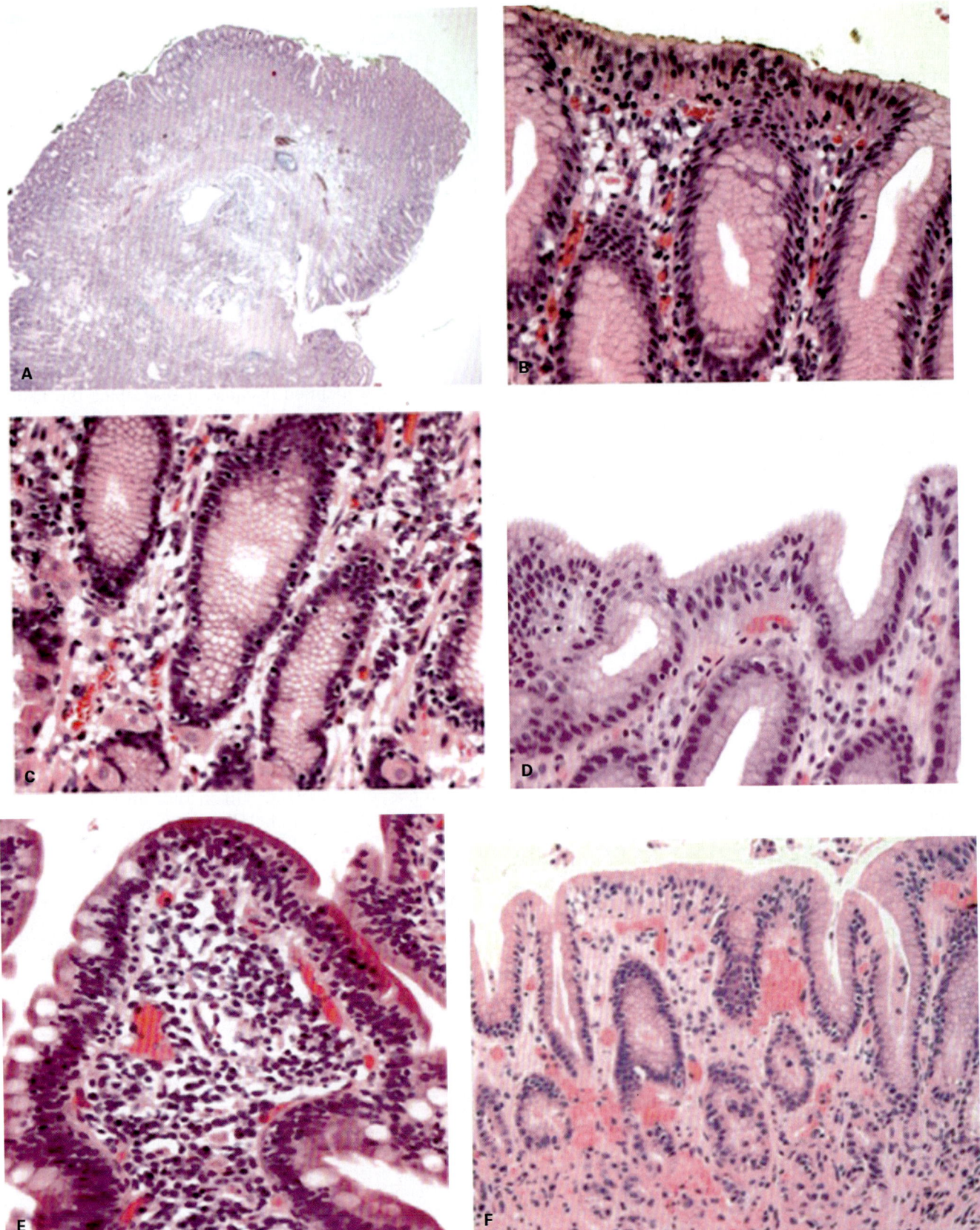

Figure 13-62. Lymphocytic gastritis. **A–C:** Ménétrier-like disease with giant gastric folds, one of which was snared. **B,C:** There is a marked intraepithelial lymphocytosis in both surface and pit epithelium. Stains for *Helicobacter* were negative. However, the amount of lamina propria inflammation is less than expected in *Helicobacter*. **D–F:** Celiac disease–associated lymphocytic gastritis **(E)**. **D** and **F** both have an intraepithelial lymphocytosis that was focal and easily missed. The lamina propria infiltrate in **(F)** is fairly typical and less than seen in *Helicobacter*. That in **(D)** is more than usually seen in gastric celiac disease and would demand a search for *Helicobacter*.

in this setting has been controversial because serologic evidence of infection frequently occurs in the absence of demonstrable identification of the organism by stain or other means.[501,502] This has led to the speculation that lymphocytic gastritis is an abnormal immune response associated with bacterial clearance.[501,503] Likewise, the effect of *H. pylori* eradication on the severity of histologic abnormalities is controversial.[501,503,504] Multiple studies have demonstrated that *H. pylori* eradication therapy often reduces the lymphocytic infiltration, resolves dyspeptic symptoms, and anemia,[503,504] as well as resolves varioliform appearance.[502] Intraepithelial lymphocytosis of equal severity in the antrum and corpus, coupled with an absence of duodenal pathology, should prompt serologic testing for *H. pylori* and eradication therapy if positive. This needs to be made clear in the pathology report as clinicians may be completely unaware of the association or treatment.[505]

A disconcerting feature seen in a small proportion of patients with *Helicobacter* are focal lymphoepithelial lesions, which can be quite disconcerting as they are usually associated with a local lymphocytic, rather than plasmacytic infiltrate. While it is possible that these represent the earliest stages of MALTomas and some euphemistically call these "min-MALT" lesions (Fig. 13-63) (see Chapter 4). We suspect that if these are B cells then they may well represent a forme fruste of MALT but that the vast majority never evolve further, and that if they are T cells, then these are likely physiologic, but the study has, to our knowledge, never been done. Nevertheless, adding a comment such as "please ensure that eradication of *Helicobacter* was successful to ensure that these lesions disappear" is not unreasonable.

(b) *Celiac disease*. In celiac disease, there is no endoscopic abnormality, and intraepithelial lymphocytosis is relatively mild, may be quite focal, and may be subtle and needs a thorough search. The accompanying lamina propria infiltrate varies from none to mild (rarely more) (see Fig. 13-62D,F), and it is mostly antral or antral-predominant.[500] Neutrophils are absent. About one-third of patients with lymphocytic gastritis have concomitant celiac sprue; approximately 10% to 30% of patients with celiac sprue have lymphocytic gastritis (depending on the number of biopsies and the diligence of the observer).[500,505,506] The lymphocytic gastritis likely represents a host response to gluten,[507] and disappears with a gluten-free diet. Hayat et al.[503] have found similar HLA antigens in both celiac sprue and lymphocytic gastritis. An antral biopsy with a mild intraepithelial lymphocytosis but no *Helicobacter* should lead to consideration of celiac disease. However, patients with Crohn's disease and common variable immunodeficiency disease can have virtually identical lesions.

(c) *Lymphocytic gastroenterocolitis*. In a very small proportion of patients lymphocytic gastritis is part of a panenteropathy. In its mildest form it includes patients with lymphocytic gastritis associated with celiac disease, which may be associated with lymphocytic or collagenous colitis in some patients with intraepithelial lymphocytosis in all three organs.

However, some patients present with severe diarrhea that can be recalcitrant to therapy, may overlap with collagenous gastroenterocolitis, and can potentially be life-threatening. Others are associated with autoimmune enteropathy that may have variable extent of involvement of the different segments of the GI tract. Patients present with weight loss and malabsorption, and the entire GI tract may show a dense inflammatory infiltrate with intraepithelial lymphocytosis. The small bowel disease is sprue-like, but often

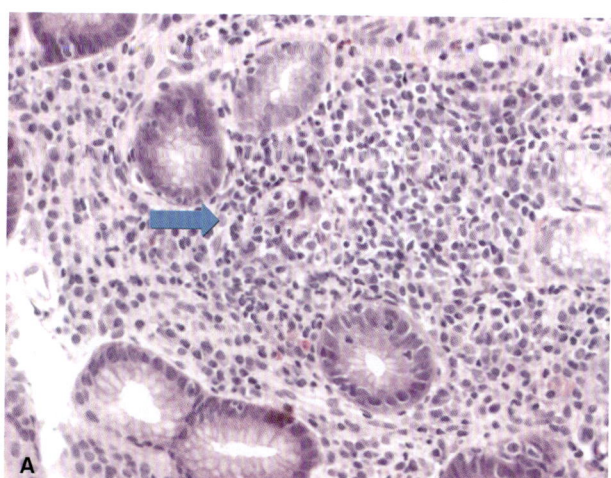
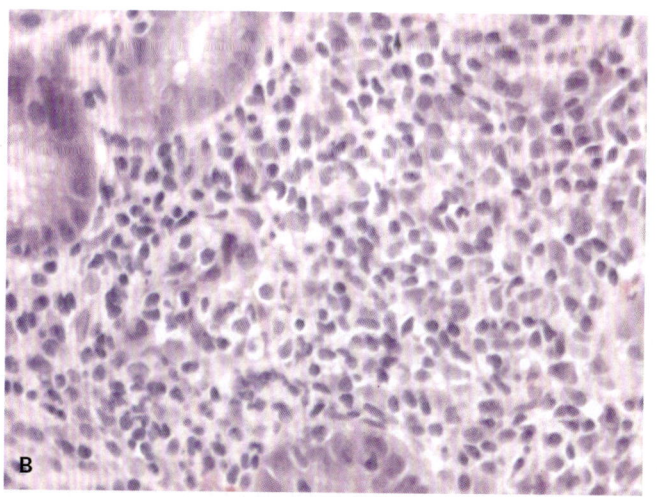

Figure 13-63. **A:** *Helicobacter* gastritis with a lymphocytic focus surrounding a pit extensively infiltrated with lymphocytes as seen in the lymphoepithelial lesions of MALT lymphoma. **B:** Detail of the lesion.

does not respond to a gluten-free diet. Patients often need steroids or other forms of immunosuppression, PPIs (unless *Helicobacter* is also present in which case it needs to be eradicated), and parental support, but may still take months to recover. Some patients are resistant to all therapies and have a high mortality. Some of these patients also have focal thickening of the subepithelial collagen band, so have a collagenous component to their disease.

- (d) *Common variable immunodeficiency*. These patients tend to have a low-grade diffuse intraepithelial lymphocytosis. The tip-off is the dearth, or relative dearth, of plasma cells in the lamina propria, although in most cases the diagnosis is already established by other means.
- (e) *Crohn's disease*. A variety of lesions can be seen in Crohn's disease (see Chapter 18), including focal intraepithelial lymphocytosis often with a focal chronic or chronic active ("focally enhanced") gastritis. There may also be a mild diffuse superficial chronic gastritis.
- (f) *Neoplasia*
  - (i) *MALT lymphoma*. In this there is increase in the IELs. Although the neoplastic B-cells produce the typical lymphoepithelial lesions and are important for the diagnosis, there is often a background of increased IELs that are normal phenotype T cells, which can be easily highlighted by CD3 stains.
  - (ii) *T-cell lymphoma*. There is a rare variant of gastric T-cell lymphoma characterized by a pattern that mimics lymphocytic gastritis, except that the intraepithelial cells are neoplastic and clonal.[508]
  - (iii) *Carcinoma*. Some carcinomas incite an intraepithelial lymphocytosis, including those associated with EBV and those that are microsatellite unstable. Data are scant and it could even be a reaction to the associated *Helicobacter*.
- (g) *Medications*. Any intraepithelial lymphocytosis should at least lead to consideration of medications as a potential cause. Ticlopidine appears to have this association as does olmesartan (see Chapter 15).[509]

Endoscopic Appearance: This depends on the underlying disease (see Table 13-12).[500] In one series of 18 patients with lymphocytic gastritis, half were normal, 5 had varioliform gastritis (raised lesions topped with a small break or depression in the mucosa), 4 had erythema and 3 erosions. None had a Ménétrier-like appearance.[510] The most severe forms of lymphocytic gastritis have large mucosal folds resembling Ménétrièr's disease, both clinically and endoscopically. The large gastric folds are frequently due to foveolar hyperplasia, as in the case of reactive gastropathy or hyperplastic polyps.[497] Irrespective of the endoscopic appearances or the distribution of the disease (oxyntic or antral mucosa or both), in the presence of severe lymphocytic gastritis one needs to carefully look for the evidence of *Helicobacter* infection.

Clinical Presentation: This is variable and depends on the underlying cause. That associated with celiac disease is that of the underlying disease. Most cases of lymphocytic gastritis have been described in asymptomatic patients older than 50 years of age. Symptoms that can occur include abdominal pain, nausea, vomiting, anorexia, weight loss,[504,511,512] iron deficiency anemia[504] with and without polypoid lesions,[502] and GI bleeding.[511] Multiple reports have attributed a protein-losing gastroenteropathy to lymphocytic gastritis.[512] The natural history of patients with lymphocytic gastritis is unclear. Healing after therapy with histamine-2 receptor blockers or PPIs, as well as without any therapy, has been described.[502–504] As indicated above, the effect of *H. pylori* eradication on the severity of histologic abnormalities is controversial, although we have seen cases where it disappeared after *H. pylori* eradication, or in case of celiac disease after gluten withdrawal.[501,503]

Morphologic diagnosis. This rests entirely on the finding of an intraepithelial lymphocytosis, which needs to be searched for routinely. Besides looking at the surface and foveolar epithelium one also needs to look carefully for other inflammatory cells, especially neutrophils, and examine the lamina propria. IELs usually have a surrounding halo, likely representing a retraction artifact. They can easily be separated from endocrine cells, which have both a better "bull's-eye" appearance in the antrum and a more open nucleus (endocrine cells usually cannot be distinguished in the oxyntic mucosa). In contrast, the nuclei of IELs are dark and hyperchromatic and have a less conspicuous cytoplasm (see Figs. 13-61 and 13-62). Special stains for *Helicobacter* tend to be remarkably good at drawing one's attention to IELs, as they are in the surface epithelium where one is looking for *Helicobacter*, and these readily stand out.

Although lymphocytic gastritis is associated with an increased prevalence of both primary gastric MALT lymphoma and gastric adenocarcinoma,[513] which may be actually related to *Helicobacter* infection rather than lymphocytic gastritis itself, at this time, there are no specific surveillance recommendations for patients with lymphocytic gastritis.

GRANULOMATOUS GASTRITIS

Granulomatous gastritis (Fig. 13-64) is not common and the incidence varies from 0.08% to 0.27% of all gastric biopsies[514] and results from a large number of infectious and noninfectious disorders (Table 13-13).[515] The underlying etiology likely differs geographically

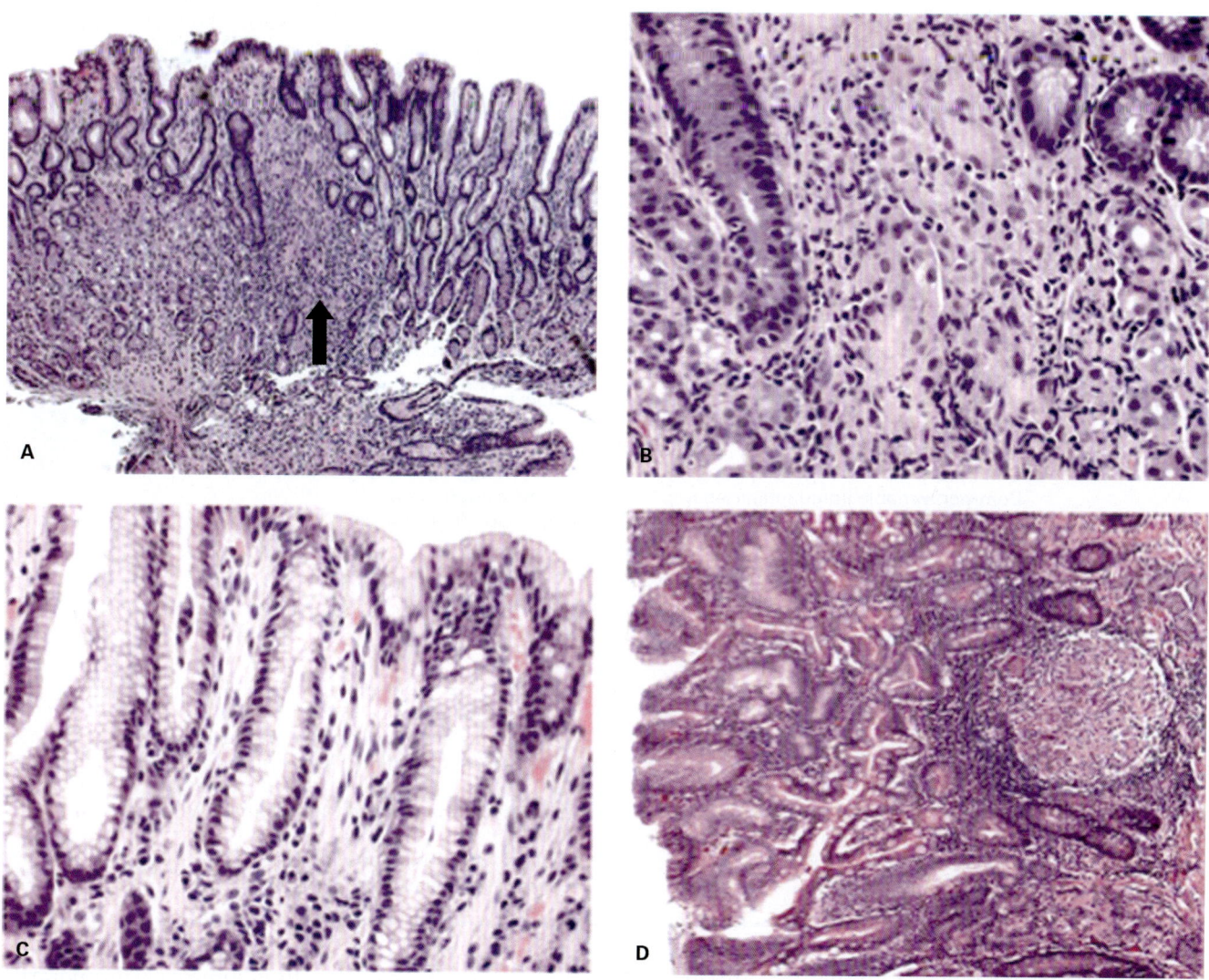

Figure 13-64. Granulomatous gastritis. **A:** A central expansion of the lamina propria can be seen (*arrow*). **B:** Detail shows a granuloma comprised of aggregates of epithelioid histiocytes and giant cells. **C:** Detail of mucosa away from the granuloma showing normal mucosa without inflammation, suggesting that this is not *Helicobacter*-related. **D:** Granulomatous gastritis on a background of *Helicobacter* with intestinal metaplasia.

throughout the world.[515-517] The most common associations is likely with *Helicobacter* infection, Crohn's disease, especially in children, and sarcoidosis, tuberculosis and idiopathic (isolated) granulomatous gastritis in adults. In a study from United States Crohn's disease followed by sarcoidosis was the most common cause, representing nearly half of the patients,[514] but this was before *Helicobacter* was recognized as a potential cause of granulomas.

Crohn's disease (CD) is most often seen in patients with an established diagnosis, but can be the presenting manifestation of the disease. Granulomas are relatively uncommon in Crohn's disease involving the stomach, and a much more common lesion is focal chronic active *Helicobacter*-negative gastritis, or a superficial diffuse chronic gastritis that resembles mild *Helicobacter* gastritis, but no organisms are found. This appears to represent an up-regulated immune system and is not specific for Crohn's disease, although no studies have (yet) been carried out to verify this (see subsequent discussion).

Studies from Asian countries show most of their granulomatous gastritides to be associated with *H. pylori*, and fewer with Crohn's disease, in concordance with a low incidence of CD in these countries. Rare causes include Langerhans cell histiocytosis, chronic granulomatous disease, common variable immunodeficiency, Whipple's disease, and systemic vasculitides. Granulomas can rarely also be seen in association with adenocarcinoma and MALT lymphoma.[518] Bacterial, fungal, and parasitic infections can also result in a granulomatous gastritis. Immunotherapy (interferon) has also been reported to produce sarcoid-like granulomas.[519] The association between granulomas

Table 13-13 Conditions Associated with Granulomatous Gastritis

DISEASE	COMMON FEATURES
Infections	
Bacterial	
Helicobacter pylori	Mucinous and nonmucinous granuloma
Tuberculosis	Necrotizing granuloma
Late syphilis	Protean
Whipple's disease	Background of diffuse histiocytes
Fungal	
Histoplasma	Foamy histiocytes more common than well-formed granulomas
Parasitic	
Anisakiasis	Relative increase of eosinophils
Strongyloidosis	
Immune-mediated disorders	
Crohn's disease	Histiocytic aggregates to granulomas
Common variable immunodeficiency	Histiocytic aggregates
Immune-mediated vasculitis	Relative lack of plasma cells
Lymphocytic enterocolitis	
Allergic granulomatosis	Churg-Strauss
Neoplasia	
Lymphoma	
Carcinoma	
Foreign body	
Sutures	Foreign body or vegetable material surrounded by foreign body–type granulomas or multinucleated giant cells, usually focal or around a few crypts
Food	
Granulomatous disease of unknown etiology	
Sarcoidosis	Extragastric nonnecrotizing granulomas
Wegener's granulomatosis	
Idiopathic isolated granulomatous gastritis	Suppurative granulomas with "dirty" necrosis and vasculitis

and neoplasia is not meant to imply that the granulomas carry or portend a greater risk of neoplasia. It may reflect the fact that the mucosa is reacting abnormally because of a neoplasm nearby or because of the precursor lesion in the vicinity.[519] Granulomas associated with a variety of immunodeficiency disorders including Whipple's disease may even represent aberrant responses to commensals.[518] Finally, mucin granulomas virtually identical to those seen in the large bowel can rarely be found in the stomach.

Helicobacter. The relationship between granulomatous gastritis and *H. pylori* infection has attracted much attention.[514,516,517,520–522] In many series, especially from Asia, *Helicobacter* was found to be one of the most common causes for granulomatous gastritis. Further, granulomas were more frequently found in the antrum, superficially located, and were related to damage within a pit in which the *H. pylori* were commonly observed.[522] These findings suggest that *H. pylori* can be causal in the pathogenesis of granulomatous gastritis. While some question this association, few studies have shown complete or partial remission following *H. pylori* eradication.[516,521,523–525] Because idiopathic granulomatous gastritis often improves temporarily after giving steroids, some have suggested that idiopathic granulomatous gastritis represents an immunologic reaction of the host against *H. pylori* infection.[516] Thus, some idiopathic granulomatous cases are speculated to undergo remission a long time after *H. pylori* eradication. However, the association of *Helicobacter* and granulomatous gastritis continues to be debated. Because this is a less well-recognized cause of gastric granulomas in Western countries, the possibility of other coexisting diseases needs to be excluded, especially other infections and CD.

Gastric sarcoidosis is said to represent between 1% and 21% of all cases of granulomatous gastritis.[526] However, involvement of the GI tract in sarcoidosis is rare, but does occur. The stomach is the most commonly affected site in sarcoidosis.[527] "Silent" granulomas were found in biopsies from fundic gland mucosa in 10% (6 of 60) of patients with disseminated sarcoidosis in one study.[528–530] The diagnosis of gastric sarcoid should never be made in the absence of evidence of the disease in other sites, and when an overt etiology is not present, chest x-ray for both sarcoid and tuberculosis is indicated. Although ulcerative gastric sarcoidosis can present throughout the stomach, it tends to occur more frequently in antral mucosa, pylorus, and lesser curvature.[531] Symptoms attributable to gastric involvement by sarcoidosis range from those of gastric outlet obstruction to UGT bleeding, possibly secondary to portal hypertension due to concomitant liver involvement. In symptomatic cases, changes in the stomach include a linitis plastica–like appearance, ulceration or erosions, and thick gastric folds.[527] Granulomas are generally found in and adjacent to these lesions. However, when a granulomatous type of inflammation is detected in gastric lesions in a patient with disseminated disease, it is essential to rule out other conditions, especially infections such as **tuberculosis**, before attributing the changes to sarcoidosis.

Idiopathic (isolated) granulomatous gastritis is a diagnosis of exclusion that refers to the histologic finding of isolated mucosal granulomas with no known association or cause and has been reported to consist 25% to 41% of all granulomatous gastritis cases. It has been described as a distinct clinico-pathologic entity; however, this concept has been questioned due to lack of adequate clinical information and follow-up in most studies.[532] As mentioned above, in some cases it may be the initial presentation of Crohn's disease, tuberculosis or sarcoidosis, and only examination of other organ systems, especially lung or other parts of the GI tract, and long-term follow-up can truly clarify their nature.

In Japan, idiopathic granulomatous gastritis is also reported as "isolated gastric sarcoidosis" because the definition of isolated granulomatous gastritis is vague.[516] Similar to other granulomatous gastritides, idiopathic granulomatous gastritis is sometimes associated with marked gross structural changes, especially in the gastric antrum. There may be narrowings or masses that simulate carcinoma and ulcerative lesions that may perforate[533,534]—findings are related to the depth of granulomas in the gastric wall.

In practice one should be careful when using idiopathic granulomatous gastritis as a pathologic diagnosis as on many occasions the etiology of the granulomatous gastritis only becomes obvious after many years of follow-up and investigations. Use of the term idiopathic granulomatous gastritis by the pathologist may create a misconception that this is a specific disorder precluding any further workup of the patient. In some of these patients the granulomas have been shown to disappear on follow-up biopsies without any treatment. Thus, it is better to use a descriptive designation of "granulomatous gastritis of uncertain etiology."

How to evaluate gastric granulomas: Aggregation of histiocytes, ideally epithelioid, is the minimum requirement of a granuloma, regardless of whether the lesion also contains necrosis, lymphocytes, plasma cells, or multinucleated giant cells. When granulomas are found unexpectedly in gastric mucosal biopsies (Fig. 13-64), the pathologist should look for clues as to why they might be there. The granulomas can be very compact, as in sarcoidosis, or be somewhat loose and ill-formed. Most cases have a background of chronic active gastritis. Some seem to be more superficial, while others are deep in the mucosa and some are clearly centered around a gland or foveolar region. There is no clear association between the superficial versus deep location of the granulomas and specific etiologies. The presence of central necrosis in the granulomas should raise a concern for an infectious etiology, especially mycobacterial and fungal infections. Presence of eosinophils in the background should raise the possibility of parasitic infection or a drug-induced mucosal injury. If there is background of moderate to severe chronic active gastritis possibilities of *Helicobacter*, sarcoidosis CD or even syphilis should be considered. If *Helicobacter* is not identified, the possibility of luetic disease should be at the back of one's mind. The *Treponemes* may be visible on a Warthin–Starry stain but may need immunohistochemistry or PCR-based assays. Positive serology or high-risk lifestyle for syphilis in such a situation should prompt further workup. However, this should come after precautionary stains for acid-fast bacilli and fungi have also been carried out. The presence of strikingly focal chronic active inflammation also suggests Crohn's disease.

Foreign body granulomas contain various types of foreign debris and might represent a reaction to some form of prior mucosal injury such as ulceration or erosion. PCR-based assays of biopsy specimens, while not a common practice, provides a faster, alternative route for diagnosis of some infectious diseases, while excluding Crohn's disease with close to 100% specificity.[535] If there is no clue as to why granulomas are present one may suggest a differential in a comment, and then the baton goes to the clinician to determine whether to proceed further with investigations for infections such as tuberculosis, immunodeficiency states, or diseases such as sarcoidosis and Crohn's disease.

Tuberculosis and *syphilis* are discussed subsequently in the section on non-*Helicobacter* gastritis (see also Chapter 19).

CARDITIS

The rising incidence of gastroesophageal junction and proximal gastric (cardia) carcinomas[536,537] has increased our interest in histopathologic changes in the gastric cardia. However, the issue has been riddled with many controversies that largely revolve around the definition of gastric cardia (anatomic vs. histologic) and significance of carditis (reflux vs. nonreflux causes). Carditis, when defined as the presence of glandular infiltration with neutrophils, is more closely related to active *H. pylori* infection than gastroesophageal reflux.[538,539] Active carditis in patients with *H. pylori* infection disappears following cure of the infection.[539] Similarly, the presence and extent of mucous glands in the gastric cardia increases with *H. pylori* infection.[181,539] The size of the region with cardiac glands is smaller in patients with GERD.[539] In contrast, carditis defined as an increase of chronic inflammatory cells (chronic carditis) should only be diagnosed in biopsies with more than a modest increase of chronic inflammatory cells. A mild increase of chronic inflammatory cells is commonly seen in cardia biopsies—perhaps secondary to physiologic reflux or yet unidentified form of injury. Though some[540] suggested that intestinal metaplasia in the cardia is most commonly part of GERD and a form of short-segment Barrett's, overall, the data support at least two if not more pathogenic mechanisms being responsible for intestinal metaplasia in the cardia[541,542] (see also Chapter 10). In one series, intestinal metaplasia of the gastric cardia secondary to GERD was uncommon (e.g., 3%) and was not found in patients with long-segment Barrett's esophagus.[539]

Interpretation of intestinal metaplasia in the cardia requires consideration of the status of the gastric mucosa elsewhere in the stomach. While intestinal metaplasia in the cardia may or may not be a form of short-segment Barrett's esophagus, it might still represent a risk of cancer. The presence of intestinal metaplasia in the cardia is also related to intestinal metaplasia and *Helicobacter* elsewhere in the more distal stomach, suggesting that these patients are at a higher risk for developing *H. pylori*–related gastric cancer.[150,539] The actual risk of patients with intestinal metaplasia in the cardia for developing cardia carcinoma can only be answered with long-term prospective studies. None of the patients in one series with intestinal metaplasia in the cardia developed carcinoma, although the median follow-up period was only 4 years.[539] Patients with intestinal metaplasia in the cardia might represent a group with more severe atrophy in the stomach and thus with a higher risk for developing *H. pylori*–related gastric cancer, as the cardia usually reflects the antrum in *Helicobacter* gastritis. Nonetheless, we all recognize the dramatic increase in the incidence of gastric cardia adenocarcinoma in developed countries and lack of intestinal metaplasia in the background mucosa of most of the patients.

Pancreatic metaplasia defined as small nests or variably sized nodules of pancreatic acinar cells has been suggested to be a metaplastic change in response to chronic atrophic gastritis,[543] a congenital feature,[544] or both. Its pathogenesis remains unclear. Apart from being seen with severe gastric atrophy associated with AIG, this is most commonly seen in the region of the gastric cardia. It is still debated whether this is metaplasia or normal variation of the gastric glandular differentiation. Immunohistochemically pancreatic type enzymes (lipase or trypsin) can be demonstrated in these foci. There is a strong correlation between pancreatic acinar metaplasia and *H. pylori* infection and no correlation with intestinal metaplasia elsewhere in the stomach.[539] The presence of pancreatic acinar cells in two infants without any background inflammatory changes has been explained as an aberration of stem cell differentiation.[545] A similar, but different pathogenic mechanism, might also play a role in pancreatic metaplasia in adults,[539] in which it seems to start in glands containing parietal cells. Immunohistochemically pancreatic-type lipase can be demonstrated in normal gastric mucosa, even in areas that morphologically do not resemble pancreatic acinar cells. Whether overt development of pancreatic-type acini is an adaptive response to gastroduodenal bile reflux is an interesting speculation that deserves further investigation.

Russell body gastritis/Carditis (Plasma cell gastritis/carditis): This is microscopically characterized by infiltration of the lamina propria by a variable number of plasma cells distended by a single round cytoplasmic eosinophilic inclusion—Russell bodies, Mott cells are similar but have multiple globules in a single cell, they are referred to as a Mott cells, but are also called grape cells or morula cells.[546] Similar staining nuclear inclusions are referred to as Dutcher bodies (Fig. 13-65). Usually the inflammatory infiltrate is dense but occasionally the chronic inflammation has resolved and only the bodies remain. At times, the nuclei of the plasma cells are barely discernible, and only extracellular eosinophilic globules are seen. Sometimes the plasma cells may contain rhomboid or needle-shaped crystalline inclusion instead. It is commonly associated with *H. pylori* infection. Its only significance is not to confuse it with something more worrisome like a plasma cell dyscrasia or a poorly differentiated carcinoma.[547] When in question, immunostains using plasma cell markers and kappa/lambda light chains or both, cytokeratin, and sometimes molecular assays can usually and easily establish its benign nature. However, some caution is warranted. While most often it is benign, occasionally we have seen cases that truly represent a plasma cell dyscrasia or underlying MALT lymphoma. In such cases presence of intranuclear inclusions in the plasma cells (Dutcher bodies), atypical morphology, or nature of the background lymphoid infiltrate are important clues to the diagnosis. Demonstration of clonality by

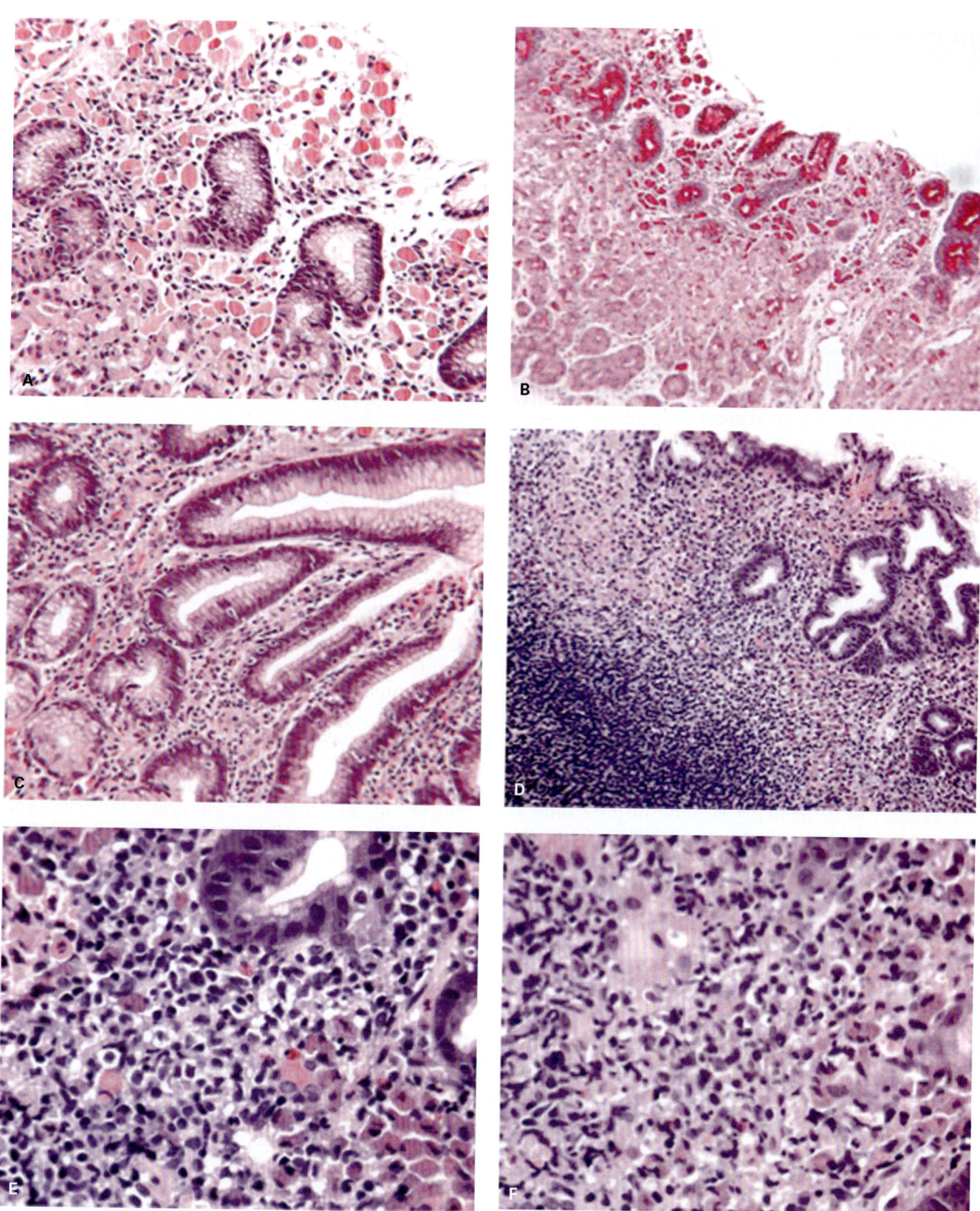

Figure 13-65. Russell body gastritis. **A:** There are myriad eosinophilic Russell bodies in the cytoplasm of plasma cells in the lamina propria. **B:** They are D-PAS positive. **C:** Mucosa elsewhere showed typical active *Helicobacter* gastritis. **D:** Second patient with Russell body gastritis and MALT lymphoma. Overview with numerous eosinophilic plasma cells containing Russell bodies. **E:** The intervening lamina propria has features of MALT lymphoma rather than the background of plasma cells seen in gastritis. **F:** Lymphoepithelial lesion in the oxyntic mucosa with the spindled nuclei of MALT lymphoma.

light chain restriction or PCR-based assays can help establish the diagnosis. In most cases this represents part of a more disseminated lymphoproliferative disease or plasma cell dyscrasia; however, we have also encountered a patient with light chain restriction in the Russell bodies, but no other evidence of a lymphoma, so its significance is uncertain. In the absence of any long-term follow-up data in such cases, at least workup to exclude any underlying lymphoproliferative disease and careful follow-up may be prudent.

NON–H. PYLORI BACTERIAL INFECTIONS

Non–H. pylori Helicobacter Species (NHPH)/"Helicobacter heilmannii"

In a minority of patients (0.17%–2.3%) with upper GI symptoms, long tightly coiled spiral bacteria, clearly distinct from the smaller gull-wing, S- or comma-shaped H. pylori, are observed in gastric biopsies[548–550] (Fig. 13-66). These unculturable bacteria were originally referred to as "Gastrospirillum hominis."[548] Analysis of the 16S rRNA gene resulted in their classification in the genus Helicobacter. They were provisionally named "H. heilmannii" after the German pathologist Konrad Heilmann, who first studied the pathology associated with these microorganisms.[549] Sequencing of several genes has shown that non–H. pylori helicobacter (NHPH) "H. heilmannii" comprise at least five different Helicobacter species (all known to colonize the stomach of animals).[551] Because of difficulties in the isolation and identification of NHPH "H. heilmannii" the epidemiology remains poorly understood. Nonetheless, current data suggest that especially pigs, dogs, and cats constitute reservoir hosts for gastric Helicobacter species with zoonotic potential.[552] A summary of NHPH "H. heilmannii" currently known to infect humans is given in Table 13-14. More than 20 species of Helicobacter have been reported to cause human infection, although most are due to H. heilmannii. This may largely be also due to the fact that on routine histology the distinction between various species in not possible, and many are possibly mixed infections. This section does not cover NHPH not currently known to infect humans.

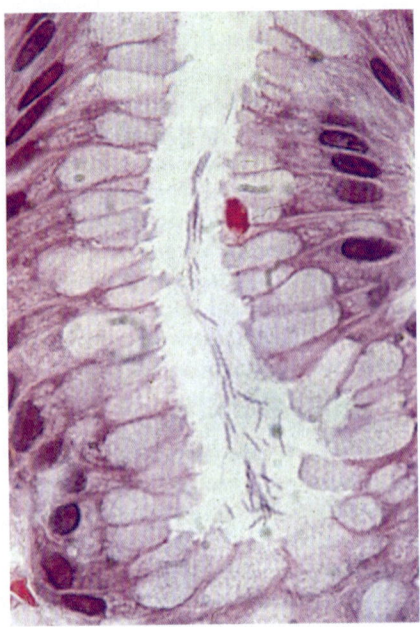

Figure 13-66. Gastrospirillum. The organisms are much longer than H. pylori.

Gastric disease associated with non–H. pylori Helicobacter species/"Helicobacter heilmannii". NHPHs ("H. heilmannii") have been implicated in the pathogenesis of gastritis,[549,550,553] gastric ulcers,[554] gastric cancer,[555] and MALT lymphoma.[553] Although "H. heilmannii"–associated gastritis is usually milder than H. pylori–associated gastritis, it is noteworthy that MALT lymphoma seems more frequent among patients infected with "H. heilmannii."[556,557] Treatment regimens are identical to those used for H. pylori as triple therapy using combinations of a PPI and two antimicrobial agents selected from clarithromycin,

Table 13-14	Non-*Helicobacter pylori* Detected in the Stomach of Humans
HELICOBACTER SPECIES	**NATURAL HOST (PREVALENCE, %)**
H. suis	Pig (60%–80% in slaughter pigs)
H. felis	Dog (47%), cat (63%), rabbit (2%–9%), cheetah
H. bizzozeronii	Dog (70%), cat (35%)
H. salomonis	Dog (9%), cat (2%), rabbit (0%–4%)
"Candidatus Helicobacter heilmannii"	Dog (20%–100%), cat (20%–100%), nonhuman primates (66%)
"Candidatus Helicobacter bovis"	Cattle (NA)

Modified from Haesebrouck F, Pasmans F, Flahou B, et al. Gastric helicobacters in domestic animals and nonhuman primates and their significance for human health. Clin Microbiol Rev. 2009;22(2):202–223, table of contents.

metronidazole, amoxicillin, and tetracycline may be effective.[558,559] Because of the low number of *in vitro* isolates available, very little data exist on the antimicrobial susceptibility and acquired resistance of gastric NHPH species. Nonetheless, acquired resistance to metronidazole may occur in *Helicobacter bizzozeronii* and *Helicobacter felis* strains of animal origin.[560]

Diagnosis. "*H. heilmannii*" infection is associated with chronic active gastritis that is usually milder than *H. pylori*–associated gastritis and a lower number of spiral organisms (0.5–1-μm-wide, 6–10-μm-long, tightly coiled spirals with up to six turns)[551] (Fig. 13-66). In some patients it may clinically and histologically present as acute gastritis. PCR and sequencing remain the gold standard for the detection of this genus.[561,562] The frequent changes in the nomenclature of gastric NHPH in the last two decades have caused considerable confusion in the literature regarding these infections. Some propose using the term "gastric NHPH" to designate gastric spirals that are morphologically different from *H. pylori*.[562] Alternatively, one can insert a comment on the diversity of this genus after a diagnosis of "*H. heilmannii*"–like organisms. Or, one can just call them all *H. heilmannii* on the grounds that it likely matters little. The main point in making the diagnosis is to appreciate that these are likely derived from animal sources, so it might be wise not to allow pets to lick one's face and mouth to prevent reinfection as far as possible.

The organisms are most easily seen with silver stains, and are sometimes stacked. Nonsilver stains make them more difficult to distinguish from *H. pylori* as they often appear far smaller than seen in silver stains. They stain with anti-*Helicobacter* antibodies, but their spiral nature is often not as apparent as in silver stains.

Tuberculosis

Tuberculosis may involve any part of the GI tract including stomach, mostly secondary to pulmonary or other systemic tuberculosis.[563] After the introduction of successful antituberculous regimens, the percentage of pulmonary tuberculosis cases with clinically evident secondary GI involvement has decreased from 38% to <5%.[564-567] Tuberculosis in general surged back with advent of AIDS,[568] but can also be seen with other immunodeficiencies, whether congenital or acquired.

Primary isolated gastric tuberculosis in immunocompetent patients is rare.[569-571] The rarity of gastric tuberculosis has been explained by the paucity of lymphatics in the gastric wall, which is not really tenable, and the effect of gastric acidity on tubercle bacilli, the rapid emptying of gastric contents, an intact gastric mucosa[572,573] and by a protective effect of *H. pylori* infection.[574] Overall, no single factor seems responsible for the resistance.

The antrum and prepyloric regions are the most common sites of tuberculous lesions in the stomach.[575,576] Nonetheless, tuberculosis can present in other sites including the gastric fundus and gastric cardia.[569,577,578]

The clinical manifestations of gastric tuberculosis are variable, so the diagnosis is easily missed. There are reports of isolated gastric tuberculosis presenting as pyrexia of unknown origin.[579] Other presentations include linitis plastica,[571,580] gastric outlet obstruction,[581] benign peptic ulcer[582] and, rarely, massive GI bleed and gastric perforation[583] or as large gastric folds. The gross appearances may be identical to those of CD, including pyloroduodenal involvement. On biopsy, granulomas can be either caseous or noncaseous. The specific diagnosis rests on the demonstration of mycobacteria in biopsy tissue and on microbiology cultures, with possible confirmation using PCR. Acid-fast bacilli are rarely seen in tissue sections, and numerous acid-fast stained levels may be required to find an organism. As the typical histology may not always be present, in the absence of demonstrable acid-fast bacilli it is important to exclude the histopathologic differentials of granulomatous diseases such as Crohn's disease, sarcoidosis, histoplasmosis, *Helicobacter*, isolated granulomatous gastritis, allergic granulomatosis and vasculitis, syphilis, gastric ulcer, and gastric cancer. PCR of biopsy specimen, especially those with visible organism on the Z-N stain, provides a faster, alternative route for diagnosis while excluding Crohn's disease if positive.[535]

Syphilis

Gastric syphilis is rare. Even though initially gastric syphilis had been viewed as a complication of tertiary syphilis, subsequent reports indicated that the stomach is commonly affected in early syphilis.[584,585-587] The gummatous reaction of tertiary syphilis in the stomach is of historical interest.[588] Many of the recent cases, but far from all, are reported in gay males or in the AIDS setting, but sporadic cases do occur, with a median age of 39 years (range 21–78).[584] In one series of affected patients, only 13% had a history of syphilis although 33% had concurrent clinical manifestations of the disease.[584]

Gastric involvement with syphilis is difficult to diagnose, because clinical presentation is protean. It can be characterized by thickened gastric folds commonly associated with a severe endoscopic gastritis with erosions. The picture may sometimes resemble a gastric malignancy with a linitis plastica pattern or a diffuse lymphoma-like pattern and thus present with nausea, vomiting or early satiety. Bleeding from ulcers or from erosive disease is a less common manifestation. Interestingly, weight loss can be prominent (65% of early disease and 53% of late disease cases).

Anorexia was reported in 15% of cases, more frequently in late disease.[584]

The histology of the gastric mucosa in secondary syphilis is also protean, hence, the term "syphilis, the great imitator." As with most unusual diagnoses the key is to think of it and look for organisms in the lamina propria with silver stains (e.g., with some hand methods for the Warthin–Starry stain, although in our experience automated methods, while good for *Helicobacter*, do not stain *Treponema* readily or strongly) when *Helicobacter* are not identified but one suspects that they should be present, or with an anti-*Treponema* antibody immunohistochemically, or by PCR. A positive serology is invariably present. The "red light" for Treponemal infection should go on when a severe diffuse gastritis is present but *Helicobacter* are not identified in the lumen when active disease (neutrophils) is present. Alternatively, an infiltrate may be present resembling lymphoma, but the infiltrate is polyclonal and lymphoepithelial lesions are not really present. The mucosa can appear amazingly atrophic, although other serologic evidence of AIG is absent. It also needs to be in the differential of granulomas when no other cause is found, so should be part of this workup.

Diffuse gastritis containing dense plasma cell or lymphocytic infiltrate is invariably observed in both early and late disease, sometimes with concomitant shallow erosions (Fig. 13-67). The inflammatory infiltrate is denser than seen in other types of gastritis. When especially dense the concern is always regarding the possibility of lymphoma, and historically lymphoma (even with resection because of this suspicion) is well-documented.[589,590] Prominent perivascular cuffing, and vasculitis, manifested as marked proliferative endarteritis or endophlebitis, typical of syphilitic involvement in other sites,

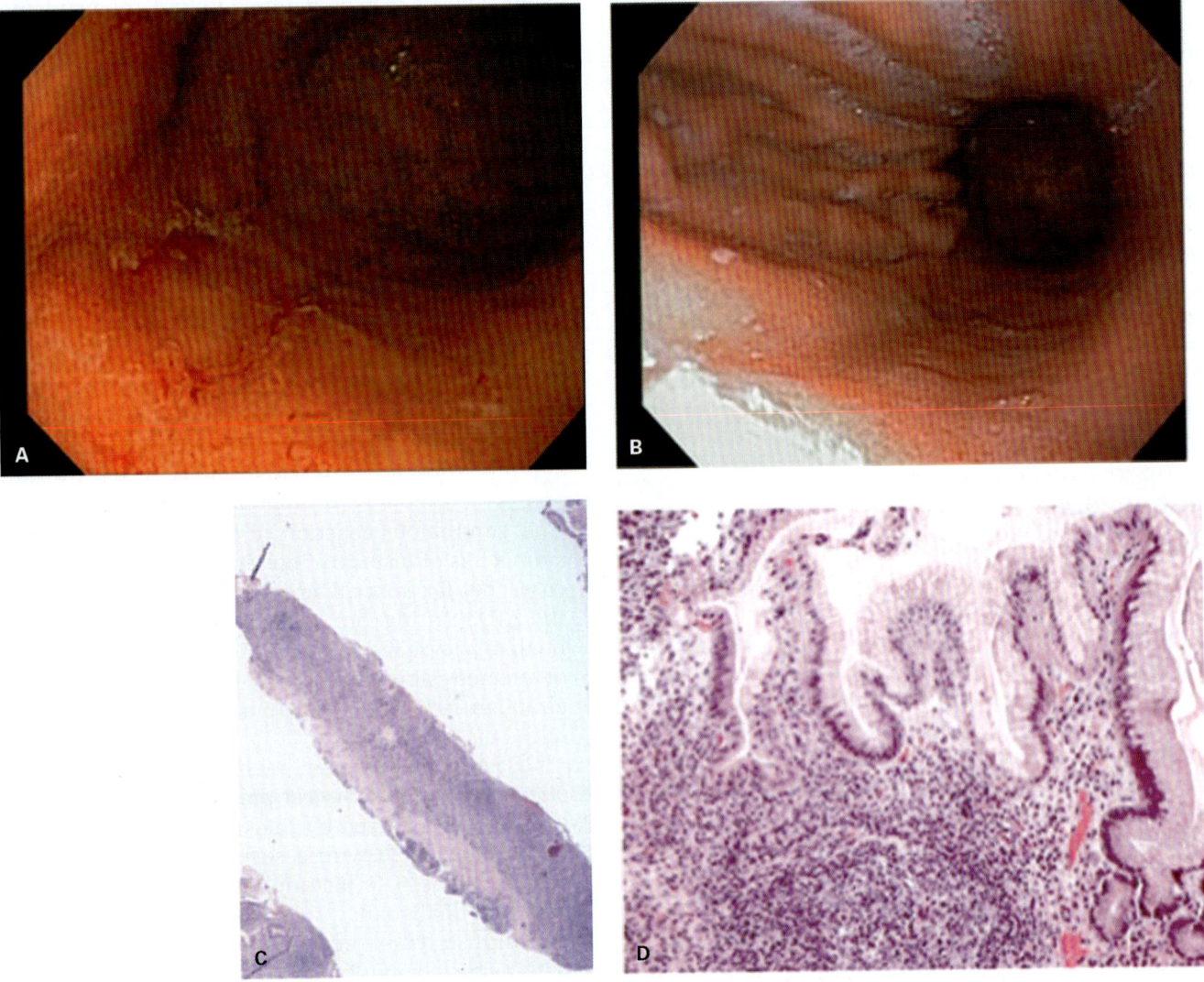

Figure 13-67. Syphilitic gastritis. **A,B:** Endoscopic appearances before and after therapy. (Courtesy of Dr. Sandy Nelles, Mississauga, Ontario.) **C:** Overview of part of one biopsy showing marked atrophy with loss of most of the pits. **D:** Lymphoid follicles (many patients are misdiagnosed as having a lymphoproliferative disorder).

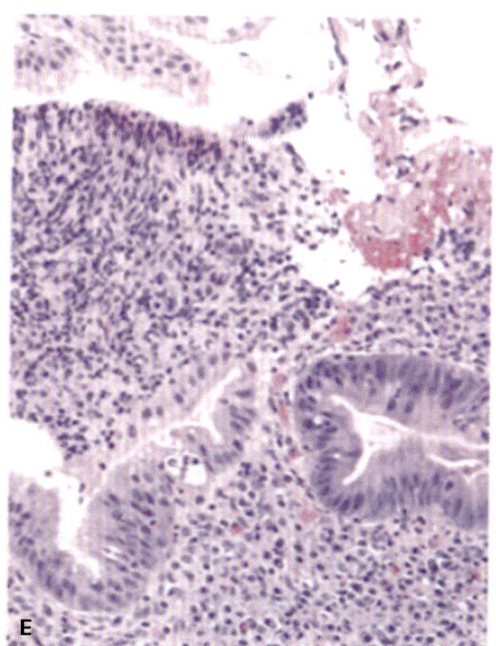
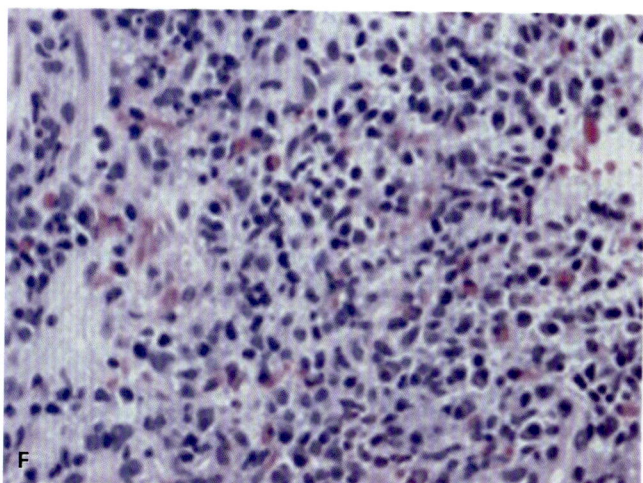
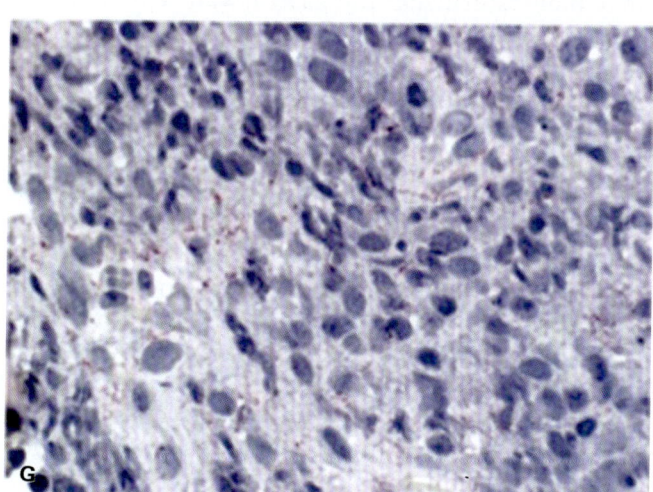

Figure 13-67. *(Continued)* **E:** A polymorphous infiltrate is present involving pits and lamina propria. **F:** Detail of the polymorphous infiltrate. **G:** Immunostain using a *T. pallidum* antibody that stain red. (Courtesy of Dr. Wun-Jiu Shieh, CDC, Atlanta GA.)

is rarely found in gastric biopsies (perhaps because most gastric biopsies do not sample the submucosa where these vessels are located). Thus, the pathologist should bear in mind the possibility of syphilitic gastritis whenever a gastric biopsy shows unusually severe chronic active gastritis with glandular destruction, or neutrophils but no *Helicobacter* are identified. These features, however, suggest only an unusual infectious or inflammatory condition; they are not diagnostic for syphilitic gastritis. Therefore, while additional histologic features including vasculitis and granuloma can also be seen, meticulous examination of the biopsy for microorganisms should be undertaken,[584,587,591,592] the key lies in thinking of the diagnosis and looking for the organism in the sections, or by PCR, or serologically.

Demonstration: *Treponema pallidum* spirochetes can be demonstrated in biopsies by silver impregnation or immunohistochemistry with standard or fluorescent antibody techniques.[591–593] *Treponema pallidum* is a gram-negative spirochete bacterium measuring 8 to 15 μm in length and 0.1 to 0.2 μm in diameter.[594] It is important to distinguish it from *H. pylori* (1–3 mm in length and 0.5–1.0 mm in diameter) and *H. heilmannii* (longer and wider than *H. pylori*, but shorter and stouter than *T. pallidum*). Practically this is less of a problem as the *Treponema* are invariably located in the lamina propria, a location where *Helicobacter* are virtually never found.[594] Detection with PCR-based assays may help confirm the diagnosis, especially when the organisms are sparse and there is a dense lymphoid infiltrate.[592,595] The proof that syphilis causes gastric lesions and symptoms rests with the demonstration of the organism in the gastric mucosa, appropriate serology, and evidence that the lesions regress after therapy. Interestingly, there is no endoscopic response to high-dose PPIs, but rapid resolution if the patient is treated for Helicobacter "on spec," as the organism remains sensitive to virtually all antibiotics. For this reason, if there is coexistent Helicobacter and syphilis, unless the patient is known to have syphilis, the latter will never be diagnosed as the former will be treated and concomitantly cure the syphilis.

Enterococcal Gastritis

There is a report of an Enterococcus-associated gastritis in a 59-year-old diabetic male detected 9 months after receiving treatment for H. pylori–associated gastritis, for ulcers. Mucosal biopsy revealed severe active but focal gastritis with surface and adjacent gram-positive coccobacilli in short to long chains with no H. pylori (see Fig. 13-15). Culture grew an Enterococcus similar to E. hirae and E. durans. No treatment was given, and endoscopy done 2 months later showed complete resolution of the gastritis and absence of H. pylori or Enterococci. The presence of NSAID gastric mucosal injury and diabetes may have been the predisposing factors.[67] This therefore needs to be in the differential diagnosis of focal chronic active Helicobacter-negative gastritis. Once this organism is recognized and not confused with Helicobacter, especially coccal forms, this organism is less uncommon than the sparse literature would suggest.

Phlegmonous and Emphysematous Gastritis

Phlegmonous gastritis (PG) is an uncommon, often fatal condition characterized by suppurative bacterial infection of the stomach, which primarily affects the submucosa but may spread to all layers of the stomach, resulting in necrosis and gangrene. The latter complication, when unassociated with thrombosis of the major vessels of the stomach, has sometimes been designated acute necrotizing gastritis.[596] Emphysematous gastritis is likely the same disease but with gas-forming organisms, and consists of bacterial infection of the deeper layers of the gastric wall.[597] Both phlegmonous and emphysematous gastritis are rare potentially life-threatening bacterial infections.[598] The distinction between them in an individual case may be arbitrary.

PG may arise from a local or a disseminated hematogenous infection and may involve either a portion (localized) of the stomach or the entire stomach (diffuse),[599] and may even extend into the small bowel. Although the pathogenesis is not precisely known, predisposing factors such as cirrhosis, alcoholism, achlorhydria, debilitation, and immune compromise have been postulated as important etiologic factors.[600–606] Nevertheless, approximately 50% of patients were previously healthy and had no significant antecedent risk factors.[599] It seems to be related to so-called spontaneous bacterial peritonitis, which may well be an extension of the same process involving the serosa and peritoneal cavity.

Strictly speaking, in order to accept a case as representing PG, bacteria should be seen (and possibly also cultured) in the submucosal exudate. The most commonly involved microorganisms are Streptococci, Escherichia coli, Pseudomonas aeruginosa, Clostridium perfringens, and Staphylococcus aureus,[596,597] and organisms are usually readily visible on a Gram stain. However, when patients with apparent PG are cured with nonoperative drainage procedures and antibiotics the classic definition of PG (demonstrable bacteria in the wall) may not be able to be fulfilled. This, of course, is fortunate for the patient because it means that antibiotic therapy may have "sterilized" the gastric wall. When submucosal swelling and gangrene are found without bacteria, another possibility is ischemia on some basis other than infection.

The typical patient presents with an acute abdomen, sometimes accompanied by hematemesis. Ultrasound or CT scan may suggest the diagnosis and endoscopy may reveal an edematous lesion suggesting a submucosal lesion with erosions or ulcers.[607,608] Histologically, there is an acute purulent inflammation of the submucosa characterized by an intense neutrophilic infiltrate, edema, congestion, and frequently necrosis. Typically, sheets of bacteria are readily evident on a Gram stain. The inflammation often extends through the full thickness of the stomach. There may be small vessel thrombosis associated with the purulent infection, but the major extrinsic gastric vessels are usually patent.[608,609]

Emphysematous gastritis needs to be differentiated from benign collections of air in the gastric wall, so-called gastric emphysema, and pneumatosis cystoides intestinalis.[610–612] Gastric emphysema is a rare condition that is caused by the disruption of the mucosa, which leads to air dissecting into the gastric wall.[610] It is known to be caused by direct gastric trauma, ingestion of corrosives, penetrating gastric ulcers, vomiting, and instrumentation such as nasogastric tube placement and endoscopy.[611,612] Sometimes it is difficult to know if gas in the wall is the result of an infection or something else, like a carbonated drink.[611] The pathologists' most common encounter of air in the wall of the gut, usually the colon, most commonly is pseudolipomatosis-iatrogenic gas presumed to be introduced during colonoscopy.

VIRAL INFECTIONS

Human herpesviridae infections: In this family, there are eight distinct viruses known to cause disease in humans (HHV-1 herpes simplex virus 1, HHV-2 herpes simplex virus 2, HHV-3 varicella zoster virus, HHV-4 Epstein–Barr virus, HHV-5 cytomegalovirus, HHV-6 herpes lymphotropic virus, HHV-7 Roseolovirus, and HHV-8 Kaposi's sarcoma associated herpesvirus[613]). Herpesviruses are known for their ability to become established in a latent form following initial transmission and reactivate with physiologic or pathologic immune suppression. During latent persistence, herpesviruses are found in other tissues, for example, HSV-1, HSV-2, and VZV in neural tissues, and EBV and HHV-6 in lymphoid tissues. In the following section, we will only discuss herpesviridae infections reported in the gastric mucosa in descending order of importance or frequency.

Cytomegalovirus Infection (HHV-5)

Isolated involvement of the stomach is rare, but has been reported.[614,615] Gastric CMV disease may be asymptomatic, may be associated with nondescript dyspepsia, or may reflect symptoms of gastric outlet obstruction with nausea and vomiting. In acute infection, symptoms may reflect just that with nausea, vomiting, and abdominal pain.[616] Something about this infection in the stomach appears to alter gastric motility[616,617] and in some patients a distinct postural relationship to symptoms may be present.[618] Occult or more overt GI bleeding may result from ulcerative lesions.[619] Childhood CMV infection has attracted considerable attention because it causes a Ménétrier-like picture and occurs in apparently immunocompetent patients.[620] This is discussed subsequently in the section on Ménétrier's disease.

Endoscopic findings characteristic of CMV gastritis include erosion(s) and oozing from mucosal surface.[621] It is likely that CMV-infected endothelium narrows vascular channels inducing local ischemia[622] eventually resulting in erosions and oozing. Irregular erosions and fold thickening, though considered common manifestations of CMV in terms of distinctive appearances, are not observed in all patients.[621] When present, mucosal thickening can mimic lymphoma or linitis plastica, or cause outlet obstruction.[623] In these more distinctive settings it is presumed that CMV is the cause of the lesions; however, one needs to ensure that there is no associated neoplasm such as lymphoma or Kaposi's sarcoma. Moreover, CMV inclusions can be identified pathologically from normal appearing mucosa as well as erosions. This demonstrates the necessity of a biopsy even if endoscopy shows only normal findings.

Histology:[614,615] Apart from finding typical CMV inclusions, the associated mucosal injury may be nondescript or there may be a pattern of reactive gastropathy. Marked hyperplasia of the foveolar epithelium and pyloric glands or both may be a prominent feature in those cases associated with mucosal fold thickening or localized masses, especially the young. CMV is also associated with chronic active gastritis or gastroduodenal ulcers[624–626] and can cause severe damage. Biopsy specimens show edema and an inflammatory infiltrate that typically has a predominance of neutrophils within the lamina propria[627] (Figs. 13-16 and 13-68). Usually, there are only a few foci of pit inflammation and pit abscesses. Less common is the picture of associated lymphoid hyperplasia.[628] If CMV-infected cells are in the antral glands they are easier to spot at low power than when they occur in the lamina propria or in endothelial cells. When CMV is associated with gastric ulcers, the typical inclusions are found in endothelial cells, fibroblasts, or histiocytes within granulation tissue, or in the mucosa adjacent to the ulcers.[629] In the latter instance, they are commonly present deep (Fig. 14-21) in the gland zones (see Fig. 13-16).

Herpes Viruses (HHV-1,2)

Though GI herpes simplex virus (HSV) infection most commonly involves the esophagus, HSV is rarely recognized in the stomach in association with gastric erosions in the immunocompromised host.[630–633] Endoscopy varies from shallow superficial ulcers that may coalesce in later stages,[631] raised erythematous nodules,[634] to an exceptional case report of Ménétrier's disease associated with HSV.[635] Herpetic gastritis is not necessarily accompanied with concomitant stomatitis or esophagitis.[630,631,634] Histologic findings can include acute and chronic inflammation with regenerative epithelial hyperplasia, areas of necrosis-like degeneration, and ulceration with fibrinopurulent exudates. Herpetic inclusions rarely have been demonstrated by H&E stain in the gastric mucosa.[630] In most cases, HSV inclusions were not seen on H&E sections but were demonstrated by tissue culture of gastric biopsies[634] or immunohistochemistry.[635] Herpetic gastritis may be more common than once believed. Because HSV infections can effectively be treated with antiviral medications, patients with infections of more visible site may already be on treatment that may prevent spread to the gastric mucosa. Prophylactic antiviral treatment, often given to prevent CMV infection, may also prevent HSV infections.[634]

Most medical literature regarding HSV and the stomach revolves around the possible role of HSV in some patients with PUD.[636–644] Although most PUD is attributable to *H. pylori* or the use of NSAIDs, a significant minority of ulcers and erosions have no clear

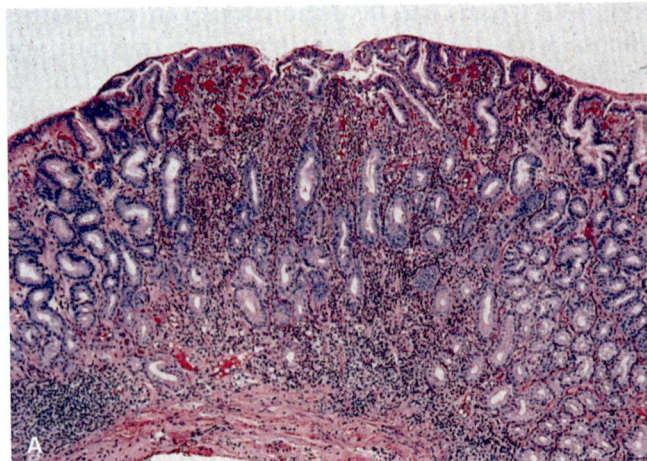
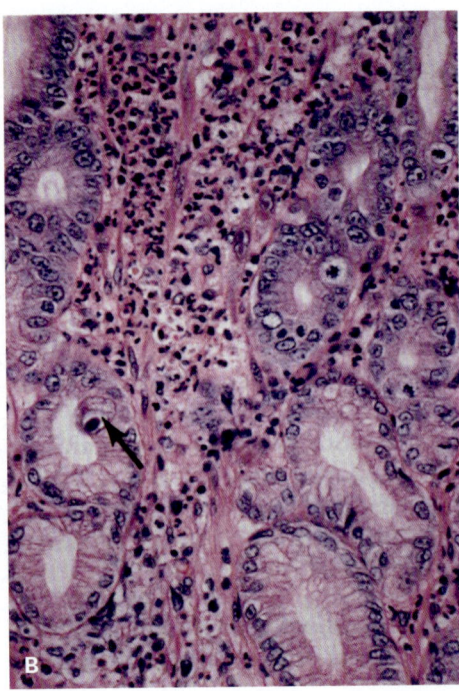

Figure 13-68. Cytomegalovirus gastritis. **A:** Low-power view showing intense panmucosal inflammation in the center of the biopsy specimen. **B:** High-power view showing the large number of neutrophils and a typical cytomegalic cell with its large intranuclear inclusion deep in an antral gland (*arrow*).

etiology. DNA of HSV-1 has been detected in human vagal[645] and celiac ganglia,[646] which provide the neural network to gastric tissue. In one study, many HSV-positive cells costained for cholecystokinin. The investigators hypothesized that HSV migrates from the vagal and celiac ganglia, initially infecting neuroendocrine cells.[636] Proponents further argue that the notable reduction in recurrent ulcers and erosions following vagotomy is caused by an interruption of HSV-1 migration from ganglia to gastric mucosa thus preventing recurrence.[636] This finding has intriguing implications if confirmed and extended.

Epstein–Barr Virus (EBV — HHV-4)

EBV typically presents as infectious mononucleosis in children and young adults; over 90% of the world's population gets exposed to EBV and has the latent viral DNA.[647] Rarely, the virus can affect the GI tract including stomach, leading to ulcerative and hemorrhagic lesions.[647–650] Patients can present with nausea, sense of early satiety, bloating, and epigastric pain.[647–650] The endoscopic differential includes NSAID-induced injury, *H. pylori* infection, marginal zone lymphoma, syphilis, and malignancy.[648] Biopsies show epithelial ulcerations and a marked expansion of the lamina propria with a diffuse lymphoid infiltrate[648] including atypical immunoblasts that can simulate gastric lymphoma.[647] Despite the presence of surface erosions and necrosis, neutrophils are not prominent. There are only a few foci of pititis and pit abscesses.[647] The presence of EBV is most frequently determined by in situ hybridization for EBV-encoded small RNA-1 (EBER-1).[651] Importantly, expression of EBER-1 should not be considered a true positive unless there is diffuse staining.[648] Prior studies on colonic resections from cases of IBD have shown isolated EBER-1 positivity in 60% of cases.[652] This finding most likely represents chronically EBV-infected B lymphocytes that happen to circulate within intestinal inflammatory infiltrates.[648] Of greatest importance in recognizing ulcerative gastritis secondary to EBV infection is to identify a self-limited condition that can potentially be mistaken for gastric lymphoma. EBV should be considered in the clinical scenario such as severe chronic active gastritis unexplicably negative for *H. pylori*, or rapid resolution without treatment, particularly in clinical scenarios suggestive of infectious mononucleosis.

EBV has also been associated with gastric carcinomas, which is a separate issue and has been discussed in Chapter 14.

Other HHV Viruses

HHV-6–positive cells (HHV-6 herpes lymphotropic virus) are frequently found in the gastroduodenal mucosa of liver transplant recipients and of immunocompetent patients undergoing gastroscopic examination because of dyspeptic symptoms.[653,654] Their significance is unclear. HHV-8 can be demonstrated in Kaposi sarcoma involving the stomach.

Other Viruses

Occasionally patients are biopsied in the prodromal phase of a disease such as measles. Biopsies may show the classical Warthin–Finkeldey giant cells (Fig. 13-17).

FUNGAL INFECTIONS

Candida albicans

Candida albicans and, to a lesser extent, *Candida tropicalis*, and *Candida glabrata*[655] (formerly known as *Torulopsis glabrata*) are commonly found in gastric ulcer or erosion beds in immunocompetent and immunocompromised hosts.[656,657] In studies of treatment of peptic ulcer with modalities other than *H. pylori* eradication there has been general,[657,658] but not unanimous[659] agreement that the healing process was unaffected by the presence of *Candida* in the ulcer bed. With the eradication of *H. pylori* as the backbone of ulcer therapy and with the use of modern potent antisecretory agents it is likely that healing can progress at the same rate whether *Candida* is colonizing or not. Organisms resembling *Candida* can also be found amongst a variety of organisms found in the stomach of patients on long-term PPIs, but presumably none stays long enough to colonize the stomach.

Smears of exudates combined with cultures, and examination of biopsies from ulcer edges for the presence of mycelia, establish the diagnosis. If gastric erosions or ulcers are seen in an immunocompromised host, it is worthwhile to look for an associated fungal infection and to treat it, if present, in conjunction with providing therapy for the peptic ulcer. The rationale is to minimize the risk of dissemination or of vascular invasion in the bed of the ulcer, especially in the neutropenic patient (see esophagus chapter). In immunocompetent patients who have biopsies taken to rule out cancer in gastric ulcers it is not required to do special stains on sections from the ulcer base to detect fungi because therapy will by unaffected by the presence of fungal organisms given how commonly they can be found in garden-variety ulcers.[655]

Histoplasmosis

GI histoplasmosis is reported primarily in association with AIDS, even in nonendemic areas.[660–662] In the AIDS setting the colon seems to be a more favored site than any other. Disseminated histoplasmosis rarely involves the stomach, and when it does, the usual feature is bleeding from gastric ulcers or from erosions on giant gastric folds that are infiltrated with numerous histiocytes usually including the granulomas of *Histoplasma capsulatum*.[663,664] However, histologic demonstration of the organisms in tissue does not necessarily imply that the organisms are viable or that the infection is active. Active infection must be proven by culture of the organism from biopsy tissue or sometimes resections.[664] *H. duboissii* is a much rarer type of histoplasma and has been reported in a case from Africa, mimicking a gastric cancer.[665]

Mucormycosis (Zygomycosis)

Mucormycosis, one of the phycomycetes class, are widely distributed fungi, and may become pathogenic in debilitated patients.[666] Many of the reports of gastric involvement come from Africa, and in some of these patients there is no underlying debility. The stomach is the most frequently affected part of the GI tract in mucormycosis and may be unassociated with rhinocerebral involvement.[667,668] Other parts of the GI tract seem more vulnerable in the immunocompromised patient than just the stomach.[669,670] Neonates and children may also have involvement of the GI.[671]

The typical lesion is a perforated or deep bleeding ulcer with black, indurated edges. The vessels at the ulcer base are thrombosed and contain the broad, nonseptate hyphae. The diagnosis has typically been made at autopsy or surgery but some are now made endoscopically.[672] Earlier recognition and institution of antifungal therapy with or without partial gastrectomy, is the best chance to avoid perforation.[673] In the past most cases were lethal, primarily because of the associated angioinvasion and dissemination.

Aspergillosis

This infection is extremely rare in the stomach.[674,675] Vascular thrombosis with resultant ischemic necrosis account for some of the ulcerations that are normally seen (Fig. 13-69).

PARASITES AND NEMATODES

Cryptosporidium

Though in a small study, *Cryptosporidium* were more commonly found in the antrum than the gastric body, and more likely in areas exhibiting reactive change,[676] it appears that gastric cryptosporidiosis does not produce gastric mucosal injury or if it does the injury is similar to that expected in the AIDS stomach without the organism. In general, GI opportunistic infections with advanced immunodeficiency occur in a small number of HIV-infected patients under highly active antiretroviral therapy. Although GI opportunistic infections

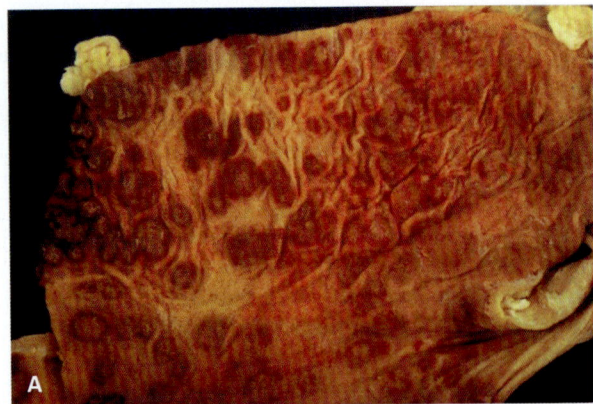
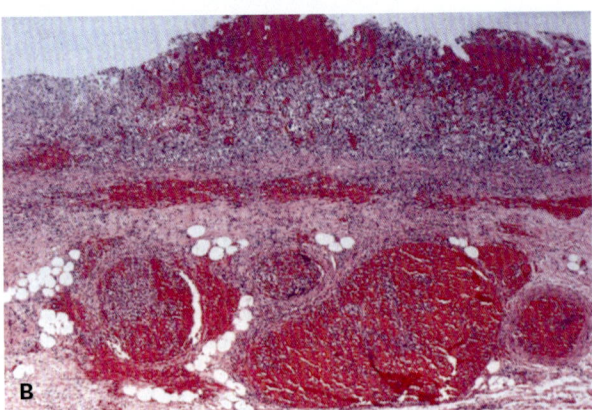
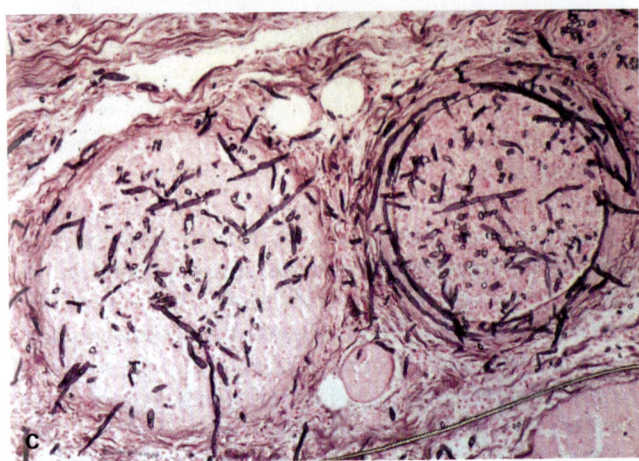

Figure 13-69. Gastric aspergillosis. **A:** Autopsy specimen from a patient with GVHD after bone marrow transplantation. The *brownish patches* represent collections of the fungus. **B:** Necrosis of the gastric wall. **C:** Septate hyphal forms inside and outside occluded blood vessels.

were detected exclusively in dyspeptic patients, they are unlikely to be related to these symptoms. To correctly diagnose opportunistic infections, multiple biopsy specimens may be necessary even from normal-appearing mucosa.[677]

Anisakiasis

This infection represents one of the risks of eating sushi and other types of raw fish.[678–680] The *Ascaris*-like larvae embed themselves in the gastric mucosa. The condition is usually short-lived and self-limited with abdominal pain, or more rarely chest pain,[681] as the main feature. It is claimed that the pain subsides within hours of endoscopic removal of the worms (Fig. 13-70A),[682] but in most cases the symptoms last several days and are attributed to some food reaction or toxin and likely go undiagnosed. Thickened gastric folds may be seen with ultrasonography.[683] The putative spectrum of injury has broadened with its finding in the esophagus, presumed due to reflux.[684,685] The infected site is inflamed with chronic inflammation and eosinophils and remnants of organisms may be present, and can even be identified by sequencing. However, usually the worms are identified and removed endoscopically as they are about 2 cms long, so they are easily seen.

The life cycle is complex, the initial host being small crustations (shrimps, krill) that are either eaten directly by mammals such as whales, but usually progress through increasing sizes of fish and ultimately by (sea) mammals (dolphins, seals, man) where the life cycle is completed. As the organism is killed by freezing at –20° C for 24 h most sushi places either do this deliberately, or rely on the fish being quick-frozen immediately after being caught to (paradoxically) keep it fresh. Nematode-free sushi is therefore actually healthier if "fresh frozen" for 24 h before serving. Undercooked or home-pickled fish are both also a potential hazards.

Other Parasites and Nematodes

Other GI hazards may occur from eating raw or poorly cooked fish—*eustrongylidiasis* is an example.[686]

Strongyloides stercoralis is common in many parts of the world, including parts of the United States. In a healthy host, the parasite usually does not cause any symptoms. In immunocompromised patients it may lead to overwhelming dissemination, if it goes unrecognized.[687] It predominates in the small bowel, and the diagnosis is made by the examination of stools and duodenal aspirates. Rarely, *Strongyloides* is found in the gastric mucosa or elsewhere in the gastric wall

Chapter 13 Stomach and Proximal Duodenum: Inflammatory and Miscellaneous Disorders

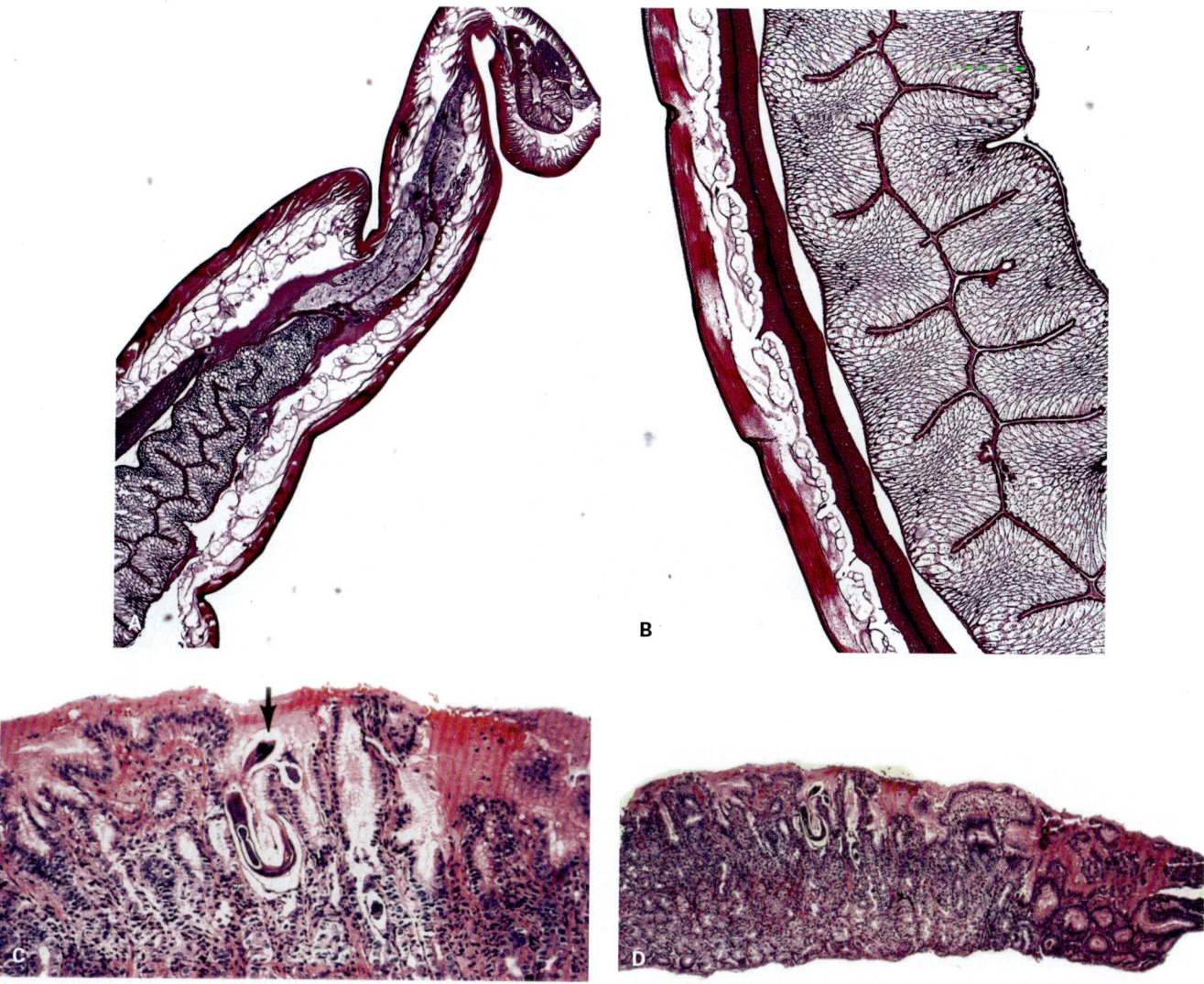

Figure 13-70. Gastric anasikiasis and strongyloides. **A:** Head of Anisakis worm identified and removed endoscopically. **B:** It consists of a large central digestive tube (esophagus). Externally there is a thick protective cuticle and underlying muscle and beneath this the excretory duct. Focally the lateral cords may also be visible. **C:** Biopsy specimen from the proximal stomach from a subepithelial hemorrhage in a patient from El Salvador after bone marrow transplantation. The worm is shown at both high (*arrow*) and low power in the pit region **(D)**.

(Fig. 13-70), usually in immunosuppressed patients.[688] While the worms are easy to see, the larvae can be extremely difficult. Where a heavy eosinophilia is present a critical look for these is required.

Other parasites. The finding of trophozoites of *Giardia lamblia* in gastric biopsies is not as rare as one might imagine but one sees what one is looking for and review of gastric biopsies in patients with Giardiasis is sometimes rewarding.[689] The possible mechanisms for its survival and presence include intestinal metaplasia, hypo- or achlorhydria (pathologic or iatrogenic), or duodenogastric reflux.[690] There are also isolated reports of gastric *toxoplasmosis*,[691] gastric involvement by *Ascaris*,[692] *taeniasis*,[693] *leishmaniasis*,[694] *schistosomiasis*,[695] *amebiasis*,[696] *Acanthamoeba* infection,[697] *toxoplasmosis*,[698,699] *Necator americanus*,[700] and hydatid disease.[701]

OTHER GASTRITIDES

INFLAMMATORY BOWEL DISEASES Crohn's Disease and Ulcerative Colitis predominantly affect the colon, ileum, jejunum, perianal area, and the oral cavity. Upper GI tract (UGT) involvement has become increasingly recognized, even in the absence of specific localizing symptoms, as patients more frequently undergo upper endoscopy. This is discussed in detail in Chapter 18.

Recognizing its importance, the revised Montreal 2005 system classifies upper GI involvement in CD, independent of other locations.[702] As such, CD L-1 to L-3 corresponds to disease involvement in the terminal ileum, colon, and ileocolon, respectively. The UGT is classified as L-4 but can accompany other

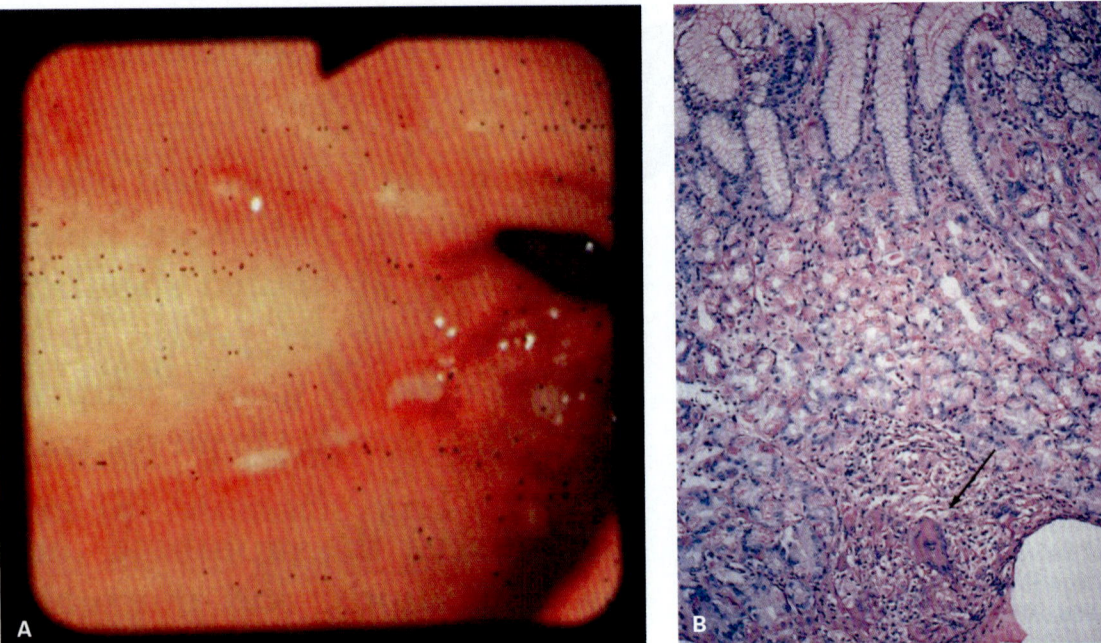

Figure 13-71. Gastric Crohn's disease. **A:** Endoscopic view of aphthous-type white-based erosions in the distal antrum near the pylorus. **B:** Isolated granuloma deep in a fundic gland biopsy specimen (*arrow*). Inflammatory cells are otherwise absent.

locations.[702] However, the Montreal classification does not specify definitions of upper tract "involvement." Obvious stenosis or ulcerations should prompt L-4 classification; however, aphthous ulcerations are recognized as reappearing sporadically.

Clinical features. Symptomatic macroscopic CD in the esophagus, stomach, and duodenum is between 1% and 5% among adults.[703,704] In contrast to earlier literature suggesting higher prevalence among children, two large studies suggest similar prevalence in adults and children.[705,706] Symptoms attributed specifically to gastroduodenal involvement are peptic ulcer-like pain and symptoms of delayed gastric emptying. Sometimes, UGT involvement may be the presenting manifestation. Nonetheless, usually, when the stomach is affected symptoms and signs of ileal or colonic involvement—diarrhea and focal colitis—are more prominent than gastric involvement. Gastric fistulas are rare but may arise from CD in the transverse colon, the small bowel (especially ileum), and ileocolonic anastomoses. Much rarer are fistulas between the esophagus and the stomach.[707] Deforming gastric involvement in this disease is uncommon and is usually confined to the antrum or pylorus. When there is deforming involvement with narrowing in the distal antrum it also commonly coexists with disease in the proximal duodenum. Stenotic or transmural disease of the stomach is uncommon in CD.

Endoscopic features. Endoscopy detects the aphthoid and serpiginous erosions, ulcerations, and mucosal irregularities[708] (Fig. 13-71). Less striking endoscopic and histologic changes may occur anywhere in the stomach but more biopsies are generally taken in the antrum. In general, at least two biopsies from each of the esophagus, antrum, and duodenum should be considered, with 2 more from oxyntic mucosa if *Helicobacter* has not been excluded.[709] Our suggestion in such instances is to use a long endoscope to get into the proximal jejunum and to take random biopsies from the small bowel, concentrating on the descending duodenum and, of course, any target lesions. In the stomach we take prepyloric and midantral biopsies as well as biopsies from one site in the body, usually the midbody greater curve. Whenever gastric erosions or ulcers are encountered in a patient with CD one must attempt to rule out other causes. It may be difficult to do so, for example, if there is erosive gastritis and the patient takes NSAIDs. Similarly, in patients who have large gastric ulcers[710] or gastric antral narrowing, malignancy must always be ruled out.[711] Endoscopy with biopsy is useful if there are suggestive but not definitive features of IBD and where corticosteroid or other long-term therapy is contemplated. In children, upper GI endoscopy may facilitate early diagnosis to avoid delayed growth. Imaging studies are more useful to define the stenotic or fistulizing type of disease.[712]

Histologic features

Crohn's Disease Highly focal inflammation, especially if chronic active inflammation, which is most often *H. pylori*–negative, should raise the possibility of Crohn's disease as in other parts of the GI tract (Figs. 13-72 and 13-73). While the term "focally enhanced" has been applied to this,[713] in our view it is not a helpful term as it refers primarily to chronic inflammation and histiocytes whereas focal chronic active inflammation is often the hallmark of this disease. "Focal chronic active gastritis" is a better term as it correctly described the pathology and most are more familiar with this system of gastritis nomenclature. A large cohort of patients with CD undergoing endoscopy were likely to have "focal lesions" (37% in the oxyntic mucosa, 41% antrum, and 12% in the duodenum and duodenal bulb). Other studies looked either specifically for chronic inflammation,[714] or for acute and chronic inflammation in *Helicobacter*-negative patients,[715] so the results are difficult to compare. We think the concept is equally well expressed by simply calling it *Helicobacter*-negative focal chronic active gastritis.

The presence of concomitant *Helicobacter* tends to obscure the focal lesions of CD, such that it may be impossible to suggest the diagnosis. Studies show a decreased prevalence of *H. pylori* in CD patients compared with controls, but this varies hugely depending on the infection rate in the population under study. The rate is also decreased in ulcerative colitis (UC) patients but not as much as CD.

In all likelihood the specificity for CD goes up if there is chronic active inflammation rather than just chronic inflammation, as lesions that include neutrophils are being used as a marker. However, there are other causes of both chronic active inflammation and granulomas, so that while these histologic features are suggestive of gastric and duodenal involvement by CD, they are not specific. Gastroduodenal involvement with CD therefore needs to be strongly considered when the following are present.

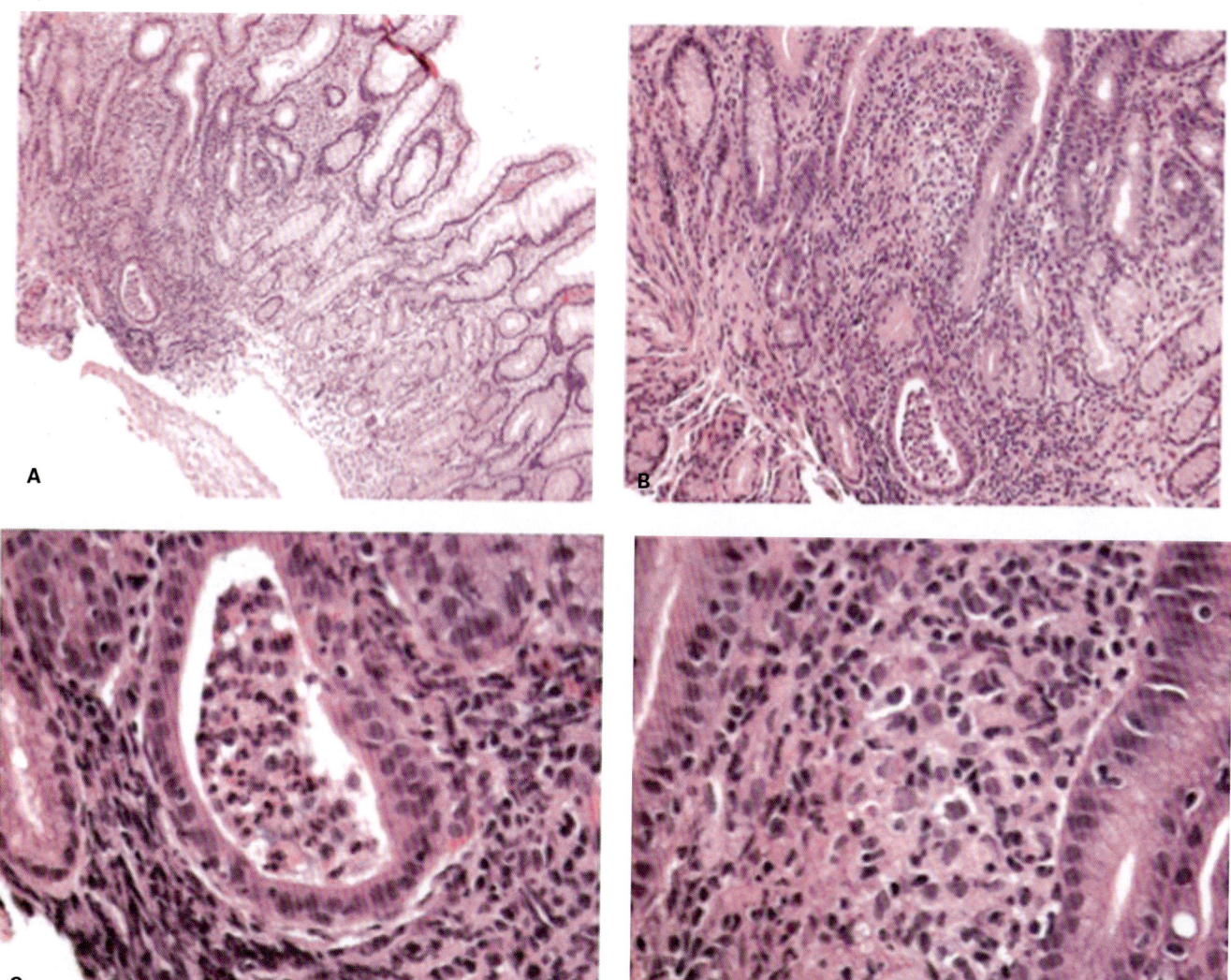

Figure 13-72. Gastric Crohn's disease. Biopsy with focal *Helicobacter* negative chronic active gastritis highly suggestive of CD. **A:** There is an obvious disparity between the inflammation in the left half of the biopsy compared to the right half that is essentially normal. **B:** Detail of the inflamed mucosa, which by itself would suggest *Helicobacter* infection. **C:** Pit abscess and surrounding chronic inflammation. **D:** Detail of center of (B) showing an aggregate of histiocytes, yet not a granuloma. Histiocytic foci can also be seen in CD.

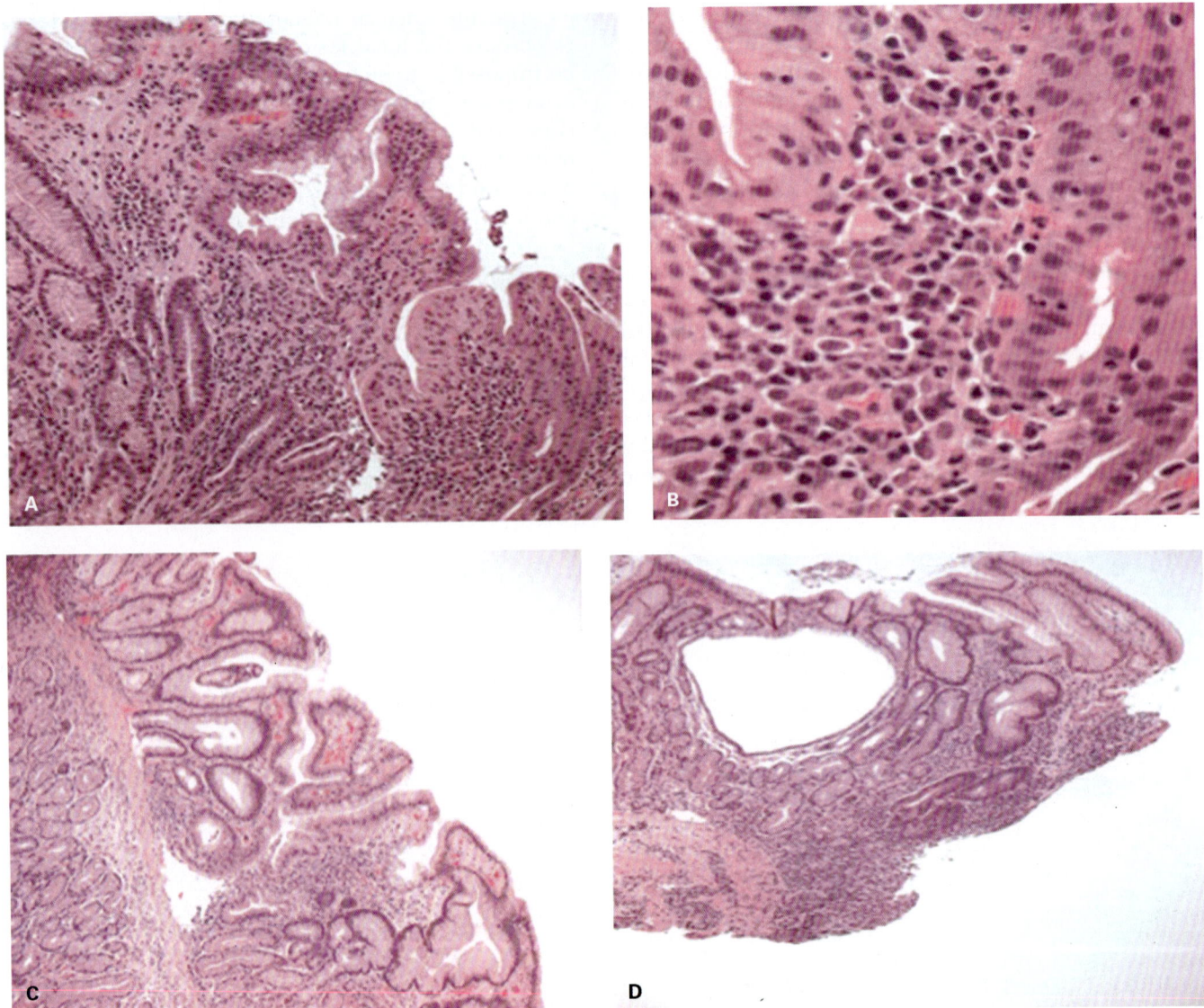

Figure 13-73. Crohn's disease. Three further biopsies that should suggest the possibility of CD. All biopsies (A/B, C, and D) have focal *Helicobacter* negative chronic active gastritis that tends to be the hallmark of gastric CD. **A:** Marked disparity in the inflammation from the chronic active disease (red detail in **B**) in the lower right corner compared to the left upper corner. In **(C)** and **(D)** comparison of the affected areas allow comparison between the inflamed and noninflamed parts of the same biopsy. This type of disparity should at least raise the question of whether this could be gastric CD. Note that none of these biopsies have granulomas.

1. Focal chronic active *Helicobacter*-negative gastritis or duodenitis, with or without eosinophils.

Neutrophils unrelated to *H. pylori* can be found in about 30% to 60% of patients with CD (likely depending on how many biopsies are taken) in both the stomach and the duodenum.[715] Nevertheless, in a large retrospective study, 34 cases of "focal enhanced gastritis" were found among 971 gastric biopsies from 927 patients. Only four were found to have IBD (two Crohn's, one UC, and one chronic colitis, type indeterminate) and the most common association (5/34) was in patients post bone marrow transplantation.[716] However, these changes are far from specific and in one study were found in 8/14 of patients with CD, 4/19 patients with UC, 2/6 patients with IBDU, 2/8 of patients with microscopic colitis, and 2/5 patients without IBD.[717]

2. Focal chronic gastritis/duodenitis.
3. Granulomas—however, these are found in no more than about 10% of patients, and in our experience the figure is much lower.
4. A diffuse but quite definite mild superficial chronic *Helicobacter*-negative gastritis is very common in both CD and UC; in one pediatric/adolescent study this was 92% in CD and 75% in UC,[718] which we suspect reflects an up-regulation of the mucosa-associated immune system. Nevertheless, we have also found that it is the rule in most adults.

There seems to be little difference in disease distribution (antrum vs. gastric body). The focality is not just between biopsies from different sites, but within a single biopsy and it often occurs in mucosa that is otherwise endoscopically uninflamed.[715] Increased macrophages have been reported in noninflamed mucosa.[719]

Ulcerative Colitis The notion that any inflammation in the UGT precludes the diagnosis of UC is no longer accepted as approximately two-thirds of CD patients and half of UC patients have microscopic abnormalities in the UGT, irrespective of the presence of symptoms, and especially in the pediatric population.[720–722] However, mucosal changes in UC are typically mild,[720,723] especially in the stomach, but may be much more severe in the duodenum and reflect the activity in the large bowel. Severe disease in the UGT is therefore most uncommon in quiescent UC and other possible causes of the inflammation need to be considered. Obvious ulcerations are more characteristic of CD.[722] Detecting granulomas at upper endoscopy (esophagus, antrum, and duodenum) appears to be the only pathologic abnormality that is useful in the discrimination between CD and UC—40% versus 0%, respectively.[720] Nonetheless, a consensus regarding the definition of what qualifies as significant "involvement" is still lacking. The North American IBD Genetics Consortium (arbitrarily) allows up to 10 minor lesions without indicating significant disease in a given location.[705] Overall, abnormal histology, including granulomatous inflammation, in otherwise normal-appearing mucosa should not be considered sufficient to be classified as gastroduodenal CD—just as such findings in the colon would not alone indicate colonic CD. For example, focal inflammation can also be seen in *H. pylori* gastritis following PPI therapy, recent eradication, or just single antibiotic therapy. Similarly, erosions or ulcers in a CD patient may be due to other causes.

Eosinophilic Gastritis

One of the major issues in discussion of any eosinophilic disorder involving the GI tract is that the criteria defining what constitutes an increase in eosinophils are not well-established. Eosinophilic gastritis is therefore considered when eosinophils dominate the biopsy. Despite this caveat, increased eosinophils or eosinophil-rich inflammatory infiltrate can be seen in the stomach in several distinct scenarios (Fig. 13-74). However, while this is often overt (Fig. 13-74A), it may be subtle when there is degranulation (Fig. 13-74B). In practice, increased eosinophils are most commonly associated with other specific inflammatory disorders. While they are often numerous in *H. pylori* infection, eosinophils do not dominate the inflammatory infiltrate and often pass unnoticed. Eosinophilic pit abscesses are rare, but sometimes they catch our attention.

When focal, and in association with a severe reactive gastropathy, by far the most common association appears to be medications such as NSAIDs/ASA, etc. (see Fig. 13-47), and then potential allergies. With medications, other changes of reactive gastropathy may be present, often with neutrophils, but usually little chronic inflammation. In some cases the reactive gastropathy may be absent or not represented in the biopsy, but the lamina propria may show a sprinkling of eosinophils that can be easily missed on a superficial examination, together with lamina propria fibrosis or hyalinization. Other medications that can cause an eosinophilia include sulfonamides, penicillin, cephalosporin, carbamazepine, azathioprine, L-tryptophan, gold salts), celiac disease, and lymphoma (see review[724]). Vasculitides (Churg–Strauss syndrome, polyarteritis nodosa) may also need to be considered (Fig. 13-74D–F). The other condition of note is CD, although other lesions are more common (see previous section) and are shown in Table 13-11.

Hypersensitivity to specific food or protein may be another scenario where eosinophils may be increased in the stomach. This happens more frequently in children where modest numbers of eosinophils can be seen as a reaction to cow's milk, or soy protein, or other allergens, but can also occasionally occur in adults.[725] Unlike eosinophilic gastroenteritis, eosinophils are scattered and are not grouped in clumps. Interestingly, although the cardia can be involved in eosinophilic esophagitis, the remainder of the stomach is usually (not always) spared, although eosinophils may reappear in the duodenum. However, occasionally eosinophilic esophagitis is accompanied by a marked excess of eosinophils, for example, in the distal antrum, with very few in the proximal duodenum. The reason for these associations is unclear.

Scant deep eosinophils (close to the muscularis mucosae) are seen with some degree of regularity especially in the antrum. When this happens, it is difficult to know whether to ignore them or include them in the report and state that the cause is not known, in case it is part of submucosal eosinophilic gastroenteritis. Rarely this is associated with collagen vascular disorders but the vast majority of the time it is unclear if this is even physiological or pathological. One should always correlate this with the peripheral eosinophil count. It can be part of a generalized eosinophilic gastroenteritis or isolated involvement of the stomach.

There are other associations, many of which are apparent once put in the clinical context, for example, parasites such as Anisakiasis that may be visible grossly (see previous discussion), involvement with neoplastic lesions such as systemic mastocytosis, although patients usually have skin and other manifestations of the disease. Practically it is often necessary to work through these causes of eosinophilic infiltration so that correlation with other clinical and endoscopic features is frequently required.

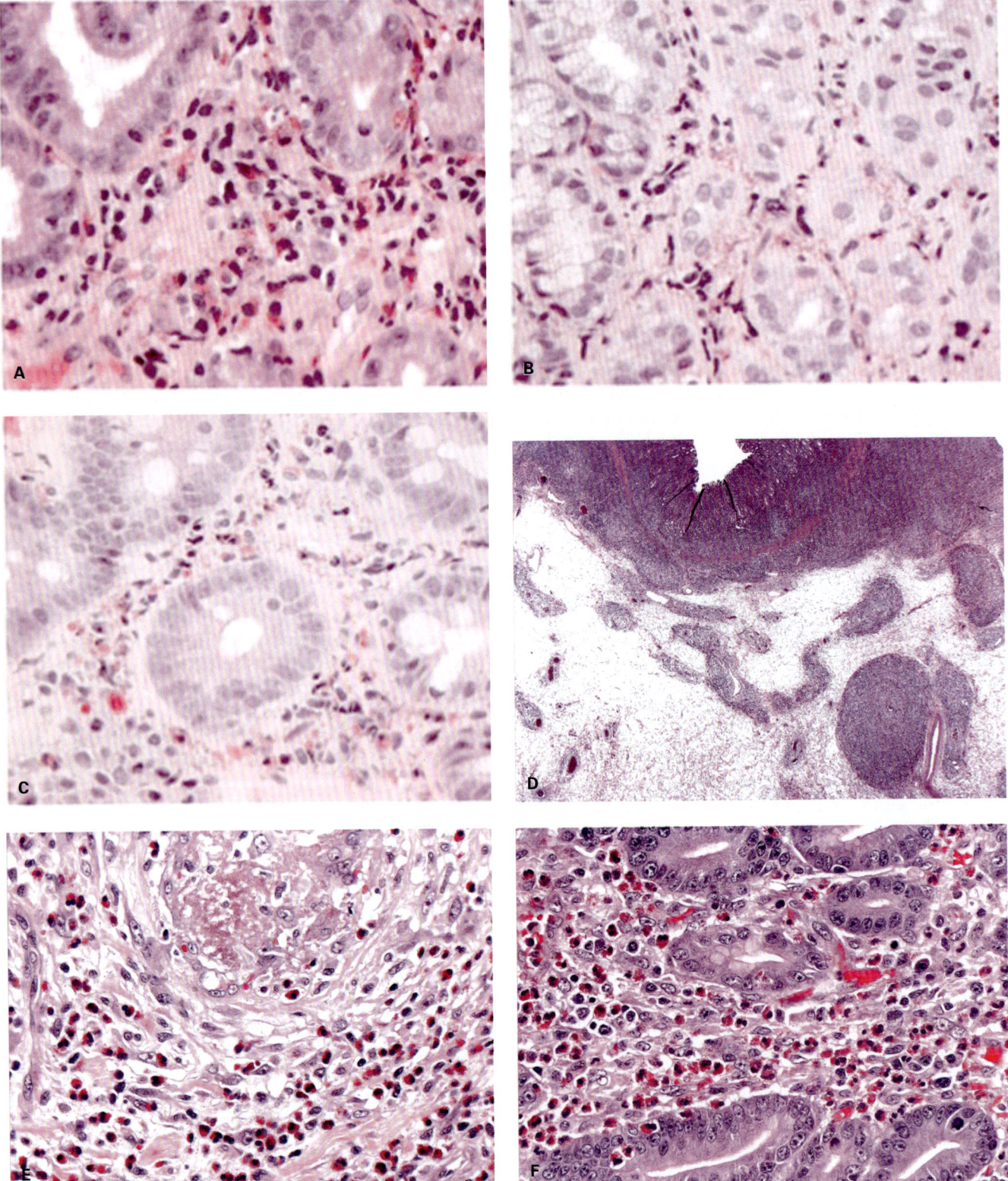

Figure 13-74. Eosinophilic gastritis. **A:** "Classical" eosinophilic gastritis. **B:** When the eosinophils degranulate, it is the faint red granularity in the lamina propria that suggests the diagnosis. **C:** Same patient as (B) showing that the eosinophilia in this patient carried over into the duodenum, typical of eosinophilic gastroenteritis. Churg Strauss syndrome. **D:** Overview of gastric wall showing an overt submucosal vasculitis—in this case primarily a phlebitis. **E:** Detail of submucosa vein with thrombosis and numerous surrounding eosinophils. **F:** Mucosa with chronic inflammation, marked reactive changes and sheets of eosinophils in the mucosa and submucosa (Courtesy of Dr Rana Bokhary, Jeddah Saudi Arabia).

Eosinophilic gastritis as part of gastric involvement in eosinophilic gastroenteritis. This is almost certainly an allergic condition that is characterized by eosinophilic infiltration of the GI tract (discussed in more detail in Chapter 18). The stomach, especially the antrum, is often involved.[726-729] All layers of the gastric wall may be involved, but there may be selective predominance of eosinophilic infiltrates in the mucosa, the muscle layers, or the subserosa, making biopsy diagnosis difficult in many cases. Histologic subclassification of eosinophilic gastroenteritis is determined according to the layer of the GI tract involved (mucosa, muscularis, or serosa). The clinical manifestation also varies depending on the layers affected. Patients presenting with vomiting, abdominal pain, diarrhea, bloody stools, failure to thrive, and iron deficiency anemia often have mucosal involvement, while patients with obstructive symptoms or dysphagia tend to have muscularis involvement. Patients with serosal involvement present with eosinophilic ascites.[728,730-733]

For a definitive diagnosis of eosinophilic gastroenteritis, four of the following criteria must be met[727]:

1. The presence of GI symptoms
2. Demonstration of eosinophilic infiltration (often >20 eosinophils per high-power field) in one or more areas of the GI tract
3. An absence of alternative causes of eosinophilia (drug reactions, parasitic infections, malignancies)
4. No involvement outside of the GI tract (i.e., no systemic eosinophilic pathology)
5. Patients are often atopic, there may be a family history, IgE levels are often elevated, and food-specific IgE antibodies may be present; these may become apparent on skin testing.[734-736] Mast cell degranulation may also occur.

This diagnosis is challenging as eosinophilic infiltration with eosinophils can be patchy.[737] When the diagnosis is suspected, careful examination of the stomach with targeting of lesions as well as uninvolved mucosa may reveal the characteristic sheets of eosinophils. Though spontaneous cure is common, some patients require steroid therapy (see Chapter 18). Some patients require surgery because of persistent gastric outlet obstruction.

Differential diagnosis. The real problem is that there are no specific numbers or distribution criteria of eosinophils on which the diagnosis should be based (Table 13-15). Most often the diagnosis is entertained when eosinophils are striking and predominate. Extensive infiltration of the gastric and often the small intestinal mucosa by eosinophils with/without peripheral eosinophilia can be seen in eosinophilic gastroenteritis, although often a peripheral eosinophilia is present. The pathogenesis remains unclear. As the presenting features overlap with more common GI diseases (such as IBD)[730,738] the differential includes all conditions with presenting features similar to those described above (i.e., IBD), as well as those that produce eosinophilia (Table 13-11). Table 13-16 summarizes a diagnostic workup for eosinophilic gastroenteritis.

Of note, in the past, the term *eosinophilic gastritis* or submucosal granuloma with eosinophilic infiltration was used to refer to inflammatory fibroid polyps (Vanek tumor).[740] These isolated polypoid

Table 13-15 Differential Diagnosis of Eosinophilic Gastroenteritis

Primary eosinophilic gastroenteritis (mucosal, muscular, and serosal forms)
  Atopic
  Nonatopic
  Familial
Secondary
  Eosinophilic disorders
  Hypereosinophilic syndrome
Diseases associated with increased eosinophils
  Celiac disease
  Connective tissue disease (scleroderma)
  Iatrogenic
  Infection
  Inflammatory bowel disease
  Vasculitis (Churg–Strauss syndrome)

Table 13-16 Diagnostic Workup for Eosinophilic Gastroenteritis

General
  Complete blood count and differential
  Serum albumin
  Total IgE
  Erythrocyte sedimentation rate
  Skin prick tests and IgE RASTs
  Skin patch testing
Infection workup (stool and colonic aspirate analysis)
Upper and lower GI endoscopy with biopsies from multiple sites
Evaluation and biopsy of any other potentially involved tissue
In the presence of hypereosinophilia (>1,500/mL)
  Peripheral blood smear
  Bone marrow analysis
  Serum tryptase
  Vitamin B_{12}
  Cardiac troponin, EKG, and echocardiogram
  Serum antineutrophil cytoplasmic antibody
  CT chest/abdomen

lesions are similar to those that occur in the ileum (see Chapter 25) and are discussed in more detail in Chapter 7.[740,741] The rare disorder allergic granulomatosis appears to be distinct from eosinophilic gastroenteritis.[742]

Collagenous Gastritis

Collagenous gastritis is a rare GI disorder characterized by an irregular thickened collagenous subepithelial band, entrapped dilated capillaries, a predominantly mononuclear infiltrate with few neutrophils, and eosinophils that may or may not be associated with intraepithelial inflammatory cells (Fig. 13-75). The subepithelial collagen band is >10 μm, but is usually massive and obvious. However, when subtle it is also easy to misinterpret it simply as hyalinization of the lamina propria, possibly the site of a previous erosion.

Although rare, collagenous gastritis has two phenotypes: pediatric-onset and adult-onset, both of which may be associated with collagenous colitis, but even less frequently as part of a gastroenterocolitis. A genetic predisposition to adult phenotype collagenous gastritis has not been established, but familial examples of collagenous colitis have been observed.[743] No etiology has been identified in the pediatric form. In adult-onset disease, autoimmune, infectious, and medication-induced causes have been considered as possible triggers.[743] In general, disease associations seem to support an immune-mediated basis. Occasionally, the differential diagnosis may include amyloidosis with subepithelial deposits (Fig. 13-76).

In children, collagenous gastritis is often not associated with collagenous colitis. It is characterized by severe anemia and abdominal pain with a nodular stomach. The anemia found in pediatric-onset collagenous gastritis is believed to be due to hemorrhage from dilated capillaries entrapped in the abnormal collagenous matrix.[744]

Adult-onset collagenous gastritis is associated with collagenous colitis and presents with voluminous watery diarrhea. Nonetheless, this subdivision may be arbitrary as the adult-onset phenotype has been described in the pediatric population[745] with a case report of collagenous gastritis progressing to collagenous gastroenterocolitis in a 12-year follow-up.[746]

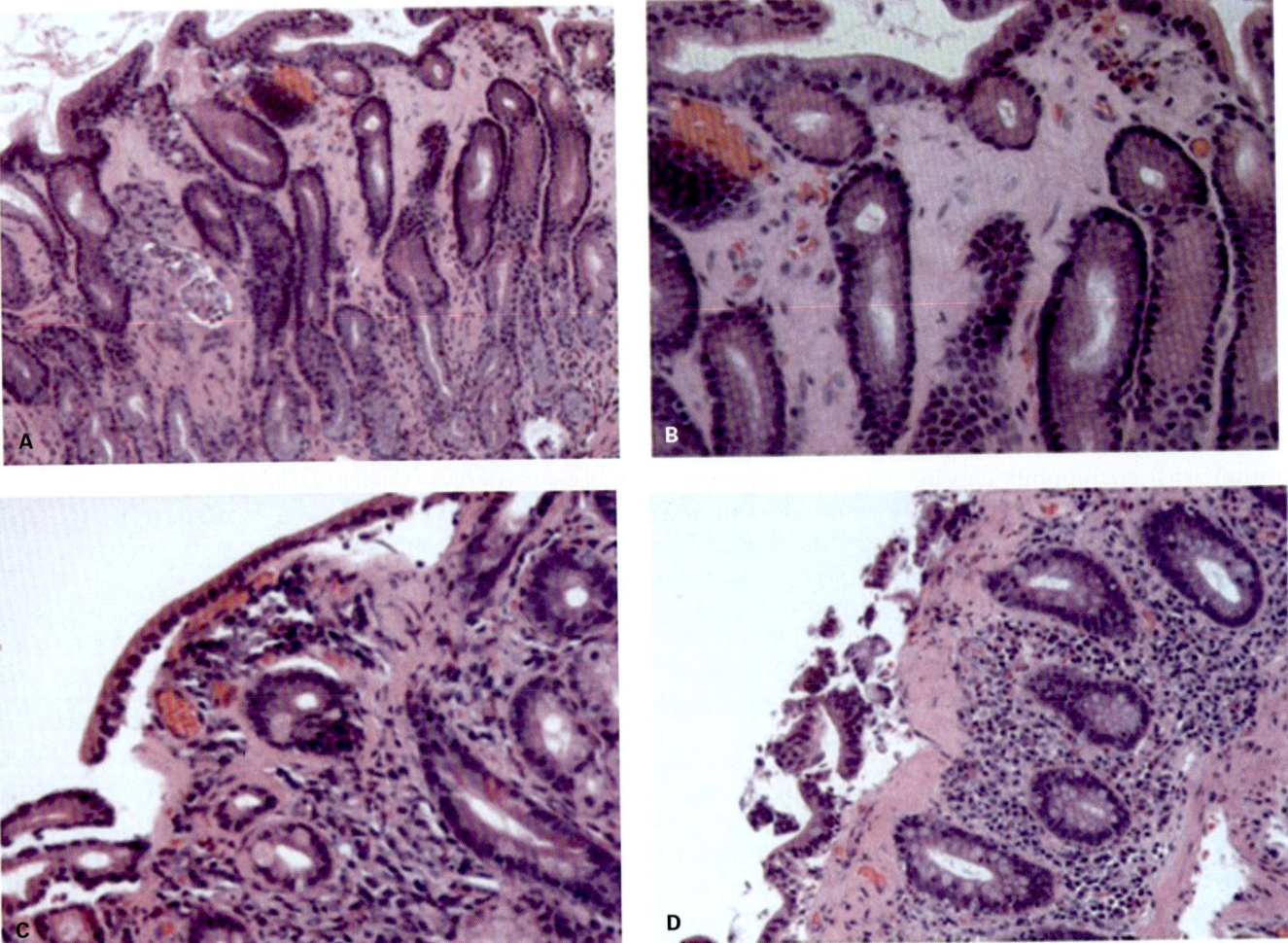

Figure 13-75. Collagenous gastritis **(A,B)**, enteritis **(C)**, and colitis **(D)** in the same patient. This can be a life-threatening combination.

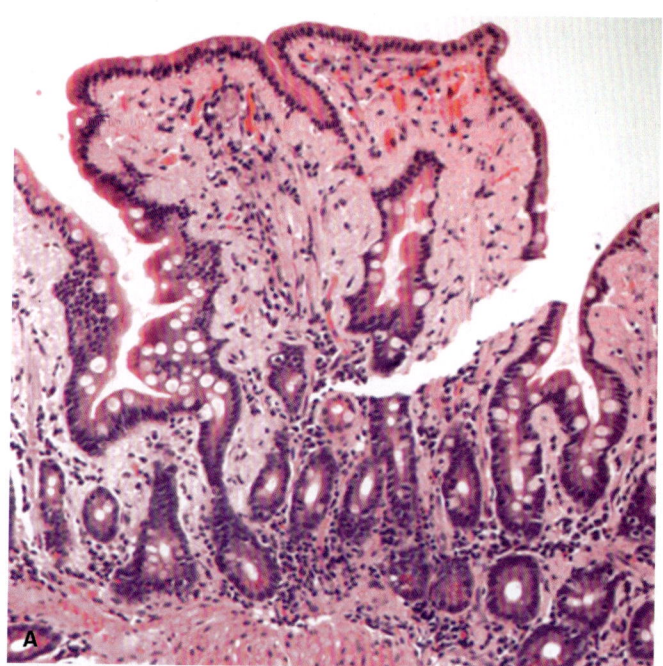

Figure 13-76. **A:** Subepithelial/lamina propria amyloid deposition—here in the duodenum, but similar deposits can be seen in any part of the GI tract. **B:** Apple-green birefringence of amyloid deposits using polarized light on Congo red stain.

The natural history of the collagenous gastritis with or without colitis is not clear. In adults, a chronic intermittent course characterizes the majority of patients[747] with no significant mortality risk or periods of severe deterioration. Furthermore, diarrhea may resolve with or without treatment, although relapses can occur.

Diffuse collagenous gastroenterocolitis. A more refractory disease seems to characterize patients presenting either as young children and early adults,[745,747] and also when part of a diffuse collagenous gastroenterocolitis, which can be life-threatening requiring hospitalization and enteral and or intravenous support that may go on for months (see Fig. 13-75). It responds poorly to most medications, including steroids and other anti-inflammatory agents, which are, nevertheless, inevitably given as a potential life-saving intervention. Following therapy the collagen band may resolve and an appearance resembling lymphocytic gastritis/enteritis (sprue) or colitis may persist for a considerable period of time. Other than severe small bowel disease, there seems nothing to distinguish this from the more typical pediatric or adult forms. Interestingly, the few examples we have seen seem to follow a well-documented infectious enteritis or colitis, which in one of our patients was *C. difficile*. The infection itself appeared to have largely resolved when the symptoms recurred necessitating hospitalization. The timing inevitably makes one think about an immune reaction to the bacterium or toxin cross reacting with antigens in the GI tract, but why the sub-epithelial unless it is all long term effects of toxin throughout the GI tract in susceptible individuals. We have also noted collagenous colitis following overt infections, possibly a similar mechanism.

Gastric Malakoplakia

Gastric involvement, particularly isolated gastric involvement in malakoplakia, is extremely rare.[748] Several reports have emphasized the presence of concomitant diseases associated with GI malakoplakia such as leukemia/lymphoma, alpha chain disease, immunodeficiency, miliary tuberculosis, multiple hemangiomas, neurofibromatosis. While in the large bowel it is associated with villous adenomas and perforating cancers, this seems not to occur in the stomach unless from direct extension.[749] To date only five cases of gastric malakoplakia have been reported in the world literature, of which only three cases had isolated involvement of the stomach (Fig. 13-77). Of these, one had a concomitant colonic adenocarcinoma with an associated inflammatory infiltrate, similar but not identical to the gastric malakoplakia.

Drug- and Chemotherapy-induced Gastritis

Gastric mucosal damage related to various drugs is common. The pattern of injury may lead to a suspicion of medications while some result in a characteristic histologic pattern.[750] In the general population,

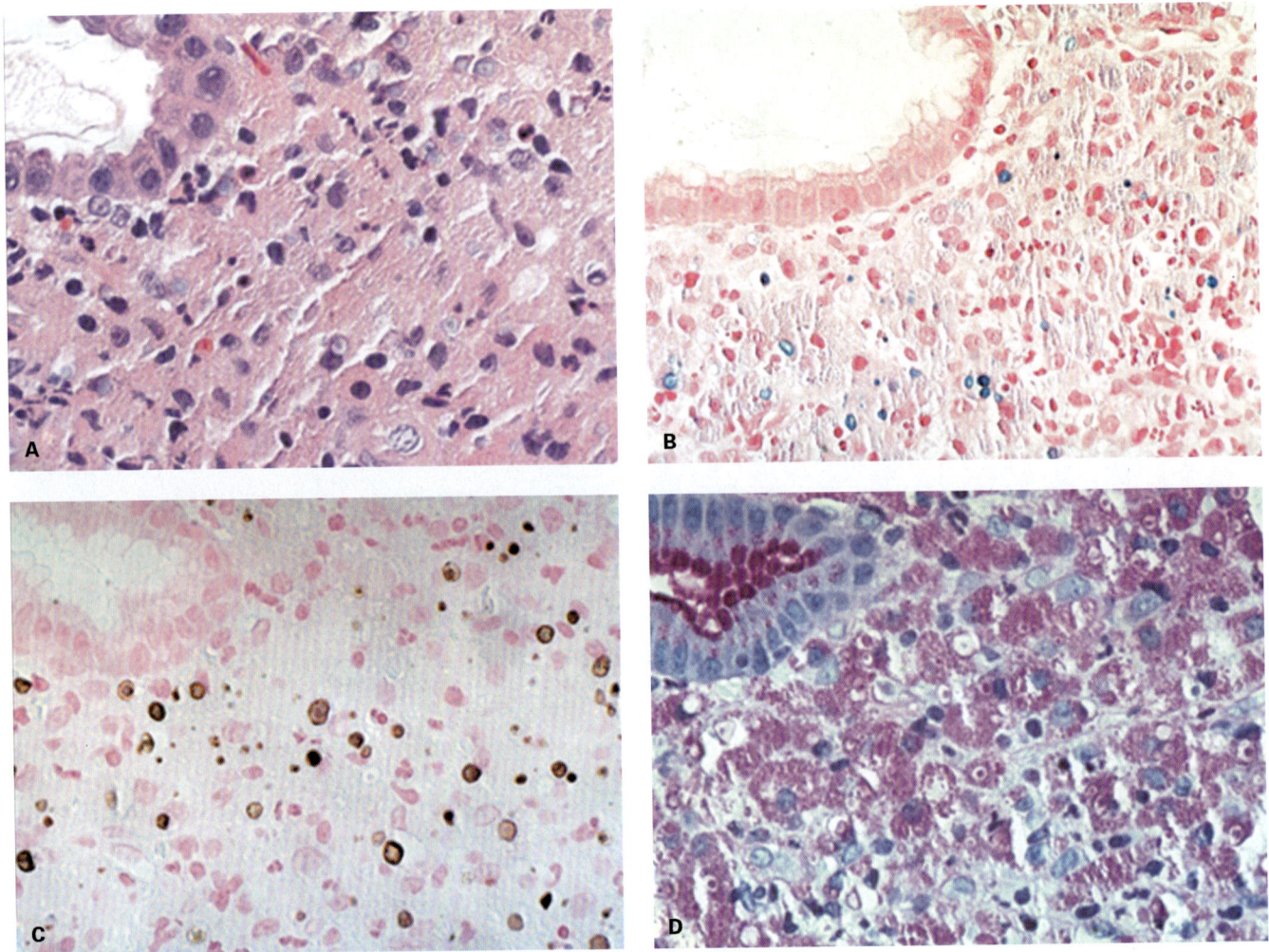

Figure 13-77. A: Gastric malacoplakia in which the concentric blue-ringed Michaelis Gutmann bodies can be identified in large histiocytes admixed with neutrophils—the characteristic combination. **B–D:** Iron, von Kossa (calcium) and D-PAS stains showing that the inclusions contain iron, calcium and that the macrophages are D-PAS-positive.

many drug-related mucosal lesions remain undiagnosed or unspecified.

1. **NSAIDs/ASA:** These are used abundantly and can elicit gastric mucosal changes in 30%/antiplatelet medications to 40% of patients[751,752] causing erosions and ulcers, especially unassociated with *Helicobacter*. Erosions with adjacent severe reactive changes, without adjacent chronic inflammation but with neutrophils or eosinophils or both with lamina propria fibrosis and hyalinization, should all lead to consideration of this class of medication (see Fig. 13-47). It is discussed in more detail previously. Various histologic changes include acute/chronic gastritis, ulcer or reactive gastropathy (see previous sections reactive regarding reactive gastropathy and eosinophilic gastritis, and *Helicobacter* and its distinction from NSAIDs). Other medications, especially **bisphosphonates** used for osteopenia, can cause similar problems from esophagus to duodenum.

2. **Chemotherapy/radiation-associated gastritis:** A wide variety of *chemotherapeutic agents* can cause gastritis and gastropathy. Gastric mucosal damage has been associated with numerous drugs including mitomycin C, 5-fluoro-2-deoxyuridine, and floxuridine.[35,753] Mucosal ulceration and bizarre epithelial atypia can be seen in association with prominent eosinophilia, vacuolization, and pleomorphic nuclei. However, "the" characteristic lesion is that in which normal pits and adjacent pits in various stages of restitution and repair are present side by side (see Fig. 13-10). Although much of the injury must be apoptosis related, when biopsies are taken this is rarely observed. Atypical reactive changes can be seen in endothelial cells and fibroblasts.

Newer therapies like **Ipilimumab** (antibodies against cytotoxic T lymphocyte antigen-4) have been reported to initiate severe panenteritis, including gastritis (see subsequent section and also Chapter 18).[754]

Gastric mucosal injury can also be seen following radiation therapy[755,756] (see Chapter 2). The changes can be noted as early as 8 to 10 days after irradiation, including nuclear karyorrhexis and cytoplasmic eosinophilia of the gastric foveolar epithelium. Inflammation is usually not prominent. Glandular necrosis with characteristic radiation-induced nuclear atypia usually follows. In severe cases, mucosal ulceration and hemorrhage, with possible late radiation effects such as endothelial proliferation and fibrinoid necrosis of the vessel walls, can be seen. Mucosal recovery is usually complete within 2 to 3 months.

Gastritis or ischemic-type gastric ulceration can be seen when the beads used for *selective intra-artery radiation therapy (SIRT)* with *selective intra-artery radiation therapy (SIRT)* inadvertently enter the arteries supplying the stomach.[757] SIRT is performed with biocompatible resin-based *yttrium-90* (^{90}Y)-labeled microspheres administered via hepatic artery branches (Fig. 13-78A,B and see Chapter 2). In the gastric mucosa, the changes range from nuclear atypia, apoptosis, epithelial flattening, and glandular cystic dilatation to capillary ectasia and prominent endothelial cells. Ulceration and ischemic gastritis often occurs. Most often the characteristic purple-colored spherical beads are easily identified in the sections. Notably, these adverse effects have been reported with an incidence of up to 10% to 29% of patients, generally within the first 2 months after the procedure.

3. **Iron pill gastritis:** Mucosal injury can be observed in patients taking iron-containing pills.[758,759] Often the indication for iron pills is iron deficiency anemia; however, iron pills can themselves result in ulceration resulting in chronic blood loss. In some cases they possibly may exacerbate a preexisting ulcer resulting in iron deficiency. The mucosal damage is believed to be mediated by oxygen metabolites secondary to ferrous and ferric ion metabolism. The mucosa frequently shows reactive gastropathy-like changes. The key to the diagnosis is recognition of a crystalline form of iron deposited in the superficial part of mucosa or luminal surface (see Fig. 13-5). The crystalline iron has a characteristic appearance that varies from golden to dirty green to some shade of purple on H&E stains. The Prussian blue stain is helpful in establishing their ferrous nature. Although it is not hemosiderin, some hemosiderin deposition in the adjacent epithelium or macrophages can be seen. The iron crystals can be embedded in granulation tissue, encrust the damaged epithelium, or get entrapped in stromal cells, or even in vessel walls in the superficial lamina propria. The changes should be differentiated from gastric glandular siderosis, in which hemosiderin accumulation is seen predominantly in the glandular epithelial cells, and is associated with systemic iron overload or hemochromatosis. Treatment consists of either withdrawing the causative iron pills or possibly replacing them with less toxic formulations. Interestingly, the mucosal injury is only seen with the pill form of the medication and not the suspension form, which could be the replacement in most situations.

4. **Colchicine:** These changes are seen in patients with altered renal or hepatic function in whom colchicine reaches toxic levels. The epithelium shows nuclear pseudostratification, increased apoptoses, and loss of polarity that can mimic dysplasia.[760] Mitotic figures arrested in metaphase, with the chromosomes often arranged as "ring" mitoses, can be seen, which is characteristic of Colchicine toxicity (Fig. 13-78). Taxol can produce identical changes, as it also inhibits microtubule formation (Fig. 13-78 C,D). Interestingly the effects in this example predominate in the intestinal metaplasia whether complete or incomplete rather than in the native foveolar mucosa.

5. **Gastric mucosal calcinosis:** This is usually seen in orthotopic transplant and chronic renal failure patients receiving either aluminum-containing antacids or sucralfate. It may also be seen with parathyroid disorders resulting in abnormalities of calcium metabolism (see later, also see Chapter 8).

6. **Kayexalate:** This drug is used in the management of hyperkalemia in renal failure patients. The main changes are seen in the large bowel, but it has also been associated with superficial gastric and duodenal ulceration with crystals admixed with fibrinous exudate as seen in the large bowel (see also Chapter 2). However, in other patients, less specific damage can be seen.[761]

HYPERTROPHIC GASTROPATHIES AND MÉNÉTRIER'S DISEASE

Hypertrophic gastropathy refers simply to thickened gastric folds, irrespective of associated symptoms or underlying pathology. There are numerous causes of giant gastric folds, which can be focal or diffuse and range from primary epithelial hyperplasia of the mucosa ("classical" Ménétrier's disease), ZES, or secondary disorders such as tumor infiltration (e.g., lymphoma), infections (CMV, histoplasmosis, syphilis), and granulomatous diseases.[517] The underlying cause for giant gastric folds often cannot be determined from gross (endoscopic) appearance.

It should be noted that much confusion surrounding these disorders is partly due to the plethora of

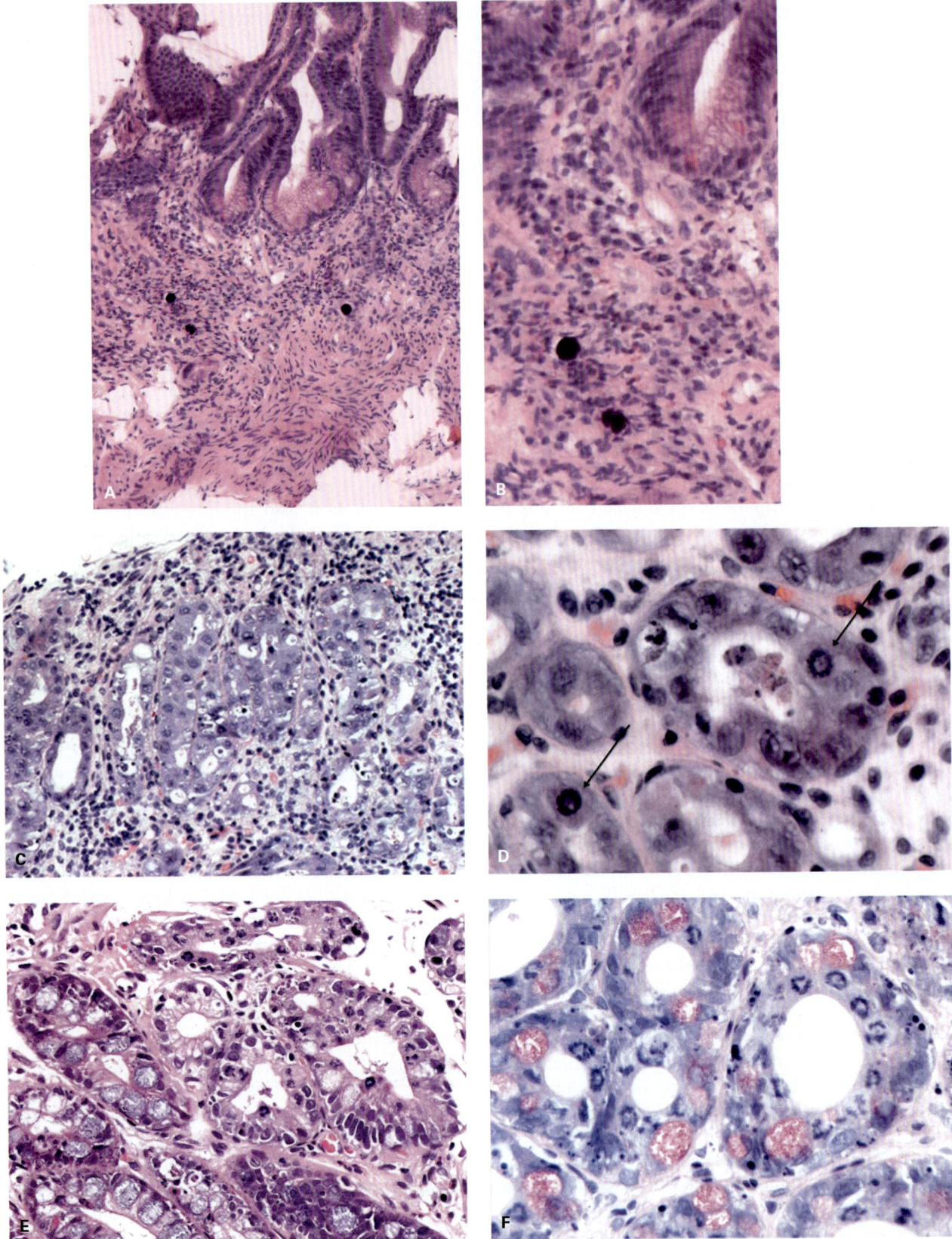

Figure 13-78. Yttrium-90 and microtubule inhibitors. **A:** Gastric mucosa with damage from Yttrium-90, the small beads of which are seen impacted in the small vessels in the lamina propria (Courtesy of Dr Liesbeth Ferdinande, Ghent, Belgium). **C:** Colchicine toxicity: low magnification shows marked reactive changes in the gastric glands in background of moderate chronic gastritis. The nuclei of the glandular epithelium look atypical and can be easily confused for dysplasia. The increase in apoptosis in the glandular epithelium is obvious even at this magnification. **D:** Detail shows nuclear atypia and few apoptotic bodies. In addition, two cells arrested in metaphase showing "ring" mitoses (*arrows*), which is a hallmark of colchicine toxicity, are seen. **E:** Numerous ring mitoses in the proliferative compartment of this gastric mucosa with intestinal metaplasia of a patient with prostate carcinoma on taxol therapy. **F:** Detail of **E** on DPAS stain (Courtesy Dr Cord Langner, Graz, Austria).

names given to them, which include *giant hypertrophic gastritis, giant fold gastritis, giant rugal hypertrophy, chronic hypertrophic proliferative gastritis, and chronic hypertrophic glandular gastritis*.[7,762-764] Table 13-17 summarizes how we believe hypertrophic gastropathies should be defined in pathology reports and in the literature.

Ménétrier's Disease: It is a rare condition named after a French physician Pierre Eugene Ménétrier (1859–1935), who described the condition in 1888. However, this name has been applied to so many entities that it is difficult to know what "true" Ménétrier's disease really is. It is associated with a protein-losing state. This has included anything with large gastric folds in a diffuse distribution, affecting the corpus (oxyntic) mucosa, infrequently the antral mucosa, and rarely both. When both antral and oxyntic mucosa may be involved, it is important to ensure that it does not continue into the rest of the bowel as seen in Cronkhite–Canada syndrome.

In his original 1888 paper Ménétrier described two different conditions:

(a) "Polyadenomes polypeux"—many adenomatous polyps—bearing in mind that all polyps of gland-forming mucosa were called adenomas in 1888. His description was that of antral and oxyntic polyps with grossly normal intervening gastric mucosa. This fits what would now be called hyperplastic (or very likely juvenile) polyposis that is sometimes restricted to the stomach (see Chapter 20). Interestingly, in these polyps Ménétrier did describe an inflammatory infiltrate of "migratory cells" ("infiltre de cellules migratrices"), the current interpretation being that these were likely neutrophils, almost certainly associated with *Helicobacter*, which Ménétrier likely did not know existed. The distinction of multiple polyps with nonpolypoid apparently normal-appearing intervening mucosa is actually a critical distinction, as multiple hyperplastic polyps can have erosions and ooze sufficiently to cause a protein-losing state, or anemia, or both. The presence of relatively normal mucosa between polyps is therefore the first part of the diagnostic algorithm in this variation of his disease.

(b) "Polyadenomes en nappes:" "En nappe" is best translated as "flowing" and therefore describes a diffuse disease. Again, Ménétrier noted "des phenomenes de gastritis chronique," so many of these were likely *Helicobacter* related (unknown by Ménétrier). Whether any corresponded to what we would now call "lymphocytic gastritis," which in some patients is also associated with *Helicobacter*, is unclear as this entity also either did not exist or was buried with chronic gastritis in 1888.

The other feature associated with Ménétrier's disease initially described was increased gastric protein loss. However, this is occasionally found in many other disorders that are associated with large gastric folds, and is not seen universally in any of the disorders that have been reported as satisfying criteria for Ménétrier's disease. Ideally, there should be loss of the secretory cells of the oxyntic mucosa and cystic dilatation of the pits (Fig. 13-79). The diagnosis of "Ménétrier's disease" therefore depends on different authors' interpretation of its diagnostic criteria.

Ménétrier's disease therefore appears not to be a distinct entity, but an admixture of a variety of conditions, and as such we tend to regard it as a descriptive diagnosis (analogous to pseudomembranes or eosinophilic infiltration that have numerous causes) but we are left with the historical fallout, as well as successive authors' attempts to "clarify" the issue (including that stated here!). Patients need to be worked up for disease mimics such as hyperplastic polyposis, isolated gastric juvenile polyposis, past/current *Helicobacter* infections (which can cause a Ménétrier-like picture and likely formed the bulk of Ménétrier's "polyadenomes en nappe"—including lymphocytic gastritis in which organisms may be rare or invisible. Diffusely infiltrating diseases) also need to be excluded. At this point, "Ménétrier's disease" becomes vanishingly rare (Fig. 13-79).

It may be better to call these as hypertrophic gastropathies (or hypertrophic hypersecretory gastropathies), and stratify them further as localized or diffuse, with and without a protein-losing state and with known underlying etiology or idiopathic

Table 13-17 Hypertrophic Gastropathies

1. **Ménétrier-"primary"**: Mucous cell hyperplasia—epithelial hyperplasia of surface and foveolar mucous cells; oxyntic glands can be normal or atrophic.
2. **Protein-losing hypertrophic conditions** "secondary Ménétrier"
   a. CMV-associated hypertrophic gastritis
   b. Hypertrophic lymphocytic gastritis
   c. *Helicobacter pylori*-associated hypertrophic gastritis
   d. HIV-associated hypertrophic gastropathy
3. **Zollinger–Ellison**: PC hypertrophy; expanded glandular compartment due to an excess of PCs
4. **Foveolar hyperplasia without gland loss** "reactive"—possibly forme fruste
5. **Some polyposis syndrome**, Cronkhite–Canada syndrome,[782] or juvenile or hyperplastic polyposis may present with a giant fold appearance.[802]
6. **Inflammatory**: syphilis, histoplasmosis, and granulomatous diseases involving the mucosa and submucosa

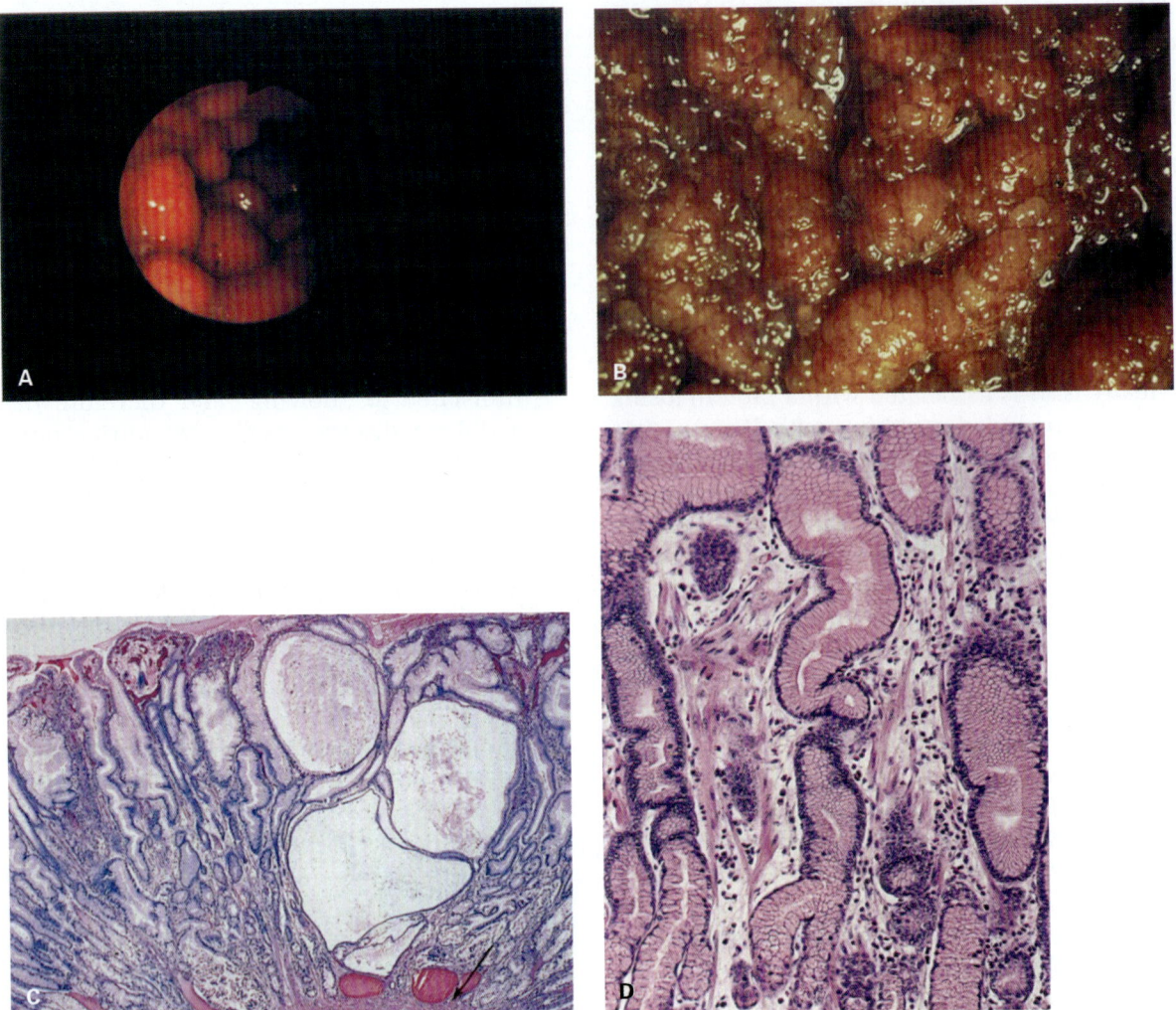

Figure 13-79. Ménétrier's disease. **A:** Endoscopic photograph showing the markedly thickened folds, which did not flatten with air insufflation. **B:** Surgical resection specimen showing the polypoid, almost bubbly excrescences. **C:** Electrocautery snare biopsy specimen from the midbody region on the greater curvature. All the fundic mucosa has been replaced down to the muscularis mucosae (*arrow*) by foveolar hyperplasia and mucous gland metaplasia. Dilated mucosal cysts are seen on the right. **D:** Higher-power view showing that foveolae and mucus glands have replaced fundic glands.

(Fig. 13-62A–C). Whatever remains in the "idiopathic" group of hypertrophic gastropathies may be what one may label as "idiopathic" Ménétrier's disease (see Fig. 13-79). With this philosophy we have classified hypertrophic gastropathy as shown in Table 13-17, which is our starting point.

We therefore attempt to make sense of this by regarding Ménétrier's disease as

1. idiopathic/primary when there is no associated inflammation, and all other features of the disease are present
2. hypertrophic gastritis with and without protein-losing states, which conceptually could also be thought of as secondary Ménétrier's disease, when there is clearly an association that can be treated. It is relatively easy to call these hypertrophic gastritis,

or secondary Ménétrier's disease, and add the cause, for example, *Helicobacter*-associated hypertrophic gastritis.

Primary/Idiopathic Ménétrier's Disease

By definition, this is idiopathic, so the etiology is unknown. However, there is a suggestion that it is related to release of transforming growth factor alpha (TGF-α) by the gastric mucosa.[765,766] TGF-α is the ligand for the EGFR tyrosine kinase, and acts an epithelial cell mitogen that inhibits gastric acid secretion, increases gastric mucin content, and appears to be increased in patients with Ménétrier's disease.[765,766] Interestingly, the mucosal hypertrophy even in the secondary forms of Ménétrier's disease is also mediated by TGF-α. This is discussed subsequently.

Ménétrier's disease is characterized by the following features:

1. Giant folds, especially in the fundus and body of the stomach, although rarely the antrum appears involved, and may be the only site (Fig. 13-79)
2. Diminished acid secretory capacity
3. A protein-losing state with hypoalbuminemia (and sometimes anemia)

Clinical Presentation

Given that Ménétrier's disease as reported in the literature has been a collection of different diseases, it is something of a moot point to suggest that there is a typical age or sex of presentation, yet such seems to be the case. Typically, the disease presents in men between ages 30 and 60, and, on rare occasions, shows a familial predisposition.[767] Ménétrier's disease causes a decrease in gastric acidity resulting from a reduction in acid-producing parietal cells. Symptoms include nausea, vomiting, postprandial abdominal pain, diarrhea, swelling, poor appetite, peripheral edema, anemia (secondary to blood loss), and weight loss.[768] It tends to be a progressive disorder with virtually no reports of spontaneous regression in patients with symptoms longer than 6 months' duration.[769,770-776]

Endoscopic features and gross pathology: The enlarged gastric folds are often centered along the greater curvature of the stomach in the fundus and body, with frequent sparing of the antrum. These folds are large and bulky and have been likened to cerebral convolutions (Fig. 13-79). They have a polypoid or nodular configuration and may have associated superficial ulcerations. The altered gastric mucosa secretes massive amounts of protein-containing mucus, which together with protein loss through superficial erosions and ulcerations explains the hypoalbuminemia and sometimes anemia.[777,778]

Pathology of Primary Ménétrier's Disease

The histologic hallmark is a marked elongation and tortuosity of the foveolar (pits), often associated with prominent cystic dilations (Fig. 13-79). These cysts may penetrate the muscularis mucosae and extend into the submucosa. The surface mucosa may be acutely inflamed and may contain erosions or ulcers, so that all the usual causes of this need to be excluded. The lamina propria is often markedly edematous, sometimes with a loose fibroblastic proliferation, and contains increased numbers of eosinophils and mononuclear cells, especially in the pit regions. However, anything resembling the chronic inflammation of Helicobacter type, or the presence of Helicobacter organisms themselves, or the presence of an intraepithelial lymphocytosis, suggests that a secondary form is likely. As expected, in the face of the marked foveolar hyperplasia, there is an accompanying extensive reduction in the number of parietal and chief cells, with replacement by mucous glands (pseudopyloric metaplasia). The reduction in parietal cells causes a decrease in gastric acidity.[768] In some cases, there may be residual pockets of relatively intact fundic glands.[779,780] When the process involves the antrum, antral gland atrophy may also be present. Submucosal lymphangiectasia may also be present and may contribute to the protein-losing gastropathy.[781] Intestinal metaplasia is not characteristic, although patches of it may be found, as it is found in many adult stomachs. Given the atrophy that is present, one would expect there to be a degree of hypergastrinemia, and therefore potentially ECL hyperplasia, but this potential facet of the disease tends to be overlooked.

In general, in patients with hypertrophic gastropathies, one needs to document the anatomic distribution and the epithelial component involved (superficial, mid, deep or combinations), and there needs to be some documentation if inflammation contributed to an overall increase in mucosal thickness, and whether it is lamina propria of intraepithelial or both.

Differential Diagnosis of Ménétrier's Disease and Clinical Implications: The biggest initial distinction is that Ménétrier's should be a diffuse disease that is usually limited to the oxyntic mucosa. The first issue then is whether this is really the case or whether there really are numerous polyps of the oxyntic mucosa (inflammatory, juvenile polyposis) in which the intervening mucosa is normal. The possibility of juvenile polyposis can be excluded by looking for evidence of family history, large intestinal involvement, and genetic mutational analysis (see Chapter 20). The distinction from the isolated gastric form associated with SMAD4 mutations is virtually impossible without the mutational analysis or presence of other known associated disorders like hereditary hemorrhagic telangiectasia. It is unclear whether mutation-negative cases represent true Ménétrier's disease or variants of gastric juvenile polyposis.

The antrum should be uninvolved, but if it is, the issue is whether this is really part of more diffuse GI disease such as Cronkhite–Canada syndrome that can present initially with similar symptoms. The histology of Ménétrier's may be identical to that seen in gastric lesions of Cronkhite–Canada syndrome but the differentiation on clinical grounds, ectodermal changes, and involvement of the small and large bowel should help, even though these are likely a manifestation of the low protein/albumen.[782] In the young especially, the question of CMV infection should immediately come to mind.

Endoscopic biopsies, even with large forceps or snares may not sample the full thickness of the mucosa, and thus may suggest the diagnosis but may not prove it. In these biopsy specimens, foveolar hyperplasia and marked edema may be evident but the sampling is usually not deep enough to document gland atrophy and accompanying cystic changes. In our experience when gastric body folds are diffusely thickened some patients who have a histologic abnormality have impressive foveolar hyperplasia but without total replacement of oxyntic glands. The main issue in differential diagnosis is

1. To exclude an infiltrating neoplasm, such as a diffuse carcinoma or lymphoma. If the lesion is clinically suspicious of malignancy, an electrocautery snare biopsy can be done. Fortunately, malignancy is uncommonly detected in large series of electrocautery snare biopsies for thick folds.[780]
2. To detect and treat other etiologies including lymphocytic gastritis and *Helicobacter* disease, rare infections such as CMV, syphilis or if erosions are present to exclude medications that can cause these.
3. The other types of epithelial hyperplasia of the stomach that produce giant gastric folds are rare but must be considered in the differential diagnosis of Ménétrier's disease, but must include ZES. These are discussed subsequently.

Pathogenesis While the pathogenesis of Ménétrier's is not completely understood, gastric mucosa hypertrophy appears to be due to EGFR activation linked with overexpression of TGF-α.[766,783] Under normal conditions, TGF-α maintains gastric homeostasis by inhibiting acid secretion and increasing gastric mucous production.[784] Indeed, a transgenic mouse model that secretes excess TGF-α developed gastric lesions that are very similar to the human disease.[765,766] TGF-α is the ligand for the EGFR tyrosine kinase, and acts as an epithelial cell mitogen that inhibits gastric acid secretion and increases gastric mucin content. In Ménétrier, overexpression of TGF-α increases gastric epithelial cell proliferation, stimulates gastric mucin production, and suppresses gastric acidity.[765,783–785] This is supported by reports of clinical improvement following treatment with a monoclonal antibody directed against the EGFR.[766,769,786] Theoretically, immunostaining for TGF-α could be diagnostic on biopsies but controlled studies with other disorders with large folds are required. Various forms of gastric inflammatory and reparative responses can also show increased foveolar TGF-α, suggesting that this finding may not be specific.[787] Also, immunostaining often gives equivocal results that are "consistent with" Ménétrier's disease, but it is often unclear if that actually adds anything to the differential diagnosis.

Treatment: There is currently no effective treatment for idiopathic/primary form of Ménétrier's disease. Patients with few symptoms and minimal hypoalbuminemia may require no specific therapy. Treatment may include medications to relieve nausea and pain. Invariably high-dose PPIs, *Helicobacter* eradication therapy, or other immunosuppressive agents are considered, but data for their use are inevitably lacking. Ultimately some patients require gastrectomy for persistent abdominal symptoms, hypoalbuminemia, and concern about gastric cancer.[776] However, cure is not guaranteed, there being one report of disease recurrence in the retained stomach following partial gastrectomy.[788] Different remedies are used for treating Ménétrier's disease depending upon disease stage. Other than steroids, this form of gastropathy can be difficult to treat and the number of different types of treatment that are said to occasionally work. Cetuximab appears to have been effective in one patient. A high-protein diet is prescribed to offset the loss of protein. Treatment with a monoclonal antibody against the EGFR has been reported to result in marked reduction in the frequency of nausea and vomiting, an increase in serum albumin concentration, and an improvement in endoscopic gastric abnormalities.[766,769,786] As with any putative increased risk of carcinoma, periodic endoscopic surveillance is mandated.

Carcinoma Complicating Ménétrier's Disease

Though a small number of carcinomas have been reported either coincidentally at the time of diagnosis or later in the course of the disease,[770–773] it is difficult to estimate the true incidence of carcinoma. In a disease that seems to be associated with intrinsic production of TGF-α that seems to drive cell proliferation, it would be surprising if gastric carcinomas were not occasionally found complicating Ménétrier's disease. The term Ménétrier's disease has been misused for other forms of hypertrophic gastropathies, and because of the reasons mentioned above, it is difficult to exclude the possibility that some of the published reports of carcinoma associated with Ménétrier's disease probably are secondary to *H. pylori* gastritis.[770] Nonetheless, the cancer incidence is likely not higher than in ordinary atrophic gastritis.[774–776] In patients with Ménétrier's who have persistent large folds after therapy, but do not require gastrectomy, some form of follow-up for this complication would seem prudent. If treated with resolution of the disease it is presumed that this risk returns to baseline, but there are no data regarding this.

Secondary Ménétrier's Disease

There are several clinicopathologic syndromes that need to be sought in potential Ménétrier's disease as many of these indicate an underlying condition that is treatable.

HYPERTROPHIC GASTROPATHY-ASSOCIATED WITH PROTEIN LOSS

Protein-losing hypertrophic gastropathy (gastritis) may complicate a variety of diseases (Table 13-17) for which the term Ménétrier's disease has been misused in the literature. Conditions associated with protein loss and giant gastric folds include CMV gastritis, lymphocytic gastritis, H. pylori gastritis, and HIV gastritis.

Cytomegalovirus-associated Hypertrophic Gastropathy

In the pediatric population, abnormal growth of gastric epithelium is most frequently triggered by an infection (usually CMV, especially in children). Its mechanism may also involve TGF-α.[783] It affects boys and girls equally with no familial transmission. It should also be recalled that while rare, this can occur in adults, and that even in children occasional patients have a Ménétrier-like disease that seems not to be CMV-related.[789] Childhood CMV-associated hypertrophic gastritis is frequently referred to as "childhood Ménétrier's"[790,791]—an example of misuse of the term.

Hypertrophic Lymphocytic Gastritis

There are several reports of the association between lymphocytic gastritis with hypertrophic gastropathy reported as "Ménétrier's disease."[792,793] There has been a suggestion that those with lymphocytic gastritis have less foveolar hyperplasia whereas those without lymphocytic gastritis had more foveolar hyperplasia, a thicker mucosa, and more mucosal edema[794] (see Fig. 13-62A–C). In a study of 23 patients who had been diagnosed with "Ménétrier's disease" H. pylori was present in 30% to 40% in both those with and without lymphocytic gastritis. Given the difficulty in detecting Helicobacter in lymphocytic gastritis (see that section) the true positive rate is likely considerably higher. The authors proposed that Ménétrier refers only to those who did not have the lymphocytic gastritis and proposed the term hypertrophic lymphocytic gastritis for the others.[794] Helicobacter pylori infection may be a treatable cause of at least some cases of hypertrophic lymphocytic gastritis[502] and should therefore be carefully sought in any patient with this condition. It may require serology and, because it is relatively innocuous, a trial of Helicobacter eradication therapy seems justified, whether the organisms can be found or not.

Helicobacter pylori–associated Hypertrophic Gastritis

Large gastric folds have also been described in H. pylori gastritis.[795–797] Anti–H. pylori therapy led to normalization of gastric fold size.[795–797] It is likely that some patients with H. pylori have thick gastric folds that may occasionally be associated with protein loss.[798] The thick folds in these patients may have histologic changes of inflammation and foveolar hyperplasia that may be associated with minimal to severe gland loss. It is noteworthy that in two of these reports,[796,797] the term "Ménétrier's disease" has been used. One patient had granulomatous gastritis associated with a Ménétrier'-like appearance.[517] It is also documented that some regress to a state of apparent atrophic gastritis, which we suspect is end-stage Helicobacter gastritis.

HIV-associated Hypertrophic Gastritis

HIV has been rarely reported with a Ménétrier-like syndrome.[799,800] The authors[800] proposed a mechanism whereby HIV may upregulate TGF production.

Large Gastric Folds Associated with Other Conditions

Large gastric folds have also been described in a variety of other conditions including infections such as histoplasmosis, syphilis, and granulomatous diseases involving the mucosa and submucosa. Neoplasms, particularly lymphoma, adenocarcinoma, and carcinoid tumors (although the latter really are multiple diffuse polyps), should be excluded in patients with enlarged gastric folds.[801] In addition, some polyposis syndrome, such as juvenile polyposis[802] and Cronkhite–Canada syndrome,[782] may present with a giant fold appearance. Juvenile polyposis has normal intervening mucosa, although sometimes polyps are so numerous that the normal intervening mucosa may be difficult to find, especially endoscopically.

Other Types of Large Gastric Folds

Some patients have large gastric folds, often antral, which on biopsy show either an apparently normal mucosa or a thickened mucosa (Fig. 13-80). Figure 13-80D clearly

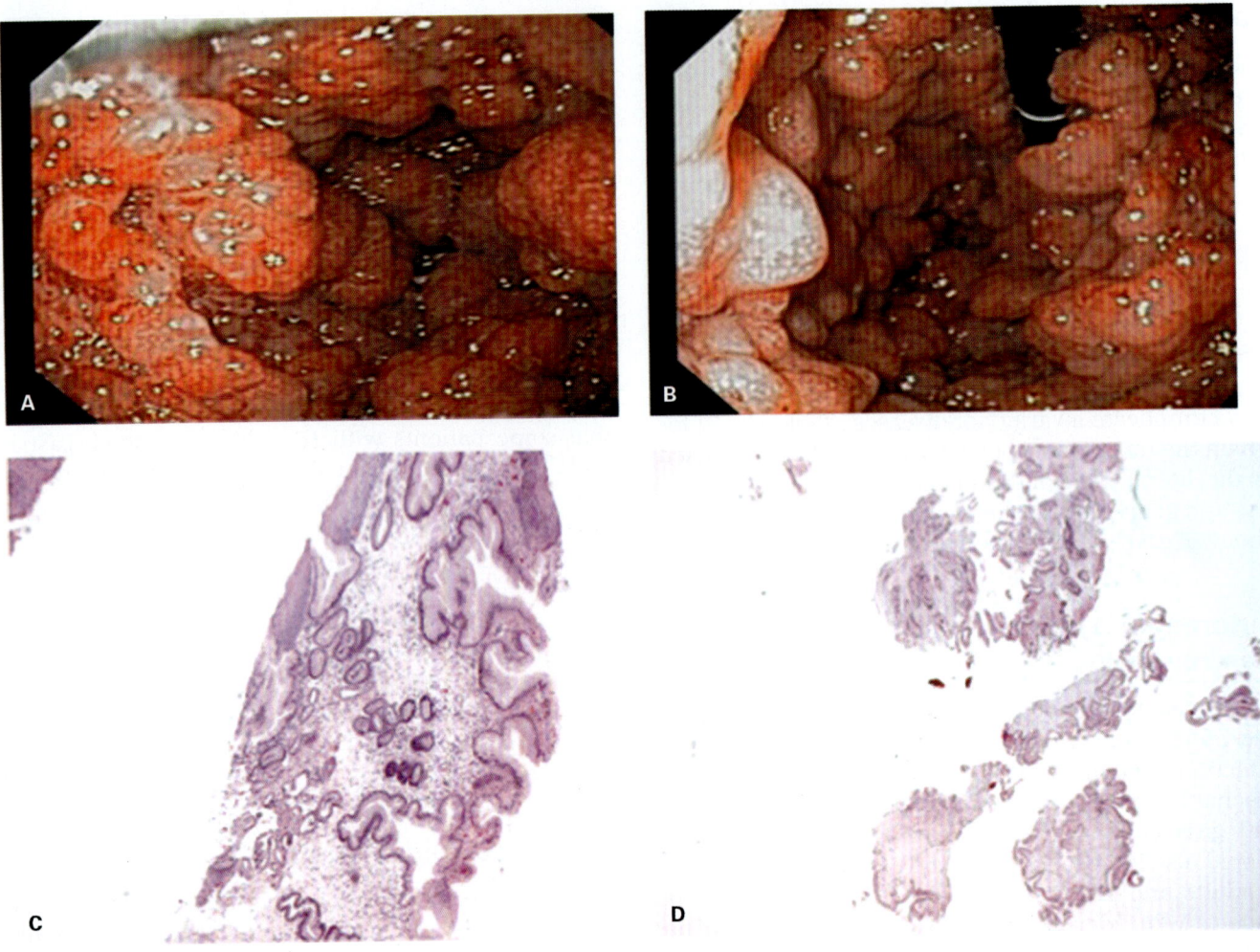

Figure 13-80. Cronkhite–Canada syndrome. **A,B:** Body and fundus. (Courtesy of Dr. Sandy Nelles, Mississauga.) **C:** Biopsy from cardia showing edematous lamina propria. **D,E:** Biopsies from gastric body showing loss of specialized mucosa and a markedly edematous stroma. The entire GI tract was similar in this patient.

has a chronic gastritis, suggesting that this may well be a variant of *Helicobacter* gastritis.

Zollinger–Ellison Syndrome was first described by Zollinger and Ellison in 1955 to describe patients with ulceration of the upper jejunum, hypersecretion of gastric acid, and non–beta islet cell tumor of the pancreas.[803] It is a secondary cause of large gastric folds, but that is where any similarity to Ménétrier's disease stops.

Clinical Presentation: ZES is a rare disorder characterized by one or more gastrin-releasing tumors (gastrinomas) in the pancreas, duodenum, or both, and rarely other locations such as the biliary tract. Gastrinomas release abnormal amounts of gastrin that acts as a trophic or growth hormone that induces ECL and PC hyperplasia resulting in an excess of gastric acid in the stomach and duodenum.[297,804] The excess acid eventually causes peptic ulcers, which may be single or multiple, and may occur in the esophagus, stomach, and duodenal bulb, or in atypical locations, such as the postbulbar portion of the duodenum or even the jejunum.[257] In about 10% of patients with ZES, the presenting symptom is diarrhea, and ulcers are absent.[257] ZES is more common among men 30 to 50 years old, but patients as young as 7 and as old as 90 have been identified.[805] Gastrinomas can be either sporadic or associated with MEN I. There is also secondary ECL cell hyperplasia (see Chapter 5). Near 25% of patients with gastrinomas have MEN I.[806] Children who have a parent with MEN1 have a 50% chance of inheriting the MEN1 gene and are, therefore, also at increased risk of ZES.[804]

Endoscopic Features and Gross Pathology: The clinical correlate of parietal cells hyperplasia is rugal hypertrophy with prominent gastric folds, which is observed in up to 90% of patients with ZES. Grossly, the thickened folds are confined to the body and fundus. The surface folds may be coarsely granular due to localized areas of mucosal expansion alternating with mucosal depressions where glands are not expanded. As discussed above, the excess acid causes refractory ulcers in atypical locations.[257] It is important to remember that thick folds in the fundus and body of the stomach (Fig. 13-81) may be observed in the ZES and in some patients with *H. pylori* or NSAID-associated duodenal ulcer disease; the latter conditions lack hypergastrinemia and gastrin-producing tumors.

Histologic Features: In ZES mucosal hyperplasia primarily affects the secretory portion of fundic glands with a large increase in the number of parietal cells. Histologic examinations of expanded areas reveal elongated glands crowded with an increased number of parietal cells which may also appear larger, and have the typical tongues seen in hypergastrinemic states, and which renders the lumen serrated rather than round. The glandular compartment of the body mucosa becomes enlarged, so that the pit gland ratio changes from the usual 1 to 3 to 1 to 4 or even 1 to 5.[807] There is also hyperplasia of the fundic ECL cells and,

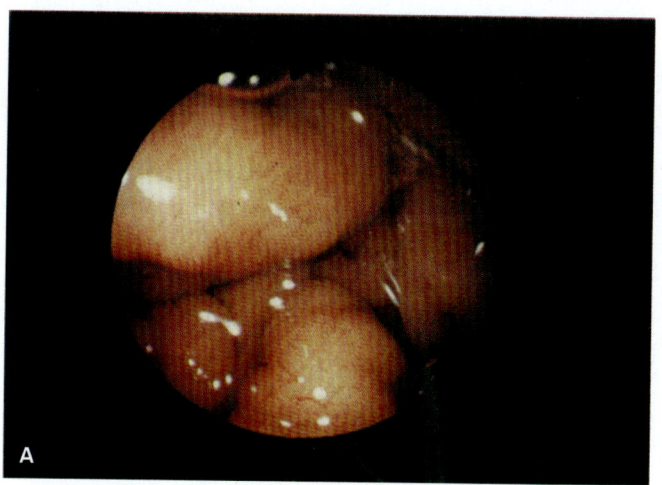

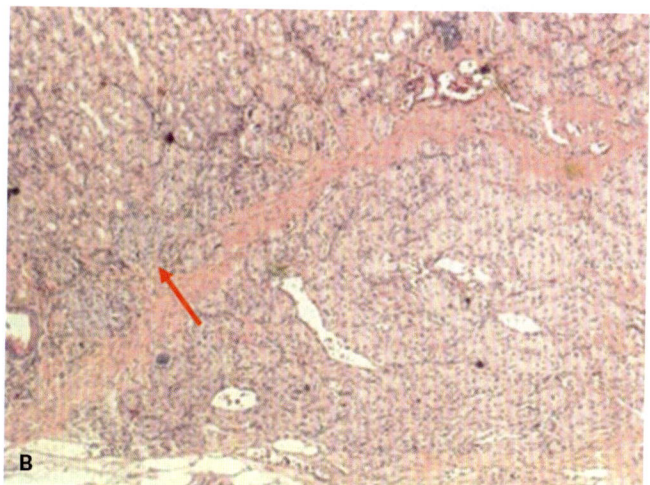

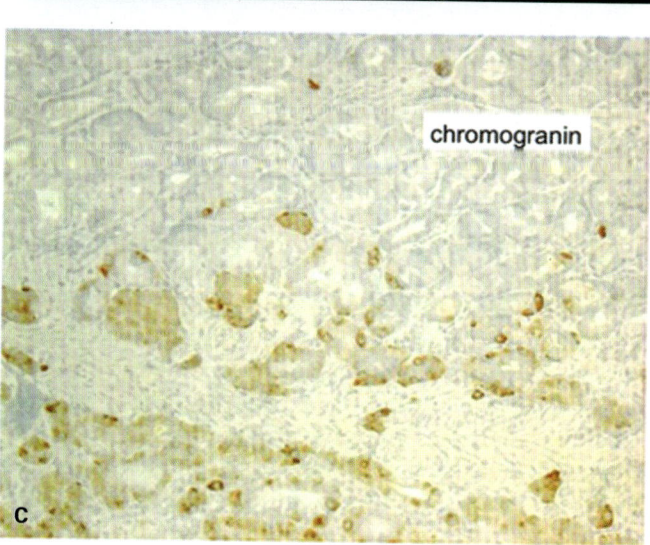

Figure 13-81. A: Zollinger–Ellison syndrome. Gastric body folds that did not flatten with air insufflation at endoscopy. **B:** Gastric carcinoid in MEN1 (Zollinger–Ellison). There is a thickened specialized zone above the muscularis mucosae, at the base of which there is endocrine (ECL) cell hyperplasia and microcarcinoids (*arrow*). However, the carcinoid extends across the muscularis mucosae into the submucosa. These tumors rarely metastasize and even if they do are incredibly slow-growing. **C:** Chromogranin immunostain reveals the same sort of ECL hyperplasia (and a deep carcinoid) seen in autoimmune gastritis, but in a hypertrophic rather than atrophic stomach.

rarely, multiple carcinoids, fundic gland polyps, and intramucosal cysts.[808] Thus the combination of a thick PC zone with underlying ECL hyperplasia, microcarcinoids, or carcinoids is virtually diagnostic of ZES (Fig. 13-81). The only differential diagnosis is the rare patient on longterm PPIs with similar features, or the exceedingly rare patients who cannot make protons and shows identical changes in the oxyntic mucosa, but has no gastrinoma. Theoretically, while ZES should have atrophy of antral G-cells, those unable to make protons have markedly increased numbers of G-cells (see Chapter 5). Some degree of foveolar hyperplasia may occasionally be seen in ZES and may result in transient confusion with Ménétrier's disease.

Differential Diagnosis: The clinical and histologic pictures are very different from those seen in Ménétrier's disease. Similar degrees of localized parietal cells hypertrophy have been observed in patients on long-term PPI therapy. Fasting serum gastrin should be measured in any patient suspected of having ZES. Measurement of gastric pH on a single specimen can be important to exclude secondary hypergastrinemia due to achlorhydria (e.g., gastric atrophy patients with atrophic gastritis, pernicious anemia, or patients receiving potent antisecretory drugs), or a primary inability to secrete protons. In Cronkhite–Canada syndrome the entire GI tract is involved (Fig. 13-80) but within the stomach both body and antrum are involved and the mucosa is massively edematous with loss of specialized glands.

Treatment: When Zollinger and Ellison described the triad,[803] most patients died from peptic ulcer complication (bleeding, perforation, and postoperative complications) rather than the underlying malignancy.[257,809] Today, acid hypersecretion can be controlled safely with PPIs, and the primary determinant of morbidity and mortality is tumor progression, although often very high doses of PPI are required.[810,811] An increasing number of patients are being diagnosed with the ZES before the development of peptic ulcer complications or spread of a malignant gastrinoma.[812] Of note, the true incidence of ZES may be an underestimate as symptoms are similar to those caused by typical *H. pylori*–associated or NSAID-associated PUD. In some of these, symptoms may be controlled by standard doses of antisecretory drugs and the patient may not be tested for hypergastrinemia.[813] Removal of the causal gastrinoma cures the syndrome provided excision is complete and there is no metastatic disease.

DISTINCTIVE ENDOSCOPIC ENTITIES

The endoscopic classification of gastritis is based on the predominant macroscopic appearance if there is an endoscopic abnormality, combined with the histologic findings. When there are endoscopic abnormalities, biopsies inevitably come from these regions and should also be taken from the background mucosa to determine if this is a focal or generalized condition. Endoscopic abnormalities include erythematous/exudative gastritis, flat erosive gastritis, raised erosive gastritis, atrophic gastritis, hemorrhagic gastritis, rugal hyperplastic gastritis, enterogastric reflux gastritis, and congestive gastropathy. Nonetheless, the endoscopic appearance correlates poorly with histologic abnormalities seen on biopsy.[814] For example, gastric mucosa that appears "normal" on endoscopy is associated with impressive and diagnostic histologic abnormalities in approximately one-third of cases.[814] Conversely, "abnormal"-appearing gastric mucosa (e.g., red, nodular, irregular, thickened, or raised) is a nonspecific finding. These endoscopic abnormalities are compatible with many different gastropathies or gastritides and can be associated with normal histology in approximately 25% of cases.[814] For these reasons, many experts advocate taking gastric biopsies in every patient undergoing upper GI endoscopy[498,507] and reserve final diagnosis following the histologic findings. We will address endoscopic findings in its broadest sense, which classifies them into three categories (erosive, nonerosive, and distinctive).

IIC. DISTINCTIVE ENDOSCOPIC ENTITIES

1. Erosive and hemorrhagic
   a. Varioliform gastritis
   b. Watermelon stomach
   c. Portal gastropathy
   d. Hemorrhagic gastritis
2. Nonerosive
   a. Nodular gastritis, children
   b. Atrophic front, adults
3. Distinctive
   a. Hypertrophic gastropathy

MISCELLANEOUS DISORDERS OF THE STOMACH

Foreign Bodies usually (90%) pass out of the stomach, without incident, into the intestinal tract. They may then become lodged in the intestines, especially if they are sharp. Larger or sharper objects must be removed endoscopically, sometimes as a combined laparoscopic approach.[815] Gastric perforation is rare. One should always bear in mind that a foreign body that does not pass may be impeded by a structural lesion such as a stricture or diaphragm.[816]

Bezoars of the stomach are hardened collections of foreign material (Fig. 13-82) that consist most

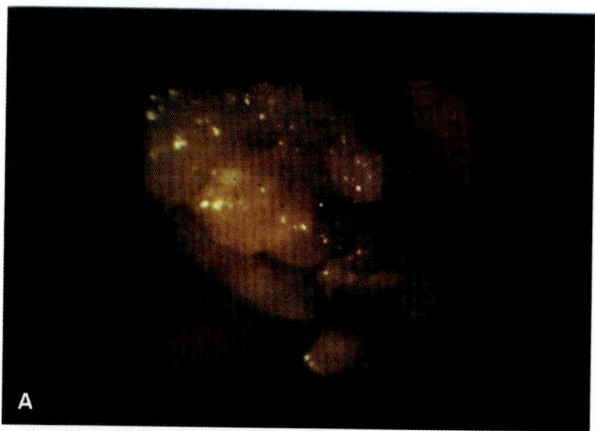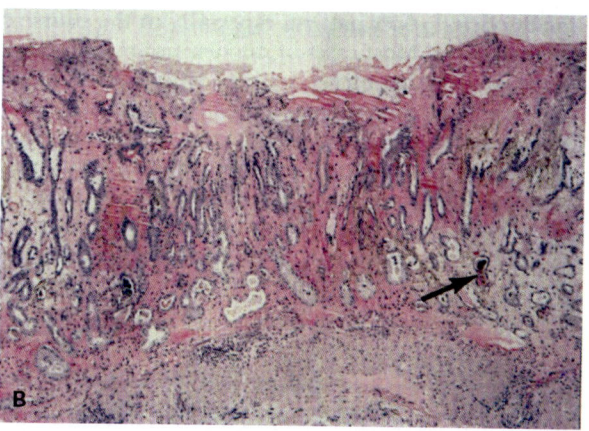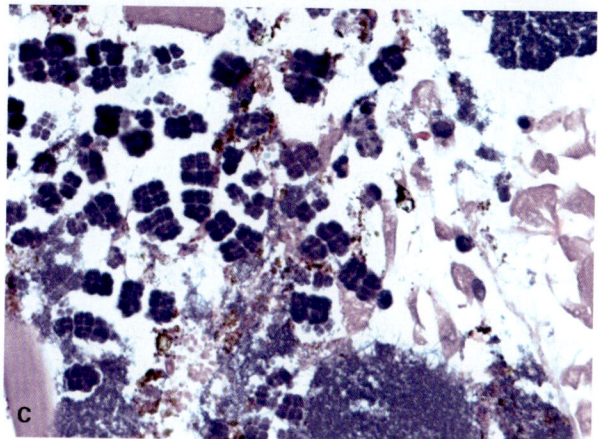

Figure 13-82. **A:** Gastric bezoar. **B:** Erosion with gland loss (ischemic appearance) underlying a bezoar. The dark-pigmented material seen especially at the right (*arrow*) presumably represents food debris. **C:** On the surface of some bezoars, organisms can be found, including the tetrads associated with Sarsinia.

commonly of plant (including the often noted persimmon seeds—diospyrobezoar) materials (phytobezoars), hair (trichobezoars), and a variety of other materials including medications, other chemicals, and fungus balls.[817,818] There seems to be no end to the variation in the composition of bezoars.[819,820] Bezoars are usually encountered in patients with altered gastric anatomy, for example, after gastric surgery or altered function as in gastroparesis. Predisposing conditions are the postgastrectomy state, diabetes, and any other disorder in which gastric emptying is delayed.[821] They may be discovered incidentally or with symptoms related to obstruction or mucosal ulceration (Fig. 13-82). Nonoperative treatment with intragastric N-acetylcysteine for the rapid dissolution of large gastric lactobezoars,[822] mechanical disruption at endoscopy or with other means,[823] and laparoscopically assistance for large bezoars obviates the need for laparotomy in many patients. However, when complications ensue, surgical removal from the stomach or intestine (if the object has passed from the stomach) is necessary.[824] Biopsies are invariably inflamed either directly or because of underlying diseases that may have reduced acid secretion. Sometimes they have organisms such as the tetrads of Sarcina (Fig. 13-82C).

Gastric Calcinosis

Gastric mucosal calcification is rarely encountered in routine biopsies. In general, gastric mucosal calcification (calcinosis) can be classified into metastatic, dystrophic, and idiopathic. While metastatic calcification is said to be the most frequently encountered those that we have seen appear to be dystrophic, and the reason for their formation has been completely unclear, with no evidence that they are occurring in vessels, and no hint of prior granulomas or organisms. Metastatic calcification is the deposition of calcium salts on largely normal mucosa in the setting of clinical conditions associated with hypercalcemia or hypophosphatemia or both. Dystrophic calcification is the deposition of calcium salts in inflamed, fibrotic, or otherwise altered tissue serum (given normal serum levels for calcium and phosphate). Gastric biopsies reveal pale blue to purple amorphous, sometimes partially calcified refractile material beneath the surface epithelium. Stains for calcium (von Kossa or alizarin red) may help in confirming its nature. Other microscopic features frequently associated include foveolar hyperplasia and mucosal edema.

The presence of mucosal calcifications may indicate generalized metastatic calcification, especially in organs where they may be fatal, such as the heart; systemic calcification is potentially reversible.[825,826] Gastric mucosal calcinosis has also been described in patients on long-term aluminum-containing antacids or sucralfate.[827] The deposition of the calcium occurs just underneath the epithelium at the tips of the foveolae and tinctorially appears similar to CMV inclusions ranging in size from 40 to 250 µm. Most of the patients in this study were organ transplant or chronic renal failure patients, and it was much less commonly seen in patients with gastric ulcer, likely requiring long-term use of the medications. X-ray analysis of the material suggested it contained aluminum, phosphorus, calcium, and chlorine.

Gastric Glandular Siderosis

Deposition of hemosiderin in gastric glandular epithelium, antral or fundic, has been referred to as gastric glandular siderosis.[759] This needs to be differentiated from deposition of crystalline iron and mucosal injury secondary to iron-containing pills (iron pill gastritis) and deposition of hemosiderin in macrophages and lamina propria secondary to prior hemorrhage/inflammation.[759] While in these "nonglandular" patterns of siderosis some deposition of hemosiderin in the epithelium can be seen, it is a minor component. In gastric glandular siderosis the deposition of hemosiderin is predominantly or exclusively in the glandular epithelium and is found in <1% of all gastric biopsies. When marked it may be obvious on H&E stains; however, more subtle deposition can only be picked up with special stains (Prussian blue stain). Special stains are also helpful in differentiating hemosiderin from lipofuscin-like pigment present in the glandular epithelium that can look similar on a H&E stain. The presence of gastric glandular siderosis has been associated with the presence of systemic iron overload/hemochromatosis in some patients. Older literature suggested that this could be also associated with alcohol abuse, although it is unclear if this is due to cirrhosis or simply secondary to portal hypertension from any cause. In some cases, however, the etiology remains unclear. The pathogenesis of hemosiderin deposition in the glandular epithelium and its functional significance with regard to stomach remains unknown at this time.

Approach to the Interpretation of Gastric Biopsies

The most important task for the pathologist is to ensure that clinical colleagues know the meaning and significance of the terms used. The general approach to biopsy diagnosis is outlined in Table 13-18. The purpose is to give the type of mucosa present based on gland type, including gland status (atrophic, metaplastic) an overview of the depth, degree, and nature of inflammation (i.e., superficial, panmucosal, or atrophic), and to note any special features present. So, from a pathology viewpoint, the following questions should be addressed with each biopsy:

1. Where is the biopsy from (anatomic compartment)?
2. Is it normal?
3. If not normal, is it a gastritis or a gastropathy or is there a focal lesion?
4. If gastropathy, is it primarily epithelial reactive changes or vascular dilatation? Are there inflammatory cells (eosinophils or neutrophils)?
5. If gastritis what is the distribution?—antral-, oxyntic-, or cardiac-predominant, or is it pangastritis (antral-predominant, oxyntic-predominant, equal in both), superficial or deep?

Surface epithelium

6. Is there an excess of IELs?
7. Are there other intraepithelial inflammatory cells?
8. Are there other inflammatory cells in the surface epithelium?—or the lamina propria—granulomas, neutrophils, eosinophils, plasma cells, lymphocytes?
9. Is there a thickened subepithelial collagen band?
10. Is there pseudopyloric or intestinal metaplasia?
11. Are there other forms of atrophy?—simple absence of glands
12. Is there dysplasia?
13. Is there endocrine cell hyperplasia?
14. Are organisms present?—*H. pylori*, other *Helicobacter* species, or other microorganisms (including spirochetes, viral, etc.)

HISTOLOGY

Site: In order to make an accurate histologic diagnosis, the first question is where does the biopsy specimen come from? The reason is that if a biopsy labeled "body" and the specimen appears phenotypically "antrum" it would prompt us to examine carefully the possibility of atrophy presenting as "pseudopyloric metaplasia." Conversely, in some patients, antral biopsies contain numerous parietal cells which should prompt a search for G-cells to confirm that this is a variation of normal. In some patients the antrum contains numerous parietal cells.

Biopsy specimens from the lesser curvature of the body and from the distal body or proximal antrum often consist of transitional or mixed gland mucosa

Table 13-18 The Differential Diagnosis in Gastric Pathology

A. PREDOMINANTLY NONINFLAMMATORY
1. Normal
2. Predominantly epithelial changes
   (a) Foveolar and smooth muscle hyperplasia with a relative paucity of inflammatory cells.. Chemical/reflux gastropathy
   (b) Variable degrees of grand loss with increased apoptosis............... GVHD
   (c) Reactive features (a and b above) with glandular atypia "thick and thin" glands and sometimes abnormal mitoses .... Radiation/chemotherapy
3. Predominant vascular pathology
   (a) Telangiectatic vessels with fibrin thrombi...................................... GAVE
   (b) Mucosal vascular ectasia.. Portal hypertension
   (c) Hemorrhage at tip of mucosal folds... Hemorrhagic/shock gastropathy

B. PREDOMINANTLY INFLAMMATORY
I. Focal inflammation
  1. Focal enhanced inflammation in CD
  2. Focal carditis in reflux gastropathy
  3. Next to an erosion in chemical gastropathy
  4. No obvious association
II. Diffuse inflammation
  1. Predominantly acute inflammatory cells
     (a) Viral, for example, CMV
     (b) Acute bacterial gastroenteritis—usually not biopsied
     (c) Early *H. pylori* infection—rarely biopsied
  2. Predominantly chronic inflammatory cells
     (a) *Helicobacter pylori* infection (patterns of gastritis and atrophy)

GASTRITIS PATTERN	INFLAMMATION	GLANDS
Antral-predominant	Antral inflammation Corpus inflammation limited to pit region	Intact
Pangastritis	Antral inflammation Deep corpus inflammation that extends beyond pit region	Intact
Atrophic pangastritis	Antral inflammation Deep corpus inflammation with variable extension into gland zones	Variable gland loss
Corpus-predominant	Minimal antral inflammation Deep corpus inflammation with variable extension into gland zones	

   (b) Autoimmune gastritis (corpus-predominant atrophic gastritis)
   (c) Other infections (syphilis)
III. Special forms of gastritis (descriptive gastritis)—see also Table 13.1, for example
  1. Lymphocytic gastritis
  2. Eosinophilic gastritis (Churg–Strauss, parasites)
  3. Granulomatous gastritis
  4. Big folds/"Ménétrier's" disease

*Chronic active if neutrophils present, chronic if neutrophils are absent.

---

containing both antral and fundic glands, or a zone of thin but otherwise unremarkable oxyntic mucosa (see Chapter 12 and earlier in this chapter). The endoscopist should be encouraged (or cajoled) to provide accurate site information. The general biopsy site designations are antrum, body, fundus, or cardia. If biopsy specimens are taken from the cardia region just below the gastroesophageal junction, the best site designation is in terms of the number of centimeters above the upper end of the gastric folds, which is far more meaningful than cms from the incisors, which varies with the length of the esophagus. In the case of antrum and body specimens, it can be important to know which curvature or wall the specimens come from as the oxyntic mucosa is thicker on the greater curve. If biopsy specimens are taken to prove that atrophic gastritis of the fundic gland mucosa is present, the best zone to sample is that where atrophy is first appreciated. This corresponds to biopsies midway between the midbody and antral corpus junction (recommended by the Sydney system) on both the lesser and the greater curvature of the stomach.

Severe atrophic gastritis at the greater curve midbody biopsy (currently recommended by the updated Sydney system) indicates a diffuse process with a high risk for concomitant dysplasia and carcinoma.

Acute Injury: Any of the previously described lesions may have histopathologic changes of acute (recent) injury. These include neutrophil infiltrate, cytoplasmic mucus depletion of surface epithelium and foveolar cells, attenuated (restituting) mucosa with erosions, or ulcers. Occasionally a mild infiltrate of lymphocytes and plasma cells occupying the superficial portion of the gastric mucosa may be present. With acute bacterial gastroenteritis (often unbiopsied) the mucosa may undergo complete healing within 4 days.

Surface and pit epithelium. A common abnormality of the epithelium in acute injury is a loss of mucin with a basophilic or purplish hue (Fig. 14-4). Cells may be cuboidal, with hyperchromatism and pleomorphism. In the pit region, mitotic figures may be increased, and when the epithelial abnormalities are severe, they may even be seen in the surface epithelium. When the pit epithelium is very abnormal, another common finding is pit lengthening, namely, foveolar hyperplasia. Foveolar hyperplasia is a common pattern of mucosal abnormality in a number of disorders, and can be seen endoscopically as thick folds or nodularity. These include hyperplastic polyps, *H. pylori* gastritis, healed ulcer sites, the stomal area of the postgastrectomy stomach, and NSAID-induced mucosal injury. In the antrum especially, foveolar hyperplasia may be accompanied by disorganization and irregularity of the foveolae, resulting in a corkscrew appearance. It is distinct from the precancerous lesion, dysplasia, as discussed in Chapter 17.

Inflammatory cells. Except at the edges of some erosions that are usually associated with medications such as NSAIDs, ASA, bisphosphonates, etc., neutrophils are rarely present without an increase in the number of mononuclear cells. Scattered eosinophils may also be seen, and can be the dominant cell.

Intestinal metaplasia is a reaction to a mucosal injury in which epithelial cells, usually beginning in the pit region, acquire the features of intestinal epithelium. These range from goblet cells to well-developed absorptive cells in various stages of maturation, including some with well-developed brush borders, and differentiated cells such as Paneth and endocrine cells. The endocrine cells in the metaplastic areas contain a variety of peptides that are normally found in the small intestine, as well as those normally found in the stomach. Areas of intestinal metaplasia can be detected more readily with Alcian blue at pH 2.5, which stains sialomucins (Fig. 14-15A), mucicarmine, or MUC2. Intestinal metaplasia that stains positively for colon-type sulfomucins (demonstrable with the high iron diamine or Alcian blue stain, pH 1.0) and may contain poorly developed brush borders has been related to gastric adenocarcinoma. CD10 or villin may be immunoreactive at the luminal border of the cells. The implications of these findings were discussed earlier. Because of sampling error, subtyping intestinal metaplasia is not useful in clinical specimens.

Endocrine cells. Hyperplasia of endocrine cells may occur in the antrum or body. An increase in the number of gastrin cells in the antrum may occur when there is hypo- or achlorhydria associated with atrophic fundic gland gastritis, but most commonly in patients taking long-term PPIs. In the gastric body, hyperplasia of endocrine cells is also associated with long-term hypergastrinemia, but hyperplasia is most prominent in association with severe atrophic fundic gland gastritis. The hyperplastic cells are primarily ECL cells, located in glands exhibiting mucous gland (pseudopyloric) metaplasia, or as tiny free collections in the lamina propria. Silver stains were once widely used to demonstrate endocrine cell hyperplasia; however, synaptophysin and chromogranin stains, or specific antibodies such as gastrin, are now used instead.

Gastric Metaplasia. The arrival of unneutralized acid in the first part of the duodenum has certain consequences. Notable among these is gastric metaplasia, the presence of gastric-type mucus-secreting cells in the surface epithelium of the duodenum. However, it is a common observation that gastric metaplasia exists without inflammation. The change probably develops as an adaptive response to acid, a suggestion that is supported by animal experiments with induced hyperchlorhydria, and in human subjects by the correlation between the presence and extent of metaplasia and maximal acid output. Furthermore, gastric metaplasia is extensive in patients with the ZES, has a lower prevalence following truncal and proximal selective vagotomy, and is not seen in patients with AIG and achlorhydria.

Interpretation. When the sites and morphology have been stated, the interpretation is by far the most important aspect of any report. It is all too easy to provide descriptions without interpretation. While this suffices if an etiology is apparent (e.g., chronic active *Helicobacter* gastritis), it becomes even more important when, for example, there is inflammation without *Helicobacter* as this has a differential diagnosis, for example, lymphocytic gastritis that has therapeutic implications, or atrophic gastritis that has implications for subsequent follow-up. Descriptive diagnoses are really descriptions and not diagnoses, so need serious consideration of an interpretation. The pathologist is the person that (should) have this knowledge, and it should not be left to the clinician to interpret the findings, or being told that "clinical correlation is required." Most do not have this specialist knowledge.

References

1. Wood MW. Essential thrombocytopenia, gastrointestinal haemorrhages, and peptic ulceration as a diagnostic problem. *Br Med J.* 1951;1(4710):799–800.
2. Reveiz L, Guerrero-Lozano R, Camacho A, et al. Stress ulcer, gastritis, and gastrointestinal bleeding prophylaxis in critically ill pediatric patients: a systematic review. *Pediatr Crit Care Med.* 2010;11(1):124–132.
3. Boukthir S, Mazigh SM, Kalach N, et al. The effect of non-steroidal anti-inflammatory drugs and *Helicobacter pylori* infection on the gastric mucosa in children with upper gastrointestinal bleeding. *Pediatr Surg Int.* 2010;26(2):227–230.
4. Desai JC, Sanyal SM, Goo T, et al. Primary prevention of adverse gastroduodenal effects from short-term use of non-steroidal anti-inflammatory drugs by omeprazole 20 mg in healthy subjects: a randomized, double-blind, placebo-controlled study. *Dig Dis Sci.* 2008;53(8):2059–2065.
5. Schindler R. Chronic gastritis. *Bull N Y Acad Med.* 1939;15(5):322–337.
6. Doig RK, Wood IJ. Gastritis: a study of 112 cases diagnosed by gastric biopsy. *Med J Aust.* 1952;1(18):593–600.
7. Schindler R. On hypertrophic glandular gastritis, hypertrophic gastropathy, and parietal cell mass. *Gastroenterology.* 1963;45:77–83.
8. Whitehead R, Truelove SC, Gear MW. The histological diagnosis of chronic gastritis in fibreoptic gastroscope biopsy specimens. *J Clin Pathol.* 1972;25(1):1–11.
9. Marshall BJ, Armstrong JA, McGechie DB, et al. Attempt to fulfil Koch's postulates for pyloric *Campylobacter. Med J Aust.* 1985;142(8):436–439.
10. Sobala GM, King RF, Axon AT, et al. Reflux gastritis in the intact stomach. *J Clin Pathol.* 1990;43(4):303–306.
11. Correa P. Chronic gastritis: a clinico-pathological classification. *Am J Gastroenterol.* 1988;83(5):504–509.
12. Price AB. The Sydney system: histological division. *J Gastroenterol Hepatol.* 1991;6(3):209–222.
13. Dixon MF, Genta RM, Yardley JH, et al. Classification and grading of gastritis. The updated Sydney system. International Workshop on the Histopathology of Gastritis, Houston 1994. *Am J Surg Pathol.* 1996;20(10):1161–1181.
14. Kirk RM, Jeffery PJ. Development of surgery for peptic ulcer: a review. *J R Soc Med.* 1981;74(11):828–830.
15. Riddell RH (ed.). *Pathology of Drug-Induced and Toxic Disease.* New York, NY: Churchill Livingstone; 1982.
16. Hawkey CJ. Non-steroidal anti-inflammatory drug gastropathy: causes and treatment. *Scand J Gastroenterol Suppl.* 1996;220:124–127.
17. Dixon MF, O'Connor HJ, Axon AT, et al. Reflux gastritis: distinct histopathological entity? *J Clin Pathol.* 1986;39(5):524–530.
18. Frezza M, Gorji N, Melato M. The histopathology of non-steroidal anti-inflammatory drug induced gastroduodenal damage: correlation with *Helicobacter pylori*, ulcers, and haemorrhagic events. *J Clin Pathol.* 2001;54(7):521–525.
19. Zhang X, Ouyang J, Wieczorek R, et al. Iron medication-induced gastric mucosal injury. *Pathol Res Pract.* 2009;205(8):579–581.
20. El-Zimaity HM, Genta RM, Graham DY. Histological features do not define NSAID-induced gastritis. *Hum Pathol.* 1996;27(12):1348–1354.
21. Weinstein WM, Buch KL, Elashoff J, et al. The histology of the stomach in symptomatic patients after gastric surgery: a model to assess selective patterns of gastric mucosal injury. *Scand J Gastroenterol Suppl.* 1985;109:77–89.
22. Hoare AM, Jones EL, Alexander-Williams J, et al. Symptomatic significance of gastric mucosal changes after surgery for peptic ulcer. *Gut.* 1977;18(4):295–300.
23. Kato Y, Sugano H, Rubio CA. Classification of intramucosal cysts of the stomach. *Histopathology.* 1983;7(6):931–938.
24. Bogomoletz WV, Potet F, Barge J, et al. Pathological features and mucin histochemistry of primary gastric stump carcinoma associated with gastritis cystica polyposa. A study of six cases. *Am J Surg Pathol.* 1985;9(6):401–410.
25. Stolte M, Panayiotou S, Schmitz J. Can NSAID/ASA-induced erosions of the gastric mucosa be identified at histology? *Pathol Res Pract.* 1999;195(3):137–142.
26. Vieth M, Muller H, Stolte M. Can the diagnosis of NSAID-induced or Hp-associated gastric ulceration be predicted from histology? *Z Gastroenterol.* 2002;40(9):783–788.
27. Laine L, Weinstein WM. Histology of alcoholic hemorrhagic "gastritis": a prospective evaluation. *Gastroenterology.* 1988;94(6):1254–1262.
28. Sharma R, Hudak ML, Tepas JJ III, et al. Prenatal or postnatal indomethacin exposure and neonatal gut injury associated with isolated intestinal perforation and necrotizing enterocolitis. *J Perinatol.* 2010;30(12):786–793.
29. Klotz AP, Kirsner JB, Palmer WL. An evaluation of gastroscopy. *Gastroenterology.* 1954;27(2):221–226.
30. Lowe JE, Graham DY, Boisaubin EV Jr, et al. Corrosive injury to the stomach: the natural history and role of fiberoptic endoscopy. *Am J Surg.* 1979;137(6):803–806.
31. Cello JP, Fogel RP, Boland CR. Liquid caustic ingestion. Spectrum of injury. *Arch Intern Med.* 1980;140(4):501–504.
32. Snover DC. Graft-versus-host disease of the gastrointestinal tract. *Am J Surg Pathol.* 1990;14(suppl 1):101–108.
33. Galati JS, Wisecarver JL, Quigley EM. Inflammatory polyps as a manifestation of intestinal graft versus host disease. *Gastrointest Endosc.* 1993;39(5):719–722.
34. Washington K, Bentley RC, Green A, et al. Gastric graft-versus-host disease: a blinded histologic study. *Am J Surg Pathol.* 1997;21(9):1037–1046.
35. Doria MI Jr, Doria LK, Faintuch J, et al. Gastric mucosal injury after hepatic arterial infusion chemotherapy with floxuridine. A clinical and pathologic study. *Cancer.* 1994;73(8):2042–2047.
36. Bourdages R, Prentice RS, Beck IT, et al. Atheromatous embolization to the stomach: an unusual cause of gastrointestinal bleeding. *Am J Dig Dis.* 1976;21(10):889–894.
37. Shepherd HA, Patel C, Bamforth J, et al. Upper gastrointestinal endoscopy in systemic vasculitis presenting as an acute abdomen. *Endoscopy.* 1983;15(5):307–311.
38. Duclos B, Baumann R, Sondag D, et al. Specific gastric localization of Wegener's disease. *Gastroenterol Clin Biol.* 1987;11(2):154–157.
39. Hojgaard L, Krag E. Chronic ischemic gastritis reversed after revascularization operation. *Gastroenterology.* 1987;92(1):226–228.
40. Tomomasa T, Hsu JY, Itoh K, et al. Endoscopic findings in pediatric patients with Henoch–Schonlein purpura and gastrointestinal symptoms. *J Pediatr Gastroenterol Nutr.* 1987;6(5):725–729.
41. Suit PF, Petras RE, Bauer TW, et al. Gastric antral vascular ectasia. A histologic and morphometric study of "the watermelon stomach." *Am J Surg Pathol.* 1987;11(10):750–757.
42. Al-Haddad M, Ward EM, DeVault KR, et al. Vascular ectasia of the proximal stomach. *Dig Dis Sci.* 2007;52(5):1367–1369.
43. Goel A, Christian CL. Gastric antral vascular ectasia (watermelon stomach) in a patient with Sjogren's syndrome. *J Rheumatol.* 2003;30(5):1090–1092.
44. Lecleire S, Ben-Soussan E, Antonietti M, et al. Bleeding gastric vascular ectasia treated by argon plasma coagulation: a comparison between patients with and without cirrhosis. *Gastrointest Endosc.* 2008;67(2):219–225.
45. Stefanidis I, Liakopoulos V, Kapsoritakis AN, et al. Gastric antral vascular ectasia (watermelon stomach) in patients with ESRD. *Am J Kidney Dis.* 2006;47(6):e77–e82.

46. Raja K, Kochhar R, Sethy PK, et al. An endoscopic study of upper-GI mucosal changes in patients with congestive heart failure. *Gastrointest Endosc.* 2004;60(6):887–893.
47. Wyatt JI, Dixon MF. Chronic gastritis—a pathogenetic approach. *J Pathol.* 1988;154(2):113–124.
48. Thuluvath PJ, Yoo HY. Portal hypertensive gastropathy. *Am J Gastroenterol.* 2002;97(12):2973–2978.
49. Quintero E, Pique JM, Bombi JA, et al. Gastric mucosal vascular ectasias causing bleeding in cirrhosis. A distinct entity associated with hypergastrinemia and low serum levels of pepsinogen I. *Gastroenterology.* 1987;93(5):1054–1061.
50. McCormack TT, Sims J, Eyre-Brook I, et al. Gastric lesions in portal hypertension: inflammatory gastritis or congestive gastropathy? *Gut.* 1985;26(11):1226–1232.
51. Laine L, Weinstein WM. Subepithelial hemorrhages and erosions of human stomach. *Dig Dis Sci.* 1988;33(4):490–503.
52. Schiessel R, Feil W, Wenzl E. Mechanisms of stress ulceration and implications for treatment. *Gastroenterol Clin North Am.* 1990;19(1):101–120.
53. Reusser P, Gyr K, Scheidegger D, et al. Prospective endoscopic study of stress erosions and ulcers in critically ill neurosurgical patients: current incidence and effect of acid-reducing prophylaxis. *Crit Care Med.* 1990;18(3):270–274.
54. Lucas CE, Sugawa C, Riddle J, et al. Natural history and surgical dilemma of "stress" gastric bleeding. *Arch Surg.* 1971;102(4):266–273.
55. Czaja AJ, McAlhany JC, Andes WA, et al. Acute gastric disease after cutaneous thermal injury. *Arch Surg.* 1975;110(5):600–605.
56. Larson GM, Koch S, O'Dorisio TM, et al. Gastric response to severe head injury. *Am J Surg.* 1984;147(1):97–105.
57. Pruitt BA Jr, Foley FD, Moncrief JA. Curling's ulcer: a clinical-pathology study of 323 cases. *Ann Surg.* 1970;172(4):523–539.
58. Lev R. Letter: stress erosions. *Am J Dig Dis.* 1973;18(12):1099–1100.
59. Shuman RB, Schuster DP, Zuckerman GR. Prophylactic therapy for stress ulcer bleeding: a reappraisal. *Ann Intern Med.* 1987;106(4):562–567.
60. Czaja AJ, McAlhany JC, Pruitt BA Jr. Acute gastroduodenal disease after thermal injury. An endoscopic evaluation of incidence and natural history. *N Engl J Med.* 1974;291(18):925–929.
61. Oktedalen O, Lunde OC, Opstad PK, et al. Changes in the gastrointestinal mucosa after long-distance running. *Scand J Gastroenterol.* 1992;27(4):270–274.
62. Schwartz AE, Vanagunas A, Kamel PL. Endoscopy to evaluate gastrointestinal bleeding in marathon runners. *Ann Intern Med.* 1990;113(8):632–633.
63. Cooper BT, Douglas SA, Firth LA, et al. Erosive gastritis and gastrointestinal bleeding in a female runner. Prevention of the bleeding and healing of the gastritis with H2-receptor antagonists. *Gastroenterology.* 1987;92(6):2019–2023.
64. Menguy R, Masters YF. Mechanism of stress ulcer. IV. Influence of fasting on the tolerance of gastric mucosal energy metabolism to ischemia and on the incidence of stress ulceration. *Gastroenterology.* 1974;66(6):1177–1186.
65. Gaudin C, Zerath E, Guezennec CY. Gastric lesions secondary to long-distance running. *Dig Dis Sci.* 1990;35(10):1239–1243.
66. Choi SC, Choi SJ, Kim JA, et al. The role of gastrointestinal endoscopy in long-distance runners with gastrointestinal symptoms. *Eur J Gastroenterol Hepatol.* 2001;13(9):1089–1094.
67. El-Zimaity HM, Ramchatesingh J, Clarridge JE, et al. Enterococcus gastritis. *Hum Pathol.* 2003;34(9):944–945.
68. Konturek JW. Discovery by Jaworski of *Helicobacter pylori* and its pathogenetic role in peptic ulcer, gastritis and gastric cancer. *J Physiol Pharmacol.* 2003;54(suppl 3):23–41.
69. Marshall B. Gastric spirochaetes: 100 years of discovery before and after Kobayashi. *Keio J Med.* 2002;51(suppl 2):33–37.
70. Marshall B. *Helicobacter* connections. *ChemMedChem.* 2006;1(8):783–802.
71. Rigas B, Feretis C, Papavassiliou ED. John Lykoudis: an unappreciated discoverer of the cause and treatment of peptic ulcer disease. *Lancet.* 1999;354(9190):1634–1635.
72. Morris A, Nicholson G. Ingestion of *Campylobacter pyloridis* causes gastritis and raised fasting gastric pH. *Am J Gastroenterol.* 1987;82(3):192–199.
73. Marshall BJ, McGechie DB, Rogers PA, et al. Pyloric *Campylobacter* infection and gastroduodenal disease. *Med J Aust.* 1985;142(8):439–444.
74. Morgan D, Kraft W, Bender M, et al. Nitrofurans in the treatment of gastritis associated with *Campylobacter pylori*. The Gastrointestinal Physiology Working Group of Cayetano Heredia and The Johns Hopkins Universities. *Gastroenterology.* 1988;95(5):1178–1184.
75. Glupczynski Y, Burette A, Labbe M, et al. *Campylobacter pylori*-associated gastritis: a double-blind placebo-controlled trial with amoxycillin. *Am J Gastroenterol.* 1988;83(4):365–372.
76. Ramsey EJ, Carey KV, Peterson WL, et al. Epidemic gastritis with hypochlorhydria. *Gastroenterology.* 1979;76(6):1449–1457.
77. Gledhill T, Leicester RJ, Addis B, et al. Epidemic hypochlorhydria. *Br Med J (Clin Res Ed).* 1985;290(6479):1383–1386.
78. Torres J, Perez-Perez G, Goodman KJ, et al. A comprehensive review of the natural history of *Helicobacter pylori* infection in children. *Arch Med Res.* 2000;31(5):431–469.
79. Malaty HM, El-Kasabany A, Graham DY, et al. Age at acquisition of *Helicobacter pylori* infection: a follow-up study from infancy to adulthood. *Lancet.* 2002;359(9310):931–935.
80. Lam SK, Talley NJ. Report of the 1997 Asia Pacific Consensus Conference on the management of *Helicobacter pylori* infection. *J Gastroenterol Hepatol.* 1998;13(1):1–12.
81. Malfertheiner P, Megraud F, O'Morain C, et al. Current concepts in the management of *Helicobacter pylori* infection: the Maastricht III Consensus report. *Gut.* 2007;56(6):772–781.
82. Dore MP, Malaty HM, Graham DY, et al. Risk factors associated with *Helicobacter pylori* infection among children in a defined geographic area. *Clin Infect Dis.* 2002;35(3):240–245.
83. Sung JJ, Kuipers EJ, El-Serag HB. Systematic review: the global incidence and prevalence of peptic ulcer disease. *Aliment Pharmacol Ther.* 2009;29(9):938–946.
84. Perez-Perez GI, Taylor DN, Bodhidatta L, et al. Seroprevalence of *Helicobacter pylori* infections in Thailand. *J Infect Dis.* 1990;161(6):1237–1241.
85. Ricuarte O, Gutierrez O, Cardona H, et al. Atrophic gastritis in young children and adolescents. *J Clin Pathol.* 2005;58(11):1189–1193.
86. Malaty HM, Evans DG, Evans DJ Jr, et al. *Helicobacter pylori* in Hispanics: comparison with blacks and whites of similar age and socioeconomic class. *Gastroenterology.* 1992;103(3):813–816.
87. Tan HJ, Goh KL. Changing epidemiology of *Helicobacter pylori* in Asia. *J Dig Dis.* 2008;9(4):186–189.
88. Yim JY, Kim N, Choi SH, et al. Seroprevalence of *Helicobacter pylori* in South Korea. *Helicobacter.* 2007;12(4):333–340.
89. Pounder RE, Ng D. The prevalence of *Helicobacter pylori* infection in different countries. *Aliment Pharmacol Ther.* 1995;9(suppl 2):33–39.
90. Blaser MJ. Epidemiology and pathophysiology of *Campylobacter pylori* infections. *Rev Infect Dis.* 1990;12(suppl 1):S99–S106.

91. Kumagai T, Malaty HM, Graham DY, et al. Acquisition versus loss of *Helicobacter pylori* infection in Japan: results from an 8-year birth cohort study. *J Infect Dis.* 1998;178(3):717-721.
92. Bourke B, Ceponis P, Chiba N, et al. Canadian Helicobacter Study Group Consensus Conference: update on the approach to *Helicobacter pylori* infection in children and adolescents—an evidence-based evaluation. *Can J Gastroenterol.* 2005;19(7):399-408.
93. Caselli M, Zullo A, Maconi G, et al. "Cervia II Working Group Report 2006": guidelines on diagnosis and treatment of *Helicobacter pylori* infection in Italy. *Dig Liver Dis.* 2007;39(8):782-789.
94. Drumm B, Perez-Perez GI, Blaser MJ, et al. Intrafamilial clustering of *Helicobacter pylori* infection. *N Engl J Med.* 1990;322(6):359-363.
95. Malaty HM, Kumagai T, Tanaka E, et al. Evidence from a nine-year birth cohort study in Japan of transmission pathways of *Helicobacter pylori* infection. *J Clin Microbiol.* 2000;38(5):1971-1973.
96. Azevedo NF, Guimaraes N, Figueiredo C, et al. A new model for the transmission of *Helicobacter pylori*: role of environmental reservoirs as gene pools to increase strain diversity. *Crit Rev Microbiol.* 2007;33(3):157-169.
97. Nurgalieva ZZ, Malaty HM, Graham DY, et al. *Helicobacter pylori* infection in Kazakhstan: effect of water source and household hygiene. *Am J Trop Med Hyg.* 2002;67(2):201-206.
98. Fujimura S, Kato S, Watanabe A. Water source as a *Helicobacter pylori* transmission route: a 3-year follow-up study of Japanese children living in a unique district. *J Med Microbiol.* 2008;57(pt 7):909-910.
99. Bockelmann U, Dorries HH, Ayuso-Gabella MN, et al. Quantitative PCR monitoring of antibiotic resistance genes and bacterial pathogens in three European artificial groundwater recharge systems. *Appl Environ Microbiol.* 2009;75(1):154-163.
100. Yamaoka Y. *Helicobacter pylori* typing as a tool for tracking human migration. *Clin Microbiol Infect.* 2009;15(9):829-834.
101. Falush D, Wirth T, Linz B, et al. Traces of human migrations in *Helicobacter pylori* populations. *Science.* 2003;299 (5612):1582-1585.
102. Linz B, Balloux F, Moodley Y, et al. An African origin for the intimate association between humans and *Helicobacter pylori*. *Nature.* 2007;445(7130):915-918.
103. Moodley Y, Linz B, Yamaoka Y, et al. The peopling of the Pacific from a bacterial perspective. *Science.* 2009; 323(5913):527-530.
104. Linz B, Schuster SC. Genomic diversity in *Helicobacter* and related organisms. *Res Microbiol.* 2007;158(10):737-744.
105. Baldwin DN, Shepherd B, Kraemer P, et al. Identification of *Helicobacter pylori* genes that contribute to stomach colonization. *Infect Immun.* 2007;75(2):1005-1016.
106. Kusters JG, van Vliet AH, Kuipers EJ. Pathogenesis of *Helicobacter pylori* infection. *Clin Microbiol Rev.* 2006;19(3): 449-490.
107. Backert S, Selbach M. Role of type IV secretion in *Helicobacter pylori* pathogenesis. *Cell Microbiol.* 2008;10(8):1573-1581.
108. Viala J, Chaput C, Boneca IG, et al. Nod1 responds to peptidoglycan delivered by the *Helicobacter pylori* cag pathogenicity island. *Nat Immunol.* 2004;5(11):1166-1174.
109. Baldwin MP. Subject to empire: married women and the British nationality and status of Aliens Act. *J Br Stud.* 2001;40(4):522-556.
110. Faber K. Chronic gastritis: its relation to achlorhydria and ulcer. *Lancet.* 1927;2:15.
111. Stemmermann GN, Hayashi T. Intestinal metaplasia of the gastric mucosa: a gross and microscopic study of its distribution in various disease states. *J Natl Cancer Inst.* 1968;41(3):627-634.
112. Lambert R. Chronic gastritis. A critical study of the progressive atrophy of the gastric mucosa. *Digestion.* 1972;7(1):83-126.
113. Faber K. Chronic gastritis: its relation to achlorhydria and ulcer. *Lancet.* 1927;2:902-917.
114. Graham DY. *Helicobacter pylori*: its epidemiology and its role in duodenal ulcer disease. *J Gastroenterol Hepatol.* 1991;6(2):105-113.
115. Dixon MF. *Helicobacter pylori* and peptic ulceration: histopathological aspects. *J Gastroenterol Hepatol.* 1991;6(2): 125-130.
116. Graham DY. *Campylobacter pylori* and peptic ulcer disease. *Gastroenterology.* 1989;96(2 pt 2 suppl):615-625.
117. Burstein M, Monge E, Leon-Barua R, et al. Low peptic ulcer and high gastric cancer prevalence in a developing country with a high prevalence of infection by *Helicobacter pylori*. *J Clin Gastroenterol.* 1991;13(2):154-156.
118. Meining A, Stolte M, Hatz R, et al. Differing degree and distribution of gastritis in *Helicobacter pylori*-associated diseases. *Virchows Arch.* 1997;431(1):11-15.
119. Malaty HM, Kim JG, El-Zimaity HM, et al. High prevalence of duodenal ulcer and gastric cancer in dyspeptic patients in Korea. *Scand J Gastroenterol.* 1997;32(8):751-754.
120. El-Zimaity HMT, Gutierrez O, Kim JG, et al. Geographic differences in the distribution of intestinal metaplasia in duodenal ulcer patients. *Am J Gastroenterol.* 2001;96(3):666-672.
121. Recavarren-Arce S, Leon-Barua R, Cok J, et al. *Helicobacter pylori* and progressive gastric pathology that predisposes to gastric cancer. *Scand J Gastroenterol Suppl.* 1991;181:51-57.
122. Sipponen P. Gastric cancer—a long-term consequence of *Helicobacter pylori* infection? *Scand J Gastroenterol Suppl.* 1994;201:24-27.
123. Weeks DL, Eskandari S, Scott DR, et al. A H^+-gated urea channel: the link between *Helicobacter pylori* urease and gastric colonization. *Science.* 2000;287(5452):482-485.
124. Mobley HL, Cortesia MJ, Rosenthal LE, et al. Characterization of urease from *Campylobacter pylori*. *J Clin Microbiol.* 1988;26(5):831-836.
125. Schreiber S, Konradt M, Groll C, et al. The spatial orientation of *Helicobacter pylori* in the gastric mucus. *Proc Natl Acad Sci U S A.* 2004;101(14):5024-5029.
126. Meyer-Rosberg K, Scott DR, Rex D, et al. The effect of environmental pH on the proton motive force of *Helicobacter pylori*. *Gastroenterology.* 1996;111(4):886-900.
127. McGowan CC, Cover TL, Blaser MJ. *Helicobacter pylori* and gastric acid: biological and therapeutic implications. *Gastroenterology.* 1996;110(3):926-938.
128. Greig MA, Neithercut WD, Hossack M, et al. Harnessing of urease activity of *Helicobacter pylori* to induce self-destruction of the bacterium. *J Clin Pathol.* 1991;44(2):157-159.
129. Neithercut WD, Williams C, Hossack MS, et al. Ammonium metabolism and protection from urease mediated destruction in *Helicobacter pylori* infection. *J Clin Pathol.* 1993;46(1):75-78.
130. Williams C, Neithercut WD, Hossack M, et al. Urease-mediated destruction of bacteria is specific for *Helicobacter* urease and results in total cellular disruption. *FEMS Immunol Med Microbiol.* 1994;9(4):273-280.
131. Graham DY, Opekun AR, Osato MS, et al. Challenge model for *Helicobacter pylori* infection in human volunteers. *Gut.* 2004;53(9):1235-1243.
132. Collins JS, Hamilton PW, Watt PC, et al. Superficial gastritis and *Campylobacter pylori* in dyspeptic patients—a quantitative study using computer-linked image analysis. *J Pathol.* 1989;158(4):303-310.

133. Bujanover Y, Konikoff F, Baratz M. Nodular gastritis and *Helicobacter pylori*. *J Pediatr Gastroenterol Nutr*. 1990;11(1):41–44.
134. Hassall E, Dimmick JE. Unique features of *Helicobacter pylori* disease in children. *Dig Dis Sci*. 1991;36(4):417–423.
135. Siurala M, Sipponen P, Kekki M. *Campylobacter pylori* in a sample of Finnish population: relations to morphology and functions of the gastric mucosa. *Gut*. 1988;29(7):909–915.
136. el-Zimaity HM, al-Assi MT, Genta RM, et al. Confirmation of successful therapy of *Helicobacter pylori* infection: number and site of biopsies or a rapid urease test. *Am J Gastroenterol*. 1995;90(11):1962–1964.
137. El-Zimaity HM, Graham DY. Evaluation of gastric mucosal biopsy site and number for identification of *Helicobacter pylori* or intestinal metaplasia: role of the Sydney system. *Hum Pathol*. 1999;30(1):72–77.
138. Broussard CS, Goodman KJ, Phillips CV, et al. Antibiotics taken for other illnesses and spontaneous clearance of *Helicobacter pylori* infection in children. *Pharmacoepidemiol Drug Saf*. 2009;18(8):722–729.
139. Sobala GM, Crabtree JE, Dixon MF, et al. Acute *Helicobacter pylori* infection: clinical features, local and systemic immune response, gastric mucosal histology, and gastric juice ascorbic acid concentrations. *Gut*. 1991;32(11):1415–1418.
140. Yamauchi K, Choi IJ, Lu H, et al. Regulation of IL-18 in *Helicobacter pylori* infection. *J Immunol*. 2008;180(2):1207–1216.
141. Sugimoto M, Furuta T, Yamaoka Y. Influence of inflammatory cytokine polymorphisms on eradication rates of *Helicobacter pylori*. *J Gastroenterol Hepatol*. 2009;24(11):1725–1732.
142. Nakajima S, Bamba N, Hattori T. Histological aspects and role of mast cells in *Helicobacter pylori*-infected gastritis. *Aliment Pharmacol Ther*. 2004;20(suppl 1):165–170.
143. Genta RM, Graham DY. Comparison of biopsy sites for the histopathologic diagnosis of *Helicobacter pylori*: a topographic study of *H. pylori* density and distribution. *Gastrointest Endosc*. 1994;40(3):342–345.
144. Graham DY, Opekun A, Lew GM, et al. *Helicobacter pylori*-associated exaggerated gastrin release in duodenal ulcer patients. The effect of bombesin infusion and urea ingestion. *Gastroenterology*. 1991;100(6):1571–1575.
145. Fitzgibbons PL, Dooley CP, Cohen H, et al. Prevalence of gastric metaplasia, inflammation, and *Campylobacter pylori* in the duodenum of members of a normal population. *Am J Clin Pathol*. 1988;90(6):711–714.
146. Sipponen P. Atrophic gastritis as a premalignant condition. *Ann Med*. 1989;21(4):287–290.
147. Vaananen H, Vauhkonen M, Helske T, et al. Non-endoscopic diagnosis of atrophic gastritis with a blood test. Correlation between gastric histology and serum levels of gastrin-17 and pepsinogen I: a multicentre study. *Eur J Gastroenterol Hepatol*. 2003;15(8):885–891.
148. Sipponen P, Ranta P, Helske T, et al. Serum levels of amidated gastrin-17 and pepsinogen I in atrophic gastritis: an observational case-control study. *Scand J Gastroenterol*. 2002;37(7):785–791.
149. Siurala M, Sipponen P, Kekki M. Chronic gastritis: dynamic and clinical aspects. *Scand J Gastroenterol Suppl*. 1985;109:69–76.
150. El-Zimaity HM, Ota H, Graham DY, et al. Patterns of gastric atrophy in intestinal type gastric carcinoma. *Cancer*. 2002;94(5):1428–1436.
151. Lamberts R, Creutzfeldt W, Struber HG, et al. Long-term omeprazole therapy in peptic ulcer disease: gastrin, endocrine cell growth, and gastritis. *Gastroenterology*. 1993;104(5):1356–1370.
152. Kuipers EJ, Uyterlinde AM, Pena AS, et al. Increase of *Helicobacter pylori*-associated corpus gastritis during acid suppressive therapy: implications for long-term safety. *Am J Gastroenterol*. 1995;90(9):1401–1406.
153. Moayyedi P, Wason C, Peacock R, et al. Changing patterns of *Helicobacter pylori* gastritis in long-standing acid suppression. *Helicobacter*. 2000;5(4):206–214.
154. Kim HY, Kim YB, Park CK, et al. Co-existing gastric cancer and duodenal ulcer disease: role of *Helicobacter pylori* infection. *Helicobacter*. 1997;2(4):205–209.
155. Ricci C, Holton J, Vaira D. Diagnosis of *Helicobacter pylori*: invasive and non-invasive tests. *Best Pract Res Clin Gastroenterol*. 2007;21(2):299–313.
156. Liston R, Pitt MA, Banerjee AK. IgG ELISA antibodies and detection of *Helicobacter pylori* in elderly patients. *Lancet*. 1996;347(8996):269.
157. Nardone G, Coscione P, D'Armiento FP, et al. Cirrhosis negatively affects the efficiency of serologic diagnosis of *Helicobacter pylori* infection. *Ital J Gastroenterol*. 1996;28(6):332–336.
158. Feldman M, Cryer B, Lee E, et al. Role of seroconversion in confirming cure of *Helicobacter pylori* infection. *JAMA*. 1998;280(4):363–365.
159. Elitsur Y, Tolia V, Gilger MA, et al. Urea breath test in children: the United States prospective, multicenter study. *Helicobacter*. 2009;14(2):134–140.
160. Braden B, Teuber G, Dietrich CF, et al. Comparison of new faecal antigen test with (13)C-urea breath test for detecting *Helicobacter pylori* infection and monitoring eradication treatment: prospective clinical evaluation. *BMJ*. 2000;320(7228):148.
161. Trevisani L, Sartori S, Galvani F, et al. Evaluation of a new enzyme immunoassay for detecting *Helicobacter pylori* in feces: a prospective pilot study. *Am J Gastroenterol*. 1999;94(7):1830–1833.
162. Vaira D, Malfertheiner P, Megraud F, et al. Diagnosis of *Helicobacter pylori* infection with a new non-invasive antigen-based assay. HpSA European study group. *Lancet*. 1999;354(9172):30–33.
163. Bravo LE, Realpe JL, Campo C, et al. Effects of acid suppression and bismuth medications on the performance of diagnostic tests for *Helicobacter pylori* infection. *Am J Gastroenterol*. 1999;94(9):2380–2383.
164. Gatta L, Vakil N, Ricci C, et al. Effect of proton pump inhibitors and antacid therapy on 13C urea breath tests and stool test for *Helicobacter pylori* infection. *Am J Gastroenterol*. 2004;99(5):823–829.
165. Laine L, Lewin D, Naritoku W, et al. Prospective comparison of commercially available rapid urease tests for the diagnosis of *Helicobacter pylori*. *Gastrointest Endosc*. 1996;44(5):523–526.
166. Gisbert JP, Abraira V. Accuracy of *Helicobacter pylori* diagnostic tests in patients with bleeding peptic ulcer: a systematic review and meta-analysis. *Am J Gastroenterol*. 2006;101(4):848–863.
167. Wang XI, Zhang S, Abreo F, et al. The role of routine immunohistochemistry for *Helicobacter pylori* in gastric biopsy. *Ann Diagn Pathol*. 2010;14(4):256–259.
168. El-Zimaity HM, Segura AM, Genta RM, et al. Histologic assessment of *Helicobacter pylori* status after therapy: comparison of Giemsa, Diff-Quik, and Genta stains. *Mod Pathol*. 1998;11(3):288–291.
169. El-Zimaity HM, Wu J, Akamatsu T, et al. A reliable method for the simultaneous identification of *H. pylori* and gastric metaplasia in the duodenum. *J Clin Pathol*. 1999;52(12):914–916.
170. Genta RM, Robason GO, Graham DY. Simultaneous visualization of *Helicobacter pylori* and gastric morphology: a new stain. *Hum Pathol*. 1994;25(3):221–226.
171. Gutierrez O, Akamatsu T, Cardona H, et al. *Helicobacter pylori* and hetertopic gastric mucosa in the upper esophagus (the inlet patch). *Am J Gastroenterol*. 2003;98(6):1266–1270.

172. Anim JT, Al-Sobkie N, Prasad A, et al. Assessment of different methods for staining *Helicobacter pylori* in endoscopic gastric biopsies. *Acta Histochem.* 2000;102(2):129–137.
173. el Zimaity HM, Wu J, Graham DY. Modified Genta triple stain for identifying *Helicobacter pylori*. *J Clin Pathol.* 1999;52(9):693–694.
174. Mendoza ML, Martin-Rabadan P, Carrion I, et al. *Helicobacter pylori* infection. Rapid diagnosis with brush cytology. *Acta Cytol.* 1993;37(2):181–185.
175. Seo TH, Lee SY, Uchida T, et al. The origin of non-*H. pylori*-related positive Giemsa staining in human gastric biopsy specimens: a prospective study. *Dig Liver Dis.* 2011;43(1):23–27.
176. Vartanian RK, Leung JK, Davis JE, et al. A novel Alcian yellow-toluidine blue (Leung) stain for *Helicobacter* species: comparison with standard stains, a cost-effectiveness analysis, and supplemental utilities. *Mod Pathol.* 1998;11(1):72–78.
177. Chey WD, Wong BC. American College of Gastroenterology guideline on the management of *Helicobacter pylori* infection. *Am J Gastroenterol.* 2007;102(8):1808–1825.
178. Bytzer P, Teglbjaerg PS. *Helicobacter pylori*-negative duodenal ulcers: prevalence, clinical characteristics, and prognosis—results from a randomized trial with 2-year follow-up. *Am J Gastroenterol.* 2001;96(5):1409–1416.
179. Jonkers D, Stobberingh E, de Bruine A, et al. Evaluation of immunohistochemistry for the detection of *Helicobacter pylori* in gastric mucosal biopsies. *J Infect.* 1997;35(2):149–154.
180. Andersen LP, Rasmussen L. *Helicobacter pylori*-coccoid forms and biofilm formation. *FEMS Immunol Med Microbiol.* 2009;56(2):112–115.
181. Kimura K. Chronological transition of the fundic-pyloric border determined by stepwise biopsy of the lesser and greater curvatures of the stomach. *Gastroenterology.* 1972;63(4):584–592.
182. El-Zimaity HM, Ramchatesingh J, Saeed MA, et al. Gastric intestinal metaplasia: subtypes and natural history. *J Clin Pathol.* 2001;54(9):679–683.
183. Tarpila S, Kekki M, Samloff IM, et al. Morphology and dynamics of the gastric mucosa in duodenal ulcer patients and their first-degree relatives. *Hepatogastroenterology.* 1983;30(5):198–201.
184. Correa P. A human model of gastric carcinogenesis. *Cancer Res.* 1988;48(13):3554–3560.
185. Correa P, Cuello C, Duque E. Carcinoma and intestinal metaplasia of the stomach in Colombian migrants. *J Natl Cancer Inst.* 1970;44(2):297–306.
186. Correa P. *Helicobacter pylori* and gastric carcinogenesis. *Am J Surg Pathol.* 1995;19(suppl 1):S37–S43.
187. Begue RE, Gonzales JL, Correa-Gracian H, et al. *Helicobacter pylori* infection in children with abdominal ailments in a developing country. *Am J Med Sci.* 1997;314(5):279–283.
188. Oi M, Oshida K, Sugimura S. The location of gastric ulcer. *Gastroenterology.* 1959;36(1):45–56.
189. Graham DY, Opekun AR, Yamaoka Y, et al. Early events in proton pump inhibitor-associated exacerbation of corpus gastritis. *Aliment Pharmacol Ther.* 2003;17(2):193–200.
190. Stolte M, Vieth M. Gastritis and gastric cancer: which morphological type of *Helicobacter* gastritis is a precancerous risk? *Chin J Dig Dis.* 2005;6(3):110–111.
191. Kelly EJ, Lagopoulos M, Primrose JN. Immunocytochemical localisation of parietal cells and G cells in the developing human stomach. *Gut.* 1993;34(8):1057–1059.
192. Cornaggia M, Capella C, Riva C, et al. Electron immunocytochemical localization of pepsinogen I (PgI) in chief cells, mucous-neck cells and transitional mucous-neck/chief cells of the human fundic mucosa. *Histochemistry.* 1986;85(1):5–11.
193. Wright NA, Pike C, Elia G. Induction of a novel epidermal growth factor-secreting cell lineage by mucosal ulceration in human gastrointestinal stem cells. *Nature.* 1990;343(6253):82–85.
194. Helpap B, Hattori T, Gedigk P. Repair of gastric ulcer. A cell kinetic study. *Virchows Arch A Pathol Anat Histol.* 1981;392(2):159–170.
195. Hattori T, Helpap B, Gedigk P. The morphology and cell kinetics of pseudopyloric glands. *Virchows Arch B Cell Pathol Incl Mol Pathol.* 1982;39(1):31–40.
196. Savage A, Jones S. Histological appearances of the gastric mucosa 15–27 years after partial gastrectomy. *J Clin Pathol.* 1979;32(2):179–186.
197. Filipe MI, Munoz N, Matko I, et al. Intestinal metaplasia types and the risk of gastric cancer: a cohort study in Slovenia. *Int J Cancer.* 1994;57(3):324–329.
198. Rokkas T, Filipe MI, Sladen GE. Detection of an increased incidence of early gastric cancer in patients with intestinal metaplasia type III who are closely followed up. *Gut.* 1991;32(10):1110–1113.
199. Huang CB, Xu J, Huang JF, et al. Sulphomucin colonic type intestinal metaplasia and carcinoma in the stomach. A histochemical study of 115 cases obtained by biopsy. *Cancer.* 1986;57(7):1370–1375.
200. Filipe MI, Potet F, Bogomoletz WV, et al. Incomplete sulphomucin-secreting intestinal metaplasia for gastric cancer. Preliminary data from a prospective study from three centres. *Gut.* 1985;26(12):1319–1326.
201. Silva S, Filipe MI, Pinho A. Variants of intestinal metaplasia in the evolution of chronic atrophic gastritis and gastric ulcer. A follow up study. *Gut.* 1990;31(10):1097–1104.
202. Siurala M, Lehtola J, Ihamaki T. Atrophic gastritis and its sequelae. Results of 19-23 years' follow-up examinations. *Scand J Gastroenterol.* 1974;9(5):441–446.
203. Rosch W, Demling L, Elster K. Is chronic gastritis a reversible process? Follow-up study of gastritis by step-wise biopsy. *Acta Hepatogastroenterol (Stuttg).* 1975;22(4):252–255.
204. Maaroos HI, Salupere V, Uibo R, et al. Seven-year follow-up study of chronic gastritis in gastric ulcer patients. *Scand J Gastroenterol.* 1985;20(2):198–204.
205. Ihamaki T, Kekki M, Sipponen P, et al. The sequelae and course of chronic gastritis during a 30- to 34-year bioptic follow-up study. *Scand J Gastroenterol.* 1985;20(4):485–491.
206. Villako K, Kekki M, Maaroos HI, et al. Chronic gastritis: progression of inflammation and atrophy in a six-year endoscopic follow-up of a random sample of 142 Estonian urban subjects. *Scand J Gastroenterol Suppl.* 1991;186:135–141.
207. Niemela S, Karttunen T, Kerola T. *Helicobacter pylori*-associated gastritis. Evolution of histologic changes over 10 years. *Scand J Gastroenterol.* 1995;30(6):542–549.
208. Valle J, Kekki M, Sipponen P, et al. Long-term course and consequences of *Helicobacter pylori* gastritis. Results of a 32-year follow-up study. *Scand J Gastroenterol.* 1996;31(6):546–550.
209. Kato I, Tominaga S, Ito Y, et al. Atrophic gastritis and stomach cancer risk: cross-sectional analyses. *Jpn J Cancer Res.* 1992;83(10):1041–1046.
210. Graham DY, Lew GM, Lechago J. Antral G-cell and D-cell numbers in *Helicobacter pylori* infection: effect of *H. pylori* eradication. *Gastroenterology.* 1993;104(6):1655–1660.
211. Fry J. Peptic ulcer: a profile. *Br Med J.* 1964;2(5412):809–812.
212. Greibe J, Bugge P, Gjorup T, et al. Long-term prognosis of duodenal ulcer: follow-up study and survey of doctors' estimates. *Br Med J.* 1977;2(6102):1572–1574.
213. Kato Y, Kitagawa T, Yanagisawa A, et al. Site-dependent development of complete and incomplete intestinal metaplasia types in the human stomach. *Jpn J Cancer Res.* 1992;83(2):178–183.

214. Ramesar KC, Sanders DS, Hopwood D. Limited value of type III intestinal metaplasia in predicting risk of gastric carcinoma. *J Clin Pathol.* 1987;40(11):1287–1290.
215. Oohara T, Tohma H, Aono G, et al. Intestinal metaplasia of the regenerative epithelia in 549 gastric ulcers. *Hum Pathol.* 1983;14(12):1066–1071.
216. Boparai V, Rajagopalan J, Triadafilopoulos G. Guide to the use of proton pump inhibitors in adult patients. *Drugs.* 2008;68(7):925–947.
217. Kuipers EJ, Lundell L, Klinkenberg-Knol EC, et al. Atrophic gastritis and *Helicobacter pylori* infection in patients with reflux esophagitis treated with omeprazole or fundoplication. *N Engl J Med.* 1996;334(16):1018–1022.
218. Stolte M, Meining A, Schmitz JM, et al. Changes in *Helicobacter pylori*-induced gastritis in the antrum and corpus during 12 months of treatment with omeprazole and lansoprazole in patients with gastro-oesophageal reflux disease. *Aliment Pharmacol Ther.* 1998;12(3):247–253.
219. Stolte M, Bethke B. Elimination of *Helicobacter pylori* under treatment with omeprazole. *Z Gastroenterol.* 1990;28(6):271–274.
220. Klinkenberg-Knol EC, Festen HP, Jansen JB, et al. Long-term treatment with omeprazole for refractory reflux esophagitis: efficacy and safety. *Ann Intern Med.* 1994;121(3):161–167.
221. Meining A, Bosseckert H, Caspary WF, et al. H2-receptor antagonists and antacids have an aggravating effect on *Helicobacter pylori* gastritis in duodenal ulcer patients. *Aliment Pharmacol Ther.* 1997;11(4):729–734.
222. Schenk BE, Kuipers EJ, Nelis GF, et al. Effect of *Helicobacter pylori* eradication on chronic gastritis during omeprazole therapy. *Gut.* 2000;46(5):615–621.
223. Berstad AE, Hatlebakk JG, Maartmann-Moe H, et al. *Helicobacter pylori* gastritis and epithelial cell proliferation in patients with reflux oesophagitis after treatment with lansoprazole. *Gut.* 1997;41(6):740–747.
224. Eissele R, Brunner G, Simon B, et al. Gastric mucosa during treatment with lansoprazole: *Helicobacter pylori* is a risk factor for argyrophil cell hyperplasia. *Gastroenterology.* 1997;112(3):707–717.
225. Furuta T, Baba S, Takashima M, et al. Effect of *Helicobacter pylori* infection on gastric juice pH. *Scand J Gastroenterol.* 1998;33(4):357–363.
226. Kuipers EJ, Uyterlinde AM, Pena AS, et al. Increase of *Helicobacter pylori*-associated corpus gastritis during acid suppressive therapy: implications for long-term safety. *Am J Gastroenterol.* 1995;90(9):1401–1406.
227. Unge P, Gad A, Gnarpe H, et al. Does omeprazole improve antimicrobial therapy directed towards gastric *Campylobacter pylori* in patients with antral gastritis? A pilot study. *Scand J Gastroenterol Suppl.* 1989;167:49–54.
228. Klinkenberg-Knol EC, Nelis F, Dent J, et al. Long-term omeprazole treatment in resistant gastroesophageal reflux disease: efficacy, safety, and influence on gastric mucosa. *Gastroenterology.* 2000;118(4):661–669.
229. Chourasia D, Misra A, Pandey R, et al. Gastric atrophy and intestinal metaplasia in a patient on long-term proton pump inhibitor therapy. *Trop Gastroenterol.* 2008;29(3):172–174.
230. Logan RP, Walker MM, Misiewicz JJ, et al. Changes in the intragastric distribution of *Helicobacter pylori* during treatment with omeprazole. *Gut.* 1995;36(1):12–16.
231. Graham DY, Opekun AR, Hammoud F, et al. Studies regarding the mechanism of false negative urea breath tests with proton pump inhibitors. *Am J Gastroenterol.* 2003;98(5):1005–1009.
232. Cohen H, Weinstein WM, Carmel R. Heterogeneity of gastric histology and function in food cobalamin malabsorption: absence of atrophic gastritis and achlorhydria in some patients with severe malabsorption. *Gut.* 2000;47(5):638–645.
233. Hirschowitz BI, Worthington J, Mohnen J. Vitamin B_{12} deficiency in hypersecretors during long-term acid suppression with proton pump inhibitors. *Aliment Pharmacol Ther.* 2008;27(11):1110–1121.
234. Cote GA, Howden CW. Potential adverse effects of proton pump inhibitors. *Curr Gastroenterol Rep.* 2008;10(3):208–214.
235. Graham DY. *Helicobacter pylori* infection in the pathogenesis of duodenal ulcer and gastric cancer: a model. *Gastroenterology.* 1997;113(6):1983–1991.
236. Graham DY. *Helicobacter pylori* infection is the primary cause of gastric cancer. *J Gastroenterol.* 2000;35(suppl 12):90–97.
237. Iijima K, Abe Y, Kikuchi R, et al. Serum biomarker tests are useful in delineating between patients with gastric atrophy and normal, healthy stomach. *World J Gastroenterol.* 2009;15(7):853–859.
238. Dan YY, So JB, Yeoh KG. Endoscopic screening for gastric cancer. *Clin Gastroenterol Hepatol.* 2006;4(6):709–716.
239. Inoue T, Uedo N, Ishihara R, et al. Autofluorescence imaging videoendoscopy in the diagnosis of chronic atrophic fundal gastritis. *J Gastroenterol.* 2010;45(1):45–51.
240. Derakhshan MH, El-Omar E, Oien K, et al. Gastric histology, serological markers and age as predictors of gastric acid secretion in patients infected with *Helicobacter pylori*. *J Clin Pathol.* 2006;59(12):1293–1299.
241. Kokkola A, Louhimo J, Puolakkainen P, et al. *Helicobacter pylori* infection and low serum pepsinogen I level as risk factors for gastric carcinoma. *World J Gastroenterol.* 2005;11(7):1032–1036.
242. Storskrubb T, Aro P, Ronkainen J, et al. Serum biomarkers provide an accurate method for diagnosis of atrophic gastritis in a general population: the Kalixanda study. *Scand J Gastroenterol.* 2008;43(12):1448–1455.
243. Miki K, Ichinose M, Shimizu A, et al. Serum pepsinogens as a screening test of extensive chronic gastritis. *Gastroenterol Jpn.* 1987;22(2):133–141.
244. Kekki M, Samloff IM, Varis K, et al. Serum pepsinogen I and serum gastrin in the screening of severe atrophic corpus gastritis. *Scand J Gastroenterol Suppl.* 1991;186:109–116.
245. Varis K, Kekki M, Harkonen M, et al. Serum pepsinogen I and serum gastrin in the screening of atrophic pangastritis with high risk of gastric cancer. *Scand J Gastroenterol Suppl.* 1991;186:117–123.
246. Korstanje A, van Eeden S, Offerhaus JA, et al. Comparison between serology and histology in the diagnosis of advanced gastric body atrophy: a study in a Dutch primary community. *J Clin Gastroenterol.* 2008;42(1):18–22.
247. Meining A, Bayerdorffer E, Muller P, et al. Gastric carcinoma risk index in patients infected with *Helicobacter pylori*. *Virchows Arch.* 1998;432(4):311–314.
248. Rugge M, Meggio A, Pennelli G, et al. Gastritis staging in clinical practice: the OLGA staging system. *Gut.* 2007;56(5):631–636.
249. Graham DY, Nurgalieva ZZ, El-Zimaity HM, et al. Noninvasive versus histologic detection of gastric atrophy in a Hispanic population in North America. *Clin Gastroenterol Hepatol.* 2006;4(3):306–314.
250. de Vries AC, Haringsma J, de Vries RA, et al. The use of clinical, histologic, and serologic parameters to predict the intragastric extent of intestinal metaplasia: a recommendation for routine practice. *Gastrointest Endosc.* 2009;70(1):18–25.
251. Shimoyama T, Fukuda S, Tanaka M, et al. Evaluation of the applicability of the gastric carcinoma risk index for intestinal type cancer in Japanese patients infected with *Helicobacter pylori*. *Virchows Arch.* 2000;436(6):585–587.

252. Matsuhisa T, Miki M, Yamada N, et al. *Helicobacter pylori* infection, glandular atrophy, intestinal metaplasia and topography of chronic active gastritis in the Nepalese and Japanese population: the age, gender and endoscopic diagnosis matched study. *Kathmandu Univ Med J (KUMJ)*. 2007;5(3):295-301.
253. Uemura N, Okamoto S, Yamamoto S, et al. *Helicobacter pylori* infection and the development of gastric cancer. *N Engl J Med*. 2001;345(11):784-789.
254. Imagawa S, Yoshihara M, Ito M, et al. Evaluation of gastric cancer risk using topography of histological gastritis: a large-scaled cross-sectional study. *Dig Dis Sci*. 2008;53(7):1818-1823.
255. Longman RJ, Douthwaite J, Sylvester PA, et al. Coordinated localisation of mucins and trefoil peptides in the ulcer associated cell lineage and the gastrointestinal mucosa. *Gut*. 2000;47(6):792-800.
256. Capelle LG, de Vries AC, Haringsma J, et al. The staging of gastritis with the OLGA system by using intestinal metaplasia as an accurate alternative for atrophic gastritis. *Gastrointest Endosc*. 2010;71(7):1150-1158.
257. Ellison EH, Wilson SD. The Zollinger-Ellison syndrome: re-appraisal and evaluation of 260 registered cases. *Ann Surg*. 1964;160:512-530.
258. Laine L, Takeuchi K, Tarnawski A. Gastric mucosal defense and cytoprotection: bench to bedside. *Gastroenterology*. 2008;135(1):41-60.
259. Yoshida M, Wakabayashi G, Ishikawa H, et al. A possible defensive mechanism in the basal region of gastric mucosa and the healing of erosions. *Clin Hemorheol Microcirc*. 2003;29(3-4):301-312.
260. Murphy KD, Lee JO, Herndon DN. Current pharmacotherapy for the treatment of severe burns. *Expert Opin Pharmacother*. 2003;4(3):369-384.
261. Guth PH. Pathogenesis of gastric mucosal injury. *Annu Rev Med*. 1982;33:183-196.
262. Ritchie WP Jr. Acute gastric mucosal damage induced by bile salts, acid, and ischemia. *Gastroenterology*. 1975;68(4, pt 1):699-707.
263. Cherry RD, Jabbari M, Goresky CA, et al. Chronic mesenteric vascular insufficiency with gastric ulceration. *Gastroenterology*. 1986;91(6):1548-1552.
264. Shimizu T, Akamatsu T, Sugiyama A, et al. *Helicobacter pylori* and the surface mucous gel layer of the human stomach. *Helicobacter*. 1996;1(4):207-218.
265. Shimizu T, Akamatsu T, Ota H, et al. Immunohistochemical detection of *Helicobacter pylori* in the surface mucous gel layer and its clinicopathological significance. *Helicobacter*. 1996;1(4):197-206.
266. Allen A, Flemstrom G. Gastroduodenal mucus bicarbonate barrier: protection against acid and pepsin. *Am J Physiol Cell Physiol*. 2005;288(1):C1-C19.
267. Farrell JJ, Taupin D, Koh TJ, et al. TFF2/SP-deficient mice show decreased gastric proliferation, increased acid secretion, and increased susceptibility to NSAID injury. *J Clin Invest*. 2002;109(2):193-204.
268. Hoffmann W, Jagla W, Wiede A. Molecular medicine of TFF-peptides: from gut to brain. *Histol Histopathol*. 2001;16(1):319-334.
269. Poulsom R, Wright NA. Trefoil peptides: a newly recognized family of epithelial mucin-associated molecules. *Am J Physiol*. 1993;265(2, pt 1):G205-G213.
270. Taupin D, Podolsky DK. Trefoil factors: initiators of mucosal healing. *Nat Rev Mol Cell Biol*. 2003;4(9):721-732.
271. Isenberg JI, Selling JA, Hogan DL, et al. Impaired proximal duodenal mucosal bicarbonate secretion in patients with duodenal ulcer. *N Engl J Med*. 1987;316(7):374-379.
272. Robert A. Cytoprotection by prostaglandins. *Gastroenterology*. 1979;77(4, pt 1):761-767.
273. Redfern JS, Feldman M. Role of endogenous prostaglandins in preventing gastrointestinal ulceration: induction of ulcers by antibodies to prostaglandins. *Gastroenterology*. 1989;96(2 pt 2 suppl):596-605.
274. Soll AH, Kurata J, McGuigan JE. Ulcers, nonsteroidal anti-inflammatory drugs, and related matters. *Gastroenterology*. 1989;96(2 pt 2 suppl):561-568.
275. Silen W. What is cytoprotection of the gastric mucosa? *Gastroenterology*. 1988;94(1):232-235.
276. Gisbert JP, Calvet X. Review article: *Helicobacter pylori*-negative duodenal ulcer disease. *Aliment Pharmacol Ther*. 2009;30(8):791-815.
277. Schwartz K. Uber penetrierende magen and jejunalgeschwuve. *Beitr Klin Chir*. 1910;67:32.
278. Isenberg JI, Spector H, Hootkin LA, et al. An apparent exception to Schwarz's dictum, "no acid—no ulcer". *N Engl J Med*. 1971;285(11):620.
279. Reid J, Taylor TV, Holt S, et al. Benign gastric ulceration in pernicious anemia. *Dig Dis Sci*. 1980;25(2):148-149.
280. Marshall BJ, Warren JR. Unidentified curved bacilli in the stomach of patients with gastritis and peptic ulceration. *Lancet*. 1984;1(8390):1311-1315.
281. Dragstedt LR, Woodward ER, Linares CA, et al. The pathogenesis of gastric ulcer. *Ann Surg*. 1964;160:497-511.
282. Linares CA, Delarosa C, Woodward ER, et al. Experimental gastric ulcer. effect of gastroenterostomy and pyloroplasty on chronic gastric ulcers produced by vagotomy in rabbits. *Arch Surg*. 1964;88:932-938.
283. Vesely KT, Kubickova Z, Dvorakova M. Clinical data and characteristics differentiating types of peptic ulcer. *Gut*. 1968;9(1):57-68.
284. Johnson AG. Proximal gastric vagotomy: does it have a place in the future management of peptic ulcer? *World J Surg*. 2000;24(3):259-263.
285. Jones DB, Howden CW, Burget DW, et al. Acid suppression in duodenal ulcer: a meta-analysis to define optimal dosing with antisecretory drugs. *Gut*. 1987;28(9):1120-1127.
286. Osefo N, Ito T, Jensen RT. Gastric acid hypersecretory states: recent insights and advances. *Curr Gastroenterol Rep*. 2009;11(6):433-441.
287. Wormsley KG, Grossman MI. Maximal histalog test in control subjects and patients with peptic ulcer. *Gut*. 1965;6(5):427-435.
288. Johnson HD, Love AH, Rogers NC, et al. Gastric ulcers, blood groups, and acid secretion. *Gut*. 1964;5:402-411.
289. Lam SK. Pathogenesis and pathophysiology of duodenal ulcer. *Clin Gastroenterol*. 1984;13(2):447-472.
290. Grossman MI, Elashoff J. Antrectomy and maximal acid output. *Gastroenterology*. 1980;78(1):165-168.
291. Kirkpatrick PM Jr, Hirschowitz BI. Duodenal ulcer with unexplained marked basal gastric acid hypersecretion. *Gastroenterology*. 1980;79(1):4-10.
292. Feldman M, Richardson CT, Fordtran JS. Effect of sham feeding on gastric acid secretion in healthy subjects and duodenal ulcer patients: evidence for increased basal vagal tone in some ulcer patients. *Gastroenterology*. 1980;79(5, pt 1):796-800.
293. Kohn A, Annibale B, Suriano G, et al. Gastric acid and pancreatic polypeptide responses to modified sham feeding: indication of an increased basal vagal tone in a subgroup of duodenal ulcer patients. *Gut*. 1985;26(8):776-782.
294. Johansen A, Hansen OH. Heterotopic gastric epithelium in the duodenum and its correlation to gastric disease and acid level. *Acta Pathol Microbiol Scand A*. 1973;81(5):676-680.
295. Johansen A, Hansen OH. Macroscopically demonstrable heterotopic gastric mucosa in the duodenum. *Scand J Gastroenterol*. 1973;8(1):59-63.

296. Carrick J, Lee A, Hazell S, et al. Campylobacter pylori, duodenal ulcer, and gastric metaplasia: possible role of functional heterotopic tissue in ulcerogenesis. Gut. 1989;30(6):790–797.
297. Andersson N, Rhedin M, Peteri-Brunback B, et al. Gastrin effects on isolated rat enterochromaffin-like cells following long-term hypergastrinaemia in vivo. Biochim Biophys Acta. 1999;1451(2–3):297–304.
298. Wang TC, Dockray GJ. Lessons from genetically engineered animal models. I. Physiological studies with gastrin in transgenic mice. Am J Physiol. 1999;277(1, pt 1):G6–G11.
299. Saeed ZA, Evans DJ Jr, Evans DG, et al. Helicobacter pylori and Zollinger–Ellison syndrome. Dig Dis Sci. 1991;36(1):15–18.
300. Fich A, Talley NJ, Shorter RG, et al. Zollinger–Ellison syndrome. Relation to Helicobacter pylori-associated chronic gastritis and gastric acid secretion. Dig Dis Sci. 1991;36(1):10–14.
301. Wiersinga WM, Tytgat GN. Clinical recovery owing to target parietal cell failure in a patient with Zollinger–Ellison syndrome. Gastroenterology. 1977;73(6):1413–1417.
302. Orloff SL, Debas HT. Advances in the management of patients with Zollinger–Ellison syndrome. Surg Clin North Am. 1995;75(3):511–524.
303. Waxman I, Gardner JD, Jensen RT, et al. Peptic ulcer perforation as the presentation of Zollinger–Ellison syndrome. Dig Dis Sci. 1991;36(1):19–24.
304. Laine L, Marin-Sorensen M, Weinstein WM. Nonsteroidal antiinflammatory drug-associated gastric ulcers do not require Helicobacter pylori for their development. Am J Gastroenterol. 1992;87(10):1398–1402.
305. Blaser MJ. Gastric Campylobacter-like organisms, gastritis, and peptic ulcer disease. Gastroenterology. 1987;93(2):371–383.
306. Goodwin CS, Armstrong JA, Marshall BJ. Campylobacter pyloridis, gastritis, and peptic ulceration. J Clin Pathol. 1986;39(4):353–365.
307. Meikle DD, Taylor KB, Truelove SC, et al. Gastritis duodenitis, and circulating levels of gastrin in duodenal ulcer before and after vagotomy. Gut. 1976;17(9):719–728.
308. Greenlaw R, Sheahan DG, DeLuca V, et al. Gastroduodenitis. A broader concept of peptic ulcer disease. Dig Dis Sci. 1980;25(9):660–672.
309. Hui WM, Lam SK, Ho J, et al. Chronic antral gastritis in duodenal ulcer. Natural history and treatment with prostaglandin E1. Gastroenterology. 1986;91(5):1095–1101.
310. Ohkusa T, Okayasu I, Miwa H, et al. Helicobacter pylori infection induces duodenitis and superficial duodenal ulcer in Mongolian gerbils. Gut. 2003;52(6):797–803.
311. El-Serag HB, Sonnenberg A. Opposing time trends of peptic ulcer and reflux disease. Gut. 1998;43(3):327–333.
312. Banatvala N, Mayo K, Megraud F, et al. The cohort effect and Helicobacter pylori. J Infect Dis. 1993;168(1):219–221.
313. Redeen S, Petersson F, Kechagias S, et al. Natural history of chronic gastritis in a population-based cohort. Scand J Gastroenterol. 2010;45(5):540–549.
314. Larkai EN, Smith JL, Lidsky MD, et al. Gastroduodenal mucosa and dyspeptic symptoms in arthritic patients during chronic nonsteroidal anti-inflammatory drug use. Am J Gastroenterol. 1987;82(11):1153–1158.
315. Graham DY, Agrawal NM, Roth SH. Prevention of NSAID-induced gastric ulcer with misoprostol: multicentre, double-blind, placebo-controlled trial. Lancet. 1988;2(8623):1277–1280.
316. Langman MJ. Epidemiologic evidence on the association between peptic ulceration and antiinflammatory drug use. Gastroenterology. 1989;96(2 pt 2 suppl):640–646.
317. Fries JF, Miller SR, Spitz PW, et al. Toward an epidemiology of gastropathy associated with nonsteroidal anti-inflammatory drug use. Gastroenterology. 1989;96(2 pt 2 suppl):647–655.
318. Levy M. Aspirin use in patients with major upper gastrointestinal bleeding and peptic-ulcer disease. A report from the Boston Collaborative Drug Surveillance Program, Boston University Medical Center. N Engl J Med. 1974;290(21):1158–1162.
319. Elashoff JD, Grossman MI. Trends in hospital admissions and death rates for peptic ulcer in the United States from 1970 to 1978. Gastroenterology. 1980;78(2):280–285.
320. Laine L. Proton pump inhibitor co-therapy with nonsteroidal anti-inflammatory drugs—nice or necessary? Rev Gastroenterol Disord. 2004;4(suppl 4):S33–S41.
321. Cryer B. NSAID-associated deaths: the rise and fall of NSAID-associated GI mortality. Am J Gastroenterol. 2005;100(8):1694–1695.
322. Straube S, Tramer MR, Moore RA, et al. Mortality with upper gastrointestinal bleeding and perforation: effects of time and NSAID use. BMC Gastroenterol. 2009;9:41.
323. Lanas A, Perez-Aisa MA, Feu F, et al. A nationwide study of mortality associated with hospital admission due to severe gastrointestinal events and those associated with nonsteroidal antiinflammatory drug use. Am J Gastroenterol. 2005;100(8):1685–1693.
324. Langman MJ. Ulcer complications associated with anti-inflammatory drug use. What is the extent of the disease burden? Pharmacoepidemiol Drug Saf. 2001;10(1):13–19.
325. Gibson T. Nonsteroidal anti-inflammatory drugs—another look. Br J Rheumatol. 1988;27(2):87–90.
326. Wolfe MM, Lichtenstein DR, Singh G. Gastrointestinal toxicity of nonsteroidal antiinflammatory drugs. N Engl J Med. 1999;340(24):1888–1899.
327. Conn HO, Blitzer BL. Nonassociation of adrenocorticosteroid therapy and peptic ulcer. N Engl J Med. 1976;294(9):473–479.
328. Messer J, Reitman D, Sacks HS, et al. Association of adrenocorticosteroid therapy and peptic-ulcer disease. N Engl J Med. 1983;309(1):21–24.
329. Koek GH, Vos R, Sifrim D, et al. Mechanisms underlying duodeno-gastric reflux in man. Neurogastroenterol Motil. 2005;17(2):191–199.
330. Fein M, Fuchs KH, Bohrer T, et al. Fiberoptic technique for 24-hour bile reflux monitoring. Standards and normal values for gastric monitoring. Dig Dis Sci. 1996;41(1):216–225.
331. Fuchs KH, Fein M, Maroske J, et al. The role of 24-hr gastric pH-monitoring in the interpretation of 24-hr gastric bile monitoring for duodenogastric reflux. Hepatogastroenterology. 1999;46(25):60–65.
332. Dai F, Gong J, Zhang R, et al. Assessment of duodenogastric reflux by combined continuous intragastric pH and bilirubin monitoring. World J Gastroenterol. 2002;8(2):382–384.
333. Keane FB, Dimagno EP, Malagelada JR. Duodenogastric reflux in humans: its relationship to fasting antroduodenal motility and gastric, pancreatic, and biliary secretion. Gastroenterology. 1981;81(4):726–731.
334. Nakos A, Zezos P, Liratzopoulos N, et al. The significance of histological evidence of bile reflux gastropathy in patients with gastro-esophageal reflux disease. Med Sci Monit. 2009;15(6):CR313–CR318.
335. Thomas WE. The possible role of duodenogastric reflux in the pathogenesis of both gastric and duodenal ulcers. Scand J Gastroenterol Suppl. 1984;92:151–155.
336. Niemela S, Heikkila J, Lehtola J. Duodenogastric bile reflux in patients with gastric ulcer. Scand J Gastroenterol. 1984;19(7):896–898.

337. Brillantino A, Monaco L, Schettino M, et al. Prevalence of pathological duodenogastric reflux and the relationship between duodenogastric and duodenogastrooesophageal reflux in chronic gastroesophageal reflux disease. *Eur J Gastroenterol Hepatol.* 2008;20(12):1136–1143.
338. Stiel D, Piper DW. Duodenogastric reflux and chronic gastric ulcer. *Aust N Z J Med.* 1981;11(2):207.
339. Ritchie WP Jr, Felger TS. Differing ulcerogenic potential of dihydroxy and trihydroxy bile acids in canine gastric mucosa. *Surgery.* 1981;89(3):342–347.
340. Marshall R, Owen WJ. Role of duodenal juice in the pathogenesis of gastroesophageal reflux disease. *Ann Surg.* 1997;225(1):135–136.
341. Tack J, Koek G, Demedts I, et al. Gastroesophageal reflux disease poorly responsive to single-dose proton pump inhibitors in patients without Barrett's esophagus: acid reflux, bile reflux, or both? *Am J Gastroenterol.* 2004;99(6):981–988.
342. Champion G, Richter JE, Vaezi MF, et al. Duodenogastroesophageal reflux: relationship to pH and importance in Barrett's esophagus. *Gastroenterology.* 1994;107(3):747–754.
343. Kauer WK, Peters JH, DeMeester TR, et al. Mixed reflux of gastric and duodenal juices is more harmful to the esophagus than gastric juice alone. The need for surgical therapy re-emphasized. *Ann Surg.* 1995;222(4):525–531; discussion 531–533.
344. Lawson HH. Effect of duodenal contents on the gastric mucosa under experimental conditions. *Lancet.* 1964;1(7331):469–472.
345. Lorusso D, Pezzolla F, Linsalata M, et al. Duodenogastric reflux and gastric mucosal cell proliferation after cholecystectomy or Billroth II gastric resection. *Gastroenterol Clin Biol.* 1994;18(11):927–931.
346. Sundbom M, Hedenstrom H, Gustavsson S. Duodenogastric bile reflux after gastric bypass: a cholescintigraphic study. *Dig Dis Sci.* 2002;47(8):1891–1896.
347. Brough WA, Taylor TV, Torrance HB. The surgical factors influencing duodenogastric reflux. *Br J Surg.* 1984;71(10):770–773.
348. Lorusso D, Misciagna G, Mangini V, et al. Duodenogastric reflux of bile acids, gastrin and parietal cells, and gastric acid secretion before and 6 months after cholecystectomy. *Am J Surg.* 1990;159(6):575–578.
349. Lorusso D, Pezzolla F, Cavallini A, et al. A prospective study on duodenogastric reflux and on histological changes in gastric mucosa after cholecystectomy. *Gastroenterol Clin Biol.* 1992;16(4):328–333.
350. Friedman GD, Siegelaub AB, Seltzer CC. Cigarettes, alcohol, coffee and peptic ulcer. *N Engl J Med.* 1974;290(9):469–473.
351. McCarthy DM. Smoking and ulcers—time to quit. *N Engl J Med.* 1984;311(11):726–728.
352. Ainley CC, Forgacs IC, Keeling PW, et al. Outpatient endoscopic survey of smoking and peptic ulcer. *Gut.* 1986;27(6):648–651.
353. Eastwood GL. Is smoking still important in the pathogenesis of peptic ulcer disease? *J Clin Gastroenterol.* 1997;25(suppl 1):S1–S7.
354. Endoh K, Leung FW. Effects of smoking and nicotine on the gastric mucosa: a review of clinical and experimental evidence. *Gastroenterology.* 1994;107(3):864–878.
355. Satyanarayana MN. Capsaicin and gastric ulcers. *Crit Rev Food Sci Nutr.* 2006;46(4):275–328.
356. Feldman M, Walker P, Green JL, et al. Life events stress and psychosocial factors in men with peptic ulcer disease. A multidimensional case-controlled study. *Gastroenterology.* 1986;91(6):1370–1379.
357. Oh TY, Yeo M, Han SU, et al. Synergism of *Helicobacter pylori* infection and stress on the augmentation of gastric mucosal damage and its prevention with alpha-tocopherol. *Free Radic Biol Med.* 2005;38(11):1447–1457.
358. Levenstein S. The very model of a modern etiology: a biopsychosocial view of peptic ulcer. *Psychosom Med.* 2000;62(2):176–185.
359. Kim YS, Park SW, Kim MH, et al. Novel single nucleotide polymorphism of the VEGF gene as a risk predictor for gastroduodenal ulcers. *J Gastroenterol Hepatol.* 2008;23(suppl 2):S131–S139.
360. Doll R, Kellock TD. The separate inheritance of gastric and duodenal ulcers. *Ann Eugen.* 1951;16(3):231–240.
361. Ellis A, Woodrow JC. HLA and duodenal ulcer. *Gut.* 1979;20(9):760–762.
362. Goedhard JG, Biemond I, Pena AS, et al. HLA and duodenal ulcer in the Netherlands. *Tissue Antigens.* 1983;22(3):213–218.
363. Schwarz S, Morelli G, Kusecek B, et al. Horizontal versus familial transmission of *Helicobacter pylori*. *PLoS Pathog.* 2008;4(10):e1000180.
364. Nahar S, Kibria KM, Hossain ME, et al. Evidence of intrafamilial transmission of *Helicobacter pylori* by PCR-based RAPD fingerprinting in Bangladesh. *Eur J Clin Microbiol Infect Dis.* 2009;28(7):767–773.
365. Rotter JI, Sones JQ, Samloff IM, et al. Duodenal-ulcer disease associated with elevated serum pepsinogen I: an inherited autosomal dominant disorder. *N Engl J Med.* 1979;300(2):63–66.
366. Ammann RW, Vetter D, Deyhle P, et al. Gastrointestinal involvement in systemic mastocytosis. *Gut.* 1976;17(2):107–112.
367. Shaw JM. Genetic aspects of urticaria pigmentosa. *Arch Dermatol.* 1968;97(2):137–138.
368. Neuhauser G, Daly RF, Magnelli NC, et al. Essential tremor, nystagmus and duodenal ulceration. A "new" dominantly inherited condition. *Clin Genet.* 1976;9(1):81–91.
369. Van Allen MW, Frohlich JA, Davis JR. Inherited predisposition to generalized amyloidosis. Clinical and pathological study of a family with neuropathy, nephropathy, and peptic ulcer. *Neurology.* 1969;19(1):10–25.
370. Lam SK, Hui WK, Ho J, et al. Pachydermoperiostosis, hypertrophic gastropathy, and peptic ulcer. *Gastroenterology.* 1983;84(4):834–839.
371. Halal F, Gervais MH, Baillargeon J, et al. Gastro-cutaneous syndrome: peptic ulcer/hiatal hernia, multiple lentigines/cafe-au-lait spots, hypertelorism, and myopia. *Am J Med Genet.* 1982;11(2):161–176.
372. Langman MJ, Cooke AR. Gastric and duodenal ulcer and their associated diseases. *Lancet.* 1976;1(7961):680–683.
373. Hirasuna JD, Shelub I, Bolt RJ. Hyperhistaminemia and peptic ulcer. *West J Med.* 1979;131(2):140–143.
374. Olinger EJ, McCarthy DM, Young RC, et al. Hyperhistaminemia and hyperchlorhydria in basophilic granulocytic leukemia. *Gastroenterology.* 1976;71(4):667–669.
375. Kang JY, Wu AY, Sutherland IH, et al. Prevalence of peptic ulcer in patients undergoing maintenance hemodialysis. *Dig Dis Sci.* 1988;33(7):774–778.
376. Abram K, Silm H, Maaroos HI, et al. Risk factors associated with rosacea. *J Eur Acad Dermatol Venereol.* 2010;24(5):565–571.
377. Baron JH, Sonnenberg A. Early history of dyspepsia and peptic ulcer in the United States. *Am J Gastroenterol.* 2009;104(12):2893–2896.
378. Kurata JH, Haile BM. Epidemiology of peptic ulcer disease. *Clin Gastroenterol.* 1984;13(2):289–307.
379. Kurata JH, Honda GD, Frankl H. The incidence of duodenal and gastric ulcers in a large health maintenance organization. *Am J Public Health.* 1985;75(6):625–629.

380. Pulvertaft CN. Peptic ulcer in twon and country. *Br J Prev Soc Med*. 1959;13:131–138.
381. Bonnevie O. The incidence of duodenal ulcer in Copenhagen county. *Scand J Gastroenterol*. 1975;10(4):385–393.
382. Drumm B, Rhoads JM, Stringer DA, et al. Peptic ulcer disease in children: etiology, clinical findings, and clinical course. *Pediatrics*. 1988;82(3, pt 2):410–414.
383. Cucino C, Sonnenberg A. The long-term time trends of peptic ulcer and ulcerative colitis are interrelated. *Am J Gastroenterol*. 2002;97(10):2657–2662.
384. Baron JH, Sonnenberg A. Hospital admissions for peptic ulcer and indigestion in London and New York in the 19th and early 20th centuries. *Gut*. 2002;50(4):568–570.
385. Post PN, Kuipers EJ, Meijer GA. Declining incidence of peptic ulcer but not of its complications: a nation-wide study in the Netherlands. *Aliment Pharmacol Ther*. 2006;23(11):1587–1593.
386. Groenen MJ, Kuipers EJ, Hansen BE, et al. Incidence of duodenal ulcers and gastric ulcers in a Western population: back to where it started. *Can J Gastroenterol*. 2009;23(9):604–608.
387. Higham J, Kang JY, Majeed A. Recent trends in admissions and mortality due to peptic ulcer in England: increasing frequency of haemorrhage among older subjects. *Gut*. 2002;50(4):460–464.
388. Weil J, Langman MJ, Wainwright P, et al. Peptic ulcer bleeding: accessory risk factors and interactions with non-steroidal anti-inflammatory drugs. *Gut*. 2000;46(1):27–31.
389. Gabriel SE, Jaakkimainen L, Bombardier C. Risk for serious gastrointestinal complications related to use of non-steroidal anti-inflammatory drugs. A meta-analysis. *Ann Intern Med*. 1991;115(10):787–796.
390. Garcia Rodriguez LA, Barreales Tolosa L. Risk of upper gastrointestinal complications among users of traditional NSAIDs and COXIBs in the general population. *Gastroenterology*. 2007;132(2):498–506.
391. Rocca B, Davi G. Should patients with osteoarthritis be treated with COX2 inhibitors rather than traditional NSAIDs? *Nat Clin Pract Rheumatol*. 2007;3(6):316–317.
392. Yaghoobi M, Farrokhyar F, Yuan Y, et al. Is there an increased risk of GERD after *Helicobacter pylori* eradication?: a meta-analysis. *Am J Gastroenterol*. 2010;105(5):1007–1013.
393. Borody TJ, Cole P, Noonan S, et al. Recurrence of duodenal ulcer and *Campylobacter pylori* infection after eradication. *Med J Aust*. 1989;151(8):431–435.
394. Pounder R. Silent peptic ulceration: deadly silence or golden silence? *Gastroenterology*. 1989;96(2 pt 2 suppl):626–631.
395. Malone DE, McCormick PA, Daly L, et al. Peptic ulcer in rheumatoid arthritis—intrinsic or related to drug therapy? *Br J Rheumatol*. 1986;25(4):342–344.
396. Freston MS, Freston JW. Peptic ulcers in the elderly: unique features and management. *Geriatrics*. 1990;45(1):39–42, 45.
397. Texter EC Jr, Baylin GJ, Ruffin JM, et al. Pyloric channel ulcer. *Gastroenterology*. 1953;24(3):319–327.
398. Strom M, Bodemar G, Lindhagen J, et al. Cimetidine or parietal-cell vagotomy in patients with juxtapyloric ulcers. *Lancet*. 1984;2(8408):894–897.
399. Nussbaum MS, Schusterman MA. Management of giant duodenal ulcer. *Am J Surg*. 1985;149(3):357–361.
400. Lumsden K, MacLarnon JC, Dawson J. Giant duodenal ulcer. *Gut*. 1970;11(7):592–599.
401. Klamer TW, Mahr MM. Giant duodenal ulcer: a dangerous variant of a common illness. *Am J Surg*. 1978;135(6):760–762.
402. Barragry TP, Blatchford JW III, Allen MO. Giant gastric ulcers. A review of 49 cases. *Ann Surg*. 1986;203(3):255–259.
403. Jaszewski R, Crane SA, Cid AA. Giant duodenal ulcers. Successful healing with medical therapy. *Dig Dis Sci*. 1983;28(6):486–489.
404. Cooke L, Hutton CF. Postbulbar duodenal ulceration. *Lancet*. 1958;1(7024):754–757.
405. Zollinger RM, Moore FT. Zollinger–Ellison syndrome comes of age. Recognition of the complete clinical spectrum and its management. *JAMA*. 1968;204(5):361–365.
406. Schade RO. The morbid anatomy of peptic ulceration. *Schweiz Z Pathol Bakteriol*. 1958;21(2):372–388.
407. Johnson HD. The special significance of concomitant gastric and duodenal ulcers. *Lancet*. 1955;268(6858):266–270.
408. McCray RS, Ferris EJ, Herskovic T, et al. Clinical differences between gastric ulcers with and without duodenal deformity. *Ann Surg*. 1968;168(5):821–823.
409. Zukerman GR, Mills BA, Koehler RE, et al. Nodular duodenitis. Pathologic and clinical characteristics in patients with end-stage renal disease. *Dig Dis Sci*. 1983;28(11):1018–1024.
410. Paoluzi P, Pallone F, Zaccardelli E, et al. Outcome of ulcer-associated duodenitis after short-term medical treatment. *Dig Dis Sci*. 1985;30(7):624–629.
411. Steer HW. Surface morphology of the gastroduodenal mucosa in duodenal ulceration. *Gut*. 1984;25(11):1203–1210.
412. Jonsson KA, Bodemar G, Norrby K, et al. Are endoscopic and/or histologic findings in gastroduodenal mucosa a predictor of clinical outcome in peptic ulcer disease? A 1-year follow-up study after initial healing with either cimetidine or medium-dose antacid. *Scand J Gastroenterol*. 1988;23(2):199–208.
413. Sircus W. Duodenitis: a clinical, endoscopic and histopathologic study. *Q J Med*. 1985;56(221):593–600.
414. Paoluzi P, Pallone F, Palazzesi P, et al. Frequency and extent of bulbar duodenitis in duodenal ulcer, endoscopic and histological study. *Endoscopy*. 1982;14(6):193–195.
415. Kekki M, Sipponen P, Siurala M. Progression of antral and body gastritis in patients with active and healed duodenal ulcer and duodenitis. *Scand J Gastroenterol*. 1984;19(3):382–388.
416. Cheli R, Giacosa A. Duodenal ulcer and chronic gastritis. *Endoscopy*. 1986;18(4):125–126.
417. Wyatt JI, Rathbone BJ, Dixon MF, et al. *Campylobacter pyloridis* and acid induced gastric metaplasia in the pathogenesis of duodenitis. *J Clin Pathol*. 1987;40(8):841–848.
418. Shousha S, Parkins RA, Bull TB. Chronic duodenitis with gastric metaplasia: electron microscopic study including comparison with normal. *Histopathology*. 1983;7(6):873–885.
419. Shousha S, Spiller RC, Parkins RA. The endoscopically abnormal duodenum in patients with dyspepsia: biopsy findings in 60 cases. *Histopathology*. 1983;7(1):23–34.
420. Kreuning J, vd Wal AM, Kuiper G, et al. Chronic nonspecific duodenitis. A multiple biopsy study of the duodenal bulb in health and disease. *Scand J Gastroenterol Suppl*. 1989;167:16–20.
421. Gormally SM, Kierce BM, Daly LE, et al. Gastric metaplasia and duodenal ulcer disease in children infected by *Helicobacter pylori*. *Gut*. 1996;38(4):513–517.
422. Shousha S, Keen C, Parkins RA. Gastric metaplasia and *Campylobacter pylori* infection of duodenum in patients with chronic renal failure. *J Clin Pathol*. 1989;42(4):348–351.
423. Shiotani A, Yamaoka Y, El-Zimaity HM, et al. NSAID gastric ulceration: predictive value of gastric pH, mucosal density of polymorphonuclear leukocytes, or levels of IL-8 or nitrite. *Dig Dis Sci*. 2002;47(1):38–43.
424. Blaser MJ. *Helicobacter pylori* and the pathogenesis of gastroduodenal inflammation. *J Infect Dis*. 1990;161(4):626–633.

425. Tytgat GN, Rauws EA. *Campylobacter pylori* and its role in peptic ulcer disease. *Gastroenterol Clin North Am.* 1990;19(1):183–196.
426. Gear MW, Truelove SC, Whitehead R. Gastric ulcer and gastritis. *Gut.* 1971;12(8):639–645.
427. Aukee S. Gastritis and acid secretion in patients with gastric ulcers and duodenal ulcers. *Scand J Gastroenterol.* 1972;7(6):567–574.
428. Zaterka S, Vieira FE, Neves P, et al. Chronic gastritis and peptic ulcer. *Acta Hepatogastroenterol (Stuttg).* 1977;24(5):381–385.
429. Soll AH, Weinstein WM, Kurata J, et al. Nonsteroidal anti-inflammatory drugs and peptic ulcer disease. *Ann Intern Med.* 1991;114(4):307–319.
430. Matsui T, Iida M, Fujishima M, et al. Linear erosions on Kerckring's folds may be diagnostic of Zollinger–Ellison syndrome. *J Clin Gastroenterol.* 1989;11(3):278–281.
431. McColl KE. How I manage *H. pylori*-negative, NSAID/aspirin-negative peptic ulcers. *Am J Gastroenterol.* 2009;104(1):190–193.
432. Botsford TW, Crowe P, Crocker DW. Tumors of the small intestine. A review of experience with 115 cases including a report of a rare case of malignant hemangioendothelioma. *Am J Surg.* 1962;103:358–365.
433. Memeo L, Jhang J, Hibshoosh H, et al. Duodenal intraepithelial lymphocytosis with normal villous architecture: common occurrence in *H. pylori* gastritis. *Mod Pathol.* 2005;18(8):1134–1144.
434. Elashoff JD, Greenfield S, Henderson D, et al. Physician recommendations of elective surgery for duodenal ulcer patients: a comparision of surgeons and medical specialists. *Gastroenterology.* 1980;79(4):750–753.
435. Wang YR, Richter JE, Dempsey DT. Trends and outcomes of hospitalizations for peptic ulcer disease in the United States, 1993 to 2006. *Ann Surg.* 2010;251(1):51–58.
436. Strickland RG. The Sydney system: auto-immune gastritis. *J Gastroenterol Hepatol.* 1991;6(3):238–243.
437. Perasso A, Testino G, de Angelis P, et al. Gastric chief cell mass in chronic gastritis. Count and relationships to parietal cell mass and functional indices. *Hepatogastroenterology.* 1991;38(suppl 1):63–66.
438. Marignani M, Delle Fave G, Mecarocci S, et al. High prevalence of atrophic body gastritis in patients with unexplained microcytic and macrocytic anemia: a prospective screening study. *Am J Gastroenterol.* 1999;94(3):766–772.
439. De Block CE, Van Campenhout CM, De Leeuw IH, et al. Soluble transferrin receptor level: a new marker of iron deficiency anemia, a common manifestation of gastric autoimmunity in type 1 diabetes. *Diabetes Care.* 2000;23(9):1384–1388.
440. Davidson RJ, Atrah HI, Sewell HF. Longitudinal study of circulating gastric antibodies in pernicious anaemia. *J Clin Pathol.* 1989;42(10):1092–1095.
441. Irvine WJ. Immunoassay of gastric intrinsic factor and the titration of antibody to intrinsic factor. *Clin Exp Immunol.* 1966;1(1):99–118.
442. Rose MS, Chanarin I. Dissociation of intrinsic factor from its antibody: application to study of pernicious anaemia gastric juice specimens. *Br Med J.* 1969;1(5642):468–470.
443. Sourial NA. Rapid protein A assay for intrinsic factor and its binding antibody. *J Clin Pathol.* 1988;41(5):568–572.
444. Desai HG, Dighe PK, Borkar AV. Parietal cell and intrinsic-factor antibodies in Indian subjects. *Scand J Gastroenterol.* 1968;3(3):321–326.
445. Hudak J, Berger Z, Varga L. An assay for serum vitamin-B_{12} and for intrinsic factor antibody type I by means of hog intrinsic factor. *Acta Med Acad Sci Hung.* 1980;37(2):157–165.
446. Appelmelk BJ, Faller G, Claeys D, et al. Bugs on trial: the case of *Helicobacter pylori* and autoimmunity. *Immunol Today.* 1998;19(7):296–299.
447. Amedei A, Bergman MP, Appelmelk BJ, et al. Molecular mimicry between *Helicobacter pylori* antigens and H^+, K^+–adenosine triphosphatase in human gastric autoimmunity. *J Exp Med.* 2003;198(8):1147–1156.
448. Uibo R, Vorobjova T, Metskula K, et al. Association of *Helicobacter pylori* and gastric autoimmunity: a population-based study. *FEMS Immunol Med Microbiol.* 1995;11(1):65–68.
449. Vorobjova T, Faller G, Maaroos HI, et al. Significant increase in antigastric autoantibodies in a long-term follow-up study of *H. pylori* gastritis. *Virchows Arch.* 2000;437(1):37–45.
450. Vorobjova T, Maaroos HI, Uibo R. Immune response to *Helicobacter pylori* and its association with the dynamics of chronic gastritis in the antrum and corpus. *APMIS.* 2008;116(6):465–476.
451. Faller G, Winter M, Steininger H, et al. Decrease of antigastric autoantibodies in *Helicobacter pylori* gastritis after cure of infection. *Pathol Res Pract.* 1999;195(4):243–246.
452. Carmel R. Reassessment of the relative prevalences of antibodies to gastric parietal cell and to intrinsic factor in patients with pernicious anaemia: influence of patient age and race. *Clin Exp Immunol.* 1992;89(1):74–77.
453. Jhala NC, Montemor M, Jhala D, et al. Pancreatic acinar cell metaplasia in autoimmune gastritis. *Arch Pathol Lab Med.* 2003;127(7):854–857.
454. Chlumska A, Boudova L, Benes Z, et al. Autoimmune gastritis. A clinicopathologic study of 25 cases. *Cesk Patol.* 2005;41(4):137–142.
455. Sjoblom SM, Sipponen P, Karonen SL, et al. Mucosal argyrophil endocrine cells in pernicious anaemia and upper gastrointestinal carcinoid tumours. *J Clin Pathol.* 1989;42(4):371–377.
456. Carmel R. Pepsinogens and other serum markers in pernicious anemia. *Am J Clin Pathol.* 1988;90(4):442–445.
457. Brinton LA, Gridley G, Hrubec Z, et al. Cancer risk following pernicious anaemia. *Br J Cancer.* 1989;59(5):810–813.
458. Hsing AW, Hansson LE, McLaughlin JK, et al. Pernicious anemia and subsequent cancer. A population-based cohort study. *Cancer.* 1993;71(3):745–750.
459. Zafad S, Madani A, Harif M, et al. Pernicious anemia associated with autoimmune hemolytic anemia and alopecia areata. *Pediatr Blood Cancer.* 2007;49(7):1017–1018.
460. Dahshan A, Poulick J, Tolia V. Special feature: pathological case of the month. Pernicious anemia and gastric atrophy in an adolescent female with multiorgan problems. *Arch Pediatr Adolesc Med.* 2001;155(5):609–610.
461. Guilloteau M, Bertrand Y, Lachaux A, et al. Pernicious anemia: a teenager with an unusual cause of iron-deficiency anemia. *Gastroenterol Clin Biol.* 2007;31(12):1155–1156.
462. Maonou H, Domenech E, Navarro-Llavat M, et al. Pernicious anaemia in triplets. A case report and literature review. *Gastroenterol Hepatol.* 2007;30(10):580–582.
463. Jacobson DL, Gange SJ, Rose NR, et al. Epidemiology and estimated population burden of selected autoimmune diseases in the United States. *Clin Immunol Immunopathol.* 1997;84(3):223–243.
464. De Block CE, De Leeuw IH, Van Gaal LF. High prevalence of manifestations of gastric autoimmunity in parietal cell antibody-positive type 1 (insulin-dependent) diabetic patients. The Belgian Diabetes Registry. *J Clin Endocrinol Metab.* 1999;84(11):4062–4067.
465. Lewin KJ, Dowling F, Wright JP, et al. Gastric morphology and serum gastrin levels in pernicious anaemia. *Gut.* 1976;17(7):551–560.

466. Rubio CA. My approach to reporting a gastric biopsy. *J Clin Pathol*. 2007;60(2):160–166.
467. Carmel R. Ethnic and racial factors in cobalamin metabolism and its disorders. *Semin Hematol*. 1999;36(1):88–100.
468. Carmel R, Green R, Jacobsen DW, et al. Serum cobalamin, homocysteine, and methylmalonic acid concentrations in a multiethnic elderly population: ethnic and sex differences in cobalamin and metabolite abnormalities. *Am J Clin Nutr*. 1999;70(5):904–910.
469. De Aizpurua HJ, Cosgrove LJ, Ungar B, et al. Autoantibodies cytotoxic to gastric parietal cells in serum of patients with pernicious anemia. *N Engl J Med*. 1983;309(11):625–629.
470. Wangel AG, Schiller KF. Diagnostic significance of antibody to intrinsic factor. *Br Med J*. 1966;1(5498):1274–1276.
471. Doniach D, Roitt IM. An evaluation of gastric and thyroid auto-immunity in relation to hematologic disorders. *Semin Hematol*. 1964;93:313–343.
472. Munichoodappa C, Kozak GP. Diabetes mellitus and pernicious anemia. *Diabetes*. 1970;19(10):719–722.
473. Davis RE, McCann VJ, Stanton KG. Type 1 diabetes and latent pernicious anaemia. *Med J Aust*. 1992;156(3):160–162.
474. Farnam J, Jorizzo JL, Grant JA, et al. Sjogren's syndrome presenting with hypereosinophilia, lymphopenia and circulating immune complexes. *Clin Exp Rheumatol*. 1984;2(1):41–46.
475. De Block CE, De Leeuw IH, Van Gaal LF. Autoimmune gastritis in type 1 diabetes: a clinically oriented review. *J Clin Endocrinol Metab*. 2008;93(2):363–371.
476. Paul I, Reichard RR. Subacute combined degeneration mimicking traumatic spinal cord injury. *Am J Forensic Med Pathol*. 2009;30(1):47–48.
477. Carmel R, Aurangzeb I, Qian D. Associations of food-cobalamin malabsorption with ethnic origin, age, *Helicobacter pylori* infection, and serum markers of gastritis. *Am J Gastroenterol*. 2001;96(1):63–70.
478. Andres E, Federici L, Serraj K, et al. Update of nutrient-deficiency anemia in elderly patients. *Eur J Intern Med*. 2008;19(7):488–493.
479. Allen LH. How common is vitamin B-12 deficiency? *Am J Clin Nutr*. 2009;89(2):693S–696S.
480. Graham DY, Malaty HM, Evans DG, et al. Epidemiology of *Helicobacter pylori* in an asymptomatic population in the United States. Effect of age, race, and socioeconomic status. *Gastroenterology*. 1991;100(6):1495–1501.
481. Dehesa M, Dooley CP, Cohen H, et al. High prevalence of *Helicobacter pylori* infection and histologic gastritis in asymptomatic Hispanics. *J Clin Microbiol*. 1991;29(6):1128–1131.
482. Meshkinpour H, Orlando RA, Arguello JF, et al. Significance of endoscopically visible blood vessels as an index of atrophic gastritis. *Am J Gastroenterol*. 1979;71(4):376–379.
483. Stockbrugger RW, Menon GG, Beilby JO, et al. Gastroscopic screening in 80 patients with pernicious anaemia. *Gut*. 1983;24(12):1141–1147.
484. Borch K. Epidemiologic, clinicopathologic, and economic aspects of gastroscopic screening of patients with pernicious anaemia. *Scand J Gastroenterol*. 1986;21(1):21–30.
485. Hirota WK, Zuckerman MJ, Adler DG, et al. ASGE guideline: the role of endoscopy in the surveillance of premalignant conditions of the upper GI tract. *Gastrointest Endosc*. 2006;63(4):570–580.
486. Borch K, Renvall H, Liedberg G, et al. Relations between circulating gastrin and endocrine cell proliferation in the atrophic gastric fundic mucosa. *Scand J Gastroenterol*. 1986;21(3):357–363.
487. Rode J, Dhillon AP, Papadaki L, et al. Pernicious anaemia and mucosal endocrine cell proliferation of the non-antral stomach. *Gut*. 1986;27(7):789–798.
488. Bordi C, Ferrari C, D'Adda T, et al. Ultrastructural characterization of fundic endocrine cell hyperplasia associated with atrophic gastritis and hypergastrinaemia. *Virchows Arch A Pathol Anat Histopathol*. 1986;409(3):335–347.
489. Solcia E, Bordi C, Creutzfeldt W, et al. Histopathological classification of nonantral gastric endocrine growths in man. *Digestion*. 1988;41(4):185–200.
490. Borch K, Renvall H, Liedberg G. Gastric endocrine cell hyperplasia and carcinoid tumors in pernicious anemia. *Gastroenterology*. 1985;88(3):638–648.
491. Schafer LW, Larson DE, Melton LJ III, et al. Risk of development of gastric carcinoma in patients with pernicious anemia: a population-based study in Rochester, Minnesota. *Mayo Clin Proc*. 1985;60(7):444–448.
492. Moses RE, Frank BB, Leavitt M, et al. The syndrome of type A chronic atrophic gastritis, pernicious anemia, and multiple gastric carcinoids. *J Clin Gastroenterol*. 1986;8(1):61–65.
493. Arnold R, Hulst MV, Neuhof CH, et al. Antral gastrin-producing G-cells and somatostatin-producing D-cells in different states of gastric acid secretion. *Gut*. 1982;23(4):285–291.
494. Flejou JF, Bahame P, Smith AC, et al. Pernicious anaemia and *Campylobacter* like organisms; is the gastric antrum resistant to colonisation? *Gut*. 1989;30(1):60–64.
495. Jevremovic D, Torbenson M, Murray JA, et al. Atrophic autoimmune pangastritis: a distinctive form of antral and fundic gastritis associated with systemic autoimmune disease. *Am J Surg Pathol*. 2006;30(11):1412–1419.
496. Mitomi H, Tanabe S, Igarashi M, et al. Autoimmune enteropathy with severe atrophic gastritis and colitis in an adult: proposal of a generalized autoimmune disorder of the alimentary tract. *Scand J Gastroenterol*. 1998;33(7):716–720.
497. Owen DA. Gastritis and carditis. *Mod Pathol*. 2003;16(4):325–341.
498. Sipponen P, Stolte M. Clinical impact of routine biopsies of the gastric antrum and body. *Endoscopy*. 1997;29(7):671–678.
499. Vakiani E, Yantiss RK. Lymphocytic gastritis: clinicopathological features, etiologic associations and pathogenesis. *Pathol Case Review*. 2008;13(5):167–171.
500. Wu TT, Hamilton SR. Lymphocytic gastritis: association with etiology and topology. *Am J Surg Pathol*. 1999;23(2):153–158.
501. Sundaram KK, Mendall MA. Lymphocytic gastritis and *Helicobacter pylori*: reluctant mucosal partners? *Helicobacter*. 2000;5(4):248–249.
502. Hachem CY, El-Zimaity H. A man with rheumatoid arthritis and iron-deficiency anemia. *MedGenMed*. 2007;9(3):64.
503. Hayat M, Arora DS, Dixon MF, et al. Effects of *Helicobacter pylori* eradication on the natural history of lymphocytic gastritis. *Gut*. 1999;45(4):495–498.
504. Shimoyama Y, Mukai M, Asato Y, et al. Clinical and endoscopic improvement of lymphocytic gastritis with eradication of *Helicobacter pylori*. *Gastrointest Endosc*. 2001;54(2):251–254.
505. Hayat M, Arora DS, Wyatt JI, et al. The pattern of involvement of the gastric mucosa in lymphocytic gastritis is predictive of the presence of duodenal pathology. *J Clin Pathol*. 1999;52(11):815–819.
506. Feeley KM, Heneghan MA, Stevens FM, et al. Lymphocytic gastritis and coeliac disease: evidence of a positive association. *J Clin Pathol*. 1998;51(3):207–210.
507. Carpenter HA, Talley NJ. Gastroscopy is incomplete without biopsy: clinical relevance of distinguishing gastropathy from gastritis. *Gastroenterology*. 1995;108(3):917–924.
508. Nga ME, Tan SH, Teh M, et al. Lymphocytic gastritis-like T cell lymphoma: molecular evidence of an unusual recurrence. *J Clin Pathol*. 2004;57(11):1222–1224.

509. Ruget O, Burtin P, Cerez H, et al. Chronic diarrhea associated with villous atrophy and lymphocytic gastritis, caused by ticlopidine. *Gastroenterol Clin Biol*. 1992;16(3):290.
510. Lynch DA, Sobala GM, Dixon MF, et al. Lymphocytic gastritis and associated small bowel disease: a diffuse lymphocytic gastroenteropathy? *J Clin Pathol*. 1995;48(10): 939-945.
511. Weiss AA, Yoshida EM, Poulin M, et al. Massive bleeding from multiple gastric ulcerations in a patient with lymphocytic gastritis and celiac sprue. *J Clin Gastroenterol*. 1997;25(1):354-357.
512. Amenomori M, Umemoto T, Kushima R, et al. Spontaneous remission of hypertrophic lymphocytic gastritis associated with hypoproteinemia. *Intern Med*. 1998;37(12):1019-1022.
513. Griffiths AP, Wyatt J, Jack AS, et al. Lymphocytic gastritis, gastric adenocarcinoma, and primary gastric lymphoma. *J Clin Pathol*. 1994;47(12):1123-1124.
514. Shapiro JL, Goldblum JR, Petras RE. A clinicopathologic study of 42 patients with granulomatous gastritis. Is there really an "idiopathic" granulomatous gastritis? *Am J Surg Pathol*. 1996;20(4):462-470.
515. Renault M, Goodier A, Subramony C, et al. Age-related differences in granulomatous gastritis: a retrospective, clinicopathological analysis. *J Clin Pathol*. 2010;63(4):347-350.
516. Yamane T, Uchiyama K, Ishii T, et al. Isolated granulomatous gastritis showing discoloration of lesions after *Helicobacter pylori* eradication. *Dig Endosc*. 2010;22(2):140-143.
517. Kim YS, Lee HK, Kim JO, et al. A case of *H. pylori*-associated granulomatous gastritis with hypertrophic gastropathy. *Gut Liver*. 2009;3(2):137-140.
518. Daniels JA, Lederman HM, Maitra A, et al. Gastrointestinal tract pathology in patients with common variable immunodeficiency (CVID): a clinicopathologic study and review. *Am J Surg Pathol*. 2007;31(12):1800-1812.
519. Pavic M, Debourdeau P, Vacelet V, et al. Sarcoidosis and sarcoid reactions in cancer. *Rev Med Interne*. 2008;29(1): 39-45.
520. Miyamoto M, Haruma K, Yoshihara M, et al. Isolated granulomatous gastritis successfully treated by *Helicobacter pylori* eradication: a possible association between granulomatous gastritis and *Helicobacter pylori*. *J Gastroenterol*. 2003;38(4):371-375.
521. Dhillon AP, Sawyerr A. Granulomatous gastritis associated with *Campylobacter pylori*. *APMIS*. 1989;97(8):723-727.
522. Maeng L, Lee A, Choi K, et al. Granulomatous gastritis: a clinicopathologic analysis of 18 biopsy cases. *Am J Surg Pathol*. 2004;28(7):941-945.
523. Koyama S, Nagashima F. Idiopathic granulomatous gastritis with multiple aphthoid ulcers. *Intern Med*. 2003;42(8): 691-695.
524. Suzuki T, Shinoda M, Takaoshi H, et al. A case of gastric sarcoidosis with remarkable imaging features on multislice CT. *Nippon Shokakibyo Gakkai Zasshi*. 2004;101(12): 1340-1343.
525. Yokoyama A, Kondo K, Nakajima M, et al. Prognostic value of circulating KL-6 in idiopathic pulmonary fibrosis. *Respirology*. 2006;11(2):164-168.
526. Croxon S, Chen K, Davidson AR. Sarcoidosis of the stomach. *Digestion*. 1987;38(3):193-196.
527. Afshar K, BoydKing A, Sharma OP, et al. Gastric sarcoidosis and review of the literature. *J Natl Med Assoc*. 2010;102(5):419-422.
528. Palmer ED. Note on silent sarcoidosis of the gastric mucosa. *J Lab Clin Med*. 1958;52(2):231-234.
529. Liang DB, Price JC, Ahmed H, et al. Gastric sarcoidosis: case report and literature review. *J Natl Med Assoc*. 2010;102(4):348-351.
530. Mukhopadhyay S, Gal AA. Granulomatous lung disease: an approach to the differential diagnosis. *Arch Pathol Lab Med*. 2010;134(5):667-690.
531. Panella VS, Katz S, Kahn E, et al. Isolated gastric sarcoidosis. Unique remnant of disseminated disease. *J Clin Gastroenterol*. 1988;10(3):327-331.
532. Sandmeier D, Bouzourene H. Does idiopathic granulomatous gastritis exist? *Histopathology*. 2005;46(3):352-353.
533. Weinstock JV. Idiopathic isolated granulomatous gastritis: spontaneous resolution without surgical intervention. *Dig Dis Sci*. 1980;25(3):233-235.
534. Compton CC, Von Lichtenberg F. Necrotizing granulomatous gastritis and gastric perforation of unknown etiology: a first case report. *J Clin Gastroenterol*. 1983;5(1):59-65.
535. Lau CF, Wong AM, Yee KS, et al. A case of colonic tuberculosis mimicking Crohn's disease. *Hong Kong Med J*. 1998;4(1): 63-66.
536. Antonioli DA, Goldman H. Changes in the location and type of gastric adenocarcinoma. *Cancer*. 1982;50(4):775-781.
537. Pera M, Cameron AJ, Trastek VF, et al. Increasing incidence of adenocarcinoma of the esophagus and esophagogastric junction. *Gastroenterology*. 1993;104(2):510-513.
538. Petersson F, Franzen LE, Borch K. Characterization of the gastric cardia in volunteers from the general population. Type of mucosa, *Helicobacter pylori* infection, inflammation, mucosal proliferative activity, p53 and p21 expression, and relations to gastritis. *Dig Dis Sci*. 2010;55(1): 46-53.
539. El-Zimaity HM, Verghese VJ, Ramchatesingh J, et al. The gastric cardia in gastro-oesophageal disease. *J Clin Pathol*. 2000;53(8):619-625.
540. Spechler SJ, Zeroogian JM, Antonioli DA, et al. Prevalence of metaplasia at the gastro-oesophageal junction. *Lancet*. 1994;344(8936):1533-1536.
541. Hirota WK, Loughney TM, Lazas DJ, et al. Specialized intestinal metaplasia, dysplasia, and cancer of the esophagus and esophagogastric junction: prevalence and clinical data. *Gastroenterology*. 1999;116(2):277-285.
542. Hackelsberger A, Gunther T, Schultze V, et al. Intestinal metaplasia at the gastro-oesophageal junction: *Helicobacter pylori* gastritis or gastro-oesophageal reflux disease? *Gut*. 1998;43(1):17-21.
543. Doglioni C, Laurino L, Dei Tos AP, et al. Pancreatic (acinar) metaplasia of the gastric mucosa. Histology, ultrastructure, immunocytochemistry, and clinicopathologic correlations of 101 cases. *Am J Surg Pathol*. 1993;17(11):1134-1143.
544. Wang HH, Zeroogian JM, Spechler SJ, et al. Prevalence and significance of pancreatic acinar metaplasia at the gastroesophageal junction. *Am J Surg Pathol*. 1996;20(12):1507-1510.
545. Luque-Barona RJ, Pereda-Salguero T, Fernandez-Alonso J. So-called pancreatic acinar metaplasia of the gastric mucosa in two infants: a post-mortem study. *Eur J Pediatr*. 1999;158(3):267-268.
546. Pizzolitto S, Camilot D, DeMaglio G, et al. Russell body gastritis: expanding the spectrum of *Helicobacter pylori*-related diseases? *Pathol Res Pract*. 2007;203(6):457-460.
547. Erbersdobler A, Petri S, Lock G. Russell body gastritis: an unusual, tumor-like lesion of the gastric mucosa. *Arch Pathol Lab Med*. 2004;128(8):915-917.
548. McNulty CA, Dent JC, Curry A, et al. New spiral bacterium in gastric mucosa. *J Clin Pathol*. 1989;42(6):585-591.
549. Heilmann KL, Borchard F. Gastritis due to spiral shaped bacteria other than *Helicobacter pylori*: clinical, histological, and ultrastructural findings. *Gut*. 1991;32(2):137-140.
550. Boyanova L, Lazarova E, Jelev C, et al. *Helicobacter pylori* and *Helicobacter heilmannii* in untreated Bulgarian children

over a period of 10 years. *J Med Microbiol.* 2007;56(pt 8):1081-1085.
551. Kivisto R, Linros J, Rossi M, et al. Characterization of multiple *Helicobacter bizzozeronii* isolates from a Finnish patient with severe dyspeptic symptoms and chronic active gastritis. *Helicobacter.* 2010;15(1):58-66.
552. Haesebrouck F, Pasmans F, Flahou B, et al. Gastric helicobacters in domestic animals and nonhuman primates and their significance for human health. *Clin Microbiol Rev.* 2009;22(2):202-223, table of contents.
553. Okiyama Y, Matsuzawa K, Hidaka E, et al. *Helicobacter heilmannii* infection: clinical, endoscopic and histopathological features in Japanese patients. *Pathol Int.* 2005;55(7):398-404.
554. Debongnie JC, Donnay M, Mairesse J, et al. Gastric ulcers and *Helicobacter heilmannii. Eur J Gastroenterol Hepatol.* 1998;10(3):251-254.
555. Yang H, Li X, Xu Z, et al. "Helicobacter heilmannii" infection in a patient with gastric cancer. *Dig Dis Sci.* 1995;40(5):1013-1014.
556. Joo M, Kwak JE, Chang SH, et al. *Helicobacter heilmannii*-associated gastritis: clinicopathologic findings and comparison with *Helicobacter pylori*-associated gastritis. *J Korean Med Sci.* 2007;22(1):63-69.
557. Stolte M, Kroher G, Meining A, et al. A comparison of *Helicobacter pylori* and *H. heilmannii* gastritis. A matched control study involving 404 patients. *Scand J Gastroenterol.* 1997;32(1):28-33.
558. De Bock M, Van den Bulck K, Hellemans A, et al. Peptic ulcer disease associated with *Helicobacter felis* in a dog owner. *Eur J Gastroenterol Hepatol.* 2007;19(1):79-82.
559. van Loon S, Bart A, den Hertog EJ, et al. *Helicobacter heilmannii* gastritis caused by cat to child transmission. *J Pediatr Gastroenterol Nutr.* 2003;36(3):407-409.
560. Van den Bulck K, Decostere A, Gruntar I, et al. In vitro antimicrobial susceptibility testing of *Helicobacter felis, H. bizzozeronii,* and *H. salomonis. Antimicrob Agents Chemother.* 2005;49(7):2997-3000.
561. Baele M, Decostere A, Vandamme P, et al. Isolation and characterization of *Helicobacter suis* sp. nov. from pig stomachs. *Int J Syst Evol Microbiol.* 2008;58(pt 6):1350-1358.
562. Baele M, Pasmans F, Flahou B, et al. Non-*Helicobacter pylori* helicobacters detected in the stomach of humans comprise several naturally occurring *Helicobacter* species in animals. *FEMS Immunol Med Microbiol.* 2009;55(3):306-313.
563. Marshall JB. Tuberculosis of the gastrointestinal tract and peritoneum. *Am J Gastroenterol.* 1993;88(7):989-999.
564. Abramson ES, Katsene ME. Clinical forms of tuberculosis in children. *Vopr Okhr Materin Det.* 1965;10:33-38.
565. Thoeni RF, Margulis AR. Gastrointestinal tuberculosis. *Semin Roentgenol.* 1979;14(4):283-294.
566. Bhansali SK. Abdominal tuberculosis. Experiences with 300 cases. *Am J Gastroenterol.* 1977;67(4):324-337.
567. Mehta JB, Dutt A, Harvill L, et al. Epidemiology of extrapulmonary tuberculosis. A comparative analysis with pre-AIDS era. *Chest.* 1991;99(5):1134-1138.
568. Brody JM, Miller DK, Zeman RK, et al. Gastric tuberculosis: a manifestation of acquired immunodeficiency syndrome. *Radiology.* 1986;159(2):347-348.
569. Liu PF, Chang CS, Wang J, et al. Primary gastric tuberculosis. *Endoscopy.* 2009;41(suppl 2):E327-E328.
570. Khan FY, AlAni A, Al-Rikabi A, et al. Primary gastric fundus tuberculosis in immunocompetent patient: a case report and literature review. *Braz J Infect Dis.* 2008;12(5):453-455.
571. Talukdar R, Khanna S, Saikia N, et al. Gastric tuberculosis presenting as linitis plastica: a case report and review of the literature. *Eur J Gastroenterol Hepatol.* 2006;18(3):299-303.
572. Gupta B, Mathew S, Bhalla S. Pyloric obstruction due to gastric tuberculosis—an endoscopic diagnosis. *Postgrad Med J.* 1990;66(771):63-65.
573. Misra RC, Agarwal SK, Prakash P, et al. Gastric tuberculosis. *Endoscopy.* 1982;14(6):235-237.
574. Perry S, de Jong BC, Solnick JV, et al. Infection with *Helicobacter pylori* is associated with protection against tuberculosis. *PLoS One.* 2010;5(1):e8804.
575. Subei I, Attar B, Schmitt G, et al. Primary gastric tuberculosis: a case report and literature review. *Am J Gastroenterol.* 1987;82(8):769-772.
576. Wig JD, Vaiphei K, Tashi M, et al. Isolated gastric tuberculosis presenting as massive hematemesis: report of a case. *Surg Today.* 2000;30(10):921-922.
577. Lin OS, Wu SS, Yeh KT, et al. Isolated gastric tuberculosis of the cardia. *J Gastroenterol Hepatol.* 1999;14(3):258-261.
578. Amarapurkar DN, Patel ND, Amarapurkar AD. Primary gastric tuberculosis—report of 5 cases. *BMC Gastroenterol.* 2003;3:6.
579. Salpeter SR, Shapiro RM, Gasman JD. Gastric tuberculosis presenting as fever of unknown origin. *West J Med.* 1991;155(4):412-413.
580. Okoro EO, Komolafe OF. Gastric tuberculosis: unusual presentations in two patients. *Clin Radiol.* 1999;54(4):257-259.
581. Woudstra M, van Tilburg AJ, Tjen JS. Two young Somalians with gastric outlet obstruction as a first manifestation of gastroduodenal tuberculosis. *Eur J Gastroenterol Hepatol.* 1997;9(4):393-395.
582. Chowdhary GN, Dawar R, Misra MC. Coexisting carcinoma and tuberculosis of stomach. *Indian J Gastroenterol.* 1999;18(4):179-180.
583. Geo SK, Harikumar R, Varghese T, et al. Isolated tuberculosis of gastric cardia presenting as perforation peritonitis. *Indian J Gastroenterol.* 2005;24(5):227-228.
584. Mylona EE, Baraboutis IG, Papastamopoulos V, et al. Gastric syphilis: a systematic review of published cases of the last 50 years. *Sex Transm Dis.* 2010;37(3):177-183.
585. Butz WC, Watts JC, Rosales-Wuintana S, et al. Erosive gastritis as a manifestation of secondary syphilis. *Am J Clin Pathol.* 1975;63(6):895-900.
586. Morin ME, Tan A. Diffuse enlargement of gastric folds as a manifestation of secondary syphilis. *Am J Gastroenterol.* 1980;74(2):170-172.
587. Tamura S, Takimoto Y, Hoshida Y, et al. A case of primary oropharyngeal and gastric syphilis mimicking oropharyngeal cancer. *Endoscopy.* 2008;40(suppl 2):E235-E236.
588. Willeford G, Childers JH, Hepner WR Jr. Gumma of the stomach in congenital syphilis. *Pediatrics.* 1952;10(2):162-168.
589. Long BW, Johnston JH, Wetzel W, et al. Gastric syphilis: endoscopic and histological features mimicking lymphoma. *Am J Gastroenterol.* Case Reports. 1995;90(9):1504-1507.
590. Wetzel WJ, Tharp M, Long B, et al. Hemorrhagic gastritis due to syphilis. An unusual condition simulating lymphoma. *J Miss State Med Assoc.* [Case Reports]. 1995;36(6):161-163.
591. Kim JS, Kang MS, Sagong C, et al. An unusual extensive secondary syphilis: condyloma lata on the umbilicus and perineum and mucous patches on the lips. *Clin Exp Dermatol.* 2009;34(7):e299-e301.
592. Chen CY, Chi KH, George RW, et al. Diagnosis of gastric syphilis by direct immunofluorescence staining and real-time PCR testing. *J Clin Microbiol.* 2006;44(9):3452-3456.
593. Martin-Ezquerra G, Fernandez-Casado A, Barco D, et al. *Treponema pallidum* distribution patterns in mucocutaneous lesions of primary and secondary syphilis: an immunohistochemical and ultrastructural study. *Hum Pathol.* 2009;40(5):624-630.

594. Neafie RC, Marty AM. Unusual infections in humans. *Clin Microbiol Rev.* 1993;6(1):34–56.
595. Palmer HM, Higgins SP, Herring AJ, et al. Use of PCR in the diagnosis of early syphilis in the United Kingdom. *Sex Transm Infect.* 2003;79(6):479–483.
596. Strauss RJ, Friedman M, Platt N, et al. Gangrene of the stomach: a case of acute necrotizing gastritis. *Am J Surg.* 1978;135(2):253–257.
597. Jung JH, Choi HJ, Yoo J, et al. Emphysematous gastritis associated with invasive gastric mucormycosis: a case report. *J Korean Med Sci.* 2007;22(5):923–927.
598. Munroe CA, Chen A. Suppurative (phlegmonous) gastritis presenting as a gastric mass. *Dig Dis Sci.* 2010;55(1):11–13.
599. Kim GY, Ward J, Henessey B, et al. Phlegmonous gastritis: case report and review. *Gastrointest Endosc.* 2005;61(1):168–174.
600. Mittleman RE, Suarez RV. Phlegmonous gastritis associated with the acquired immunodeficiency syndrome/pre-acquired immunodeficiency syndrome. *Arch Pathol Lab Med.* 1985;109(8):765–767.
601. Blei ED, Abrahams C. Diffuse phlegmonous gastroenterocolitis in a patient with an infected peritoneo-jugular venous shunt. *Gastroenterology.* 1983;84(3):636–639.
602. Guo J, Young SK, Lorenzo CR, et al. Phlegmonous gastritis in a patient with myeloid sarcoma: a case report. *Appl Immunohistochem Mol Morphol.* 2009;17(5):458–462.
603. Miller AI, Smith B, Rogers AI. Phlegmonous gastritis. *Gastroenterology.* 1975;68(2):231–238.
604. Stein LB, Greenberg RE, Ilardi CF, et al. Acute necrotizing gastritis in a patient with peptic ulcer disease. *Am J Gastroenterol.* 1989;84(12):1552–1554.
605. Schultz MJ, van der Hulst RW, Tytgat GN. Acute phlegmonous gastritis. *Gastrointest Endosc.* 1996;44(1):80–83.
606. Lee BS, Kim SM, Seong JK, et al. Phlegmonous gastritis after endoscopic mucosal resection. *Endoscopy.* 2005;37(5):490–493.
607. Lifton LJ, Schlossberg D. Phlegmonous gastritis after endoscopic polypectomy. *Ann Intern Med.* 1982;97(3):373–375.
608. Kan-no Y, Irisawa A, Takagi T, et al. Endosonographic diagnosis and follow-up of phlegmonous gastritis. *J Clin Ultrasound.* 2007;35(9):524–526.
609. Hommel S, Savoye G, Lorenceau-Savale C, et al. Phlegmonous gastritis in a 32-week pregnant woman managed by conservative surgical treatment and antibiotics. *Dig Dis Sci.* 2007;52(4):1042–1046.
610. Zenooz NA, Robbin MR, Perez V. Gastric pneumatosis following nasogastric tube placement: a case report with literature review. *Emerg Radiol.* 2007;13(4):205–207.
611. Moon SW, Lee SW, Choi SH, et al. Gastric emphysema after methyl ethyl ketone peroxide ingestion. *Clin Toxicol (Phila).* 2010;48(1):90–91.
612. Kalina M, Rubino M. Recurrent gastric emphysema. *Am Surg.* 2009;75(11):1149–1151.
613. Davison AJ. Herpesvirus systematics. *Vet Microbiol.* 2010;143(1):52–69.
614. Bobak DA. Gastrointestinal infections caused by cytomegalovirus. *Curr Infect Dis Rep.* 2003;5(2):101–107.
615. Vachon GC, Brown BS, Kim C, et al. CMV gastric ulcer as the presenting manifestation of AIDS. *Am J Gastroenterol.* 1995;90(2):319–321.
616. Nowak TV, Goddard M, Batteiger B, et al. Evolution of acute cytomegalovirus gastritis to chronic gastrointestinal dysmotility in a nonimmunocompromised adult. *Gastroenterology.* 1999;116(4):953–958.
617. Van Thiel DH, Gavaler JS, Schade RR, et al. Cytomegalovirus infection and gastric emptying. *Transplantation.* 1992;54(1):70–73.
618. Giladi M, Lembo A, Johnson BL Jr. Postural epigastric pain: a unique symptom of primary cytomegalovirus gastritis? *Infection.* 1998;26(4):234–235.
619. Kim JJ, Simpson N, Klipfel N, et al. Cytomegalovirus infection in patients with active inflammatory bowel disease. *Dig Dis Sci.* 2010;55(4):1059–1065.
620. Megged O, Schlesinger Y. Cytomegalovirus-associated protein-losing gastropathy in childhood. *Eur J Pediatr.* 2008;167(11):1217–1220.
621. Kakugawa Y, Kami M, Matsuda T, et al. Endoscopic diagnosis of cytomegalovirus gastritis after allogeneic hematopoietic stem cell transplantation. *World J Gastroenterol.* 2010;16(23):2907–2912.
622. Roberts WH, Sneddon JM, Waldman J, et al. Cytomegalovirus infection of gastrointestinal endothelium demonstrated by simultaneous nucleic acid hybridization and immunohistochemistry. *Arch Pathol Lab Med.* 1989;113(5):461–464.
623. Lagasse JP, Causse X, Legoux JL, et al. Cytomegalovirus gastritis simulating cancer of the linitis plastica type on endoscopic ultrasonography. *Endoscopy.* 1998;30(9):S101–S102.
624. Murray RN, Parker A, Kadakia SC, et al. Cytomegalovirus in upper gastrointestinal ulcers. *J Clin Gastroenterol.* 1994;19(3):198–201.
625. Varsky CG, Correa MC, Sarmiento N, et al. Prevalence and etiology of gastroduodenal ulcer in HIV-positive patients: a comparative study of 497 symptomatic subjects evaluated by endoscopy. *Am J Gastroenterol.* 1998;93(6):935–940.
626. Chiu HM, Wu MS, Hung CC, et al. Low prevalence of *Helicobacter pylori* but high prevalence of cytomegalovirus-associated peptic ulcer disease in AIDS patients: comparative study of symptomatic subjects evaluated by endoscopy and CD4 counts. *J Gastroenterol Hepatol.* 2004;19(4):423–428.
627. Megarbane B, Resiere D, Ferrand J, et al. Difficulties in assessing cytomegalovirus-associated gastric perforation in an HIV-infected patient. *BMC Infect Dis.* 2005;5(1):28.
628. Zucker GM, Otis C, Korowski K, et al. Cytomegalovirus gastritis associated with pseudolymphoma. *J Clin Gastroenterol.* 1994;18(3):222–226.
629. Andrade Jde S, Bambirra EA, Lima GF, et al. Gastric cytomegalic inclusion bodies diagnosed by histologic examination of endoscopic biopsies in patients with gastric ulcer. *Am J Clin Pathol.* 1983;79(4):493–496.
630. Sperling HV, Reed WG. Herpetic gastritis. *Am J Dig Dis.* 1977;22(11):1033–1034.
631. Howiler W, Goldberg HI. Gastroesophageal involvement in herpes simplex. *Gastroenterology.* 1976;70(5, pt 1):775–778.
632. McDonald GB, Shulman HM, Sullivan KM, et al. Intestinal and hepatic complications of human bone marrow transplantation. Part II. *Gastroenterology.* 1986;90(3):770–784.
633. Alexander JA, Cuellar RE, Fadden RJ, et al. Cytomegalovirus infection of the upper gastrointestinal tract before and after liver transplantation. *Transplantation.* 1988;46(3):378–382.
634. Nelson AC, Crippin JS. Gastritis secondary to herpes simplex virus. *Am J Gastroenterol.* 1997;92(11):2116–2117.
635. Jun DW, Kim DH, Kim SH, et al. Ménétrier's disease associated with herpes infection: response to treatment with acyclovir. *Gastrointest Endosc.* 2007;65(7):1092–1095.
636. Tsamakidis K, Panotopoulou E, Dimitroulopoulos D, et al. Herpes simplex virus type 1 in peptic ulcer disease: an inverse association with *Helicobacter pylori*. *World J Gastroenterol.* 2005;11(42):6644–6649.
637. Kang JY, Lee TP, Guan R, et al. Antibody to herpes simplex virus type 1 in peptic ulcer patients. *J Gastroenterol Hepatol.* 1990;5(4):387–390.
638. Archimandritis A, Markoulatos P, Tjivras M, et al. Herpes simplex virus types 1 and 2 and cytomegalovirus in peptic

ulcer disease and non-ulcer dyspepsia. *Hepatogastroenterology*. 1992;39(6):540–541.
639. Rand KH, Jacobson DG, Cottrell CR, et al. Antibodies to herpes simplex type 1 in patients with active duodenal ulcer. *Arch Intern Med*. 1983;143(10):1917–1920.
640. van der Merve CF, Alexander JJ. Herpes simplex virus and duodenal ulceration. *Lancet*. 1982;2(8301):762.
641. Vestergaard BF, Rune SJ. Type-specific herpes-simplex-virus antibodies in patients with recurrent duodenal ulcer. *Lancet*. 1980;1(8181):1273–1274.
642. Toljamo KT, Niemela SE, Karttunen TJ, et al. The role of herpes simplex and *Helicobacter pylori* infection in the etiology of persistent or recurrent gastric erosions: a follow-up study. *Dig Dis Sci*. 2002;47(4):818–822.
643. Lohr JM, Nelson JA, Oldstone MB. Is herpes simplex virus associated with peptic ulcer disease? *J Virol*. 1990;64(5):2168–2174.
644. Kemker BP Jr, Docherty JJ, De Lucia A, et al. Herpes simplex virus: a possible etiologic agent in some gastroduodenal ulcer disease. *Am Surg*. 1992;58(12):775–778.
645. Warren KG, Brown SM, Wroblewska Z, et al. Isolation of latent herpes simplex virus from the superior cervical and vagus ganglions of human beings. *N Engl J Med*. 1978;298(19):1068–1069.
646. Rand KH, Berns KI, Rayfield MA. Recovery of herpes simplex type 1 from the celiac ganglion after renal transplantation. *South Med J*. 1984;77(3):403–404.
647. Chen ZM, Shah R, Zuckerman GR, et al. Epstein-Barr virus gastritis: an underrecognized form of severe gastritis simulating gastric lymphoma. *Am J Surg Pathol*. 2007;31(9):1446–1451.
648. Toll AD, Malik S, Tuluc M. Ulcerative gastritis secondary to Epstein-Barr viral infection. *Dig Dis Sci*. 2010;55(1):218–219.
649. Kitayama Y, Honda S, Sugimura H. Epstein-Barr virus-related gastric pseudolymphoma in infectious mononucleosis. *Gastrointest Endosc*. 2000;52(2):290–291.
650. Zhang Y, Molot R. Severe gastritis secondary to Epstein-Barr viral infection. Unusual presentation of infectious mononucleosis and associated diffuse lymphoid hyperplasia in gastric mucosa. *Arch Pathol Lab Med*. 2003;127(4):478–480.
651. Gulley ML. Molecular diagnosis of Epstein-Barr virus-related diseases. *J Mol Diagn*. 2001;3(1):1–10.
652. Clayton RA, Malcomson RD, Gilmour HM, et al. Profuse gastrointestinal haemorrhage due to delayed primary Epstein-Barr virus infection in an immunocompetent adult. *Histopathology*. 2005;47(4):439–441.
653. Ljungman P. Beta-herpesvirus challenges in the transplant recipient. *J Infect Dis*. 2002;186(suppl 1):S99–S109.
654. Wang FZ, Larsson K, Linde A, et al. Human herpesvirus 6 infection and cytomegalovirus-specific lymphoproliferative responses in allogeneic stem cell transplant recipients. *Bone Marrow Transplant*. 2002;30(8):521–526.
655. Fidel PL Jr, Vazquez JA, Sobel JD. *Candida glabrata*: review of epidemiology, pathogenesis, and clinical disease with comparison to *C. albicans*. *Clin Microbiol Rev*. 1999;12(1):80–96.
656. Katzenstein AL, Maksem J. Candidal infection of gastric ulcers. Histology, incidence, and clinical significance. *Am J Clin Pathol*. 1979;71(2):137–141.
657. Gotlieb-Jensen K, Andersen J. Occurrence of *Candida* in gastric ulcers. Significance for the healing process. *Gastroenterology*. 1983;85(3):535–537.
658. Di Febo G, Miglioli M, Calo G, et al. *Candida albicans* infection of gastric ulcer frequency and correlation with medical treatment. Results of a multicenter study. *Dig Dis Sci*. 1985;30(2):178–181.
659. Zwolinska-Wcislo M, Budak A, Trojanowska D, et al. Fungal colonization of the stomach and its clinical relevance. *Mycoses*. 1998;41(7–8):327–334.
660. Hung CC, Wong JM, Hsueh PR, et al. Intestinal obstruction and peritonitis resulting from gastrointestinal histoplasmosis in an AIDS patient. *J Formos Med Assoc*. 1998;97(8):577–580.
661. Halline AG, Maldonado-Lutomirsky M, Ryoo JW, et al. Colonic histoplasmosis in AIDS: unusual endoscopic findings in two cases. *Gastrointest Endosc*. 1997;45(2):199–204.
662. Wheat J. Histoplasmosis in the acquired immunodeficiency syndrome. *Curr Top Med Mycol*. 1996;7(1):7–18.
663. Fisher JR, Sanowski RA. Disseminated histoplasmosis producing hypertrophic gastric folds. *Am J Dig Dis*. 1978;23(3):282–285.
664. Orchard JL, Luparello F, Brunskill D. Malabsorption syndrome occurring in the course of disseminated histoplasmosis: case report and review of gastrointestinal histoplasmosis. *Am J Med*. 1979;66(2):331–336.
665. Sanguino JC, Rodrigues B, Baptista A, et al. Focal lesion of African histoplasmosis presenting as a malignant gastric ulcer. *Hepatogastroenterology*. 1996;43(9):771–775.
666. Lyon DT, Schubert TT, Mantia AG, et al. Phycomycosis of the gastrointestinal tract. *Am J Gastroenterol*. 1979;72(4):379–394.
667. Cherney CL, Chutuape A, Fikrig MK. Fatal invasive gastric mucormycosis occurring with emphysematous gastritis: case report and literature review. *Am J Gastroenterol*. 1999;94(1):252–256.
668. Knoop C, Antoine M, Vachiery JL, et al. Gastric perforation due to mucormycosis after heart-lung and heart transplantation. *Transplantation*. 1998;66(7):932–935.
669. Hosseini M, Lee J. Gastrointestinal mucormycosis mimicking ischemic colitis in a patient with systemic lupus erythematosus. *Am J Gastroenterol*. 1998;93(8):1360–1362.
670. Margolis PS, Epstein A. Mucormycosis esophagitis in a patient with the acquired immunodeficiency syndrome. *Am J Gastroenterol*. 1994;89(10):1900–1902.
671. Reimund E, Ramos A. Disseminated neonatal gastrointestinal mucormycosis: a case report and review of the literature. *Pediatr Pathol*. 1994;14(3):385–389.
672. Sheu BS, Lee PC, Yang HB. A giant gastric ulcer caused by mucormycosis infection in a patient with renal transplantation. *Endoscopy*. 1998;30(5):S60–S61.
673. Sanchez J, Noskin GA. Recent advances in the management of fungal infections. *Cancer Treat Res*. 1998;96:167–182.
674. Rex JH, Walsh TJ, Anaissie EJ. Fungal infections in iatrogenically compromised hosts. *Adv Intern Med*. 1998;43:321–371.
675. Minamoto GY, Rosenberg AS. Fungal infections in patients with acquired immunodeficiency syndrome. *Med Clin North Am*. 1997;81(2):381–409.
676. Rivasi F, Rossi P, Righi E, et al. Gastric cryptosporidiosis: correlation between intensity of infection and histological alterations. *Histopathology*. 1999;34(5):405–409.
677. Werneck-Silva AL, Prado IB. Gastroduodenal opportunistic infections and dyspepsia in HIV-infected patients in the era of Highly Active Antiretroviral Therapy. *J Gastroenterol Hepatol*. 2009;24(1):135–139.
678. Muraoka A, Suehiro I, Fujii M, et al. Acute gastric anisakiasis: 28 cases during the last 10 years. *Dig Dis Sci*. 1996;41(12):2362–2365.
679. Kakizoe S, Kakizoe H, Kakizoe K, et al. Endoscopic findings and clinical manifestation of gastric anisakiasis. *Am J Gastroenterol*. 1995;90(5):761–763.
680. Bouree P, Paugam A, Petithory JC. Anisakidosis: report of 25 cases and review of the literature. *Comp Immunol Microbiol Infect Dis*. 1995;18(2):75–84.
681. Sugano S, Suzuki T, Kagesawa M, et al. Noncardiac chest pain due to acute gastric anisakiasis. *Dig Dis Sci*. 1993;38(7):1354–1356.

682. Sugimachi K, Inokuchi K, Ooiwa T, et al. Acute gastric anisakiasis. Analysis of 178 cases. *JAMA*. 1985;253(7): 1012–1013.
683. Okai T, Mouri I, Yamaguchi Y, et al. Acute gastric anisakiasis: observations with endoscopic ultrasonography. *Gastrointest Endosc*. 1993;39(3):450–452.
684. Urita Y, Nishino M, Koyama H, et al. Esophageal anisakiasis accompanied by reflux esophagitis. *Intern Med*. 1997;36(12):890–893.
685. Kim HJ, Park C, Cho SY. A case of extragastrointestinal anisakiasis involving a mesocolic lymph node. *Korean J Parasitol*. 1997;35(1):63–66.
686. Wittner M, Turner JW, Jacquette G, et al. Eustrongylidiasis—a parasitic infection acquired by eating sushi. *N Engl J Med*. 1989;320(17):1124–1126.
687. Grove DI. Human strongyloidiasis. *Adv Parasitol*. 1996;38: 251–309.
688. Yaldiz M, Hakverdi S, Aslan A, et al. Gastric infection by *Strongyloides stercoralis*: a case report. *Turk J Gastroenterol*. 2009;20(1):48–51.
689. Misra V, Misra SP, Dwivedi M, et al. *Giardia lamblia* trophozoites in gastric biopsies. *Indian J Pathol Microbiol*. 2006;49(4):519–523.
690. Oberhuber G, Kastner N, Stolte M. Giardiasis: a histologic analysis of 567 cases. *Scand J Gastroenterol*. 1997;32(1):48–51.
691. Merzianu M, Gorelick SM, Paje V, et al. Gastric toxoplasmosis as the presentation of acquired immunodeficiency syndrome. *Arch Pathol Lab Med*. 2005;129(4):e87–e90.
692. Pontes JM, Leitao MC, Portela F, et al. Gastric ascariasis: a rare cause of upper gastrointestinal bleeding. *Endoscopy*. 1996;28(9):792–793.
693. Uygur-Bayramicli O, Yavuzer D, Dolapcioglu C, et al. Granulomatous gastritis due to taeniasis. *J Clin Gastroenterol*. 1998;27(4):351–352.
694. Balkhair A, Ben Abid F. Gastric and cutaneous dissemination of visceral leishmaniasis in a patient with advanced HIV. *Int J Infect Dis*. 2008;12(1):111–113.
695. Hoare M, Gelson WT, Davies SE, et al. Hepatic and intestinal schistosomiasis after orthotopic liver transplant. *Liver Transpl*. 2005;11(12):1603–1607.
696. Otrakji CL, Albores-Saavedra J, Martinez AJ. Gastric malignant lymphoma with superimposed amebiasis. *Am J Gastroenterol*. 1990;85(1):72–75.
697. Thamprasert K, Khunamornpong S, Morakote N. *Acanthamoeba* infection of peptic ulcer. *Ann Trop Med Parasitol*. 1993;87(4):403–405.
698. Alpert L, Miller M, Alpert E, et al. Gastric toxoplasmosis in acquired immunodeficiency syndrome: antemortem diagnosis with histopathologic characterization. *Gastroenterology*. 1996;110(1):258–264.
699. Kofman E, Khorsandi A, Sarlin J, et al. Gastric toxoplasmosis: case report and review of the literature. *Am J Gastroenterol*. 1996;91(11):2436–2438.
700. Dumont A, Seferian V, Barbier P. Endoscopic discovery and capture of *Necator americanus* in the stomach. *Endoscopy*. 1983;15(2):65–66.
701. Thomas S, Mishra MC, Kriplani AK, et al. Hydatidemesis: a bizarre presentation of abdominal hydatidosis. *Aust N Z J Surg*. 1993;63(6):496–498.
702. Silverberg MS, Satsangi J, Ahmad T, et al. Toward an integrated clinical, molecular and serological classification of inflammatory bowel disease: report of a Working Party of the 2005 Montreal World Congress of Gastroenterology. *Can J Gastroenterol*. 2005;19(suppl A):5–36.
703. Wagtmans MJ, Verspaget HW, Lamers CB, et al. Clinical aspects of Crohn's disease of the upper gastrointestinal tract: a comparison with distal Crohn's disease. *Am J Gastroenterol*. 1997;92(9):1467–1471.
704. Freeman HJ. Long-term clinical behavior of jejunoileal involvement in Crohn's disease. *Can J Gastroenterol*. 2005;19(9):575–578.
705. Nguyen GC, Torres EA, Regueiro M, et al. Inflammatory bowel disease characteristics among African Americans, Hispanics, and non-Hispanic Whites: characterization of a large North American cohort. *Am J Gastroenterol*. 2006; 101(5):1012–1023.
706. Heyman MB, Kirschner BS, Gold BD, et al. Children with early-onset inflammatory bowel disease (IBD): analysis of a pediatric IBD consortium registry. *J Pediatr*. 2005;146(1):35–40.
707. Rholl JC, Yavorski RT, Cheney CP, et al. Esophagogastric fistula: a complication of Crohn's disease—case report and review of the literature. *Am J Gastroenterol*. 1998;93(8):1381–1383.
708. Alcantara M, Rodriguez R, Potenciano JL, et al. Endoscopic and bioptic findings in the upper gastrointestinal tract in patients with Crohn's disease. *Endoscopy*. 1993;25(4): 282–286.
709. Paerregaard A. What does the IBD patient hide in the upper gastrointestinal tract? *Inflamm Bowel Dis*. 2009;15(7): 1101–1104.
710. Moonka D, Lichtenstein GR, Levine MS, et al. Giant gastric ulcers: an unusual manifestation of Crohn's disease. *Am J Gastroenterol*. 1993;88(2):297–299.
711. Patel M, Banerjee B, Block JG, et al. Gastric Crohn's disease complicated by adenocarcinoma of the stomach: case report and review of the literature. *Am J Gastroenterol*. 1997;92(8):1368–1371.
712. Yamamoto T, Bain IM, Connolly AB, et al. Gastroduodenal fistulas in Crohn's disease: clinical features and management. *Dis Colon Rectum*. 1998;41(10):1287–1292.
713. Oberhuber G, Puspok A, Oesterreicher C, et al. Focally enhanced gastritis: a frequent type of gastritis in patients with Crohn's disease. *Gastroenterology*. 1997;112(3):698–706.
714. Parente F, Cucino C, Bollani S, et al. Focal gastric inflammatory infiltrates in inflammatory bowel diseases: prevalence, immunohistochemical characteristics, and diagnostic role. *Am J Gastroenterol*. 2000;95(3):705–711.
715. Wright CL, Riddell RH. Histology of the stomach and duodenum in Crohn's disease. *Am J Surg Pathol*. 1998;22(4):383–390.
716. Xin W, Greenson JK. The clinical significance of focally enhanced gastritis. *Am J Surg Pathol*. 2004;28(10): 1347–1351.
717. Danelius M, Ost A, Lapidus AB. Inflammatory bowel disease-related lesions in the duodenal and gastric mucosa. *Scand J Gastroenterol*. 2009;44(4):441–445.
718. Kundhal PS, Stormon MO, Zachos M, et al. Gastral antral biopsy in the differentiation of pediatric colitides. *Am J Gastroenterol*. 2003;98(3):557–561.
719. Yao K, Iwashita A, Yao T, et al. Increased numbers of macrophages in noninflamed gastroduodenal mucosa of patients with Crohn's disease. *Dig Dis Sci*. 1996;41(11): 2260–2267.
720. Tobin JM, Sinha B, Ramani P, et al. Upper gastrointestinal mucosal disease in pediatric Crohn disease and ulcerative colitis: a blinded, controlled study. *J Pediatr Gastroenterol Nutr*. 2001;32(4):443–448.
721. Abdullah BA, Gupta SK, Croffie JM, et al. The role of esophagogastroduodenoscopy in the initial evaluation of childhood inflammatory bowel disease: a 7-year study. *J Pediatr Gastroenterol Nutr*. 2002;35(5):636–640.
722. Lemberg DA, Clarkson CM, Bohane TD, et al. Role of esophagogastroduodenoscopy in the initial assessment of children with inflammatory bowel disease. *J Gastroenterol Hepatol*. 2005;20(11):1696–1700.

723. Rubenstein J, Sherif A, Appelman H, et al. Ulcerative colitis associated enteritis: is ulcerative colitis always confined to the colon? *J Clin Gastroenterol.* 2004;38(1):46–51.

724. Straumann A, Simon HU. The physiological and pathophysiological roles of eosinophils in the gastrointestinal tract. *Allergy.* 2004;59(1):15–25.

725. Katz AJ, Twarog FJ, Zeiger RS, et al. Milk-sensitive and eosinophilic gastroenteropathy: similar clinical features with contrasting mechanisms and clinical course. *J Allergy Clin Immunol.* 1984;74(1):72–78.

726. Johnstone JM, Morson BC. Eosinophilic gastroenteritis. *Histopathology.* 1978;2(5):335–348.

727. Klein NC, Hargrove RL, Sleisenger MH, et al. Eosinophilic gastroenteritis. *Medicine (Baltimore).* 1970;49(4):299–319.

728. Cello JP. Eosinophilic gastroenteritis—a complex disease entity. *Am J Med.* 1979;67(6):1097–1104.

729. Talley NJ, Shorter RG, Phillips SF, et al. Eosinophilic gastroenteritis: a clinicopathological study of patients with disease of the mucosa, muscle layer, and subserosal tissues. *Gut.* 1990;31(1):54–58.

730. Steffen RM, Wyllie R, Petras RE, et al. The spectrum of eosinophilic gastroenteritis. Report of six pediatric cases and review of the literature. *Clin Pediatr (Phila).* 1991;30(7):404–411.

731. Rothenberg ME. Eosinophilic gastrointestinal disorders (EGID). *J Allergy Clin Immunol.* 2004;113(1):11–28; quiz 9.

732. Yun MY, Cho YU, Park IS, et al. Eosinophilic gastroenteritis presenting as small bowel obstruction: a case report and review of the literature. *World J Gastroenterol.* 2007;13(11):1758–1760.

733. Matsushita M, Hajiro K, Morita Y, et al. Eosinophilic gastroenteritis involving the entire digestive tract. *Am J Gastroenterol.* 1995;90(10):1868–1870.

734. Khan S, Orenstein SR. Eosinophilic gastroenteritis: epidemiology, diagnosis and management. *Paediatr Drugs.* 2002;4(9):563–570.

735. Khan S, Orenstein SR. Eosinophilic gastroenteritis. *Gastroenterol Clin North Am.* 2008;37(2):333–348, v.

736. Spergel JM, Brown-Whitehorn T. The use of patch testing in the diagnosis of food allergy. *Curr Allergy Asthma Rep.* 2005;5(1):86–90.

737. Katoulis AC, Bozi E, Samara M, et al. Idiopathic bullous eosinophilic cellulitis (Wells' syndrome). *Clin Exp Dermatol.* 2009;34(7):e375–e376.

738. Kristopaitis T, Neghme C, Yong SL, et al. Giant antral ulcer: a rare presentation of eosinophilic gastroenteritis—case report and review of the literature. *Am J Gastroenterol.* 1997;92(7):1205–1208.

739. Audicana MT, Kennedy MW. *Anisakis simplex*: from obscure infectious worm to inducer of immune hypersensitivity. *Clin Microbiol Rev.* 2008;21(2):360–379, table of contents.

740. Johnstone JM, Morson BC. Inflammatory fibroid polyp of the gastrointestinal tract. *Histopathology.* 1978;2(5):349–361.

741. Ishikura H, Sato F, Naka A, et al. Inflammatory fibroid polyp of the stomach. *Acta Pathol Jpn.* 1986;36(3):327–335.

742. Abell MR, Limond RV, Blamey WE, et al. Allergic granulomatosis with massive gastric involvement. *N Engl J Med.* 1970;282(12):665–668.

743. Temmerman F, Baert F. Collagenous and lymphocytic colitis: systematic review and update of the literature. *Dig Dis.* 2009;27(suppl 1):137–145.

744. Cote JF, Hankard GF, Faure C, et al. Collagenous gastritis revealed by severe anemia in a child. *Hum Pathol.* 1998;29(8):883–886.

745. Suskind D, Wahbeh G, Murray K, et al. Collagenous gastritis, a new spectrum of disease in pediatric patients: two case reports. *Cases J.* 2009;2:7511.

746. Winslow JL, Trainer TD, Colletti RB. Collagenous gastritis: a long-term follow-up with the development of endocrine cell hyperplasia, intestinal metaplasia, and epithelial changes indeterminate for dysplasia. *Am J Clin Pathol.* 2001;116(5):753–758.

747. Leung ST, Chandan VS, Murray JA, et al. Collagenous gastritis: histopathologic features and association with other gastrointestinal diseases. *Am J Surg Pathol.* 2009;33(5):788–798.

748. Gustavo LC, Robert ME, Lamps LW, et al. Isolated gastric malakoplakia: a case report and review of the literature. *Arch Pathol Lab Med.* 2004;128(11):e153–e156.

749. McClure J. Malakoplakia of the gastrointestinal tract. *Postgrad Med J.* 1981;57(664):95–103.

750. Parfitt JR, Driman DK. Pathological effects of drugs on the gastrointestinal tract: a review. *Hum Pathol.* 2007;38(4):527–536.

751. Haber MM, Lopez I. Gastric histologic findings in patients with nonsteroidal anti-inflammatory drug-associated gastric ulcer. *Mod Pathol.* 1999;12(6):592–598.

752. Quinn CM, Bjarnason I, Price AB. Gastritis in patients on non-steroidal anti-inflammatory drugs. *Histopathology.* 1993;23(4):341–348.

753. Choi HY, Takeda M. Gastric epithelial atypia following hepatic arterial infusion chemotherapy. *Diagn Cytopathol.* 1985;1(3):241–244.

754. Oble DA, Mino-Kenudson M, Goldsmith J, et al. Alpha-CTLA-4 mAb-associated panenteritis: a histologic and immunohistochemical analysis. *Am J Surg Pathol.* 2008;32(8):1130–1137.

755. Novak JM, Collins JT, Donowitz M, et al. Effects of radiation on the human gastrointestinal tract. *J Clin Gastroenterol.* 1979;1(1):9–39.

756. Berthrong M, Fajardo LF. Radiation injury in surgical pathology. Part II. Alimentary tract. *Am J Surg Pathol.* 1981;5(2):153–178.

757. Ogawa F, Mino-Kenudson M, Shimizu M, et al. Gastroduodenitis associated with yttrium 90-microsphere selective internal radiation: an iatrogenic complication in need of recognition. *Arch Pathol Lab Med.* 2008;132(11):1734–1738.

758. Abraham SC, Yardley JH, Wu TT. Erosive injury to the upper gastrointestinal tract in patients receiving iron medication: an underrecognized entity. *Am J Surg Pathol.* 1999;23(10):1241–1247.

759. Marginean EC, Bennick M, Cyczk J, et al. Gastric siderosis: patterns and significance. *Am J Surg Pathol.* 2006;30(4):514–520.

760. Iacobuzio-Donahue CA, Lee EL, Abraham SC, et al. Colchicine toxicity: distinct morphologic findings in gastrointestinal biopsies. *Am J Surg Pathol.* 2001;25(8):1067–1073.

761. Abraham SC, Bhagavan BS, Lee LA, et al. Upper gastrointestinal tract injury in patients receiving kayexalate (sodium polystyrene sulfonate) in sorbitol: clinical, endoscopic, and histopathologic findings. *Am J Surg Pathol.* 2001;25(5):637–644.

762. Ritter MM, Richter WO, Schwandt P. Ménétrier disease. Hypertrophic, hypersecretory protein-losing gastropathy. *Fortschr Med.* 1987;105(11):201–203.

763. Fraisse H, Meley J, Baril A, et al. Contribution to the study of Ménétrier's disease (polyadenoma in patches; hypertrophic gastropathy with giant folds), particularly to its radiological aspects. Apropos of 4 unpublished cases. *Arch Fr Mal App Dig.* 1966;55(9):777–796.

764. Engelsing B. Gigantic hypertrophic gastropathy (Ménétrier's disease). *Med Klin.* 1971;66(47):1597–1602.

765. Takagi H, Jhappan C, Sharp R, et al. Hypertrophic gastropathy resembling Ménétrier's disease in transgenic

mice overexpressing transforming growth factor alpha in the stomach. *J Clin Invest.* 1992;90(3):1161–1167.
766. Coffey RJ, Washington MK, Corless CL, et al. Ménétrier disease and gastrointestinal stromal tumors: hyperproliferative disorders of the stomach. *J Clin Invest.* 2007;117(1):70–80.
767. Larsen B, Tarp U, Kristensen E. Familial giant hypertrophic gastritis (Ménétrier's disease). *Gut.* 1987;28(11):1517–1521.
768. Wilkerson ML, Meschter SC, Brown RE. Ménétrier's disease presenting with iron deficiency anemia. *Ann Clin Lab Sci.* 1998;28(1):14–18.
769. Fiske WH, Tanksley J, Nam KT, et al. Efficacy of cetuximab in the treatment of Ménétrier's disease. *Sci Transl Med.* 2009;1(8):8ra18.
770. Johnson MI, Spark JI, Ambrose NS, et al. Early gastric cancer in a patient with Ménétrier's disease, lymphocytic gastritis and *Helicobacter pylori. Eur J Gastroenterol Hepatol.* 1995;7(2):187–190.
771. Wood MG, Bates C, Brown RC, et al. Intramucosal carcinoma of the gastric antrum complicating Ménétrier's disease. *J Clin Pathol.* 1983;36(9):1071–1075.
772. Simson JN, Jass JR, McColl I. Ménétrier's disease and gastric carcinoma. *J R Coll Surg Edinb.* 1987;32(3):134–136.
773. Schindler R. Ménétrier's disease-giant fold gastritis. *Gastrointest Endosc.* 1969;15(4):206–207.
774. Hsu CT, Ito M, Kawase Y, et al. Early gastric cancer arising from localized Ménétrier's disease. *Gastroenterol Jpn.* 1991;26(2):213–217.
775. Scharschmidt BF. The natural history of hypertrophic gastropy (Ménétrier's disease). Report of a case with 16 year follow-up and review of 120 cases from the literature. *Am J Med.* 1977;63(4):644–652.
776. Searcy RM, Malagelada JR. Ménétrier's disease and idiopathic hypertrophic gastropathy. *Ann Intern Med.* 1984;100(4):565–570.
777. Pacheco EJ, Moreno AJ, Ramos A, et al. Diagnosis of Ménétrier's disease with Tc-99m human serum albumin scintigraphy. *Clin Nucl Med.* 1995;20(2):114–116.
778. Kelly DG, Miller LJ, Malagelada JR, et al. Giant hypertrophic gastropathy (Ménétrier's disease): pharmacologic effects on protein leakage and mucosal ultrastructure. *Gastroenterology.* 1982;83(3):581–589.
779. Palmer ED. What Ménétrier really said. *Gastrointest Endosc.* 1968;15(2):83–90 passim.
780. Komorowski RA, Caya JG. Hyperplastic gastropathy. Clinicopathologic correlation. *Am J Surg Pathol.* 1991;15(6):577–585.
781. Miura S, Asakura H, Tsuchiya M. Lymphatic abnormalities in protein-losing gastropathy, especially in Ménétrier's disease. *Angiology.* 1981;32(5):345–354.
782. Daniel ES, Ludwig SL, Lewin KJ, et al. The Cronkhite-Canada syndrome. An analysis of clinical and pathologic features and therapy in 55 patients. *Medicine (Baltimore).* 1982;61(5):293–309.
783. Sferra TJ, Pawel BR, Qualman SJ, et al. Ménétrier disease of childhood: role of cytomegalovirus and transforming growth factor alpha. *J Pediatr.* 1996;128(2):213–219.
784. Dempsey PJ, Goldenring JR, Soroka CJ, et al. Possible role of transforming growth factor alpha in the pathogenesis of Ménétrier's disease: supportive evidence form humans and transgenic mice. *Gastroenterology.* 1992;103(6):1950–1963.
785. Coffey RJ, Romano M, Polk WH, et al. Roles for transforming growth factor-alpha in gastric physiology and pathophysiology. *Yale J Biol Med.* 1992;65(6):693–704; discussion 621–623.
786. Burdick JS, Chung E, Tanner G, et al. Treatment of Ménétrier's disease with a monoclonal antibody against the epidermal growth factor receptor. *N Engl J Med.* 2000;343(23):1697–1701.
787. Bluth RF, Carpenter HA, Pittelkow MR, et al. Immunolocalization of transforming growth factor-alpha in normal and diseased human gastric mucosa. *Hum Pathol.* 1995;26(12):1333–1340.
788. Gold BM, Meyers MA. Progression of Ménétrier's disease with postoperative gastrojejunal intussusception. *Gastroenterology.* 1977;73(3):583–586.
789. Drut RM, Gomez MA, Lojo MM, et al. Cytomegalovirus-associated Ménétrier's disease in adults. Demonstration by polymerase chain reaction (PCR). *Medicina (B Aires).* 1995;55(6):659–664.
790. Kovacs AA, Churchill MA, Wood D, et al. Molecular and epidemiologic evaluations of a cluster of cases of Ménétrier's disease associated with cytomegalovirus. *Pediatr Infect Dis J.* 1993;12(12):1011–1014.
791. Occena RO, Taylor SF, Robinson CC, et al. Association of cytomegalovirus with Ménétrier's disease in childhood: report of two new cases with a review of literature. *J Pediatr Gastroenterol Nutr.* 1993;17(2):217–224.
792. Haot J, Bogomoletz WV, Jouret A, et al. Ménétrier's disease with lymphocytic gastritis: an unusual association with possible pathogenic implications. *Hum Pathol.* 1991;22(4):379–386.
793. Wolber RA, Owen DA, Anderson FH, et al. Lymphocytic gastritis and giant gastric folds associated with gastrointestinal protein loss. *Mod Pathol.* 1991;4(1):13–15.
794. Wolfsen HC, Carpenter HA, Talley NJ. Ménétrier's disease: a form of hypertrophic gastropathy or gastritis? *Gastroenterology.* 1993;104(5):1310–1319.
795. Badov D, Lambert JR, Finlay M, et al. *Helicobacter pylori* as a pathogenic factor in Ménétrier's disease. *Am J Gastroenterol.* 1998;93(10):1976–1979.
796. Kaneko T, Akamatsu T, Gotoh A, et al. Remission of Ménétrier's disease after a prolonged period with therapeutic eradication of *Helicobacter pylori. Am J Gastroenterol.* 1999;94(1):272–273.
797. Shimoyama T, Fukuda S, Tanaka M, et al. Healing of cimetidine-resistant Ménétrier's disease by eradication of *Helicobacter pylori* infection. *J Clin Gastroenterol.* 1998;27(4):348–350.
798. Bayerdörffer E, Ritter MM, Hatz R, et al. Healing of protein losing hypertrophic gastropathy by eradication of *Helicobacter pylori*—is *Helicobacter pylori* a pathogenic factor in Ménétrier's disease? *Gut.* 1994;35(5):701–704.
799. Sanchez C, Brody F, Pucci E, et al. Laparoscopic total gastrectomy for Ménétrier's disease. *J Laparoendosc Adv Surg Tech A.* 2007;17(1):32–35.
800. Duprey KM, Ahmed S, Mishriki YY. Ménétrier disease in an acquired immunodeficiency syndrome patient. *South Med J.* 2010;103(1):93–95.
801. Komorowski RA, Caya JG, Geenen JE. The morphologic spectrum of large gastric folds: utility of the snare biopsy. *Gastrointest Endosc.* 1986;32(3):190–192.
802. Pintiliciuc OG, Heresbach D, de-Lajarte-Thirouard AS, et al. Gastric involvement in juvenile polyposis associated with germline SMAD4 mutations: an entity characterized by a mixed hypertrophic and polypoid gastropathy. *Gastroenterol Clin Biol.* 2008;32(5, pt 1):445–450.
803. Zollinger RM, Ellison EH. Primary peptic ulcerations of the jejunum associated with islet cell tumors of the pancreas. *Ann Surg.* 1955;142(4):709–723; discussion, 724–728.
804. Jensen RT. Management of the Zollinger-Ellison syndrome in patients with multiple endocrine neoplasia type 1. *J Intern Med.* 1998;243(6):477–488.

805. Norton JA, Fraker DL, Alexander HR, et al. Surgery to cure the Zollinger–Ellison syndrome. *N Engl J Med.* 1999;341(9):635–644.
806. Jensen RT. Gastrinomas: advances in diagnosis and management. *Neuroendocrinology.* 2004;80(suppl 1):23–27.
807. Appelman H. Non-neoplastic tumor-like lesions, predominantly epithelial. In: Lewin KA, ed. *Atlas of Tumor Pathology.* 3rd ed. Washington, DC: Armed Forces Institute of Pathology; 1995:183–232.
808. Aprile MR, Azzoni C, Gibril F, et al. Intramucosal cysts in the gastric body of patients with Zollinger–Ellison syndrome. *Hum Pathol.* 2000;31(2):140–148.
809. Fox PS, Hofmann JW, Wilson SD, et al. Surgical management of the Zollinger–Ellison syndrome. *Surg Clin North Am.* 1974;54(2):395–407.
810. McArthur KE, Collen MJ, Maton PN, et al. Omeprazole: effective, convenient therapy for Zollinger–Ellison syndrome. *Gastroenterology.* 1985;88(4):939–944.
811. Maton PN, Vinayek R, Frucht H, et al. Long-term efficacy and safety of omeprazole in patients with Zollinger–Ellison syndrome: a prospective study. *Gastroenterology.* 1989;97(4):827–836.
812. Metz DC, Pisegna JR, Fishbeyn VA, et al. Control of gastric acid hypersecretion in the management of patients with Zollinger–Ellison syndrome. *World J Surg.* 1993;17(4):468–480.
813. Berna MJ, Hoffmann KM, Serrano J, et al. Serum gastrin in Zollinger–Ellison syndrome: I. Prospective study of fasting serum gastrin in 309 patients from the National Institutes of Health and comparison with 2229 cases from the literature. *Medicine (Baltimore).* 2006;85(6):295–330.
814. Khakoo SI, Lobo AJ, Shepherd NA, et al. Histological assessment of the Sydney classification of endoscopic gastritis. *Gut.* 1994;35(9):1172–1175.
815. Chu P, Crosthwaite GL. Gastric foreign bodies: no longer a cross to bear. *Aust N Z J Surg.* 1999;69(5):393–394.
816. Oak S, Bhatnagar M, Kulkarni B, et al. Prepyloric diaphragm detected following foreign body ingestion. *Indian J Gastroenterol.* 1996;15(3):109–110.
817. Lee J. Bezoars and foreign bodies of the stomach. *Gastrointest Endosc Clin N Am.* 1996;6(3):605–619.
818. Phillips MR, Zaheer S, Drugas GT. Gastric trichobezoar: case report and literature review. *Mayo Clin Proc.* 1998;73(7):653–656.
819. Bakken DA, Abramo TJ. Gastric lactobezoar: a rare cause of gastric outlet obstruction. *Pediatr Emerg Care.* 1997;13(4):264–267.
820. Battin M, Kennedy J, Singh S. A case of plastikophagia. *Postgrad Med J.* 1997;73(858):243–244.
821. Koulas SG, Zikos N, Charalampous C, et al. Management of gastrointestinal bezoars: an analysis of 23 cases. *Int Surg.* 2008;93(2):95–98.
822. Heinz-Erian P, Klein-Franke A, Gassner I, et al. Disintegration of large gastric lactobezoars by N-acetylcysteine. *J Pediatr Gastroenterol Nutr.* 2010;50(1):108–110.
823. Muguruma N, Okamura S, Okahisa T, et al. Electrohydraulic lithotripsy treatment for persimmon bezoars. *Endoscopy.* 1998;30(5):S60.
824. Ersoy YE, Ayan F, Ersan Y. Gastro-intestinal bezoars: thirty-five years experience. *Acta Chir Belg.* 2009;109(2):198–203.
825. Gorospe M, Fadare O. Gastric mucosal calcinosis: clinicopathologic considerations. *Adv Anat Pathol.* 2007;14(3):224–228.
826. Kim TH, Yang SY. Stomach calcification revealed by gastrofibroscopy in a haemodialysis patient. *Nephrology (Carlton).* 2010;15(5):592–593.
827. Greenson JK, Trinidad SB, Pfeil SA, et al. Gastric mucosal calcinosis. Calcified aluminum phosphate deposits secondary to aluminum-containing antacids or sucralfate therapy in organ transplant patients. *Am J Surg Pathol.* 1993;17(1):45–50.
828. Strickland RG, Mackay IR. A reappraisal of the nature and significance of chronic atrophic gastritis. *Am J Dig Dis.* 1973;18(5):426–440.
829. Pitchumoni CS, Glass GB. Patterns of gastritis in alcoholics. *Biol Gastroenterol (Paris).* 1976;9(1):11–16.
830. Baggett HC, Parkinson AJ, Muth PT, et al. Endemic iron deficiency associated with *Helicobacter pylori* infection among school-aged children in Alaska. *Pediatrics.* 2006;117(3):e396–e404.
831. Yokota S, Konno M, Mino E, et al. Enhanced Fe ion-uptake activity in *Helicobacter pylori* strains isolated from patients with iron-deficiency anemia. *Clin Infect Dis.* 2008;46(4):e31–e33.
832. Sandven I, Abdelnoor M, Nesheim BI, et al. *Helicobacter pylori* infection and hyperemesis gravidarum: a systematic review and meta-analysis of case-control studies. *Acta Obstet Gynecol Scand.* 2009;88(11):1190–1200.
833. Vilchis J, Duque X, Mera R, et al. Association of *Helicobacter pylori* infection and height of Mexican children of low socioeconomic level attending boarding schools. *Am J Trop Med Hyg.* 2009;81(6):1091–1096.
834. El-Zimaity HM, Ota H, Scott S, et al. A new triple stain for *Helicobacter pylori* suitable for the autostainer: carbol fuchsin/Alcian blue/hematoxylin-eosin. *Arch Pathol Lab Med.* 1998;122(8):732–736.
835. El-Zimaity HM. Modified triple stain (carbol fuchsin/Alcian blue/hematoxylin-eosin) for the identification of *Helicobacter pylori.* *Arch Pathol Lab Med.* 2000;124(10):1416–1417.
836. Chamberlain CE, Peura DA. *Campylobacter (Helicobacter) pylori.* Is peptic disease a bacterial infection? *Arch Intern Med.* 1990;150(5):951–955.
837. Ford AC, Talley NJ. Does *Helicobacter pylori* really cause duodenal ulcers? Yes. *BMJ.* 2009;339:b2784.
838. Hobsley M, Tovey FI, Bardhan KD, et al. Does *Helicobacter pylori* really cause duodenal ulcers? No. *BMJ.* 2009;339:b2788.
839. Nimo RE, Carmel R. Increased sensitivity of detection of the blocking (type I) anti-intrinsic factor antibody. *Am J Clin Pathol.* 1987;88(6):729–733.
840. Veijola LI, Oksanen AM, Sipponen PI, et al. Association of autoimmune type atrophic corpus gastritis with *Helicobacter pylori* infection. *World J Gastroenterol.* 2010;16(1):83–88.

Gastric Epithelial Polyps and Tumors

14

Chapter Outline

ADENOMA/DYSPLASIA/ INTRAEPITHELIAL NEOPLASIA
Definitions and Terminology
Special Stains for Characterizing Gastrointestinal Epithelial cells
Classification of Gastric Adenomas
  Intestinal-type adenomas
  Gastric-type adenomas
  Pyloric gland adenoma
  Foveolar adenoma
  Fundic gland adenoma
Grading of Adenoma/Dysplasia/ Intraepithelial Neoplasia
  Low-grade adenoma/dysplasia/ intraepithelial neoplasia
  High-grade adenoma/dysplasia/ intraepithelial neoplasia
Differential Diagnosis
  Distinction of regenerative changes from adenoma (dysplasia/ intraepithelial neoplasia)
  Distinction of high-grade dysplasia/ adenoma/intraepithelial neoplasia) from invasive carcinoma
GASTRIC CARCINOMA
Introduction
Gastric Cardia Carcinoma
Carcinoma of the Gastric Antrum and Body
Pathogenesis
Risk Factors
  Helicobacter pylori infection
  Epstein Barr virus, CIMP-H and K-ras
  JC virus
  Dietary factors
  Smoking
  Genetic factors
  Hereditary gastric cancer predisposition syndromes
  Other genetic abnormalities predisposing to gastric cancer
  Polymorphism in genes

Predisposing Conditions
  H. pylori–related chronic atrophic gastritis
  Postgastrectomy
  Immunodeficiency disorders
  Menetrièr's disease
Premalignant Lesions of the Stomach
  Adenoma/dysplasia/intraepithelial neoplasm
  Gastric polyps
Gross Features of Gastric Carcinoma
Gross Features of Superficial Cancers and Their Subdivision
Classification and Natural History of Early and Late (Advanced) Gastric Carcinoma
  Early gastric carcinoma/cancer
  Advanced gastric cancer
Histologic Classification of Gastric Carcinomas
  Lauren classification
  Nakamura classification
  Ming classification
  WHO histologic classification and grading of gastric cancer
HISTOLOGICAL SUBTYPES OF CARCINOMA
Tubular Adenocarcinoma
Well-differentiated Adenocarcinoma
Moderately Well-differentiated Adenocarcinoma
Poorly Differentiated Adenocarcinoma
Papillary Adenocarcinoma
Mucinous Adenocarcinoma (syn. Mucoid, Mucus, Colloid, and Muconodular Adenocarcinoma)
Signet-ring Cell Carcinoma
Endocrine Cell Tumors
Rare Variants of Gastric Carcinoma
  Gastric carcinoma with lymphoid stroma (syn. medullary carcinoma, gastric lymphoepithelioma-like carcinoma)
  α-Fetoprotein-producing gastric carcinoma and hepatoid adenocarcinoma

  Adenosquamous and squamous cell carcinoma
  Choriocarcinoma (syn. chorioepithelioma)
  Yolk sack tumor (syn. endodermal sinus tumor)
  Paneth cell carcinoma
  Micropapillary carcinoma
  Gastric adenocarcinoma of fundic gland type (fundic gland carcinoma, combined parietal and chief cell carcinoma) including parietal cell carcinoma and chief cell carcinoma
  Fundic gland adenoma
  Extremely well-differentiated adenocarcinoma
  Pyloric gland carcinoma
  Composite adenocarcinoma and endocrine tumor with pancreatic differentiation and pancreatic type tumors
  Undifferentiated carcinoma
  Serrated dysplasia and carcinoma
  Gastric teratoma
  Carcinosarcoma
  Gastroblastoma
Growth Pattern of Gastric Adenocarcinoma
  Superficial (spreading) carcinoma
  Organoid differentiation
  Stromal reaction
Differential Diagnosis and Clinical Implications
  Early gastric cancer
  Distinction from histiocytic lesions
  Lymphoma
  Metastatic carcinoma
  Neuroendocrine (NET— carcinoid) tumors
  Granular cell tumors
  Bizarre undifferentiated cells (pseudosarcomatous changes)
  Radiation therapy and chemotherapy
Spread of Gastric Carcinoma and Prognostic Factors

Prognosis of Gastric Carcinoma
  Early gastric cancer
  Risk of nodal metastases in early gastric carcinoma
  Gastric remnant carcinoma
  Advanced gastric cancer
  Neoadjuvant therapy
  Her2 status
  K-ras status
Biopsy Diagnosis of Gastric Carcinoma
  Biopsy before surgical resection
  Misreading of biopsies for carcinoma
Value of Cytology in the Diagnosis of Gastric Carcinoma
Handling of Gastric Specimens and Intraoperative Evaluation
  Polypectomy specimens
  Endoscopic mucosal or submucosal specimens
  Resection specimens
NONNEOPLASTIC POLYPS
Classification
Biopsy and Excision of Gastric Polyps: Role of the Pathologist
  Approach to the biopsy diagnosis of gastric polyps

Fundic Gland Polyps
  Pathology
  Clinical implications
Hyperplastic and Inflammatory Polyps
  Pathology
  Dysplasia/carcinoma in hyperplastic polyps
  Clinical implications for inflammatory/hyperplastic polyps
Differential Diagnosis
  Single polyps
  Multiple gastric polyps
Juvenile Polyps
  Pathology
Peutz–Jeghers Polyps
  Pathology
PTEN Hamartoma Tumor Syndrome
Familiar Gastric Hyperplastic Polyposis
Cronkhite–Canada Syndrome–Associated Polyps
  Pathology
Polypoid Gastritis
Gastric Xanthomas (Xanthelasmas, Lipid Islands)
  Pathology

Mucosal Bumps and Nodules
Solitary Polypoid Hamartoma (Gastric Hamartoma with Myxoid Stroma, Hamartomatous Inverted Polyp, Heterotopic Inverted Polyp)
  Pathology
Gastritis Cystica Polyposa (Gastric Stomal Polypoid Hyperplasia, Gastric Stomal Polypoid Hypertrophic Gastritis)
  Pathology
  Mucosal and Submucosal Cysts
Gastritis Cystica Profunda
  Pathology
  Differential diagnosis
Heterotopic Pancreas (Ectopic Pancreas, Pancreatic Rests, Adenomyoma, Adenomyomatous Hamartoma, Myoglandular Hamartoma, Myoepithelial Hamartoma)
  Pathology
  Differential Diagnosis
Brunner Gland Heterotopia/Nodule
Heterotopic Antral Mucosa in Oxyntic Mucosa

ADENOMA/DYSPLASIA/INTRAEPITHELIAL NEOPLASIA

Definitions and Terminology

Gastric epithelial neoplastic lesions, which do not fit the criteria for an adenocarcinoma, have traditionally been referred to as *adenomas* when they are raised, elevated, nodular, or overtly polypoid, or *dysplasia* when they involve flat mucosa. On the other hand, particularly in Japan, the concept of adenoma/dysplasia is considered as a single entity (adenoma) based on the notion that the cytologic features of adenoma and dysplasia are the same, whether they are elevated, flat, or depressed. The concept of intraepithelial neoplasia (IEN) (low-grade and high-grade) merges these concepts, but has the disadvantage that, in the gastrointestinal (GI) tract, many apparent benign tumors have abnormalities in genes traditionally associated with neoplasia, including some overt syndromes known to be complicated by neoplasia (juvenile polyposis syndrome [JPS], Peutz–Jeghers syndrome [PJS]). Consequentially, the term "intraepithelial neoplasia" can also be viewed conceptually in a broader sense for lesions that have features of a neoplasm but are not (yet) overtly dysplastic, as well as a synonym for dysplastic lesions.[1] When used for the latter, like dysplasia, it refers to gastric epithelial neoplastic lesions without lamina propria invasion, irrespective of their gross appearance (elevated, flat, and depressed). From a practical viewpoint, adenoma/dysplasia/IEN is a subjective interpretation of a series of morphologic changes when compared to the normal or metaplastic gastric mucosa.

In this section, we use the following definitions.[1]

Adenoma—a circumscribed benign neoplasm composed of tubular or villous structures lined by dysplastic epithelium whether elevated, flat, or depressed. It represents interpretation of a series of morphologic changes when compared to the normal or metaplastic gastric mucosa.

Dysplasia is used as the defining characteristic of adenomas. However, it is also used generically for lesions found incidentally on biopsy in which no endoscopic lesion was identified, usually in biopsies showing intestinal metaplasia, fully acknowledging that this may well be dependent on the generation of endoscope used, its resolution, the availability of high-definition monitors, the expertise of the endoscopist together with the care and time taken looking for lesions, and whether tools for accentuating lesions such as narrow-band imaging or chromoendoscopy are used.

Dysplasia is subjectively graded into *low-grade dysplasia (LGD)* and *high-grade dysplasia (HGD)*, the latter having either loss of polarity or architectural distortion in the absence of invasion in the lamina propria (some may call this carcinoma in situ; it also conforms to what is included as "cancer" in Japan).

Intramucosal carcinoma has invasion into the lamina propria and is also included in the Japanese term "cancer."

Invasive carcinoma in the stomach refers to any tumor that has invaded into the lamina propria or beyond.

The major problems in dealing with these are as follows:

1. The distinction of dysplasia/IEN from atypical regenerative and hyperplastic features.
2. Grading when and if this is necessary.
3. The distinction of high-grade lesions from minimally invasive (intramucosal) adenocarcinoma.

Special Stains for Characterizing Gastrointestinal Epithelial cells

The importance of analyzing phenotypic expression of tumor cells using cell lineage markers has been demonstrated in the GI tract.[2] The GI mucosa is covered by mucin-producing cells that produce cell-specific mucins. Mucins are highly glycosylated glycoproteins and their core proteins (mucin core proteins: MUC) have been named according to the corresponding genes (mucin gene).[3] MUC5AC (sometimes abbreviated simply to MUC5), MUC6, and MUC2 are expressed in gastric surface mucous cells, gastric gland mucous cells (cardiac gland cells, mucous neck cells, and pyloric gland cells), and intestinal goblet cells, respectively.[4,5]

Histochemically, gastric mucous cells have neutral mucins (glycoproteins) and show strong reactivity with periodic acid–Schiff (PAS) reaction—usually carried out with diastase to remove any glycogen present—diastase PAS, or D-PAS. On the other hand, intestinal mucous cells, and intestinal metaplasia in the stomach, have acid mucins and show reactivity with Alcian blue (AB) stain or high iron diamine stain for specifically demonstrating acid sialomucins and sulfated mucins (a subgroup of acid mucins), respectively, and also weakly with PAS. A combined AB/DPAS stain demonstrates them both. AB stain can also be used as a substitute for sulfomucin stain depending on the pH at which the stain is carried out. Staining at pH 2.5 detects acid mucins (both sialomucins and sulfated mucins) but at pH 1.0 it detects sulfated mucins but not sialomucins.

In addition to mucins, CD10, a 100-kD surface metalloendopeptidase, and other brush border proteins such as villin, is specifically expressed on the brush border of small intestinal epithelial cells in the GI tract.[6] The expression of these mucins and intestinal enzyme are cell type specific; hence, they are useful phenotypic indicators of cell differentiation in normal, metaplastic, or neoplastic epithelial cells in the GI tract.[2]

The endocrine cells can be demonstrated using either specific markers (e.g., gastrin, somatostatin, serotonin, ghrelin) or nonspecific markers (synaptophysin, chromogranin A, CD56, CD57) while vesicular monoamine transporter 2 (VMAT2) stains enterochromaffin-like cells. These are discussed further in Chapters 5 and 12.

Classification of Gastric Adenomas

Architecturally, gastric adenomas are categorized as tubular, tubulovillous, or villous adenoma.[1] Tubular adenomas consist of tubules covered by dysplastic epithelium and surrounded by lamina propria. The dysplastic epithelium lining these tubules often remains relatively superficial, but sometimes can extend from the surface to the crypt base. They appear as rounded or oval structures on cross section. Villous adenoma consists of villi with a core of lamina propria covered by dysplastic epithelium and often shows a papillary configuration with branching. Tubulovillous adenoma has a mixture of tubular and villous structures, each contributing at least 25% to the tumor.[1]

Phenotypically, gastric adenoma can be classified as follows:

1. Intestinal-type adenoma
2. Gastric-type adenoma
    i. Pyloric gland adenoma
    ii. Foveolar adenoma
    iii. Fundic gland adenoma

In practice, it is probably more accurate to think of intestinal, foveolar, and pyloric gland dysplasia, so that if they occur in association with other polyps/lesions they are recognized. The majority of gastric adenomas belong to the intestinal type, and gastric-type adenomas are less common, but not rare, although foveolar adenomas far outnumber pyloric gland adenomas. There are clinical and morphologic differences between intestinal-type and gastric-type adenoma.

Intestinal-type adenomas. Intestinal-type adenomas are composed of varying admixtures of goblet cells, intestinal-type absorptive cells, Paneth cells, and occasional endocrine cells, or columnar cells with varying degrees of differentiation.

Clinical Features Intestinal-type adenomas occur predominantly in the sixth to seventh decades of life, more frequently in males than in females (3:1) and are associated with chronic gastritis with atrophy and intestinal metaplasia[7] and often also with *Helicobacter pylori* infection in the nonmetaplastic mucosa.[8] They tend to arise more frequently in the lesser curvature of the antrum and angulus.

The frequency of carcinoma arising in adenomas depends on tumor size and histologic grade. In the study by Kamiya et al.,[9] 85 mostly small adenomas were followed for up to 12 years. During the follow-up, many adenomas grew little and sometimes even diminished in size; however, focal carcinomas (carcinoma in situ) were detected in 11% (nine lesions) and seven invasive carcinomas developed in those more than 2 cm in diameter.[9] Increasing size of the adenoma was helpful in predicting the development of carcinoma in these lesions.[9] Saraga et al.[10] found that low-grade adenomas remained stable for many years, whereas high-grade adenomas were frequently associated with cancer. Another study from Italy showed that about 90% of adenomas with LGD did not become invasive carcinoma in 5 years, whereas 80% with HGD did.[11]

Clinical implications: It is usually best to remove all adenomas endoscopically, by polypectomy, endoscopic mucosal resection (EMR), or endoscopic submucosal dissection (ESD). Alternatively, while low-grade adenoma should ideally be removed endoscopically, if impractical, patients require at least subsequent endoscopic checkups since the lesion may evolve into an invasive cancer. This is the case when there are multiple adenomas and all cannot be definitively removed. Hence the endoscopist usually focuses on the largest lesions with the rationale being the correlation between size and malignant potential. High-risk adenomas (larger than 2 cm in diameter,[9] high-grade adenomas[10-12]) should be removed endoscopically unless there are good contraindications.

Pathologic Findings In the elevated (sessile polypoid) form, typically adenomatous epithelium is confined to the upper to mid mucosa overlying non-neoplastic mucosa with normal or more often cystically dilated glands. In flat and depressed adenomas, the adenomatous epithelium occupies almost the entire thickness of the mucosa.

Intestinal-type adenomas can be subdivided into exclusively intestinal phenotype (complete intestinal type) (Fig. 14-1) and mixed gastric and intestinal phenotype (incomplete intestinal type) (Fig. 14-2) using immunostaining for GI cell lineage markers (see below).[13,14] The majority of low-grade adenomas are the complete intestinal type and this type seems to be stable.[14] On the other hand, mixed gastric and intestinal phenotype adenomas predominate over the complete intestinal type in high-grade adenomas and also in intramucosal carcinomas.[14] In addition, a long-term follow-up study revealed that adenomas that developed into adenocarcinoma frequently displayed gastric-type differentiation (incomplete metaplasia).[15]

Thus a gastric phenotype in gastric adenoma suggests higher malignant potential.

Histologically, dysplastic glands of complete intestinal-type adenomas tend to be straight and are lined by columnar cells with acidophilic cytoplasm similar to intestinal absorptive cells with scattered goblet cells and sometimes Paneth cells near the mid-part or the base of the dysplastic glands (Fig. 14.1A–D). Superficially, nuclei are elongated and the nuclei are less stratified (Fig.14-1B). In the deeper part of the glands the nuclei tend to be larger with more stratification and scattered mitoses, seemingly forming a generative zone (Fig. 14-1C). Toward the base, the dysplastic cells have basally oriented, enlarged nuclei containing tiny nucleoli (Fig. 14-1D).

Dysplastic glands of the mixed gastric and intestinal-type adenoma show more architectural distortion with irregular crypts lined by goblet cell–type cells, columnar mucous cells showing variable stages of differentiation, and less frequent Paneth cells (Fig.14.2A–C).

Rarely, in atrophic stomachs, intestinal-type carcinoid tumors arise in gastric tubular adenoma (Fig. 14-3).[16,17]

Immunohistochemically, in complete intestinal-type adenoma, CD10 is expressed on the luminal surface of intestinal absorptive-type cells (Fig. 14-1E), MUC2 (Fig. 14-1F) is expressed in the goblet cells, and MUC5AC (Fig. 14-1G) and MUC6 (Fig. 14-1H) are negative, resembling the phenotype of complete intestinal metaplasia or small intestinal epithelium. MUC2-positive cells tend to be distributed more superficially (Fig. 14-1F). Ki-67-positive proliferating cells are densely distributed beneath the superficial layer, the generative zone. In mixed gastric and intestinal-type adenoma, resembling phenotype of incomplete intestinal metaplasia, goblet cells and columnar cells show varying degrees of reactivity for MUC5AC (Fig. 14-2D), MUC6 (Fig. 14-2E), and MUC2 (Fig. 14-2F), but not for CD10 (Fig. 14-2G). MUC5AC-positive cells, MUC2-positive cells, and MUC6-positive cells tend to be distributed in the upper or deeper layers, respectively (Fig. 14-2D–F). The Ki-67-positive proliferating cells are more concentrated in the deeper parts.

Gastric-type adenomas. Gastric-type adenomas are composed of cells native to normal gastric mucosa, and there are two subtypes. Pyloric gland adenomas predominantly consist of pyloric gland mucous cells (Fig. 14-4), whereas foveolar adenomas are predominantly composed of mucous cells resembling the mucous cells of the gastric surface epithelium and foveolae (Fig. 14-5). By definition, both are dysplastic, although the nuclear atypia often tends to be quite subtle. Dysplasia arising in other polyps (hyperplastic, fundic gland, hamartomas) tends to be of foveolar or intestinal type if intestinal metaplasia is present.

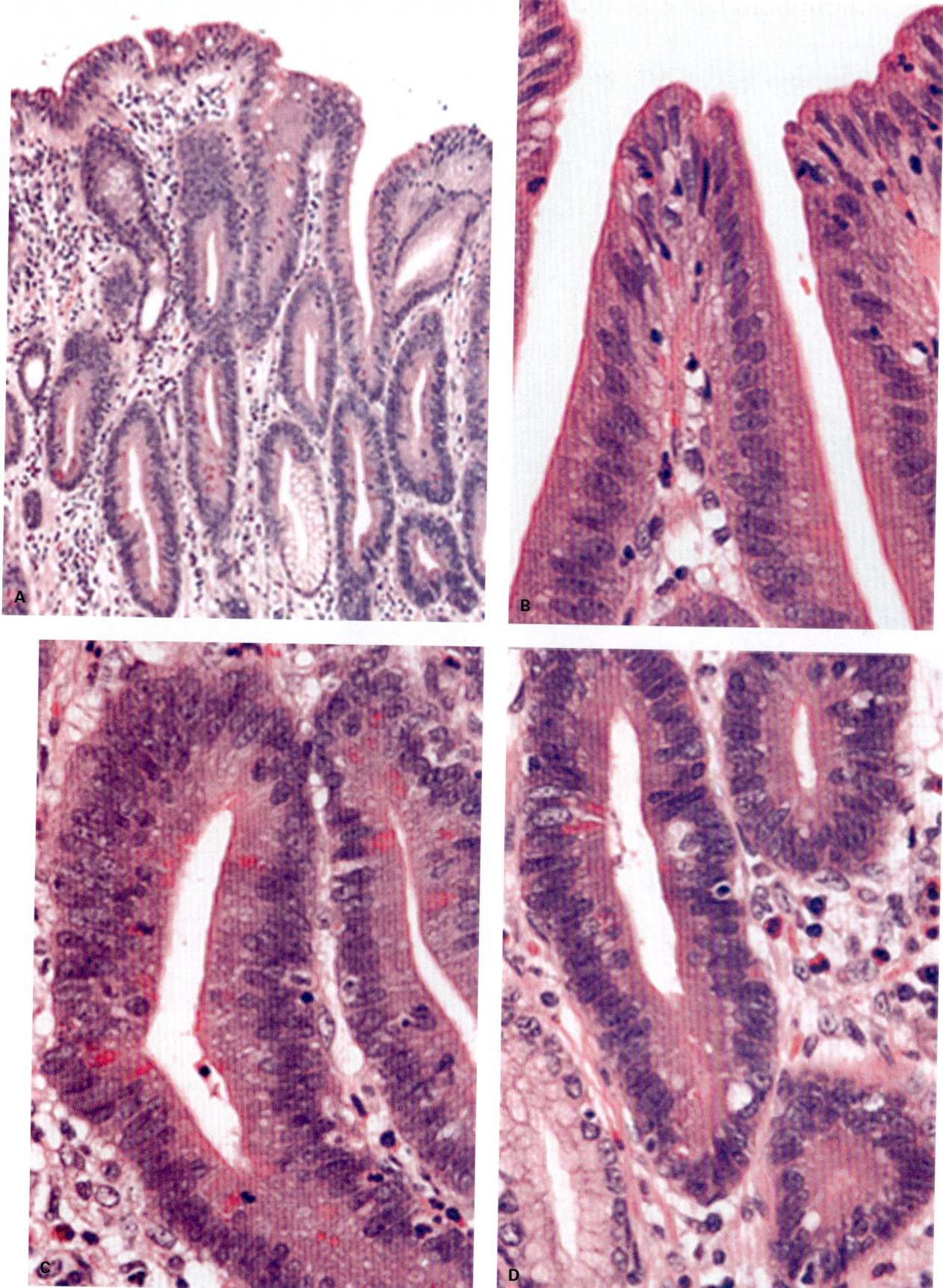

Figure 14-1. Intestinal-type adenomas (complete intestinal type). **A:** The structure of dysplastic glands of complete intestinal-type adenomas tends to be straight and similar to that of the normal small intestine. **B:** Superficially, adenoma glands are lined by columnar cells with a brush border and nuclei are elongated and the nuclei are less stratified at the gastric luminal surface. **C:** In the mid part, the nuclei are stratified, mitotic figures are found and Paneth cells are distributed among columnar cells. **D:** The bases of adenoma glands are lined by cells with basally oriented, enlarged nuclei containing tiny nucleoli.

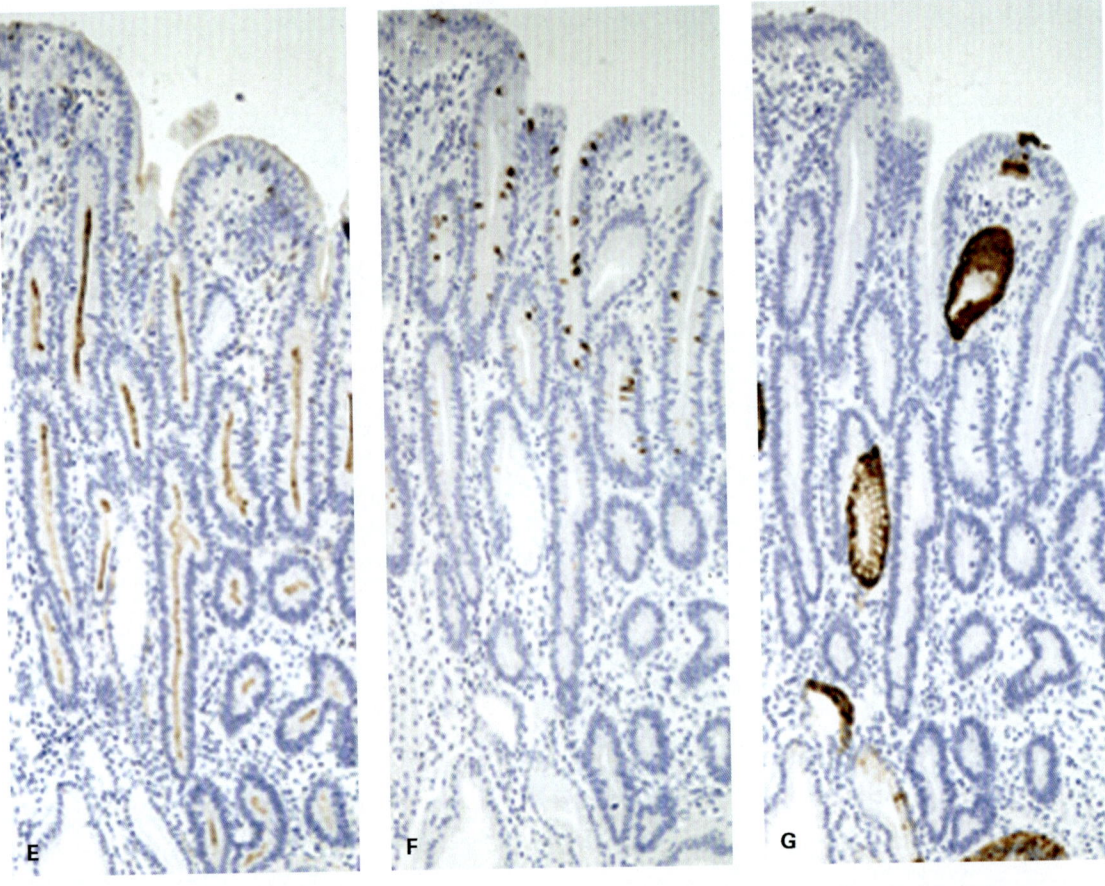
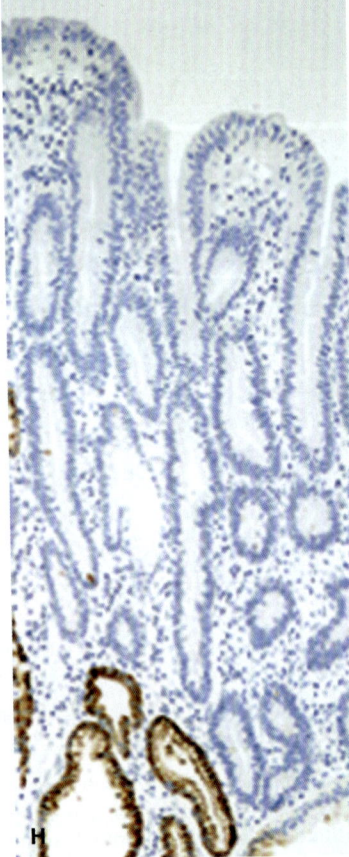

Figure 14-1. *(Continued)* E: CD10 is expressed on the luminal surface along the apical membrane of adenoma cells and (F) MUC2-positive goblet cells are distributed in the upper portion of adenoma glands. G: Adenoma cells show no immunoreactivity for MUC5AC, those staining being residual nondysplastic foveolar cells. H: Residual nondysplastic glands are positive. Adenoma cells show no immunoreactivity for MUC6.

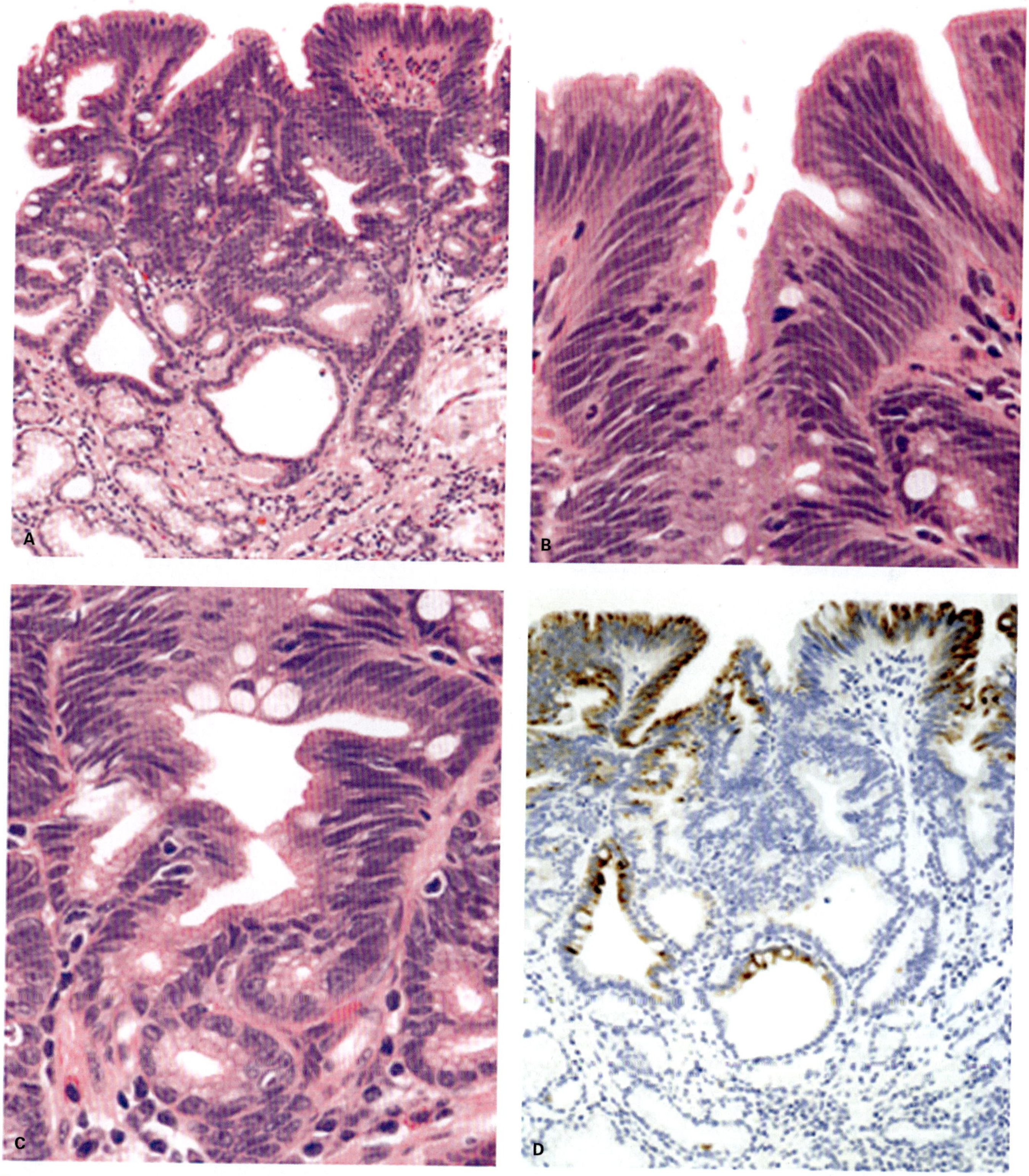

Figure 14-2. Mixed gastric and intestinal-type adenoma (incomplete intestinal type). **A:** The structure of dysplastic glands of mixed gastric and intestinal-type adenomas tend to be complex and similar to that of incomplete intestinal metaplasia. **B:** Superficially, dysplastic glands are lined by columnar cells and goblet cells and shows differentiation toward the gastric luminal surface. **C:** In the crypt bases, dysplastic glands are lined by cuboidal cells with basally oriented round nuclei with small nucleoli. **D:** Most of the MUC5AC-positive adenoma cells and

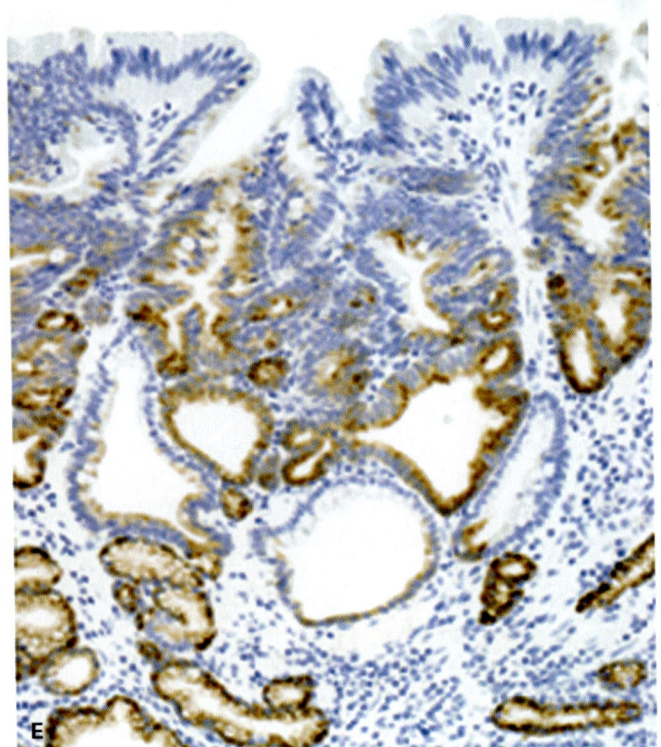
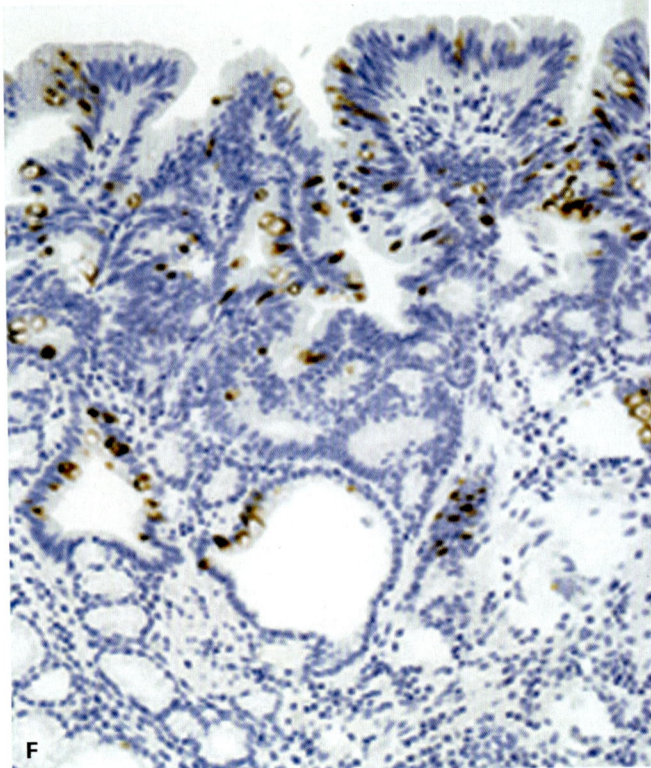
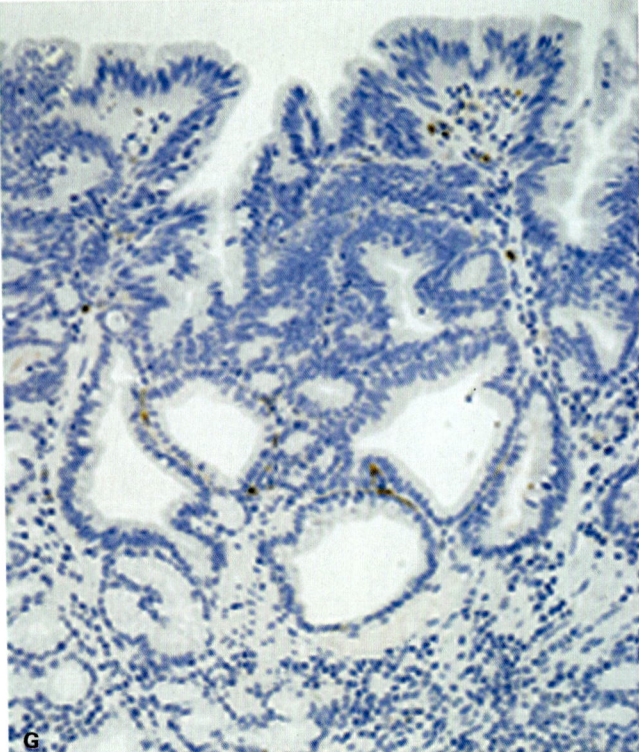

Figure 14-2. *(Continued)* **(E)** MUC6-positive adenoma cells are distributed superficially and basally, respectively. **F:** Most of the MUC2-positive adenoma goblet cells are distributed in the mid to superficial part. **G:** CD10 is negative in adenoma tissue.

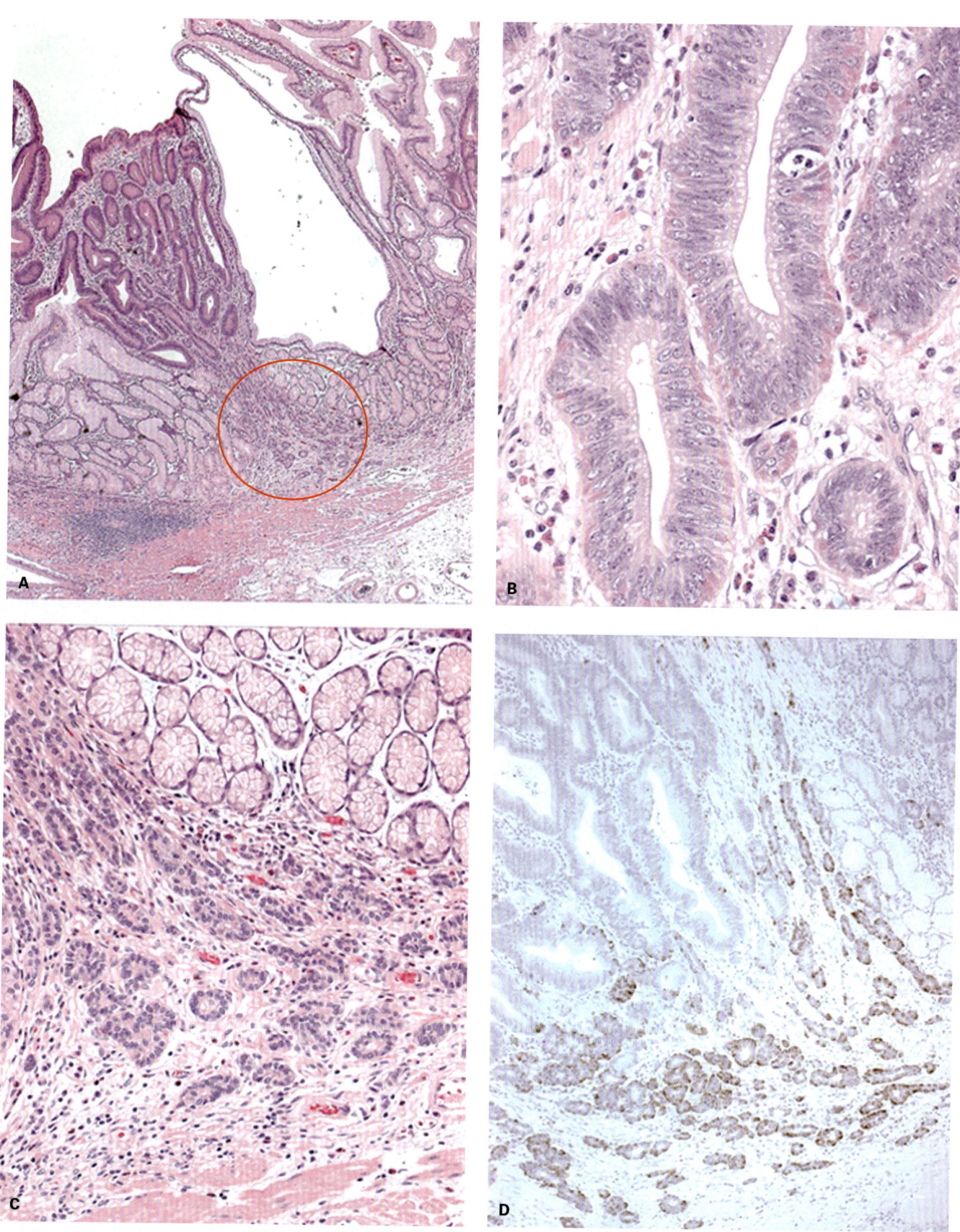

Figure 14-3. Carcinoid (well-differentiated neuroendocrine tumor) arising in a gastric tubular adenoma. **A:** Overview showing well-differentiated neuroendocrine tumor immediately above the muscularis mucosae (*circled area*) arising in gastric tubular adenoma that can be seen top left. **B:** Detail of tubular adenoma showing that endocrine cells are admixed with tall columnar glandular epithelium. Their subnuclear orange-red granules (serotonin-producing enterochromaffin cells) can be seen at the periphery of adenomatous glands. **C:** Detail of well-differentiated endocrine component. **D:** Immunoreactivity with serotonin in the endocrine component as well as scattered cells in the tubular adenoma.

Pyloric gland adenoma. The phenotypic characteristics of pyloric gland adenoma were first described by Borchard et al.[18] and by Watanabe et al.[19] in 1990. Since then, Vieth et al.[20] and Kushima et al.[21] reported a more detailed clinicopathologic analysis of pyloric gland adenoma.

Clinical Features Pyloric gland adenomas of the stomach are said to account for about 2.7% of all gastric polyps and occur commonly in the elderly, the mean age being around 73 ± 12.8 years, and invariably occur in corpus mucosa (64%). This is a little surprising as one would expect them to arise in the antrum where pyloric glands are normally present. However, while they are mainly associated with atrophic gastritis and gastric atrophy, they can be found anywhere between the lower esophagus and duodenum, gallbladder, and presumably wherever there is pyloric metaplasia. The male-to-female ratio is 1:3. In the European population, they are often found in patients with autoimmune gastritis (36%).[20]

Pathologic Findings Macroscopically, pyloric gland adenomas usually present as nodular and dome-like lesions primarily in the oxyntic mucosa, although there is no reason why they should not occur wherever gastric-type mucosa is found.[22,23]

Microscopically, they are principally composed of lobules containing closely packed pyloric-type glands lined by columnar or cuboidal epithelial cells connected to gastric foveola-like structures confined superficially (Fig. 14-4A). These glandular cells show clear or pale eosinophilic cytoplasm and small and oval to round-shaped nuclei with small but conspicuous nucleoli (Fig. 14-4B,D).[21] However, the changes are quite subtle, and unless one deliberately compares normal pyloric gland nuclei with those seen in these lesions and looks for the open chromatin and small nucleoli they are easy to miss. In one study, adenocarcinoma was found in 30% of gastric pyloric adenomas and a possibility of pyloric gland adenoma–adenocarcinoma sequence has been raised.[21] Although these adenomas can clearly be seen to infiltrate adjacent tissue, their metastasizing potential is still unclear. This creates a problem when these extend to polypectomy margins and complete removal entails major resections, for example, duodenal pyloric gland adenomas abutting onto pancreas (see subsequent section on pyloric gland carcinomas).

Immunohistochemically, most glandular cells are positive for MUC6 (gastric pyloric/antral gland mucous cell marker) (Fig. 14-4E); on the other hand, cells of the foveolar-like structure and some glandular cells are positive for MUC5AC (gastric surface and foveolar cell marker) (Fig. 14-4F).[21] Considering that MUC5AC is expressed in mucous cells of gastric epithelium in fetal gastric mucosa,[24] colocalization of MUC5AC and MUC6 in cells of gastric pyloric gland adenoma suggests an immature phenotype of these cells. MUC2 and CD10 are generally negative.[21] These tumors are often considered to be tumors with a predominantly mucous neck cell phenotype. The Ki-67-positive proliferating cells are distributed in the deeper parts of the foveolar structures and in the superficial parts of pyloric-type glands.

Foveolar adenoma. Foveolar adenomas are composed predominantly of dysplastic surface or foveolar-type cells with an apical cap of neutral mucin. They express gastric surface mucous cell–type mucin (MUC5AC) but not intestinal mucin.[25–27a-c] There is an increased incidence of foveolar adenoma in patients with familial adenomatous polyposis.[25] Sporadic foveolar adenomas are uncommon, but not rare.

Pathologic Findings This type of adenoma may have a papillary/villous structure (Fig. 14-5). On biopsy specimens, tumors showing papillary/villous structure composed of columnar or cuboidal cells with clear cytoplasm rich in neutral mucins are often difficult to differentiate from well-differentiated adenocarcinoma of gastric type.[21]

Adenocarcinoma of gastric foveolar type are superficially very similar, often having papillary/villous projections in the upper portion but also irregular branching/fusion (Fig. 14-6) and an intramucosal carcinoma in the middle to deeper portion.[21] In the foveolae of both, adenoma and the well-differentiated adenocarcinoma of gastric type, the upper portions of the papillary/villous structures are lined by tall columnar cells with enlarged cell size and low nuclear–cytoplasmic ratio (Figs. 14-5A–C and 14-6A,B) and resemble the surface and foveolar epithelium (Fig. 14-5D), whereas the deeper portions are lined by cuboidal cells resembling pyloric gland cells (Fig. 14-5E). These cells have varying degrees of mucinous cytoplasm and basally situated nuclei, which are slightly larger than those of normal gastric mucosa and are hyperchromatic.

Immunohistochemically, foveolar adenoma and well-differentiated adenocarcinoma of gastric type show similar mucin phenotypes. They show immunoreactivity for MUC5AC (Fig. 14-5F) and MUC6 (Fig. 14-5G) in the upper and lower portions of the papillary structures, respectively, showing differentiation similar to gastric pyloric mucosa. MUC2-reactive cells may be only focal or sporadic, if present (Fig. 14-5H), and CD10 is generally negative. The Ki-67-positive proliferating cells are distributed in the lower parts of the foveolar structures and in the upper parts of pyloric-type glands.

Fundic gland adenoma. We include this section cautiously as these are still poorly understood and characterized. Lesions are encountered such as those seen in fundic gland carcinoma (see subsequently), but without any evidence of submucosal invasion. Some of such lesions encountered consist of multilayered fundic gland epithelium that have been described as chief cell adenomas, parietal cell adenomas, and also as mucous neck gland adenomas. Some consider the chief cell predominant type as an intermediate phenotype between mucous neck cell and chief cell (immature chief cell).[27a-c] The lesions are well circumscribed and appear to be able to differentiate along both parietal and chief cell lineages, and the term used depends on the dominant cell type, unless one uses an all inclusive term such as fundic gland (or mucous neck) adenoma. Because of their similarity to fundic gland carcinomas they are illustrated with that section to allow easy comparison in Figure 14-27. These lesions are rare but clearly different from fundic gland polyps, and their natural history is unknown.

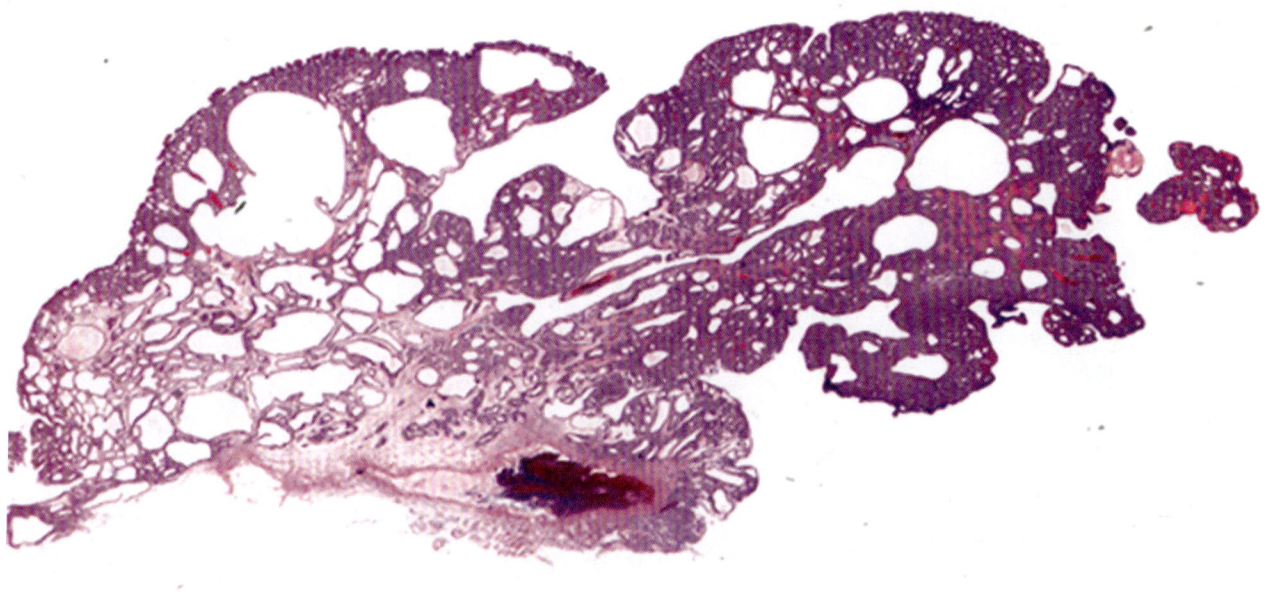

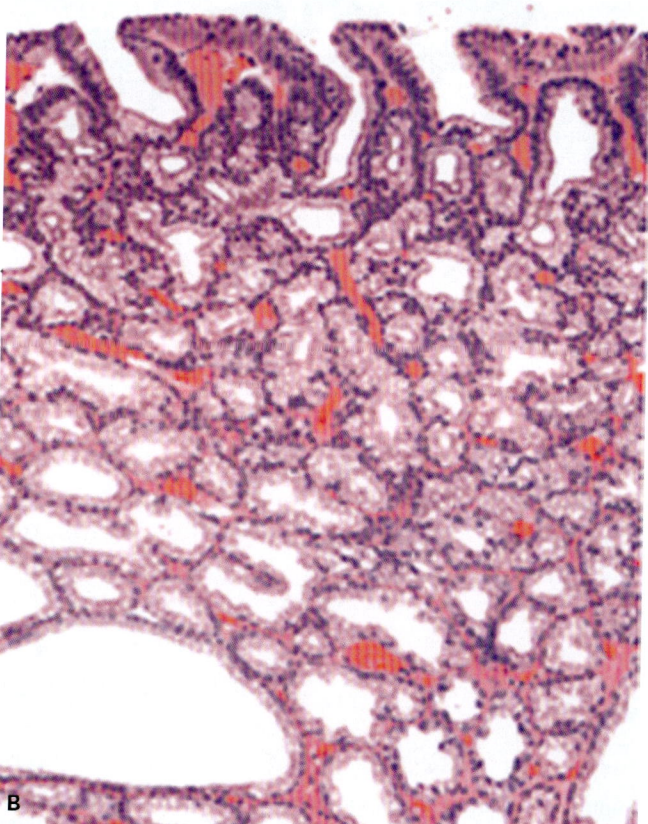

Figure 14-4. Pyloric gland adenoma. **A:** Pyloric gland adenoma showing sessile configuration containing dilated glands. **B:** They are composed of closely packed, pyloric-type glands, some of which are cystically dilated and foveolar-like structures on the surface **(B)**.

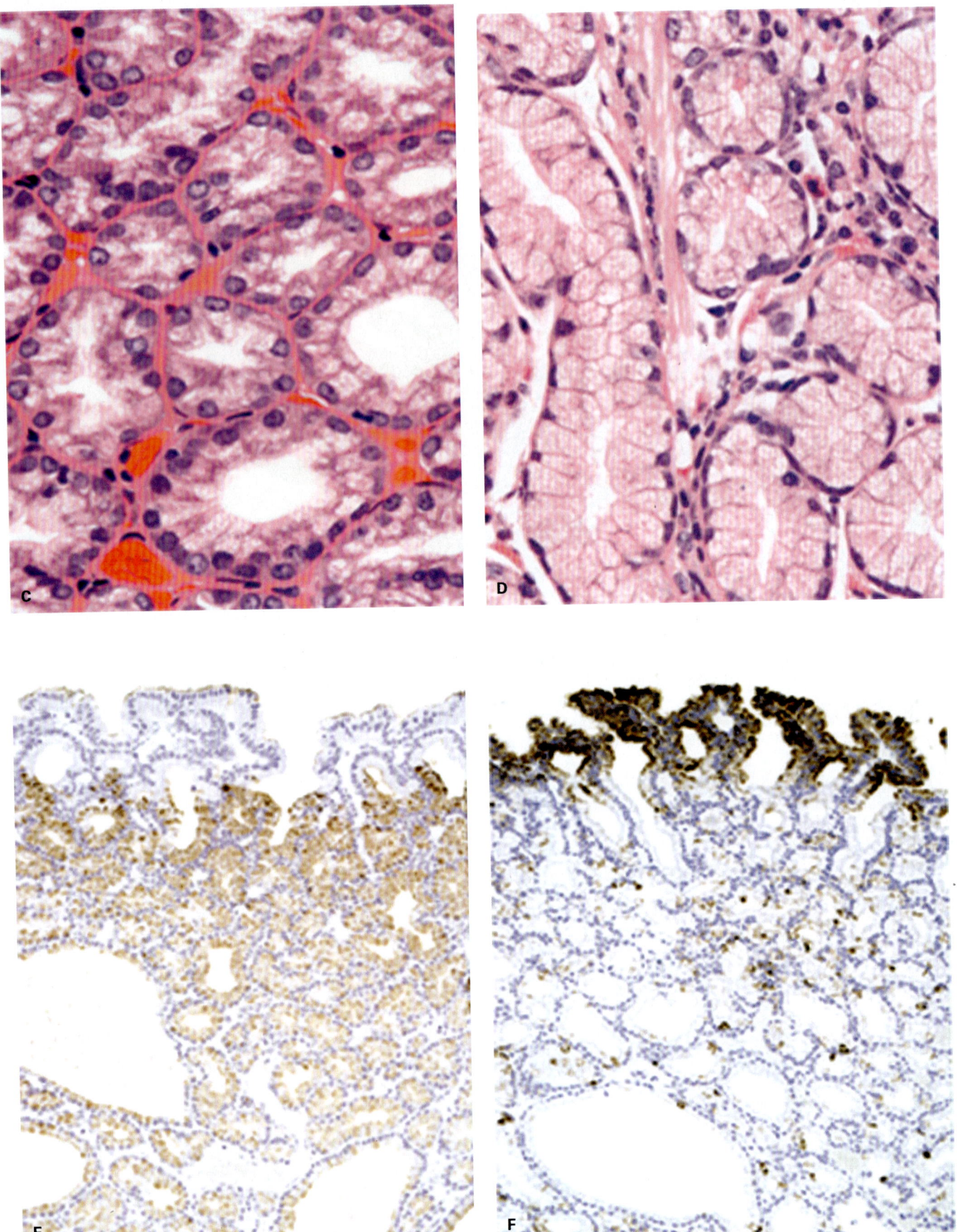

Figure 14-4. *(Continued)* Pyloric-type glands are lined by cuboidal epithelial cells showing oval- to round-shaped nuclei, which are enlarged **(C)** compared to those of normal pyloric gland cells, with small but conspicuous nucleoli **(D)**. **E:** MUC6 is strongly positive in pyloric-type glands **(F)**. MUC5AC is positive in the foveolae on the surface and in some cells in pyloric-type glands.

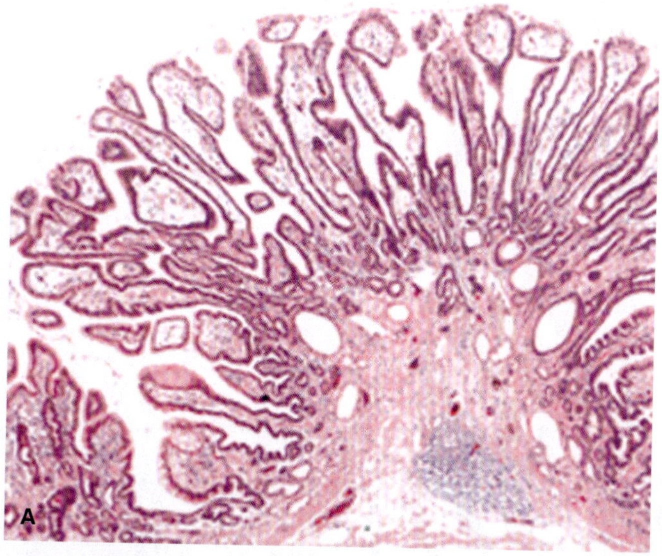

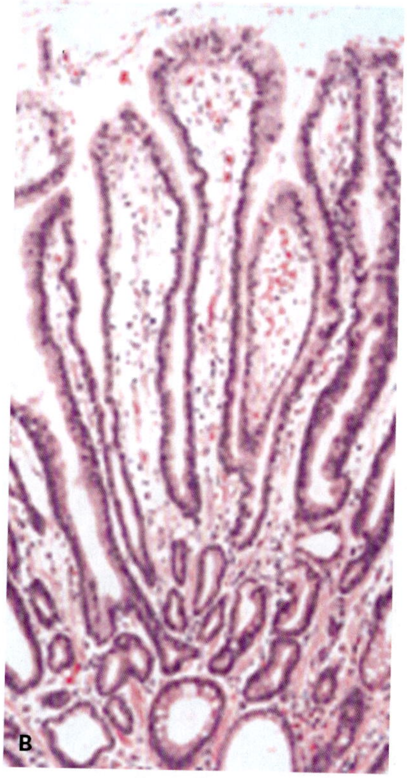

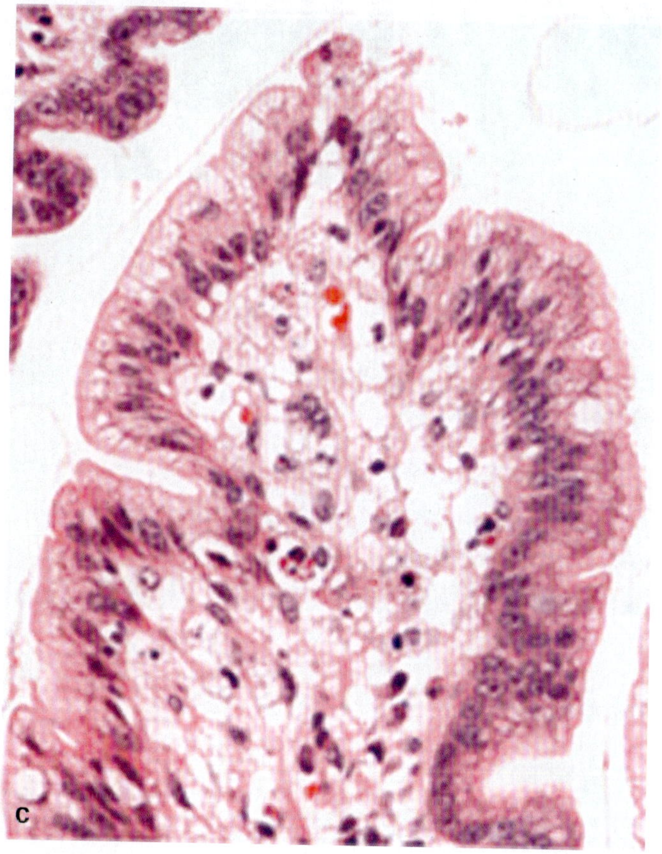

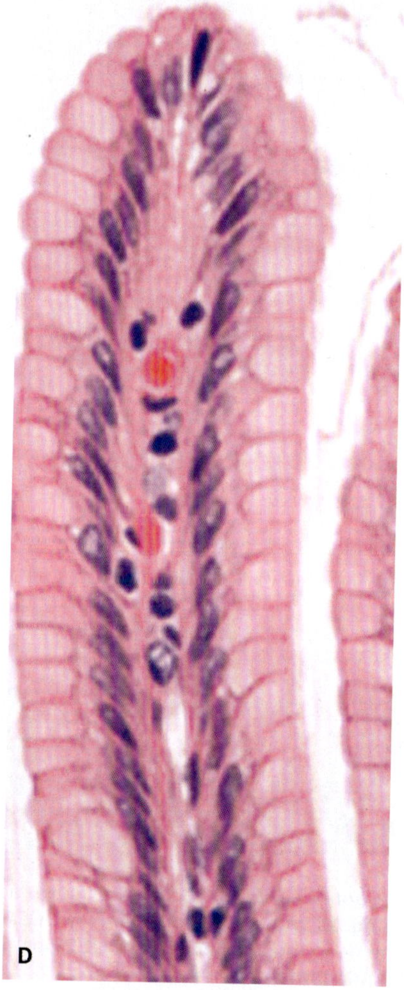

Figure 14-5. Foveolar adenoma. **A,B:** Foveolar type adenomas frequently have papillary projections. **C:** A papillary projection is lined by columnar cells with clear mucin-containing cytoplasm and basally oriented nuclei with small nucleoli. **D:** This is in contrast to the nuclei of normal foveolar epithelial cells, which have evenly distributed chromatin with inconspicuous nucleoli.

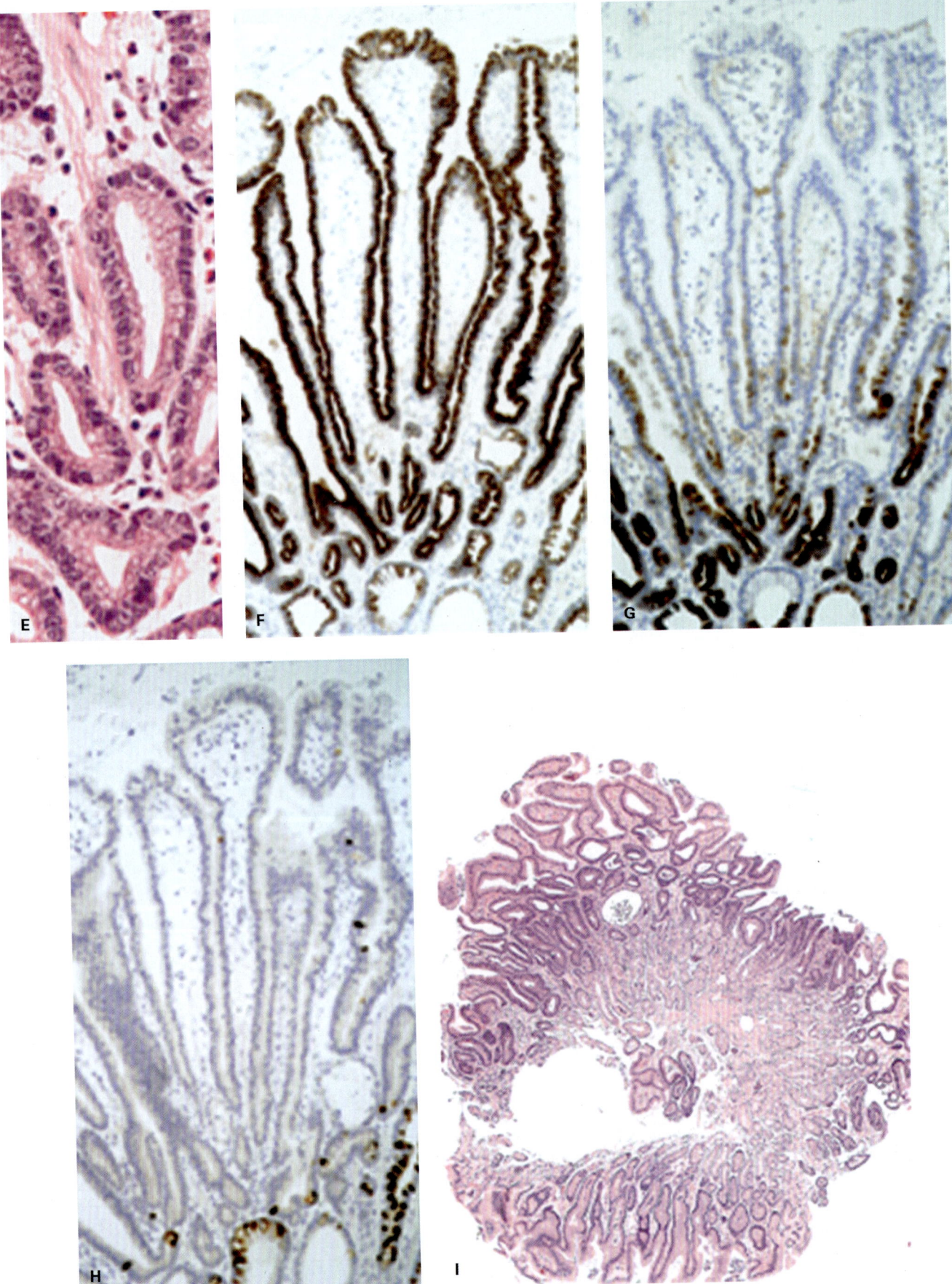

Figure 14-5. *(Continued)* **E:** In the deep mucosa, adenoma glands resemble pyloric glands and are lined by cuboidal cells with basally oriented nuclei with small nucleoli. **F:** MUC5AC is positive in tumor cells lining papillae and glands. **G:** MUC6 is positive in tumor cells in the deep mucosal level. **H:** MUC2-positive cells are found in intestinal metaplasia and are also scattered in adenoma. **I:** Antral foveolar adenoma.

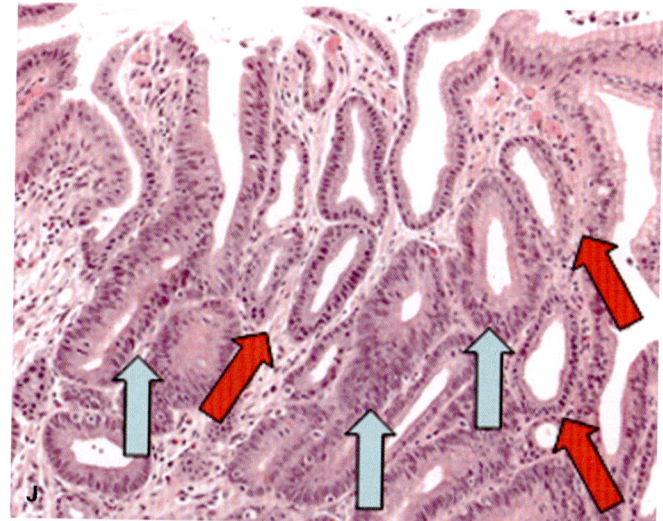

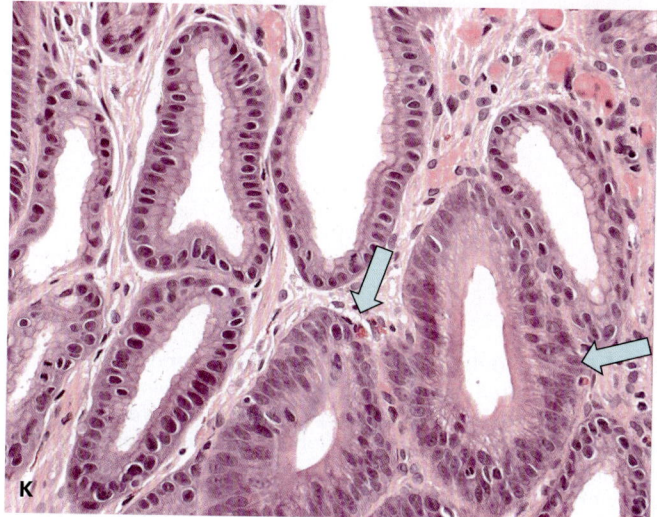

Figure 14-5. *(Continued)* **J:** Detail that has a combination of dysplastic glands with nuclear stratification (low grade, *blue arrows*) and reactive changes with basal nuclei and little overlap (*red arrows*). **K:** Detail of (J) showing the contrast between reactive glands (**left**) and dysplastic glands (*blue arrows*).

Grading of Adenoma/Dysplasia/Intraepithelial Neoplasia

Adenomas can be subjectively graded into low grade and high grade; indeed, there are numerous classifications of dysplasia/intraepithelial (noninvasive) neoplasia, but the two-grade (high and low grade) system is most consistent.[28–32] There is no real utility in using an older three-grade system (mild, moderate, severe dysplasia), as the current literature even for other sites, including other parts of the GI tract, uses a two-grade system, so there is no "action" plan that addresses a three-grade system. Also, more objective criteria can be applied to a two-grade system, which should therefore result in greater reproducibility. Nevertheless, it has to be appreciated that this is a continuum of changes as well as focality within the lesion (we grade the highest), so that in the midrange there will inevitably be less reproducibility. However, as all adenomas need to be removed endoscopically where possible, and, surprisingly, in practice most adenomas seem to classify fairly readily, this tends to be less of an issue than might be expected.

Low-grade adenoma/dysplasia/intraepithelial neoplasia. In intestinal-type adenomas, most cells have deeply staining eosinophilic or amphophilic columnar cytoplasm but goblet cells are common, particularly in lower grades of dysplasia. Enterochromaffin cells and, less frequently, Paneth cells may be present. Tumor cells have closely packed elongated nuclei with dense chromatin. If they show nuclear pseudostratification, the nuclei retain their polarity and they are confined to the basal half or two-third of the cell (Fig. 14-7). In low-grade adenomas, mitoses are usually limited to the superficial third of the mucosa.

High-grade adenoma/dysplasia/intraepithelial neoplasia. High-grade adenomas are graded primarily in intestinal epithelium, where it has more marked architectural and cytologic atypia, but having "more" changes states overtly that this is a subjective evaluation, and where LGD stops and HGD starts is subjective. The ends of the spectrum have relatively little interobserver variability when both are classical in either the metaplastic or the foveolar pathway. The architectural changes produce crowded glands that may be irregularly shaped with frequent branching and budding. In extreme cases, cribriforming may also be found.

Cytologically, high-grade adenoma consists of two main types. In the intestinalized variant, nuclei may be elongated and hyperchromatic and of irregular size. In this type, nuclear stratification may regularly extend to the cell surface, failing to mature into recognizable cell types, and nuclear polarity may be lost (Fig. 14-8). In foveolar dysplasia, tumor cells often are paler and cuboidal rather than having elongated cytoplasm and have ovoid to round and vesicular nuclei with irregular contours and prominent nucleoli. In these cases, nuclear stratification may be less prominent than in low-grade adenoma, but frequently with loss of polarity (an observation that, in Japan, is included as diagnostic criteria of "carcinoma") (Fig. 14-9). Mitoses are often numerous, and atypical mitoses may be noted. In foveolar dysplasia, the grading of dysplasia can be very difficult as the nuclei may be basal (low-grade) but the cytological detail high-grade, with loss of polarity that is again very subjective. Fortunately as they all need to be removed

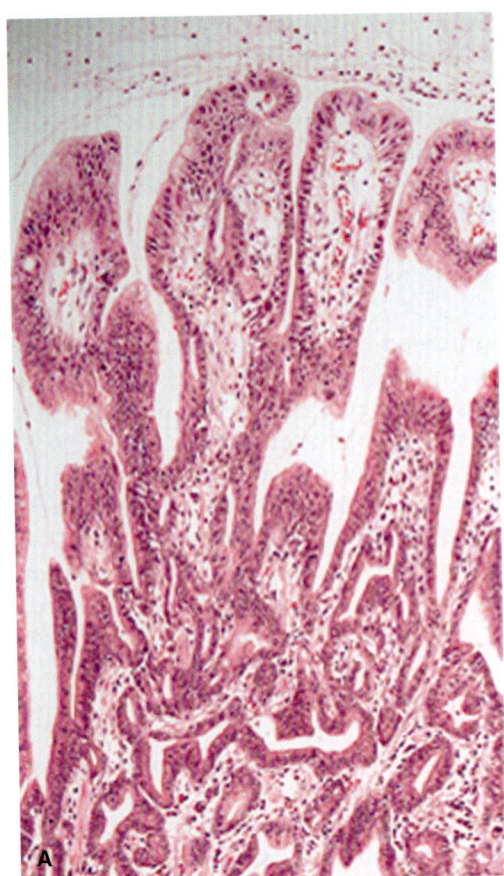
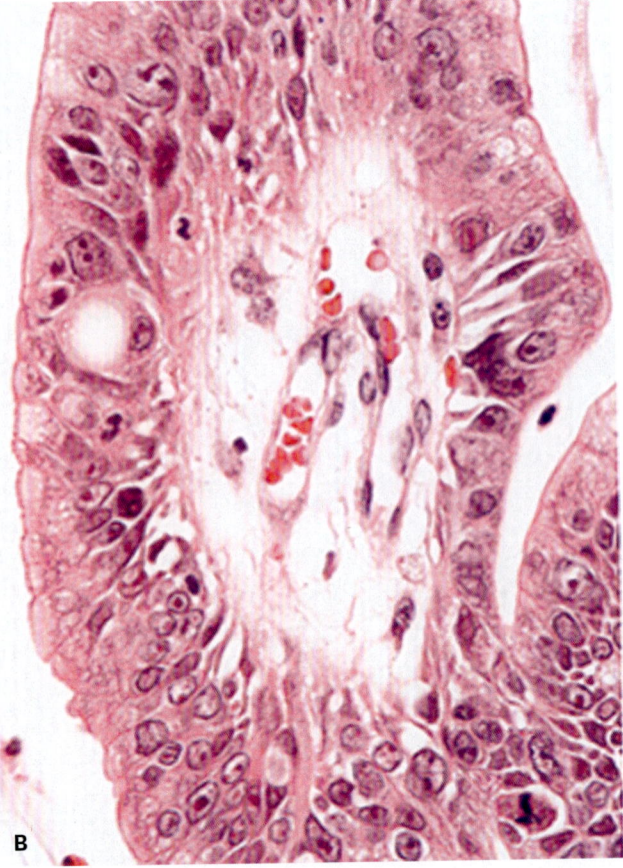
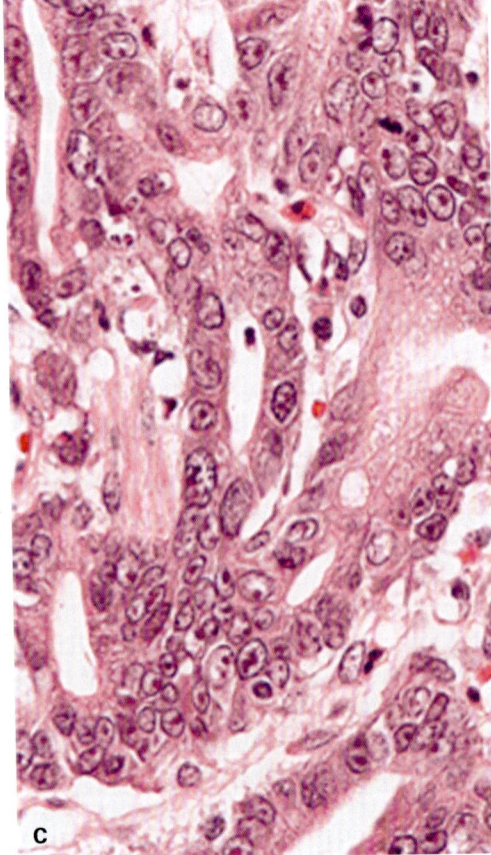

Figure 14-6. Well-differentiated gastric-type adenocarcinoma. **A:** Well-differentiated gastric-type adenocarcinoma showing papillary projections in the upper portion and irregular branching/fusion in the deeper portion. **B:** A papillary projection is lined by columnar cells with clear staining cytoplasm and basally oriented enlarged vesicular nuclei with prominent nucleoli. In contrast, the nuclei of normal foveolar epithelial cells have evenly distributed chromatin with inconspicuous nucleoli in Figure 14-5D. In the deeper portion, tumor shows irregular fusion indicative of invasion of the lamina propria **(C)**.

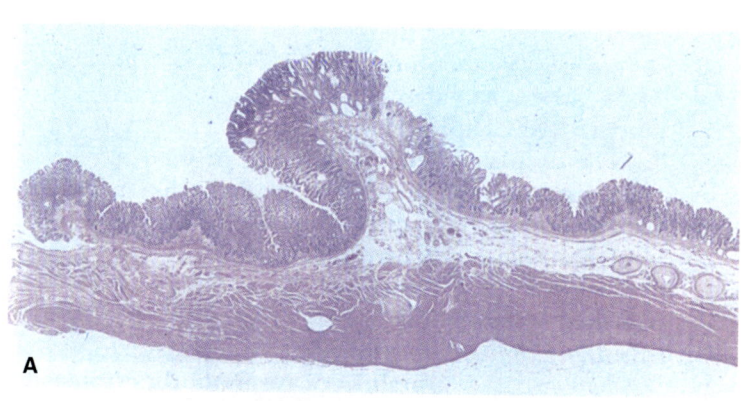
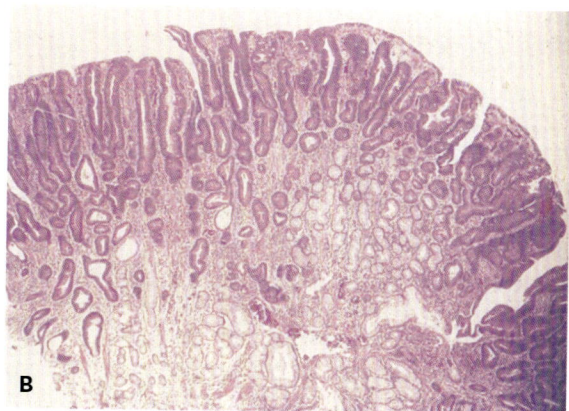
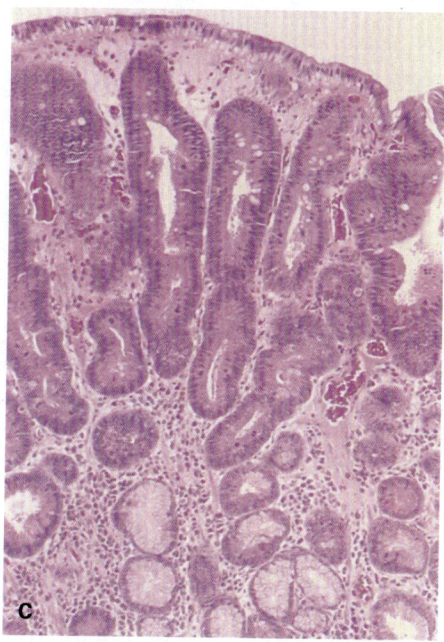
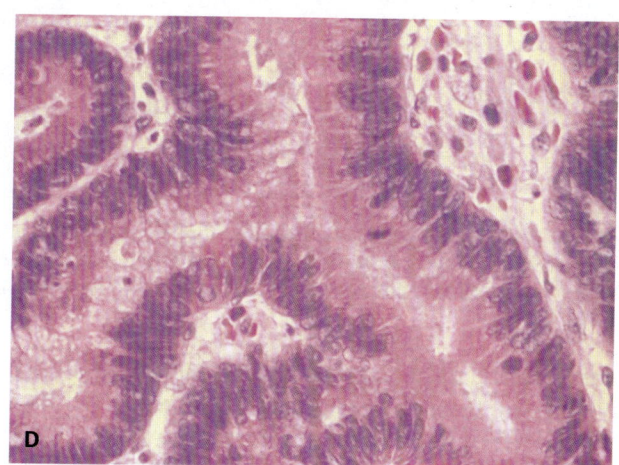

Figure 14-7. Low-grade dysplasia (intraepithelial neoplasia/adenoma). Gastric adenoma. **A:** Whole mount showing a small-stalked polyp. **B:** At low power, the diffusely eosinophilic cytoplasm resulting from failure to differentiate into mucin-producing cells is apparent, together with a prominent rim of nuclei around each gland resulting from the dysplasia present. **C:** Detail contrasts the features of the adenomatous glands superficially with the remaining normal foveolae beneath. **D:** Typical dysplasia with enlarged, hyperchromatic, stratified nuclei in cells that appear like intestinal absorptive cells but are actually just immature.

endoscopically (if possible), the distinction matters less when treated this way.

Differential Diagnosis

Distinction of regenerative changes from adenoma (dysplasia/intraepithelial neoplasia). Reparative changes in the stomach are common. Most occur in native foveolar mucosa, but variants include those arising in intestinal metaplasia, both complete and incomplete, and each is different morphologically. The latter can be recognized by the presence of the metaplasia in the adjacent mucosa, or goblet cells within the regenerating mucosa. However, complete intestinal metaplasia starts with intestinal nuclei that are already considerably larger than native mucosa, so this needs to be taken into account, while nuclei in incomplete intestinal metaplasia are more open and vesicular with distinct small nucleoli. Reactive changes therefore enhance all of these features. All forms of reactive mucosa have "acute" mucin depletion and enlarged pleomorphic nuclei occupying most of the cell (see Chapter 13 and Fig. 14-5K), and may be accompanied by erosions or ulcers. The tip-off is the presence of the following features:

1. Restituting (regenerating) mucosa (low cuboidal or columnar) with nuclei that are usually more widely separated than in normal mucosa, especially superficially. These may be totally devoid of mucin and

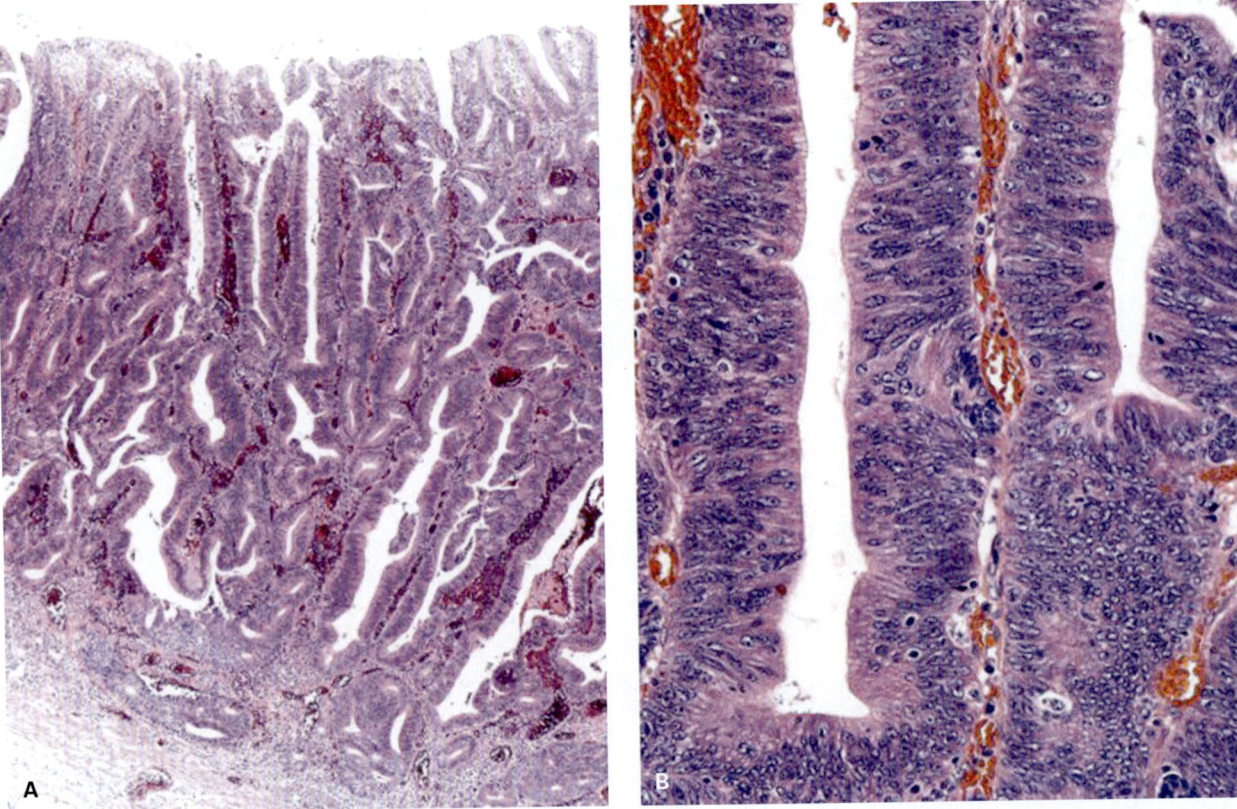

Figure 14-8. High-grade dysplasia (intraepithelial neoplasia/ adenoma) in intestinal epithelium. **A:** Overview with closely packed irregular pits. **B:** Tumor cells have elongated and hyperchromatic nuclei of irregular size. Nuclear stratification extends to the cell surface, with failure of maturation into recognizable cell types, and nuclear polarity is lost.

nuclei make up virtually the entire cell. Mitoses may be present on the surface and high in the pits. Vesicular nuclei with a thin nuclear membrane and prominent nucleoli may be present. Adjacent nuclei may vary in size and shape, but do not have the marked uniform hyperchromatism, the heavy chromatin rim, or the marked overlapping that characterizes dysplasia, although an occasional uniformly hyperchromatic nucleus may be seen.

2. Usually a degree of maturation superficially, to the degree that a diagnosis of dysplasia should be made very cautiously in the presence of active restitution. Cytoplasm may remain very eosinophilic.
3. In the bases of these pits nuclei can overlap and be stratified and hyperchromatic, and cause problems and are therefore likely to be confused with adenoma.
4. The lamina propria can show a variety of changes from chronic reactive features (capillary dilatation, hypertrophy of smooth muscle, an assortment of inflammatory cells), but sometimes it is densely hyalinized and acellular. This immediately suggests that the lack of inflammation makes *Helicobacter* unlikely and that the etiology is therefore very likely to be medications (see below).

There are some diagnostic problems. In some cases, especially in polyps, enlarged nuclei that are often stratified are found in which there is little or no ulceration or inflammation; these nuclei therefore cannot be ignored, yet they are not blatantly dysplastic. They can be handled in a variety of ways; the only mandatory procedure is to take multiple levels to ensure that an underlying carcinoma is not lurking elsewhere in the polyp. It is usually best to utilize the terms *atypical changes* or *indefinite for dysplasia*, but if the polyps have been removed it is of no clinical significance, and this needs to be stated. Because the regenerative pattern itself may produce a back-to-back appearance, albeit rarely, care must be taken not to add a little nuclear aberration to the architectural abnormality and make a diagnosis of carcinoma in situ.

The causes of reactive changes and its morphology are described in more detail in Chapter 13 (Gastritis) and include proximity to gastric ulcers and erosions, ingestion of medications such as nonsteroidal (NSAID) anti-inflammatory drugs and alcohol, and in the duodenogastric reflux, particularly following a Billroth II anastomosis, *H. pylori*–associated gastritis, and also shock.

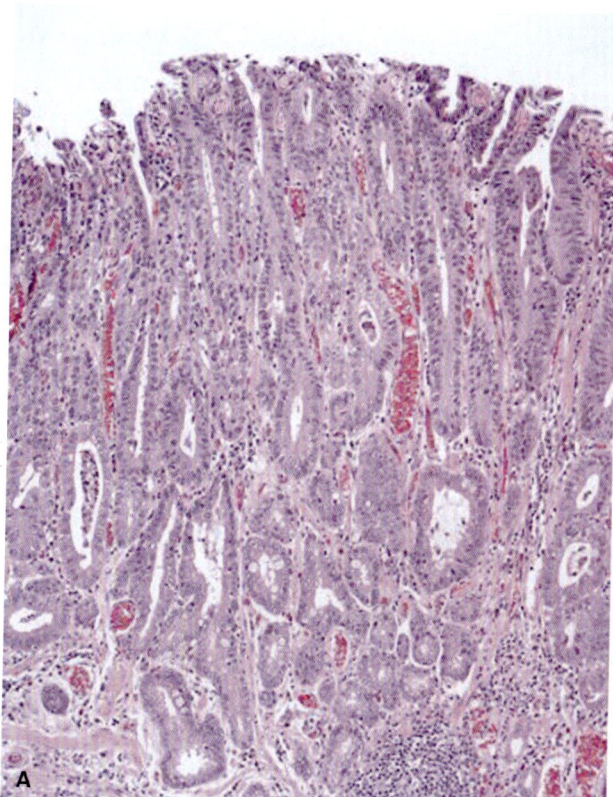 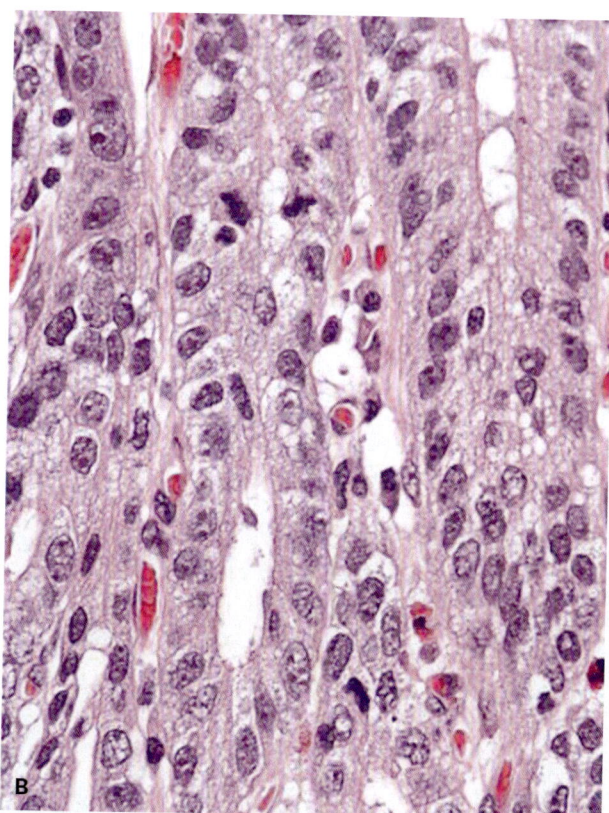

Figure 14-9. High-grade dysplasia (intraepithelial neoplasia/ adenoma) in nonmetaplastic mucosa. **A:** Tightly packed irregular but orderly pits. **B:** Tumor cells show paler and cuboidal rather than elongated cytoplasm and ovoid to round and vesicular nuclei with irregular contours and prominent nucleoli. Nuclear stratification is less prominent than in low-grade adenoma, but nuclear polarity is lost. The tightly placed glands make it very difficult to determine whether there is intramucosal carcinoma, and interobserver variability regarding this is poor, but largely irrelevant as such lesions need removing endoscopically where possible to determine whether there has been submucosal invasion and to assess all of the margins.

Distinction of high-grade dysplasia/adenoma/ intraepithelial neoplasia) from invasive carcinoma.

Criteria for the distinction of high-grade adenoma from carcinoma are different between the Western viewpoint and the Japanese viewpoint.[33] Because of the abundant lymphatic and capillary supply in the gastric mucosa, infiltration into the lamina propria has a low but definite metastasizing potential. For this reason, infiltration into the lamina propria warrants a diagnosis of intramucosal carcinoma from the Western viewpoint, but is just included as "cancer" from the Japanese (Fig. 14-10),[33] which is based on cytologic and architectural criteria and on the assumption that carcinoma cells must be present within an epithelial layer before beginning stromal invasion. The proliferating tubules of infiltrating carcinoma are often smaller than the adjacent dysplastic tubules and may sometimes infiltrate as irregular glands, small clusters of cells with or without lumina, and ultimately single cells. The most difficult cases are those in which there is proliferation of a small number of regular dysplastic tubules budding into the lamina propria. Sometimes these are a little irregular and may have small papillary projections. However, the tubules do share common walls, so that the term *gland within gland* or *back-to-back* is applicable. In these cases, it is a subjective decision as to whether the lesion should be called high-grade adenoma (dysplasia/IEN) that includes carcinoma in situ, with or without invasion of the lamina propria. Interestingly, three-dimensional reconstruction study of adenocarcinoma showed that one of the distinctive features of invasive growth of well-differentiated adenocarcinoma into the lamina propria is an anastomosis among the tubules, producing loops, which is responsible for generating patterns resembling X, Y, and H shapes (lateral fusion) on two-dimensional sections.[34]

GASTRIC CARCINOMA

Introduction

Gastric carcinomas occur in two main parts of the stomach: Cardia and the distal stomach (antrum and

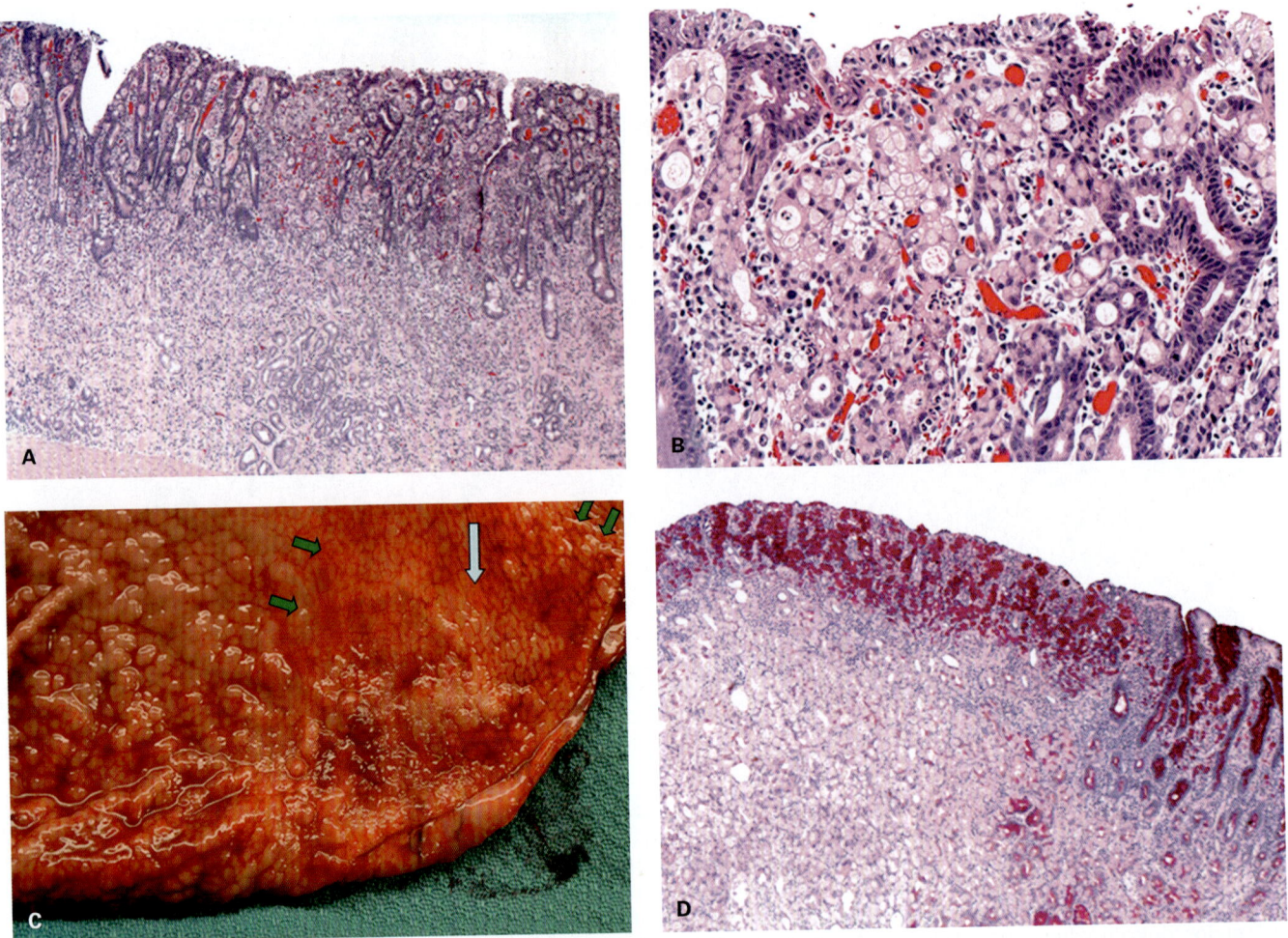

Figure 14-10. Intramucosal carcinoma. Although this large (8 cm) superficial spreading carcinoma was entirely intramucosal, there were eight positive nodes. **A:** The upper part of the mucosa has overt architectural distortion indicative of intramucosal carcinoma. **B:** Detail showing mucin-depleted carcinoma on both sides and an aggregate of mucin-producing cells with signet rings centrally. **C:** Fresh specimen in which the visible lesion is lower right (*blue arrow*) but intramucosal carcinoma extends well into the minimally irregular distortion (*green arrows*). **D:** When the entire area was blocked, mucin producing tumors could be easily detected using a PAS stain rather than an H&E. This is useful when the entire stomach needs to be embedded (as here) to determine extent or multiplicity of carcinomas, and when prophylactic gastrectomy is carried out for CDH1 (E-cadherin) germ-line mutations.

lesser curvature of the body). They occur more frequently in the latter.

Gastric Cardia Carcinoma

Carcinoma of the cardia differs clinicopathologically from those of the rest of the stomach (noncardia cancer) and appears to have different predisposing causes from noncardia cancer and some similarities to esophageal adenocarcinomas.[35] Contrary to a decline in noncardia cancer, the incidence of cardia cancer is increased, especially in the Western countries.[35,36]

This slightly awkward term is used for carcinomas at the gastroesophageal junction, the problem being exactly what that is. Conceptually, this is where the esophagus ends and the stomach begins, but in practice there are no universally accepted reproducible landmarks that identify exactly where this is. In practice it is usually identified endoscopically as the top of the gastric folds, or the lower end of the vascular arcades, although these are not always the same (see chapter on normal stomach). However, when tumors are large it can be impossible to know precisely where they originated and often their epicenter is used to classify them. One popular classification system is the Siewart system in which carcinomas more than 3 cm above the upper end of the gastric folds are Barrett's associated cancers, those more than 2 cm below (sub-cardial) are gastric, and the remainder are cardiac. The problem is that as the tumors get smaller those in the subcardiac region are clearly gastric, while those in the cardia that touch the gastroesophageal junction (GEJ) can be either of gastric or of Barrett's origin (unless a rare histologic type that makes it gastric).

As per the current AJCC classification tumors that are either clearly below the GEJ and not involving it or those that are more than 5 cm below the GEJ when GEJ is involved are considered cardiac. Despite, problems in the classification, they are worth separating because subcardial cancers have a better prognosis. Nevertheless, the morphology is the same as for other gastric carcinomas. When compared with subcardia cancers, cardiac cancers had a higher male-to-female ratio, tended to be elevated, and had a higher incidence of mediastinal node metastasis, a higher tumor, node, metastasis (TNM) stage, and a significantly lower patient survival rate.[37,38] On immunohistochemical staining, loss of p16 and SMAD 4 and overexpressions of carcinoembryonic antigen (CEA) and CD44 were more frequent in cardia carcinoma than in noncardia carcinoma, as was Epstein–Barr virus (EBV) infection.[37] Many tend to lump gastric cardia cancers with distal esophageal adenocarcinomas, however, these also have important differences despite some similarities.

Carcinoma of the Gastric Antrum and Body

The incidence and mortality of gastric cancer have fallen worldwide.[39] However, gastric cancer remains the fourth most common cancer and the second leading cause of cancer-related death in the world.[40,41] Its incidence varies greatly from country to country. High-incidence areas include Eastern Asia, East Europe, and Central and South America.[41] Low incidence rates are found in North America, Northern Europe, North and East Africa, and Southeastern Asia.[41]

Gastric carcinomas do not consist of a homogeneous group of tumors. There are several distinct clinicopathologic entities with different predisposing conditions and probably etiologies. They can be divided into two major histologic types: Those arising in native mucosa and those arising in metaplastic (intestinal) mucosa. These were called *intestinal or differentiated type* (in metaplastic mucosa) and *diffuse or undifferentiated type*, corresponding to carcinomas arising in native gastric mucosa, although there is an overlap of patterns in some and others defy classification. Intestinal-type carcinomas predominate in high-incidence geographic areas for gastric carcinoma[42] and its incidence has decreased.[43,44] Conversely, diffuse-type carcinoma has a more uniform geographic distribution and is relatively more common in low-incidence areas[44] and its incidence has been stable[43] or has increased.[44] To some extent, they appear to have different underlying causes, precursor lesions, and rates of growth. While these fundamental histologic types have stood the test of time generally, more useable classifications are now in place (discussed subsequently).

Pathogenesis

Pathogenetic factors will be discussed in terms of risk factors, predisposing conditions, and premalignant lesions.

Risk Factors

A *risk factor* is an attribute that confers a higher than expected incidence of cancer on a population. In gastric carcinoma, there are marked geographic variations, possibly due to environmental factors. Genetic predisposition may also be a factor. Epidemiologic studies have clearly shown that migration from a high-risk area (e.g., Japan) to a low-risk region (e.g., Hawaii) is associated with a decline in the incidence of gastric cancer, most notably in the second generation.[45–47] Similar findings have been reported from Colombia.[46] These studies have also shown that environmental factors are important in the genesis of carcinoma.

***Helicobacter pylori* infection.** Epidemiologic studies have revealed a strong association of *H. pylori* infection with intestinal or diffuse type of gastric cancer development.[48] However, the absolute risk is only about twice that of the non–*H. pylori*–infected population, even though *H. pylori* is designated as a major (Class 1) risk factor. Supporting this, animal models with *H. pylori* infection showed promotion of gastric carcinogenesis.[49–51] Prospective cohort studies have shown the strongest evidence to support the role of *H. pylori* infection in gastric cancer development, although the relative risk (RR) is only a little over two. Yet with so many in the world being infected, this is a significant risk on a worldwide basis. In a prospective study of 1,526 Japanese participants, gastric cancers developed in 2.9% of *H. pylori*–infected people and in none of the *H. pylori*–noninfected individuals.[52] Furthermore, it has been demonstrated that *H. pylori* eradication reduced the incidence of metachronous gastric carcinoma after endoscopic resection of early gastric cancer.[53] It is involved in both types of carcinoma, although the association with intestinal-type carcinomas appears most marked.

H. pylori is involved in the development of gastric cancer through two major pathways: The indirect action on gastric epithelial cells through inflammation and the direct action on epithelial cells through the induction of protein modulation[54,55] and gene mutation.[56] Inflammation is found especially with organisms containing CpG island methylator phenotype (CIMP), responsible for production of CagA and VacA toxins (see next section).

In the indirect pathway of chronic *H. pylori* gastritis, enhancement of helper Th1-type CD4 T-cell infiltration and their products, interferon gamma, and a variety of proinflammatory cytokines have been demonstrated and play a crucial role in the induction of gastritis.[57-59] Among proinflammatory cytokines enhanced in H. pylori–related gastritis, both interleukin (IL)-1β and tissue necrosis factor alpha (TNFα) enhance nuclear factor-κB (NF-κB) activation in epithelial, inflammatory, and mesenchymal cells. NF-κB functions as a tumor promoter in inflammation-associated cancer[60] and exerts an antiapoptotic action[61] with the production of various cytokines[61] and cyclooxygenase-2.[62]

In the direct pathway, H. pylori directly perturbs intracellular signaling events by delivering bacterial agents into the cells through a bacterial type IV secretion apparatus, encoded by the HP *cag* pathogenicity island (*cag*PAI).[54,55] H. pylori also directly activates NF-κB in the gastric epithelial cells and induces gene mutations in epithelial cells by enhancing the expression of activation-induced cytidine deaminase (AID) in gastric epithelial cells through NF-κB activation.[56] AID, a member of the cytidine deaminase family, is essential for somatic hypermutation and class-switch recombination of immunoglobulin genes in B lymphocytes by acting as an editor of DNA and RNA.[63]

In addition, H. pylori infection enhances aberrant DNA methylation in the gastric mucosa through direct action of H. pylori on epithelial cells or H. pylori–induced inflammation, and the methylation may cause gastric carcinogenesis by silencing the tumor suppressor gene.[64]

Epstein–Barr virus, CIMP-H, and K-ras. EBV is a double-stranded DNA virus that is associated with about 10% of gastric carcinomas, yet the data are a little conflicting. Cancers occur predominantly in a slightly younger male population. Nevertheless,

1. Gastric carcinomas with lymphoid stroma[65-67] have a strong association with EBV, and in about 85% of these tumors, by in situ hybridization.[67]
2. If one looks at an unselected series of gastric carcinomas, about 8% to 10% of those will also contain EBV, and these are fairly equally distributed between intestinal and diffuse types. This suggests either that the lymphoepithelial variant may transform into regular variants or that regular variants are by far the most common EBV-associated carcinomas, but that when the rare lymphoepithelial variant occurs it is much more likely to be EBV associated.

Whether EBV infection of gastric stem cells occurs from the associated lymphoid cells or occurs directly is unclear, but data suggest that the virus is found only in the epithelial cells. Nevertheless, the mechanism of EBV carcinogenesis appears to be through methylation of the promoter region of many cancer-related genes, and subsequent transformation and selection of the predominant clones.[67] Interestingly, the CpG island methylator phenotype (CIMP), which is characterized by simultaneous methylation of the CpG islands of multiple genes, is related to EBV infection. When carcinomas that had high CIMP methylation (CIMP-H) were compared with tumors that had low CIMP methylation (CIMP-L) or negative CIMP methylation (CIMP-N), EBV-associated tumors were found to be associated strongly with CIMP-H, with hypermethylation of tumor-related genes, but there was an inverse relationship with p53 and K-ras mutations, with none of the latter in one study being detected among CIMP-H tumors. Carcinomas that have wild-type K-ras can therefore be expected to be enriched with EBV-associated carcinomas. CIMP-H tumor was also associated with proximal location, diffuse type, and less advanced pathologic TNM status. Patients who had CIMP-N gastric tumors had a significantly worse survival than patients who had CIMP-H tumors or CIMP-L tumors. In addition, among EBV-negative gastric carcinoma subgroups, CIMP-H gastric carcinoma showed comparatively higher frequency of methylation than CIMP-I or CIMP-N, especially of p16 and hMLH1. CIMP-N gastric carcinoma predominantly consisted of advanced carcinoma with significantly higher frequency of lymph node metastasis.[68]

Finally, one study found that mixed-type carcinomas, which have both diffuse and intestinal components, had more methylated genes than either "pure" diffuse or intestinal carcinomas, and were present in both components of these mixed tumors. Further, this trend was also observed when EBV-positive or microsatellite instability (MSI)-positive carcinomas were excluded from the analysis. and was significantly higher than was found in either intestinal or diffuse carcinomas. These findings suggest that the mixed intestinal-diffuse type of carcinoma may be a distinct subgroup characterized by enhanced CpG island hypermethylation of promoters.[69]

JC virus. JC virus (JCV) is a polyomavirus that infects humans worldwide, with more than 80% of the adult population having antibodies against it. JCV sequences are frequently present throughout the normal human GI tract and in colorectal and gastric cancers. JCV expresses the T-Ag protein, which in one study was found in half of 90 gastric cancer tissues, but was independent of EBV expression. However, T-Ag expression was detected in a significantly lower percentage of MSI-H cancers (14%) than in non–MSI-H cancers. T-Ag-positive gastric cancers showed a significant increase in the allelic losses and aberrant methylation compared with T-Ag–negative gastric cancers.[70]

Dietary factors. The dietary factors implicated are high salt consumption, associated with salted fish and meat, smoked foods, and low caloric intake. Smoking and alcohol consumption may also contribute. Nitrosamines, resulting from the conversion of dietary nitrates in the acid milieu of the stomach, have also been proposed but are unconfirmed as important carcinogenic agents in gastric carcinoma.[71] Consequently, there has been an interest in the possible role of antioxidants (which can prevent the conversion of nitrates to nitrosamine), such as vitamins C and E and selenium, in lowering the risk of gastric cancer.[72]

Smoking. Smoking is significantly associated with gastric cancer, especially noncardia cancer, in a dose-dependent manner.[73–75] Moist snuff or smokeless tobacco, which is commonly used in Scandinavia as an alternative to cigarettes, has been shown to enhance noncardia gastric cancer.[76]

Genetic factors. Individual risk from carcinogen exposure varies as a function of both environmental and inherited genetic factors. Inherited genetic susceptibility is involved in gastric carcinogenesis in two ways: (a) germline mutations involved in hereditary gastric cancer predisposing to either syndromes or other genetic abnormalities that predisposing to gastric cancer and (b) polymorphism in genes.

Hereditary gastric cancer predisposition syndromes. These contribute a small population of gastric cancers and include hereditary nonpolyposis colon cancer syndrome (HNPCC, GAPPS syndrome, Lynch's syndrome), hereditary diffuse gastric cancer (HDGC), Li–Fraumeni syndrome, familial adenomatous polyposis, Peutz–Jeghers syndrome, and juvenile polyposis (with or without hereditary hemorrhagic telangiectasia (HHT) syndrome), and there are doubtless others with a clear familial trait waiting to be discovered.

HNPCC results from germline mutations in one of the mismatch repair genes (e.g., MLH1, MSH2, MSH6, PMS1, and PMS2) and tumors that arise in association with HNPCC are characterized by MSI. Gastric cancers are said to arise in 11% of HNPCC families and the majority of these cancers are of intestinal type.[77]

HDGC is the currently known autosomal dominantly inherited disorder characterized by early onset of diffuse gastric cancer (DGC) of signet-ring cell type.[78,79] In prophylactic gastrectomy specimens performed in at-risk family members, "in-situ signet-ring cell carcinoma" (putative precursor lesions for HDGC), sometimes with pagetoid spread along the gastric glands or foveolae, is commonly identified.[79] Female mutation carriers have a risk also for lobular breast cancer.[71] HDGC must fulfill one of the following criteria:

1. Two or more cases of documented DGCs in first- or second-degree relatives under the age of 50, or
2. Three or more cases of documented DGC in first- or second-degree relatives independent of the age of diagnosis.[80]

A germline mutation in the E-cadherin (*CDH1*) gene has been identified in 30% to 40% of HDGC families.[80] *CDH1* germline mutation carriers in HDGS have a >70% lifetime risk of developing diffuse-type gastric cancers.[81] The inactivation of *CDH1* is caused by heterozygous germline mutations of *CDH1* and the somatic inactivation of the second *CDH1* allele by mechanisms that include DNA promoter hypermethylation.[82,83] The *CDH1* gene encodes for E-cadherin, which is a transmembrane protein expressed at the baso-lateral cell surface of the epithelial cells. E-cadherin plays an important role in cell-to-cell adhesion through its extracellular domain and also in tumor suppressor function through the interaction of its intracellular cytoplasmic domain with the catenins. The loss of cell-to-cell adhesion and promotion of tumor invasiveness may follow the loss of E-cadherin.[84]

GAPPS syndrome (gastric adenocarcinoma and proximal polyposis of the stomach) has proximal fundic gland polyposis but there is nothing else to suggest FAP in this autosomal dominant syndrome, although it seems likely to be the result of activation of the wnt signalling pathway.

Over 50% of families with Li–Fraumeni syndrome have an identifiable germline TP53 mutation[85,85a] and patients with Li–Fraumeni syndrome are at increased risk for developing multiple primary cancers. Classic Li–Fraumeni syndrome is defined by the following criteria:

1. A proband with a sarcoma diagnosed before 45 years of age.
2. A first-degree relative with any cancer under 45 years of age.
3. A first- or second-degree relative with any cancer under 45 years of age or a sarcoma at any age.

Familial adenomatous polyposis (FAP) results from germline mutations in the FAP (adenomatous polyposis coli [APC]) tumor suppressor gene on chromosome 5q21-q22. In stomachs of FAP patients, fundic gland polyps are the most common gastric lesions and adenomas are less common. FAP families occasionally develop gastric cancers, particularly in Japanese families.[86,87] However, while occasional cases do develop either from antral adenomas or from dysplastic fundic gland polyps in the West,[88] they are vanishingly rare so that no significant increased risk is found for gastric cancer in FAP patients in Western countries.[87,89]

LGD in fundic gland polyps is quite frequent, but HGD and carcinomas arising in fundic gland polyps seem extremely rare. Interestingly, inflammation and H. pylori are rare in fundic gland polyps whether sporadic or syndromic.

Peutz–Jeghers syndrome is an autosomal-dominant disorder characterized by mucocutaneous pigmentation, hamartomatous polyps, and an increased risk of associated malignancies; germline mutations of the tumor suppressor gene LKB1/STK11 are responsible for this syndrome. A meta-analysis of Peutz–Jeghers syndrome showed that cancers having a statistically significant increased RR compared with the general population include esophagus (57), stomach (213), small intestine (520 because small bowel cancer is rare), colon (84), pancreas (132), lung (17), breast (15), endometrium (16), and ovary (27), but not testicular or cervical malignancies.[90] These markedly decrease longevity compared to the general population—see Chapter 20.

Juvenile polyposis is usually associated with large bowel polyps, but those with SMAD4 germline abnormalities are associated with gastric juvenile polyps and an increased risk of gastric carcinoma, which may develop as early as the fourth decade of life. Forests of polyps may be present (see subsequent section in this chapter). Carcinoma develops in dysplastic juvenile polyp. Germline testing becomes important for follow-up as surveillance endoscopy is required with this group of patients. It should also be remembered that a combined syndrome of JPS and HHT (termed JPS/HHT) may be present in 15% to 22% of individuals with an *SMAD4* mutation, so that the possibility of juvenile polyps and their sequelae need to be considered in patients with HHT and a germline SMAD4.[1]

Other genetic abnormalities predisposing to gastric cancer. These include DNA aneuploidy, decreased expression of tumor suppressor or protective genes due to promoter hypermethylation (*p16, p27, TFF1,* and *MLH1*), amplification of oncogenes, or overexpression of growth factors (Cox-2, HGF, VEGF, EGFR/EGFR, c-Met, and amplified breast cancer-1 or AIB-1).[91]

Polymorphism in genes. Molecular cancer epidemiology has revealed that genetic polymorphisms influence both response and susceptibility to carcinogens and that these gene–environmental interactions could explain the high variation in gastric cancer incidence around the world.[92,93] Genetic polymorphisms found to be associated with gastric cancer risk include genes in (a) mucosal protection (mucin gene), (b) inflammatory responses (proinflammatory cytokine genes including IL-1β, IL-10, and TNF-α, TLR4, and HLA), (c) carcinogen metabolisms, (d) oxidative damage, and (e) DNA repair.[92] Among these, a meta-analysis showed the most consistent results associated with increased gastric cancer risk were IL-1β and NAT1 (involved in the metabolism of aromatic and heterocyclic amine carcinogens) variants and that polymorphisms in HLA-DQ, TNF-α, CYP2E (involved in the metabolism of low-molecular-weight toxins and N-nitrosamines) might confer some protective effect against gastric cancer.[92]

Predisposing Conditions

These are pathologic processes associated with an increased risk of cancer. These include atrophic gastritis, subtotal gastrectomy, immunodeficiency syndromes, chronic gastric ulceration, and Menetriér's disease. It should be stressed that the association of these disorders is controversial and that some conditions, such as atrophic gastritis and postgastrectomy states, may be more relevant to high-risk countries, and that Menetriér's disease is very poorly defined and likely involves several different entities.

The association of *chronic gastric ulceration* with carcinoma is controversial and often difficult to prove. In order to demonstrate this association convincingly, it is necessary to demonstrate the typical features of a chronic gastric ulcer with a carcinoma arising from it, usually at one margin. This may be difficult in advanced cases, in which the tumor may have overrun much of the ulcer.

Early studies from Japan frequently reported cancers around ulcers, but now these cancers are rarely seen.[47,94] It is also noteworthy to remember that early gastric cancer may closely resemble a benign peptic ulcer, and heal temporarily with proton pump inhibitors (PPIs).

***H. pylori*–related chronic atrophic gastritis.** This is by far the most important precursor of gastric cancer. Long-term follow-up studies in Finland on patients with atrophic gastritis, with or without pernicious anemia, have shown a 9% incidence of gastric cancer.[95] Furthermore, studies in Japan have shown that 80% of gastric cancers arise in atrophic gastric mucosa,[96] specifically in areas of *incomplete intestinal metaplasia* characterized by combined foveolar mucin cells and intestinal goblet cells, the latter having poorly developed microvilli, secretion of sulfomucins, and a lack of Paneth cells.[47,97] This increased risk of gastric carcinoma in patients with severe atrophic gastritis does not appear to be borne out in countries that have lower prevalence rates in general for gastric cancer. The key factor seems to be multifocal intestinal metaplasia on a background of chronic atrophic gastritis. The whole concept of an advancing front of atrophy in chronic *H. pylori* gastritis, previously thought to be just an aging change, is discussed further in Chapter 13.

A prospective study of 1,526 Japanese participants showed that patients with *H. pylori* infection and severe atrophic gastritis, corpus-predominant gastritis, or both, along with intestinal metaplasia were at high risk for intestinal-type gastric cancer, and that many of the patients with diffuse-type gastric cancer had atrophic changes and pangastritis.[52] Cancers tend to be located in the gastric antrum and lesser curve.

A possible association of diffuse-type gastric cancer in young adults with nodular gastritis has also been suggested from observations in Japanese.[98–101] Nodular gastritis is characterized by the presence of *H. pylori* infection and follicular gastritis and shows a predilection for females and young adults.[98,99,101]

Postgastrectomy. The risk of carcinoma developing in the gastric remnant following subtotal gastrectomy (almost always in peptic ulcer disease) has been estimated at 5% to 10%. It is said to occur much more frequently following partial gastric resection with Billroth II anastomosis[47,102] and has been blamed on reflux of bile that also contains activated pancreatic juice and ensures reflux of small intestinal bacteria into a stomach secreting little acid, as the G-cell–rich antral area has been removed with consequent atrophy of oxyntic mucosa. It appears to be a late complication, occurring 15 to 25 years after gastrectomy.[47,102] The tumors may occur anywhere in the residual stump or at the stoma and are invariably adenocarcinoma histologically, although there is one report of a squamous cell carcinoma.[103] These findings have been disputed by some,[104] who in their long-term follow-up studies in the United States have found that the incidence of gastric cancer is no more common among patients with prior gastric surgery for ulcer disease than in the general population. Nevertheless, inflammatory polyps with marked reactive change are common at the anastomotic line, and this tends to be where carcinomas occur. It should also be recalled that as the gastrectomy was likely carried out for "peptic ulcer disease"— a somewhat archaic term that now embraces both *H. pylori* and medication (NSAIDs, ASA, etc.), many of these patients may well still be harboring *H. pylori* in their proximal stomach, although the role that this plays in the carcinomas, which are usually much more distal, is unclear and may be minimal.

Immunodeficiency disorders. The risk of cancer in the primary immunodeficiency disorders ranges from 2% to 10%.[45] Many of the tumors are lymphomas, but gastric carcinoma also occurs (see Chapter 3). Because the association is usually recognized and patients are clinically followed up, predisposing factors such as *H. pylori* are invariably eradicated, but carcinomas may still arise in the noninflamed mucosa.

Menetriér's disease. (See also Chapter 13). There are a number of case reports describing the association of Menetriér's disease with gastric cancer,[105] and we have seen several apparent examples of this (Fig. 14-11). The problem with Menetriér's disease is that it is a poorly defined disorder in the literature, often merely referring clinically to giant gastric folds. Thus more accurate information about the specific lesions is needed before this condition can be labeled a premalignant condition. In classic forms it is limited to the oxyntic mucosa, and is diffuse without areas of intervening normal mucosa,

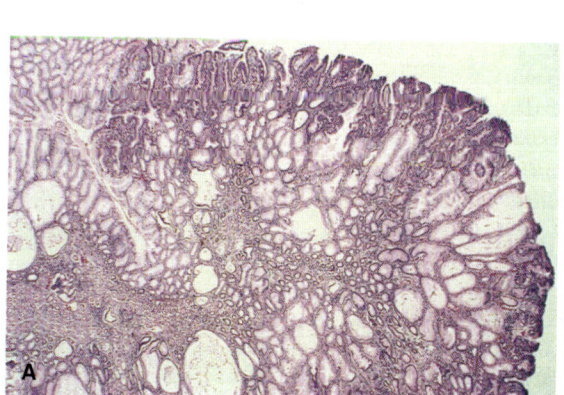
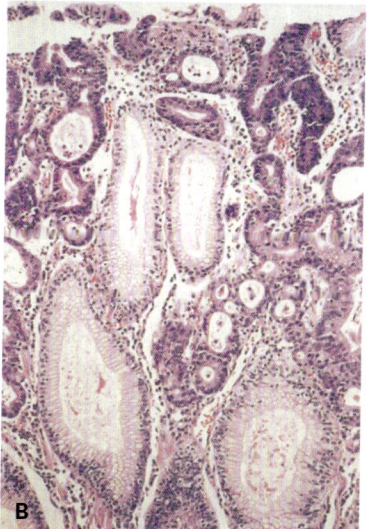

Figure 14-11. Dysplasia and carcinoma associated with Menetrier's disease. **A:** Gastric mucosa showing marked thickening resulting from foveolar hyperplasia, elongation of glands, and cystic formation. There is dysplasia of the superficial glands. **B:** Higher-power magnification of part (A) showing infiltrating neoplastic glands.

thus excluding multiple hyperplastic-type polyps from this diagnosis. However, at least some patients with cancer and a diagnosis of Menetrier's disease are very likely examples of juvenile polyposis with predominant or isolated gastric involvement. As with most gastric diseases there are two questions: (a) Is *Helicobacter* present, and if it is then eradicate it, and see if the underlying disease improves. If not (b) is there a lymphocytic gastritis that may indicate undetected *H. pylori* requiring serology. If so again it should be eradicated. Prolonged antisecretory therapy may be required after eradication. If there is no *H. pylori* infection or inflammation and serology is negative, then PPIs are often given "on spec." This condition is discussed further in Chapter 13. More recently, TGF-α or epidermal growth factor was shown to be significantly up-regulated in Menetrier's disease.[106] This resulted in selective expansion of surface mucus cells in the fundus and the body of stomach. These patients have been successfully treated with a blocking monoclonal antibody specific to EGFR (C225).

Premalignant Lesions of the Stomach

Premalignant lesions have morphologic features of neoplasia and have the potential to become cancerous. They usually arise in individuals who have one or two predisposing conditions and probably represent the final common pathway through which these conditions give rise to cancer.

Adenoma/dysplasia/intraepithelial neoplasm. Gastric adenomas are considered to carry an unusually high risk of carcinoma. The larger the polyp, and higher the grade of dysplasia, the higher is the frequency of malignant transformation. Overall about 35% of gastric adenomatous polyps show intramucosal carcinoma/high grade dysplasia, in contrast to 4% to 5% of hyperplastic polyps.[107] This is discussed in detail in the previous section on adenomas.

Gastric polyps. Gastric polyps other than adenomas, such as fundic gland polyps, especially in patients with FAP and those of familial juvenile polyposis, may also on occasion show dysplasia and malignant transformation, as may a small proportion of sporadic hyperplastic polyps (see subsequent discussion).

Gross Features of Gastric Carcinoma

Macroscopically, a number of classifications have been proposed for gastric carcinoma, but the most widely adopted or modified is that of Borrmann (Fig. 14-12).[108] Although a fifth category is sometimes added for those that do not fit (unclassifiable).

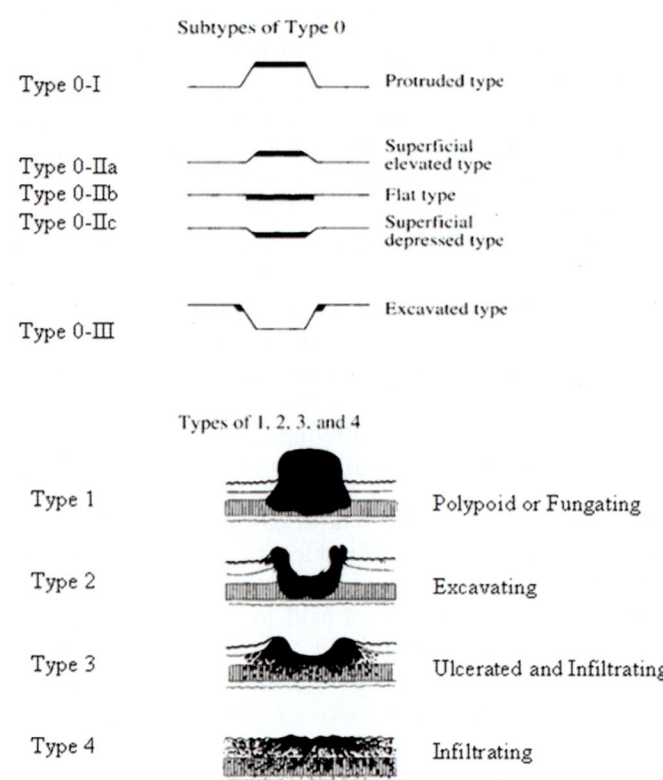

Figure 14-12. Macroscopic types of gastric cancer. The original Borrmann classification are the types 1 to 4, while the subtypes of early gastric carcinoma (superficial flat carcinomas, type 0) were added subsequently and reflect the same principles. (Reprinted from Japanese Gastric Cancer Association. Japanese Classification of Gastric Carcinoma, 2nd English edition. *Gastric Cancer* 1998;10–24, p. 12 Figs. 3 and 4, with permission.)

Type 0 was also added for superficial tumors (Fig. 14-12)[109,110]:

Type 0—Superficial, flat tumors with or without minimal elevation or depression
Type 1—Polypoid tumors
Type 2—Ulcerated carcinoma with sharply determined and raised margins
Type 3—Ulcerated carcinoma without definite limits, infiltrating into the wall
Type 4—Diffusely infiltrating carcinomas in which ulceration is usually not marked
Type 5—Unclassifiable carcinomas that do not fit into any of the above types

Types 1, 2, 3, and 4 correspond to the four classes found in Borrmann's classification for advanced gastric cancer.[108]

Advanced gastric carcinomas are characterized by exophytic intraluminal or infiltrative growth patterns modified by surface erosion and ulceration.[47,94] Some advanced carcinomas reveal macroscopically superficial flat tumors resembling early gastric cancers and they are also described as subtypes of type 0 (Fig. 14-13).

Type 0-IIb—flat

Type 0-IIc—slightly depressed due to surface erosion or mucosal atrophy (Fig. 14-13)

The excavated type 0-III is characterized by a deep ulcer with a rim of narrow margin of cancer. In the combined superficial types, the type occupying the largest area is described first, followed by the next type, for example, IIc + III.

Although there is an overall correlation between these subtypes and long-term prognosis, with type 0-I having the best prognosis and type 0-III the worst, the ultimate prognosis is related to the depth of invasion of the tumor (see next section). With the exception of the ulcerating and diffusely infiltrating tumors, which do appear to behave in a more aggressive manner, there is little evidence that the gross morphology of gastric adenocarcinomas is of any prognostic significance. Thus a too precise macroscopic classification of gross lesions is of limited practical value, especially since there is often a mixture of gross types in any one case.

Classification and Natural History of Early and Late (Advanced) Gastric Carcinoma

Early gastric carcinoma/cancer. Early gastric cancer has been defined as a gastric neoplasm confined to the mucosa and submucosa, irrespective of whether lymph node metastases are present. Histologically, both early and advanced gastric cancer shows the same histologic spectrum. Tsukuma et al.[112] followed 43 cases of early gastric cancers from 6 to 88 months in patients refusing resection. They found that 16 (37%) remained unchanged, while the remaining 27 developed into advanced carcinomas. These results and those of similar studies by others suggest that the two types of cancer are the same entity but at different stages of development.

Early gastric carcinoma can be subdivided histologically into *intramucosal* carcinoma, in which there is invasion into the lamina propria or muscularis mucosae, and *submucosal* invasion. Most of the tumors occur in the antrum and lesser curvature, and about 10% are multifocal. In Japan, approximately 50% of all gastric cancers fall into this category.[113,114] In Western series, the incidence of early gastric cancer is reported to be around 10% to 20% of all gastric carcinomas.[115]

There is a rough correlation between the subtypes of early gastric cancer and advanced cancers. Polypoid early lesions tend to give rise to advanced polypoid carcinomas, and type II lesions, with the exception of the large eroded type, give rise to ulcerative infiltrating carcinomas. The large eroded type and the excavated types may result in a wider variety of advanced cancers, ranging from the ulcerative infiltrating to the diffusely infiltrative carcinomas.[47]

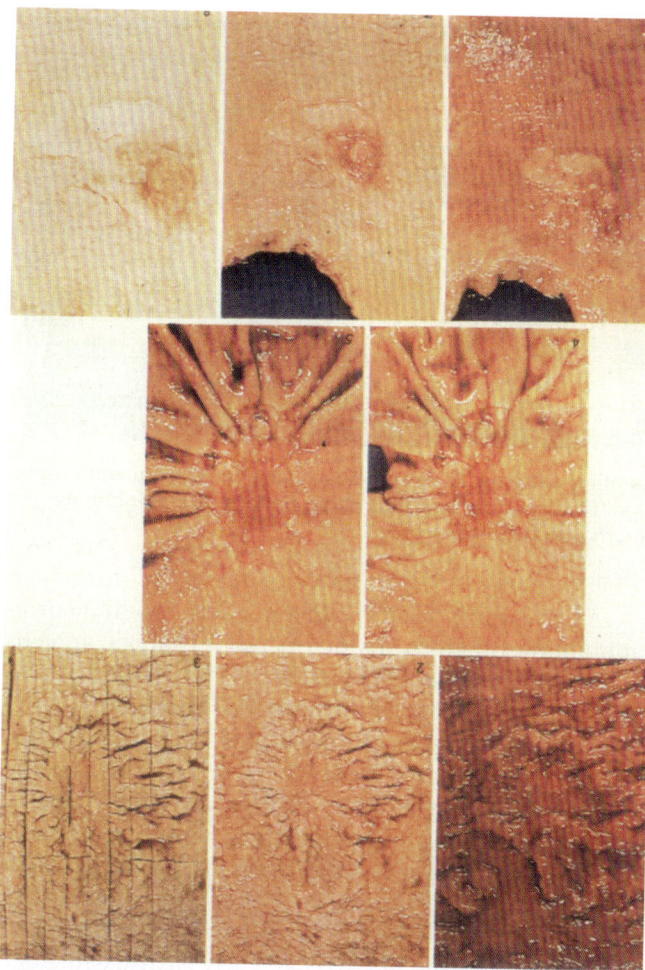

Figure 14-13. Early gastric carcinoma. Composite of gross appearances. The **top panels** shows types I and IIa (elevated and polypoid). The **middle panels** shows types IIc + III (depressed and excavated pattern), and the **bottom panels** shows types IIa + IIc (elevated and depressed pattern). (Courtesy T. Mochizuki.)

Gross Features of Superficial Cancers and Their Subdivision

These tumors are sometimes referred to as "type 0 gastric cancers," especially in Japan, and can also be divided into the usual three main groups:

Protruded type (type 0-I)
Superficial type (type 0-II) with yet three further subdivisions, 0-IIa, 0-IIb, and 0-IIc
Excavated type (type 0-III) (Fig. 14-13)[110]

The superficial type of tumor is by far the most common, accounting for just under 80% of early gastric cancer; the other two types account for about 10% each.[47,111]

The subdivisions of type 0-II are

Type 0-IIa—superficial elevated that has a mucosa approximately up to twice as thick as the surrounding mucosa (practically 2–3 mm in thickness)

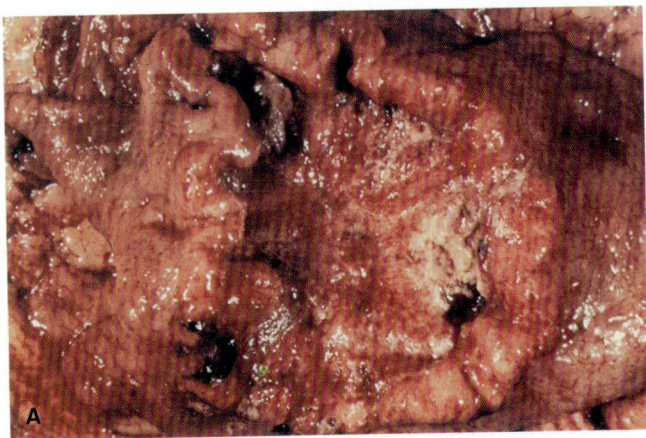
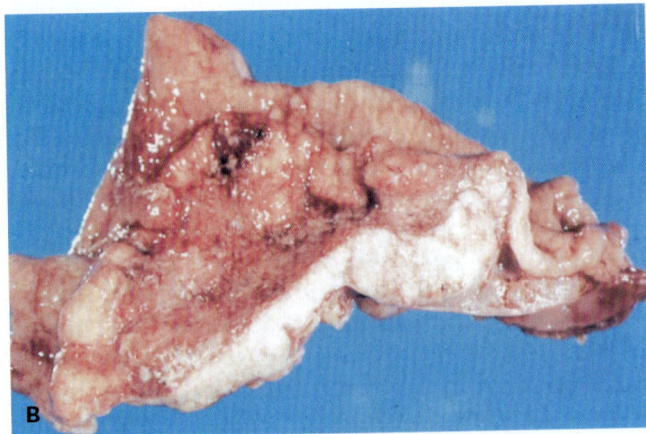

Figure 14-14. Advanced gastric cancer showing infiltrative and ulcerating patterns. **A:** Exophytic excavating type showing markedly raised, rolled margins and central ulceration with crater formation. **B:** Ulcerating and infiltrating pattern. The longitudinal cut through the tumor shows diffuse infiltration and thickening of the stomach wall by tumor.

There is also a fairly close correlation between macroscopic appearance, histologic type, and depth of invasion.[47,116] Polypoid or elevated lesions are usually well differentiated, whereas excavated and large, depressed lesions are often poorly differentiated. Similarly, small lesions (<3 cm) with demarcated margins are usually well differentiated and show no or little invasion, whereas larger lesions with serrated margins are often poorly differentiated, with signet-ring cells, and invade into the submucosa.[47,117]

Advanced gastric cancer. Advanced gastric cancer is defined as a gastric neoplasm invading the gastric wall beyond the submucosa (into the muscularis propria or beyond)

At the time of presentation, advanced gastric cancer is usually readily visible endoscopically, forming obvious lesions that still form the bulk of resections (Fig. 14-14), and is often associated with vague symptoms such as weight loss and anemia. Other modes of presentation consist of ulcer-type pain, occult or overt GI bleeding, or gastric outlet obstruction if the tumors are near the pylorus. Some patients present with widely metastatic disease.

Linitis plastica (leather bottle stomach) is a diffusely infiltrative carcinoma, usually involving the greater part of the stomach, associated with a marked desmoplastic reaction and resulting in a grossly thickened stomach, which has been likened to a leather bottle (Fig. 14-15). Frequently there is also a concomitant giant hypertrophy of the mucosal folds. Because of the intense fibrosis, the often undifferentiated nature of the tumor cells, and the associated mucosal ulceration, these tumors can be misdiagnosed as chronic peptic ulcer. The exact origin of these tumors within the stomach can be impossible to find.

As with early gastric cancers, there is some correlation between gross characteristics, histologic appearances, and the age of the patient. The exophytic and expanding lesions tend to be well or moderately well-differentiated, associated with intestinal metaplasia, and found in elderly patients, whereas the diffusely thickened and infiltrative lesions are often poorly differentiated and tend to occur in younger patients. Superficial spreading carcinomas make up about 3% of gastric cancers. As stated previously, they can measure up to 10 cm in diameter, but are confined to the mucosa and submucosa and behave like early gastric cancers.

The size of advanced gastric cancers at the time of diagnosis can vary from <2 to more than 15 cm in diameter and can affect the entire stomach (linitis plastica). The majority are in the 2- to 6-cm (44%) and 6- to 10-cm range (30%).[118]

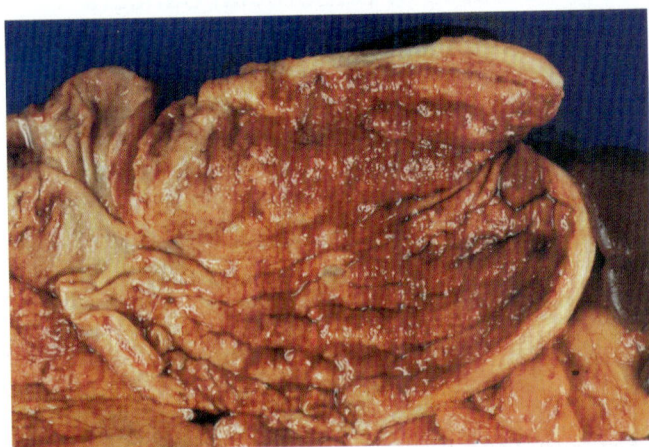

Figure 14-15. Linitis plastica (diffusely infiltrative gastric carcinoma). The whole stomach is involved, and the gastric wall is thickened. The mucosa appears swollen and covered in blood but is otherwise intact.

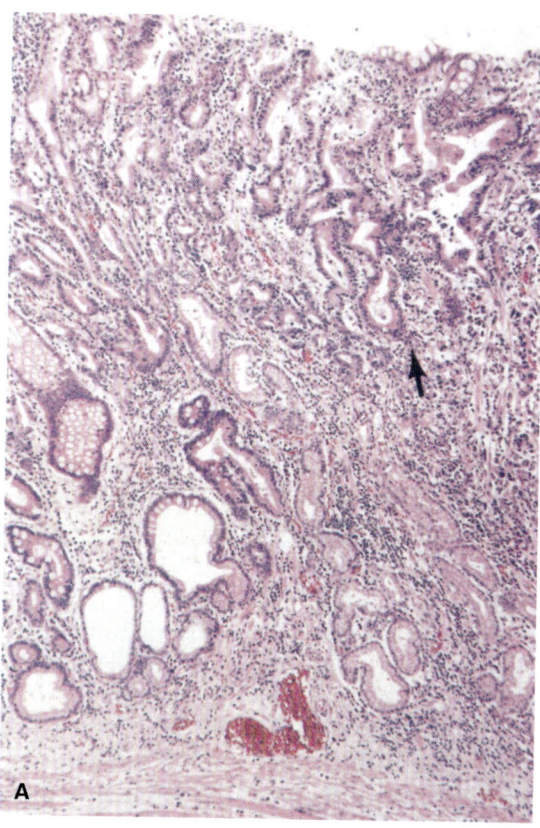
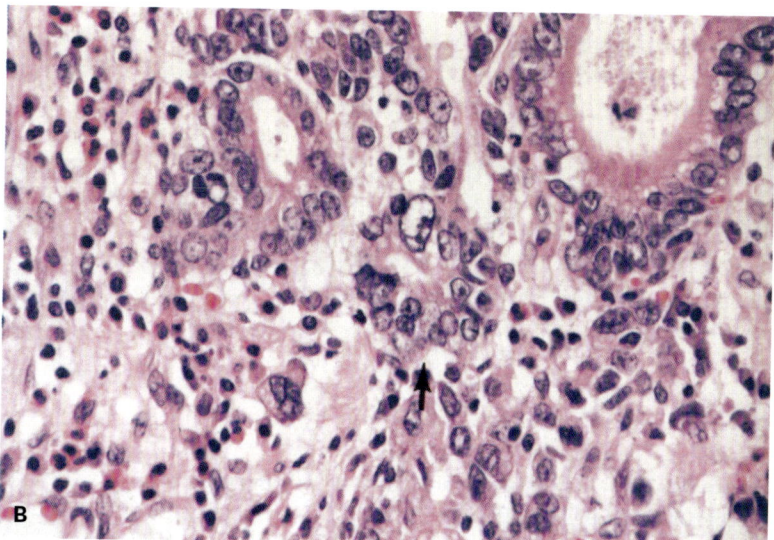

Figure 14-16. Intramucosal carcinoma of the stomach. **A:** Antral mucosa showing chronic gastritis, intestinal metaplasia, and high-grade dysplasia (*arrow*). **B:** Higher-power magnification of the arrowed area in part (A) showing infiltration of the lamina propria by poorly differentiated epithelial cells.

Histologic Classification of Gastric Carcinomas

Lauren classification. Because of the limitations of the morphologic classifications in regard to reproducibility and clinical outcome, a number of simplified classifications have been proposed. Lauren[119] proposed classifying advanced gastric carcinomas into two types: *intestinal* and *diffuse*.

The intestinal type (presumed to be derived from intestinalized gastric mucosa) is more common in males and older age groups. It usually has a polypoid or fungating gross appearance and often an expansile growth pattern. Histologically, it is characterized by well-defined glandular structures and is almost invariably associated with intestinal metaplasia and variable degree of atrophic gastritis (Fig. 14-16). It shows preferential metastasis to the liver.

In contrast, the diffuse type (thought to arise from native gastric cells) shows a more equal male-to-female ratio and is more frequent in younger individuals. It has an ulcerative or infiltrative gross appearance and a diffuse, infiltrative growth pattern. Histologically, it is usually a poorly differentiated adenocarcinoma, often with signet-ring cells (see subsequent discussion) and features of linitis plastic (Fig.14-17). It tends to metastasize to the peritoneal cavity. While Lauren's

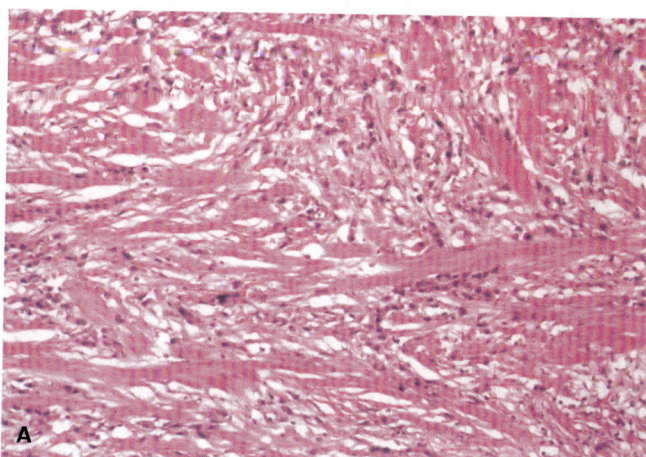
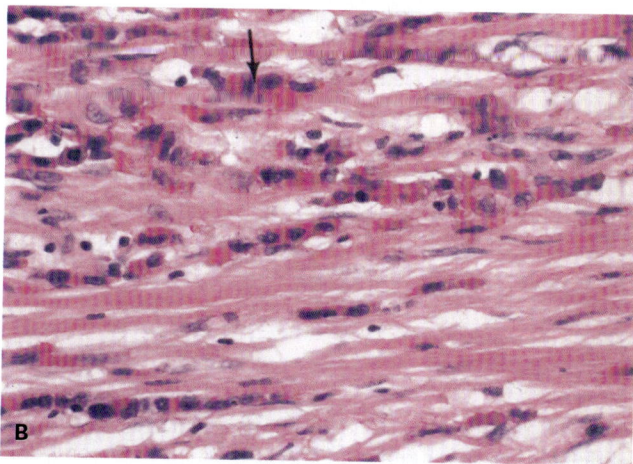

Figure 14-17. Linitis plastica. **A:** There is a dense desmoplastic reaction with interspersed atypical cells. **B:** PAS stain showing mucin-positive malignant cells (*arrow*) infiltrating the desmoplastic stroma in a single-file pattern.

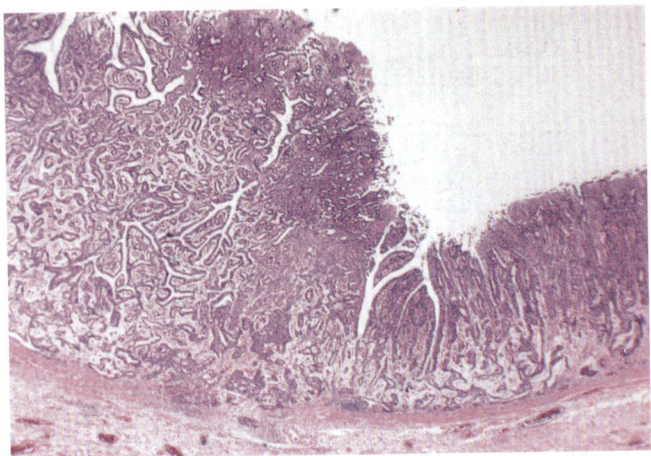

Figure 14-18. Gastric adenocarcinoma, expanding type, with a uniform pushing lower margin.

classification has not revealed differences in survival, it has proven useful for comparative epidemiologic studies, although about 15% of cases show an overlap of patterns and are impossible to classify.[119]

Nakamura classification. Nakamura et al. classified gastric carcinoma into two types based on the histogenesis and biologic characteristics: differentiated and undifferentiated carcinoma.[120,121] They correspond to Lauren's intestinal and diffuse tumor types, respectively.

Ming classification. Ming[122] divided advanced gastric cancer into expansile and infiltrative types according to their microscopic growth patterns (Figs. 14-18 and 14-19). In general, Ming's expansile and infiltrative tumors correspond to Lauren's intestinal and diffuse tumor types, with a similar number of cases showing overlap in patterns.

WHO histologic classification and grading of gastric cancer. The World Health Organization (WHO) divides gastric carcinoma into four main histologic types of adenocarcinoma (papillary, tubular, mucinous, and signet-ring carcinoma) (Fig. 14-20) and rare variants (see below).[1] The diagnosis is based on the predominant histologic type. It is still uncertain whether, stage for stage, the different types of gastric adenocarcinoma affect the prognosis. This may in part be due to variation in the histologic type of gastric cancer from one area to another. For example, an adenocarcinoma may have a papillary pattern superficially and may be mucinous in the deeper portions.

HISTOLOGICAL SUBTYPES OF CARCINOMA

Tubular Adenocarcinoma

This type is composed predominantly of branching tubules resembling colonic epithelium and, less commonly, small glandular structures resembling *antral glands* (Fig. 14-20A). The glands may be cystically dilated with mucus. The tumor cells are columnar, cuboidal, or flattened and contain variable amounts of intracytoplasmic mucin.

The WHO classification of tumor differentiation is based on the grades of glandular differentiation. Thus this grading system also applies primarily to tubular adenocarcinoma as follows.

Well-differentiated Adenocarcinoma

These tumors show well-developed glands lined by tall columnar cells. Ultrastructurally, they have well-defined cell junctions. They are rich in capillaries and sparse in stroma, and basically resemble colorectal tumors (Fig. 14-20A).

Moderately Well-differentiated Adenocarcinoma

These tumors are intermediate in appearance between well- and poorly differentiated adenocarcinomas. The glandular origin of these tumors is obvious, but the glands are less well formed with cribriform or acinar forms. The amount of stroma is variable.

Poorly Differentiated Adenocarcinoma

In these tumors, gland formation is poor and the dominant pattern is one of anastomosing trabeculae, small or large solid clusters, or single cells (Fig. 14-20B,C). Cytologically, the tumor cells are small and immature, and ultrastructurally have scant microvilli

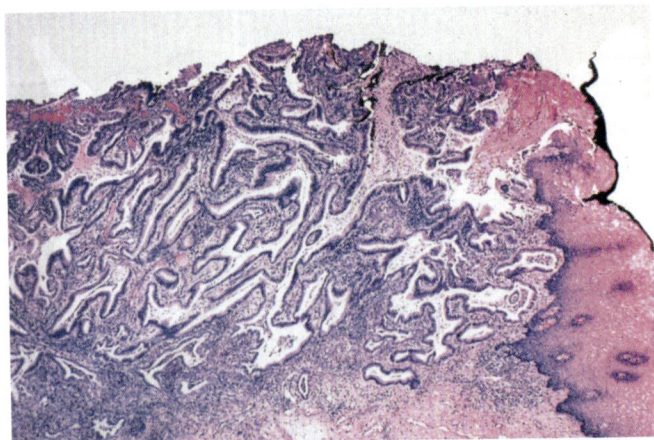

Figure 14-19. Gastric adenocarcinoma, infiltrative type, with an irregular margin of tumor infiltration. This tumor arose from the gastric cardia.

and small mucin granules and lack tight junctions. As a rule, these tumors arise in nonmetaplastic gastric mucosa, and tend to infiltrate the stroma diffusely, eliciting a dense desmoplastic reaction.

Papillary Adenocarcinoma

This type is composed of villous-like epithelial processes with fibrovascular cores. The tumor cells are cylindrical or cuboidal, with or without well-formed, striated borders, and frequently secrete mucus as small droplets (intestinal type), or cylindrical or cuboidal mucous cells (gastric type). They may also contain goblet cells. These tumors typically grow as polypoid masses protruding into the gastric lumen, and deeply in an expansile manner, with pushing margins (Fig. 14-20D).

Mucinous Adenocarcinoma (syn. Mucoid, Mucus, Colloid, and Muconodular Adenocarcinoma)

These tumors produce abundant intracellular and extracellular mucus, which may be visible grossly. By definition, mucinous stroma occupies more than 50% of the tumor. They may show two growth patterns: (a) glands lined by mucus-secreting carcinoma cells with extracellular mucus (Fig. 14-20E) and (b) scant fragments of disrupted glands or cell clusters floating in extracellular mucus pool (Fig. 14-20F). Signet-ring cells may be found in some of these tumors, but do not dominate carcinoma tissue.

Signet-ring Cell Carcinoma

In this type of carcinoma, more than 50% of the tumor consists of carcinoma cells with varying degrees of intracytoplasmic mucin that may present in isolated or small groups. They may consist of the following types of cells independently or in combination within any one tumor[123]: (a) surface mucous cell type (foveolar cell type) that has a small- to medium-sized faintly reticular cytoplasm rich in neutral mucins (surface mucous cell–type mucins), (b) gland mucous cell type that has a small- to medium-sized faintly eosinophilic granular cytoplasm rich in neutral or acid mucins (gland mucous cell–type mucins), (c) goblet cell type that has medium-sized to large clear cytoplasm rich in acid mucin, (d) microcystic type that has intracellular microcyst or intracellular lumina with small amount

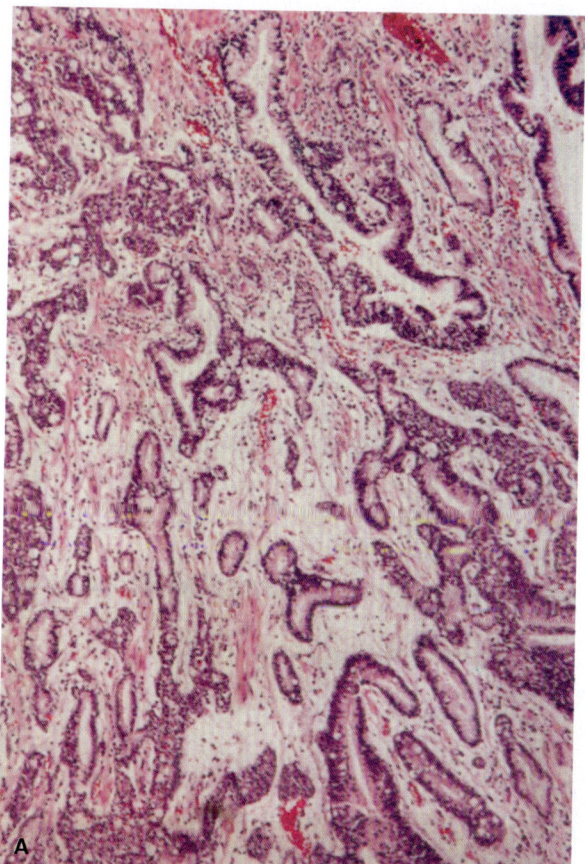
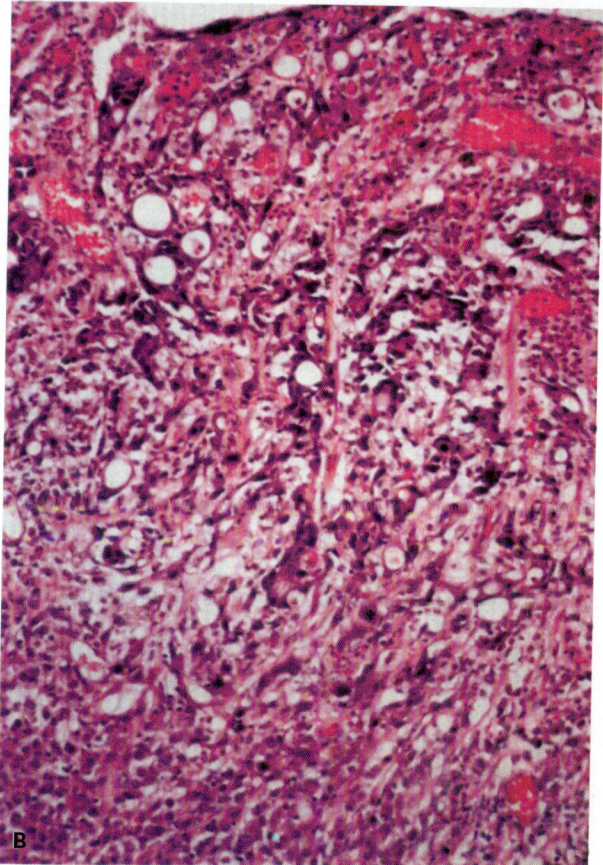

Figure 14-20. Histologic spectrum of gastric carcinoma. **A:** Well-differentiated tubular adenocarcinoma. **B:** Poorly differentiated adenocarcinoma containing anastomosing tubules of tumor cells.

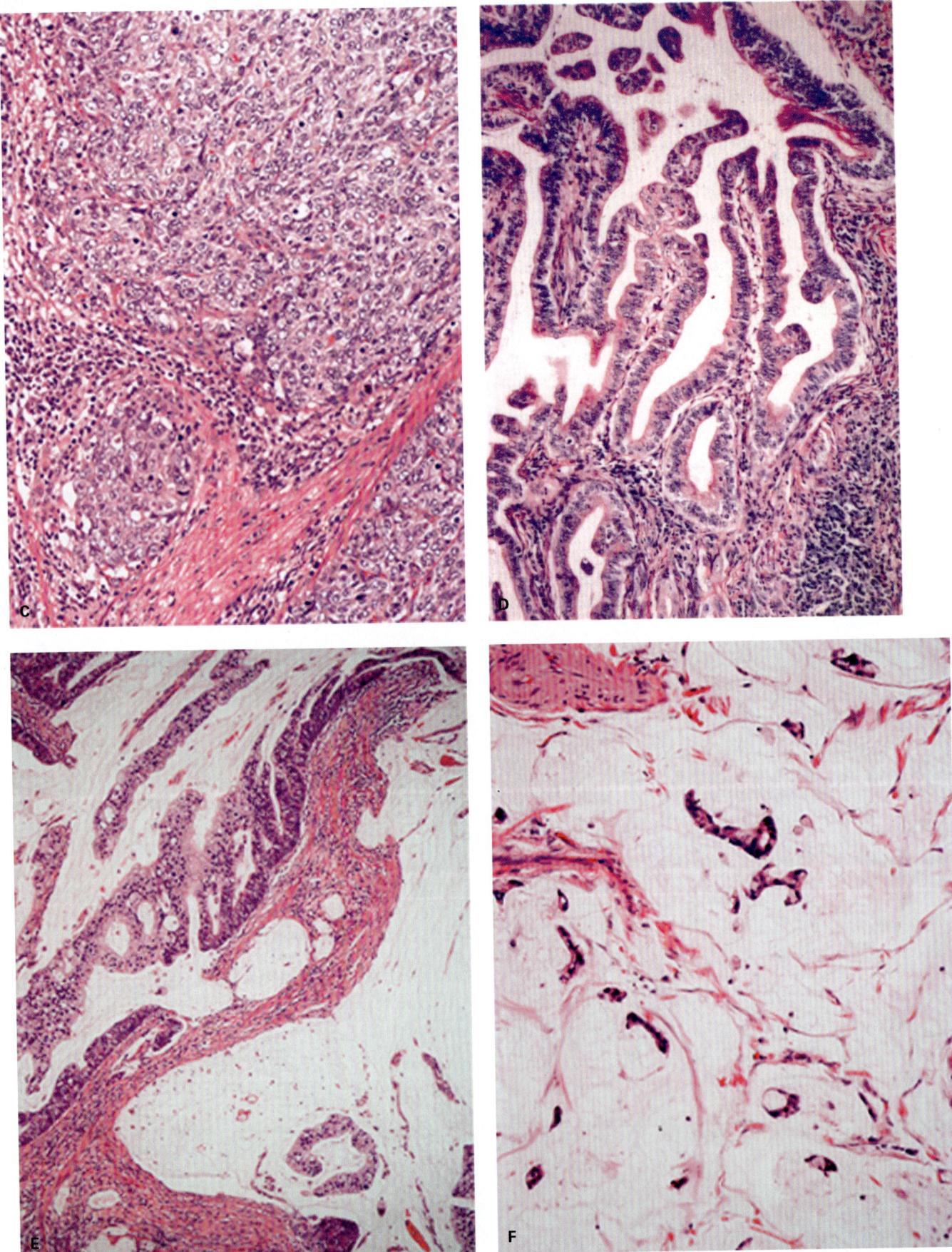

Figure 14-20. *(Continued)* **C:** Poorly differentiated adenocarcinoma showing solid clusters of malignant cells. **D:** Papillary adenocarcinoma. **E:** Mucinous carcinoma consisting of glands lined by mucus-secreting carcinoma cells with extracellular mucus. **F:** Mucinous carcinoma containing scant fragments of disrupted glands or cell clusters floating in extracellular mucus pool.

of mucins lining the inner surface of microcysts, and (e) immature type that has a small cytoplasm containing only a small amount of mucins and exhibiting a high N/C ratio (Figs. 14-10 and 14-21).

The detection of these malignant cells is sometimes subtle and they are easily missed, as they may occur in otherwise normal mucosa. They can be enhanced using mucin stains, ideally PAS stain, with or without AB at pH 2.5, the latter staining acid mucins (Fig. 14-21B,J). PAS stains both neutral and acid mucins found in normal superficial and deep glands in the stomach. Many signet-ring carcinomas would be expected to contain only neutral mucins, and this is sometimes the case. However, they may also contain acid mucins typically found in goblet cells; so they sometimes also stain with mucicarmine or AB (AB pH 2.5) stains or a combined AB-PAS stain. However, sometimes they contain only acid mucin, as is typically seen in normal gastric mucosa; so they do not stain with either AB or mucicarmine. If mucicarmine is used as "the" mucin stain, it will not stain tumor cells only producing neutral mucins, leading to a false-negative mucin stain, and so is best avoided,) unless used with a PAS stain. Immunostaining for low molecular weight or pancytokeratin is also helpful in highlighting tumor cells in the lamina propria, and is preferred as some diffuse and signet-ring carcinomas can lose most or all of their mucin in the deeper part of the mucosa. In fact, immunostains have largely replaced traditional mucin stains when available due to their higher sensitivity and specificity.

When signet-ring cells infiltrate the submucosa and deeper tissues, they frequently provoke a dense fibrous reaction often resulting in linitis plastica (Fig. 14-17). However, this lesion is not unique to signet-ring cell carcinomas; any poorly differentiated adenocarcinomas can elicit a similar desmoplastic reaction. Further, some of the diffusely infiltrating, poorly differentiated carcinomas do not always evoke this reaction. A number of these tumors contain numerous admixed endocrine cells. These are discussed in Chapter 5.

Endocrine Cell Tumors

These include the low-grade (neuro) endocrine tumors (carcinoids), small cell carcinomas (poorly differentiated endocrine neoplasm), and mixed exocrine–endocrine carcinomas. These tumors are discussed under endocrine cell tumors in Chapter 5.

Rare Variants of Gastric Carcinoma

Gastric carcinoma with lymphoid stroma (syn. medullary carcinoma, gastric lymphoepithelioma-like carcinoma). These are uncommon and account for approximately 4% (or less) of all gastric carcinomas.[124] They are considered separately from the usual gastric carcinomas because they are considerably less aggressive and are morphologically distinctive. The significance of these lesions for the pathologist is that they may be confused with lymphomas.

The patient's age at presentation and the presenting symptoms of gastric carcinomas with lymphoid stroma are similar to those of the usual gastric cancers. However, there is a higher male-to-female ratio (~3:1 compared to the usual 2:1).[124]

Grossly, the tumors can occur throughout the body and antrum, although they are most frequent at the junction of the antrum and body. They may present either as an early gastric cancer or, more commonly in the United States, as advanced gastric cancer. The early cancers have the gross features of any of the types of early gastric cancer previously described. The advanced cancers are usually centrally ulcerated, circumscribed lesions with eversion of the mucosa at the ulcer margin. On cut sections the tumor has an expansive growth pattern with a homogeneous gray or gray-white moist surface, resembling lymphoma.

Histologically, gastric carcinoma with lymphoid stroma is characterized by nests of tumor widely separated by an inconspicuous stroma with a dense lymphoplasmacytic infiltrate (Fig. 14-22A). The latter consists of mature lymphocytes with CD8+ T cells being predominant, plasma cells, and occasional neutrophils and eosinophils. The epithelial component consists of trabeculae, small alveoli, and primitive tubuloglandular patterns. At the stage of intramucosal carcinoma, gastric carcinoma with lymphoid stroma frequently shows "lace pattern" showing irregular tubular structure with the connection and fusion of neoplastic glands resembling lacework.[125] The tumor cells are small, regular, and polygonal, with clear or slightly eosinophilic cytoplasm. They may contain PAS-positive material and gastric mucins.[125] The nuclei are usually regular, vesicular with small nucleoli, and normally scant mitoses. The metastatic lesions show similar morphologic changes. EBV-encoded small RNA-1 (EBER-1) is demonstrated uniformly in the nuclei and nucleoli of carcinoma cells and rarely in inflammatory cells around the carcinoma (Fig. 14-22D). However, all such tumors are not related to EBV, some are micro satellite instability high (MSI-H), and few are neither EVB positive or MSI-H. Interestingly, the EBV virus is also not restricted to this subgroup of carcinomas and may be found in a small proportion of other types if searched for. However, EBV-associated carcinomas seem to represent a different pathway characterized by promoter methylation of a variety of genes, thus preventing transcription, but seem not to be related to Her2 status, at least in initial publications.[126–128]

The major confusion histologically may be with malignant lymphoma. The demonstration of cytoplasmic mucin by the PAS stain is usually sufficient. If this stain is equivocal, immunohistochemical

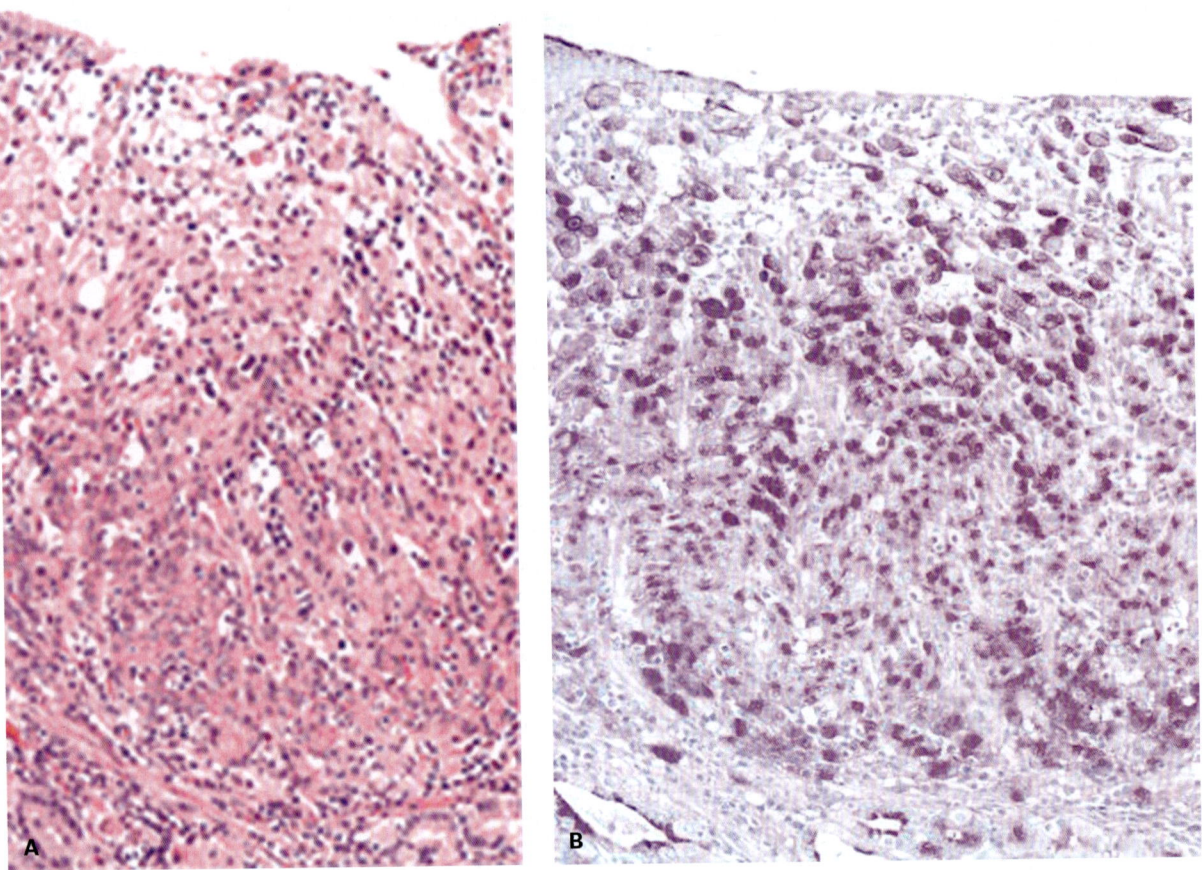
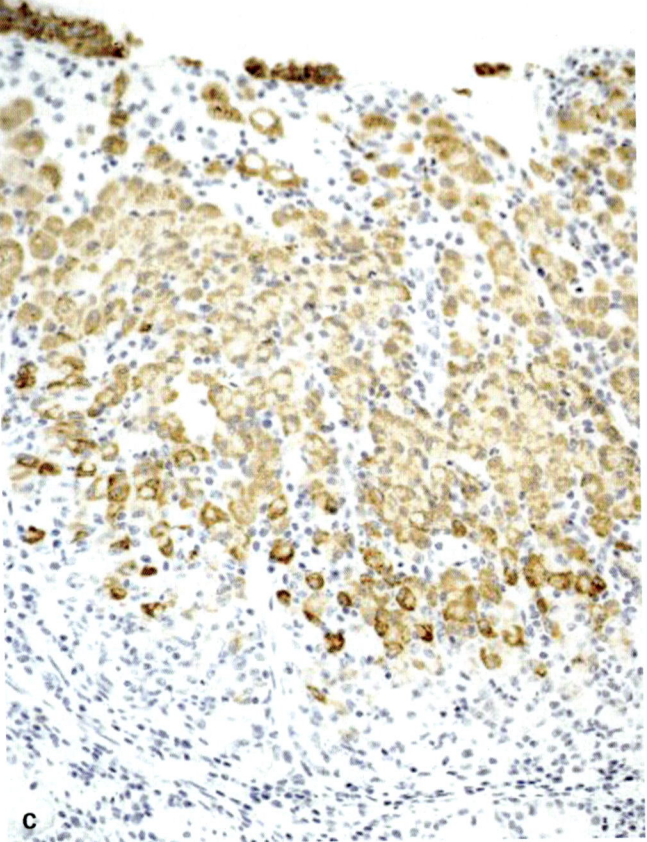

Figure 14-21. Histologic spectrum of signet-ring cell carcinoma. Figures 14-21A–E and 14-21I–K were prepared from serial sections. **A:** Intramucosal signet-ring carcinoma replicating the typical "layering" of pyloric mucosa. It should be noted that these changes tend to be lost once there is submucosal invasion. **B:** Carcinoma cells contain neutral mucin only (AB-PAS stain). **C:** The upper layer contains carcinoma cells showing properties of the surface mucous cells positive for MUC5AC, which stains foveolar mucin. In the middle layer, there are immature carcinoma cells having relatively little cytoplasm and having a higher nuclear–cytoplasmic (N/C) ratio.

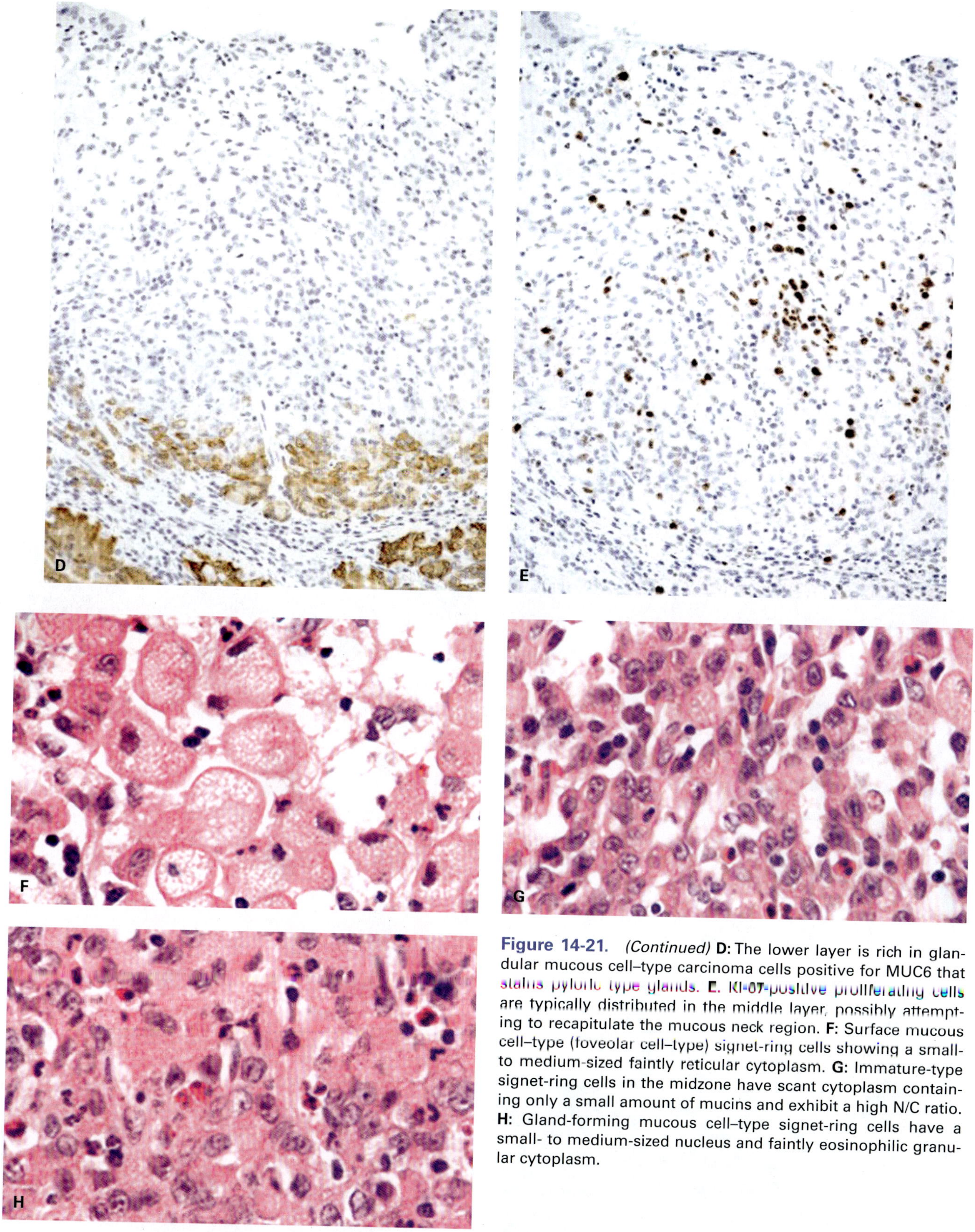

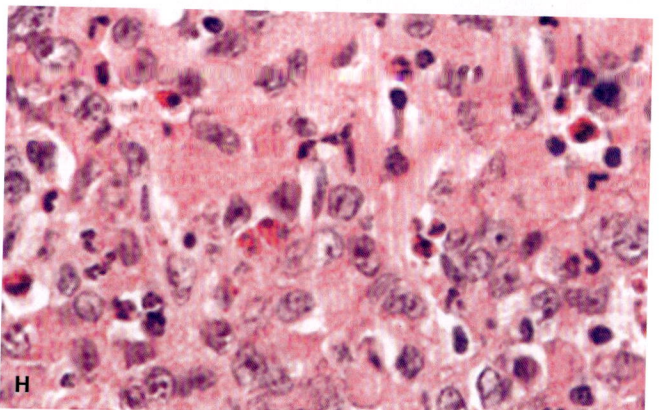

Figure 14-21. *(Continued)* **D:** The lower layer is rich in glandular mucous cell–type carcinoma cells positive for MUC6 that stains pyloric type glands. **E:** Ki-67–positive proliferating cells are typically distributed in the middle layer, possibly attempting to recapitulate the mucous neck region. **F:** Surface mucous cell–type (foveolar cell–type) signet-ring cells showing a small- to medium-sized faintly reticular cytoplasm. **G:** Immature-type signet-ring cells in the midzone have scant cytoplasm containing only a small amount of mucins and exhibit a high N/C ratio. **H:** Gland-forming mucous cell–type signet-ring cells have a small- to medium-sized nucleus and faintly eosinophilic granular cytoplasm.

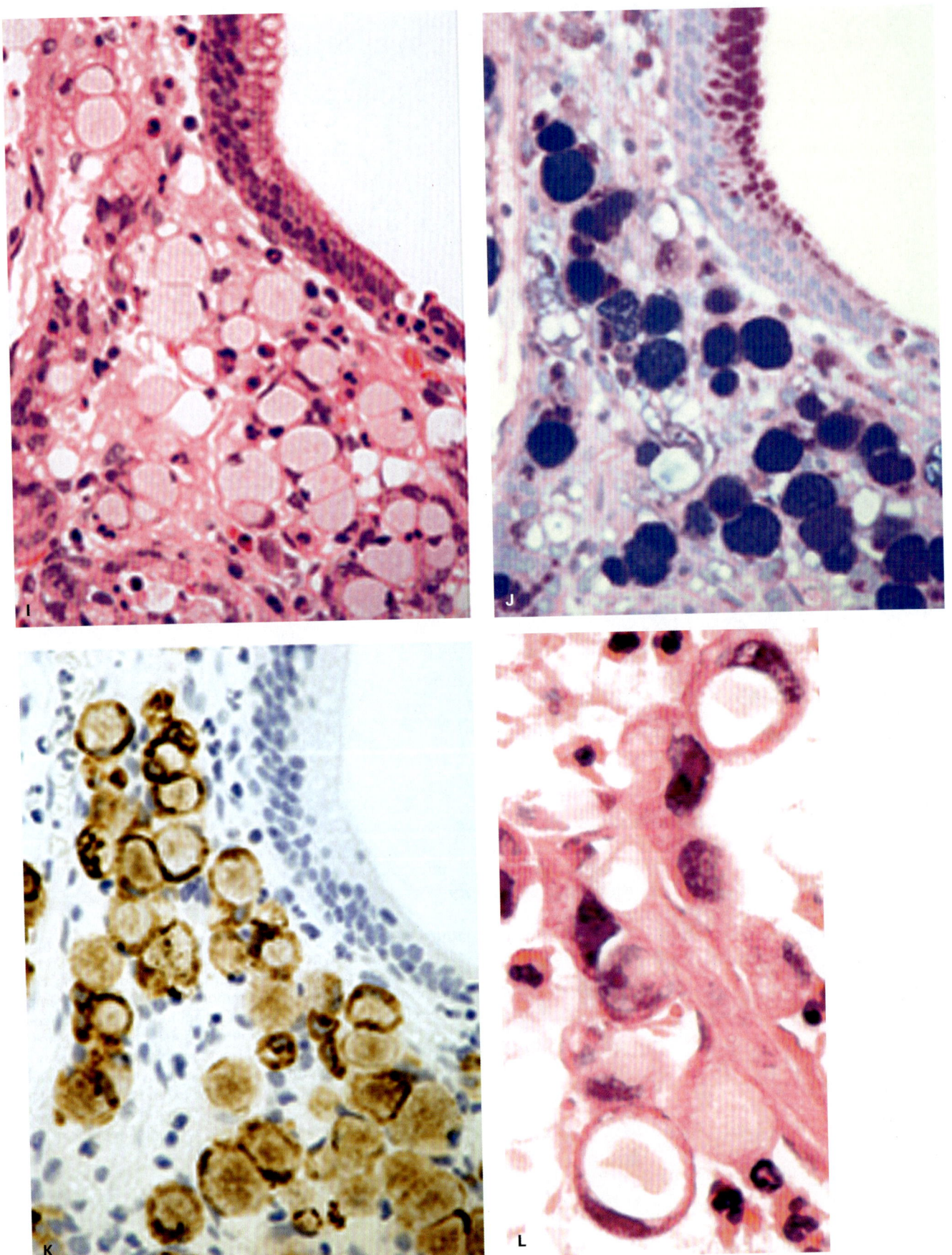

Figure 14-21. *(Continued)* **I:** Goblet cell–type signet-ring cells have medium-sized to large clear cytoplasm rich in acid mucin (**J**, AB-PAS stain) and MUC2-positive mucin (**K**). **L:** Microcystic signet-ring cells have intracellular microcysts or intracellular lumina.

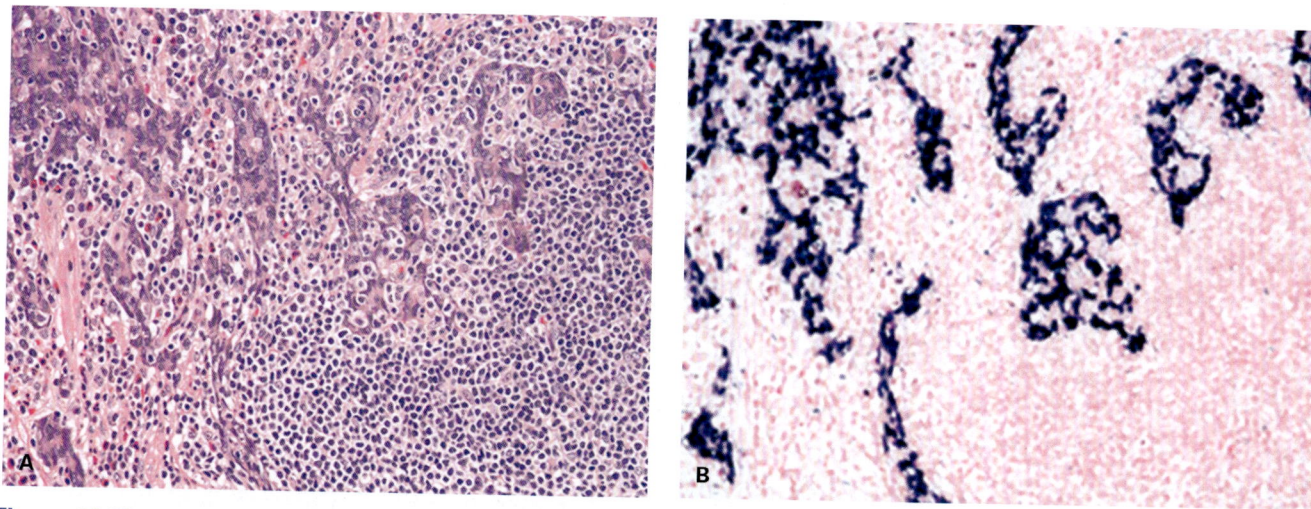

Figure 14-22. Gastric carcinoma with lymphoid stroma. **A:** Syncytial nests of tumor cells separated by a nondesmoplastic lymphoid stroma. **B:** EBV DNA is demonstrated uniformly in the nuclei and nucleoli of carcinoma cells by in situ hybridization for EBV.

demonstration of CEA and keratin will confirm the epithelial nature of the tumor cells.

The behavior of the early gastric cancers with lymphoid stroma, namely, those confined to the mucosa and submucosa, is similar to that of the usual gastric cancers. However, the 5-year survival of patients with tumors infiltrating into the muscularis propria or serosa is considerably better for those with lymphoid stroma, that is, 97% to 76% and 77% to 30% respectively. Comparable figures for metastatic lesions are not available.[124]

α-Fetoprotein-producing gastric carcinoma and hepatoid adenocarcinoma.

α-Fetoprotein (AFP)-producing gastric carcinoma is a distinctive but rare type of gastric carcinoma and patients also have high levels of serum AFP. AFP-producing carcinoma foci might evolve through genetic progression or genetic divergence or both from ordinary adenocarcinoma.[129]

Clinically, patients present with the usual features of advanced gastric cancer and are found to have high serum AFP levels (in the thousands). The prognosis is poor, with rapid and widespread dissemination, attributed to extensive vascular dissemination.

Histologically, the tumor may contain a combination of areas with tubular, tubulopapillary adenocarcinoma foci, poorly differentiated carcinoma, primitive enterocyte-like enteroblastic and hepatoid foci (Fig. 14-24).[130–132] The enteroblastic areas show tubular or tubulopapillary carcinoma with clear cytoplasm similar to those of the developing gut epithelium (Fig. 14-23A,B).[130,131] The hepatoid areas show the full spectrum of hepatocellular carcinomas, including sinusoidal structure and bile production (Fig. 14-23A,C). AFP is demonstrated in enteroblastic and hepatoid foci (Fig. 14-23D).[130,131] Hepatic differentiation can be further established immunohistochemically by the demonstration of albumin, AFP (the immunoreactivity of which, along with CEA, is much higher in hepatoid carcinoma than hepatocellular carcinoma, while HepPar-1 only stains in a minority), α-1-antitrypsin, and HepPar1,[133] or by in situ hybridization for albumin mRNA. The diagnosis of AFP-producing gastric carcinoma is easy if hepatoid areas are clearly distinguishable within the gastric tumor. Histological findings of gastric tumor coupled with the high serum AFP levels are helpful. However, differentiation from metastatic hepatocellular carcinoma can be problematic because of histologic and immunophenotypic overlap. Histologically, the presence of an adenocarcinomatous component and the clinical absence of a hepatic mass are important clues to the diagnosis. SALL4 is reported to be a sensitive marker for AFP-producing gastric carcinoma and could also be useful to distinguish hepatoid gastric carcinoma from primary hepatocellular carcinoma.[134]

Adenosquamous and squamous cell carcinoma.

These are very rare tumors, accounting for <0.5% of all gastric cancers.[103] Clinically and on gross examination they are indistinguishable from the usual adenocarcinomas.[135] Two-thirds of them are found in the distal half of the stomach. Pure squamous cell carcinomas are vanishingly rare; it has been shown that meticulous study usually reveals at least small foci of adenocarcinoma.[135] These tumors are believed to arise from foci of squamous metaplasia, although it is possible that they may also arise from primitive cells with the ability to differentiate toward both glandular and squamous epithelium or from heterotopic mucosa or potentially squamous metaplasia in the stomach.[135]

Histologically, poorly differentiated adenocarcinomas may sometimes resemble squamous carcinomas. Thus it is imperative to demonstrate unequivocal features of squamous differentiation, namely, squamous pearls or definite prickles. Ultrastructurally, squamous

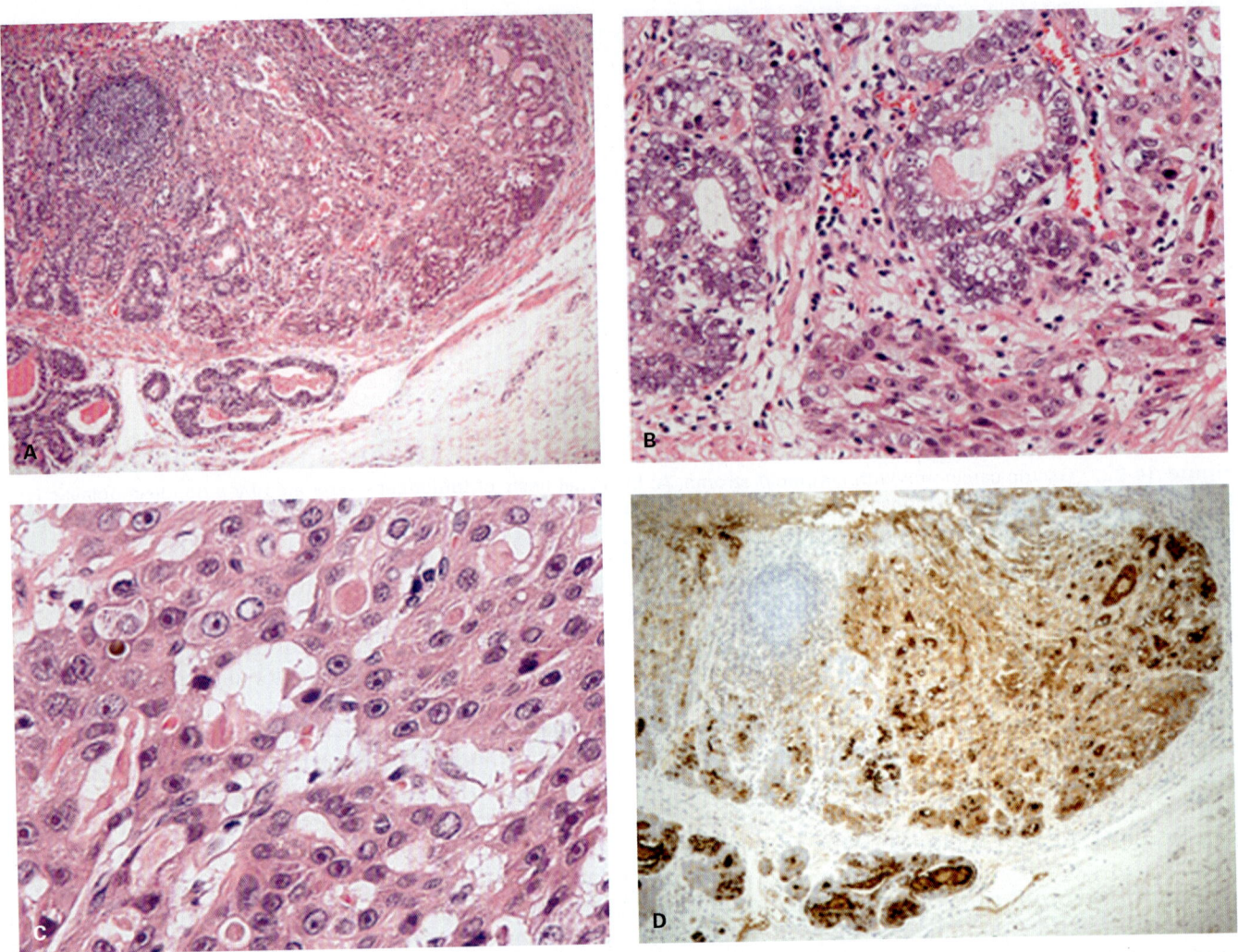

Figure 14-23. α-Fetoprotein-producing gastric carcinoma. **A:** Adenocarcinoma consisting of tumor cells forming tubular structure penetrating into the submucosa in the left (enteroblastic type) and tumor cells forming trabecular or solid nest in the right (hepatoid type). **B:** The enteroblastic type showing tubular carcinoma with clear cytoplasm similar to those of the developing gut epithelium. **C:** The hepatoid type showing similar features of hepatocellular carcinomas, including sinusoidal structure and bile production. **D:** α-Fetoprotein is demonstrated in enteroblastic and hepatoid type.

areas show the typical features of squamous cells, with tonofibrils and keratinization. The amounts of squamous and glandular components are variable and may range from virtually pure squamous cell carcinomas to only microscopic foci.[103] Occasionally, individual cells containing both tonofibrils and mucous vacuoles are observed.[136]

Unusual patterns, such as a mucoepidermoid carcinoma[136] and a collision tumor at the esophagogastric junction consisting of squamous cell carcinoma and adenocarcinoma, have also been described.[136,137]

Adenosquamous carcinomas behave in a more aggressive manner than adenocarcinomas because of their greater invasiveness and their lymphatic and vascular dissemination.[135]

Choriocarcinoma (syn. chorioepithelioma). These are exceedingly rare gastric tumors that occur in the absence of gonadal tumors or other primary sites of choriocarcinoma, and identical to similar tumors that occur in esophagus or intestines. They are almost invariably associated with foci or adenocarcinoma, supporting the hypothesis that these tumors are derived by dedifferentiation of neoplastic mucosal epithelial cells rather than primary germ cell tumors, and choriocarcinoma-like carcinoma is probably a better term.[138,139]

The patients range in age from 30 to 80, but tend to be elderly, and there is a 2:1 male-to-female preponderance.[140,141] The tumors can occur anywhere in the stomach but predominate in the antrum.[142]

Histologically, these tumors are almost always associated with adenocarcinoma, varying from microscopic foci to large portions of the tumor. They show the characteristic features of choriocarcinoma with syncytial and cytotrophoblastic elements (Fig. 14-24A,B), and in one reported case there

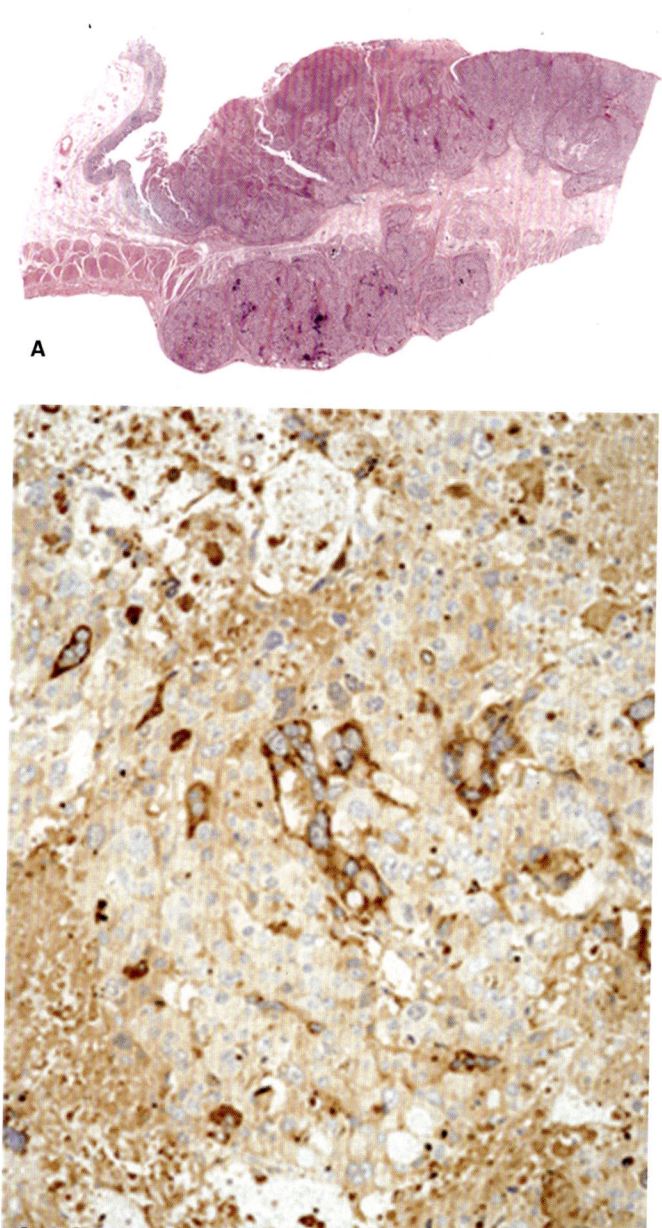
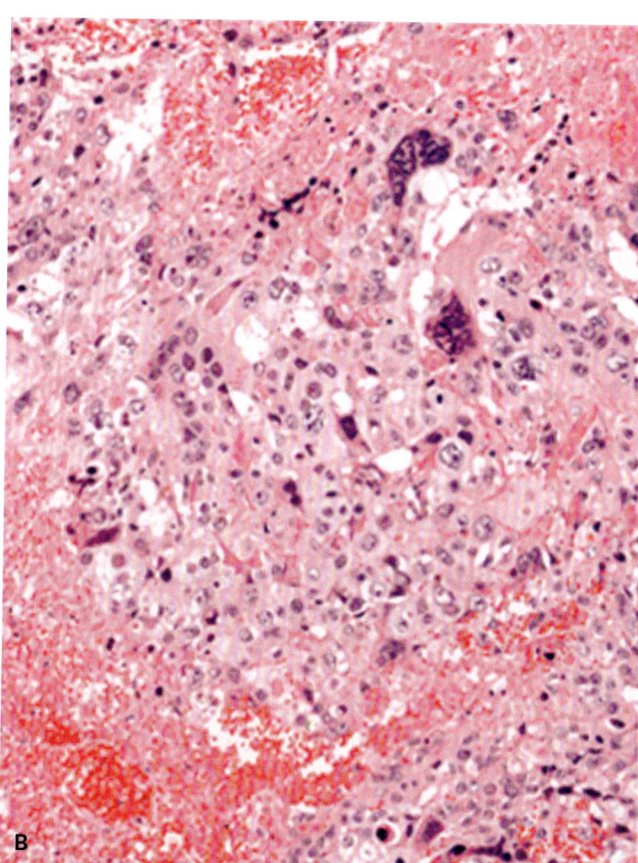

Figure 14-24. Choriocarcinoma. **A:** Carcinoma massively penetrating into the subserosa. **B:** Carcinoma consists of cytotrophoblastic cells and scattered syncytiotrophoblastic giant cells and **(C)** shows immunoreactivity for β-HCG. (Courtesy M. Fukushima, MD, Shinshu University, Japan.)

were foci of *yolk sac tumor*.[140] Beta subunits of human chorionic gonadotropin (hCG) (Fig. 14-24C), placental lactogen, and pregnancy-specific glycoprotein have all been demonstrated immunohistochemically within the trophoblastic elements of the tumor. Serum hCG levels are commonly elevated.[141,143] It is also noteworthy that hCG has been reported in gastric carcinomas without choriocarcinomatous foci.[144]

The prognosis of this tumor is grim, with many patients having widespread metastases at the time of diagnosis.

Yolk sack tumor (syn. endodermal sinus tumor). This is another vanishingly rare tumor of the stomach, which, like choriocarcinoma, may be associated with foci of gastric adenocarcinoma.

Histologically, it has all the features of endodermal sinus tumors, including Schiller–Duval bodies and hyaline droplets.[130]

Patients have raised serum AFP levels, and AFP can be demonstrated immunohistochemically within the tumor. The tumor is highly aggressive and metastasizes rapidly to regional lymph nodes, liver, peritoneum, and the lungs.

Paneth cell carcinoma. Gastric carcinomas rich in Paneth cell–type cells have been reported.[145-147] Paneth cell-type gastric carcinomas are variants of intestinal carcinomas and are characterized by cytoplasmic eosinophilic coarse granular and they show immunoreactivity for lysozyme and human defensin-5 (HD5).[145-147]

Micropapillary carcinoma. These are rare in the stomach and virtually identical in their morphology and prognosis to their colonic counterparts (See Chapter 20).

Gastric adenocarcinoma of fundic gland type (fundic gland carcinoma, combined parietal, and chief cell carcinoma) including parietal cell carcinoma and chief cell carcinoma. Gastric adenocarcinoma of fundic gland type has been proposed for tumors that clearly are differentiating into the parietal and chief cells of the oxyntic mucosa. They can be classified into three categories based on the predominant tumor cells: parietal cell predominant type, chief cell predominant type, and mixed type.[148,149] Similar tumors have been reported as a variant of fundic gland polyp with chief cell hyperplasia.[150,151]

Parietal Cell Predominant Type (Parietal Cell Carcinoma and Oncocytic Carcinoma) This is a very rare gastric carcinoma with the morphologic features of parietal cells.[152-154]

Histologically, they are composed of solid sheets of polygonal cells with abundant eosinophilic cytoplasm. Like parietal cells, they show immunoreactivity for H/K-ATPase and human milk fat globule-2 (HMFG-2).[154] Ultrastructurally, they are characterized by abundant mitochondria, tubulovesicles, and intracellular canaliculi, features typical of parietal cells (Fig. 14-25).[152,154]

There is some suggestion that these tumors may behave less aggressively than the usual gastric cancers.[152,153] In a report by Capella et al.[152] of three patients, two with only one lymph node metastasis and one with four, it was stated that two were alive and well 1 and 2 years postoperatively. The third patient (with only one positive node) died 5 months postoperatively of intestinal obstruction of uncertain etiology. However, more information is needed before the prognosis of these lesions can be accurately determined. Gastric carcinomas, which have morphologic features that are similar to those of parietal cell carcinomas, but are negative with anti H/K-ATPase antibody, were reported as gastric oncocytoma.[155] If the H/K-ATPase antibody is not available, then platelet-derived growth factor receptor-a or MUC1 demonstrated the intercellular secretory apparatus beautifully—see chapter 12. As these tumors arise from fundic gland mucosa they should not have atrophy or metaplasia in the adjacent mucosa.

Chief Cell Predominant Type (Gastric Adenocarcinoma with Chief Cell Differentiation) These are low-grade carcinomas located in the upper third of the stomach.[148,149]

Histologically, they are well-differentiated adenocarcinomas predominantly composed of mildly atypical columnar or cuboidal tumor cells with pale basophilic cytoplasm or coarse eosinophilic cytoplasmic granules with basally situated nuclei, resembling gastric chief cells (Fig. 14-26).[148,149] In most cases, no intestinal metaplasia, atrophic change, and chronic gastritis are found in the background mucosa of the tumors.[149] Immunohistochemically, they are positive for pepsinogen I, pepsinogen II, MUC6, and Runt-related transcription factor gene 3 (RUNX3) in their cytoplasm (Fig. 14-26), and some tumor cells are positive for H/K-ATPase alpha subunit, but negative for defensin-5, CD10, and Cdx2, showing gastric phenotype.[148,149]

Mixed Parietal and Chief Cell Type These are incredibly rare. Anecdotally, we have seen few of these with a gradation from hyperplastic to dysplastic to intramucosal carcinoma to submucosaly invasive tumors; these were all resected endoscopically (Fig. 14-27). There was no clinical evidence of metastasis (nodal or distant) and with a limited follow-up of several years.

Fundic gland adenoma. Occasionally very disorganized but non-infiltrating nodules of fundic gland mucosa are seen, in which nuclei are larger than usual but also exhibit a degree of multilayering and no invasive carcinoma is identified. Some regard them as fundic gland adenomas or fundic gland nodules. One consisting largely of parietal cells that was located immediately below the Z-line is shown in Figure 14-27C–E.

Extremely well-differentiated adenocarcinoma. There are variants of gastric adenocarcinoma designated as extremely well-differentiated adenocarcinoma (EWDA), which are classified into gastric type and intestinal type.[156,157] EWDA distributes predominantly in the middle or upper third of the stomach. Macroscopically, early gastric-type EWDA shows protruded or superficial elevated type. On the other hand, early intestinal-type EWDA shows preferentially superficial elevated or superficial depressed type. Advanced EWDAs in both types are polypoid lesions.

Histologically, in gastric type EWDA, most of the glands and tumor cells are very bland and difficult to discriminate from benign foveolar epithelial hyperplasia or pyloric glands except that when deeper invasion, metastasis, or both are present when the diagnosis becomes obvious (Fig. 14-28, see also Fig. 14-6). But compared to normal epithelium, their foveolar structures are frequently elongated and the tumor cells and their nuclei are slightly larger and more hyperchromatic (Fig. 14-28). Cystic dilatation of the glands sometimes containing luminal debris may be seen, especially in the deeper parts of the lamina propria, which should alert pathologists of this possibility. Intestinal-type EWDA resembles intestinal metaplasia with minimal nuclear atypia and irregular tubular structures showing branching, tortuous, anastomosing, and plexiform structures, which are more

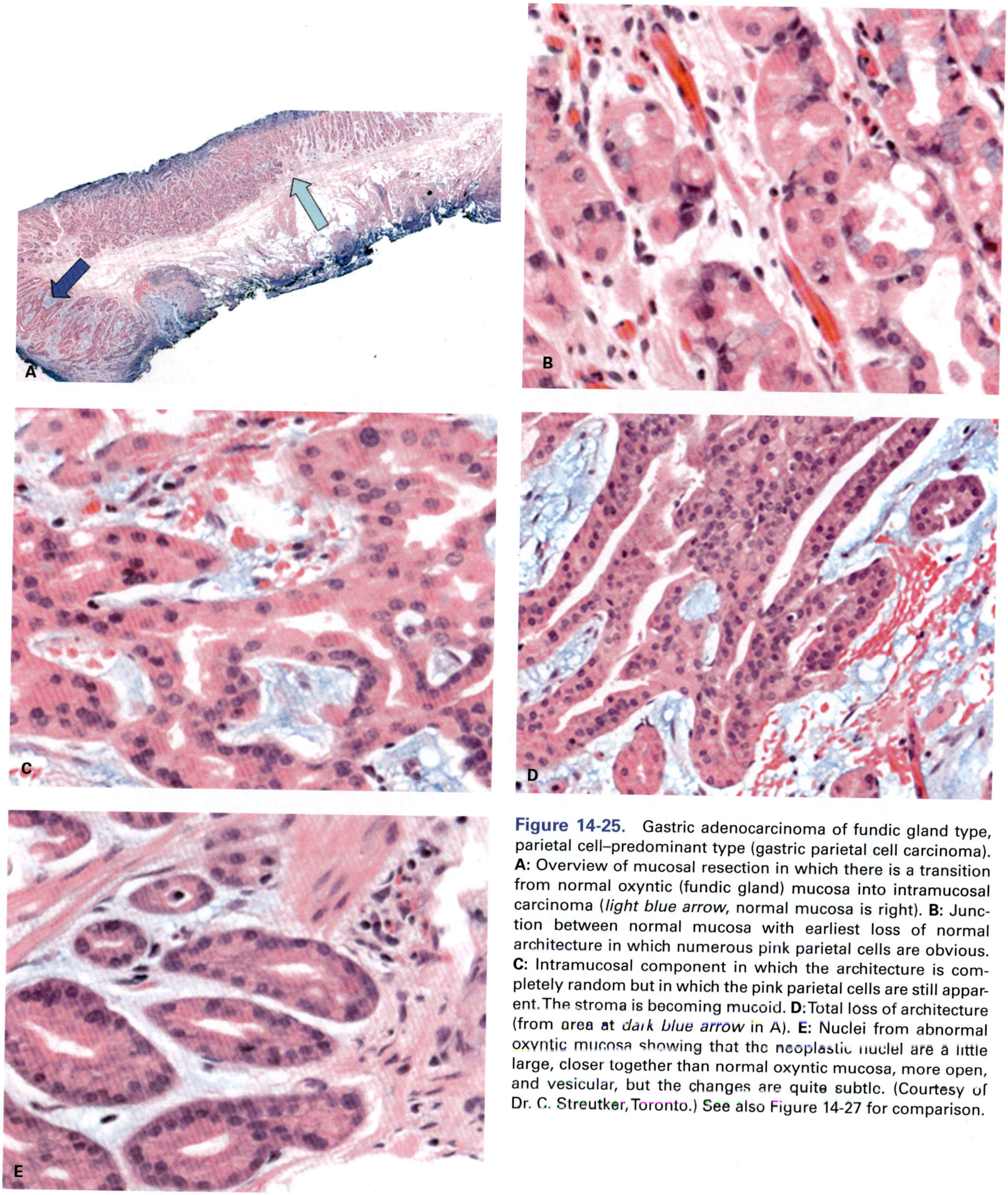

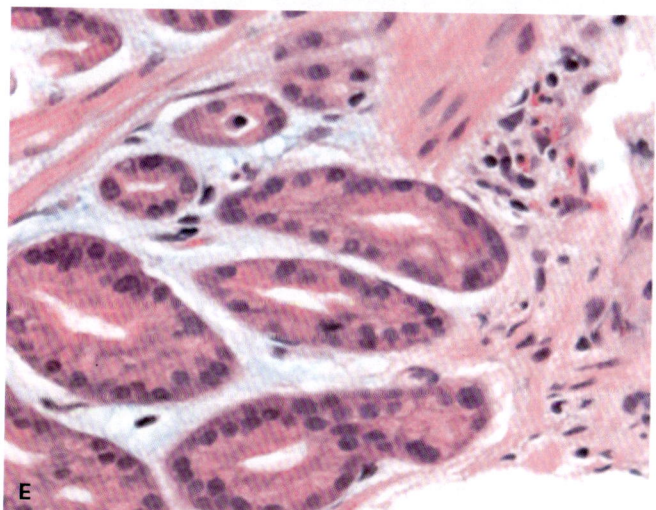

Figure 14-25. Gastric adenocarcinoma of fundic gland type, parietal cell–predominant type (gastric parietal cell carcinoma). **A:** Overview of mucosal resection in which there is a transition from normal oxyntic (fundic gland) mucosa into intramucosal carcinoma (*light blue arrow*, normal mucosa is right). **B:** Junction between normal mucosa with earliest loss of normal architecture in which numerous pink parietal cells are obvious. **C:** Intramucosal component in which the architecture is completely random but in which the pink parietal cells are still apparent. The stroma is becoming mucoid. **D:** Total loss of architecture (from area at *dark blue arrow* in A). **E:** Nuclei from abnormal oxyntic mucosa showing that the neoplastic nuclei are a little large, closer together than normal oxyntic mucosa, more open, and vesicular, but the changes are quite subtle. (Courtesy of Dr. C. Streutker, Toronto.) See also Figure 14-27 for comparison.

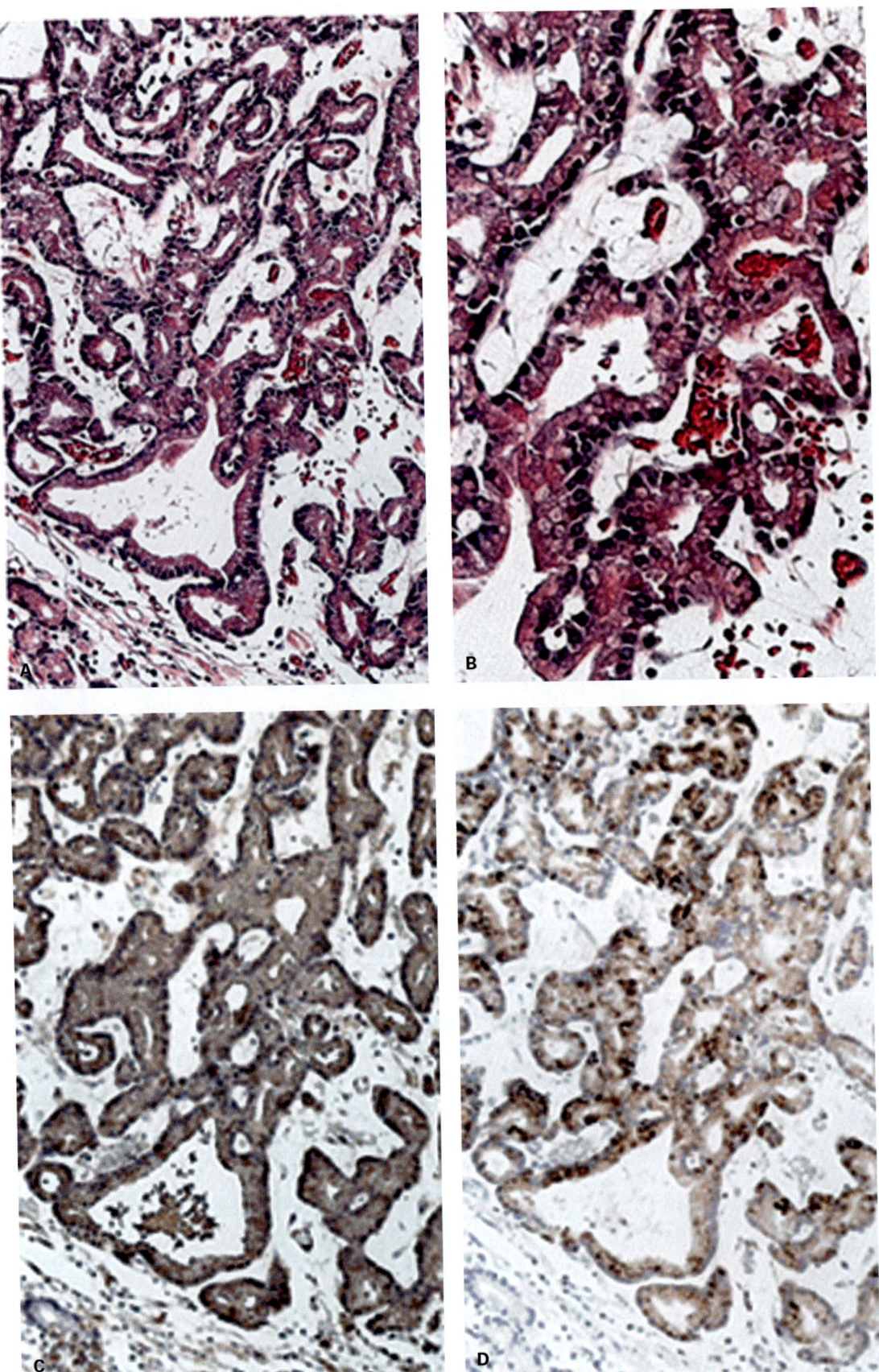

Figure 14-26. Gastric adenocarcinoma of fundic gland type, chief cell–predominant type (gastric adenocarcinoma with chief cell differentiation). Tubular adenocarcinoma **(A)** predominantly composed of mildly atypical columnar or cuboidal tumor cells with pale basophilic cytoplasm or coarse eosinophilic cytoplasmic granules and basally situated nuclei **(B)**. Tumor cells are diffusely positive for pepsinogen I **(C)**, MUC6 **(D)**, and RUNX3 **(E)**.

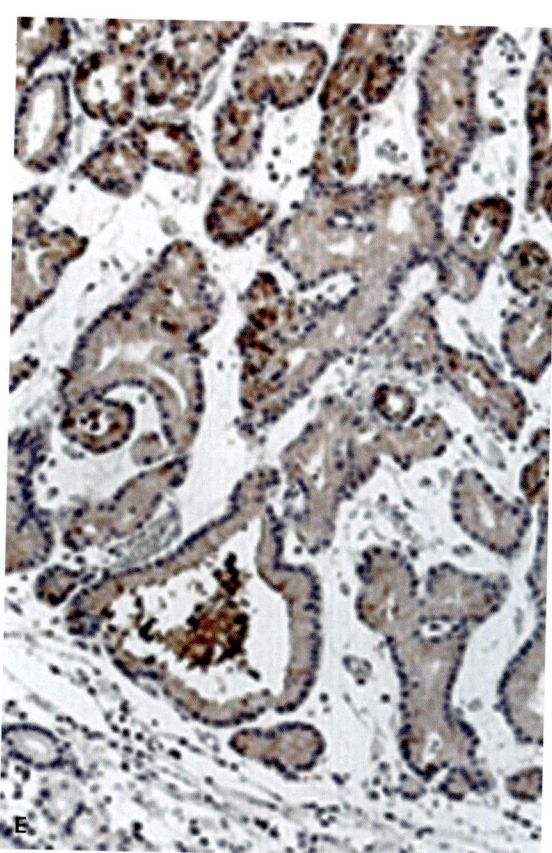

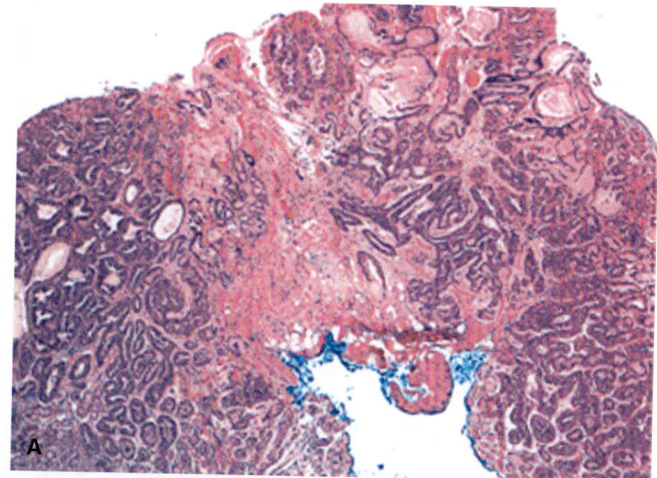

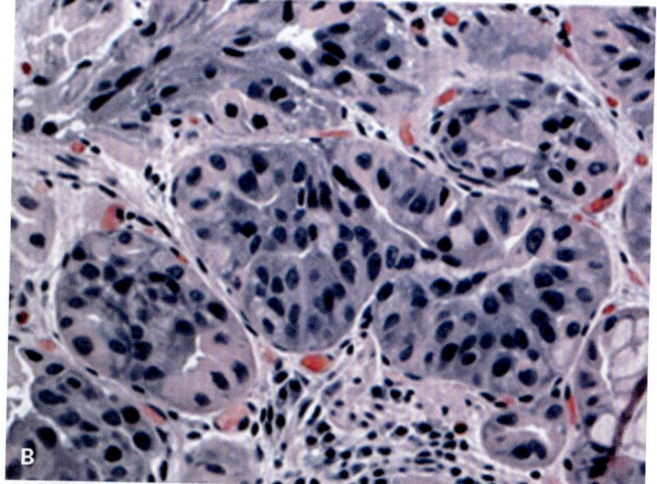

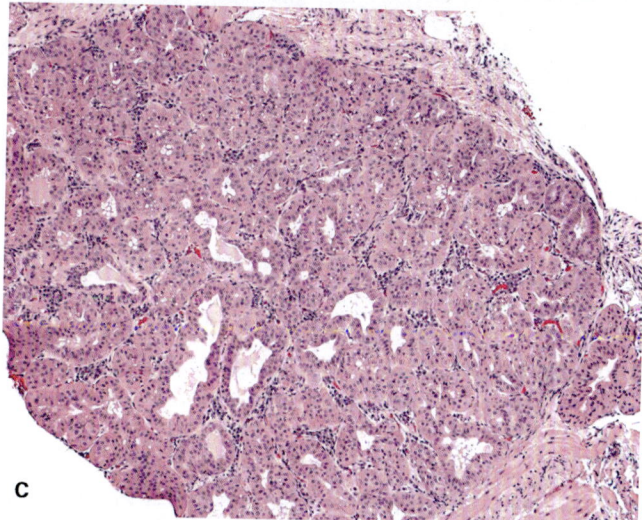

Figure 14-26. *(Continued)* (A–C, E. Modified from Tsukamoto T, Yokoi T, Maruta S, et al. Gastric adenocarcinoma with chief cell differentiation. *Pathol Int.* 2007;57:517–522, Fig 2 in p. 518, with permission. D. Courtesy T. Tsukamoto, MD, Mie University, Japan.)

pathognomonic than cytologic features (Fig. 14-29). Phenotypically, intestinal-type EWDA demonstrates complete intestinal type (small intestinal type), or incomplete intestinal type (gastric and intestinal mixed type). Because of its resemblance to hyperplastic pylori mucosa or intestinal metaplasia, EWDAs are often overlooked or misdiagnosed. However, multifocal and repeated biopsies may be useful to recognize more atypical areas suggesting malignancy, because most EWDAs have foci of pathognomonic features with higher degree of atypia. In this respect, they resemble other "minimal deviation" carcinomas such as the adenoma malignum seen in the uterine cervix.

Pyloric gland carcinoma. This term can be confusing as formerly "pylorocardiac gland carcinoma" was applied to a tumor that would now be best classified as a tubular or well-differentiated carcinoma of foveolar type. The introduction of MUC stains made it clear that some of these were primarily of foveolar origin, arising from mucosa that was similar to the superficial and mid parts of the mucosa in being predominantly

Figure 14-27. Gastric adenocarcinoma of fundic gland type, mixed chief and parietal cell type. **A:** The mucosa has the same architectural distortion as seen in the previous two figures, but **(B)** the tumor is a mixture of parietal and chief cells. **C–E:** Fundic gland adenoma. **C:** Overview showing a well circumscribed but haphazard group of pits.

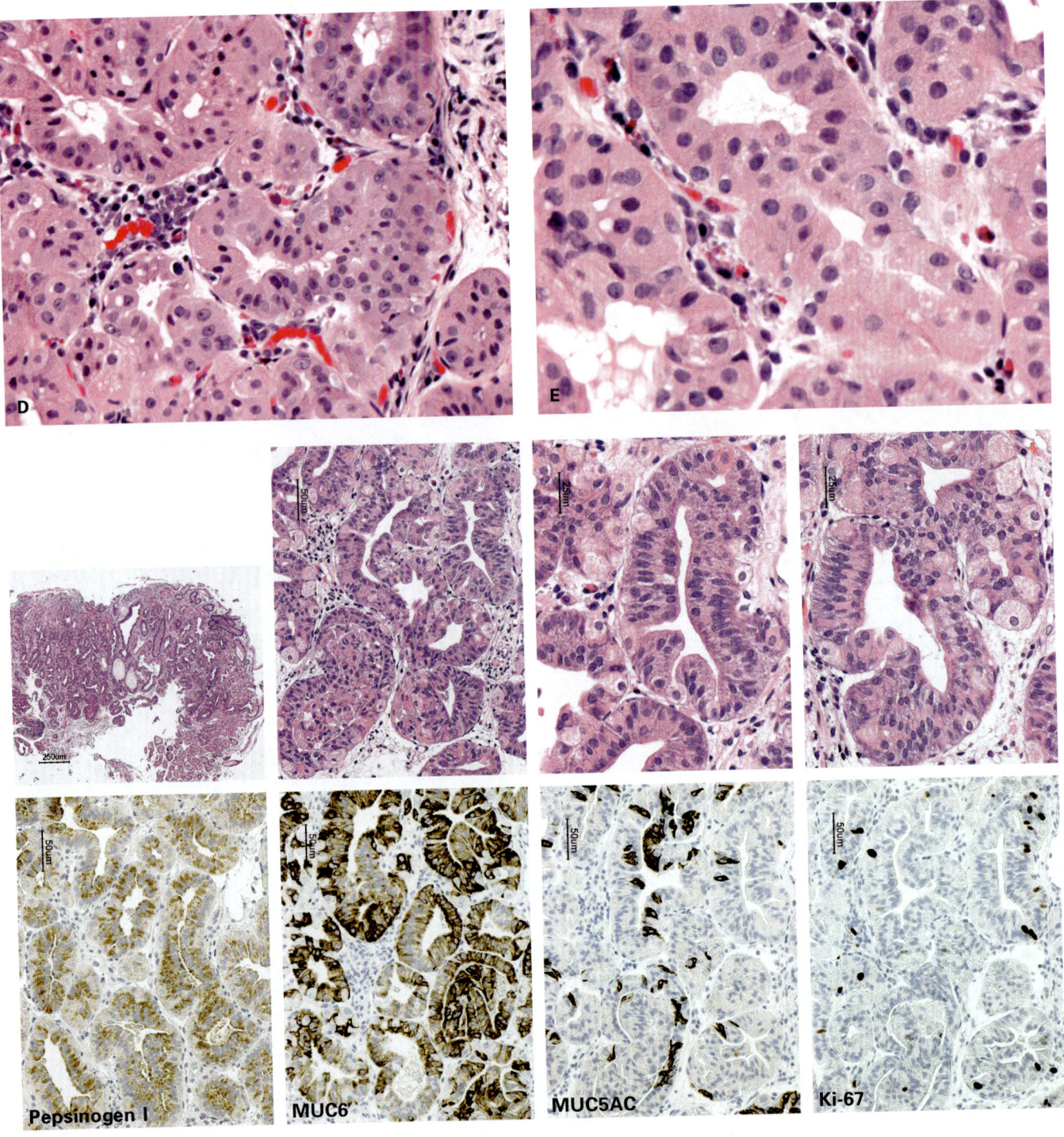

Figure 14-27. (Continued) D: Most appear to be parietal cells but they are multilayered, and on the right there is a hint of chief cell differentiation with more amphophilic staining cells. E: In this part almost all are parietal cells. F: Further example that includes immunohistochemistry. Pepsinogen indicates chief cell differentiation, MUC5AC foveolar, MUC6 pyloric gland mucin, so indicates the type of mucin as cells differentiate towards the muscularis mucosae from the mucous neck region (Courtesy of Drs. Michael Vieth, Bayreuth, Germany and Hidenabu Watanabe, Japan).

MUC5-immunoreactive. However, some were predominantly MUC 6-immunoreactive, implying an origin from the pyloric or deep parts of the mucosa, and some of these carcinomas clearly had an origin in pyloric gland adenomas (see preceding discussion). The term pyloric gland carcinoma is now applied to a carcinoma arising from a pyloric gland adenoma, although theoretically it could also be applied to any carcinoma in which the MUC 5AC and 6 replicated that seen in pyloric gland adenomas. In fact, some tumors that are in the EWDAs category show pyloric gland phenotype and are diffusely positive for MUC6.

However, the diagnosis of pyloric gland carcinoma and pyloric gland adenoma is also not easy. Sometimes the edges of a pyloric gland carcinoma can be seen to infiltrate into the adjacent structures, and this can be brought out using proliferation markers such as Mib-1. Some may show early lamina propria invasion.[21]

Although these tumors that seem to be arising in a pyloric gland adenoma may well have metastasizing potential, at the time of writing there appear to be no examples of this. The other group of pyloric gland carcinomas comprise of tumors that are often made of varying size glandular structures, often with inspissated secretions or luminal debris that despite the well-differentiated morphology often are highly invasive and high stage at the time of diagnosis. The cytologic dysplasia is quite subtle so that architectural abnormalities may be the best way of making the diagnosis, especially on biopsies. Cytologically, nuclei need to be compared with normal pyloric glands until one gets to see the more open and vesicular nuclei and the small but definite nucleoli that characterize these tumors (Fig. 14-30). The overlying surface may have gastric foveolar or phenotype or contain intestinal metaplasia, and the in-situ component also typically has low grade dysplasia.

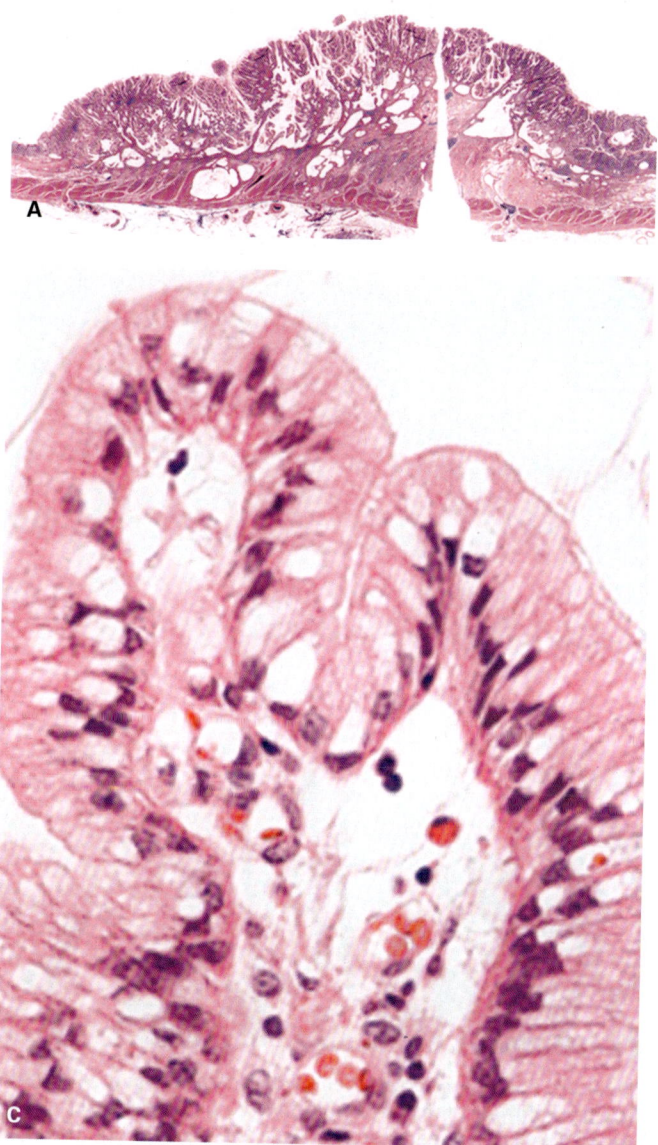

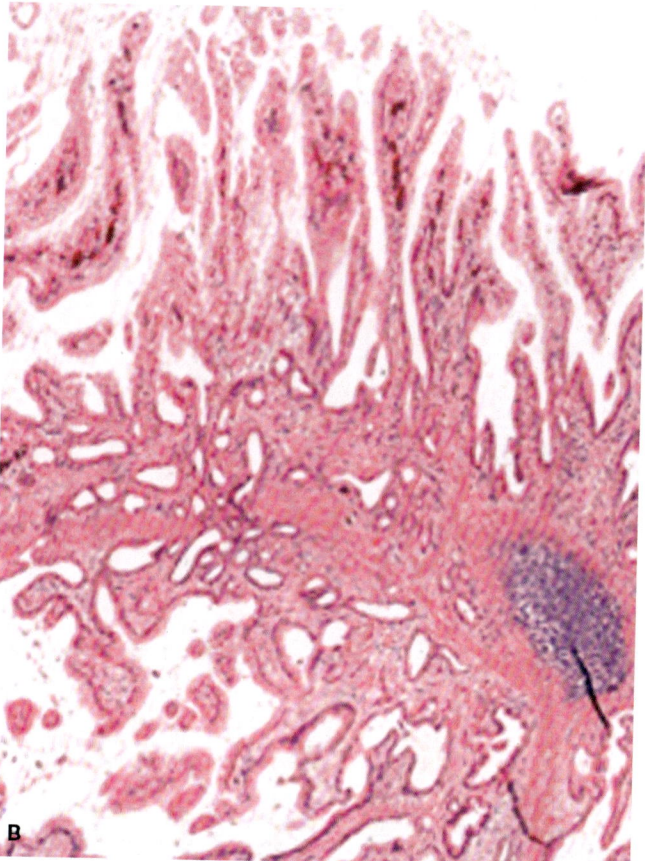

Figure 14-28. Extremely well-differentiated adenocarcinoma, gastric type. **A,B:** Tumor glands proliferate haphazardly with papillary configuration at the surface and invading into the muscularis propria. **C:** A papillary projection at the superficial mucosal level is lined by clear columnar cells with basally located small nuclei with fine nuclear chromatin and resembles hyperplastic foveolar epithelium.

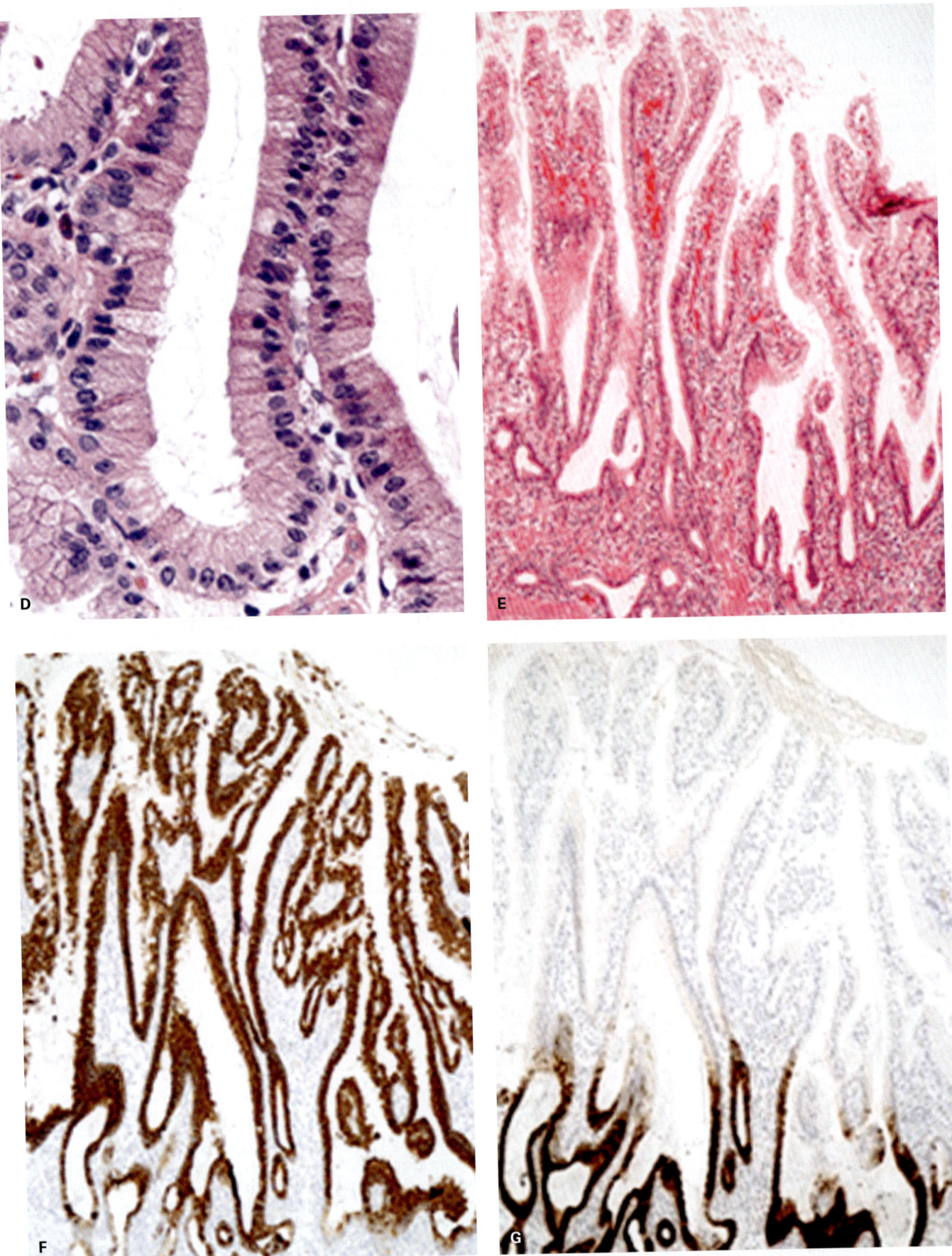

Figure 14-28. *(Continued)* **D:** Cancer glands in the deep mucosal level are lined by cuboidal cells with eosinophilic fine granular cytoplasm and basally oriented small round nuclei with fine nuclear chromatin and they resemble pyloric gland cells. **E,F:** In the papillary projection, MUC5AC is positive in most of the tumor cells and MUC6 is positive in tumor cells in the basal potion **(E,G)**.

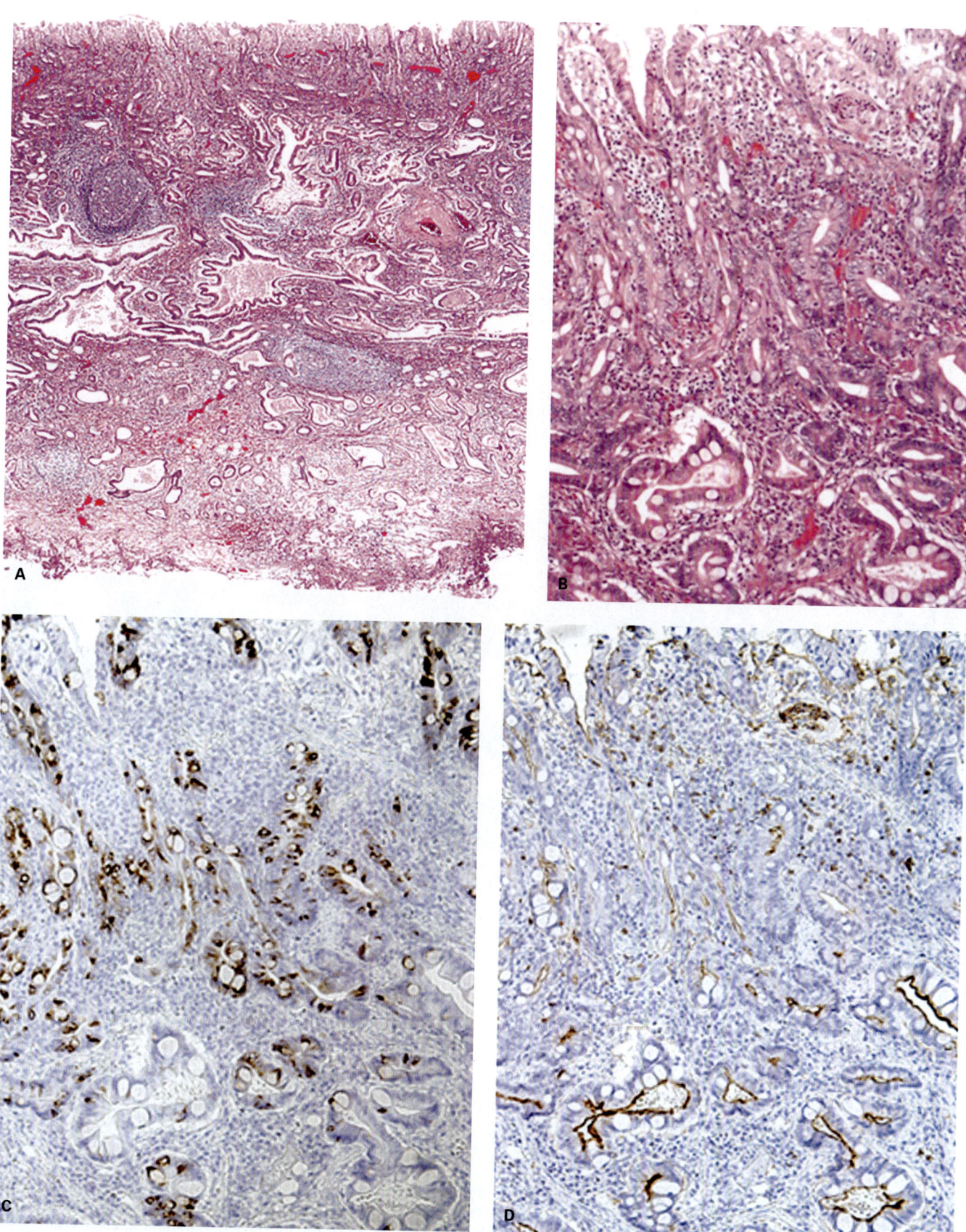

Figure 14-29. Extremely well-differentiated adenocarcinoma of the stomach, small intestinal (complete intestinal type). **A,B:** Carcinoma showing the irregular arrangement of glands mimicking that of complete-type intestinal metaplasia penetrates into the submucosal layer. **C:** They show immunoreactivity for MUC2 in the goblet cells and **(D)** CD10 along the luminal surfaces of atypical glands.

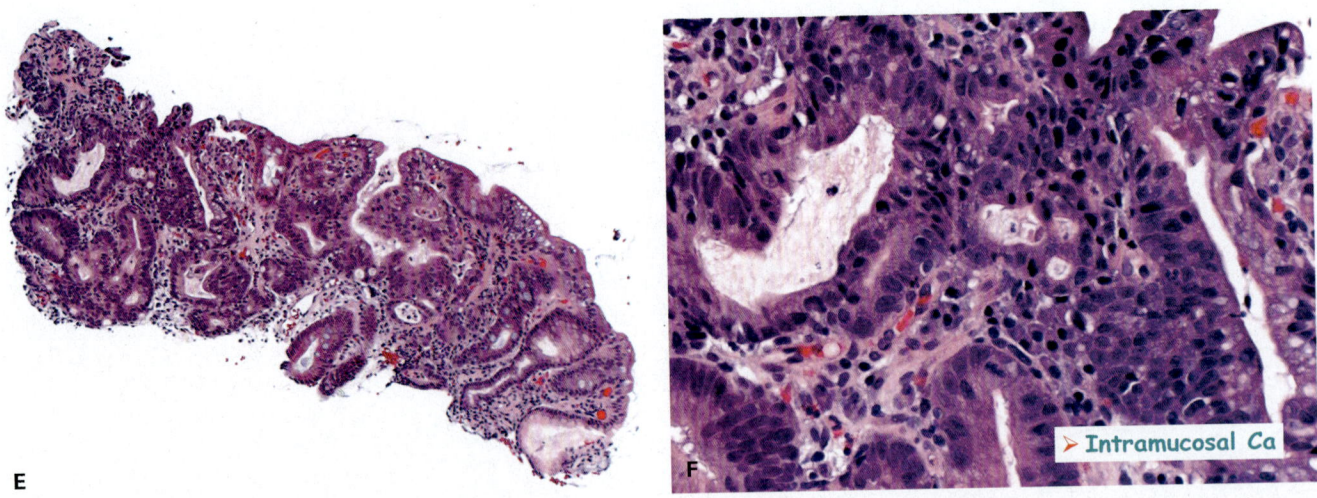

Figure 14-29. *(Continued)* **E and F:** Biopsy of very well-differentiated intestinal type adenocarcinoma. Note that the main changes are architectural and the nuclear changes are relatively subtle and not typical of adenomatous dysplasia, although goblet cells are readily seen.

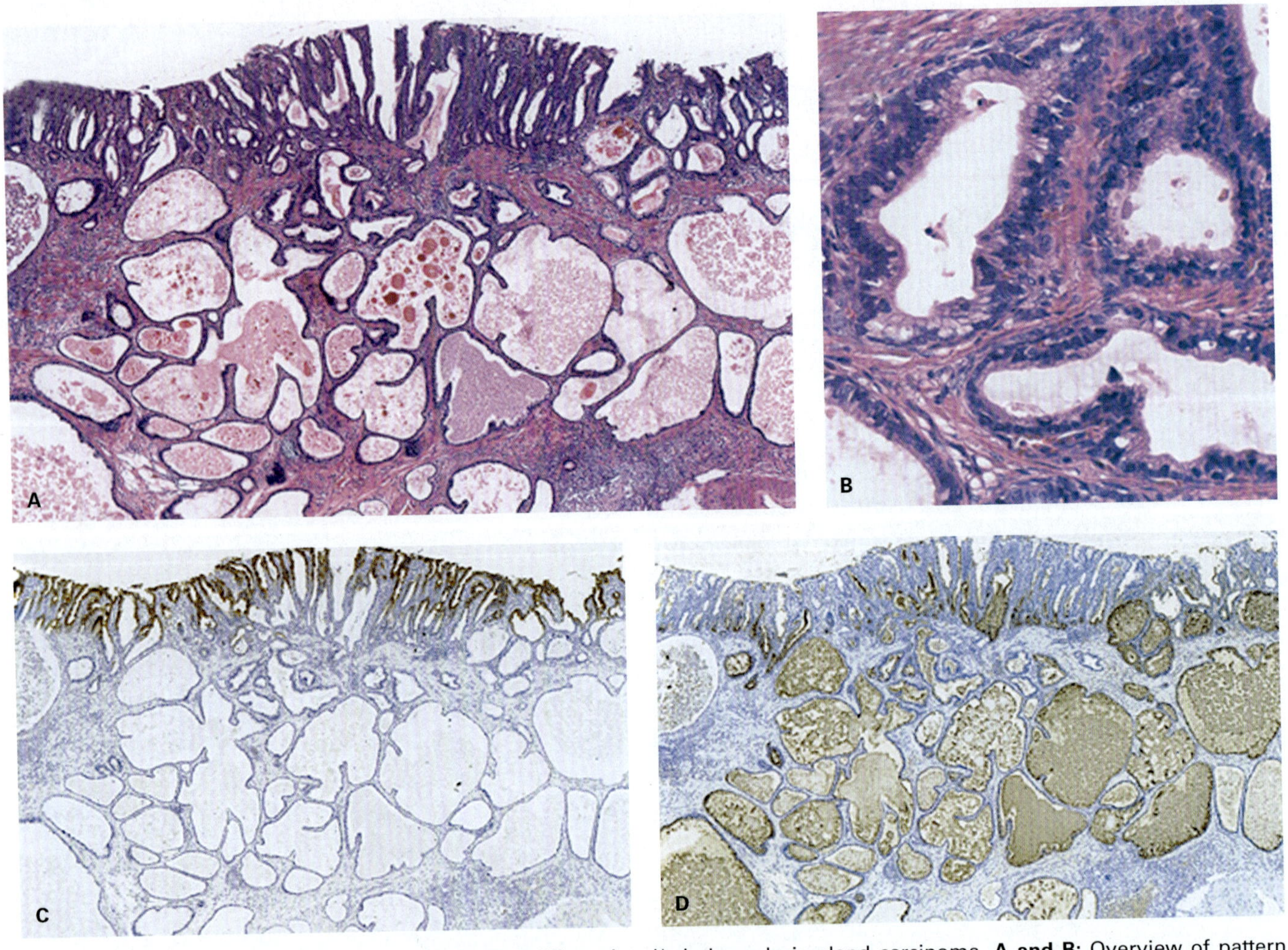

Figure 14-30. Pyloric gland carcinoma. **A–D:** Well-differentiated/tubular pyloric gland carcinoma. **A and B:** Overview of pattern and detail of the cells in which small supranuclear mucin vacuoles are present in many of the cells. **C and D:** MUC5AC which stains superficial foveolar gastric mucin, and MUC6, which stains pyloric gland mucin, show the invasive component to consist entirely of pyloric type glands, while the surface consists of foveolar type epithelium with low grade dysplasia.

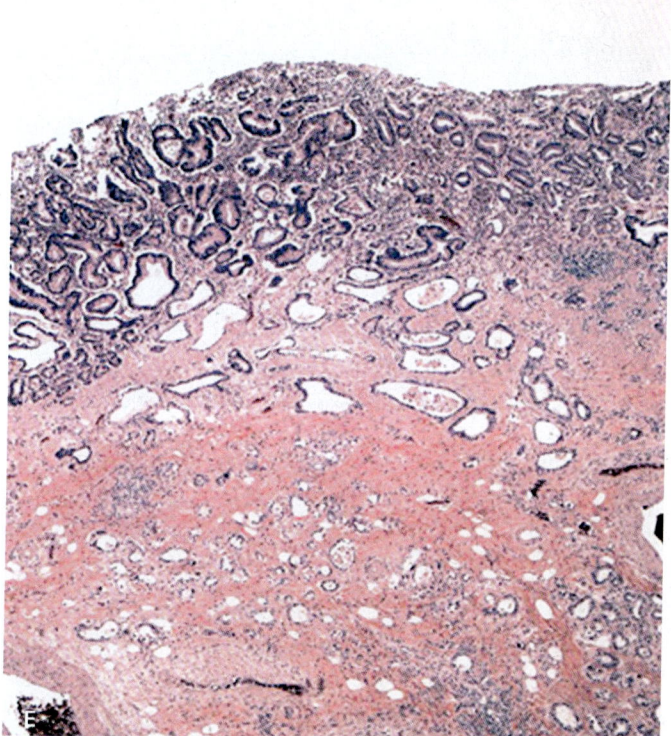
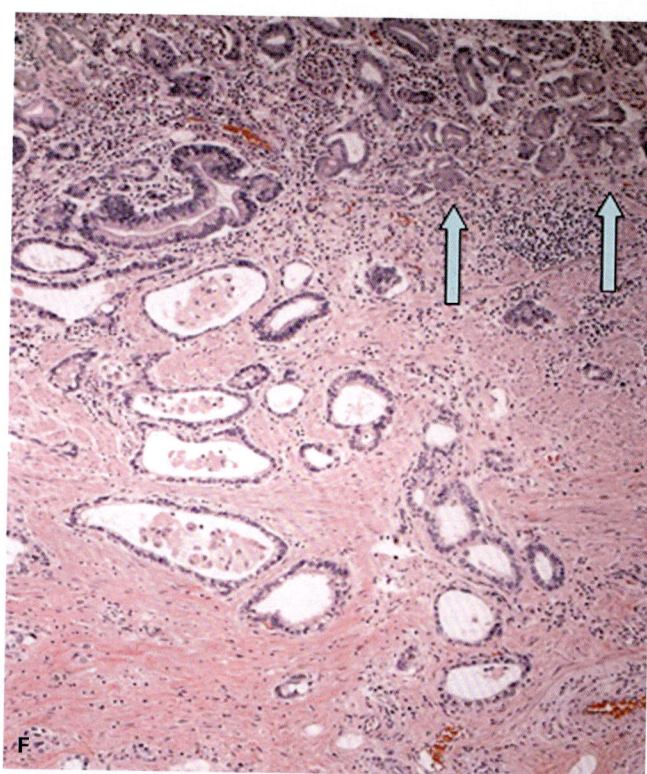

Figure 14-30. *(Continued)* **E** and **F:** Overview of a second tumor again with the typical appearances of glands dropping off from the bases of the dysplastic gastric pits. Note the mucosal pyloric type glands (*arrows*) and the difficulty that might be encountered in making a diagnosis of invasion in a biopsy.

Composite adenocarcinoma and endocrine tumor with pancreatic differentiation and pancreatic type tumors. Rare cases of pancreatic-type endocrine, acinar, and mixed tumors have been reported to arise in the stomach, mostly in cases with pancreatic heterotopia or metaplasia.[158–160] The tumors are often located in the submucosa and lack a surface dysplastic component. The histology of the tumors is identical to their pancreatic counterparts; however, in biopsies, the diagnosis can be problematic unless one thinks of this possibility and performs appropriate immunostains. Rare cases of mixed adenocarcinoma–endocrine tumor with pancreatic differentiation have been also reported that lacked any recognizable pancreatic heterotopias (Fig. 14-31).[161] In reported cases the glandular component consisted of columnar epithelial cells resembling gastric foveolar or intestinal goblet cells, consistent with a well-differentiated adenocarcinoma. The endocrine component was histologically well differentiated, carcinoid-like, and stained with the usual endocrine markers (chromogranin A and synaptophysin), while the glandular component stained variably for cytokeratins (7 and 20), CEA, and mucin core peptides (MUC2 and MUC5AC). At least one pancreatic acinar-type enzyme (trypsin, chymotrypsin, or lipase) was demonstrated in the glandular- as well as endocrine-appearing components, with some amphicrine differentiation. One patient with abdominal pain also had an elevated serum lipase level, clinically mimicking acute pancreatitis. Nodal metastasis similar to the primary tumors was seen in two of the cases. The long-term outcome of these tumors remains unknown.

Undifferentiated carcinoma. A small number of gastric tumors, which are composed of solid sheets of spheroidal or polygonal cells, lack any histologic features of differentiation, such as mucin production or gland formation, to determine their cell of origin. They probably represent a heterogeneous group of tumors, since special studies sometimes help to elucidate their cell of origin. For example, the demonstration of keratin or CEA immunohistochemically in some tumors indicates a tumor of the epithelial type. Some have an overt inflammatory component (Fig. 14-32), and immunohistochemistry may be needed to define their true nature. Some, especially those with a lymphoid stroma (Fig. 14-22), may need immunohistochemistry to distinguish them from a lymphoproliferative lesion. Electron microscopy may also help sometimes, primarily in poorly differentiated endocrine cell tumors, by finding dense core granules within the tumor.

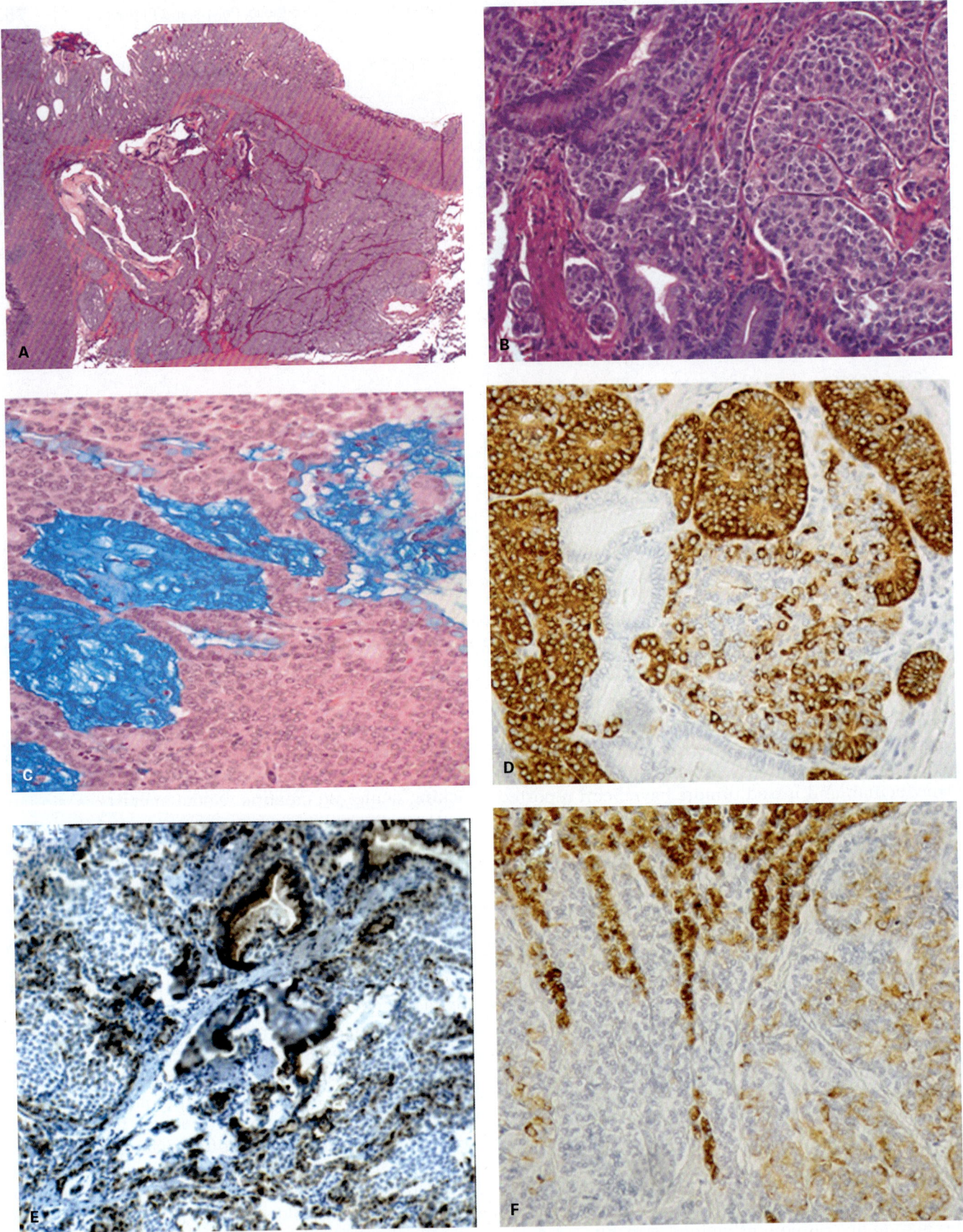

Figure 14-31. Composite adenocarcinoma and endocrine tumor with pancreatic differentiation. **A:** Overview showing that the tumor is predominantly a submucosal tumor with focal extension into the mucosa. Few mucin pools are visible even at this magnification. **B:** Detail showing the admixture of glandular with a well-differentiated endocrine component. Goblet cells are admixed with tall columnar glandular epithelium. **C:** Alcian blue stain demonstrating mucin pools. **D:** Immunoreactivity with chromogranin A in the endocrine component as well as scattered cells in the glandular component. **E,F:** Immunoreactivity with lipase and trypsin is seen in the endocrine as well as acinar and glandular components.

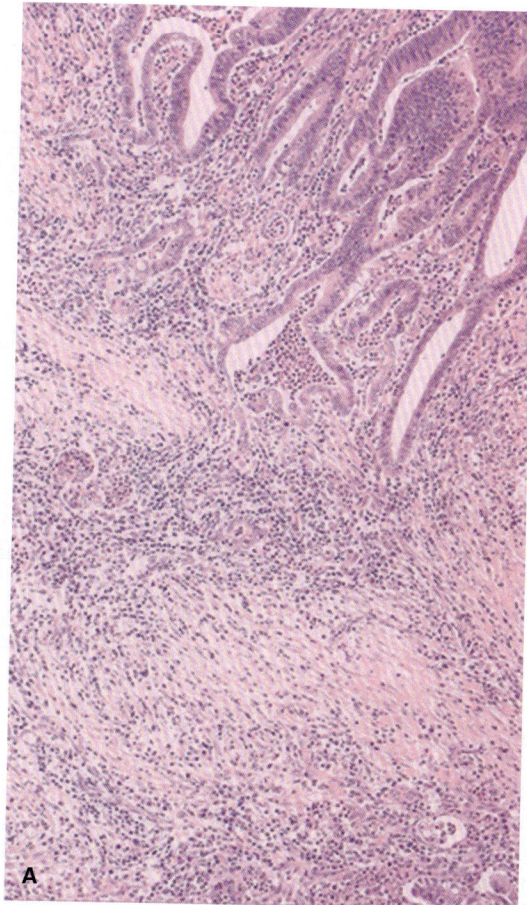
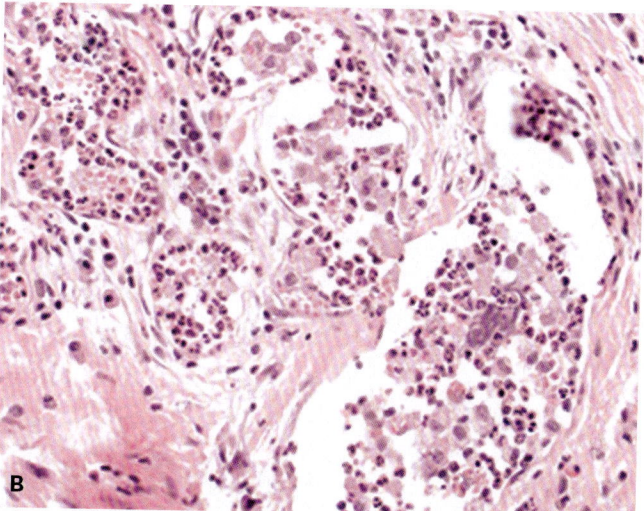
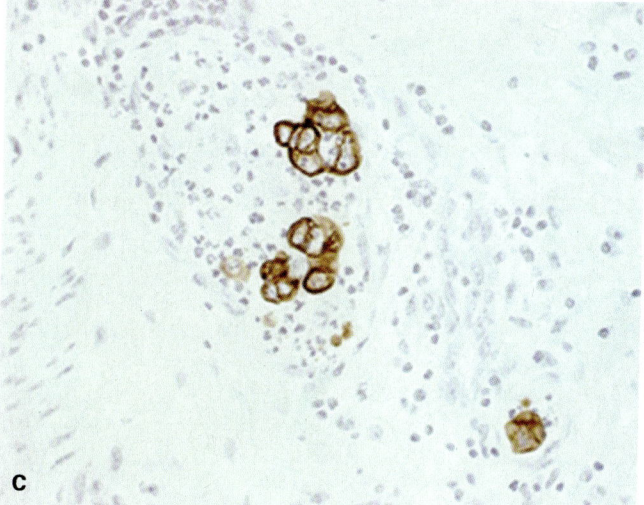

Figure 14-32. A,B: Undifferentiated inflammatory carcinoma with extensive endothelial channel permeation in which neutrophils predominate. **C:** Low molecular weight cytokeratin highlights the carcinoma cells.

Serrated dysplasia and carcinoma. Serrated lesions, both invasive and noninvasive, have been described in the cardia and elsewhere in the stomach.[162,163] It is difficult to know if these are really distinctive lesions or whether a serrated pattern is a basic pattern to which intestinal epithelium reverts under stress, as is seen in Barrett's esophagus, in the cardia, in gastric polyps (Fig. 14-33), in flat small bowel mucosa, in serrated polyps of the large bowel, and in inflammatory bowel disease (IBD). Further, in all of these lesions and locations they can also have dysplasia and a spectrum of changes up to and including carcinoma (Fig. 14-33). The lesion shown in Figure 14-33 could be interpreted as a hyperplastic polyp with dysplasia and intramucosal carcinoma, albeit with serrations, or a serrated polyp exhibiting a range of serrated changes from nondysplastic to carcinoma. It remains to be seen whether these will prove to be distinctive lesions or simply a variation on a theme. Further, in inflammatory polyps consisting of granulation tissue that is undergoing reepithelialization, the superficial pits frequently have a corkscrew or hyperplastic-polyp–like appearance, irrespective of where they occur in the glandular GI tract.

Gastric teratoma. These occur primarily in male infants who present with GI bleeding. The infants commonly have a palpable mass.[164]

Histologically, gastric teratomas are benign and morphologically similar to benign teratomas elsewhere. They are characterized by mature elements of all three germ layers, especially skin, ciliated epithelium, smooth muscle, cartilage, and neural tissue.[165] The tumors are benign and are cured by simple excision.[166]

Carcinosarcoma. Carcinosarcomas of the GI tract are rare tumors composed of epithelial and mesenchymal elements, the most common site of occurrence being the esophagus.

Clinically, gastric carcinosarcomas tend to occur primarily in males and in a younger age group (fifth decade) than gastric adenocarcinoma. Although lymph node metastases seem to occur late, the mortality rate is high.[167]

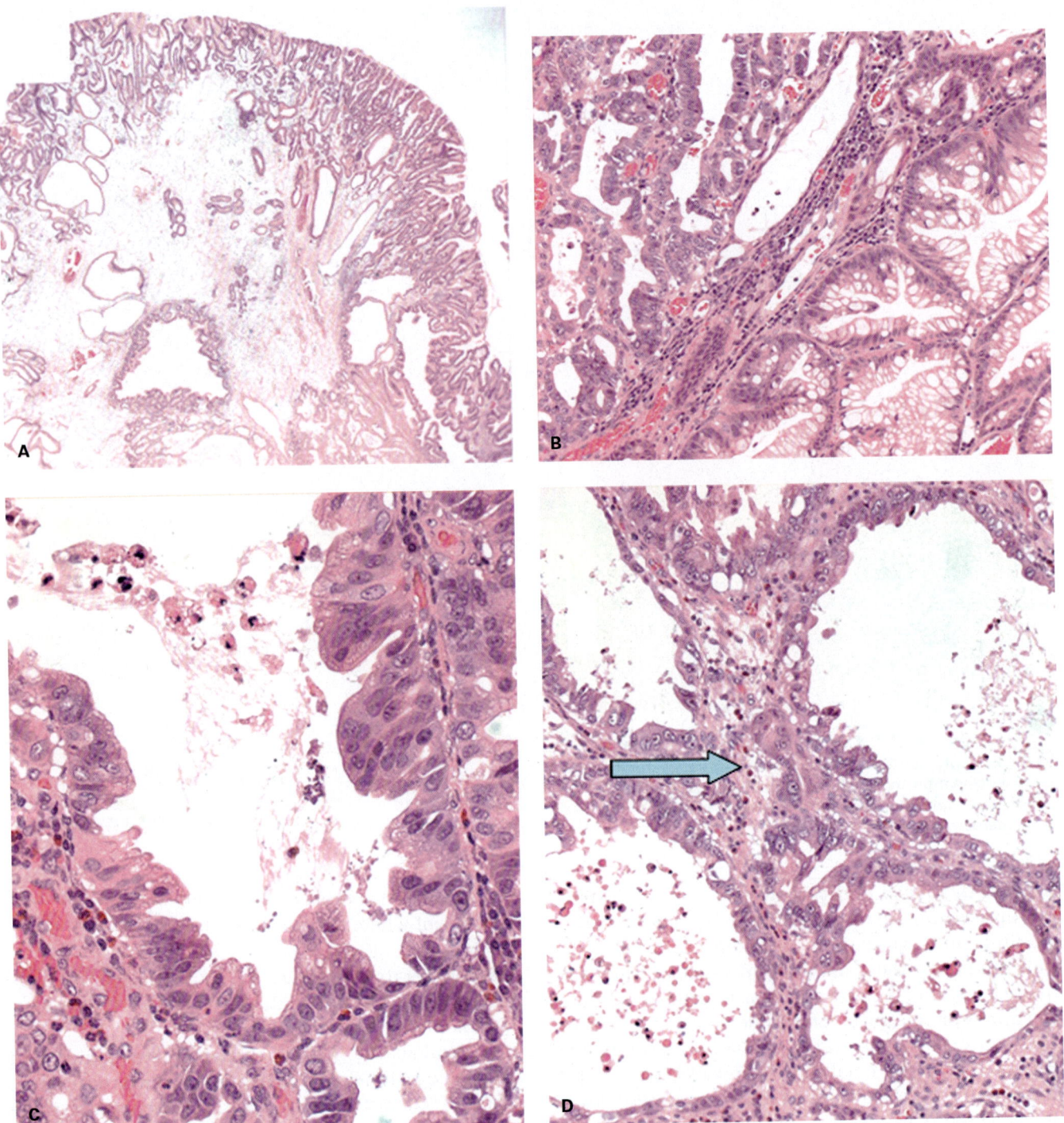

Figure 14-33. Serrated dysplasia and carcinoma. **A:** Overview of a polypoid lesion that has the overall appearances of a hyperplastic polyps. **B:** Part of a polypoid lesion with overserrations in the low-grade dysplasia (*right*) and adjacent high-grade dysplasia/carcinoma (*left*). **C:** Detail showing the nuclear features. **D:** Focus of lamina propria invasion (*arrow*).

The histogenesis of carcinosarcomas is now fairly well established, being of epithelial origin with spindle cell change and, in some, mesenchymal differentiation (smooth or striated muscle, malignant cartilage or bone, etc.). The sarcomatous component of the tumor is often, but not always cytokeratin immunoreactive. On gross examination, the tumors are found to be located most commonly in the pyloric region and are large polypoid[168] or ulcerated tumors.[169]

Histologically, the tumor consists of an admixture of randomly mixed epithelial and mesenchymal components. The epithelial component is mostly tubular or papillary adenocarcinoma and cases with adenosquamous[170] and neuroendocrine components[171] have also been reported. In most reported cases, the sarcomatous component of the tumor was poorly differentiated and was not adequately characterized. However, in some reports, there was clear-cut evidence of smooth muscle differentiation by transmission electron microscopy and immunohistochemistry,[172] rhabdomyosarcomatous,[169] osteosarcomatous,[169] and chondrosarcomatous differentiation.[173] However, care has to be taken as synovial sarcomas, which can also be biphasic, and rarely gastroblastoma, also occur in the stomach (see Chapter 7).

Gastroblastoma. These are also distinct types of biphasic tumors and discussed in more detail in Chapter 7.

Growth Pattern of Gastric Adenocarcinoma

Superficial (spreading) carcinoma. These carcinomas are early gastric carcinomas that frequently produce gastric symptoms over a long period. They often measure up to 10 cm in diameter but remain confined to the mucosa and submucosa (see Fig. 14-10).[174,175]

Organoid differentiation. Organoid differentiation is defined as the organization of intramucosal carcinoma into distinct patterns.[123,176] Disturbance in this pattern of organoid differentiation is closely related to the submucosal invasion. It is divided into two major types—gastric and intestinal metaplastic type. The former is classified into three subtypes: pyloric mucosal subtype, foveolar subtype, and glandular subtype. One of these is illustrated in Figure 14-21

Stromal reaction. Tumors can be further defined by their stromal content. Cellular tumors with minimal intervening stroma are called *medullary*, whereas those that elicit a dense desmoplastic reaction are referred to as *scirrhous* (Fig. 14-18). Scirrhous carcinomas that involve the entire stomach result in *linitis plastica*, the so-called leather bottle stomach (Fig. 14-15).

Differential Diagnosis and Clinical Implications

Early gastric cancer. Some of the major problems are the discrimination between benign *gastric erosions* and *ulcers* from ulcerating carcinomas, as well as the differentiation of signet-ring cell carcinoma from *histiocytes, muciphages,* and *gastric lipid islands*.

The appearances of early carcinomas may be difficult to differentiate from those of benign erosions and ulcers. The endoscopist should at least suspect malignancy whenever a gastric erosion or ulcer looks atypical (e.g., heaped margins) and should take multiple biopsy specimens from the margins of the lesion (at least four). It is also important for him or her to be aware that extensive invasion may occur with extremely small carcinomas, and that these therefore require the same definitive surgery as more advanced cancers.[177]

For the pathologist, there are two major issues. First, if the tissue is so small, poorly oriented, and distorted that adequate evaluation is impossible, then it is imperative that levels be cut and examined throughout all biopsy specimens; if necessary, more tissue should be requested without hesitation. The second issue is the interpretation of bland-appearing tumor cells, including signet-ring cells, lying singly or in clusters in the lamina propria.

Distinction from histiocytic lesions. Small collections of carcinoma cells may be overlooked or may sometimes be confused with histiocytes or muciphages and, less commonly, with gastric lipid islands. Muciphages in the stomach are vanishingly rare; therefore, from a practical point of view, atypical goblet cells and signet-ring cells indicate carcinoma until proven otherwise. We have also encountered cases in which the finding of signet-ring cells caused confusion with metabolic disorders. Cytokeratin immunohistochemistry demonstrating these cells in the lamina propria resolves the issue. Although the involvement of the stomach in metabolic storage disorders with infiltration of macrophages mimicking carcinoma cells is possible, it is highly unlikely and we have not encountered any such cases. See also the section on histiocytic tumors discussed subsequently.

Langerhans cell histiocytosis of the stomach is a very rare condition.[178] It should not cause confusion with carcinoma because the cells lack mucin and have the typical bean-shaped nuclei described in Langerhans cell histiocytosis. Gastric lipid islands may on occasion bear a superficial resemblance to signet-ring cell carcinoma. However, closer examination reveals clusters of bland-appearing, foamy cells with small, regular, centrally located nuclei within the lamina propria (see gastric xanthoma). If for any reason there is still doubt following a PAS stain (mucicarmine may not stain these cells if they contain only neutral mucin), a keratin stain or a histiocytic marker (CD68 or CD163), or both, resolves the issue. Conversely, if the cells are devoid of mucin and if fresh tissue is available, cytoplasmic lipid can be demonstrated by frozen section.

Lymphoma. Occasionally it is difficult to differentiate poorly differentiated carcinoma from diffuse, large cell *lymphoma*. Multiple sections for evidence of mucin production or glandular differentiation need to be examined for diagnostic confirmation. However, this is often done without success. Good markers are now available for epithelial cells (keratin or CEA) and for lymphoid cells (common leukocyte antigen), making the distinction between them easy most of the time. Fortunately, the immunohistochemistry panel for lymphoma always includes a keratin stain both to avoid this trap and to demonstrate lymphoepithelial lesions.

Metastatic carcinoma. Metastatic carcinoma of the stomach is rare, occurring in approximately 2% of patients with extraintestinal primaries in one autopsy study.[179] The most common tumors to metastasize to the stomach are breast cancer, lung cancer, and melanoma, and these may mimic primary carcinoma if they involve the mucosa. Direct extension from pancreatic or transverse colon primaries may also occur and form submucosal nodules budding into the lumen initially; these nodules may later break down and form fistula tracts. Clues to the metastatic nature of the lesion are multicentricity and, particularly in small lesions, an absence of metaplastic or dysplastic changes in the gastric mucosa, although this may not be seen in diffuse gastric carcinoma anyway. Sometimes the bulk of the tumor appears to lie deep within the stomach wall, and it is apparent that the mucosa is secondarily involved from below. Metastatic carcinoma may produce polyps and, rarely, may give a linitis plastica appearance to the stomach; this is most commonly seen in metastatic breast carcinoma, usually of the lobular type,[180] and, rarely, in other signet-ring tumors, particularly those of large bowel origin. Differentiation of a metastatic lobular carcinoma of the breast from primary diffuse-type gastric cancer can be problematic as the morphology is very similar and immunohistochemically poorly differentiated gastric carcinomas may express estrogen and progesterone receptors.[181] The situation can be further complicated by the fact that some patients with germline CDH-1 mutations with inherited predisposition to these tumors may develop both tumors. However, the typical single-file pattern of lobular carcinoma[180] and positivity for gross cystic disease fluid protein (GCDFP)[182] or mammoglobin may support a breast primary, while CDX2 expression would support a gastric primary.[182] Immunohistochemistry for HMB-45, tyrosinase, and Melan-A will identify metastatic melanoma.[183]

Neuroendocrine (NET—carcinoid) tumors. The distinction of *well-differentiated* NETs from carcinoma is usually easy. Difficulty may occur in the rare islet cell tumors, metastatic to the stomach or arising from ectopic pancreas in the stomach, as these are morphologically indistinguishable from carcinoid tumors. These are discussed further in Chapters 5 and 13.

Granular cell tumors. These tumors occasionally mimic poorly differentiated carcinomas. They are usually located in the submucosa, may be multiple, and

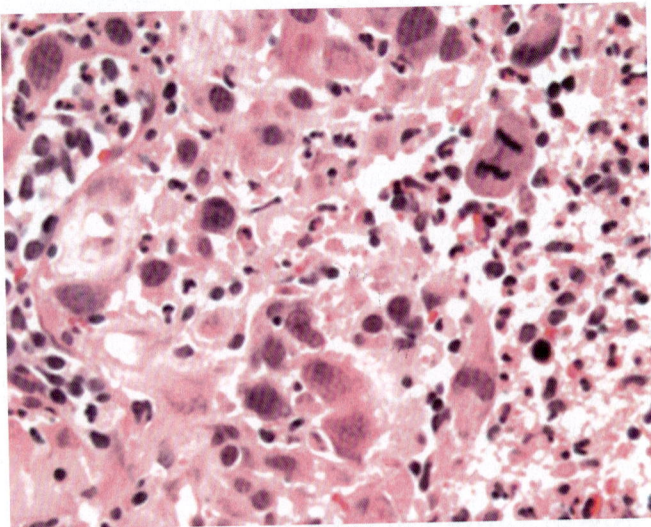

Figure 14-34. Bizarre undifferentiated cells in a chronic gastric ulcer mimicking carcinoma. There are many bizarre cells with hyperchromatic nuclei set in a background of inflammation and fibrosis. Mitoses may also be found but vary from none to prominent.

may show a mild desmoplastic response. Histologically, they are characterized by small, bland nuclei, lack of mitoses, granular eosinophilic cytoplasm, absence of mucin, and S100 positivity (see Chapter 7).

Bizarre undifferentiated cells (pseudosarcomatous changes). Degenerative changes associated with gastric erosions and ulcers may sometimes contain numerous bizarre, undifferentiated cells that can mimic undifferentiated carcinoma (Fig. 14-34). Features that distinguish these reactive lesions from carcinoma are the admixed granulation tissue, the presence of ulcers, and the gradual merging of the lesions with the adjacent normal tissue.[184] They are essentially similar to the pseudosarcomatous stroma seen in inflammatory polyps; indeed, granulation tissue at the edges of erosions and ulcers may be polyploid. These cells can be very bizarre and have numerous atypical-appearing mitoses, and are immunoreactive only for vimentin, and often CD10, but are negative for cytokeratin. They are entirely reactive in nature.

On frozen sections, granulation tissue with plump endothelial cells lining vascular channels may occasionally mimic well-differentiated adenocarcinoma, but the associated inflammatory cells help differentiate it from carcinoma.

Radiation therapy and chemotherapy. These forms of therapy may sometimes induce ulceration and epithelial atypia with architectural distortion, pleomorphism, and hyperchromasia, which can be confused with carcinoma. A history of prior irradiation and chemotherapy, lack of mitoses, and features of radiation injury, such as bizarre fibroblasts and arterial vascular changes, will help differentiate the two. Gastric pits at all stages of repair with adjacent normal pits or intermixed pits that are actively restituting will also help. (See also Chapter 2.)

Spread of Gastric Carcinoma and Prognostic Factors

Gastric tumors characteristically progress by *local extension* from the mucosa to the submucosa through muscularis propria to subserosal tissues, and sometimes into surrounding organs and throughout the peritoneal cavity. They also grow upward or downward intramurally, sometimes involving the entire stomach. Tumors of the cardia frequently extend into the lower esophagus to the point where it may sometimes be difficult to be certain whether they originated in the stomach or esophagus. These tumors will be discussed subsequently. Tumor in the distal antrum usually appears to stop abruptly at the pyloric sphincter on gross examination. However, microscopically there can be subserosal invasion sometimes, especially within lymphatics.[185] Microscopically, lymphatic invasion is common, but venous invasion is uncommonly demonstrated, although it must occur fairly often in view of the frequency of liver metastases.

These tumors also frequently recur in the gastric remnant following gastrectomy (20%–50% of cases), usually because of tumor left behind at the time of the original surgery.[186] Spread beyond the stomach is by *peritoneal seeding* and by *lymphatic* and *vascular dissemination*. Peritoneal dissemination occurs in about 40% of patients,[187] with involvement of the omentum, peritoneum, and serosa of the intestines.

Lymph node metastases are very common, occurring in up to 90% of advanced gastric cancers.[187] The superior gastric nodes are usually involved, but the pancreatic and splenic lymph nodes may also be affected, especially in tumors of the midportion of the stomach. In 15% of cases, metastases to Virchow's node (left supraclavicular nodes) are found.[187]

Bloodborne metastases are also fairly common, usually to liver or lung (35% of cases),[187] but no organs are spared. Ovarian metastases occur in approximately 10% of gastric tumors, usually of the infiltrative type.[188] Grossly they are characterized by bilateral smooth enlargement of the ovaries and microscopically by diffuse tumor infiltration, usually by signet-ring cells (Krukenberg tumors, Krukenberg being an ophthalmologist at Halle who published his paper on ovarian tumors when he was 25). These ovarian metastases could present before the primary and may be associated with ovarian dysfunction, such as virilization.[188]

The manner of *tumor dissemination* is not usually random but appears to be related to tumor type.[47] Thus bulky tumors are usually well differentiated (Lauren's intestinal type),[119] have a pushing margin, and disseminate most commonly to the liver and lymph nodes and, less commonly, to the peritoneal cavity. In contrast, the poorly differentiated or signet-ring cell carcinomas (Lauren's diffuse type) are *infiltrative*, commonly elicit a dense desmoplastic reaction, and tend to spread most commonly to the peritoneal cavity and lymph nodes and, less frequently, to the liver. The mucinous tumors behave in a manner similar to infiltrative tumors. In all three types of tumor, dissemination to other sites occurs in about 10% of cases.

Prognosis of Gastric Carcinoma

Survival rate of gastric cancer patients has continued to improve: In a recent British report the number of curative resections increased from 33% to 41% and 5-year survival increased from 15% to 41% over a 20-year period.[189] Similar improvement has been reported from United States[190,191] and Germany.[192]

Early gastric cancer. In Japan, the prognosis of early gastric cancer after surgery is excellent with a reported 5-year survival of 95%.[193] In the United States, it is in the region of 90%.[191] The pattern of invasion in early gastric carcinoma varies from a few cells into the lamina propria to large, well-demarcated cancerous masses that occupy a large portion of the submucosa and press the muscularis propria down. The 10-year survival rate is lowest in the latter, being about 65%.[193]

A number of studies have analyzed the factors responsible for death from early gastric cancers, which are due primarily to local recurrences or liver metastases.[177,194-196] There is no relationship between invasion and cellular differentiation. For example, signet-ring cell carcinomas are as frequent in intramucosal as in submucosal lesions. In contrast, tumor size and depth of invasion are significant predictors of spread. There is almost a direct correlation between the size of the tumor and the degree of invasion. In one study, approximately 30% of early gastric carcinomas <2 cm in diameter showed submucosal invasion, whereas 65% and 90% of lesions measuring 3 and 4 cm, respectively, showed submucosal extension.[117] In turn, depth of invasion is related to the probability of regional lymph node metastasis and a reduced 5-year survival. Thus, for intramucosal carcinomas, the likelihood of lymph node metastases is 0% to 4%; the 5-year survival is approximately 94% without lymph node metastases and 92% with metastases. The likelihood of lymph node metastases in early gastric cancers with submucosal invasion is about 15%, and the 5-year survival with these cancers, with and without lymph node metastases, is 89% and 80%, respectively.

Risk of nodal metastases in early gastric carcinoma. In a retrospective study performed by Gotoda et al.,[197] the likelihood of lymph node metastases was studied in patients with early gastric cancers who had previously undergone gastrectomy.

1. In patients with differentiated *intramucosal* carcinoma (papillary carcinoma, well-differentiated tubular carcinoma, moderately differentiate tubular adenocarcinoma) measuring <30 mm in diameter without lymphovascular invasion there were no lymph node metastases detected in 1,230 patients (Table 14-1) In this study, the Japanese definition of intramucosal carcinoma was applied in which both HGD and invasion into the lamina propria are included. Surprisingly, to date there appear to be no data for prognosis when vascular invasion is present, the assumption being that they all likely require resection. However, similar data in large bowel carcinomas suggest that invasion into the submucosa <1 mm in depth, even with endothelial channel invasion, has virtually no metastasizing potential (3%)[198] so that a degree of caution is appropriate in managing these lesions.

2. Tumors with invasion into the submucosa limited to a depth of 500 μm (SM1) were not associated with lymph node metastases (n = 145; Table 14-1). In a separate study, patients with well-differentiated SM1 tumors measuring <30 mm in diameter without lymphovascular invasion also did not demonstrate any lymph node metastases (n = 117).[199] However, a further study suggested that SM1 tumors that fulfill these criteria (differentiated tumors, lack of lymphovascular invasion, diameter <30 mm) may still be at risk. In a study by Ishikawa et al.,[200] 2 of 15 patients fulfilling these criteria had lymph node metastases at the time of gastrectomy. The authors concluded that superficial invasion into the submucosa may still present a risk for lymph node metastasis. In a separate case series, two patients were reported to have developed node metastasis after endoscopic resection of well-differentiated SM1 tumors measuring <15 mm in diameter.[200] Although no submucosal lymphovascular invasion was present in either of these cases, lymphatic invasion was detected in one of the cases in the muscularis mucosae, a finding that underscores the importance of identifying lymphatic invasion in the mucosal compartment. Again, there appear to be no data for prognosis when lymphovascular invasion is present.

It is important to be aware that extensive invasion may occur with extremely small carcinomas. These lesions therefore require the same definitive surgery as more advanced cancers.[201]

Expanded histologic criteria for endoscopic resection of EGC have been recommended for tumors fulfilling the following criteria (Table 14-1).[197,202] All tumors must be differentiated and without evidence of lymphovascular invasion. Intramucosal carcinomas without ulceration or intramucosal carcinomas <30 mm in diameter with ulceration are amenable to endoscopic resection. Superficial invasion (SM1 ≤ 500 μm; SM2 > 500 μm) into the submucosa can also be considered for endoscopic resection in tumors <30 mm in diameter, although the studies by Ishikawa et al. and Nagano et al. would suggest that there may be a slightly increased risk in this group of patients.[200,203]

Gastric remnant carcinoma. Residual or recurrent cancer in the gastric remnant following resection appears to be most likely in the superficial depressed lesions (type 0-IIc). These cancers often have poorly defined lateral margins, and there is a danger that the primary resection may not encompass the entire neoplasm. Kodama et al.[195] have identified another type of early gastric cancer with aggressive behavior. This lesion is usually elevated and well differentiated histologically, with an expansile growth pattern causing destruction of the muscularis mucosae and filling of the subjacent submucosa. According to the authors, 25%

Table 14-1 Lymph Node Metastasis in Patients with D2 Gastrectomy Surgery for Early Gastric Cancer

		DIFFERENTIATED		UNDIFFERENTIATED	
Depth	Ulcer	<3 cm	>3 cm	<2 cm	>2 cm
M	−	0/742	0/187	0/141	6/214 (2.8%)
M	+	0/488	7/230 (3.0%)	8/271 (3.0%)	44/743 (5.9%)
SM1	±	0/145	2/78 (2.6%)	NR	NR

M, mucosa; SM1, submucosal invasion <500 μm; NR, not reported.
Modified from Gotoda T, Yanagisawa A, Sasaoka M, et al. Incidence of lymph node metastasis from early gastric cancer: estimation with a large number of cases at two large centers. *Gastric Cancer.* 2000;3:219–225.
Differentiated adenocarcinoma includes papillary carcinoma, well-differentiated tubular carcinoma, and moderately differentiate tubular adenocarcinoma. Undifferentiated carcinoma includes poorly differentiated carcinoma and signet-ring cell carcinoma.

of these lesions had venous invasion, 40% had tumor invasion into the submucosal lymphatics, and 25% had metastases in the perigastric nodes. The overall 10-year survival of these tumors was 65%. They appear to have an increased likelihood of being EBV associated. Extensive reactive changes, cystic dilatation of glands and inflammatory polyps are frequent in the adjacent mucosa, all of which are secondary to the longstanding duodeno-gastric reflux.

Advanced gastric cancer. Several prognostic factors have been stated to be important, such as tumor stage, type, differentiation, size, and growth pattern.

The tumor stage (TNM classification) is the most important in the estimation of the prognosis and management of gastric cancer patients (UICC TNM Classification of Malignant Tumors; Table 14-2).[191,204] Patients die primarily because of venous invasion resulting in hepatic metastases, although data and examination and significance of these are not regularly documented or analyzed; serosal spread results in peritoneal dissemination, while nodal metastases ultimately can drain into the thoracic duct and disseminate to the lungs. It is also used as a surrogate marker, especially for the likelihood of vascular invasion.

Lymph node status is the most important prognostic factor in gastric cancer patients with curative resection.[189,191] The best survival occurs with gastric tumors without lymph node involvement. Survival drops off steeply once the lymph nodes are involved[189,191]; so the 5-year survival for gastric cancer of patients with pN1 (one to two nodes involved), pN2 (three to six nodes involved), and pN3 (more than six nodes involved) are 76%, 57%, and 26%, respectively in Korea, and 62%, 33%, and 17%, respectively, in the United States.[191] Unfortunately, most advanced gastric cancers already have lymph node involvement at presentation.[205] Thus patients with early gastric cancers confined to the mucosa and submucosa have a 5-year survival of about 95%. With invasion into the muscularis propria this falls to about 60% to 80%, and to <50% if the tumor invades the subserosa and serosa.[206,207]

Tumor grade may also significantly affect survival. Thus the overall 5-year survival of patients with highly differentiated carcinomas is 50%, with moderately and poorly differentiated carcinomas 18%, and with linitis plastica only 3%.[208] Similarly, patients who have adenocarcinomas with massive lymphoid stroma do about twice as well, stage for stage, as those with other advanced gastric cancers.[124]

It is still unclear whether the variations in the behavior of gastric tumors due to stage and grade are caused by independent factors or are interrelated; that is, are the more undifferentiated tumors more likely to be associated with more advanced stages? In one study, it was found that patients with highly differentiated adenocarcinoma had a much better prognosis than those with moderately or poorly differentiated adenocarcinoma and that patients with linitis plastica did very poorly indeed. It was also found that when the duration of symptoms was analyzed, the growth rate of the better-differentiated tumors was found to be slow compared to that of the poorly differentiated tumors. However, when the stage was taken into consideration, the authors could not show statistically significant differences in survival between the histologic groups.[208] Hermanek[209] has demonstrated differences in survival according to grade of tumor in advanced gastric cancer (but not in early gastric cancer). Thus, in surgically resectable advanced gastric cancer, stage for stage, the 5-year survival rates for the intestinal type of carcinoma was significantly better than those for the diffuse type—for example, T_2, 64% versus 45%; T_3, 42% versus 17%. Further studies are needed to clarify this matter.

Neoadjuvant therapy. In patients receiving adjuvant therapy, it is usual to grade the response to the therapy. There are numerous staging systems, and as expected, the fewer the grades, the greater the reproducibility. A typical four-grade system is given in Table 14-3 (grade 0, complete response; grade 1, single cells or small groups of tumor cells remaining; grade 2, residual cancer outgrown by fibrosis; grade 3, minimal response and extensive residual cancer, poor response). Other four-grade systems are no tumor, >0% response, <50% response, and no response. The important thing is communication.

Her2 status. It is apparent from the TOGa ("triumph over gastric cancer") trial that patients with advanced carcinomas may respond to trastuzumab (Herceptin), in patients with amplification of Her2. However, cases that are positive (score of 3+) are eligible for the treatment, as are those that are equivocal (score 2+) are treated if found positive on FISH/SISH analysis. Overall, about 20% of cancers are positive, especially intestinal type, and likely have a poorer prognosis, that is improved a little with Her2 antibodies. Her2 IHC is therefore standard in gastroesophaeal adenocarcinomas.[210,211]

K-ras status. Given the introduction of K-ras testing in colorectal cancer to predict response to the EGFR antibodies cetuximab (Erbitux) or panitumumab (Vectibix), it is inevitable that the same parallels will be drawn for gastric cancer. Yet preliminary data in end-stage patients at the end of the chemotherapy algorithm are not convincing.[69] Nevertheless, its introduction into earlier stages of therapy in patients with wild-type K-ras, especially in association with other chemotherapeutic agents such as irinotecan, can be expected.

Table 14-2 TNM Classification and Staging of Gastric Carcinoma (Seventh Edition)

TNM Clinical Classification

Primary Tumor (T)

TX	Primary tumor cannot be assessed
T0	No evidence of primary tumor
Tis	Carcinoma in situ: intraepithelial tumor without invasion of the lamina propria
T1	Tumor invades the lamina propria, muscularis mucosae, or submucosa
	T1a Tumor invades the lamina propria or muscularis mucosae
	T1b Tumor invades submucosa
T2	Tumor invades the muscularis propria[1]
T3	Tumor penetrates subserosal connective tissue without invasion of visceral peritoneum or adjacent structures[1,2]
T4	Tumor invades serosa (visceral peritoneum) or adjacent structures[1,2]
	T4a Tumor invades serosa (visceral peritoneum)[1–3]
	T4b Tumor invades adjacent structures[1–3]

Notes:
1. The adjacent structures of the stomach include the spleen, transverse colon, liver, diaphragm, pancreas, abdominal wall, adrenal gland, kidney, small intestine, and retroperitoneum.
2. Intramural extension to the duodenum or esophagus is classified by the depth of greatest invasion in any of these sites, including the stomach.
3. A tumor may penetrate the muscularis propria with extension into the gastrocolic or gastrohepatic ligaments, or into the greater or lesser omentum, without perforation of the visceral peritoneum covering these structures. In this case, the tumor is classified T3. If there is perforation of the visceral peritoneum covering the gastric ligaments or the omentum, the tumor should be classified T4.

Regional Lymph Nodes (N)

NX	Regional lymph node(s) cannot be assessed
N0	No regional lymph node metastasis
N1	Metastasis in one to two regional lymph nodes
N2	Metastasis in three to six regional lymph nodes
N3	Metastasis in seven or more regional lymph nodes
	N3a Metastasis in 7–15 regional lymph nodes
	N3b Metastasis in 16 or more regional lymph nodes

Distant Metastasis (M)

M0	No distant metastasis
M1	Distant metastasis

pTNM Pathologic Classification

The pT and pN categories correspond to the T and N categories.

The stages are as follows:

Stage	T	N	M
Stage 0	Tis	N0	M0
Stage IA	T1	N0	M0
Stage IB	T2	N0	M0
	T1	N1	M0
Stage IIA	T3	N0	M0
	T2	N1	M0
	T1	N2	M0
Stage IIB	T4a	N0	M0
	T3	N1	M0
	T2	N2	M0
	T1	N3	M0
Stage IIIA	T4a	N1	M0
	T3	N2	M0
	T2	N3	M0
Stage IIIB	T4b	N0	M0
	T4b	N1	M0
	T4a	N2	M0
	T3	N3	M0
Stage IIIC	T4b	N2	M0
	T4b	N3	M0
	T4a	N3	M0
Stage IV	Any T	Any N	M1

Reprinted from Stomach. In: Edge SB, Byrd DR, Compton CC. *AJCC Cancer Staging Manual.* 7th ed. New York, NY: Springer, 2010:117–226, with permission.

Table 14-3 Grading of the Effects of Neoadjuvant Therapy	
TUMOR REGRESSION GRADE DESCRIPTION	TUMOR REGRESSION GRADE
No viable cancer cells	0 (complete response)
Single cells or small groups of cancer cells	1 (moderate response)
Residual cancer outgrown by fibrosis	2 (minimal response)
Minimal or no tumor kill; extensive residual cancer	3 (poor response)

After Ryan R, Gibbons D, Hyland JMP, et al. Pathological response following long-course neoadjuvant chemoradiotherapy for locally advanced rectal cancer. *Histopathology.* 2005;47:141–146.

Table 14-4 Causes of Errors in the Biopsy Diagnosis of Gastric Carcinoma

Preanalytical—specimen mix-ups, wrong biopsy, inappropriate labeling
  Carryover of tissue
  Tumor inadequately sampled
Analytical—False positives
  Misinterpretation of reactive/regenerative changes, bizarre stromal fibroblasts
  Radiation/chemotherapy changes
False negatives
  Failure to recognize tumor cells, for example, bland nuclei, scant nuclei (e.g., linitis plastica)
  Failure to recognize abnormal architecture
  Failure to section block adequately
  Tissue crushed or necrotic
  Wrong slide picked up inadvertently
Postanalytical—wrong slide, or wrong case number dictated/reported

Biopsy Diagnosis of Gastric Carcinoma

In the case of gastric ulcers, most of the biopsies should be concentrated at the edges, right at the interface between ulcer and mucosal edge.[212] One specimen can be taken from the base of the ulcer, providing that it is not so deep as to carry a major risk of perforation. In the case of sessile polypoid lesions, several specimens should be taken from the base, in addition to those obtained from the top of the lesion. When areas are difficult to target for biopsy (e.g., high lesser curvature of the cardia) or when tissue is very gritty, yielding only tiny fragments, then more should be taken.

More important than the specific number of specimens is their quality. The endoscopist or endoscopy assistant should examine the specimens before they are placed in the fixative container. This helps to ensure that adequate samples are being submitted. Not infrequently, fragments of mucus or blood clot are obtained; these should not count as part of the total number of biopsies planned in a given case (see Chapter 1).

Biopsy before surgical resection. Biopsies are sometimes taken proximal to the planned resection zone prior to resection of gastric cancer for cure. The rationale for this practice is to minimize the risk of leaving behind a tumor that has spread intramucosally, of leaving behind HGD, or both. However, it is important not to be lulled into a false sense of security by negative results. Some gastric adenocarcinomas, notably the poorly differentiated variants, are notorious for spreading diffusely through the stomach in the submucosa and beyond. Thus it is important to examine carefully the margins of gastric resections. Increasingly some form of gastric mapping may be carried out prior to surgery, for example, 16 biopsies: 4 from antrum, 3 from lesser curvature, 3 from greater curvature, 2 from incisura (angularis), 4 from cardia (usually on retroflexion).

Misreading of biopsies for carcinoma. Although this applies to all organs, at least in our consultation practices, the stomach is the major site for both false-positive and -negative biopsy interpretations. There are a number of reasons for *false-negative* biopsy results; these are listed in Table 14-4. The major reason is *inadequate sampling* of the tumor. Rarely, the lesion may be in a difficult location to biopsy. The specimens may be small and crushed, and thus inadequate technically, or the tumor may be necrotic superficially. A less common but important cause of a false-negative result is *failure to recognize the tumor*. This is especially true in

1. Some cases of poorly differentiated carcinoma, which may mimic histiocytes in gastritis. In these cases, there is a diffuse accompanying inflammation with infiltration of single cells, often between apparently normal-looking gastric glands. Immunohistochemistry, especially cytokeratins, is most helpful in identifying the infiltrating tumor cells and the threshold for using them should be low, especially if there is clinical suspicion as well.
2. Well-differentiated tumors in which there is little cytologic atypia, when the infiltrative pattern can be difficult to appreciate (see, e.g., section on very well-differentiated carcinoma). This pattern of infiltration is also well appreciated on cytokeratin staining, and can help in appreciating both the infiltrative pattern and the presence of isolated tumor cells in the lamina propria, both of which provide strong evidence as to the diagnosis.

In addition to false-negative results there may be *false-positive* diagnoses (Table 14-4). *Regenerating mucosa* at the margins of ulcers may be confused with carcinoma as may pseudosarcomatous changes, both dealt with previously. See also the preceding chapter.

Value of Cytology in the Diagnosis of Gastric Carcinoma

Brush cytology is now rarely used and has been replaced by multiple biopsies, unless there is a major pathology or clinical interest in making the diagnosis by this method.

Handling of Gastric Specimens and Intraoperative Evaluation

Polypectomy specimens. These are handled similar to colonic polyps (see Chapter 20). If a stalk is present and the resection margin at the base identified, with ink or dye if not apparent, the polyp is serially sectioned in the vertical axis and submitted in toto.

Endoscopic mucosal or submucosal specimens. It has become increasingly clear that most patients with early gastric cancers may be treated effectively with endoscopic resection or endoscopic polypectomy and may not require surgery with lymph node dissection. Differentiated intramucosal carcinomas (papillary carcinoma, well-differentiated tubular adenocarcinoma, and moderately differentiated tubular adenocarcinoma) without submucosal invasion and measuring < 30 mm may be suitable for EMR or ESD (see Chapter 1). EMRs are performed by injecting saline into the submucosa to raise the lesion. The raised mucosa is then snared and cut using electrocautery. Ideally, the mucosa is removed in one piece but frequently lesions are excised piecemeal. However, the technique of submucosal mucosal dissection (ESD) is a more precise technique in which the mucosa to be removed is marked, and an electric scalpel used to dissect the entire lesion in toto in the submucosal plane. The latter takes longer to perform but the ensuing specimen is easy to examine histologically as it is one piece so the margins are easy to examine. This contrasts with EMR in which the lesion is often removed piecemeal and the fragments can be virtually impossible to put back together, assuming they are all retrieved from the stomach after the EMR. In a study by Hamanaka et al., patients with early gastric cancers who received EMR or ESD had a lower incidence of residual disease or local recurrence if the gastric tumors were excised in one piece (Table 14-5).

Both types of endoscopic procedures can be performed for intramucosal carcinoma provided there are no poor prognostic histologic factors present. A multicenter retrospective review of EMR and ESD was performed on a total of 714 patients with EGC, with excellent results.[199] Over a median follow-up period of 3.2 years (range 6–60 month), the 3-year cumulative residual or recurrence-free rate was 94.4% and the overall survival rate was 99.2% for both EMR and ESD combined.

Endoscopic mucosal resection or submucosal dissection specimens may be received for treatment of adenoma or early gastric cancer. Orientation of the specimen can be difficult although an attempt to orient the specimen should be made. This may be especially difficult, if not impossible, if the specimen is received piecemeal as is the case with most EMRs. However, in some endoscopy units, the lesion to be resected is tattooed periorally to mark the proposed margin of endoscopic resection, and this aids considerably in identifying margins. After orientation, the deep margin should be inked with dye. Accordingly, the peripheral margins can be inked a different color. The specimen if not fragmented can be pinned out to a corkboard and immersed in formalin for overnight fixation. The specimen should be sectioned in 3-mm increments and submitted in its entirety (Fig. 14-35). The objective of the gross handling of the specimen should be to assess the presence and depth of invasion and to provide feedback to the gastroenterologist of the adequacy of the resection margins.

Resection specimens. Table 14-6 summarizes our method of handling stomachs removed for gastric

Table 14-5 One-Piece and Piecemeal EMR in Early Gastric Cancer

	ONE–PIECE EMR		PIECEMEAL EMR	
	n = 1,115(%)	Residual tumor and local recurrence	n = 326(%)	Residual tumor and local recurrence
Curative	911 (82)	0	146 (45)	7
Noncurative	160 (14)	16	80 (25)	26
Not evaluable	44 (4)	8	100 (30)	17

Modified from Hamanaka H, Gotoda T. EMR for early gastric cancer. *Pathol Clin Med.* 2003;21:1086–1091. (Ref. 292.)

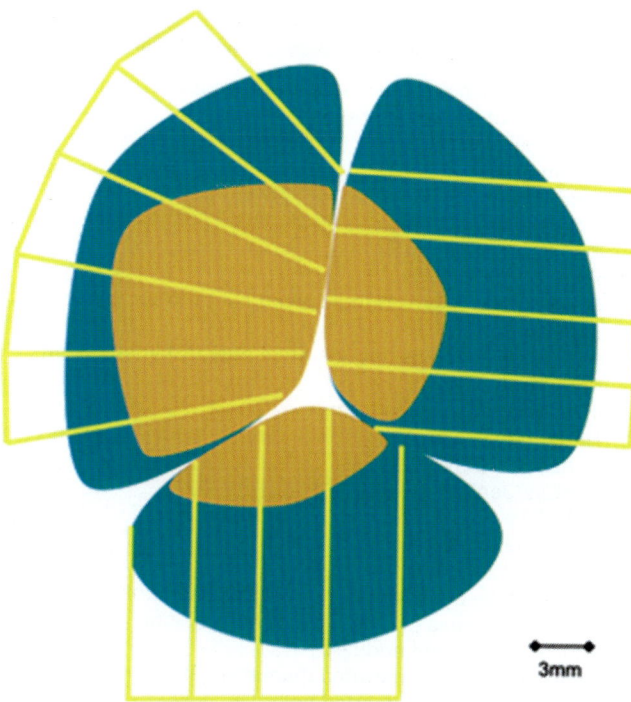

Figure 14-35. Handling of endoscopic mucosal resection. After orientation and inking of the peripheral and deep margins, the specimen should be sectioned in 3-mm increments and submitted in toto. (With kind permission from Dr. Masanori Tanaka, Japan.)

cancer. The resected specimen should be carefully opened, pinned out, photographed, and fixed in neutral buffered formalin. The most critical features in the reporting of gastric cancers are the determination of the tumor stage (extent of tumor invasion and lymph node invasion) and of whether the resection margins are involved for staging and prognosis of these tumors. Thus, the size and extent of tumor penetration should be carefully assessed, particularly whether there has been invasion of the muscularis propria and beyond. It is also important to sample all perigastric lymph nodes in order to determine the number containing metastases. The other pathologic features, such as the associated lesions, are primarily of epidemiologic interest, other than *Helicobacter* for which eradication therapy reduces the risk of subsequent new carcinomas, or features indicative of etiology (e.g., germline abnormalities).

The handling of gastric resections for palliation only (e.g., in cases with liver metastases or extensive intra-abdominal spread) obviously need not be as detailed. Sections should be taken to confirm the diagnosis, assess the depth of invasion, and determine whether there is tumor involvement of the resection margins. In addition, it is important to confirm the presence of metastases by biopsy, because on rare occasions lesions that are thought to be metastatic prove to be something else, for example, granulomata.

Table 14-6 Examination of Gastric Resection Specimens

INTRAOPERATIVE SPECIMENS
1. Measure distance of tumor from proximal resection margin in the fresh unstretched specimen
2. If required, do frozen section study of proximal resection margin to exclude tumor at any level (i.e., mucosa to serosa)
3. Photograph

FIXED SPECIMEN
Extent of surgery
  1. Stomach
  2. Other tissues and organs
Location
Gross pathology
  Growth patterns
    Type 0 Superficial, flat tumors with or without minimal elevation or depression.
    Type 1—Polypoid or fungating
    Type 2—Excavating
    Type 3—Ulcerated and infiltrating
    Type 4—Diffusely infiltrating
Depth of penetration and involvement of other structures
Histology
  1. Tumor
    Type (e.g., WHO classification) and differentiation
    Lauren's classification (intestinal, diffuse, unclassified)
  2. Lymphatic infiltration, venous infiltration, or both, especially extramural
  3. Depth of invasion
  4. Resection margins
  5. Lymph nodes site, involvement and number
Associated lesions
  Gastritis, intestinal metaplasia, dysplasia, and polyps
Summary statement
  Pathologic staging (pTNM, AJCC—state edition used)
  Likely behavior of tumor and prognosis

Gastrectomy for early gastric cancer requires the same meticulous attention as advanced gastric cancer. It is important to determine the gross configuration and histologic type of the tumor. The carcinoma should be examined histologically in its entirety, and particular attention should be paid in sampling all the regional lymph nodes, and in the search for submucosal vessel invasion (Fig. 14-36).

NONNEOPLASTIC POLYPS

This section excludes gastric adenoma and carcinoma (see previous sections on gastric adenoma and carcinoma), endocrine hyperplasia, microcarcinoids, and neoplasia (see Chapters 5 and 13), lymphoid tumors (see Chapter 4), and mesenchymal tumors including inflammatory fibroid polyps (see Chapter 7).

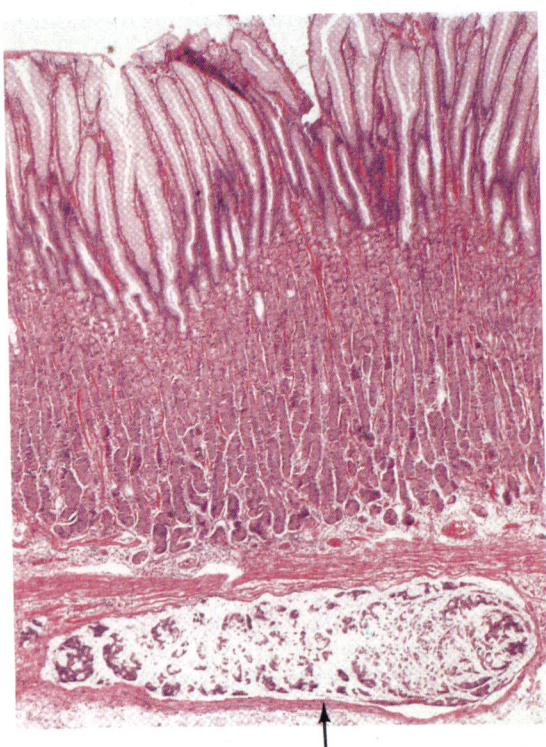

Figure 14-36. Gastric carcinoma showing submucosal lymphatic tumor dissemination (*arrow*). This section came from the resection margin, which appeared grossly uninvolved.

Classification

The classification of gastric polyps in the literature is confusing because there are numerous systems of classification but few reproducible criteria for diagnosis. Our classification of gastric polyps and tumors encompasses many of these and is given in Table 14-7. The separation of neoplastic epithelial polyps, primarily adenomas, from nonneoplastic mucosal polyps (primarily hyperplastic) is a fundamental distinction that must be made in classifying gastric polyps. We recognize that it may be impossible to distinguish hyperplastic, inflammatory, regenerative, juvenile, Cronkhite–Canada polyps, on morphologic grounds alone and Menetriér's disease particularly on biopsies.

The distinction of adenomas from other polyps is made by the presence of dysplastic epithelium in adenomas as their defining characteristic; adenomas are therefore neoplasms without evidence of invasion.

Biopsy and Excision of Gastric Polyps: Role of the Pathologist

The vast majority of gastric polyps are fundic gland polyps, followed by hyperplastic/inflammatory polyps,[213] and have a very low risk of containing a carcinoma. Fundic gland polyps are usually obvious endoscopically, while with hyperplastic polyps,

Table 14-7 Gastric Polyps

MUCOSAL (epithelium±lamina propria±muscularis mucosa)
Neoplasms of epithelial origin
   Adenoma
   Carcinoma
     Primary
     Secondary
   Carcinoids (Chapter 5)
Nonneoplastic polyps
   Fundic gland polyps (fundic gland hamartoma, cystic hamartoma)
   Hyperplastic polyps (regenerative polyps, hyperplasiogenous polyps)
Polyps in polyposis syndromes
   Hereditary
     Juvenile polyps
     Peutz–Jeghers polyps
     PTEN hamartoma tumor syndrome
     Familial hyperplastic polyposis
   Non-Hereditary
     Cronkhite–Canada syndrome–associated polyps
Gastric xanthomas (xanthelasmas, lipid islands)
Mucosal bumps and nodules
Solitary polypoid hamartoma (hamartomatous inverted polyp, heterotopic inverted polyp)
Gastritis cystica polyposa (gastric stomal polypoid hyperplasia)
Mucosal and submucosal cysts
   Cystic dilatation of gastric glands
   Gastritis cystica profunda
Heterotopic tissue
   Heterotopic pancreas (ectopic pancreas, pancreatic rests, adenomyoma, adenomyomatous hamartoma, myoglandular hamartoma, myoepithelial hamartoma)
   Brunner gland heterotopia
Some forms of gastritis
LYMPHOID (Chapter 4)
   Hyperplasia and lymphoid nodules
   Lymphoma
MESENCHYMAL AND STROMAL TUMORS (Chapter 7)
   GI stromal tumor
   Smooth muscle tumor
   Glomus tumor and hemangiopericytoma
   Inflammatory fibroid polyp
   Plexiform fibromyxoid tumor
   Neurogenic tumor
   Granular cell tumor
   Lipoma
   Vascular and lymphangiomatous tumor
COMBINED TUMORS

the onus is on the endoscopist and the pathologist to establish that the polyp is benign by simple biopsy or polypectomy, to assess whether there is background *H. pylori* (which may be causative) or sometimes atrophic gastritis (possibly with endocrine cell nests) or other pathology is present in the adjacent mucosa. Biopsy of the adjacent mucosa also serves as a control when the architectural abnormality of the polyp is relatively subtle. Because adenomas tend to have maximal dysplasia superficially, biopsy is an easy method of distinguishing the major subtypes of gastric polyps, although it may miss foci of invasion into the lamina propria or submucosa should invasion be present.

The mucosa overlying submucosal lesions may be biopsied to prove that it is nonneoplastic and normal, inferring the submucosal nature of the tumor, particularly in smaller polyps. In larger lesions, an attempt may be made to establish a diagnosis either by performing multiple biopsies at the same site or by aspiration biopsy endoscopically.

Approach to the biopsy diagnosis of gastric polyps.
In dealing with biopsies or excised gastric polyps, the approach is initially to decide whether an overt neoplasm is present, often with sheets of malignant tumor cells such as seen in carcinoma, lymphoma, metastases, carcinoid, and stromal tumors. The next question is whether, at low power whether there is abnormal architecture or not—random glands and lamina propria, excess of lamina propria, muscle fibers, and then whether the epithelium is unequivocally dysplastic; if so, is it focal—suggesting superimposed dysplasia (or carcinoma) in a pre-existing polyp, or diffuse, involving the entire lesion. The picture may be confusing if dysplasia occurs in another type of polyp. If the polyp is not dysplastic, then other specific and usually obvious types of polyps must be excluded. These include fundic gland polyps, myoepithelial hamartomas, and Peutz–Jeghers polyps, xanthomas, and lesions characterized by an eosinophilic infiltrate (inflammatory fibroid polyp or eosinophilic gastroenteritis), and the spectrum of inflammatory/hyperplastic polyps that includes juvenile polyps.

If the biopsy specimen appears to consist of normal gastric mucosa and a specific diagnosis cannot be made, then the possibility that the lesion is submucosal should be considered. Sometimes areas of patchy gastritis may be biopsied as mucosal bumps/polyps. Levels through the block may be required to exclude the latter. However, if the tissue is clearly polypoid, without architectural distortion, and the foveolar region is of increased length, it is likely focal foveolar hyperplasia—likley a variant of hyperplastic polyp. This then leaves the group of polyps characterized by an excess of mucosa, often with an increased content of inflammatory cells, and invariably with architectural distortion and often cystic dilatation of some of the glands. This includes the group of polyps that have variously been called *hyperplastic, retention, inflammatory,* or *hyperplasiogenous*. If numerous, it may also include hyperplastic, juvenile, and Cronkhite–Canada polyps, although diffuse GI polyposis and associated clinical features distinguish the latter. Juvenile polyposis may have other stigmata, although rare types that have isolated gastric involvement are also known to occur. Menetrier's disease is the final differential diagnosis in this group.

Fundic Gland Polyps

Most fundic gland polyps are sporadic, but they may be associated with FAP. Between sporadic fundic gland polyps and FAP-associated fundic gland polyps, some differences are observed in age, sex, and radiologic and endoscopic features, although the polyps are histologically similar.[214] Sporadic fundic gland polyps have a strong female predominance (most common in middle-aged females).[215] In FAP patients, fundic gland polyps are present in about half of the patients, may develop as early as the first decade, and show an equal gender distribution.[216]

There have been reports of PPIs being associated with fundic gland polyps.[217,218] While this potential link is still controversial,[219] nevertheless, longitudinal studies show that on long-term PPIs the frequency of both fundic gland polyps and hyperplastic polyps increases while the prevalence of *H. pylori* deceases.[220,221] The lack of association of fundic gland polyps with *H. pylori* and any form of gastritis has long been recognized, and it has been suggested that these polyps may produce an excess of lysozyme, which acts as an antibacterial to suppress growth of *H. pylori*.[222] Organisms leave the antrum and move proximally seeking acid to neutralize the cloud of ammonium produced by their urease. Nevertheless, most fundic gland polyps biopsied now have changes associated with proton pump therapy, and most patients taking long-term PPIs have fundic gland polyps exhibiting the typical parietal cell hypertrophy associated with them.

Sporadic fundic gland polyps are mostly linked to activating beta-catenin (91%) and it raises the question of whether this makes fundic gland polyps neoplasms. Clearly, they are not histologically neoplastic; neither is it surprising that histologic lesions have such mutations, for they have to grow to their size by a mechanism that promotes their growth. In the broadest sense they could be regarded as "intraepithelial neoplasm mutations." The concept that these polyps may be molecular, but not histologic, neoplasms is embedded in the 2010 WHO "Blue Book." Beta-catenin mutations are found infrequently in APC (8%)[210,211] whereas FAP-associated fundic gland polyps are caused by second somatic hits in *APC* gene, but not beta-catenin mutations.[223] Similar mutations are found in PPI-associated polyps, but it is reversible with cessation of the PPIs. The relationship between fundic gland polyps and FAP needs to be put in context, for in nonreferral centers, one might be lucky to find a single patient with fundic gland polyps that has FAP, but most patients with FAP will have fundic gland polyps. Gastric carcinomas are rarely associated with FGPs, although an hereditary syndrome of gastric adenocarcinoma associated with proximal polyposis (GAPPS) is discussed previously.

Pathology. Grossly, fundic gland polyps are small (usually a few millimeters and rarely more than 1 cm) and sessile lesions with a smooth surface contour and present as single or multiple (Fig. 14-37A,B). They occur in the parietal/chief cell–bearing region of the stomach in otherwise normal oxyntic mucosa.[224]

Microscopically, the diagnosis is usually very straightforward and made at low power (Figs. 14-37A,C and 14-38A,C). Cysts appear to be the result of cystic dilatation of pits deep to the mucous neck cells, so that the cysts that form are lined by mucous cells, chief cells, and parietal cells. These cells gradually become atrophic as the cysts dilate, and cuboidal cells in which occasional flattened parietal cells can still be identified predominate. In patients taking PPIs, hypertrophied parietal cells with apical snouts can be identified and can vary from modest as shown here to flamboyant in some patients on lifetime PPIs (Fig. 14-37E,F). Superficial mucin-producing cells may also line some of the cysts, particularly those closer to the lumen. Inflammation is characteristically absent, rasing the question of whether inflammation is protective for the formation of these polyps, and therefore the mutations that are associated with them.

When looking at fundic gland polyps there are two questions

1. Are there parietal cell changes as seen in long-term ingestion of PPIs?
2. Is dysplasia or changes indefinite for dysplasia present in the mucous neck regions? Most but not all of these polyps with dysplasia will be found in patients with FAP and the dysplasia is rarely more than low grade, likely because most of these polyps are small.

Dysplasia in fundic gland polyps have been found in 1% of sporadic cases[224] and up to 44% of FAP-associated cases.[224–226] They occur in the foveolar compartment of fundic gland polyps (Fig. 14-38).[224–226] HGD is rare and has been described in non-FAP patients[227] as well as in patients with FAP.[226] The dysplasia tends to be of gastric foveolar type with subtle low grade dysplasia. Indeed some may be called "indefinite for dysplasia" when, in a patient with FAP, in the absence of any other cause, any "atypia" really has to be the very earliest changes of dysplasia. This is analogous to adenomas with only a few crypts in the large bowel in FAP, when virtually all abnormal crypts in resections are adenomas. In patients with FAP, gastric adenocarcinoma arising from fundic gland polyps is incredibly rare but has also been reported.[228,229]

Clinical implications. This poses a problem of how to handle fundic gland polyps in patients with FAP and other inherited disease predisposing to fundic gland polyps (Lynch's syndrome, attenuated familial polyposis coli, *MUTYH*-associated polyposis). If they are present should they be examined or ignored, biopsied or removed? There are not good data that sporadic fundic gland polyps with low grade dysplasia have any risk of progressing to carcinoma, probably because most are removed when small and seem to have little growth potential. Because the incidence of carcinoma is almost zero, a good argument can be made for ignoring them altogether, especially as the high incidences of dysplasia will frequently lead to concern, and, if done properly, an end-viewing scope is needed for this part, and then a side-viewing scope for the duodenum, which is the prime purpose of the endoscopy. There are no guidelines, so many take a quick peek on the way down, and if there are any polyps that are unduly large or disconcerting go on to examine the duodenum, but then insert a forward-viewing scope to remove or biopsy the offending polyp. In the lack of any guidelines or data, most gastroenterologists will have some concern once a diagnosis of dysplasia is made, and will follow-up these patients depending on other risk factors including age, at arbitrarily chosen intervals, removing (better than biopsying as it may be impossible to know which one was biopsied) any large or worrisome polyp. Gastrectomy is only really indicated when unequivocal invasive carcinoma is demonstrated extending beyond the stalk of the polyp or is grossly malignant. Intramucosal carcinoma in polyps has virtually no metastasizing potential so polypectomy is adequate local treatment.

Hyperplastic and Inflammatory Polyps

Inflammatory and hyperplastic polyps are considered together because while in the pure form they may be easily distinguished by the amount of inflammation, and also superficial ulceration of inflammatory polyps when present; there is so much overlap that in many instances they probably represent the same polyp at different points in time. Inflamed hyperplastic polyps may therefore be indistinguishable from inflammatory polyps, while when the inflammation resolves from inflammatory polyps they may resemble hyperplastic (or juvenile) polyps.

Hyperplastic polyps are benign, nonneoplastic polyps, and therefore are characterized by an overgrowth of nondysplastic epithelium and often an excess of lamina propria. They are the second most common polyps encountered in the stomach,[213] although prior to PPIs they made up about 75% of all gastric polyps. They have a wide age range but are more common with increasing age. Most are incidental findings at endoscopy, where they are presumed to represent a reaction to previous gastric mucosal

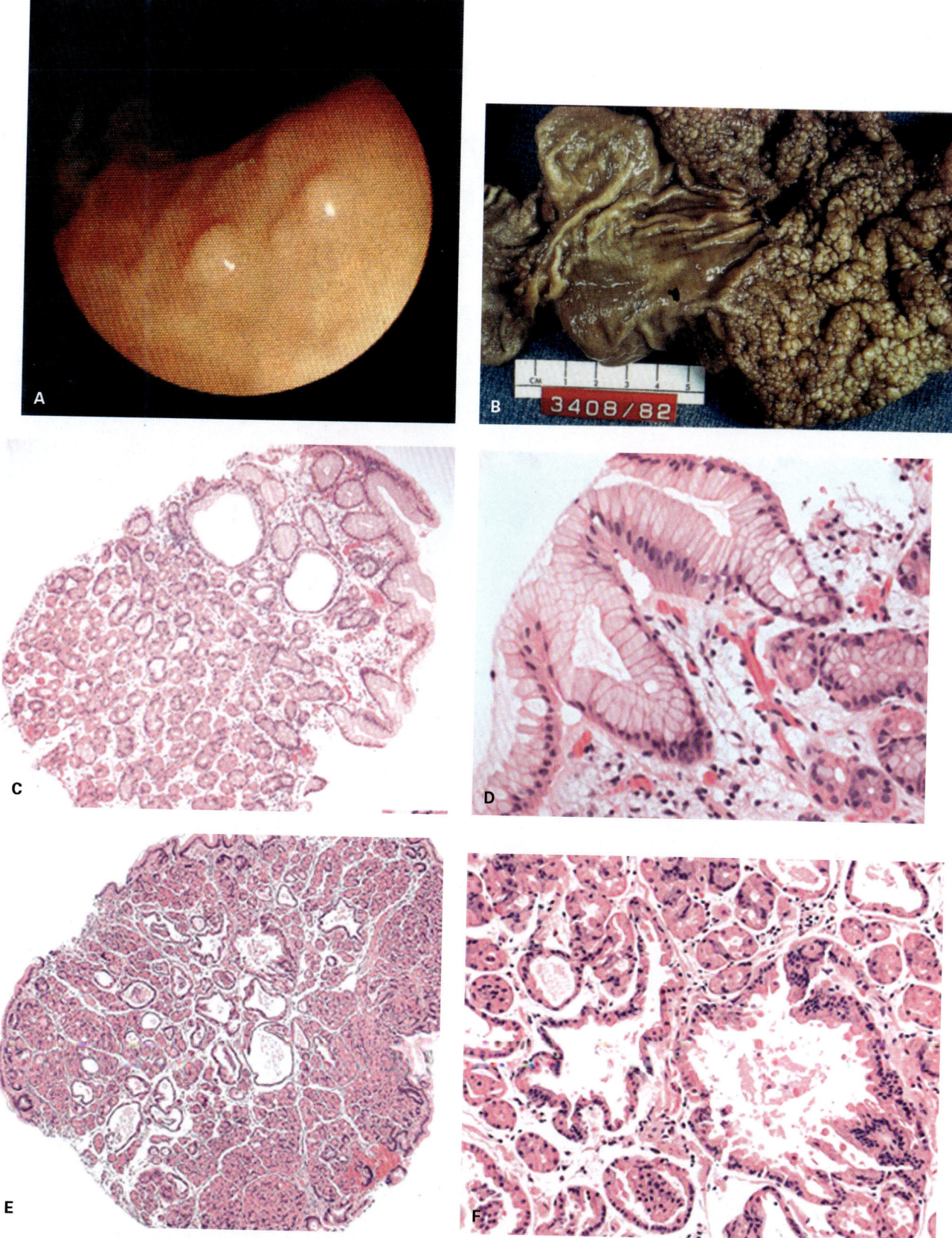

Figure 14-37. Gastric fundic gland polyps. **A:** Endoscopic appearance with several small bumps in the body mucosa. **B:** Part of a gastroduodenostomy in a patient with familial adenomatous polyposis (Gardner's syndrome), demonstrating myriad small polyps carpeting, but limited to, the gastric body. **C,D:** Typical very early fundic gland polyp in which mucosa is expanded by small cystic dilatations in many of the glands. Note that the surface mucosa has absolutely normal foveolar epithelium, while the lack of inflammation in the lamina propria is also typical. **E:** More typical fundic gland polyp readily recognizable at low power. **F:** Detail showing some cysts lined by mucus-producing cells, others by parietal and chief cells. However, the parietal cells are large and have apical snouts as seen in long-term antisecretory therapy, invariably proton pump inhibitors.

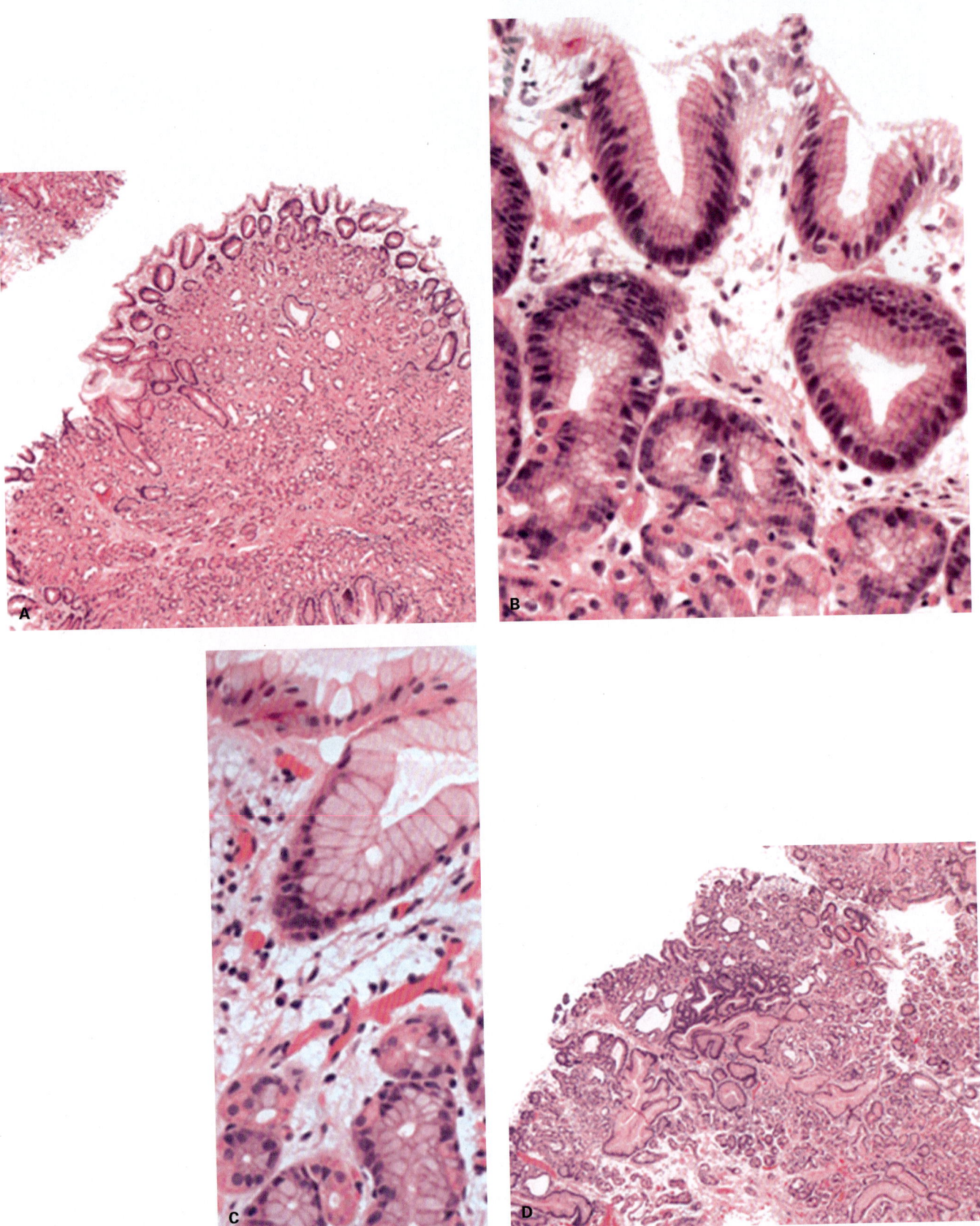

Figure 14-38. Dysplasia in fundic gland polyps. **A:** Overview of typical fundic gland polyps that looks unremarkable. **B:** Detail of surface shows that nuclei in the mucous neck region are enlarged and hyperchromatic in the absence of any inciting inflammatory cause. However, it may need comparison with normal foveolar mucosa **(C)** to make the diagnosis. This patient had familial adenomatous polyposis. **D:** More overt area of low-grade dysplasia readily visible at low power.

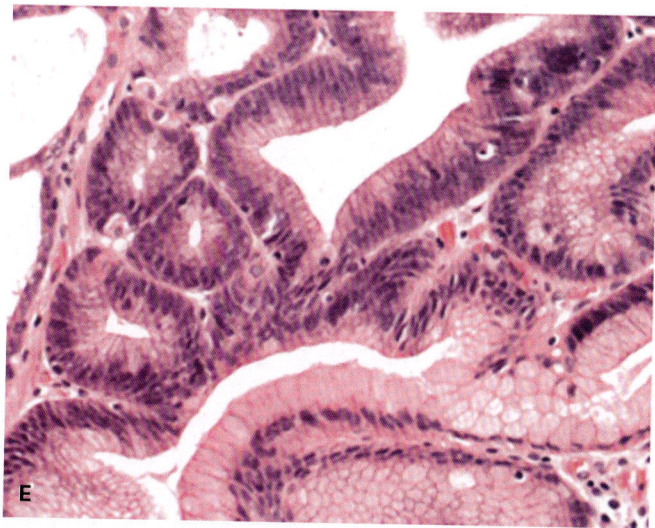

Figure 14-38. *(Continued)* **E:** Detail in which adjacent dysplastic and nondysplastic mucosa can be compared.

injury. They are most commonly associated with *H. pylori*, chemical gastropathy or, infrequently, autoimmune-associated chronic gastritis.[217,218]

While hyperplastic polyps are found anywhere in the stomach, they are most common in the antrum and at the junction of antral and body mucosa. They range from a few millimeters to a few centimeters in size; their distinction endoscopically from other polyps such as adenomas is not possible. Hyperplastic polyps seem to change their forms from sessile and semispherical, semipedunculated, and consequently to pedunculated as they grow larger (Figs. 14-39 and 14-40).

Pathology. This spectrum of polyps is characterized by marked elongation and architectural distortion of the pits, often with a focal superficial corkscrew appearance and usually accompanied by cysts. At the inflammatory polyp end of the spectrum of the hyperplastic polyp, there may be marked excess of lamina propria, particularly in heavily inflamed polyps, with granulation tissue at the surface (Fig. 14-40). Occasionally, lymphoid nodules, with or without germinal centers, are also present. The epithelium is often mucin depleted, attenuated, and very eosinophilic. Active reepithelialization over an ulcerated surface is manifested by attenuated cuboidal to low columnar epithelium with widely separated vesicular nuclei containing prominent eosinophilic nucleoli. Superficial mitotic figures may be seen, but are rare and are not indicative of malignant transformation. Mucin-producing cells do not appear until the cells are columnar and may be intestinalized. Invagination of the surface mucosa occurs with budding, which may produce a back-to-back appearance, which is distinguished from carcinoma in situ by the absence of dysplasia (Fig. 14-40).

Cystic dilatation of the pits is common, a stage that some prefer to call a *retention polyp*, a term we prefer not to use for simplicity or confusion with juvenile polyps (which are morphologically identical). It is because of this new pit formation that some object to the term *hyperplastic polyp*, as it is far more than a simple hyperplasia. Interestingly, the pits immediately beneath the ulcerated surface often have a characteristic (serrated) corkscrew appearance and resemble the crypts seen in colonic hyperplastic polyps. Nevertheless, this corkscrew change is seen frequently in any gut epithelium, particularly polyps, immediately beneath an ulcerated surface, irrespective of the nature of the polyp itself. However, there is no other similarity between hyperplastic polyps of the stomach and large bowel lesions.

Immediately beneath the surface epithelium, stromal mesenchymal cells may sometimes be extremely bizarre, resembling radiation fibroblasts and mimicking sarcoma (pseudosarcomatous change) (Fig. 14-34).[230] Nevertheless, there is no evidence that these are anything other than reactive fibroblasts. They are immunoreactive only with vimentin and often CD10, even though precautionary stains especially for carcinoma and melanoma may be contemplated. Rarely, food or other foreign debris may be present (Fig. 14-40H).

The other end of the inflammatory/hyperplastic polyp spectrum typical hyperplastic polyps, consist of similar epithelial changes during or following resolution of the inflammatory component. There is much less lamina propria and inflammation, so that most of the polyp is epithelial and consists of mature foveolar mucus-producing cells (Fig. 14-40). Smooth muscle fibers are commonly seen between the gastric pits, arising from thickened, split, and fragmented muscularis mucosae and occasionally from venules. The thick arborizing muscle bundles so characteristic

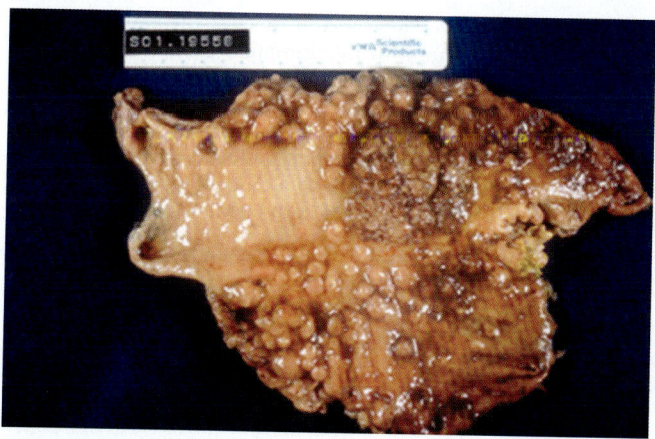

Figure 14-39. Hyperplastic polyps. Gastrectomy with a carcinoma but numerous hyperplastic polyps restricted to the oxyntic mucosa, which was also atrophic. These polyps are also too large for fundic gland polyps.

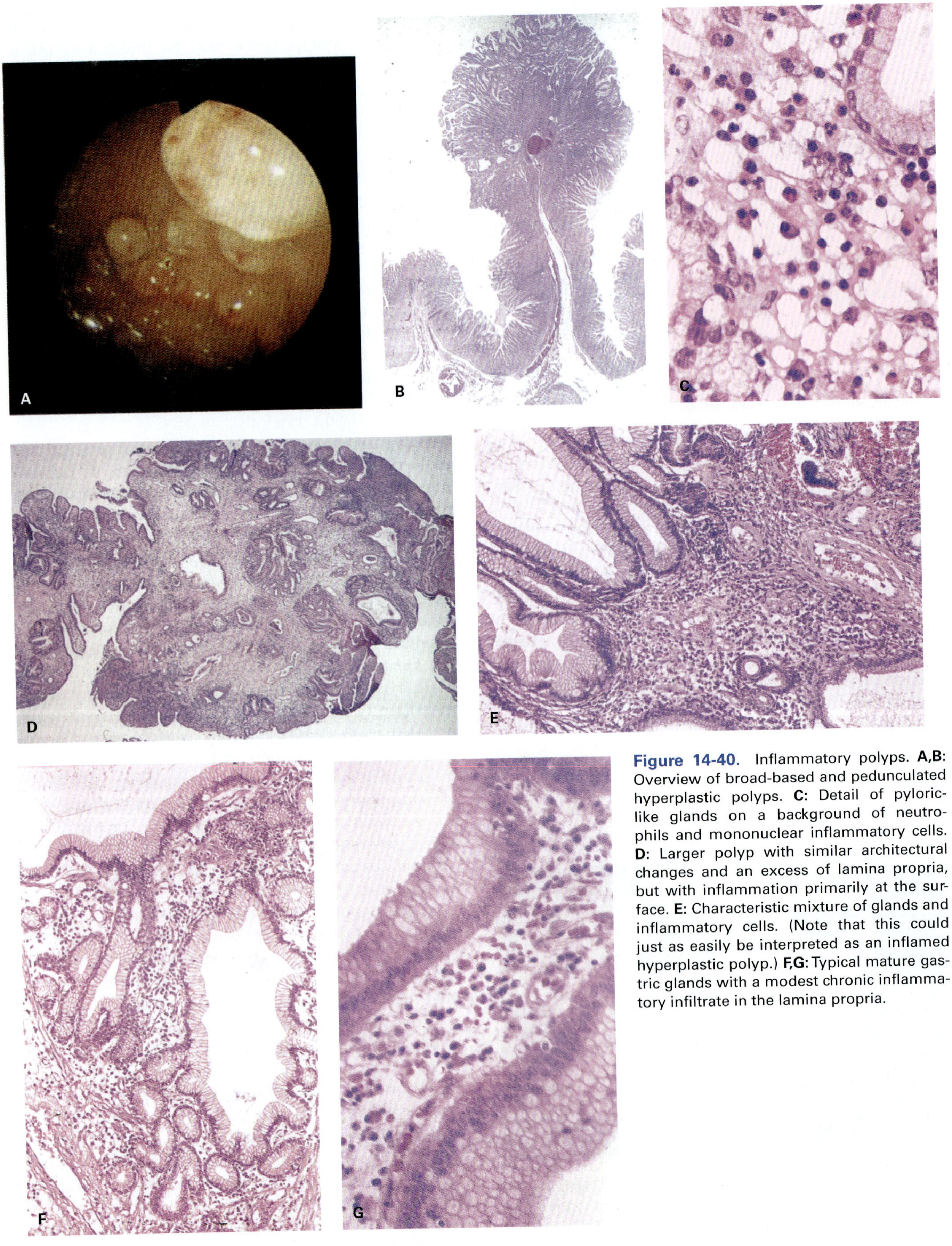

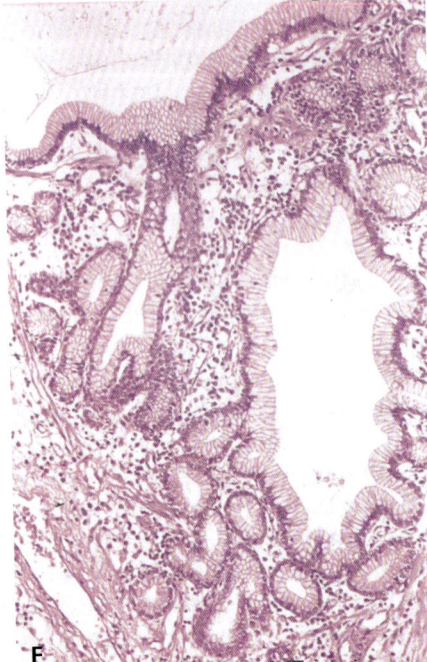
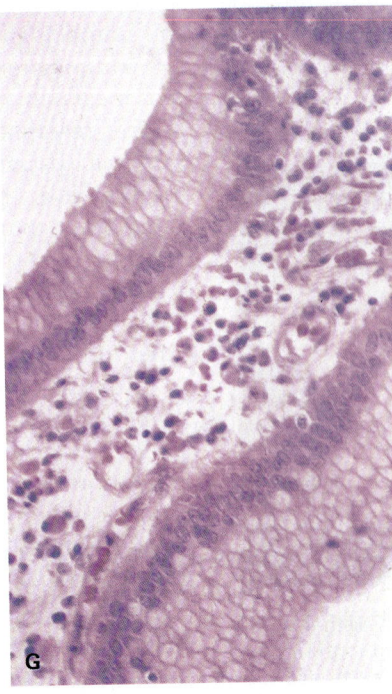

Figure 14-40. Inflammatory polyps. **A,B:** Overview of broad-based and pedunculated hyperplastic polyps. **C:** Detail of pyloric-like glands on a background of neutrophils and mononuclear inflammatory cells. **D:** Larger polyp with similar architectural changes and an excess of lamina propria, but with inflammation primarily at the surface. **E:** Characteristic mixture of glands and inflammatory cells. (Note that this could just as easily be interpreted as an inflamed hyperplastic polyp.) **F,G:** Typical mature gastric glands with a modest chronic inflammatory infiltrate in the lamina propria.

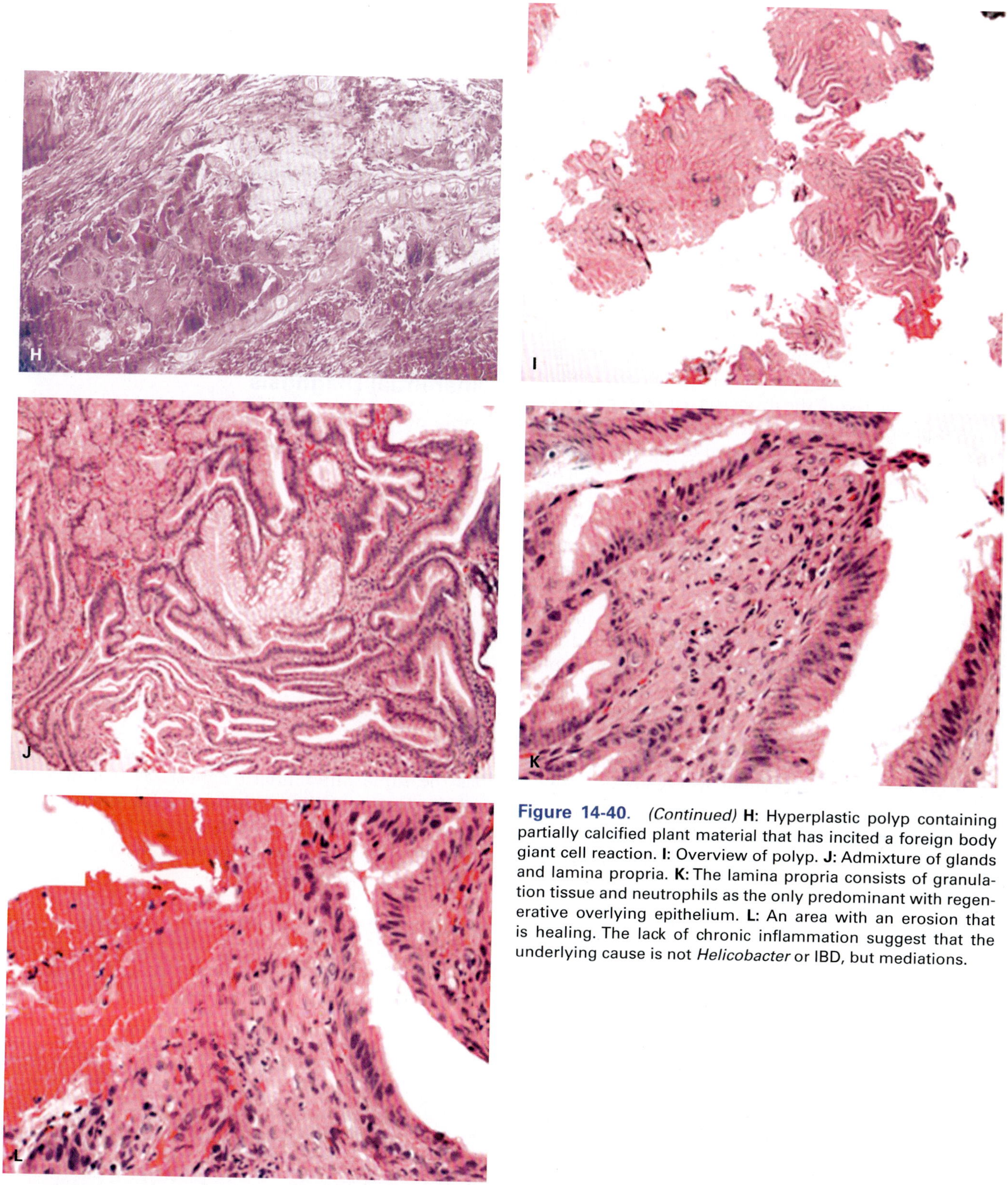

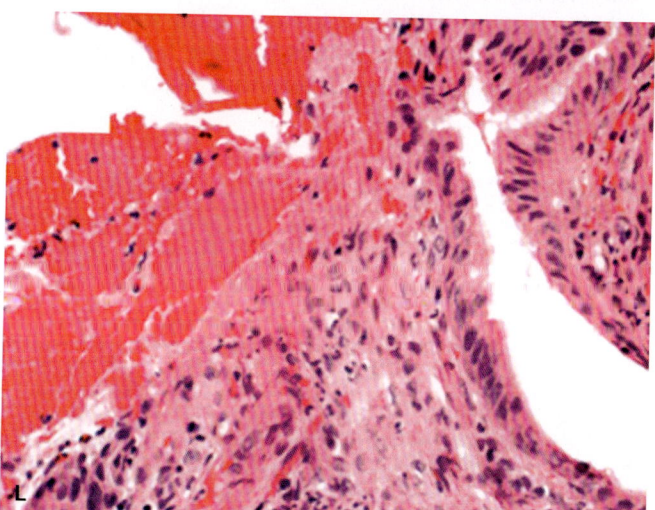

Figure 14-40. *(Continued)* **H:** Hyperplastic polyp containing partially calcified plant material that has incited a foreign body giant cell reaction. **I:** Overview of polyp. **J:** Admixture of glands and lamina propria. **K:** The lamina propria consists of granulation tissue and neutrophils as the only predominant with regenerative overlying epithelium. **L:** An area with an erosion that is healing. The lack of chronic inflammation suggest that the underlying cause is not *Helicobacter* or IBD, but mediations.

of Peutz–Jeghers polyps are usually absent, and in the rare examples in which this occurs, PJ polyps are architecturally normal, unlike inflammatory polyps in which the architecture is totally haphazard. Rarely, metaplastic bone may be present.[231]

Intestinal metaplasia is relatively common in hyperplastic polyps in both the incomplete and complete forms; it does not seem to be related to the development of carcinoma in those few polyps in which carcinoma has been encountered. Rarely, squamous morules may be present.[232]

Dysplasia/carcinoma in hyperplastic polyps.
The frequency of dysplasia and carcinoma foci in hyperplastic polyps is 0.2% to 10% for dysplasia (probably about 5%), and 0.6% to 3.7% for carcinoma, respectively.[233-238] The risk of the dysplasia/carcinoma arising in hyperplastic polyps appears to increase in polyps larger than 1 cm and is not related to the age or sex of patients, the number, location, or gross appearance of polyps.[237] Dysplasia/carcinomas are frequently located at the head or the surface of the polyps (Fig. 14-41, see also 14-33). Carcinomas arising in hyperplastic polyp are often well or moderately differentiated tubular carcinoma or papillary intramucosal carcinomas;[237,238] however, some cases of poorly differentiated and signet-ring cell carcinoma have also been reported.[239,240] Phenotypically, dysplasia/carcinoma arising in hyperplastic polyp has gastric-type mucin or mixed gastric- and intestinal-type mucin.[241] In hyperplastic polyps with neoplastic foci, dysplastic glands are usually present adjacent to adenocarcinomas and dysplasia and adenocarcinoma often show the overexpression of p53 protein and high Ki-67 index, suggesting the malignant transformation through the hyperplasia–dysplasia–carcinoma sequence in the gastric hyperplastic polyp.[238]

Clinical implications for inflammatory/hyperplastic polyps.
There are two main issues with these polyps. The first is their etiology. If the patient is *Helicobacter*-positive, then consideration should be given to eradicating them as it will likely prevent the formation of further polyps, unless the cause is not *Helicobacter* but something else such as medications and autoimmune gastritis.

The second is the neoplastic potential of these polyps. Although a degree of referral or selection bias may be involved, the figures given above are disconcerting, especially when follow-up is instituted instead of endoscopically removing them, and underlying causes are not treated. An argument can therefore be made for removing hyperplastic or inflammatory polyps.

Differential Diagnosis

Single polyps.
The lack of distinctive features, such as dysplasia or those associated with fundic gland polyps, or the known history of juvenile polyposis leaves the diagnosis firmly in the spectrum between inflammatory and hyperplastic polyps including focal foveolar hyperplasia. The distinction is arbitrary, depending on the degree of inflammation, with those in which it is marked being called inflammatory polyps and those in which it is not being considered hyperplastic polyps. A further diagnosis of focal foveolar hyperplasia can also be made when no architectural distortion is present. Some may prefer not to make these distinctions, as they are without clinical significance.

Multiple gastric polyps.
The presence of a few polyps has the same differential diagnosis as that of single polyps. However, difficulties can arise when part or all of the stomach has polyps that are large and multiple or numerous; the differential diagnosis is that

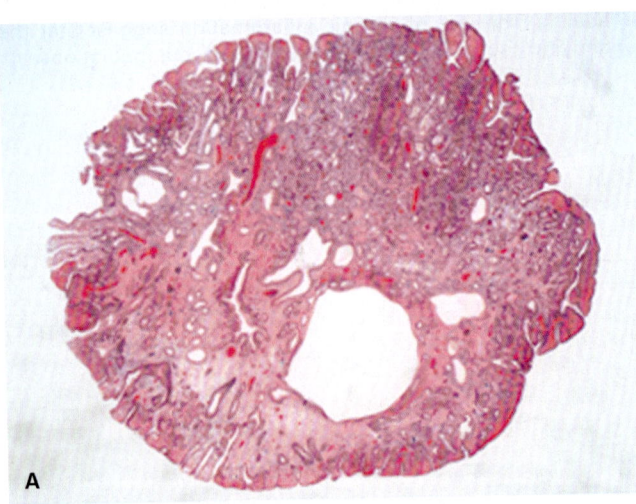
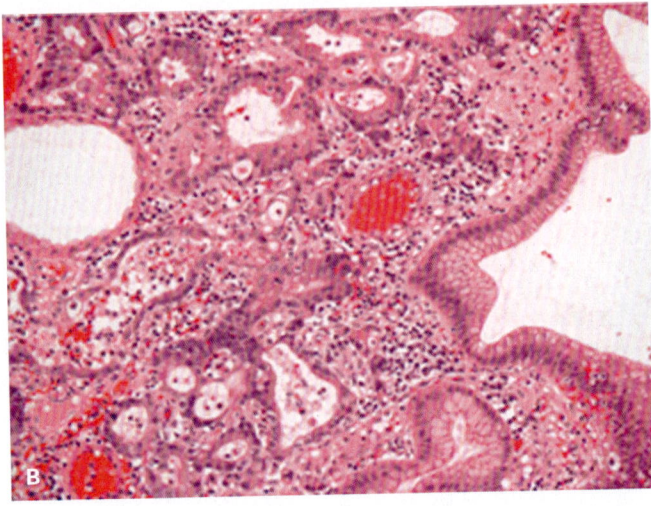

Figure 14-41. Carcinoma in hyperplastic polyp with intramucosal carcinoma at the head of the polyp. Overview **(A)** and detail **(B)**. Notice that the luminal mucosa (right) is normal, but the architectural complexity of the neoplastic component to its left is apparent.

of Menetrier's disease, Cronkhite–Canada syndrome, and juvenile polyposis. The latter two types can usually be distinguished from Menetrier's disease by their smaller size and the presence of intervening normal mucosa as well as a history of juvenile polyposis. However, we have seen examples of hyperplastic polyposis with numerous large polyps and erosions presenting as a protein-losing enteropathy, thereby mimicking both juvenile polyposis and Menetrier's disease clinically.

The distinction from juvenile polyposis rests on the demonstration of juvenile polyposis in the large bowel, although rare examples of isolated gastric involvement have been recognized and genetic testing may help (see Chapter 20). The differentiation from Cronkhite–Canada syndrome may be difficult morphologically, but the disease is clinically very distinct and invariably involves the GI tract diffusely; typical ectodermal features may also be present.

Juvenile Polyps

Gastric juvenile polyps occur either as a part of a generalized juvenile polyposis syndrome[242,243] or as a part of gastric familial juvenile polyposis (Fig. 14-42).[244] Juvenile polyposis syndrome is a dominantly inherited disorder characterized by predisposition for juvenile polyps in which affected individuals develop upper or lower GI polyps, or both, and have a predisposition to cancer of the GI tract.[242,243] Juvenile polyps develop from infancy through adulthood and most individuals with juvenile polyposis syndrome have some polyps by age 20.[245] Gastric polyps affect the antrum and extend to the fundus, eventually becoming more numerous, larger, and more pedunculated.[246]

In patients with juvenile polyposis syndrome, the incidence of colorectal cancer is 17% to 22% by age 35 years and approaches 68% by age 60 years, while the incidence of gastric cancer is 21% in those with gastric polyps.[247] It is also noteworthy that adenoma or adenocarcinoma can be found in these polyps.[246,248] It is therefore reasonable to suggest that patients with juvenile polyposis should undergo periodic upper as well as lower endoscopy with a view to removing these polyps (see Chapter 21).

Germline mutations in BMPR1A/ALK3[249,250] and SMAD4/DPC4,[239] which are involved in the TGF-B signaling pathway, have each been identified in 20% of patients with juvenile polyposis syndrome, but those with the mutations seem most prone toward gastric polyps and therefore dysplasia and carcinoma arising in them.[249,250] Some patients also have HHT, a condition that appears to have a mutation in the SMAD4 gene identical to that seen in juvenile polyposis syndrome; so it is not surprising that they coexist, and perhaps only surprising that this relationship was not found much sooner.[251]

Pathology. Juvenile polyps are histologically indistinguishable from hyperplastic polyps (Fig. 14-42), from which they can be separated only by a history of juvenile polyposis, with typical polyps in the large bowel and sometimes other congenital anomalies (see also Chapter 20). It is said that those with associated HHT have thickened and more prominent vessels, but we are unconvinced.

Peutz–Jeghers Polyps

Peutz–Jeghers syndrome is characterized by the association of GI hamartomatous polyposis and mucocutaneous pigmentation (see Chapter 20 for more details). Peutz–Jeghers polyps are most prevalent in the small intestine, but also occur in the stomach and large bowel in the majority of affected individuals. Gastric polyps occur in 25% to 50% of patients with this syndrome,[252] but they may also occur sporadically.[253] For details of the genetics see Chapter 20.

A meta-analysis of Peutz–Jeghers syndrome showed that GI cancers showed a statistically significant excess in this syndrome in the stomach (the relative risk, RR, of cancer in patients with Peutz–Jeghers syndrome compared with the general population: of 213), small intestine (RR = 520), and colon (RR = 84).[90] However, the origin of cancers in patients with Peutz–Jeghers syndrome is still disputed. Some reported the hamartoma–adenoma–carcinoma sequence in the stomach, small intestine, and colorectal polyps,[254–261] or the hamartoma–carcinoma sequence.[262]

Peutz–Jeghers polyps are usually small and commonly pedunculated rather than sessile polyps with a villiform surface (classical type) or smooth surface. They may grow to a large size and ulcerate or bleed. While they may develop at any site in the stomach, they may preferentially affect the antrum; however, gastric outlet obstruction is rare.

Pathology. Classical gastric Peutz–Jeghers polyps are identical to their counterparts elsewhere in the GI tract, an arborizing framework of smooth muscle extending from the muscularis mucosae into lamina propria, which is covered with fundic or antral-type mucosa (Fig. 14-43). However, they can be very difficult to diagnose when small, as the smooth muscle component is not an early feature, so small P–J polyps can resemble hyperplastic polyps. Other features can include foveolar hyperplasia with cystic change, lamina propria edema, congestion, and inflammation with relatively inconspicuous smooth muscle. Unlike gastric mucosa with hyperplastic polyps in which the background mucosa often has either H. pylori or reactive gastropathy, the interpolypoid gastric mucosa in PJS is usually normal. Complications include dysplasia (Fig. 14-43B–D), carcinoma, and misplaced glands that

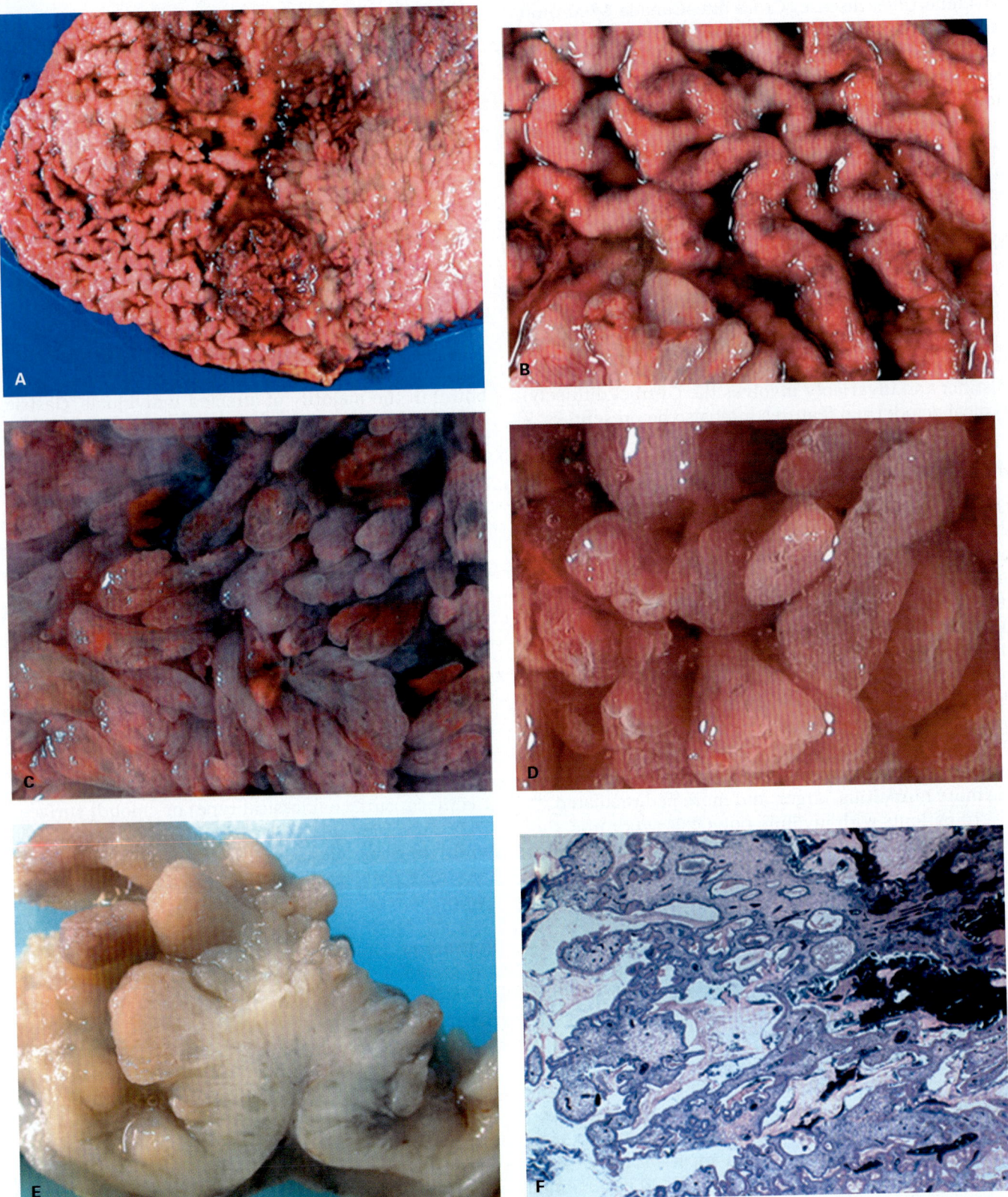

Figure 14-42. Gastric juvenile polyposis. **A–D:** Resected specimen from a patient with SMAD4 mutation revealing diffuse polyps throughout the entire stomach. It is impossible to distinguish them from hyperplastic polyps but interpret them as juvenile polyps in patients with juvenile polyposis of the large bowel or known mutation. **E:** Section through a larger fixed polyp showing the "retention" cysts. **F:** Overview showing typical admixture of glands and lamina propria.

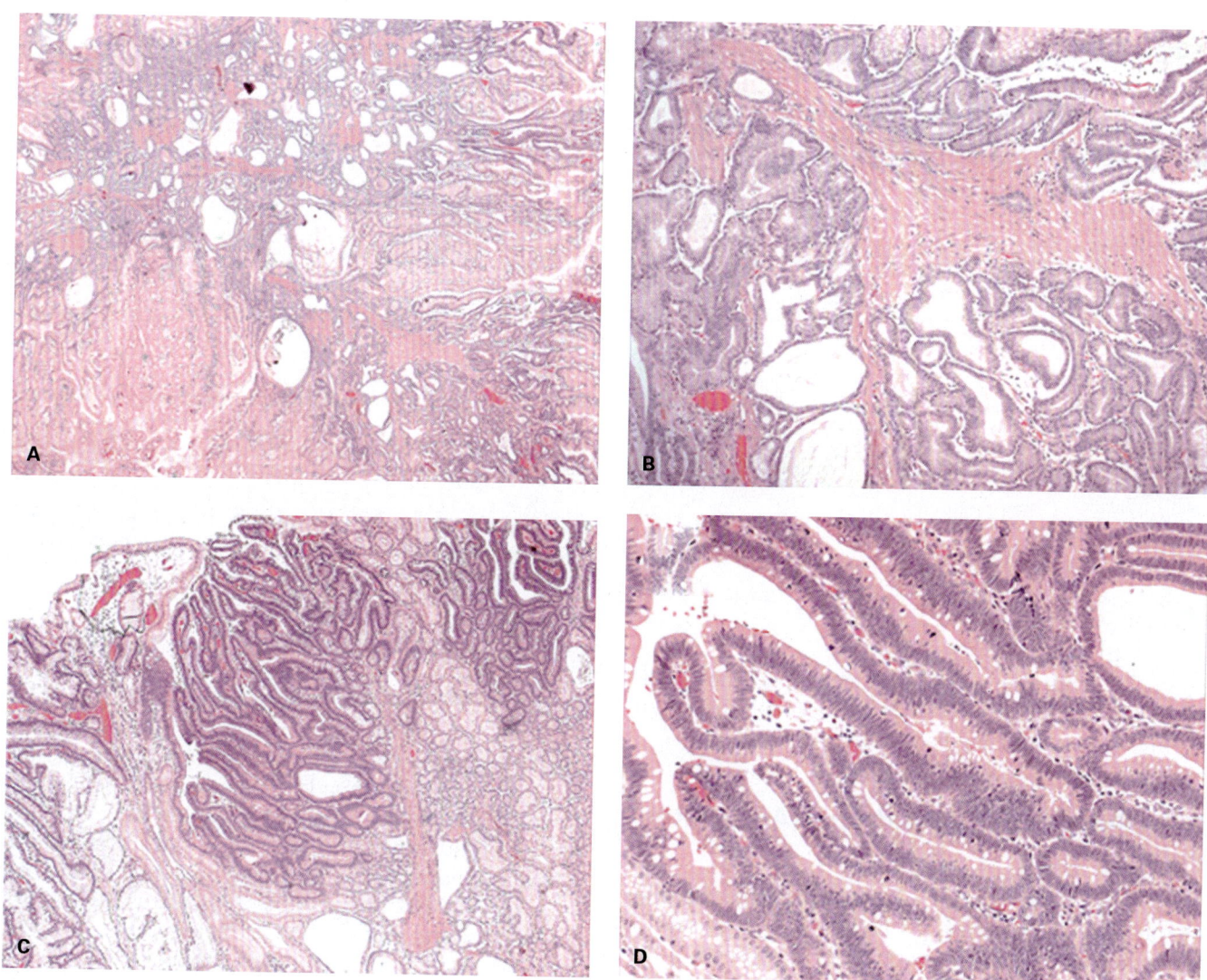

Figure 14-43. Peutz-Jeghers syndrome gastric polyps. **A:** PJ polyp showing the typical arborizing muscular framework. **B–D:** Dysplasia in gastric PJ polyp.

can go into the submucosa and even muscularis propria (see also Chapter 20). Fortunately, these are rarely dysplastic as the diagnosis between invasion depends on a combination of the dysplasia, invasive pattern, and desmoplasia if present. Even if minimally dysplastic they have no metastasizing potential.

PTEN Hamartoma Tumor Syndrome

The *PTEN* hamartoma tumor syndrome, which is caused by germline mutations of the *PTEN* tumor suppressor gene, unifies the heterogeneous group of disorders including Cowden's syndrome (CS), Bannayan–Riley–Ruvalcaba syndrome (BRRS), Proteus syndrome (PS), and Proteus-like syndrome (see Chapter 20 for more details).

CS is a multiple hamartoma syndrome with a high risk of benign and malignant tumors of the breast, thyroid, and endometrium. Other characteristic features of CS are mucocutaneous manifestations, macroencephaly, and GI lesions (hamartomatous polyps and esophageal glycogenic acanthosis). The diagnosis guideline for CS is updated annually by the National Comprehensive Cancer Network (http://www.nccn.org). Most gastric polyps are histologically similar to sporadic hyperplastic polyps (Fig. 14-44).[263]

Familiar Gastric Hyperplastic Polyposis

In patients of familiar gastric hyperplastic polyposis, more than 50 genetically acquired gastric hyperplastic polyps are found[264–266] and this is in association with GI neoplasia (gastric carcinoma,[265] colorectal adenoma, and carcinomas[266,267]) and cutaneous psoriasis.[264,265] Autosomal dominant inheritance of this syndrome was reported.[264,265] Since these cases were reported prior to wide availability of genetic testing for *SMAD4* mutation it is unclear if they are separate from juvenile

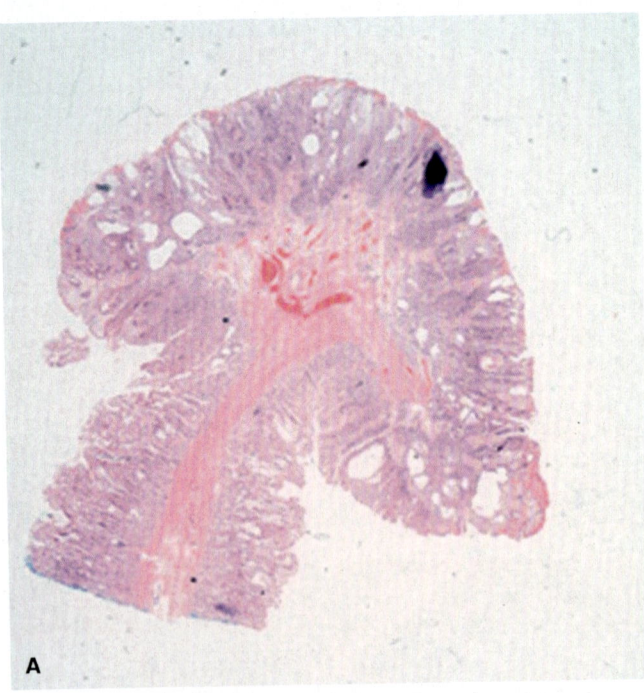
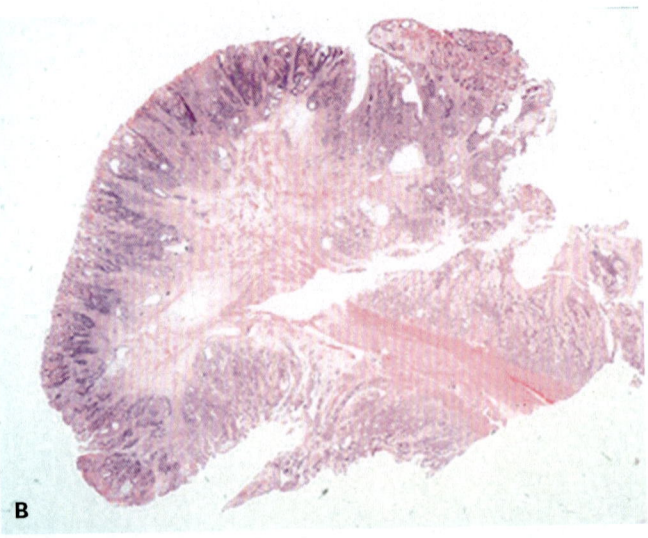
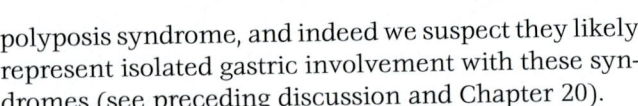

Figure 14-44. Cowden's syndrome. **A:** Oxyntic mucosa with a polyp virtually indistinguishable from a hyperplastic polyp. **B:** Adjacent polyp with overt dysplasia.

polyposis syndrome, and indeed we suspect they likely represent isolated gastric involvement with these syndromes (see preceding discussion and Chapter 20).

Cronkhite–Canada Syndrome–Associated Polyps

This rare syndrome is a nonhereditary disorder characterized by diffuse GI polyposis that is said to be hamartomatous, but more likely represents a diffuse inflammatory process (see also Chapter 20). It is characterized clinically by a severe protein-losing enteropathy causing hypoalbuminemia, by wasting, alopecia, hyperpigmentation, and characteristic nail changes; it presents in middle adulthood and has a slight male predominance.[268,269]

There is marked polypoid thickening of the mucosa of the entire GI tract. The gastric disease may resemble a carpet of juvenile polyps; indeed, they are often indistinguishable.[269] Gastric Cronkhite–Canada polyps are sessile and superimposed on the enlarged gastric fold. Unlike Menetriér's disease, the entire stomach (and usually the entire intestinal tract) is affected and the entire mucosa may be thickened (Fig. 14-45A). Typical ectodermal changes are usually present (alopecia, onychogryphosis, and hyperpigmentation). Occasional instances of gastric carcinoma supervening have been reported.[268,269]

Pathology. CCS is characterized by foveolar hyperplasia with corkscrewed or cystic change, an excess of edematous lamina propria with an inflammatory infiltrate both in the polypoid and interpolypoid mucosa (Fig. 14-45C,D).[269,270] The specialized cells of the gastric body and fundus virtually disappear, and the cysts are lined by tail mucus-producing columnar epithelium. Surface erosions may also be present. Histologic features of Cronkhite–Canada polyps, juvenile polyps, and hyperplastic polyps show considerable overlap. They are often indistinguishable, except that in Cronkhite–Canada syndrome the interpolypoid mucosa is also involved.[270,271] Extension of polyps diffusely into the duodenum and rest of the GI tract distinguishes CCS from other syndromes (see also Chapter 20).

Polypoid Gastritis

It should be remembered that simple gastritis, as well as eosinophilic infiltration, can sometimes cause a distinctly polypoid appearance to the mucosa (see Chapter 13). In severe gastritis, the body mucosa may be studded with tiny little hyperplastic polyps that many times obscure the background atrophy in the intervening mucosa.

Gastric Xanthomas (Xanthelasmas, Lipid Islands)

These are relatively common small white to yellow lesions or excrescences seen in up to 60% of residual stomachs of patients who have undergone partial gastrectomy. The incidence increases with time, and is usually at least 5 years earlier,[272] when they are usually found at the stoma. In the unoperated stomach they have been found in up to 6% of patients. They are usually antral and at the lesser curve, but

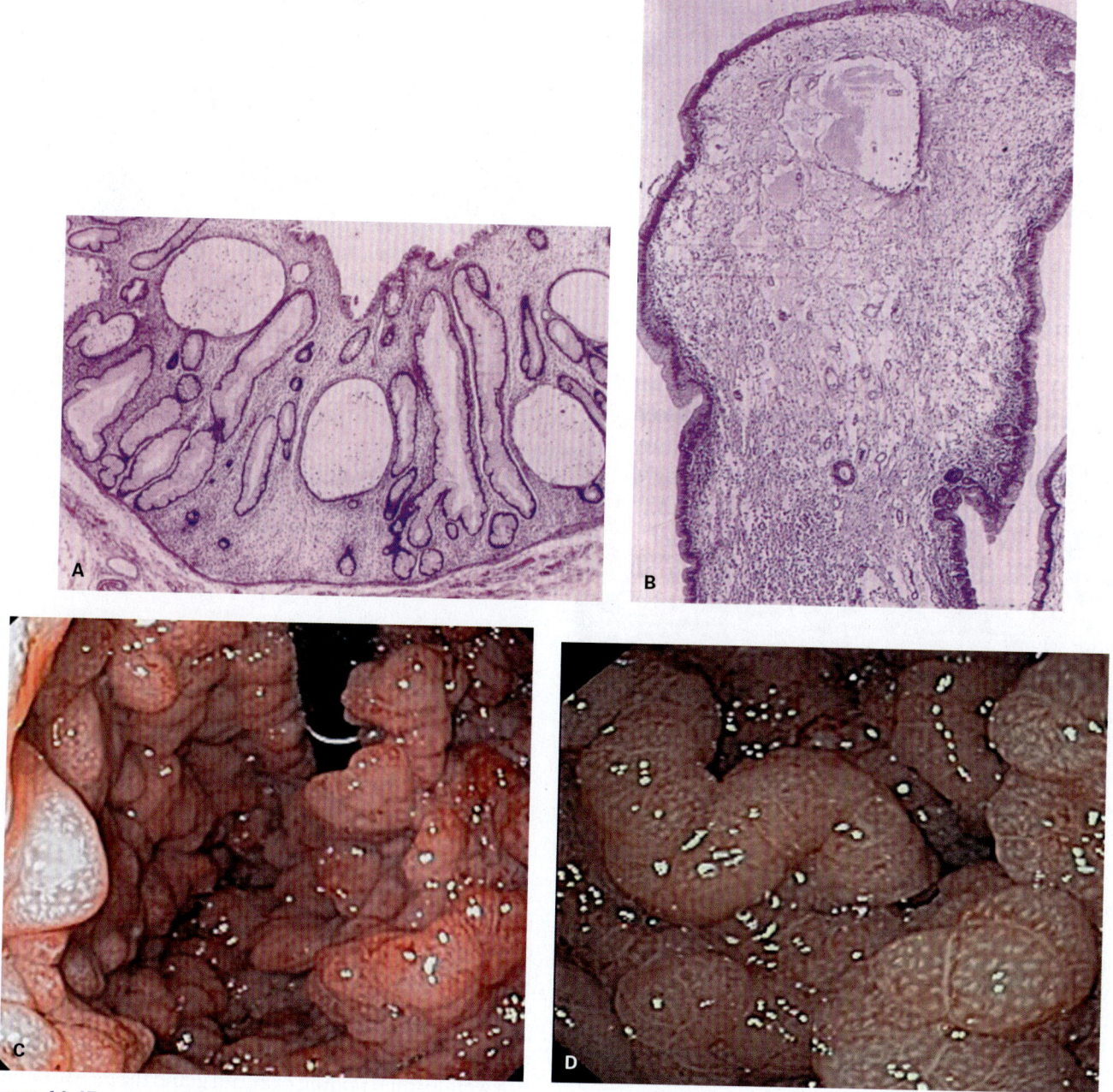

Figure 14-45. Cronkhite–Canada syndrome. **A,B:** Gastric mucosa with no specialized or pyloric glands, cystically dilated pits with overt architectural distortion and an edematous lamina propria. **C,D:** Endoscopic appearances. The stomach is diffusely involved—changes that extended diffusely throughout the GI tract. (Courtesy Dr. Sandra Nelles, Mississauga, Ontario.)

occasionally body or fundic in position, and may be multiple. They are sometimes associated with *H. pylori*–infected chronic active gastritis.[273] They are unrelated to systemic diseases characterized by hyperlipoproteinemia or hypercholesterolemia, or to other diseases characterized by an excess of macrophages in the lamina propria, but are likely related to bile reflux into the stomach. More recently, dyslipidemia (lower HDL–cholesterol and higher LDL–cholesterol) and atrophic gastritis are found to be related to gastric xanthoma, but *H. pylori* infection is not.[272]

Pathology. They consist of numerous foamy macrophages that virtually replace the lamina propria, particularly its upper half (Fig. 14-46). The nuclei are small and central. The major differential diagnosis is signet-ring carcinoma, which is strongly diastase-PAS and often, but not always, mucicarmine- and keratin-positive. Lipid islands can be stained with Sudan black, oil red O, and some histiocytic markers but do not contain mucin. Rod-shaped bacteria positive with anti–*H. pylori* antibody was reported in the phagosome of the xanthoma cells.[273] Rarely,

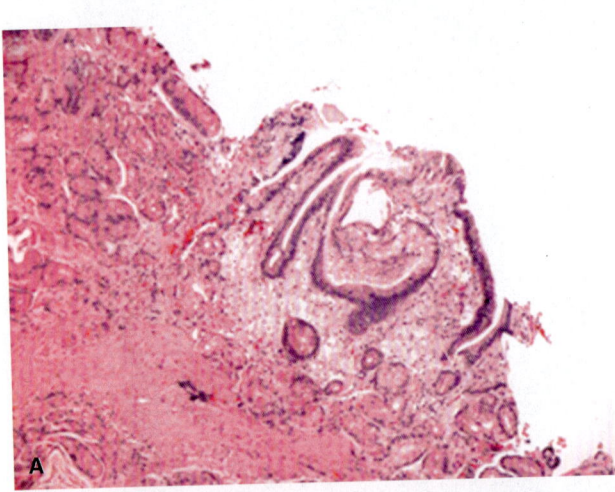
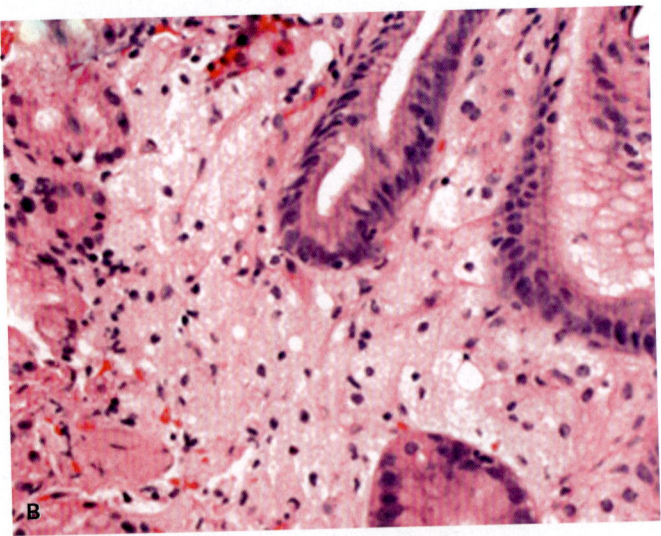
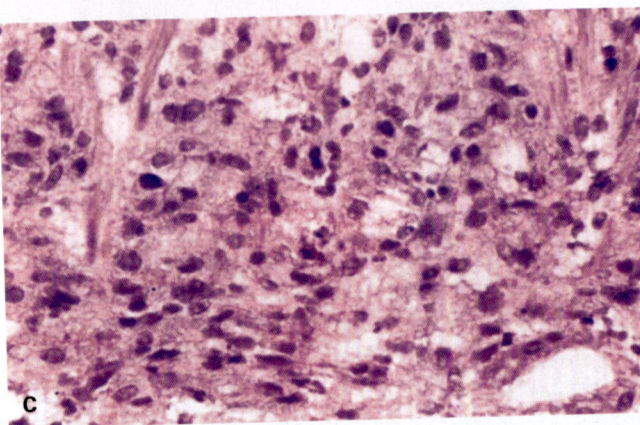

Figure 14-46. Gastric xanthoma (xanthelasma, lipid island). **A,B:** Numerous large, pale-staining, and faintly vacuolated macrophages are present in the lamina propria. **B:** PAS stain shows lack of mucin. **C:** Bland-appearing histocyte-like gastric carcinoma for contrast.

they may need to be distinguished from granular cell tumors, Langerhans histiocytosis (histiocytosis X), or malacoplakia. Immunohistochemistry for cytokeratins (negative) and CD68 (immunoreactive) are the easiest way of distinguishing carcinoma and histiocytes.

Mucosal Bumps and Nodules

It is not uncommon for a mucosal bump or nodule to be visualized endoscopically and biopsied, only for the pathology report to come back as "normal mucosa" or a similar comment. This may be caused by the following:

1. Sampling error during endoscopy.
2. The focal presence of a lesion in the material submitted but not on the actual slide(s) examined (either the technologist cut through it or it is still in the block).
3. A submucosal lesion.
4. Irregular but normal gastric mucosa producing small bumps or nodules.

The last is often seen easily in resected stomachs, particularly when they have been pinned out and fixed overnight, a process that tends to accentuate mucosal irregularities. In the gastric body, the mucosa appears absolutely normal microscopically; in the antrum, the appearance may be that of otherwise unremarkable antral tissue, but sometimes the entire nodule consists of a well-formed nodule of antral gland tissue. We believe these appearances to be a variant of normal rather than an adenoma or hamartoma. They are sometimes associated with antral gastritis. Inflamed mucosa may similarly be polypoid (see Chapter 13), but it is unclear whether the bump preceded or accompanied the inflammation or whether it might resolve with the inflammation. If there is a real increase in mucosal thickness, focal foveolar hyperplasia is the likely diagnosis. The possibility of a submucosal lesion causing the bump is usually implied if biopsy of the bump reveals normal mucosa.

Rebiopsy is rarely necessary for small lesions unless there is a high degree of suspicion that a clinically significant lesion is present, such as a tumor that may directly affect patient management.

Solitary Polypoid Hamartoma (Gastric Hamartoma with Myxoid Stroma, Hamartomatous Inverted Polyp, Heterotopic Inverted Polyp)

This lesion occurs preferentially in the fundic mucosa as a pedunculated polyp mimicking a submucosal tumor (Fig. 14-47A).[274,275] They are considered to be acquired as they occur in older adults (mean age, 59 years) and represent the inverted growth of gastric mucosa through breaks in the muscularis mucosae into submucosa (heterotopic inverted polyp), but are thought not to be hamartomatous in nature.[274,275]

Pathology. There is overlying gastric mucosa and a submucosal mass of lobulated mucosa of similar gastric type. Each lobule has a centrally located lumen and is surrounded by smooth muscle (Fig. 14-47B,C).[274,275] The submucosal glands may contain cysts or mucous glands resembling cardiac or pyloric glands.[264] However, parietal cells can also be found (Fig. 14-47G). The stroma can sometimes be myxoid (Fig. 14-47D–F).

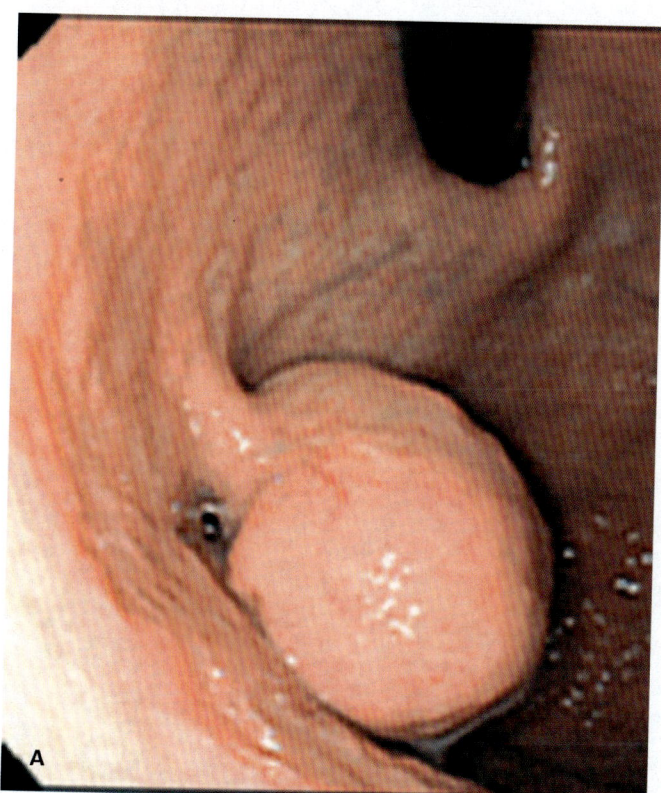
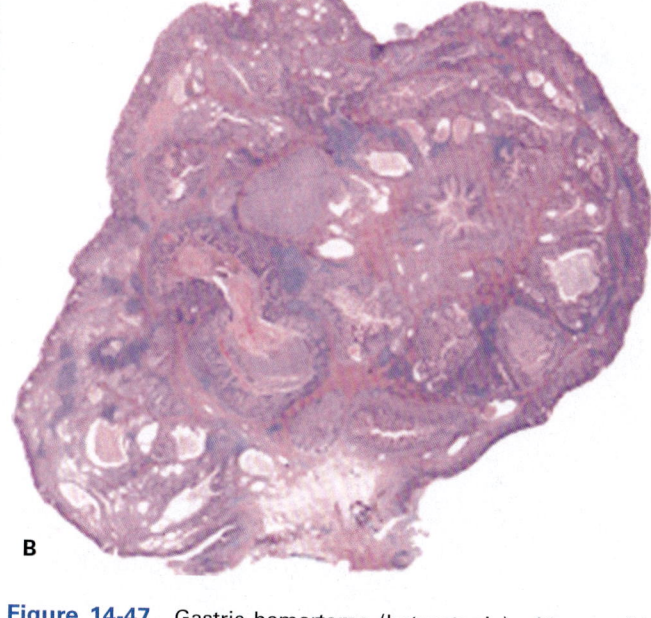
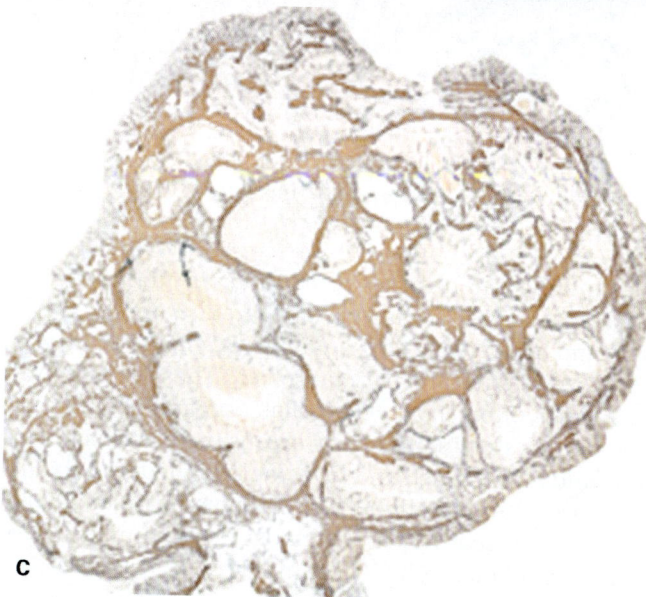

Figure 14-47. Gastric hamartoma (heterotopia) with myxoid stroma. **A:** Endoscopic appearance with a pedunculated polyp. (Courtesy H. Yokozawa, MD, Shinshu University, Japan.) **B:** Polyp consisting of the overlying gastric mucosa and a submucosal mass with centrally located lumen. **C:** αSMA staining showing that polyp is lobulated by smooth muscle bundles.

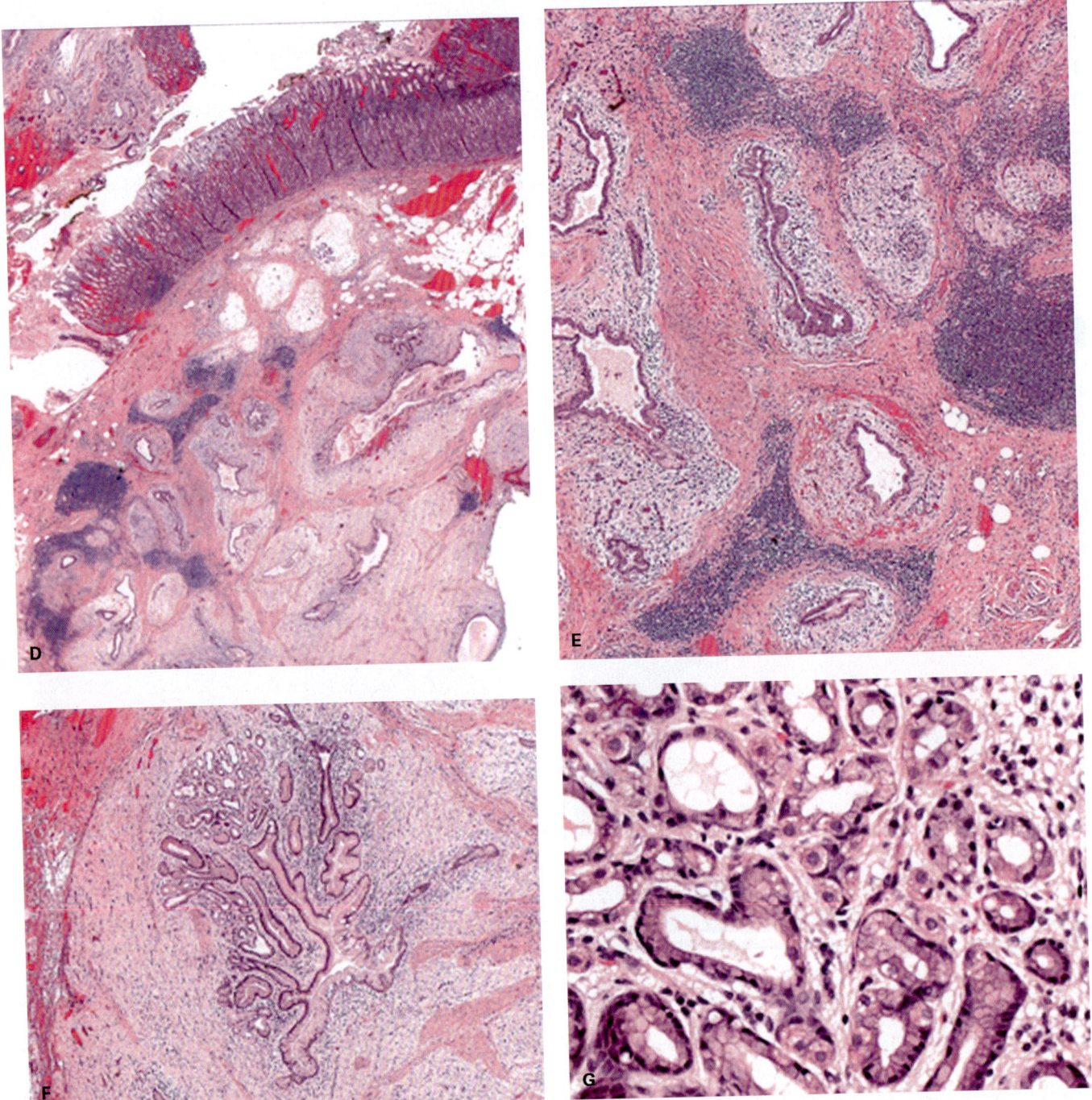

Figure 14-47. *(Continued)* **D–F:** Detail showing inverted fundic mucosa with a myxoid stroma. **G:** Detail shows mature parietal, chief, and mucous-producing cells.

Gastritis Cystica Polyposa (Gastric Stomal Polypoid Hyperplasia, Gastric Stomal Polypoid Hypertrophic Gastritis)

Gastritis cystica polyposa appear as sessile polypoid lesions, either multiple or confluent, on the gastric side of gastroenteric anastomoses along the line of anastomoses, especially near the greater curvature (Fig. 14-48).[276] Bile reflux[276,277] and prolapse of mucosa through the stoma[278] are involved in their pathogenesis.

Pathology. The distinctive features are the elongated foveolae with a corkscrew appearance of the gastric pits and hyperplasia of pseudopyloric glands along with decrease of chief and parietal cells.[276] These pseudopyloric glands often show cystic dilatation and occasionally these cysts show submucosal extension (gastritis cystica profunda).[279] Surface and foveolae are lined by cuboidal or short columnar epithelial cells showing mucin depletion and nuclear hyperchromatism with similar regenerative epithelial cells. The lamina propria is somewhat

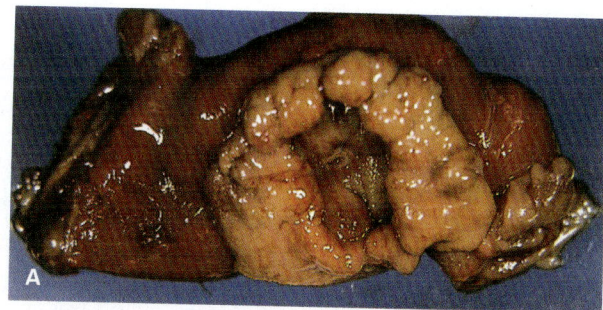
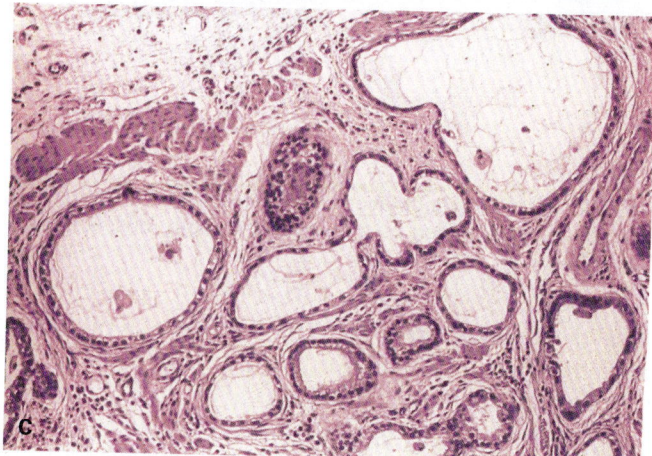
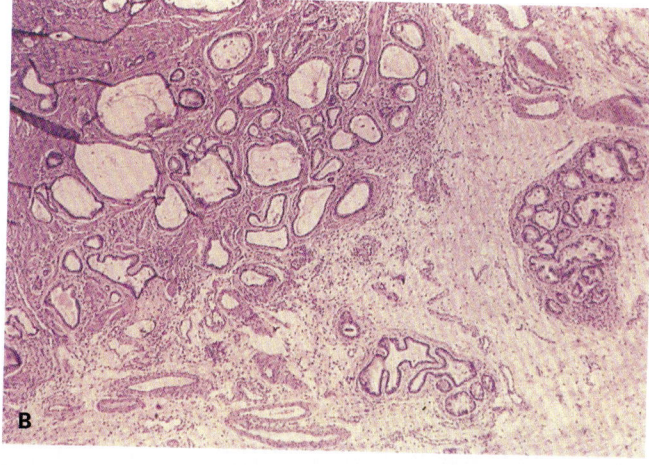

Figure 14-48. Gastritis cystica polyposa. **A:** Gastroenterostomy site in which, apart from an anastomotic ulcer in the jejunum, the gastric side is multinodular. **B,C:** The nodules consist of inflammatory polyps with dilated glands, inflammatory cells, often admixed with muscle, presumably representing prolapse changes. It is in these lesions that neoplastic changed can occur.

broadened and slightly edematous with mild to moderate degree of inflammatory infiltrates. Thin bundles of smooth muscle originate from muscularis mucosae and extend toward the mucosal surface (Fig. 14-48B,C). A gradual morphologic transition is observed between the protuberant lesions and the surrounding mucosa.

Mucosal and Submucosal Cysts

Cystic dilatation of gastric glands These cysts are usually incidental findings in resections and are virtually never large enough to be visible endoscopically, although they may be the only change visible in an endoscopic "bump."

Cystic dilatation of glands is very common in the stomach, especially the cardia, and seems to occur under a variety of conditions. Terms such as *gastritis cystica superficialis* are now outmoded and may be misleading because inflammation is not always a component of these lesions; if a term is required, *cystic dilatation* (or *intramucosal cysts*) is preferred. Cysts appear to form when the outlet of the gland is obstructed leading to secondary atrophic changes in the epithelium lining some of these cysts. Cysts may occur as isolated findings when they appear to be of no significance, but they seem to occur with increased frequency particularly in the background mucosa of a variety of gastric lesions: adenoma, adenocarcinoma, or peptic ulcer.[280] In the last, they are presumably the result of chronic inflammation with atrophy and distortion of glands.[280] Interestingly, ciliated metaplasia can be found in some of these dilated antral glands in up to 40% of patients with cysts accompanying plaque-like areas of dysplasia (*borderline lesion*).[281] Cysts are also part of a variety of polypoid lesions in the stomach, particularly in fundic gland polyps and hyperplastic polyps, but also in the much less common juvenile polyps, Menetriér's disease, and the Cronkhite–Canada syndrome.

Gastritis Cystica Profunda

In gastritis cystica profunda, gastric glands are displaced into the submucosa and they form submucosal cysts, resembling the features of colitis cystica profunda. They were found in 10.7% of 1,500 resected stomachs under several different circumstances: 15% in gastric ulcer, 9.9% in gastric carcinoma, 4% in duodenal ulcer, and 11% in chronic gastritis,[282] and they occur particularly immediately proximal to gastroenterostomy anastomosis lines.[268,279] Macroscopically, they may present as a submucosal tumor. They can be congenital or acquired (i.e., epithelial components enter the submucosal layer as a result of reactive proliferation) in nature. The latter is supported by that they occur in middle-aged and elderly individuals, and that *H. pylori* infection has been shown to induce the inverted growth of gastric mucosa into submucosa in Mongolian gerbils.[283]

Pathology. In the submucosa, irregularly dilated cysts arising from displaced gastric glands that are often pyloric or cardiac type are present, surrounded

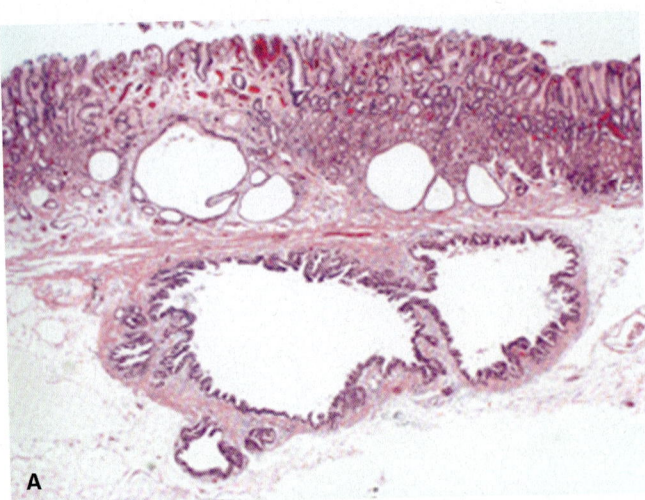 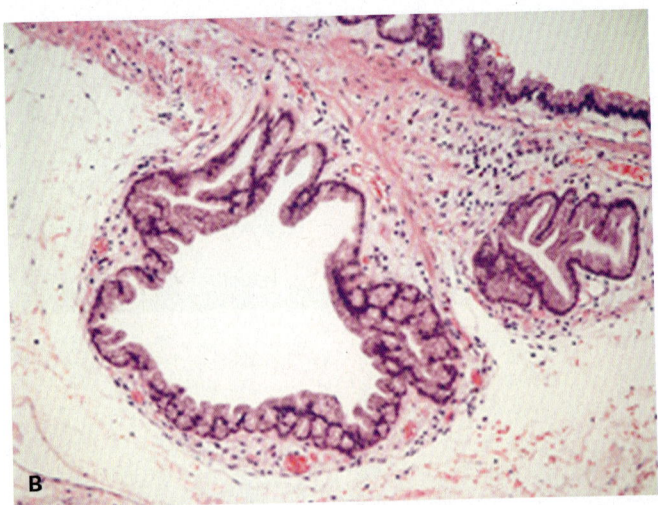

Figure 14-49. Gastritis cystica profunda. **A:** Cysts are noted from the mucosa to the submucosa. **B:** Dilated submucosal glands surrounded by lamina propria-like stroma and the displaced gastric mucosa is surrounded by a bundle of smooth muscle but no duplication of the muscularis mucosae or fibrosis to suggest prior inflammation.

by lamina propria–like stroma (Fig. 14-49). The displaced gastric mucosa is rimmed by bundles of smooth muscle extending from the muscularis mucosae. Over the heterotopic glands, the muscularis mucosae were irregularly thickened and gastric mucosa occasionally appears to connect with the submucosal displaced mucosa through interrupted parts of the muscularis mucosae.

Differential Diagnosis. Potential confusion between gastric cystica profunda lesions and invasive carcinoma exists in both directions. Lesions previously described as superficial gastric carcinoma with submucosal cysts are much more likely to represent relative maturation of the deeper portion of an adenocarcinoma than gastric cystica profunda, but this differential diagnosis depends on the demonstration of direct continuity between overlying carcinoma and underlying cysts and the presence of dysplasia, however mild, in the submucosal cysts. Occasionally, the submucosal tissue is mature by all criteria despite the presence of overlying carcinoma.[284] Under these circumstances, while we generally prefer not to use the term *superficial carcinoma with submucosal cysts* because it is entirely descriptive and avoids an interpretation, there are rare occasions where it may be appropriate.

Minimal deviation carcinomas (very well-differentiated carcinoma as described previously), while relatively rare, can also cause real problems. These are infiltrating carcinomas that are very well differentiated, with good gland formation and very little nuclear pleomorphism but with a clearly infiltrative pattern that may be apparent by destruction of the muscularis propria and sometimes an infiltrating edge with smaller irregular glands, although few of these may be present. Occasional glands may have a focal desmoplastic reaction. Uncommonly, lymphatic, perineural, or capillary infiltration may be present. Cytologically, the nuclei may have so little dysplasia that careful comparison of adjacent nuclei is necessary to notice their changing polarity or variation in chromatin content from cell to cell. Thus, they clearly behave like a carcinoma but lack most of the characteristic nuclear morphologic features. These are described and illustrated previously. Unless the muscularis propria is infiltrated, the distinction between carcinoma and gastric cystica profunda is almost completely subjective and, fortunately, is of virtually no significance to the patient. In these instances there is little doubt about the morphologic features, but opposing views regarding the interpretation occur. Because in most of these instances tumor is limited to the submucosa or superficial muscularis propria, the prognosis is good and metastases have not yet been convincingly demonstrated.

Heterotopic Pancreas (Ectopic Pancreas, Pancreatic Rests, Adenomyoma, Adenomyomatous Hamartoma, Myoglandular Hamartoma, Myoepithelial Hamartoma)

These lesions occur at all ages and have been reported in the literature under a variety of names, but are uncommon. They are usually found on the greater curve of the antrum, although they may be located within a few centimeters of either side of the gastroduodenal junction.[285] They are thought to arise during rotation of the foregut when fragments of pancreas become separated. They appear as submucosal tumors endoscopically, forming a dome-shaped mass protruding into the antrum; they may be several centimeters or larger in size and sometimes have central umbilication through which secretions drain. Most are incidental findings, but some are large enough to cause gastric outlet obstruction. Although most diseases of the pancreas can occur in these polyps, they are very uncommon; for example, carcinoma is rare.[286,287] Some ulcerate and bleed, and they may rarely cause obstructive jaundice. Occasionally they occur high in the oxyntic mucosa, and have central umbilication. They are invariably interpreted as gastrointestinal stromal tumors (GISTs), mucosal biopsies generally are unhelpful, but sometimes fine-needle aspiration can provide the diagnosis. Although benign, they often end up being resected for a variety of reasons (Fig. 14-50). They can contain all elements of the pancreas, and besides acute pancreatitis, a whole range of pancreatic tumors have been described in these lesions. The vast majority of the time these lesions are clinically irrelevant.

Pathology. They consist of a mixture of tissues that may be found in the pancreas, but usually consist primarily of ducts and surrounding simple mucin-producing glands, often admixed with thick bundles of smooth muscle. The ducts are lined by tall columnar epithelium that is usually mucin-producing but occasionally consists of absorptive type cells and occasionally squamous metaplasia. Pancreatic parenchyma that usually includes islets of Langerhans can be found in about a third of these cases.[288] Adenomyoma is a condition similar to heterotopic pancreas but they are composed of smooth muscle, cysts, and pancreatico-biliary-type ducts, Brunner's glands, and sometimes pancreatic tissue.[289]

Differential Diagnosis. The major problem with these tumors occurs if a frozen section is requested, when a mixture of ducts or simple glands and muscles may be readily misinterpreted as well-differentiated invasive carcinoma. The combination of bland cytology, and awareness of these lesions and their morphology is a prerequisite for avoiding this trap.

These tumors can rarely develop features of acute pancreatitis or malignancy (see above).

Brunner Gland Heterotopia/Nodule

The most frequently affected site with this lesion in the stomach is the prepyloric antrum.

Histologically, this forms a submucosal (and rarely mucosal) (Fig. 14-51) mass resembling Brunner

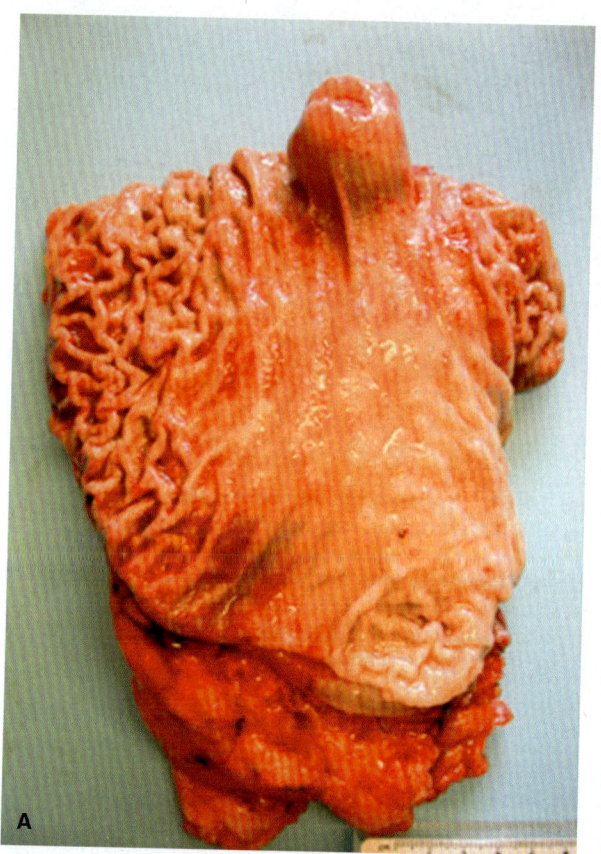
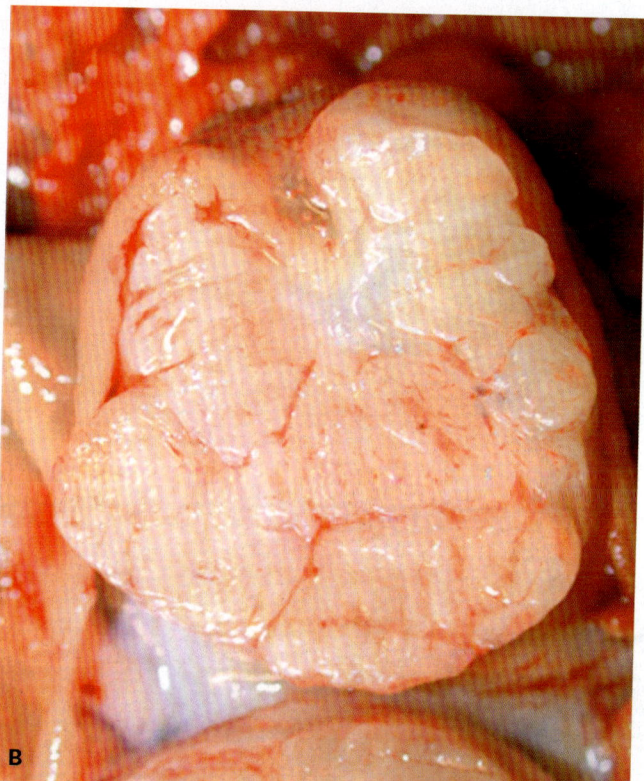

Figure 14-50. Heterotopic pancreas resected as GIST. **A,B:** Submucosal nodule toward the cardia, diagnosed confidently as a GIST given the central umbilication, which actually represents the draining duct from the pancreatic tissue. This had exocrine and endocrine components.

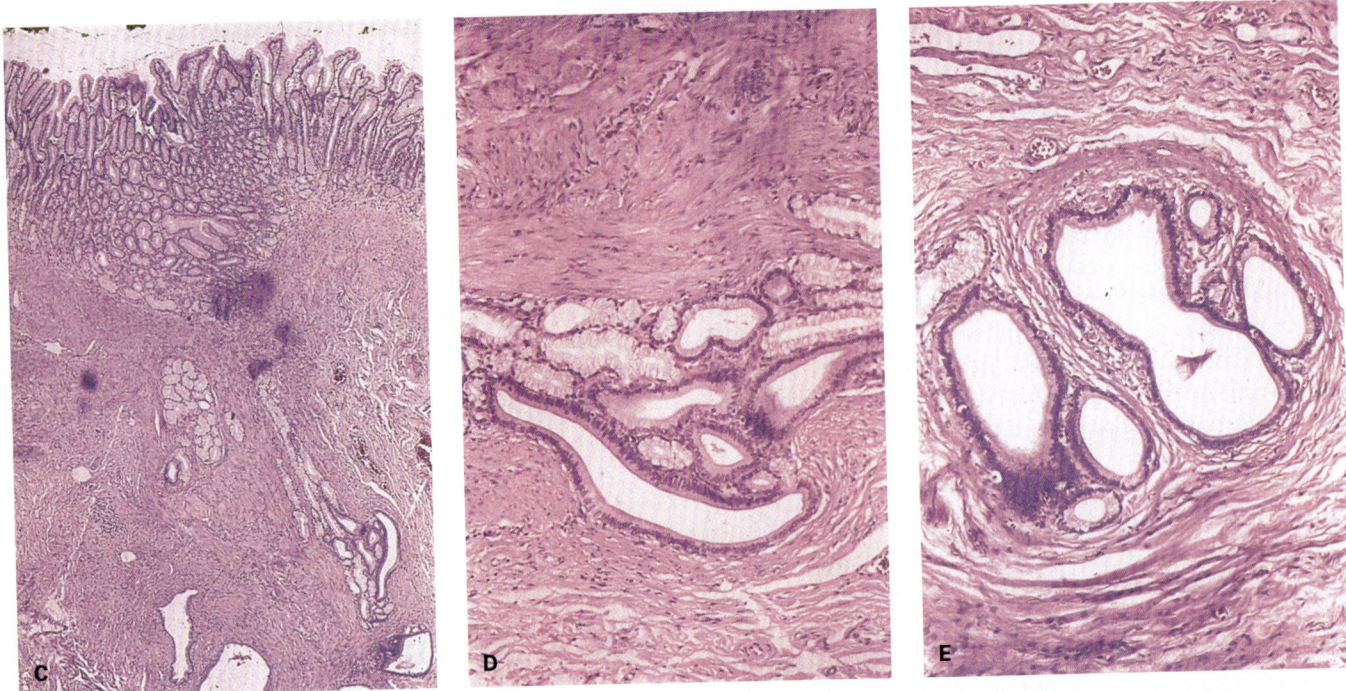

Figure 14-50. *(Continued)* **C–E:** Heterotopic pancreas/myoepithelial hamartoma. Polyp in the gastric antrum in which numerous duct-like structures surrounded by a sling of smooth muscles are present in the submucosa, mimicking pancreatic ducts.

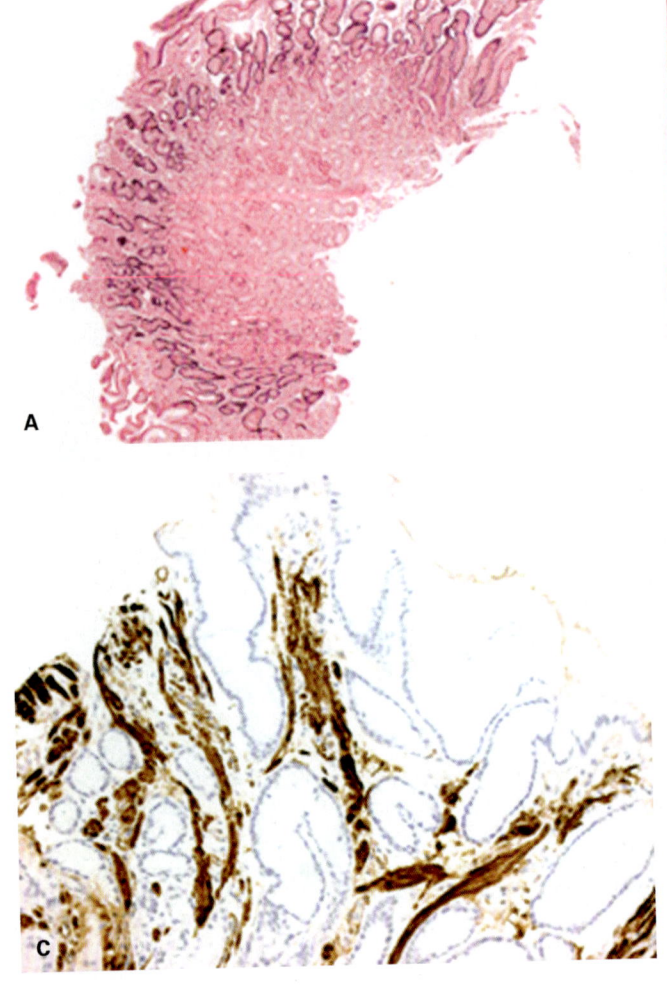

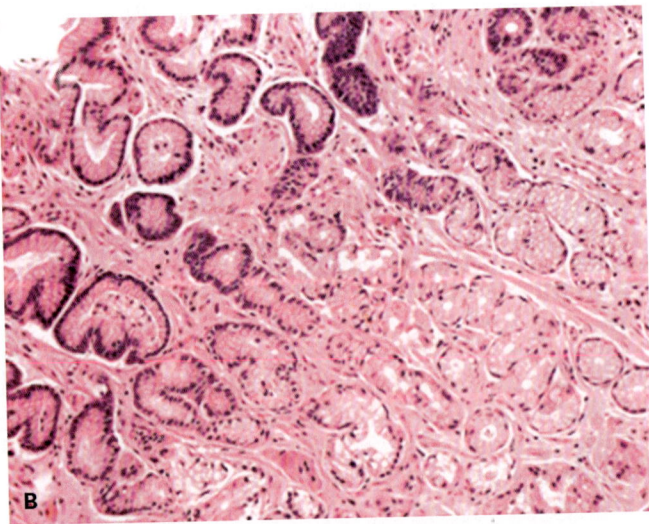

Figure 14-51. Brunner's gland nodule. **A,B:** Antral polyp consisting of a hypertrophied nodule of mucous-producing glands ("Brunner's glands"), although here it is mucosal. However, mucous-producing glands are both mucosal and submucosal so occasionally the nodule is mucosal rather than submucosal. **C:** Actin stain showing the proliferation of smooth muscle, likely representing prolapse changes, that is frequently present.

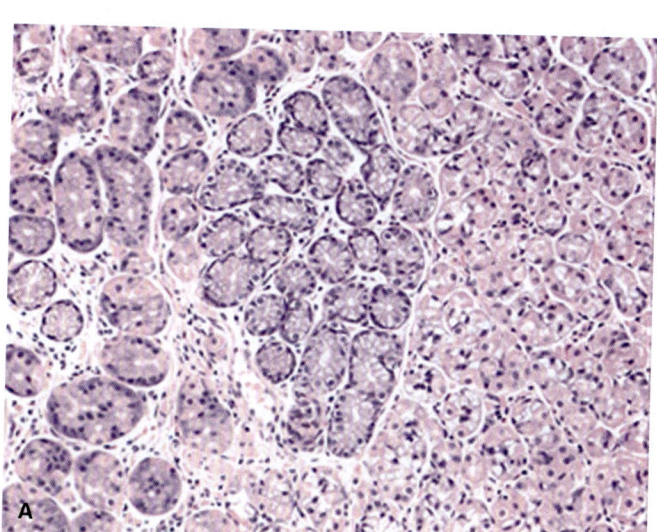 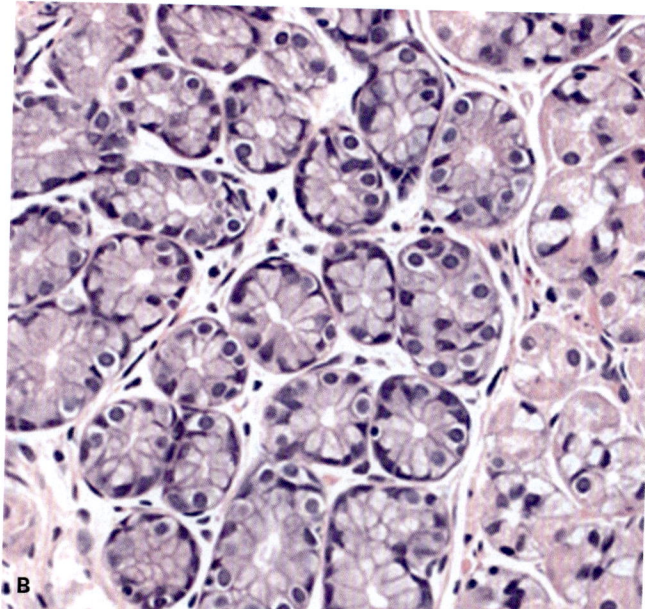

Figure 14-52. **A,B:** Nodule of antral mucosa in the middle of oxyntic mucosa. In (B) the "halo" endocrine cells are clearly visible.

gland nodules.[290,291] Care needs to be taken to compare the nuclei with normal Brunner's gland nuclei to ensure that the lesion is not a pyloric gland adenoma, which can be quiet subtle. In larger polyps there are frequently prolapse changes resulting in thick bundles of muscle (Fig. 14-51C).

Heterotopic Antral Mucosa in Oxyntic Mucosa

Rarely small nodules are found in the oxyntic mucosa that appear to have all of the features of the antral mucosa including the presence of regularly distributed G-cells (Fig. 14-52).

References

1. Lauwers G, Carneiro F, Graham D, et al. Gastric carcinoma. In: Bosman F, Carneiro F, Hruban R, eds. WHO Classification of Tumours of the Digestive System. Lyon, France: IARC Press, 2010.48–68.
2. Tatematsu M, Tsukamoto T, Inada K. Stem cells and gastric cancer: role of gastric and intestinal mixed intestinal metaplasia. Cancer Sci. 2003;94:135–141.
3. Moniaux N, Escande F, Porchet N, et al. Structural organization and classification of the human mucin genes. Front Biosci. 2001;6:D1192–D1206.
4. Buisine MP, Devisme L, Maunoury V, et al. Developmental mucin gene expression in the gastroduodenal tract and accessory digestive glands. I. Stomach. A relationship to gastric carcinoma. J Histochem Cytochem. 2000;48:1657–1666.
5. Buisine MP, Devisme L, Degand P, et al. Developmental mucin gene expression in the gastroduodenal tract and accessory digestive glands. II. Duodenum and liver, gallbladder, and pancreas. J Histochem Cytochem. 2000;48:1667–1676.
6. Trejdosiewicz LK, Malizia G, Oakes J, et al. Expression of the common acute lymphoblastic leukaemia antigen (CALLA gp100) in the brush border of normal jejunum and jejunum of patients with coeliac disease. J Clin Pathol. 1985;38:1002–1006.
7. Nakano H, Persson B, Slezak P. Study of the gastric mucosal background in patients with gastric polyps. Gastrointest Endosc. 1990;36:39–42.
8. Komoto K, Haruma K, Kamada T, et al. Helicobacter pylori infection and gastric neoplasia: correlations with histological gastritis and tumor histology. Am J Gastroenterol. 1998;93:1271–1276.
9. Kamiya T, Morishita T, Asakura H, et al. Long-term follow-up study on gastric adenoma and its relation to gastric protruded carcinoma. Cancer. 1982;50:2496–2503.
10. Saraga EP, Gardiol D, Costa J. Gastric dysplasia. A histological follow-up study. Am J Surg Pathol. 1987;11:788–796.
11. Rugge M, Cassaro M, Di Mario F, et al. The long term outcome of gastric non-invasive neoplasia. Gut. 2003;52:1111–1116.
12. Nakamura S, Matsumoto T, Ishikawa T, et al. Long term clinical course of gastric adenoma: a retrospective analysis of tumors with enlargement and those with malignant transformation. Stomach Intest. 2002;37:1009–1100.
13. Oya M, Yao T, Nakamura T, et al. Intestinal phenotypic expression of gastric depressed adenomas and the surrounding mucosa. Gastric Cancer. 2003;6:179–184.
14. Tsukashita S, Kushima R, Bamba M, et al. MUC gene expression and histogenesis of adenocarcinoma of the stomach. Int J Cancer. 2001;94:166–170.
15. Kolodziejczyk P, Yao T, Oya M, et al. Long-term follow-up study of patients with gastric adenomas with malignant transformation. An immunohistochemical and histochemical analysis. Cancer. 1994;74:2896–2907.
16. Ito H, Ito M, Tahara E. Minute carcinoid arising in gastric tubular adenoma. Histopathology. 1989;15:96–99.
17. Harada T, Imura M, Masutani M, et al. Carcinoid tumor detected in gastric adenoma during long-term follow-up. Gastrointest Endosc. 2001;53:804–806.

18. Borchard F, Ghanei A, koldovsky U, et al. Gastrale differenzierung in adenomen der magenschleimhaut. Immunocytochemische und elektronenmikroskopische untersuchungen. *Verh Ges Pathol.* 1990;74:528.
19. Watanabe H, Jass J, Sobin L. *Histological Classification of Gastric Tumours. Histological Typing of Oesophageal and Gastric Tumours.* Berlin, Germany: Springer-Verlag; 1990:34–38.
20. Vieth M, Kushima R, Borchard F, et al. Pyloric gland adenoma: a clinico-pathological analysis of 90 cases. *Virchows Arch.* 2003;442:317–321.
21. Kushima R, Vieth M, Borchard F, et al. Gastric-type well-differentiated adenocarcinoma and pyloric gland adenoma of the stomach. *Gastric Cancer.* 2006;9:177–184.
22. Kushima R, Ruthlein HJ, Stolte M, et al. "Pyloric gland-type adenoma" arising in heterotopic gastric mucosa of the duodenum, with dysplastic progression of the gastric type. *Virchows Arch.* 1999;435:452–457.
23. Kushima R, Vieth M, Mukaisho K, et al. Pyloric gland adenoma arising in Barrett's esophagus with mucin immunohistochemical and molecular cytogenetic evaluation. *Virchows Arch.* 2005;446:537–541.
24. Lopez-Ferrer A, Barranco C, de Bolos C. Apomucin expression and association with Lewis antigens during gastric development. *Appl Immunohistochem Mol Morphol.* 2001;9:42–48.
25. Abraham SC, Montgomery EA, Singh VK, et al. Gastric adenomas: intestinal-type and gastric-type adenomas differ in the risk of adenocarcinoma and presence of background mucosal pathology. *Am J Surg Pathol.* 2002;26:1276–1285.
26. Abraham SC, Park SJ, Lee JH, et al. Genetic alterations in gastric adenomas of intestinal and foveolar phenotypes. *Mod Pathol.* 2003;16:786–795.
27a. Kushima R, Muller W, Stolte M, et al. Differential p53 protein expression in stomach adenomas of gastric and intestinal phenotypes: possible sequences of p53 alteration in stomach carcinogenesis. *Virchows Arch.* 1996;428:223–227.
27b. Kushima R, Sekine S, Matsubara A, Taniguchi H, Ikegami M, Tsuda H. Gastric adenocarcinoma of the fundic gland type shares common genetic and phenotypic features with pyloric gland adenoma. *Pathol Int.* 2013;63:318–325.
27c. Singhi AD, Lazenby AJ, Montgomery EA. Gastric adenocarcinoma with chief cell differentiation: a proposal for reclassification as oxyntic gland polyp/adenoma. *Am J Surg Pathol.* 2012;36:1030–1035.
28. Cuello C, Lopez J, Correa P, et al. Histopathology of gastric dysplasias: correlations with gastric juice chemistry. *Am J Surg Pathol.* 1979;3:491–500.
29. Goldstein NS, Lewin KJ. Gastric epithelial dysplasia and adenoma: historical review and histological criteria for grading. *Hum Pathol.* 1997;28:127–133.
30. Rubio CA, Hirota T, Itabashi T. Atypical mitoses in elevated dysplasias of the stomach. *Pathol Res Pract.* 1985;180:372–376.
31. Lauwers GY, Riddell RH. Gastric epithelial dysplasia. *Gut.* 1999;45:784–790.
32. Misdraji J, Lauwers GY. Gastric epithelial dysplasia. *Semin Diagn Pathol.* 2002;19:20–30.
33. Schlemper RJ, Itabashi M, Kato Y, et al. Differences in diagnostic criteria for gastric carcinoma between Japanese and Western pathologists. *Lancet.* 1997;349:1725–1729.
34. Takahashi T, Iwama N. Three-dimensional morphology of gastric adenocarcinoma. Atypical glands as a basis for histopathologic diagnosis. *Tohoku J Exp Med.* 1984;143:451–465.
35. Antonioli DA, Goldman H. Changes in the location and type of gastric adenocarcinoma. *Cancer.* 1982;50:775–781.
36. Blot WJ, Devesa SS, Kneller RW, et al. Rising incidence of adenocarcinoma of the esophagus and gastric cardia. *JAMA.* 1991;265:1287–1289.
37. Kim MA, Lee HS, Yang HK, et al. Clinicopathologic and protein expression differences between cardia carcinoma and noncardia carcinoma of the stomach. *Cancer.* 2005;103:1439–1446.
38. Ichikura T, Chochi K, Sugasawa H, et al. Proposal for a new definition of true cardia carcinoma. *J Surg Oncol.* 2007;95:561–566.
39. Parkin DM, Pisani P, Ferlay J. Estimates of the worldwide incidence of eighteen major cancers in 1985. *Int J Cancer.* 1993;54:594–606.
40. Parkin DM, Bray FI, Devesa SS. Cancer burden in the year 2000. The global picture. *Eur J Cancer.* 2001;37(suppl 8):S4–S66.
41. Parkin DM. International variation. *Oncogene.* 2004;23:6329–6340.
42. Munoz N. Gastric carcinogenesis. In: Reed PI, Hill MJ, eds. *Gastric Carcinogenesis: Proceedings of the 6th Annual Symposium of the European Organization for Cooperation in Cancer Prevention Studies (ECP).* Amsterdam, The Netherlands: Elsevier Science; 1988: 51–69.
43. Kaneko S, Yoshimura T. Time trend analysis of gastric cancer incidence in Japan by histological types, 1975–1989. *Br J Cancer.* 2001;84:400–405.
44. Henson DE, Dittus C, Younes M, et al. Differential trends in the intestinal and diffuse types of gastric carcinoma in the United States, 1973-2000: increase in the signet ring cell type. *Arch Pathol Lab Med.* 2004;128:765–770.
45. Haas J, Schottenfield D. *Epidemiology of Gastric Cancer.* New York, NY: Plenum; 1978.
46. Correa P, Haenszel W, Tannenbaum S. Epidemiology of gastric carcinoma: review and future prospects. *Natl Cancer Inst Monogr.* 1982;62:129–134.
47. Nagayo T. *Histogenesis and Precursors of Human Gastric Cancer.* Berlin, Germany: Springer-Verlag; 1986.
48. Tatemichi M, Sasazuki S, Inoue M, et al. Different etiological role of *Helicobacter pylori* (Hp) infection in carcinogenesis between differentiated and undifferentiated gastric cancers: a nested case-control study using IgG titer against Hp surface antigen. *Acta Oncol.* 2008;47:360–365.
49. Sugiyama A, Maruta F, Ikeno T, et al. *Helicobacter pylori* infection enhances N-methyl-N-nitrosourea-induced stomach carcinogenesis in the Mongolian gerbil. *Cancer Res.* 1998;58:2067–2069.
50. Shimizu N, Inada K, Nakanishi H, et al. *Helicobacter pylori* infection enhances glandular stomach carcinogenesis in Mongolian gerbils treated with chemical carcinogens. *Carcinogenesis.* 1999;20:669–676.
51. Maruta F, Ota H, Genta RM, et al. Role of N-methyl-N-nitrosourea in the induction of intestinal metaplasia and gastric adenocarcinoma in Mongolian gerbils infected with *Helicobacter pylori. Scand J Gastroenterol.* 2001;36:283–290.
52. Uemura N, Okamoto S, Yamamoto S, et al. *Helicobacter pylori* infection and the development of gastric cancer. *N Engl J Med.* 2001;345:784–789.
53. Fukase K, Kato M, Kikuchi S, et al. Effect of eradication of *Helicobacter pylori* on incidence of metachronous gastric carcinoma after endoscopic resection of early gastric cancer: an open-label, randomised controlled trial. *Lancet.* 2008;372:392–397.
54. Asahi M, Azuma T, Ito S, et al. *Helicobacter pylori* CagA protein can be tyrosine phosphorylated in gastric epithelial cells. *J Exp Med.* 2000;191:593–602.
55. Higashi H, Nakaya A, Tsutsumi R, et al. *Helicobacter pylori* CagA induces Ras-independent morphogenetic response

through SHP-2 recruitment and activation. *J Biol Chem.* 2004;279:17205–17216.
56. Matsumoto Y, Marusawa H, Kinoshita K, et al. *Helicobacter pylori* infection triggers aberrant expression of activation-induced cytidine deaminase in gastric epithelium. *Nat Med.* 2007;13:470–476.
57. Itoh T, Wakatsuki Y, Yoshida M, et al. The vast majority of gastric T cells are polarized to produce T helper 1 type cytokines upon antigenic stimulation despite the absence of *Helicobacter pylori* infection. *J Gastroenterol.* 1999;34:560–570.
58. Itoh T, Seno H, Kita T, et al. The response to *Helicobacter pylori* differs between patients with gastric ulcer and duodenal ulcer. *Scand J Gastroenterol.* 2005;40:641–647.
59. Smythies LE, Waites KB, Lindsey JR, et al. *Helicobacter pylori*-induced mucosal inflammation is Th1 mediated and exacerbated in IL-4, but not IFN-gamma, gene-deficient mice. *J Immunol.* 2000;165:1022–1029.
60. Pikarsky E, Porat RM, Stein I, et al. NF-kappaB functions as a tumour promoter in inflammation-associated cancer. *Nature.* 2004;431:461–466.
61. Sun XF, Zhang H. NFKB and NFKBI polymorphisms in relation to susceptibility of tumour and other diseases. *Histol Histopathol.* 2007;22:1387–1398.
62. Leung WK, Wu KC, Wong CY, et al. Transgenic cyclooxygenase-2 expression and high salt enhanced susceptibility to chemical-induced gastric cancer development in mice. *Carcinogenesis.* 2008;29:1648–1654.
63. Honjo T, Kinoshita K, Muramatsu M. Molecular mechanism of class switch recombination: linkage with somatic hypermutation. *Annu Rev Immunol.* 2002;20:165–196.
64. Maekita T, Nakazawa K, Mihara M, et al. High levels of aberrant DNA methylation in *Helicobacter pylori*-infected gastric mucosae and its possible association with gastric cancer risk. *Clin Cancer Res.* 2006;12:989–995.
65. Tokunaga M, Land CE, Uemura Y, et al. Epstein–Barr virus in gastric carcinoma. *Am J Pathol.* 1993;143:1250–1254.
66. Oda K, Tamaru J, Takenouchi T, et al. Association of Epstein–Barr virus with gastric carcinoma with lymphoid stroma. *Am J Pathol.* 1993;143:1063–1071.
67. Uozaki H, Fukayama M. Epstein–Barr virus and gastric carcinoma–viral carcinogenesis through epigenetic mechanisms. *Int J Clin Exp Pathol.* 2008;1:198–216.
68. Chang MS, Uozaki H, Chong JM, et al. CpG island methylation status in gastric carcinoma with and without infection of Epstein–Barr virus. *Clin Cancer Res.* 2006;12:2995–3002.
69. Park IH, Kim SY, Kim YW, et al. Clinical characteristics and treatment outcomes of gastric cancer patients with isolated para-aortic lymph node involvement. *Cancer Chemother Pharmacol.* 2011;67:127–136.
70. Yamaoka S, Yamamoto H, Nosho K, et al. Genetic and epigenetic characteristics of gastric cancers with JC virus T-antigen. *World J Gastroenterol.* 2009;15:5579–5585.
71. Schlag P, Bockler R, Peter M. Nitrite and nitrosamines in gastric juice: risk factors for gastric cancer? *Scand J Gastroenterol.* 1982;17:145–150.
72. Weisburger JH, Reddy BS, Hill P, et al. Nutrition and cancer—on the mechanisms bearing on causes of cancer of the colon, breast, prostate, and stomach. *Bull N Y Acad Med.* 1980;56:673–696.
73. Chao A, Thun MJ, Henley SJ, et al. Cigarette smoking, use of other tobacco products and stomach cancer mortality in US adults: the Cancer Prevention Study II. *Int J Cancer.* 2002;101:380–389.
74. Gonzalez CA, Pera G, Agudo A, et al. Smoking and the risk of gastric cancer in the European Prospective Investigation Into Cancer and Nutrition (EPIC). *Int J Cancer.* 2003;107:629–634.
75. Koizumi Y, Tsubono Y, Nakaya N, et al. Cigarette smoking and the risk of gastric cancer: a pooled analysis of two prospective studies in Japan. *Int J Cancer.* 2004;112:1049–1055.
76. Zendehdel K, Nyren O, Luo J, et al. Risk of gastroesophageal cancer among smokers and users of Scandinavian moist snuff. *Int J Cancer.* 2008;122:1095–1099.
77. Aarnio M, Salovaara R, Aaltonen LA, et al. Features of gastric cancer in hereditary non-polyposis colorectal cancer syndrome. *Int J Cancer.* 1997;74:551–555.
78. Huntsman DG, Carneiro F, Lewis FR, et al. Early gastric cancer in young, asymptomatic carriers of germ-line E-cadherin mutations. *N Engl J Med.* 2001;344:1904–1909.
79. Carneiro F, Huntsman DG, Smyrk TC, et al. Model of the early development of diffuse gastric cancer in E-cadherin mutation carriers and its implications for patient screening. *J Pathol.* 2004;203:681–687.
80. Suriano G, Yew S, Ferreira P, et al. Characterization of a recurrent germ line mutation of the E-cadherin gene: implications for genetic testing and clinical management. *Clin Cancer Res.* 2005;11:5401–5409.
81. Oliveira C, Seruca R, Carneiro F. Genetics, pathology, and clinics of familial gastric cancer. *Int J Surg Pathol.* 2006;14:21–33.
82. Grady WM, Willis J, Guilford PJ, et al. Methylation of the CDH1 promoter as the second genetic hit in hereditary diffuse gastric cancer. *Nat Genet.* 2000;26:16–17.
83. Pinheiro H, Bordeira-Carrico R, Seixas S, et al. Allele-specific CDH1 downregulation and hereditary diffuse gastric cancer. *Hum Mol Genet.* 2010;19:943–952.
84. Milne AN, Carneiro F, O'Morain C, et al. Nature meets nurture: molecular genetics of gastric cancer. *Hum Genet.* 2009;126:615–628.
85. Nichols KE, Malkin D, Garber JE, et al. Germ-line p53 mutations predispose to a wide spectrum of early-onset cancers. *Cancer Epidemiol Biomarkers Prev.* 2001;10:83–87.
85a. Worthley DL, Phillips KD, Wayte N, et al. Gastric adenocarcinoma and proximal polyps of the stomach (GAPPS): a new autosomal dominant syndrome. *Gut* 2012;61:774–779.
86. Iwama T, Mishima Y, Utsunomiya J. The impact of familial adenomatous polyposis on the tumorigenesis and mortality at the several organs. Its rational treatment. *Ann Surg.* 1993;217:101–108.
87. Wallace MH, Phillips RK. Upper gastrointestinal disease in patients with familial adenomatous polyposis. *Br J Surg.* 1998;85:742–750.
88. Hofgartner WT, Thorp M, Ramus MW, et al. Gastric adenocarcinoma associated with fundic gland polyps in a patient with attenuated familial adenomatous polyposis. *Am J Gastroenterol.* 1999;94:2275–2281.
89. Offerhaus GJ, Giardiello FM, Krush AJ, et al. The risk of upper gastrointestinal cancer in familial adenomatous polyposis. *Gastroenterology.* 1992;102:1980–1982.
90. Giardiello FM, Brensinger JD, Tersmette AC, et al. Very high risk of cancer in familial Peutz-Jeghers syndrome. *Gastroenterology.* 2000;119:1447–1453.
91. Stemmermann G, Heffelfinger SC, Noffsinger A, et al. The molecular biology of esophageal and gastric cancer and their precursors: oncogenes, tumor suppressor genes, and growth factors. *Hum Pathol.* 1994;25:968–981.
92. Gonzalez CA, Sala N, Capella G. Genetic susceptibility and gastric cancer risk. *Int J Cancer.* 2002;100:249–260.

93. Vineis P, Perera F. Molecular epidemiology and biomarkers in etiologic cancer research: the new in light of the old. *Cancer Epidemiol Biomarkers Prev.* 2007;16:1954–1965.
94. Ming S. *Tumors of the Esophagus and Stomach.* Washington, DC: Armed Forces Institute of Pathology; 1973.
95. Siurala M, Lehtola J, Ihamaki T. Atrophic gastritis and its sequelae. Results of 19–23 years' follow-up examinations. *Scand J Gastroenterol.* 1974;9:441–446.
96. Nagayo T. *Precursors of Human Gastric Cancer: Their Frequencies and Histological Characteristics.* Baltimore, MD: University Park Press; 1977.
97. Ming SC, Bajtai A, Correa P, et al. Gastric dysplasia. Significance and pathologic criteria. *Cancer.* 1984;54:1794–1801.
98. Miyamoto M, Haruma K, Yoshihara M, et al. Five cases of nodular gastritis and gastric cancer: a possible association between nodular gastritis and gastric cancer. *Dig Liver Dis.* 2002;34:819–820.
99. Miyamoto M, Haruma K, Yoshihara M, et al. Nodular gastritis in adults is caused by *Helicobacter pylori* infection. *Dig Dis Sci.* 2003;48:968–975.
100. Hirahashi M, Yao T, Matsumoto T, et al. Intramucosal gastric adenocarcinoma of poorly differentiated type in the young is characterized by *Helicobacter pylori* infection and antral lymphoid hyperplasia. *Mod Pathol.* 2007;20:29–34.
101. Shiotani A, Kamada T, Kumamoto M, et al. Nodular gastritis in Japanese young adults: endoscopic and histological observations. *J Gastroenterol.* 2007;42:610–615.
102. Toftgaard C. Gastric cancer after peptic ulcer surgery. A historic prospective cohort investigation. *Ann Surg.* 1989;210:159–164.
103. Ruck P, Wehrmann M, Campbell M, et al. Squamous cell carcinoma of the gastric stump. A case report and review of the literature. *Am J Surg Pathol.* 1989;13:317–324.
104. Schafer LW, Larson DE, Melton LJ III, et al. The risk of gastric carcinoma after surgical treatment for benign ulcer disease. A population-based study in Olmsted County, Minnesota. *N Engl J Med.* 1983;309:1210–1213.
105. Scharschmidt BF. The natural history of hypertrophic gastrophy (Menetrier's disease). Report of a case with 16 year follow-up and review of 120 cases from the literature. *Am J Med.* 1977;63:644–652.
106. Coffey RJ, Washington MK, Corless CL, et al. Menetrier disease and gastrointestinal stromal tumors: hyperproliferative disorders of the stomach. *J Clin Invest.* 2007;117:70–80.
107. Laxen F, Sipponen P, Ihamaki T, et al. Gastric polyps; their morphological and endoscopical characteristics and relation to gastric carcinoma. *Acta Pathol Microbiol Immunol Scand A.* 1982;90:221–228.
108. Borrman R. *Geschwulste des Magens and Duodenums.* Vol. 4, Pt. 1. Berlin, Germany: Springer; 1926.
109. Murakami T. Pathomorphological diagnosis. Definition and gross classification of early gastric cancer. In: Murakami T, ed. *Early Gastric Cancer. Gann Monograph on Cancer Research.* Vol. 11. Tokyo, Japan: University of Tokyo Press; 1971:53–55.
110. Japanese Gastric Cancer Association. Japanese classification of gastric carcinoma—2nd English Edition. *Gastric Cancer.* 1998;1:10–24.
111. Sakita T, Yoshimori M. *Early Diagnosis of Gastric Cancer.* Baltimore, MD: University Park Press; 1976.
112. Tsukuma H, Mishima T, Oshima A. Prospective study of "early" gastric cancer. *Int J Cancer.* 1983;31:421–426.
113. Hisamichi S, Sugawara N. Mass screening for gastric cancer by X-ray examination. *Jpn J Clin Oncol.* 1984;14:211–223.
114. Xuan ZX, Ueyama T, Yao T, et al. Time trends of early gastric carcinoma. A clinicopathologic analysis of 2846 cases. *Cancer.* 1993;72:2889–2894.
115. Everett SM, Axon AT. Early gastric cancer in Europe. *Gut.* 1997;41:142–150.
116. Morson B. *The Japanese Classification of Early Gastric Cancer.* Baltimore, MD: Williams & Wilkins; 1977.
117. Johansen AA. Early gastric cancer. *Curr Top Pathol.* 1976;63:1–47.
118. Monafo WW Jr, Krause GL Jr, Medina JG. Carcinoma of the stomach. Morphological characteristics affecting survival. *Arch Surg.* 1962;85:754–763.
119. Lauren P. The two histological main types of gastric carcinoma: diffuse and so-called intestinal-type carcinoma. An attempt at a histo-clinical classification. *Acta Pathol Microbiol Scand.* 1965;64:31–49.
120. Nakamura K, Sugano H, Takagi K. Carcinoma of the stomach in incipient phase: its histogenesis and histological appearances. *Gann.* 1968;59:251–258.
121. Sugano H, Nakamura K, Kato Y. Pathological studies of human gastric cancer. *Acta Pathol Jpn.* 1982;32(suppl 2): 329–347.
122. Ming SC. Gastric carcinoma. A pathobiological classification. *Cancer.* 1977;39:2475–2485.
123. Akamatsu T, Katsuyama T. Histochemical demonstration of mucins in the intramucosal laminated structure of human gastric signet ring cell carcinoma and its relation to submucosal invasion. *Histochem J.* 1990;22: 416–425.
124. Watanabe H, Enjoji M, Imai T. Gastric carcinoma with lymphoid stroma. Its morphologic characteristics and prognostic correlations. *Cancer.* 1976;38:232–243.
125. Moritani S, Kushima R, Sugihara H, et al. Phenotypic characteristics of Epstein–Barr-virus-associated gastric carcinomas. *J Cancer Res Clin Oncol.* 1996;122:750–756.
126. Geddert H, Zur Hausen A, Gabbert HE, et al. EBV-infection in cardiac and non-cardiac gastric adenocarcinomas is associated with promoter methylation of p16, p14 and APC, but not hMLH1. *Cell Oncol (Dordr).* 2011;34(3):209–214.
127. Uozaki H, Barua RR, Minhua S, et al. Transcriptional factor typing with SOX2, HNF4aP1, and CDX2 closely relates to tumor invasion and Epstein–Barr virus status in gastric cancer. *Int J Clin Exp Pathol.* 2011;4:230–240.
128. Haas M, Buttner M, Rau TT, et al. Inflammation in gastric adenocarcinoma of the cardia: how do EBV infection, Her2 amplification and cancer progression influence tumor-infiltrating lymphocytes? *Virchows Arch.* 2011;458: 403–411.
129. Fujii H, Ichikawa K, Takagaki T, et al. Genetic evolution of alpha fetoprotein producing gastric cancer. *J Clin Pathol.* 2003;56:942–949.
130. Motoyama T, Aizawa K, Watanabe H, et al. Alpha-Fetoprotein producing gastric carcinomas: a comparative study of three different subtypes. *Acta Pathol Jpn.* 1993;43:654–661.
131. Matsunou H, Konishi F, Jalal RE, et al. Alpha-fetoprotein-producing gastric carcinoma with enteroblastic differentiation. *Cancer.* 1994;73:534–540.
132. Ritter JH, Mills SE, Gaffey MJ, et al. Clear cell tumors of the alimentary tract and abdominal cavity. *Semin Diagn Pathol.* 1997;14:213–219.
133. Terracciano LM, Glatz K, Mhawech P, et al. Hepatoid adenocarcinoma with liver metastasis mimicking hepatocellular carcinoma: an immunohistochemical and molecular study of eight cases. *Am J Surg Pathol.* 2003;27: 1302–1312.
134. Ushiku T, Shinozaki A, Shibahara J, et al. SALL4 represents fetal gut differentiation of gastric cancer, and is diagnostically useful in distinguishing hepatoid gastric carcinoma from hepatocellular carcinoma. *Am J Surg Pathol.* 2010;34:533–540.

135. Mori M, Iwashita A, Enjoji M. Adenosquamous carcinoma of the stomach. A clinicopathologic analysis of 28 cases. *Cancer.* 1986;57:333–339.
136. Mori M, Fukuda T, Enjoji M. Adenosquamous carcinoma of the stomach. Histogenetic and ultrastructural studies. *Gastroenterology.* 1987;92:1078–1082.
137. Majmudar B, Dillard R, Susann PW. Collision carcinoma of the gastric cardia. *Hum Pathol.* 1978;9:471–473.
138. Liu AY, Chan WY, Ng EK, et al. Gastric choriocarcinoma shows characteristics of adenocarcinoma and gestational choriocarcinoma: a comparative genomic hybridization and fluorescence in situ hybridization study. *Diagn Mol Pathol.* 2001;10:161–165.
139. Kobayashi A, Hasebe T, Endo Y, et al. Primary gastric choriocarcinoma: two case reports and a pooled analysis of 53 cases. *Gastric Cancer.* 2005;8:178–185.
140. Garcia RL, Ghali VS. Gastric choriocarcinoma and yolk sac tumor in a man: observations about its possible origin. *Hum Pathol.* 1985;16:955–958.
141. Mori H, Soeda O, Kamano T, et al. Choriocarcinomatous change with immunocytochemically HCG-positive cells in the gastric carcinoma of the males. *Virchows Arch A Pathol Anat Histol.* 1982;396:141–153.
142. Krulewski T, Cohen LB. Choriocarcinoma of the stomach: pathogenesis and clinical characteristics. *Am J Gastroenterol.* 1988;83:1172–1175.
143. Ramponi A, Angeli G, Arceci F, et al. Gastric choriocarcinoma; an immunohistochemical study. *Pathol Res Pract.* 1986;181:390–396.
144. Fukayama M, Hayashi Y, Koike M. Human chorionic gonadotropin in gastric carcinoma. An immunohistochemical study suggesting independent regulation of subunits. *Virchows Arch A Pathol Anat Histopathol.* 1987;411:205–212.
145. Kazzaz BA, Eulderink F. Paneth cell-rich carcinoma of the stomach. *Histopathology.* 1989;15:303–305.
146. Ooi A, Nakanishi I, Itoh T, et al. Predominant Paneth cell differentiation in an intestinal type gastric cancer. *Pathol Res Pract.* 1991;187:220–225.
147. Inada KI, Mizoshita T, Tsukamoto T, et al. Paneth type gastric cancer cells exhibit expression of human defensin-5. *Histopathology.* 2005;47:330–331.
148. Tsukamoto T, Yokoi T, Maruta S, et al. Gastric adenocarcinoma with chief cell differentiation. *Pathol Int.* 2007;57:517–522.
149. Ueyama H, Yao T, Nakashima Y, et al. Gastric adenocarcinoma of fundic gland type (chief cell predominant type): proposal for a new entity of gastric adenocarcinoma. *Am J Surg Pathol* 2010;34:609–619.
150. Muller-Hocker J, Rellecke P. Chief cell proliferation of the gastric mucosa mimicking early gastric cancer: an unusual variant of fundic gland polyp. *Virchows Arch.* 2003;442:496–500.
151. Matsukawa A, Kurano R, Takemoto T, et al. Chief cell hyperplasia with structural and nuclear atypia: a variant of fundic gland polyp. *Pathol Res Pract.* 2005;200:817–821.
152. Capella C, Frigerio B, Cornaggia M, et al. Gastric parietal cell carcinoma—a newly recognized entity: light microscopic and ultrastructural features. *Histopathology.* 1984;8:813–824.
153. Byrne D, Holley MP, Cuschieri A. Parietal cell carcinoma of the stomach: association with long-term survival after curative resection. *Br J Cancer.* 1988;58:85–87.
154. Yang GY, Liao J, Cassai ND, et al. Parietal cell carcinoma of gastric cardia: immunophenotype and ultrastructure. *Ultrastruct Pathol.* 2003;27:87–94.
155. Takubo K, Honma N, Sawabe M, et al. Oncocytic adenocarcinoma of the stomach: parietal cell carcinoma. *Am J Surg Pathol.* 2002;26:458–465.
156. Endoh Y, Tamura G, Motoyama T, et al. Well-differentiated adenocarcinoma mimicking complete-type intestinal metaplasia in the stomach. *Hum Pathol.* 1999;30:826–832.
157. Yao T, Utsunomiya T, Oya M, et al. Extremely well-differentiated adenocarcinoma of the stomach: clinicopathological and immunohistochemical features. *World J Gastroenterol.* 2006;12:2510–2516.
158. Chetty R, Weinreb I. Gastric neuroendocrine carcinoma arising from heterotopic pancreatic tissue. *J Clin Pathol.* 2004;57:314–317.
159. Fukunaga M. Gastric carcinoma resembling pancreatic mixed acinar-endocrine carcinoma. *Hum Pathol.* 2002;33:569–573.
160. Sun Y, Wasserman PG. Acinar cell carcinoma arising in the stomach: a case report with literature review. *Hum Pathol.* 2004;35:263–265.
161. Jain D, Eslami-Varzaneh F, Takano AM, et al. Composite glandular and endocrine tumors of the stomach with pancreatic acinar differentiation. *Am J Surg Pathol.* 2005;29:1524–1529.
162. Rubio CA. Serrated adenoma of the duodenum. *J Clin Pathol.* 2004;57:1219–1221.
163. Rubio CA. Serrated neoplasia of the stomach: a new entity. *J Clin Pathol.* 2001;54:849–853.
164. Siegel MJ, Shackelford GD. Gastric teratomas in infants: report of two cases. *Pediatr Radiol.* 1978;7:197–200.
165. Moriuchi A, Nakayama I, Muta H, et al. Gastric teratoma of children—a case report with review of the literature. *Acta Pathol Jpn.* 1977;27:749–758.
166. Haley T, Dimler M, Hollier P. Gastric teratoma with gastrointestinal bleeding. *J Pediatr Surg.* 1986;21:949–950.
167. Bansal M, Kaneko M, Gordon RE. Carcinosarcoma and separate carcinoid tumor of the stomach. A case report with light and electron microscopic studies. *Cancer.* 1982;50:1876–1881.
168. Kayaselcuk F, Tuncer I, Toyganozu Y, et al. Carcinosarcoma of the stomach. *Pathol Oncol Res.* 2002;8:275–277.
169. Teramachi K, Kanomata N, Hasebe T, et al. Carcinosarcoma (pure endocrine cell carcinoma with sarcoma components) of the stomach. *Pathol Int.* 2003;53:552–556.
170. Sato Y, Shimozono T, Kawano S, et al. Gastric carcinosarcoma, coexistence of adenosquamous carcinoma and rhabdomyosarcoma: a case report. *Histopathology.* 2001;39:543–544.
171. Randjelovic T, Filipovic B, Babic D, et al. Carcinosarcoma of the stomach: a case report and review of the literature. *World J Gastroenterol.* 2007;13:5533–5536.
172. Kuroda N, Oonishi K, Iwamura S, et al. Gastric carcinosarcoma with neuroendocrine differentiation as the carcinoma component and leiomyosarcomatous and myofibroblastic differentiation as the sarcomatous component. *APMIS.* 2006;114:234–238.
173. Cho KJ, Myong NH, Choi DW, et al. Carcinosarcoma of the stomach. A case report with light microscopic, immunohistochemical, and electron microscopic study. *APMIS.* 1990;98:991–995.
174. Okabe H. *Growth of Early Gastric Cancer. Clinical Study of Growth and Invasive Patterns of Early Gastric Cancer. Its Position in the Natural History of Gastric Cancer.* Vol. 11. Tokyo, Japan: University of Tokyo Press; 1972.
175. Levin K, Appeleman H. *Tumors of the Esophagus and Stomach.* Vol. Fascicle 18, 3rd Series. Washington, DC: Armed Forces Institute of Pathology; 1995.

176. Fujimori Y, Akamatsu T, Ota H, et al. Proliferative markers in gastric carcinoma and organoid differentiation. *Hum Pathol.* 1995;26:725-734.
177. Ohta H, Noguchi Y, Takagi K, et al. Early gastric carcinoma with special reference to macroscopic classification. *Cancer.* 1987;60:1099-1106.
178. Nozaki Y, Oshiro H, Nakajima A. Langerhans cell histiocytosis of the stomach mimicking early gastric cancer. *Clin Gastroenterol Hepatol.* 2010;8(9):A18.
179. Menuck LS, Amberg JR. Metastatic disease involving the stomach. *Am J Dig Dis.* 1975;20:903-913.
180. Cormier WJ, Gaffey TA, Welch JM, et al. Linitis plastica caused by metastatic lobular carcinoma of the breast. *Mayo Clin Proc.* 1980;55:747-753.
181. Zhao XH, Gu SZ, Liu SX, et al. Expression of estrogen receptor and estrogen receptor messenger RNA in gastric carcinoma tissues. *World J Gastroenterol.* 2003;9:665-669.
182. O'Connell FP, Wang HH, Odze RD. Utility of immunohistochemistry in distinguishing primary adenocarcinomas from metastatic breast carcinomas in the gastrointestinal tract. *Arch Pathol Lab Med.* 2005;129:338-347.
183. Geller SA, Dhall D, Alsabeh R. Application of immunohistochemistry to liver and gastrointestinal neoplasms: liver, stomach, colon, and pancreas. *Arch Pathol Lab Med.* 2008;132:490-499.
184. Isaacson P. Biopsy appearances easily mistaken for malignancy in gastrointestinal endoscopy. *Histopathology.* 1982;6:377-389.
185. Majima S, Yamaguchi I, Yoshida K, et al. Duodenal extension of carcinoma of the stomach. *Tohoku J Exp Med.* 1964;83:159-167.
186. Ming S. *Tumors of the Esophagus and Stomach.* Washington, DC: Armed Forces Institute of Pathology; 1984.
187. Ringertz N. The pathology of gastric carcinoma. *Natl Cancer Inst Monogr.* 1967;25:275-285.
188. Lewin KJ, Appleman HD. *Carcinoma of the stomach. Tumors of the Esophagus and Stomach. Atlas of Tumor Pathology*, 3rd Series, Fascicle 18. Washington, DC: Armed Forces Institute of Pathology; 1996:245-330.
189. Desai AM, Pareek M, Nightingale PG, et al. Improving outcomes in gastric cancer over 20 years. *Gastric Cancer.* 2004;7:196-201,discussion 201-203.
190. Brennan MF, Karpeh MS Jr. Surgery for gastric cancer: the American view. *Semin Oncol.* 1996;23:352-359.
191. Strong VE, Song KY, Park CH, et al. Comparison of gastric cancer survival following R0 resection in the United States and Korea using an internationally validated nomogram. *Ann Surg.* 2010;251:640-646.
192. Siewert JR, Bottcher K, Stein HJ, et al. Relevant prognostic factors in gastric cancer: ten-year results of the German Gastric Cancer Study. *Ann Surg.* 1998;228:449-461.
193. Kidokoro T. *Frequency of Resection, Metastasis, and Five-Year Survival Rate of Early Gastric Carcinoma in a Surgical Clinic.* Vol. 11. Tokyo, Japan: University of Tokyo Press; 1972.
194. Antonioli D. Current concepts in carcinoma of the stomach. In: Appleman H, ed. *Pathology of the Esophagus, Stomach and Duodenum.* New York, NY: Churchill Livingstone; 1984.
195. Kodama Y, Inokuchi K, Soejima K, et al. Growth patterns and prognosis in early gastric carcinoma. Superficially spreading and penetrating growth types. *Cancer.* 1983;51:320-326.
196. Matsusaka T, Kodama Y, Soejima K, et al. Recurrence in early gastric cancer: a pathologic evaluation. *Cancer.* 1980;46:168-172.
197. Gotoda T, Yanagisawa A, Sasako M, et al. Incidence of lymph node metastasis from early gastric cancer: estimation with a large number of cases at two large centers. *Gastric Cancer.* 2000;3:219-225.
198. Tateishi Y, Nakanishi Y, Taniguchi H, et al. Pathological prognostic factors predicting lymph node metastasis in submucosal invasive (T1) colorectal carcinoma. *Mod Pathol.* 2010;23:1068-1072.
199. Gotoda T, Sasako M, Ono H, et al. Evaluation of the necessity for gastrectomy with lymph node dissection for patients with submucosal invasive gastric cancer. *Br J Surg.* 2001;88:444-449.
200. Ishikawa S, Togashi A, Inoue M, et al. Indications for EMR/ESD in cases of early gastric cancer: relationship between histological type, depth of wall invasion, and lymph node metastasis. *Gastric Cancer.* 2007;10:35-38.
201. Hirota T, Itabashi M, Suzuki K, et al. *Clinicopathologic Study of Minute and Small Early Gastric Cancer: Histogenesis of Gastric Cancer.* Vol. 15, (Pt. 2). New York, NY: Appleton-Century-Crofts; 1980.
202. Gotoda T, Yamamoto H, Soetikno RM. Endoscopic submucosal dissection of early gastric cancer. *J Gastroenterol.* 2006;41:929-942.
203. Nagano H, Ohyama S, Fukunaga T, et al. Two rare cases of node-positive differentiated gastric cancer despite their infiltration to sm1, their small size, and lack of lymphatic invasion into the submucosal layer. *Gastric Cancer.* 2008;11:53-57,discussion 57-58.
204. UICC. *TNM Classification of Malignant Tumours.* 6th ed. New York, NY: Wiley-Blackwell; 2009.
205. Brennan MF. Current status of surgery for gastric cancer: a review. *Gastric Cancer.* 2005;8:64-70.
206. Yoshikawa K, Maruyama K. Characteristics of gastric cancer invading to the proper muscle layer—with special reference to mortality and cause of death. *Jpn J Clin Oncol.* 1985;15:499-503.
207. Ishigami S, Natsugoe S, Miyazono F, et al. Clinical merit of subdividing gastric cancer according to invasion of the muscularis propria. *Hepatogastroenterology.* 2004;51:869-871.
208. Ohman U, Wetterfors J, Moberg A. Histologic grading of gastric cancer. *Acta Chir Scand.* 1972;138:384-390.
209. Hermanek P. Clinical significance of histologic classification in accordance with Lauén as an addition to pTNM. *Scand J Gastroenterol.* 1987;22(suppl 133):33-35.
210. De Vita F, Giuliani F, Silvestris N, et al. Human epidermal growth factor receptor 2 (HER2) in gastric cancer: a new therapeutic target. *Cancer Treat Rev.* 2010;36(suppl 3):S11-S15.
211. Bang YJ, Van Cutsem E, Feyereislova A, et al. Trastuzumab in combination with chemotherapy versus chemotherapy alone for treatment of HER2-positive advanced gastric or gastro-oesophageal junction cancer (ToGA): a phase 3, open-label, randomised controlled trial. *Lancet.* 2010;376:687-697.
212. Hatfield AR, Slavin G, Segal AW, et al. Importance of the site of endoscopic gastric biopsy in ulcerating lesions of the stomach. *Gut.* 1975;16:884-886.
213. Carmack SW, Genta RM, Schuler CM, et al. The current spectrum of gastric polyps: a 1-year national study of over 120,000 patients. *Am J Gastroenterol.* 2009;104:1524-1532.
214. Nishiura M, Hirota T, Itabashi M, et al. A clinical and histopathological study of gastric polyps in familial polyposis coli. *Am J Gastroenterol.* 1984;79:98-103.
215. Declich P, Tavani E, Ferrara A, et al. Sporadic fundic gland polyps: clinico-pathologic features and associated diseases. *Pol J Pathol.* 2005;56:131-137.
216. Jarvinen HJ, Sipponen P. Gastroduodenal polyps in familial adenomatous and juvenile polyposis. *Endoscopy.* 1986;18:230-234.

217. Choudhry U, Boyce HW Jr, Coppola D. Proton pump inhibitor-associated gastric polyps: a retrospective analysis of their frequency, and endoscopic, histologic, and ultrastructural characteristics. *Am J Clin Pathol.* 1998;110:615–621.
218. el-Zimaity HM, Jackson FW, Graham DY. Fundic gland polyps developing during omeprazole therapy. *Am J Gastroenterol.* 1997;92:1858–1860.
219. Vieth M, Stolte M. Fundic gland polyps are not induced by proton pump inhibitor therapy. *Am J Clin Pathol.* 2001;116:716–720.
220. Hongo M, Fujimoto K. Incidence and risk factor of fundic gland polyp and hyperplastic polyp in long-term proton pump inhibitor therapy: a prospective study in Japan. *J Gastroenterol.* 2010;45(6):618–624.
221. Hsu WH, Wu IC, Kuo CH, et al. Influence of proton pump inhibitor use in gastrointestinal polyps. *Kaohsiung J Med Sci.* 2010;26:76–83.
222. Rubio CA. Lysozyme overexpression in fundic gland polyps. *Anticancer Res.* 2010;30:1021–1024.
223. Abraham SC, Nobukawa B, Giardiello FM, et al. Fundic gland polyps in familial adenomatous polyposis: neoplasms with frequent somatic adenomatous polyposis coli gene alterations. *Am J Pathol.* 2000;157:747–754.
224. Wu TT, Kornacki S, Rashid A, et al. Dysplasia and dysregulation of proliferation in foveolar and surface epithelia of fundic gland polyps from patients with familial adenomatous polyposis. *Am J Surg Pathol.* 1998;22:293–298.
225. Bertoni G, Sassatelli R, Nigrisoli E, et al. Dysplastic changes in gastric fundic gland polyps of patients with familial adenomatous polyposis. *Ital J Gastroenterol Hepatol.* 1999;31:192–197.
226. Bianchi LK, Burke CA, Bennett AE, et al. Fundic gland polyp dysplasia is common in familial adenomatous polyposis. *Clin Gastroenterol Hepatol.* 2008;6:180–185.
227. Jalving M, Koornstra JJ, Gotz JM, et al. High-grade dysplasia in sporadic fundic gland polyps: a case report and review of the literature. *Eur J Gastroenterol Hepatol.* 2003;15:1229–1233.
228. Zwick A, Munir M, Ryan CK, et al. Gastric adenocarcinoma and dysplasia in fundic gland polyps of a patient with attenuated adenomatous polyposis coli. *Gastroenterology.* 1997;113:659–663.
229. Garrean S, Hering J, Saied A, et al. Gastric adenocarcinoma arising from fundic gland polyps in a patient with familial adenomatous polyposis syndrome. *Am Surg.* 2008;74:79–83.
230. Dirschmid K, Walser J, Hugel H. Pseudomalignant erosion in hyperplastic gastric polyps. *Cancer.* 1984;54:2290–2293.
231. Elster K, Carson W, Eidt H, et al. Significance of gastric polypectomy (histological aspect). *Endoscopy.* 1983;15(suppl 1):148–149.
232. Schlosnagle DC, Hardin RD. Squamous morules in gastric mucosa. *J Clin Gastroenterol.* 1988;10:332–334.
233. Abraham SC, Nobukawa B, Giardiello FM, et al. Sporadic fundic gland polyps: common gastric polyps arising through activating mutations in the beta-catenin gene. *Am J Pathol.* 2001;158:1005–1010.
234. Daibo M, Itabashi M, Hirota T. Malignant transformation of gastric hyperplastic polyps. *Am J Gastroenterol.* 1987;82:1016–1025.
235. Orlowska J, Jarosz D, Pachlewski J, et al. Malignant transformation of benign epithelial gastric polyps. *Am J Gastroenterol.* 1995;90:2152–2159.
236. Zea-Iriarte WL, Sekine I, Itsuno M, et al. Carcinoma in gastric hyperplastic polyps. A phenotypic study. *Dig Dis Sci.* 1996;41:377–386.
237. Han AR, Sung CO, Kim KM, et al. The clinicopathological features of gastric hyperplastic polyps with neoplastic transformations: a suggestion of indication for endoscopic polypectomy. *Gut Liver.* 2009;3:271–275.
238. Terada T. Malignant transformation of foveolar hyperplastic polyp of the stomach: a histopathological study. *Med Oncol.* 2011;28(4):941–944.
239. Hirano H, Yoshida T, Yoshimura H, et al. Poorly differentiated adenocarcinoma with signet-ring cell carcinoma in a hyperplastic polyp of the stomach: report of a case. *Surg Today.* 2007;37:901–904.
240. Hirasaki S, Suzuki S, Kanzaki H, et al. Minute signet ring cell carcinoma occurring in gastric hyperplastic polyp. *World J Gastroenterol.* 2007;13:5779–5780.
241. Yao T, Kajiwara M, Kuroiwa S, et al. Malignant transformation of gastric hyperplastic polyps: alteration of phenotypes, proliferative activity, and p53 expression. *Hum Pathol.* 2002;33:1016–1022.
242. Stemper TJ, Kent TH, Summers RW. Juvenile polyposis and gastrointestinal carcinoma. A study of a kindred. *Ann Intern Med.* 1975;83:639–646.
243. Howe JR, Mitros FA, Summers RW. The risk of gastrointestinal carcinoma in familial juvenile polyposis. *Ann Surg Oncol.* 1998;5:751–756.
244. Watanabe A, Nagashima H, Motoi M, et al. Familial juvenile polyposis of the stomach. *Gastroenterology.* 1979;77:148–151.
245. Desai DC, Neale KF, Talbot IC, et al. Juvenile polyposis. *Br J Surg.* 1995;82:14–17.
246. Hizawa K, Iida M, Yao T, et al. Juvenile polyposis of the stomach: clinicopathological features and its malignant potential. *J Clin Pathol.* 1997;50:771–774.
247. Haidle J, Howe J. Juvenile Polyposis Syndrome. In: Pagon R, Bird T, Dolan C, et al., eds. *GeneReviews* (Internet). Seattle, WA: University of Washington; 2003 (updated 2008).
248. Yoshida T, Haraguchi Y, Tanaka A, et al. A case of generalized juvenile gastrointestinal polyposis associated with gastric carcinoma. *Endoscopy.* 1988;20:33–35.
249. Sayed MG, Ahmed AF, Ringold JR, et al. Germline SMAD4 or BMPR1A mutations and phenotype of juvenile polyposis. *Ann Surg Oncol.* 2002;9:901–906.
250. Howe JR, Sayed MG, Ahmed AF, et al. The prevalence of MADH4 and BMPR1A mutations in juvenile polyposis and absence of BMPR2, BMPR1B, and ACVR1 mutations. *J Med Genet.* 2004;41:484–491.
251. Gallione C, Aylsworth AS, Beis J, et al. Overlapping spectra of SMAD4 mutations in juvenile polyposis (JP) and JP-HHT syndrome. *Am J Med Genet A.* 2010;152A:333–339.
252. Utsunomiya J, Gocho H, Miyanaga T, et al. Peutz-Jeghers syndrome: its natural course and management. *Johns Hopkins Med J.* 1975;136:71–82.
253. Oncel M, Remzi FH, Church JM, et al. Course and follow-up of solitary Peutz-Jeghers polyps: a case series. *Int J Colorectal Dis.* 2003;18:33–35.
254. Foley TR, McGarrity TJ, Abt AB. Peutz-Jeghers syndrome: a clinicopathologic survey of the "Harrisburg family" with a 49-year follow-up. *Gastroenterology.* 1988;95:1535–1540.
255. Estrada R, Spjut HJ. Hamartomatous polyps in Peutz-Jeghers syndrome. A light-, histochemical, and electron-microscopic study. *Am J Surg Pathol.* 1983;7:747–754.
256. Perzin KH, Bridge MF. Adenomatous and carcinomatous changes in hamartomatous polyps of the small intestine (Peutz-Jeghers syndrome): report of a case and review of the literature. *Cancer.* 1982;49:971–983.
257. Miller LJ, Bartholomew LG, Dozois RR, et al. Adenocarcinoma of the rectum arising in a hamartomatous polyp in a patient with Peutz-Jeghers syndrome. *Dig Dis Sci.* 1983;28:1047–1051.

258. Konishi F, Wyse NE, Muto T, et al. Peutz-Jeghers polyposis associated with carcinoma of the digestive organs. Report of three cases and review of the literature. *Dis Colon Rectum.* 1987;30:790–799.
259. Narita T, Eto T, Ito T. Peutz-Jeghers syndrome with adenomas and adenocarcinomas in colonic polyps. *Am J Surg Pathol.* 1987;11:76–81.
260. Hizawa K, Iida M, Matsumoto T, et al. Neoplastic transformation arising in Peutz-Jeghers polyposis. *Dis Colon Rectum.* 1993;36:953–957.
261. Flageole H, Raptis S, Trudel JL, et al. Progression toward malignancy of hamartomas in a patient with Peutz-Jeghers syndrome: case report and literature review. *Can J Surg.* 1994;37:231–236.
262. Spigelman AD, Murday V, Phillips RK. Cancer and the Peutz-Jeghers syndrome. *Gut.* 1989;30:1588–1590.
263. Hizawa K, Iida M, Matsumoto T, et al. Gastrointestinal manifestations of Cowden's disease. Report of four cases. *J Clin Gastroenterol.* 1994;18:13–18.
264. Seruca R, Carneiro F, Castedo S, et al. Familial gastric polyposis revisited. Autosomal dominant inheritance confirmed. *Cancer Genet Cytogenet.* 1991;53:97–100.
265. Carneiro F, David L, Seruca R, et al. Hyperplastic polyposis and diffuse carcinoma of the stomach. A study of a family. *Cancer.* 1993;72:323–329.
266. Niv Y, Delpre G, Sperber AD, et al. Hyperplastic gastric polyposis, hypergastrinaemia and colorectal neoplasia: a description of four cases. *Eur J Gastroenterol Hepatol.* 2003;15:1361–1366.
267. Davion T, Lescanne-Darchis I, Maunoury V, et al. Hyperplastic gastric polyposis and familial colonic adenomas. Apropos of a case. *Gastroenterol Clin Biol.* 1996;20:298–302.
268. Cronkhite LW Jr, Canada WJ. Generalized gastrointestinal polyposis; an unusual syndrome of polyposis, pigmentation, alopecia and onychotrophia. *N Engl J Med.* 1955;252:1011–1015.
269. Daniel ES, Ludwig SL, Lewin KJ, et al. The Cronkhite-Canada Syndrome. An analysis of clinical and pathologic features and therapy in 55 patients. *Medicine (Baltimore).* 1982;61:293–309.
270. Yokoyama A, Yamashita H, Moriuchi A, et al. Chronkheit-Canada syndrome associated with adenosquamous carcinoma in gastric polyps. Report of a an autopsy case. *Stomach Intest.* 1983;18:981–990.
271. Sagara K, Fujiyama S, Kamuro Y, et al. Cronkhite-canada syndrome associated with gastric cancer: report of a case. *Gastroenterol Jpn.* 1983;18:260–266.
272. Domellof L, Eriksson S, Helander HF, et al. Lipid islands in the gastric mucosa after resection for benign ulcer disease. *Gastroenterology.* 1977;72:14–18.
273. Hori S, Tsutsumi Y. *Helicobacter pylori* infection in gastric xanthomas: immunohistochemical analysis of 145 lesions. *Pathol Int.* 1996;46:589–593.
274. Carfagna G, Pilato FP, Bordi C, et al. Solitary polypoid hamartoma of the oxyntic mucosa of the stomach. *Pathol Res Pract.* 1987;182:326–330.
275. Itoh K, Tsuchigame T, Matsukawa T, et al. Unusual gastric polyp showing submucosal proliferation of glands: case report and literature review. *J Gastroenterol.* 1998;33: 720–723.
276. Koga S, Watanabe H, Enjoji M. Stomal polypoid hypertrophic gastritis: a polypoid gastric lesion at gastroenterostomy site. *Cancer.* 1979;43:647–657.
277. Kondo K. Duodenogastric reflux and gastric stump carcinoma. *Gastric Cancer.* 2002;5:16–22.
278. Owen D, Kelly J. *Reflux Gastritis. Atlas of Gastrointesitnal Pathology.* Philadelphia, PA: W.B. Saunders; 1994:36–37.
279. Franzin G, Novelli P. Gastritis cystica profunda. *Histopathology.* 1981;5:535–547.
280. Rubio CA, Kato Y, Sugano H, et al. The intramucosal cysts of the stomach. VII: a pathway of gastric carcinogenesis? *J Surg Oncol.* 1986;32:214–219.
281. Rubio CA, Serck-Hanssen A. Ciliated metaplasia in the gastric mucosa. II. In a European patient with gastric carcinoma. *Pathol Res Pract.* 1986;181:382–384.
282. Yamagiwa H, Matsuzaki O, Ishihara A, et al. Heterotopic gastric glands in the submucosa of the stomach. *Acta Pathol Jpn.* 1979;29:347–350.
283. Ikeno T, Ota H, Sugiyama A, et al. *Helicobacter pylori*-induced chronic active gastritis, intestinal metaplasia, and gastric ulcer in Mongolian gerbils. *Am J Pathol.* 1999;154: 951–960.
284. Iwanaga T, Koyama H, Takahashi Y, et al. Diffuse submucosal cysts and carcinoma of the stomach. *Cancer.* 1975;36:606–614.
285. Zarling EJ. Gastric adenomyoma with coincidental pancreatic rest: a case report. *Gastrointest Endosc.* 1981;27: 175–177.
286. Al Jitawi SA, Hiarat AM, Al-Majali SH. Diffuse myoepithelial hamartoma of the duodenum associated with adenocarcinoma. *Clin Oncol.* 1984;10:289–293.
287. Tanimura A, Yamamoto H, Shibata H, et al. Carcinoma in heterotopic gastric pancreas. *Acta Pathol Jpn.* 1979;29: 251–257.
288. Nickels J, Laasonen E. Pancreatic heterotopia. *Duodecim.* 1970;86:133–140.
289. Lasser A, Koufman WB. Adenomyoma of the stomach. *Am J Dig Dis.* 1977;22:965–969.
290. Johnson CD, Bynum TE. Brunner gland heterotopia presenting as gastric antral polyps. *Gastrointest Endosc.* 1976;22:210–211.
291. Jacob CO, Batt L, Horovitz A, et al. Myoepithelial hamartoma of Brunner's gland in the stomach. *Gastrointest Endosc.* 1982;28:48–49.
292. Hamanaka H, Gotoda T. EMR for early esophageal cancer. *Pathol Clin Med.* 2003;21:1086–1091.

Index

Pages in italic refer to figures
Pages in italic followed by "t" refer to tables

A

Abdominal cocoon, 918–919
Abdominal colon tumor, 211
Abdominothoracic dorsal enteric diverticula, 913
Aberrant crypt foci, 1468–1469
Abetalipoproteinemia
　apoprotein B deficiency, 971
　pathogenesis, 971
　pathology, 971, 971–972
Abnormal deposits
　barium granuloma, 1182, 1183
　mercury, 1183
　oleogranulomas (paraffinomas), 1182–1183
　radiologic masses, baroliths, and acute appendicitis, 1183
Abscesses
　and appendiceal stump complications, 818, 819
　hepatic, 817
　periappendiceal, 816–817
Acanthosis, 1564, 1564
Acanthosis nigricans, 399
Acetyl cholinesterase stains, 269, 271
Achalasia/cardiospasm
　barium examination, 248
　gross appearance, 247, 248
　histology, 247–248, 248
　prevalence, 246–247
　secondary, 248–249
Acid dumping, 959–960, 960, 961
Acid secretion, in stomach, 564, 566
Acquired aganglionosis, 247
Acquired esophageal stenosis/stricture. see Esophageal webs and rings
Acquired immunodeficiency syndrome (AIDS), 167–168
　enteropathy, 112, 112
　GI complications, 110
　　chronic diarrhea, 111
　　highly active antiretroviral therapy, 111
　　infections, 113, 113t
　　neoplasms, 113–115, 115
　　severity and duration of symptoms, 111–112
　with giardiasis, 113
　infection identification, pathologist role, 110–111
　Kaposi's sarcoma, 167
　　clinical features, 113
　　pathology, 113–114, 114
　　rectum, 114
　　therapy, 114
　lymphoma
　　Hodgkin's lymphomas, 115
　　non-Hodgkin's lymphomas, 114, 115

pathogenesis and clinical features, 111–113, 112
and small bowel mucosal disease, 957
surveillance, 111
Acquired jejunal diverticulosis, 276
Acquired visceral neuropathies
　with Chagas' disease
　　causes, 274–275
　　differential diagnosis, 275
　　gross appearance, 275
　　histology, 275
　gastrointestinal hemorrhage, 275
　inflammatory visceral neuropathy, 274
　miscellaneous visceral neuropathies, 275
　paraneoplastic neuropathy, 275
　toxic/drug-induced visceral neuropathy, 274
Acrodermatitis enteropathica, 960
Acromegaly, 389
Actinomyces
　A. israelii, 1271–1272, 1272
　characteristics, 1271–1272, 1272
　diagnosis, 1271–1272, 1272
　Rhodococcus equi/Corynebacterium equi, 1272–1273
　sulfur granules, 1271, 1272
Actinomycosis, 822
Acute appendicitis. see Appendicitis
Acute enteritis, 820
Acute esophageal necrosis, 439
Acute HIV infection, 486–487
Acute infectious/self-limited colitis and proctitis
　and biopsy diagnosis, 1220–1221, 1220–1222, 1223
　causes, 1226–1227
　diagnosis, 1228
　gross and endoscopic appearances, 1227
　histology, 1227–1228
　iatrogenic and drug-associated inflammatory changes, 1156, 1157
　inflammatory bowel disease exacerbations, 1227
　pathogenesis and clinical features, 1227
Acute intestinal pseudoobstruction, 252
Acute mesenteric ischemia
　causes of, 35, 37t
　coagulation disorders, 35
　diagnosis, 37
　mortality, 37–38
　symptoms and signs of, 37
Acute necrotizing and esophagitis, 491
Acute radiation reaction, 969–970, 970
Acute renal failure, 390
Acute terminal ileitis, 1243, 1244
Adenoacanthoma, 533–534

Adenocarcinoid. see Goblet cell carcinoma (GCC)
Adenocarcinoma, 175
　adenoacanthoma, 533–534
　adenoid cystic carcinoma, 532
　adenosquamous carcinoma, 533–534
　in anal canal, 1577–1579, 1578
　choriocarcinoma, 534
　comparative survival, 849t, 864
　composite, 753, 754
　differential diagnosis and clinical implications
　　bizarre undifferentiated cells, 758, 758
　　early gastric cancer, 757
　　granular cell tumors, 758
　　histiocytic lesions, distinction from, 757
　　lymphoma, 757–758
　　metastatic carcinoma, 758
　　neuroendocrine (NET–carcinoid) tumors, 758
　　radiation therapy and chemotherapy, 758–759
　of esophagus
　　biopsy diagnosis of, 534–536, 534–544, 539–544
　　definition, 525
　extremely well-differentiated, 744, 747, 749–752
　grading appendiceal carcinomas, 853, 854, 856, 857
　growth pattern, 757
　hepatoid adenocarcinoma, 534
　in heterotopic gastric mucosa, 532, 533
　large bowel-type carcinoma, 851, 853, 854, 855–856
　in Meckel's diverticulum, 918, 918
　moderately well-differentiated, 734
　mucinous differentiation, 735
　mucoepidermoid carcinoma, 532
　papillary differentiated, 735
　poorly differentiated, 734–735
　stomach
　　biopsy diagnosis, 763–764
　　clinical implications, 757–759
　　cytology, 764
　　differential diagnosis, 757
　　expanding type, 734
　　fundic gland type, 744, 745–747
　　gastric specimens handling, 764t, 765–765, 765t
　　growth pattern, 757
　　infiltrative type, 734
　　prognostic factors, 759–763, 760t–762t
　　spread, 759
　TNM staging, 857
　tubular, 734, 735–736
　unusual variants of, 532–534, 533

I-1

Adenocarcinoma (*Continued*)
  variants, 851
  well-differentiated, 734, *735–736*
Adenoid cystic carcinoma, 1579
Adenoma-carcinoma/dysplasia-carcinoma sequence
  continued growth, 1467–1468
  critical mass and invasion, 1468
  development, 1467
  molecular abnormalities, 1466–1467
  progression, 1466
Adenomas
  in anal canal, *1577*, 1577–1579
  and anal gland hidrocystoma, 1577
  Brunner's gland, 1331–1333, *1331–1333*
  and colorectal carcinoma, *1460*
  columnar cells, 215–216, *216*
  columnar dysplasias, 1579
  composite, 216–217, *217*, 1503–1504, *1506*
  diminutive, 1386
  with endocrine cell nests/neoplasm, 1389, *1390*
  endocrine cells, 215–216, *216*
  flat and depressed, *1388*, 1388–1389
  foveolar, 714, *717–719*
  fundic gland, 714–715, *747–748*
  in gastric epithelial polyps and tumors
    classification, 707–720
    definition, 706
    differential diagnosis, 721–723
    grading, 719, 721
    phenotypic expression, 707
    terminology, 706–707
  gastric-type adenomas, 708, *711*, *712*
  growth and development, 1466–1470
  high-grade adenoma, 719, 721, *722*
  HNPCC, 1452
  intestinal-type adenomas
    characteristics, 708, *709*, *710*
    clinical features, 707–708
    implications, 708
    pathologic findings, 708
  large bowel
    age, sex, and distribution, 1375–1376
    definition, 1375
    diminutive polyps, 1376
    gross and endoscopic appearances, 1377, *1378t*, *1381*
    histology, 1377, *1380–1385*, 1381, 1384
    natural history, 1376
    synchronous and metachronous, 1376
    tubular adenoma, 1385
    tubular vs. villous patterns, 1384–1385
    tubulovillous adenoma, 1385–1386
    villous adenoma, 1385
  low-grade adenoma, 719, *721*
  microscopic, 1386
  papillary, 1337
  pituitary, 389
  pyloric gland, 714, *715–716*
  sessile serrated polyps/adenoma, 1355, 1358–1359, *1358–1360*
  small bowel
    clinical features, 1336–1337
    gross and endoscopic appearances, 1337, *1337*, *1338*
    histology, 1338–1339, *1339*
    management, 1339–1340
  stomach
    classification, 707–720
    definition, 706
    differential diagnosis, 721–723
    grading, 719, 721
    phenotypic expression, 707
    terminology, 706–707
  surface colorectal-type, *1577*, 1577
  traditional serrated
    clinical features, 1363
    differential diagnosis, 1368–1369, 1371–1372, *1371–1373*
    gross and endoscopic features, 1363
    histology, 1363–1364, *1364–1367*
    immunophenotype and molecular pathology, 1365–1368, *1366–1367*, *1368t*
    interobserver variability, 1368
    treatment and follow-up, 1373, 1375
  tumors of, appendix
    diffuse mucosal hyperplasia, 832, *834*, 835, 836
    growth patterns, 830
    hyperplastic polyps, *835*, 836
    polyps with dysplasia, *837*, 838
    serrated hyperplasia and polyps, *830t*, *832t*, 833
    sessile serrated polyps, 836, *837*, 838
    tubular and tubulovillous, 830–831, *831*
    villous, *831*, 832
Adenomyoma, 1335, *1336*
Adenosine monophosphate (AMP), 1229
Adenosquamous carcinoma, 741–742
Adenoviruses
  enteric, 1287–1288, *1287–1288*
  infection, and acute appendicities, 819, *819*
Adhesions, 62
Adipocytic lesions
  angiolipoma, 343
  atypical lipoma, 342–343
  fatty tumors, differential diagnosis of, 344
  lipohyperplasia, of ileocecal valve, 340–341, *341*
  lipomatous polyposis and epiploic lipomatosis, 343, *343*
  liposarcoma, 343–344
  submucosal lipoma, 341–342, *342*
Adrenal gland, 388
Adult pyloric stenosis, 251
Advanced gastric cancer, 761
Aeromonas
  A. hydrophila, 1242–1243
  A. shigelloides, 1243
African visceral myopathy, 261
Aganglionic segment of colon, 268, *269*
Agenesis, of appendix, 801
Agranulocytic appendicitis, 813, *814*
AIG. see Autoimmune gastritis (AIG)
Alcohol
  and esophageal squamous cell carcinoma, 507
  laxatives, 1163
Allergic disorders, selective IgA deficiency, 101
Allergic granulomatous angiitis, 54, *55*, *56*
Allergies, food hypersensitivity, 952
Allografts, *111t*
Alpha-heavy chain disease, 400
Aluminum silicate titanium-containing pigment in terminal ileum, 1180
Amelanotic spindled cell melanomas, 360
American trypanosomiasis. see Chagas' disease
Amines, biogenic, 191
Amoebic infection
  ameboma (amoebic pseudotumor), 1294
  complications, 1293
  diagnosis and treatment, 1294
  epidemiology, 1289–1290
  fulminant colitis, 1294
  gross and endoscopic pathology, 1290–1291, *1291*
  histology, 1291, *1292–1293*, 1293
  pathogenesis and clinical features, 1290
Amoebic pseudotumor, 1294
AMP. see Adenosine monophosphate (AMP)
Amyloid deposition, gastrointestinal involvement
  classification, 403–404
  clinical features, 404–405, *405*
  clinical implications, 405
  diagnosis, 405
  histologic features, *404*, 405
  properties, 403–404
Amyloidosis
  and hypothyroidism, 276
  and small bowel, normal villous architecture of, 972
Anal canal
  anorectal anomalies, classification of, *1558t*
  blood supply, 1554, *1555*, *1556*
  definitions and associated problems, 1547, *1548–1549*, *1549–1552*, *1550–1552*
  developmental abnormalities, 1557–1558, *1558t*
  hemorrhoids
    clinical features, 1559, *1560*
    description, *1558*, 1558–1559
    hemorrhoidectomy specimens dealing, 1559–1560
    histologic features, 1559, *1560*
    pathogenesis, 1559
  Hirschsprung's disease, 1557
  inflammatory cloacogenic polyps, 1562–1563, *1563*
  inflammatory lesions
    fissures and fistulae, 1560–1561, *1562*
    granuloma inguinale, 1562
    lymphogranuloma venereum, 1562
    syphilis, *1561*, 1561–1562
    viral infections, 1561
  lesions of
    basal cell carcinoma, 1581
    bowenoid papulosis, 1581
    Bowen's disease, 1581
    hidradenitis suppurativa, 1582

invasive squamous cell carcinoma, 1581
keratoacanthoma, 1581
lichen sclerosus, 1582
Paget's disease, 1581–1582, *1582*
lymphatic supply, 1554
microscopic anatomy
anal transition zone, *1550–1551*, 1557
columnar zone, *1550–1549*, 1554, 1557
ducts and glands, *1555*, 1557
perianal skin, *1553*, 1557
squamous zone, *1552*, 1557
musculature, *1548*, *1553*, 1554
nerves and biopsy implications, 1557
perianal hematoma, 1560
prolapse, 1562–1563, *1563*
surface anatomy, *1548–1549*, *1552*, *1553*, 1554
tags of, 1563, *1563*
tumors of
adenocarcinoma, 1577–1579, *1578*
adenoid cystic carcinoma, 1579
adenomas, *1577*, 1577–1579
anal gland carcinoma, 1579
anal gland hidrocystoma, 1577
anal intraepithelial neoplasia, 1567–1569, *1568–1569*, *1570*
Bowen's disease, 1569–1570
condyloma acuminatum, 1564–1565, *1565*, *1566*
dysplasias, 1567, *1568–1569*
epithelial hyperplasia without dysplasia, *1564*, 1564
invasive squamous cell carcinoma, 1570–1576, *1572*, *1573*, *1574*, *1576*
malignant melanoma, 1579–1580, *1580*
mesenchymal, 1580
mucoepidermoid carcinoma, 1579
small cell carcinoma, 1579
surface colorectal-type adenomas, *1577*, 1577
unusual adenoma-like columnar dysplasias, 1579
verrucous carcinoma, 1565, *1566*, 1567
Anal disease, 1061–1063, *1063*, *1064*
Anal gland carcinoma, 1579
Anal gland hidrocystoma, 1577
Anal intraepithelial neoplasia (AIN)
biomarkers in, 1567–1569
and Bowen's disease of perianal skin, 1567, *1568–1569*
and dysplasias, *1564*, 1567
invasive squamous cell carcinoma, 1571, 1575–1576, *1576*
minor surgical specimens, 1569
Anal tags, 1563, *1563*
Anal transition zone (ATZ), 1549–1551, *1550–1551*, 1557
Anal tumors, biopsy technique, 24
Anal/perianal symptoms, 1218
Anaphylactoid purpura, 55–56, *58*
Anaplastic large-cell lymphoma, 173
ANCAs. *see* Antineutrophil cytoplasmic antibodies (ANCAs)
Ancylostomiasis, 1300, *1300*

Anemia, pernicious, 199
autoimmune gastritis, 635
H. pylori–related chronic atrophic gastritis, 728
predominant antibody defects, 728
selective IgA deficiency, 101
Angiitis, 54, *55*, *56*
Angiodysplasia, 73–74. *see also* Vascular ectasia
Angiofollicular hyperplasia, 132–133
Angiography, ischemia following, 1152–1153
Angioimmunoblastic lymphadenopathy, 175–176
Angiolipoma, 343
Angioma, 73
Angiomyolipoma, 354
Angiosarcoma, *73t*, 345, *346*, 347
Angiostrongylus costaricensis, 1300–1301
Angle of His, 422
Anisakiasis, 660, *661*, *1301*, 1301–1302
Anorectal anomalies, classification of, *1558t*
Antibiotic-associated colitis, 1255
Anticoagulant-associated hemorrhage, 1153, *1153*
Anticoagulants, 35, 65, 66
Antineoplastic agents, 66
Antineutrophil cytoplasmic antibodies (ANCAs)
Churg-Strauss syndrome, 54, *55*, *56*
microscopic polyarteritis nodosa, 54–55, *57*, *58*
Wegener's granulomatosis, 53
Antiretroviral therapies, 114
Antral gland of stomach, *561*, 563
Antral mucosa, of stomach, 560, *561*, *562*, *562*, 563
Antrum, in stomach, 554, *554*
Anus, GI problem in AIDS patients, 113. *see also* Anal canal
Apc-β-catenin gene complex, 1462–1463
Apoptotic bodies, 108
Appendectomy, 1007–1008
Appendicitis
appendiceal stump complications
abscess formation, 818, *819*
endoscopic excision, 818
hemorrhage, 818
intussusception, 818
polyps, 818–819
recurrent, 817
xanthogranulomatous and malacoplakia, 818, *819*
clinical features, 806–808, *807*
complications of
appendiceal epithelium, 815–816, *816*
escaped fecalith, 817
fistula, 817
hepatic abscess formation, 817
multiple lumina formation, 817
perforation, 815
periappendiceal abscesses and productive periappendiceal fibrosis, 816–817
suppuration and suppurative pyelophlebitis, 817
Crohn's disease, 824–828, *825*, *826*, *827*, *828*

definition, 806
granulomatous appendicitis, 824–828, *825*, *826*, *827*, *828*
gross appearance, 808, *809*
histology, 808–809, *810*, *811*
infections
bacterial, 820–823, *821*, *822*
parasites, *823*, 823–824
viral, 819–820, *820*
issues with, 814–815
resolution, 811–812, *812*
terminology, 812–814, *813*, *814*
Appendix
acquired structural abnormalities
diverticula, 803–805, *804–805*
intussusception, 805–806
torsion and volvulus, 805
adenocarcinomas
grading appendiceal carcinomas, 853, 854, 856, 857
large bowel-type carcinoma, 851, 853, *854*, 855–856
TNM staging, 857
variants, 851
anatomy, normal, *797*, 797–798, *798*
biopsy technique, 24
combined tumors, 864, *865–866*
congenital structural abnormalities
agenesis, 801
duplication, 801–802, *802–803*, *802t*
fistula, 803
helicus and horseshoe, 803
heterotopic tissue, 803
Crohn's disease, 824–828, *825*, *826*, *827*, *828*
and cystic fibrosis, 828, *829*
dilated appendices, 801
epithelium of, 798
function of, 797
goblet cell carcinoma
clinical features, 859
gross pathology, 859
histology, *858–859*, 859–860
immunohistochemistry, 860
poorly differentiated, 860, *861*, *862*
prognosis and treatment, 864
signet ring carcinoma, 862, *862–863*, 864
terminology and histogenesis, 857, *858–859*, 859
granulomatous appendicitis, 824–828, *825*, *826*, *827*, *828*
and Hirschsprung's disease, 828
histology, *798*, 798–799, *799*, *800*
iatrogenic use of, 806
lamina propria of, 798, *799*
and malacoplakia, 827
metastatic disease involving, 866, 868
mucinous neoplasms
clinical features, 841
gross appearances, 841, *841*, *842*
histology, 841–843, *843*, *844*, *845*, 845
incidence, 841
issues with, 845–849, *846*
molecular pathology and immunohistochemistry, 845
terminology, 839–840, *840t*

Appendix (Continued)
   mucosa of, 798, *798*
   obstruction of, 807–808
   other rare tumors and lesions, 864–866, 866–868
   porcelain, 841
   practical approach and issues
      cystadenomas and cystadenocarcinomas, 839
      hybrid lesions, 839
      mucocele, 839
      terminology and differential diagnosis, 838–839
   pseudomyxoma peritonei
      gross appearances, 849–850
      microscopic appearance, 850
      pathology of cytoreduction, 850
      terminology and classification, 849, *849t*
   routine pathologic examination, 799–801
   submucosa of, 799
   tumors of
      adenomas, 830–838
      large bowel tumors, 828–830
      polyps and other benign lesions, 830, *830t, 831*
   variants of, *813*, 813–814, *814*
Appendix helicus, 803
APUD system, 190–192
Arc of Riolan, 32
Argentaffin cells, 190, 889
Argyrophil cells, 190
Arterial spasm
   hypotensive and hypovolemic agents, 1155
   vasopressin, 1155
Arterial supply
   in anal canal, 1554, *1555, 1556*
   muscularis mucosae, 30
   stomach of, 555
Arterial/venous thrombosis
   drug-induced vasculitis, 1153–1155, *1154*
   estrogen and oral contraceptives, 1153–1155, *1154*
   oral contraceptive and IBD, 1155
Arteriovenous malformations (AVMs), 73, 77, 78, *78*
Arteritis, 828, *828*
   giant cell, 51–52
   polyarteritis nodosa, 49, *49t, 50t,* 53, 53–55, *57, 58*
   Takayasu, 51–52
Arthritis, rheumatoid
   and connective tissue disorders, 383
   vasculitis, 54, *57*
Ascariasis (round worm), 1302
Ascaris lumbricoides infection with AIDS, 113
Aspergillosis, 1310, *1311*, 1312
Aspergillus, 489
Ataxia telangiectasia, 165, 167
   DiGeorge's syndrome, 105
   selective IgA deficiency, 101
Atherosclerosis, 33, 38, 60
Atresia
   bowel structures
      associations, 910
      classification of, 909–910, *910t*
      etiology, 909
      gross appearance, 909–910
      pathogenesis, 910
      pathology, 910, *911*
   esophageal, 429–430, *430, 430t*
Atrophic gastritis, *605*, 605–606
   primary immunodeficiency disorders, 100
   staging
      Baylor system, 613, *614*
      endoscopic screening, 612
      Erasmus index, 613–614
      gastritis risk index, 612–613
      histopathology staging systems, 612
      OLGA system, 613, *613t*
      serology, 612
Atypical lipoma, 342–343
Auerbach's myenteric plexus, 242, *242*
Autofluorescence imaging (AFI), 8
Autoimmune enteropathy (AIE)
   clinical features, 951
   description, 949, 950
   pathogenesis, 951
   pathology, 951, *952*
   prognosis, 951–952
   treatment, 951–952
Autoimmune gastritis (AIG), 199–202, *200*
   clinical features, 637–638
   pathogenesis, 635
   pathology, 638–643
   subtypes, 636–637
Autoimmune hepatitis, 393
Autoimmune polyendocrinopathy syndrome type 1, 389–390
Autoimmune thyroid disease, 385

B

Bacteria
   Actinomyces, 1271–1272, *1272*
   actinomycosis, 822
   acute enteritis, 820
   antibiotic-associated colitis, 1255
   bacterial flora, 1214
   Brucella, 1271
   Campylobacter
      clinical and endoscopic features, 1240
      gross and endoscopic findings, 1240
      histology, 1241, *1241*
      pathogenesis, 1240
   Chlamydia, 1273–1274, *1274–1275*
   Chlamydial proctitis, 1273–1274, *1274–1275*
   Clostridium botulinum, 1256, 1257–1258
   Clostridium difficile
      clinical features, 1252
      complications, 1254–1255
      description, 1250
      diagnosis and differential diagnosis, 1254
      epidemiology, 1250–1251
      gross and endoscopic appearances, 1252, *1253*, 1254
      histology, *1253*, 1254
      and inflammatory bowel disease, 1255
      pathogenesis, 1251–1252
      Pseudomembranous enteritis, 1254
      treatment, 1254–1255
   Clostridium perfringens
      description, 1255
      enteritis necroticans, 1255–1256, *1256–1257*
   Escherichia coli
      characteristics, 1229
      clinical features, 1232
      enteroadherent *E. coli* (EAEC)/ diffusely adherent or enteroadherent, 1230–1231, *1232*
      enterohemorrhagic *E. coli* (EHEC), 1231–1232
      enteroinvasive *E. coli* (EIEC), 1230
      enteropathogenic *E. coli* (EPEC), 1230, *1232*
      enterotoxigenic *E. coli* (ETEC), 1230
      gross and endoscopic appearances, 1232, *1233*
      hemolytic uremic syndrome, 1234
      histology, 1232, *1233*, 1234
      pathotypes, *1230t*
      thrombotic thrombocytopenic purpura, 1234
      verotoxin, 1234
   and esophagitis, 489
   gonococcal proctitis, 1266, 1266–1267
   granuloma inguinale, 1249, *1250*
   and immunohistochemical applications in gastrointestinal disorders, 21
   lymphogranuloma venereum, 1273
   Mycobacterium avium - intracellulare
      description, 1263, 1264
      differential diagnosis, 1264, 1266
      pathology, 1264, *1264–1265*
   Mycobacterium tuberculosis
      description, 1260
      gross and endoscopic findings, 1261, *1261*
      histology and differential diagnosis, *1261*, 1261–1263
      pathogenesis and clinical features, 1260–1261
   neutropenic enterocolitis/typhlitis, 1257–1258, *1259*
   phlegmonous enterocolitis, 1258
   Rhodococcus equi, 1272–1273
   rickettsial disease, 1274–1275
   Salmonella
      characteristics, 1235–1236
      classification, 1236–1237
      S. enterocolitis, 1237–1238
      typhoid fever, 1238–1240, *1239*
   Shigella
      clinical features, 1235
      diagnosis, 1235
      gross and endoscopic appearances, 1235
      histology, 1235, *1236*
      pathogenesis, 1234–1235
      treatment, 1235
   spirochetes, *1267–1268, 1267–1271, 1270–1271*
   spirochetosis, 821, *821*
   tuberculosis and mycobacterial infection, 821–822
   Vibrios
      clinical features, 1228

diagnosis, 1229
epidemiology, 1228
pathogenesis, 1228–1229
pathology, 1229
treatment and follow-up, 1229
Whipple's disease, 822–823
Yersinia, 821, *822*
description, 1243–1244
endoscopic findings, 1245, *1246*, *1247*
gross pathology, 1245
histology, 1245, *1246*, *1247*, 1247–1248
pathogenesis and clinical features, 1244–1245
Y. pseudotuberculosis, *1248*, 1248–1249, *1249*
Bacterial overgrowth syndrome, 959, *959*
Balantidium coli, 1293, 1294, *1295*
Balloon mesh cytology, 7, *7*
Barium granuloma, 1182, *1183*
Barrett's carcinoma, *217*
Barrett's esophagus
adenocarcinoma in
adenoacanthoma, 533–534
adenoid cystic carcinoma, 532
adenosquamous carcinoma, 533–534
and aneuploidy, 528
back-to-back appearance, 536, *538*
basal cell hyperplasia, 535
biopsy diagnosis of, 534–536, *534–544*, 539–544
choriocarcinoma, 534
clinical features, 529
and dysplasia, 526–527
endoscopic ablation techniques, 530–531
endoscopic appearance, *529*, 529–530
endoscopic mucosal resection, 531, *531*
granulation tissue, 535–536, *537*
gross appearance, *529*, 529–530
hepatoid adenocarcinoma, 534
in heterotopic gastric mucosa, 532, *533*
microscopic appearance, 530, *530*
mucoepidermoid carcinoma, 532
pathogenesis, 525–526
prognosis, 531–532
and radiation therapy, 535
regenerated glands, 536, *538*
risk of, 525–526
short segment, 528, *528*
squamous mucosa, 535, *536*, *537*
of submucosa, 532–533
unusual variants of, 532–534, *533*
ancillary techniques, 484
biopsies postablation, 476, *476*
carcinoma
goblet cells, 472–473
intramucosal, *479*, 482–483
invasive, 483
chromoendoscopy, 8–9
definition, 468–469, 471
diagnosis, 469–471, *470–472*, 476–479
dysplasia
associated with adenocarcinoma, 526–527
diagnosis, 479
high grade, 482
indefinite for, 479–480

inter- and (intra) observer variability, 483–484
low-grade, *477*, *478*, 480–481, *482*
second opinion need, 483–484
endoscopic grading, 474
epidemiology and pathophysiology, 473–474
histology, *474*, 474–476, *475*
morphologic development, 474
mucosal types encounter, 476–477
neoplasia associated with, 477–479, *477–480*
postendoscopic resection, 476, *476*
risk, of carcinoma, 473
specimen handling, 8–9
Basal cell
carcinoma, 1581
in esophagus, 425
Basaloid squamous cell carcinoma, *524*, 525
β-catenin, 333
B-cell disorders, 102
Beef tapeworm, 1307, *1307*. see also *Taenia saginata*
Behçet's disease, 57, 60, 497
connective tissue disorder, 383, 384
IBD
clinical features, 1086–1087
epidemiology, 1086–1088, *1087*
pathology, *1087*, 1087–1088
Benign disorders involving histiocytes
associated with drug use
gross and endoscopic appearances, 1172–1173
histology, 1173, *1173*
iron-containing macrophages, 1171–1172, *1173*
pseudomelanosis coli (melanosis coli), 1172, *1175–1176*
associated with infections
malakoplakia and xanthogranulomatous inflammation, 1174–1176, *1176–1177*, 1178
Mycobacterium avium-intracellulare, 1173
Whipple's disease, 1173
associated with miscellaneous disorder
iron-containing macrophages, 1179, *1179t*
muciphages, 1179–1180, *1181–1182*
xanthoma/xanthelasma, 1179–1180, *1182*
associated with storage disease, 1178, *1178t*, *1179t*
black pigments in terminal ileum and large bowel
aluminum silicate titanium-containing pigment in, 1180
injected India ink as a tattoo, 1180
normal histiocytes, 1171, *1172*, *1172t*
Benign fibroblastic polyp, *326*
Benign mucous membrane pemphigoid, 397
Benign unclassifiable mucosal bumps (BUMPS), 1412, *1413*, *1414*, 1415
Bezoar formation, 386, *386*
BI/NAP1/027, 1251
Biopsy
of anal canal, 1574–1575

cutting process, 13, *13*, 15, *15*
dissection
depth of tumor penetration, 25
incidental findings, 26
lymph node, 25
resected margins sections of, 26
of tumors, 25
venous invasion by tumor, 25–26
electrocautery snare
endoscopic mucosal resection, 5
endoscopic submucosal dissection, 5, 6
shave biopsy technique, 5
snare polypectomy, 4, *4*
snare polypectomy after submucosal injection, 4–5
submucosal lesions, 5
embedding process, 13–14, *14*
endoscopic findings, description, 16
fine-needle aspirates, 6, *7*
forceps, pinch
cold biopsies, 3
en face, 3, *3*
hinged jaws, 2, 3
hot biopsy technique, 3
jumbo, 2, 3
in pediatrics, 2, 3
size and shape, 2, 3
skinny, 2, 3
turn-and-suction biopsy technique, 3
frozen sections, 23
guide to sites for taking, *12t*
insufflation with fixative, 24–25
interpretation, technical problems
intraepithelial spaces, 20, *20*
mucosal hemorrhage and edema, 18–19
pseudoerosions, 19, *19*
irradiated tumors, 1574–1575
microscopic examination approach, 17–18
mucosal, 1
pathologist's interpretation
mild nonspecific chronic inflammation, 20–21
review, 17
photography, 23
polyps handling, 11–12
processing techniques
embedding on edge, 13
multiple serial sections, 15
poor, *13*
sectioning specimens, 13
small-piece histology, *2t*
quality improvement, 1
rectal, 15, 19
reexamination, fixed specimen, 25
routine fixation, 12
special fixatives
immunohistochemical applications, gastrointestinal disorders, 21
immunohistochemical stains, 21
infections, *18t*, 22–23
tuberculosis and *Mycobacterium avium-intracellulare*, 23
specimen
handling, 11

Biopsy (*Continued*)
  location, 16
  number, 16–17
  opening, 23–24
  size, 16–17
  surgically resected, 23
  transport, 6
storage conditions, 21–23
systematic approach, specimen interpretation, 18, *18t*
tissue processing technique, 12–13, *13*
Biopsy, diagnosis
  of adenocarcinoma, esophageal, 534–536, *534–544*, 539–544
  and enteric infections
    acute infectious (self-limited) colitis, 1220, *1220–1222*, 1222
    cholera, 1220
    cytopathic changes/detection of, *1217t*, 1222
    electron microscopy, 1223
    histochemical stains, 1222–1223, *1223t*
    histologic pattern, 1222
    mild acute/chronic inflammation, 1222
    molecular tests, 1223, *1223t*
  gastric, 69, 75
  of gastric polyps and tumors, 763–764
  GI bleeding, 64, *64*
  ischemic colitis, 47, 60
  mucosal, 54, *56, 57*, 74, 78
  polypoid neural lesions, 327–328
  specimens, 80
  spindle cell carcinoma, 522
Biphasic epithelial–mesenchymal esions
  gastroblastoma, 357, *358, 359*, 359
  spindle cell carcinoma/carcinosarcoma, 356–357, *356–357*
  synovial sarcoma, 354–356, *355*
Black esophagus, 437, 439, 491
Blastocystis hominis, 1295
  infection with AIDS, 113
Blood supply
  in anal canal, 1554, *1555, 1556*
  bowel, large and small, 900
  in esophagus, 29, 423
  small and large intestine, 32, *32, 33*
  in stomach, 30, *30*, 555
Blood vessels, in stomach
  arterial supply, 555
  venous drainage, 555
Bloodborne metastases, 759
Blue rubber-bleb nevus syndrome, *73t*
Blunt trauma, 38, 67
Bochdalek hernias, 907
Boerhaave's syndrome, 435, *435t*
Bone marrow transplantation
  characteristics, 106
  chronic GVHD, 110
  GI infections, *107t*
  graft versus host disease
    clinical presentation, 107–108
    diagnosis, 110
    gross appearance, 108
    histology, 108, *109*
    pathogenesis, 107
  infections, 106
  parasitic infestations, *107t*
  transplantation regimen, 106
Botulism, 1256
Bouin's solution, fixative, 12
Bowel, large and small. *see also* Large intestine; Small intestine; specific diseases of
  atresia
    associations, 910
    classification of, 909–910, *910t*
    etiology, 909
    gross appearance, 909–910
    pathogenesis, 910
    pathology, 910, *911*
  bone marrow transplantation, GVHD, 108, *109*
  complications of
    abdominal cocoon, 918–919
    abdominothoracic dorsal enteric diverticula, 913
    hemorrhage and infarction, 913
    infarcted appendix epiploica-peritoneal mouse, 919
    malignancy, 913
    Meckel's diverticulum, 913–918, *916, 917, 918*
    metabolic diseases, 919
    mucous cast, 918, *918*
    peritoneal encapsulation, 918, *918*
    vascular malformations, 919
  congenital anomalies
    diaphragmatic hernias, 907
    duodenal bands, 908
    fixation, lack of, 905
    gastroschisis, 907
    heterotopia, *904*, 904–905
    intestinal musculature, *908*, 908–909, *909*
    malrotation, 905
    mesenterium ileocolicum commune, 908
    metaplasia, 905, *905*
    Morgagni hernia/Morgagni-Larrey hernia, 907–908
    omphaloceles, 907
    retroperitoneal hernias, 907
    volvulus, 905–906, *906*
  diaphragms, 910–912, *911*
  diverticular disease
    definition, 227
    terminology, 227
  enteric duplications, 912
  mechanical disorders and disorders of propulsion
    cystic fibrosis, 919
    hypoplastic left colon syndrome, 919
    meconium ileus, 919
    megacystis-microcolon-intestinal hypoperistalsis syndrome, 919–920
    neonatal necrotizing enterocolitis, 920–922
    obstruction, 919–920
  simple duplications
    characteristic features, 912
    gross appearance, 912, *913, 914*
    histology, 912–913, *913, 914*
    site, 912
    split notochord theory, 912
  stenoses, 910–912
  structure
    blood vessels, 900
    endocrine cells, *881*, 888–890, *889*
    external appearance, 875–877, *876*
    goblet cells, 890, *890*
    ileocecal valve, 884–885, *885*
    and immune system, 889, 893–895, *894*
    internal appearance, 877–879, *877–879*
    interstitial cells of Cajal, *897*, 897–899, *899*
    kinetics, 891, *892*
    lamina propria, 889, 893–895, *894*
    lymphatics, 900, *900*
    microfold cells, 891
    mucosa, large intestine, *882*, 885–887, *886, 888, 889*
    mucosa, small intestine, 880–884, *880–885*
    muscularis mucosae, 895
    muscularis propria, 895
    myenteric plexus, *896*, 896–897, *897*
    nerve supply, *896*, 896–897, *897*
    paneth cells, *882*, 887–888
    pericrypt fibroblast sheath, 891, 893, *893*
    serosa, 899–900
    stem cells, 891, *892*
    submucosa, *882*, 895, *895*
  webs, 910–912, *911*
Bowenoid papulosis, 1581
Bowen's disease
  in anal canal, 1569–1570
  anal intraepithelial neoplasia, 1567, *1568–1569*
  invasive squamous cell carcinoma, 1571
  lesions of anal canal, 1581
  tumors in, 1569–1570
BRAF mutations, 305
Bronchoesophageal fistula, 430–431
Bronchogenic cysts, 432
Brown bowel syndrome, 498, 973, *974*
Brucella, 1271
Brucellosis, 1271
Brunner's gland
  adenoma, 1331–1333, *1331–1333*
  heterotopia/ nodule, 785, *786*, 787
  nodules and polyps, 1329, 1330, *1330*
Bruton's agammaglobulinemia, 102
Buerger's disease, 52
Bullous disorders, 394, 397
BUMPS. *see* Benign unclassifiable mucosal bumps (BUMPS)
Burkitt's lymphoma
  clinical presentation, 155, *156*
  immunophenotype and molecular genetics, 156
  incidence, 155
  pathology, 155–156, *156*
  prognosis and treatment, 156

C

Calcifying fibrous tumor, 339, *341*
Cameron's ulcer, 468, *468*

Campylobacter, 1242
   C. jejuni, 125, 152
      clinical and endoscopic features, 1240
      gross and endoscopic findings, 1240
      histology, 1241, *1241*
      idiopathic inflammatory bowel disease, 1242
      pathogenesis, 1240
Cancer, inflammatory bowel disease, malignancy in
   anal carcinoma, 1125
   carcinoma after surgery, 1126
   carcinoma complicating ulcerative colitis, 1123–1124
   carcinoma in indeterminate colitis, 1125
   colorectal cancer in colitis, *1120*, 1121–1123, *1122–1124*
   Crohn's disease, 1124–1125
   malignancies, 1125–1126
   molecular pathogenesis of, *1099*, 1099–1101, *1100t*
Candida
   C. albicans, 487
      immunodeficient patients, 115
Candidiasis, 1308
   intestinal host defences, 89
Capillaria philippinensis, *1302*, 1302–1303
Capillariasis, *1302*, 1302–1303
Carcinoid syndrome, 206, 208, 221
Carcinoid tumors, *195*
   classification, 198
   definition of, 194
   duodenum
      gangliocytic paraganglioma, 205
      gastrinomas, 204, *205*
      somatostatinomas, 204, *206*
   glandular pattern, *195*, *206*
   gross examination
      appearance, 196, *197*
      appendectomy, 196, *197*
      dissection recommendations for, 196–197
      polypectomies, 197
      resections, 196
   growth patterns, *195*, *195*, 196
   in Meckel's diverticulum, 917
   metastatic risk for, 196
   midgut, 206–208, *206–208*
   occurrence, 196
   ribbon-like pattern, 221
   in specific sites
      abdominal colon, 211
      appendix, 208–211, *209*, *210*
      cecum/terminal ileum, 208
      duodenum, 204–206, *205*, *206*
      esophagus, 198–199
      ileum, 206–208, *206–208*
      jejunum, 206–208, *206–208*
      rectum, 211–212, *212*
      stomach, 199–204, *199t*, *200–203*
   staging and grading, 197–198
   stomach, *199t*
      type I, 199–202, *200–202*
      type II, 202–203
      type III, 203, *203*
      type IV, 204
   well-differentiated, 194–198

Carcinoids, *849t*, 864
Carcinoma. *see also* Adenoma-carcinoma/ dysplasia-carcinoma; Colorectal carcinoma
   adenoid cystic, 532, 1579
   adenosquamous and squamous cell, 741–742
   anal gland, 1579
   basal cell, 1581
   basaloid squamous cell, 524, 525
   biopsy diagnosis
      error in, causes of, *763t*
      misreading, 763–764, *763t*
      before surgical resection, 763
   brush cytology, 764
   carcinosarcoma, 755–757
   chief cell predominant type, 744, *745–746*
   choriocarcinoma, 742–743, *743*, 1503
   classification
      Lauren classification, *733*, 733–734
      Ming classification, 734, *734*
      Nakamura classification, 734
      WHO histologic classification and grading of gas-tric cancer, 734, *735*
   clear cell, 1500, *1501*, *1501*
   cytology role in, 764
   desmoplastic, *358*
   diffuse-type signet ring, 1496
   in diverticular polyps, 237
   dysplasia/adenomas and, *1424*, 1428–1430
   endocrine, 213–215, *213–215*
   α-fetoprotein-producing gastric, 741, *741*, *742*
   gastric teratoma, 755
   goblet cell, 1497, *1497*
   invasive, 1391
   lymphocytic gastritis, 645–646
   medullary, 389–390
   micropapillary colon, 1497–1499, *1498*
   minimally invasive/superficial carcinoma, 1575
   MLH1-deficient, 1451–1452
   MSI-H, 1492–1493
   mucinous/colloid, 1494–1495, *1496*
   mucoepidermoid, 532, 1579
   mucosal, 511
   neuroendocrine (*see* Endocrine carcinomas)
   nonanal basaloid/cloacogenic, 1502, *1503*
   one-piece and piecemeal EMR, *764t*
   Paneth cell-type, 743
   parietal cell predominant type, 744
   prognosis
      advanced gastric cancer, 761
      early gastric cancer, 759
      factors, 759
      gastric remnant carcinoma, 760–761
      Her2 status, 761
      K-ras status, 761
      lymph node status, 761
      neoadjuvant therapy, 761, *763t*
      nodal metastases risk, 760, *760t*
      tumor grade, 761
   pyloric gland, 747, 749, 752–753
   radiation therapy, 72
   risk factors, gastric
      CIMP-H, 726

      dietary factors, 727
      Epstein-Barr virus, 726
      genetic factors, 727
      Helicobacter pylori infection, 725–726
      hereditary gastric cancer predisposition syndromes, 727–728
      JC virus, 726
      K-ras, 726
      polymorphism in genes, 728
      smoking, 727
   serrated dysplasia and, 755, *756*
   short segment Barrett's esophagus, 528, *528*
   signet-ring cell, 35, 45, 735, 737, *738–740*
   small bowel
      clinical features, 1343
      diagnosis and management, 1348–1349
      gross and endoscopic appearances, 1343–1345, *1344*
      histology, 1345, *1345–1347*
      immunophenotype and molecular pathology, 1347–1348, *1348*
      pathogenesis, 1341, *1342*, *1343*
      staging and prognosis, 1349–1350, *1349t*, *1350t*
      treatment, 1349
   small cell, 522–525, *523*, 1503–1504, *1506*, 1579
   specimen handling and intraoperative evaluation
      endoscopy mucosal/submucosal specimens, 764, *764t*, 765
      polypectomy specimens, 764
      resection specimens examination, 764–765, *765t*
   spindle cell, 356–357, *356–357*
   squamous, 1502, *1503*
   squamous carcinoma *in situ*, 1569–1570
   stomach
      classification, 731–732, *732*
      features of, 730
      gastric antrum and body, 725
      gastric cardia, 724–725
      histologic classification, 733–734
      natural history, 731–732, *732*
      pathogenesis, 725
      predisposing conditions, 728–730
      premalignant lesions, 730
      risk factors, 725–728
      superficial cancers and subdivision, 731
      variants of, 737–757
   superficial, 511
   thyroid, medullary, 389–390
   types, 730, *730*
   undifferentiated, 753, 755
   varicoid, 512
   verrucous, 1565, *1566*, 1567
   yolk sack tumor, 743
Carcinosarcoma, 356–357, *356–357*, 1502–1503
Cardia region, in stomach, 552, 554, 555, *555*
Cardiac disease
   congestive cardiac failure, 399–400
   infective endocarditis, 400
   open-heart surgery, gastrointestinal complications, 400

Cardiac glands
  in esophagus, 426
  mucosa, 557–558, *558*
Cardiac transplantation, 400
Carditis, 649–652, *651*
  gastritis, 650, *651*, 652
Carney's triad, 307, *308–309*, 309
Carney-Stratakis syndrome, 309
Cathartic colon, 1162, *1164*
CD4 cells, 112
CD117, for gastrointestinal stromal tumors, 303–304, *303t*
CDK8, 1463
CDKN2A gene, 1464
Cecal volvulus, 63, 906
Cecum and proximal colon, diverticulosis of
  clinical features, 238
  pathogenesis, 238
  pathology, 238–239, *239*
Celiac axis compression syndrome, 38
Celiac disease, 1341
Celiac sprue
  diagnosis, 13
  and endocrine cell hyperplasia, 219
  and esophageal tumors, 508
  immune mechanisms in, 90
  and small bowel mucosal disease, with severe flat mucosa
    with acute dramatic metabolic derangements, 945–946
    associations of, 940
    biopsy in untreated, 940–943, *942–943*, *944*
    clinical features, 938–940
    collagenous, *936t*, 949, *950*
    complications of, 943–944
    and dermatitis herpetiformis, 944, *944–945*
    endoscopic appearance, 940–943, *942–943*, *944*
    IgA deficiency, associated with, 940
    latent, 945
    lymphocytic gastritis, associated with, 940
    pathogenesis, 936–938, *939*
    preclinical disease, 945
    rebiopsy in, *944*, 946–947
    refractory, 947–949
    relatives of patients with, 945
    small bowel ulceration, 944
    tropical, 953–954, *954*
    tumors, 943–944
    unclassified, 949
  specimen handling, 13
Celiac trunk, 31
Cestodes
  Diphyllobothrium latum (fish tapeworm), 1307
  Hymenolepsis nana (dwarf tapeworm), 1308
  Taenia saginata (beef tapeworm), 1307, *1307*
  Taenia solium (pork tapeworm), 1307–1308
Chagas' disease, 248–249
  causes, 274–275
  differential diagnosis, 275

gross appearance, 275
histology, 275
Chemotherapy
  esophageal, squamous cell carcinoma, 515–516
  invasive squamous cell carcinoma, 1575
  small bowel mucosal disease, with variably severe lesions, 969–970, *970*
Childhood kwashiorkor, 954, *954*
Chlamydia, 1273–1274, *1274–1275*
  chlamydial proctitis
    clinical features, 1273–1274
    gross and endoscopic features, 1274, *1274*
    histology, 1274, *1275*
  enteric infections, 1218
  infection, 824–825
  lymphogranuloma venereum, 1273
Chlamydial proctitis, 1273–1274, *1274–1275*
Cholera
  diagnosis, 1229
  epidemiology, 1228
  pathogenesis, 1228–1229
  pathology, 1229
  treatment and follow-up, 1229
Cholera toxin, 1216
Choriocarcinoma, 534, 742–743, *743*
Choriocarcinoma-like carcinoma, 1503
Choristomas, 540
Chromoendoscopy
  autofluorescence imaging, 8
  Barrett's esophagus, 7, 8–9
  confocal endomicroscopy, 8
  dye spraying technique, 9
  inflammatory bowel disease, 7, *8*, 9–10, *10*
  inflammatory (pseudo) polyps, 10
  narrow band imaging, 8
  ulcerative colitis, 9–10, *10*
Chromosomal alterations, 305
Chronic atrophic gastritis
  H. pylori-related, 728–729
  immunodeficiency disorder, 729
  Menetrièr's disease, 729–730
  postgastrectomy, 729
Chronic diarrhea. *see* Diarrhea
Chronic granulomatous disease, 828, *829*
  granulomatous disorders, 407
  phagocytic and cell dysfunction, 106
  small bowel mucosal disease, 973
Chronic GVHD, 110
Chronic idiopathic inflammatory bowel diseases
  colitis associated with primary sclerosing cholangitis, 1078–1079
  Crohn's disease
    anal and perianal disease, 1061–1063, *1063*, *1064*
    clinical features and classification, 1045, *1046t*
    definition, 1044–1045
    endoscopic features and gross pathology, 1045–1046, *1046–1050*, *1048–1049*
    management, 1063
    microscopic pathology, 1049, *1050–1055*, *1051–1053*, *1053t*, 1055–1057, *1056t*, *1057–1061*, 1060, 1061

    and small intestinal transplantation, 1078–1079
    and ulcerative colitis, 1071–1072
  epidemiology, 1000–1001
  etiology and pathogenesis
    appendectomy, 1007–1008
    environmental factors, 1004–1007
    genetic factors, 1001, 1002, *1003t–1004t*, 1004
    immune system, 1008–1009
    smoking and, 1007
  extragastrointestinal manifestations, 1077–1078, *1077t*
  indeterminate colitis/IBD-unclassified
    characteristics, 1067
    pathology, 1068–1071, *1073*
    treatment and prognosis, 1078
  ulcerative colitis
    appendiceal involvement, 1028, *1028*
    in children, 1030, *1031*
    clinical features, 1010–1011
    cuffitis, 1044
    dysplasia and cancer, *1040*, 1042–1043
    endoscopic features and gross pathology, 1011, *1012–1015*, 1013
    focality/patchiness, *1027*, 1027–1028
    fulminant colitis and toxic megacolon, *1032–1034*, 1032–1036, *1034t*, 1035
    ileal involvement, *1029*, 1029–1030
    ileal pouches and complications, 1037–1041, *1039–1041*, 1041
    medical therapy, 1036–1037, *1037*
    microscopic pathology, *1015*, 1015–1027, *1017–1019*, *1020*, *1021t*, *1022t*, *1023–1027*
    pouch biopsies, 1041–1042
    pouch problems, 1041
    prepouch ileitis, 1043–1044
    proctitis/ulcerative proctitis, 1030–1032, *1030t*
    rectal sparing, 1028–1029
    rectum in ulcerative proctocolitis, following ileorectal anastomosis, 1036
  ulcerative colitis vs. Crohn's disease
    macroscopic differences, 1064–1066, *1065t*
    microscopic differences, 1066–1067, *1066t*, 1068–1072
  upper gastrointestinal tract involvement, 1072, *1073*, *1074*, *1075*, 1075–1076, *1076*
Chronic idiopathic intestinal pseudoobstruction (CIIP)
  African visceral myopathy, 261
  causes, *254t*
  clinical features, 253
  clinicopathologic implications, 253–254
  complications, 261
  desmin myopathy, 261
  examining erections
    fibrosis, 255, *255*
    hypertrophied muscularis propria, 254, *255*
    loss of ICCs, 257
    myenteric plexus, *256*
    rudimentary muscle layer, *256*

submucosal muscle layer, *257*
trichrome staining, 255, *255*
familial/sporadic visceral myopathy
  gross appearance, 256–257, *258*
  histology, 257, *258*, *259*
  pathology, 256
  with SMA-positive inclusion bodies, 260–261
α-smooth muscle actin deficiency, 259–260
submucosal muscle layer, *257*
Chronic inflammation with/without focal active colitis
  iatrogenic and drug-associated inflammatory changes
    cimetidine, 1159
    5-flucytosine, 1159
    gold enteritis and colitis, 1159, *1160*
    ipilimumab and anti PD-1, 1158, *1158*
    isotretinoin, 1159
    mycophenolate mofetil, 1158
    penicillamine, 1159
    rituximab, 1158
Chronic inflammatory bowel diseases, differential diagnosis of
  diversion colitis, 1081–1082, *1082*
  diverticular colitis, 1079, *1080*, 1081, *1081*
  drug-induced mucosal injury, 1095–1096
  ileal endometriosis, 1096
  infections, 1093–1095, *1093t*, *1095*
  ischemia, 1096, *1096*
  sarcoidosis, 1096, *1097*
Chronic intestinal pseudoobstruction
  with acquired jejunal diverticulosis, 276
  with amyloidosis and hypothyroidism, 276
  clinical features, 253
  clinicopathologic implications, 253–254
  electron microscopy, 254
  immunostains, 253–254
  molecular and genetic studies, 254
  with myotonic muscular dystrophy, 276
  with progressive muscular dystrophy, 276
  with scleroderma, 276
Chronic mesenteric ischemia, 38
Chronic mucocutaneous candidiasis, 103, *105*
Chronic renal failure, 390–392
Churg-Strauss syndrome (CSS), 54, *55*, *56*, 966
Cicatricial pemphigoid, 397
Cimetidine, 1159
CIMP-H, 726
Circulatory anatomy
  anastomotic connections, 31
  arc of Riolan, 32
  blood supply
    esophagus, 29
    small and large intestine, 32, *32*
    stomach, 30, *30*
  inferior mesenteric artery, 32, *32*
  superior mesenteric artery, 31–32, *32*
Circumferential margins, 877
Clear cell, 190
  carcinoma, 1500, 1501, *1501*
  sarcoma, 348, 350, *351*
Clofazimine (Lamprene), 1156

Clostridial infections, 1250. *see also Clostridium*
Clostridial toxins, 1216
Clostridium
  C. botulinum, 1256, 1257–1258
  C. difficile, 44, *48*
    clinical features, 1252
    complications, 1254–1255
    description, 1250
    diagnosis and differential diagnosis, 1254
    epidemiology, 1250–1251
    gross and endoscopic appearances, *1252*, *1253*, 1254
    histology, *1253*, 1254
    and inflammatory bowel disease, 1255
    pathogenesis, 1251–1252
    pseudomembranous colitis, 1251
    pseudomembranous enteritis, 1254
    toxins, 1251
    treatment, 1254–1255
  C. perfringens
    clinical features, 1256
    description, 1255
    enteritis necroticans, 1255–1257, *1256*
    pathogenesis, 1255–1256
    pathology, 1256, *1256*
Clotted venous saccule, 1560
CMUSE. *see* Cryptogenic multifocal ulcerous stenosing enteritis (CMUSE)
C-MYC, 1463
Coagulation disorders, 401
Cobblestoning, 39, 42, 44
Cocaine, *33t*, 42, 43, 64
Coccidiosis, 1295, 1298, *1298*
  Cryptosporidium, 1295–1298, *1296–1297*
  Cystoisospora belli (Coccidiosis), 1298, *1298*
  microsporidiosis, 1298, *1299*
  Toxoplasma, 1298
  trypanosomiasis (Chagas' disease), 1300
Colchicine, 671, *672*
Cold biopsies, 1391
Colitis, 1276
  acute infectious-type, 1156, *1157*
  antibiotic-associated, 1255
  associated with primary sclerosing cholangitis, 1079
  chronic inflammation with/without focal active
    cimetidine, 1159
    5-flucytosine, 1159
    gold enteritis and colitis, 1159, *1160*
    ipilimumab and anti PD-1, 1158, *1158*
    isotretinoin, 1159
    mycophenolate mofetil, 1158
    penicillamine, 1159
    rituximab, 1158
  CMV-associated, *1281–1282*
  Crohn's, *1053*, *1071*, 1158
  cystica profunda, 1563
  cystica profunda, inflammatory bowel disease, 1168–1169, *1169*
  definition, 1218
  and enteritis cystica superficialis, 1170, *1170t*

eosinophilic, *1091*, 1091–1092, *1091t*
focal active, 1082–1083
granulomatous and eosinophilic enteritis, 1156–1158
and herpes simplex virus, 1276
ischemia
  aortofemoral bypass surgery, *47*
  Clostridium difficile toxin, 44, *48*
  colon, ischemic stricture, 45, *48*
  colonic ischemia, 42–43
  endoscopic biopsy, *47*
  etiology, 43, *43t*
  hemosiderin-laden macrophages, 45, *49*
  large bowel infarction, *46*
  massive bowel infarction, 42
  microscopy, 44–45, *46–48*
  pathology, 43–44, *43–46*
  transient/evanescent, 43
left-sided, *1013*, 1029
lymphocytic, 90, 994–996, *995*
microscopic, 994–995, *995*
neutropenic colitis, 66
obstructive, 1088–1089, *1089*
primary immunodeficiency disorders, 101
pseudomembranes and ischemic, 1156
Salmonella, *1237*, 1237–1238
ulcerative
  appendiceal involvement, 1028, *1028*
  in children, 1030, *1031*
  clinical features, 1010–1011
  dysplasia and cancer, *1040*, 1042–1043
  endoscopic features and gross pathology, 1011, *1012–1015*, 1013
  focality/patchiness, *1027*, 1027–1028
  fulminant colitis and toxic megacolon, *1032–1034*, 1032–1036, *1034t*, *1035*
  ileal involvement, *1029*, 1029–1030
  ileal pouches and complications, 1037–1041, *1039–1041*, *1041*
  medical therapy, 1036–1037, *1037*
  microscopic pathology, *1015*, 1015–1027, *1017–1019*, *1020*, *1021t*, *1022t*, *1023–1027*
  pouch biopsies, 1041–1042
  pouch problems, 1041
  proctitis/ulcerative proctitis, 1030–1032, *1030t*
  rectal sparing, 1028–1029
  rectum in ulcerative proctocolitis, following ileorectal anastomosis, 1036
Collagenous colitis
  associations, 988
  clinical features, 988
  definition, 988
  differential diagnosis, 994
  endoscopic appearance, 988
  histology, 405
  immune mechanisms in, 90
  and microscopic colitis, 988–994, *989–992*
  pathogenesis, 986–988
  perforation, 993
  prognosis, 996–997
Collagenous sprue, *936t*, 949, *950*

Colon
  cancer, in young, 1506–1507, 1509
  diverticular disease of (see Large bowel diverticular disease)
  GI problem in AIDS patients, 112
  MALT lymphomas, 161
  mantle cell lymphoma
    clinical presentation, 161
    differential diagnosis, 162
    immunophenotype and molecular genetics, 162
    pathology, 161–162, *162*
    treatment and prognosis, 162
  multiple lymphomatous polyposis, 162–163
  rectum and anal canal, 160–161
  ulcerative colitis, 161
Colonic elastosis and elastofibroma, 1410, *1411*
Colonic endocrine cells, 219
Colonic mucosal perineurioma, *326*
Colonic mucosal-submucosal elongated polyp/mucosubmucosal polyp, *1409*, 1409–1410
Colonic pseudoobstruction, 252
Colonization, 1215
Colonoscopy, 10–11
Colorectal carcinoma
  adenoma and progression, *1460*
  biopsy diagnosis
    grading and histologic typing, 1482
    infiltrating pattern, 1481
    inflammatory infiltrate, 1489
    invasive carcinoma, 1480
    lymphovascular invasion, 1486, 1488
    mucin and lectin changes, 1482–1483
    nodal involvement and peritumoral deposits, 1490–1492
    perineural invasion, 1488
    radial surgical margin involvement, 1486
    serosal involvement, 1483, 1485–1486
    tumor budding, 1489–1490
    tumor desmoplasia, 1481–1482
    tumor differentiation, 1483
  chronic infection, 1456
  de novo carcinoma, 1470
  growth and kinetics, 1469–1470
  incidence and demographics, 1453–1454
  molecular genetics and pathogenesis
    apc-β-catenin gene complex, 1462–1463
    CDKN2A gene, 1464
    chromosomal instability pathway, 1458, 1460
    cytogenetic abnormalities, 1465
    deleted in colon cancer (DCC) gene, 1464
    genes and signaling pathways, 1462
    genotype–phenotype correlations, 1465–1466
    methylation pathways, 1461–1462
    microsatellite instability pathway, 1460–1461
    p53 signaling, 1464
    pathologic staging, *1510t*
    PTEN protein, 1464
    RAS-MAPK and PI3K signaling pathway, 1463–1464
    sequential molecular changes, 1458
    telomerase activity, 1465
    TGF-β signaling pathway, 1464
    Wnt signaling pathway, 1462–1463
  MSI-H carcinoma, 1492–1493
  MSS with CpG island methylation, 1493
  polyposis syndromes and family history, 1456
  predisposing factors, 1454–1456
  premalignant lesions, 1457
  prior cholecystectomy, 1457
  prior colorectal neoplasia, 1456
  prior local irradiation, 1456–1457
  prior ureterosigmoidostomy, 1457
  prognosis of
    clinical factors, 1509
    pathologic features, 1509–1515
  specimen resection, 1473–1474
  spontaneous disappearance, 1470
  terminology, 1453
  treatment
    adjuvant therapy, 1515
    postoperative adjuvant chemotherapy, 1515
    recurrence and metastases, 1516–1517
    targeted therapy, 1515–1516
  usual/conventional-type, 1478–1480
Columnar dysplasias, 1579
Columnar zone, in anal canal, *1550–1549*, 1554, 1557
Columnar-lined esophagus (CLE), 469
Common variable hypogammaglobulinemia, *955*, 956–957, *958*
Common variable immunodeficiency (CVID), 95, 99
Composite adenoma/carcinoma-carcinoid tumors, 1503–1504, *1506*
Computed tomography (CT), 37, 230, 292, 293
Condyloma acuminatum, 1564–1565, *1565*, *1566*
Condylomalatum, perianal, *1561*
Confocal endomicroscopy, 8
Congenital agammaglobulinemia, 102
Congenital cysts, of esophagus, 431–432
Congenital duplications, esophageal, 431–432, *432*
Congenital fistula, 803
Congenital hypertrophic pyloric stenosis, 250–251
Congenital microvillus atrophy. *see* Microvillus inclusion disease
Congenital tufting enteropathy, 955–956, *956*
Congestive cardiac failure, 399–400
Congestive gastropathy, 585, *586*
Connective tissue diseases (CTDs)
  gastrointestinal manifestation of arthritis, rheumatoid, 383
    Behçet's disease, 383
    clinical features, 379–380
    dermatomyositis, 382
    hereditary, 384
    miscellaneous, 383–384
    mixed, 383
    overlap syndrome, 383
    pathology, 380–382
    scleroderma, 379–384
    systemic lupus erythematosus, 383
  vasculitis, 54, 55
Contaminated bowel syndrome. *see* Stasis syndrome
Contrast media, 1155
Conventional dysplasia, 1362–1363
Corpus gland mucosa, 558–560, *559*, *560*
Corrosive and esophagitis, 493–494
Corynebacterium equi, 1272–1273
Cowden's syndrome, 399, 1430–1431, *1431–1432*, 1432
Cow's milk allergy, 1007, 1091
COX pathway, 267
Cribriform/comedocarcinoma, 1505
Crohn's disease, 1341
  in anal canal, *1562*
  appendix, 824–828, *825*, *826*, *827*, *828*
  arteritis, 828, *828*
  chronic idiopathic inflammatory bowel diseases
    anal and perianal disease, 1061–1063, *1063*, *1064*
    clinical features and classification, 1045, 1046t
    definition, 1044–1045
    endoscopic features and gross pathology, 1045–1046, *1046–1050*, 1048–1049
    management, 1063
    microscopic pathology, 1049, *1050–1055*, 1051–1053, *1053t*, 1055–1057, *1056t*, *1057–1061*, 1060, 1061
    and small intestinal transplantation, 1078–1079
  endocrine tumors, 217
  histiocytic diseases
    decidualization, 827, *827*
    sarcoidosis, 828
  inherited disorders, 828, *829*
  invasive squamous cell carcinoma, 1571
  involvement, 497, *498*
  isolated appendiceal, 826
  in large bowel, 905, *905*
  lymphocytic esophagitis in, 497
  lymphoid hyperplasia, 825, *825*
  morphologic appearance, 824
  resections and biopsy techniques, 23
  selective IgA deficiency, 101
  small bowel mucosal disease, with variably severe lesions, 967, *967*
  vs. tuberculosis, 1262, 1263, *1263t*
  ulcerative colitis, 826, *827*
    IBD, 662–665, *663*, *664*
    macroscopic differences, 1064–1066, *1065t*
    microscopic differences, 1066–1067, *1066t*, *1068–1072*
    synchronous and metachronous, 1071–1072
Cronkhite-Canada syndrome, *678*
  clinical features, *1433*, 1433–1434
  differential diagnosis, 1434, 1436

gross and endoscopic appearances, *1433*, 1434
histology, 1434, *1435*
pathogenesis and molecular genetics, 1434
treatment, 1436
Cronkhite-Canada syndrome-associated polyps, 778, *779*
Crypt cell carcinoma. *see* Goblet cell carcinoma (GCC)
Cryptococcosis, 1310
Cryptogenic multifocal ulcerous stenosing enteritis (CMUSE), 1083–1084, *1084*, 1088
Cryptosporidium, 659–660, 1295–1298, *1296–1297*
  description, 1295
  diagnosis, 1298
  infection
    with AIDS, 113
    immunodeficient patients, 115
    and small bowel mucosal disorders, small bowel biopsy in, 932
  pathogenesis and clinical features, 1295–1296
  pathology, *1296–1297*, *1296–1297*, 1296–1298
Crystal deposition
  barium granuloma, 1182, *1183*
  mercury, 1183
  oleogranulomas (paraffinomas), 1182–1183
  radiologic masses, baroliths, and acute appendicitis, 1183
CTDs. *see* Connective tissue diseases (CTDs)
Cuffitis, 1044
Cup cells, 890
Curvature of stomach, 552–554, *553*
Cyclin E, 1463
Cystadenocarcinomas, 839
Cystadenomas, 839
Cystic dilatation, 783
Cystic fibrosis
  and appendix, 828, *829*
  and bowel, mechanical disorders of, 919
Cystic profunda, 783, *784*
Cystica superficialis, 783
Cystoisospora belli, 1298, *1298*
Cysts
  bronchogenic, 432
  congenital, 431–432
  mucosal, 783
  neurenteric, 432
  retention, 443–444, *444*, 839
Cytology
  balloon mesh, 7, *7*
  direct-vision brush, 7
  fine-needle aspirates, *6*, *7*
Cytomegalovirus (CMV)
  and esophagitis, 486, *486*
  immunodeficient patients, 115
  infection
    description, 1278
    gastric disease associated with, 657, *658*
    pathogenesis, 1278
    primary infection, 1278–1279
    reactivated infection, 1279–1280, *1279–1282*, 1282–1283

D

Darier's disease, 398
Deleted in colon cancer (DCC) gene, 1464
Deletions, 304
Delhi belly/Montezuma's revenge, 1224
Dentate line of anal canal, 1549, 1550
Dermal papillae, 425
Dermatitis herpetiformis, 944, *944–945*
Dermatogenic enteropathy, 398–399
Dermatomyositis, 382, 399
Descending duodenum, 875
Desmin myopathy, 261
Desmoid tumor/intraabdominal fibromatosis, 331–333, *332*
Desmoplastic carcinoma, *358*
Diabetes mellitus
  description, 487, 498
  gastrointestinal manifestation of
    clinical manifestations, 386–387
    pathogenesis, 386–387
    pathology, 387
Diaphragms, 910–912, *911*
  diseases of, *1150*
  hernias in, 907
Diarrhea
  GI problem in HIV patients, 111
  inflammatory bowel disease
    chemotherapeutic agents, 1170–1171
    mycophenolate mofetil, 1171
    proton pump inhibitors, 1171
  mechanisms of, 1216
  pathogenic enteric viruses, 1284
  traveler's, 1224, *1225t*
  watery, 388
Diathermy
  acellular mucin pools, 1397, *1398*
  cold biopsies, 1391
  depth of invasion, 1395
  extravasated mucin pools vs. invasive mucinous carcinoma, 1397, *1397*
  gross and endoscopic appearances, 1393–1394
  histology, 1395
  hot biopsies, 1389, *1391*
  invasive carcinoma, 1391
  malignant polyps, 1398–1399, *1399*, *1400*, 1401–1403
  misplaced glands vs. invasive carcinoma, 1397–1398
  misplaced submucosal adenomatous glands, 1395, *1396*, 1397
  pathology, 1394, *1394*
  prognosis and management, *1046t*, 1403–1406, *1405*
  snare biopsy and polypectomy, 1389, 1391, *1391*
Dientamoeba fragilis, 1294
Diet, and esophageal squamous cell carcinoma, 507
Dieulafoy lesion, *76*, 76–77
Diffuse eosinophilic infiltrate, 266, *267*
Diffuse esophageal spasm, 249, *250*
Diffuse ganglioneuromatosis, 320, 321, 323
Diffuse large B-cell lymphoma (DLBCL)
  classification, 148
  immunophenotype of, 149
  microscopic findings, 148, *148*
  occurrence, 149
  survival of, 149
Diffuse lymphoid infiltration, 266, *266*
Diffuse lymphoid tissue, distribution, 89
Diffuse nodular lymphoid hyperplasia, 136–139, *137*, *138*
Diffuse-type signet ring carcinomas, 1496
DiGeorge's syndrome
  ataxia telangiectasia, 105
  characteristics, 105
  22q11 chromosomal deletion, 105
  transcobalamin II deficiency, 105
  Wiskott–Aldrich syndrome, 105
Digestive tract ischemia, mechanical obstruction and
  adhesions, 62
  hernias, 62–63
  intussusception, *63*, 63–64
  pathogenesis, 61–62
  volvulus, 63
Digestive tract vascularization
  esophagus
    esophageal veins, 29
    extramural arterial supply, 29
    intramural arterial pattern, 29
  stomach, small and large intestine
    collateral blood supply, 33
    extramural circulation, 31–33, *32*
    intramural circulation, *30*, 30–31
    venous drainage, 33
Digitalis, *33t*
Diminutive polyps, 1376
Diphyllobothrium latum, 1307
Direct-vision brush, cytology, 7
Disaccharidase deficiencies, 973
Dissection, biopsy
  depth of tumor penetration, 25
  incidental findings, 26
  lymph node, 25
  sections of resected margins, 26
  of tumors, 25
  venous invasion by tumor, 25–26
Disseminated lymphoma, 175
Diverticula
  abdominothoracic dorsal enteric, 913
  of appendix, 803–805, *804–805*
  in esophagus
    atypical, in scleroderma, 443
    esophageal intramural pseudodiverticulosis, 443–444, *444*
    lower, 442–443, *443*
    mid, 442–443, *443*
    retention cysts, 443–444, *444*
    upper, 442, *442*
  uncomplicated, *916*
Diverticular disease
  of colon (*see* Large bowel diverticular disease)
  and endometriosis, 237
  and IBD (diverticular colitis)
    clinical presentation and features, 237, 237–238
    differential diagnosis, 238
  small and large intestines
    definition, 227
    terminology, 227

Diverticular polyps
    carcinoma in, 237
    inverted diverticulum, 236–237, 237
Diverticulitis
    appendiceal, 813
    definition, 227, 228
Diverticulosis
    of cecum and proximal colon
        clinical features, 238
        pathogenesis, 238
        pathology, 238–239, 239
    definition, 227, 228
    of duodenum and small intestine, 239, 239–240
DLBCL. see Diffuse large B-cell lymphoma (DLBCL)
DNA ploidy, 516
DOG1 immunostain, 265, 265
Downhill varices, 438
Down's syndrome
    and bowel, atresia, 910
    and Zellweger's syndromes, 905
Drinking water, contamination of, 1224
Drug-associated and iatrogenic vascular injuries
    anticoagulant-associated hemorrhage, 1153, 1153
    arterial spasm
        hypotensive and hypovolemic agents, 1155
        vasopressin, 1155
    arterial/venous thrombosis
        drug-induced vasculitis, 1153–1155, 1154
        estrogen and oral contraceptives, 1153–1155, 1154
        oral contraceptive and IBD, 1155
    changes secondary to contrast media, 1155
    ischemia following angiography
        embolization, 1152–1153
        trauma to the vessel wall, 1152
    neonatal perforation, 1155
    perforation, 1155
    retroperitoneal hematomas, 1153
    Stevens–Johnson syndrome, 1156
Drug-induced esophagitis, 494
Drug-induced vasculitis, 64, 64–66, 66
Drugs and chemicals, changes due to
    colitis (see Chronic inflammation)
    enemas and laxatives
        glutaraldehyde, hydrogen peroxide/peracetic acid, 1160–1161, 1161–1162
        hypertonic saline enemas, 1160
        polyethylene glycol, 1162
        soap, 1161–1162, 1161
        sodium phosphate (fleets enemas) and bisacodyl, 1159, 1161
    iatrogenic gas introduced at endoscopy (pseudolipomatosis), 1166–1167
        gross and endoscopic appearances, 1167
        histology, 1167, 1167
    ingested drugs, 1163–1164
    laxatives
        alcohol, 1163
        cathartic colon, 1162, 1164
    foreign material, injected, 1163
    myenteric plexus damage, pseudoobstruction, and stercoral ulceration, 1162–1163
    pneumatosis cystoides intestinalis
        clinical features, 1165
        gross and endoscopic disease, 1165
        histology, 1165, 1166
        pathogenesis, 1164–1165
        prognosis, 1165–1166
Duodenal bands, 908
Duodenal biopsy specimen, 15, 15
Duodenal bulb. see Duodenitis
Duodenal diverticula, 239, 239–240
Duodenal mucosal bumps, 1335
Duodenal paraganglioma, 328
Duodenal ulcer, 628, 628–630
Duodenitis
    clinical features, 627–630
    complications, 633–634, 634
    fundic gland heterotopia, 630–631
    pathogenesis, 627–630
    pathology
        differential diagnosis, 632–633, 633
        gross pathology, 630
        healing and healed ulcers, 633
        histology, 631, 631–632, 632
    salt and pepper appearance, 630, 630
    treatment, 635
Duodenum
    biopsy technique, 24
    carcinoid tumors
        gangliocytic paraganglioma, 205
        gastrinomas, 204, 205
        somatostatinomas, 204, 206
    granular cell tumor, 329
    in stomach, 553
Duplications
    in appendix, 801–802, 802–803, 802t
    and bowel, large and small
        enteric duplications, 912
        simple duplications, 912–914, 913, 914
    in esophagus, 431–432, 432
    in small bowel carcinoma, 1341
Dwarf tapeworm, 1308. see also Hymenolepsis nana
Dysplasia, 200
    and anal intraepithelial neoplasia, 1564, 1567
    with Barrett's esophagus
        adenocarcinoma in, 526–527
        diagnosis, 479
        high grade, 482
        indefinite for, 479–480
        inter- and (intra) observer variability, 483–484
        low-grade, 477, 478, 480–481, 482
        second opinion need, 483–484
    and cancer, 1040, 1042–1043
    columnar, unusual adenoma-like, 1579
    gastric epithelial polyps and tumors
        definition, 706
        grading, 719, 721
        grading of, 1386, 1387
    hereditary thymic, 102–103
    inflammatory bowel disease, malignancy in
        classification and grading, 1114, 1114–1115
        clinical implications, 1119, 1119–1121, 1120
        grading dysplasia, 1115–1116, 1115t
        gross pathology, 1102–1103, 1103–1104, 1103t
        immunohistochemistry, 1117–1119, 1118
        issues of, 1116–1117
        lesions management, 1101–1102
        microscopic pathology, 1103–1112, 1105–1112
        reactive changes, distinction from, 1112, 1113, 1114
    invasive squamous cell carcinoma, 1571
    predominant cell-mediated immunodeficiency, 102–103
    in squamous cell carcinoma, 508–509, 510
Dysplasia-associated lesion or mass (DALM), 1101
Dysplastic mucosal polyps
    clinical features, 1336–1337
    gross and endoscopic appearances, 1337, 1337, 1338
    histology, 1338–1339, 1339
    management, 1339–1340
Dysproteinemias, 400

E
EAEC organisms. see Enteroadherent Escherichia coli (EAEC)
ECL-cell, 218
Ectasia, vascular
    colon, 77, 77
    dysplasia distinction, GVHD, 583, 585
    GAVE, 74–76, 75
    histologic examination, 74
    mucosa, 73
    prevalence, 74
Ectopic pancreas, 784–785, 785–786, 1335, 1336
Edema, during biopsy, 18–19
Edwardsiella tarda, 1242–1243, 1243
Ehlers–Danlos syndrome, 79–80, 384
Elastofibroma, 340
Electrocautery snare biopsy
    endoscopic mucosal resection, 5
    endoscopic submucosal dissection, 5, 6
    shave biopsy technique, 5
    snare polypectomy, 4, 4
    snare polypectomy after submucosal injection, 4–5
    submucosal lesions, 5
Elongated dermal papillae, 459, 460
Embolization, 35, 64, 64
    ischemia following angiography, 1152–1153
Embryonal rhabdomyosarcoma, 350
Emphysematous gastritis, 656
Endocrine carcinomas
    colon, 215, 215
    esophageal, 214
    large cell, 213, 214
    non-small cell, 213

rectum, 215, *215*
small cell, 213, *213*
Endocrine cell hyperplasia
  with celiac sprue, 219
  G cell, primary, 218
Endocrine cell tumors, 206
Endocrine cells
  APUD system, 190–192
  argentaffin, 190
  argyrophil, 190
  basigranulated, 190
  and bowel, structure of, *881*, 888–890, *889*
  clear, 190
  clinical implications, 192–193, *193t*
  in colorectal polyps, 216
  cytoplasms, 190, *191*
  D cells, 192
  dysgenesis, 219–220
  ECL cells, 192
  enterochromaffin, 190
  eosinophilic granules, 190, *191*
  in esophagus, 424
  G cells, 192
  gastric, stomach of, 564, *565t*
  gastrin, 192
  peptide hormones, 191
  silver stains, 192
  of stomach, *557t*
Endocrine disorders
  adrenal gland, 388
  autoimmune thyroid disease, 385
  endocrine pancreas, 386–387
  gastrinoma, 387
  gonads, 388
  hyperparathyroidism, 385
  hyperthyroidism, 384–385
  hypoparathyroidism, 385–386
  hypothalamus and pituitary, 388–389
  hypothyroidism, 385
  islets of Langerhans, hyperfunction of, 387
  somatostatinoma, 388
  thyroid neoplasms, 385
  VIPoma syndrome, 387–388
Endocrine mucosa, *567t*
Endocrine pancreas
  clinical manifestations, 386–387
  pathogenesis, 386–387
  pathology, 387
Endocrine tumors, 79
  abnormalities, 221–222
  carcinoid, *195*
    abdominal colon, 211
    appendectomy, 196, 197
    appendix, 208–211, *209*, *210*
    cecum/terminal ileum, 208
    classification, 198
    definition of, 194
    dissection recommendations for, 196–197
    duodenum, 204–206, *205*, *206*
    esophagus, 198–199
    gangliocytic paraganglioma, 205
    gastrinomas, 204, *205*
    glandular, 206
    gross appearance, 196, *197*
    growth patterns, 195, *195*, 196
    ileum, 206–208, *206–208*
    jejunum, 206–208, *206–208*
    metastatic risk for, 196
    midgut, 206–208, *206–208*
    occurrence, 196
    polypectomies, 197
    rectum, 211–212, *212*
    resections, 196
    somatostatinomas, 204, *206*
    staging and grading, 197–198
    stomach, 199–204, *199t*, *200–203*
    type I, 199–202, *200–202*
    type II, 202–203
    type III, 203, *203*
    type IV, 204
  classification of, *193t*
  clinical implications, 192–193, *193t*
  Crohn's disease, 217
  genetics of, 194
  metastatic, *220*, 220–221
  multiple endocrine neoplasia type I, 194
  neurofibromatosis type I, 194
  ulcerative colitis, 217
Endodermal sinus tumor, 743
Endolimax nana infection, 113
Endometrial stromal sarcoma, 351, *353*
Endometriosis, 1518, 1520, *1521–1522*, 1523
  diverticular disease and, 237
  gastrointestinal involvement, 407–408, *408–409*
Endoscopic banding, 439
Endoscopic mucosal resection (EMR), 5, 531, *531*
Endoscopic sclerotherapy, 438–439
Endoscopic submucosal dissection (ESD), 5, *6*
Endoscopic variceal ligation (EVL), 438–439
Endoscopy techniques
  accessories used, 6, *6*
  aspiration, 6, *6*
  benign-appearing lesions, *16t*
  chromoendoscopy, 7–11, *8*, *10*
  cytology, 6, *7*
  infections diagnosis, 6, 6–7, *7*
  mucosal biopsy, 1
  recommended approach, *17t*
  suction trap, 6, *7*
  virtual histology, 11, *12t*
Endothelial and vascular tumors
  angiosarcoma, 345, *346*, 347
  hemangioma, 344, 344, 345, 345
  intestinal vascular lesions associated with clinical syndromes, 348
  Kaposi's sarcoma, *346*, 347
  lymphangioma, 347–348, *347–349*
Enemas, drugs and chemicals changes in
  glutaraldehyde, hydrogen peroxide/ peracetic acid, 1160–1161, *1161–1162*
  hypertonic saline enemas, 1160
  polyethylene glycol, 1162
  soap, *1161–1162*, 1161
  sodium phosphate (fleet)s enemas and bisacodyl, 1159, *1161*
Entamoeba coli infection, 113
Entamoeba histolytica
  differential diagnosis, 1293
  epidemiology, 1289–1290
Enteric adenoviruses, 1287–1288, *1287–1288*
  other causes of viral diarrhea, 1288
Enteric duplications, 912
Enteric infections
  acute infectious/self-limited colitis and proctitis
    causes, 1226–1227
    diagnosis, 1228
    gross and endoscopic appearances, 1227
    histology, 1227–1228
    inflammatory bowel disease exacerbations, 1227
    pathogenesis and clinical features, 1227
  bacteria
    Actinomyces, 1271–1273, *1272*
    Aeromonas hydrophila, 1242–1243
    antibiotic-associated colitis, 1255
    Brucella, 1271
    Campylobacter, 1240–1242
    Chlamydia, 1273–1274, *1274–1275*
    clostridial infections, 1250–1255, *1253*
    Clostridium botulinum, 1256, 1257–1258
    Clostridium perfringens, 1255–1256, *1256–1257*
    Edwardsiella tarda, 1242–1243
    Escherichia coli, 1229–1234
    gonococcal proctitis, *1266*, 1266–1267
    granuloma inguinale, 1249, *1250*
    Legionella, 1243
    mycobacterial infections, 1260–1263
    neutropenic enterocolitis/typhlitis, 1257–1258, *1259*
    Phlegmonous enterocolitis, 1258
    Plesiomonas shigelloides, 1242–1243
    rickettsial disease, 1274–1275
    Salmonella, 1235–1238
    Shigella, 1234–1235
    spirochetes, *1267–1268*, 1267–1271, *1270–1271*
    toxic megacolon, 1241–1242, *1242*, *1246*
    typhoid fever, 1238–1240
    Vibrios, 1228–1229
    Yersinia, 1243–1249, *1246–1249*
  biopsy diagnosis of, *1217t*, 1220–1222, *1220–1223*, *1223t*
  classification, *1211t–1213t*
  fungi
    aspergillosis, *1310*, *1311*, 1312
    candidiasis, 1308
    histoplasmosis, 1308, *1309*, 1310
    pneumocystis, 1312
    South American blastomycosis, 1312, *1312*
  GI infections
    biopsy diagnosis, 1220–1223, *1222*, *1223t*, *1224t*
    cellular changes, *1217t*
    clinical conditions, 1224–1226, *1225t*
    clinical features, 1218

Enteric infections (*Continued*)
  clinical presentation, *1211t–1213t*
  diagnostic methods, *1211t–1213t*
  endoscopic and gross findings, 1218
  morbidity and mortality rate, 1210
  pathogens, *1217t*
  stool examination and culture, 1219–1220
 host defense mechanisms, 1210
 mechanisms
  adherence and initial attachment, 1215
  colonization, 1215
  diarrhea, enteroadherent and, 1216
  infection, 1215–1216
  persistence of infection, 1216
  tissue invasion, 1215
  toxin production, 1215–1216
 parasites
  amoeba, 1289–1294, *1291–1293*
  ancylostomiasis, 1300, *1300*
  Angiostrongylus costaricensis, 1300–1301
  anisakiasis, *1301*, 1301–1302
  ascariasis, 1302
  Balantidium coli, 1293, 1294, *1295*
  Blastocystis hominis, 1295
  capillariasis, *1302*, 1302–1303
  cestodes, *1307*, 1307–1308
  coccidiosis, 1295–1300, *1296–1299*
  Dientamoeba fragilis, 1294
  enterobiasis, 1303
  esophagostomiasis, 1303
  nematodes, 1300–1305
  protozoa, 1288–1300
  strongyloidiasis, 1303–1304, *1304*
  trematodes, 1305–1307, *1306–1307*
  trichinosis, 1304
  trichuriasis, 1305, *1305*
 virus
  enteric adenoviruses, 1287–1288, *1287–1288*
  enteric viruses, 1284
  herpes simplex virus, 1276–1278, *1277*
  herpesvirus infections, 1276–1283
  norovirus, 1285–1287
  rotavirus infections, 1285, *1286*
Enteric nervous system
 interstitial cells of cajal, 244, 244–245, *245*
 microscopy, 242–243
 muscle layers innervation, *243*, 243–244
 myenteric plexus, 243, *243*
 nerve plexuses, 242
Enteric viruses
 adenoviruses, 1287–1288, *1287–1288*
 nonpathogenic, 1284
 pathogenic, 1284
Enteritis
 acute, 820
 and colitis cystica superficialis, 1170, *1170t*
 cystica profunda, inflammatory bowel disease, 1168–1169, *1169*
 definition, 1218
 necroticans
  clinical features, 1256
  Darmbrand, 1255

  pathogenesis, 1255–1256
  pathology, 1256, *1256*
  pseudomembranous, 1254
Enteroadherent *Escherichia coli* (EAEC)
 diffusely adherent/enteroadherent, 1230–1231, *1232*
 organisms, 1215, 1229, 1230, 1271
Enterobiasis, 1303
Enterochromaffin cells, 190
Enterochromaffin-like cell (ECL-cell), 199, *199t*, 200, *201*
Enterococcal gastritis, 656
 distinctive (specific) types, 587, *587*
 gastric disease associated with, 656
Enterocolic lymphocytic phlebitis, 57, *59*
Enterocolitis
 hemorrhagic, 38, *39*, 43
 neutropenic/typhlitis, 1257–1258, *1259*
 phlegmonous, 1258
 Salmonella, *1237*, 1237–1238
Enterohemorrhagic *Escherichia coli* (EHEC), 1215, 1216, 1229, 1231–1232, *1233*
Enteroinvasive *Escherichia coli* (EIEC), 1215, 1230
Enteropathogenic *Escherichia coli* (EPEC), 1230, *1232*
Enteropathy-type T-cell lymphoma (ETL)
 classification, 157
 clinical presentation, 157–158
 immunophenotype and molecular genetics, 160
 incidence, 157
 pathogenesis, 157
 pathology, 158–160, *159*
 treatment and prognosis, 160
Enterotoxigenic *Escherichia coli* (ETEC), 1216, 1229, 1230
Enzyme deficiency states
 disaccharidase deficiencies, 973
 ornithine transcarbamylase deficiency, 973
Eosinophilic colitis, *1091*, 1091–1092, *1091t*
Eosinophilic esophagitis (EoE)
 biopsy sites, 492–493
 characteristics, 491
 clinical history, 492, *492*
 differential diagnosis, 493
 pathogenesis, 492
 pathology, 492, 493, *493*
 symptoms, 492
Eosinophilic gastritis
 differential diagnosis, 667, *667t*
 gastric involvement in, 667
Eosinophilic gastroenteritis
 Churg–Strauss vasculitis, 54, 56
 small bowel mucosal disease, with variably severe lesions
  clinical and differential diagnosis, 965
  clinical features, 965
  diagnosis, 964
  differential diagnosis, 965–967
  endoscopic findings and gross pathology, 965, *966*
  pathogenesis, 965
  pathology, 965, *966*

Eosinophils
 and eosinophilic gastroenteritis, 964–967, *966*
 and food hypersensitivity, 952–953
 immune mechanisms in, 90
Epidermolysis bullosa, 394, 397
Epidermolysis bullosa acquisita (EBA), 397
Epigastric hernias, 62
Epiphrenic diverticulum, *443*
Epiploic lipomatosis, 343, *343*
Epiploic tenia, 876
Epiploica–peritoneal mouse, infarcted appendix, 919
Epithelial biphasic tumor, of young adults, 357, *358*, 359, *359*
Epithelial cell replacement, impaired small intestine, 969–970, *970*
Epithelial differentiation. see Adenomas
Epithelial hyperplasia without dysplasia, 1564, *1564*
Epithelioid GIST, *297*
Epithelioid stromal tumors
 frozen section diagnosis, 294
 microscopic appearances, 294, *297*
Epstein-Barr virus (EBV), 129, 155, 157, 167, 168, 170, 172, 173, 726
 associated smooth muscle tumors, 314, 316
 gastric disease associated with, 658
Ergot, 43, 64, 65
Ergotamine, *33t*
Erosions
 biopsy, 456
 eosinophils, 457, *458*
 neutrophils, 457, *457*
 reactive epithelial changes, 458, *458*
 and sequela, 456, *456–457*
Erosive esophagitis, 461–462, *462*
Escherichia coli
 characteristics, 1229
 clinical features, 1232
 enteroadherent *E. coli* (EAEC)/diffusely adherent or enteroadherent, 1230–1231, *1232*
 enterohemorrhagic *E. coli* (EHEC), 1231–1232
 enteroinvasive *E. coli* (EIEC), 1230
 enteropathogenic *E. coli* (EPEC), 1230, *1232*
 enterotoxigenic *E. coli* (ETEC), 1230
 gross and endoscopic appearances, 1232, *1233*
 hemolytic uremic syndrome, 1234
 histology, 1232, *1233*, 1234
 pathotypes, *1230t*
 thrombotic thrombocytopenic purpura, 1234
 verotoxin, 1234
Esophageal atresia, 429–430, *430*, *430t*
Esophageal cardiac glands, 426
Esophageal intramural pseudodiverticulosis
 pathogenesis and clinical features, 443–444, *444*
 pathology, 444, *444*
Esophageal ischemia., 35, *35*
Esophageal leiomyomatosis, 316

Esophageal motility disorders
  achalasia/cardiospasm
    barium examination, *248*
    gross appearance, 247, *248*
    histology, 247–248, *248*
    prevalence, 246–247
  diffuse esophageal spasm, 249, *250*
  idiopathic hypertrophy, 249–250
  idiopathic muscular hypertrophy, 249, *249*
  secondary achalasia, 248–249
Esophageal polyps and tumors
  Barrett's esophagus (*see* Barrett's esophagus)
  choristomas, 540
  classification, 505, *506t*
  fibrovascular polyps, 540, *541*
  hamartomas, 540
  inflammatory polyps, 539
  melanoma, malignant, 540–541, *542*
  mesenchymal, 543–544, *544*
  mucosal tags, 539–540
  parathyroid rests, 540
  pathologist's diagnostic role, 506
  secondary, 542–543, *543*
  squamous cell carcinoma (*see* Squamous cell carcinoma)
  squamous papilloma, *538*, 539, *539*
  squamous papillomatosis, 539
  thyroid rests, 540
Esophageal tears
  pathogenesis and clinical features, 437
  pathology, *437*, 437–438
Esophageal varices
  acute esophageal necrosis, 439
  endoscopic sclerotherapy, 438–439
  pathogenesis and clinical features, 438, *438*
  pathology, *438*, 439
Esophageal webs and rings
  description, 439–440
  lower, *441*, 441–442
  mid, 441
  multiple, 440, *440*
  single, 440, *440*
  upper, 440–441, *441*
Esophageal xanthelasma, 445
Esophagitis
  and acute necrotizing, 491
  and bacterial, 489
  and corrosive, 493–494
  and cytomegalovirus, 486, *486*
  drug-induced, 494
  EoE (*see* Eosinophilic esophagitis (EoE))
  and exfoliative, 490–491, *491*
  and herpes, 484, *485*
  herpes simplex virus, 484–486, *485*
  and lymphocytic, 489–490, *490*
  and pill, 494
Esophagostomiasis, 1303
Esophagus
  anatomy, 422–423, *423*, *424*
  angle of His, 422
  and black, 491
  blood supply, 423
  bone marrow transplantation, GVHD, 108, *109*

  candidiasis, 89
  carcinoid tumors, 198–199
  carcinosarcoma, 356–357, *356–357*
  chronic GVHD, 110
  developmental and congenital anomalies
    bronchoesophageal fistula, 430–431
    bronchogenic cysts, 432
    congenital cysts, 431–432
    duplication, 431–432, *432*
    esophageal atresia, 429–430, *430*, *430t*
    gastric heterotopia, *433*, 433–434
    heterotopias, *433*, 433–434
    neurenteric cysts/remnants, 432
    pulmonary sequestrations, 434–435
    short esophagus, 434
    stenosis/stricture, 434, *434t*
    tracheoesophageal fistulas, 429–430, *431*
  digestive tract vascularization
    blood supply, 29
    esophageal veins, 29
    extramural arterial supply, 29
    intramural arterial pattern, 29
  diverticula and pseudodiverticula
    atypical, in scleroderma, 443
    esophageal intramural pseudodiverticulosis, 443, 444–443
    lower, 442–443, *443*
    mid, 442–443, *443*
    retention cysts, 443–444, *444*
    upper, 442, *442*
  embryology and development of, *427–428*, 427–429, *429*
  esophageal fistula, *439*, 439–442
  esophageal hemorrhage
    esophageal tears, *437*, 437–438
    esophageal varices, *438*, 438–439
  esophageal perforation
    causes of, *435t*
    nonspontaneous rupture and penetration, 435–437, *436*
    spontaneous rupture, 435
  esophageal tumors, 24
  esophageal webs and rings
    description, 439–440
    lower, *441*, 441–442
    mid, 441
    multiple, 440, *440*
    single, 440, *440*
    upper, 440–441, *441*
  esophageal xanthelasma, 445
  functions of, 426
    age-dependent changes, 426
  GI problem in AIDS patients, 112
  glycogenic acanthosis, 444–445, *445*
  granular cell tumor, 329–330, *329–330*
  hiatal hernia, 422
  histology
    mucosa, 423–426, *425*, *426*
    muscularis propria, *425*, 426
    submucosa, *425*, 426
  leiomyomas of, 313–314, *315*
  lymphomas, 138–139
  monophasic synovial sarcoma, 355, *355*
  mucosal bridge, 444
  radiation injury, 68, 70, 72

  rhabdomyosarcoma, 348
  small cell carcinoma, 213, *213*, 214
  stenosis/stricture, 434, *434t*
  submucosal lesions, 5
Estrogen, 35, 65
ETL. *see* Enteropathy-type T-cell lymphoma (ETL)
Exfoliative and esophagitis, 490–491, *491*
Exomphalos, 907
External hemorrhoids, 1560
External hernias, 62
Extraintestinal tumors, 410, *410*
Extraluminal duodenal diverticulum, 239, *239*
Extrinsic nervous system, 242

F

Fabry's disease, 405–406
Familial adenomatous polyposis (FAP)
  attenuated variants
    clinical features, 1441
    colectomy, 1443
    genotypes, 1440
    pathology, 1441
    prenatal diagnosis, 1443
    screening of, 1441–1443
    treatment, 1441
    upper GI disease, 1443
  molecular genetics and pathogenesis, 1439, *1439t*
  pathogenesis, 1341, *1342*
  variants
    Gardner's syndrome, 1439–1440
    Turcot's syndrome, 1440
Familial enteropathy, 954, *955*
Familial gastrointestinal stromal tumors, 399
Familial GIST syndrome, 306–307, *308*
Familial mediterranean fever (FMF), 409–410
Familial mitochondrial neurogastrointestinal encephalomyopathy (MNGIE), 263, *264*
Familial visceral neuropathy, 262–263, *263*, *264*
Familial/sporadic visceral myopathy
  gross appearance, 256–257, *258*
  histology, 257, *258*, *259*
  pathology, 256
  with SMA-positive inclusion bodies, 260–261
Familial gastric hyperplastic polyposis, 777–778
Fasciolopsis buski, 1305–1307
Fatty tumors, differential diagnosis of, 344
Femoral hernias, 62
α-Fetoprotein-producing gastric carcinomas, 741, *741*, *742*
Fibroblastic polyps, 325, *326*, 327
Fibroblastic/myofibroblastic tumors
  calcifying fibrous tumor, 339, *341*
  desmoid tumor/intraabdominal fibromatosis, 331–333, *332*
  elastofibroma, 340
  inflammatory fibroid polyp, 333–335, *333–335*

Fibroblastic/myofibroblastic tumors (Continued)
  inflammatory myofibroblastic tumor, 337, 338, 339
  plexiform fibromyxoma of gastric antrum, 335–336, 336, 337
  solitary fibrous tumor/hemangiopericytoma, 339, 340
Fibroepithelial polyps, 1563, 1563
Fibromuscular arterial dysplasia, 60
Fibrosing lesions
  idiopathic retroperitoneal fibrosis, 363–365, 364
  sclerosing mesenteritis, 362, 362–363, 363
  sclerosing peritonitis, 363
  Weber–Christian disease, 365
Fibrosis
  CIIP, 255, 255
  intestines (see Idiopathic ulcers, intestines)
  large bowel diverticular disease, 234
Fibrous histiocytoma, malignant, 353
Fibrovascular polyps, 540, 541
Fine-needle aspirates, in biopsy, mucosal, 6, 7
First-degree hemorrhoids in anal canal, 1559
Fish tapeworm, 1307. see also Diphyllobothrium latum
Fissures
  in anal canal inflammatory lesions, 1560–1561, 1562
  invasive squamous cell carcinoma, 1571
Fistulas
  in anal canal inflammatory lesions, 1560–1561, 1562
  bronchoesophageal, 430–431
  congenital, 803
  esophageal, 439, 439–442
  invasive squamous cell carcinoma, 1571
  tracheoesophageal, 429–430, 431
Fixation
  lack of, 905
  routine, 12
Fixatives
  biopsy, insufflation with, 24–25
  Bouin's solution, 12
  Hollande's, 12
  special
    immunohistochemical applications, gastrointestinal disorders, 21
    immunohistochemical stains, interpretation, 21
Flat and depressed adenomas, 1388, 1388–1389
Florid squamous hyperplasia, 1564, 1564
5-Flucytosine, 1159
Flush-type adenomas, 1388, 1388–1389
Focal active colitis, 1082–1083
Focal mucosal erosion, large bowel diverticular disease, 234, 234
Folds of Kerckring, 877, 877
Folic acid deficiency, 969–970, 970
Follicular dendritic cell sarcoma, 360–361, 361
Follicular lymphomas
  clinical presentation, 163
  differential diagnosis, 163–164, 165t

immunophenotype and molecular genetics, 163
  incidence, 163
  pathology, 163, 164
  treatment and prognosis, 164–165
Food hypersensitivity
  eosinophils, 952–953
  gastrointestinal reactions, 952
  nonspecific lesions, 952, 953
Forceps, endoscopic pinch biopsy
  cold biopsies, 3
  en face, 3, 3
  hinged jaws, 2, 3
  hot biopsy technique, 3
  jumbo, 2, 3
  in pediatrics, 2, 3
  size and shape, 2, 3
  skinny, 2, 3
  turn-and-suction biopsy technique, 3
Fourth-degree hemorrhoids in anal canal, 1559
Foveolar adenoma, 714, 717–719
Frozen section diagnosis, 23, 294
Fulminant colitis
  and amoebic infection, 1294
  and toxic megacolon, 1032–1034, 1032–1036, 1034t, 1035
Fundic gland
  adenoma, 714–715, 747–748
  heterotopia, duodenitis, 630
  mucosa, 558–560, 559, 560
  polyps, 767–768, 769–771
Fundus, in stomach, 554, 554
Fungi
  aspergillosis, 659, 660, 1310, 1311, 1312
  Candida albicans, 487, 659
  candidiasis, 1308
  clinic symptoms and prognosis, 489
  diabetes mellitus, 487
  histoplasmosis, 659
    causative agent, 1308, 1309, 1310
    cryptococcosis, 1310
    phycomycosis/mucormycosis, 1310, 1310–1311
  intestinal host defences, 89
  mucor, 488, 488
  mucormycosis, 659
  pneumocystis, 1312
  South American blastomycosis, 1312, 1312

G

GALT. see Gut-associated lymphoid tissue (GALT)
Gamma-heavy chain disease, 400
Gangliocytic paraganglioma, 205
Ganglioneuroma
  diffuse ganglioneuromatosis, 320, 321, 323
  ganglioneuromatous polyposis, 320
  multiple endocrine neoplasia, 322
  neuromatous proliferation, 323
  polypoid ganglioneuromas, 320, 321
Ganglioneuromatous polyposis, 320
Gardner's syndrome, 1341, 1342
Gastric antral vascular ectasia (GAVE), 74–76, 75

Gastric antrum
  and body carcinoma, 725
  plexiform fibromyxoma of, 335–336, 336, 337
Gastric arterial supply, in stomach, 555
Gastric calcinosis, 681–682
Gastric cardia carcinoma, 724–725
Gastric endocrine cells, 564, 565t
Gastric epithelial polyps and tumors
  adenocarcinoma
    biopsy diagnosis, 763–764
    clinical implications, 757–759
    cytology, 764
    differential diagnosis, 757
    gastric specimens handling, 764t, 765–765, 765t
    growth pattern, 757
    prognostic factors, 759–763, 760t–762t
    spread, 759
  adenoma in
    classification, 707–720
    definition, 706
    differential diagnosis, 721–723
    grading, 719, 721
    phenotypic expression, 707
    terminology, 706–707
  Brunner gland heterotopia/nodule, 785, 786, 787
  carcinomas
    classification, 731–732, 732
    features of, 730
    gastric antrum and body, 725
    gastric cardia, 724–725
    histologic classification, 733–734
    natural history, 731–732, 732
    pathogenesis, 725
    predisposing conditions, 728–730
    premalignant lesions, 730
    risk factors, 725–728
    superficial cancers and subdivision, 731
    variants of, 737–757
  Cronkhite-canada syndrome-associated polyps, 778, 779
  familiar gastric hyperplastic polyposis, 777–778
  gastric xanthomas, 778–780, 780
  gastritis cystic profunda
    differential diagnosis, 784, 784
    pathology, 783–784, 784
  heterotopic pancreas, 784–785, 785–786
  juvenile polyps, 775, 776
  mucosal bumps and nodules, 780
  mucosal cysts, 786
  nonneoplastic polyps
    biopsy and excision, 766–767
    classification, 766, 766t
    differential diagnosis, 774–775
    fundic gland polyps, 767–768, 769–771
    hyperplastic polyps, 768, 771, 771–773, 774
    inflammatory polyps, 768, 771, 771–773, 774
    multiple gastric polyps, 774–775
    pathology, 771, 774, 774
    single polyps, 774
  Peutz–Jeghers polyps, 775, 777, 777

polypoid gastritis, 778
PTEN hamartoma tumor syndrome, 777, 778
solitary polypoid hamartoma, 781, 781–782
Gastric folds
  clinical presentation, 678–679
  differential diagnosis, 680
  histologic features, 679–680
  large, 677
  treatment, 680
  Zollinger-Ellison syndrome, 678, 679
Gastric GIST, 293, 299
Gastric glandular siderosis, 682
Gastric glomus tumor, 316–317, 317
Gastric heterotopia, in esophagus
  pathogenesis and clinical features, 433–434
  pathology, 433, 434
Gastric lymphoid hyperplasia, 131–132, 132
Gastric malakoplakia, 669, 670
Gastric measles, 1283, 1283–1284
Gastric mucins, 563–564
Gastric mucosal calcinosis, 671
Gastric oxyntic heterotopias, 629
Gastric polyps. *see* Non-neoplastic polyps
Gastric surfaces, in stomach, 554
Gastric ulcer, 629
Gastric xanthomas, 778–780, 780
Gastrin cells (G cells), 218, 218, 219
Gastrinomas, 204, 205. *see also* Zollinger-Ellison syndrome
  gastrointestinal manifestation of, 387
Gastritis
  atrophic, 605, 605–606
  autoimmune
    clinical features, 637–638
    pathogenesis, 635–636
    pathology, 638–643
    subtypes, 636–637
  bezoars, 680, 681
  biopsy interpretation, 682
  calcification, 681–682
  carditis, 649–652, 651
  classification, 571
    ABC classification, 571, 572t
    historical prospective, 572, 573t
    predominant histologic change, 573–574, 574t
    Sydney system, 572–573, 573t
    Whitehead's classification, 571–572
  clinical features, 629–630
  collagenous, 668, 668–669
  distinctive endoscopic entities, 680
  distinctive (specific) type
    atrophic gastritis and gastric atrophy, 605–612
    atypical clinical presentations, 621
    endoscopic appearance, peptic erosions and ulcers, 621–627
    epidemiology, 620–621
    gastroduodenal erosions and ulcers, 615
    H. pylori diagnosis, 595
    H. pylori infection, 587–589, 589t
    H. pylori-associated gastritis histology, 591, 592, 593–595, 594
    infections, 587, 588, 589
    invasive methods, 595–602
    noninvasive methods, 595–596
    pathogenetic factors, 615–620
    staging gastric atrophy, 612–614
  drug- and chemotherapy-induced
    chemotherapy/radiation-associated gastritis, 670–671
    colchicine, 671, 672
    gastric mucosal calcinosis, 671
    iron pill gastritis, 671
    kayexalate, 671
    NSAIDs/ASA, 670
  emphysematous, 656
  endoscopic features, 680
  enterococcal, 656
  eosinophilic, 665–668, 666, 667t
    differential diagnosis, 667, 667t
    gastric involvement in, 667
  foreign bodies, 680
  fungal infections
    aspergillosis, 659, 660
    Candida albicans, 659
    histoplasmosis, 659
    mucormycosis, 659
  gastric biopsies interpretation, 682
  gastric calcinosis, 681–682
  gastric glandular siderosis, 682
  granulomatous, 646–649
  histology
    acute injury, 684
    endocrine cells, 684
    gastric metaplasia, 684
    inflammatory cells, 684
    intestinal metaplasia, 684
    site, 682
    surface and pit epithelium, 684
  inflammatory bowel diseases, 661–671
  large gastric folds, 677–680
  lymphocytic
    description, 643
    etiologies, 643–646
  Ménétrier's disease, 673–677
  non-*H. pylori* helicobacter species
    diagnosis, 653
    emphysematous, 656
    enterococcal gastritis, 656
    phlegmonous, 656
    in stomach of humans, 652t
    syphilis, 653–656, 654–655
    tuberculosis, 653
  parasites and nematodes
    anisakiasis, 660
    cryptosporidium, 659–660
    Strongyloides stercoralis, 660–661, 661
  phlegmonous, 656
  polypoid, 778
  primary immunodeficiency disorders, 100
  protein-losing hypertrophic gastropathy, 677
  serology, 595–596
  stool antigen, 596
  types, 587–627
  urea breath tests, 596
  viral infections, 657–659
Gastritis cystic profunda
  differential diagnosis, 784, 784
  pathology, 783–784, 784
Gastroblastoma, 357, 358, 359, 359

Gastroenteritis, 957–959, 964–967, 966
Gastroesophageal junction (GEJ), 452
Gastroesophageal reflux disease (GERD), 525
  biopsy and criteria uses
    cardia, 458–459
    erosions, 456–458, 456–460, 460t
    traditional sites, 458
  classification, of esophagitis by etiology, 451, 451t
  correlation, 452
  definition, 451
  endoscopy, 452, 453, 454
  etiology, 452–453, 453
  GEJ, 452
  gross/endoscopic appearances, 455–456
  histologic diagnosis and criteria
    dilated intercellular space, 461
    evaluating reactive changes, 460
    grading reactive epithelial changes, 461
    less reliable criteria, 460, 460–461
    signing out reactive changes, 461–462, 462
  inflammatory cells
    cameron's ulcer, 468, 468
    complications, 467–468
    manifestation, 464–465, 467, 467
    progression, 467
    related strictures, 468
  long-term therapy, 42
  Los Angeles grading system, 453–455, 454
  nonerosive, 455, 455
  pathogenesis, 452–453, 453
  prognosis, 452
  symptoms, 452
  therapy, 452
Gastrointestinal disorders, 21
Gastrointestinal (GI) hemorrhage, 275
Gastrointestinal (GI) infections
  biopsy diagnosis
    acute infectious (self-limited) colitis, 1220, 1220–1222, 1222
    electron microscopy, 1223
    mild acute/chronic inflammation, 1222
    molecular tests, 1223, 1223t, 1224t
    no change, 1220
    organisms and cytopathic changes detection, 1222
    special stains, 1222–1223, 1223t
    specific histologic pattern, 1222
  cellular changes, 1217t
  clinical conditions
    health care-associated/nosocomial/infection, 1225
    localized outbreaks, 1224–1225
    oral-anal sexual practices, 1225–1226
    traveler's diarrhea, 1224, 1225t
  clinical features, 1218
  clinical presentation, 1211t–1213t
  diagnostic methods, 1211t–1213t
  endoscopic and gross findings, 1218
  morbidity and mortality rate, 1210
  pathogens, 1217t
  stool examination and culture, 1219–1220

Gastrointestinal ischemia
  etiology
    acute mesenteric ischemia, 35, 37–38, *37t*
    chronic mesenteric ischemia, 38
    esophageal ischemia., 35, *35*
    gastric ischemia, 35, *36*
  pathology
    diffuse mucosal flattening, 40, *41*
    ileum, focal segmental infarction, 38, *39*
    inflammatory bowel disease, 41–42
    ischemic colitis, 42–45
    ischemic proctitis, 45–46
    mesenteric vein thrombosis, 38, 41, *42*
    microscopy, 40–42
    mucosal ulceration, 39, *39*
    small intestinal ischemic necrosis, 41, *41*
    thumbprinting, 39, *40*
    villi, Gruenhagen–Mingazzini space, 40, *40*
  pathophysiology
    causes of, 33–34, *33t*
    cellular effects, 34
    mucosa, 34
    reperfusion injury, 34–35
Gastrointestinal manifestation
  coagulation disorders, 401
  hematologic disorders, 400–403
  hemolytic uremic syndrome, 400–401
  skin disorders (*see* Skin disorders)
Gastrointestinal neuroectodermal tumor (GINECT), 350–351, *352*
Gastrointestinal stromal tumors (GISTs), 265
  CD117- and DOG1-positive tumors, 303–304, *303t*
  demography and clinical aspects, 292
  diagnostic procedures, 292–293, *293*
  differential diagnosis, 310, *310t–312t*, 313
  frozen section diagnosis, 294
  GIST syndromes
    Carney's triad, 307, *308–309*, 309
    familial GIST syndrome, 306–307, *308*
    GIST-paraganglioma syndrome/Carney–Stratakis syndrome, 309
    neurofibromatosis type 1/von Recklinghausen's disease, 307
    pediatric GIST, 309
    small GIST, 309–310
    sporadic multiple GIST, 309
  gross examination and appearances, 294, *295*
  histogenesis, 292
  immunohistochemistry
    CD117-negative, 303
    DOG1, 301
    false-positive immunoreactivity, 301, *302*, 303
    membrane staining, 301
  microscopic appearances
    epithelioid, *297*
    histological changes, 294, *297*
    pleomorphic, *298*
    posttreatment changes, 301
    spindle cell, *296*
    unusual morphologic variants, 297, *300*, 301

  molecular features and mutational analysis
    CD117 negative, 304
    chromosomal alterations, 305
    classification, 307t
    KIT and *PDGFRA*, 304
    SDHB expression, NF1 and BRAF mutations, 305
    SDHB-deficient, 305, *308*
  predicting behavior, 305–306, *306t*
  reporting GIST, 313, *313t*
  surgery, 294
  targeted therapy with imatinib, 293–294
Gastrointestinal (GI) tract
  functional anatomy, 89–94
  gut-associated lymphoid tissue distribution
    Carnoy's fixative, 90
    dome region, 92–93
    follicular area, 93
    intramucosal cellular infiltrate, 90
    intramucosal lamina propria, 90
    mucosal lamina propria macrophages, 90
    mucosal mast cells, 90
    neutrophils, 90
    parafollicular zone, 93
    Peyer's patch, 91, *91*
    solitary lymphoid follicles, 91
Gastrointestinal motility disorders
  gut, musculature, 241
  gut, normal motility apparatus, 240–241
  smooth muscle demonstration, 241–242
Gastrointestinal neuromuscular disorders
  classification, *246t*
  London classification, *247t*
Gastroparesis, 251
Gastropathy
  chemical/reflux-associated, reactive, 575–583
  classification, 571
  congestive, 585, *586*
  distinctive (specific) types
    predominantly vascular changes, 583–587
    reactive (predominant epithelial) changes, 575–583
  hemorrhagic, 585–587
  hypertrophic, 571
  types, 574–587
Gastroschisis, 907
GAVE. *see* Gastric antral vascular ectasia (GAVE)
Gay bowel disease, 1226
Genital tract cancers, 1571
GERD. *see* Gastroesophageal reflux disease (GERD)
Giant cell arteritis, 51–52
Giant condyloma of Bushke and Lowenstein, 1565, *1566*, 1567
Giardia, 1288–1289, *1289*
  epidemiology, 1288
  G. lamblia, 932
  pathogenesis and clinical features, 1288–1289, *1289*

Giardiasis
  with AIDS, 113
  primary immunodeficiency disorders, 100
Giemsa stain, 23
GIST syndromes
  Carney's triad, 307, *308–309*, 309
  familial GIST syndrome, 306–307, *308*
  GIST-paraganglioma syndrome/Carney–Stratakis syndrome, 309
  neurofibromatosis type 1/von Recklinghausen's disease, 307
  pediatric GIST, 309
  small GIST, 309–310
  sporadic multiple GIST, 309
Glandular carcinoid tumor, *206*
Glandular zone, of stomach, 557
Glomus tumor, 316–317, *317*
Glove powder peritonitis, 1156
Glutaraldehyde, hydrogen peroxide/peracetic acid, 1160–1161, *1161–1162*
Gluten free diet, 946–947
Glycogenic acanthosis, 444–445, *445*
Goblet cell carcinoma (GCC), 1497, *1497*
  clinical features, 859
  gross pathology, 859
  histology, 858–859, *859–860*
  immunohistochemistry, 860
  poorly differentiated, 860, *861*, 862
  prognosis and treatment, 864
  signet ring carcinoma, 862, *862–863*, 864
  terminology and histogenesis, 857, *858–859*, 859
  tumor, 209
Goblet cell hyperplastic polyps (GCHP), 1354, *1357*
Goblet cells, 890, *890*
Gold enteritis and colitis, 1159, *1160*
Golgi zone, 301, *302*
Gonads, 388
Gonococcal proctitis, 1266, 1266–1267
  gross and endoscopic appearances, 1266, *1266*
  histology, *1266*, 1266–1267
Graft versus host disease (GVHD), 496
  chronic GVHD, 110
  clinical presentation, 107–108
  diagnosis, 110
  gross appearance, 108
  histology, 108, *109*
  pathogenesis, 107
Granular cell tumor, 329–330, *329–330*
Granulation tissue, 535–536, *537*
Granulocytic sarcoma, *176*, 176–177, *177*
Granuloma inguinale, 1249, *1250*
  in anal canal, 1562
  differential diagnosis, 1249
  gross appearance, *1250*
  prognosis, 1249
  ulceration and fibrosis, *1250*
Granulomatosis, Wegener's 51, 53
Granulomatous and eosinophilic enteritis/colitis, 1156–1158
Granulomatous appendicitis
  arteritis, 828, *828*
  histiocytic diseases
    decidualization, 827, *827*
    sarcoidosis, 828

inherited disorders, 828, *829*
isolated appendiceal, 826
lymphoid hyperplasia, 825, *825*
morphologic appearances, 824
ulcerative colitis, 826, *827*
Granulomatous disease, chronic, 828, *829*
  small bowel mucosal disease, 973
Granulomatous disorders
  chronic granulomatous disease, 407
  sarcoidosis, 406–407
Granulomatous esophagitis and sarcoid, 497–498
Granulomatous gastritis
  characteristics, 646–647, *647*
  conditions associated with, 647, *648t*
  evaluation of, *647*, 649
  gastric sarcoidosis, 648–649
  H. pylori infection, 648
  idiopathic (isolated) granulomatous gastritis, 649
Gut
  cellular immune system, 94
  intestinal host defences, 88–89
  musculature, 241
  normal motility apparatus, 240–241
Gut-associated immune system, 1214
Gut-associated lymphoid tissue (GALT), 891
  Carnoy's fixative, 90
  distribution, 89
  dome region, 92–93
  follicular area, 93
  intramucosal cellular infiltrate, 90
  intramucosal lamina propria, 90
  mucosal lamina propria macrophages, 90
  mucosal mast cells, 90
  neutrophils, 90
  parafollicular zone, 93
  Peyer's patch, 91, *91*
  solitary lymphoid follicles, 91
GVHD. *see* Graft *versus* host disease (GVHD)

H

Hamartomas
  and esophageal, polyps and tumors, 540
  myoepithelial, 784–785, *785–786*, 1335, *1336*
  polyps, 1328
Heat-induced epitope retrieval (HIER), 303
Helicobacter pylori
  biopsy site(s) role, 602
  epidemiology, 589–590
  and esophageal squamous cell carcinoma, 508
  gastritis
    diagnosis, 595
    disorders associated with, 614
    distribution and severity, 590–591
    histology, 591, *592*, 593–595, *594*
    infection, 587–589, *589t*
  in heterotopia, 905
  infection, 725–726
    diagnosis, 15
  invasive methods
    culture, 596–597
    detection method, 595–602
    hematoxylin and eosin, 597–598

histology, 597
rapid urease test, 596
nonsteroidal anti-inflammatory drugs and synergy with, 629
stains, identification of
  description, 598–599, *599t*
  immunohistochemistry, 601–602
  non-silver-based stains, *600*, 601
  silver-based stains, 600–601
Helminths, 23
Hemangioma, *73t*, 344, 344–345, *345*
Hemangiopericytoma, 339, *340*
Hematologic disorders, gastrointestinal manifestation of
  coagulation disorders, 401
  dysproteinemias, 400
  hemolytic uremic syndrome, 400–401
  mastocytosis, 401–403
  Rosai–Dorfman disease, 403
Hematomas
  intramural, 66, 67, 435
  perianal, 1560
  retroperitoneal, 1153
Hemicolectomy, 1132, *1133*
Hemochromatosis, 1179
Hemodialysis, 391
Hemolytic uremic syndrome (HUS), 400–401, 1234
Hemophilia, 401
Hemopoeitic stem cell transplantation
  characteristics, 106
  chronic GVHD, 110
  GI infections, *107t*
  graft versus host disease
    clinical presentation, 107–108
    diagnosis, 110
    gross appearance, 108
    histology, 108, *109*
    pathogenesis, 107
  infections, 106
  parasitic infestations, *107t*
  transplantation regimen, 106
Hemorrhage
  during biopsy, 18–19
  gastrointestinal, 66–67
  large bowel diverticular disease, 236
Hemorrhagic enterocolitis, 38, *39*, 43
Hemorrhagic gastropathy, 585–587
Hemorrhagic infarction, 913
Hemorrhoidectomy, 1559–1560
Hemorrhoids, in anal canal
  clinical features, 1559, *1560*
  description, *1558*, 1558–1559
  hemorrhoidectomy specimens dealing, 1559–1560
  histologic features, 1559, *1560*
  pathogenesis, 1559
Henle's plexus, 242
Henoch–Schönlein purpura, 55–56, *58*
Hepatic disorders, gastrointestinal manifestation of
  autoimmune hepatitis, 393
  liver transplantation, 394
  portal hypertension, 393
  primary sclerosing cholangitis, 393
Hepatobiliary disorders, 1077–1078, *1077t*
Hepatoid adenocarcinoma, 534

Her2 status, 761
Hereditary connective tissue disorders, 384
Hereditary gastric cancer predisposition syndromes, 727–728
Hereditary nonpolyposis colon cancer (HNPCC)
  adenomas uses, 1452
  clinical features, 1446
  immunohistochemistry, 1447, 1449–1450
  lymphoid polyposis with reactive lymphoid hyperplasia, 1453
  management and follow-up, 1452
  MLH1-deficient carcinomas, 1451–1452
  molecular genetics and pathogenesis, 1445–1446
  Muir-Torre syndrome, 1452–1453
  multiple adenomas, 1453
  pathogenesis, 1341
  pathology and diagnosis, 1446–1447
  penetrance and extracolonic disease, 1446
  post resection management, 1452
  prognosis, 1452
  screening, 1450–1451
Hereditary thymic dysplasia, 102–103
Hermansky–Pudlak syndrome, 1085–1086, *1086*
Hernias
  anterior abdominal wall, 62
  diaphragmatic, 63
  epigastric, 62
  external, 62
  hiatal, 453
    esophagus in, 422, *423*
    sliding, 453, *453*
  incisional, 62
  inguinal and femoral, 62
  internal, 62–63
  Richter's, 62
  umbilical, 62
  ventral, 62
Herpes simplex virus (HSV)
  colitis, 1276
  complications, 485
  cytomegalovirus infection
    description, 1278
    pathogenesis, 1278
    primary infection, 1278–1279
    reactivated infection, 1279, *1279–1282*, 1279–1283
  and esophagitis, 404, *405*
  gastrointestinal manifestation of, 398
  measles, *1283*, 1283–1284
  proctitis
    description, 1276
    gross appearance, 1276, *1277*
    histology, 1276–1277, *1277*
  varicella zoster, 485, 486
Herpesvirus infections, 1276–1283
  in anal canal, 1561
  colitis, 1276
  complications, 485
  cytomegalovirus infection (*see* Cytomegalovirus (CMV))
  diagnosis, 6

Herpesvirus infections (Continued)
  and esophagitis, 484, *485*
  gastric disease associated with, 657–658
  inflammatory response, 115
  measles, *1283*, 1283–1284
  proctitis, 1276, *1277*
  varicella zoster, 485, *486*
Heterotopias
  and bowel, large and small, *904*, 904–905
  gastric heterotopia
    pathogenesis and clinical features, 433–434
    pathology, *433*, 434
  in Meckel's diverticulum, 904, *905*
  in small bowel carcinoma, 1341
  tracheobronchial remnants, 434
Heterotopic appendiceal tissue, 803
Heterotopic gastric mucosa, 1333, *1334–1334*, 1335
Heterotopic mesenteric ossification, 365
Heterotopic pancreas, 784–785, *785–786*, 1335, *1336*
Hiatal hernia, 422, *423*, 453
  reflux disease, 453
  sliding, 453, *453*, *453*
Hidradenitis suppurativa, 1582
Hidrocystoma, 1577
High-grade adenoma, 719, *721*, *722*
High-grade dysplasia, 706, *707*
Highly active antiretroviral therapy (HAART), 111
Hilton's white line, 1549, 1552
Hirschsprung's disease
  anal canal, 1557
  and appendix, 828
  biopsy techniques, 22t
  clinical presentation and features, 268
  diagnosis
    biopsy types, 271–272
    immunohistochemical staining, 270
    intraoperative frozen section, 272
  etiology and pathogenesis, 268–269
  gross appearance, 269, *269*
  histology
    acetyl cholinesterase stains, 269, *271*
    aganglionic segment of colon, 268, *269*
    hypertrophied myenteric nerve, 269, *270*
    mucosa and submucosa, 269, *270*
    rectum, 269, *271*
  mural eosinophils in, 274
  variants, 272, 272t
Histiocytes, benign disorders involving
  associated with drug use
    gross and endoscopic appearances, 1172–1173
    histology, 1173, *1173*
    iron-containing macrophages, 1171–1172, *1173*
    pseudomelanosis coli (melanosis coli), 1172, *1175–1176*
  associated with infections
    malakoplakia and xanthogranulomatous nflammation, 1174–1176, *1176–1177*, 1178
    Mycobacterium avium-intracellulare, 1173
    Whipple's disease, 1173

  associated with miscellaneous disorder
    iron-containing macrophages, 1179, *1179t*
    muciphages, 1179–1180, *1181–1182*
    xanthoma/xanthelasma, 1179–1180, *1182*
  associated with storage disease, 1178, *1178t*, *1179t*
  black pigments in terminal ileum and large bowel
    aluminum silicate titanium-containing pigment in terminal ileum, 1180
    injected India ink as a tattoo, 1180
  normal histiocytes, 1171, *1172*, *1172t*
Histiocytic diseases, 826–828, *827*
Histiocytic sarcoma, 174–175
Histiocytosis X, 175
Histogenesis, gastrointestinal stromal tumors, 292
Histoplasmosis
  causative agent, 1308, *1309*, 1310
  cryptococcosis, 1310
  phycomycosis/mucormycosis, 1310, *1310–1311*
Hodgkin's lymphomas, 115, 174
Hollande's fixative, 12
Hollow visceral myopathy, 256
Homosexuality, 1570–1571
Hookworm, 1300, *1300*
Host defense mechanisms
  immune mechanisms, 1210
    gut-associated immune system, 1214
    host infection, 1214
  nonimmune mechanisms, 1210
    gastric juices, acidity of, 1210–1211
    intestinal motility, 1211
    mucus, 1211, 1214
    normal resident bacterial flora, 1214
Hot biopsies, 1389, *1391*
Human herpesviridae infections, 1276. see also Herpesvirus infections
Human immunodeficiency virus (HIV), 167t. see also Acquired immunodeficiency syndrome (AIDS)
Human papillomavirus (HPV), 486, *487*
  of esophagus, 486, *487*
  infection
    anal intraepithelial neoplasia, 1567
    and esophageal squamous cell carcinoma, 508
Hymenolepsis nana (dwarf tapeworm), 1308
Hypercoagulable states, 33t, 43
Hypercoagulation, 65
Hypereosinophilic syndrome, 967
Hyperganglionosis, 273
Hypergastrinemia, 199, 202, 203, 204, 218
Hyperkeratosis plantaris et palmaris, 398
Hyperkeratotic disorders, 398
Hyperparathyroidism, 385
Hyperplasias, 218, 218–219, *219*, 265, 265–266
  endocrine cells, disorders of, 219, *219*
  epithelial hyperplasia without dysplasia, 1564, *1564*
  florid squamous, 1564, *1564*

  mesenteric veins, 57, *59*
  pseudoepitheliomatous, 1564, *1564*
Hyperplastic polyps, 768, 771, *771–773*, 774
  clinical features, 1353
  gross and endoscopic appearances, 1353, *1353*, *1354*
  histology, 1354–1355, *1355–1357*
  tumors of, appendix
    adenomas, *835*, 836
Hypersecretory conditions, 616–617
Hypersensitivity vasculitis, 66
Hypertension, 60, 65, 67
Hyperthyroidism, 384–385
Hypertonic saline enemas, 1160
Hypertrophic gastropathy. see also Gastric folds
  description, 671
  and Ménétrier's disease (see Ménétrier's disease)
  with protein loss
    Helicobacter pylori-associated, 677
    HIV, 677
Hypertrophied muscularis propria, 254, *255*
Hypobetalipoproteinemia, *971*, 971–972
Hypogammaglobulinemia
  diffuse nodular lymphoid hyperplasia, 136–139, *137*, *138*
  secondary (acquired) immunodeficiency disorders, 106
  and small bowel mucosal disease, *955*, 956–957, *958*
Hypogammaglobulinemic sprue, 100
Hypoganglionosis, 273
Hypoparathyroidism, 385–386
Hypoperfusion, 33, 35, 43
Hypopituitarism, 389
Hypoplastic left colon syndrome, 919
Hypoplastic villous syndrome. see Microvillus inclusion disease
Hypotension, 33
Hypotensive and hypovolemic agents, 1155
Hypothalamus and pituitary, 388–389
Hypothyroidism
  and chronic intestinal pseudoobstruction, 276
  gastrointestinal manifestation of, 385
Hypovolemia, 33, 42

I

Iatrogenic and drug-associated inflammatory changes
  acute infectious-type colitis, 1156, *1157*
  chronic inflammation with/without focal active colitis
    cimetidine, 1159
    5-flucytosine, 1159
    gold enteritis and colitis, 1159, *1160*
    ipilimumab and anti PD-1, 1158, *1158*
    isotretinoin, 1159
    mycophenolate mofetil, 1158
    penicillamine, 1159
    rituximab, 1158
  granulomatous and eosinophilic enteritis/colitis, 1156–1158

methyldopa, 1156, *1157*
pseudomembranes and ischemic colitis, 1156
signet-ring changes, 1156
Iatrogenic disorders, vascular system
  gastrointestinal hemorrhage, 66–67
  iatrogenic intestinal ischemia
    arterial obstruction/constriction, 64, *64*
    drug-induced vascular lesion, 64–66, *65*, *66*
    neutropenic colitis, 66
  radiation injury
    acute, 68–69, *69*
    chronic, 69–70, *71*, *72*, 72
    incidence of, 67
    pathophysiology, 67–68, 68t
Iatrogenic gas, at endoscopy, drugs and chemicals changes, 1166–1167
  gross and endoscopic appearances, 1167
  histology, 1167, *1167*
IBD. see Inflammatory bowel disease (IBD)
Idiopathic acute appendicits. see Appendicitis
Idiopathic hypertrophy, 249–250
Idiopathic inflammatory bowel disease (IIBD)
  complications of
    anal disease, 1061–1063, *1063*, *1064*
    backwash ileitis, 1011
    benign strictures, *1015*
    in *Campylobacter*, 1242
    Campylobacter enterocolitis, 1242
    diffuse colitis, 1151
    diversion colitis, 1081–1082
    diversion proctocolitis
    enteritis cystica profunda, 1168–1169, *1169*
    fulminant colitis, *1032–1034*, 1032–1036, 1034t, *1035*
    indeterminate colitis, 1067–1071, *1073*
    inflammatory polyps, 1025
    list of, 1077, 1077t
    perianal disease, 1061–1063, *1063*, *1064*
    pouchitis, 1037–1038
    toxic megacolon, *1032–1034*, 1032–1036, 1034t, *1035*
  definition, 999
  gross pathology, 1011, 1013, 1045–1046, 1048–1049
  and inflammatory bowel disease and microscopic colitis, 999
Idiopathic megacolon, 274
Idiopathic muscular hypertrophy, 249, *249*
Idiopathic retroperitoneal fibrosis, 363–365, *364*
Idiopathic ulcers, intestines
  CMUSE, 1083–1084, *1084*, 1088
  gross and endoscopic appearances, 1144t, 1145–1146, *1146–1147*
  histology, *1146–1147*, 1146–1148
  nonsteroidal anti-inflammatory drugs
    clinical features, 1148
    and diverticular disease, 1151
    idiopathic IBD, 1151–1152
    and large intestinal disease, 1151
    left-sided colonic increase of eosinophils, 1152

pathogenesis, 1148–1149
  and small intestinal disease, 1149, *1149–1150*, 1151
pathogenesis and clinical features, 1144–1145
potassium chloride, 1152
IgA deficiency syndromes, 957
Ileal conduits, 1517
Ileitis, acute terminal, 1243, *1244*
Ileocecal valve, 340–341, *341*, 884–885, *885*
Ileostomy stomas, pouches, and conduits, 1341, *1343*
Ileum, 875, *899*
  carcinoid tumors, 206–208, *206–208*
  ileal endometriosis, 1096
  involvement in, *1029*, 1029–1030
  pouches and complications, 1037–1041, *1039–1041*, 1041
Imatinib, gastrointestinal stromal tumors, 293–294
Immotile cilia syndrome, 905
Immune system, gastrointestinal
  and bowel, large and small, *889*, 893–895, *894*
  cellular, 94
  function, 89–94
  humoral, 93–94, *94*
  intestinal host defense mechanisms, 88–89
  lymphoid tissue distribution, *89*, 89–90
  nonimmunologic factors, 89
  T-cell system, 94
Immunodeficiency disorders. see also Hypogammaglobulinemia
  chronic granulomatous disease, 106
  DiGeorge's syndrome
    ataxia telangiectasia, 105
    characteristics, 105
    22q11 chromosomal deletion, 105
    transcobalamin II deficiency, 105
    Wiskott–Aldrich syndrome, 105
  intestinal host defences, 88–89
  intestinal tract
    common variable immunodeficiency, 95
    intrinsic and associated morphologic changes, 97–98
    mucosal lesions, infections, 96–97
    neoplasms, 98, 98t
    no significant alteration, 96, *96*
    pathologist's diagnostic role, 94
    primary immunodeficiency disorders, 95, 95t, 96t
    secondary immunodeficiency disorders, 95
  invasive squamous cell carcinoma, 1571
  lymphoma
    AIDS, 167–168, *167t*
    inflammatory bowel disease, 170–171
    methotrexate-associated, 171
    primary immunodeficiency-associated, 165–167
    PTLD, 168–170, *169*
  nonimmunologic defects, 105
  in patients, workup, 115
  phagocytic and cell dysfunction, 106

primary disorders
  predominant antibody defects, 99–102
  predominant cell-mediated immunodeficiency, 102–105
  World Health Organization (WHO) classification, 98, 99t
secondary (acquired) disorders
  acquired immunodeficiency syndrome (AIDS), 110–115
  B-cell dysfunction with dysgammaglobulinemia, 106
  bone marrow transplantation, 106–110
  hypogammaglobulinemia, 106
  iatrogenic complications, 106
  intestinal transplantation, 110
  malnutrition, 106
  morphologic changes, 106
  pathologic manifestations, 106
  and small bowel mucosal disease, *955*, 956–957, *958*
  systemic mastocytosis, 106
Immunoglobulin (IgA), 93
  deficiency
    B-cell disorders, 102
    histology, 101–102
    infantile X-linked agammaglobulinemia, 102
    pathogenesis and clinical features, 101
    secretory component deficiency, 102
  intestinal host defenses, 88–89
Immunohistochemistry
  gastrointestinal stromal tumors
    CD117-negative, 303
    DOG1, 301
    false-positive immunoreactivity, 301, *302*, 303
    membrane staining, 301
  stains, 21
  tissue handling
    fixation, 12
    transport, 6
Immunoproliferative small intestinal disease (IPSID)
  clinical presentation, 152–153
  diagnosis and differential diagnosis, 154–155
  etiopathogenesis, 152
  immunophenotype and molecular genetics, 154
  incidence of, 151–152
  occurrence, 152
  pathology, 153–154, *153t*, *154*
  treatment and prognosis, 155
Immunostains, 253–254
Impaired epithelial cell replacement, 969–970, *970*
Incisional hernias, 62
Incomplete intestinal metaplasia, 610, 728
Indeterminate colitis
  carcinoma in, 1125
  definition, 999, 1067
  microscopic features, 1066t
  pathology, 1068–1071, *1073*
Infant botulism, 1256
Infantile pyloric stenosis (IPS), 250–251
  circular muscle, 250
  ganglion cells, 250, *251*

Infantile pyloric stenosis (IPS) (Continued)
neurotransmitters, 251
prevalence, 250
Infantile X-linked agammaglobulinemia, 102
Infarcted appendix epiploica–peritoneal mouse, 919
Infarction
and duplication, complications of, 913
segmental, 39, 39
Infection
in acute appendicitis, 808
agents
in situ hybridization assays, 1223t
monoclonal/polyclonal antibodies, 1223t
PCR assays, 1224t
in anal canal
granuloma inguinale, 1562
lymphogranuloma venereum, 1562
syphilis, 1561, 1561–1562
virus, 1561
bacteria, 489
during biopsy, 22–23
bone marrow transplantation, 106
fungal
candida albicans, 487
clinic symptoms and prognosis, 489
diabetes mellitus, 487
mucor, 488, 488
GI problems in AIDS patient, 113, 113t
and inflammatory bowel disease, 1227
mechanisms of
adherence and initial attachment, 1215
colonization, 1215
diarrhea, enteroadherent and, 1216
persistence of infection, 1216
tissue invasion, 1215
nosocomial, 1225
and oral–anal sexual practices, 1225–1226, 1226t
outbreaks of, 1224–1225
and small bowel mucosal disease, 968
toxin production mechanisms
cholera toxin, 1216
clostridial toxins, 1216
shiga and shiga-like toxins, 1216
staphylococcal enterotoxins, 1216
verotoxin, 1216
viruses (see also Viruses)
acute HIV, 486–487
CMV, 486, 486
HPV, 486, 487
HSV type I, 484–486, 485
Yersinia pseudotuberculosis, 1248, 1248–1249, 1249
Infectious gastroenteritis, 587, 587, 957–959
Infectious mononucleosis, 820
Infective endocarditis, 400
Inferior mesenteric artery, 32, 32
Inflammation, large bowel diverticular disease, 234, 234
Inflammatory bowel disease (IBD), 41, 45, 57, 60. see also Idiopathic inflammatory bowel disease (IIBD); Ulcerative colitis
adaptation to prolapse, 1169–1170
apoptotic bodies, 108
Behçet's disease
clinical features, 1086–1087
epidemiology, 1086
pathology, 1087, 1087–1088
cancer
anal carcinoma, 1125
carcinoma after surgery, 1126
carcinoma complicating ulcerative colitis, 1123–1124
carcinoma in indeterminate colitis, 1125
colorectal cancer in colitis, 1120, 1121–1123, 1122–1124
Crohn's disease, 1124–1125
malignancies, 1125–1126
molecular pathogenesis of, 1099, 1099–1101, 1100t
chromoendoscopy, 9–10, 10
and *Clostridium difficile*, 1255
colitis (and enteritis) cystica profunda, 1168–1169, 1169
collagenous gastritis, 668, 668–669
compensatory changes, 1167–1168
Crohn's disease and ulcerative colitis
clinical features, 662
endoscopic features, 662
histologic features, 662–665, 663, 664
diarrhea
chemotherapeutic agents, 1170–1171
mycophenolate mofetil, 1171
proton pump inhibitors, 1171
diversion colitis, 1081–1082, 1082
diverticular disease
clinical presentation and features, 237, 237–238
differential diagnosis, 238
diverticular colitis, 1079, 1080–1081, 1081
drug- and chemotherapy-induced gastritis
chemotherapy/radiation-associated gastritis, 670–671
colchicine, 671, 672
gastric mucosal calcinosis, 671
iron pill gastritis, 671
kayexalate, 671
NSAIDs/ASA, 670
drug-associated, 1134–1136, 1135t
dysplasia
classification and grading, 1114, 1114–1115
clinical implications, 1119, 1119–1121, 1120
grading dysplasia, 1115–1116, 1115t
gross pathology, 1102–1103, 1103–1104, 1103t
immunohistochemistry, 1117–1119, 1118
issues of, 1116–1117
lesions management, 1101–1102
microscopic pathology, 1103–1112, 1105–1112
reactive changes, distinction from, 1112, 1113, 1114
enteritis and colitis cystica superficialis, 1170, 1170t
eosinophilic colitis, 1091, 1091–1092, 1091t
eosinophilic gastritis, 665–668, 666, 667t
Escherichia coli, verotoxin, 1234
extrinsic damage to bowel, 1168
focal active colitis, 1082–1083
gastric malakoplakia, 669, 670
Hermansky–Pudlak syndrome, 1085–1086, 1086
iatrogenic diseases, 1134–1136
incidental terminal ileitis, 1083–1084, 1084
instrumentation, 1168
large-bowel disease in acute pancreatitis, 1168
malabsorption, 1170
neoplasms (following immune suppression and radiation), 1171
neutrophil function defects, 1084–1085, 1085
NK cell enteropathy, 1089, 1090, 1091
obstructive colitis, 1088–1089, 1089
pathologist, role of, 1136
rectal mucosal prolapse, 1170
reporting ileitis, 1083–1084
Inflammatory cells
basal hyperplasia vs. squamous dysplasia, 463, 464
eosinophils, 462
GERD (see also Gastroesophageal reflux disease (GERD))
cameron's ulcer, 468, 468
complications, 467–468
manifestation, 464–465, 467, 467
related strictures, 468
IEM, 462, 462–463
marked hyperplasia of rete pegs vs. invasive squamous carcinoma, 464, 465
neutrophils, 462
polyps, 463, 463
squamous mucosa, atypical in, 464, 466
Inflammatory cloacogenic polyps, 1562–1563, 1563
Inflammatory fibroid polyp, 333–335, 333–335
Inflammatory lesions, of anal canal
fissures and fistulae, 1560–1561, 1562
granuloma inguinale, 1562
lymphogranuloma venereum, 1562
syphilis, 1561, 1561–1562
viral infections, 1561
Inflammatory myofibroblastic tumor, 337, 338, 339
Inflammatory polyps, 539, 540, 768, 771, 771–773, 774, 1407, 1408, 1409
Inflammatory pseudo polyps. see Inflammatory polyps
Inflammatory vascular disorders. see Vasculitis
Inflammatory visceral neuropathy, 274
Inguinal hernia, 62
Injected India ink as a tattoo, 1180
Instrumentation of inflammatory bowel disease, 1168
Insular carcinoids, endocrine tumors, 209, 209, 210

Internal anal sphincter, 1554
Internal hemorrhoids, 1560
Internal hernias, 62–63
Internal sphincter achalasia/ultrashort hirschsprung's disease, 273
Interstitial cells of Cajal (ICC), 292
  abnormalities of
    DOG1 immunostain, 265, *265*
    hyperplasia, *265*, 265–266
    prognosis and therapy, 266
  and bowel, structure of, *897*, 897–899, *899*
  enteric nervous system, *244*, 244–245, *245*
  of stomach, 566–567
Intestinal arteries, 32
Intestinal diverticula, 227
Intestinal ischemia
  arterial obstruction/constriction, *64*, 64
  collateral circulation, 34
  drug-induced vascular lesion, 64–66, *65*, *66*
  neutropenic colitis, 66
Intestinal lymphangiectasia, *968*, 968–969
Intestinal lymphocytic epithelioganglionitis, 265
Intestinal lymphoma, 967–968
Intestinal metaplasia, *610*, 610–611
Intestinal motility, 1211
Intestinal musculature, *908*, 908–909, *909*
Intestinal neuronal dysplasia, 272–273
Intestinal pseudoobstruction
  acute intestinal pseudoobstruction, 252
  biopsies, of muscularis propria, 253
  clinical features, 253
  definition, 251–252
  Ogilvie's syndrome, 252
Intestinal spirochetosis
  description, 1269
  histology, 1270–1271, *1270–1271*
  pathogenesis and clinical features, 1269–1270
Intestinal tract, diffuse lymphoid tissue, *89*, 89
Intestinal transplantation
  acute cellular rejection, grading scheme, 111t
  secondary (acquired) immunodeficiency disorders, 110
Intestinal tumors, biopsy technique, 24
Intestinal type carcinoma, 851
Intestinal vascular lesions associated with clinical syndromes, 348
Intestinal-type adenomas
  characteristics, 708, *709*, *710*
  clinical features, 707–708
  clinical implications, 708
  pathologic findings, 708
Intolerance, food, 952
Intraepithelial lymphocytes (IELs), 89
  diffuse lymphoid tissue, *89*, 89
  intestinal host defences, 88–89
Intraepithelial lymphocytosis, small bowel mucosal disease, with variably severe lesions
  acrodermatitis enteropathica, 960
  bacterial overgrowth syndrome, 959

celiac disease, 645
description, *937t*, 956
immunodeficiency syndromes, 956–957
infectious gastroenteritis, 957–959
Zollinger–Ellison syndrome, 959–960
Intraepithelial neoplasia, 508–509
Intraluminal duodenal diverticulum, 239–240
Intramucosal carcinoma, gastric epithelial polyps and tumors
  definition, 707
  grading, 719, 721
Intramucosal cysts, 783
Intramural hematoma, 435
Intranuclear neuronal inclusions, *263*, 263
Intrinsic nervous system. *see* Enteric nervous system
Intussusception, *63*, 63–64
  of appendix, 805–806, 814, 818
  and Burkitt's-like lymphoma, 155, *156*
  mechanical obstruction, *63*, 63–64
Intussusceptum, 63
Intussuscipiens, 63
Invasive carcinoma, 707
Invasive squamous cell carcinoma
  in anal canal
    chemotherapy and radiotherapy, 1575
    cigarette smoking, 1571
    clinical features, 1571
    Crohn's disease, 1571
    fissures and fistulas, 1571
    gross appearances, 1571–1572, *1572*
    histologic features, 1572, *1573*, 1574, *1574*
    homosexuality and sexually transmitted diseases, 1570–1571
    immunodeficiency, 1571
    intraepithelial anal squamous neoplasia, 1575–1576, *1576*
    irradiated tumors, biopsy of, 1574–1575
    low socioeconomic status, 1570
    lymphogranuloma venereum, 1571
    minimally invasive/superficial carcinoma, 1575
    multiparity and genital tract cancers, 1571
    premalignant lesions, 1571
    prior irradiation, 1571
    spindle cell variant, 1574
    spread and staging, 1575
    treatment and prognosis, 1575
  lesions of anal canal, 1581
Inverted diverticulum, 236–237, *237*
IPEX syndrome, 199, 220, 389–390
  autoimmune enteropathy, 950
  predominant cell-mediated immunodeficiency, 103
Ipilimumab and anti PD-1, 1158, *1158*
IPSID. *see* Immunoproliferative small intestinal disease (IPSID)
Iron pill gastritis, drug- and chemotherapy-induced gastritis, 671
Iron-containing macrophages, histiocytes
  associated with drug use, 1171–1172, *1173*
  associated with miscellaneous disorder, 1179–1180, *1181–1182*

Irradiation, and squamous cell carcinoma, 508, 515–516
Irritable bowel syndrome, 65, 282
Ischemia
  from atherosclerosis, 33
  digestive tract (*see* Digestive tract ischemia, mechanical obstruction and)
  following angiography, drug-associated injuries
    embolization, 1152–1153
    vessel wall trauma, 1152
  gastrointestinal (*see* Gastrointestinal ischemia)
Ischemic colitis
  aortofemoral bypass surgery, *47*
  clinical manifestations, 42–45
  Clostridium difficile toxin, 44, *48*
  colonic ischemia, 42–43
  endoscopic biopsy, *47*
  etiology, 43, 43t
  healing phase, 45
  hemosiderin-laden macrophages, 45, *49*
  ischemic stricture, 45, *48*
  large bowel infarction, *46*
  massive bowel infarction, 42
  microscopy, 44–45, *46–48*
  pathology, 43–44, *43–46*
  resection specimens, 44
  thumbprinting, 43
  transient/evanescent, 43
Ischemic proctitis, 45–46
Ischemic strictures, 41, 45, 48
Islets of Langerhans, hyperfunction of, 387
Isospora belli, 113. *see also Cystoisospora belli*
Isotretinoin, 1159

J

JC virus (JCV), 726
Jejunoileal diverticula
  gross appearance, *239*, 240
  histology, 240
  pathogenesis and clinical features, 240
Jejunoileitis, ulcerative, 158, *159*
Jejunum, 875
  carcinoid tumors, 206–208, *206–208*
Jumbo biopsy forceps, 2
Juvenile polyps and and juvenile polyposis syndrome, 775, *776*
  clinical features, 1422
  diagnosis and differential diagnosis, 1429–1430
  dysplasia/adenomas and carcinoma, 1424, 1428–1430
  gross and endoscopic appearances, 1423–1428, *1423–1428*
  histology, 1424–1425, *1425–1428*, 1428
  of infancy, 1422–1423
  molecular genetics, 1423
  treatment, 1430

K

Kaposi's sarcoma, *346*, 347
  AIDS associated, 167
  clinical features, 113

Kaposi's sarcoma (Continued)
  pathology, 113–114, *114*
  rectum, *114*
  therapy, 114
Kawasaki's disease, 52–53
Keratoacanthoma, lesions of anal canal, 1581
Ki-1lymphoma, 173
Kinetics, of bowel, 891, *892*
KIT mutation, 304
Kohlmeier–Degos Syndrome, 60
K-ras, 726
Kwashiorkor, childhood, 954, *954*

L

Lactase deficiency, 973
Lamina propria, *889*, 893–895, *894*
  in esophagus, 426
  of stomach, 564, 566
Langerhans cells, 175, 424
Laparoscopic surgery, GIST, 294
Large bowel adenomas
  age, sex, and distribution, 1375–1376
  definition, 1375
  diminutive polyps, 1376
  gross and endoscopic appearances, 1377, *1378t*, *1381*
  histology, 1377, *1380–1385*, 1381, 1384
  natural history, 1376
  synchronous and metachronous, 1376
  tubular adenoma, 1385
  tubular vs. villous patterns, 1384–1385
  tubulovillous adenoma, 1385–1386
  villous adenoma, 1385
Large bowel diverticular disease
  clinical features, 229–230
  complication, 229
  definitions, 227–228
  diverticular colitis, 227–236, *230–236*
  endoscopy, 230
  gross pathology
    mucosal ridges, 230, *232*
    muscularis propria, *232*
    prediverticular disease, 231–232, *232*, *233*
    specimen handling, 232–233
    teniae, 230, *231*
  histology
    fibrosis, 234
    focal mucosal erosion, 234, *234*
    hemorrhage, 236
    inflammation, 234, *234*
    mucosa herniations, 233, *233*
    perforated diverticulum, 235, *235*
  imaging, 230, *231*
  pathogenesis
    bowel wall weakness, 229
    incidence, 228
    intraluminal pressure, of colon, 228–229
    prevalence, 228
    terminology, 227
Large bowel tumors
  serrated/hyperplastic polyps (see Serrated/hyperplastic polyps)
  urinary conduits tumors
    endometriosis, 1518, 1520, *1521–1522*, 1523
    ileal conduits, 1517
    secondary tumors of large bowel, 1518, *1519–1520*
    ureterosigmoidostomy sites, 1517–1518
Large intestine. *see also* Bowel, large and small; specific diseases of
  embryology and development, 900–904, *901*, *902*, *903*
  external appearance of, *876*, 876–877
  internal appearance of, *878*, 878–879, *879*
  mucosa, *882*, 885–887, *886*, *888*, *889*
  peritonealized and nonperitonealized surfaces, 877
Latent celiac sprue, 945
Late-onset immunodeficiency syndromes, *955*, 956–957, *958*
Lauren classification, 733, *733*–734
Laxatives, drugs and chemicals, changes due to
  alcohol, 1163
  cathartic colon, 1162, *1164*
  foreign material, injected, 1163
  glutaraldehyde, hydrogen peroxide/peracetic acid, 1160–1161, *1161–1162*
  hypertonic saline enemas, 1160
  myenteric plexus damage, pseudoobstruction, and stercoral ulceration, 1162–1163
  polyethylene glycol, 1162
  soap, *1161–1162*, 1161
  sodium phosphate (fleet)s enemas and bisacodyl, 1159, *1161*
Leather bottle stomach, 732, 757
Left-sided diverticula, 227–228
Legionella, 1243
Leiomyomas, 313–314, *315*
  in Meckel's diverticulum, 917, *918*
Leiomyomatosis, 316
Leiomyomatosis peritonealis disseminata (LPD), 316
Leiomyosarcoma, 317–318, *318*. *see also* Mesenchymal tumors
Leukemia, *176*, 176–177, *177*
Leukoplakia
  in anal canal, 1559
  definition, 496
LGV. *see* Lymphogranuloma venereum (LGV)
Lichen planus, 398
Lichen sclerosus, lesions of anal canal, 1582
Lift-and-cut technique
  bleb formation, 4
  non lifting sign, 5
Ligament of Treitz, 875
Linear hyperplasia, *201*
Linitis plastica, 732, *732*, 733, 737
Lipid islands of stomach, 778–780, *780*
Lipid metabolism, disorders
  Fabry's disease, 405–406
  Tangier disease, 406
  Wolman's disease, 406
Lipid storage diseases, *972*, 972–973
Lipocytes, tumors of
  lipomatous polyposis and epiploic lipomatosis, 343, *343*
  submucosal lipomas, *342*
Lipohyperplasia, of ileocecal valve, 340–341, *341*
Lipomatous polyposis and epiploic lipomatosis, 343, *343*
Liposarcoma, 343–344
Liver transplantation, gastrointestinal manifestation of, 394
Los Angeles grading system, 453–455, *454*
Lower esophageal diverticulum. *see* Mid esophageal diverticulum
Lower esophageal sphincter (LES), 422
Lower esophageal webs and rings. *see* Schatzki rings
Low-grade adenoma adenoma, 719, 721, *722*
Low-grade dysplasia (LGD), 706, *707*
Luetic infection, 489
Luminal obliteration, 812, *812*
Lymph node metastases, 759, *760t*
Lymphangiectasia, intestinal, *968*, 968–969
Lymphangioma, 347–348, *347–349*
Lymphatic dissemination, 759
Lymphatics
  in anal canal, 1554
  in bowel, large and small, 900, *900*
  in esophagus, 423
  in stomach, 555
Lymphocytes
  diffuse lymphoid tissue, 90
  in esophagus, 425, *426*
Lymphocytic and esophagitis, 489–490, *490*
Lymphocytic colitis, 994–995, *995*. *see also* Collagenous colitis; Microscopic colitis
Lymphocytic dysplasia, 125
Lymphocytic gastritis
  associations, 643t
  description, 643
  etiologies
    celiac disease, 645
    clinical presentation, 646
    Crohn's disease, 646
    endoscopic appearance, 646
    Helicobacter, 643, *644*, 645
    immunodeficiency, 646
    lymphocytic gastroenterocolitis, 645–646
    medications, 646
    morphologic diagnosis, 646
    neoplasia, 646
Lymphocytic phlebitis, enterocolic, 57, *59*
Lymphogranuloma venereum (LGV), 1273
  in anal canal, 1562
  invasive squamous cell carcinoma, 1571
Lymphoid hyperplasia
  angiofollicular hyperplasia, 132–133
  Helicobacter gastritis, 130–131
  occurrence, 130
  pseudolymphoma
    diagnosis, 131
    pathology, 131–132, *132*
  rectum, 135–136, *136*
  small intestine
    diffuse nodular, 136–139, *137*, *138*
    duodenum, 133, 135, *135*
    ileum and appendix, 133, *134*, 135
Lymphoid nodules and tumors, 1335

Lymphoid tissue
  diffuse, 89, 89–90
  distribution, 89–94
  GALT (see Gut-associated lymphoid tissue (GALT))
  gut-associated distribution, 89
  intraepithelial lymphocytes, 89, 89–90
  lymphoid follicles
    mast cells, 90
    overlying epithelium and, 133, 134
    zones, 91, 91, 138–140, 153
  M cells, 92, 92
  macrophages, 90
Lymphoma, 362
  AIDS associated
    Hodgkin's lymphomas, 115
    non-Hodgkin's lymphomas, 114, 115
  classification, 126–127, 126t, 127t
  clinical presentation, 127–128, 128t
  colon (see Colon)
  definition, 125
  diagnostic workup of, 130
  enteropathy-associated T-cell, 126, 126t, 159, 160
  esophagus, 138–139
  follicular center cell, 93
  gastric (see Stomach)
  incidence of, 125
  lymphoepithelium, 124
  lymphoid hyperplasia (see Lymphoid hyperplasia)
  lymphoproliferative disorders (see Lymphoproliferative disorders)
  MALT, 139–143, 161
  Mantle-zone, 161
  marginal zone, 139–143, 161
  molecular diagnosis
    clonal B-cell proliferation, 129–130
    lymphoma-associated translocation, 129
    molecular techniques, 128–129
    viral infection and cDNA chip, 129
  pathogenesis, 125–126
  primary intestinal, 967–968
  small intestine (see Small intestine)
  stomach (see Stomach)
Lymphomatoid granulomatosis, 172
Lymphoplasmacytic lymphomas, 165, 166
Lymphoproliferative disorders, 124.
  see also Lymphoid hyperplasia; Lymphoma; Small intestine; Stomach; specific lymphoproliferative disorders
  miscellaneous, 163–177
Lynch's syndrome
  adenomas uses, 1452
  clinical features, 1446
  immunohistochemistry, 1447, 1449–1450
  lymphoid polyposis with reactive lymphoid hyperplasia, 1453
  management and follow-up, 1452
  MLH1-deficient carcinomas, 1451–1452
  molecular genetics and pathogenesis, 1445–1446
  Muir-Torre syndrome, 1452–1453
  multiple adenomas, 1453
  pathogenesis, 1341

pathology and diagnosis, 1446–1447
penetrance and extracolonic disease, 1446
postresection management, 1452
prognosis, 1452
screening, 1450–1451

M
Macroglobulinemia, 969
Malabsorption
  inflammatory bowel disease, 1170
  small bowel mucosal disease, 949
  syndrome, tropical sprue, 953–954, 954
Malacoplakia/Malakoplakia
  and appendix, 827
  gastric, 669, 670
  inflammatory bowel diseases, 669, 670
  and xanthogranulomatous inflammation, 1174–1176, 1176–1177, 1178
Malformations
  arteriovenous, 73, 77, 78, 78
  vascular, 919
Malignant fibrous histiocytoma, 353
Malignant gastrointestinal neuroectodermal tumor (GINECT), 350–351, 352
Malignant lymphoma, 918
Malignant peripheral nerve sheath tumor (MPNST), 330–331, 331
Malignant-atrophic papulosis, 60
Mallory–Weiss tears
  pathogenesis and clinical features, 437
  pathology, 437, 437–438
Malnutrition, secondary (acquired) immunodeficiency disorders, 106
Malrotation, 905
MALT lymphoma. see Mucosa-associated lymphoid tissue (MALT) lymphoma
Mantle cell lymphoma
  clinical presentation, 161
  differential diagnosis, 162
  immunophenotype and molecular genetics, 162
  pathology, 161–162, 162
  treatment and prognosis, 162
Mantoux test, 1262
Marginal artery, 30–32
Marsh type 1 lesion, 930, 933, 934
Marsh type 3 lesion, 934, 934–935, 939, 941–945
Mastocytic enterocolitis, 282
Mastocytosis
  gastrointestinal manifestation of, 401–403
  systemic, 106
Matrix metalloproteinases (MMPs), 516
Measles, 1283, 1283–1284
Mechanical obstruction. see also Digestive tract ischemia, mechanical obstruction and
  adhesions, 62
  hernias, 62–63
  intussusception, 63, 63–64
  pathogenesis and clinical features, 61–62
  volvulus, 63
Meckel's diverticulum, 240
  in adenocarcinomas, 918, 918
  clinical features, 915

description, 913, 914
pathology, 915–916, 917, 918
tumors in, 916
  adenocarcinomas, 918, 918
  carcinoid, 917
  malignant lymphoma, 918
  mesenchymal, 917, 918
and vitelline duct, 914, 915
Meconium ileus, 919
Medullary carcinoma, 389–390
Megacolon, 1032–1034, 1032–1036, 1034t, 1035, 1241–1242, 1242, 1246
Megacystis-microcolon-intestinal hypoperistalsis syndrome (MMIHS), 260
  and bowel, mechanical disorders of, 919–920
  diagnosis, 273
  immature ganglia, 274
  mural eosinophils in Hirschsprung's disease, 274
Megaduodenum, 254, 256
Megaesophagus, 275
Megajejunum, 254
Meissner's submucosal plexus, 242
Melanocytes, in esophagus, 424
Melanoma, 360, 360, 540–541, 542, 1564–1565, 1565, 1566, 1579–1580, 1580
Melanosis coli, 424. see also Pseudomelanosis coli
Melanotic adenocarcinoma and malignant melanoma, 1504–1505
Ménétrier's disease, 729–730
  carcinoma complicating, 676
  clinical presentation, 675
  differential diagnosis, 675–676
  endoscopic appearance, 674, 675
  pathogenesis, 676
  pathology, 675–676
  polyadenomes en nappes, 673–674
  polyadenomes polypeux, 673
  primary/idiopathic, 674–675
  secondary, 677
  treatment, 676
Mercury, 1183
Merkel cells, 425, 425
Mesenchymal tumors. see also Gastrointestinal stromal tumors; Neurogenic tumors
  adipocytic lesions
    angiolipoma, 343
    atypical lipoma, 342–343
    fatty tumors, differential diagnosis of, 344
    lipohyperplasia, of ileocecal valve, 340–341, 341
    lipomatous polyposis and epiploic lipomatosis, 343, 343
    liposarcoma, 343–344
    submucosal lipoma, 341–342, 342
  in anal canal, 1580
  biphasic epithelial-mesenchymal lesions
    gastroblastoma, 357, 358, 359, 359
    spindle cell carcinoma/carcinosarcoma, 356–357, 356–357
    synovial sarcoma, 354–356, 355

Mesenchymal tumors. see also
Gastrointestinal stromal tumors;
Neurogenic tumors (Continued)
endothelial and vascular tumors
angiosarcoma, 345, 346, 347
hemangioma, 344, 344–345, 345
intestinal vascular lesions associated
with clinical syndromes, 348
Kaposi's sarcoma, 346, 347
lymphangioma, 347–348, 347–349
fibroblastic/myofibroblastic tumors
calcifying fibrous tumor, 339, 341
desmoid tumor/intraabdominal
fibromatosis, 331–333, 332
elastofibroma, 340
inflammatory fibroid polyp, 333–335,
333–335
inflammatory myofibroblastic tumor,
337, 338, 339
plexiform fibromyxoma of gastric
antrum, 335–336, 336, 337
solitary fibrous tumor/
hemangiopericytoma, 339, 340
fibrosing lesions
idiopathic retroperitoneal fibrosis,
363–365, 364
sclerosing mesenteritis, 362, 362–363,
363
sclerosing peritonitis, 363
Weber-Christian disease, 365
in Meckel's diverticulum, 917, 918
miscellaneous sarcomas
clear cell sarcoma, 348, 350, 351
endometrial stromal sarcoma, 351, 353
malignant gastrointestinal
neuroectodermal tumor, 350–351, 352
undifferentiated high grade
pleomorphic sarcoma/malignant
fibrous histiocytoma, 353
undifferentiated sarcoma, 353
non-mesenchymal tumors
follicular dendritic cell sarcoma,
360–361, 361
lymphoma, 362
melanoma, 360, 360
sarcomatoid adult granulosa cell
tumor, 362
non-neoplastic lesions
heterotopic mesenteric ossification, 365
mycobacterial spindle cell
pseudotumor, 368
pseudosarcomatous granulation
tissue, 365, 366–367
reactive nodular fibrous pseudotumor,
365, 366
xanthogranulomatous pseudotumor,
367–368, 368
perivascular epithelioid cell umors
angiomyolipoma, 354
PEComa, 353–354, 354
smooth muscle tumors
Epstein–Barr Virus-associated, 314, 316
glomus tumor, 316–317, 317
leiomyomas, 313–314, 315
leiomyomatosis, 316
leiomyomatosis peritonealis
disseminata, 316

leiomyosarcoma, 317–318, 318
smooth muscle hamartoma, 316
striated muscle tumors
rhabdomyoma, 348
rhabdomyosarcoma, 348, 350
Mesenchymal tumors, esophageal,
543–544, 544
Mesenteric artery
inferior, 32, 32
superior, 31–32, 32
Mesenteric fibromatosis, 362, 364
Mesenteric ischemia, acute
causes of, 35, 37t
coagulation disorders, 35
diagnosis, 37
mortality, 37–38
symptoms and signs of, 37
Mesenteric ossification, heterotopic, 365
Mesenteric venous thrombosis, 38, 41, 42
Mesenterium ileocolicum commune, 908
Mesocolic hernias, 907
Mesocolic tenia, 876
Mesorectal excision, 877
Metabolic disorders, 22t, 919
Metaplasia
Barrett esophagus, 10
and bowel, large and small, 905, 905
colonic, 1341
gastric, 1335
pyloric, 803
squamous, 1384, 1384
Metastatic endocrine tumors, 220,
220–221
Methyldopa, 1156, 1157
Microcarcinoids, 217
Microfold (M) cells, 891
Microglandular goblet cell carcinoma. see
Goblet cell carcinoma (GCC)
Microglandular mucinous carcinoma. see
Goblet cell carcinoma (GCC)
Micropapillary colon carcinoma,
1497–1499, 1498
Microsatellite instability pathway,
1460–1461
Microscopic appearances, gastrointestinal
stromal tumors
epithelioid, 297
histological changes, 294, 297
pleomorphic, 298
post treatment changes, 301
spindle cell, 296
unusual morphologic variants, 297,
300, 301
Microscopic colitis
Brainerd diarrhea, 998
in children, 998–999
clinical features, 988
collagenous colitis, 988–994, 989–992
and endoscopic findings, 988
epidemiology, 986
etiology and pathogenesis, 986–988,
986t, 987t
and idiopathic inflammatory bowel
diseases, 999
lymphocytic colitis, 994–995, 995
lymphocytic colitis, differential
diagnosis of, 996

perforation, 993
small intestine, microscopic colitis and
involvement of, 996, 996, 997
treatment and prognosis, 996–997
variants, 997–998
Microsporidiosis, 1298, 1299
Microsporidium infection, 113
Microvesicular hyperplastic polyp
(MVHP), 1354, 1355–1356
Microvillus inclusion disease, 954, 955
Mid esophageal diverticulum
pathogenesis and clinical features,
442–443, 443
pathology, 443
Mid esophageal webs and rings, 441
Midgut carcinoids, 206–208, 206–208
Mild chronic inflammation, 20–21
Mild mucosal lesion, 974–975
Milk protein, 952, 953
Milroy's syndrome, 968
Ming classification, 734, 734
Miscellaneous visceral neuropathies, 275
Missense mutations, 304
Mixed connective tissue disorder, 383
Mixed neuronal glial tumor, 331
Mixed polyposis syndrome, 1437
MLH1, heritable promoter
hypermethylation of, 1449
Mononucleosis, infectious, 820
Montezuma's revenge, 1224
Montreal 2005 system classification, 662
Morgagni hernia/Morgagni-Larrey hernia,
907–908
Motility disorders
of esophagus (see Esophageal motility
disorders)
of stomach
gastroparesis, 251
pyloric stenosis, 250–251
MSH2
EPCAM mutations and loss of, 1449
heritable promoter hypermethylation
of, 1449
MSI-H carcinoma, 1492–1493
Mucin, 1211
Mucinous carcinoid. see Goblet cell
carcinoma (GCC)
Mucinous neoplasms
clinical features, 841
gross appearances, 841, 841, 842
histology, 841–843, 843, 844, 845, 845
incidence, 841
issues with, 845–849, 846
dysplasia and distinction of, LAMN,
845–849, 846
follow-up and therapy, 848–849
perforation, 847
rupture and mucin extravasation,
847–848
unusual variations, 848
molecular pathology and
immunohistochemistry, 845
terminology, 839–840, 840t
Mucinous/colloid carcinoma, 1494–1495,
1496
Mucin-poor hyperplastic polyps (MDHP),
1354, 1357

Muciphages, histiocytes associated with miscellaneous disorder, 1179–1180, 1181–1182
Mucocutaneous lymph node syndrome, 52–53
Mucoepidermoid carcinoma, 1579
Mucor, 488, *488*, 498
Mucormycosis, 1310, *1310–1311*
Mucosa
  of appendix, 798, *798*
  of esophagus
    basal cells, 424, 425, *425*
    endocrine cells, 424
    lamina propria, *425*, 426
    Langerhans cells, 424
    lymphocytes, 425, *426*
    melanocytes, 424
    Merkel cells, 424, *425*
    mitoses, 424
    muscularis mucosae, 426, *426*
    squamous epithelium, 424, *425*
  large intestine, *882*, 885–887, *886*, *888*, *889*
  prolapsed, anal canal in, 1562–1563, *1563*
  small intestine
    epithelium, *880*, 880–882, *881*, *882*, *883*
    ileal pigment, 882–883, *884*, *885*
    jejunal villi, 880, *880*, *881*
    lamina propria, 882–883, *884*
  of stomach
    acid secretion, 564, *566*
    antral mucosa, 560, *561*, *562*, 562, *563*
    cardiac gland mucosa, 557–558, *558*
    gastric endocrine cells, 564, 565t
    gastric mucins, 563–564
    glandular zone, 557
    lamina propria, 564, *566*
    muscularis mucosae, 566
    neck zone, 557, *557*
    oxyntic mucosa, 558–560, *559*, *560*
    pit epithelium, *556*, 556–557
    pit pattern, 556
    superficial zone, *556*, 556–557
    transition zones, 562–563, *563*
Mucosa herniations, 233, *233*
Mucosa-associated lymphoid tissue (MALT) lymphoma, 891, 895
  characterization, 141, *142–144*
  clinical presentation, 140, *140*
  clinical reports, 145–146
  colon, 161
  differential diagnosis
    vs. chronic gastritis, 147
    clinical management, 146–147
    mini-MALT, 147
    small lymphocytic lymphoma, 147–148
  gastric, 139–143, 161
  genetic and epigenetic abnormalities, 143–145
  limitation, 141
  lymphocytic gastritis, 645
  microscopic findings, 141, *142*, *143*
  pathogenesis, *139*, 139–140
  pathologist's role, 146
  pathology
    plasma cell population, 143, *143*
    types of lymphocytes, 142–143
    ulcers, 140, *141*
    vague nodular architecture, 142, *143*
  patients follow-up, 146
  prognosis, 145
  small intestine, 150–151, *151*, *152*
  treatment, 145
Mucosal biopsy, 1
Mucosal bridge, in esophagus, 444
Mucosal bumps
  duodenal, 1335
  and nodules, 780
Mucosal changes, apoptotic colopathy
  abnormal mitosis, 1142, *1142*
  acute toxic injury, 1137–1142, *1138–1141*
  Dysplasia mimics related to medication, 1140, 1142
  neutropenic enterocolitis (typhlitis, neutropenic appendicitis), 1143
Mucosal hemorrhage, during biopsy, 18–19
Mucosal neuroma/Schwann cell hamartoma, 323, *324–325*, 325
Mucosal prolapse syndromes. *see* Solitary rectal ulcer syndrome
Mucosal tags, 539–540
Mucosal transition zones, 562–563, *563*
Mucous cast, 918, *918*
Mucous cell hyperplasia, 606, *608*, 608–609
Muir–Torre syndrome, 1452–1453
Multiple endocrine neoplasia (MEN), 322
  and medullary carcinoma of thyroid, 389–390
  syndromes, 389–390
  type I (MEN-I)
    endocrine tumors, 194
    gastrinomas, 204, *205*
    type II carcinoid tumors, 202, 203
  type IIB (MEN IIB), 273
  Zollingerer–Ellison syndrome, 202, 203
Multiple gastric polyps, 774–775
Multiple lymphomatous polyposis, 162–163
Mural eosinophils, in Hirschsprung's disease, 274
Muscularis mucosae, 241, 895
  in esophagus, 426, *426*
  of stomach, 566
Muscularis propria, 241, 895
  biopsies, 253
  of esophagus, *425*, *426*
  large bowel diverticular disease, 232
  of stomach, 566–567
Musculature
  in anal canal, *1548*, *1553*, *1554*
  gastrointestinal, *908*, 908–909, *909*
MUTYH-associated polyposis, 1443–1444
Mycobacterial infections
  and acute appendicitis, 821–822
  incidence of, 1260
  mycobacterium avium-intracellulare
    differential diagnosis, 1264, 1266
    pathology, 1264, *1264*, *1265*
  mycobacterium tuberculosis
    gross and endoscopic findings, 1261, *1261*
    histology and differential diagnosis, 1261, *1261–1263*
    pathogenesis and clinical features, 1260–1261
    of terminal ileum, *1261*
Mycobacterial spindle cell pseudotumor, 368
Mycobacterium avium-intracellare (MAI)
  biopsy technique, 23
  description, 1263, 1264
  differential diagnosis, 1264, 1266
  enteric infections, 1218
  histiocytes associated with infections, 1173
  pathology, 1264, *1264–1265*
  vs. Whipple's disease, 964, 964t
Mycobacterium tuberculosis
  description, 1260
  gross and endoscopic findings, 1261, *1261*
  histology and differential diagnosis, 1261, *1261–1263*
  pathogenesis and clinical features, 1260–1261
Mycophenolate mofetil, 1158
Mycosis fungoides, 172–173
Myenteric plexus, *896*, 896–897, *897*
  CIIP, 256
  damage, 1162–1163
  enteric nervous system, 243, *243*
Myoepithelial hamartoma, 1335, *1336*
Myotonic muscular dystrophy, 276

N

Nakamura classification, carcinomas, 734
Narrow band imaging (NBI), chromoendoscopy, 8
Natural killer (NK) cell
  enteropathy, IBD, 1089, *1090*, 1091
  properties, diffuse lymphoid tissue, 90
  T-cell lymphoma, 173–174
Neck zone/middle zone, of stomach, 557, *557*
Necrosis, acute esophageal, 439
Necrotic mucosa, 35, 39, 44, *44*
Nematodes, 1300–1305
Neonatal left colon syndrome, 919
Neonatal necrotizing enterocolitis (NEC)
  and bowel, mechanical disorders of
    clinical features, 920–921
    description, 920
    pathogenesis, 920
    pathology, 921, *921–922*
Neonatal perforation, drug-associated and iatrogenic vascular injuries, 1155
Neoplasms
  ataxia telangiectasia, 105
  biopsy technique, 22t, 24
  following immune suppression and radiation, inflammatory bowel disease, 1171
  gastrointestinal problems in AIDS patients, 113–115, *115*
  immunodeficiency disorders, 98, 98t
  primary immunodeficiency disorders, 101

Neoplastic disease, gastrointestinal involvement, 410, *410*
Nerve plexuses, enteric nervous system, 242
Nerve stain, 253
Nerve supply, 556, *896*, 896–897, *897*
Neural nitric oxide synthase enzyme (nNOS), 251
Neural plexi, *896*, 896–897, *897*
Neurenteric cysts, 432
Neuroendocrine. *see* Endocrine carcinomas
Neuroendocrine tumors (NETs), *195*
- classification, 198
- definition of, 194
- duodenum
  - gangliocytic paraganglioma, 205
  - gastrinomas, 204, *205*
  - somatostatinomas, 204, *206*
- glandular pattern, *195*, *206*
- gross examination
  - appearance, 196, *197*
  - appendectomy, 196, *197*
  - dissection recommendations for, 196–197
  - polypectomies, 197
  - resections, 196
- growth patterns, 195, *195*, 196
- in Meckel's diverticulum, 917
- metastatic risk for, 196
- midgut, 206–208, *206–208*
- occurrence, 196
- ribbon-like pattern, 221
- in specific sites
  - abdominal colon, 211
  - appendix, 208–211, *209*, *210*
  - cecum/terminal ileum, 208
  - duodenum, 204–206, *205*, *206*
  - esophagus, 198–199
  - ileum, 206–208, *206–208*
  - jejunum, 206–208, *206–208*
  - rectum, 211–212, *212*
  - stomach, 199–204, *199t*, *200–203*
- staging and grading, 197–198
- stomach, *199t*
  - type I, 199–202, *200–202*
  - type II, 202–203
  - type III, 203, *203*
  - type IV, 204
- well-differentiated, 194–198
Neurofibroma, 320
Neurofibromatosis, 194, 204
Neurofibromatosis type 1/von Recklinghausen's disease, 307
Neurogenic disorders, classification, *246t*
Neurogenic tumors
- fibroblastic polyps, 325, *326*, 327
- ganglioneuroma
  - diffuse ganglioneuromatosis, 320, 321, *323*
  - ganglioneuromatous polyposis, 320
  - multiple endocrine neoplasia, 322
  - neuromatous proliferation, 323
  - polypoid ganglioneuromas, 320, *321*
- granular cell tumor, 329–330, *329–330*
- malignant peripheral nerve sheath tumor, 330–331, *331*
- mixed neuronal glial tumor, 331
- mucosal neuroma/Schwann cell hamartoma, 323, *324–325*, *325*
- neurofibroma, 320
- paraganglioma, *328*, 328–329
- perineurioma, 325, 327
- polypoid neural lesions, biopsy diagnosis of, 327–328
- schwannoma, 318, *319*, 320
Neurologic disorders, *246t*, 275–276
Neuromuscular disorders, *246t*
Neuronal hyperplasia, 812, *812*
Neurotransmitters
- chronic intestinal pseudoobstruction, 254
- infantile pyloric stenosis, 251
Neutropenic appendicitis, 813, *814*
Neutropenic colitis, 66
Neutropenic enterocolitis
- clinical features, 1258
- gross appearances, 1258, *1259*
- histology, 1258, *1259*
- pathogenesis, 1257–1258
Neutrophils
- function defects, IBD, 1084–1085, *1085*
- immune mechanisms in, 90
Nezelof syndrome, *99t*
NF1 mutations, 305
Nodal metastases risk, 760
Nodular duodenitis, 392
Non-anal basaloid (cloacogenic) carcinoma, 1502, *1503*
Nondysplastic mucosal polyps
- small bowel polyps
  - Brunner's gland adenoma, 1331–1333, *1331–1333*
  - Brunner's gland nodules and polyps, 1329, 1330, *1330*
  - duodenal mucosal bumps, 1335
  - heterotopic gastric mucosa, 1333, *1334–1334*, 1335
  - heterotopic pancreatic tissue, 1335, *1336*
  - lymphoid nodules and tumors, 1335
Non-enteropathogenic viruses, 1284
Non-erosive, nonspecific gastritis, 588
Non-*Helicobacter pylori* helicobacter species
- diagnosis, 653
- gastric disease associated with
  - emphysematous, 656
  - enterococcal gastritis, 656
  - phlegmonous, 656
  - in stomach of humans, *652t*
  - syphilis, 653–656, *654–655*
  - tuberculosis, 653
Non-Hodgkin's lymphomas, AIDS associated lymphoma, 114, *115*
Non-mesenchymal tumors
- follicular dendritic cell sarcoma, 360–361, *361*
- lymphoma, 362
- melanoma, 360, *360*
- sarcomatoid adult granulosa cell tumor, 362
Non-neoplastic lesions
- heterotopic mesenteric ossification, 365
- mycobacterial spindle cell pseudotumor, 368
- pseudosarcomatous granulation tissue, 365, *366–367*
- reactive nodular fibrous pseudotumor, 365, *366*
- xanthogranulomatous pseudotumor, *367–368*, 368
Non-neoplastic polyps, 1412, *1413–1415*, 1415
- gastric epithelial polyps and tumors
  - biopsy and excision, 766–767
  - classification, 766, *766t*
  - differential diagnosis, 774–775
  - fundic gland polyps, 767–768, *769–771*
  - hyperplastic polyps, 768, 771, *771–773*, 774
  - inflammatory polyps, 768, 771, *771–773*, 774
  - multiple gastric polyps, 774–775
  - pathology, 771, 774, *774*
  - single polyps, 774
- large bowel, 1412, *1413–1415*, 1415
- serrated/hyperplastic polyps, 1412, *1413–1415*, 1415
- small bowel
  - Brunner's gland adenoma, 1331–1333, *1331–1333*
  - Brunner's gland nodules and polyps, 1329, 1330, *1330*
  - duodenal mucosal bumps, 1335
  - heterotopic gastric mucosa, 1333, *1334–1334*, 1335
  - heterotopic pancreatic tissue, 1335, *1336*
  - lymphoid nodules and tumors, 1335
- stomach
  - biopsy and excision, 766–767
  - classification, 766, *766t*
  - differential diagnosis, 774–775
  - fundic gland polyps, 767–768, *769–771*
  - hyperplastic and inflammatory polyps, 768, 771, *771–773*, 774
  - pathology, 771, 774, *774*
Non-polypoid, plaque-like adenomas, *1388*, 1388–1389
Non-reflux esophagitis, 484
Nonspecific colitis. *see* Microscopic colitis
Nonspecific ulcers, 967
Non-spontaneous rupture
- pathogenesis and clinical features, 435–436, *436*
- pathology, 436–437
Non-steroidal anti-inflammatory drugs (NSAIDs)
- and duodenum, 581
- and esophagus, 614
- and gastric, 670
- and IBD, 670
- idiopathic ulcers, intestines
  - clinical features, 1148
  - diaphragm disease, *1150*
  - and diverticular disease, 1151
  - idiopathic IBD, 1151–1152
  - and large intestinal disease, 1151
  - left-sided colonic increase of eosinophils, 1152

pathogenesis, 1148–1149
and small intestinal disease, 1149, 1149–1150, 1151
and rectum, 282
and stomach, 42
Norovirus infections, 1285–1287
Norovirus/Norwalk virus, 1285–1287
Nosocomial infection, 1225
NSAIDs. *see* Non-steroidal anti-inflammatory drugs (NSAIDs)

O

Obstruction
  of appendix, 807–808
  and bowel, mechanical disorders of
    cystic fibrosis, 919
    hypoplastic left colon syndrome, 919
    meconium ileus, 919
    megacystis-microcolon-intestinal hypoperistalsis syndrome, 919–920
Obstructive colitis, 1088–1089, *1089*
Obstructive enteritis, *1089*
Ogilvie's syndrome, 252
Oleogranulomas (paraffinomas), crystal deposition, 1182–1183
Omphaloceles and bowel, congenital anomalies, 907
Onychodystrophy, 1433, *1433*
Open-heart surgery, gastrointestinal complications, 400
Oral contraceptives
  and arterial/venous thrombosis, 1153–1155, *1154*
  and thrombosis, 1153–1155, *1154*
Oral sodium phosphate, 1145
Oral-anal sexual practices, 1225–1226, *1226t*
Organisms. *see also* Bacteria; Fungi; Parasites; Spirochetes; Viruses
  adherence, 1215
  colonization, 1215
  enteroadherent/enteroaggregative, 1215, 1216, 1229, 1230
  enterohemorrhagic, 1215, 1216, 1229, 1231–1232, *1233*
  enteroinvasive, 1215
  enterotoxigenic, 1216, 1229, 1230
  initial attachment, 1215
  and mechanisms of infection, 1215–1216
  persistence of infection, 1216
  tissue invasion, 1215
  toxin production, 1215–1216
Ornithine transcarbamylase deficiency, small bowel mucosal disease, 973
Overlap syndrome, 383
Oxyntic mucosa, of stomach, 558–560, *559, 560*

P

p53 signaling, 1464
Paget's disease, lesions of anal canal, 1581–1582, *1582*
PAN. *see* Polyarteritis nodosa (PAN)
Pancolitis, 1010, *1071*
Pancreas, ectopic, 784–785, *785–786*, 1335, *1336*
Pancreatic rests, 784–785, *785–786*

Pancreatitis, acute, 1168
Paneth cells, and bowel, structure of, *882*, 887–888, 1338
Paneth cell-type carcinomas, 743
Panmucosal gastritis, *658*
Papillae
  dermal, 425
  elongated dermal, 459, *460*
Papillary adenocarcinoma, 735
Papillary adenoma, 1337
Papillomavirus infections, in anal canal, 1561
Papulosis, malignant-atrophic, 60
Paracoccidioides brasiliensis, 1312, *1312*
Paraduodenal hernias. *see* Mesocolic hernias
Paraganglioma, 328, *328–329*
Paraneoplastic neuropathy, 275
Paraneoplastic syndromes, gastrointestinal involvement, 263, *265*, 410, *410*
Paraneoplastic vasculitis, 56
Parasites
  and acute appendicitis, *823*, 823–824
  and enteric infections
    amoeba, 1294
    ancylostomiasis, 1300, *1300*
    Angiostrongylus costaricensis, 1300–1301
    anisakiasis, *1301*, 1301–1302
    ascariasis, 1302
    Balantidium coli, 1293, 1294, *1295*
    Blastocystis hominis, 1295
    capillariasis, *1302*, 1302–1303
    cestodes, *1307*, 1307–1308
    coccidiosis, 1295–1300, *1296–1300*
    Dientamoeba fragilis, 1294
    enterobiasis, 1303
    esophagostomiasis, 1303
    nematodes, 1300–1305
    protozoa, 1288–1289, *1289*
    strongyloidiasis, 1303–1304, *1304*
    trematodes, 1305–1307, *1306–1307*
    trichinosis, 1304
    trichuriasis, 1305, *1305*
  and immunohistochemical applications in gastrointestinal disorders, 21
  and nematodes
    anisakiasis, 660
    Cryptosporidium, 659–660
    Giardia lamblia, 661
    Strongyloides stercoralis, 660–661, *661*
Parasitic infections
  amoeba
    ameboma (amoebic pseudotumor), 1294
    complications, 1293
    diagnosis and treatment, 1294
    epidemiology, 1289–1290
    fulminant colitis, 1294
    gross and endoscopic pathology, 1290–1291, *1291*
    histology, 1291, *1292–1293*, 1293
    pathogenesis and clinical features, 1290
  ancylostomiasis, 1300, *1300*
  Angiostrongylus costaricensis, 1300–1301
  anisakiasis, *1301*, 1301–1302

  ascariasis (round worm), 1302
  Balantidium coli, 1293, 1294, *1295*
  Blastocystis hominis, 1295
  capillariasis, *1302*, 1302–1303
  cestodes
    Diphyllobothrium latum (fish tapeworm), 1307
    Hymenolepsis nana (dwarf tapeworm), 1308
    Taenia saginata (beef tapeworm), 1307, *1307*
    Taenia solium (pork tapeworm), 1307–1308
  coccidiosis
    Cryptosporidium, 1295–1298, *1296–1297*
    Cystoisospora belli (Coccidiosis), 1298, *1298*
    microsporidiosis, 1298, *1299*
    toxoplasma, 1298
    trypanosomiasis (Chagas' disease), 1300
  Dientamoeba fragilis, 1294
  enterobiasis, 1303
  esophagostomiasis, 1303
  nematodes, 1300–1305
  potentially pathogenic protozoa
    Balantidium coli, 1293, 1294, *1295*
    Blastocystis hominis, 1295
    Dientamoeba fragilis, 1294
  protozoa, *Giardia*, 1288–1289, *1289*
  strongyloidiasis, 1303–1304, *1304*
  trematodes
    Fasciolopsis buski, 1305–1307
    schistosomiasis, 1305–1306, *1306–1307*
  trichinosis, 1304
  trichuriasis, 1305, *1305*
Parathyroid, 385
Parathyroid rests, 540
Parietal cell carcinoma, 35, *36*, 744, *745*
Parkinson's disease, 499
Paterson-Kelly syndrome, 440
Pathologist endoscopist dialogue, *2t*
PDGFRA mutation, 304
PEComa, 353–354, *354*
Pecten of anal canal, 1549, 1550, *1552*
Pectinate line of anal canal, 1549, 1550
Pediatric GIST, 309
Pedunculated polyps, 1394, *1394*
Pellagra, gastrointestinal involvement, 409
Pemphigus vulgaris, gastrointestinal manifestation of, 397
Penicillamine, chronic inflammation with/without focal active colitis, 1159
Peptic ulcer disease (PUD)
  atypical clinical presentations., 621
  bicarbonate secretion, 615
  endoscopic appearance, peptic erosions and ulcers, 621, *622*, 623
  epidemiology, 620–621
  gastric mucosal blood flow, 615
  with *H. pylori* gastritis, 614, *614t*
  histology, gastroduodenal ulcers, 623–627, *624–627*
  mucus, 615
  pathogenetic factors
    acid and pepsin, 616

Peptic ulcer disease (PUD) (Continued)
  associated diseases, 620
  drugs, 618–619
  duodenal ulcer, 618t
  duodenogastric reflux, 619
  environmental factors, 619
  heredity, 619–620
  hypersecretory conditions associated with peptic ulcer, 616–617
  psychological stress, 619
  retained antrum syndrome, 617
  Zollinger-Ellison syndrome, 616–617
  prostaglandins, 615
Perforated diverticulum, large bowel diverticular disease, 235, 235
Perforation
  and acute appendicitis, 813, 813
  drug-associated and iatrogenic vascular injuries, 1155
  mucinous neoplasms, issues with, 847
Perianal alveolar rhabdomyosarcoma, 350
Perianal disease, chronic idiopathic inflammatory bowel diseases, 1061–1063, 1063, 1064
Perianal hematomas, anal canal, 1560
Perianal herpes infections, 1561
Perianal rhabdomyosarcoma, 350
Perianal skin
  in anal canal, 1553, 1557
  Bowen's disease of, 1567, 1568–1569, 1569–1570
  lesions of
    basal cell carcinoma, 1581
    bowenoid papulosis, 1581
    Bowen's disease, 1581
    hidradenitis suppurativa, 1582
    invasive squamous cell carcinoma, 1581
    keratoacanthoma, 1581
    lichen sclerosus, 1582
    Paget's disease, 1581–1582, 1582
  squamous carcinoma *in situ*, 1569–1570
Periappendiceal abscesses, 816–817
Pericrypt fibroblast sheath, 891, 893, 893
Perineurioma, 325, 327
Peritoneal encapsulation, 918, 918
Peritoneal seeding, 759
Perivascular epithelioid cell tumors
  angiomyolipoma, 354
  PEComa, 353–354, 354
Pernicious anemia (PA), 199
  selective IgA deficiency, 101
Petechial hemorrhages, 405, 405
Peutz-Jeghers polyps and polyposis
  clinical features, 1415, 1417, 1417
  differential diagnosis, 1420
  gastric, 775, 777, 777
  gross and endoscopic appearances, 1418, 1419
  histology, 1418, 1420
  molecular genetics, 1418
  treatment, 1420, 1422
Peutz-Jeghers syndrome, 775, 777, 777, 1341
Peyer's patches, 91, 91
  immunohistochemistry, 93
  small bowel mucosal disease, 931
  and small intestine
    internal appearance, 877, 877
    mucosa, 881, 882, 883
Phagocytic and cell dysfunction, 106
Phlebectasia, 78–79
Phlebitis, enterocolic lymphocytic, 57, 59
Phlegmonous enterocolitis, 1258
Phlegmonous gastritis (PG), 656
Photography, biopsy technique, 23
Phycomycosis/mucormycosis, 1310, 1310–1311
Pig-Bel disease, 1255, 1256
Piles, 1558
Pill and esophagitis, 494
Pill-induced esophagitis, 494
Pinworm/threadworm. *see* Enterobiasis
Pit epithelium cells, of stomach, 556, 556–557
Pituitary adenoma, 389
Pituitary gland, 388
Plasmacytic colitis, 994
Plasmacytomas, solitary, 171, 171–172
Plasmids, 1043, 1216, 1230, 1244
Pleomorphic carcinoma, 1505
Pleomorphic GIST, 298
Pleomorphic sarcomas, 353
Plesiomonas shigelloides, 1242–1243, 1243
Plexiform fibromyxoma, of gastric antrum, 335–336, 336, 337
Plicae circulares, 877
Plummer–Vinson syndrome, 403, 440
Pneumatosis cystoides intestinalis, drugs and chemicals, changes due to
  clinical features, 1165
  gross and endoscopic disease, 1165
  histology, 1165, 1166
  pathogenesis, 1164–1165
  prognosis, 1165–1166
Pneumocystis, 1312
Pneumocystis carinii, 111
Polyarteritis nodosa (PAN)
  characterization, 53, 53
  classification, 49, 49t, 50t
  definition, 53
  microscopic, 54–55, 57, 58
Polyethylene glycol enemas, 1162
Polymyositis, 382
Polyp(s)
  fibrovascular, 540, 541
  inflammatory, 539
  inflammatory cloacogenic, 1562–1563, 1563
  multiple gastric, 774–775
  and neoplasms, diverticula associated carcinoma in, 237
    inverted diverticulum, 236–237, 237
  pedunculated, 354, 781, 1393, 1394, 1394
  serrated/hyperplastic
    adenoma with endocrine cell nests/neoplasm, 1389, 1390
    adenomas, growth and development, 1466–1470
    carcinosarcoma, 1502–1503
    choriocarcinoma-like carcinoma, 1503
    classification, 1352t
    clear cell carcinoma, 1500, 1501, 1501
    clinical features, 1470–1471
    colon cancer, in young, 1506–1507, 1509
    colonic elastosis and elastofibroma, 1410, 1411
    colonic mucosal–submucosal elongated polyp (mucosubmucosal polyp), 1409, 1409–1410
    colorectal carcinoma, 1453–1466, 1509–1515, 1511t, 1512t
    composite adenoma/carcinoma-carcinoid tumors, 1503–1504, 1506
    Cowden's syndrome, 1430–1431, 1431–1432, 1432
    cribriform/comedocarcinoma, 1505
    Cronkhite-Canada syndrome, 1433, 1433–1434, 1435, 1436
    diathermy, 1389, 1391, 1391
    diffuse-type signet ring carcinomas, 1496
    distribution, 1471
    dysplasia, grading of, 1386, 1387
    familial adenomatous polyposis, 1437, 1439–1443, 1439t
    flat and depressed adenomas, 1388, 1388–1389
    goblet cell carcinoma, 1497, 1497
    gross and endoscopic appearances, 1471, 1472–1476, 1473–1478
    histology, 1478–1483, 1479–1481, 1484, 1485, 1485, 1486, 1487–1492, 1488–1493
    hyperplastic polyps, 1352–1355, 1353–1357
    inflammatory polyps, 1407, 1408, 1409
    juvenile polyps and juvenile polyposis syndrome, 1422–1425, 1423–1428, 1428–1430
    large bowel adenomas, 1375–1377, 1381, 1384–1386, 1388, 1389, 1391
    Lynch's syndrome, 1444–1453
    melanotic adenocarcinoma and malignant melanoma, 1504–1505
    micropapillary colon carcinoma, 1497–1499, 1498
    mixed polyposis syndrome, 1437
    mucinous/colloid carcinoma, 1494–1495, 1496
    MUTYH-associated polyposis, 1443–1444
    nomenclature and classification, 1351–1352
    non-anal basaloid (cloacogenic) carcinoma, 1502, 1503
    nonneoplastic polyps, 1412, 1413–1415, 1415
    Peutz-Jeghers polyps and polyposis, 1415, 1417, 1417
    polypoid prolapsing mucosal fold, 1410, 1410
    post–chemotherapy and radiation changes, 1493–1494
    rhabdoid tumors, 1505
    serrated adenocarcinoma, 1499–1500
    serrated polyps with dysplasia, 1359–1360, 1361–1362, 1362–1363
    serrated/hyperplastic polyposis syndrome, 1436, 1436–1437

sessile serrated polyps/adenoma, 1355, 1358-1359, *1358-1360*
small cell carcinoma, 1503-1504, *1506*
squamous carcinoma, 1502, *1503*
traditional serrated adenomas, 1363-1364, *1364-1367*
treatment and prognosis, 1515-1517
sessile, 1394, *1394*
single, 774
small bowel
  Brunner's gland adenoma, 1331-1333, *1331-1333*
  Brunner's gland nodules and polyps, 1329, 1330, *1330*
  duodenal mucosal bumps, 1335
  heterotopic gastric mucosa, 1333, *1334-1334*, 1335
  heterotopic pancreatic tissue, 1335, *1336*
  lymphoid nodules and tumors, 1335
Polypectomy, snare polypectomy, 4, *4*
Polypoid carcinoma, *855*, 1342, 1391
Polypoid ganglioneuromas, 320, *321*
Polypoid gastritis, 778
Polypoid neural lesions, biopsy diagnosis of, 327-328
Polypoid prolapsing mucosal fold, 1410, *1410*
Polyposis syndromes, 830, 1415, *1416t*
Polyserositis, recurring, 409-410
Poorly differentiated endocrine neoplasms. see Endocrine carcinomas
Pork tapeworm. see *Taenia solium*
Portal hypertension, 79, 393, 585, *586*
Post transplant lymphoproliferative disorders (PTLD)
  clinical presentation, 168-169
  etiology and pathogenesis, 168
  incidence, 168
  pathology, *169*, 169-170
Postbulbar ulcer, 621
Postgastrectomy, 729
Postoperative stomach, 578, *579*
Potassium chloride, idiopathic ulcers, intestines, 1152
Pouchitis, 1037-1038
  diagnosis, 1039, *1039*
  etiology and pathogenesis, 1038-1039
  histology, 1039, *1040-1041*, 1041, *1042*
Prediverticular disease, large bowel diverticular disease, 231-232, *232*, *233*
Predominant antibody defects
common variable hypogammaglobulinemia, 99
common variable immunodeficiency, 99
diffuse nodular lymphoid hyperplasia, 100, *100*
histology, 100-101
pathogenesis and clinical features, 98-100
pathologist role, 101
X-linked agammaglobulinemia, 99
Predominant cell-mediated immunodeficiency
chronic mucocutaneous candidiasis, 103, *105*

hereditary thymic dysplasia, 102-103
IPEX syndrome, 103
pathogenesis and clinical findings, 102
severe combined immunodeficiency disease, 102
Swiss-type agammaglobulinemia, 102-103
Pregnancy, gastrointestinal symptoms, 388
Primary gastric T-cell lymphoma, 149-150
Primary histiocytosis X, 175
Primary immunodeficiency disorders
predominant antibody defects
  common variable hypogammaglobulinemia, 99
  common variable immunodeficiency, 99
  diffuse nodular lymphoid hyperplasia, 100, *100*
  histology, 100-101
  pathogenesis and clinical features, 98-100
  pathologist's diagnostic role, 101
  X-linked agammaglobulinemia, 99
predominant cell-mediated immunodeficiency
  chronic mucocutaneous candidiasis, 103, *105*
  hereditary thymic dysplasia, 102-103
  IPEX syndrome, 103
  pathogenesis and clinical findings, 102
  severe combined immunodeficiency disease, 102
  Swiss-type agammaglobulinemia, 102-103
selective IgA deficiency
  B-cell disorders, 102
  histology, 101-102
  infantile X-linked agammaglobulinemia, 102
  pathogenesis and clinical features, 101
  secretory component deficiency, 102
World Health Organization (WHO) classification, 98, *99t*
Primary sclerosing cholangitis (PSC), 393
Primary visceral neuropathies
diffuse eosinophilic infiltrate, 266, *267*
diffuse lymphoid infiltration, 266, *266*
familial visceral neuropathy, 262-263, *263*, *264*
interstitial cells of cajal, abnormalities of
  DOG1 immunostain, 265, *265*
  hyperplasia, *265*, 265-266
  prognosis and therapy, 266
paraneoplastic syndromes, 263, *265*
slow transit constipation, 266-267
sporadic visceral neuropathy, 263
Prior irradiation, invasive squamous cell carcinoma, 1571
Proctitis
chlamydial, 1273-1274, *1274-1275*
definition, 1218
gonococcal, *1266*, 1266-1267
gross appearance, 1276, *1277*
and herpes simplex virus
  description, 1276
  gross appearance, 1276, *1277*
  histology, 1276-1277, *1277*

histology, 1276-1277, *1277*
ischemic, 45-46
radiation, 70
Proctitis/localized colitis cystica profunda
gross and endoscopy, 280
inflammatory cloacogenic polyp, 281, 281-282
nuclear atypicality, dysplasia, and carcinoma, 280-281
pathogenesis and histology, 280, *280*
Proctitis/ulcerative proctitis, 1030-1032, *1030t*
Progressive muscular dystrophy
Progressive muscular dystrophy, chronic intestinal pseudoobstruction with, 276
Progressive systemic sclerosis. see Scleroderma
Prolapse of anal canal, 1562-1563, *1563*
Prostaglandins, 615
Protein-calorie malnutrition. see Childhood kwashiorkor
Protein-losing enteropathy, 973
Proton pump inhibitors (PPIs), in *H. pylori* infection, *611*, 611-612
Protozoa, 1288-1300
  Giardia, 1288-1289, *1289*
pathogenic
  Balantidium coli, 1293, 1294, *1295*
  Blastocystis hominis, 1295
  Dientamoeba fragilis, 1294
Protozoal infections. see Parasites
Proximal duodenum. see Duodenitis
Psammoma bodies, 204, *206*
Pseudodiverticula, in esophagus
atypical, in scleroderma, 443
esophageal intramural pseudodiverticulosis, 443-444, *444*
lower, 442-443, *443*
mid, 442-443, *443*
retention cysts, 443-444, *444*
upper, 442, *442*
Pseudodiverticulosis, esophageal intramural, 443-444, *444*
Pseudoepitheliomatous hyperplasia, 496, *1564*
Pseudolipomatosis, drugs and chemicals
gross and endoscopic appearances, 1167
histology, 1167, *1167*
Pseudolymphoma
diagnosis, 131
pathology, 131-132, *132*
Pseudomelanosis coli, 1172, *1175-1176*
Pseudomelanosis, in esophagus, 424
Pseudomembranes, 41, 44, *46*, *48*
enteritis, 1156
and ischemic colitis, 1156
Pseudomyxoma peritonei
gross appearances, 849-850
microscopic appearance, 850
pathology of cytoreduction, 850
terminology and classification, 849, *849t*
Pseudoobstruction
acute intestinal, 252
chronic intestinal
with acquired jejunal diverticulosis, 276

Pseudoobstruction (Continued)
  with amyloidosis and hypothyroidism, 276
  clinical features, 253
  clinicopathologic implications, 253–254
  electron microscopy, 254
  immunostains, 253–254
  molecular and genetic studies, 254
  with myotonic muscular dystrophy, 276
  with progressive muscular dystrophy, 276
  with scleroderma, 276
  colonic, 252
  intestinal
    acute intestinal pseudoobstruction, 252
    biopsies, of muscularis propria, 253
    clinical features, 253
    definition, 251–252
    Ogilvie's syndrome, 252
  laxatives, 1162–1163
Pseudopolyps. see Inflammatory polyps
Pseudopyloric metaplasia, in metaplasia, 905
Pseudosarcomatous granulation tissue, 365, 366–367
Pseudotumors, inflammatory, 1176
Pseudoxanthoma elasticum, 79, 384
PTEN hamartoma tumor syndrome, 777, 778
PTEN protein, 1464
PTLD. see Post transplant lymphoproliferative disorders (PTLD)
Puborectalis, in anal canal, 1554
Pulmonary sequestrations, in esophagus, 434–435
Pulsion, diverticulum of esophagus, 442
Pyelophlebitis, suppurative, 817
Pyloric canal, 554, *554*
Pyloric channel ulcer, 621
Pyloric gland adenoma, 714, *715–716*
Pyloric metaplasia, 803
Pyloric sphincter region, 554, *554*
Pyloric stenosis
  adult pyloric stenosis, 251
  infantile pyloric stenosis, 250–251
Pyloro-cardiac cell carcinoma, 530, 747
Pylorus, 554, *554*

Q

22q11 chromosomal deletion, 105. see also DiGeorge's syndrome

R

Radial margins, 877
Radiation Injury
  acute
    colon, 69
    complications, 69
    esophagus, 68
    small intestine, 69
    stomach, 68–69, *69*
  chronic
    clinical presentation, 70, *72*
    esophagus, 70, *72*
    small and large intestines, 70, *72*
    stomach, 70, *71*
    symptoms, 69–70, *71*
  and eosinophilic colitis etiology, 68, 70, 72
  incidence of, 67
  pathophysiology, 67–68
  vascular lesions, 68
Radiotherapy, invasive squamous cell carcinoma, 1575
Rapid urease test, 596
RAS-MAPK and PI3K signaling pathway, 1463–1464
Reactivated cytomegalovirus infection
  gross appearance, 1279–1280, *1279–1280, 1279–1280*
  histology, 1280, *1281–1282*, 1282, 1282–1283
Reactive (chemical/reflux-associated) gastropathy
  acute reactive gastropathy
    acute phase, 576–577
    chronic phase, 577, 577–578, *578*
    toxic gastropathy, 578, *580*
  characteristics, 575
  distinction of, dysplasia, 578–580, *580*
    alcoholic gastropathy, 581–582
    bottom-up dysplasia, 578–579
    caustic-induced injury, 582
    chemotherapy and radiation, 582
    clinical implications, 581
    graft versus host disease, 582
    in intestinal metaplasia, 580
    ischemia, 582–583, *583*, *584*
    regenerative atypia, 579
    reporting chronic changes, 581
    reporting reactive gastropathy, 580
  with erosions in *Helicobacter*, 578
  histology, 575–576
  pathogenesis, 575
Reactive nodular fibrous pseudotumor, 365, *366*
Rectal biopsy, 48, *53*, 72
Rectal mucosal prolapse, 1170
Rectal (anal) tonsil, 135
Rectum
  AIDS associated Kaposi's sarcoma, 114
  carcinoid tumors, 211–212, *212*
  GI problem in AIDS patients, 113
  sparing, 1028–1029
  terms of, 878
  in ulcerative proctocolitis, following ileorectal anastomosis, 1036
Recurrent appendicitis, 817
Reed-Sternberg cells, 154, 155, 158, 167, 173, 174, 820
Refractory celiac sprue, small bowel mucosal disease
  case examples, 973–974
  clinical perspectives, 948
  enteropathy-associated T-cell lymphoma, 157–160
  histopathology perspectives, 948–949
  symptoms of, 947
  T cells, 947, 948
  types of, *945*, 947, 948
Regenerative hyperplasia, 440, 442, 1114
Reiter's syndrome, 384

Remnants, 432
Renal disease
  clinical implications, 393
  endoscopic and histologic appearances, 392
  findings, 392
  gastrointestinal manifestation of
    acute renal failure, 390
    chronic renal failure, 390–392
    pathogenesis, 390
  pathologist role, 393
  renal transplantation, 392–393
Renal failure
  acute, 390
  chronic, 390–392
  pathogenesis, 390
Renal transplantation, 392–393
Rendu-Osler-weber Syndrome, 77, 77–78
Reperfusion injury, 34–35
Resection specimens, polyarteritis nodosa, 44
Retention cysts, 839
  in esophagus, 443–444, *444*
Retroperitoneal hematomas, 1153
Retroperitoneal hernias, 907
Revised European American Lymphoma (REAL), 126, 127
Rhabdoid tumors, 1505
Rhabdomyoma, 348
Rhabdomyosarcoma, 348, *350*
Rheumatoid arthritis (RA)
  and connective tissue disorders, 383
  vasculitis, 383, *384*
Rhodococcus equi, 1272–1273
Rhodococcus equi/corynebacterium equi, 1272–1273
Richter's hernia, 62
Rickettsial disease, 1274–1275
  rocky mountain spotted fever, 1274–1275
Right-sided diverticula, 228
Right-sided diverticulosis
  clinical features, 238
  pathogenesis, 238
  pathology, 238–239, *239*
Rituximab, 1158
Rocky mountain spotted fever, 1274–1275
Rosai-Dorfman disease, 403
Rotavirus infections
  clinical features, 1285
  pathogenesis, 1285
  pathology, 1285, *1286*
Round worm. see Ascariasis
Russell body gastritis/carditis, 650, *651*, 652

S

Salmonella
  characteristics, 1235–1236
  classification, 1236–1237
Salmonella enterocolitis
  clinical features, 1237
  endoscopic appearances, 1237
  fulminant infections, 1238
  histology, 1237–1238
  inflammatory bowel disease, 1238
  salmonella infection in inflammatory, 1238

typhoid fever
    gross appearance, 1239, *1239*
    histology, 1239–1240
    pathogenesis and clinical features, 1238–1239
Salt and pepper appearance, duodenitis, 630, *630*
Sarcoidosis
    chronic inflammatory bowel diseases, differential diagnosis of, 1096, 1097
    granulomatous disorders, 406–407
Sarcomas, miscellaneous
    clear cell sarcoma, 348, 350, *351*
    endometrial stromal sarcoma, 351, *353*
    malignant gastrointestinal neuroectodermal tumor, 350–351, *352*
    undifferentiated high grade leomorphic sarcoma/malignant fibrous histiocytoma, 353
    undifferentiated sarcoma, 353
Sarcomatoid adult granulosa cell tumor, 362
Schatzki rings
    clinical features, *441*, 441–442
    pathogenesis, *441*, 441–442
    pathology, *441*, 442
Schistosomiasis, 1305–1306, *1306–1307*
Schwann cell hamartoma, 323, *324–325*, 325
Schwannoma, 318, *319*, 320
Scleroderma
    atypical esophageal diverticulum, *443*
    chronic intestinal pseudoobstruction with, 276
    gastrointestinal manifestation of
        clinical features, 379–380
        clinical implications, 382
        gross pathology, 380–382
        histology, 380–382
        pathogenesis, 379–380
Sclerosing encapsulating peritonitis, 918–919
Sclerosing mesenteritis, *362*, 362–363, *363*
Sclerosing peritonitis, 363
Scurfin, autoimmune enteropathy, 950
SDHB. *see* Succinyl dehydrogenase subunit B (SDHB)
Secondary achalasia, 248–249
Secondary (acquired) immunodeficiency disorders
    acquired immunodeficiency syndrome (AIDS)
        gastrointestinal AIDS infections, 113, 113t
        gastrointestinal complications, 110
        gastrointestinal neoplasms in, 113–115, *115*
        pathogenesis and clinical features, 111–113, *112*
        pathologist's diagnostic role, 110–111
    B-cell dysfunction with dysgammaglobulinemia, 106
    bone marrow transplantation
        characteristics, 106
        chronic GVHD, 110
        graft *versus* host disease, 106–110, *109*
        infections, 106
        transplantation regimen, 106
    hypogammaglobulinemia, 106
    iatrogenic complications, 106
    intestinal transplantation, 110
    malnutrition, 106
    morphologic changes, 106
    pathologic manifestations, 106
Secondary tumors
    esophageal, 542–543, *543*
    of large bowel, 1518, *1519–1520*
Second-degree hemorrhoids in anal canal, 1559
Secretory component deficiency, 102
Secretory IgA, 93
Selective IgA deficiency
    B-cell disorders, 102
    histology, 101–102
    pathogenesis and clinical features, 101
Selective intra-artery radiation therapy (SIRT), 671
Serosa
    of bowel, large and small, 899–900
    of stomach, 566–567
Serrated adenocarcinoma, 1499–1500
Serrated adenomas, 836, *837*, 838
Serrated polyps with dysplasia, 1359–1360, *1361–1362*, 1362–1363
Serrated/hyperplastic polyposis syndrome, *1436*, 1436–1437
Serrated/hyperplastic polyps
    adenoma
        with endocrine cell nests/neoplasm, 1389, *1390*
        growth and development, 1466–1470
    carcinosarcoma, 1502–1503
    choriocarcinoma-like carcinoma, 1503
    classification, 1352t
    clear cell carcinoma, 1500, 1501, *1501*
    clinical features, 1470–1471
    colon cancer, in young, 1506–1507, 1509
    colonic elastosis and elastofibroma, 1410, *1411*
    colonic mucosal–submucosal elongated polyp (mucosubmucosal polyp), 1409, 1409–1410
    colorectal carcinoma, 1453–1466
        prognosis of, 1509–1515, 1511t, 1512t
    composite adenoma/carcinoma-carcinoid tumors, 1503–1504, *1506*
    Cowden's syndrome, 1430–1431, *1431–1432*, 1432
    cribriform/comedocarcinoma, 1505
    Cronkhite-Canada syndrome, *1433*, 1433–1434, *1435*, 1436
    diathermy, 1380, 1391, *1391*
    diffuse-type signet ring carcinomas, 1496
    distribution, 1471
    dysplasia, grading of, 1386, *1387*
    familial adenomatous polyposis, 1437, 1439–1443, 1439t
    flat and depressed adenomas, *1388*, 1388–1389
    goblet cell carcinoma, 1497, *1497*
    gross and endoscopic appearances, 1471, *1472–1476*, 1473–1478
    histology, 1478–1483, *1479–1481*, *1484*, 1485, *1485*, *1486*, *1487–1492*, 1488–1493
    hyperplastic polyps, 1352–1355, *1353–1357*
    inflammatory polyps, 1407, *1408*, 1409
    juvenile polyps and juvenile polyposis syndrome, 1422–1425, *1423–1428*, 1428–1430
    large bowel adenomas, 1375–1377, 1381, 1384–1386, 1388, 1389, 1391
    Lynch's syndrome, 1444–1453
    melanotic adenocarcinoma and malignant melanoma, 1504–1505
    micropapillary colon carcinoma, 1497–1499, *1498*
    mixed polyposis syndrome, 1437
    mucinous/colloid carcinoma, 1494–1495, *1496*
    MUTYH-associated polyposis, 1443–1444
    nomenclature and classification, 1351–1352
    non-anal basaloid (cloacogenic) carcinoma, 1502, *1503*
    nonneoplastic polyps, 1412, *1413–1415*, 1415
    Peutz-Jeghers polyps and polyposis, 1415, 1417, *1417*
    polypoid prolapsing mucosal fold, 1410, *1410*
    post–chemotherapy and radiation changes, 1493–1494
    rhabdoid tumors, 1505
    serrated adenocarcinoma, 1499–1500
    serrated polyps with dysplasia, 1359–1360, *1361–1362*, 1362–1363
    serrated/hyperplastic polyposis syndrome, *1436*, 1436–1437
    sessile serrated polyps/adenoma, 1355, 1358–1359, *1358–1360*
    small cell carcinoma, 1503–1504, *1506*
    squamous carcinoma, 1502, *1503*
    traditional serrated adenomas, 1363–1364, *1364–1367*
    treatment and prognosis, 1515–1517
Sessile adenoma, 215, *215*, 1337, *1337*
Sessile polyps, 1394, *1394*
Sessile serrated polyps/adenoma, 1355, 1358–1359, *1358–1360*
Severe combined immunodeficiency disease, 165
    predominant cell-mediated immunodeficiency, 102
Severe idiopathic constipation, 266–267, 274
Sexually transmitted diseases, 1570–1571
Shave biopsy technique, 5
Shiga and Shiga-like toxins, 1216
Shigella
    clinical features, 1235
    diagnosis, 1235
    gross and endoscopic appearances, 1235
    histology, 1235, *1236*
    pathogenesis, 1234–1235
    treatment, 1235
Short esophagus, 434
Short segment Barrett's esophagus, 528, *528*
Signet-ring cell carcinomas, 735, 737, *738–740*

Signet-ring changes, 1156
Simple duplications and bowel
   characteristic features, 912
   gross appearance, 912, *913*, *914*
   histology, 912–913, *913*, *914*
   site, 912
   split notochord theory, 912
Single polyps, 774
Sinus histiocytosis with massive lymphadenopathy, 403
Sjogren's syndrome, 383–384
Skin disorders
   acrodermatitis enteropathica, 960
   dermatitis herpetiformis, 944, *944–945*
   and esophageal inflammation
     glycogenic acanthosis, 495, *495*
     lichen planus, 495, *495*
     pemphigus vulgaris, 495, *495*
   gastrointestinal manifestation of, *395t–396t*
     acanthosis nigricans, 399
     acrodermatitis enteropathica, 398
     bullous disorders, 394, 397
     cicatricial pemphigoid, 397
     Cowden's disease, 399
     Darier's disease, 398
     dermatogenic enteropathy, 398–399
     dermatomyosis, 399
     epiderolysis bullosa acquisita, 397
     familial gastrointestinal stromal tumors, 399
     herpes simplex virus infection, 398
     hyperkeratotic disorders, 398
     malignant disease, 399
     pemphigus vulgaris, 397
     Stevens-Johnson syndrome, 397
     tylosis, 398
   primary, *395–396t*
Skinny forceps, 2, *3*
Slow transit constipation (STC), 266–267
Small bowel
   allografts, acute cellular rejection, 111t
   bone marrow transplantation, GVHD, 108, *109*
   diverticular disease
     definition, 227
     terminology, 227
Small bowel mucosal disease
   abnormal appearance, 933–936, *933t*, *936t*
   alternative terminology, 935, *944–945*
   approach to, 930
   evaluation of, 932–933
   miscellaneous disorders
     brown bowel syndrome, 973, *974*
     enzyme deficiency states, 973
     protein-losing enteropathy, 973
   normal appearance, *930–931*, 930–935
   normal villous architecture
     abetalipoproteinemia, *971*, 971–972
     amyloidosis, 972
     chronic granulomatous disease, 973
     duodenal biopsies, *930–931*, 931–932
     geographic variation, 932
     histology, 930, *930–931*, 930–932
     hypobetalipoproteinemia, *971*, 971–972
     lipid storage diseases, *972*, 972–973
     mild chronic inflammation, 932
     regional variations in, *930–931*, 930–932
     tangential artifact, *930–931*, 932
     traumatic artifact, 932
   with severe flat mucosa
     autoimmune enteropathy, 949, 951–952, *952*
     case examples, 973–975
     celiac sprue, 936–947, *936t*, *939*, *941*, *942–943*, *944–945*
     childhood kwashiorkor, 954, *954*
     collagenous sprue, *936t*, 949, *950*
     congenital tufting enteropathy, 955–956, *956*
     description, *936t*
     familial enteropathy, 954, *955*
     food hypersensitivity, 952–953, *953*
     microvillus inclusion disease, 954, *955*
     refractory celiac sprue, 947–949
     tropical sprue, 953–954, *954*
     unclassified sprue, 949
   thin and flat mucosa, 935
   with variably severe lesions, diagnostic/distinctive histology
     Crohn's disease, 967, *967*
     description, *937t*, 960
     eosinophilic gastroenteritis, 964–967, *966*
     impaired epithelial cell replacement, 969–970, *970*
     intestinal lymphangiectasia, *966*, *968*, 968–969
     intestinal lymphoma, 967–968
     nonspecific ulcers, 967
     Waldenstrom's macroglobulinemia, 969, *969*
     Whipple's disease, 960–964, *962–964*, *964t*
   with variably severe lesions, intraepithelial lymphocytosis
     acrodermatitis enteropathica, 960
     bacterial overgrowth syndrome, 959
     description, *937t*, 956
     immunodeficiency syndromes, 956–957
     infectious gastroenteritis, 957–959
     Zollinger-Ellison syndrome, 959–960
   villous atrophy, 935, *944–945*
Small bowel polyps
   nondysplastic mucosal polyps
     Brunner's gland adenoma, 1331–1333, *1331–1333*
     Brunner's gland nodules and polyps, 1329, 1330, *1330*
     duodenal mucosal bumps, 1335
     heterotopic gastric mucosa, 1333, *1334*, 1335
     heterotopic pancreatic tissue, 1335, *1336*
     lymphoid nodules and tumors, 1335
   serrated polyps, of small bowel, 1340
   small bowel adenomas
     clinical features, 1336–1337
     gross and endoscopic appearances, 1337, *1337*, *1338*
     histology, 1338–1339, *1339*
     management, 1339–1340
Small bowel tumors
   carcinoma
     clinical features, 1343
     diagnosis and management, 1348–1349
     gross and endoscopic appearances, 1343–1345, *1344*
     histology, 1345, *1345–1347*
     immunophenotype and molecular pathology, 1347–1348, *1348*
     pathogenesis, 1341, *1342*, *1343*
     staging and prognosis, 1349–1350, *1349t*, *1350t*
     treatment, 1349
   polyps
     nondysplastic mucosal polyps, 1329–1335, *1330–1336*
     serrated polyps of small bowel, 1340
     small bowel adenomas, 1336–1340, *1337–1339*
   secondary tumors, 1350–1351
   tumors and tumor-like conditions, 1351
Small cell carcinoma, 522–525, *523*, 1503–1504, *1506*
   in anal canal, 1579
Small GIST, 309–310
Small intestine. *see also* Bowel, large and small; specific diseases of
   Burkitt's lymphoma
     clinical presentation, 155, *156*
     immunophenotype and molecular genetics, 156
     incidence, 155
     pathology, 155–156, *156*
     prognosis and treatment, 156
   CD4+ phenotype, 160
   digestive tract vascularization
     collateral blood supply, 33
     extramural circulation, 31–33, *32*
     intramural circulation, *30*, 30–31
     venous drainage, 33
   diverticulosis of, *239*, 239–240
   embryology and development, 900–904, *901*, *902*, *903*
   enteropathy-type T-cell lymphoma
     classification, 157
     clinical presentation, 157–158
     immunophenotype and molecular genetics, 160
     incidence, 157
     pathogenesis, 157
     pathology, 158–160, *159*
     treatment and prognosis, 160
   external appearance of, 875
   GI problem in AIDS patients, 112
   internal appearance of, *877*, 877–878, *878*
   IPSID
     clinical presentation, 152–153
     diagnosis and differential diagnosis, 154–155
     etiopathogenesis, 152
     immunophenotype and molecular genetics, 154
     incidence of, 151–152
     occurrence, 152

pathology, 153–154, *153t*, *154*
treatment and prognosis, 155
lymphoid hyperplasia
diffuse nodular, 136–139, *137*, *138*
duodenum, 133, 135, *135*
ileum and appendix, 133, *134*, *135*
MALT lymphoma, 150–151, *151*, *152*
mucosa
epithelium, *880*, 880–882, *881*, *882*, *883*
ileal pigment, 882–883, *884*, *885*
jejunal villi, 880, *880*, *881*
lamina propria, 882–883, *884*
primary immunodeficiency disorders, 100
of volvulus, 905–906, *906*
Smoking
and anal tumors, 1571
and chronic idiopathic inflammatory bowel diseases, 1007
and esophageal squamous cell carcinoma, 507
Smooth muscle
demonstration, 241–242
hamartoma, 316
α-smooth muscle, 254
actin deficiency, 259–260
tumors
Epstein–Barr Virus-associated, 314, 316
glomus tumor, 316–317, *317*
leiomyomas, 313–314, *315*
leiomyomatosis, 316
leiomyomatosis peritonealis disseminata, 316
leiomyosarcoma, 317–318, *318*
smooth muscle hamartoma, 316
Smooth muscle actin (SMA), 259–260, 301
Snare biopsy and polypectomy, 1389, 1391, *1391*
Snare polypectomy, 4, *4*
after submucosal injection, 4–5
Soap enemas, 1162
Solitary fibrous tumor/hemangiopericytoma, 339, *340*
Solitary plasmacytomas, *171*, 171–172
Solitary polypoid hamartoma, 781, *781–782*
Solitary rectal ulcer syndrome (SRUS), 46
differential diagnosis, *278*, *279*
gross and endoscopic appearances, 277, *280*
histology, *277–278*, *277–279*
irritable bowel syndrome, 282
pathogenesis, 277
proctitis/localized colitis cystica profunda
gross and endoscopy, 280
inflammatory cloacogenic polyp, *281*, *281–282*
nuclear atypicality, dysplasia, and carcinoma, 280–281
pathogenesis and histology, 280, *280*
Somatostatinomas, 204, *206*
gastrointestinal manifestation of, 388
South American blastomycosis, 1312, *1312*
Spindle cell carcinoma
biopsy diagnosis, 522
gross appearance, 520, *521*
histogenesis, 522
microscopic appearances, 520, *521*, 522

Spindle cell carcinoma/carcinosarcoma, 356–357, *356–357*
Spindle cell GIST, *296*
Spindle cell variant of squamous cell carcinoma, 1574
Spirochetes
and immunohistochemical applications in gastrointestinal disorders, 21
intestinal spirochetosis
description, 1269
histology, 1270–1271, *1270–1271*
pathogenesis and clinical features, 1269–1270
syphilis
clinical features, 1267–1268, *1267–1268*
pathology, *1267–1268*, 1268–1269
prevalence of, 1267
Spontaneous rupture, in esophageal perforation
pathogenesis and clinical features, 435, *435t*
pathology, 435
Sporadic (type III) carcinoid, 203, *203*
Sporadic multiple GIST, 309
Sporadic visceral neuropathy, 263
Sporotrichum, 489
Squamocolumnar junction, in stomach, 555, *555*
Squamous carcinoma, 1502, *1503*
Squamous carcinoma *in situ*. *see* Bowen's disease
Squamous cell carcinoma, 533–534
AIDS associated, 113
esophageal
adenocarcinoma (*see* Adenocarcinoma)
and alcohol, 507
basaloid squamous cell carcinoma, 524, *525*
bronchopneumonia, 517
celiac sprue, 508
and chemotherapy, 515–516
clinical features, 506
definition, 506
and diet, 507
DNA ploidy, 516
dysplasia in, 508–509, *510*
endoscopic appearance, 509, *511*, 511–512, *512*
endoscopic mucosal resection, 517, *518*, *519*
genetic factors, 507–508
gross appearance, 509, *511*, 511–512, *512*
H. pylori, 508
haematogenous dissemination, 517
human papillomavirus infection, 508
intraepithelial neoplasia, 508–509
intramural metastases, 515
and irradiation, prior, 508
lymph node metastasis, 515
lymphovascular invasion, 515
microscopic appearance, *513*, 513–514, *514*
pathogenesis, 506
and predisposing conditions, 508

premalignant lesions, 508–509
prognosis, 514–517
protective factors, 508
radial margin, 515
risk factors, 507–508
small cell carcinoma, 522–525, *523*
and smoking, 507
spindle cell carcinoma, 520, *521*, 522
spread of, 514–517
staging, 514–517
superficial esophageal carcinoma, 517–518, *518*, *519*
superficial spreading carcinoma, 517–518
T stage, 515
TNM classification, 514–515
tylosis palmaris et plantaris., 508
unusual variants of, 517, 518, *518–521*, *520*, 522–525, *523*, *524*
verrucous carcinoma, 518, 520, *520*
invasive (*see* Invasive squamous cell carcinoma)
verrucous, 1565, *1566*, 1567
Squamous epithelial hyperplasia, 1564, *1564*
Squamous metaplasia, 905, *905*
Squamous mucosa
biopsy and criteria uses
cardia, 458–459
erosions, 456–458, *456–460*, *460t*
traditional sites, 458
endoscopy, 453
gross/endoscopic appearances, 455–456
Los Angeles grading system, 453–455, *454*
nonerosive, 455, *455*
reactive changes, 458, *459*
and sequela, 456, *456–457*
Squamous papilloma, 538, *539*, *539*
Squamous papillomatosis, 539
Squamous zone distal the dentate line, *1552*, 1557
Staphylococcal enterotoxins, 1216
Stasis syndrome, 959, *959*
Steatorrhea, 106, 111
Stem cell transplantation
characteristics, 106
chronic GVHD, 110
GI infections, *107t*
graft versus host disease
clinical presentation, 107–108
diagnosis, 110
gross appearance, 108
histology, 108, *109*
pathogenesis, 107
infections, 106
parasitic infestations, *107t*
transplantation regimen, 106
Stem cells and bowel, structure of, 891, *892*
Stenosis
acquired (*see* Esophageal webs and rings)
and bowel, large and small, 910–912
congenital esophageal, 434, *434t*
Stercoral ulceration, 1162–1163
Stercoral ulcers, 60–61, *61*

Stevens-Johnson syndrome
  drug-associated and iatrogenic vascular
      injuries, 1156
  gastrointestinal manifestation of, 397
Stomach
  adult orientation of, 552, 553
  anatomy
    antrum, 554, 554
    blood vessels and lymphatics, 555
    cardia region, 554, 555, 555
    curvatures of, 553, 553, 554
    fundus, 554, 554
    gastric surfaces, 554
    nerve supply, 556
    pyloric region, 554, 554
    squamocolumnar junction, 555, 555
  biopsy technique, 24
  bone marrow transplantation, GVHD,
      108, 109
  cardia region of, 552
  developmental abnormalities of, 565t,
      567, 567
  diffuse large B-cell lymphoma
    classification, 148
    immunophenotype of, 149
    microscopic findings, 148, 148
    occurrence, 149
    survival of, 149
  digestive tract vascularization
    collateral blood supply, 33
    extramural circulation, 31–33, 32
    intramural circulation, 30, 30–31
    venous drainage, 33
  duodenum region of, 553
  endocrine cells of, 557t
  GI problem in AIDS patients, 112
  ICCs, 566–567
  MALT lymphoma
    characterization, 141, 142–144
    clinical presentation, 140, 140
    clinical reports, 145–146
    differential diagnosis, 146–148
    genetic and epigenetic abnormalities,
        143–145
    limitation, 141
    microscopic findings, 141, 142, 143
    pathogenesis, 139, 139–140
    pathologist's role, 146
    pathology, 140–143
    patients follow-up, 146
    plasma cell population, 143, 143
    prognosis, 145
    treatment, 145
    types of lymphocytes, 142–143
    ulcers, 140, 141
    vague nodular architecture, 142, 143
  motor disorders of
    gastroparesis, 251
    pyloric stenosis, 250–251
  mucosa (see Mucosa)
  muscularis propria, 566–567
  premalignant lesions, 730
  primary gastric t-cell lymphoma,
      149–150
  primary immunodeficiency disorders, 100
  serosa, 566–567
  submucosa, 566

Striated muscle tumors
  rhabdomyoma, 348
  rhabdomyosarcoma, 348, 350
Strictures
  esophageal, 434, 434t
  intestines (see Idiopathic ulcers,
      intestines)
Stromal and smooth muscle tumors
  Epstein–Barr Virus–associated, 314, 316
  glomus tumor, 316–317, 317
  leiomyomas, 313–314, 315
  leiomyomatosis, 316
  leiomyomatosis peritonealis
      disseminata, 316
  leiomyosarcoma, 317–318, 318
  smooth muscle hamartoma, 316
Strongyloides stercoralis, 660–661, 661
  infection with AIDS, 113
Strongyloidiasis, 115, 1303–1304, 1304
Submucosa
  and bowel, structure of, 882, 895, 895
  of esophagus, 425, 426
  of stomach, 566
Submucosal lesions biopsy, 5
Submucosal lipoma, 341–342, 342
Submucosal plexus, 242, 242
Subtotal villous atrophy, 934, 944–945
Succinyl dehydrogenase subunit B (SDHB)
  deficient, 305, 308
  expression, 305
Sucrose deficiency, 973
Suction biopsy technique, 3
Suction trap, 115
Sulfur granules, 1271, 1272
Superficial carcinoma, 511
Superficial esophageal carcinoma, 517–518
Superficial zone, of stomach, 556, 556–557
Superior mesenteric artery, 31–32, 32
  syndrome, 38
Suppurative pyelophlebitis, 817
Surface colorectal-type adenomas, 1577,
    1577
Surface epithelial cells, 782
Surgical anal canal, 1551
Swiss-type agammaglobulinemia, 102–103
Synovial sarcoma, 354–356, 355
Syphilis, 653–654
  in anal canal, 1561, 1561–1562
  clinical features, 1267–1268, 1267–1268
  gastric disease associated with, 653–656,
      654–655
  pathology, 1267–1268, 1268–1269
  prevalence of, 1267
  rectal, 1267
Systemic disease
  Behçet's disease, 497
  Brown bowel syndrome, 498
  Crohn's disease
    involve, 497, 498
    lymphocytic esophagitis in, 497
  diabetes mellitus, 498
  granulomatous esophagitis and sarcoid,
      497–498
  GVHD, 496
  leukoplakia, 496
  Parkinson's disease, 499
  pseudoepitheliomatous hyperplasia, 496

  skin diseases and esophageal
      inflammation
    glycogenic acanthosis, 495, 495
    lichen planus, 495, 495
    pemphigus vulgaris, 495, 495
  ulcerative colitis, 498
Systemic lupus erythematosus (SLE)
  and connective tissue disorders, 383
  polyarteritis nodosa, 54
  selective IgA deficiency, 101
Systemic mastocytosis, 106

T

Taenia saginata (beef tapeworm), 1307, 1307
Taenia solium (pork tapeworm), 1307–1308
Takayasu arteritis, 52
Talc granulomas, 1156
Tangier disease, 406
Tapeworms. *see* Cestodes
T-cell
  intestinal host defenses, 88–89
  lymphocytic gastritis, 645
Telangiectasias, 77, 77–78
Teniae, 230, 231
TGF-β signaling pathway, 1464
Third-degree hemorrhoids in anal canal,
    1559
Thromboangiitis obliterans, 52
Thrombocytopenia, 35, 55, 66
Thrombocytosis, 401
Thrombolytic agents, 66
Thrombosis
  drug-induced vasculitis, 1153–1155, 1154
  estrogen and oral contraceptives,
      1153–1155, 1154
  oral contraceptive and IBD, 1155
Thrombotic thrombocytopenic purpura,
    1234
Thumbprinting, 39, 40, 43, 60
Thymic dysplasia, 102–103
Thyroid, 389–390
Thyroid neoplasms, 385
Thyroid rests, 540
Tissue specimens, gastrointestinal tract, 1
TNM classification
  ampullary and nonampullary small
      bowel tumors, 1349t
  esophageal, squamous cell carcinoma,
      514–515
Torsion, 805
Torulopsis glabrata, 489
Toxic megacolon, 1241–1242, 1242, 1246
  in *Campylobacter*, 1241–1242, 1242
Toxic vasculitis, 66
Toxic/drug-induced visceral neuropathy, 274
Toxin production, 1215–1216
  cholera toxin, 1216
  clostridial toxins, 1216
  shiga and shiga-like toxins, 1216
  staphylococcal enterotoxins, 1216
  verotoxin, 1216
Toxoplasma, 1298
Toxoplasma gondii, 1295
Tracheobronchial remnants, 434
Tracheoesophageal fistulas, 429–430, 431
Traction, divetticulum of esophagus, 442
Traditional serrated adenomas

clinical features, 1363
differential diagnosis, 1368–1369, 1371–1372, *1371–1373*
gross and endoscopic features, 1363
histology, 1363–1364, *1364–1367*
immunophenotype and molecular pathology, 1365–1368, *1366–1367*, 1368t
interobserver variability, 1368
treatment and follow-up, 1373, 1375
Transcobalamin II deficiency syndrome, 105
Transplantation
bone marrow
characteristics, 106
chronic GVHD, 110
GI infections, 107t
graft versus host disease, 107–108, *109*, 110
infections, 106
parasitic infestations, 107t
cardiac, 400
renal, 392–393
transplantation regimen, 106
Transverse band, 555
Trauma
abdominal, 35, 66
blunt, 38, 67
Traveler's diarrhea, 1224, *1225t*
Trematodes
Fasciolopsis buski, 1305–1307
schistosomiasis, 1305–1306, *1306–1307*
Trichinella spiralis, 1304
Trichinosis, 1304
Trichrome staining, 255, *255*
Trichuriasis, 1305, *1305*
Trichuris trichiura. see Trichuriasis
Tropical sprue
immune mechanisms in, 90
small bowel mucosal disease, 953–954, *954*
Trypanosoma cruzi, 249, 274
Trypanosomiasis (Chagas' disease), 1300
Tuberculosis, 653
and acute appendicitis, 821–822
biopsy technique, 23
description, 1260
gastric disease associated with, 653
gross and endoscopic findings, 1261, *1261*
histology and differential diagnosis, *1261*, 1261–1263
pathogenesis and clinical features, 1260–1261
pathologic features, 1263t
Tubular adenomas, 830–831, *831*
Tubular carcinoids, 210, *210*
Tubulovillous adenomas, 830–831, *831*
Tuft cells, 890
Tumor dissemination, 759
Tumor stage (TNM classification), 761, 762t
Tumors
adenomas of, appendix
diffuse mucosal hyperplasia, 832, *834, 835*, 836
growth patterns, 830
hyperplastic polyps, *835*, 836
polyps with dysplasia, *837*, 838

serrated hyperplasia and polyps, 830t, 832t, 833
sessile serrated polyps, 836, *837*, 838
tubular and tubulovillous, 830–831, *831*
villous, *831*, 832
of anal canal
adenocarcinoma, 1577–1579, *1578*
adenoid cystic carcinoma, 1579
adenomas, *1577*, 1577–1579
anal gland carcinoma, 1579
anal gland hidrocystoma, 1577
anal intraepithelial neoplasia, 1567–1569, *1568–1569, 1570*
Bowen's disease, 1569–1570
condyloma acuminatum, 1564–1565, *1565, 1566*
description, 1563, 1564
dysplasias, 1567, *1568–1569*
epithelial hyperplasia without dysplasia, 1564, *1564*
invasive squamous cell carcinoma, 1570–1576, *1572, 1573, 1574, 1576*
malignant melanoma, 1579–1580, *1580*
mesenchymal, 1580
mucoepidermoid carcinoma, 1579
small cell carcinoma, 1579
surface colorectal-type adenomas, 1577, *1577*
unusual adenoma-like columnar dysplasias, 1579
verrucous carcinoma, 1565, *1566*, 1567
of appendix
adenomas, 830–838
hyperplastic polyps, *835*, 836
large bowel tumors, 828–830
polyps and other benign lesions, 830, 830t, 831
calcifying fibrous, 339, *341*
endocrine, 79
endothelial and vascular
angiosarcoma, 345, *346*, 347
hemangioma, 344, 344–345, *345*
intestinal vascular lesions associated with clinical syndromes, 348
Kaposi's sarcoma, *346*, 347
lymphangioma, 347–348, *347–349*
epithelioid stromal, 294, *297*
esophagus, biopsy technique, 24
fatty, 344
fibroblastic/myofibroblastic
calcifying fibrous tumor, 339, *341*
desmoid tumor/intraabdominal fibromatosis, 331–333, *332*
elastofibroma, 340
inflammatory fibroid polyp, 333–335, *333–335*
inflammatory myofibroblastic tumor, 337, *338*, 339
plexiform fibromyxoma of gastric antrum, 335–336, *336, 337*
solitary fibrous tumor/hemangiopericytoma, 339, *340*
gastrointestinal, 112
gastrointestinal stromal (*see* Gastrointestinal stromal tumors)
glomus, 316–317, *317*

granular cell, 329–330, *329–330*
inflammatory myofibroblastic, 337, *338*, 339
mesenchymal (*see* Mesenchymal tumors)
mixed neuronal glial, 331
neurogenic
fibroblastic polyps, 325, *326*, 327
ganglioneuroma, 320, 321, *321–323*, 323
granular cell tumor, 329–330, *329–330*
malignant peripheral nerve sheath tumor, 330–331, *331*
mixed neuronal glial tumor, 331
mucosal neuroma/Schwann cell hamartoma, 323, *324–325*, 325
neurofibroma, 320
paraganglioma, *328*, 328–329
perineurioma, 325, 327
polypoid neural lesions, biopsy diagnosis of, 327–328
schwannoma, 318, *319*, 320
nonmesenchymal
follicular dendritic cell sarcoma, 360–361, *361*
lymphoma, 362
melanoma, 360, *360*
sarcomatoid adult granulosa cell tumor, 362
perivascular epithelioid cell
angiomyolipoma, 354
PEComa, 353–354, *354*
smooth muscle
Epstein–Barr Virus–associated, 314, 316
glomus tumor, 316–317, *317*
leiomyomas, 313–314, *315*
leiomyomatosis, 316
leiomyomatosis peritonealis disseminata (LPD), 316
leiomyosarcoma, 317–318, *318*
smooth muscle hamartoma, 316
specimen examination
assessing depth of penetration, 25
opening, 23–24
striated muscle
rhabdomyoma, 348
rhabdomyosarcoma, 348, *350*
Turner syndrome, 77
Tylosis, 398
Tylosis palmaris et plantaris., 508
Typhlitis. see Neutropenic enterocolitis
Typhoid fever
clinical features, 1238–1239
enteric infections, histologic features, 1222
gross appearance, 1239, *1239*
histology, 1239–1240
pathogenesis, 1238–1239

U

Ulcer. see also Peptic ulcer disease (PUD)
Cameron's, 468, *468*
healing and healed, 633
idiopathic, intestines
gross and endoscopic appearances, 1144t, 1145–1146, *1146–1147*
histology, 1146–1147, *1146–1148*
nonsteroidal anti-inflammatory drugs, 1148–1149, 1148–1152, *1149–1150*, 1150–1152

Ulcer. see also Peptic ulcer disease (PUD) (Continued)
  pathogenesis and clinical features, 1144–1145
  potassium chloride, 1152
  ileum, 39, 39
  intestinal, 52, 54
  mucosa, 44, 46, 66
  nonspecific, 1146–1147
  stercoral, 60–61
  stomach, 49
Ulcer-associated cell lineage and bowel, 905, 905
Ulcerated diverticulum, 237
Ulcerative colitis (UC), 498
  chromoendoscopy, 9–10, 10
  chronic idiopathic inflammatory bowel diseases
    appendiceal involvement, 1028, 1028
    in children, 1030, 1031
    clinical features, 1010–1011
    cuffitis, 1044
    dysplasia and cancer, 1040, 1042–1043
    endoscopic features and gross pathology, 1011, 1012–1015, 1013
    focality/patchiness, 1027, 1027–1028
    fulminant colitis and toxic megacolon, 1032–1034, 1032–1036, 1034t, 1035
    ileal involvement, 1029, 1029–1030
    ileal pouches and complications, 1037–1041, 1039–1041, 1041
    medical therapy, 1036–1037, 1037
    microscopic pathology, 1015, 1015–1027, 1017–1019, 1020, 1021t, 1022t, 1023–1027
    other diseases affecting, 1043–1044
    pouch biopsies, 1041–1042
    pouch problems, 1041
    proctitis/ulcerative proctitis, 1030–1032, 1030t
    rectal sparing, 1028–1029
    rectum in ulcerative proctocolitis, following ileorectal anastomosis, 1036
  Churg-Strauss syndrome, 51
  vs. Crohn's disease
    macroscopic differences, 1064–1066, 1065t
    microscopic differences, 1066–1067, 1066t, 1068–1072
  endocrine tumors, 217
  and eosinophilic colitis, cause of, 1091–1092, 1091t
  and follicular proctitis, 1024
  perinuclear ANCA, 51
  selective IgA deficiency, 101
  specimen handling, 9–10, 10
Umbilical hernia, 62
Unclassified celiac sprue, 949
Undifferentiated high grade leomorphic sarcoma, 353
Undifferentiated sarcoma, 353
Upper esophageal diverticula. see Zenker's diverticulum
Upper esophageal webs and rings, 440–441, 441
Urea breath test, 596

Ureterosigmoidostomy sites, 1517–1518
Urinary conduits tumors
  endometriosis, 1518, 1520, 1521–1522, 1523
  ileal conduits, 1517
  secondary tumors of large bowel, 1518, 1519–1520
  ureterosigmoidostomy sites, 1517–1518

V

Valvulae conniventes, 877, 877
Varicella zoster infection, 485, 486
Varicoid carcinoma, 512
Vascular disorders. see also specific vascular disorders
  arteriovenous malformation, 78, 78
  classification, 72, 73
  clinical presentation, 73
  dieulafoy lesion, 76, 76–77
  Ehlers–Danlos syndrome, 79–80
  GAVE, 74–76, 75
  incidence of, 72
  phlebectasia, 78–79
  portal hypertension, 79
  pseudoxanthoma elasticum, 79
  specimen handling, 80, 80–81
  telangiectasias, 77, 77–78
  vascular ectasia, 73–74
Vascular dissemination, 759
Vascular ectasia
  colon, 77, 77
  GAVE, 74–76, 75
  histologic examination, 74
  mucosa, 73
  prevalence, 74
Vascular malformations and bowel, complications of, 919
Vascular tumors, endothelial and angiosarcoma, 345, 346, 347
  hemangioma, 344, 344–345, 345
  intestinal vascular lesions associated with clinical syndromes, 348
  Kaposi's sarcoma, 346, 347
  lymphangioma, 347–348, 347–349
Vascularization, digestive tract. see Digestive tract vascularization
Vasculitis
  ANCA- associated
    Churg-Strauss syndrome, 54, 55, 56
    microscopic polyarteritis nodosa, 54–55, 57, 58
    Wegener's granulomatosis, 53
  biological screening, 47, 50t
  biopsy diagnosis, 60
  classification
    antineutrophil cytoplasmic antibodies, 51
    caliber blood vessel, 47, 50, 50t
    etiological, 51
    histological pattern, 47, 49t
    hypersensitivity, 49
  clinical presentation, 47, 50t, 51
  differential diagnosis, 60
  Henoch-Schönlein purpura, 55–56, 58
  infectious, 52
  large vessel
    Buerger's disease, 52

giant cell arteritis, 51–52
Takayasu arteritis, 52
malignant-atrophic papulosis, 60
medium vessel
  Kawasaki's disease, 52–53
  polyarteritis nodosa, 53, 53
microscopic diagnosis, 48
miscellaneous condition
  Behçet's disease, 57, 60
  enterocolic lymphocytic phlebitis, 57, 59
  paraneoplastic vasculitis, 56
  stercoral ulcers, 60–61, 61
  vasculopathy, 49
vasculopathy, 49
Vasoconstrictor drugs, 64
Vasopressin, 64
  arterial spasm, 1155
Venous drainage
  in anal canal, 1554, 1555, 1556
  of stomach, 555
Ventral hernias, 62
Verotoxin, 1216, 1234
Verrucous carcinomas, 518, 520, 520
  tumors, anal canal in, 1564, 1565, 1566, 1567
Verrucous squamous cell carcinoma, 1565, 1566, 1567
Vessel wall trauma, 1152
Vibrios
  clinical features, 1228
  diagnosis, 1229
  epidemiology, 1228
  pathogenesis, 1228–1229
  pathology, 1229
  treatment and follow-up, 1229
Villous adenoma, 831, 832
VIPoma syndrome, 387–388
Virtual histology, 11
Viruses, 1276
  adenovirus, 819, 819
  in anal canal, 1561
  cytomegalovirus, 819
    infection (HHV-5), 657, 658
  enteric adenoviruses, 1287–1288, 1287–1288
  enteric viruses
    nonpathogenic, 1284
    pathogenic, 1284
  Epstein-Barr virus, 658
  herpes simplex virus (see Herpes simplex virus)
  herpesviruses, 657–658, 1276–1283, 1561
  HHV-6-positive cells, 658
  and immunohistochemical applications in gastrointestinal disorders, 21
  infection (see also Infection)
    acute HIV, 486–487
    CMV, 486, 486
    HPV, 486, 487
    HSV type I, 484–486, 485
  infectious mononucleosis, 820
  measles, 659, 819–820, 820
  norovirus, 1285–1287
  papillomavirus, 1561
  rotavirus

pathogenesis and clinical features, 1285
pathology, 1285, *1286*
Vitamin B$_{12}$ deficiency, 969–970, *970*
Volvulus, 805
    and bowel, large and small, 905–906, *906*
    occurence, 63
    stomach and small intestine, 63
von Recklinghausen's disease, 307

W

Waldenström's macroglobulinemia, 165, *166*, 400, 969, *969*
Watermelon stomach, 74
Weber–Christian disease, 365
Webs, 910–912, *911*
Wegener's granulomatosis, 51, 53
Western-type lymphomas, 155
Whipple's disease, 822–823
    and acute appendicitis, 822–823
    histiocytes associated with infections, 1173
    small bowel mucosal disease, with variably severe lesions
        clinical features, 960–961
        differential diagnosis, 964
        endoscopic findings, 961–962, *962*
        pathogenesis, 960–961
        pathology, 962, *963–964*
Whipworm, 1305, *1305*
White line of anal canal, 1551
Wiskott-Aldrich syndrome, 105, 165–167
Wnt signaling pathway, 1462–1463
Wolman's disease, 406

X

Xanthelasma, esophageal, 445
Xanthogranulomatous pseudotumor, 367–368, 368
Xanthoma/xanthelasma, 1179–1180, *1182*
X-linked agammaglobulinemia (XLAG), 99

Y

Yersinia infections
    and acute appendicitis, 821, *822*
    description, 1243–1244
    endoscopic findings, 1245, *1246*, *1247*
    enteric infections, histologic features, 1222
    gross pathology, 1245, *1247*
    histology, 1245, *1246*, 1247–1248, 1247–1248 *1247*
    pathogenesis and clinical features, 1244–1245
    Y. pseudotuberculosis, *1248*, 1248–1249, *1249*
Yolk sack tumor, 743

Z

Zenker's diverticulum, 442, *442*
Ziehl-Neelsen technique, 23, 1262
Zinc deficiency syndrome, 960
Z-line
    in esophagus, 422, 423, *423*
    GERD, 452
Zollinger-Ellison syndrome (ZES), 196
    gastric folds, 678, *679*
    from gastrinomas, 204
    and multiple endocrine neoplasia, 202, 203
    and small bowel mucosal disease, 959–960, *960*, *961*
    type I carcinoid tumor/NET, 199–202, *200–202*
    type II carcinoid tumor/NET, 202–203
    type III carcinoid tumor/NET, 203 *203*
    type IV carcinoid tumor/NET, 204
    well differentiated, 196
Zonal aganglionosis, 273